Anesthetic Pharmacology

Second Edition

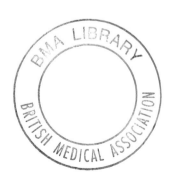

Anesthetic Pharmacology

Second Edition

Edited by

Alex S. Evers

Mervyn Maze

Evan D. Kharasch

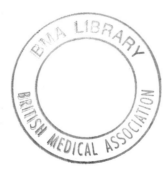

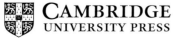

CAMBRIDGE
UNIVERSITY PRESS

CAMBRIDGE UNIVERSITY PRESS
Cambridge, New York, Melbourne, Madrid, Cape Town, Singapore,
São Paulo, Delhi, Dubai, Tokyo, Mexico City

Cambridge University Press
The Edinburgh Building, Cambridge CB2 8RU, UK

Published in the United States of America by
Cambridge University Press, New York

www.cambridge.org
Information on this title: www.cambridge.org/9780521896665

First edition published by Churchill Livingstone 2004
Second edition published by Cambridge University Press 2011

Printed in the United Kingdom at the University Press, Cambridge

A catalog record for this publication is available from the British Library

Library of Congress Cataloging in Publication Data
Anesthetic pharmacology / edited by Alex S. Evers, Mervyn Maze, Evan D.
Kharasch. – 2nd ed.
    p. ; cm.
  Includes bibliographical references and index.
  ISBN 978-0-521-89666-5 (hardback)
1. Anesthetics. I. Evers, Alex S. II. Maze, M. (Mervyn) III. Kharasch, Evan D.
  [DNLM: 1. Anesthetics–pharmacology. 2. Analgesics–pharmacology. QV 81]
  RD82.A687 2011
  615′.781–dc22
                                                                        2010028676
ISBN 978-0-521-89666-5 Hardback

Contents

Section 4 – Clinical applications: evidence-based anesthesia practice

Contributors

Waiel Almoustadi, MBBS
Department of Anesthesiology
University of Manitoba
Winnipeg, Manitoba, Canada

Brian J. Anderson, PhD, FANZCA, FJFICM
Associate Professor of Anesthesiology
University of Auckland
Auckland, New Zealand

David B. Auyong, MD
Staff Anesthesiologist
Department of Anesthesiology
Virginia Mason Medical Center
Seattle, WA, USA

Michael Avidan, MBBCh, FCASA
Associate Professor, Anesthesiology
and Cardiothoracic Surgery
Department of Anesthesiology
Washington University School of Medicine
St. Louis, MO, USA

Michael J. Avram, PhD
Associate Professor of Anesthesiology
Director of the Mary Beth Donnelley
Clinical Pharmacology Core Facility
Northwestern University Feinberg School of Medicine
Chicago, IL, USA

Roland J. Bainton, MD
Associate Professor
Department of Anesthesia and Perioperative Care
University of California
San Francisco, CA, USA

Jeffrey R. Balser, MD, PhD
The James Tayloe Gwathmey Professor of Anesthesiology
and Pharmacology
Vice Chancellor for Health Affairs and Dean
Vanderbilt University School of Medicine
Nashville, TN, USA

Juliana Barr, MD
Associate Professor in Anesthesia
Stanford University School of Medicine
Staff Anesthesiologist and Acting ICU
Medical Director
Veterans Administration Palo Alto
Health Care System
Palo Alto, CA, USA

W. Scott Beattie, MD, PhD, FRCPC
R. Fraser Elliot Chair in Cardiac Anesthesia
Director of Anesthesia Research
University Health Network
Department of Anesthesia
University of Toronto
Toronto, Canada

Manfred Blobner, MD
Klinik für Anaesthesiologie der Technischen
Universität München
Klinikum rechts der Isar
Munich, Germany

T. Andrew Bowdle, MD, PhD
Professor of Anesthesiology and
Adjunct Professor of Pharmaceutics
Chief of the Division of Cardiothoracic
Anesthesiology
University of Washington
Seattle, WA, USA

Walter A. Boyle, MD
Professor of Anesthesiology, Developmental
Biology and Surgery
Washington University School of Medicine
St. Louis, MO, USA

Eugene B. Campbell, MB, ChB
Consultant Gastroenterologist
Erne Hospital
Enniskillen, County Fermanagh, UK

Laura F. Cavallone, MD
Assistant Professor of Anesthesiology
Washington University School of Medicine
St. Louis, MO, USA

Mario Cibelli, MD
Department of Anaesthesia
St. George's Healthcare NHS Trust
London, UK

C. Michael Crowder, MD, PhD
Professor of Anesthesiology and Developmental Biology
Washington University School of Medicine
St. Louis, MO, USA

Ola Dale, MD, PhD
Department of Circulation and Medical Imaging
Norwegian University of Science and Technology
Trondheim, Norway

M. Frances Davies, PhD
Anesthesia Service
Stanford University
Palo Alto, CA, USA

Mark Dershwitz, MD, PhD
Professor of Anesthesiology
Department of Anesthesiology
University of Massachusetts Medical School
Worcester, MA, USA

George Despotis, MD
Associate Professor, Pathology, Immunology
and Anesthesiology
Department of Anesthesiology
Washington University School of Medicine
St. Louis, MO, USA

Clifford S. Deutschman, MD, FCCM
Professor of Anesthesiology and Critical Care
Director, Stavropoulos Sepsis Research Program
University of Pennsylvania School of Medicine
Philadelphia, PA, USA

Brian S. Donahue, MD, PhD
Associate Professor of Anesthesiology
Vanderbilt University School of Medicine
Nashville, TN, USA

Marcel E. Durieux, MD, PhD
Professor of Anesthesiology
and Neurological Surgery
University of Virginia
Charlottesville, VA, USA

Thomas J. Ebert, MD, PhD
Professor and Program Director
Department of Anesthesiology
Medical College of Wisconsin
Milwaukee, WI, USA

Talmage D. Egan, MD
Professor and Staff Physician
Director of Neuroanesthesia
Department of Anesthesiology
University of Utah School of Medicine
Salt Lake City, UT, USA

Helge Eilers, MD
Associate Professor
Department of Anesthesia and Perioperative Care
University of California
San Francisco, CA, USA

E. Wesley Ely, MD, MPH
Department of Medicine
Health Services Research Center
Vanderbilt University School of Medicine
Nashville, TN, USA

Charles W. Emala, MD
Associate Professor of Anesthesiology
College of Physicians and Surgeons
Columbia University
New York, NY, USA

Alex S. Evers, MD
Henry E. Mallinckrodt Professor of Anesthesiology
Professor of Internal Medicine and
Developmental Biology
Washington University School of Medicine
St. Louis, MO, USA

Heidrun Fink, MD
Klinik für Anaesthesiologie der Technischen
Universität München
Klinikum rechts der Isar
Munich, Germany

Pierre Foëx, DM, MA
Professor of Anesthetics
Nuffield Department of Anesthetics
University of Oxford
The John Radcliffe Hospital
Oxford, UK

Stuart A. Forman, MD, PhD
Associate Professor of Anesthesiology
Harvard Medical School
Department of Anesthesia & Critical Care

Massachusetts General Hospital
Boston, MA, USA

Helen F. Galley, PhD
Senior Lecturer in Anaesthesia and Intensive Care
University of Aberdeen
Aberdeen, UK

Josephine M. Garcia-Ferrer, PhD
Department of Anesthesiology
Washington University School of Medicine
St. Louis, MO, USA

Robert W. Gereau IV, PhD
Professor of Anesthesiology
Washington University Pain Center and Department
of Anesthesiology
Washington University School of Medicine
St. Louis, MO, USA

Tony Gin, MD, FANZCA, FRCA
Anesthesia and Intensive Care and Paediatrics
The Chinese University of Hong Kong
Prince of Wales Hospital
Shatin, Hong Kong

David Glick, MD
Associate Professor of Anesthesia and Critical Care
Medical Director of the Postanesthesia Care Unit
Anesthesia and Critical Care
The University of Chicago
Chicago, IL, USA

B. Joseph Guglielmo, PharmD
Department of Clinical Pharmacy
University of California
San Francisco, CA, USA

Dhanesh K. Gupta, MD
Associate Professor of Anesthesiology
and Neurological Surgery
Northwestern University Feinberg School of Medicine
Chicago, IL, USA

Howard B. Gutstein, MD
Professor, Department of Anesthesiology
and Pain Management
Department of Biochemistry and Molecular Biology
The University of Texas – MD Anderson Cancer Center
Houston, TX, USA

Robert G. Hahn, MD, PhD
Professor of Anesthesiology
Department of Anaesthesia

University of Linköping
Linköping, Sweden

Greg B. Hammer, MD
Professor of Anesthesia and Pediatrics
Lucile Packard Children's Hospital
Stanford University Medical Center
Stanford, CA, USA

Brian P. Head, PhD
Department of Anesthesiology
University of California
San Diego, CA, USA

Helen Higham, MB, ChB
Nuffield Department of Anaesthetics
John Radcliffe Hospital
Oxford, UK

Laureen Hill, MD
Associate Professor and Vice Chair of Anesthesiology
Associate Professor of Surgery
Washington University School of Medicine
St. Louis, MO, USA

Kirk Hogan, MD, JD
Professor of Anesthesiology
Department of Anesthesiology
University of Wisconsin School of Medicine
and Public Health
Madison, WI, USA

Charles W. Hogue Jr., MD
Associate Professor of Anesthesiology
and Critical Care Medicine
The Johns Hopkins Medical Institutions
The Johns Hopkins Hospital
Baltimore, MD, USA

Christopher G. Hughes, MD
Department of Anesthesiology
Vanderbilt University Medical Center
Nashville, TN, USA

Eric Jacobsohn, MBChB, MHPE, FRCPC
Professor and Chairman of Anesthesiology
University of Manitoba
Winnipeg, Manitoba, Canada

Roger A. Johns, MD, MHS
Professor of Anesthesiology and Critical Care Medicine
The John Hopkins Medical Institutions
The John Hopkins Hospital
Baltimore, MD, USA

Dean R. Jones, MD, FRCPC
Assistant Professor of Anesthesiology
Department of Anesthesiology
Columbia University
New York, NY, USA

Max Kelz, MD, PhD
Assistant Professor of Anesthesiology and Critical Care
University of Pennsylvania
Philadelphia, PA, USA

Evan D. Kharasch, MD, PhD
Russell D. and Mary B. Shelden
Professor of Anesthesiology
Vice-Chancellor for Research
Washington University
St. Louis, MO, USA

Ellen W. King, MD
Associate in the Department of Anaesthesia
University of Iowa
Iowa City, IA, USA

W. Andrew Kofke, MD, MBA, FCCM
Professor, Director of Neuroanesthesia
Department of Anesthesiology and Critical Care
University of Pennsylvania
Philadelphia, PA, USA

Tom C. Krejcie, MD
Professor of Anesthesiology and Associate
Chair for Research
Northwestern University Feinberg School of Medicine
Chicago, IL, USA

Richard M. Langford, FRCA, FFPMRCA
Professor of Anaesthesia and Pain Medicine
Pain and Anaesthesia Research Centre
Barts and the London NHS Trust
London, UK

H. T. Lee, MD, PhD
Assistant Professor of Anesthesiology
and Vice-Chair for Laboratory Research
Columbia University
New York, NY, USA

Isobel Lever, PhD
Department of Anaesthetics, Pain Medicine
and Intensive Care
Imperial College London
Chelsea and Westminster Hospital
London, UK

Jerrold H. Levy, MD, FAHA
Professor and Deputy Chair for Research
Director of Cardiothoracic Anesthesiology
Emory University School of Medicine
Atlanta, GA, USA

J. Lance Lichtor, MD
Professor of Anesthesiology
University of Massachusetts Medical School
Worcester, MA, USA

Larry Lindenbaum, MD
Resident
Department of Anesthesiology
Medical College of Wisconsin
Milwaukee, WI, USA

Hung Pin Liu, MD
Department of Anesthesiology
Washington University School of Medicine
St. Louis, MO, USA

Geoff Lockwood, MBBS, PhD
Consultant Anaesthetist
Hammersmith Hospital
London, UK

Alex Macario, MD, MBA
Professor of Anesthesia & Health Research and Policy
Department of Anesthesia
Stanford University School of Medicine
Stanford, CA, USA

Conan MacDougall, PharmD, MAS
Department of Clinical Pharmacy
University of California
San Francisco, CA, USA

M. B. MacIver, MSc, PhD
Professor of Anesthesiology
Department of Anesthesia
Stanford University Medical Center
Stanford, CA, USA

Aman Mahajan, MD, PhD
Chief, Cardiac Anesthesiology
Associate Professor
David Geffen School of Medicine at UCLA
Los Angeles, CA, USA

Nándor Marczin, MD, PhD
Department of Academic Anaesthetics
Imperial College
Chelsea and Westminster Hospital
London, UK

J. A. Jeevendra Martyn, MD, FRCA, FCCM
Department of Anesthesia, Critical Care and Pain Medicine
Harvard Medical School, Massachusetts General Hospital
and Shriners Hospitals for Children
Boston, MA, USA

George A. Mashour, MD, PhD
University of Michigan Medical School
Ann Arbor, MI, USA

Mervyn Maze, MB, ChB, FRCP, FRCA, FMedSci
Chair, Department of Anesthesia
University of California, San Francisco
San Francisco, CA, USA

Thomas McDowell, MD, PhD
Associate Professor of Anesthesiology
University of Wisconsin School of Medicine and Public Health
Madison, WI, USA

Stuart McGrane, MD
Department of Anesthesiology and Division of Critical Care
Vanderbilt University Medical Center
Nashville, TN, USA

Berend Mets, MB, ChB, PhD
Eric A. Walker Professor and Chair
Department of Anesthesiology
Penn State College of Medicine
Hershey, PA, USA

Patrick Meybohm, MD
University Hospital Schleswig-Holstein
Campus Kiel, Germany

Charles F. Minto, MB, ChB
Staff Anaesthetist
Department of Anaesthesia and Pain Management,
Royal North Shore Hospital
Senior Lecturer, University of Sydney
Sydney, Australia

Jonathan Moss, MD, PhD
Professor and Vice-Chairman of Anesthesia & Critical Care
Chairman of the Institutional Review Board
Anesthesia and Critical Care
University of Chicago
Chicago, IL, USA

Mohamed Naguib, MD
Department of General Anesthesiology
Institute of Anesthesiology
Cleveland Clinic
Cleveland, OH, USA

Istvan Nagy, MD, PhD
Department of Anaesthetics, Pain Medicine
and Intensive Care
Faculty of Medicine
Imperial College
Chelsea and Westminster Hospital
London, UK

Nick Oliver, MBBS, MRCP
Clinical Research Fellow
Faculty of Medicine
Imperial College
London, UK

Paul S. Pagel, MD, PhD
Professor of Anesthesiology
Medical College of Wisconsin
Milwaukee, WI, USA

Pratik P. Pandharipande, MD, MSCI
Department of Anesthesiology and Division of Critical Care
Vanderbilt University Medical Center
Nashville, TN, USA

Piyush Patel, MD, FRCPC
Professor, Department of Anesthesioloogy
University of California
San Diego, CA, USA

Andrew J. Patterson, MD, PhD
Associate Professor
Department of Anesthesia
Stanford University Medical Center
Stanford, CA, USA

Robert A. Pearce, MD, PhD
Professor and Chair of Anesthesiology
University of Wisconsin School of Medicine and Public Health
Madison, WI, USA

Ronald G. Pearl, MD, PhD
Professor of Anesthesiology
Department of Anesthesiology
Stanford University School of Medicine
Stanford, CA, USA

Misha Perouansky, MD
Professor of Anesthesiology
University of Wisconsin School of Medicine
and Public Health
Madison, WI, USA

Kristof Racz, MD
Department of Academic Anaesthetics
Imperial College

Chelsea and Westminster Hospital
London, UK

Chinniampalayam Rajamohan, MBBS, MD, FRCA, FRCPC
University of Manitoba
Department of Anesthesiology
Winnipeg, Manitoba, Canada

Nilesh Randive, MD, FRCA
Lecturer in Academic Anaesthesia
Pain and Anaesthesia Research Centre
Barts and the London NHS Trust
London, UK

Imre Redai, MD
Assistant Professor
Department of Anesthesiology
College of Physicians and Surgeons
Columbia University
New York, NY, USA

Stephen Robinson, MD, FRCP
Consultant Physician and Endocrinologist
Imperial College NHS Trust
London, UK

Richard W. Rosenquist, MD
Professor of Anesthesia
Director, Pain Medicine Division
University of Iowa
Iowa City, IA, USA

Carl E. Rosow, MD, PhD
Professor of Anesthesiology
Department of Anesthesia and Critical Care
Massachusetts General Hospital
Boston, MA, USA

Uwe Rudolph, MD
Associate Professor of Psychiatry
Director, Laboratory of Genetic Neuropharmacology
Mailman Research Center
Harvard Medical School
Belmont, MA, USA

Francis V. Salinas, MD
Staff Anesthesiologist
Department of Anesthesiology
Virginia Mason Medical Center
Seattle, WA, USA

Robert D. Sanders, BSc, MBBS, FRCA
Department of Anaesthetics, Pain Medicine
and Intensive Care
Imperial College
London, UK

Sunita Sastry, MD
Department of Anesthesia
Stanford University School of Medicine
Stanford, CA, USA

Michael Schäfer, MD
Department of Anesthesiology and Intensive Care Medicine
Charité University
Berlin, Germany

Jens Scholz, MD, PhD
Department of Anesthesiology
University Hospital of Eppendorf
Hamburg, Germany

Thomas W. Schnider, Prof. Dr. med.
Institut for Anasthesiologie
Kantonsspital
St. Gallen, Switzerland

Mark A. Schumacher, PhD, MD
Associate Professor
Department of Anesthesia and Perioperative Care
University of California
San Francisco, CA, USA

John W. Sear, MA, PhD, MBBS, FFARCS, FANZCA
Nuffield Department of Anaesthetics
John Radcliffe Hospital, Headington
Oxford, UK

Frédérique S. Servin, MD
Département d'Anesthésie et de Réanimation Chirurgicale
CHU Bichat Claude Bernard
Paris, France

Jeffrey H. Silverstein, MD
Professor of Anesthesiology, Surgery, and Geriatrics & Adult
Development
Department of Anesthesiology
Mount Sinai School of Medicine
New York, NY, USA

Tom De Smet, MSc
Department of Anesthesia
University Medical Center Groningen
and University of Groningen
Groningen, The Netherlands

Martin Smith, MBBS, FRCP
Consultant Physician and Endocrinologist
Salisbury NHS Foundation Trust
Salisbury, UK

Joe Henry Steinbach, PhD
Russell and Mary Shelden Professor of Anesthesiology
Department of Anesthesiology

Washington University School of Medicine
St. Louis, MO, USA

Markus Steinfath, MD, PhD
Department of Anaesthesiology and Intensive
Care Medicine
University Hospital Schleswig-Holstein
Campus Kiel, Kiel, Germany

David F. Stowe, MD, PhD
Professor of Anesthesiology
Medical College of Wisconsin
Milwaukee, WI, USA

Gary R. Strichartz, PhD
Professor of Anesthesia (Pharmacology)
Harvard Medical School
Boston, MA, USA

Michel M. R. F. Struys, MD, PhD
Professor and Chairman
Department of Anesthesia
University Medical Center Groningen
and University of Groningen
Groningen, The Netherlands

Isao Tsuneyoshi, MD
Department of Anesthesiology
Faculty of Medicine
University of Miyazaki
Miyazaki-shi, Japan

Robert A. Veselis, MD
Associate Professor
Department of Anesthesiology
Memorial Sloan-Kettering Cancer Center
New York, NY, USA

Arthur Wallace, MD, PhD
Professor of Anesthesiology and
Perioperative Care
University of California, San Francisco
San Francisco, CA, USA

Robert P. Walt, MD, FRCP
Department of Gastroenterology
Queen Elizabeth Hospital
Edgbaston
Birmingham, UK

David C. Warltier, MD, PhD
Chairman, Department of Anesthesiology
Medical College of Wisconsin
Milwaukee, WI, USA

Nigel R. Webster, MD
Anaesthesia and Intensive Care
Institute of Medical Sciences
University of Aberdeen
Aberdeen, UK

Jeanine Wiener-Kronish, MD
Henry Isiah Dorr Professor of Anesthesia
Department of Anesthesia and Critical Care
Massachusetts General Hospital
Boston, MA, USA

Troy Wildes, MD
Assistant Professor of Anesthesiology
Washington University School of Medicine
St. Louis, MO, USA

Paul Wischmeyer, MD
Professor of Anesthesiology
University of Colorado School of Medicine
Denver, CO, USA

Ling-Gang Wu, MD, PhD
Senior Investigator
National Institute of Neurological Disorders and Stroke
Bethesda, MD, USA

Stephen Yang, MD
Department of Anesthesia
Mount Sinai Hospital Medical Center
New York, NY, USA

Preface

Recent years have seen the beginning of a revolution in our understanding of how anesthesia is produced and how the drugs used by perioperative practitioners work at a molecular level. Concomitantly, the clinical practice of anesthesia has become increasingly more complex and demanding. As a result of these developments, there continues to be a growing chasm between clinically sophisticated anesthesiologists who may be inadequately versed in basic and molecular pharmacology, and anesthetic researchers who are well versed in the mechanistic details of anesthetic drug action, but inadequately informed about the clinical context in which these drugs are used. The first edition of *Anesthetic Pharmacology: Physiologic Principles and Clinical Practice* was assembled with the aim of bridging this chasm.

Since then, the understanding of molecular mechanisms of drug action has grown, mechanisms of interindividual variability in drug response are better understood, and the practice of anesthesiology has expanded to the preoperative environment, locations out of the operating room and out of the hospital, and into various intensive care units. Consequently, *Anesthetic Pharmacology* has been significantly revised into a second edition. Significant changes include the addition of a third editor, expansion from three to four sections, and enhanced organization and readability to make the material accessible to a wide range of trainees, practitioners, and pharmacologists.

Anesthetic Pharmacology is designed to be a sophisticated, accessible, reliable, and user-friendly primer of fundamental and applied pharmacology that is targeted for use by the full spectrum of those providing care in the perioperative period.

The book is organized into four fully integrated sections. The first two sections consider the principles and targets of anesthetic drug action, and the last two sections address the pharmacology and therapeutic use of the drugs themselves. Section one, "Principles of drug action," provides detailed theoretical and practical information about anesthetic pharmacokinetics and about cell signaling pathways involved in anesthetic drug action. Section two, "Physiologic substrates of drug action," is conveniently arranged by organ systems and presents the molecular, cellular, and integrated physiology of the organ or functional system, highlighting targets and substrates. Section three, "Essential drugs in anesthetic practice," presents the pharmacology and toxicology of major classes of drugs that are used perioperatively. A fourth section, "Clinical applications: evidence-based anesthesia practice," has been added to this edition to provide integrated and comparative pharmacology, and the practical therapeutic application of drugs for specific perioperative indications.

The layout of the chapters accommodates to the varying needs of the readership. Each chapter contains the fundamental body of knowledge needed by practitioners, as well as more in-depth information, including basic research directions and sophisticated clinical applications. The chapters all conclude with a concise summary of the material deemed to be essential knowledge for trainees and those seeking recertification. Through the judicious use of illustrations, boxes, and tables, information is presented in a comprehensible fashion for all levels of readership.

Principles of drug action

Pharmacodynamic principles of drug action

Stuart A. Forman

Introduction

The effects of drugs on patients in the operating room vary with drug dosage, from patient to patient, and with time. Different doses of drugs result in different concentrations in various tissues, producing a range of therapeutic and sometimes undesirable responses. Responses depend on drug pharmacokinetics (the time course of drug concentration in the body) and drug pharmacodynamics (the relationship between drug concentration and drug effect). These processes may be influenced by factors including pre-existing disease, age, and genetic variability. Patient responses to drugs may also be dynamically altered by factors such as temperature, pH, circulating ion and protein concentrations, levels of endogenous signaling molecules, and coadministration of other drugs in the operating room environment. Pharmacodynamics, the focus of this chapter, is the study of where and how drugs act to produce their effects, encompassing drug actions on biological systems ranging from molecules to organisms and their responses from conformational changes to behavior and emotional states [1,2].

Developments in pharmacology have been greatly affected by the rapid growth in our understanding of biology at the molecular level. Molecular targets for many drugs used in the practice of anesthesia are now known in varying degrees of detail. This knowledge enables development of efficient assays to identify new potential drugs and, in some cases, structure-based design of improved therapeutic drugs. The practice of anesthesiology requires an understanding of human pharmacodynamics and pharmacokinetics, but real expertise, and particularly the ability to innovate, demands deeper understanding of the scientific basis of our practical knowledge. The first and larger part of this chapter focuses on central concepts of molecular drug–receptor interactions. In actuality, most drugs affect more than one molecular target, and the impact of drug actions at the cellular, tissue, and organism levels are the result of integrated effects at these higher system levels. The latter part of the chapter covers pharmacodynamic concepts pertinent to drug responses in animals and humans. Some of the terms used, including *potency, efficacy,* and *selectivity,* have parallel meanings at both the molecular and organism levels.

Throughout this chapter, molecular pharmacodynamics concepts are illustrated both with cartoons and with simple chemical reaction schemes, which lend themselves to quantitative algebraic analyses. This quantitative formalism is provided to encourage a deeper understanding of important pharmacodynamic concepts for those who make the small additional effort.

Drug receptors

Drugs are exogenous chemical substances used to alter a physiological system. A drug may be identical to an endogenous compound, such as a peptide, amino acid, nucleotide, carbohydrate, steroid, fatty acid, or gas. Examples of endogenous factors used in anesthesiology include potassium for diuretic-induced hypokalemia, insulin for diabetes, clotting factor VIII for hemophilia, and nitric oxide for pulmonary hypertension.

Receptors versus drug targets

Pharmacologic receptors are defined as macromolecular proteins on the cell membrane or within the cytoplasm or cell nucleus that bind to specific endogenous factors (drugs), such as neurotransmitters, hormones, or other substances, and initiate cellular responses to these drugs. Protein drug targets also encompass circulating enzymes, non-chemically stimulated (e.g., voltage- or mechanically activated) membrane channels, and membrane transporters. The definition of drug targets can be further broadened to include DNA, RNA, and epigenetic control molecules, components of pathogenic or commensal microbes, toxins, etc. Drug receptor proteins may consist of one or more peptide chains.

Receptor protein structure can be characterized by features at multiple levels:

(1) Primary structure – the amino acid sequence.
(2) Secondary structure – the peptide subdomain folding pattern (e.g., α-helix, β-sheet, random).
(3) Tertiary structure – the entire peptide folding, including domain–domain interactions and disulfide bridges.

Anesthetic Pharmacology, 2nd edition, ed. Alex S. Evers, Mervyn Maze, Evan D. Kharasch. Published by Cambridge University Press. © Cambridge University Press 2011.

(4) Quaternary structure – assembly of multiple peptides, including peptide–peptide interactions and disulfide bridges.

(5) Post-translational peptide modifications – including phosphorylation, lipidation, biotinylation, glycosylation, etc.

Physicochemical forces that determine receptor structure are intrapeptide, interpeptide, and with surrounding water or lipid. These forces include:

(1) Covalent bonds – sharing of electron pairs between atoms.

(2) Ionic bonds – attraction between oppositely charged ion pairs (repulsion can also affect structure).

(3) Hydrogen bonds – weak dipole–dipole forces between electronegative atoms and hydrogen, usually bonded to oxygen or nitrogen. Solvent water provides many hydrogen bonds for proteins.

(4) Van der Waals interactions – close-range attractive and repulsive forces between atoms.

(5) Hydrophobic interactions – forces arising from the energetically favorable interaction between nonpolar molecular domains that repel (i.e., do not hydrogen-bond with) solvent water.

Enzymes (circulating or intracellular) are in an aqueous environment. Hydrophobic interactions tend to make these proteins have hydrophilic exteriors and hydrophobic interiors.

Transmembrane proteins have at least one hydrophobic domain that crosses the lipid bilayer [3]. They may have multiple hydrophobic domains within the membrane and hydrophilic domains in the extracellular and intracellular spaces.

Receptor nomenclature and categorization

Classically, drug receptors have been categorized based on their sensitivity to various drugs (endogenous or otherwise). For example, **nicotinic** acetylcholine (nACh) receptors in muscle, neurons, and glia are strongly activated (agonized) by acetylcholine and nicotine (an alkaloid from tobacco), and less so by muscarine (an alkaloid from *Amanita muscaria* mushrooms), whereas **muscarinic** acetylcholine (mACh) receptors in smooth and cardiac muscle are strongly activated by acetylcholine and muscarine, but weakly by nicotine. Other receptors named for drugs widely used in anesthesia include opioid receptors and adrenergic receptors (adrenoceptors).

Drug receptor categorization by molecular structure – Analysis of genes and messenger RNA that encode proteins has provided an enormous quantity of data on protein **families** and **superfamilies**, which represent different classes of drug receptors. The *British Journal of Pharmacology*'s "Guide to Receptors and Channels" [4] lists seven classes of pharmacologic protein targets based upon similar structure and function: seven-transmembrane (7TM) receptors, ligand (transmitter)-gated channels, ion channels, catalytic receptors, nuclear receptors, transporters, and enzymes. Nomenclature for this ever-growing list is maintained by the International Union of Basic and Clinical Pharmacology (www.iuphar-db.

org). Building upon the example given for classical receptor nomenclature, nicotinic acetylcholine receptors are classified as transmitter-gated channels. More specifically, nicotinic ACh receptors on fetal muscle consist of five homologous polypeptide subunits, $\alpha_1/\alpha_1/\beta_1/\gamma/\delta$, surrounding a transmembrane cation channel. The genes for these subunits were first cloned in the 1980s, providing a complete primary amino acid sequence [5]. Genetic analysis has subsequently identified more than a dozen closely related polypeptides (α_{1-10}, β_{1-4}, γ, δ, and ε) that combine to form a variety of nACh receptors, constituting a **receptor family**. The subunit types and stoichiometry for native pentameric nACh receptors in muscle and neural tissues remains an area of intensive research [6]. In adult muscle nACh receptors, the ε subunit replaces δ, but ε may re-emerge in muscle receptors formed during pathological conditions such as after burn or denervation injury. Neuronal and glial nACh receptors consist mostly of either α_7 subunits or α_4/β_2 combinations, while postsynaptic nACh receptors in autonomic ganglia consist of α_3/β_4 and $\alpha_3/\alpha_4/\beta_2/\beta_4$ combinations.

Muscarinic ACh receptors are distinguished from nicotinic ACh receptors not only by their distinct pharmacology and tissue distribution; they belong to an entirely separate superfamily of receptors, the seven-transmembrane G-protein-coupled receptors. Genetic analysis has revealed five distinct types of muscarinic receptors in a family (M_1 through M_5) [7].

Receptor superfamilies of related cellular receptors have been identified based on structural analyses (mostly peptide sequence homologies from genetic data, but also x-ray crystallography) and functional studies. Receptors within superfamilies are thought to have evolved from common ancestor receptors. This chapter provides a broad overview of several chemoreceptor superfamilies (Fig. 1.1). Following chapters contain detailed discussion of some of these superfamilies.

(1) **The seven-transmembrane receptors**, also known as G-protein-coupled receptors (GPCRs) are the largest superfamily of drug targets, containing over 60 families of proteins [8–11]. Some genes encode seven-transmembrane receptors with yet undefined physiological roles, known as orphan receptors. These are membrane proteins formed by a single peptide containing seven transmembrane helices with an extracellular N-terminal domain and an intracellular C-terminal domain. Endogenous GPCR agonists include neurotransmitters, small peptide hormones, neurotransmitters, prostanoids, and nucleotides. The intracellular domains of these receptors interact with a heterotrimeric G-protein complex that includes a GTPase domain. Activation of GPCRs leads to generation of second messengers such as cAMP, cGMP, and intracellular calcium. Persistent activation leads to a drop-off in activity, termed **desensitization**, via several mechanisms. Intracellular domains may be

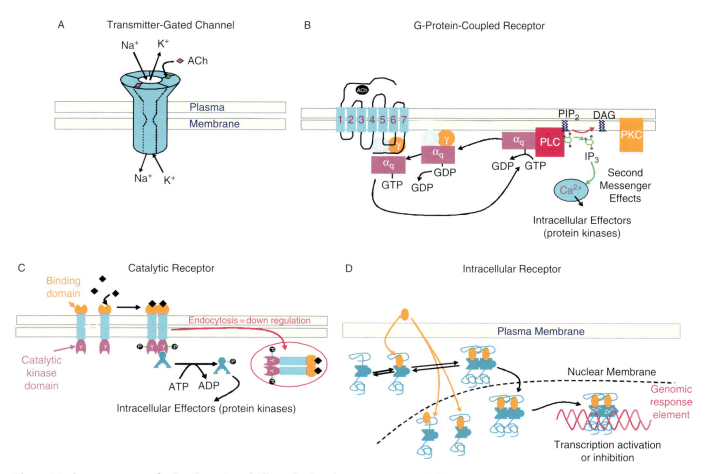

Figure 1.1. Drug receptor superfamilies. Illustrations of different families of receptor proteins, including (A) transmitter-gated ion channels, (B) G-protein-coupled receptors, (C) catalytic receptors, and (D) intracellular receptors.

modified by intracellular enzymes, blocking interactions with G-protein complexes. In addition, these receptors may be removed from the cell surface via endocytosis. This superfamily is described in detail in Chapter 2. Drugs used in anesthesia that target GPCRs include atropine and glycopyrollate (muscarinic ACh receptors), antihistamines (histamine receptors), opioids (opioid receptors), adrenergic drugs (adrenoceptors), adenosine (adenosine receptors), and some antiemetics (dopamine receptors).

(2) **The Cys-loop ligand-gated ion channel** superfamily (LGICs) are transmitter-gated channels. This superfamily includes four families of membrane proteins that are fast neurotransmitter receptors: nicotinic ACh receptors, γ-aminobutyric acid type A (GABA$_A$) receptors, glycine receptors, and serotonin type 3 (5-HT$_3$) receptors [12,13]. All of these ligand-gated ion channels contain five subunits arranged around a transmembrane ion pore. All subunits in this superfamily have structures that include a large N-terminal extracellular domain containing a Cys-X$_{13}$-Cys motif (the Cys-loop), four transmembrane

(TM) helical domains, and a large intracellular domain between TM3 and TM4. Activating drugs (neurotransmitters) bind to sites formed at the interface between extracellular domains [14]. These binding events are coupled to gating of the ion-conductive pore, and opening of this ion channel leads to altered electrical potential within cells. Persistent activation of these receptors leads to desensitization via a conformational change in the receptor that reduces response to neurotransmitter. This superfamily is described in detail in Chapter 3. Drugs used in anesthesia that target Cys-loop LGICs include neuromuscular blockers (nicotinic ACh receptors), intravenous and volatile general anesthetics (GABA$_A$ and glycine receptors), and antiemetics (5-HT$_3$ receptors).

(3) **Catalytic receptors** contain an extracellular drug-binding domain, one (typically) or more transmembrane domains, and an intracellular enzyme domain. There are several classes of these receptors: receptor tyrosine kinases (RTKs) [15,16], tyrosine kinase associated receptors (TKARs), receptor serine/threonine kinases (RSTKs),

receptor guanylate cyclases, and receptor tyrosine phosphatases (RTPs). Drugs include growth factors (e.g., insulin), trophic factors, activins, inhibins, cytokines, lymphokines such as tumor necrosis factor [17,18], and natriuretic peptide. Toll-like receptors, which recognize molecular markers on invasive pathogens and activate cellular immune defenses, are also in this class. Drug binding to catalytic receptors usually causes receptor dimerization with accompanying activation. Intracellular enzymatic activity triggers a variety of functional changes. Active dimer forms undergo endocytosis as a mechanism of desensitization.

(4) **Intracellular receptors – Nuclear receptors** are a superfamily of intracellular transcription factors that interact with small hydrophobic molecules such as steroids, vitamin D, thyroid hormones, and retinoid hormones (retinoic acid and vitamin A) [19]. Receptor–drug complexes either form in the nucleus or translocate from cytoplasm to nucleus. Genomic DNA response elements bind to dimeric receptor–drug complexes at 60-amino-acid domains that also coordinate zinc ions. Nuclear receptors regulate gene transcription.

(5) **Endocytotic receptors** are transmembrane receptors that bind extracellular drugs and then translocate into the cell by endocytosis, a process of clathrin-coating, invagination, and vesicle formation. These receptors take up essential cell nutrients such as cholesterol (bound to low-density lipoprotein or LDL) and iron (bound to ferritin). Other cell-surface receptors may undergo endocytosis as a mechanism of receptor downregulation, usually following persistent activation.

(6) **Other protein drug targets.** The above list of receptors is truncated for simplicity. Other drug receptor superfamilies include many ion channels such as transient receptor potential (TRP) ion channels (important in peripheral sensory transduction) and voltage-gated ion channels, including sodium channels, potassium channels, chloride channels, and calcium channels (important in myocardium, skeletal muscle and nerve excitability, and propagation of electrical signals). Other transmitter-gated ion channels include N-methyl-D-aspartate (NMDA)-sensitive and kainite-sensitive glutamate receptor ion channels, purinergic receptors, and zinc-activated channels. Drug targets also include a variety of transmembrane pumps and transporters for ions (e.g., the $Na^+/K^+/2Cl^-$ cotransporter target of the diuretic furosemide), neurotransmitters, and other molecules. Intracellular and circulating enzymes represent another large class of drug targets, including cyclooxygenase, lipoxygenases, phosphodiesterases, and hemostatic factors.

There are several **common themes** in the physiology of drug receptor superfamilies. First, receptor–effector coupling is often a multiple-step process, providing these systems with both positive (amplification) and negative feedback. Second,

active receptors usually are formed from multiple peptides. Drug-gated ion channels exist as multimers with multiple sites for their endogenous drugs, and in most cases more than a single drug must bind in order to activate these channels. G-protein-coupled receptors are multimeric complexes that dissociate upon activation. Both enzyme-linked receptors and intracellular receptors dimerize as they activate following drug binding. Third, most receptor molecules undergo desensitization following persistent activation.

Drug–receptor interactions
Drug–receptor binding
The first step in the chain of events leading to a drug effect in a physiological system is binding to a site on its receptor. Drug binding sites on receptor molecules are classified as **orthosteric** (the site where endogenous activators bind) or **allosteric**. The term *allosteric* literally means *other place*, and was originally applied to modulatory sites on enzymes that are distinct from active (substrate) sites. When applied to receptors, the term may have multiple meanings. In particular, the orthosteric sites of chemoreceptors "allosterically" alter activity of the "active sites," which may be enzymatic sites where substrates bind, sites where other proteins (e.g. G proteins) bind, or ion pores.

Drug binding studies on receptors are used to characterize their affinities. Measuring binding in tissue, cells, or purified receptor proteins requires the ability to accurately measure receptor-bound drug independently from free (unbound) drug, and correction for nonspecific binding to other components of tissues, cells, and even experimental equipment. Whereas drug binding to receptors will display saturation as all of the receptor sites become occupied, **nonspecific binding** is characterized by low affinity and is therefore usually linear and nonsaturable over the drug concentration range relevant for receptor binding (Fig. 1.2).

Reversible interactions between drugs and their receptor sites are determined by the same noncovalent biophysical forces that affect protein structure: ionic bonds, hydrogen bonds, van der Waals interactions, and the hydrophobic effect. At the molecular level, initial drug–receptor binding is a bimolecular association process, and the drug concentration (in moles/liter, M) is an independent (controllable) variable in in-vitro experiments. The bimolecular association rate is $[D] \times k_{on}$, where k_{on} is the on-rate in units of $M^{-1} s^{-1}$. Drug dissociation is a unimolecular process, characterized by an off-rate, k_{off}, with units of s^{-1} (Eq. 1.1). The strength of reversible interactions between a drug and its site(s) on a receptor is reflected in its **equilibrium binding affinity**, which is usually reported as a **dissociation constant**, K_D, with units in moles/liter (M). When the drug concentration $[D] = K_D$, association and dissociation rates are equal. High affinity is associated with a low K_D, and low affinity with a high K_D.

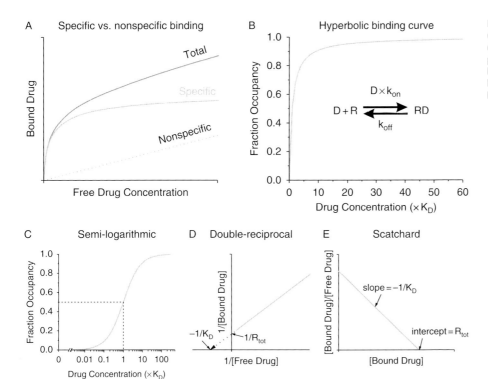

Figure 1.2. Drug binding graphical analysis. (A) Illustration of specific vs. nonspecific binding. (B) Correcting total binding for nonspecific binding produces a saturable hyperbolic binding curve on linear axes (Eq. 1.4). (C) Semilogarithmic plot with logarithmic concentration axes. (D) Lineweaver–Burke double-reciprocal plot. (E) Scatchard plot.

Drug binding

A quantitative treatment of this concept should be familiar from chemical equilibrium theory. In the simplest case with a single drug binding site:

$$D + R \underset{k_{\mathrm{off}}}{\overset{[D] \times k_{\mathrm{on}}}{\rightleftharpoons}} RD \qquad (1.1)$$

where $K_{\mathrm{D}} \equiv \dfrac{k_{\mathrm{off}}}{k_{\mathrm{on}}} = \dfrac{[R] \times [D]}{[RD]}$ (1.2)

Thus $[RD] = [R] \times \dfrac{[D]}{K_{\mathrm{D}}}$ (1.3)

Assuming the total number of receptors $R_{\mathrm{tot}} = R + RD$ is constant (the law of mass action), then the fraction of bound receptors is:

$$\frac{[RD]}{[R_{\mathrm{tot}}]} = \frac{[RD]}{[R] + [RD]} = \frac{[R] \times \frac{[D]}{K_{\mathrm{D}}}}{[R] \times \left(1 + \frac{[D]}{K_{\mathrm{D}}}\right)} = \frac{[D]}{[D] + K_{\mathrm{D}}} \qquad (1.4)$$

Equation 1.4 is a **Langmuir isotherm** or a hyperbolic binding curve (Fig. 1.2B). Site occupancy is ~1% at $[D] = 0.01 \times K_{\mathrm{D}}$, 10% at $0.11 \times K_{\mathrm{D}}$, 50% at K_{D}, 90% at $9 \times K_{\mathrm{D}}$, and 99% at $99 \times K_{\mathrm{D}}$. Because of the wide range (four orders of magnitude) of drug concentrations needed to span from low occupancy to nearly saturated, binding curves are frequently plotted with drug concentration on a logarithmic axis (Fig. 1.2C).

The semilog plot displays a sigmoid shape. The midpoint of this curve (50% occupancy) corresponds to K_{D}.

Linear transformations of Eq. 1.4 are frequently used to provide easier graphical analysis (common before computerized nonlinear regression analysis). The Lineweaver–Burke or double-reciprocal plot (Fig. 1.2D) is readily derived from Eq. 1.4:

$$\frac{[R_{\mathrm{tot}}]}{[RD]} = \frac{[D] + K_{\mathrm{D}}}{[D]} = 1 + \frac{K_{\mathrm{D}}}{[D]}, \text{ thus } \frac{1}{[RD]} = \frac{1}{[R_{\mathrm{tot}}]} + \frac{1}{[D]} \times \frac{K_{\mathrm{D}}}{[R_{\mathrm{tot}}]} \qquad (1.5a)$$

Plotting $1/[RD]$ vs. $1/[D]$ (i.e., reciprocal of bound drug vs. reciprocal of free drug) gives a line with slope $= K_{\mathrm{D}}/[R_{\mathrm{tot}}]$ and intercept on the y-axis $= 1/[R_{\mathrm{tot}}]$. The extrapolated x-axis intercept is $-1/K_{\mathrm{D}}$.

Equation 1.5a can be rearranged to give:

$$\frac{[RD]}{[D]} = \frac{[R_{\mathrm{tot}}]}{K_{\mathrm{D}}} - \frac{[RD]}{K_{\mathrm{D}}} \qquad (1.5b)$$

Equation 1.5b is the basis for another common linear transformation of binding data, the Scatchard plot (Fig. 1.2E). For Scatchard analysis, the ratio of bound to free drug ($[RD]/[D]$) is plotted against bound drug ($[RD]$), resulting in a line with slope $= -1/K_{\mathrm{D}}$ and x-axis intercept $= R_{\mathrm{tot}}$.

Stoichiometry of drug binding may be greater than one site per receptor, especially for multi-subunit receptors. When more than one site is present, there may be different binding affinities associated with different receptor subsites. In addition there may be cooperative interactions between different subsites. **Binding cooperativity** may be positive or negative.

Positive cooperativity is when occupancy of one site enhances binding at another site. Negative cooperativity is when occupancy of one site reduces affinity at another site.

Selectivity – Drug receptor sites display variable degrees of **selectivity** for drugs with slightly different molecular structures [20–22]. An important example of this concept is the selectivity for different adrenoceptor subtypes (α_1, α_2, β_1, and β_2) to various derivatives of the endogenous transmitters epinephrine and norepinephrine (e.g., phenylephrine, dopamine, isoproterenol, terbutaline, etc.) [23]. Another common feature of many drug sites is **stereoselectivity**. Drugs often have one or more chiral centers. A single chiral center means that the drug can exist as a pair of enantiomers (mirror images, R- or S-, *d-* or *l-*), while multiple chiral centers results in diastereomers. Drug enantiomers (and diastereomers) may interact differently with receptor sites and with other sites. If a high-affinity stereoisomer can be isolated, it may act as a more potent, more efficacious, and less toxic drug. Examples used in anesthesia include etomidate, a general anesthetic used as a pure R(+) stereoisomer [24], levobupivacaine, the L-isomer of bupivacaine [25], and cisatracurium, the *cis*-diastereomer of atracurium.

Specificity – Many drugs bind to more than one molecular target at clinically relevant concentrations. One receptor may mediate the desired therapeutic action, while binding to other targets may be associated with side effects or toxicity. Specificity of binding is therefore usually a desirable feature of drugs. High specificity means that the drug interacts with only one or a small number of target sites.

Small hydrophilic drugs can diffuse rapidly and are exploited for rapid cell-to-cell signaling (e.g., neurotransmission). Small drugs have limited ability to form noncovalent binding interactions, so are generally lower affinity and lower specificity than large drugs. In some cases, two or more small drugs are required for effect (e.g., neurotransmitters). Large drugs diffuse more slowly, but can generate more binding affinity and specificity.

Consequences of drug–receptor interactions

The previous section examined drug binding to receptors. This section now examines the consequences of drug binding, that is, drug response or drug effects. Drugs may either increase or decrease various functions of biological systems. **Drug effects** may be studied in molecules, cells, or tissues under conditions of well-defined free drug concentration, resulting in concentration–response relationships [26]. Drug responses are typically **graded** within an experimentally established minimum to maximum range, and may be mediated directly by the drug receptor (e.g., an ionic current due to activation of an ion channel chemoreceptor) or by a second messenger (e.g., cAMP concentration) or other downstream cellular processes (e.g., muscle contraction force).

Most drug effects are **reversible**, ending when drug concentration and occupation of receptor binding sites diminish to zero. Drug effects may also be **irreversible**. Irreversible drugs form covalent bonds with receptors (e.g., aspirin acetylates cyclooxygenase, irreversibly inactivating the enzyme). **Pseudoirreversible** drugs are high-affinity noncovalent drugs that unbind so slowly that they are effectively irreversible. Antibodies and certain toxins that bind with sub-nanomolar affinity behave pseudoirreversibly.

Agonists

Agonists are drugs that bind to and activate receptors, resulting in a biological response. Agonist effects are described by two fundamental characteristics, **efficacy** and **potency** (Fig. 1.3A) [27]. Efficacy reflects the ability of the agonist to activate the receptor, and is the maximal response or effect possible when all receptor sites are fully occupied (sometimes called E_{max}). Agonists may be classified as **full agonists** (high efficacy) or **partial agonists** (low efficacy). Full agonists elicit a maximum possible response from a system, while partial agonists elicit less than a full response, even when all receptors are occupied. At the receptor level, full agonists activate nearly all receptors, while partial agonists activate only a fraction of receptors [28,29]. Partial agonism can be a desirable feature of drugs, particularly when full agonism is associated with toxicity. For example, full opioid receptor agonists can cause profound respiratory depression, whereas partial agonists that cause less respiratory depression may provide a safety advantage, while also limiting antinociceptive efficacy.

Potency refers to the concentration (or amount) of a drug needed to produce a defined effect. The most common measure of agonist potency is the **half-maximal effective concentration** (EC_{50}), the concentration at which a drug produces 50% of its maximal possible response in a molecule, cell, or tissue [27]. Potency and EC_{50} are inversely related: when EC_{50} is low, potency is high, and vice versa. At the molecular level, agonist potency is related to its affinity for the receptor, but is not exactly equal to it, because **receptor activation is not equivalent to agonist binding**. Quantitatively, an agonist's EC_{50} is a function of both its binding affinity, K_A (the subscript A designates an agonist drug) and its efficacy, which depends on the series or network of linked responses that follow binding. A simple example is a two-step model for activation of a receptor-ion channel target, where efficacy is represented by a second monomolecular transition from inactive (nonconductive) to the active (conductive) state (Eq. 1.6). Agonist (A) binding to the inactive receptor (R) is defined by the equilibrium binding site affinity K_A, and channel activation is characterized by the equilibrium between inactive and active drug-bound receptors (RA and RA*, respectively). If the inactive $\leftrightarrow$ active equilibrium strongly favors the RA* state, then the RA state is depopulated, which results in more receptor binding. When this happens, EC_{50} is lower than K_A (Fig. 1.3B).

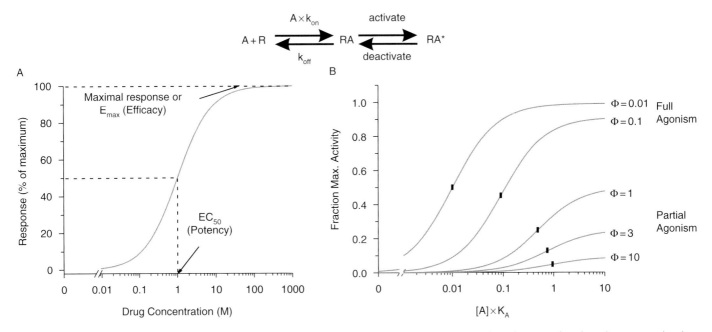

Figure 1.3. Agonist efficacy and apparent potency (EC_{50}). (A) This panel appears similar to Fig. 1.2C, except that the ordinate is a physiological response, rather than binding-site occupancy. The maximal response is drug efficacy. The concentration producing half-maximal response is the EC_{50}. (B) Lines were generated using Eq. 1.7. Affinity for inactive receptors, K_A, was held constant. ϕ is defined as the equilibrium constant for activation: $\phi = [RA]/[RA^*]$. Thus, a low ϕ value is associated with full agonism and a high ϕ is associated with partial agonism. The midpoints of the curves, EC_{50}, are indicated by vertical bars. Note that EC_{50} approximates K_A only when ϕ is much larger than 1.

$$A + R \underset{k_{off}}{\overset{[A] \times k_{on}}{\rightleftharpoons}} RA \underset{k_{deactivate}}{\overset{k_{activate}}{\rightleftharpoons}} RA \qquad (1.6)$$

where K_A is the dissociation constant for A binding to R and $\phi \equiv \dfrac{k_{deactivate}}{k_{activate}} = \dfrac{[RA]}{[RA^*]}$. The fraction of *active receptors* is:

$$\frac{[RA^*]}{[R_{tot}]} = \frac{[R] \times \dfrac{[A]}{\phi K_A}}{[R] \times \left(1 + \dfrac{[A]}{K_D} + \dfrac{[A]}{\phi K_A}\right)} = \frac{[A]}{[A] + \phi[A] + \phi K_A}$$
$$= \left(\frac{1}{1+\phi}\right) \times \left(\frac{[A]}{[A] + \frac{\phi K_A}{1+\phi}}\right) \qquad (1.7)$$

Equation 1.7 has the same form as Eq. 1.4, with a maximum amplitude of $(1 + \phi)^{-1}$ and half-maximal concentration (K_A^{app} or EC_{50}) $= \phi K_A / (1 + \phi)$. The amplitude factor $(1 + \phi)^{-1}$ is agonist **intrinsic efficacy**, often designated as ε [27]. When ϕ is large (inactive state favored), efficacy is low (partial agonism) and when ϕ is small, efficacy is high (full agonism). The EC_{50} is only close to K_A when $\phi \gg 1$ (i.e., for weak partial agonists). When efficacy is high (i.e., $\phi < 1$), EC_{50} is less than K_A (Fig. 1.3B).

Note that the serial binding → activation scheme in Eq. 1.6 does not allow nondrugged receptors to activate. The conformational change triggered by agonist binding is presumed to be due to "induced fit," wherein agonist binding to the inactive receptor induces or allows a conformational change that both activates the receptor and tightens agonist binding. Agonist binding to active receptors is characterized by a dissociation constant of ϕK_A.

Multiple agonist sites and the Hill equation – When occupancy of more than one drug-binding site is required to activate a receptor, concentration–response curves often display a steeper dependence on drug concentration. The case with two equivalent sites is:

$$D + R \underset{k_{off}}{\overset{2[A] \times k_{on}}{\rightleftharpoons}} RA \underset{2k_{off}}{\overset{[A] \times k_{on}}{\rightleftharpoons}} RA_2 \qquad (1.8)$$

Dissociation constants at each step reflect the different binding and unbinding rates depending on the number of binding sites. Thus:

$$[RA] = [R] \times \frac{2 \times [A]}{K_A} \qquad (1.9)$$

and

$$[RA_2] = [RA] \times \frac{[A]}{2 \times K_A} = [R] \times \frac{[A]^2}{K_A^2} \qquad (1.10)$$

The fraction of activatable RA_2 receptors is:

$$\frac{[RA_2]}{[R_{tot}]} = \frac{[RA_2]}{[R] + [RA] + [RA_2]}$$
$$= \frac{[R] \times \dfrac{[A]^2}{K_A^2}}{[R] \times \left(1 + \dfrac{2[A]}{K_A} + \dfrac{[A]^2}{K_A^2}\right)} = \left(\frac{[A]}{[A] + K_A}\right)^2 \qquad (1.11)$$

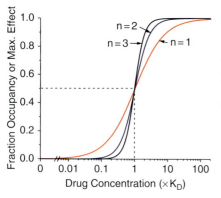

Figure 1.4. Hill analysis for multiple agonists. Semilogarithmic logistic dose–response curves, generated using Eq. 1.13, with $n = 1$, 2, and 3. Note that the midpoint of the curves (EC_{50}) is not dependent on the Hill-slope, n.

The general form of this equation for n equivalent drug (D) sites is:

$$\frac{RD_n}{R_{tot}} = \left(\frac{D}{D + K_D}\right)^n \qquad (1.12)$$

Note that when $D = K_D$, $RD_n/R_{tot} = (0.5)^n$. The half-maximal occupancy/activity concentration, EC_{50}, is no longer proportional to K_D (K_A). A closely related equation that is often used for graphical/parametric analysis of concentration–response data is the **Hill equation** [30], also known as the **logistic equation**:

$$\text{Response} = (E_{max} - E_{min}) \times \frac{[D]^n}{[D]^n + EC_{50}^n} + E_{min} \qquad (1.13)$$

E_{max} and E_{min} are respectively, maximum and minimum responses. In Eq. 1.13, the half-maximal effect concentration (EC_{50}) is independent of n (Fig. 1.4). Values of the **Hill coefficient** (n) larger than 1 indicate more than one drug site and possible positive cooperativity. Values of n lower than 1 may also indicate multiple drug sites (heterogeneous binding) with possible negative cooperativity.

Indirect agonists act through mechanisms that do not involve binding to the target receptor. A common example in anesthesia is the use of acetylcholinesterase inhibitors such as neostigmine and pyridostigmine to reverse neuromuscular blockade. By slowing the breakdown of acetylcholine (ACh) in motor synapses, these drugs increase the ACh concentration, increasing the activation of postsynaptic nicotinic ACh receptors.

Antagonists

Antagonists are drugs that inhibit receptor activity [31]. Receptor antagonists can be classified as **competitive** or **noncompetitive** (Fig. 1.5).

Competitive antagonists bind at the orthosteric (agonist) sites, but do not activate receptors. As a result, they prevent agonists from occupying those sites and inhibit receptor activation. In other words, competitive antagonists and agonists

display **mutually exclusive binding**. Binding assays with increasing concentrations of competitive antagonists result in reduced agonist binding, and vice versa. Thus, addition of a reversible competitive antagonist results in a rightward shift of the agonist dose–response (toward higher doses), decreasing the apparent potency (increased EC_{50}) of the agonist. Reversible competitive antagonist binding and effects are **surmountable** – increasing the concentration of agonist displaces inhibitor from binding sites and restores full agonist occupancy and response – and therefore agonist efficacy is unchanged (Fig. 1.6B).

$$\begin{array}{c} A + I + R \xrightleftharpoons{K_A} RA \\[4pt] k_I \Big\updownarrow \\[4pt] RI \end{array} \qquad (1.14)$$

In Eq. 1.14, A is an agonist, while I is a reversible competitive antagonist with dissociation constant K_I (the subscript I is for inhibitor). We eliminate receptor activation for simplicity. The fraction of activatable RA receptors is:

$$\frac{[RA]}{[R_{tot}]} = \frac{[RA]}{[R] + [RA] + [RI]} = \frac{[R] \times \dfrac{[A]}{K_A}}{[R] + [R] \times \left(\dfrac{[A]}{K_A} + \dfrac{[I]}{K_I}\right)}$$

$$= \frac{[A]}{[A] + K_A \times \left(1 + \dfrac{[I]}{K_I}\right)} \qquad (1.15)$$

This equation again has the general form of a Langmuir isotherm with a constant maximum occupancy of 1.0 and half occupancy at $[A] = K_A \times (1 + [I]/K_I)$. Thus, as [I] increases, agonist concentration–responses shift rightward in a parallel fashion and EC_{50} increases as a linear function of [I] (Fig. 1.6). **Schild analysis** [32] is based on this relationship: the ratio of agonist concentrations needed to evoke an equal response (e.g., 50% of maximum) in the presence vs. absence of a competitive inhibitor is:

$$\frac{[EC_X]_I}{[EC_X]_0} = 1 + \frac{[I]}{K_I} \qquad (1.16)$$

A similar relationship exists for the competitive inhibitor when the agonist is varied. The **IC_{50}** for inhibitors is the concentration that inhibits half of the control response with no inhibitor. Thus:

$$\frac{[A]}{[A] + K_A \times \left(1 + \dfrac{IC_{50}}{K_I}\right)} = \frac{1}{2} \times \frac{[A]}{[A] + K_A} \qquad (1.17)$$

Solving for IC_{50}, one obtains:

$$IC_{50} = K_I \times \left(1 + \frac{[A]}{K_A}\right) \qquad (1.18)$$

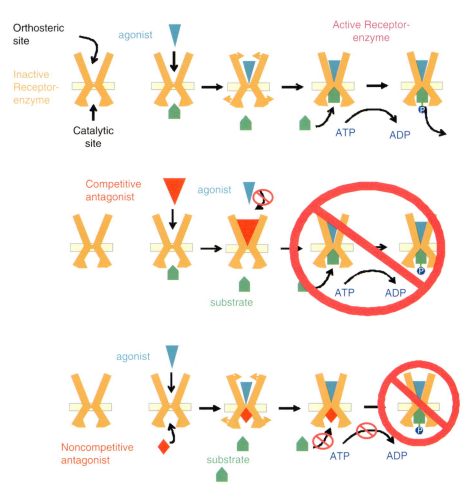

Figure 1.5. Model receptor illustration of agonism and antagonism. Top: A simple catalytic receptor model is illustrated, depicting agonist (blue triangle) binding, which induces a conformational change allowing substrate (green) binding and phosphorylation. Middle: A competitive inhibitor (red triangle) binds to the agonist (orthosteric) site, preventing agonist binding and activation of the receptor. Bottom: A noncompetitive inhibitor (red diamond) does not block agonist binding, but binds at the active site, preventing substrate binding and thereby reducing activity whether or not agonist binds.

Partial agonists as competitive antagonists – In the presence of full agonists, partial agonists appear to inhibit receptors like competitive antagonists. Partial agonists bind at orthosteric sites, preventing occupancy by full agonists, and reducing activation. Partial agonists do not produce full inhibition, because high concentrations activate a fraction of receptors. Their inhibitory effect is surmountable with increased concentrations of full agonist.

Noncompetitive antagonists bind at sites other than the orthosteric site (allosteric sites). Thus, noncompetitive antagonists can bind to receptors whether or not orthosteric sites are occupied by agonist. In the simplest case of noncompetitive inhibition, agonist binding is unaffected, but receptor activation is blocked. Thus, addition of noncompetitive antagonists will not alter agonist binding affinity or the number of agonist sites, but result in a reduced number of activatable receptors. In the presence of noncompetitive antagonism, agonist concentration–responses display reduced agonist efficacy with unaltered EC_{50} (Fig. 1.7). Inhibition by noncompetitive antagonists is not surmountable with high agonist concentrations.

Equation 1.19 and Figure 1.7 illustrate noncompetitive antagonism when the affinities of agonists and antagonists are independent:

$$A + I + R \xrightleftharpoons{K_A} RA$$
$$k_I \big\updownarrow \qquad k_I \big\updownarrow \qquad (1.19)$$
$$RI \xrightleftharpoons{K_A} RAI$$

Thus:

$$\frac{[RA]}{R_{tot}} = \frac{[RA]}{[R] + [RA] + \|RI\| + [RAI]} =$$

$$\frac{[R] \times \dfrac{[A]}{K_A}}{[R] \times \left(1 + \dfrac{[A]}{K_A} + \dfrac{[I]}{K_I} + \dfrac{[A]\cdot[I]}{K_I}\right)} = \left(\frac{K_I}{[I]+K_I}\right) \times \frac{[A]}{[A]+K_A} \quad (1.20)$$

This equation again is a Langmuir isotherm with amplitude $= K_I/([I] + K_I)$ and $EC_{50} = K_A$. (We have again simplified the math by eliminating receptor activation steps.) In this case, $IC_{50} = K_I$. Note that agonist EC_{50} is independent of inhibitor concentration and IC_{50} is independent of agonist concentration.

Irreversible antagonists, whether they act at the orthosteric site (competitive) or not, reduce the number of activatable receptors, while the remaining unbound receptors behave normally. This is another form of insurmountable inhibition,

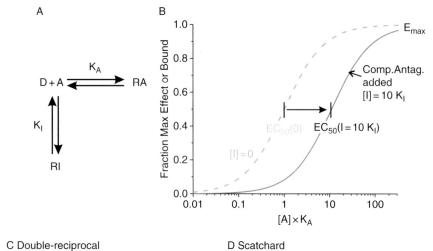

Figure 1.6. Competitive inhibition. (A) Mutually exclusive receptor occupation is depicted schematically. The RA state can activate, but the RI state cannot. (B) Agonist concentration–response curves were generated with Eq. 1.13. Addition of a competitive inhibitor reduces agonist binding and effects at low agonist concentrations, while increasing agonist EC_{50} (shifting agonist concentration–response rightward). The inhibition is surmountable, as E_{max} remains unchanged. (C) A double-reciprocal plot for agonist binding experiments in the presence of a reversible competitive inhibitor shows an altered slope and a change in apparent K_A, but the same number of receptors. (D) A Scatchard plot for agonist binding depicting the change in slope in the presence of a competitive inhibitor.

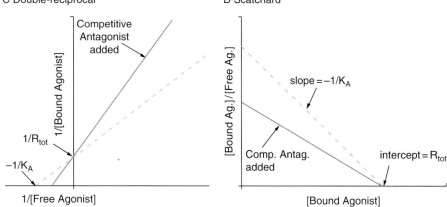

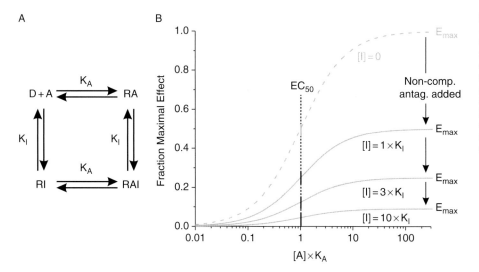

Figure 1.7. Noncompetitive inhibition. Left: A scheme depicting binding of inhibitor (I) to receptors whether or not agonist is bound. Right: The panel shows the effect of non-competitive inhibitor on agonist concentration–response curves. Noncompetitive and irreversible antagonists reduce apparent agonist efficacy (E_{max}) without changing apparent K_A (EC_{50}), indicated by the vertical bars. Note that agonist binding studies in the presence of a noncompetitive inhibitor of this type will not show any change, because the inhibitor does not compete with agonist or alter its affinity.

and concentration–response data in receptors exposed to irreversible antagonists appear similar to those for noncompetitive antagonists. Competitive binding studies can reveal whether an irreversible antagonist binds at the orthosteric site, which would lead to reduced agonist binding, or allosteric sites, which would not reduce agonist binding.

Indirect antagonism occurs without receptor binding. One mechanism of indirect antagonism is direct binding to agonist (or drug), making it unable to bind to its receptor. An example is the use of protamine to bind and inactivate heparin, preventing activation of its molecular target, antithrombin.

Allosteric receptor activation models

A more general treatment of drug–receptor interactions enables formal description of situations that are frequently observed in molecular pharmacology, but which are poorly described by serial binding-activation models. These receptor models, introduced in 1965 by Monod, Wyman, and Changeux, are referred to as allosteric models, based on the fact that agonist binding sites for receptors are distinct from their active sites (ion channels or enzyme domains, etc.) [33]. The major difference between allosteric activation models and the serial binding-activation models described above is that allosteric models allow for receptor activation in the absence of agonists. This adds a fourth state, R^*, and results in a cyclic scheme (Eq. 1.20). Many receptors, including many GPCRs, are indeed partially active in the absence of agonists, indicating a pre-existing equilibrium between active and inactive receptors [34]. Agonist binding shifts this equilibrium further toward the active state, and, by implication, agonists bind more tightly to the active state than to the inactive state. The existence of the R^* state differs fundamentally from the induced-fit hypothesis implied by serial binding-activation models. In practice, serial binding-activation represents a subset of conditions that can be described by allosteric models, specifically when the fraction of R^* is extremely small relative to R.

The simplest allosteric model for agonism is shown in Eq. 1.21.

$$\begin{array}{ccc} A + R & \xrightarrow{K_A} & RA \\ L_0 \updownarrow & & \updownarrow L_1 \\ R^* & \xrightarrow{K_A^*} & RA^* \end{array} \qquad (1.21)$$

Note that undrugged R can convert to an active state R^* without agonist binding. An equilibrium constant (L_0) characterizes this monomolecular transition: $L_0 = [R]/[R^*]$. L_1 is equivalent to ϕ in Eqs. 1.6 and 1.7. Equation 1.21 also explicitly shows that agonist binding to active receptors is different from binding to inactive receptors. Furthermore, because of the cyclic nature of the scheme, there is a constraint on the system, $K_A \times L_1 = L_0 \times K_A^*$, so:

$$\frac{L_1}{L_0} = \frac{K_A^*}{K_A} \qquad (1.22)$$

Thus, this system is defined by only three equilibrium constants.

The ratio $K_A^*/K_A \equiv c$ is the allosteric agonist efficacy. Highly efficacious agonists ($c << 1$) shift the equilibrium strongly toward the active state by binding much more tightly to active than to inactive receptors.

The fraction of active receptors is:

$$\frac{[R^*] + [RA^*]}{R_{tot}} = \frac{1}{1 + L_0 \times \left(\frac{1 + [A]/K_A}{1 + [A]/K_A^*}\right)} \qquad (1.23)$$

When $[A] = 0$, the minimum fraction of active receptors is $(1 + L_0)^{-1}$ and when $[A]$ is very high (occupying all agonist sites), the fraction of active receptors approaches $(1 + cL_0)^{-1}$.

Also implicit in the allosteric gating concept is that there are conformational changes in the agonist binding site that are coupled to activation of the receptor. These conformational changes are associated with tighter binding to agonist at the orthosteric site, but are not necessarily "induced" by agonist binding, because they may occur in the absence of agonists.

Using the formalism of allosteric gating, **full agonists** and **partial agonists** are redefined (Fig. 1.8B) [35]. Agonists shift the equilibrium toward active states, so **for all agonists, $c < 1$**. Full agonists are those for which $c \times L_0 << 1$, and partial agonists are those for which $c \times L_0 > 1$ (i.e., less than 50% activation is induced). An interesting feature of this concept is that agonist efficacy is dependent on L_0, so when L_0 is small, an agonist that only modestly shifts the activation equilibrium can stimulate a large fraction of receptors to activate. Conversely, if L_0 is extremely large (i.e., the receptor has extremely low spontaneous activity), agonists need to shift the activation equilibrium a great deal to activate a significant fraction of receptors (Fig. 1.8C).

The concept of **inverse agonism** can be understood in the context of allosteric activation schemes. Inverse agonists are drugs that bind to the orthosteric site, and where $c > 1$ (Fig. 1.8D) [36]. Thus, inverse agonists stabilize the inactive state relative to the active state by binding to inactive receptors more strongly than to active receptors. Indeed, upon careful study, many drugs that are categorized as competitive antagonists are found to be inverse agonists or extremely weak partial agonists. In the context of allosteric schemes, a truly competitive antagonist binds both active and inactive receptors with equal affinity and has no impact on the activation equilibrium; that is, $c = 1$.

Allosteric gating schemes are useful for modeling multisubunit receptors with multiple agonist sites. For example, with two homologous subunits and only two receptor states (inactive R and active R^*), agonist sites are all identical and couple equally to activation:

$$\begin{array}{ccccc} 2A + R & \xrightleftharpoons{1/2K_A} & RA & \xrightleftharpoons{2K_A} & RA_2 \\ L_0 \updownarrow & & cL_0 \updownarrow & & c^2L_0 \updownarrow \\ 2A + R^* & \xrightleftharpoons{1/2K_A^*} & RA^* & \xrightleftharpoons{2K_A^*} & RA_{2^*} \end{array} \qquad (1.24)$$

The fraction of active receptors is:

$$\frac{[R^*] + [RA^*] + [RA_2^*]}{R_{tot}} = \frac{1}{1 + L_0 \times \left(\frac{1 + [A]/K_A}{1 + [A]/cK_A}\right)^2} \qquad (1.25)$$

Allosteric concepts are also useful for modeling interactions between different drugs on a single receptor. Some drugs are

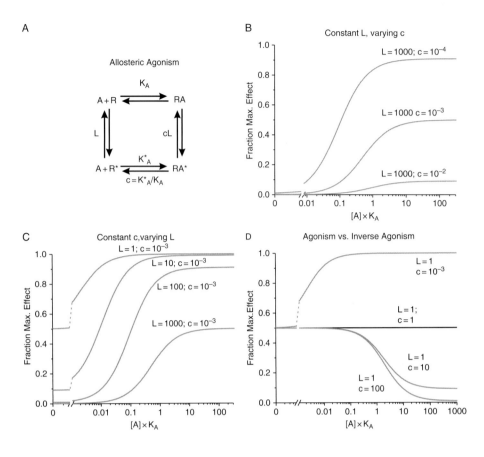

Figure 1.8. Allosteric models: agonism and inverse agonism. (A) A simple allosteric activation scheme is depicted showing inactive (R) and active (R*) receptor forms with different affinities for agonist. Agonist–response curves in panels B–D were generated using Eq. 1.23. (B) L_0 is held constant, c (efficacy) varies. Note how this panel looks just like Fig. 1.3B, because when L_0 is large the allosteric model behaves like a serial binding-activation model. (C) Efficacy (c) is constant, L_0 varies. Note spontaneous activity and higher apparent efficacy and potency of agonist as L_0 decreases. (D) Inverse agonism (reduced activity) is observed when spontaneous activity is present and $c > 1$. Pure competitive antagonism is present when $c = 1$.

allosteric enhancers. Examples include classic benzodiazepines like diazepam and midazolam that sensitize $GABA_A$ receptors to GABA, shifting GABA concentration–responses for $GABA_A$ receptors leftward. This effect could be due to allosteric effects on the GABA binding site (reducing K_A) or due to effects on receptor activation (i.e., reducing L_0). Studies on spontaneously active mutant $GABA_A$ receptors demonstrate that benzodiazepines directly enhance receptor activation in the absence of GABA, indicating that benzodiazepines are in fact weak **allosteric agonists** [37].

Spare receptors

Spare receptors exist if a maximal cellular or tissue response is elicited when receptors are not fully occupied by agonist. Formally, the presence of spare receptors is equivalent to very high drug efficacy for agonists, while reducing the apparent effect of inhibitors (Fig. 1.9). Neuromuscular transmission is characterized by spare receptors. Critical neuromuscular junctions, such as those in the diaphragm and major muscle groups, have an extremely high density of nicotinic ACh receptors. In most cases, activation of a small fraction of nACh receptors is adequate to fully activate postsynaptic muscle fascicles. With administration of nondepolarizing muscle relaxants that competitively block ACh receptor activation, symptoms of weakness typically are first seen in ocular and pharyngeal muscles, which

have smaller degrees of spareness for neurotransmission. Weakness in trunk muscles typically occurs when over 80% of receptors are blocked. Agonist concentration–responses in tissues or cells with spare receptors are shifted toward lower concentrations relative to molecular responses (Fig. 1.9A). In contrast, antagonist concentration–responses are shifted toward higher concentrations, because a maximal response may be present until a large fraction of receptors are inhibited (Fig. 1.9B). When noncompetitive inhibitors are studied in experimental systems with spare receptors, they may produce rightward shifts in agonist concentration–response without decreasing apparent efficacy. This occurs because they reduce the degree of spareness. Thus, noncompetitive inhibitors may appear to act competitively in systems exhibiting spare receptors, whereas binding studies can reveal the underlying noncompetitive interaction with agonists.

Signal amplification

Signal amplification is typical of receptors that are coupled to enzymes. Amplification is another mechanism that mimics spare receptors. Drug binding to GPCRs triggers G-protein activation that persists much longer than drug binding at the receptor. Each G protein can catalyze the production of many second-messenger molecules before deactivation. In turn, second messengers can trigger additional cascades of intracellular signal activation.

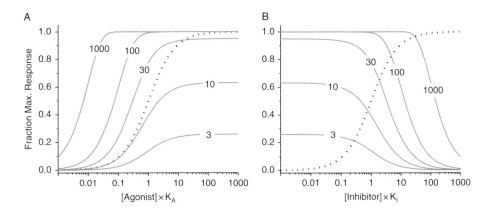

Figure 1.9. Spare receptors. (A) Spare receptors cause an apparent increase in potency and efficacy of agonists. In this model, approximately 35 receptors must be activated for a maximal cellular response and the number of receptors per cell is labeled on each curve. If there are less than 35 receptors in the cell, a sub-maximal response is observed and apparent K_A (EC_{50}) is fairly constant. When there are spare receptors (i.e., more than 35 receptors per cell), low agonist concentrations are needed to achieve the maximum response (whatever concentration activates 35 receptors). EC_{50} is therefore significantly reduced. The dotted line represents fractional agonist occupation (binding) of receptors. (B) Spare receptors cause an apparent decrease in the potency of antagonists. In this case, no inhibition occurs until noncompetitive inhibitor binding has reduced the number of active receptors to less than 35. Thus, higher fractional antagonist occupancy is required as the number of receptors per cell increases. The dotted line represents fractional antagonist occupation (binding).

Thus, GPCR activation is amplified in both space and time and occupation of a small fraction of receptors can result in a maximal cellular or tissue response that outlasts drug binding to the receptor. Similarly, the enzyme-linked surface receptors initiate cascades of phosphorylation or dephosphorylation which amplify the initiating receptor activation.

Signal damping

Signal damping or negative feedback is often present to limit physiological drug responses. This is usually observed as a diminishing response to equal drug doses over time. The term for rapidly (hours) diminishing responses to repeated drug administration is **tachyphylaxis**. Resistance to drug effects that develops over longer periods (days to months) is termed **tolerance**. Tachyphylaxis may be linked to receptor desensitization in some cases, such as the phase II neuromuscular block associated with prolonged succinylcholine administration. Ligand-gated ion channels, when persistently exposed to high agonist concentrations, go through a monomolecular conformational change that reduces channel opening even while agonist is bound. Many voltage-gated ion channels go through a similar process (inactivation). Mechanisms that involve other molecules can also damp responses. Synapses such as the neuromuscular junction show altered structure and activity within hours after physiological changes such as reduced presynaptic motor neuron activity or profound blockade of postsynaptic activity [38]. Some downstream proteins activated following GPCR agonism (receptor kinases) are feedback inhibitors that phosphorylate GPCRs and reduce their activity. Similarly, protein phosphatases (both surface receptor-linked and cytoplasmic) can be mechanisms that oppose various protein kinase enzymes. Other, slower negative feedback mechanisms include depletion of neurotransmitters or metabolites, expression of regulatory factors, receptor downregulation, and transcriptional changes.

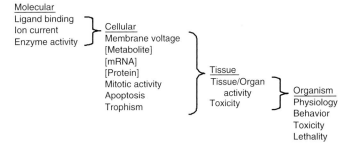

Figure 1.10. Integration of drug responses from molecules to organism.

Drug effects on organisms

Integration of drug effects – Drug responses show different concentration-dependent patterns in molecules vs. cells vs. tissues vs. animals, because the spatial and temporal integration of effects is altered at different system levels (Fig. 1.10). As a result, small changes in occupancy or efficacy at one step in a signal transduction cascade may have large effects on the overall system. Moreover, variability in individual responses at different system levels, due to genetics, environment, drug interactions, and other factors, can lead to significant interindividual differences in response to drugs. Therefore, assessing dose–response relationships in individuals provides different information than studies in populations.

Drug–response analysis in individual organisms is analogous to that in molecular pharmacology, because organism responses are the integration of multiple molecular events, governed by similar underlying relationships, and thus molecular and organism concentration–response curves have similar sigmoidal shapes. However, analysis of drug effects in organisms is usually **parametric** (descriptive), and difficult to relate quantitatively to underlying mechanisms [27]. Clinical concentration–response determinations most commonly

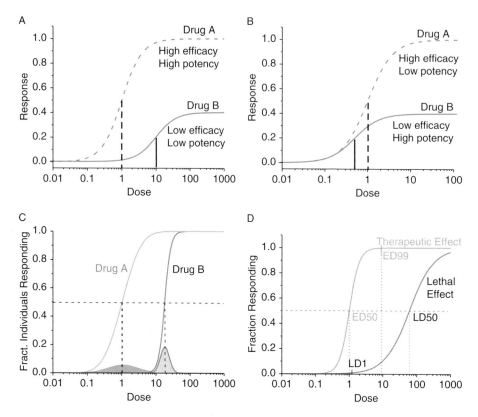

Figure 1.11. Clinical dose–response concepts. (A, B) These panels illustrate the concepts of efficacy and absolute potency in comparing drugs with similar effects. Efficacy is the maximum response. Absolute potency is the inverse of ED_{50}. A drug with low absolute potency but high efficacy may be more effective than an equal dose of a drug with higher absolute potency but lower efficacy. (C) Population dose–response studies are based on quantal (yes/no) outcomes at different drug doses. Quantal responses are often distributed in a classical bell-shaped probability curve on semilogarithmic axes (filled curves). Cumulative response curves (lines) generated from the quantal response data are sigmoidal and can be described using the Hill equation. Note that the slopes of the cumulative curves are determined by the variability (width) of the population response distributions. (D) Toxicity ratios are usually reported as the ratio of the mid-points of toxicity vs. therapeutic dose–responses. Here, the 50% lethal dose in a group of animals (LD50) is 60 times higher than the half-effect dose (ED50). However, the dose that is effective for 99% (ED99) is also lethal for about 10%. The certain safety factor (ED99/LD1) for this drug is low, about 0.1.

measure drug concentrations in blood (plasma or serum) because of its accessibility, although certain exceptions are well-known (e.g., end-tidal volatile anesthetic concentrations). Recognizing that blood is not the real site of drug action, the concept of **effect-site concentration** has been applied in pharmacokinetic/pharmacodynamic (PK/PD) models (see Chapter 5). Frequently, **dosage** rather than concentration is the independent variable used for pharmacological studies in organisms when biophase drug concentrations are not measured.

Pharmacodynamic **responses** in animals can be therapeutic, toxic, or lethal. **Graded** log drug concentration–response or dose–response curves for an individual subject measure responses on a **continuous scale** from minimum to maximum. Examples of graded responses include pupil size, blood pressure, heart rate, temperature, intracranial pressure, or pain relief. Pharmacodynamic analysis of graded concentration–response curves in individual subjects therefore parallels that in molecular, cellular, and tissue studies. The independent concepts of drug potency and efficacy are applied similarly (Fig. 1.11A–B). **Efficacy** is the maximal response in an individual achievable at the highest drug dose and **absolute drug potency** for graded responses is defined as the reciprocal of the ED_{50} (the dose producing half-maximal response). Figure 1.11A and B illustrate the comparison of drug pairs with respect to their potency and efficacy for the same effect.

Drug–response analysis in populations – In anesthesiology, it is easy to observe that responses to the same drug dose vary widely among patients. Part of the art of delivering anesthesia is titrating drug doses to provide optimal therapy for a specific patient, particularly when the drug has significant toxicities. At the same time, anesthesiologists must know dosing ranges that are appropriate for broad populations of patients, to provide dosing guidelines. For populations of patients, what matters is determining drug doses that result in important clinical (therapeutic or toxic) endpoints. As a result, characterizing dose–response relationships in populations is based on **quantal responses** and **quantal dose–response curves**. Quantal responses are either/or outcomes in individuals, such as awake/asleep, stroke/no stroke, alive after five years, etc. Graded responses may also be quantized. For example, a 20 mmHg decrease in blood pressure (yes/no), or a 50% decrease in pain (yes/no). Thus the y-axis on a quantal dose–response curve is the fraction (or percentage) of the population that exhibits the defined response (Fig. 1.11C–D). The minimum dose required to achieve the specified quantal response in a population of study subjects is usually distributed in a bell-shaped probability curve (Fig. 1.11C). The cumulative fraction of subjects that respond at a given dose (i.e., responding at that dose or lower) appears as a sigmoid curve on semilogarithmic axes. It is important to note that the shape, particularly the slope, of cumulative dose–response relationships derived from quantal data reflects the heterogeneity of the population studied rather than the underlying physiology of drug action (Fig. 1.11C).

Parameters used to describe graded dose–response curves, such as potency and efficacy, have analogs for quantal dose–response curves. Thus the dose producing a therapeutic effect in 50% of the population studied is the **ED50**, and the maximum fraction of the population displaying the specified response at high drug doses represents **population efficacy**. Note that the nomenclature for quantal (ED50) and graded (ED$_{50}$) dose–response curves differs, with the subscript numeral used only in the latter case.

In an organism or patient, a single drug may have (in fact usually has) multiple effects, and each effect may have a different dose–response relationship, depending on the mechanisms underlying each effect. Quantal dose–response curves can be used to describe multiple drug effects, such as therapeutic response, drug toxicity, or even drug lethality (more commonly in animals, for toxicity and safety testing). For example, the dose producing a particular toxicity in half the population is the **TD50**, and that causing lethality in half the population is the **LD50**. A more useful measure of drug safety than just the LD50 or TD50 is the distance between the concentration–response curves (Fig. 1.11D). The **therapeutic index** is defined as the LD50/ED50 (or sometimes TD50/ED50). Another, more stringent measure of drug safety is the **certain safety factor**, defined as the LD1/ED99 (or TD1/LD99). Compared with the therapeutic index, certain safety factor is less dependent on assuming similar slopes of the therapeutic and toxic effect curves.

Summary

Pharmacodynamics is the study of how drugs alter physiological functions, which is initiated by drug interactions with molecular targets. Drugs used in anesthesiology interact with a variety of receptors, which are proteins within or on the surface of cells that are activated by endogenous drugs, resulting in altered cell function. Receptors are categorized both by the drugs that activate them and by their structure and function. Families and superfamilies of receptors (e.g., G-protein-coupled receptors and ligand-gated ion channels) are defined by the degree of structural and functional similarity among groups of receptors. Receptors display varying degrees of selectivity for drugs with similar chemical structures. Conversely, drugs show varying degrees of specificity for the plethora of receptors in organisms. Drug–receptor binding can be understood as a simple bimolecular interaction process, which is characterized by an equilibrium dissociation constant, K_D. Saturable drug binding to receptors with one site appears graphically as a hyperbolic Langmuir isotherm. Graphs of bound drug against log[free drug] appears as a sigmoidal (s-shaped) curve. Drug effects are classified as agonism (activation) or antagonism (inhibition of activity). Drug effects in molecules, cells, and tissues are displayed using concentration–response curves, which are characterized by a maximal effect (efficacy), and a half-maximal effect concentration (EC$_{50}$).

Receptor responses to drugs at the molecular level are not necessarily proportional to drug binding. Intrinsic efficacy describes the fraction of receptors activated when fully bound by an agonist, which is modeled as a second equilibrium between inactive and active agonist-bound receptors. Full agonists and partial agonists activate, respectively, a high fraction or a low fraction of bound receptors, and the EC$_{50}$ of a full agonist will be lower than that of a partial agonist with the same binding affinity for inactive receptors. Cells and tissues may possess spare receptors, implying that activation of a fraction of receptors produces a maximal response, resulting in increased apparent sensitivity to agonists and decreased apparent sensitivity to antagonists. Antagonism may be due to competitive binding at the agonist (orthosteric) site or noncompetitive binding at other (allosteric) sites. The effect of reversible competitive antagonism is surmountable with increasing agonist concentrations, while noncompetitive antagonism and irreversible antagonism are insurmountable. Many receptors display partial activity in the absence of agonists, and these may be described using allosteric activation models that incorporate an undrugged active receptor state. In these models, agonists shift the inactive ↔ active equilibrium toward active states. Inverse agonists are defined in the context of allosteric models as drugs that stabilize inactive more than active receptors, reducing spontaneous activity.

Drug responses in animals and humans are the result of integrated effects, including signal amplification and dampening (negative feedback) mechanisms at cellular, tissue, and physiological systems levels. Tachyphylaxis and tolerance are terms for declining responses to repeated drug dosing over short (hours) or long (days to months) time periods. When drug concentration is not defined, graded dose–response studies in individual animals often display the familiar sigmoid shape and are described by efficacy (maximal effect at high doses) and potency, defined as the inverse of the half-maximal effect dose (ED$_{50}$). Population studies generally specify quantal (yes/no) drug responses such as a therapeutic endpoint and toxic side effects, including lethality, displaying the fraction of individuals reaching these endpoints at each dose. A single drug may be characterized by different potencies for multiple actions, including ED50 for therapeutic action, TD50 for toxicity, and LD50 for lethality.

References

1. Buxton I. Pharmacokinetics and pharmacodynamics. In: Brunon L, Lazo J, Parker K, eds., *Goodman & Gilman's The Pharmacological Basis of Therapeutics*, 11th edn. New York, NY: McGraw Hill, 2006: 1–40.

2. Bourne H, von Zastrow M. Drug receptors and pharmacodynamics. In: Katzung B, ed., *Basic and Clinical Pharmacology*, 10th edn. New York, NY: McGraw Hill, 2007: 11–33.

3. Nyholm TK, Ozdirekcan S, Killian JA. How protein transmembrane segments

sense the lipid environment. *Biochemistry* 2007; **46**: 1457–65.

4. Alexander SPH, Mathie A, Peters JA. Guide to receptors and channels (GRAC), 4th edn. *Br J Pharmacol* 2009; **158** (Suppl. 1): S1–S254.

5. Noda M, Takahashi H, Tanabe T, *et al.* Structural homology of *Torpedo californica* acetylcholine receptor subunits. *Nature* 1983; **302**: 528–32.

6. Arneric SP, Holladay M, Williams M. Neuronal nicotinic receptors: a perspective on two decades of drug discovery research. *Biochem Pharmacol* 2007; **74**: 1092–101.

7. Wess J, Eglen RM, Gautam D. Muscarinic acetylcholine receptors: mutant mice provide new insights for drug development. *Nat Rev Drug Discov* 2007; **6**: 721–33.

8. Pierce KL, Premont RT, Lefkowitz RJ. Seven-transmembrane receptors. *Nat Rev Mol Cell Biol* 2002; **3**: 639–50.

9. Kristiansen K. Molecular mechanisms of drug binding, signaling, and regulation within the superfamily of G-protein-coupled receptors: molecular modeling and mutagenesis approaches to receptor structure and function. *Pharmacol Ther* 2004; **103**: 21–80.

10. Christopoulos A, Kenakin T. G protein-coupled receptor allosterism and complexing. *Pharmacol Rev* 2002; **54**: 323–74.

11. Luttrell LM. Reviews in molecular biology and biotechnology: transmembrane signaling by G protein-coupled receptors. *Mol Biotechnol* 2008; **39**: 239–64.

12. Ortells MO, Lunt GG. Evolutionary history of the drug-gated ion-channel superfamily of receptors. *Trends Neurosci* 1995; **18**: 121–7.

13. Connolly CN, Wafford KA. The Cys-loop superfamily of drug-gated ion channels: the impact of receptor structure on function. *Biochem Soc Trans* 2004; **32**: 529–34.

14. Unwin N. Refined structure of the nicotinic acetylcholine receptor at 4A resolution. *J Mol Biol* 2005; **346**: 967–89.

15. Schlessinger J. Cell signaling by receptor tyrosine kinases. *Cell* 2000; **103**: 211–25.

16. Saltiel AR, Kahn CR. Insulin signalling and the regulation of glucose and lipid metabolism. *Nature* 2001; **414**: 799–806.

17. Locksley RM, Killeen N, Lenardo MJ. The TNF and TNF receptor superfamilies: integrating mammalian biology. *Cell* 2001; **104**: 487–501.

18. Hehlgans T, Pfeffer K. The intriguing biology of the tumour necrosis factor/tumour necrosis factor receptor superfamily: players, rules and the games. *Immunology* 2005; **115**: 1–20.

19. Gronemeyer H, Gustafsson JA, Laudet V. Principles for modulation of the nuclear receptor superfamily. *Nat Rev Drug Discov* 2004; **3**: 950–64.

20. Taylor P, Talley TT, Radic Z, *et al.* Structure-guided drug design: conferring selectivity among neuronal nicotinic receptor and acetylcholine-binding protein subtypes. *Biochem Pharmacol* 2007; **74**: 1164–71.

21. Brancaccio D, Bommer J, Coyne D. Vitamin D receptor activator selectivity in the treatment of secondary hyperparathyroidism: understanding the differences among therapies. *Drugs* 2007; **67**: 1981–98.

22. Boeckler F, Gmeiner P. Dopamine D3 receptor drugs: recent advances in the control of subtype selectivity and intrinsic activity. *Biochim Biophys Acta* 2007; **1768**: 871–87.

23. Muntz KH, Zhao M, Miller JC. Downregulation of myocardial beta-adrenergic receptors. Receptor subtype selectivity. *Circ Res* 1994; **74**: 369–75.

24. Belelli D, Muntoni AL, Merrywest SD, *et al.* The in vitro and in vivo enantioselectivity of etomidate implicates the GABAA receptor in general anaesthesia. *Neuropharmacology* 2003; **45**: 57–71.

25. Foster RH, Markham A. Levobupivacaine: a review of its pharmacology and use as a local anaesthetic. *Drugs* 2000; **59**: 551–79.

26. Colquhoun D. The quantitative analysis of drug-receptor interactions: a short history. *Trends Pharmacol Sci* 2006; **27**: 149–57.

27. Neubig RR, Spedding M, Kenakin T, Christopoulos A. International Union of Pharmacology Committee on Receptor Nomenclature and Drug Classification. XXXVIII. Update on terms and symbols in quantitative pharmacology. *Pharmacol Rev* 2003; **55**: 597–606.

28. Del Castillo J, Katz B. Interaction at end-plate receptors between different choline derivatives. *Proc R Soc Lond B Biol Sci* 1957; **146**: 369–81.

29. Colquhoun D. Binding, gating, affinity and efficacy: the interpretation of structure–activity relationships for agonists and of the effects of mutating receptors. *Br J Pharmacol* 1998; **125**: 924–47.

30. Hill A. The possible effects of the aggregation of the molecules of hemoglobin on its dissociation curves. *J Physiol* 1910; **40**: iv–vii.

31. Gaddum JH. Theories of drug antagonism. *Pharmacol Rev* 1957; **9**: 211–18.

32. Schild HO. Drug antagonism and pAx. *Pharmacol Rev* 1957; **9**: 242–6.

33. Monod J, Wyman J, Changeux J. On the nature of allosteric transitions: a plausible model. *J Mol Biol* 1965; **12**: 88–118.

34. Milligan G. Constitutive activity and inverse agonists of G protein-coupled receptors: a current perspective. *Mol Pharmacol* 2003; **64**: 1271–6.

35. Ehlert FJ. Analysis of allosterism in functional assays. *J Pharmacol Exp Ther* 2005; **315**: 740–54.

36. Kenakin T. Efficacy as a vector: the relative prevalence and paucity of inverse agonism. *Mol Pharmacol* 2004; **65**: 2–11.

37. Rusch D, Forman SA. Classic benzodiazepines modulate the open-close equilibrium in $\alpha 1\beta 2\gamma 2L$ γ-aminobutyric acid type A receptors. *Anesthesiology* 2005; **102**: 783–92.

38. Akaaboune M, Culican SM, Turney SG, Lichtman JW. Rapid and reversible effects of activity on acetylcholine receptor density at the neuromuscular junction in vivo. *Science* 1999; **286**: 503–7.

Principles of drug action
G-protein-coupled receptors

Marcel E. Durieux

Introduction

G-protein-coupled receptors (GPCRs) are involved in the transduction of signals from a variety of extracellular signaling molecules, including hormones, neurotransmitters, and cytokines. The diversity of the effector pathways which may couple to GPCRs gives rise to considerable signaling flexibility. Furthermore, tissue-specific expression of various downstream targets allows for specificity, and signaling regulation may occur at multiple levels. Consequently, there is a range of potential opportunities for pharmacologic intervention, and GPCRs are extremely important in anesthesiology; for example, α- and β-adrenergic agonists and opiates all act on GPCRs. Tolerance to drugs like opiates poses a significant clinical challenge, and an understanding of the mechanisms underlying desensitization may help identify future targets for intervention. This chapter deals with the general principles of signal transduction and the specifics of GPCR signaling pathways and common second-messenger systems, as well as exploring the mechanisms for receptor desensitization.

General principles

Signal transduction

The terms **signal transduction** and **cell signaling** refer to the mechanisms by which biologic information is transferred between cells. Intercellular and intracellular signaling pathways are essential to the growth, development, metabolism, and behavior of the organism [1,2], which helps explain why the human genome includes at least 3775 genes (or 14.3% of genes) involved in signal transduction [3]. More than 2% of genes encode GPCRs.

The cellular response to an extracellular signaling molecule requires its binding to a specific receptor (Table 2.1), which then transduces this information to changes in the functional properties of the target cell. The particular receptors expressed by the target cell determine its sensitivity to various signaling molecules and determine the specificity involved in cellular responses to various signals. Receptors can be classified by their cellular localization (Fig. 2.1). The majority of hormones and neurotransmitters, including peptides, catecholamines, amino acids, and their derivatives, are water-soluble (hydrophilic) signaling molecules that interact with cell-surface receptors. Prostaglandins are an exception, in that they are lipid-soluble (hydrophobic) signaling molecules that interact with cell-surface receptors. Most hydrophobic signaling molecules diffuse across the plasma membrane and interact with intracellular receptors. Steroid hormones, retinoids, vitamin D, and thyroxine are examples. These molecules are transported in the blood bound to specific transporter proteins, from which they dissociate in order to diffuse across cell membranes to bind to specific receptors in the nucleus or cytosol. The hormone–receptor complex then acts as a transcription factor to modulate gene expression. However, recent evidence suggests that receptors for the steroid estrogen also act at the plasma membrane, modulating intracellular Ca^{2+} and cyclic adenosine $3'$-$5'$-monophosphate (cAMP) levels through G-protein interactions. Nitric oxide (NO), and possibly carbon monoxide (CO), are members of a class of gaseous signaling molecules that readily diffuse across cell membranes to affect neighboring cells. NO, which is unstable and has a short half-life (5–10 seconds), is able to diffuse only a short distance before breaking down, and therefore acts as a paracrine signal only. Cell-surface receptors can also bind to insoluble ligands, such as the extracellular matrix of cell adhesion molecules, interactions which are crucial to cell development and migration.

Properties of signal transduction pathways

Signal transduction pathways have a number of common properties with important functional implications [4]. **Signal amplification** occurs as a result of sequential activation of catalytic signaling molecules. This enables sensitive physiologic responses to small physical (several photons) or chemical (a few molecules of an odorant) stimuli, as well as graded responses to increasingly larger stimuli. **Specificity** is imparted by specific receptor proteins and their association with cell-type-specific signaling pathways and effector mechanisms. Additional specificity is imparted by the existence of distinct

Anesthetic Pharmacology, 2nd edition, ed. Alex S. Evers, Mervyn Maze, Evan D. Kharasch. Published by Cambridge University Press. © Cambridge University Press 2011.

Table 2.1. Receptor classification

Cell-surface receptors	

G-protein-coupled	Receptors for hormones, neurotransmitters (biogenic amines, amino acids), and neuropeptides
	  Activate/inhibit adenylate cyclase
	  Activate phospholipase C
	  Modulate ion channels

Ligand-gated ion channels	Receptors for neurotransmitters (biogenic amines, amino acids, peptides) Mediate fast synaptic transmission
Enzyme-linked cell-surface receptors	
Receptor guanylate cyclases	Receptors for atrial natriuretic peptide, Escherichia coli heat-stable enterotoxin
Receptor serine/threonine kinases	Receptors for activin, inhibin, transforming growth factor β (TGFβ)
Receptor tyrosine kinases	Receptors for peptide growth factors
Tyrosine kinase-associated	Receptors for cytokines, growth hormone, prolactin
Receptor tyrosine phosphatases	Ligands unknown in most cases
Intracellular receptors	
Steroid receptor superfamily	Receptors for steroids, sterols, thyroxine (T_3), retinoic acid, and vitamin D

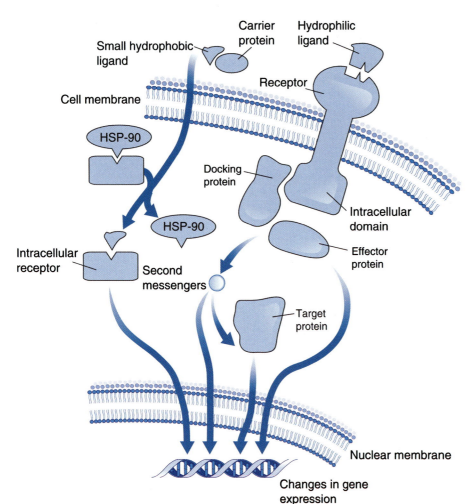

Figure 2.1. Extracellular signaling. Ligands bind to either cell-surface receptors or intracellular receptors. Most signaling molecules are hydrophilic and therefore unable to cross the plasma membrane. They bind to cell-surface receptors, which in turn generate one or more intracellular signals (second messengers) inside the target cell or change the activity of effector proteins (e.g., G proteins, protein kinases, ion channels) through their intracellular effector domains. Receptor activation can result in direct changes in the intrinsic enzymatic activities of the receptor intracellular domain, or it can work indirectly through association of the receptor with intracellular mediators, which in turn regulate the activity of effector proteins. Some effectors translocate to the nucleus to control gene expression (e.g., transcription factors) or to other subcellular compartments. Some small signaling molecules, by contrast, diffuse across the plasma membrane and bind to receptors inside the target cell, either in the cytosol (as shown) or in the nucleus. Many of these small signaling molecules are hydrophobic and nearly insoluble in aqueous solutions; therefore, they are transported in the bloodstream and other extracellular fluids bound to carrier proteins, from which they dissociate before entering the target cell. HSP-90, heat shock protein-90.

receptors coupled to different intracellular signaling pathways that respond to the same extracellular signal. Thus a single extracellular signal can elicit different effects on different target cells depending on the receptor subtype and the signaling mechanisms present. A good example is the neurotransmitter acetylcholine, which stimulates contraction of skeletal muscle, but relaxation of smooth muscle. Differences in the intracellular signaling mechanisms also allow the same receptor to produce different responses in different target cells. **Pleiotropy** results from the ability of a single extracellular signal to generate multiple responses in a target cell: for example, the opening of some ion channels, the closing of others, activation or inhibition of many enzymes, modification of the cytoskeleton, or changes in gene expression.

G-protein-coupled receptors

A variety of signals (hormones, neurotransmitters, cytokines, pheromones, odorants, photons) produce their intracellular actions by a pathway that involves interaction with receptors that activate G proteins [5,6]. G proteins act as molecular switches to relay information from activated receptors to the appropriate effectors [7,8]. An agonist-stimulated receptor can activate several hundred G proteins, which in turn activate a variety of downstream effectors [9]. GPCRs have a particularly important role in pharmacology – more than two-thirds of all nonantibiotic drugs target GPCRs – and are thus critical to anesthesiology [10]. Genetical disruption in their function is involved in a number of disease states [11].

The GPCR signaling pathway

G-protein-coupled signal transduction begins with receptor proteins in the plasma membrane, which sense changes in the extracellular environment. As a result of the interactions between these receptors and their ligands, signals are transduced across the plasma membrane (Fig. 2.1). Ligand binding to a GPCR causes a change in the shape (conformation) of the receptor, which is transmitted to the cell interior. This results in a change in the activity of a coupled intracellular guanine nucleotide (GTP)-binding protein (**G protein**), which subsequently activates or inhibits intracellular enzymes or ion channels. Through this mechanism, the activation of many GPCRs leads to changes in the concentration of intracellular signaling molecules, termed **second messengers**. These changes are usually transient, a result of the tight regulation of the synthesis and degradation (or release and reuptake) of these intracellular signals. Important second messengers include cAMP, cyclic guanosine $3'$-$5'$-monophosphate (cGMP), 1,2-diacylglycerol, inositol 1,4,5-trisphosphate (IP_3), and Ca^{2+}. Changes in the concentrations of these second messengers following receptor activation modulate activities of important regulatory enzymes and effector proteins. The most important second-messenger-regulated enzymes are protein kinases and phosphatases, which catalyze the phosphorylation and dephosphorylation,

respectively, of key enzymes and proteins in target cells. Reversible phosphorylation alters the function or localization of specific proteins. It is the predominant effector mechanism involved in mediating cellular responses to almost all extracellular signals.

GPCR structure and function

GPCRs form a large and functionally diverse receptor superfamily; more than 500 (more than 2% of total genes) members have been identified, and a large number of **orphan receptors** (receptors identified as GPCRs by amino acid structure, for which the ligand is not known) brings the total of GPCRs over a thousand.

The G proteins, coupled to by the receptors, are heterotrimeric structures, that is, they consist of three distinct protein subunits: a large α subunit and a smaller βγ subunit dimer. The βγ complex is so tightly bound that it is usually considered a single unit. The binding of extracellular signals to their specific receptors on the cell surface initiates a cycle of reactions to promote guanine nucleotide exchange on the G-protein α subunit. This involves three major steps: (1) the signal (ligand) activates the receptor and induces a conformational change in the receptor; (2) the activated receptor "turns on" a heterotrimeric G protein in the cell membrane by forming a high-affinity ligand–receptor–G-protein complex, which promotes exchange of guanosine triphosphate (GTP) for guanosine diphosphate (GDP) on the α subunit of the G protein, followed by dissociation of the α subunit and the βγ subunit dimer from the receptor and each other; and (3) the appropriate effector protein(s) is then regulated by the dissociated G-protein α or βγ (or both) subunits, which thereby transduces the signal. The dissociation of the G protein from the receptor reduces the affinity of the receptor for the agonist. The system returns to its basal state as the GTP bound to the α subunit is hydrolyzed to GDP by a catalytic activity (or GTPase) inherent in the α subunit, and the trimeric G-protein complex reassociates and turns off the signal.

A number of different isoforms of G-protein α, β, and γ subunits have been identified that mediate the stimulation or inhibition of functionally diverse effector enzymes and ion channels (Table 2.2). Among the effector molecules regulated by G proteins are adenylate cyclase, phospholipase C, phospholipase A_2, cGMP phosphodiesterase, and Ca^{2+} and K^+ channels. These effectors then produce changes in the concentrations of a variety of second-messenger molecules or in the membrane potential of the target cell.

Despite the diversity in the extracellular signals that stimulate the various effector pathways activated by G-protein-coupled receptors, these receptors are structurally homologous, which is consistent with their common mechanism of action. Molecular cloning and sequencing have shown that these receptors are characterized by seven hydrophobic transmembrane α helical segments of 20–25 amino acids connected by alternating intracellular and extracellular loops. Therefore, GPCRs cross the membrane seven times (hence the alternative terms

Table 2.2. Diversity of G-protein-coupled receptor signal transduction pathways: G proteins and their associated receptors and effectors

G protein	Representative receptors	Effectors	Effect
G_s	β_1, β_2, β_3 adrenergic; D_1, D_5 dopamine	Adenylate cyclase Ca^{2+} channels	Increased cAMP; increased Ca^{2+} influx
G_i	α_2 adrenergic; D_2; M_2, M_4 muscarinic; μ, δ, κ opioid	Adenylate cyclase Phospholipase A_2 K^+ channels	Decreased cAMP; eicosanoid release; hyperpolarization
G_k	Atrial muscarinic	K^+ channel	Hyperpolarization
G_q	M_1, M_3 muscarinic; α_1 adrenergic	Phospholipase C β	Increased IP_3, DG, Ca^{2+}
G_{olf}	Odorants	Adenylate cyclase	Increased cAMP (olfactory)
G_t	Photons	cGMP phosphodiesterase	Decreased cGMP (vision)
G_o	?	Phospholipase C Ca^{2+} channels	Increased IP_3, DG, Ca^{2+}; decreased Ca^{2+} influx

cAMP, adenosine 3′-5′-monophosphate; cGMP, guanosine 3′-5′-monophosphate; DG, 1,2,-diacylglycerol; G_s, stimulation; G_i, inhibition; G_k, potassium regulation; G_q, phospholipase C regulation; G_{olf}, olfactory; G_t, transducin; G_o, other; IP_3, inositol trisphosphate.

seven-transmembrane domain, heptahelical, or serpentine receptors; Fig. 2.2). The structural domains of G-protein-coupled receptors involved in ligand binding and in interactions with G proteins have been analyzed by deletion analysis (in which segments of the receptor are sequentially deleted), by site-directed mutagenesis (in which specific single amino acid residues are deleted or mutated), and by constructing chimeric receptor molecules (in which recombinant chimeras are formed by splicing together complementary segments of two related receptors). For example, the agonist isoproterenol binds among the seven transmembrane α helices of the β_2-adrenoceptor near the extracellular surface of the membrane. The intracellular loop between α helices 5 and 6 and the C-terminal segments is important for specific G-protein interactions.

Heterogeneity within the GPCR signaling pathway exists both at the level of the receptors and at the level of the G proteins. A single extracellular signal may activate several closely related receptor subtypes. For example, six genes for α-adrenoceptors and three genes for β-adrenoceptors have been identified, all of which can be activated by the ligand norepinephrine. Likewise, G proteins consist of multiple subtypes. Sixteen homologous α-subunit genes are classified as subtypes (G_s, G_i, G_k, G_q, and so on) based on structural similarities. The different α subunits have distinct functions, coupling with different effector pathways. The different β- and γ-subunit isoforms may also couple with distinct signaling pathways. Heterogeneity in effector pathways makes divergence possible within GPCR-activated pathways. This effector pleiotropy can arise from two distinct mechanisms: (1) a single receptor can activate multiple G-protein types, and/or (2) a single G-protein type can activate more than one second-messenger pathway. Thus a single type of GPCR can activate several different effector pathways within a given cell, whereas the predominant pathway may vary between cell types. All together, this ability of a single agonist to activate multiple receptor subtypes, which in turn can interact with multiple G-protein subtypes and thereby activate various effectors, allows a tremendous amount of flexibility in signaling, as well as many opportunities for regulation.

The structure and function of the α- and β-adrenoceptors for epinephrine and norepinephrine and their associated G proteins exemplify some of these principles (Fig. 2.2). β-adrenoceptors are coupled to the activation of adenylate cyclase, a plasma-membrane-associated enzyme that catalyzes the synthesis of cAMP. cAMP was the first second messenger identified and has been found to exist in all prokaryotes and animals. The G protein that couples β-adrenoceptor stimulation to adenylate cyclase activation is known as G_s, for stimulatory G protein. Epinephrine-stimulated cAMP synthesis can be reconstituted in phospholipid vesicles using purified β-adrenoceptors, G_s, and adenylate cyclase, which demonstrates that no other molecules are required for the initial steps of this signal transduction mechanism. In the resting state, G_s exists as a heterotrimer consisting of α_s and $\beta\gamma$ subunits, with GDP bound to α_s. Agonist binding to the β-adrenoceptor alters the conformation of the receptor and exposes a binding site for G_s. The GDP-G_s complex binds to the agonist-activated receptor, thereby reducing the affinity of α_s for GDP, which dissociates, allowing GTP to bind. The α_s subunit bound to GTP then dissociates from the G-protein complex, and binds to and activates adenylate cyclase. The affinity of the receptor for agonist is reduced following dissociation of the G-protein complex, leading to agonist dissociation and a return of the receptor to its inactive state. Activation of adenylate cyclase is rapidly reversed following agonist dissociation from the receptor because the lifetime of active α_s is limited by its intrinsic GTPase activity. The bound GTP is thereby hydrolyzed to GDP, which returns the α subunit to its inactive conformation. The α_s subunit then dissociates from adenylate cyclase, rendering it inactive, and reassociates with $\beta\gamma$ to reform G_s.

Nonhydrolyzable analogs of GTP, such as GTPγS or GMPPNP, prolong agonist-induced adenylate cyclase activation

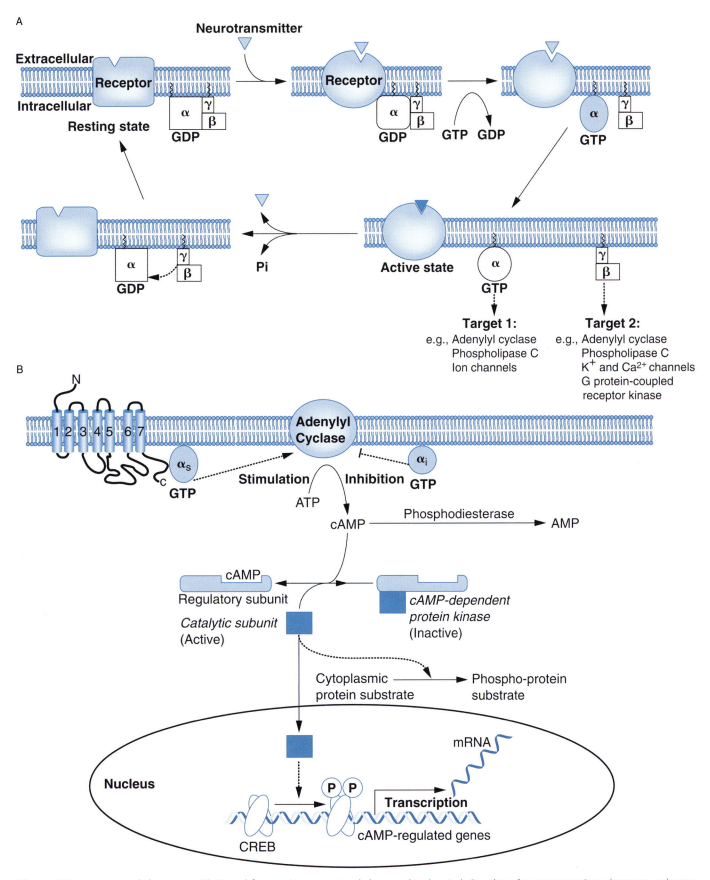

Figure 2.2. G-protein-coupled receptors. (A) General features. Many receptors belong to this class, including those for neurotransmitters, hormones, odorants, light, and Ca²⁺. These receptors associate with heterotrimeric G proteins composed of three subunits: α, β, and γ. They are not transmembrane proteins but are

by preventing inactivation of active α_s. Such compounds are important research tools, but the mechanism also has clinical implications. Cholera toxin and pertussis toxin are adenosine diphosphate (ADP)-ribosyltransferases, and induce selective ADP ribosylation of α_s or α_i, respectively, which inhibits its GTPase activity and results in prolonged $G_s\alpha$ activation or $G_i\alpha$ inactivation.

The activity of adenylate cyclase can be negatively regulated by receptors coupled to the inhibitory G protein, G_i. An example is the α_2-adrenoceptor, which is coupled to inhibition of adenylate cyclase through G_i. Thus the same extracellular signal, epinephrine in this example, can either stimulate or inhibit the formation of the second messenger cAMP, depending on the particular G protein that couples the receptor to the cyclase. G_i, like G_s, is a heterotrimeric protein consisting of an α_i subunit and a $\beta\gamma$ subunit. Activated α_2 receptors bind to G_i and lead to GDP dissociation, GTP binding, and complex dissociation, as occurs with G_s. Both the released α_i and the $\beta\gamma$ complex are thought to contribute to adenylate cyclase inhibition, α_i by direct inhibition, and $\beta\gamma$ by direct inhibition and indirectly, by binding to and inactivating any free α_s subunits. Activated G_i can also open K^+ channels, an example of how a single G protein can regulate multiple effector molecules.

Receptor desensitization

The number and function of cell-surface receptors are subject to regulation by several mechanisms [9]. Many receptors undergo receptor desensitization in response to prolonged exposure to a high concentration of ligand, a process by which the number or function of receptors is reduced, so that the physiologic response to the ligand is attenuated (tachyphylaxis). This process is often responsible for decreased response to administered drugs (such as adrenergic agonists or opiates). At times, however, it can have beneficial consequences: for example, it appears that the analgesic action of cannabinoids may result in part from their ability

to desensitize transient receptor potential vanilloid 1 (TRPV1) receptors [12], and the prolonged effect of the antiemetic palonosetron may be explained in part by its ability to desensitize 5-HT_3 receptors.

Receptor desensitization can occur by several mechanisms, including receptor internalization, downregulation, and modulation (Fig. 2.3). Receptor **internalization** by endocytosis is a common mechanism for desensitization of hormone receptors (e.g., insulin, glucagon, epidermal growth factor), and may be the manner in which palonosetron desensitizes 5-HT_3 receptors. The agonist–receptor complex is sequestered by receptor-mediated endocytosis, which results in translocation of the receptor to intracellular compartments (endosomes) that are inaccessible to ligand. This is a relatively slow process. Cessation of agonist stimulation allows the receptor to recycle to the cell surface by exocytosis. In other cases the internalized receptors are degraded and are no longer available for recycling, a process known as receptor **downregulation**. Receptors must then be replenished by protein synthesis. Receptor downregulation in response to prolonged agonist stimulation can also occur at the level of receptor protein synthesis or of receptor mRNA regulation caused by changes in gene transcription, mRNA stability, or both. These processes are of great importance in modulating the effects of drugs, e.g., opiates [13].

A more rapid and transient form of receptor desensitization involves receptor **modulation** by phosphorylation, which can rapidly change receptor affinity, signaling efficiency, or both. For example, the β-adrenoceptor is desensitized as a result of phosphorylation of a number of sites in its intracellular carboxy-terminal domain by cAMP-dependent protein kinase, protein kinase C (PKC), and β-adrenergic receptor kinase (βARK), a G-protein-coupled receptor kinase (GRK). The former kinase is activated as a result of β-receptor stimulation of adenylate cyclase and results in homologous or heterologous desensitization, whereas the latter kinase is active only on

Caption for Figure 2.2. (*cont.*) associated with the membrane by covalently bound fatty acid molecules. In the resting state, GDP is bound to the α subunit, which is closely attached to the βγ complex. When the neurotransmitter binds to the receptor, the conformation of the receptor changes, inducing a change in the conformation of the α subunit, which expels GDP and replaces it by GTP. The GTP-bound α subunit is no longer capable of interacting with the receptor or γ. GTP-bound α and γ interact with specific targets that differ for each isoform α or γ subunits. After a short time GTP is hydrolyzed to GDP and α-GDP reassociates with γ. At about the same time, the neurotransmitter leaves its receptor, which returns to its resting state. G protein, guanine nucleotide-binding protein; Pi, inorganic phosphate. (B) The adenylate cyclase/protein kinase A (PKA) pathway. cAMP is formed from ATP by a class of transmembrane enzymes, adenylate cyclases. A cytosolic form of adenylate cyclase has also been described recently. Transmembrane adenylate cyclases are activated by two related subtypes of G-protein α subunits, α_s (stimulatory, which is ubiquitous) and α_{off} (olfactory, which is found in olfactory epithelium and a subset of neurons). Adenylate cyclases are inhibited by α_i (inhibitory). In addition, some adenylate cyclases can be stimulated or inhibited by βγ, or Ca^{2+} combined with calmodulin. Cyclic adenosine 3'-5'-monophosphate (cAMP) is inactivated by hydrolysis into AMP by phosphodiesterases, a family of enzymes that is inhibited by theophylline and related methylxanthines. cAMP has only two known targets in vertebrates: one is a cAMP-gated ion channel that is most prominently found in olfactory neurons, and the other is cAMP-dependent protein kinase that is present in all cells. cAMP-dependent protein kinase is a tetramer composed of two catalytic subunits and two regulatory subunits (only one of each is shown). When cAMP binds to the regulatory subunits (two molecules of cAMP bind to each regulatory subunit), they dissociate from the catalytic subunits. The free active catalytic subunit phosphorylates numerous specific substrates including ion channels, receptors, and enzymes. In addition, the catalytic subunit can enter the nucleus, where it phosphorylates transcription factors. One well-characterized transcription factor phosphorylated in response to cAMP is cAMP response element-binding protein (CREB). In the basal state, CREB forms a dimer that binds to a specific DNA sequence in the promoter region of cAMP-responsive genes, called CRE (cAMP-responsive element). CREB is unable to promote transcription when it is not phosphorylated, whereas phospho-CREB strongly stimulates transcription. Genes regulated by CREB include immediate-early genes *c-Fos* and c-Jun. CREB is also activated by Ca^{2+} calmodulin-dependent protein kinase.

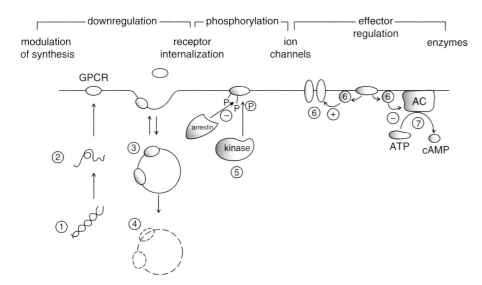

Figure 2.3. Receptor desensitization. A multitude or systems regulates GPCR signaling. Synthesis and expression of receptors can be regulated at the DNA (1) and RNA (2) level, i.e., at the levels of gene transcription as well as translation, post-translational modification, and trafficking to the membrane. Expressed receptors can be removed from the membrane by internalization (3); internalized receptors can either be recycled to the membrane or degraded (4). All the processes are relatively slow, and referred to as receptor downregulation. Faster modulation of receptor functioning often involves phosphorylation of the receptor by one of a variety of kinases (5). Commonly, this phosphorylation allows interaction between the receptor and a member of the arrestin family, thereby blocking receptor functioning. Additional possibilities for regulation exist downstream of the receptor itself. Both ion channels and enzymes such as adenylate cyclase (AC) can be modulated to counteract the effects of GPCR on their signaling. For exampale, whereas opioid receptor signaling normally results in a decrease in cAMP levels because of inhibition of AC, modulating AC into a hyperactive state can induce cellular tolerance to opiate signaling. G, G protein; +, activates; −, inhibits; P, phosphorylates.

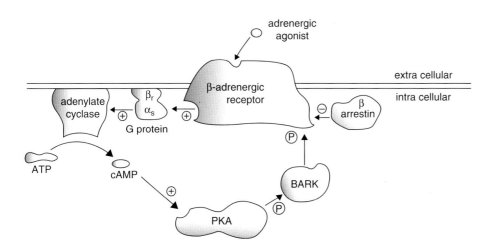

Figure 2.4. Modulation of β-adrenoceptor functioning by β-adrenergic receptor kinase (βARK) and β-arrestin. Ligand binding to the β-adrenoceptor results in activation of its associated G protein. The α_s G-protein subunit in turn activates adenylate cyclase, which converts ATP to cAMP, resulting in increased intracellular levels of this second messenger. One of the enzymes regulated by cAMP is protein kinase A (PKA), and one of its phosphorylation targets is βARK. Once phosphorylated, βARK in turn selectively phosphorylates serine and threonine residues on activated β-adrenoceptor molecules. As a result, these phosphorylated receptors become accessible for interaction with β-arrestin, which binds to the receptor and blocks further signaling. Together, this system forms a feedback loop that prevents over-activated β-adrenoceptor signaling. Similar systems exist for other GPCRs. +, activates; −, inhibits; P, phosphorylates.

β receptors occupied by ligand and therefore results in only homologous desensitization. Phosphorylation by βARK leads to the binding of β-arrestin to the receptor [14]. Arrestins are a group of proteins that sterically hinder the coupling between a GPCR and its associated G protein [15]. These processes both serve to uncouple the active ligand–receptor complex from interacting with the G_s protein, creating a negative feedback loop for modulation of β-receptor activity (Fig. 2.4). In other instances, receptor phosphorylation can affect ligand affinity or associated ion-channel kinetics rather than G-protein coupling.

Signaling regulation is an area of very active research, and a variety of molecular systems involved in this process have been identified. In addition to those mentioned above, these include systems that affect ligand binding specificity and affinity, and coupling between receptors, G proteins, and effectors [9].

These systems all provide potential drug targets, many of which could be of use in anesthesiology. A particularly relevant, yet complex, example is the regulation of opiate signaling. All anesthesiologists are familiar with the profound tolerance that can occur during chronic opiate treatment, at times requiring more than 100 times normal doses for a clinically relevant effect [16]. On the other hand, a degree of tolerance develops to opiates administered during the course of a single anesthetic, and results in increased analgesic requirements postoperatively, an effect most clearly demonstrated with use of remifentanil [17]. The latter primarily results from desensitization and internalization of the μ-opioid receptor itself. Desensitization occurs by a mechanism similar to that described above for adrenoceptors: the opioid receptor is phosphorylated by a G-protein-coupled receptor kinase, increasing the affinity for an arrestin. This subsequently leads to decreased effector coupling, and induces internalization of the receptor. Chronic tolerance to opiates results from desensitizing effects throughout the various opiate signaling pathways. Opioid receptors couple to G_i and G_o proteins, with the main effectors being an inwardly rectifying potassium channel, voltage-gated calcium channels, and adenylate cyclase (see also Chapters 3 and 4). Each of these effector systems can be regulated to counteract the effects of opiates. Prolonged opiate exposure induces changes in the coupling between the receptor and the coupled potassium channel, resulting in less effect of the drug. However, the magnitude of this effect is insufficient to explain clinically observed increases in tolerance, and indeed other parts of the signaling pathway are affected as well. The intracellular result of opioid receptor signaling is a decrease in cAMP levels (see next section), and cellular tolerance can develop by hyperactivation of adenylate cyclase (possibly induced by G-protein $\beta\gamma$ units) that counteracts this opiate-induced decrease. Yet further desensitization of the system can occur because of changes in feedback from other cells in the network, which functionally counteract the opiate effect. All of these desensitizing actions are in principle amenable to modulation by drugs.

An area of particular interest is the synaptic plasticity induced by opiates, which in essence makes the nervous system "learn" to be less responsive to the drugs. This process, which occurs after both short-term and long-term opiate administration, is highly dependent on changes in glutamate receptor expression, and therefore opiate tolerance can be modulated significantly by drugs that affect glutamate signaling. In the context of anesthesiology, ketamine (an NMDA receptor antagonist) has found a place in preventing or even reversing opiate tolerance. For example, in rats, fentanyl administration reduces the effectiveness of a subsequent morphine bolus. This desensitizing effect can be completely prevented by ketamine pretreatment. In addition, fentanyl induces a long-term hyperalgesia of several days' duration. This hyperalgesia is similarly prevented by ketamine. Hence, it appears the drug has beneficial effects on both short-term and long-term desensitizing processes [18]. However, it is not clear if these findings always translate to the clinical setting, as ketamine did not affect opiate requirements after remifentanil-based anesthesia for major spine surgery [19].

The desensitizing processes mentioned here do not exhaust the list. A number of other systems change their functioning in response to opioid receptor signaling: protein kinase A (PKA), adrenergic systems in the locus coeruleus, γ-aminobutyric acid (GABA) signaling, MAP kinases, and phosphoinositide-3 kinases have all been shown to be affected, although their role in the clinical symptomatology of opiate tolerance remains to be determined. In addition, there are well-described roles of opiates that are not directly associated with pain pathways, but are similarly modulated by desensitization. μ-Opioid receptor activation induces a proinflammatory response, in part by modulating cytokine and chemokine receptors. In contrast,

activation of κ-opioid receptors is able to reverse this effect by downregulating these receptor systems [20].

So, even for a single pharmacologic class such as the opiates, we already find a remarkably large number of potential targets for interference with desensitization processes. Only very few of these have been explored outside the cellular laboratory. We may expect, however, that the future will bring us novel classes of drugs, specifically targeted to modulating desensitization of G-protein-coupled receptor systems.

Second messengers

Cyclic adenosine 3′-5′-monophosphate

cAMP, the first intracellular messenger identified, operates as a signaling molecule in all eukaryotic and prokaryotic cells. A variety of hormones and neurotransmitters have been found to regulate the levels of cAMP. Adenylate cyclases form a class of membrane-bound enzymes that catalyze the formation of cAMP, usually under the control of receptor-mediated G-protein-coupled stimulation (by α_s and α_{olf}) and inhibition (by α). The rapid degradation of cAMP to adenosine 5′-monophosphate by one of several isoforms of cAMP phosphodiesterase provides the potential for rapid reversibility and responsiveness of this signaling mechanisms. Most of the actions of cAMP are mediated through the activation of cAMP-dependent protein kinase (PKA) and the concomitant phosphorylation of substrate protein effectors on specific serine or threonine residues.

Substrates for cAMP-dependent protein kinase are characterized by two or more basic amino acid residues on the amino-terminal side of the phosphorylated residue. The various substrates for cAMP-dependent protein kinase present in different cell types explain the diverse tissue-specific effects of cAMP. They include ion channels, receptors, enzymes, cytoskeletal proteins, and transcription factors (e.g., cAMP response element-binding protein [CREB]).

Calcium ion and inositol trisphosphate

Along with cAMP, Ca^{2+} controls a wide variety of intracellular processes [21]. Ca^{2+} entry through Ca^{2+} channels or its release from intracellular stores triggers hormone and neurotransmitter secretion, initiates muscle contraction, and activates many protein kinases and other enzymes. The concentration of free Ca^{2+} is normally maintained at a very low level in the cytosol of most cells ($< 10^{-6}$ M) compared with the extracellular fluid ($\sim 10^{-3}$ M) by a number of homeostatic mechanisms. A Ca^{2+} ATPase in the plasma membrane pumps Ca^{2+} from the cytosol to the cell exterior at the expense of adenosine triphosphate (ATP) hydrolysis, a Ca^{2+} ATPase in the endoplasmic and sarcoplasmic reticulum concentrates Ca^{2+} from the cytosol into intracellular storage organelles, and a Na^+/Ca^{2+} exchanger, which is particularly

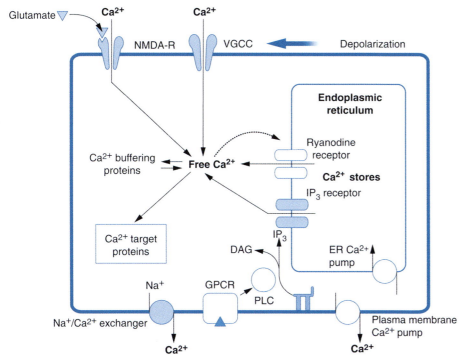

Figure 2.5. Pathways by which Ca^{2+} can enter the cytosol as a second messenger in response to extracellular signals. Ca^{2+} enters a nerve terminal from the extracellular fluid through voltage-gated Ca^{2+} channels when the nerve terminal membrane is depolarized by an action potential. Binding of an extracellular signaling molecule to a cell-surface receptor generates inositol 1,4,5-trisphosphate (IP_3), which stimulates the release of Ca^{2+} from the endoplasmic reticulum. Ca^{2+} is a divalent cation whose concentrations are relatively high in the extracellular space (approximately 1.2 mM) and more than 10 000 times lower within the cytosol (approximately 100 nM). In resting conditions, the plasma membrane is impermeable to Ca^{2+}. In neurons, it can penetrate through specific channels that include voltage-gated Ca^{2+} channels (VGCC) and glutamate receptors of the N-methyl-D-aspartate (NMDA) subtype. When these channels are open, in response to depolarization in the case of VGCC or in the presence of glutamate in the case of NMDA receptor, Ca^{2+} flows readily into the cytosol following both its concentration gradient and the electrical potential. Ca^{2+} can also be released into the cytosol from internal stores (the endoplasmic reticulum). Two types of Ca^{2+} channels are responsible for the release of Ca^{2+} from internal stores: one is the IP_3 receptor, the opening of which is triggered by IP_3, a second messenger generated by phospholipase C from phosphatidylinositol 4,5-bisphosphate; and the other is the ryanodine receptor, named after ryanodine, a drug that triggers its opening. Opening of ryanodine receptors is triggered by Ca^{2+} itself by a mechanism called Ca^{2+}-induced Ca^{2+} release, which can give rise to propagation of waves of Ca^{2+} release along the endoplasmic reticulum. In the cytosol, Ca^{2+} is mostly bound to specific binding proteins. Some of them function as buffering proteins, preventing excessive increases in cytosolic free Ca^{2+}. Others are the actual targets of Ca^{2+}, which account for the potent biologic effects of this cation. Among the best-characterized targets are calmodulin and calmodulin-related proteins, which undergo a conformational change enabling them to interact with, and activate, a number of enzymes. Ca^{2+} can also bind to another type of protein domain called C2. Free Ca^{2+} in the cytosol is maintained at very low levels by several highly active processes that include Ca^{2+} pumps and Ca^{2+} exchangers. The Ca^{2+} pumps have a high affinity but a low capacity for Ca^{2+} and are used for fine tuning of Ca^{2+} levels. They are located on the plasma membrane and the membrane of the endoplasmic reticulum, and their energy is provided by adenosine triphosphate (ATP) hydrolysis. Na^+/Ca^{2+} exchangers, whose driving force is provided by the Na^+ gradient, have a large capacity, but a low affinity for Ca^{2+}. DAG, diacylglycerol; ER, endoplasmic reticulum; GPCR, G-protein-coupled receptor; NMDA-R, N-methyl-D-aspartate subtype of glutamate receptor; PLC, phospholipase C.

active in excitable plasma membranes, couples the electro-chemical potential of Na^+ influx to the efflux of Ca^{2+} (Na^+-driven Ca^{2+} antiport). Although mitochondria have the ability to take up and release Ca^{2+}, they are not widely believed to play a major role in cytosolic Ca^{2+} homeostasis during normal conditions.

Changes in intracellular free Ca^{2+} concentration can be induced directly by depolarization-evoked Ca^{2+} entry down its electrochemical gradient through voltage-gated Ca^{2+} channels (as in neurons and muscle), by extracellular signals that activate Ca^{2+}-permeable ligand-gated ion channels (e.g., the NMDA glutamate receptor), or directly by extracellular signals coupled to the formation of IP_3 (Fig. 2.5). IP_3 is formed in response to a number of extracellular signals that interact with G-protein-coupled cell-surface receptors (G_q, G_{11}) coupled to the activation of phospholipase C [22].

Phospholipase C hydrolyzes phosphatidylinositol 4,5-bisphosphate to IP_3 and diacylglycerol; further degradation of diacylglycerol by phospholipase A_2 can result in the release of arachidonic acid. All three of these receptor-regulated metabolites are important second messengers. IP_3 increases intracellular Ca^{2+} by binding to specific IP_3 receptors on the endoplasmic reticulum, which are coupled to a Ca^{2+} channel that allows Ca^{2+} efflux into the cytosol. IP_3 receptors are similar to the Ca^{2+} release channels (ryanodine receptors) of muscle sarcoplasmic reticulum that release Ca^{2+} in response to excitation. Diacylglycerol remains in the plasma membrane where it activates PKC, whereas arachidonic acid, in addition to its metabolism to biologically active prostaglandins and leukotrienes, can also activate PKC. The Ca^{2+} signal is terminated by hydrolysis of IP_3 and by the rapid reuptake or extrusion of Ca^{2+}.

Ca^{2+} carries out its second-messenger functions primarily after binding to intracellular Ca^{2+} binding proteins, of which calmodulin is the most important. Calmodulin is a ubiquitous multifunctional Ca^{2+} binding protein, highly conserved between species, which binds four atoms of Ca^{2+} with high affinity. Ca^{2+} can also bind to C2 domains found in several proteins (PKC, phospholipase A_2, synaptotagmin).

PKC is a family of serine/threonine protein kinases consisting of 12 structurally homologous phospholipid-dependent isoforms with conserved catalytic domains, which are distinguished by their variable N-terminal regulatory domains and cofactor dependence [23]. The Ca^{2+}-dependent or conventional isoforms of PKC (cPKC) are components of the phospholipase C/diacylglycerol signaling pathway. They are regulated by the lipid second messenger 1,2-diacylglycerol, by phospholipids such as phosphatidylserine, and by Ca^{2+} through specific interactions with the regulatory region. Binding of diacylglycerol to the C1 domain of cPKC isoforms (α, β_1, β_2, γ) increases their affinity for Ca^{2+} and phosphatidylserine, facilitates PKC translocation and binding to cell membranes, and increases catalytic activity. The novel PKC isoforms (nPKC; δ, ϵ, η, θ, μ) are similar to cPKCs, but lack the C2 domain and do not require Ca^{2+}. The atypical isoforms (aPKC; ζ, λ) differ considerably in the regulatory region, and do not require Ca^{2+} or diacylglycerol for activity.

Summary

Cell signaling pathways are important for multiple biological functions. The role of the receptor is to bind signaling molecules and transduce this information into a functional response. Receptor expression determines tissue and cell sensitivity to a variety of signaling molecules. Receptors may be expressed at the cell surface, where they typically interact with insoluble ligands or hydrophilic molecules – an exception being prostaglandins, which are hydrophobic. Intracellular receptors interact with hydrophobic signaling molecules which cross the plasma membrane by diffusion. Signal transduction pathway organization can facilitate signal amplification, specificity, and pleiotropy.

The G-protein-coupled receptor (GPCR) superfamily is large and functionally diverse, and constitutes an important pharmacologic target. These receptors have seven transmembrane domains, and are coupled to an intracellular heterotrimeric guanine nucleotide (GTP)-binding protein (G protein). Ligand binding induces a conformational change in the GPCR, and GTP replaces GDP on the G protein. The

$\beta\gamma$ subunit and the GTP-bound α subunit of the G protein then dissociate from the receptor. Different isoforms of the G-protein subunits are coupled to diverse effector pathways which alter the concentration of second-messenger molecules or produce changes in the membrane potential of the cell. Effectors activated or inhibited by G-protein subunits include adenylate cyclase, phospholipase C, phospholipase A_2, cyclic GMP (cGMP) phosphodiesterase, and calcium and potassium ion channels. Pleiotropy at multiple stages in GPCR signal transduction gives rise to flexibility in signaling and regulation.

Common second-messenger molecules include cyclic adenosine $3'$-$5'$-monophosphate (cAMP), inositol 1,4,5-trisphosphate (IP_3), 1,2-diacylglycerol (DAG), and calcium ions (Ca^{2+}). Certain G-protein subunits can stimulate or inhibit membrane-bound adenylate cyclase, which catalyzes cAMP formation. cAMP activates cAMP-dependent protein kinase, which in turn phosphorylates a variety of targets such as ion channels, enzymes, and transcription factors, which are present in different cell types. Some G-protein subunits activate phospholipase C to hydrolyze phosphatidylinositol 4,5-bisphosphate to IP_3 and DAG. IP_3 binds receptors on the endoplasmic reticulum, causing release of Ca^{2+} into the cytosol. Calcium signaling pathways are mediated by Ca^{2+} binding proteins such as calmodulin. DAG and its metabolite, arachidonic acid, activate protein kinase C. Second-messenger-regulated enzymes such as kinases and phosphatases modulate the function and localization of downstream proteins to produce a cellular response. Changes in second-messenger concentration are usually transient by virtue of tightly regulated degradation, synthesis, release, and reuptake.

Dissociation of the G protein from the receptor reduces receptor–ligand affinity, and the agonist is released. The α subunit of the G protein has intrinsic GTPase activity, which hydrolyses the bound GTP to GDP. The GDP-bound α subunit rejoins the $\beta\gamma$ subunit, returning the G protein to its resting state.

Receptor desensitization following prolonged exposure to high-concentration agonist is one mechanism of regulation, which can cause decreased responses to drugs, including adrenoceptor agonists and opiates. Receptors may be internalized by endocytosis, their expression may be downregulated by increased degradation or decreased synthesis, or the receptor may be modulated by phosphorylation to achieve rapid, transient desensitization. Receptor modulation can lead to the binding of arrestins, which hinder coupling to the associated G protein, as occurs in the desensitization of the β-adrenoceptor; modulation can also affect ligand affinity or ion channel kinetics. Pharmacologic intervention in the processes underlying desensitization has the potential to reduce tolerance to drugs such as opiates.

References

1. Alberts B, Bray D, Lewis J, *et al.* Cell signaling. In: *Molecular Biology of the Cell*, 3rd edn. New York, NY: Garland, 1994: 721–85.

2. Lodish H, Baltimore D, Berk A, *et al.* Cell-to-cell signaling: hormones and receptors. In: Lodish H, Baltimore D, Berk A, *et al.*, eds., *Molecular Cell Biology*, 3rd edn. New York, NY: Scientific American Books, 1995: 853–924.

3. Hemmings HC. Cell signaling. In: Hemmings HC, Hopkins PM, eds., *Foundations of Anesthesia: Basic and Clinical Sciences*. London: Mosby, 2000: 21–36.

4. Venter JC, Adams MD, Myers EW, *et al.* The sequence of the human genome. *Science* 2001; **291**: 1304–51.

5. Carroll RC, Beattie EC, von Zastrow M, Malenka RC. Role of AMPA receptor endocytosis in synaptic plasticity. *Nat Rev Neurosci* 2001; **2**: 315–24.

6. Hepler JR, Gilman AG. G proteins. *Trends Biochem Sci* 1992; **17**: 383–7.

7. Exton JH. Cell signalling through guanine-nucleotide-binding regulatory proteins (G proteins) and phospholipases. *Eur J Biochem* 1997; **243**: 10–20.

8. Hamm HE, Gilchrist A. Heterotrimeric G proteins. *Curr Opin Cell Biol* 1996; **8**: 189–96.

9. Luttrell LM. Transmembrane signaling by G protein-coupled receptors. *Methods Mol Biol* 2006; **332**: 3–49.

10. Coleman DE, Sprang SR. How G proteins work: a continuing story. *Trends Biochem Sci* 1996; **21**: 41–4.

11. Thompson MD, Percy ME, McIntyre Burnham W, Cole DE. G protein-coupled receptors disrupted in human genetic disease. *Methods Mol Biol* 2008; **448**: 109–37.

12. Patwardhan AM, Jeske NA, Price TJ, *et al.* The cannabinoid WIN 55,212-2 inhibits transient receptor potential vanilloid 1 (TRPV1) and evokes peripheral antihyperalgesia via calcineurin. *Proc Natl Acad Sci U S A* 2006; **103**: 11393–8.

13. Martini L, Whistler JL. The role of mu opioid receptor desensitization and endocytosis in morphine tolerance and dependence. *Curr Opin Neurobiol* 2007; **17**: 556–64.

14. Barki-Harrington L, Rockman HA. Beta-arrestins: multifunctional cellular mediators. *Physiology* 2008; **23**: 17–22.

15. DeWire SM, Ahn S, Lefkowitz RJ, Shenoy SK. Beta-arrestins and cell signaling. *Annu Rev Physiol* 2007; **69**: 483–510.

16. Christie MJ. Cellular neuroadaptations to chronic opioids: tolerance, withdrawal and addiction.

Br J Pharmacol 2008; **154**: 384–96.

17. Joly V, Richebe P, Guignard B, *et al.* Remifentanil-induced postoperative hyperalgesia and its prevention with small-dose ketamine. *Anesthesiology* 2005; **103**: 147–55.

18. Laulin JP, Maurette P, Corcuff JB, *et al.* The role of ketamine in preventing fentanyl-induced hyperalgesia and subsequent acute morphine tolerance. *Anesth Analg* 2002; **94**: 1263–9.

19. Engelhardt T, Zaarour C, Naser B, *et al.* Intraoperative low-dose ketamine does not prevent a remifentanil-induced increase in morphine requirement after pediatric scoliosis surgery. *Anesth Analg* 2008; **107**: 1170–5.

20. Finley MJ, Happel CM, Kaminsky DE, Rogers TJ. Opioid and nociceptin receptors regulate cytokine and cytokine receptor expression. *Cell Immunol* 2008; **252**: 146–54.

21. Moncada S, Higgs A. The L-arginine-nitric oxide pathway. *N Engl J Med* 1993; **329**: 2002–12.

22. Berridge MJ, Lipp P, Bootman MD. The versatility and universality of calcium signalling. *Nat Rev Mol Cell Biol* 2000; **1**: 11–21.

23. Divecha N, Irvine RF. Phospholipid signaling. *Cell* 1995; **80**: 269–78.

**Section 1
Chapter**

3

Principles of drug action

Ion channels

Thomas McDowell, Misha Perouansky, and Robert A. Pearce

Introduction

Ion channels are integral membrane proteins that form an aqueous channel in the lipid bilayer through which charged particles can pass. There are many different types of ion channels, and they may be classified according to the factors that regulate channel opening and closing (gating), as well as the types of ions allowed to traverse the pore (selectivity). This chapter reviews the structure and function of the major classes of channels, focusing on those that are essential to neuronal and cardiac function and signaling. These include the voltage-gated ion channels, which open and close in response to changes in the voltage across the cell membrane, and the ligand-gated ion channels, which open in the presence of extracellular ligands (e.g., neurotransmitters). Included in the discussion of voltage-gated ion channels are the background or baseline K^+ channels, some of which are activated by anesthetics and thus may contribute to the anesthetic state.

Basic membrane electrophysiology

Membrane potential is determined by ionic conductances

Whether ions go into or out of the cell when a channel opens depends on both the membrane potential and the concentration gradient for that ion at the time the channel is open. Under physiologic conditions, Na^+, Ca^{2+}, and K^+ ions generally flow down their respective concentration gradients. Thus when their respective channels are opened, Na^+ and Ca^{2+} ions flow into the cell, whereas K^+ ions flow out of the cell. However, Na^+ and Ca^{2+} ions will be repelled from entering the cell if the interior of the cell is very positively charged, whereas K^+ ions tend to be retained in the cell if it is very negatively charged. The membrane potential at which net flow for a particular ion through its channel is zero, and beyond which the direction of flow reverses, can be calculated using the Nernst equation [1], which is based on thermodynamic principles and is shown in a simplified form as:

$$E_{ion} = \frac{60\,mV}{z_{ion}} \log \frac{[ion]_{extracellular}}{[ion]_{intracellular}} \tag{3.1}$$

In this equation, E_{ion} is the Nernst potential or reversal potential for the ion of interest, z_{ion} is the charge number for the ion, and the log term is the ratio of extracellular to intracellular concentrations of the ion. For the K^+ ion, for example, the ratio of extracellular to intracellular concentrations is approximately 5 mM/150 mM ($= 0.033$), making E_K about –90 mV. This means that at membrane potentials more positive than –90 mV, K^+ ions will flow out of the cell, whereas at potentials more negative than –90 mV, K^+ ions will flow into the cell. Conversely, the reversal potentials for Na^+ and Ca^{2+} are about +60 mV and +200 mV, respectively, because the concentrations of these ions are greater outside than inside the cell (especially Ca^{2+}, which has a resting intracellular concentration of about 100 nM).

The Nernst equation is used to determine the membrane potential at which no current will flow when the membrane is permeable to only one ion. Excitable cell membranes, however, are permeable to several different ions, mainly Na^+, Ca^{2+}, K^+, and Cl^-. In cells, the membrane potential at which no current flows is the resting membrane potential, and it can be estimated if the concentration gradients and resting conductances of the major permeant ions are known by using the following equation [2]:

$$E_m = \left[\left(\frac{g_{Na}}{g_{total}}\right)E_{Na} + \left(\frac{g_{Ca}}{g_{total}}\right)E_{Ca} + \left(\frac{g_k}{g_{total}}\right)E_K + \left(\frac{g_{Cl}}{g_{total}}\right)E_{Cl} \right] \tag{3.2}$$

E_m is the resting potential of the membrane, g stands for conductance (the reciprocal of resistance), g_{total} is the sum of all individual ionic conductances, and E_{Na}, E_{Ca}, and so on are the Nernst potentials for each permeant ion. The resting membrane potential is determined by the weighted sum of the Nernst potentials for all permeant ions, the weighting term being the conductance of each ion relative to the total conductance. Therefore, it is easy to see that the membrane potential will trend toward the Nernst potential for a particular ion

Anesthetic Pharmacology, 2nd edition, ed. Alex S. Evers, Mervyn Maze, Evan D. Kharasch. Published by Cambridge University Press. © Cambridge University Press 2011.

when the conductance for that ion is large relative to other ionic conductances in the membrane. In normal neurons at rest, E_m is dominated by E_K and E_{Cl} because of the relatively large resting conductances for these ions, and the membrane is hyperpolarized at rest. When Na^+ and Ca^{2+} channels open, however, the membrane depolarizes toward the positive Nernst potentials for these ions.

Voltage-gated ion channels

Three types of voltage-gated ion channels

Voltage-gated channels are found in neurons, muscle, and endocrine cells. At normal resting membrane potentials (usually –60 to –80 mV), these channels are closed. When the membrane is depolarized (becomes less negative), the channels undergo a conformational change, which opens the pore of the channel allowing ions to pass through. The type of ion that is allowed to traverse the channel is determined by the structure of the pore and is used to classify the channel. The three main classes of voltage-gated channels are the Na^+, Ca^{2+}, and K^+ channels. Although they share some physical characteristics that determine their voltage sensitivity, other differences in their structures and ionic selectivities contribute to their unique physiologic functions.

Opening and closing of individual ion channels are modeled as nearly instantaneous state transitions of the channel protein that are both voltage-dependent and time-dependent. In the simplest model, the channel can switch from the closed, nonconducting state (C) to the open, conducting state (O), and then transition either back to the closed state or to an inactivated, nonconducting state (I).

$$C \leftrightarrow O \leftrightarrow I \qquad (3.3)$$

After the channel reaches the inactivated state, it cannot open again until the membrane is hyperpolarized, allowing a transition back to the closed state from which it can once again open. This is referred to as recovery from inactivation.

How do voltage-gated channels affect neuronal activity and signaling?

When a channel opens, ions flow passively according to the driving electrical and chemical gradients as described earlier. For Na^+ and K^+ channels, approximately 10^4 to 10^5 ions pass through a single channel each millisecond, and during an action potential, thousands of channels may open. This massive flux of ions, however, may represent only about 0.1% of the total number of ions inside a cell, so the concentration gradients for Na^+ and K^+ do not change much during periods of normal neuronal activity. Conversely, because of the ability of the cell membrane to separate and store electrical charge (the capacitance of the lipid bilayer is about 1 $\mu F/cm^2$), ionic shifts of this magnitude produce enormous changes in membrane potential. It is through these changes in membrane potential that information is coded and rapidly transferred from one part of the cell to another.

For example, consider a peripheral sensory neuron that responds to mechanical deformation of the skin. When the sensory terminal associated with the Ruffini ending in the skin is deformed, a generator potential is evoked in the nerve ending. This is a passive electrical response, in that the ionic shifts that produced the depolarization are short-lived and the depolarization will dissipate as the ions travel through their aqueous environment to areas of lower potential energy. If, however, the depolarization reaches a critical threshold level, it will trigger an action potential, a series of complex voltage-dependent and time-dependent changes in ionic conductances. Voltage-gated Na^+ channels in the membrane open, which then produce a rapid depolarization that reaches a peak near the Nernst potential for Na^+. Ca^{2+} and K^+ channels may also be activated at this time. As Na^+ channels inactivate, the membrane potential returns to its resting level and other voltage-gated channels close or inactivate. The action potential is an active, regenerative, all-or-none response of constant magnitude and duration that does not dissipate over space or time. Deformation of the distal sensory nerve terminal, originally sensed as a generator potential, is converted by voltage-gated ion channels to an action potential, which can be propagated from the skin to the spinal cord, and from there to higher brain centers (via chemical synapses) where the skin deformation is sensed.

As described for Na^+ and K^+ channels, opening of voltage-gated Ca^{2+} channels also produces changes in membrane potential as charged Ca^{2+} ions enter the cell. However, Ca^{2+} channels also signal through a different mechanism. Because the intracellular Ca^{2+} concentration is normally maintained at very low levels (about 100 nM) compared with Na^+ (about 10 mM) and K^+ (about 150 mM) ions, the influx of even a small number of Ca^{2+} ions can transiently increase the intracellular Ca^{2+} concentration by several fold. This is particularly true in neuronal presynaptic terminals, because of their small volume and high density of Ca^{2+} channels. Increases in intracellular Ca^{2+} can cause neurotransmitter release, open Ca^{2+}-activated ion channels, and regulate Ca^{2+}-dependent kinases and phosphatases.

General structure of voltage-gated ion channels

The voltage-gated ion channels are protein complexes formed by the association of several individual subunits. The largest subunit of each channel is termed the α subunit ($α_1$ for the Ca^{2+} channel) (Fig. 3.1). The three-dimensional structure and function of the α subunits of the voltage-gated channels are strikingly similar, reflecting similarities in their voltage-dependent gating and high ionic conductance. If the α subunit of a voltage-gated ion channel is expressed in the absence of other subunits,

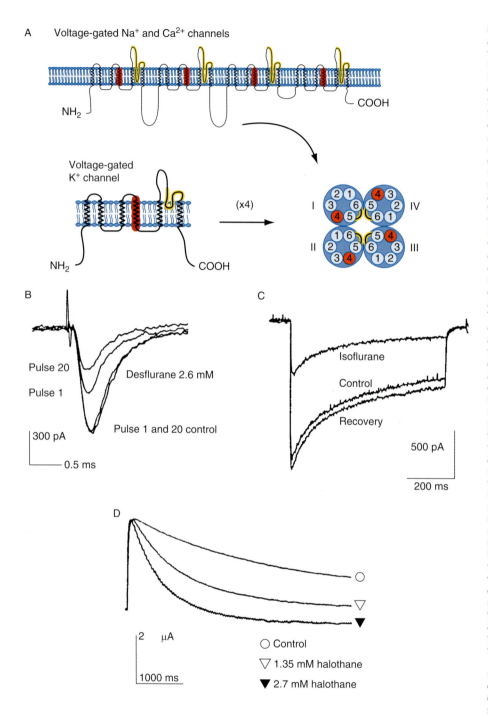

A Voltage-gated Na$^+$ and Ca^{2+} channels

NH$_2$

COOH

Voltage-gated K$^+$ channel

NH$_2$

COOH

(x4)

B

Pulse 20

Pulse 1

Desflurane 2.6 mM

Pulse 1 and 20 control

300 pA

0.5 ms

C

Isoflurane

Control

Recovery

500 pA

200 ms

D

2 μA

○ Control

▽ 1.35 mM halothane

▼ 2.7 mM halothane

1000 ms

Figure 3.1. Structure of voltage-gated ion channels and the effects of anesthetics. (A) The main subunits of the voltage-gated ion channels. The α subunit of the Na$^+$ channel and the α$_1$ subunit of the Ca^{2+} channel have similar structures, shown schematically by the drawing at the top. A single protein is segregated into four repeating homologous domains (I–IV), each containing six membrane-spanning segments (S1–S6). The α subunit of the voltage gated K$^+$ channel (A, *bottom left*) contains only one domain of six membrane-spanning segments. In each domain of all three types of channels, the fourth transmembrane segment (shown in red) is highly charged and is the voltage sensor. The long extracellular loop between the fifth and sixth transmembrane segments (shown in yellow) forms the outer vestibule of the pore of the channel. In the membrane, four domains aggregate to form the main structure of the channel, as shown in an "end-on" view (A, *bottom right*). (B) Currents through voltage-gated Na$^+$ channels recorded from a Chinese hamster ovary cell stably transfected with the gene coding for rat brain IIA (Na$_v$1.2) sodium channels [3]. Twenty depolarizing voltage steps from –85 to 0 mV were applied at a frequency of 5 Hz to elicit Na$^+$ currents. The large downward deflections represent inward ionic currents. In control conditions, Na$^+$ current activated and inactivated rapidly during the short depolarizations. The magnitude of the Na$^+$ current did not change after repetitive stimulation (compare pulse 1 and pulse 20). After exposing the cell to a solution containing desflurane (2.6 mM), the Na$^+$ current was immediately reduced (pulse 1) and decreased even more after repetitive stimulation (compare pulse 1 to pulse 20 in the presence of desflurane), indicating both tonic and phasic block of Na$^+$ channels. (C) Currents through voltage-gated Ca^{2+} channels recorded from an isolated rat hippocampal pyramidal neuron in response to a depolarizing voltage step from –90 to –10 mV [4]. Downward deflections in the traces indicate inward currents. The control current increased rapidly after the voltage step and decayed over time, representing inactivation of Ca^{2+} channels. Open channels closed rapidly at the end of the voltage step. Exposure of the cell to extracellular solution equilibrated with isoflurane 2.5% in the gas phase reduced the magnitude of the Ca^{2+} current evoked by the same voltage step. This inhibition was reversed after washout of anesthetic-containing solution (recovery). (D) Currents through voltage-gated K$^+$ channels recorded from *Xenopus* oocytes injected with cRNA for the voltage gated K$^+$ channel K$_v$ 2.1 [5]. The membrane potential was rapidly stepped from –50mV to +50 mV at the beginning of the trace and held at +50mV for 10 seconds. Upward deflections indicate outward membrane current. In control conditions, the K$^+$ current increased rapidly and showed a slow decay over the long depolarization, representing slow inactivation of these K$^+$ channels. Exposure of the cell to extracellular solution containing increasing concentrations of halothane (1.35 and 2.7 mM) markedly accelerated the current inactivation. The current traces are normalized to emphasize inactivation rates.

it forms a channel with ionic selectivity and voltage-dependent behaviors that are similar to those of the native channel. The other subunits that associate with α subunits to form functional channels in vivo are much smaller proteins and are thought to stabilize the α subunit and modulate its function.

The α subunits of the Na$^+$ and Ca^{2+} channels were the first to be cloned, and their primary amino acid sequences were the first to be deduced. These α subunits are large proteins containing four repeating homologous domains (I–IV) separated by long cytoplasmic loops, which allow the four domains to aggregate in the membrane, forming a central pore through which the ions pass (Fig. 3.1). Each domain consists of six membrane-spanning α-helical segments (S1–S6) that anchor the protein in the membrane. The fourth transmembrane segment (S4) of each domain is considered to be the voltage sensor because it contains several positively charged amino acids in an otherwise hydrophobic α-helix. Movement of these positive charges during changes in transmembrane potential produces conformational changes in the protein that ultimately lead to voltage-dependent gating of the channel. The segment of the protein that connects the fifth and sixth transmembrane segments, sometimes called the P loop, forms part of the outer portion, or outer vestibule, of the pore. The amino acids within the P loop are important in determining the ionic selectivity of the channel. The overall structure of the pore-forming part of the voltage-gated K^+ channel is almost identical to that of the Na^+ and Ca^{2+} channels, the only exception being that each of the four domains is a separate protein. K^+ channels are thus formed by the aggregation of four individual α subunits into either a homotetramer or, with different α subunits, a heterotetramer.

Individual voltage-gated ion channels
Na^+ channels
The voltage-gated Na^+ channel is composed of an α subunit and one or more auxiliary β subunits. The α subunit is the largest subunit and contains both the pore region of the channel and the voltage sensor. Nine different genes encoding functional Na^+ channel α subunit have been identified ($Na_v1.1$–1.9), as well as splice variants. These different isoforms are preferentially expressed in different tissues or at different times of development. The cytoplasmic linker between domains III and IV of the α subunit is responsible for inactivation of the Na^+ channel. After the channel opens, this segment of the protein is drawn to the inner surface of the channel like a "hinged lid," where it is thought to physically block ions from passing through the pore [6,7].

Four different protein isoforms comprise the family of Na^+ channel β subunits. These β subunits are each about one-tenth of the mass of the α subunit and are anchored in the cell membrane through one transmembrane segment. Their extracellular domains are large and have structures similar to those of immunoglobulins. Beta subunits regulate the expression and subcellular targeting of Na^+ channels, and modulate the function of the α subunit [6,8].

The effects of local anesthetics on Na^+ channel function are described in Chapter 36. Unlike local anesthetics, general anesthetics were initially thought to have little effect on voltage-gated Na^+ channels. More recent evidence has revealed important effects of anesthetics on central nervous system (CNS) Na^+ channels at concentrations similar to those required for clinical anesthesia [3, 9–11]. Both volatile and intravenous anesthetics decrease Na^+ currents by enhancing voltage-dependent inactivation of the channel. Volatile anesthetics

inhibit resting Na^+ channels but actually bind more strongly to the inactivated state of the channel, leading to a use-dependent block of Na^+ currents similar to that described for local anesthetics (Fig. 3.1B; see also Chapter 36). This Na^+ channel inhibition does not alter axonal conduction, but inhibition of Na^+ currents in central glutamatergic presynaptic terminals may lead to changes in the action potential waveform and thereby reduce excitatory neurotransmitter release [11,12].

Ca^{2+} channels
The voltage-gated Ca^{2+} channel is composed of 4–5 different subunits. The pore-forming and voltage-sensing portions of the voltage-gated Ca^{2+} channel are contained in the largest subunit, the $α_1$ subunit. Ten isoforms of the $α_1$ subunit exist, and according to current nomenclature are arranged into three subfamilies based on amino acid sequence homology [13,14]. $Ca_v1.1$–1.4 include all the dihydropyridine-sensitive high-voltage-activated L-type Ca^{2+} channels expressed in muscle, heart, endocrine cells, and neuronal tissue. $Ca_v2.1$–2.3 include the N-type, P/Q-type, and R-type high-voltage-activated Ca^{2+} channels found primarily in neurons and neuroendocrine cells. $Ca_v3.1$–3.3 include the three types of low-voltage-activated rapidly inactivating T-type channels. Each subfamily, and in some cases the isoforms within a subfamily, can be identified by its biophysical properties and sensitivities to blockers and toxins. Splice variants of these subunits also exist [13].

Four accessory Ca^{2+} channel subunits that interact with the $α_1$ subunit have been described [6,14,15]. The β subunit of the Ca^{2+} channel, unlike that of the Na^+ channel, is a cytoplasmic protein. There are four gene products and several splice variants, all with similar structure and function. The β subunit associates with the cytoplasmic linker between domains I and II of the $α_1$ subunit and regulates both the trafficking of the channel to the membrane and the kinetics of channel activation and inactivation. The $α_2$ and δ subunits are derived from a single preprotein that is post-translationally divided into the two subunit proteins, which are then linked together by a disulfide bond. The $α_2$ subunit is entirely extracellular, whereas the δ subunit contains a transmembrane segment that anchors the $α_2δ$ complex in the membrane. Four different genes encode $α_2δ$ subunits, and splice variants of these exist. The $α_2δ$ subunits regulate expression of Ca^{2+} channels, and may modulate channel gating [16]. Finally, eight types of γ subunit have been discovered, as well as splice variants. All have four transmembrane segments and intracellular amino and carboxy termini. The first γ subunit was found to associate with Ca^{2+} channel $α_1$ subunits in skeletal muscle, and others have since been shown to associate with different $α_1$ subunits in other tissues. Interestingly, some γ subunits associate with and regulate the trafficking and gating of AMPA-type glutamate receptors instead of Ca^{2+} channels. When associated with Ca^{2+} channel subunits, γ subunits have variable effects on gating [15,17].

The α_1 subunits of Ca_v2 channels display two interesting structural features not found in other α_1 subunits. The first is in the cytoplasmic loop linking domains I and II, which contains a site that interacts with the $\beta\gamma$ subunits of inhibitory GTP-binding proteins (G proteins) [14]. This molecular interaction is responsible for the well-known inhibition of these Ca^{2+} channels by agonists of G-protein-coupled receptors (e.g., opioids, norepinephrine, baclofen). The second interesting feature of Ca_v2 α_1 subunits is that the cytoplasmic linker between domains II and III interacts with the soluble N-ethylmaleimide-sensitive attachment factor receptor (SNARE) proteins syntaxin, SNAP-25, and synaptotagmin, which are part of the cellular machinery involved in synaptic vesicle exocytosis and neurotransmitter release [18–20]. This interaction segregates Ca^{2+} channels to parts of the membrane where vesicle docking and release occur, allowing Ca^{2+} entry to be localized to these areas where it can initiate rapid neurotransmitter release.

Most Ca^{2+} channels gate over the same range of voltages as Na^+ channels, although the rate of inactivation is much slower. Ca^{2+} channels prolong the duration of the action potential and provide Ca^{2+} entry during depolarization, an effect seen particularly in cardiac ventricular myocytes. Ca_v3 channels are somewhat unique in that they activate at more hyperpolarized membrane potentials and inactivate more quickly than other types of Ca^{2+} channels. These distinct biophysical properties allow Ca_v3 channels to provide different functions, such as increasing the magnitude of low threshold potentials, neuronal pacemaking, and burst firing [21].

The effects of general anesthetics on voltage-gated Ca^{2+} channels have been studied in a variety of tissues. Almost all anesthetics tested inhibit Ca^{2+} channels to some extent (Fig. 3.1C). The volatile anesthetics reduce native Ca^{2+} currents in many types of neuronal tissue [4,22–29], although the magnitude and concentration dependence of the effects are somewhat variable. All families of voltage-gated Ca^{2+} channels have been shown to be sensitive to anesthetics. As with voltage-gated Na^+ channels, anesthetics appear to stabilize the inactivated state of Ca^{2+} channels. For some Ca_v1 and 2 channels, volatile anesthetics increase the rate of Ca^{2+} current inactivation, slow recovery from inactivation, and cause hyperpolarizing shifts in the voltage dependence of inactivation [28]. Further evidence comes from single channel recordings, in which open channel lifetimes were decreased and closed channel lifetimes were increased by halothane, suggesting stabilization of nonconducting (closed, inactivated, or both) states of the channel [27].

K^+ channels

Four individual α-subunit proteins aggregate in the cell membrane to create the pore-forming segment of the voltage-gated K^+ channel (Fig. 3.1A). Forty genes encode voltage-gated K^+ channel α subunits, which are divided into 12 families (K_v1–12) each with between one and eight members [30]. Additional variability is produced by alternative splicing of many of these subunit transcripts. Individual α subunits form either homotetramers or heterotetramers, which then associate with at least three different types of accessory proteins.

Three intracellular $K_v\beta$ subunit isoforms exist, which pair with the α subunits of K_v1 channels in a 1:1 stoichiometry and regulate membrane expression and channel gating [6,30]. In addition, the N-terminus of the β_1 subunit forms the inactivation gate for the pore formed by K_v1 α subunits [31]. Recent studies have shown that β subunits also act as aldo-keto reductases, thus coupling the redox state of the cell to K^+ channel activity [32]. Four isoforms of the K^+ channel interacting protein (KChIP) regulate K_v4 channels. Five types of minK-like subunits or minK-related peptides (MiRPs) associate with and regulate K_v7, K_v10, K_v11, and perhaps other K_v families [6].

The structure of several types of K^+ channels, including a mammalian $K_v1.2$, have been deduced using x-ray crystallography [33,34]. The shapes of the conducting portions of the channels are similar, shaped like an "inverted teepee" with the narrowest external diameter on the cytoplasmic side. Conversely, the internal pore region is widest at the cytoplasmic end, forming a large water-filled cavity. The gate is formed from the inner helices of the four S6 segments of K_v, which bend near the inner surface of the membrane to allow channel opening. The selectivity filter is the narrowest region of the pore, formed by the P loops from the S5–6 linker at the extracellular end of the channel. The highly conserved amino acids in this region, known as the "signature sequence," provide rapid and selective passage to K^+ ions but exclude other ions [1,34,35].

The N-terminal portion of some K_v α and β subunits is mobile in the cytoplasm and is responsible for rapid "N-type" inactivation by blocking the pore in a "ball and chain" type of model. The N-terminal "ball" interacts with the small cytoplasmic linker between transmembrane segments 5 and 6 of the α subunit, where it prevents flow of K^+ ions through the pore of the channel [31]. Only one of the four N-terminal regions is required to produce inactivation, although the rate of inactivation is four times slower if only one subunit retains its N-terminus.

As with Na^+ and Ca^{2+} channels, voltage-gated K^+ channels open in response to depolarization of the cell membrane. Historically, K^+ channel currents have been classified according to their rates and voltage dependences of activation and inactivation. These biophysical attributes (i.e., how the channel responds to voltage over time) define the role that each K^+ channel has in the cell. For example, delayed rectifier-type K^+ channels activate rapidly and show little or no inactivation, whereas fast transient, or A-type K^+ channels, inactivate rapidly during a depolarization. Delayed rectifiers from the K_v1 family are found on nerve axons, where they keep axonal action potentials short so Na^+ channels can recover from inactivation and initiate the next action potential as quickly as possible. Conversely, A-type K^+ channels, such as those from the K_v4 family, are located at axon hillocks, dendrites, and other regions of the neuron where action potentials are generated. In these areas, passive membrane depolarizations produced by synaptic potentials and receptor potentials

A Different classes of K⁺ channels

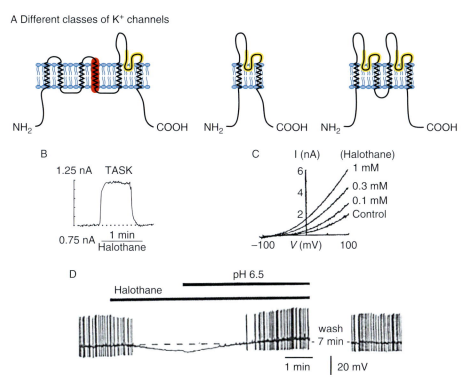

Figure 3.2. Structures of the main classes of K⁺ channels and the effects of anesthetics. (A) The three main classes of K⁺ selective channels, differing in the number of transmembrane (TM) segments and the number of P loop (P) segments in each subunit. Left to right: the 6TM/1P class of voltage-gated K⁺ channels (reproduced from Fig. 3.1A to facilitate comparison among the K⁺ channel classes); the 2TM/1P class (including K_{ir} and K_{ATP} channels); and the 4TM/2P class, also known as the K_{2P} or tandem-pore-domain K⁺ channels. (B) Membrane current measured at a holding potential of 0 mV in a COS cell transfected with DNA containing the human *TASK* gene [38]. Application of halothane (1 mM) rapidly and reversibly increased outward currents, indicating activation of the TASK channel by halothane. (C) Membrane current–voltage relations in a COS cell transfected with DNA containing the human *TREK-1* gene [38]. Current was recorded during a rapid linear increase in membrane potential in the absence (control) and the presence of various concentrations of halothane in solution. Outward current is positive. Halothane increased currents through the TREK-1 channel. (D) Membrane potential recorded from a rat locus coeruleus neuron in the presence of bicuculline and strychnine to block γ-aminobutyric acid type A (GABA_A) receptors and glycine receptors, respectively, in a brain slice preparation [39]. These neurons contain mRNA for TASK-1 [40]. Spontaneous action potential firing is seen at the beginning of the trace. Halothane (0.3 mM) hyperpolarized the membrane and inhibited action potential firing. Acidifying the extracellular solution (pH 6.5) reversed the hyperpolarization, as would be expected if the effect of halothane was caused by activation of the TASK-1 channel, which is inhibited by acidic solutions.

are converted to action potentials in a graded fashion, such that larger depolarizations are coded as a higher frequency of action potential firing. A-type K⁺ channels contribute to this frequency modulation of passive electrical potentials. If A-type K⁺ channels were not present, all depolarizations above the threshold for action potential generation would elicit the same high frequency of action potential firing, regardless of magnitude [1].

Voltage-gated K⁺ channels are generally insensitive to anesthetics. Delayed rectifier-type K⁺ channels, from squid giant axon [36] and a $K_v2.1$ channel cloned from mammalian brain [35] are inhibited by relatively high concentrations of anesthetics. Interestingly, these normally sustained currents displayed rapid inactivation in the presence of anesthetics (Fig. 3.1D). A-type K⁺ currents recorded from ventricular myocytes also show enhanced inactivation, a prolongation of recovery from inactivation, and a hyperpolarizing shift in the inactivation curve [37]. These effects are all consistent with anesthetics stabilizing the inactivated state of K⁺ channels.

Voltage-gated K⁺ channels account for about half of all known mammalian K⁺ selective ion channels [30]. Both voltage-gated and non-voltage-gated K⁺ channels share the highly conserved "signature sequence" within the pore region that defines the K⁺ selectivity of the channel. Large differences in channel structure (Fig. 3.2) and gating define three major classes of mammalian K⁺ channels [35].

Channels with six transmembrane segments and one pore (6TM/1P)

K⁺ channels in this family include the voltage-gated channels K_v1–12 and most Ca^{2+}-activated K⁺ channels (K_{Ca}) [30,35,41]. There are eight K_{Ca} channels organized into five families, each with unique conductances and Ca^{2+} sensitivity [41]. The α subunits of 6TM/1P channels form tetramers, and may associate with various auxiliary subunits to form a native channel [6]. K_v channels were described in detail earlier in this chapter.

Channels with two transmembrane segments and one pore (2TM/1P)

There are 15 known K⁺ channels with this simple structure, including the inwardly rectifying K⁺ channels ($K_{ir}1$–5; $K_{ir}7$)

and adenosine-triphosphate (ATP)-sensitive K^+ channels (K_{ATP}, or $K_{ir}6.1-2$) [35,42]. K_{ir} channels conduct K^+ into the cell during hyperpolarization, but K^+ efflux during depolarization is limited by intracellular Mg^{2+} and polyamines, which block the pore. These channels function primarily to maintain a hyperpolarized membrane potential. K_{ATP} channels are formed from a complex of four inwardly rectifying K^+ channel subunits and four sulfonylurea receptors. K_{ATP} channels close with increases in the intracellular ATP/adenosine diphosphate (ADP) ratio, thus coupling membrane potential and electrical excitability to the metabolic state of the cell. In pancreatic β cells, inhibition of K_{ATP} channels causes insulin secretion. In myocardium and neuronal tissues, activation of K_{ATP} channels protects cells from ischemic or hypoxic insults, or both. In vascular smooth muscle, K_{ATP} channel activation produces vasodilation and may mediate autoregulation in the coronary and cerebral circulations. Volatile anesthetics activate K_{ATP} channels, which may be a mechanism for their protective effects during cerebral and myocardial ischemia [43].

Channels with four transmembrane segments and two pores (4TM/2P)

Channels with four transmembrane segments and two pores are variously referred to as 4TM/2P, K_{2P}, two-pore-domain, or tandem-pore-domain channels. Fifteen mammalian genes encode K_{2P} subunits, which combine as either hetero- or homodimers to form functional channels. Common names include TWIK1–2 (tandem of P domains in weak inward-rectifier K^+ channels; $K_{2P}1$, $K_{2P}6$), TREK1–2 (TWIK-related K^+ channels; $K_{2P}2$, $K_{2P}10$), TASK1–3 (TWIK-related acid-sensitive K^+ channels; $K_{2P}3$, $K_{2P}5$, $K_{2P}9$), TRAAK (TWIK-related arachidonic-acid-stimulated K^+ channels; $K_{2P}4$), and TRESK (TWIK-related spinal cord K^+ channels; $K_{2P}18$) [44]. The primary function of K_{2P} channels seems to be maintenance of a hyperpolarized membrane potential by providing a background or baseline potassium "leak" conductance, though they can be individually regulated by stretch, temperature, pH, arachidonic acid, and phospholipds [45].

Tandem-pore-domain K^+ channels are also activated by anesthetics. In 1982, Nicoll and Madison [46] reported that anesthetics hyperpolarized rat hippocampal neurons, likely by increasing a K^+ conductance. Franks and Lieb [47] later confirmed that anesthetics activated a background K^+ channel in certain neurons of the pond snail *Lymnaea stagnalis*. This channel was recently cloned and confirmed to be a K_{2P} channel similar to human TASK channels [48], which, along with TREK and TRESK channels, are also activated by volatile anesthetics (Fig. 3.2B–D) [38–40,48]. In rat hypoglossal motoneurons and locus coeruleus neurons, which both contain mRNA for TASK-1, anesthetics activate a potassium conductance with properties similar to those of expressed TASK-1 [39]. Anesthetics hyperpolarize these neurons by up to 13 mV and inhibit their spontaneous electrical activity at clinically appropriate concentrations [39].

Ligand-gated ion channels
Ionotropic and metabotropic receptors

Neurotransmitters, hormones, and other small molecules released as intercellular messengers influence the activity of ion channels through two types of receptors. In the case of **ionotropic** receptors, such as the nicotinic acetylcholine receptor (nAChR) found at the neuromuscular junction, the transmitter binding site and the transmembrane ion channel are integral to a single protein (or protein complex, because most ion channels are formed as multimers of homologous or heterologous subunits). Binding of the transmitter directly alters the activity of the ion channel, allowing the flow of cations across the membrane for nAChR, which results in depolarization. Receptors that operate in this fashion are responsible for rapid synaptic transmission (over a time scale of milliseconds), although these may also display sustained or tonic activity. In the case of **metabotropic** receptors, such as the β-adrenoceptor found in cardiac myocytes, the transmitter receptor (binding site) and the effector (Ca^{2+} channels) are separate molecules. They are coupled through GTP-binding proteins (G proteins), either indirectly through cascades of intracellular signaling pathways, or more directly through membrane-delimited pathways where subunits of the G protein directly alter ion-channel activity (see Chapter 2). The time course of action through metabotropic receptors is much slower than through ionotropic receptors, typically operating over a time scale of seconds or even minutes, although in rare cases activation and deactivation occur as rapidly as 50 ms. G-protein-coupled pathways are dealt with more extensively in Chapter 2, so the discussion in this chapter is limited primarily to ionotropic receptors. However, it should be noted that many of the ligand-gated as well as voltage-gated ion channels discussed in this chapter are subject to modulation through second messengers initiated by metabotropic receptors.

Five families of ionotropic receptors

Just as voltage-gated channels are grouped into families on the basis of sequence similarities between the genes that encode different members, ligand-gated ion channels also have been grouped into separate families based on sequence homology. The largest and most diverse family includes the nAChR, the ionotropic serotonin (5-HT_3) receptor, the γ-aminobutyric acid type A (GABA_A) receptor, and the glycine receptor. The N-terminus of each subunit of these receptors contains a characteristic 15-member loop that is formed by the disulfide linkage between a pair of cysteines, and consequently this family has been referred to as the **Cys-loop** family [49]. Each of these receptors is a pentamer, composed of five homologous subunits, each with four transmembrane (TM) segments and an extracellular N-terminus segment that contains residues that form the neurotransmitter binding site

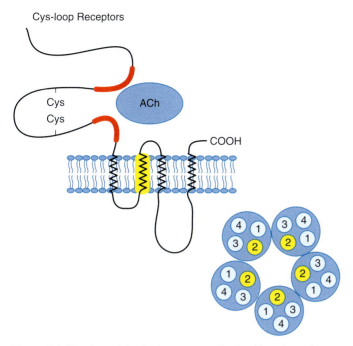

Cys-loop Receptors

Figure 3.3. Topology of the Cys-loop receptor family of ligand-gated receptors. Each subunit contains four membrane-spanning segments, designated TM1–TM4. The second segment, TM2 (shown in yellow), lines the pore of the channel. Functional receptors are composed of five subunits in a pseudosymmetrical arrangement (inset). The transmitter-binding site (shown in red) is formed by several discontiguous loops formed by the large extracellular N-terminal domain.

(Fig. 3.3; see also Chapters 18, 24, and 29). Two of these receptors are cation-selective and excitatory (nAChR and 5-HT$_3$) and two are anion-selective and inhibitory (GABA$_A$ and glycine).

A second family of receptors is activated by **glutamate**, the major excitatory neurotransmitter in the brain. Different combinations of subunits form channels that are activated by the selective ligands N-methyl-D-aspartate (NMDA), α-amino-3-hydroxy-5-methylisoxazole-4-propionic acid (AMPA), and kainate (KA). Each of these receptors is composed of four subunits, each of which has four transmembrane segments and a P loop that is structurally similar to that of voltage-activated channels. A third family of ionotropic receptors, termed **P2X receptors**, binds ATP in the extracellular space. Like the other ionotropic receptors, P2X receptors are multimers. Each subunit is thought to possess only two membrane-spanning segments, with three subunits combining to form a functional channel (but in the absence of a crystal structure for P2X receptors this structure should be considered tentative). The last two classes of ionotropic receptors, the **transient receptor potential** (TRP) receptors and **cyclic nucleotide-gated** (CNG) channels, are structurally similar to the members of the voltage-activated ion channel superfamily. They are formed as tetramers of six transmembrane-spanning units with a pore loop between the fifth and six segments. The TRP family is notable for its great diversity in activation

mechanisms and ion selectivities, exceeding those of any other group of ion channels. A common theme is that these receptors play important roles in generating responses to all major classes of external stimuli (light, sound, temperature, touch, and taste) as well as the local environment (osmolarity, other chemical sensation).

Cys-loop receptor family (nAChR, GABA$_A$, glycine, and 5-HT$_3$)

These ion channels exist as pentamers, with the transmitter binding sites for all receptors in this family located at the interfaces between subunits [50]. At least two transmitter molecules are required to produce full channel activation, as reflected in Hill coefficients greater than 1 [51]. It has proved difficult to determine the precise stoichiometry and subunit composition of the majority of receptors in the brain, but it seems clear that the majority of receptors are heteromeric, composed of subunits from multiple classes, and even multiple subunits from a single class for some receptors [52,53].

The detailed structure of this receptor class has emerged recently through a combination of two approaches: determination of the crystal structure of the molluscan acetylcholine-binding protein (AChBP), a structural and functional homolog of the amino-terminal ligand-binding domain of an nAChR α subunit [54]; and the elucidation of the structure of the membrane-spanning region through cyro-electron microscopy of crystalline postsynaptic membranes derived from the electric organ of the *Torpedo* electric ray [55]. Molecular models based on these structures, mutagenesis studies, and the development of affinity labels are yielding unprecendented insights into many features of channel function and anesthetic modulation.

One TM2 segment from each subunit lines the ion-conducting pore of the channel; the other TM segments form rings around this central pore in contact with membrane lipids [55]. Mutation of the channel-facing residues of TM2 leads to alterations in conductance and ion selectivity, and it has even been possible to change normally cation-selective channels to anion-selective channels and vice versa in chimeric receptors and through mutation of selected residues [56–58]. Whereas in the voltage-gated K$^+$ channel the P loop located at the extracellular end of the channel confers charge selectivity, in the Cys-loop family an analogous coiled-loop structure located at the cytoplasmic end of the channel may serve a similar function [57]. The location of the "gate" also appears to be close to the cytoplasmic end of the channel. The mechanism by which ligand binding becomes transduced to channel gating involves interactions between ligand-binding loops and residues at the extracellular ends of the transmembrane domains [59,60], with stepwise transitions propagating through the transmembrane segments [61].

In this chapter only the glycine and 5-HT$_3$ receptors of the Cys-loop family will be described. The other members are described in Chapters 18 (nAChR), 24, and 29 (GABA$_A$ receptor).

Glycine receptors

Glycine receptors (GlyRs) are inhibitory receptors that are selectively permeable to anions. They mediate rapid inhibitory synaptic transmission, primarily in the spinal cord and brainstem. Glycinergic synapses do exist elsewhere, however, including in the cerebellum, hippocampus, and retina, and extrasynaptic GlyRs are also widely distributed throughout the CNS [62]. A total of five GlyR subunits (α_{1-4} and β) have been identified. In adults, two α and three β subunits combine to form a functional channel. α_3-subunit-containing GlyRs mediate inhibitory neurotransmission onto spinal nociceptive neurons. These receptors are inhibited by inflammatory mediators, suggesting that they may play a role in inflammatory pain sensitization. Drugs that potentiate GlyRs may act as muscle relaxants and analgesics, so they remain interesting targets for development of novel therapeutic drugs [63].

Like GABA$_A$ receptors, the activity of glycine receptors is enhanced by volatile anesthetics and alcohols [64]. This effect may play a role in the suppression of movement through a spinal action of these drugs. Nevertheless, the inability to reverse anesthetic effects through spinal administration of glycine receptor antagonists suggests that this is not the entire mechanism by which movement is abolished by volatile drugs [65].

5-HT$_3$ receptors

Many subtypes of serotonin (5-hydroxytryptophan or 5-HT) receptors exist, but with the exception of the ionotropic 5-HT$_3$ subtype all are metabotropic (G-protein-coupled) [62]. Ionotropic 5-HT$_3$ receptors are excitatory, selectively permeable to cations, and may play a variety of roles in the CNS, including anxiolytic [66], analgesic [67], and emetic [68]. 5-HT$_3$ antagonists, such as ondansetron and dolasetron, have been widely used in the prevention and treatment of postoperative nausea and vomiting [69] and may also be useful in the treatment of irritable bowel syndrome [70].

P2X receptor family

ATP is used not only as a cellular fuel but also as a signaling molecule (see Jarvis and Khakh [71] for a recent review). Specialized receptors that respond to extracellular ATP, termed purinergic type 2 (P2) receptors to distinguish them from adenosine-sensitive purinergic type 1 (P1) receptors, exist as metabotropic (P2Y) and ionotropic (P2X) receptors. Seven different P2X receptor subunits have been identified to date. It is known that they combine to form homomultimers and heteromultimers, but as no crystal structure is available for these channels, the number of subunits that are required to form functional channels and other aspects of their structure are not known with certainty. These subunits appear to be structurally much simpler than the other ligand-gated channels, with only two transmembrane domains per subunit. A large cysteine-rich extracellular loop forms the ligand-binding domain. Channels are permeable to cations, but show little selectivity, with approximately equal permeability to Na$^+$ and K$^+$ and significant permeability to Ca^{2+}.

P2X receptors are found in a diverse range of organisms, ranging from parasitic worms through mammals, suggesting that signaling by ATP through P2X receptors is a general mechanism. In mammals, they are found throughout the body and brain, and they play physiological roles in neuron-to-muscle and neuron-to-neuron communication, including smooth muscle constriction, breathing, and taste [72–74]. Accumulating evidence indicates that they are also involved in a number of pathophysiological processes, including chronic and inflammatory pain, bone formation and resorption, and blood pressure regulation [75–78]. Because of the relatively recent identification of this family of receptors and the lack of subtype-specific antagonists, our understanding of the roles that are played by these receptors remains somewhat limited. However, given their wide distribution, and accumulating evidence for their involvement in a wide range of physiological and pathophysiological processes, further research in this area will undoubtedly lead to important advances and novel therapeutic strategies.

Glutamate receptor family
Glutamate as a neurotransmitter

Glutamate's role as an excitatory neurotransmitter is detailed in Chapter 14. In addition, glutamate and its receptors provide an important molecular interface for neuron–glia interaction – ionotropic and metabotropic glutamate receptors are widely expressed in various types of glial cells [79]. Glutamate released from neurons can activate these receptors and cause several effects including modulation of transmitter uptake into glial cells, thereby affecting synaptic transmission [80], modulation of K$^+$ conductances within glial cells and consequent changes in the extracellular ion composition, and release of neuroactive substances from glia that can feedback and modulate synaptic transmission [81].

Glutamic acid is found in very high levels in the CNS. Because it does not cross the blood–brain barrier, it must originate from local metabolism. It participates in intermediary glucose metabolism in addition to its role in intercellular communication and therefore shares with GABA the problem of dissociating neurotransmitter from metabolic roles. Glutamate is formed through two distinct pathways: either from glucose in the Krebs cycle and transamination of α-ketoglutarate or directly from glutamine. Inactivation of released glutamate is mainly through reuptake by dicarboxylic acid transporters, and enzymatic inactivation does not play a significant role. Glutamate also serves as the substrate source for glutamic acid decarboxylase, the GABA synthesizing enzyme (Fig. 3.4A).

A
(Glutamate)

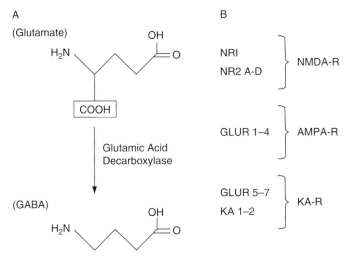

B

NRI
NR2 A-D
} NMDA-R

GLUR 1–4 } AMPA-R

GLUR 5–7
KA 1–2
} KA-R

(GABA)

Figure 3.4. Glutamate in the central nervous system (CNS). (A) l-glutamate ((S)-glutamate according to the official IUPAC nomenclature) has an acidic side chain that carries a negative charge at physiologic pH. In the CNS, it serves as the only substrate for the γ-aminobutyric acid (GABA) synthesizing enzyme glutamic acid decarboxylase. (B) The ionotropic glutamate receptors are classified into three subtypes according to the most selective agonist available: N-methyl-d-aspartate (NMDA), α-amino-3-hydroxy-5-methylisoxazole-4-propionic acid (AMPA, formerly quisqualate), and kainate (KA). Each subtype comprises several subunits and different splice variants exist for numerous subunits. Native receptors are likely to be heteromultimers.

Three types of ionotropic glutamate receptors

The ionotropic family of glutamate receptors comprises three classes of receptors based on agonist specificities: AMPA, kainate, and NMDA receptors. (Note that glutamate can act through metabotropic receptors (mGluR) as well; this topic is covered in Chapter 2.) The former two families were collectively referred to as non-NMDA receptors, because neither agonists nor antagonists clearly (until recently) distinguished between them. Cloning studies have demonstrated, however, that AMPA and kainate activate distinct receptor complexes (Fig. 3.4B).

The ionotropic glutamate receptors are tetrameric proteins – four subunits assemble to form a functional receptor-channel complex. Each subunit consists of a large extracellular N-terminus domain, three hydrophobic transmembrane segments (M1, M3, M4), and an intracellular C-terminus (Fig. 3.5). The pore region is formed by the amphipathic reentrant hairpin loop M2, similar in structure to the pore-forming region of K^+ channels. The ligand binds to two regions one before M1, the other between M3 and M4 [85].

AMPA receptors

Alpha-amino-3-hydroxy-5-methylisoxazole-4-propionic acid (AMPA) receptors mediate fast excitatory transmission at most synapses in the CNS. The four subunits that combine to form these receptors, GluR1–GluR4, are encoded by four closely related genes. Each subunit exists in two alternative splice variants: flip and flop. In the rodent embryonic brain,

AMPA receptors are expressed predominantly as flip variants. Adult levels of the flop variant, which carries most of the excitatory transmission in the adult brain, are reached by the 14th postnatal day. AMPA receptors are either homomeric or heteromeric tetramers composed of these multiple subunits, which results in a marked functional diversity of the native receptors.

AMPA receptor channels are permeable to cations. Glutamate and AMPA elicit rapidly desensitizing responses in the AMPA receptor, whereas AMPA-receptor-mediated responses to kainate do not desensitize [86,87]. The speed of desensitization depends on the subunit composition and on the splice variant (flip or flop), and can vary by more than an order of magnitude [40,88].

Three different binding sites can be identified on AMPA receptors: a site that binds agonist (glutamate), a site that binds drugs that alter desensitization, and an intra-ion channel binding site that binds channel blockers. The binding site for glutamate and competitive antagonists is formed by two discontiguous segments located between the N-terminus and M1 and between M3 and M4, respectively [89]. A separate site binds aniracetam (a pyrrolidine) and CTZ (cyclothiazide, a benzothiadiazine). Binding of these drugs removes desensitization in the flip variants [90–92]. A third binding site located near the intracellular entrance to the channel pore binds a variety of spider and wasp toxins, all of which act as channel blockers.

The AMPA-receptor-mediated component of the glutamatergic excitatory postsynaptic current (EPSC) is characterized by its fast time course. As at other fast chemical synapses, this is the result of a brief (~1ms) high concentration (~1mM) transient of transmitter in the cleft [93]. Diffusion of transmitter away from the synaptic cleft appears to be very rapid (estimated time constant = 1.2 ms [93]), and deactivation rather than desensitization of receptors determines the time constant of EPSC decay [94,95]. At certain synapses, however, desensitization may be the determining factor [96].

Typically, postsynaptic Ca^{2+} entry at a glutamatergic synapse takes place through NMDA receptor channels, with AMPA-receptor-mediated depolarization of the postsynaptic membrane relieving the voltage-dependent block of NMDA receptor channels by Mg^{2+}. Recently, mice lacking the GluR2 subunit have been produced by gene targeting [97]. Despite the increased Ca^{2+} permeability and the ensuing physiologic changes in vitro, these mice survive into adulthood without obvious deficits except for reduced anesthetic drug requirements for certain anesthetic endpoints [98,99].

Kainate receptors

The kainate receptor family (KAR) comprises two groups of subunits (GluR5, GluR6, GluR7 and KA1, KA2), which differ in molecular size, percentage of sequence identity, affinity for kainate, and distribution throughout the CNS.

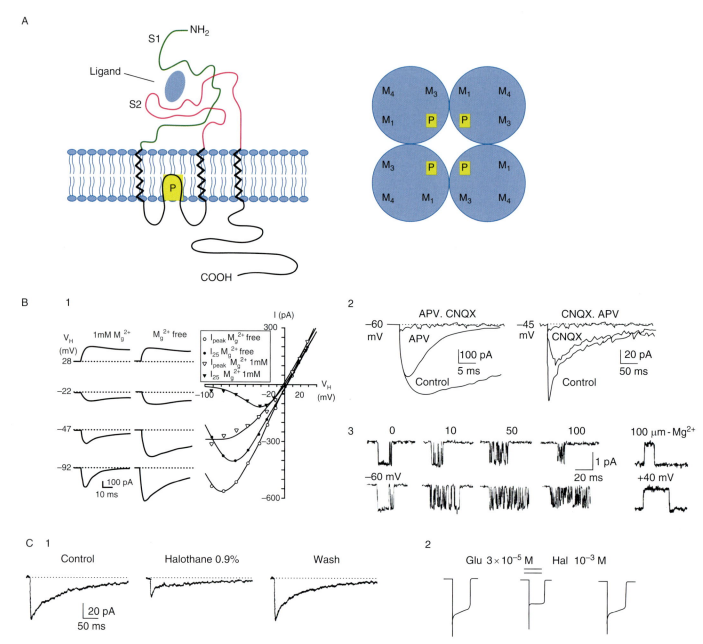

Figure 3.5. Glutamate receptors. (A) Schematic drawing of a glutamate receptor subunit, based on the proposed structure of NMDA receptor subunits [82]. Clam shell-like S1 and S2 domains create binding sites (ligand) for glutamate on AMPA, and glutamate (NR2) or glycine (NR1) on the NMDA receptor subunits, respectively. Note the presence of the hairpin loop P, which is a characteristic of all glutamate receptor subunits. On the right, the three transmembrane domains (M1, M3, M4) and the pore-lining P loop are arranged in a heterotetrameric structure with the P loop lining the pore region. (B) Basic physiology and pharmacology of glutamate-receptor-mediated excitatory postsynaptic currents (glu-EPSCs). Glu-EPSCs consist typically of a non-NMDA- and an NMDA-receptor-mediated component. (B1) In Mg^{2+}-containing solution, glu-EPSCs have a fast time course at negative holding potentials, determined mainly by the non-NMDA-receptor-mediated component. Depolarization of the holding potential removes the voltage-dependent block of the NMDA receptor channels by Mg^{2+} and recruits a slow glu-EPSC component. In Mg^{2+}-free saline, the slow, NMDA-receptor-mediated component is present at all holding potentials. Plotting the current–voltage relationship of this glu-EPSC graphically illustrates these issues. The non-NMDA-receptor-mediated component of the EPSC shows a linear current-voltage relationship across a wide range of voltages in the presence (*open triangles*) and absence (*open circles*) of Mg^{2+}. The NMDA-receptor-mediated component, by contrast, displays a nonlinear behavior at voltages more negative than –20 mV in the presence of Mg^{2+} (*closed triangles*, negative slope conductance) that is rectified in nominally "Mg^{2+}-free" saline (*closed circles*). The nonlinearities of the I/V relationships in "Mg^{2+}-free" saline at negative holding potentials are probably caused by residual Mg^{2+} [83]. (B2) Selective antagonists were instrumental in delineating the physiologic roles of the glu-EPSC components. The slow, NMDA-receptor-mediated component can be blocked by aminophosphonovaleric acid (APV), leaving the non-NMDA-receptor-mediated component that is sensitive to 6-cyano-7-nitroquinoxaline-2,3-dione (CNQX), which does not distinguish between α-amino-3-hydroxy-5-methylisoxazole-4-propionic acid (AMPA) and kainate receptors. Conversely, application of CNQX leaves a slow APV-sensitive component [83]. (B3) The Mg^{2+} block is further illustrated in two single-channel recordings: long channel openings induced by NMDA are dose-dependently blocked by increasing Mg^{2+} concentrations at –60 mV, evidenced by increasing "flickering" of the channel. Flickering is absent at +40 mV [84]. (C1) EPSCs recorded from hippocampal CA1 pyramidal cells in acute mouse slices [83]. (C2) Recordings obtained from cultured mouse central neurons.

Although AMPA and kainate receptor subunits can coexist in the same neuron [97], they do not coassemble with each other [100].

Our understanding of the physiologic role of KARs lags behind that of the other ionotropic glutamate receptors, in large part because kainic acid, the agonist most frequently used to activate KARs, elicits large nondesensitizing currents at AMPA receptors and small desensitizing responses at native KARs, thereby obscuring kainate channel activity in native preparations. Conversely, AMPA activates certain KARs; hence the encompassing term non-NMDA receptors. Currently available KAR-selective drugs are either difficult to use in the slice preparation (e.g., concanavalin A, a lectin that removes KAR desensitization [101,102]) or are selective for certain subunits (e.g., GluR5) with limited expression in the CNS [103], making it difficult to assess the roles of specific subunit combinations in native receptors present at different sites in the CNS.

Despite these difficulties, a physiologic role for KARs has been demonstrated in rat hippocampus. Whereas rapid synaptic transmission does not seem to involve postsynaptic kainate receptors [104], they do play an important role in modulation of transmitter release [105]. In the hippocampal CA3 region, release of GABA onto pyramidal cells and interneurons appears to be differentially regulated by kainate receptors. Functional native kainate receptors also have been demonstrated in dorsal root ganglion neurons [106]. Certain brain regions, e.g., the hippocampal CA3 area, show particularly high levels of kainate receptor expression [107]. It has been noted earlier that these areas are particularly susceptible to excitotoxic injury, and it has been proposed that kainate receptors may play a causal role.

NMDA receptors

The N-methyl-D-aspartate (NMDA) receptor family comprises five subunits: the "fundamental" NR1 and the "modulatory" NR2A–NR2D. The NR1 subunit can form homomeric receptor channels with the basic NMDA receptor channel properties but small amplitude current responses [108]. NR2 subunits do not form functional receptors on their own but their coexpression with NR1 amplifies the current responses through the heteromeric receptors by several orders [109]. As for the other glutamate receptors, diversity is increased with alternative splicing – eight splice variants have been reported for the NR1 subunit [109]. In-situ hybridization and immunohistochemistry have determined that the NR1 subunit is ubiquitous in the rodent brain. The NR2 subunits show distinct regional patterns and developmental changes in subunit expression [110,111]. NMDA receptor channels mediate excitatory neurotransmission in a way that is different from and complementary to the frequently colocalized AMPA receptors. AMPA receptors have a low affinity to glutamate, fast binding, and unbinding kinetics. NMDA receptors, by contrast, have high affinity to glutamate ($K_D \approx$ 100-fold lower than AMPA receptors), prolonged binding, and repeated channel openings.

Moreover, NMDA receptors can be activated by glutamate released from neighboring synapses [112]. The 10–90% rise time of NMDA-receptor-gated currents is ~ 10 ms, which means that the AMPA-receptor-mediated component of the synaptic current has mostly decayed before the NMDA component reaches its peak. The desensitization of NMDA receptors varies depending on the experimental conditions but is always significantly slower than the desensitization of AMPA receptors [113–115].

In contrast to AMPA receptors, a high permeability for Ca^{2+} is the rule rather than the exception for NMDA receptor channels. The Ca^{2+} permeability is characteristically combined with a voltage-dependent block of the channel by Mg^{2+}. Single-channel studies have shown that the NMDA receptor channel has a conductance of 40–50 pS in saline containing no Mg^{2+}. Addition of Mg^{2+} causes the single-channel currents to occur in bursts of short-lasting openings separated by brief closures, implicating a block of the open channel [84,116]. In addition, the degree of sensitivity to block by Mg^{2+} is determined by the type of NR2 subunit that forms the receptor–channel complex [117,118].

Glycine is an essential coagonist of glutamate at the NMDA receptor. It binds to the NR1 subunit at a region that corresponds to the glutamate recognition site at the NR2 subunits and has been termed the strychnine-insensitive glycine binding site. The ED_{50} of glycine is 0.1–0.7 μM [119]. D-Serine and D-alanine are naturally occurring agonists at the glycine site. Considering that the extracellular concentration of D-serine in rodent frontal cortex is 6.5 μM, enough to saturate the glycine-binding site of the NMDA receptor, D-serine may also act as an endogenous coagonist [120]. In addition, drugs affecting the NMDA receptor can bind at the intra-ion channel binding site and at multiple modulatory sites, such as the redox, the H^+, the Zn^{2+}, and the polyamine binding sites [121].

The NMDA receptor plays a special role in synaptic transmission. At resting membrane potential the channel is blocked by Mg^{2+} and current flows only when the neuronal membrane is depolarized and the Mg^{2+} block is relieved (Fig. 3.5B). This depolarization is provided in the *post*natal brain typically by AMPA receptors, which have been shown to colocalize at the same synapses [122]. In the *pre*natal brain, glutamatergic synapses may lack AMPA receptors. There, the depolarization necessary to remove the Mg^{2+} block can be provided by $GABA_A$ receptors, because of a more depolarized reversal potential for Cl^- [123]. Once current flows, extracellular Ca^{2+} enters the cell through the NMDA receptor channel. Once activated, NMDA-receptor-mediated synaptic currents last for prolonged periods of time. Taken together, these properties enable the NMDA receptor channel to function as a "coincidence detector" of presynaptic activity and postsynaptic depolarization and, through the injection of Ca^{2+}, to play a critical role in synaptogenesis and to initiate plastic changes in the strength of synaptic connections. Long-term potentiation (the strengthening of synaptic connections) [124–126] and long-term depression (the weakening of synaptic connections) [127,128] are changes that depend on the temporal pattern of synaptic activity and are mediated through glutamate receptors.

Receptor localization

In addition to the classic (pre- and post-) synaptic locations, functional glutamate receptors can be also found at peri- and extrasynaptic sites [129]. Together with intracellular pools, these receptors are in a constant dynamic equilibrium with the synaptic receptors, an arrangement that allows rapid changes in receptor numbers in response to plasticity-inducing events. Extrasynaptic GluR2 AMPA receptors, for example, can enter the synaptic region and therefore act as a readily available pool to supply synapses.

Ionotropic glutamate receptors of all three classes can be found in presynaptic locations, on excitatory as well as on inhibitory terminals, where they typically (but not exclusively) facilitate transmitter release [130]. The functional role of this presynaptic modulation of transmitter release awaits clarification.

It is not surprising that the most important excitatory neurotransmitter system is also involved in a number of important pathologic processes in the nervous system. Even though no pathogenic mutation has yet been demonstrated in a human glutamate receptor gene (mouse knockout mutations of these genes produce mild to severe neurologic symptoms), changes in the expression patterns of glutamate receptors seem to contribute to drug-induced behavioral adaptations, as evidenced by increased GluR1 levels in some parts of the brain that are found with chronic alcohol, cocaine, and morphine use. Mutations in GluR6 may influence the age of onset of Huntington disease. Better understood is the relationship between activation of the glutamatergic system during abnormal conditions or abnormal activation of the glutamatergic transmitter system leading to neuronal injury and cell death, collectively referred to as "excitotoxicity." Typical examples include focal and global ischemia, hypoglycemia and physical trauma, metabolic poisoning, drug abuse, certain food toxicities, and epilepsy. Glutamate, acting at its various receptors, induces neuronal death by (1) an increase in intracellular free Ca^{2+}, which activates a number of proteases, phospholipases, and endonucleases; (2) generation of free radicals that destroy cellular membranes; and (3) induction of apoptosis [131]. The ability of certain anesthetic drugs to block the NMDA receptor has opened up the possibility that there are some anesthetics for which NMDA block contributes importantly to their anesthetic action. This class of anesthetic, exemplified by xenon [132], nitrous oxide [133], and ketamine [134,135], reduce the efficacy of excitatory neurotransmission by "inhibiting" glutamate receptors. These anesthetic drugs also have been used in pathologic settings in which the excitotoxic action of glutamate on NMDA receptors plays a prominent role [136].

TRP and CNG channel families

The TRP (transient receptor potential) family of cation channels is notable for its great diversity in activation mechanisms and ion selectivities, exceeding those of any other group of ion channels (for a review, see Venkatachalam and Montell [137]). The mammalian branch alone of the TRP superfamily consists of 28 members. They can be subdivided into six main subfamilies organized into two groups. Group 1 consists of TRPC ("Canonical"), TRPV ("Vanilloid"), TRPM ("Melastatin"), and TRPA ("Ankyrin"); group 2 includes TRPP ("Polycystin," mutated in the autosomal dominant form of polycystic kidney disease) and TRPML ("Mucolipin," mutated in mucolipidosis type IV). Mutations in four of the group 1 TRP proteins also underlie several human diseases.

The CNG (cyclic nucleotide-gated) channels are found in several types of cells, but they have been studied primarily in photoreceptors and olfactory sensory neurons (for a review, see Kaupp and Seifert [138]). They are gated by the second messengers of the visual and olfactory signaling cascades, cAMP and cGMP respectively, and play critical roles in vision and olfaction by operating as the transduction channels that generate stimulus-induced receptor potentials [139].

Structurally, the TRP and CNG channels, which are not generally considered members of the same family but do nevertheless share common structural and functional features, resemble the superfamily of voltage-activated channels (i.e., Na^+, K^+, and Ca^{2+} channels). Both TRP and CNG channels incorporate six transmembrane segments, with a pore loop between the fifth and sixth transmembrane segments, and both are permeable to cations.

A highly unusual characteristic of the TRP channels is the impressive diversity of cation selectivities and specific activation mechanisms: even a single TRP channel can be activated through a number of seemingly disparate mechanisms [137,140]. The CNG channels are all nonselective cation channels that have substantial Ca^{2+} permeability under physiological conditions, and like other Ca^{2+}-permeable channels, they are subject to feedback regulation via Ca^{2+}-mediated mechanisms.

The TRPV subfamily comprises channels that are critically involved in nociception and thermosensing (TRPV1, TRPV2, TRPV3, TRPV4; see Chapter 16 for additional detail) as well as highly Ca^{2+}-selective channels involved in Ca^{2+} absorption/reabsorption in mammals (TRPV5, TRPV6). A unifying theme in this group is that TRP proteins play critical roles in sensory physiology, which include contributions to vision, taste, olfaction, hearing, touch, and thermo- and osmosensation [141]. Surprisingly, even single receptors can respond to disparate types of signals. For example, TRPV1 responds to heat as well as botanical and proinflammatory compounds. In this regard TRP channels can be considered multiple signal integrators.

Recently, it was found that several inhaled and injected general anesthetics can activate TRPA1, a key ion channel in the pain pathway. Interestingly, this property was limited to drugs that are clinically considered to be pungent when inhaled (isoflurane, desflurane) or painful when injected (propofol, etomidate) [142]. The absence of these effects in genetically modified animals that lack TRPA1 receptors supports a causal role for TRPA1 channel activation in the irritating properties of these drugs.

Summary

Ion channels are integral membrane proteins that form an aqueous channel in the lipid bilayer through which charged particles can pass. There are many different types of ion channels, and they may be classified according to the factors that regulate channel opening and closing (gating), as well as the types of ions allowed to traverse the pore (selectivity). When a channel opens, ions flow passively down their electrochemical gradients as described by the Nernst equation. Whether ions go into or out of the cell when a channel opens depends on both the membrane potential and the concentration gradient for that ion at the time the channel is open.

Voltage-gated ion channels are found in neurons, muscle, and endocrine cells and consist of three main classes: the Na^+, Ca^{2+}, and K^+ channels. At normal resting membrane potentials these channels are closed. When the membrane is depolarized (becomes less negative), the channels open, allowing ions to pass through. The type of ion that is allowed to traverse the channel is determined by the structure of the pore and is used to classify the channel. The voltage-gated ion channels are protein complexes formed by the association of several individual subunits. The α subunit comprises the channel pore and confers both its ion-selectivity and its voltage-sensitivity. The other associated subunits stabilize the α subunit and modulate its function. The α subunits of Na^+ and Ca^{2+} channels contain four repeating homologous domains each consisting of six membrane-spanning segments. The four domains aggregate in the cell membrane to form a central pore through which ions pass. The α subunit of the voltage-gated K^+ channel is almost identical to the Na^+ and Ca^{2+} channels except that each of the four domains is a separate protein and the channels are formed by aggregation of four individual α subunits.

There are nine different genes that encode α subunits of voltage-gated Na^+ channels and four different β subunits with which they associate. These different combinations of Na^+ channel isoforms have different functional properties and are expressed in different tissues and at different times of development. There are 10 isoforms of the voltage-gated Ca^{2+} channels that are categorized into three families: high-voltage-activated l-type Ca^{2+} channels, expressed in muscle, heart,

endocrine cells, and neuronal tissue; N-type, P/Q-type, and R-type high-voltage-activated Ca^{2+} channels, found primarily in neurons; and low-voltage-activated rapidly inactivating T-type channels. Forty genes encode voltage-gated K^+ channel α subunits, which are divided into 12 families each with between one and eight members. There are also a large number of accessory subunits that associate with the K^+ channel α subunits, creating an enormous array of subunit combinations and functional variety. In addition to the voltage-gated K^+ channels, there are a variety of other K^+-selective ion channels, including the K_{ATP} channels and the two-pore-domain K^+ channels.

Neurotransmitters, hormones, and other small molecules released as intercellular messengers influence the activity of ion channels through two types of receptors. In metabotropic receptors the transmitter receptor (binding site) and the effector (ion channel) are separate molecules. In ionotropic receptors (ligand-gated ion channels) the transmitter binding site and the transmembrane ion channel are integral to a single protein. There are five families of ionotropic receptors that are responsible for rapid synaptic transmission:

- **Cys-loop receptor family (nAChR, GABA$_A$, glycine, and 5-HT$_3$)** – Each of these receptors is composed of five homologous subunits, each with four transmembrane segments and an extracellular segment that contains the neurotransmitter binding site.
- **Glutamate receptor family (AMPA, kainate, NMDA)** – Each receptor is composed of four subunits, each of which has four transmembrane segments.
- **The P2X receptor family** – Bind ATP in the extracellular space.
- **Transient receptor potential (TRP) receptors** and **cyclic nucleotide-gated (CNG) channels** – These receptors transduce responses to many external stimuli (light, sound, temperature, touch, and taste).

The great variety of ion channels present in excitable tissue endows cells with the potential for tremendous flexibility in integrating and transmitting information, transducing extracellular signals into cellular responses, and responding to changing environmental conditions. Many of the drugs that are used clinically act by modulating ion-channel activity, in many cases acting on multiple types of channels to produce desirable actions as well as undesirable side effects. Traditional classification schemes based on pharmacologic characteristics are being supplemented or supplanted by schemes based on an emerging understanding of the underlying structures and molecular components. In many cases these approaches have become integrated, but in others there remains a separation that awaits fuller characterization of the pharmacologic properties of various gene products. It is hoped that more specific drugs will result from our emerging understanding of the roles played by the various channels in normal function and in pathologic conditions.

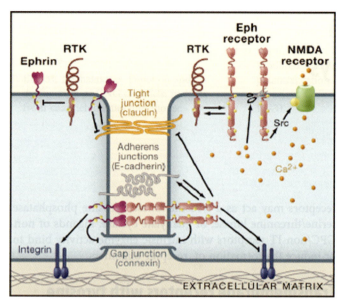

Figure 4.1. Receptor tyrosine kinases (RTK) are activated by two types of extracellular signaling molecule. The first includes certain growth factors, and the second, molecules bound to cells, such as ephrins. Cell-surface-bound signaling molecules regulate cell adhesion and migration. The diagram shows the positioning of RTK and ephrins at the cell surface and cross-talk that can occur between different receptor groups (yellow circles indicate tyrosine phosphorylation, scissors indicate proteolytic cleavage). Reproduced with permission from Pasquale [4].

serine or threonine residues in proteins, including voltage- and ligand-gated ion channels and G-protein-coupled receptors. Through these processes, cellular responses are modified within seconds to minutes after receptor activation.

RTKs, through PI3K, induce the formation of docking sites for more than 200 intracellular proteins in humans, including a few PKC isoforms and protein kinase B (PKB). PKB promotes cell survival by inhibiting the activity and transcription of certain molecules involved in programmed cell death, apoptosis (see more details on apoptosis later in this chapter). Through these effects RTKs evoke long-term changes in cell behavior.

The adaptor protein Grb2 links the activity of RTKs to their major downstream signaling cascade, the three-step mitogen-activated protein kinase (MAP kinase) cascade [6]. The third member of the MAP kinase cascade (MAP kinases such as the extracellular signal-regulated protein kinase 1/2, ERK1/2) phosphorylates various cytoplasmic proteins, including ribosomal kinases and MAP-kinase-activated protein kinases. In addition, MAP kinases can enter the nucleus, where they phosphorylate a series of transcription factors. Hence, RTKs induce transcriptional, translational, and post-translational changes in the cells by initiating MAP kinase cascade activity.

Activated RTKs can also phosphorylate STATs, which then dissociate from the receptor. STATs form homo- or hetero-dimers, which translocate to the nucleus, where they bind to DNA response elements and, similarly to MAP kinases, regulate gene transcription.

One of the best-known RTKs is the receptor tyrosine kinase A (trkA), which together with its high-affinity ligand, NGF, is particularly important in perioperative care [7]. NGF is one of the most important inflammatory mediators, which in addition to inflamed tissues is also produced in tissues subjected to surgical interventions [8]. TrkA is expressed by a major sub-population of nociceptive primary sensory neurons [9]. On the one hand, trkA activation induces PLCγ and PI3K activity, which result in increased responsiveness of the cells [10]. On the other hand, the NGF-trkA complex is internalized and transported to the perikarya, where it induces transcription of various genes [11,12].

Transmembrane receptors with phosphatase activity

Non-GPC/non-IT receptors with intrinsic enzyme activity may have intrinsic phosphatase activity. These molecules are called **receptor protein tyrosine phosphatases** (R-PTPs). In addition to RTKs, R-PTPs are also involved in the regulation of tyrosine phosphorylation of many proteins, which is a major signaling event in many intracellular signaling pathways.

The intracellular part of R-PTPs usually has two catalytic domains [13–15]. R-PTPs have a high number of splice variants and their extracellular parts are highly variable. The extracellular part of some of these receptors contains immunoglobulin-like domains, and fibronectin type III domains indicating the role of R-PTPs in cell recognition and adhesion. At present there are more than 30 R-PTPs, which are assigned into seven groups. The type I R-PTP, CD45, is expressed on hematopoietic cells, while other R-PTPs are expressed either exclusively on neurons or both on neurons and on various non-neuronal cells.

The great majority of R-PTPs are orphan receptors, at present. Some of them seem to be activated by homophylic interactions. Others, such as CD45, could be activated by heterophylic ligands, such as galectin 1 [16]. Interestingly, while dimerization of other non-GPC/non-IT receptors with intrinsic enzyme activity activates the receptor, the same process seems to inhibit the activity of R-PTPs [17].

Cytoplasmic tyrosine kinases have been shown to be the substrate of various R-PTPs. It has been demonstrated that R-PTP-mediated dephosphorylation of inhibitory phosphorylation contributes to the activation of the tyrosine kinases. In addition, RTKs, including the insulin and epithelial growth factor receptors, may also be the substrates for R-PTPs.

Within the nervous system, R-PTPs are involved in neuronal development, nerve regeneration, and signal transduction. At the peripheral tissues, CD45 is the best-known R-PTP [17]. CD45 is involved in a series of physiological and pathological processes, including the development of hematologic malignancies, autoimmune diseases, and allograft

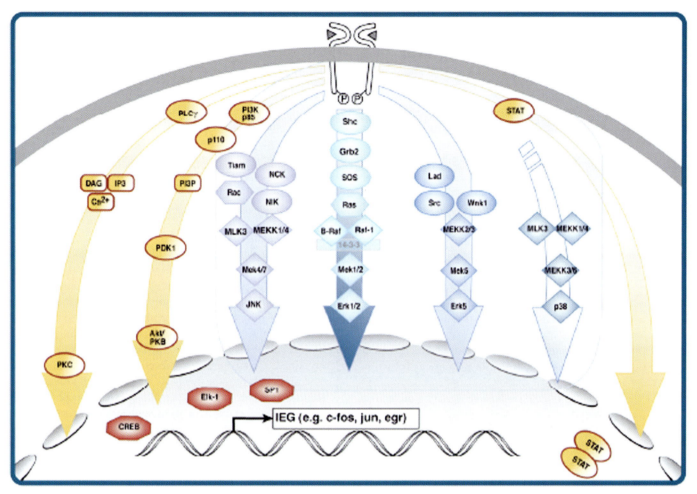

Figure 4.2. Growth factors are extracellular signaling factors that bind to receptor tyrosine kinases (RTKs) to activate intracellular signaling pathways, including the mitogen-activated protein kinase (MAPK), phosphatidylinositol-3-kinase (PI3K), protein kinase C (PKC) and signal transducers and activators of transcription (STAT) signaling pathways. Reproduced with permission from Katz *et al.* [2].

rejection [17]. The involvement of CD45 in this latter process makes this receptor a particularly interesting in the perioperative care of transplant patients. The earlier finding that antibodies raised against the CD45 isoform CD45RB produce lifetime protection from allograft rejection [18], together with recent preclinical findings [19], suggests that targeting CD45RB signaling in transplant patients with adequate thymic function may provide a long-term allograft tolerance.

Transmembrane receptors with intrinsic serine/threonine kinase activity

Non-GPC/non-IT receptors in the plasma membrane may also have intrinsic serine/threonine kinase activity. These receptors can be activated by members of the transforming growth factor β (TGFβ) superfamily of polypeptides [20,21]. There are two types of **TGFβ receptors**, the type I and type II receptors. The majority of the TGFβ ligands bind to the type II receptor. Ligand binding then attracts type I receptors into the complex. Within the complex, serine residues in the cytoplasmic domain of the type I receptor are phosphorylated. The phosphorylated

type I receptor then binds to, and activates, one of the 5 "R" isoforms of the latent gene regulatory protein, Smad. After dissociation from the receptor complex, R-Smad binds to another isoform of Smad (Smad4), and the R-Smad-Smad4 complex is translocated into the nucleus. There, the R-Samd-Smad4 complex regulates gene transcription. In addition to R-Smad, TGFβ receptors can also activate the MAP kinase pathways, inducing additional transcriptional and post-translational regulatory processes through TGFβ receptor activation.

TGFβ receptors are expressed by virtually every cell in the human body, and are involved in a variety of cellular functions, including regulation of apoptosis, cell proliferation, differentiation and migration, and extracellular matrix production. Through these cellular functions TGFβ receptors are involved in the regulation of immune responses and tissue repair. Congenital dysfunctions of signaling through various TGFβ receptors result in a series of hereditary conditions, such as hereditary hemorrhagic telangiectasia, primary pulmonary hypertension, and congestive heart failure, which may underlie many perioperative complications [21].

A recombinant TGFβ, the bone morphogenic protein, is licensed for treating fractures.

Transmembrane receptors with intrinsic guanylate cyclase activity

At least seven transmembrane non-GPC/non-IT receptors with intrinsic guanylate cyclase activity have been identified in mammals [22]. Four of these **receptor guanylate cyclases** (rGC) are orphan receptors, at present. Three rGCs, the GC-A, GC-B, and GC-C receptors, have established ligands GC-A is activated by A-type natriuretic peptide (ANP) and B-type NP (BNP), GC-B is activated by C-type NP (CNP), while GC-C is responsive to the heat-stable enterotoxin and the intestinal peptides uroguanylin, guanylin, and lymphoguanylin [23–25].

The catalytic domains of rGCs are separated in the receptor dimers in resting condition. Ligand binding induces the assembly and subsequent activation of the two guanylate cyclases, which results in the formation of cyclic guanosine monophosphate (cGMP). cGMP activates the cGMP-dependent serine/threonine protein kinase G (PKG), cGMP-binding phosphodiesterases (PDEs), and cyclic nucleotide-gated ion channels [23]. These cGMP-responsive molecules can also be activated by cytosolic guanylate cyclases, which in turn are activated by the gaseous transmitters nitric oxide (NO) and carbon monoxide (CO) [26,27]. Thus, cGMP-responsive signaling molecules provide a major hub in intracellular signaling.

GC-C and its ligands regulate cell proliferation in the intestine, and may prevent the growth and spread of colon cancer. GC-A is expressed in the heart, kidney, adrenal gland, smooth muscle, and endothelial cells of vessels, as well as in neurons. The GC-A ligands ANP and BNP are predominantly cardiac hormones synthesized in the atrium and ventricle, respectively, when the pressure or stretch in the heart is increased [28]. While ANP modulates blood pressure and volume, BNP protects against cardiac hypertrophy and fibrosis by inhibiting extracellular matrix production, promoted for example by TFGβ [22]. Serum BNP level is used as a marker for acute cardiac events, such as heart failure and myocardial infarction. Nesiritide is a recombinant human BNP expected to act on GC-A, and improve haemodynamic profile in severe heart failure.

CNP is produced predominantly by endothelial cells, while GC-B is expressed by adipose tissues, fibroblasts, and neurons in certain areas of the brain. CNP, through GC-B, inhibits smooth muscle and fibroblast proliferation and extracellular matrix production [22]. However, it promotes endothelial proliferation. It is believed that through these effects CNP and GC-B regulate vascular and tissue remodeling.

Plasma membrane receptors linked to cytoplasmic enzymes

Many plasma membrane receptors do not have their own enzyme activity. Instead, ligand binding induces the activity of independent enzymes coupled to the receptors. These independent enzymes, which may have tyrosine, serine/threonine, or caspase activity, then initiate the activity of various intracellular signaling pathways.

Transmembrane receptors coupled to cytosolic tyrosine kinases

Ligands of these receptors include a large number of extracellular signaling molecules, the great majority of which are cytokines. Some of the plasma membrane non-GPC/non-IT receptors that are coupled to cytosolic tyrosine kinases bind to extracellular matrix molecules. These receptors are called **integrins**.

Cytokine receptors

Cytokines include a variety of molecules, such as interferons, interleukins (IL-2, IL-6, IL-9, IL-10, IL-15), and hormones including leptin, somatotropin, prolactin, erythropoietin, granulocyte colony-stimulating factor, granulocyte–macrophage colony-stimulating factor, and thrombopoietin. Because of the variety of ligands, cytokine receptors form the most diverse family of receptors. Cytokine receptors bind members of the Janus kinase (JAK) family, a subset of tyrosine kinases [29]. Ligand binding brings the two JAKs within the cytokine receptor dimer into close proximity, which allows cross-phosphorylation of tyrosine residues both in JAKs and in the receptor dimer itself. Phosphorylated tyrosine residues in the receptor serve as docking sites for members of the STAT family. As in the case of RTKs, activated STATs are released from the receptor, form dimers, translocate to the nucleus, and bind to specific enhancer elements [30].

Because of their diversity, cytokine receptors are involved in a huge array of physiological and pathological processes [31]. The effect of interferons, interleukins, and hormones acting on blood cell production is particularly important in perioperative care. For example, interleukin signaling in white blood cells regulates all aspects – initiation, propagation, and resolution – of inflammatory reactions. Moreover, several drugs used in treating malignancies, or in the treatment of patients after bone marrow transplantation, act through JAK-STAT pathways.

Immunoreceptors

A group of non-GPC/non-IT receptors are coupled to members of the so-called Src family of cytoplasmic tyrosine kinases [32,33]. These immunoreceptors are expressed on various lymphocytes and other hematopoeitic cells, and consist of T-cell, B-cell, and natural killer cell immunoreceptors (TCR, BCR, and NCR, respectively) and receptors for the Fc portion of immunoglobulins. The intracellular domain of the immunoreceptors expresses the tyrosine-based activation motif (ITAM), which is phosphorylated by Src after ligand binding. The phosphotyrosines then serve as docking sites for other tyrosine kinases. Phosphorylation of these kinases then attracts adaptor proteins, through which downstream signaling molecules, including PI3K and the MAP kinase pathways, are activated. These signaling molecules induce effects similar to those induced when they are activated by RTKs. As a result, cells respond to immunoreceptor activation with transcriptional changes and secretion of various mediators.

Immunoreceptors are involved in the generation of inflammatory, including allergic, reactions, and thus they may be involved in the development of various postoperative complications. At present only a very few drugs targeting immunoreceptors are available.

Integrins

Integrins are bidirectional transmembrane signaling molecules that conduct mechanical information between the two sides of the plasma membrane [34–37]. They detect changes in forces acting on the cell surface, by binding to the extracellular matrix and cell-surface molecules and the cytoskeleton.

The currently known 18 α- and 8 β-integrin subunits form 24 different types of integrins. The αβ composition of integrins shows certain tissue and ligand specificity. Based on ligand specificity, integrins are classified as laminin-binding, collagen-binding, leukocyte, and arginine–glycine–aspartic acid (RGD)-recognizing integrins. Integrins, in addition to the extracellular matrix and cytoskeleton, also associate with molecules in the plasma membrane, which include other receptors, such as growth-factor tyrosine kinases.

Bidirectional signaling through integrins includes extracellular matrix-binding-evoked changes in cellular behavior (*outside-in signaling*) and intracellular signaling-molecule-evoked changes in integrin behavior, such as changes in the affinity of integrins to extracellular ligands (*inside-out signaling*). Moreover, the outside-in and inside-out signalings also influence each other. Binding an extracellular matrix molecule to integrins initiates clustering of integrins, and recruitment of cytoplasmic molecules into cell-matrix adhesion structures. The recruited molecules include integrin-binding proteins, adaptor/scaffolding proteins, which bind integrins to the cytoskeleton, and enzymes, such as the tyrosine kinase focal adhesion kinase (FAK) and Src. Tyrosine phosphorylation attracts kinases, including several isoforms of PKC and PI3K, and the MAP kinase cascade activating enzyme. PKC, PI3K, and the MAP kinase cascade initiate signaling similar to that evoked by RTK activation.

Integrins are involved in a series of physiological and pathological functions, including wound healing, thrombus formation, angiogenesis, and inflammation. Furthermore, the function of many other receptors depends on integrin activity. Thus, the activity of integrins may influence the length of perioperative care. A few drugs used in clinics target integrins. For example, abciximab is an anti-β3 antibody, which inhibits the ligand binding of the α4β7 integrin on thrombocytes, and it is used to prevent thrombosis.

Transmembrane receptors coupled to cytosolic serine/threonine kinases

Many receptors involved in the fast and nonspecific innate immune response to pathogens are non-GPC/non-IT plasma membrane receptors coupled to cytoplasmic serine/threonine kinases [38,39]. The extracellular part of these receptors have characteristic immunoglobulin-like domains, while their intracellular part contains the also characteristic Toll/IL-1 receptor domain (TIR). Based on the presence of the TIR domain, these receptors form the family of the **TIR receptors**.

The TIR receptor family consists of subfamilies, which include receptors for the proinflammatory cytokines, IL-1 (IL-1R), and IL-18 (IL-18R), and the Toll-like receptors (TLR). These latter receptors are responsible for recognizing pathogen-associated structures. In addition, the TIR family also includes orphan receptors. While the IL-1 receptor subfamily contains at least 10 molecules, the TLR subfamily has at least 11.

Binding of IL-1 or IL-18 to their respective cognate receptors, IL-1RI or IL-1Rrp1, initiates the binding of respective coreceptors (IL-1RAcP or AcPL) to the receptor–ligand complex. Only the receptor–ligand–coreceptor complexes can initiate intracellular signaling. Soluble forms of IL-1 and IL-18 receptors also exist, which may also bind IL-1 or IL-18, resulting in sequestration of these ligands and inhibiting their activity. Formation of the IL-1R dimers results in bringing the two TIR domains into close proximity.

In contrast to IL-1Rs, TLRs present as hetero- or homodimers in the inactive state. TLR hetero- and homodimers show certain ligand-specificity. Ligand binding to TLRs induces conformational changes, resulting again in the two TIR domains in close proximity.

In both types of ligated receptors, the TIR domains serve as a platform for adaptor proteins. The adaptor protein recruits type 4 of the serine/threonine kinase, IL-1 receptor-associated kinase 4 (IRAK-4), which in turn recruits and phosphorylates type 1 IRAK (IRAK-1). After dissociation from the receptor, the activated IRAK-1 forms a so-called signalosome with adaptor molecules, through which it activates downstream signaling pathways. The activity of these downstream signaling events results in the activity of some MAP kinases and the transcription factor, nuclear factor κB (NFκB) (Fig. 4.3).

Members of the NFκB family are one of the major transcription factors [40–42]. NFκB is activated by a variety of stimuli, including exposure of the cell to bacteria, viruses, and factors that induce cellular stress, such as ultraviolet (UV) illumination. NFκB is present in cells in an inactive form. NFκB activation involves the dissociation of the inhibitory unit from the molecule, which then translocates into the nucleus, where it binds to specific 10-base-pair DNA sites called κB sites. NFκB regulates the transcription

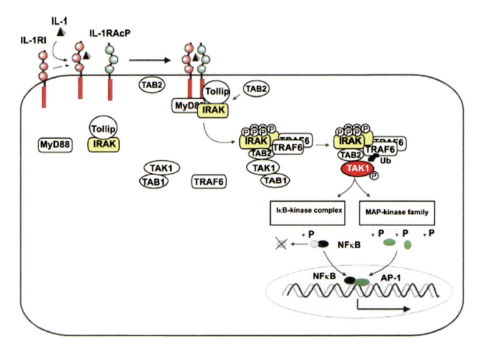

Figure 4.3. Receptors for the cytokine interleukin 1 (IL-1R) mediate the fast and nonspecific innate immune response to pathogens. IL-Rs are non-GPC/non-IT plasma membrane receptors coupled to cytoplasmic serine/threonine kinases. The intracellular part of IL-Rs contains the Toll/IL-1 receptor domain (TIR). TIR forms a platform for adaptor proteins, such as TAB2, which then recruit the type 4 serine/threonine kinase, IL-1 receptor-associated kinase 4 (IRAK-4), which in turn recruits and phosphorylates type 1 IRAK (IRAK-1). Activated IRAK-1 dissociates from the receptor to activate downstream signaling pathways, such as those involving mitogen-activated protein kinases (MAPKs) and the transcription factor nuclear factor κB (NFκB). Reproduced with permission from Martin and Wesche [38].

of hundreds of genes, including those which encode cytokines, immunoreceptors, enzymes involved in immune and inflammatory responses, plasma membrane receptors, and growth factors. Given the fast response of NFκB after an encounter with a pathogen or cellular stress, its activation is vital for the development of appropriate cellular responses.

Because of the pivotal role of TIR receptors in the innate immune response, they are involved in the development of a series of conditions that may complicate perioperative care. While IL-1Rs are involved in the development of pain associated with tissue and nerve injury, TLRs are involved in allergic reactions of the airways. TLRs seem to regulate lung injury and repair. Moreover, TLRs may be involved in acute allograft rejection, particularly in thoracic organ transplantation. Not surprisingly, TIR receptors are also involved in the development of sepsis [43].

Transmembrane receptors coupled to caspases and NFκB

A group of cytokines, the members of the tumor necrosis factor (TNF) superfamily, act as yet another type of non-GPC/non-IT plasma membrane receptors, the **TNF receptors** (TNFRs). Human TNFs form a family of 19 trimeric membrane-bound or soluble proteins, which are produced by various cells, including macrophages, monocytes, lymphocytes, keratinocytes, fibroblasts, and neurons. For the 19 TNFs, there are 29 TNFRs. TNFRs are also trimers. While each ligand–receptor pair is considered as a

system, there is a considerable cross-affinity between the ligands and receptors [44].

Based on the signaling pathways, TNFRs are divided into three groups. The first group, including one of the receptors (TNFR1) for the prototypic TNF, TNFα, contains the so-called death domain (DD). Ligand binding to TNFR with the DD results in the formation of death-inducing signaling complex through the recruitment of an adaptor protein to the DD and the protease, caspase 8, to the adaptor protein. Activated caspase 8 initiates the hierarchical caspase cascade, which is in the center of the apoptotic process [45,46]. As a result, executor caspases (caspase 3, 6, and 7) are activated which then cleave an array of cellular proteins, including structural and regulatory proteins.

The second group of TNFRs, including the second receptor for TNFα, TNFR2, contains a domain (TIM) which, after ligand-binding-induced trimerization of the intracellular part of the receptor, enables binding members of the adaptor protein, TNFR-associated factor (TRAF), family [47]. Some members of the TRAF family serve as adaptor proteins to IRAK, which is activated also by members of the TIR family. Hence, it is not surprising that the result of activation of members of this second group of TNFRs is similar to that of the TIRs, and it includes induction of NFκB, MAP kinase, and PI3K activity.

Members of the third group of TNFRs do not contain domains that bind enzymes or adaptor proteins to start intracellular signaling. These are called TNF decoy receptors, and they inhibit TNF binding to members of the first and second groups of TNFRs, thus inhibiting the initiation of signaling.

TNFs and their receptors play a major role in the development of hair follicles and mammary glands, and in the regulation of bone homeostasis. Moreover, TNFs are involved in the development of pain [48,49]. However, the main role of TNFs is to coordinate the development and function of the adaptive immune system. TNFs, together with TIRs, are major players in the development of sepsis [43]. Moreover, TNFs also play an important role in the development of stretch-induced lung injury [50]. Thus, it could be expected that drugs targeting TNF signaling will appear soon to treat perioperative complications.

Cytoplasmic enzymes

The gaseous extracellular signaling molecules, NO and CO, act on soluble guanylate cyclase (sGC). Thus sGC acts as a receptor, responding directly to extracellular signals. Activation of sGC, similarly to that of rGCs, results in cGMP production. cGMP then activates PKG, cGMP-binding PDE, and cyclic nucleotide-gated ion channels. At the periphery, NO- and CO-evoked activation of sCG results in vasodilation and platelet disaggregation. In the nervous system, both NO and CO act as transmitters. NO has been shown to be involved in the development of pain associated with tissue and nerve injury [51].

NO-sGC signaling contributes to the development of systemic inflammation-induced refractory hypotension [52,53]. NO production is initiated by the release of inflammatory mediators, such as histamine, platelet activating factor, or TNFα, which act on endothelial cells. Ca^{2+} released from the intracellular stores and bound to the Ca^{2+}-binding protein, calmodulin, activates endothelial NO synthase. NO then, through inducing cGMP production in smooth muscle cells, evokes relaxation of blood vessels. Methylene blue blocks sGC activity, and it has successfully been used to treat anaphylactic hypotension [52].

Nuclear receptors

Nuclear receptors (NRs) are ligand-activated transcription factors which play a key role in a wide variety of physiological processes, including development, control, and maintenance of homeostasis and blood pressure as well as cellular proliferation, differentiation, and death [54]. The nuclear receptor superfamily comprises receptors for steroids, thyroid hormones, vitamin D_3, and retinoids. Dysfunction of NR signaling leads to reproductive, proliferative, and metabolic diseases, such as infertility, cancer, and diabetes [55].

The most common mechanisms through which NRs mediate their effects is the initiation of gene expression by direct binding to specific DNA sequences of target genes. This mechanism is referred to as **transactivation**. NR activation can also inhibit gene expression by binding to transcription factors. This process is called **transrepression** [56].

Since the majority of NRs are dispersed in the cytosol, their ligands must diffuse or be transported into the cell. Many NRs are orphan receptors at present. However, since many of them mediate the transcription of an array of diverse detoxifying derivatives of the supergene family of cytochrome P450, they have become targets of drug development in a host of diseases.

NRs are modular proteins with a conserved structure, consisting of an amino-terminal domain, a central DNA-binding domain, a linker domain, and a ligand-binding carboxy-terminal domain [57]. The amino-terminal domain, which is recognized by coactivators and other transcription factors, is a heterogenic, ligand-independent, regulatory region containing the so-called *activating function 1 (AF-1) site* [58]. The role of AF-1 is to mediate the binding of NR to coactivators, which facilitate or inhibit transcriptional activation of target genes. AF-1-mediated gene activation requires synergism with another activating function site, AF-2, harbored in the C-terminal domain [59].

The central domain, also known as the C domain or DNA-binding domain, is crucial for DNA recognition and binding. The structure of the C domain is a highly conserved. It contains the so-called *zinc fingers*, which are two finger-shaped structures the stability of which is contributed by zinc ions. Zinc fingers are crucial for recognition and binding to the *hormone response element* (HRE) genes, which code for the downstream effectors of NR. Differences in amino-acid sequences of the C domain in various NRs account for the binding specificity of the receptors to either a 5′-AGAACA-3′ or a 5′-AGCTCA-3′ site. Dimerization between two C domains is often necessary for recognition of complementary DNA sequences [60].

Studies on unligated (*apo-*) and ligated (*holo-*) NRs have revealed that ligand-binding domains of the NR share a common structure [61,62]. It consists of a ligand-binding pocket covered by a "lid." The pocket itself contains residues, which are important contributors for the functioning of the AF-2 [63]. Hence, AF-2 becomes competent for transcription initiation only following binding of a specific ligand and a subsequent sequential modification of the ligand-binding domain, which results in the stabilization of the ligand-binding pocket and its closure by the "lid" [64,65].

The NRs are classified into four classes. The classification is based on the mechanism of action and subcellular localization of the receptor in the absence of the ligand. Class I receptors are expressed in the cytosol, and mostly bound to heat shock proteins. This class of NR is activated mainly by steroids. The interaction of class I NRs with their ligand results in the dissociation of the receptor from the heat shock protein, followed by homodimerization of the receptor and translocation of the homodimer into the nucleus. Class II NRs, in contrast to the class I receptors, are always expressed in the nucleus. Class II receptors form complex with a corepressor molecule until the receptor binds to its ligand. The binding induces dissociation of the corepressor and subsequent recruitment of a coactivator. Class III NRs share most of the features of typical class I NRs, except that they only bind to inverted HRE. Finally, class IV NRs are different from other NRs in that they bind only to half-site HRE because they have only one functional DNA-binding domain [66].

Compounds acting on NRs are used very often in anesthesiology and intensive care. Steroids, for example, in addition to their anti-inflammatory effects are also used for other indications. Dexamethasone is often used as an antiemetic in the pre-induction phase of general anesthesia. A recent study demonstrated that dexamethasone reduces postoperative nausea and vomiting by 26%, which is comparable to that of ondansetron, which has specifically been designed for that purpose [67].

Recently, NRs have been investigated for their role in the mechanisms of pain relief. The cannabinoid receptor-mediated analgesic effects have been thought to depend on opioid receptor-mediated upregulation of spinal cannabinoid receptors. However, it has been demonstrated that cannabinoid receptor upregulation depends on a glucocorticoid-receptor pathway [68]. These findings could have important implications in the development of new approaches aimed to control perioperative pain.

Summary

Non-G-protein-coupled and non-ionotropic (non-GPC/non-IT) receptors are expressed in the plasma membrane, in the cytoplasm, and in the nucleus. They may have a role in the development of complications that impact perioperative care.

Single transmembrane domain receptors expressed at the cell surface may have intrinsic tyrosine kinase, tyrosine phosphatase, serine/threonine kinase, or guanylate cyclase activity. Tyrosine kinase A (trkA) is the receptor for nerve growth factor (NGF), an inflammatory mediator produced in response to surgery. A number of other receptor tyrosine kinases (RTK) transduce signals from a variety of growth factors, as well as cell-surface-bound signaling molecules which regulate adhesion and migration. CD45 is a receptor protein tyrosine phosphatase (R-PTP) which is expressed on hematopoietic cells and may be a potential therapeutic target in the prevention of allograft rejection. Whilst the ligands for many R-PTPs remain unknown, there is evidence of a role for R-PTPs in the activation of tyrosine kinases. Transforming growth factor β (TGFβ) receptors have intrinsic serine/threonine kinase activity. Hereditary conditions arising from TGFβ signaling dysfunction could contribute to perioperative complications. Ligands for receptor guanylate cyclases include natriuretic peptides (NP), A-type NP (ANP), B-type NP (BNP), and C-type NP (CNP), as well as certain bacterial toxins and intestinal peptides. ANP and

BNP are predominantly cardiac hormones, and serum levels of BNP can reveal acute cardiac events. CNP produced by endothelial cells may regulate vascular and tissue remodeling.

Plasma membrane receptors without intrinsic enzyme activity may be coupled to intracellular tyrosine kinases, serine/threonine kinases, or caspases. The actions of tyrosine-kinase-coupled receptors such as cytokine receptors and immunoreceptors have important implications for postoperative inflammatory or allergic reactions. Signaling pathways downstream of cytokine receptors are targeted by drugs used following bone marrow transplantation or in the treatment of malignancies. Integrins are important tyrosine-kinase-coupled receptors in healing and inflammation and have been targeted in pharmacologic prevention of thrombosis. Transmembrane receptors coupled to serine/threonine kinases include Toll-like receptors, which recognize molecular patterns expressed by pathogens, and receptors for several proinflammatory cytokines; both receptor types belong to the Toll/IL-1 (TIR) receptor family. As key receptors in the innate immune response, TIRs are involved in pain, allergic reactions, lung injury and repair, sepsis, and acute allograft rejection. Some tumor necrosis factor receptors (TNFRs) act via caspases. The caspase signaling cascade culminates in the activation of proteases which cleave cellular proteins to bring about apoptosis. Some TNFRs are linked to signaling pathways which activate nuclear factor κB (NFκB). TNFRs are involved in pain, the development of sepsis, stretch-induced lung injury, and possibly postoperative cognitive dysfunction.

Extracellular signaling molecules which cross the plasma membrane to act on receptors in the cytoplasm include nitric oxide (NO) and carbon monoxide (CO), which activate soluble guanylate cyclase. Both ligands cause vasodilation and platelet disaggregation in the periphery, and NO is involved in the development of pain resulting from injury and the development of inflammation-induced refractory hypotension.

Some ligands, including steroids, thyroid hormones, vitamin D_3, and retinoids, enter the cell to interact directly with transcription factors, known as nuclear receptors (NRs). NRs mediate transactivation or transrepression of gene expression, affecting transcription of genes involved in wide-ranging physiological processes. NRs are divided into four classes: class I NRs reside in the cytosol, often sequestered there by heat shock proteins until ligand binding; class II receptors are expressed in the nucleus, complexed with a corepressor molecule until activation; class III and class IV receptors are distinguished by their distinct DNA-binding specificities. Steroids have anti-inflammatory properties and can also have antiemetic effects. Furthermore, NR pathways may have implications in the development of therapeutics for perioperative pain control.

References

1. Li E, Hristova K. Role of receptor tyrosine kinase transmembrane domains in cell signaling and human pathologies. *Biochemistry* 2006; **45**: 6241–51.

2. Katz M, Amit I, Yarden Y. Regulation of MAPKs by growth factors and receptor tyrosine kinases. *Biochim Biophys Acta* 2007; **1773**: 1161–76.

3. Müller-Sieburg CE, Townsend K, Weissman IL, Rennick D. Proliferation and differentiation of highly enriched mouse hematopoietic stem cells and progenitor cells in response to defined growth factors. *J Exp Med* 1988; **167**: 1825–40.

4. Pasquale EB. Eph-ephrin bidirectional signaling in physiology and disease. *Cell* 2008; **133**: 38–52.

5. Nakae J, Kido Y, Accili D. Distinct and overlapping functions of insulin and IGF-I receptors. *Endocr Rev* 2001; **22**: 818–35.

6. Raman M, Chen W, Cobb MH. Differential regulation and properties of MAPKs. *Oncogene* 2007; **26**: 3100–12.

7. Chao MV, Rajagopal R, Lee FS. Neurotrophin signalling in health and disease. *Clin Sci (Lond)* 2006; **110**: 167–73.

8. Banik RK, Subieta AR, Wu C, Brennan TJ. Increased nerve growth factor after rat plantar incision contributes to guarding behavior and heat hyperalgesia. *Pain* 2005; **117**: 68–76.

9. Averill S, McMahon SB, Clary DO, Reichardt LF, Priestley JV. Immunocytochemical localization of trkA receptors in chemically identified subgroups of adult rat sensory neurons. *Eur J Neurosci* 1995; **7**: 1484–94.

10. Shu X, Mendell LM. Nerve growth factor acutely sensitizes the response of adult rat sensory neurons to capsaicin. *Neurosci Lett* 1999; **274**: 159–62.

11. Fang X, Djouhri L, McMullan S, Berry C, Okuse K, Waxman SG, Lawson SN. trkA is expressed in nociceptive neurons and influences electrophysiological properties via $Na_v1.8$ expression in rapidly conducting nociceptors. *J Neurosci* 2005; **25**: 4868–78.

12. Kuruvilla R, Zweifel LS, Glebova NO, Lonze BE, Valdez G, Ye H, Ginty DD. A neurotrophin signaling cascade coordinates sympathetic neuron development through differential control of TrkA trafficking and retrograde signaling. *Cell* 2004; **118**: 243–55.

13. Bixby JL. Ligands and signaling through receptor-type tyrosine phosphatases. *IUBMB Life* 2001; **51**: 157–63.

14. Chiarugi P, Buricchi F. Protein tyrosine phosphorylation and reversible oxidation: two cross-talking posttranslation modifications. *Antioxid Redox Signal* 2007; **9**: 1–24.

15. Paul S, Lombroso PJ. Receptor and nonreceptor protein tyrosine phosphatases in the nervous system. *Cell Mol Life Sci* 2003; **60**: 2465–82.

16. Walzel H, Schulz U, Neels P, Brock J. Galectin-1, a natural ligand for the receptor-type protein tyrosine phosphatase CD45. *Immunol Lett* 1999; **67**: 193–202.

17. Hermiston ML, Xu Z, Weiss A. CD45: a critical regulator of signaling thresholds in immune cells. *Annu Rev Immunol* 2003; **21**: 107–37.

18. Lazarovits AI, Poppema S, Zhang Z, *et al.* Prevention and reversal of renal allograft rejection by antibody against CD45RB. *Nature* 1996; **380**: 717–20.

19. Deng S, Moore DJ, Huang X, *et al.* Antibody-induced transplantation tolerance that is dependent on thymus-derived regulatory T cells. *J Immunol* 2006; **76**: 2799–807.

20. de Caestecker M. The transforming growth factor-beta superfamily of receptors. *Cytokine Growth Factor Rev* 2004; **15**: 1–11.

21. Gordon KJ, Blobe GC. Role of transforming growth factor-beta superfamily signaling pathways in human disease. *Biochim Biophys Acta* 2008; **1782**: 197–228.

22. Garbers DL, Chrisman TD, Wiegn P, *et al.* Membrane guanylyl cyclase receptors: an update. *Trends Endocrinol Metab* 2006; **17**: 251–8.

23. Potter LR, Abbey-Hosch S, Dickey DM. Natriuretic peptides, their receptors, and cyclic guanosine monophosphate-dependent signaling functions. *Endocr Rev* 2006; **27**: 47–72.

24. Quian X, Prabhakar S, Nandi A, Visweswariah SS, Goy MF. Expression of GC-C, a receptor-guanylate cyclase, and its endogenous ligands uroguanylin and guanylin along the rostrocaudal axis of the intestine. *Endocrinology* 2000; **141**: 3210–24.

25. Sindić A, Schlatter E. Cellular effects of guanylin and uroguanylin. *J Am Soc Nephrol* 2006; **17**: 607–16.

26. Bellamy TC, Garthwaite J. Pharmacology of the nitric oxide receptor, soluble guanylyl cyclase, in cerebellar cells. *Br J Pharmacol* 2002; **136**: 95–103.

27. Ryter SW, Otterbein LE. Carbon monoxide in biology and medicine. *Bioessays* 2004; **26**: 270–80.

28. Kuhn M. Molecular physiology of natriuretic peptide signalling. *Basic Res Cardiol* 2004; **99**: 76–82.

29. Haan C, Kreis S, Margue C, Behrmann I. Jaks and cytokine receptors–an intimate relationship. *Biochem Pharmacol* 2006; **72**: 1538–46.

30. Schindler C, Levey DE, Decker T. JAK-STAT signalling: from interferons to cytokines. *J Biol Chem* 2007; **282**: 20059–63.

31. O'Sullivan LA, Liongue C, Lewis RS, Stephenson SEM, Ward AC. Cytokine receptor signalling through the Jak-Stat-Socs pathway in disease. *Mol Immunol* 2007; **44**: 2497–506.

32. Abram CL, Lowell CA. Convergence of immunoreceptor and integrin signaling. *Immunol Rev* 2007; **218**: 29–44.

33. Underhill DM, Goodridge HS. The many faces of ITAMs. *Trends Immunol* 2007; **28**: 66–73.

34. Alenghat FJ, Ingber DE. Mechanotransduction: all signals point to cytoskeleton, matrix, and integrins. *Sci STKE* 2002; **2002**: PE6.

35. Berrier AL, Yamada KM. Cell-matrix adhesion. *J Cell Physiol* 2007; **213**: 565–73.

36. Hynes RO. Integrins: bidirectional, allosteric signaling machines. *Cell* 2002; **110**: 673–87.

37. Takada Y, Ye X, Simon S. The integrins. *Genome Biol* 2007; **8**: 215.

38. Martin MU, Wesche H. Summary and comparison of the signaling mechanisms of the Toll/interleukin-1 receptor family. *Biochim Biophys Acta* 2002; **1592**: 265–80.

39. O'Neill LA, Bowie AG. The family of five: TIR-domain-containing adaptors in Toll-like receptor signalling. *Nat Rev Immunol* 2007; **7**: 353–64.

40. Carmody RJ, Chen YH. Nuclear factor-kappaB: activation and regulation during toll-like receptor signaling. *Cell Mol Immunol* 2007; **4**: 31–41.

41. Pahl HL. Activators and target genes of Rel/NF-kappaB transcription factors. *Oncogene* 1999; **18**: 6853–66.

42. Tergaonkar V. NFkappaB pathway: a good signaling paradigm and therapeutic target. *Int J Biochem Cell Biol* 2006; **38**: 1647–53.

43. Cavaillon JM, Adib-Conquy M. Bench-to-bedside review: endotoxin tolerance as a model of leukocyte reprogramming in sepsis. *Crit Care* 2006; **10**: 233.

44. Hehlgans T, Pfeffer K. The intriguing biology of the tumour necrosis factor/tumour necrosis factor receptor superfamily: players, rules and the games. *Immunology* 2005; **115**: 1–20.

45. Chowdhury I, Tharakan B, Bhat GK. Current concepts in apoptosis: the physiological suicide program revisited. *Cell Mol Biol Lett* 2006; **11**: 506–25.

46. Shi Y. Apoptosome: the cellular engine for the activation of caspase-9. *Structure* 2002; **10**: 285–8.

47. Arron JR, Walsh MC, Choi Y. TRAF-mediated TNFR-family signaling. *Curr Protoc Immunol.* 2002; Chapter 11: Unit 11.9D.

48. Ji RR, Strichartz G. Cell signaling and the genesis of neuropathic pain. *Sci STKE* 2004; **2004**: reE14.

49. Zimmermann M. Pathobiology of neuropathic pain. *Eur J Pharmacol* 2001; **429**: 23–37.

50. Wilson MR, Choudhury S, Takata M. Pulmonary inflammation induced by high-stretch ventilation is mediated by tumor necrosis factor signaling in mice. *Am J Physiol Lung Cell Mol Physiol* 2005; **288**: L599–607.

51. McMahon SB, Cafferty WB, Marchand F. Immune and glial cell factors as pain mediators and modulators. *Exp Neurol* 2005; **192**: 444–62.

52. Evora PR, Simon MR. Role of nitric oxide production in anaphylaxis and its relevance for the treatment of anaphylactic hypotension with methylene blue. *Ann Allergy Asthma Immunol* 2007; **99**: 306–13.

53. Stawicki SP, Sims C, Sarani B, Grossman MD, Gracias VH. Methylene blue and vasoplegia: who, when, and how? *Mini Rev Med Chem* 2008; **8**: 472–90.

54. Olefsky JM. Nuclear receptor minireview series. *J Biol Chem* 2001; **276**: 36863–4.

55. Laudet V, Gronemeyer H. *The Nuclear Receptors Factbook*. San Diego, CA: Academic Press, 2001.

56. Pascual G, Glass CK. Nuclear receptors versus inflammation: mechanisms of transrepression. *Trends Endocrinol Metab* 2006; **17**: 321–7.

57. Wrange O, Gustafsson JA. Separation of the hormone- and DNA-binding sites of the hepatic glucocorticoid receptor by means of proteolysis. *J Biol Chem* 1978; **253**: 856–65.

58. Warnmark A, Treuter E, Wrighr AP, Gustafsson JA. Activation functions 1 and 2 of nuclear receptors: molecular strategies for transcriptional activation. *Mol Endocrinol* 2003; **17**: 1901–9.

59. Tora L, White J, Brou C, Tasset D, Webster N, Scheer E, Chambon P. The human estrogen receptor has two independent nonacidic transcriptional activation functions. *Cell* 1989; **59**: 477–87.

60. Freedman LP, Luisi BF, Korszun ZR, Basavappa R, Sigler PB, Yamamoto KR. The function and structure of the metal coordination sites within the glucocorticoid receptor DNA binding domain. *Nature* 1988; **334**: 543–6.

61. Bourguet W, Ruff M, Chambon P, Gronemeyer H, Moras D. Crystal structure of the ligand-binding domain of the human nuclear receptor RXRα. *Nature* 1995; **375**: 377–82.

62. Moras D, Gronemeyer H. The nuclear receptor ligand-binding domain: structure and function. *Curr Opin Cell Biol* 1998; **10**: 384–91.

63. Brzozowski AM, Pike ACW, Dauter Z, *et al.* Molecular vasis of agonism and antagonism in the owstrogen receptor. *Nature* 1997; **389**: 753–8.

64. Vivat V, Zechel C, Wurtz J-M, *et al.* A mutation mimics the ligand-induced transconformation of the retinoid X receptor. *EMBO J* 1997; **16**: 5697–709.

65. Wurtz H-M, Bourguet W, Renaud JP, Vivat V,Vhambon P, Moras D, Gronemeyer H. A canonical structure for the ligand-binding domain in nuclear receptors. *Nat Struct Biol* 1996; **3**: 87–94.

66. Novac N, Heinzel T. Nuclear receptors: overview and classification. *Curr Drug Targets Inflamm Allergy* 2004; **3**: 335–46.

67. Apfel CC, Korttila K, Abdalla M, *et al.* A factorial trial of six interventions for the prevention of postoperative nausea and vomiting. *N Engl J Med* 2004; **350**: 2441–51.

68. Lim G, Wang S, Mao J. Central glucocorticoid receptors modulate the expression of spinal cannabinoid receptors induced by chronic morphine exposure. *Brain Res* 2005; **1059**: 20–7.

Principles of drug action

Principles of pharmacokinetics

Thomas W. Schnider and Charles F. Minto

Introduction

Achieving the appropriate drug effects at any time during surgery, at the end of surgery, and after surgery is an important objective of anesthesia. The main drugs used to induce general anesthesia are the hypnotics, analgesics, and muscle relaxants, which are given to ensure unconsciousness, to provide analgesia and suppress the hemodynamic response, and to suppress reflex movements, respectively. The dose of each drug is titrated against the individual patient's response to achieve the intraoperative therapeutic goals. The patient should lose consciousness rapidly after induction, the level of analgesia should follow closely the level of surgical stimulation, and at the end of the operation the drug effect should dissipate so that the patient wakes up, has no residual muscle relaxation, and is pain-free. Unfortunately, at the end of an operation the desired intraoperative drug effects are viewed as "side effects," e.g., excessive sedation and respiratory depression.

From a pharmacologic perspective, anesthesia is concerned with controlling the time course of drug effect. This is dependent on the site and rate of input of the drug, the distribution of the drug within the body, the elimination of the drug from the body, and the sensitivity of the patient to the drug. Innumerable anatomic, physiologic, and chemical factors influence these processes. If we knew quantitatively all of the factors affecting the distribution, elimination, and sensitivity to a drug in an individual patient, we could predict the time course of drug effect exactly. However, we only know a minority of all the aspects of the dose–response relationship and, unfortunately, an understanding of one important factor generally does not explain the bigger picture. For example, the higher lipid solubility of fentanyl is sometimes used to explain its faster onset of effect compared with morphine. Although it is not possible to quantify the speed of onset with this knowledge, it might be tempting to categorize opioids based on this property. However, we know that there must be other important factors because alfentanil has a faster onset of effect than fentanyl, despite its lower lipid solubility.

Mathematic models are commonly used to relate the administered drug dose to the measured drug concentration (a **pharmacokinetic** model) and to relate the measured drug concentrations to the measured drug effects (a **pharmacodynamic** model). After a model that describes the time course of effect in an individual patient has been developed, factors that are responsible for an individual's deviation from the average response are included in the model, that is if they are statistically justifiable. With such models the time course of the drug effect for other dosing regimens and other patients can be predicted. Inversely, the dose, dose interval, or infusion rate that is required to achieve a desired concentration and desired effect level can also be calculated.

This chapter focuses on the pharmacokinetic and pharmacodynamic (PK/PD) principles necessary for understanding the time course of drug effect.

Basic pharmacokinetic parameters

The first basic PK parameter considered here is volume of distribution (V_d). In the simplest case, the amount of drug administered intravenously is related to the concentration measured in the plasma. Thus the apparent V_d can be calculated with the formula $V_d = \frac{\text{Amount}}{\text{Concentration}}$, which assumes that the drug is administered into a single well-mixed compartment. If a drug remains unbound in the plasma and does not distribute into other tissues, the V_d would be the same as the plasma volume. However, most drugs leave the plasma and distribute into and bind to other tissues. If the binding capacity of the tissue is very high, the relative amount of drug circulating in the plasma will be low. It is possible for the calculated V_d to be much larger than the whole-body volume. For instance, the V_d of furosemide is 7.7 L/70 kg, but chloroquine is 13 000 L/70 kg. Therefore it is better to refer to this volume as an *apparent* V_d because it does not correspond with a real anatomic volume. Usually the apparent *initial* volume of distribution is reported, which, for an intravenous bolus dose, is calculated according to the above formula using the concentration "back-extrapolated" to time zero.

The second basic pharmacokinetic parameter is clearance (*CL*). Clearance is often defined as the volume of plasma that

Anesthetic Pharmacology, 2nd edition, ed. Alex S. Evers, Mervyn Maze, Evan D. Kharasch. Published by Cambridge University Press. © Cambridge University Press 2011.

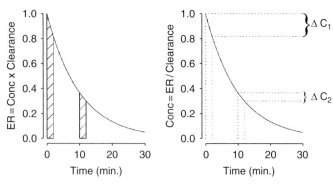

Figure 5.1. Intravenous bolus for a one-compartment model; volume of distribution = 10 L, clearance (Cl) = 1 L/min, elimination rate constant, $k = Cl/V = 0.1$ min^{-1}, dose = 10 mg. The elimination rate (ER) decreases over time (left). ER = k × amount remaining in the central compartment at any time. The amount in the central compartment equals the concentration multiplied by the volume of the central compartment. The area under the curve shaded between 0 and 2 minutes (left) equals the amount of drug eliminated in this interval. The area under the curve shaded between 10 and 12 minutes (left) equals the amount of drug eliminated in this interval. The total area under the elimination rate (mg/min) against time (min) curve equals the dose administered (mg). The graph on the right shows the concentration changing over time. The total area under the concentration (mg mL^{-1}) against time (min) curve equals the dose divided by clearance (right). At any time, the rate of decrease of concentration (the slope of the concentration vs. time curve) divided by the concentration is a constant, i.e., it is an exponential process. Note that the change in the concentration in the interval from 0 to 2 minutes (ΔC_1) is greater than in the interval from 10 to 12 minutes (ΔC_2).

must be completely cleared of the drug per unit time; that is, clearance has the same units as flow. Figure 5.1 shows the elimination rate and concentrations for 30 minutes after an intravenous bolus dose. More drug is cleared from the plasma per unit of time at the beginning when the concentration is high, i.e., *the elimination rate is proportional to the concentration* (ER ∞ C). From this relationship, we obtain another helpful definition: clearance is the proportionality constant, which relates the rate of elimination to the measured concentration (ER = $CL \cdot C$). The amount of drug (A) eliminated during any time interval Δt is given by the equation: $A_{\Delta t} = ER \cdot = CL \cdot C \cdot \Delta t$. Note that $C \cdot \Delta t$ is the area under the concentration curve in the Δt interval. By summing all the $C \cdot \Delta t$ elements, the complete area under the concentration time curve (AUC) will be the result. Mathematically, this is expressed by the integral: $AUC = \int_0^\infty C(t) \cdot dt$. The total amount of drug eliminated between time zero and infinity must be the same as the dose. Therefore we can rewrite the above equation as follows:

$$Dose = CL \cdot AUC \tag{5.1}$$

which gives us an estimate of clearance obtained using non-compartment methods:

$$CL = \frac{Dose}{AUC} \tag{5.2}$$

We can also calculate the V_d by noncompartment methods, using so-called "moment analysis." The first moment is given

by $t \cdot C(t)$, which is the product of the elapsed time, t, and the concentration at time t. Analogous to the calculation of AUC, the area under the moment curve is $AUMC = \int_0^\infty t \cdot C(t) \cdot dt$, from which we can calculate V_d as:

$$V_d = CL \cdot \frac{AUMC}{AUC} = CL \cdot MRT \tag{5.3}$$

This term AUMC/AUC provides the mean residence time (MRT), defined as the arithmetic average of the times that each drug molecule remains in the body. Practically, moment analysis makes only minimal assumptions about how the drug is distributed and eliminated, because the parameters are estimated based on the measured concentrations. However, the analysis theoretically requires concentration measurements until "infinite time." Because a limited number of concentration measurements are available, the area under the curve from the last measurement until infinity must be extrapolated, which introduces some assumptions. If the extrapolated area under the curve forms a significant percentage of the total area under the curve (area under data + area under extrapolated curve), then we have less confidence in the estimated parameters. To analyze data after different types of drug input, e.g., oral dosing or intravenous infusions, modifications to the above formulae are necessary.

The determination of the basic pharmacokinetic parameters clearance, volume of distribution, and mean residence time by noncompartment methods represents the gold standard by which the estimates of other approaches should be compared. Unfortunately, these parameters alone are insufficient. To facilitate rational drug selection and the development of rational dosing guidelines, a thorough understanding of several other important concepts is required.

Compartment models

It is helpful to think of compartment models in terms of a hydraulic model [1]. The cross-sectional area of the bucket represents the volume of distribution, the height of water in the bucket represents the drug concentration, and the amount of water added to the bucket represents the amount of drug added to the body. Thus for a given amount of water added to the bucket (dose), the water level (concentration) will be higher when the cross-sectional area (volume of distribution) is smaller, and the water level (concentration) will be lower when the cross-sectional area (volume of distribution) is larger. If a single hole is made in the bucket (representing drug elimination), the water level will decrease in an exponential manner, i.e., the rate of change in the height of water will be proportional to the height of water at any time.

The pharmacokinetics of many drugs are poorly described by a single bucket, because many drugs used in anesthesia distribute extensively into different body compartments. We can make a better model by connecting other buckets to the central bucket by means of small connecting hoses of different

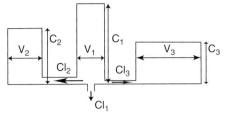

Figure 5.2. Two-dimensional representation of a hydraulic model. The width of each box is proportional to the volume of the respective compartment. The height of the box is proportional to the concentration of the compartment. The size of the intercompartmental and metabolic clearances corresponds to the width of the tubes.

diameters. When water is now added to the central bucket, the water level decreases because of two processes: water runs out the bottom of the central bucket (drug elimination) and water runs between the central bucket and the peripheral buckets (drug distribution). With regard to pharmacokinetics the drug moves always along the concentration gradient. As long as the concentration in the central compartment is higher than in the peripheral compartments the drug distributes into the peripheral compartments. Once the concentration in the central compartment is lower the drug will redistribute back into the central compartment, from which it is eliminated (Fig. 5.2).

It is customary to differentiate between different phases of the decrease in concentration following an intravenous bolus dose. The "distribution phase" usually refers to the initial rapid decrease in concentrations, and the "elimination phase" usually refers to the later slower decline in concentrations. However, as is apparent from the hydraulic model, these two processes actually occur simultaneously, rather than sequentially. As described above, the rate of elimination is proportional to the concentration. Thus it is during the initial high concentrations of the "distribution phase" (when the drug is moving from the central to the peripheral compartments) that the *elimination rate* is greatest. Also, it is during the "elimination phase" that the rate of decline of concentrations is slowed by the distribution of drug from the peripheral compartments back into the central compartment.

To derive the parameters of a compartment model, assumptions must be made about the structure of the model. The compartment models that are normally used are called *mammillary models*. This means that the drug is administered into the central compartment; the peripheral compartments are connected to the central compartment; drug is eliminated from the central compartment; and no drug is eliminated from the peripheral compartments. Other types of models exist (e.g., catenary models) in which the compartments are connected in a chainlike manner. Because the shape of the curve changes with the number of compartments, the model that best fits the data must be selected based on objective statistical criterion. Nonlinear regression is used to estimate the model parameters, so that the model predictions accurately describe the measured concentrations.

Compartment models can be parameterized in several different ways. A common method involves ordinary differential

equations. The underlying idea is that drug elimination and drug distribution between the compartments is described by rate constants (k), which are commonly assigned subscripts to indicate the direction of drug movement. The central volume of distribution (V_1) and five rate constants (k_{10}, k_{12}, k_{13}, k_{21}, k_{31}) describe a three-compartment model. Another common method is to use a polyexponential equation, e.g., $C(t) = \text{Dose} \cdot (A_1 \cdot e^{-\lambda^1} + A_2 \cdot e^{-\lambda^2} + A_3 \cdot e^{-\lambda^3})$. In this case, a plot of the natural logarithm of the concentrations that are observed after an intravenous bolus versus time reveals three distinct slopes, which are equal to λ_1, λ_2, and λ_3. Although a different equation is required to describe the concentrations after an intravenous infusion, the same coefficients (A_1, A_2, A_3) and hybrid-rate constants (λ_1, λ_2, and λ_3) are used. Another common method is to use three volumes (V_1, V_2, V_3) and three clearances (CL_1, CL_2, CL_3). Other combinations of parameters are possible. However, for a one-, two-, or three-compartment model, the number of parameters required is always twice the number of compartments. With one full set of parameters, all of the other parameters can be calculated.

Figure 5.3 illustrates two drugs, which both have a steady-state volume of distribution (V_{dss}) of 100 L. However, the drug on the left is described by a one-compartment model and the drug on the right is described by a two-compartment model. Both drugs also have the same clearance ($CL = CL_1$). The two-compartment model has a volume of distribution at steady state, V_{dss}, which is divided between two compartments and is given by $V_{dss} = V_1 + V_2$, whereas the one-compartment model has a V_{dss} equal to its initial volume of distribution (in this case, labeled V_d). As illustrated in Fig. 5.3 (*bottom*), the measured drug concentrations for the two-compartment model (drug elimination and distribution) are different from the one-compartment model (drug elimination only).

It should now be obvious that, although very important, the basic pharmacokinetic parameters (V_{dss}, CL, and MRT) obtained by noncompartment methods do not adequately describe the pharmacokinetic behavior of drugs that are best described by multicompartment models. It is possible for two drugs with identical steady-state volume of distribution and clearance to have completely different concentrations following the same dosing history. For multicompartment models, all model parameters must be known to calculate the predicted concentrations. Even when all of the parameters are available, it is nearly impossible to make correct inferences about the pharmacokinetic behavior of a drug without the aid of computer simulations [2].

So far we have not mentioned a very popular pharmacokinetic parameter: the half-time or half-life. For a one-compartment model, the meaning of the half-time is unambiguous and it can be calculated easily. Plotting the natural logarithm of the drug concentrations following an intravenous bolus on the y-axis against time on the x-axis will obtain a straight line with slope $-k$. In any time interval equal to $t_{1/2}$, the concentration, C, will decrease by one-half from C to $C/2$. Thus:

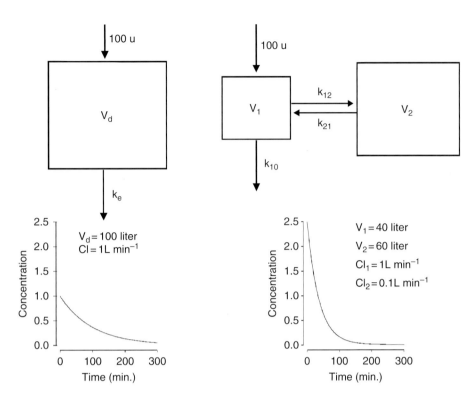

Figure 5.3. Intravenous bolus for one- and two-compartment models. The concentrations decline exponentially, shown over the first 5 hours. Both drugs have a steady-state volume of distribution (V_{dss}) of 100 L. The rate of movement of drug (mg min^{-1}) in the directions of the arrows are governed by the product of the amount of drug in the compartment (units = mg) and the rate constants (units = min^{-1}). The direction of movement is indicated by the subscripts, e.g., k_e and k_{10} are the elimination-rate constants from the central compartment (compartment one) to the outside (compartment zero), k_{12} is the rate constant governing the rate of drug movement from compartment one to compartment two (the peripheral compartment), and k_{21} is the rate constant governing the rate of drug movement from compartment two to compartment one. After administration of 100 units (u) bolus to the one-compartment model, the initial concentration is given by 100 u/100 L = 1 u L^{-1}. After administration of 100 units bolus to the two-compartment model, the initial concentration is given by 100 u/40 L = 2.5 u L^{-1} (*bottom graphs*). The drug is assumed to mix instantaneously in the central compartment. Both drugs have the same clearance. Thus the total area under the curve over all time will be identical. The predicted concentrations for the one-compartment model (*bottom left*) can be completely described by two parameters, V_d (which for the one-compartment model is the same as V_{dss}) and Cl, both of which can be estimated by noncompartment techniques. However, the predicted concentrations for the two-compartment model (*bottom right*) cannot be described by V_{dss} and Cl alone; two more parameters are required.

$$k = \frac{\Delta y}{\Delta x}$$

$$k = \frac{\log_e(C) - \log_e(C/2)}{t_{1/2}}$$

$$t_{1/2} = \frac{\log_e(2)}{k}$$

$$t_{1/2} = \frac{0.693}{k}$$

(5.4)

For a one-compartment model, $t_{1/2}$ describes the time required for the concentrations to decrease by one-half, which is unchanged for any combination of boluses or infusions, and is unchanged by the duration of drug administration. We can also call it the "elimination half-life," and quite correctly imply that it is also the time to eliminate half of the drug from the body. Thus, for a one-compartment model, the "context-sensitive half-time" (see later) equals the elimination half-life, and does not change with the duration of the infusion.

However, for drugs that are described by multicompartment pharmacokinetics, the concept of half-time is more complicated. Instead of a single exponential process with one half-time, the pharmacokinetics are described by two or more exponential processes. Thus each of the exponential terms (λ_1, λ_2, and λ_3), a half-time can be calculated as: $t_{1/2.i} = \frac{0.693}{\lambda_i}$. Often these are referred to as the α, β, γ half-lives.

Importantly, the time for the concentration to decrease by 50% is dependent on the preceding dosing history and can vary with the duration of drug administration. For multicompartment models, the time for the concentration to decrease by half does not equal the time to eliminate half of the drug from the body, and the time required to eliminate half of the drug from the body is not the same as the "elimination half-life." For this reason, the expression *terminal half-life* is preferred to *elimination half-life*. Other concepts are required, because a single parameter, such as one half-time, cannot represent the entire time course of the concentration of a drug described by multicompartment pharmacokinetics. Concepts such as *context-sensitive half-time* and *relative decrement time* are better suited, and will be discussed later in this chapter.

Several factors influence the estimated parameters, including obvious problems, such as errors in the dose, errors in the timing of the samples, and errors in measuring the drug concentrations. However, design issues are also important. Factors such as the site of sampling (e.g., arterial vs. venous), the method of administration (e.g., bolus vs. infusion), and the number and timing of samples, in particular the duration of sampling, also have an important influence on the parameter estimates. In general, the longer the sampling time the more "compartments" can be detected. Based on many hours of sampling, a three-compartment model is commonly reported for many drugs to describe their pharmacokinetics. Sometimes the three compartments are assigned physiologic significance, i.e., the central compartment is thought to correspond with the vascular space; the second compartment with the rapidly equilibrating, high-perfusion tissues, such as muscle; and the large third compartment with the slowly equilibrating, low-perfusion tissues, such as fat. Based on measurements obtained for 6–7 days after 30 minutes of isoflurane and sevoflurane, five-compartment models were reported [3]. The five compartments were referred to as: (1) the central compartment, (2) the vessel-rich group, (3) the muscle group, (4) the fourth compartment, and (5) the fat group. It is important to remember that these models were developed to describe the time course of measured concentrations at a single site (e.g., plasma or end-tidal) and that no drug concentrations were actually measured in the "vessel-rich group," "the fourth compartment," "muscle," or "fat." Conversely, in physiologic models, mathematic models for each organ are based on careful studies of measured concentrations relevant to each organ.

Special compartment models

The assumption that the rate of elimination (and drug movement between the compartments) is proportional to the concentration in the relevant compartments implies that the concentration at any time is linearly related to the dose or infusion rate, respectively. Or simply, the models imply that doubling a bolus dose or doubling an infusion rate will double the concentrations. But this might be an invalid assumption for some drugs. A prerequisite for linearity is that the elimination and transport processes are not saturated. However, when the enzyme system responsible for elimination becomes saturated, the rate of drug elimination reaches a maximum and becomes concentration-independent. The pharmacokinetics of alcohol is a well-known example for nonlinear kinetics within the "therapeutic" range.

The elimination rate (ER) for a one-compartment model with nonlinear kinetics is described as:

$$ER = \frac{V_{max} \cdot C_u(t)}{K_m + C_u(t)} \tag{5.5}$$

where $C_u(t)$ is the concentration of unbound of drug at time t and K_m is the Michaelis–Menton constant, which is the concentration at which the rate is half maximum, V_{max}. Two extremes can be distinguished. Firstly, when the C_u is much smaller than K_m, the process is not saturated and the elimination is proportional to the concentration (linear kinetics). Secondly, when C_u is much greater than K_m, the elimination rate approaches V_{max} and is concentration-independent. These extremes are expressed in Eq. 5.6:

$$\begin{aligned} \text{if}: \quad & C_u << K_m \\ \text{then}: \quad & ER = \frac{V_{max}}{K_m} \cdot C_u(t) = CL \cdot C_u(t) \\ \text{if}: \quad & C_u >> K_m \\ \text{then}: \quad & ER = V_{max} \end{aligned} \tag{5.6}$$

If the amount of drug excreted by specific routes (e.g., into the bile and urine) is also known, more complex compartment models can be developed with more than a single site of elimination. Sometimes the pharmacokinetics of a metabolite can be of interest, particularly if the metabolite is active clinically. To develop a compartment model for both the parent compound and the metabolite, it is necessary to measure the concentrations of both substances. The underlying principle is that a fraction of the parent compound is converted into the metabolite, which is then described by its own pharmacokinetic model [4]. The accuracy of the model will be improved if the kinetics of the metabolite can be investigated (by administering pure metabolite without parent compound) in the same subjects in a crossover study design.

Physiologically based pharmacokinetic (PBPK) models

The classical compartment models are coarse abstraction of the real distribution and elimination process. Still these models describe the measured and observed concentrations well. It goes without saying that by predicting the concentration in the central compartment no information is available about the time course of the concentration in the different tissues. More complex studies are required in order to develop more complex models. If such a PBPK model is based on enough detailed physiological and pharmacokinetic information it is possible to allometrically scale a model developed in rats to humans for a given anesthetic [5]. With these models it is then also possible to investigate the influence of changes in cardiac output and organ blood flow on the time course of the concentration in the blood and in various organs and tissues. Unfortunately the development of such accurate models is expensive and can only be performed in animals.

The classical compartment model is particulary weak at describing and predicting the time course of the concentration during the first one to two minutes after an intravenous bolus dose. The basic assumption of immediate mixing of the drug within the blood is clearly wrong. In order to describe this phase better, more complex (but not as complex as a full PBPK model) recirculatory models [6] or hybrid physiologic models [7] are required. These models also describe the concentrations in different parts of the circulation and helped us to have a better understanding of the pharmacokinetic process of the initial phase of drug administration. Emphasizing the importance the distribution and recirculation process on determining the adequate size of a bolus dose, Krejcie and

Avram coined the expression *front-end kinetics* [8]. Although this is very important for the peak blood concentration, the influence of the rather inaccurate description of the time course of the concentration during the first minute with traditional models is probably not as relevant with regard to onset of effect. Because anesthetics do not act in the blood, there is a delay between the time course of the concentration in the blood and the concentration at the site of drug effect.(see below). This additional transfer constant (or delay) moderates the impact of short-term variations of the blood concentration with regard to onset of drug effect.

Drug input

In theory, an intravenous bolus dose is an infusion with an infinite rate, i.e., the total amount of drug is instantaneously injected at $t = 0$. The bolus dose concept is appealing because it makes the mathematics of the pharmacokinetic model somewhat easier. Because of the assumption of instantaneous mixing of the drug within the central compartment, the concentration is maximal at $t = 0$. In reality neither the infusion rate can be infinite nor can the drug distribute throughout the central or blood compartment instantaneously. For example, a 100 mg bolus of propofol administered over 15 seconds is really an infusion rate equal to 400 mg min^{-1}. The use of "infusion rate" equations rather than "bolus dose" equations has the advantage of avoiding maximum predicted concentrations as $t = 0$. Still the mixing is not instantaneous because the drug must return to the heart, pass through the pulmonary circulation and then through the systemic circulation before it is detected at an arterial sampling site. Even during an infusion at "steady state," the drug concentrations in different parts of the circulation may not be the same, particularly if the drug is rapidly metabolized. Although traditional compartment models only poorly describe arterial concentrations during the first minute or so, they adequately model the time course of the concentration thereafter.

With a constant infusion rate, IR, the concentration rises gradually towards a steady state. This is the result of two processes, as defined in the following equation for a one-compartment model:

$$\frac{dA}{dt} = IR - ER \tag{5.7}$$

This differential equation states that rate of change in the amount (A) of drug in the compartment is equal to the rate of drug entering the compartment (the infusion rate) minus the rate of drug leaving the compartment (the elimination rate). This equation indicates how differential equations are used to describe complex models. The concentration in the compartment is then obtained by dividing the amount in the compartment by the volume of the compartment. During the infusion, the elimination rate increases in proportion to the increasing concentration, whereas the input rate is constant.

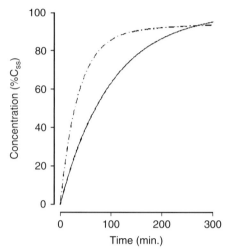

Figure 5.4. Intravenous infusion for one- and two-compartment model. Parameters for both drugs are identical to those in Fig. 5.3. The half-time for the one-compartment model is 69 minutes and the two half-times for the two-compartment model are 25 minutes and 460 minutes. Both drugs in this simulation have the same clearance, and the infusion rate is the same. The steady-state concentration (100 u L^{-1}) is given by the product of rate (100 u min^{-1}) and clearance (1 L min^{-1}). For the one-compartment model (*solid line*), the following relationship is observed: after 1, 2, 3, 4, and 5 half-lives, 50%, 75%, 87.5%, 93.75%, and 97% of steady-state concentration is achieved. For the two-compartment model (*dashed line*), this relationship is no longer true; despite the longer terminal half-time (460 minutes), the initial approach toward the steady-state level is more rapid. Without knowing the respective coefficients (see text), it is not possible to predict the relative contribution of each exponential process. In this example, A_1/λ_1 accounts for 90% of the area under the curve and A_2/λ_2 accounts for only 10% of the area under the curve. Thus the shorter half-time is of greater significance initially.

Therefore, the concentration will increase until the elimination rate equals the infusion rate (Fig. 5.4), at which time a steady-state concentration is achieved (theoretically only after an infinite time). The concentration at any time, t, during the infusion is described by the following equations:

$$C(t) = \frac{IR}{k_{10} \cdot V_1} \left(1 - e^{-k_{10} \cdot t}\right)$$

$$C(t = \infty) = \frac{IR}{k_{10} \cdot V_1} = \frac{IR}{Cl_1} \tag{5.8}$$

The first line only applies to a one-compartment model, but the second line is also true for two- and three-compartment models.

Another important category of drug administration is absorption from an extravascular site, such as the buccal area, gastrointestinal tract, the muscles, the skin, and the respiratory tract. For the intravenous route, the rate of input is precisely known. In contrast, for the extravascular routes the rate of input of the drug into the circulation is influenced by a variety of different physical and chemical processes. Factors such as the formulation of the drug, its molecular weight, its lipid solubility, its pK_a, the pH value of the tissue, and the blood supply to the site will all affect the rate of absorption. Importantly, there may be a significant delay between drug

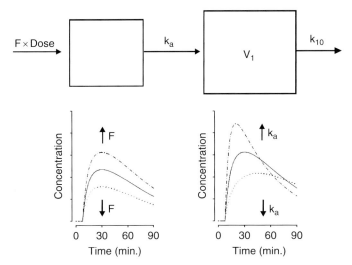

Figure 5.5. Extravascular dose and one-compartment model. The fraction of the absorbed dose is described by the bioavailability, F. Increasing the F by one-third (*dashed line*) or decreasing F by one-third (*dotted line*) will increase or decrease the concentrations proportionally (*left*). The rate of increase and decrease of the concentration in the central compartment (V_1) is determined by the absorption rate constant (k_a) and the elimination rate constant (k_{10}). Usually k_a is greater than k_{10}. (If k_a is very small compared with k_{10}, then "flip-flop" kinetics exist and the slow terminal half-time is due to the slow absorption process, rather than a slow elimination process.) Increasing the k_a (*dashed line*) will increase the maximum concentration (C_{max}), which will occur earlier (t_{max}), and decreasing k_a (*dotted line*) will decrease the maximum concentration (C_{max}), which will occur later (t_{max}) (*right*). If the dose, bioavailability, and clearance are unchanged, the area under the three curves will be the same. In both graphs, the absorption begins after a lag time (t_{lag}) of several minutes.

administration and the commencement of absorption from the site (referred to as the lag time or t_{lag}), and only some fraction of the total dose may be absorbed. The bioavailability, F, can be calculated when data are available for both intravenous (iv) and extravascular (ev) administration of the same drug. The calculation assumes that clearance remains constant when the two routes are compared:

$$Dose_{iv} = CL \cdot AUC_{iv}$$
$$F \cdot Dose_{ev} = CL \cdot AUC_{ev}$$
$$F = \left(\frac{AUC_{ev}}{AUC_{iv}}\right) \cdot \left(\frac{Dose_{iv}}{Dose_{ev}}\right) \tag{5.9}$$

Thus by definition the bioavailability of a drug given intravenously is 100%, whereas only a fraction (F) of this might reach the systemic circulation when given by an extravascular route. For example, if some of an orally administered drug passes the gastrointestinal tract without being absorbed, and some undergoes first-pass metabolism, the area under the curve for the oral route will be smaller than the intravenous route (given the same dose) and the bioavailability will be less than 100%.

Figure 5.5 shows a compartment model that describes the time course of the concentration after extravascular administration of a drug. It shows the impact of changing the bioavailability (F) or absorption rate on the concentration in the

central compartment. The mathematic expression for such a model must include two separate pharmacokinetic processes: the *absorption rate* and the *elimination rate*. The rate of decrease in the amount of drug in the extravascular site equals the rate of absorption from the site. The rate of change in the amount of drug in the central compartment equals the rate of absorption from the extravascular site minus the rate of elimination from the central compartment. This can be expressed in the following two differential equations:

$$\frac{dA_{ev}}{dt} = -k_a \cdot A_{ev}(t)$$
$$\frac{dA_1}{dt} = k_a \cdot A_{ev}(t) - k_{10} \cdot A_1(t) \tag{5.10}$$

where A_{ev} denotes amount of drug in the extravascular site, k_a represents the absorption rate constant, k_{10} represents the elimination rate constant from the central compartment, and the amount of drug in the extravascular site at $t = 0$ is $F \times Dose$. Again, the concentration in the central compartment is then obtained by dividing the amount in the compartment by the volume of the central compartment. Data from oral dose studies are often summarized with two parameters, the time (t_{max}) of the maximum concentration and the maximum concentration (C_{max}), which are compound descriptors of the absorption and distribution/elimination processes. In some circumstances it is possible to estimate the absorption half-life based on t_{max}. Often the absorption process is more complex, and adequate description requires a model with more than a single absorption-rate constant [7]. To detect the appropriate form of the absorption process, "deconvolution" methods are used to analyze data obtained after both intravenous and extravascular routes of administration in the same individuals.

Effect-compartment concept

After an intravenous bolus dose, it takes time to establish an effect. This is most obvious when substances whose effect can be measured objectively and continuously are used, such as muscle relaxants. The drug must be transported close to the site of effect, penetrate into the tissue, bind to a receptor, and elicit some intracellular process, which eventually will be called the *effect*. All of these steps are time-consuming and introduce a delay between the time course of the plasma concentration and the time course of the effect.

Figure 5.6 shows the effect of a brief remifentanil infusion on the electroencephalogram. The concentration versus effect curve forms a counterclockwise hysteresis loop. If the concentration in the central compartment produced the effect without delay, the concentration versus effect curve would be a simple curve, i.e., there would be no loop. Thus the loop is present because the concentration was measured at the wrong site, i.e., in the case of remifentanil, the blood is not the site of drug effect.

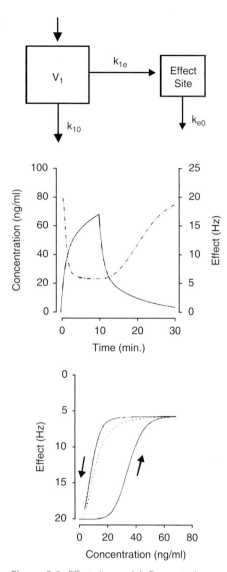

Figure 5.6. Effect-site model. Concentrations are measured in the central compartment, which is not the site of drug effect. An additional effect-site compartment (a one-compartment model) is added to the model (*top*). This model describes the delay between concentration in the central compartment and the effect without changing the pharmacokinetic model developed to describe the concentrations in the central compartment. The volume of the effect site is a tiny fraction of the volume of the central compartment and k_{1e} is a tiny fraction of k_{e0}. If the rate constant, k_{e0}, is large (a short $t_{1/2} k_{e0}$), then the effect site equilibrates rapidly with the central compartment. At steady state, the concentration in the effect site equals the concentration in the central compartment. A 10-minute remifentanil infusion (*middle*) shows the increase and decrease of remifentanil concentrations (*solid line*) and the decrease and increase in the spectral edge frequency (*dashed line*). The counterclockwise loop is seen when the effect is plotted against the concentration in the central compartment (*bottom*). For the same level of effect, the concentration is higher during onset than during offset, because central-compartment concentrations are the driving force for the movement of drug to and from the effectsite. It is important to plot the effect on the y-axis with the baseline effect at the origin, otherwise the direction of the loop is reversed. The *dashed line* shows the nonlinear static relationship between the concentration and effect in the effect site compartment, which is usually described by an E_{max} pharmacodynamic model.

Hull and colleagues [10] and Sheiner and coworkers [11] introduced the effect-compartment concept based on data from studies with muscle relaxants. Unfortunately, the effect-site concentration cannot be measured directly. It is not a real "measurable" concentration, but rather a virtual concentration in a virtual compartment. For any concentration in this virtual compartment, there is a corresponding effect. This relationship between concentration and effect in this compartment is usually nonlinear and static (does not explicitly depend on time). If the concentration in the central compartment is maintained at a constant level, the model assumes that at equilibrium the concentration in the effect site equals the concentration in the central compartment. If the blood concentration is measured, it is assumed that the effect site is in equilibrium with the blood concentrations at steady state. If the unbound plasma concentrations (likely to be different to the blood concentration) are measured, it is assumed the effect site is in equilibrium with the unbound plasma concentrations at steady state.

An important property of this virtual compartment is that it has negligible volume and contains only a negligible amount of drug. The delay is mathematically described by a single parameter, k_{e0}, the effect-site equilibration-rate constant, which is a first-order process. When k_{e0} is large, the rate of equilibration is rapid and the effect-site concentrations will rapidly approach the central-compartment concentrations. Conversely, when k_{e0} is small, the rate of equilibration is slow and the effect-site concentrations will only slowly approach the central-compartment concentrations. This can be expressed as an equilibration half-life, where $t_{1/2} k_{e0} = \frac{Log_e(2)}{k_{e0}} = \frac{0.693}{k_{e0}}$, so that a rapid rate of equilibration (a large k_{e0}) gives a short equilibration half-life and vice versa.

The concept has been depicted differently by various authors. Sometimes the rate constant k_{e0} is directed out of the effect compartment, sometimes k_{e0} is directed back to the central compartment, sometimes a rate constant k_{1e}, which is negligibly small, is used to describe the rate at which drug moves from the central compartment to the effect-site compartment. Independent of the graphical representation of the effect compartment, the key principles are the same: (1) the effect site is a hypothetical compartment where there is no delay between concentration and effect; (2) the time course of the concentration in the central compartment is not affected by the addition of the effect site to the pharmacokinetic model; and (3) at equilibrium the concentration in the effect site is equal to the concentration in the central compartment.

Predictors of onset

The time to the peak effect-site concentration (t_{peak}) is a dose-independent pharmacokinetic parameter (Fig. 5.7). It is, however, dependent on both the plasma pharmacokinetic parameters and the rate of equilibration between the plasma and the effect site. Thus t_{peak} is an important descriptor of onset of drug effect, which is particularly useful when comparing drugs of the same group. We note, however, that t_{peak} only coincides

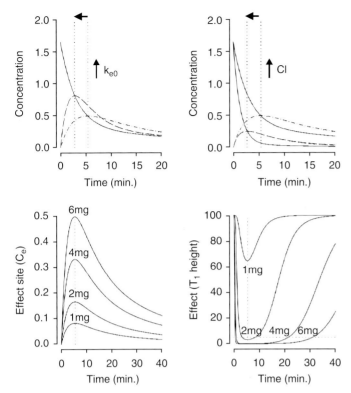

Figure 5.7. Onset of drug effect after intravenous bolus dose. A pharmacokinetic and pharmacodynamic model for vecuronium is used to illustrate the principles. An increase in k_{e0} (shorter $t_{1/2} k_{e0}$) results in a more rapid equilibration between the central compartment and the effect site (*top left*). This results in an earlier t_{peak}, the time of peak effect-site concentration (*arrow*). A more rapid decrease in concentrations in the central compartment (e.g., increase in clearance) also results in an earlier t_{peak} (*top right*; the k_{e0} is not changed in this simulation). Increasing the dose increases the effect-site C_{peak}, but does not change the effect-site t_{peak} (*bottom left*). Increasing the dose does not change the time of the maximum effect for submaximal doses (*bottom right*). However, the time to 95% depression of twitch height is shorter, and the duration of effect is longer, for doses greater than the D_{95} (the dose causing 95% suppression of the twitch height).

with the time of peak effect when a submaximal dose is given. With "supramaximal" doses, the maximum effect will occur prior to t_{peak}. However, even if a drug is administered by infusion, and supramaximal doses have been administered, it is still possible to determine t_{peak} by simulations based on the PK/PD model [12–14].

Neither the central volume (V_1) nor volume of distribution at steady state (V_{dss}) is a useful parameter for calculating the bolus dose required to achieve a desired effect. The use of V_1 or V_{dss} results in calculated loading doses that are either too small or too large, respectively. In contrast, the t_{peak} concept has been used to calculate optimal initial bolus doses [15]. The volume of distribution at the time of the peak effect-site concentration (Vd_{pe}) following an intravenous bolus dose is calculated as:

$$Vd_{pe} = \frac{V_1}{C_{peak}/C_0}, \qquad (5.11)$$

where V_1 is the central volume of distribution, C_0 is the concentration at the $t = 0$ (as predicted by the pharmacokinetic model), and C_{peak} is the predicted effect-site concentration at the time of

the peak effect-site concentration. Using Vd_{pe} we can calculate the loading dose to achieve the effect-site concentration (C_{peak}) associated with a desired effect at t_{peak} as:

$$\text{Loading dose} = C_{peak} \cdot Vd_{pe} \qquad (5.12)$$

In this way, drugs can be compared by calculating the time to a specified effect using the full PK/PD model.

Predictors of offset

Using computer simulations, Youngs and Shafer found that no single parameter of the pharmacokinetic model predicted fast recovery [16]. They showed that the implications of a change in a single parameter on the time course of onset and offset of drug effect could only be predicted if all the other parameters of the pharmacokinetic model remain unchanged. For example, if all the other parameters of the model were fixed a small V_1 or big CL_1, or both, predicted rapid recovery. However, a large CL_1 can be completely offset by other parameters of the pharmacokinetic model. Because no two drugs differ only by one parameter, comparison is not possible on a parameter by parameter basis. Nevertheless, the most commonly quoted and traditional descriptor of drug offset is the drug's "terminal" half-life [17], which using the above notation for a three-compartment model can be calculated as $\log_e(2)/\lambda_3$. Unfortunately, if we know only one (or even all three) of the half-times, we cannot calculate the rate of decline of the drug concentrations; a computer and all six parameters are necessary to complete this calculation. However, some insight into the relative contribution of each half-time can be obtained relatively easily by calculating A_1/λ_1, A_2/λ_2, and A_3/λ_3 as a percentage of the total area under the curve $A_1/\lambda_1 + A_2/\lambda_2 + A_3/\lambda_3$.

Shafer and Varvel introduced the concept of recovery curves based on simulations for the purpose of rational opioid selection [18]. Hughes and colleagues subsequently coined the expression *context-sensitive half-time* [19]. This concept provides a graphical insight into the pharmacokinetic behavior of many drugs. For many drugs the time required for the concentration to decrease by 50% increases with the duration of the infusion (Fig. 5.8). Although providing an insight into the pharmacokinetics of a drug in a way that simply is not possible by inspection of the model parameters, the context-sensitive half-time may not be clinically relevant, because the percentage decrease in concentration required for recovery from drug effect is not necessarily 50%. Bailey generalized this concept to *relative decrement times*, which incorporates the pharmacodynamic model into the simulations [20,21].

Bailey extended these concepts further by evaluating the duration of drug effect when drug effect is assessed in a binary, response/no-response fashion [20,22]. The mean effect time (MET) is the area under the probability of drug effect curve as a function of time after drug administration is discontinued, assuming that the probability of responsiveness to surgical

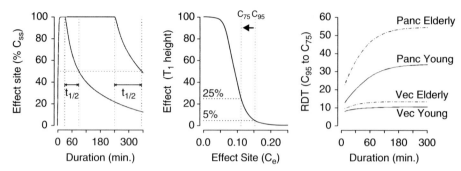

Figure 5.8. Offset of drug effect. The rate of decline of concentrations for a one-compartment model is always the same whatever the dosing history or duration of infusion. This is generally not true for drugs described by multicompartment pharmacokinetic models. Steady-state effect site concentrations (C_{ss}) are maintained for pancuronium (panc) in the elderly for 30 minutes and 240 minutes (*left*). The time taken for the concentration to decrease by half depends on the duration of the infusion. In the context of a 30-minute target-controlled infusion of pancuronium, the effect-site concentration takes about 70 minutes to decrease by half. In the context of a 240-minute target-controlled infusion of pancuronium, the effect-site concentration takes about 114 minutes to decrease by half. A series of such simulations can be performed to construct a curve showing the time taken for the concentration to decrease by half for a large range of infusion rates. The simulations can be performed for both the central-compartment concentrations and the effect-site concentrations. However, the time taken for the concentrations to decrease by half (from whatever starting value) may have absolutely no clinical relevance. For example, if the relaxant concentration is extremely high, when the concentrations decrease by half the patient may still have no recovery of neuromuscular block. The concentration response curve for vecuronium (vec) in the young is shown (*middle*). If we infuse vecuronium to maintain the single twitch at 5% of control (TOFC = 1) and we give anticholinesterase when single twitch is 25% of control (TOFC = 4), then we can use these two endpoints to calculate the clinically relevant percentage decrement for vecuronium (~27%). Relevant decrement time curves for pancuronium and vecuronium in the young and elderly are shown (*right*).

stimulation was reduced to 10% (C_{90}) during the infusion. As noted by Bailey, the pharmacodynamic analysis of binary data is mostly assessed by logistic regression of data pooled from multiple patients. With this methodology, the gradient of the pharmacodynamic model is often relatively low, reflecting high interindividual variability. If the slope of the individual concentration–response relationship is steep, and if the anesthesiologist has titrated the dose to effect, the time to offset of drug effect may be much shorter than that predicted by the MET.

Drug accumulation

When a drug is administered at regular intervals, there is always some drug remaining in the body before the next dose is given. Theoretically, some drug remains in the body forever, because the amount of drug in the body after a single intravenous bolus dose is given by $(Dose/V_1) \times e^{-(CL/V_1) \cdot t}$ (for a one-compartment model), which only equals zero at infinite time. When a fixed dose of a drug is given at frequent intervals, the concentration will gradually increase toward a steady-state concentration, and the total amount of drug in the body will accumulate. This is true for all drugs and, with regard to this behavior, claims that some drugs are "noncumulative" are misleading.

The *cumulation ratio* (CR) is defined as the ratio of the peak amount of drug in the body at the *cumulation plateau* (peak at steady state) to the peak amount of drug in the body after a single dose [23]. The following equation for CR is based on intravenous bolus dosing, and only applies to a one-compartment model:

$$CR = \frac{1}{1 - 2^{-(\tau/t_{1/2})}} \qquad (5.13)$$

Thus the CR depends entirely on the ratio of dosing interval (τ) to half-life ($t_{1/2}$). When the dosing interval equals the half-life, CR equals 2, i.e., the peak levels at steady state or plateau are twice those after a single intravenous dose. When the dosing interval is less than the $t_{1/2}$, CR is greater than 2, and when the dosing interval is more than the $t_{1/2}$, CR approaches unity. This ratio is sometimes referred to as the accumulation factor and accumulation index.

Once neuromuscular blockade recovers spontaneously, small doses of relaxant are usually administered to keep relaxation at a certain level of effect. Generally, the duration of effect of the first additional dose is shorter than that of identical doses administered later. This phenomenon has been called "cumulation" in the neuromuscular literature [24]. This is a different phenomenon to the accumulation described above. Indeed, this longer duration of effect after later doses does not occur with a one-compartment model. Rather, it is a property of drugs that are described by multicompartment pharmacokinetic models, and occurs for the same reasons that the context-sensitive half-time changes with duration of infusion.

Dose equivalence: principles of calculation

Switching from one drug to another of the same class can be desirable for different reasons. In pain therapy, changing the route of administration between the intravenous, oral, transcutaneous, epidural, and intrathecal routes is not uncommon. Sometimes, the change of route also necessitates changing the drug. Possibly a department decides that a new drug has a better risk/benefit ratio, or is just significantly cheaper with no obvious change in risk/benefit ratio, and changes to the new drug. In a whole variety of situations, it becomes necessary to calculate equipotent doses of a new drug, which unfortunately is more difficult than believed by most clinicians. Most often, recommendations regarding equivalent dosing are empirical [25,26], mostly because of lack of detailed PK/PD models. Often a "potency ratio" (between different routes or between different drugs) or observed total drug consumption are used to develop the new dosing regimen. Although both factors contain some information regarding appropriate dosing, neither alone is sufficient. The "one ampoule = equipotent dose" philosophy has caused more than one clinician to claim that the drug simply is ineffective. Obviously, the amount of drug in one ampoule is not necessarily equipotent to others in its class. However, even if one ampoule is equipotent for an intravenous bolus dose, it might not be equipotent when given by infusion. The time course of effect of two different drugs may be entirely different, even if an "equipotent bolus dose" or "equipotent infusion rate" is used.

To understand the principles involved, we will use PK/PD modeling to calculate the equipotent doses of two opioids with which anesthesiologists are familiar: fentanyl and alfentanil. For both of these drugs, an effect-site model has been developed using the electroencephalogram (EEG) as a sensitive and continuous measure of drug effect [27]. This research also provides us with the C_{50} value for each drug (the steady-state concentration required to produce 50% depression in the spectral edge of the processed EEG). We assume that this also provides us with a guide to the relative C_{50} for other clinically relevant measures of drug effect, such as the concentration associated with spontaneous respiration during anesthesia and the concentration required to obtund the response to intubation [28]. The C_{50} is 6.9 ng mL^{-1} for fentanyl and 520 ng mL^{-1} for alfentanil, which is approximately 75 times greater. If we want to give an intravenous bolus dose of alfentanil that is similar to 50 μg fentanyl, does this mean that we should give 75 times as much (3.75 mg)? Those familiar with both drugs will know from their clinical experience that a single bolus of 50 μg of fentanyl is an appropriate dose, which generally permits spontaneous breathing during general anesthesia. In contrast, 3.75 mg alfentanil will render the patient apneic and, in conjunction with a modest dose of hypnotic, is probably enough to render most patients unresponsive to intubation. These two doses are certainly not equipotent!

Based on our understanding of the effect-site concept, we can use Eq. 5.12 to determine the intravenous bolus dose required to give a concentration equal to the C_{50} for both drugs at the time of peak effect-site concentration (t_{peak}). First we must calculate the Vd_{pe}. The ratio of the peak effect-site concentration to the initial concentration in the central compartment at $t = 0$ (C_{peak}/C_0) is 0.16 for fentanyl and 0.33 for alfentanil. Dividing the central volume of distribution by this ratio gives Vd_{pe} for each drug: fentanyl, 12.7/0.16 = 76.9 L; alfentanil, 2.18/0.33 = 6.6 L. The dose to achieve the

respective C_{50} at t_{peak} is calculated as $C_{50} \times Vd_{pe}$, which gives a dose of 530 μg for fentanyl and 3.43 mg for alfentanil. Thus, based on the effect-site model and the steady-state C_{50}, we have calculated that only 6.5 times as much alfentanil as fentanyl (not 75 times!) is required for an equipotent intravenous bolus dose at the time of the peak effect-site concentration. Returning to the original example (50 μg fentanyl), we conclude that this is equipotent to an intravenous bolus dose of approximately 325 μg (6.5 × 50 μg) alfentanil at t_{peak}. Thus from the perspective of a single intravenous bolus dose, there is almost "twice as much opioid" in a 1000 μg ampoule of alfentanil compared with a 100 μg ampoule of fentanyl. However, the time course of effect is certainly different. The t_{peak} for alfentanil is much earlier at approximately 1.5 minutes compared with 3.7 minutes for fentanyl, necessitating a change in the timing of events if one wishes to compare the clinical effectiveness of these two doses at their peak. Although these two doses are equipotent at their peak effect, they are certainly not equipotent for the entire duration of a short anesthetic.

Is this equipotent bolus dose ratio (~ 6.5 : 1) also applicable for intravenous infusions, or should the steady-state C_{50} ratio of 75 : 1 be used? Based on our understanding of infusion pharmacokinetics, we can use Eq. 5.8 to determine the infusion rate that will result in a concentration equal to the C_{50} for both drugs at steady state. First we must know the clearance for each drug, which is 0.71 L min^{-1} for fentanyl and 0.19 L min^{-1} for alfentanil. Then we calculate the dose to achieve the respective C_{50} at steady state as $C_{50} \times CL$, which gives an infusion rate of approximately 300 μg h^{-1} for fentanyl and approximately 6 mg h^{-1} for alfentanil. Thus based on the steady-state C_{50} and clearance, approximately 20 times more alfentanil than fentanyl (not 75 times!) is required for an equipotent intravenous infusion at steady-state conditions. However, these infusion rates may not be particularly useful in clinical practice, because it takes about 24 hours for fentanyl, and about 5 hours for alfentanil, to attain 90% of their steady-state concentrations (Fig. 5.9, left).

To maintain equieffective steady-state concentrations of fentanyl and alfentanil, the relative infusion rates required vary over time, gradually approaching the steady-state ratio of ~ 20:1 the longer the targeted concentrations are maintained (Fig. 5.9, right). If we use a alfentanil: fentanyl infusion rate ratio of 10:1 to 20:1, based on 100 μg h^{-1} for fentanyl, we obtain an infusion rate of 1–2 mg h^{-1} for alfentanil, which agrees with clinical experience.

In this example, for which we have well-defined PK/PD models, we find that there is no simple "equipotent ratio" on which we can base "equipotent dosing" when switching between fentanyl and alfentanil. We have assumed that the relative potency based on the steady-state EEG concentration–response relationship is true for other clinical measures of drug effect. We have also assumed that the relative gradients for other measures of effect are similar for the two drugs. We have found that although the steady-state potency differs by a ratio

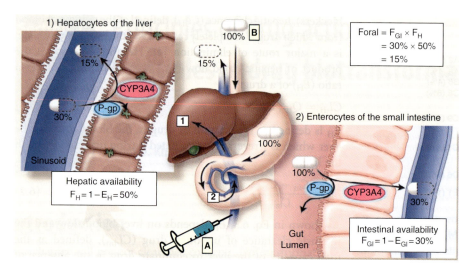

Figure 6.3. Metabolism of a theoretical drug after intravenously and oral administration. (A) An intravenously injected drug is eliminated in the liver, where it undergoes metabolism by CYP3A4 and/or transport by P-glycoprotein (P-gp) in hepatocytes (1). The hepatic extraction ratio (E_H) is 0.5, and therefore hepatic availability ($1 - E_H$) is 0.5 (50%) after each passage of blood through the liver. (B) The orally administered drug undergoes sequential first-pass elimination by CYP3A4 metabolism and/or transport by P-gp in enterocytes of the small intestine (2) and then hepatocytes of the liver (1). The intestinal extraction ratio (E_{GI}) is 0.7, and therefore intestinal availability ($1 - E_{GI}$) is 0.3 (30%). Although the drug is 100% absorbed from the gastrointestinal tract, the oral bioavailability is only 15%. Adapted with permission from Bailey and Dresser [6].

Intestinal extraction can range from < 1% to > 99%, but can be particularly important for drugs with high first-pass clearance and low oral bioavailability. Low oral bioavailability, once attributed only to hepatic first-pass extraction, is now known to result also from a quantitatively significant component of intestinal first-pass extraction. Intestinal metabolism plays a relatively minor role in systemic drug elimination.

Basic drug metabolism concepts

Several recent reviews and textbooks provide a comprehensive perspective on drug biotransformation [1,9–14]. A more in-depth, multi-part review is also available [15].

Therapeutic drugs, whether natural products or synthetic, tend to be relatively lipophilic because they typically must traverse one or more plasma membranes to reach their site of action. In general, biotransformation reactions convert compounds to more polar hydrophilic molecules that are more amenable to excretion, generally via the kidney. Traditionally, biotransformation reactions have been categorized as phase I and phase II reactions. The former are termed functionalization reactions, which introduce or uncover a functional group (hydroxyl, amine, acid) that moderately increases drug polarity and prepares it for a phase II reaction. The latter are conjugation reactions which covalently link the drug or metabolite with a highly polar molecule which renders the conjugate very water-soluble and thereby excreted. Phase I and II reactions can occur on the same molecule. Alternatively, drugs may undergo only phase I or only phase II reactions (the latter if a functional group is already present). Drugs may be eliminated unchanged, or as their phase I metabolites, or as phase II conjugates.

Phase I reactions include oxidation, reduction, dehydrogenation, and hydrolysis. They are typically (except hydrolysis) catalyzed by cytochrome P450 (CYP; see below). Most are carbon oxidations, which involve the initial insertion of an oxygen atom. Oxygen remains on the drug molecule with hydroxylation reactions, and leaves on the alkyl group as the aldehyde with dealkylation reactions. Phase I oxidative reactions include aromatic and aliphatic hydroxylation, O- and N-dealkylation (of which N-demethylation is a subset), epoxidation, and oxidative deamination and dehalogenation. N- and S-oxidation may also occur. Reduction is another type of phase I reaction, often under anaerobic conditions. Some drugs may undergo both oxidation and reduction, depending on the oxygen tension. For example, halothane undergoes (1) oxidation to a trifluoroacyl halide which can subsequently react with liver proteins to form trifluoroacetylated protein neoantigens, and (2) anaerobic reduction to a free radical which gives rise to chlorodifluoroethylene and chlorotrifluoroethane. Hydrolysis is a phase I reaction that is not catalyzed by CYP, but is catalyzed by esterases/amidases.

Enzymes of metabolism

Phase I enzymes
Cytochrome P450

Cytochrome P450 (CYP) is the main drug-metabolizing enzyme system (Fig. 6.2A) [1,16]. The CYP system is a superfamily of membrane-bound heme proteins that catalyze the biotransformation of endogenous (i.e., steroids) and exogenous compounds [17,18]. CYPs are called mixed-function oxidases or monooxygenases, because they insert one atom of molecular oxygen into the substrate and one atom into water. CYPs can also catalyze other reactions, such as reduction.

The mixed-function oxidase system involves several enzymes in addition to CYP, including the requisite participation of the flavoprotein NADPH-cytochrome P450 reductase, as well as NADPH-cytochrome b_5 reductase and cytochrome b_5. The typical oxidation reaction generally involves an initial hydroxylation, with NADPH providing two electrons to reduce one atom of molecular oxygen to water and insert the other into the substrate. The overall scheme can be represented as:

$$RH + O_2 + NADPH + H^+ \rightarrow ROH + H_2O + NADP^+$$

where RH is the substrate and ROH is the oxidized metabolite. In rare cases, NADPH-cytochrome P450 reductase itself can catalyze drug metabolism, such as nitro reduction or quinone reduction.

More than 50 human P450s have been identified, although only a small fraction are responsible for the majority of drug metabolism (Fig. 6.2) [1–3].

The individual CYPs evolved from a common ancestor protein, and are classified according to their sequence evolution [1,13]. CYPs that share > 40% sequence homology are grouped in a family (designated by an Arabic number, e.g., CYP2), those with > 55% homology are in a subfamily (designated by a letter, e.g., CYP2A), and individual CYPs are identified by a third number (e.g., CYP2A6). The majority of drugs in humans are metabolized by CYPs 1, 2, and 3 (particularly CYPs 2C, 2D6, and 3A). CYPs are predominantly "microsomal" enzymes (as are glucuronosyltransferase and glutathione transferase). Microsomes are not a physiologic organelle, but rather correspond to the smooth endoplasmic reticulum.

CYPs can have numerous genetic variants; indeed, there are several highly polymorphic CYPs. Allelic CYP variants are designated by an asterisk and number (e.g., CYP3A5*3, where the "wild-type" is always designated CYP3A5*1) [1,13]. Since identification of new genetic variants is ongoing, a website (www.cypalleles.ki.se) is updated regularly with new variants and their frequencies.

CYP isoforms can exhibit varying degrees of substrate specificity. Some, such as CYP2E1, have a relatively small and restrictive active site and accept only structurally similar substrates. Others, such as CYP3A, have a very open and accommodating active site (indeed at least two active sites) [19]. They are called promiscuous because they metabolize a large number of structurally diverse substrates. Similarly, substrates can exhibit a low degree of P450 isoform selectivity (antipyrine is metabolized by CYPs 1A2, 2A6, 2C9, 2C19, 2D6, 2E1, and 3A) [20] or a very high degree of isoform selectivity (meperidine and nifedipine are metabolized predominantly by CYP3A4, with little or no metabolism by the highly similar CYP3A5) [21]. Isoform selectivity can also exhibit an unusual oxygen dependence, as exemplified with halothane, which undergoes oxidation by CYPs 2E1 and 2A6, and reduction by 2A6 and 3A4 [22]. CYPs can also exhibit regioselectivity, specifically oxidizing only one portion of a molecule. For example, CYP1A2 catalyzes ropivacaine 3-hydroxylation, while CYP3A4 catalyzes 4-hydroxylation, 2-methyl-hydroxylation, and N-dealkylation [23].

Identification of the major CYP isoform(s) (or other enzymes) responsible for metabolizing drugs is termed *reaction phenotyping*, and is done both in vitro and in vivo [24].

Regulatory agencies now require this of all drugs in development. For each CYP isoform, prototypic selective substrates and inhibitors have been identified, and are used for reaction phenotyping [25]. This is accomplished in vitro by identifying (1) which individual cDNA-expressed CYP isoforms metabolize the drug, (2) which isoform-selective chemical inhibitors or antibodies inhibit metabolism of the drug by human liver microsomes, and (3) correlations between the metabolism of a candidate drug with either the protein content or catalytic activity of specific CYP isoforms in microsomes from a population of human livers.

The actual contribution of any individual CYP isoform to overall in-vitro microsomal metabolism will depend on the in-vitro intrinsic clearance (V_{max}/K_m, as defined in Chapter 5) by that specific isoform, the relative content of the isoform in the liver (or other organ), and the substrate concentration. Reaction phenotyping in vitro is optimally evaluated at therapeutic drug concentrations. When reactions are performed at high substrate concentrations, the results must be interpreted cautiously. It is not uncommon for more than one CYP to catalyze a metabolic pathway. The relative importance of each CYP to a specific pathway of metabolism depends on the in-vitro intrinsic clearance and the relative isoform content in organs.

Identification of a predominant CYP isoform in vivo is accomplished using analogous methods [26,27]. CYP isoform-selective inducers (drugs which increase the enzyme tissue content and/or activity) and inhibitors (often the same ones used in vitro) can be used to evaluate their effect on metabolism of the candidate drug. In a population of subjects, one can also correlate the metabolism of a candidate substrate with the subjects' CYP phenotype or genotype.

The expression of various CYPs in human liver, and the fraction of common clinically used drugs which they metabolize, are shown in Fig. 6.2. Five CYPs (1A2, 2C9, 2C19, 2D6, and 3A4) catalyze ~ 95% of CYP-mediated drug biotransformation (~ 75% of all drug metabolism). From the perspective of anesthesiology, the most important are CYPs 2B6, 2D6, 2E1, and 3A.

CYP3A

The CYP3A subfamily is the most significant group of biotransformation enzymes in clinical medicine, responsible for metabolizing over half of all drugs [28–30]. The important CYP3A isoforms are CYP3A4, the polymorphically expressed CYP3A5, and the fetal form CYP3A7. CYP3A enzymes in toto are the predominant CYP in human liver and intestine. CYP3A enzymes exhibit very broad substrate specificity (Table 6.1), with drugs ranging in size from halothane (a two-carbon alkane, mw 197) to cyclosporine (mw 1206). CYP3As also catalyze a wide variety of oxidative and reductive biotransformation reactions.

CYP3A4 is the most quantitatively abundant CYP in human liver, accounting for, on average, 30% of total hepatic CYP and as much as 60% in some livers. It is also the

Table 6.1. Representative human CYP3A substrates, inhibitors, and inducers

Substrates	
Opioids	alfentanil,[a] fentanyl, sufentanil, methadone, l-α-acetylmethadol (LAAM), buprenorphine, codeine, dextromethorphan
Benzodiazepines	midazolam,[a] triazolam, diazepam, alprazolam, temazepam
Local anesthetics	lidocaine, bupivacaine, ropivacaine, cocaine
Calcium antagonists	verapamil, diltiazem, nifedipine, nicardipine, nimodipine, felodipine, amlodipine
Immunosuppressants	cyclosporine, tacrolimus
Miscellaneous	erythromycin,[a] tamoxifen, paclitaxel, ondansetron, granisetron, lovastatin, simvastatin, atorvastatin, cortisol, terfenadine, astemizole, quinidine, cisapride, lansoprazole, imipramine, amitriptyline, cyclophosphamide, dapsone, amiodarone, testosterone

Inhibitors[b]	
Macrolides	troleandomycin,[a] erythromycin, clarithromycin
Antifungals	ketoconazole,[a] miconazole, itraconazole, fluconazole, clotrimazole
HIV drugs	indinavir, nelfinavir, ritonavir, saquinavir, amprenavir, nefazodone, delavirdine
Miscellaneous	grapefruit juice, 3A4 substrates

Inducers	
	rifampicin,[a] phenobarbital, phenytoin, carbamazepine, dexamethasone, nelfinavir, efavirenz

[a] The most widely used human in-vivo probes (selective substrates and inhibitors).
[b] Many inhibitors and inducers are also substrates.

predominant CYP in human intestine (Fig. 6.2B). Of importance in anesthesiology, CYP3A4 metabolizes all of the fentanyl-series synthetic opioids except remifentanil, most benzodiazepines, and local anesthetics. Prototype CYP3A4 substrates include midazolam and alfentanil. CYP3A4 activity is remarkably susceptible to induction and inhibition, which alter the metabolism and clearance of CYP3A substrates, often with profound clinical consequence (Table 6.1). The prototype inducer is rifampicin, but barbiturates, phenytoin, carbamazepine, glucocorticoids, and herbals such as St. John's wort also increase CYP3A4

content and activity several-fold. Prototype inhibitors are the macrolide antibiotic troleandomycin, the antifungal ketoconazole, and the protease inhibitor ritonavir, although other drugs in the same class (protease inhibitors) also inhibit CYP3A4. Drugs which are CYP3A4 substrates can competitively inhibit the metabolism of other CYP3A4 drugs. There is wide interindividual variability in CYP3A4 activity, but no clinically significant genetic polymorphisms or ethnic differences in activity have been found to date.

CYP3A5 is similar to CYP3A4 and metabolizes many but not all CYP3A4 substrates, usually with diminished activity [31]. CYP3A5 is polymorphically expressed, both in liver and intestine, in 5–15% of Caucasians, ~ 40% of Chinese, and > 50% of African-Americans. When present, it may account for more than half of the hepatic and an average of 25% of the intestinal CYP3A in some individuals [3]. CYPs 3A4 and 3A5 are induced and inhibited by many of the same drugs. Individuals expressing CYP3A5 along with 3A4 may have greater metabolism of some (alprazolam, tacrolimus) but not other (midazolam, alfentanil, verapamil) CYP3A drugs, for reasons not yet known [32]. CYP3A5 is the major CYP in human kidney [33]. Unlike the liver, in which 3A4 is ubiquitous and 3A5 is sometimes expressed, in the kidney CYP3A5 is ubiquitous and 3A4 is expressed in only about 25% of subjects. Renal CYP3A may have a role in drug metabolism.

CYP3A7 is also similar to CYP3A4. It is expressed exclusively in fetal liver, comprising 50% of total CYP. The metabolic capabilities of CYP3A7 are similar to those of 3A4 and 3A5.

CYP2D

CYP2D6, although accounting for only 2–5% of total human hepatic CYP protein, nonetheless metabolizes 20–25% of all drugs and is one of the most important human CYPs [13,34–36]. It is also of considerable historical significance, being the first identified CYP genetic polymorphism (named the "debrisoquine/sparteine polymorphism," after the two drugs whose metabolism was bimodally distributed). The prototype CYP2D6 substrate probe is dextromethorphan O-demethylation, and quinidine the standard inhibitor. CYP2D6 is not inducible by drugs or hormones. A representative sample of CYP2D6 substrates and inhibitors is listed in Table 6.2. The list is notable for a group of opioids which undergo both CYP2D6-mediated O-demethylation and CYP3A4-mediated N-demethylation (Fig. 6.4). Most pertinent is codeine, now known to be a prodrug requiring metabolic activation to morphine [36]. The genetic and drug interaction implications of codeine metabolism are discussed below.

The CYP2D6 polymorphism is an autosomal recessive trait. More than 50 variant CYP2D6 alleles have been identified, which typically result in absent or catalytically deficient CYP2D6 protein. Populations comprise efficient or extensive metabolizers (EM, wild-type, homozygotes with normal CYP activity), intermediate metabolizers (IM, heterozygotes with reduced CYP activity), poor metabolizers (PM, homozygotes with absent activity), and ultrarapid metabolizers (UM, with enhanced CYP activity due to gene duplication, up to 13 copies). The CYP2D6 genetic polymorphism exhibits ethnic and racial as well as geographic diversity. The frequency distribution in a typical European population is 70–80% EM, 10–15% IM, 7–8% PM, and 2–10% UM. The PM frequency is 7–8% in Caucasians, 2% in African-Americans, and < 1% in Asians, and the UM frequency is 30% in Ethiopians, 10% in Spanish and Italians, 1–2% in northern Europeans, and < 1% in Asians. Table 6.3 lists geographic variability in CYP2D6 phenotypes. For drugs which are inactivated by metabolism via CYP2D6, there is a higher incidence of adverse effects among PM, and a higher incidence of therapeutic failures among UM.

CYP2B

CYP2B6 is expressed primarily in liver, and also in intestine, brain, kidney, and lung [37,38]. CYP2B6 was initially considered to be a minor enzyme, expressed in only some individuals and in low levels, and not important in human drug biotransformation. This was incorrect, however, and it is now known that CYP2B6 is expressed in greater amounts (up to 6% of total CYP), in all individuals, metabolizes numerous drugs (~ 8% of total), and is clinically important [39]. The prototype probe for human CYP2B6 is bupropion hydroxylation and the inhibitor is clopidogrel. CYP2B6 is the primary enzyme catalyzing propofol hydroxylation, and N-demethylation of methadone, meperidine, and both (R)- and (S)-ketamine [40–42]. 2B6 also metabolizes benzodiazepines (diazepam, temazepam, midazolam) and other drugs such as verapamil, lidocaine, and clopidogrel. Many drugs previously considered to be metabolized predominantly by CYP3A are now known to be metabolized and cleared by both CYP2B and CYP3A, and sometimes only by CYP2B. For example, methadone clearance was formerly thought to be dependent on CYP3A, and the drug label warns against CYP3A drug interactions. Nonetheless, it is now clear that while CYP3A does metabolize methadone in vitro, it has little or no role in clinical methadone metabolism and clearance [42,43]. Rather, CYP2B6 is the primary determinant of methadone metabolism and clearance, which is susceptible to CYP2B6 drug interactions [42–44]. Both CYP2B6 and CYP3A4 are highly inducible, and by the same drugs (such as rifampicin and anticonvulsants), and thus the potential for drug interactions with these 2B/3A substrates is considerable. CYP2B6 is highly polymorphic, with a frequent (> 50% of African-Americans) allele resulting in enzyme with reduced activity (CYP2B6*6). Thus both genetic variability and susceptibility to induction/inhibition account for the > 100-fold interindividual variability in CYP2B6 activity.

Table 6.2. Representative human CYP2D6 substrates and inhibitors

Substrates

Opioids	codeine, dextromethorphan,[a] dihydrocodeine, hydrocodone, oxycodone, tramadol
Antipsychotics	haloperidol, perphenazine, risperidone, thioridazine, chlorpromazine
TCAs	amitriptyline, clomipramine, desipramine, imipramine, nortriptyline, clozapine, maprotiline, trazodone
Antiarrhythmics	encainide, flecanide, mexilitine, procainamide, sparteine
β-blockers	alprenolol, bufurolol, labetolol, metoprolol, propranolol, timolol, carvedilol
SSRIs	fluoxetine, fluvoxamine, paroxetine, sertraline, citalopram, venlafaxine
Miscellaneous	debrisoquine, selegiline, tamoxifen, dolasetron, ondansetron, tropisetron

Inhibitors

	quinidine,[a] cimetidine, haloperidol, SSRIs

[a] The most widely used human in-vivo probes (selective substrates and inhibitors).

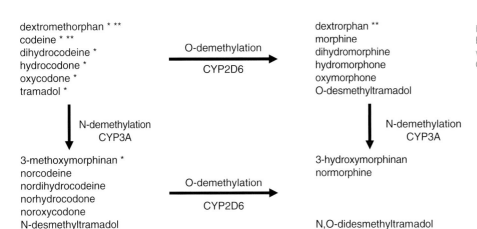

dextromethorphan * **
codeine * **
dihydrocodeine *
hydrocodone *
oxycodone *
tramadol *

→ O-demethylation CYP2D6 →

dextrorphan **
morphine
dihydromorphine
hydromorphone
oxymorphone
O-desmethyltramadol

N-demethylation CYP3A ↓

3-methoxymorphinan *
norcodeine
nordihydrocodeine
norhydrocodone
noroxycodone
N-desmethyltramadol

→ O-demethylation CYP2D6 →

N-demethylation CYP3A ↓

3-hydroxymorphinan
normorphine

N,O-didesmethyltramadol

Figure 6.4. Role of CYP2D6 and CYP3A4 in the bioactivation and inactivation of oral opioids. Pathways known to be metabolized by CYP2D6 and CYP3A4 are indicated by * and **, respectively.

Table 6.3. Geographic variability in the frequency of CYP2D6 phenotypes

Region	Poor metabolizers	Intermediate metabolizers	Extensive metabolizers	Ultrarapid metabolizers
America	0	0	93	9
Sub-Saharan Africa	2	16	77	5
North Africa	0	10	50	40
Middle East	1	10	76	12
Europe	8	5	84	2
Central/South Asia	1	6	91	1
East Asia	0	30	68	1
Oceana	0	0	75	25

Frequencies are based on data in Ingelman-Sundberg et al. [13].

Other CYPs

CYP1A2 is expressed almost exclusively in the liver, while CYP1A1 is almost exclusively found extrahepatically, particularly in the lung [45]. CYP1As are inducible by cigarette smoke, charbroiled foods, and polycyclic aromatic hydrocarbons. Overall, CYP1A2 metabolizes a small fraction of therapeutic drugs, but the list includes caffeine, phenacetin, and ropivacaine [23]. CYP1A1 metabolizes polycyclic aromatic hydrocarbons.

CYP2A6 is expressed mainly in the liver, and also in the respiratory tract [46]. CYP2A metabolizes a small number of drugs (notably methoxyflurane and halothane) and a large number of environmental toxins, carcinogens, and nicotine. It catalyzes both the aerobic oxidation and anaerobic reduction of halothane, and, although it is the minor CYP isoform responsible for human halothane oxidation, may nonetheless play a role in immune-based halothane hepatitis. There is wide interindividual variability in CYP2A6 activity.

CYP2C is a major class, containing CYPs 2C8, 2C9, 2C18, and 2C19, together accounting for about a fourth of total hepatic CYP and metabolizing approximately 15–20% of all therapeutic drugs [47]. CYP2Cs are of little relevance in anesthesia, except that they metabolize barbiturates and diazepam. A CYP2C19 polymorphism accounts for inter-racial differences in the clinical disposition and dose requirements for diazepam, particularly PM homozygotes. For perspective, the major isoform determining the elimination and clinical effects of warfarin is CYP2C9, which has highly significant genetic polymorphisms that affect clinical outcome and toxicity. In the future, patients may undergo genetic testing to determine warfarin dosing [48].

CYP2E1 comprises approximately 6% of total hepatic P450, and metabolizes few drugs (notable exceptions being paracetamol [acetaminophen] and ethanol) [49,50]. Nevertheless, it is of considerable toxicological and carcinogenic importance, because it metabolizes numerous small molecules, halogenated hydrocarbons and solvents, and it is of paramount importance in anesthesia because it metabolizes all the volatile anesthetics [51]. The prototypic substrate probe is chlorzoxazone and the standard inhibitor is disulfiram (and in vitro its primary metabolite diethyldithiocarbamate). CYP2E1 is highly inducible, both pathophysiologically (obesity, diabetes) and by numerous chemicals. There are mutant CYP2E1 alleles, but they appear to be of little clinical significance. CYP2E1 is the primary enzyme oxidizing the volatile anesthetics halothane, enflurane, isoflurane, sevoflurane, desflurane (most likely), and methoxyflurane, although the last is metabolized by several CYPs. CYP2E1 is responsible for the oxidative metabolic activation of halothane, which results in halothane hepatitis [22,52]. In humans, CYP2E1 is expressed primarily in the liver, but not in the kidney. This may explain in part why, despite hepatic metabolism and defluorination of both methoxyflurane and sevoflurane, methoxyflurane (metabolized by many CYPs) is metabolized in the kidney and is nephrotoxic, while sevoflurane (metabolized only by CYP2E1) is not metabolized in the kidney and is not nephrotoxic [51]. In contrast to the situation in humans, CYP2E1 is expressed in rat kidney. This species difference has implications for interpreting animal models of CYP2E1-mediated anesthetic metabolism and toxicity [53].

Non-P450 enzymes

Esterases

Ester/amide hydrolysis is a ubiquitous reaction catalyzed by a diverse array of enzymes in blood and tissue. Two major enzyme families catalyzing these reactions are carboxylesterases and cholinesterases, both of which are critically important in anesthetic pharmacology.

Carboxylesterases are predominantly microsomal enzymes with wide tissue distribution [54,55]. Human carboxylesterase expression is highest in the liver, and also occurs in the gastro-intestinal tract, brain, and possibly blood. They have a very nonselective substrate specificity and also hydrolyze amides, thereby converting esters and amides to more water-soluble acids, alcohols, and amines that are subsequently eliminated. Microsomal carboxylesterases are inducible by many of the compounds which induce microsomal CYP. Two broad-substrate human liver microsomal carboxylesterases have been isolated (hCE-1 and -2). For example, hCE-1 catalyzes the metabolism of cocaine to benzoylecgonine, meperidine to meperidinic acid (the major metabolite), and heroin (3,6-diacetylmorphine) to 6-monoacetylmorphine, the active metabolite. hCE-2 also hydrolyzes heroin both to 6-monoacetylmorphine and then to morphine.

Human cholinesterases include acetylcholinesterase (AChE) and plasma cholinesterase (also known as serum cholinesterase, pseudocholinesterase, butyrylcholinesterase, and nonspecific cholinesterase) [56,57]. The major function of AChE is to hydrolyze acetylcholine at the neuromuscular junction, thereby terminating synaptic transmission. Two other AChE forms are located in erythrocytes and the brain.

Plasma cholinesterase is widely distributed in blood, liver, and other tissues, and has an unknown physiologic role but great relevance to drug metabolism. It contains two active sites, the anionic site and the esteratic (catalytic) site at which ester hydrolysis actually occurs. Activity is mildly to moderately decreased by pregnancy, liver disease, renal failure, and cardiopulmonary bypass (from hemodilution), and markedly inhibited by ecothiopate, organophosphate pesticides, and reversible inhibitors of AChE (neostigmine, edrophonium, physostigmine, pyridostigmine). Plasma cholinesterase was one of the first enzymes for which pharmacogenetic variation was elucidated, based on heritable interindividual variability in the response to succinylcholine (see Chapter 10) [56].

The prototype substrate for plasma cholinesterase is succinylcholine, which is successively hydrolyzed to succinylmonocholine and to succinic acid. Hydrolysis is rapid, with 90% of a dose metabolized within one minute, and thereby presystemic clearance is substantial and robust (a 70% reduction in enzyme activity only moderately prolongs neuromuscular blockade). Mivacurium is also hydrolyzed by plasma cholinesterase, at a rate 70–90% of that of succinylcholine. Patients with cholinesterase variants respond similarly to mivacurium and succinylcholine. The ester local anesthetics cocaine, procaine, and chloroprocaine are metabolized by plasma cholinesterase. Heroin undergoes extensive deacetylation in blood to 6-monoacetylmorphine, and further hydrolysis to morphine. The former reaction is catalyzed rapidly by plasma cholinesterase, and more slowly by erythrocyte AChE, although the latter reaction accounts for the majority of hydrolysis in vivo, and only erythrocyte AChE can convert 6-monoacetylmorphine to morphine.

Other drugs, including remifentanil and esmolol, also undergo extensive biotransformation and inactivation. Remifentanil is hydrolyzed by nonspecific esterases in plasma and (more so) in tissue, but not by plasma cholinesterase [58]. Hence remifentanil elimination is not altered by pseudocholinesterase deficiency or by hepatic insufficiency [59]. In contrast, and unlike most ester drugs, esmolol metabolism in humans is catalyzed exclusively by esterases in erythrocytes rather than in plasma.

Others

Numerous other enzymes act on xenobiotics, but are quantitatively less important than those above with respect to the metabolism of therapeutic drugs. These include monoamine oxidase. flavin monooxygenase, aldehyde oxidase, alcohol and aldehyde dehydrogenases, the oxidoreductases xanthine oxidase-xanthine dehydrogenase, and epoxide hydrolases.

Phase II enzymes

There are several enzyme families including methyl- and sulfotransferases, acetyl- and acyltransferases, glucuronosyltransferases, and glutathione transferases which directly conjugate drugs, or conjugate their oxidative metabolites.

Glucuronosyltransferase

Uridine diphosphate glucuronosyltransferases (UGTs) are a family of microsomal enzymes that add glucuronic acid to a variety of lipophilic compounds containing phenolic, alcohol, amine, carboxyl, or sulfhydryl groups [60]. UGTs are expressed predominantly in the liver. Glucuronides are more water-soluble than their parent compounds, circulate freely in plasma, and are rapidly excreted in bile or urine (depending on size). Glucuronides may be more or less pharmacologically active than their parent drugs. Since the intestine contains significant amounts of β-glucuronidase, which hydrolyzes glucuronides back to their parent compounds, the free compounds can be intestinally reabsorbed and transported to the liver to undergo re-conjugation and re-excretion; this is referred to as *enterohepatic recirculation*.

There are 15 human UGTs, broadly classified into the UGT1 (phenol/bilirubin) and UGT2 (steroid/bile) families. UGT1As glucuronidate endogenous compounds and a considerable number of drugs (phenols, amines, anthraquinones, flavones). UGT2A and 2B enzymes glucuronidate bile acids, steroids, and retinoids and a few drugs. UGT2B7 has the broadest substrate specificity among 2B isoforms. Glucuronidation is inducible by barbiturates, antiepileptics, and rifampicin, and inhibited by probenecid.

Glucuronidation is an important biotransformation pathway for certain drugs in anesthesia. Glucuronidation by liver and kidney UGT1A9 is the major route of systemic propofol elimination [61]. UGT2B7 glucuronidates a number of opioids such as morphine (both the 3- and 6- positions), codeine, naloxone, nalorphine, buprenorphine, oxymorphone, and hydromorphone [62]. Morphine 6-glucuronidation is particularly important, since this metabolite is more potent than its parent drug, can play a significant role in analgesia, and the finding of UGT2B7 in human brain suggests that in-situ formation of morphine-6-glucuronide may play a role in analgesia [63,64]. The glucuronide of 1-hydroxymidazolam is pharmacologically active, circulates in high concentrations in plasma, is renally excreted, and is thought to underlie the prolonged effects of midazolam in patients with renal insufficiency when used for ICU sedation.

Glutathione-S-transferase

Glutathione-S-transferases (GST) catalyze the reaction of the tripeptide glutathione (gly-cys-glu) with chemically reactive drugs, metabolites, and environmental toxins [65]. GSTs are primarily a defensive system for detoxification and protection against oxidative stress, and hence are abundantly and ubiquitously expressed in most tissues. There are many cytosolic and a few membrane-bound microsomal GSTs. The human soluble cytosolic GSTs are largely responsible for conjugating toxins and drugs.

Conjugation to glutathione generally renders the resulting molecule more water-soluble, less chemically reactive, and more rapidly eliminated. Nonetheless, for a small number of molecules such as halocarbons, glutathione conjugation constitutes a mechanism for bioactivation and toxification, specifically nephrotoxicity [66]. These conjugates are excreted in bile and cleaved into corresponding cysteine conjugates, which may be reabsorbed from the intestine. Cysteine conjugates may be N-acetylated, forming mercapturic acid conjugates, which are nontoxic and excreted in urine. Circulating glutathione and cysteine conjugates and mercapturic acids can be actively taken up by renal proximal tubular cells, where they may undergo bioactivation by the enzyme cysteine conjugate β-lyase to highly reactive intermediates which cause proximal tubular necrosis. This complex multi-organ, multi-enzyme pathway is often referred to as the "β-lyase pathway" [66]. The haloalkene "compound A," which results from sevoflurane degradation by carbon dioxide absorbents, undergoes metabolism by this complex pathway, both in animals and in humans [67–70]. Compound-A nephrotoxicity in rats is attributed to glutathione- and β-lyase-dependent bioactivation. The absence of human compound-A toxicity has been ascribed to species differences in dose and relative metabolism by detoxication (mercapturate formation) versus toxification (β-lyase) pathways [70].

Others

N-acetyl-transferase is a phase II enzyme which N-acetylates many amine-containing drugs (such as isonizaid and procainamide). Genetic polymorphism in N-acetyl-transferase segregates populations into fast and slow acetylators, which may influence therapeutic response and toxicity of some drugs. This pathway is of little importance to anesthetic drugs. Sulfotransferases, which are cytosolic, catalyze the transfer of a sulfate group to numerous endogenous and a small number of exogenous compounds containing amine, phenol, alcohol,

or steroid functionalities. Sulfation is an important pathway in neonates for elimination of paracetamol and morphine.

Extrahepatic metabolism

Intestine

Almost all biotransformation enzymes expressed in the liver are also present in the intestine, albeit at lower content [7,8]. Principle enzymes include the CYPs, esterases, alcohol dehydrogenase, glucuronosyltransferases, sulfotransferases, N-acetyl-transferase, and glutathione transferases. Unlike the liver, which has generally uniform regional distribution of biotransformation activity, many of the enzymes (especially CYPs) are nonuniformly distributed in the intestine, with decreasing content from duodenum to ileum (75% of CYP3A is in the duodenum and jejunum), and a preferential expression at the apical portion of the intestinal villus. CYP3A (3A4, and in some persons 3A5) is the predominant CYP, accounting for most (> 70%) of total intestinal CYP (Fig. 6.2B) [3]. Total intestinal CYP3A4 content is less than that in liver, but higher than in other extrahepatic organs. Liver and gut CYP3A4 are identical proteins, although they are independently regulated and not coordinately expressed. Their substrate profiles, activities, and responses to inducers and inhibitors are generally similar. One notable exception is that grapefruit juice (except in massive doses) inhibits gut but not liver CYP3A. Intestinal metabolism accounts for a significant portion of first-pass clearance of numerous orally administered CYP3A substrates.

Kidney

Human kidneys are fully capable of oxidizing and conjugating drugs [71,72]. They express P450, GSTs, glutathione peroxidase, and glutathione reductase, and flavin monooxygenases, esterases, glucuronyltransferases, N-acetyl-transferases, and cysteine conjugate β-lyase. Most of the extrahepatic glucuronidation in the body is thought to occur in the kidney. Indeed, almost one-third of total-body propofol clearance occurs by renal elimination, probably by intrarenal glucuronidation [73,74]. Total human kidney CYP content is approximately an order of magnitude less than in the liver. CYP3A enzymes are the most abundant human renal CYPs, with 3A5 predominant and both 3A4 and 3A5 variably expressed [33,75]. Although total renal microsomal CYP3A content (per mg protein) is 2–3 orders of magnitude less than that of liver, the specific content of CYP3A in proximal tubular cells (where CYPs are exclusively located) approximates that in hepatocytes. Renal CYP3As are fully competent to metabolize hepatic CYP3A substrates, and are thought to contribute significantly to the metabolism and/or clearance of drugs such as cyclosporine and methoxyflurane [76,77].

Human and rat kidneys differ markedly in their expression of P450s and GSTs. Human kidneys express mainly CYPs 3A and 4A [72,78]. In contrast, rat kidneys express a considerable number of CYP isoforms [79]. An important difference is the absence of CYP2E1 in human kidneys, particularly in comparison to human liver, where it constitutes about 7% of total P450, and in rat kidneys, where it is highly expressed. This is important because CYP2E1 is the major isoform responsible for the metabolism of most volatile anesthetics. The ability of human kidneys to metabolize methoxyflurane but not sevoflurane, explained by the metabolism of the former by several P450s (including renal CYP3A) but the latter only by CYP2E1 (which is not present in human kidneys), is thought potentially to underlie the nephrotoxicity of methoxyflurane but not sevoflurane in humans, despite their similar hepatic metabolism [77].

Other

Human brain is known to express P450s from all three major families, although there are regioselective and isoform-selective differences in expression [80]. Cerebral P450 activity is low, does not contribute to systemic drug elimination, but may contribute to the blood–brain barrier and biosynthesis of signaling molecules, and a few studies have shown the ability of human brain to metabolize psychotropic drugs.

The lung is a major target organ for inhaled therapeutic drugs, the obvious site of inhaled anesthetics delivery, and nasal and inhaled drug delivery are an increasingly pursued alternative for systemic drug administration. The major phase I and II enzymes are expressed in human lung, and may participate in pulmonary first-pass metabolism, elimination, and toxification [72,81].

Biotransformation and age

Pediatrics

Drug disposition, dosing, response, and adverse effects are substantially different in children and adults [82], with differences in biotransformation, and consequently pharmacokinetics, a major reason [83,84]. The fetus is fully competent to metabolize hormones and drugs, and the liver is the main site of fetal biotransformation, catalyzing both phase I and phase II reactions. There are significant age-dependent differences in biotransformation, with the greatest changes occurring between birth and age 2 for phase I enzymes, and birth and adolescence for phase II pathways, with comparatively minimal changes in activity between childhood and adulthood [83].

Fetal and neonatal biotransformation is less than in infants and adults. Anesthetic drugs with reduced clearance or metabolism in neonates include diazepam, midazolam, fentanyl, morphine, paracetamol, and naloxone [85]. Total hepatic CYP concentration at birth is approximately half that of adults, and the individual CYP isoforms mature at different rates. Maturation of drug-metabolizing enzymes, rather than changes in hepatic size or blood flow, is considered to be the major factor responsible for these changes. Fetal drug metabolism is unique, because the more water-soluble metabolites produced by oxidation and conjugation do not readily cross the placenta back to the mother, thereby prolonging fetal exposure.

Information on the individual drug-metabolizing enzymes in pediatrics and the developmental aspects of biotransformation has grown exponentially in the past decade, and a detailed presentation is beyond this chapter, but generalities are addressable [83,84]. One group of enzymes (typified by CYP3A7, flavin monooxygenase, and sulfotransferases) have their highest expression in the first trimester, remain at high concentrations or decrease during gestation, and are lower or silenced by age 2. Another group (CYP3A5, CYP2C19, certain sulfotransferases) has relatively constant expression through gestation, and CYP2C19 increases within the first year. Most enzymes (CYPs 2A2, 2C9, 2D6, 2E1, 3A4, aldehyde dehydrogenase, and certain sulfotransferases) are missing or expressed minimally in the fetus, with onset of expression often in the second or third trimester, with substantial increases in expression in the first 1–2 years after birth. Increases in CYP during the neonatal period (< 4 weeks) are attributable primarily to CYP2C isoforms.

CYP3A isoforms undergo the greatest and most complex pattern of maturation, termed a "developmental switch" [84]. CYP3A7 is the major isoform present in human embryonic, fetal, and newborn liver (Fig. 6.5A) [86]. It is expressed most abundantly in gestation and declines rapidly after birth to less than 10% of newborn levels by 3–12 months. Fetal CYP3A4 expression is minimal, but it rises immediately after birth, concomitant with the decline in CYP3A7. CYP3A4 activity reaches 30–50% of adult levels in the first 2–5 years (Fig. 6.5B) [87]. CYP3A7 is also expressed in the placenta and pregnant endometrium. Although CYP3A7 has high sequence similarity to CYP3A4, and metabolizes several 3A4 substrates, activity towards most substrates and some hormones is considerably less than that of CYP3A4.

Morphine biotransformation illustrates important developmental differences in phase II metabolism, such as glucuronidation and sulfation [83]. Fetal and neonatal hepatic glucuronidation is immature, < 10–30% of adult activity, and does not mature for several years into childhood. Morphine glucuronidation and clearance increase with both gestational and postnatal age. In contrast, sulfotransferase activity is mature at birth, and can compensate for impaired glucuronidation. Morphine is preferentially sulfated in neonates, but preferentially glucuronidated in adults.

Pregnancy

Fetal drug metabolism, described above, occurs within the greater context of pregnancy [88,89]. Pregnancy increases maternal hepatic activity of CYPs 2A6, 2C9, 2D6 and 3A4, and UGTs 1A and 2B7, while CYPs 1A2 and 2C19 are decreased, altering drug disposition. The placenta is relatively devoid of phase I enzymes, but rich in phase II enzymes and drug transporters which affect fetal drug exposure.

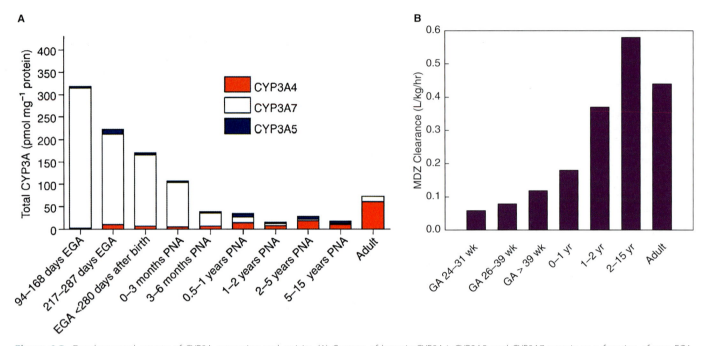

Figure 6.5. Developmental aspects of CYP3A expression and activity. (A) Content of hepatic CYP3A4, CYP3A5, and CYP3A7 protein as a function of age. EGA, estimated gestational age; PNA, postnatal age. Reproduced with permission from Stevens [86] (B) Clearance of the CYP3A4 probe midazolam (MDZ). GA, gestational age. Redrawn with permission from de Wildt et al. [87].

Geriatrics

Like many physiologic functions in geriatrics, clinical drug biotransformation represent the combined influence of normal aging, disease, environment, and drug interactions [90–92]. Hepatic size and liver blood flow decline with age, and clearance of many drugs appears to decline in healthy aging in parallel with reduced liver volume. Nonetheless, biotransformation in the aging liver does not decline similarly for all enzymes, pathways and drugs, and there is increased interindividual variability with aging. In general, the activity of phase I reactions declines with age, particularly esterases. Some, but not all, studies suggest decreased activity of hepatic CYP isoforms. In contrast, phase II reactions are considered to be relatively unchanged.

Interindividual and intraindividual variability in drug metabolism

Variability is a significant clinical issue which can markedly affect drug disposition and response [93]. Variability can often result in > 100-fold ranges in drug exposure (area under the concentration–time curve), potentially even rendering patients nonresponsive to certain drugs or causing toxicity. Causes of interindividual variability include genetics (sex, race, ethnicity, enzyme polymorphisms), age, environment (diet, smoking, ethanol, solvent or other xenobiotic exposure), disease, and drug interactions. Many of the genetic causes of variability have been addressed above.

Applied clearance concepts

Understanding the influence of disease and drug interactions on hepatic drug elimination requires further explication of the basic concept of hepatic clearance (CL_H), the product of hepatic blood flow (Q_H) and hepatic extraction ratio (E_H) of a drug (Eqs. 6.1, 6.5). Drugs can be categorized by the efficiency of their removal by the liver, as high- ($E_H > 0.7$), intermediate- ($0.3 < E_H < 0.7$), or low-extraction ($E_H < 0.3$) drugs. For high-extraction drugs, $Q_H << f_u \cdot CL_{int}$ and therefore CL_H approaches Q_H, because the efficiency of extraction is so great that Q_H is a more rate-limiting factor than metabolism. The systemic clearance of high-extraction drugs is "flow-limited," depends on Q_H, and will be sensitive to changes in Q_H but insensitive to changes in metabolism (CL_{int}). High-extraction drugs have low oral bioavailability because of extensive first-pass hepatic metabolism. For low-extraction drugs, $Q_H >> f_u \cdot CL_{int}$ and therefore CL_H approaches $f_u \cdot CL_{int}$. Thus the systemic clearance of low-extraction drugs is "capacity-limited," depends on CL_{int}, and is highly susceptible to even small changes in CL_{int}. Low-extraction drugs have a high oral bioavailability. The extraction ratios of commonly used anesthetics are shown in Table 6.4.

Drug interactions

Metabolic drug–drug and drug–diet interactions are a major source of both inter- and intraindividual variability in drug disposition, clinical response, and toxicity [7,94–96]. Such interactions are hepatic, intestinal, or both (Fig. 6.3), and occur most with phase I reactions (specifically CYP). CYP induction (usually increased expression, although decreased degradation can occur with CYP2E1) results in increased enzyme activity. CYP inhibition can be noncompetitive or competitive. CYP inhibitors and inducers are classified as weak, moderate, or strong, corresponding to a 1.25-, 2-, or 5-fold change in the plasma area under the concentration–time curve (AUC), and corresponding to a 20–50%, 50–80%, or > 80% change in clearance. Drug interactions are constantly being discovered, and review articles may not be as current as websites, such as one maintained particularly for this purpose [18].

The kinetic consequences of enzyme inhibition and induction are dependent on the extraction ratio and route of administration of the drug [4]. For example, systemic clearance of the low-extraction opioid alfentanil is exquisitely sensitive to hepatic CYP3A induction and inhibition, while that of the high-extraction opioids fentanyl and sufentanil is less affected (Fig. 6.6) [97,98]. For orally administered drugs, the changes in AUC with induction and inhibition will always be greater than those after IV administration, particularly for intermediate- and high-extraction drugs. In addition, the differences in the percentage change in the AUC after oral versus IV administration are greater for high- than with low-extraction drugs. The influence of CYP3A induction and inhibition on the metabolic elimination and clinical sedation

of midazolam, and the greater effect after oral versus IV administration, is shown in Fig. 6.7 [97,99].

The role of biotransformation, pharmacogenetics, and drug interactions in interindividual variability in drug disposition and response is illustrated by codeine, a prodrug requiring CYP2D6-mediated metabolic activation (O-demethylation) to the μ-opioid agonist morphine, and further UGT2B7-mediated metabolism to the agonist morphine-6-glucuronide [36]. CYP2D6-deficient individuals are poor metabolizers (PMs) of codeine, with markedly diminished or absent morphine formation and minimal if any analgesia (Fig. 6.8A) [100]. Conversely, individuals with CYP2D6 gene duplication (ultrarapid metabolizers) have greater morphine formation, and may be predisposed to toxicity. Ethnic variations attributable to codeine biotransformation have also been observed. For example, Chinese subjects produced less morphine from codeine, were less sensitive to the opioid effects of codeine, and might therefore experience reduced analgesia from codeine [101,102]. The metabolic drug interaction with the CYP2D6 inhibitor quinidine markedly diminishes codeine bioactivation and morphine formation (Fig. 6.8B) [103]. Interactions at pathways other than bioactivation or inactivation can also have metabolic consequence. For example, rifampicin induction of CYP3A4 increased codeine N-demethylation (Fig. 6.4), making less codeine available for O-demethylation, and thereby decreasing the formation of morphine [104].

Pharmacogenetics

It is clear from the preceding information that genetics can be a major contributor to interpatient variability in drug metabolism and drug response, both therapeutic and toxic. Clinical tests for determining CYP polymorphisms are now technologically available, and can be highly effective in individualizing drug selection and dosing, particularly of drugs with a narrow therapeutic index [105]. Nevertheless, their clinical implementation is limited and their practical utility is not yet clear [48,106]. It is likely that genetic testing will become more ubiquitous, if not required by regulatory agencies, towards the goal of "personalized medicine." Likely candidates are warfarin

Table 6.4. Hepatic extraction of some commonly used drugs

Low extraction ($E_H < 0.3$)	thiopental, diazepam, lorazepam, triazolam, theophylline, alfentanil, methadone
Intermediate extraction	methohexital, midazolam, vecuronium, rocuronium, ropivacaine, mepivacaine, hydromorphone
High extraction ($E_H > 0.7$)	etomidate, propofol, ketamine, bupivacaine, lidocaine, metoprolol, propranolol, labetolol, fentanyl, sufentanil, remifentanil, meperidine, morphine, naloxone

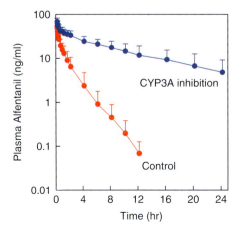

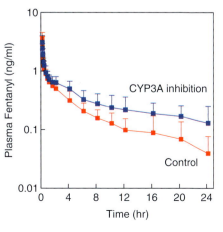

Figure 6.6. Influence of hepatic extraction ratio of the consequence of a drug interaction. CYP3A activity and intrinsic clearance were reduced by administering the CYP3A inhibitor troleandomycin prior to IV injection of the opioids alfentanil (low-extraction) or fentanyl (high-extraction). Alfentanil clearance was inhibited 88% (from 5.5 ± 2.2 to 0.6 ± 0.2 mL kg^{-1} min^{-1}) while fentanyl clearance was reduced by only 40% (from 15.3 ± 5.0 to 9.4 ± 3.1 mL kg^{-1} min^{-1}). Redrawn with permission from Ibrahim et al. [98].

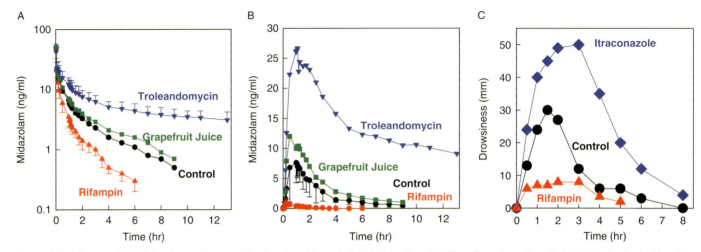

Figure 6.7. Influence of CYP3A drug interactions on midazolam disposition and clinical effects. (A and B) Effect of hepatic and intestinal CYP3A induction by rifampicin, hepatic and intestinal CYP3A inhibition by troleandomycin, and selective intestinal CYP3A inhibition by grapefruit juice on plasma of midazolam concentrations after (A) IV midazolam 1 mg and (B) oral midazolam 3 mg. Redrawn with permission from Kharasch *et al.* [97]. (C) Effect of hepatic and intestinal CYP3A induction by rifampicin, and hepatic and intestinal CYP3A inhibition by itraconazole on sedation after 15 mg oral midazolam. Redrawn with permission from Backman *et al.* [99].

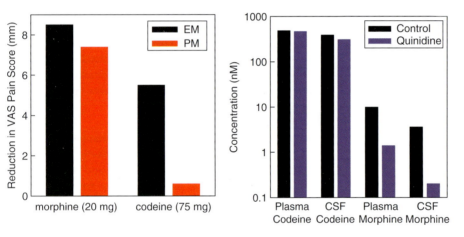

Figure 6.8. Influence of CYP2D6 activity on codeine metabolism and analgesia. (A) Pharmacogenetic effects. Shown are the median of the peak changes in peak pain during a cold pressor test in CYP2D6 extensive (EM) and poor (PM) metabolizers who received morphine or codeine. Morphine analgesia was the same in EMs and PMs. Plasma codeine concentrations were not different in PMs and EMs, but morphine and morphine-6-glucuronide were undetectable in plasma of PMs. Codeine reduced pain only in the EMs. Redrawn with permission from Poulsen *et al.* [100]. (B) Drug interaction effects. Median plasma and cerebrospinal fluid (CSF) concentrations of codeine and morphine in 17 patients 2 h after 125 mg oral codeine without or with CYP2D6 inhibition by pretreatment with 200 mg oral quinidine. Codeine concentrations were not different, but CYP2D6 inhibition reduced morphine concentrations. Redrawn with permission from Sindrup *et al.* [114].

therapy (*CYP2C9*) and antineoplastic drugs (*CYP2D6* for tamoxifen therapy of breast cancer, thiopurine methyltransferase for 6-mercaptopurine and azathioprine, and *UGT1A1* for irinotecan) [106].

Biotransformation in disease

Liver disease can markedly affect drug biotransformation, with significant clinical consequences, including for anesthesia [107]. A discussion of hepatic disease and pharmacokinetics in general is found in other chapters. Impaired drug metabolism in chronic liver disease can result from reduced liver mass, reduced enzymatic activity in remaining hepatocytes, or diminished hepatic blood flow. There is nonhomogeneous and variable reduction in the activity of various CYP isoforms with worsening liver disease, with the earliest and most profound reductions in the order CYP2C19 > 1A2 > 2D6 > 2E1, with 3A4/5 also very significantly affected [108]. CYP activity

is diminished more than phase II conjugation activity (glucuronidation) in mild–moderate cirrhosis because of greater susceptibility to the relative hypoxemia in cirrhosis, but glucuronidation is impaired in advanced disease. Worsening liver disease (based on the Child–Pugh classification) is generally associated with greater reduction in intrinsic clearance than in hepatic blood flow. Evaluation of biotransformation capabilities of orthotopic liver transplants, in comparison with age-matched controls, found the clinical activities of CYPs 2C19 and 2D6 lower, CYPs 1A2 and 3A4 unchanged, and CYP2E1 greater, measured one month after transplant [109]. The consequence of liver disease on hepatic drug clearance will depend, as it does for drug interactions, on the extraction ratio of a drug, as well as on disease severity. Hepatic clearance of low-extraction drugs (e.g., alfentanil) is diminished even with mild–moderate disease, while that of high-extraction drugs (e.g., morphine, lidocaine) is relatively unchanged. More severe liver disease, such as cirrhosis with alterations in Q_H and portosystemic shunting, will have a significant impact on the CL_H of high-extraction drugs.

Kidney disease reduces glomerular filtration rate and therefore the renal clearance of drugs which are eliminated entirely or partly by the kidney, with consequently altered pharmacokinetics. While it is well understood that such drugs require dose adjustment in patients with acute or chronic renal failure, it was widely assumed that drugs cleared by hepatic metabolism and transport (nonrenal clearance) were unaffected by renal disease. That notion has been refuted, and it is now clear that renal failure affects intestinal absorption and first-pass metabolism, hepatic metabolism and clearance, and hepatic, intestinal, and renal transport, with the clinical consequence of altered nonrenal clearance (30–90% reduction) and bioavailability (70–100% increase) [110,111]. Circulating uremic factors (some of which are dialyzable) are thought to cause chronic inflammation and cytokine upregulation, leading to downregulation of hepatic and intestinal CYP, phase II conjugation enzymes, and transporters. For example, morphine glucuronidation is significantly impaired in chronic renal failure, but midazolam clearance (reflecting hepatic CYP3A activity) is unaffected. Patients with renal insufficiency should not be assumed to have normal drug biotransformation and clearance.

Systemic diseases such as infection and inflammation diminish the expression and activity of CYPs and other drug-metabolizing enzymes, with consequently altered drug clearance [112,113]. This is thought to be secondary to increased cytokine production and suppression of transcription. Hepatic and intestinal drug metabolism can be suppressed by both acute and chronic inflammation. It appears that CYPs can be regulated by multiple cytokines, that the CYP isoforms regulated by individual cytokines differ, and thus the drugs whose disposition is altered may vary with the acute inflammatory stimulus, chronic disease, or the immunomodulatory drug.

Summary

Biotransformation, or drug metabolism, is a major determinant of drug bioavailability, clearance, clinical effect, and toxicity. This is a complex and diverse field which has undergone explosive growth in the last two decades owing to the application of molecular biology and genetic techniques to a traditionally more chemically oriented discipline. The entire process of drug disposition (pharmacokinetics) encompasses absorption, distribution, metabolism, and elimination ("ADME"), and sometimes includes toxicity ("ADMET"), because toxicity often relates to biotransformation. Drug metabolism is not an isolated pharmacokinetic phenomenon. For example, metabolism is often the major route of drug elimination, and metabolism can occur in intestinal epithelia right after drug absorption, affecting "net" absorption, or bioavailability. The liver is the primary site of biotransformation, and renal metabolism may be significant for certain drugs.

In drug development, elucidation of biotransformation pathways and mechanisms now occurs early in the development timeline, and regulatory agencies now require considerable information about drug metabolism and drug interactions. Information on the latter, which was traditionally gathered over long periods of clinical use via reports of adverse drug reactions, is now prospectively determined from in-vitro enzyme systems and clinical models of biotransformation. Far more is known about the metabolism of recently developed drugs than those developed decades ago.

Metabolism plays a prominent role in the disposition of numerous drugs used in anesthesia, including opioids (fentanyl, alfentanil, sufentanil, remifentanil, morphine, codeine, oxycodone, hydrocodone, hydromorphone, dextromethorphan, meperidine, methadone), sedative-hypnotics (propofol, fospropofol, thiopental, methohexital), benzodiazepines (midazolam, triazolam, diazepam, alprazolam), local anesthetics (lidocaine, bupivacaine, ropivacaine, procaine, chloroprocaine, cocaine), neuromuscular blockers (succinylcholine, rocuronium, vecuronium, pancuronium, mivacurium, (cis-)atracurium), and volatile anesthetics (particularly the more soluble ones). Metabolism is central to the mechanism by which methoxyflurane caused renal failure, halothane caused hepatitis, and meperidine can cause seizures.

Drug metabolism can result in bioactivation of an inactive prodrug, formation of an active or inactive metabolite, or occasionally a toxic metabolite. Phase I metabolism chemically modifies the drug structure, and phase II metabolism adds an endogenous molecule to the drug or metabolite to render it even more water-soluble for elimination. The cytochrome P450 (CYP) enzyme system is the most important for metabolizing therapeutic drugs, and the CYPs most relevant to anesthesiology are CYP2B6, CYP2D6, CYP2E1, and CYP3A. Esterases are also important in clinical anesthesia. Drug metabolism has been deliberately exploited in anesthetic development to target routes or sites of metabolism, develop prodrugs, and accelerate or retard rates of drug inactivation.

Drug metabolism is also a major determinant of interindividual variability in drug effect, due to pharmacogenetic differences and drug interactions. Indeed, pharmacogenetics as a discipline has its roots in drugs used in anesthesia. Interindividual variability in drug metabolism, potentially resulting in > 100-fold ranges in drug exposure, is a significant clinical issue which can markedly affect drug pharmacokinetics, clinical response, and toxicity. Causes of variability include genetics (sex, race, ethnicity, and genetic polymorphisms in enzyme activity), age, environment (diet, smoking, chemical exposure), disease, and drug interactions. Biotransformation activity at the extremes of age differs, increasing from fetal to age 2 and declining in the elderly. Hepatic drug biotransformation may be impaired directly in hepatic disease, and indirectly in renal disease. Understanding drug metabolism is essential for understanding anesthetic pharmacokinetics, clinical effects, and side effects, and for individualizing patient care.

References

1. Zanger UM, Turpeinen M, Klein K, Schwab M. Functional pharmacogenetics/genomics of human cytochromes P450 involved in drug biotransformation. *Anal Bioanal Chem* 2008; **392**: 1093–108.

2. Rowland-Yeo K, Rostami-Hodjegan A, Tucker GT. Abundance of cytochromes P450 in human liver: a meta analysis. *Br J Clin Pharmacol* 2004; **57**: 687–8.

3. Paine MF, Hart HL, Ludington SS, *et al.* The human intestinal cytochrome P450 "pie". *Drug Metab Dispos* 2006; **34**: 880–6.

4. Wilkinson GR. Clearance approaches in pharmacology. *Pharmacol Rev* 1987; **39**: 1–47.

5. Baker M, Parton T. Kinetic determinants of hepatic clearance: plasma protein binding and hepatic uptake. *Xenobiotica* 2007; **37**: 1110–34.

6. Bailey DG, Dresser GK. Natural products and adverse drug interactions. *CMAJ* 2004; **170**: 1531–2.

7. Kaminsky LS, Zhang QY. The small intestine as a xenobiotic-metabolizing organ. *Drug Metab Dispos* 2003; **31**: 1520–5.

8. Galetin A, Gertz M, Houston JB. Potential role of intestinal first-pass metabolism in the prediction of drug–drug interactions. *Expert Opin Drug Metab Toxicol* 2008; **4**: 909–22.

9. Levy RH, Thummel KE, Trager WF, Hansten PD, Eichelbaum M, eds. *Metabolic Drug Interactions.* Philadelphia, PA: Lippincott, Williams & Wilkins, 2000.

10. Gibson GG, Skett P. *Introduction to Drug Metabolism*, 3rd edn. Cheltenham: Nelson Thornes Publishers, 2001.

11. Wilkinson GR. Drug metabolism and variability among patients in drug response. *N Engl J Med* 2005; **352**: 2211–21.

12. Strolin Benedetti M, Whomsley R, Baltes E. Involvement of enzymes other than CYPs in the oxidative metabolism of xenobiotics. *Expert Opin Drug Metab Toxicol* 2006; **2**: 895–921.

13. Ingelman-Sundberg M, Sim SC, Gomez A, Rodriguez-Antona C. Influence of cytochrome P450 polymorphisms on drug therapies: pharmacogenetic, pharmacoepigenetic and clinical aspects. *Pharmacol Ther* 2007; **116**: 496–526.

14. Pelkonen O, Turpeinen M, Hakkola J, *et al.* Inhibition and induction of human cytochrome P450 enzymes: current status. *Arch Toxicol* 2008; **82**: 667–715.

15. Kramer SD, Testa B. The biochemistry of drug metabolism: an introduction. Part 6. Inter-individual factors affecting drug metabolism. *Chem Biodivers* 2008; **5**: 2465–578.

16. Guengerich FP. Cytochrome P450s and other enzymes in drug metabolism and toxicity. *AAPS J* 2006; **8**: E101–11.

17. Nelson DR. The cytochrome P450 homepage. *Hum Genomics* 2009; **4**: 59–65. http://drnelson.uthsc.edu/CytochromeP450.html (accessed May 11, 2010).

18. Flockhart DA. Drug interactions: cytochrome P450 drug interaction table. Indiana University School of Medicine (2007). http://medicine.iupui.edu/clinpharm/ddis/table.asp (accessed May 11, 2010).

19. Ekins S, Stresser DM, Williams JA. *In vitro* and pharmacophore insights into CYP3A enzymes. *Trends Pharmacol Sci* 2003; **24**: 161–6.

20. Sharer JE, Wrighton SA. Identification of the human hepatic cytochromes P450 involved in the *in vitro* oxidation of antipyrine. *Drug Metab Dispos* 1996; **24**: 487–94.

21. Niwa T, Murayama N, Emoto C, Yamazaki H. Comparison of kinetic parameters for drug oxidation rates and substrate inhibition potential mediated by cytochrome P450 3A4 and 3A5. *Curr Drug Metab* 2008; **9**: 20–33.

22. Kharasch ED. Adverse drug reactions with halogenated anesthetics. *Clin Pharmacol Ther* 2008; **84**: 158–62.

23. Oda Y, Furuichi K, Tanaka K, *et al.* Metabolism of a new local anesthetic, ropivacaine, by human hepatic cytochrome P450. *Anesthesiology* 1995; **82**: 214–20.

24. Harper TW, Brassil PJ. Reaction phenotyping: current industry efforts to identify enzymes responsible for metabolizing drug candidates. *AAPS J* 2008; **10**: 200–7.

25. Madan A, Usuki E, Burton LA, Ogilvie BW, Parkinson A. In vitro approaches for studying the inhibition of drug-metabolizing enzymes and identifying the drug-metabolizing enzymes responsible for the metabolism of drugs. In: Rodrigues AD, ed., *Drug–Drug Interactions.* New York, NY: Marcel Dekker, 2002: 217–94.

26. Streetman DS, Bertino JS, Nafziger AN. Phenotyping of drug-metabolizing enzymes in adults: a review of in-vivo cytochrome P450 phenotyping probes. *Pharmacogenetics* 2000; **10**: 187–216.

27. Fuhr U, Jetter A, Kirchheiner J. Appropriate phenotyping procedures for drug metabolizing enzymes and transporters in humans and their simultaneous use in the "cocktail" approach. *Clin Pharmacol Ther* 2007; **81**: 270–83.

28. Burk O, Wojnowski L. Cytochrome P450 3A and their regulation. *Naunyn Schmiedebergs Arch Pharmacol* 2004; **369**: 105–24.

29. Daly AK. Significance of the minor cytochrome P450 3A isoforms. *Clin Pharmacokinet* 2006; **45**: 13–31.

30. Plant N. The human cytochrome P450 sub-family: transcriptional regulation, inter-individual variation and interaction networks. *Biochim Biophys Acta* 2007; **1770**: 478–88.

31. Wojnowski L, Kamdem LK. Clinical implications of CYP3A polymorphisms. *Expert Opin Drug Metab Toxicol* 2006; **2**: 171–82.

32. Kharasch ED, Walker A, Isoherranen N, *et al.* Influence of CYP3A5 genotype on the pharmacokinetics and pharmacodynamics of the cytochrome P4503A probes alfentanil and midazolam. *Clin Pharmacol Ther* 2007; **82**: 410–26.

33. Haehner BD, Gorski JC, Vandenbranden M, *et al.* Bimodal distribution of renal cytochrome P450 3A activity in humans. *Mol Pharmacol* 1996; **50**: 52–9.

34. Zanger UM, Raimundo S, Eichelbaum M. Cytochrome P450 2D6: overview and update on pharmacology, genetics, biochemistry. *Naunyn Schmiedebergs Arch Pharmacol* 2004; **369**: 23–37.

35. Ingelman-Sundberg M. Genetic polymorphisms of cytochrome P450

2D6 (CYP2D6): clinical consequences, evolutionary aspects and functional diversity. *Pharmacogenomics J* 2005; **5**: 6–13.

36. Madadi P, Koren G. Pharmacogenetic insights into codeine analgesia: implications to pediatric codeine use. *Pharmacogenomics* 2008; **9**: 1267–84.

37. Zanger UM, Klein K, Saussele T, *et al.* Polymorphic CYP2B6: molecular mechanisms and emerging clinical significance. *Pharmacogenomics* 2007; **8**: 743–59.

38. Wang H, Tompkins LM. CYP2B6: new insights into a historically overlooked cytochrome P450 isozyme. *Curr Drug Metab* 2008; **9**: 598–610.

39. Turpeinen M, Raunio H, Pelkonen O. The functional role of CYP2B6 in human drug metabolism: substrates and inhibitors in vitro, in vivo and in silico. *Curr Drug Metab* 2006; **7**: 705–14.

40. Court MH, Duan SX, Hesse LM, Venkatakrishnan K, Greenblatt DJ. Cytochrome P-450 2B6 is responsible for interindividual variability of propofol hydroxylation by human liver microsomes. *Anesthesiology* 2001; **94**: 110–9.

41. Yanagihara Y, Kariya S, Ohtani M, *et al.* Involvement of CYP2B6 in N-demethylation of ketamine in human liver microsomes. *Drug Metab Dispos* 2001; **29**: 887–90.

42. Kharasch ED, Hoffer C, Whittington D, Sheffels P. Role of hepatic and intestinal cytochrome P450 3A and 2B6 in the metabolism, disposition and miotic effects of methadone. *Clin Pharmacol Ther* 2004; **76**: 250–69.

43. Kharasch ED, Bedynek PS, Park S, *et al.* Mechanism of ritonavir changes in methadone pharmacokinetics and pharmacodynamics. I. Evidence against CYP3A mediation of methadone clearance. *Clin Pharmacol Ther* 2008; **84**: 497–505.

44. Totah RA, Sheffels P, Roberts T, *et al.* Role of CYP2B6 in stereoselective human methadone metabolism. *Anesthesiology* 2007; **108**: 363–74.

45. Gunes A, Dahl ML. Variation in CYP1A2 activity and its clinical implications: influence of environmental factors and genetic polymorphisms. *Pharmacogenomics* 2008; **9**: 625–37.

46. Satarug S, Tassaneeyakul W, Na-Bangchang K, Cashman JR, Moore MR. Genetic and environmental influences on therapeutic and toxicity outcomes: studies with CYP2A6. *Curr Clin Pharmacol* 2006; **1**: 291–309.

47. Goldstein JA. Clinical relevance of genetic polymorphisms in the human CYP2C subfamily. *Br J Clin Pharmacol* 2001; **52**: 349–55.

48. Gage B, Eby C, Johnson J, *et al.* Use of pharmacogenetic and clinical factors to predict the therapeutic dose of warfarin. *Clin Pharmacol Ther* 2008; **84**: 326–31.

49. Cederbaum AI. CYP2E1–biochemical and toxicological aspects and role in alcohol-induced liver injury. *Mt Sinai J Med* 2006; **73**: 657–72.

50. Gonzalez FJ. The 2006 Bernard B. Brodie Award Lecture. CYP2E1. *Drug Metab Dispos* 2007; **35**: 1–8.

51. Kharasch ED, Thummel KE. Identification of cytochrome P450 2E1 as the predominant enzyme catalyzing human liver microsomal defluorination of sevoflurane, isoflurane and methoxyflurane. *Anesthesiology* 1993; **79**: 795–807.

52. Kharasch ED, Hankins D, Mautz D, Thummel KE. Identification of the enzyme responsible for oxidative halothane metabolism: implications for prevention of halothane hepatitis. *Lancet* 1996; **347**: 1367–71.

53. Kharasch ED, Schroeder JL, Liggitt HD, *et al.* New insights into the mechanism of methoxyflurane nephrotoxicity and implications for anesthetic development I. Identification of the nephrotoxic metabolic pathway. *Anesthesiology* 2006; **105**: 726–36.

54. Imai T, Taketani M, Shii M, Hosokawa M, Chiba K. Substrate specificity of carboxylesterase isozymes and their contribution to hydrolase activity in human liver and small intestine. *Drug Metab Dispos* 2006; **34**: 1734–41.

55. Imai T. Human carboxylesterase isozymes: catalytic properties and rational drug design. *Drug Metab Pharmacokinet* 2006; **21**: 173–85.

56. Davis L, Britten JJ, Morgan M. Cholinesterase. Its significance in anaesthetic practice. *Anaesthesia* 1997; **52**: 244–60.

57. Liederer BM, Borchardt RT. Enzymes involved in the bioconversion of ester-based prodrugs. *J Pharm Sci* 2006; **95**: 1177–95.

58. Manullang J, Egan TD. Remifentanil's effect is not prolonged in a patient with pseudocholinesterase deficiency. *Anesth Analg* 1999; **89**: 529–30.

59. Dershwitz M, Hoke JF, Rosow CE, *et al.* Pharmacokinetics and pharmacodynamics of remifentanil in volunteer subjects with severe liver disease. *Anesthesiology* 1996; **84**: 812–20.

60. Kiang TK, Ensom MH, Chang TK. UDP-glucuronosyltransferases and clinical drug–drug interactions. *Pharmacol Ther* 2005; **106**: 97–132.

61. Favetta P, Degoute CS, Perdrix JP, *et al.* Propofol metabolites in man following propofol induction and maintenance. *Br J Anaesth* 2002; **88**: 653–8.

62. Coffman BL, Rios GR, King CD, Tephly TR. Human UGT2B7 catalyzes morphine glucuronidation. *Drug Metab Dispos* 1997; **25**: 1–4.

63. King CD, Rios GR, Assouline JA, Tephly TR. Expression of UDP-glucuronosyltransferases (UGTs) 2B7 and 1A6 in the human brain and identification of 5-hydroxytryptamine as a substrate. *Arch Biochem Biophys* 1999; **365**: 156–62.

64. van Dorp EL, Romberg R, Sarton E, Bovill JG, Dahan A. Morphine-6-glucuronide: morphine's successor for postoperative pain relief? *Anesth Analg* 2006; **102**: 1789–97.

65. Frova C. Glutathione transferases in the genomics era: new insights and perspectives. *Biomol Eng* 2006; **23**: 149–69.

66. Anders MW. Formation and toxicity of anesthetic degradation products. *Annu Rev Pharmacol Toxicol* 2005; **45**: 147–76.

67. Jin L, Baillie TA, Davis MR, Kharasch ED. Nephrotoxicity of sevoflurane compound A [fluoromethyl-2,2-difluoro-1-(trifluoromethyl)vinyl ether] in rats: evidence for glutathione and cysteine conjugate formation and the role of renal cysteine conjugate

β-lyase. *Biochem Biophys Res Commun* 1995; **210**: 498–506.

68. Iyer RA, Frink EJ, Ebert TJ, Anders MW. Cysteine conjugate β-lyase-dependent metabolism of compound A (2-[fluoromethoxy]-1,1,3,3,3-pentafluoro-1-propene) in human subjects anesthetized with sevoflurane and in rats given compound A. *Anesthesiology* 1998; **88**: 611–18.

69. Kharasch ED, Thorning DT, Garton K, Hankins DC, Kilty CG. Role of renal cysteine conjugate b-lyase in the mechanism of compound A nephrotoxicity in rats. *Anesthesiology* 1997; **86**: 160–71.

70. Kharasch ED, Jubert C. Compound A uptake and metabolism to mercapturic acids and 3,3,3-trifluoro-2-fluoromethoxypropanoic acid during low-flow sevoflurane anesthesia. Biomarkers for exposure, risk assessment, and interspecies comparison. *Anesthesiology* 1999; **91**: 1267–78.

71. Lohr JW, Willsky GR, Acara MA. Renal drug metabolism. *Pharmacol Rev* 1998; **50**: 107–41.

72. Pavek P, Dvorak Z. Xenobiotic-induced transcriptional regulation of xenobiotic metabolizing enzymes of the cytochrome P450 superfamily in human extrahepatic tissues. *Curr Drug Metab* 2008; **9**: 129–43.

73. Hiraoka H, Yamamoto K, Miyoshi S, *et al*. Kidneys contribute to the extrahepatic clearance of propofol in humans, but not lungs and brain. *Br J Clin Pharmacol* 2005; **60**: 176–82.

74. McGurk KA, Brierley CH, Burchell B. Drug glucuronidation by human renal UDP-glucuronosyltransferases. *Biochem Pharmacol* 1998; **55**: 1005–12.

75. Lash LH, Putt DA, Cai H. Drug metabolism enzyme expression and activity in primary cultures of human proximal tubular cells. *Toxicology* 2008; **244**: 56–65.

76. Dai Y, Iwanaga K, Lin YS, *et al*. In vitro metabolism of cyclosporine A by human kidney CYP3A5. *Biochem Pharmacol* 2004; **68**: 1889–902.

77. Kharasch ED, Hankins DC, Thummel KE. Human kidney methoxyflurane and sevoflurane metabolism: Intrarenal fluoride production as a possible mechanism of methoxyflurane nephrotoxicity. *Anesthesiology* 1995; **82**: 689–99.

78. Cummings BS, Lasker JM, Lash LH. Expression of glutathione-dependent enzymes and cytochrome P450s in freshly isolated and primary cultures of proximal tubular cells from human kidney. *J Pharmacol Exp Ther* 2000; **293**: 677–85.

79. Cummings BS, Zangar RC, Novak RF, Lash LH. Cellular distribution of cytochromes P-450 in the rat kidney. *Drug Metab Dispos* 1999; **27**: 542–8.

80. Meyer RP, Gehlhaus M, Knoth R, Volk B. Expression and function of cytochrome P450 in brain drug metabolism. *Curr Drug Metab* 2007; **8**: 297–306.

81. Zhang JY, Wang Y, Prakash C. Xenobiotic-metabolizing enzymes in human lung. *Curr Drug Metab* 2006; **7**: 939–48.

82. Bartelink IH, Rademaker CM, Schobben AF, van den Anker JN. Guidelines on paediatric dosing on the basis of developmental physiology and pharmacokinetic considerations. *Clin Pharmacokinet* 2006; **45**: 1077–97.

83. Strolin Benedetti M, Whomsley R, Baltes EL. Differences in absorption, distribution, metabolism and excretion of xenobiotics between the paediatric and adult populations. *Expert Opin Drug Metab Toxicol* 2005; **1**: 447–71.

84. Hines RN. The ontogeny of drug metabolism enzymes and implications for adverse drug events. *Pharmacol Ther* 2008; **118**: 250–67.

85. Gow PJ, Ghabrial H, Smallwood RA, Morgan DJ, Ching MS. Neonatal hepatic drug elimination. *Pharmacol Toxicol* 2001; **88**: 3–15.

86. Stevens JC. New perspectives on the impact of cytochrome P450 3A expression for pediatric pharmacology. *Drug Discov Today* 2006; **11**: 440–5.

87. de Wildt SN, Kearns GL, Leeder JS, van den Anker JN. Cytochrome P450 3A: ontogeny and drug disposition. *Clin Pharmacokinet* 1999; **37**: 485–505.

88. Myllynen P, Pasanen M, Vahakangas K. The fate and effects of xenobiotics in human placenta. *Expert Opin Drug Metab Toxicol* 2007; **3**: 331–46.

89. Hodge LS, Tracy TS. Alterations in drug disposition during pregnancy: implications for drug therapy. *Expert Opin Drug Metab Toxicol* 2007; **3**: 557–71.

90. Kinirons MT, O'Mahony MS. Drug metabolism and ageing. *Br J Clin Pharmacol* 2004; **57**: 540–4.

91. Perucca E. Age-related changes in pharmacokinetics: predictability and assessment methods. *Int Rev Neurobiol* 2007; **81**: 183–99.

92. Strolin Benedetti M, Whomsley R, Canning M. Drug metabolism in the paediatric population and in the elderly. *Drug Discov Today* 2007; **12**: 599–610.

93. Lin JH. Pharmacokinetic and pharmacodynamic variability: a daunting challenge in drug therapy. *Curr Drug Metab* 2007; **8**: 109–36.

94. Lin JH, Lu AY. Interindividual variability in inhibition and induction of cytochrome P450 enzymes. *Annu Rev Pharmacol Toxicol* 2001; **41**: 535–67.

95. Sweeney BP, Bromilow J. Liver enzyme induction and inhibition: implications for anaesthesia. *Anaesthesia* 2006; **61**: 159–77.

96. Paine MF, Oberlies NH. Clinical relevance of the small intestine as an organ of drug elimination: drug-fruit juice interactions. *Expert Opin Drug Metab Toxicol* 2007; **3**: 67–80.

97. Kharasch ED, Walker A, Hoffer C, Sheffels P. Intravenous and oral alfentanil as in vivo probes for hepatic and first-pass CYP3A activity: noninvasive assessment using pupillary miosis. *Clin Pharmacol Ther* 2004; **76**: 452–66.

98. Ibrahim AE, Feldman J, Karim A, Kharasch ED. Simultaneous assessment of drug interactions with low- and high-extraction opioids: application to parecoxib effects on the pharmacokinetics and pharmacodynamics of fentanyl and alfentanil. *Anesthesiology* 2003; **98**: 853–61.

99. Backman JT, Kivistö KT, Olkkola KT, Neuvonen PJ. The area under the plasma concentration–time curve for oral midazolam is 400-fold larger during treatment with itraconazole than

with rifampicin. *Eur J Clin Pharmacol* 1998; **54**: 53–8.

100. Poulsen L, Brøsen K, Arendt-Nielsen L, *et al.* Codeine and morphine in extensive and poor metabolizers of sparteine: pharmacokinetics, analgesic effect and side effects. *Eur J Clin Pharmacol* 1996; **51**: 289–95.

101. Tseng CY, Wang SL, Lai MD, Lai ML, Huang JD. Formation of morphine from codeine in Chinese subjects of different CYP2D6 genotypes. *Clin Pharmacol Ther* 1996; **60**: 177–82.

102. Caraco Y, Sheller J, Wood AJ. Impact of ethnic origin and quinidine coadministration on codeine's disposition and pharmacodynamic effects. *J Pharmacol Exp Ther* 1999; **290**: 413–22.

103. Sindrup SH, Arendt-Nielsen L, Brosen K, *et al.* The effect of quinidine on the analgesic effect of codeine. *Eur J Clin Pharmacol* 1992; **42**: 587–92.

104. Caraco Y, Sheller J, Wood AJJ. Pharmacogenetic determinants of codeine induction by rifampicin: The impact on codeine's respiratory,

psychomotor and miotic effects. *J Pharmacol Exp Ther* 1997; **281**: 330–6.

105. Juran BD, Egan LJ, Lazaridis KN. The AmpliChip CYP450 test: principles, challenges, and future clinical utility in digestive disease. *Clin Gastroenterol Hepatol* 2006; **4**: 822–30.

106. Huang RS, Ratain MJ. Pharmacogenetics and pharmacogenomics of anticancer agents. *CA Cancer J Clin* 2009; **59**: 42–55.

107. Verbeeck RK. Pharmacokinetics and dosage adjustment in patients with hepatic dysfunction. *Eur J Clin Pharmacol* 2008; **64**: 1147–61.

108. Frye RF, Zgheib NK, Matzke GR, *et al.* Liver disease selectively modulates cytochrome P450–mediated metabolism. *Clin Pharmacol Ther* 2006; **80**: 235–45.

109. Liu S, Frye RF, Branch RA, *et al.* Effect of age and postoperative time on cytochrome P450 enzyme activity following liver transplantation. *J Clin Pharmacol* 2005; **45**: 666–73.

110. Nolin TD, Naud J, Leblond FA, Pichette V. Emerging evidence of the impact of kidney disease on drug metabolism and transport. *Clin Pharmacol Ther* 2008; **83**: 898–903.

111. Dreisbach AW, Lertora JJ. The effect of chronic renal failure on drug metabolism and transport. *Expert Opin Drug Metab Toxicol* 2008; **4**: 1065–74.

112. Aitken AE, Richardson TA, Morgan ET. Regulation of drug-metabolizing enzymes and transporters in inflammation. *Annu Rev Pharmacol Toxicol* 2006; **46**: 123–49.

113. Morgan ET. Impact of infectious and inflammatory disease on cytochrome P450-mediated drug metabolism and pharmacokinetics. *Clin Pharmacol Ther* 2009; **85**: 434–8.

114. Sindrup SH, Hofmann U, Asmussen J, *et al.* Impact of quinidine on plasma and cerebrospinal fluid concentrations of codeine and morphine after codeine intake. *Eur J Clin Pharmacol* 1996; **49**: 503–9.

Principles of drug action

Drug transport and transporters

Roland J. Bainton and Evan D. Kharasch

Drug transporters and localized pharmacokinetics

Xenobiotics and defining chemical space

Living organisms use biologic compartments to perform discrete biochemical processes, to localize and control the natural small molecules contained within [1]. Foreign small molecules, called xenobiotics, share the same molecular weight range and solubility characteristics as endogenous small molecules and are thus able to penetrate biologic spaces. As xenobiotics also possess potent biointeraction (i.e., drug-like) properties they are the source for nearly all clinically useful pharmaceuticals [2]. To balance the cells' needs of access to endogenous small molecules and control of xenobiotic penetration, powerful biotransformation and bioelimination pathways have evolved to control chemical space (Chapter 6). These same processes present challenges for delivering clinically useful therapies to particular organ spaces, as xenobiotics have complex and unpredictable relationships with the selectively expressed small molecule transporters or specially tuned metabolic systems [2]. Thus understanding how any one pharmaceutical interacts with biologically defined chemical space requires a closer examination of that drug's susceptibility to highly localized pharmacokinetic processes affecting chemical persistence at the site of action.

Lipid bilayers and drug localization

Lipid bilayers physically partition aqueous spaces [1] (Fig. 7.1), creating cells and specialized internal subcellular compartments. In addition, formation of cell–cell contacts in conjunction with diffusion-tight junctional complexes divides the external cellular milieu into different interstitial spaces [1] (Fig. 7.2). This biophysical boundary prevents passive diffusion of large molecules such as proteins and nucleic acids between different compartments and greatly curtails the movement of electrolytes, soluble components of metabolism, and drugs. Drugs and xenobiotics are often in equilibrium between charged and charge-neutral states (Fig. 7.2). Charge-neutral molecules more readily transit lipid bilayers and possess better penetration rates into cells by

orders of magnitude (*passive permeability*, Fig. 7.1). Cellular penetration may be augmented (*influx transport*) or opposed (*efflux transport*) by active cellular processes (see below), a feature that allows drugs to take multiple routes to a target (Fig. 7.2). To control the ability of drugs to transit freely in cellular space and still maintain chemical partition, cells organize molecular systems to contain, modify, or move endogenous and foreign lipophilic molecules from one space to another.

Small-molecule partition and transporters

Chemical partition is the sine qua non of cell biology, and cellular transport systems play a vital role in chemical compartmentalization. An enormous variety of transmembrane protein transporters are dedicated to selectively moving small molecules across membranes [3]. Their role is so broad that by some estimates 15–30% of all membrane proteins are transporters [1]. Among the many substrates that transmembrane protein transporters relocalize are glucose, anabolic intermediates, amino acids, neurotransmitters, metabolic products, and lipids [3]. The vast majority of transporters have high substrate specificity and are organized by DNA sequence relatedness and known function. They are referred to as solute carrier (SLC) proteins and include 46 different gene families with over 360 genes in humans [3]. Their enormous diversity speaks to the wide variety of intracellular environments and their highly specific needs.

The precision, specificity, and ability of these transport systems to act against concentration gradients allows small molecules to have discrete functions depending on their localization. For example, plasma membrane transporters of the SLC6 class specialize in the transport of monoamines from the interstitial space to the cytoplasm. These transporters perform two key functions for the cell: (1) providing amino acids to the cytoplasm for metabolic purposes, and (2) reducing extracelluar concentrations of monoamines when unwanted [4]. However, when the same molecule (or close derivative) is to be used as a neurotransmitter, the SLC18 transporters highly concentrate and package the molecule into synaptic vesicles. After release into the extracelluar space for signaling at the postsynaptic membrane, neurotransmitters are rapidly taken up by SLC6 class

Anesthetic Pharmacology, 2nd edition, ed. Alex S. Evers, Mervyn Maze, Evan D. Kharasch. Published by Cambridge University Press. © Cambridge University Press 2011.

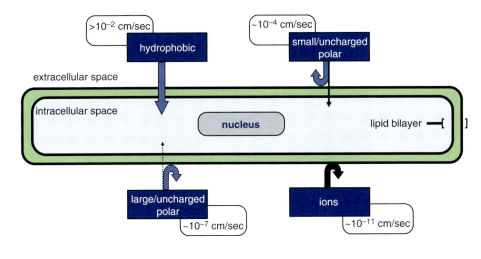

Figure 7.1. Chemical partition across bilayers. Lipid bilayers (green lines) are formed by virtue of the chemical characteristics of their constituent phospholipids: a hydrophilic phosphate head group and a hydrophobic carbon-chain tail. The head groups associate with the aqueous environment, while the tail groups self-associate and form the internal, hydrophobic core of the bilayer. This layer must be transited if nutrients as well as drugs are to reach targets inside the cell, and movement across this bilayer is also dictated by specific chemical properties. Paracellular movement refers to passage of molecules between cells, bypassing cell membrane barriers. Transcellular movement requires passage across membrane barriers. More hydrophobic chemicals and compounds can cross the barrier with relative ease and have a high permeability coefficient (expressed in the figure as cm s^{-1}) whereas chemicals with low permeability coefficients (such as ions) cannot passively transit the lipid bilayer and must cross via other means such as carrier-mediated transport. All chemicals critical to sustaining life fall along this continuum. Modified with permission from Alberts *et al.* [1].

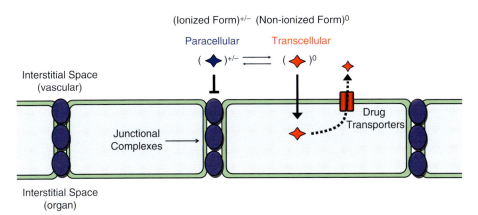

Figure 7.2. Chemical partition across cellular boundaries. Cells separate one interstitial space from another. Cellular barriers rely upon two modes of exclusion to maintain xenobiotic exclusion, as small molecules can interact with cells in two ways. Charged molecules (blue stars) are excluded by the boundary function of lipid bilayers, very low rates of endocytosis, and tight diffusion barriers provided by special lateral-border junctional complexes (blue ovals) of barrier epithelium. Small uncharged molecules (red stars) pass easily through lipid bilayers (green), but active efflux transporters (red) move them back into the humoral space, creating an active transport barrier. As drugs in aqueous solution are in equilibrium between charged and uncharged forms, a true xenobiotic barrier must maintain both properties simultaneously to manifest chemical exclusion.

transporters. Moving small molecules across cell membranes is entropically unfavorable, and thus transporters require energy expenditure either directly using adenosine triphosphate (ATP), or dissipating other existing electrochemical gradients (e.g., Na/K) by using symport or antiport mechanisms [3]. Together, transporter systems create the chemical preconditions for cellular function, restore chemical conditions after perturbation, and clear chemical space of unwanted metabolites. Thus transporters are essential actors in almost every biologic function.

Localized pharmacokinetic spaces

Acting in concert with, or after the action of, phase I and phase II metabolism (Chapter 6), to move drugs and their metabolites across lipid bilayers, transporters are often referred to as phase III metabolism. Therefore transporters are often highly expressed in organs of biotransformation such as the liver and intestine, and metabolism and transport together create formidable pharmacokinetic barriers. Different organ systems tune their biodefense systems by locally

applying phase I, II, and III mechanisms [5]. Thus, for a drug to be clinically effective, it must possess high target specificity, favorable organismal pharmacokinetics, and complementary properties for highly localized chemical partition processes at the cellular level. It is in this latter context that the special role of drug transporters and their ability to control xenobiotic chemical space in drug action are considered.

Drug transporters
Discovery of drug efflux transporters

Xenobiotic transporters were identified as a consequence of the study of multidrug resistance to chemical cancer treatment in the 1970s [6,7]. Highly efficient cytotoxic resistance to a broad spectrum of cancer drugs could occur suddenly and unexpectedly after initiation of chemotherapy [8]. Analysis of drug-resistant tumor cells determined that this new-found resilience correlated with upregulation of a few transmembrane proteins, suggesting that chemotheraputic protection systems were quite

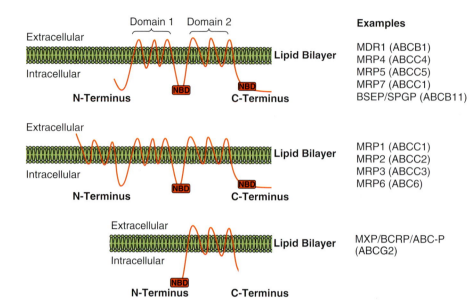

Figure 7.3. Membrane topologies of known xeno-biotic transporters. (*Top*) P-gp-like ABC transporters have 12 transmembrane (TM) domains and two nucleotide-binding domains (NBD). (*Middle*) In the ABCC class a second membrane topology preserves the core P-gp-like transporter with an additional five TMs on the N-terminus. (*Bottom*) The half-transport-ers of the ABCG class have six TMs and one NBD. They are thought to dimerize to promote drug transport function. Modified with permission from Gottesman *et al.* [12].

Examples

MDR1 (ABCB1)
MRP4 (ABCC4)
MRP5 (ABCC5)
MRP7 (ABCC1)
BSEP/SPGP (ABCB11)

MRP1 (ABCC1)
MRP2 (ABCC2)
MRP3 (ABCC3)
MRP6 (ABC6)

MXP/BCRP/ABC-P
(ABCG2)

different from the highly specific SLC transporter systems dis-cussed above. Ultimately these genes were identified as active drug efflux pumps that, unlike most SLC transporters, had surprisingly broad substrate specificity. These proteins were found to bind and transport a wide spectrum of chemothera-peutics back into the extracellular space, thus reducing the effective internal concentration of cytotoxic drugs [8]. Interest-ingly, these cells were not intrinsically more resistant to che-motherapeutics at the target sites, but had instead coopted and enhanced an endogenous chemical partition system to strengthen the chemical barrier at the membrane [8].

Whole genome sequencing methods have discovered large families of similar multidrug resistance transporter (MDR) genes in nearly all organisms [9,10]. Most of these proteins belong to a large and highly conserved class of transmembrane proteins known as ATP-binding cassette (ABC) transporters [8,11]. The archetypal ABC transporter contains two six-pass transmembrane domains and two cytoplasmic nucleotide-binding domains, although the proteins do vary structurally depending on their class (Fig. 7.3). Full transporters are large proteins with 1200–2200 amino acids, and half-transporters have 650–800 amino acids. Half-transporters are thought to function as dimers in the membrane, potentially generating additional functional heterogeneity by combining different substrate preference into one transport pocket [8].

Unfortunately, unlike other transport systems where ligand binding is well understood, only a few specifics are known about the mechanism of xenobiotic binding to ABC transporters. Efficient efflux, for example, is thought to result from conformational changes of the transporter which allow an alternating high substrate-affinity (cell-facing)/low substrate-affinity (extracellular-facing) organization [8]. This permits intracellular presentation of the drug at one interface and release (or efflux) into the extracellular milieu on the

other side. Evidence is mounting that drug binding to the major substrate-promiscuous xenobiotic transporters occurs in the membrane and not from the solution. Thus, these transporters may be designed to act at a protein/lipid-mem-brane interface [8].

The ABC gene family

The approximately 50 human ABC genes occur in seven families (A through G), although only a subset are known to play major roles in drug transport. The major xenobiotic efflux transporter familes are the B, C, and G gene classes (Table 7.1). Interestingly, while ABC gene sequence and sub-families are highly conserved from yeast to flies to humans, the specific roles of most gene products are unknown. ABC transporter localization in polarized cell interfaces is essential to chemoprotective function, as net flux of xenobiotics into or away from various interstitial spaces is determined by the type, quantity, efflux or influx orientation, and apical/basal orientation at the protective interface (e.g., the vascular endo-thelium of the blood–brain barrier, as in Figs. 7.4 and 7.5) [8,13]. Unfortunately as the best studies of ABC transporters in the animal are limited to a few genes (see below), it is not known whether or how they function as a complementary system in the biology of chemical exclusion.

Important subtypes of drug efflux transporters

ABCB$_1$ (P-glycoprotein)

P-glycoprotein (P-gp, ABCB$_1$, or the multidrug resistance transporter MDR1) was the first xenobiotic transporter discovered in multidrug-resistant cancer cells [7] and is

Table 7.1. ABC transporter genes are highly conserved. Pairwise analysis using human ABC transporters versus *Drosophila* using NCBI BLAST (http://blast.ncbi.nlm.nih.gov/Blast.cgi) demonstrates high conservation of transporter number per class and high identity among classes. Similar results are obtained from comparison with other metazoan genomes, and thus ABC genes are highly evolutionarily conserved and likely to play fundamental roles in cellular biology. The major xenobiotic transporters are from the B, C, and G classes, but A-class transporters may play roles in some cases.

Subfamily	Human	*Drosophila*	Identities (%)	Positives (%)
A	12	10	20–37	34–56
B	11	8	43–57	59–75
C	13	14	23–50	40–67
D	4	2	56–59	71–74
E	1	1	77	88
F	3	3	41–69	56–82
G	5 (+1)	15	22–54	41–71
Total	50	53		

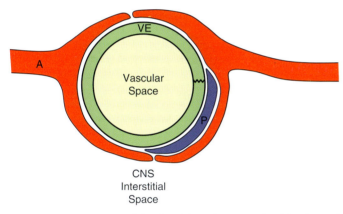

Figure 7.4. Organization of the blood–brain barrier (BBB). While chemical protection is focused at discrete epithelial layers, surrounding tissue can have essential roles in molding and assisting the localized PK potential. This is particularly true at the BBB, where properties of the vascular endothelium (VE) are induced and controlled by surrounding tissues. The BBB VE is thought to receive inductive cell-fate signals from the CNS parenchyma (not shown), while astrocytes (A) and pericytes (P) assist in and regulate localized responses to chemical and immune stress.

responsible for the most profound effects on localized xenobiotic protection of all the ABC transporter subfamily proteins. P-gp is a twelve-pass transmembrane protein of 140 kD and is highly expressed at important chemoprotective interfaces (Table 7.2). It has the broadest substrate specificity of the ABC genes, transporting a significant number of drugs, including anticancer drugs, HIV-protease inhibitors, antibiotics, antidepressants, antiepileptics, and opioids such as morphine and loperamide (Table 7.2). P-gp substrates are generally amphipathic and range in size from 300 to 2000 Da.

P-gp also functions in a wide range of environments including the GI tract, renal proximal tubule cells, the canalicular surfaces of hepatocytes, the capillary endothelial cells of testes, and the blood–brain barrier. Thus the potential for significant drug interactions is widespread [8]. For example, oral bioavailability of the anti-inflammatory drug cyclosporine A is greatly increased by amlodipine, a P-gp substrate that doubles as a P-gp inhibitor [8]. Another example is loperamide, an opioid antidiarrheal that produces no notable central nervous system (CNS) effects at normal doses because intestinal P-gp-mediated efflux retards systemic absorption [8]. However, when loperamide is given with the P-gp inhibitor quinidine, significant systemic absorption occurs, CNS delivery ensues, and side effects such as respiratory depression arise [16]. Thus localized transporter interactions can have substantial effects on drug bioavailability. This is particularly pertinent in fentanyl pharmacodynamics, based on the association between P-gp polymorphisms and fentanyl respiratory depression [17]. In patients under spinal anesthesia given intravenous fentanyl (2.5 μg kg^{-1}), there are differences in suppression of ventilatory effort between three distinct P-gp genotypes prominent in ethnically Korean populations. The presumption is that P-gp transports fentanyl at CNS barriers, and therefore P-gp polymorphisms significantly alter brain concentration despite equivalent doses. Thus, a highly localized drug partition phenomenon can affect drug responses, but they are dependent on the relationship of the specific interface (i.e., the blood–brain barrier) and the protected localization of the drug target (i.e., neurons containing opioid receptors).

ABCC transporters (MRPs)

Multidrug resistance proteins (MRPs) are the largest class of ABC transporters relevant to drug resistance and drug distribution and are ubiquitously expressed [18]. There are 12 proteins in this class with two distinct types of transmembrane protein topologies (Fig. 7.3). Although they contain only 15% sequence identity to P-gp they are predicted to posses a similar structure, with two nucleotide-binding domains and similar membrane topology to ABCB transporters (Fig. 7.3) [12]. Furthermore, like P-gp, they can extrude a wide array of amphipathic anions. Interestingly, all members of this particular subfamily, also called ABCC transporters, are lipophilic anion transporters that are broadly involved in cancer therapeutic resistance [18]. They are quite adept at effluxing methotrexate, thereby lessening the effect of an important chemotherapeutic in the brain [8]. MRP substrate specificities show a preference for glutathione and glucuronide conjugates, thus drug elimination could be greatly facilitated when transporters are locally paired with the appropriate phase II enzymes (e.g., glucuronyl transferases, Chapter 6). Nevertheless MRPs also efficiently transport unconjugated compounds such as anthracyclines,

Table 7.2. Major human drug transporters P-glycoprotein (P-gp), multidrug resistance protein (MRP), breast cancer resistance protein (BRCP), organic anion transporting polypeptide (OATP), organic cation transporter (OCT), and organic anion transporter (OAT) are the best-studied drug transporters. They can share substrates and inhibitors. Modified with permission from Loscher and Potschka [13], Dobson and Kell [14], Zhang et al. [15].

Transporter gene	Aliases	Localization	Function	Selected substrates	Selected inhibitors
ABC family					
ABCB₁	P-glycoprotein, MDR1	BBB, BRB, intestine, liver, kidney, placenta, adrenal, testis	efflux	digoxin, fexofenadine, morphine, loperamide, corticoids, cyclosporine, paclitaxel, verapamil, methotrexate	cyclosporine, verapamil, quinidine, ritonavir, ketocoanzole, itraconazole
ABCC1	MRP1	BBB, breast, lung, heart, kidney, blood cells, liver, intestines, testes, placenta	efflux	glutathione or glucuronide conjugates, leukotriene C4, etoposide, methotrexate	probenecid, sulfinpyrazone, cyclosporine
ABCC2	MRP2	intestine, liver, kidney, brain, placenta	efflux	bilirubin, indinavir, cisplatin	cyclosporine
ABCG2	BCRP	BBB, intestine, liver, breast, placenta	efflux	anthracyclines, mitoxantrone, prazosin, topotecan, methotrexate	elacridar (GF120918), cyclosporine, fumitremorgin C
SLCO family					
SLCO1A2	OATP1A2	Liver, kidney, brain, lung, colon	uptake, efflux	fexofenadine, rocuronium, enalapril, rosuvastatin	
SLCO1B1	OATP1B1	BBB, brain, kidney, liver	uptake, efflux	organic anions, bile salts, digoxin, fexofenadine, methotrexate, rifampin	cyclosporine, verapamil, rifampin, similar to P-gp
SLC family					
SLC22A1	OCT1	liver	uptake	metformin	quinidine, quinine, verapamil, cimetidine
SLC22A2	OCT2	kidney, brain	uptake	metformin, amantadine, memantine, varenicline	cimetidine
SLC22A6	OAT1	kidney, brain	uptake	acyclovir, adefovir, methotrexate, zidovudine	probenecid, cefadroxil, cefamandole, cefazolin, diclofenac
SLC22A8	OAT3	kidney, brain	uptake	cimetidine, methotrexate, zidovudine	probenecid, cefadroxil, cefamandole, cefazolin, cimetidine

BBB, blood–brain barrier; BRB, blood–retinal barrier.

epipodophyllotoxins, vinca alkaloids, and camptothecins (Table 7.2) [18]. MRPs are known to localize to both apical and basal interfaces of chemical protection interfaces and thus can participate in moving drugs in both directions between interstitial spaces (Fig. 7.5) [8,13].

ABCG2 (BCRP)

Breast cancer resistance protein (BCRP), so named for its discovery in an especially drug-resistant breast cancer cell line [21], is the second member of the five-member half-transporter ABCG subfamily (Fig. 7.3) [10]. BCRP is expressed throughout the body but most notably in the liver, intestinal epithelium, placenta, blood–brain barrier, and a variety of stem cells. Like P-gp, BCRP is quite promiscuous in its choice of substrate and is powered by the hydrolysis of ATP. BCRP substrates generally include compounds that are relatively large in molecular weight and either positively or negatively charged and amphipathic. Specific substrates for BCRP-mediated efflux include antineoplastic drugs and their metabolites (e.g., methotrexate and sulfated methotrexate),

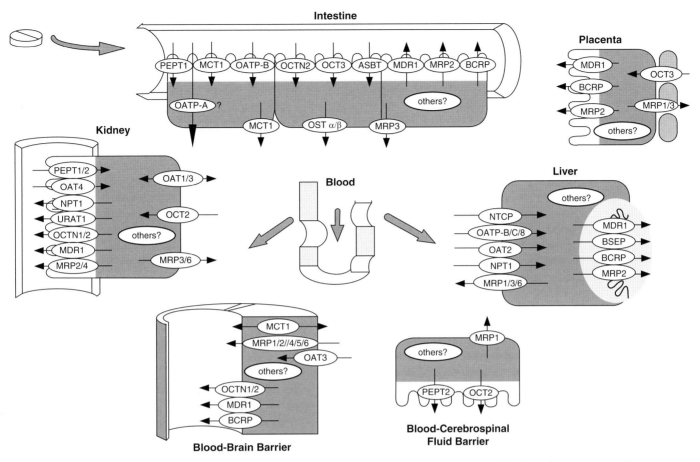

Figure 7.5. Membrane localization of drug transporters at the blood–brain barrier. Organ spaces subject to specific chemical constraints usually organize the tightest control of chemical space at one cellular layer. These chemical barriers use tight junctions and transporter content, type, and apical/basal localization to modulate the protected interstitial space to the purpose and susceptibilities of the underlying tissue [19,20]. The vascular endothelium of the BBB is one of the most potent localized pharmacokinetic interfaces and has a vast array of drug efflux and influx transporters at both vascular and CNS interfaces. Similar organization is repeated at the blood–cerebrospinal fluid barrier, renal epithelium of the kidney, intestinal epithelium, hepatocyte/bile-duct interfaces, and placenta; thus drug action at an individual organ can depend greatly on the chemoprotective efficiency of a particular exposure interface. For transcellular transport, drugs need to cross two different membranes on the basal and apical sides. In the intestine, drugs are absorbed from the luminal side (brush border membrane) and excreted into the portal blood across the basolateral membrane. In the liver, drugs are taken up into hepatocytes across the sinusoidal membrane and excreted into the bile. In the kidney, drugs undergo secretion (urinary excretion) or reabsorption. In the case of secretion, drugs are taken up from the basolateral side and excreted in the urine across the apical side. However, in the case of reabsorption, drugs are taken up from the urine and excreted in the circulating blood. Reproduced with permission from Tsuji [19].

topotecan and irinotecan (both topoisomerase I inhibitors), as well as mitoxantrone, camptothecin and flavopiridol, xenobiotic toxins, food-borne carcinogens, and endogenous compounds [8]. BCRP, unlike MRPs, is also adept at transporting glutamated folates and folate antagonists [8]. Therefore, like P-gp, BCRP is a major factor in conferring resistance to a wide range of therapeutics and is central to pharmacokinetics and toxicity considerations [8].

Other drug transporters

SLC21 transporters (organic anion transporter proteins)

Despite the relative abundance of SLC transporters at protective barrier interfaces, few are known to participate directly in

drug transport. One exception is the organic anion transporter proteins (OATPs), which are not structurally related to ABC transporters, but belong to the solute carrier transporters class 21 (SLC21/SLCO) [3]. OATPs primarily use passive transport mechanisms driven by electrochemical gradients or symport/antiport mechanisms, but interestingly show other functional similarities to P-gp. The best-characterized OATP xenobiotic transporters are OATP1A2, OATP1B1, OATP1B3, and OATP2B1 [14,15]. They are generally efflux transporters, found at chemoprotective interfaces, prominently in brain endothelial cells, and also in liver, lung, kidney, and testes. In-situ mRNA hybridization also demonstrates broad expression in central brain tissue, suggesting a role in general cellular protection as well as barrier function. In-vitro experiments suggest that OATPs can transport many structurally divergent molecules, reminiscent of P-gp. Examples include bile acids, steroids, estrogen, many anionic compounds, and glutathione or glucuronide conjugates [22]. Certain drug–food interactions (e.g., grapefruit juice) [23] may be attributable to inhibition of OATPs, but further characterization of the in-vivo role of OATPs in drug interactions is needed. Interestingly, unlike ABC transporters, some OATPs can also function as drug influx transporters (Fig. 7.4). Bidirectional transport and/or the counteracting of efflux transport occurs at numerous tissue interfaces including the gut, liver, kidney, and blood–brain barrier [19,20]. How these competing transporter processes are regulated, coordinated, and potentially circumvented or controlled will require a better understanding of drug–transporter interactions at cellular interfaces and methods for analyzing net localized pharmacokinetic disposition of drugs.

Specially protected anatomic spaces

Specialized cellular boundary systems have evolved to limit access to sensitive biologic spaces [12,24]. Transporters are critical to the processes of drug uptake, distribution, metabolism, and excretion and may play multiple roles simultaneously depending on their localization, expression levels, and activity. Transporters are especially important in highly sensitive organs such as the CNS, where they are important determinants of drug pharmacodynamics [25].

CNS drug barriers
Blood–brain barrier

The blood–brain barrier (BBB) is the largest pharmacokinetic interface within the CNS (about $20 \, m^2$) [26], and thus the primary focus of the many efforts to understand and control drug access to the brain [27]. The BBB evolved due to the brain's unique chemical sensitivity and requirement for the highest level of chemical protection. BBB drug transporters can profoundly influence the clinical effectiveness of drugs acting in the brain [13].

The BBB has a complex cellular makeup that is functionally integrated with surrounding brain tissue as part of the neurovascular unit [11,28]. The complete neurovascular unit comprises the capillary vascular endothelium, pericytes, a basement membrane, closely associated astrocytic glia, and nearby neurons [29] (Fig. 7.4). The highly polarized vascular endothelium is the primary site of chemical exclusion. It possesses very tight lateral border junctions [30] and a diverse array of apically (i.e., vascular) facing efflux drug transporters, including P-gp, MRP1, and BCRP (Fig. 7.5). The functional importance of these transporters to drug partition in the brain has been studied using gene-specific genetic null mice (knockouts) [31–35]. In single transporter loss-of-function experiments, two- to ten-fold increases in CNS penetration of specific ABC transporter substrates including chemotherapeutics can result

after IV administration [36]. That ABC transporters can so profoundly affect brain drug concentration by their presence or absence in a single endothelial layer suggests a plausible mechanism for increased drug sensitivity of the CNS in transporter-associated pharmacogenomic studies [17] (see P-gp, above). Furthermore these studies promote the idea of specifically targeting xenobiotic transporter function to more readily concentrate drugs in the brain for treating CNS illnesses such as brain cancer, multiple sclerosis, and Alzheimer's disease [27].

Astrocytic glia form a continuous circumferential and close association with the basement membrane, further isolating the vascular and CNS interstitial spaces, but their role in chemical exclusion is unclear. The astroglial cell layer is less than a micron thick and lacks very tight junctions at cell–cell contacts, and xenobiotic transporters should therefore not directly affect CNS glial cell chemopartition. Indeed, genomic data show a much lower level of xenobiotic transporter and junctional protein expression in the astroglia compared to vascular endothelium (R. Daneman and B. Barres, personal communication and [37]). Thus, while astrocytes are essential for BBB maintenance and function, their role in chemical protection may be to sense or integrate chemical, metabolic, and inflammatory stresses which must be coordinated to maintain proper physiologic balance for neurons [11]. Substantial efforts are under way to develop model systems and new methods to identify regulatory controls and chemoresponsive physiologies in the hope of specifically modulating drug barrier function at the BBB and ultimately improving clinical treatment options [27].

Blood-retinal barrier (BRB)

Transport of molecules between the vitreous/retina and systemic circulation is restricted by the blood-retinal barrier (BRB, also called the retinal BBB or RBBB), composed of retinal pigment epithelium (RPE) and endothelial cells of the retinal blood vessels. The RPE maintains a tight barrier to diffusion to the interstitial fluid of the surrounding connective tissue of the eye. Vascular access to the retina is primarily through the retinal blood vessels, which penetrate with the optic nerve and run parallel to the retinal surface. The capillary bed of the retinal vascular endothelium maintains tight junctions and apically facing transporters morphologically similar to the BBB in the central brain. A unique feature of the eye is the ability to bypass the barrier by topical application or injection into the vitreous humor. However, while drug delivery to the CNS is uniquely possible in the eye, transport processes resident at the RBBB promote very rapid removal of small molecules into the systemic circulation. For example, common topical ophthalmic drugs such as erythromycin, dexamethasone, and cyclosporine are substrates for prominent RBBB transporters and can be found in the systemic circulation after ocular administration [38]. These transporters include MDR1, MRP1, BRCP, and numerous OATPs [38]. Localized pharmacokinetic methods for measuring efflux across the BRB are limited; therefore reliable quantitative estimation of the roles of inner and outer BRB has not been well established in humans. In rabbits, however, MDR1 present at the RBBB can be selectively modulated using traditional inhibitors such as quinidine and cyclosporine A [39]. Furthermore, diffusion barrier studies have been carried out in mice, where labeled mannitol is used as a biomarker for retinal diffusion barrier integrity [40] and has shown diffusion-tight function of the BRB. Thus experimental models identify the BRB as an effective barrier similar to the BBB.

Blood–cerebrospinal fluid barrier and choroid plexus

The blood–cerebrospinal fluid barrier (B-CSFB) is derived from a special confluence of the pia mater and a single layer of CSF-facing glial cells (the ependyma). This meeting of two barrier layers is known as the choroid plexus and is the site of CSF production. Throughout the rest of the CNS, ependymal cells become diffusion-tight, utilizing the same modes of separation discussed at the capillary–brain interface above. Here, therefore, chemical exclusivity of the CNS is maintained by an anatomically simpler system than at the BBB. The CSF production cycle is completed by rapid uptake at arachnoid granulations. Together, the CSF production and brain barrier system is thought to perform cleansing functions, further augmenting the chemical protection provided by the BBB [41].

Because the diffusion of polar substances at the B-CSFB is less hindered than at the BBB [41], drug administration into CSF has been proposed to circumvent the BBB and gain access to the CNS. However, potent chemical exclusion properties are present at the B-CSFB (i.e., ependymal cells), as at the choroid plexus [42]. Specifically, transporters OAT, OATP1, OATP2, MRP1, and MDR1 are present in high levels, suggesting an explanation for why the CSF has not proven to be a dependable access point for the administration of chemotherapy or other drugs into the CNS. Nevertheless, certain drugs can overcome these barrier processes by a combination of favorable penetration chemistry and poor transportability. For example, sodium-channel blockers such as bupivicaine are used for subarachnoid block.

Gastrointestinal tract

Intestinal drug uptake usually occurs by mass action and passive permeability when high concentrations are presented to the microvillus absorption surface. An empirical set of rules, known as Lipinski's Rule of Fives, describes how small molecules passively cross the lipid bilayer. Oral drugs can violate only one of the following criteria: (1) not more than five hydrogen bond donors, (2) not more than 10 hydrogen bond acceptors, (3) molecular weight under 500 Da, and (4) an octanol/water partition coefficient log P less than 5. Pharmaceuticals that possess these properties are better at passing the chemoprotective interface of the gut, but these constraints do not allow small molecules to bypass the action of transporters.

Xenobiotic transporters are abundantly represented throughout the enteral space (Fig. 7.5) [43,44]. P-gp is apically localized in microvilli throughout the gut epithelium, found in highest amounts in the ileum and jejunum, and counteracts the passive or active absorption of xenobiotics [25]. For instance, mouse P-gp knockouts demonstrate increased absorption and bioavailability of many oral xenobiotics [45], and uptake of some drugs is markedly increased by small molecules that inhibit P-gp function [16]. BCRP is the transporter expressed in highest abundance throughout the human small intestine [46]. In addition to countering the absorption of some orally administered drugs, certain transporter systems, particularly ABCC proteins, counter the absorption of drug glucuronides that are excreted in bile. Intestinal efflux transporters act in concert with intestinal phase I metabolism to limit drug bioavailability.

Liver

Hepatic drug elimination depends on passive or active hepatic uptake, intracellular metabolism, excretion of metabolites or parent drug into bile, and/or excretion of metabolites or parent drug into sinusoidal blood. Transporters are involved in uptake, biliary excretion, and sinusoidal efflux (Fig. 7.5) [23]. SLC-type transporters in the basolateral (sinusoidal) membrane (OATPs, OATs, OCTs) mediate the uptake of organic cations, anions, bilirubin, and bile salts. ABC transporters (P-gp, BCRP, MRPs) at the canalicular membrane mediate the efflux into bile of drugs, metabolites, and bile salts. MRPs may also mediate drug and metabolite efflux back into the blood. The balance of vectorial uptake and efflux drug transport together with intracellular metabolism, determines drug elimination. Hepatic drug transporters are subject to pharmacogenetic variability, and drug–drug interactions.

In murine models, transporter disruption can effect the distribution of important anesthetic drugs such as opiates. Morphine-3-glucuronide (M3G), the most abundant metabolite of morphine, is transported in vitro by human MRP2 (ABCC2) that is present in the apical membrane of hepatocytes. Loss of biliary M3G secretion in MRP2(-/-) mice results in its increased sinusoidal transport, which can be attributed to MRP3. Combined loss of MRP2 and MRP3 leads to a substantial accumulation of M3G in the liver, resulting in low rates of sinusoidal membrane transport and the prolonged presence of M3G in plasma [47]. These results suggest that in vertebrates MRP2 and MRP3 transporters provide alternative routes for the excretion of a glucuronidated substrate from the liver in vivo. This illustrates the potential complexity of interactions between transporters and modifying enzymes intrinsic to particular chemoprotective environments.

Kidney

Transporters mediate active tubular secretion and reabsorption in the kidney, which, together with glomerular filtration, determine drug elimination (Fig. 7.5). The primary focus of renal excretion is the proximal tubule, which actively takes up organic anions and cations at the basolateral membrane and extrudes them across the apical brush border membrane into the urine; hence transepithelial flux requires two distinct sets of transporters. Many drugs (weak acids) and their phase II conjugates are organic anions. OATs 1 and 3 are the primary organic anion uptake transporters at the basolateral membrane (although they may also interact with neutral and cationic compounds), while efflux into the tubular lumen is mediated primarily by the ABC subfamily C transporters MRP2, MRP4, and BCRP [48]. Organic cations are typically transported into renal tubular cells at the basolateral membrane by OCTs 1 and 2, and effluxed into urine at the apical membrane by P-gp, OCT3, and novel organic cation transporters OCTN1 and OCTN2. Selective expression and specific localization of transporters at different apical and basal interfaces in the tubule, pharmacogenetic variability in their activity, and drug interactions play a determinative role in drug elimination.

Transporter-based drug interactions can occur in the kidney by competing for elimination. For example, probencid inhibits OATP-mediated excretion of antibiotics [49]. In addition, methotrexate has strong potential interactions with non-steroidal anti-inflammatory drugs (NSAIDs), particularly after prolonged high-dose chemotheraputic use [49].

Placenta

The placenta is the sole medium of metabolic exchange between fetus and mother; hence it protects the fetus by providing a major obstacle to chemical penetration. The important chemical properties determining placental transfer by passive diffusion are similar to other organs: molecular weight, pK_a of drug, lipid solubility, and plasma protein binding. The transport barrier in placenta is found in the syncytiotrophoblast, a multinucleated single cell layer that performs nutrient and waste exchange between mother and fetus [50]. This layer is further elaborated into two distinct interfaces: a maternal-facing brush border and a fetal-facing basal membrane [50].

It is in these two interfaces that a variety of membrane transporters perform directional fluxing of metabolites and drugs. Specifically, the brush border membrane contains all three major classes of ABC transporters (i.e., P-gp, MRP1–3, and BCRP) as well as specialized transporters such as the serotonin, norepinephrine, and carnitine transporters (SERT, NET, OCTN2) [50]. On the other side of the divide, the fetal-facing basal membrane contains transporters such as the organic anion transporters OAT4 and OATP-B in addition to the reduced folate transporter RFT-1 [50]. Combinations of genetic loss of P-gp function with specific inhibitors of BCRP markedly increase drug penetration of topetecan to the fetus, which is not seen in the genetically sensitized background alone. Thus the placenta is an essential chemical filter for the fetal protected space and exemplifies the potential for overlapping and redundant function of chemoprotective mechanisms [51].

Transporter biology: special topics

Drug transporter methods

The field of transporter biology is relatively new, and a brief description of experimental methods used to identify the role of transporters in drug disposition may be helpful. Accurate physical measurement of localized drug concentration can be difficult in very compact biologic spaces like the BBB/CNS interface, and consequently methods of measurement require some explanation [52].

In-vitro methods are most commonly used to study human transporter activity and identify candidate transporters for a given substrate. Cell culture systems amenable to transfection of influx or efflux transporter genes, or direct injection of transporter mRNA into *Xenopus* oocytes, express and localize transporter proteins to the cell surface. Isolated membrane vesicles can also be prepared. Exposure to drug on one side of a cell layer, then measurement on both sides, to determine the ratio of substrate penetration to negative controls or by using transporter inhibitors, allows individual assessment of luminal and abluminal transporters and their mechanisms. Unfortunately, heterologous systems have several problems when attributing a specific physiologic function to a transporter, because it is specifically overexpressed. Studies using membranes of confluent primary human cells can provide more information, particularly on the contribution of relevant transporters for a specific drug. Ex-vivo assays, however, lack functional context since organ-specific gross anatomy and transporter interface conditions do not mimic the animal. In addition, the transporter must function away from its normal molecular constituents, and thus potential modulators of substrate preference and functional compensations are lost.

In animals (and occasionally in humans) ex-vivo or in-situ organ perfusion allows direct measurement of drug influx and efflux concentrations. Advantages of this method are a close control of the time course of drug administration and concentration. Furthermore, drug goes directly from perfusate to the brain (or other organ studied), bypassing systemic biotransformation. Although this experimental methodology is more precise, it still requires bulk tissue concentration measurement, and hence does not provide data about discrete localization in the brain (or other organ). Calculation of the brain efflux index can be used as an indirect measure of chemical partition at the BBB. A drug is injected directly into the brain with an impermanent tracer. The ratio of test solute to the reference tracer determines the brain efflux activity. An improved method is tissue (often intracerebral) microdialysis. This method directly samples small-molecule solutes in brain interstitial fluid through a semiporous membrane. Microdialysis is difficult and costly to perform, however, and may have its own artifacts. Transgenic rodent models using knockouts or knock-ins of transporters are a common approach to identifying transporter function with respect to drug disposition and effect. However, there is still a great deal of argument surrounding the similarity of physiologic function even between highly homologous vertebrate systems.

In humans, pharmacogenomic approaches often attempt to identify transporter polymorphisms which may alter pharmacokinetics or pharmacodynamics. The use of drug probes to selectively inhibit a transporter's function, and assess the effect on pharmacokinetics or pharmacodynamics, is limited by the lack of transporter-selective inhibitor probes. This is unlike the methods used to profile cytochrome P450s in drug metabolism, where P450-selective inhibitor drugs are available.

Drug–drug interactions and transporters

Drugs themselves can act to modulate xenobotic transport, and any new pharmaceutical is a potential effector of chemical partition. While the number of current examples is small, as new therapeutics are developed the opportunity for drug–drug interactions through transporter inhibition becomes increasingly problematic. This issue is further exacerbated by the wide tissue distribution of transporters like P-gp, which makes it difficult to predict the potential for affecting drug distribution and efficacy in a site-dependent fashion. As noted above, P-gp loss of function can affect both brain and gut uptake depending on the drug in question [36,45]. This is not just a theoretical problem but occurs with many commonly used medications. For instance, verapamil and the cyclosporine analog PSC833 lead to increased brain concentration of antiepileptics such as carbamazapine, phenytoin, and phenobarbitol [13,53]. The combination of quercetin, a P-gp substrate, and digoxin also has demonstrated toxicity [53]. Lastly, β-blockers such as talinolol exhibit increased oral bioavailability when intestinal P-gp activity is reduced in both animal models and human observations [53]. Unfortunately there is no set of chemoprotective rules that can warn clinicians of potential interactions. Currently all drug–drug interactions are determined empirically, and hence the need for a more complete analysis of the organization of chemical protection in the animal.

Modulating transporter function in vivo for clinical purposes

The BBB is a dynamic structure regulated by many competing inputs [11]. In vertebrates, transcellular diffusion can be modified by adjusting either the level or the activity of transporter proteins [54]. Transcription of a number of efflux transporters including P-gp, MRP2, MRP3, and OATP2 is regulated in part by the pregnane X receptor (PXR), a nuclear receptor that is activated by naturally occurring steroids as well as a wide variety of xenobiotics [55–57]. Higher levels of transporter expression result in more efficient xenobiotic efflux and a tighter BBB [58]. The activity of some transporters can also be influenced by cell-signaling pathways. For example, binding of endothelin 1 to the ET_B receptor rapidly and reversibly inhibits transport activity of P-gp via nitric oxide synthase and protein kinase-C mediated pathways [59].

ABC transporter chemopartition function can also be modulated by drugs. In this case one drug acts as competitive substrate antagonist against more favored transport molecules (Table 7.1). This explains why many drugs are listed as both substrate and antagonist in substrate/inhibitor tables. Several clinical scenarios have attempted to introduce drugs like "selective" transport inhibitors at the BBB interface to improve penetration of chemotherapeutics, but no clinical benefit has yet been obtained [13,60]. Nevertheless the search for more selective competitive inhibitors or allosteric modulators of ABC transporters is quite active in both academic and industrial research [8].

Future directions in the study of chemical protection

The ability of an organism to protect itself against environmental threats, whether predation or chemical insult, is as essential as the ability to convert food into energy. Chemical transporters of the variety discussed in this chapter are present across evolutionary time, with the essential structure of proteins such as members of the ABC superfamily changing very little across phyla. For example, there is increasing evidence that species as distant as fruit flies and humans use very similar means to exclude xenobiotics from privileged compartments such as the CNS [61]. The decoding of the fruit fly *Drosophila melanogaster* genome has enabled investigators to identify genes and proteins that are conserved across species, including analogs of many of the ABC transporters relevant to human physiology and pathology (Table 7.1) [10]. While the component parts of chemoprotective systems are just coming to light (i.e., transporters and metabolic enzymes that are chemically organized), there is little understanding of the regulation and adaptations such a system requires. Model systems using human cell culture, animal models, and the tools of pharmacogenomics will play a large role in furthering the understanding of chemical protection. Once there are better understandings of localized cellular or subcellular drug concentrations and identification of novel modulators of chemical partition, better methods of therapeutic drug delivery can be developed to improve clinical outcomes.

Summary

Biophysical boundaries prevent passive diffusion of large molecules, such as proteins and nucleic acids, between different compartments and greatly curtail the movement of electrolytes, soluble components of metabolism, and drugs. An enormous variety of transmembrane protein transporters are dedicated to selectively moving small molecules across membranes. Transporters are essential actors in almost every biologic function, as transporter systems create the chemical preconditions for cellular function, restore chemical conditions after perturbation, and clear chemical space of unwanted metabolites. The precision, specificity, and ability of these transport systems to act against concentration gradients allow small molecules to have discrete functions depending on their localization. Drugs share the same molecular weight range and solubility characteristics as many endogenous small molecules and are subject to the same physiologic processes, and the same transporters, as endogenous molecules.

Drug (xenobiotic) transporters were initially identified during studies of multidrug cancer resistance. These proteins were efflux pumps with broad substrate specificity, capable of binding and transporting a wide spectrum of chemotherapeutics back into the extracellular space, thereby reducing the effective intracellular concentration of cytotoxic drugs. Cancer cells had coopted and enhanced an endogenous chemical partition system to strengthen the cell-membrane chemical barrier and confer drug resistance.

Cell-surface transporters are now known to be ubiquitous, present across evolutionary time with relatively conserved functions across species, and capable of influx and/or efflux transport of numerous drugs. P-glycoprotein (abbreviated P-gp, and also termed $ABCB_1$ or the multidrug resistance transporter, MDR1) was the first xenobiotic transporter discovered in multidrug-resistant cancer cells. P-gp also functions in a wide range of normal tissues such as the gastrointestinal tract, renal proximal tubule cells, the canalicular surfaces of hepatocytes, the capillary endothelial cells of testes, and the blood–brain barrier. Transporters may influence drug absorption, distribution, tissue penetration, metabolism, and excretion. There is also the potential for significant drug interactions.

How these competing transporter processes are regulated, coordinated, and potentially circumvented or controlled will require a better understanding of drug–transporter interactions at cellular interfaces and methods for analyzing net localized pharmacokinetic disposition of drugs. For a drug to be clinically effective, it must possess high target specificity, favorable organismal pharmacokinetics, and complementary properties for highly localized chemical partition processes at the cellular level. Drugs themselves can act to modulate xenobiotic transport, and any new pharmaceutical is a potential effector of chemical partition.

References

1. Alberts B, Johnson A, Lewis J, *et al.* *Molecular Biology of the Cell*. New York, NY:Garland, 2007.

2. van de Waterbeemd H, Gifford E. ADMET in silico modelling: towards prediction paradise? *Nat Rev Drug Discov* 2003; **2**: 192–204.

3. Hediger MA, Romero MF, Peng JB, *et al.* The ABCs of solute carriers: physiological, pathological and therapeutic implications of human membrane transport proteins Introduction. *Pflugers Arch* 2004; **447**: 465–8.

4. Torres GE, Gainetdinov RR, Caron MG. Plasma membrane monoamine transporters: structure, regulation and function. *Nat Rev Neurosci* 2003; **4**: 13–25.

5. Torrie LS, Radford JC, Southall TD, *et al.* Resolution of the insect ouabain paradox. *Proc Natl Acad Sci U S A* 2004; **101**: 13689–93.

6. Dano K. Active outward transport of daunomycin in resistant Ehrlich ascites tumor cells. *Biochim Biophys Acta* 1973; **323**: 466–83.

7. Juliano RL, Ling V. A surface glycoprotein modulating drug permeability in Chinese hamster ovary cell mutants. *Biochim Biophys Acta* 1976; **455**: 152–62.

8. Sarkadi B, Homolya L, Szakacs G, Varadi A. Human multidrug resistance ABCB and ABCG transporters: participation in a chemoimmunity defense system. *Physiol Rev* 2006; **86**: 1179–236.

9. Annilo T, Chen ZQ, Shulenin S, *et al.* Evolution of the vertebrate ABC gene family: analysis of gene birth and death. *Genomics* 2006; **88**: 1–11.

10. Dean M, Annilo T. Evolution of the ATP-binding cassette (ABC) transporter superfamily in vertebrates. *Annu Rev Genomics Hum Genet* 2005; **6**: 123–42.

11. Zlokovic BV. The blood–brain barrier in health and chronic neurodegenerative disorders. *Neuron* 2008; **57**: 178–201.

12. Gottesman MM, Fojo T, Bates SE. Multidrug resistance in cancer: role of ATP-dependent transporters. *Nat Rev Cancer* 2002; **2**: 48–58.

13. Loscher W, Potschka H. Blood–brain barrier active efflux transporters: *ATP-binding cassette gene family*. *NeuroRx* 2005; **2**: 86–98.

14. Dobson PD, Kell DB. Carrier-mediated cellular uptake of pharmaceutical drugs: an exception or the rule? *Nat Rev Drug Discov* 2008; **7**: 205–20.

15. Zhang L, Zhang YD, Strong JM, Reynolds KS, Huang SM. A regulatory viewpoint on transporter-based drug interactions. *Xenobiotica* 2008; **38**: 709–24.

16. Sadeque AJ, Wandel C, He H, Shah S, Wood AJ. Increased drug delivery to the brain by P-glycoprotein inhibition. *Clin Pharmacol Ther* 2000; **68**: 231–7.

17. Park HJ, Shinn HK, Ryu SH, *et al.* Genetic polymorphisms in the $ABCB_1$ gene and the effects of fentanyl in Koreans. *Clin Pharmacol Ther* 2007; **81**: 539–46.

18. Kruh GD, Belinsky MG. The MRP family of drug efflux pumps. *Oncogene* 2003; **22**: 7537–52.

19. Tsuji A. Impact of transporter-mediated drug absorption, distribution, elimination and drug interactions in antimicrobial chemotherapy. *J Infect Chemother* 2006; **12**: 241–50.

20. Shitara Y, Horie T, Sugiyama Y. Transporters as a determinant of drug clearance and tissue distribution. *Eur J Pharm Sci* 2006; **27**: 425–46.

21. Doyle LA, Yang W, Abruzzo LV, *et al.* A multidrug resistance transporter from human MCF-7 breast cancer cells. *Proc Natl Acad Sci U S A* 1998; **95**: 15665–70.

22. Petrovic V, Teng S, Piquette-Miller M. Regulation of drug transporters during infection and inflammation. *Mol Interv* 2007; **7**: 99–111.

23. Kim RB. Organic anion-transporting polypeptide (OATP) transporter family and drug disposition. *Eur J Clin Invest* 2003; **33** (Suppl 2): 1–5.

24. Abbott NJ. Dynamics of CNS barriers: evolution, differentiation, and modulation. *Cell Mol Neurobiol* 2005; **25**: 5–23.

25. Schinkel AH, Jonker JW. Mammalian drug efflux transporters of the ATP binding cassette (ABC) family: an overview. *Adv Drug Deliv Rev* 2003; **55**: 3–29.

26. Begley DJ, Brightman MW. Structural and functional aspects of the blood–brain barrier. *Prog Drug Res* 2003; **61**: 39–78.

27. Neuwelt E, Abbott NJ, Abrey L, *et al.* Strategies to advance translational research into brain barriers. *Lancet Neurol* 2008; **7**: 84–96.

28. McCarty JH. Cell biology of the neurovascular unit: implications for drug delivery across the blood-brain barrier. *Assay Drug Dev Technol* 2005; **3**: 89–95.

29. Ballabh P, Braun A, Nedergaard M. The blood–brain barrier: an overview: structure, regulation, and clinical implications. *Neurobiol Dis* 2004; **16**: 1–13.

30. Reese TS, Karnovsky MJ. Fine structural localization of a blood-brain barrier to exogenous peroxidase. *J Cell Biol* 1967; **34**: 207–17.

31. Wijnholds J, Evers R, van Leusden MR, *et al.* Increased sensitivity to anticancer drugs and decreased inflammatory response in mice lacking the multidrug resistance-associated protein. *Nat Med* 1997; **3**: 1275–9.

32. Lorico A, Rappa G, Flavell RA, Sartorelli AC. Double knockout of the MRP gene leads to increased drug sensitivity in vitro. *Cancer Res* 1996; **56**: 5351–5.

33. Schinkel AH, Smit JJ, van Tellingen O, *et al.* Disruption of the mouse mdr1a P-glycoprotein gene leads to a deficiency in the blood-brain barrier and to increased sensitivity to drugs. *Cell* 1994; **77**: 491–502.

34. Vlaming ML, Lagas JS, Schinkel AH. Physiological and pharmacological roles of ABCG2 (BCRP): recent findings in Abcg2 knockout mice. *Adv Drug Deliv Rev* 2009; **61**: 14–25.

35. Enokizono J, Kusuhara H, Ose A, Schinkel AH, Sugiyama Y. Quantitative investigation of the role of breast cancer resistance protein (Bcrp/Abcg2) in limiting brain and testis penetration of xenobiotic compounds. *Drug Metab Dispos* 2008; **36**: 995–1002.

36. Schinkel AH. Pharmacological insights from P-glycoprotein knockout mice. *Int J Clin Pharmacol Ther* 1998; **36**: 9–13.

37. Cahoy JD, Emery B, Kaushal A, *et al.* A transcriptome database for astrocytes, neurons, and oligodendrocytes: a new resource for understanding brain development and function. *J Neurosci* 2008; **28**: 264–78.

38. Mannermaa E, Vellonen KS, Urtti A. Drug transport in corneal epithelium and blood–retina barrier: emerging role of transporters in ocular pharmacokinetics. *Adv Drug Deliv Rev* 2006; **58**: 1136–63.

39. Kajikawa T, Mishima HK, Murakami T, Takano M. Role of P-glycoprotein in distribution of rhodamine 123 into aqueous humor in rabbits. *Curr Eye Res* 1999; **18**: 240–6.

40. Derevjanik NL, Vinores SA, Xiao WH, *et al.* Quantitative assessment of the integrity of the blood-retinal barrier in mice. *Invest Ophthalmol Vis Sci* 2002; **43**: 2462–7.

41. Johanson CE, Duncan JA, Stopa EG, Baird A. Enhanced prospects for drug delivery and brain targeting by the choroid plexus-CSF route. *Pharm Res* 2005; **22**: 1011–37.

42. Emerich DF, Skinner SJ, Borlongan CV, Vasconcellos AV, Thanos CG. The choroid plexus in the rise, fall and repair of the brain. *Bioessays* 2005; **27**: 262–74.

43. Dietrich CG, Geier A, Wasmuth HE, *et al.* Influence of biliary cirrhosis on the detoxification and elimination of a food derived carcinogen. *Gut* 2004; **53**: 1850–5.

44. Kusuhara H, Sugiyama Y. Role of transporters in the tissue-selective distribution and elimination of drugs: transporters in the liver, small intestine, brain and kidney. *J Control Release* 2002; **78**: 43–54.

45. Lagas JS, Sparidans RW, van Waterschoot RA, *et al.* P-glycoprotein limits oral availability, brain penetration, and toxicity of an anionic drug, the antibiotic salinomycin. *Antimicrob Agents Chemother* 2008; **52**: 1034–9.

46. Englund G, Rorsman F, Rönnblom A, *et al.* Regional levels of drug transporters along the human intestinal tract: co-expression of ABC and SLC transporters and comparison with Caco-2 cells. *Eur J Pharm Sci* 2006; **29**: 269–77.

47. van de Wetering K, Zelcer N, Kuil A, *et al.* Multidrug resistance proteins 2 and 3 provide alternative routes for hepatic excretion of morphine-glucuronides. *Mol Pharmacol* 2007; **72**: 387–94.

48. El-Sheikh AA, Masereeuw R, Russel FG. Mechanisms of renal anionic drug transport. *Eur J Pharmacol* 2008; **585**: 245–55.

49. Inui KI, Masuda S, Saito H. Cellular and molecular aspects of drug transport in the kidney. *Kidney Int* 2000; **58**: 944–58.

50. Ganapathy V, Prasad PD. Role of transporters in placental transfer of drugs. *Toxicol Appl Pharmacol* 2005; **207**: 381–7.

51. Jonker JW, Smit JW, Brinkhuis RF, *et al.* Role of breast cancer resistance protein in the bioavailability and fetal penetration of topotecan. *J Natl Cancer Inst* 2000; **92**: 1651–6.

52. Smith QR. A review of blood–brain barrier transport techniques. In: Nag S, ed., *Methods in Molecular Medicine.* Totowa, NJ:Humana Press, 2003: 193–208.

53. Balayssac D, Authier N, Cayre A, Coudore F. Does inhibition of P-glycoprotein lead to drug–drug interactions? *Toxicol Lett* 2005; **156**: 319–29.

54. Miller DS, Bauer B, Hartz AM. Modulation of P-glycoprotein at the blood-brain barrier: opportunities to improve central nervous system pharmacotherapy. *Pharmacol Rev* 2008; **60**: 196–209.

55. Kliewer SA, Goodwin B, Willson TM. The nuclear pregnane X receptor: a key regulator of xenobiotic metabolism. *Endocr Rev* 2002; **23**: 687–702.

56. Kliewer SA, Moore JT, Wade L, *et al.* An orphan nuclear receptor activated by pregnanes defines a novel steroid signaling pathway. *Cell* 1998; **92**: 73–82.

57. Bauer B, Yang X, Hartz AM, *et al.* In vivo activation of human pregnane X receptor tightens the blood–brain barrier to methadone through P-glycoprotein up-regulation. *Mol Pharmacol* 2006; **70**: 1212–19.

58. Perez-Tomas R. Multidrug resistance: retrospect and prospects in anti-cancer drug treatment. *Curr Med Chem* 2006; **13**: 1859–76.

59. Hartz AM, Bauer B, Fricker G, Miller DS. Rapid regulation of P-glycoprotein at the blood–brain barrier by endothelin-1. *Mol Pharmacol* 2004; **66**: 387–94.

60. Kemper EM, Boogerd W, Thuis I, Beijnen JH, van Tellingen O. Modulation of the blood-brain barrier in oncology: therapeutic opportunities for the treatment of brain tumours? *Cancer Treat Rev* 2004; **30**: 415–23.

61. Mayer F, Mayer N, Chinn L, *et al.* Evolutionary conservation of vertebrate blood–brain barrier chemoprotective mechanisms in Drosophila. *J Neurosci* 2009; **29**: 3538–50.

Principles of drug action

8 Target-controlled infusions and closed-loop administration

Michel M. R. F. Struys and Tom De Smet

Introduction

The goal of optimal drug dosing in anesthesia is the capability to obtain and maintain a desired time course of clinical and therapeutic drug effect as accurately as possible. Accuracy of administration is essential for effective anesthesia with minimal adverse drug effects. In current clinical practice, anesthetic drugs are predominantly still administered using standard dosing guidelines and techniques, ignoring the large interindividual variability in dose–response relationships. The application of computer-controlled continuously updated infusion rates based on mathematical models, clinical-effects feedback, or, in the absence of quantifiable effects, carefully selected surrogate measures, may yield better patient-individualized dosing.

The dose–response relationship can be divided into three parts (Fig. 8.1): the relationship between the administered dose and the plasma concentration (pharmacokinetics, PK), the relationship between blood or effect-organ concentration and clinical effect (pharmacodynamics, PD), and the coupling between pharmacokinetics and pharmacodynamics (PK/PD). If the plasma or effect-site concentration of a drug could be known, then the complexity of the dose–response relationship would be reduced to pharmacodynamics only (Fig. 8.1). The PK/PD principles required to fully understand this chapter are presented in Chapters 1 and 5.

In contrast to inhalation anesthetics, for which the inspired and end-tidal concentrations can be measured continuously in real time ("on-line"), the actual plasma or effect-organ concentration of an intravenously administered drug is not immediately measurable in clinical practice. Therefore, it is impossible to steer intravenous infusion regimens manually to maintain an on-line measured plasma concentration. It becomes even more complex if one wants to target a specific effect-site concentration. Consequently, it requires a drug model and a computer continuously updating the administration rate to maintain an estimated drug concentration in plasma or at the effect site. This technique is called **target-controlled infusion** (TCI).

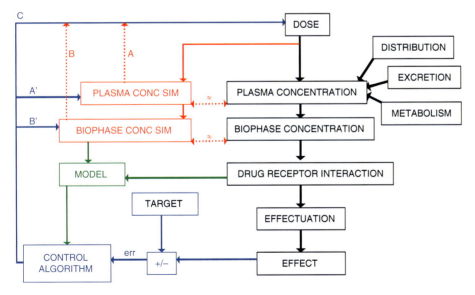

Figure 8.1. Schematic representation of the pharmacokinetic and pharmacodynamic processes determining the relationship between administered dose and resulting effect intensity of a drug (black). Pharmacokinetic factors such as distribution, metabolism, and/or excretion determine the relationship between drug dose and drug concentration in the biophase. In the biophase the drug interacts with the receptor and the pharmacologic effect is accomplished via transduction processes. Target-controlled infusion (TCI) will use a model to estimate the plasma or biophase drug concentration (red), and will calculate the dose needed to approach a target concentration in plasma (A) or biophase/effect site (B). Closed-loop feedback will measure the error between the effect and the target effect to control the dose administration (blue). Better closed-loop performance can result if, rather than using the dose as a direct actuator, the *simulated* variable of a TCI system is used as actuated variable. (A/A', B/B'). The TCI system then compensates for part of the complexity of the dose–interaction relationship. Advanced control algorithms may take into account a (continuously updated) model of the interaction (green).

Anesthetic Pharmacology, 2nd edition, ed. Alex S. Evers, Mervyn Maze, Evan D. Kharasch. Published by Cambridge University Press. © Cambridge University Press 2011.

Two methods for controlling drug administration can be distinguished: open-loop and closed-loop control. In the context of this chapter, **open-loop control** is considered to be any practice where the anesthesiologist administers a drug (either a dose or an infusion based on a desired or targeted drug concentration or clinical effect), assesses the patient's response, and makes a decision to revise the dosing accordingly. Decision-making may be assisted by information on the estimated (if using target-controlled infusion, TCI) or real (inhalational anesthetic) plasma or effect-site concentration. **Closed-loop control** (also called "feedback" control) takes the anesthesiologist "out of the loop." The anesthesiologist only enters the desired clinical or surrogate effect to be maintained (depth of hypnosis, muscle twitch, etc.). The computer program-based controller will autonomously calculate the optimal drug administration rate, based on the measured actual value of the controlled variable, the set-point and, potentially, internal models of the expected dose–response relationship in the (individual) patient.

Open-loop target-controlled infusion

History and definitions

The availability of computers embedded in syringe pumps and better knowledge of drug PK/PD models have now enabled the administration of intravenous drugs as easily as inhalation anesthetics, by applying TCI to achieve and maintain a desired plasma or effect-site concentration. The principle behind TCI techniques is to use PK/PD modeling and calculations to predict a set concentration in one of the pharmacokinetic compartments. TCI was developed to optimize the time course of drug effect by targeting a specific therapeutic drug concentration in a specific body compartment, mostly the plasma or the effect site. Multicompartment mammillary PK/PD models, derived from pharmacologic modeling studies, are used in TCI systems to calculate the infusion rates to achieve and maintain the target concentration as fast and accurately as possible without an overshoot in drug concentrations. This avoids side effects which often occur after initial bolus dosing. A microprocessor-controlled infusion pump is required to perform the complex calculations and control drug administration. It is impossible to achieve the required concentrations with the same accuracy when using manually controlled infusion systems, due to the complexity of drug PK/PD characteristics. The target concentration is set by the anesthesiologist, after having evaluated a patient's individual requirements. This technique is called open-loop controlled TCI.

TCI is based on the original theoretical approach for maintaining and achieving a steady-state blood concentration of a drug whose pharmacokinetics can be described by a two-compartment model as first published by Kruger-Thiemer [1] and clinically tested by Schwilden and coworkers [2]. The schemes developed by these pioneers for drugs conforming to a two-compartment model became known as BET (bolus, elimination, transfer) schemes, and are built on three concepts. First, the initial bolus dose of drug required to achieve the initial targeted plasma concentration (C_{pT}) is equal to $C_{pT} \cdot V_d$ (where V_d is the volume of distribution). Second, the elimination rate (k_e) is proportional to the plasma concentration, so that a constant plasma concentration in steady state results in a fixed portion of the total drug amount being eliminated per unit of time. To maintain a constant plasma concentration, elimination is compensated for by a constant-rate infusion. Third, the amount of drug distributed or transferred to peripheral tissues declines exponentially, as the gradient between the central compartment and the peripheral compartment decreases. This requires an infusion at an exponentially declining rate to replace drug "lost" from the central compartment by distribution until steady state.

Since BET schemes are relatively straightforward to calculate manually, they led to standard dosing guidelines, which are still being used. However, BET has two major drawbacks. First, it is only applicable in the absence of drug previously administered. Since changing the concentration target violates this requirement, it becomes very difficult to find equally straightforward rules in such situations. Second, it has been recognized over the years that the pharmacokinetics of most anesthetics conform best to a three- rather than a two-compartment model, requiring similar but more complex infusion strategies. Furthermore, it was understood that plasma is not the site of drug effect, and one needs to consider the temporal hysteresis of drug effect (i.e., effect lags behind blood concentration) to optimize drug delivery, making the standard infusion schemes even more complex. As a result, effect-compartment-controlled TCI was developed, targeting the effect site [3]. Continuously calculating the required infusion rate to rapidly achieve and maintain a concentration level trajectory which accurately meets the needs of surgical patients therefore requires a computer-controlled infusion pump. It is impossible to achieve similar performance when using manually controlled infusion systems.

Several academic groups have developed TCI systems to study drug optimization. Since the early 1990s the software for the systems developed in Stanford (Stanpump), Stellenbosch (Stelpump), and Gent (RUGLOOP) universities has been available on request from the authors and at times freely available over the Internet. Several pharmacokinetic simulation programs have also been available (examples include IVA-SIM, TIVATrainer). Initially, the individual academic groups referred to TCI technology by a variety of acronyms, including CATIA (computer-assisted total intravenous anesthesia) [4], TIAC (titration of intravenous agents by computer) [5], CACI (computer-assisted continuous infusion) [6], and CCIP (computer-controlled infusion pump) [7]. The term target-controlled infusion (TCI) has been used in this context most often [8] and has become the standard. The development of TCI introduced various new conceptual terminologies into anesthesia, which are listed in Table 8.1 [9].

The first commercially available TCI system was the Diprifusor (AstraZeneca, London, UK), a microprocessor module included in intravenous infusion pumps sold by several manufacturers from 1996 until 2006 (in numerous countries around the world except the USA). The development of the Diprifusor has been described in detail [10]. Its application was limited to target-controlled infusions of Diprivan (propofol; AstraZeneca), targeting plasma concentrations, and it imposed the use of pre-filled glass syringes of propofol tagged electronically for single use. More recently, pump companies have introduced more flexible so-called "open TCI" systems capable of administering propofol, but also opiates, ketamine, muscle relaxants, etc. in modes targeting either plasma or effect-compartment concentrations.

Mathematical model

As explained in Chapter 5, the pharmacokinetics of many intravenous drugs can be accurately described by mammillary multicompartment models. The concept of these models and the underlying mathematical representation is based on the theory of linear stationary systems [11]. Whenever these models are used, it is assumed that the represented processes of drug distribution and elimination in the body are linear and time-invariant, or that the applied amounts are small enough to be represented by such models. All TCI implementations apply, in one form or another, two essential principles

resulting from this assumption: the principle of *superposition*, stating that the response to a composite input is identical to the sum of the responses of the inputs separately, and the principle of *time invariance*, stating that if a signal input $x(t)$ results in an output $y(t)$, then the time-shifted input signal $x(t + T)$ results in exactly the same output $y(t + T)$, shifted over the same amount of time.

A three-compartment mammillary model including the effect-site compartment is shown in Fig. 8.2. In this model structure, intravenous drugs are delivered into and eliminated from the central (plasma) compartment only. The central compartment exchanges drug with the peripheral compartments at a rate proportional to the drug concentration gradients between them. The effect-site compartment is considered as a negligibly small fourth compartment whose drug exchange rate with the central compartment is characterized by the rate constant k_{1e}. The differential equations describing this model are expressed in terms of drug amount, not concentrations, knowing that the drug concentration in a compartment equals the drug amount divided by the compartment's volume. The following differential equations describe the model as a function of time:

$$
\begin{aligned}
dA_1(t) &= (I(t) + k_{21}.A_2(t) + k_{31}.A_3(t) + k_{e0}.A_4(t) \\
&\quad - (k_{10} + k_{12} + k_{13} + k_{1e}).A_1(t)).dt \\
dA_2(t) &= (k_{12}.A_1(t) - k_{21}.A_2(t)).dt \\
dA_3(t) &= (k_{13}.A_1(t) - k_{31}.A_3(t)).dt \\
dA_4(t) &= (k_{1e}.A_1(t) - k_{e0}.A_4(t)).dt
\end{aligned}
\tag{8.1}
$$

Since the terms $k_{e0}.A_4(t)$ and $k_{1e}.A_1(t)$ are very small, they can be ignored in the calculation of $dA_1(t)$, yielding the simplified differential equation:

$$
\begin{aligned}
dA_1(t) &= (I(t) + k_{21}.A_2(t) + k_{31}.A_3(t) \\
&\quad - (k_{10} + k_{12} + k_{13}).A_1(t)).dt
\end{aligned}
\tag{8.2}
$$

One particular feature in the ratio of compartment volumes and drug exchange constants must be taken into account. In equilibrium, the drug concentration in all compartments

Table 8.1. Terminology introduced by TCI

C_{pT}	Target plasma concentration
C_{eT}	Target effect-site concentration
C_{pM}	Measured plasma concentration
C_{pCALC}	Calculated plasma concentration
C_{eCALC}	Calculated effect-site concentration

Adapted from Glass *et al.* [9].

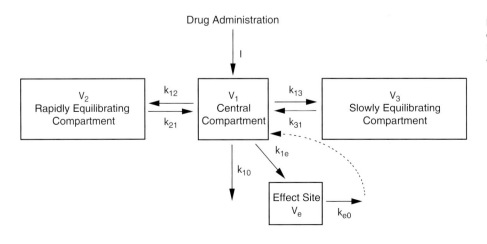

Figure 8.2. Schematic representation of a three-compartment mammillary plus effect-site compartment model for the behavior of an intravenously administered drug in the body.

Drug Administration

should be identical. At that time, there is no more net drug transfer between the central and the peripheral compartments:

$$dA_n = 0 \quad \text{or} \quad k_{1n}.A_1(t) = k_{n1}.A_n(t), \forall\, n > 1 \tag{8.3}$$

Since

$$c_n(t) = A_n(t)/V_n, c_n(\infty) = c_1(\infty), \forall\, n \tag{8.4}$$

must necessarily

$$k_{1n}.c_1(\infty).V_1 = k_{n1}.c_n(\infty).V_n \text{ or } V_n \tag{8.5}$$

$$= V_1\, k_{n1}/k_{1n}. \, \forall\, n > 1$$

so the volume of any peripheral compartment is known when the ratio of exchange rates with the central compartment is known.

The set of differential equations to calculate the drug concentration in the central compartment can be converted into an equivalent impulse response function. The impulse response for an n-compartment model, $u_n(t)$, is an n-exponential function of the form:

$$u_1(t) = P_1 e^{-a_1 t} + P_2 e^{-a_2 t} + \ldots + P_n e^{-a_n t} \tag{8.6}$$

The impulse response can be considered as the central-compartment concentration over time in response to a unit amount of drug, infused instantaneously. A derivation of the impulse response function from the differential equations is found in the specialized literature [12].

As for any linear time-invariant system, the relationship between an arbitrary drug input $r(t)$ and the resulting central compartment drug concentration can be calculated as:

$$A_1(t) = r(t)^* u_1(t) \tag{8.7}$$

where $u_1(t)$ is the impulse response function and * denotes the mathematical operation of convolution.

If pharmacodynamic data are also available for the drug of interest so that a value has been defined for k_{e0}, there exists a $n + 1$ exponential impulse response function, $u_e(t)$, for the effect compartment of the form:

$$u_e(t) = Q_1 e^{-a_1 t} + Q_2 e^{-a_2 t} + \ldots + Q_n e^{-a_n t} \tag{8.8}$$

$$+ [SQ_i].e^{-k_{e0} t}$$

$$i = 1$$

with $Q_i = -P. k_{e0}/(\alpha_i - k_{e0})$, which characterizes completely the relation between drug input into the central compartment and the resulting effect-compartment drug concentration, such that

$$A_e(t) = r(t)^*.u_e(t) \tag{8.9}$$

If the time course of the central-compartment drug concentration is known, an alternative method to calculate the effect-site concentration is the following convolution integral:

$$A_e(t) = k_{1e}.\exp(-k_{e0}.t)^* A_1(t) \tag{8.10}$$

Since the effect-site compartment is assumed to have an arbitrarily small volume, the relationship between k_{1e} and k_{e0} is known as $k_{1e} = k_{e0} \cdot V_e/V_1$.

In practice, the convolution method is too cumbersome for TCI systems using embedded microcontrollers with long drug infusion histories. Most TCI systems will apply a piecewise constant infusion rate rather than a continuously adjusted infusion rate to track the target concentration set by the anesthesiologist. A typical constant-rate interval is 10 seconds. At each multiple of the interval time, the concentration resulting from the infusion is calculated. For this evaluation, either an Euler approximation of the differential equations [13] or an analytical solution for a piecewise-continuous infusion profile in a recursive algorithm [3] is applied.

Control strategy

Theoretically, the infusion regimen required over time can be calculated using a mathematical deconvolution from the desired concentration profile:

$$r(t) = u_1(t)^{*-1} . C_{1_d} \tag{8.11}$$

where $^{*-1}$ denotes deconvolution. A (piecewise constant) concentration C_{1_d}, meaning the target concentration set by the anesthesiologist, is the desired outcome. This approach is impractical for TCI implementations in the embedded microprocessors. Instead, at each multiple of the standard interval time, the superposition principle is used to calculate the appropriate administration rate for the next interval to reach the user-set target concentration as soon as possible, as shown in Fig. 8.3A and B for plasma and effect-compartment TCI, respectively.

Plasma targeting

Since pharmacokinetic models ignore the delay in plasma concentration caused by drug mixing and initial recirculation, the maximum plasma concentration resulting from a constant infusion rate over an infusion interval in the absence of earlier drug administration is observed at the end of the infusion interval. Let $C_{pr}(t)$ be the plasma concentration resulting from a reference amount rate $r[0,T]$ applied over the infusion interval T. The superposition principle is then applied as follows (and as graphically represented in Fig. 8.3A):

$$r_1[0, T] = C_t/C_{pr}(T).r \text{ yields } C_{p1}(t), C_{p1}(T) = C_t \tag{8.12}$$

$$r_2[T, 2T] = (C_t - C_{p1}(2T))/C_{pr}(T).r \text{ yields } C_{p2}(t),$$

$$C_{p1}(2T) + C_{p2}(2T) = C_t \text{ etc.}$$

Effect-site targeting

Even with TCI control, the only way to decrease plasma concentration and "extract" an infused dose of drug from the body is by waiting for its elimination. Thus an overshoot in drug concentration leading to an overshoot in clinical effect or potentially adverse drug effects should be avoided. The delay

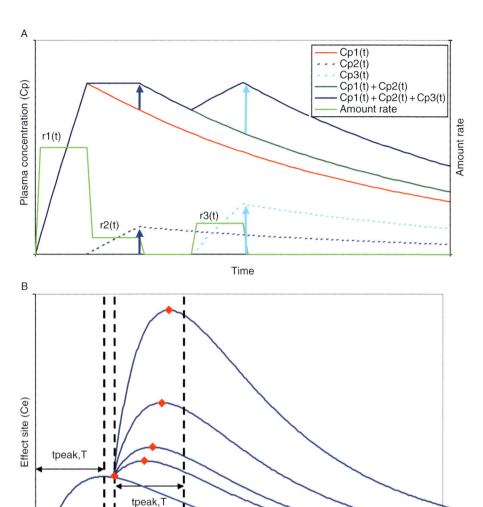

A

B

Figure 8.3. Superposition principle applied in (A) plasma and (B) effect-site targeting with a piecewise continuous infusion. In plasma targeting, the required infusion rate is readily calculated knowing the target concentration, the zero-infusion concentration decay, and the plasma concentration resulting from a unit rate infusion interval. In effect-site concentration, the maximum effect-site concentration occurs at t_{peak}, T instead of at the end of the infusion. Subsequent infusions yield a t_{peak}, T that is a function of both the infusion history and the infusion rate to be applied.

between the time course of the plasma and effect-site concentrations results in a peak effect-site concentration only some time after an instantaneous bolus infusion of drug. This time to peak effect-site concentration (t_{peak}) will cause the peak effect-site concentration induced by a constant infusion rate interval to be postponed past the end of the infusion interval (t_{peak},T). Consequently, targeting for an effect-site concentration to be reached exactly at the end of the infusion interval T results in an effect-site concentration overshoot afterwards. To attain the target effect-site concentration without overshoot, the TCI algorithms reference the concentration at t_{peak},T. There is a minor caveat, however: the time of peak effect-site concentration resulting from the superposition of two successive constant–rate infusion intervals is a nonlinear function of

the relative magnitude of the two infusions (Fig. 8.3B). When targeting the effect-site concentration, TCI systems need to take an iterative approach to calculate the required infusion rate each interval instead of the straightforward approach for targeting plasma concentration [3].

Manual infusion, plasma, or effect-compartment TCI ?

The benefits of TCI become clear when compared to manual infusion schemes. The simulations in Fig. 8.4 demonstrate the differences between various administration modes. In this virtual patient (male, 170 cm, 70 kg, 25 years), the propofol plasma and effect-site concentrations (simulated using the model published by Schnider *et al.* [14,15]) and

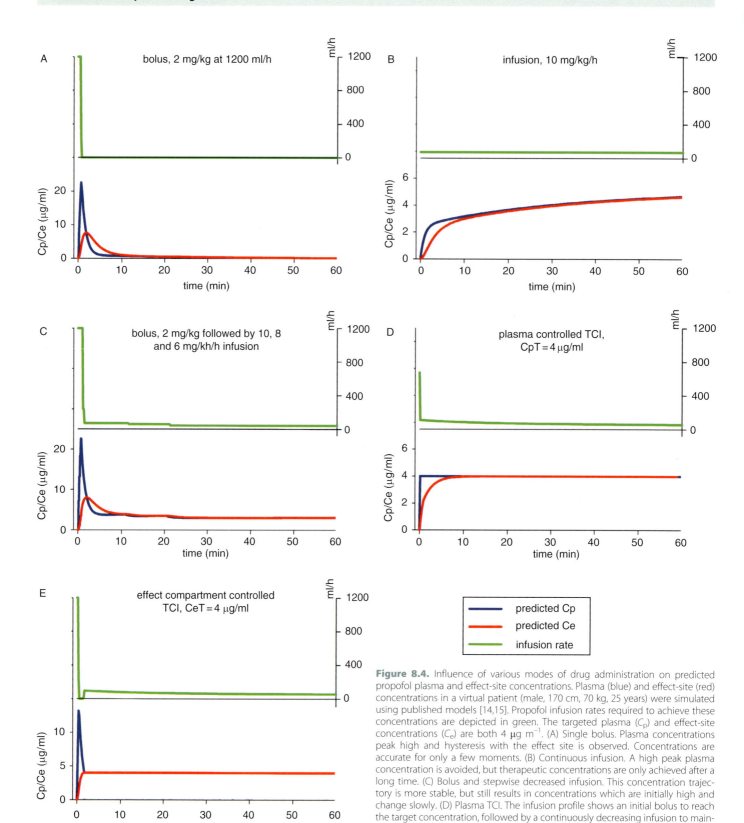

Figure 8.4. Influence of various modes of drug administration on predicted propofol plasma and effect-site concentrations. Plasma (blue) and effect-site (red) concentrations in a virtual patient (male, 170 cm, 70 kg, 25 years) were simulated using published models [14,15]. Propofol infusion rates required to achieve these concentrations are depicted in green. The targeted plasma (C_p) and effect-site concentrations (C_e) are both 4 μg m^{-1}. (A) Single bolus. Plasma concentrations peak high and hysteresis with the effect site is observed. Concentrations are accurate for only a few moments. (B) Continuous infusion. A high peak plasma concentration is avoided, but therapeutic concentrations are only achieved after a long time. (C) Bolus and stepwise decreased infusion. This concentration trajectory is more stable, but still results in concentrations which are initially high and change slowly. (D) Plasma TCI. The infusion profile shows an initial bolus to reach the target concentration, followed by a continuously decreasing infusion to maintain a stable plasma concentration. The effect-site concentration, however, still shows a slow equilibration to the target concentration. (E) Effect-compartment TCI. The initial bolus is larger, to achieve the desired effect-site concentration, but overshoots the plasma concentration. After the bolus, the pump stops infusing and waits for equilibration. Then a slowly decreasing infusion rate is needed to maintain target concentrations.

the infusion rates are depicted. When administering a single bolus (Fig. 8.4A), plasma concentration peaks high (depending on the infusion rate) and hysteresis with the effect-site concentration is observed. A bolus achieves only a few moments of accurate concentrations. With a continuous infusion (Fig. 8.4B), a high peak plasma concentration is avoided, but therapeutic concentrations are only achieved after a long time. Classically, propofol is administered as a bolus and a stepwise decreased infusion (e.g., 10 – 8 – 6 mg kg^{-1} h^{-1}) (Fig. 8.4C). This enables some stable concentration trajectory, but still results in concentrations which are initially high and change slowly, with possible accumulation during long-lasting infusions. Figure 8.4D shows a plasma-targeted TCI infusion. The infusion profile shows the need for an initial bolus to reach the target concentration, followed by a continuously decreasing infusion to maintain a stable plasma concentration. The effect-site concentration, however, still shows a slow equilibration to the target concentration. In order to reach and maintain an accurate effect-site concentration, without overshoot at the effect-site level, effect-compartment TCI is required (Fig. 8.4E). Here, the initial bolus is larger, overshooting the plasma level but not the effect-site level. After the bolus, the pump stops infusing and waits for equilibration. Then, a slowly decreasing infusion rate is needed to maintain all concentrations at the target level. The simulations in Fig. 8.4 are done with propofol, but could have been done using various other intravenous drugs.

The simulations illustrate how effect-compartment TCI offers the fastest control of clinical drug effect. When using effect-compartment TCI, two potential pitfalls should be recognized. First, the accuracy of k_{e0} is especially critical in effect-site targeting, because it will determine the overshoot and undershoot in plasma concentrations during changes in targeted effect-site concentrations. Accurate simulated concentrations demand a model developed from a study combining blood sampling with frequent measurements of drug effect, resulting in an overall model for the dose–response behavior of the drug. Historically, the time constants of PK models and the k_{e0} of PD studies without accurate blood samples (thereby lacking the PK model) were sometimes naively merged, possibly resulting in inaccurate predictions of clinical drug effect [16]. However, if no integrated PK/PD model exists, the time of peak effect after a bolus injection (t_{peak}) can be used to recalculate k_{e0} using the PK of interest to yield the correct time of peak effect [3]. Second, "the" effect-site is calculated using one typical drug effect (e.g., cerebral drug effect as measured by EEG). The time course of other (side) effects (e.g., hemodynamic effect for hypnotics) most frequently follows another trajectory, and one should therefore be careful when overshooting the plasma concentration to hasten plasma-effect-site equilibration in compromised patients to avoid the onset of side effects. Concerns about high plasma concentrations that result from

targeting the effect site can be addressed by limiting the peak plasma concentration overshoot [17].

Context-sensitive half-time and decrement time
Originally, the context-sensitive half-time was defined as the time required for the plasma concentration to decrease by 50% after an infusion that maintained a constant concentration, with the context being the duration of infusion [18]. As the effect-site is most often more relevant, the original concept was enlarged towards the *context-sensitive decrement time*, in which the decrement is calculated in the compartment of interest (plasma or effect site) [19]. TCI technology enables the user to specify an endpoint concentration, and the computer will estimate the time to reach this concentration taking into account the infusion history. This feature might help in optimizing the targets at the end of anesthesia in order to avoid delayed recovery, and it can be used for both hypnotics and analgesics. Due to the exponential decays involved in drug elimination, together with population variability, the inaccuracy of these estimates in predicting clinical endpoints is large, especially after long infusions or for low endpoint concentrations.

Performance evaluation of TCI technology
In order to select the best PK/PD model for TCI application, prospective testing is required during TCI application. For some of the drugs, research (and the controversy) is still going on. Tables 8.2 and 8.3 show the most commonly applied models and drugs in clinically available TCI devices. Investigators who have assessed the accuracy of propofol TCI report inevitable deviation of actual plasma concentrations from the targeted plasma concentrations [31]. Other than possible technical problems in both software and hardware, possible sources of variability arise during estimation of the pharmacokinetic parameters and from the TCI. For example, there is variance among the parameters of a polyexponential function fitted to a single set of concentration-time data. In addition, there is PK variation among the subjects who constituted the sample from which the averaged parameter set was derived. Often, because of cost considerations, the number of subjects in the sample is small, casting doubt as to whether the sample can be assumed to represent the population adequately. Furthermore, patients receiving TCI do not necessarily belong to the same population from whom the original pharmacokinetic model was derived, and the effect of the surgical procedure can result in PK variability within each patient [32]. All of these factors can lead to bias and inaccuracy of the concentrations achieved during TCI.

Several calculation and statistical methods are used to describe the accuracy of a specific parameter set [31]:
- *prediction error* (%) of the predicted concentration in plasma:

Table 8.2. Commonly applied PK/PD models for TCI systems for hypnotics

Drug	Propofol	Propofol	Propofol	Propofol	Ketamine
Model	Marsh [20]	Schnider [14, 15]	Paedfusor [21]	Kataria [22]	Domino [23]
Parameter					
V_1	0.228 L kg^{-1}	4.27 L	0.458 L kg^{-1}	0.52 L kg^{-1}	0.063 L kg^{-1}
V_2	0.363 L kg^{-1}	$18.9 - 0.391 \times$ (age $- 53$) L	1.34 L kg^{-1}	1.0 L kg^{-1}	0.207 L kg^{-1}
V_3	2.893 L kg^{-1}	238 L	8.20 L kg^{-1}	8.2 L kg^{-1}	1.51 L kg^{-1}
k_{10} (min^{-1})	0.119	$0.443 + 0.0107 \times$ (weight $- 77$) $- 0.0159 \times$ (LBM $- 59$) $+ 0.0062 \times$ (height $- 177$)	$70 \times$ weight $- 0.3/458.3$	0.066	0.4381
k_{12} (min^{-1})	0.112	$0.302 - 0.0056 \times$ (age $- 53$)	0.12	0.113	0.5921
k_{13} (min^{-1})	0.042	0.196	0.034	0.051	0.59
k_{21} (min^{-1})	0.055	$(1.29 - 0.024 \times$ (age $- 53$))$/$ $(18.9 - 0.391$(age $- 53$))	0.041	0.059	0.247
k_{31} (min^{-1})	0.0033	0.0035	0.0019	0.0032	0.0146
k_{e0} (min^{-1})	0.26[a]	0.456	NA	NA	NA
TPPE (min)	NA	1.69	NA	NA	NA

[a] k_{e0} derived independently from the PK model [24].
NA, not available.

Table 8.3. Commonly applied PK/PD models for TCI systems for analgesics

Drug	Remifentanil	Sufentanil	Fentanyl	Alfentanil
Model	Minto [25, 26]	Gepts [27]	Shafer [7]	Maitre [28]
Parameter				
V_1	$5.1 - 0.0201$(age $- 40$) $+ 0.072$(LBM $- 55$) L	14.3 L	6.09 L	♂ $= 0.111$ L kg^{-1} ♀ $= 1.15 \times 0.111$ L kg^{-1}
V_2	$9.82 - 0.0811$(age $- 40$) $+ 0.108$(LBM $- 55$) L	63.4 L	28.1 L	12.0 L
V_3	5.42 L	251.9 L	228 L	10.5 L
k_{10} (min^{-1})	$((2.6 - 0.0162$(age $- 40$) $+ 0.0191$(LBM $- 55$))$/V_1$	0.0645	0.083	<40 yr $= 0.356/V_1$ >40 yr $= 0.356 - (0.00269$(age $- 40$))$/V_1$
k_{12} (min^{-1})	$((2.05 - 0.0301$(age $- 40$))$/V_1$	0.1086	0.4713	0.104
k_{13} (min^{-1})	$(0.076 - 0.00113$(age $- 40$))$/V_1$	0.0229	0.22496	0.017
k_{21} (min^{-1})	$k_{12} \times V_1/V_2$	0.0245	0.1021	0.067
k_{31} (min^{-1})	$k_{13} \times V_1/V_2$	0.0013	0.00601	<40 yr $= 0.0126$ >40 yr $= 0.0126 - 0.000113$(age $- 40$)
k_{e0} (min^{-1})	$0.595 - 0.007$(age $- 40$)	NA	0.147[a]	0.77[a]
TPPE (min)[b]	NA	5.6	3.6	1.4

[a] k_{e0} is derived independently from the PK model by Scott *et al.* [29].
[b] from Shafer and Varvel [30].
NA, not available.

$$PE = (\text{measured} - \text{predicted}/\text{predicted}) \times 100\%$$

PE is an indication of the bias of the achieved concentrations, and the absolute value PE ($|PE|$) is a measure of the precision (inaccuracy).

- *Median absolute prediction error* indicates the inaccuracy of TCI in the i-th subject:

$$MDAPE_i = \text{median}\{|PE|_{ij}, \ j = 1, \ldots, N_i\}$$

  where N_i is the number of values of $|PE|$ obtained for the i-th subject.

- *Median prediction error* reflects the bias of TCI in the i-th subject:

$$MDPE_i = \text{median}\{PE_{ij}, j = 1, \ldots, N_i\}$$

- *Divergence* is a measure of how the resulting drug concentrations in a subject are affected by time. It is defined as the slope of the linear regression equation of $|PE|$ against time and is expressed in units of percentage divergence per hour. A positive value indicates progressive widening of the gap between predicted and measured concentrations, whereas a negative value reveals that the measured concentrations converge on the predicted values.

- *Wobble* is another index of the time-related changes in performance and measures the intrasubject variability in performance errors. In the i-th subject the percentage of wobble is calculated as follows:

$$\text{wobble}_i = \text{median}\{|PE_{ij} - MDPE_i|, j = 1, \ldots, N_i\}$$

Clinically applied models for TCI: model selection

For most intravenous drugs, multiple PK/PD models have been published. Propofol is the most extensively investigated drug (Table 8.2). A comparison of the available propofol PK models [33] found that the parameter sets provided by Marsh et al. [20] proved adequate with acceptable prediction errors (MDPE −7%; MDAPE 18% [20]) during TCI use. The Marsh set has been implemented in the Diprifusor (AstraZeneca) and has been validated clinically in plasma-controlled TCI mode for many years in different clinical situations [33–35]. It has the major drawback of using only weight as a model covariate. More recently, age, height, weight, and lean body mass (LBM) were evaluated as covariates in a new three-compartment PK model for propofol [14]. The large variability in the study population (18–81 years and 44–123 kg) provides a wide applicability of the model. Various authors rated the performance of the model as better than the Marsh model, but, when administered in combination with opiates, larger MDPE and MDAPE were found [36,37]. Furthermore, the inclusion of lean body mass as a covariate may lead to incorrect drug dosages in morbidly obese patients due to the quadratic behavior of the lean body mass function [38], which demonstrates that care should be taken when applying a model outside its

study population's range. Beside the classical 1% and 2% propofol known as Diprivan 1% and 2% (AstraZeneca), multiple alternative formulations have been commercialized. For some of these, kinetics are similar [14,39,40].

To optimize drug delivery, targeting the effect site is more appropriate. Accurate description of the drug transfer between the plasma and effect site requires an accurate k_{e0}, characterizing a first-order process. Previously, the Diprifusor TCI system for propofol applied a naive method of combining separate pharmacokinetic and pharmacodynamic studies, which resulted in biased results. For propofol, only the model from Schnider et al. has studied combined kinetics and dynamics [14,15] and has been widely used in clinical devices. Since both k_{e0} (0.456 min^{-1}) and t_{peak} (1.69 min) have been published for this model, the options are to use the k_{e0} as it stands or to recalculate a new k_{e0} corresponding to a t_{peak} of 1.69 minutes in a specific patient. The last approach was clinically confirmed in various studies [41–44]. This approach has also been used in combination with the Marsh kinetic, leading to a high k_{e0} value of 1.21 min^{-1} [45].

Two PK models for propofol TCI in children have been used experimentally in clinical practice. A three-compartment model for propofol in a population of children between 3 and 11 years used weight as the sole significant covariate [23]. Weight-adjusting the volumes and clearances significantly improved the accuracy of the pharmacokinetics. Adjusting the pharmacokinetics for inclusion of additional patient covariates or using a mixed-effects model did not further improve the ability of the pharmacokinetic parameters to describe the observations. This model was safely used during esophagogastroduodenoscopy in children, although no blood samples were taken [46]. A more recent test of this model found a high bias with an overall underestimation of measured propofol concentration versus the target concentration [47]. An alternative system for pediatric application of propofol TCI, called the "Paedfusor," was developed at Glasgow University. This TCI prototype system for children, incorporating one of the preliminary models developed by Schüttler et al. [48], was clinically validated and found to have an acceptable performance [21]. No effect-compartment-controlled TCI has been reported in children, due to the lack of accurate models. Preliminary work shows that propofol pharmacodynamics in children differs from that in adults [49].

Several PK/PD models for opioids are shown in Table 8.3. The covariate independent models for sufentanil have been verified, with acceptable MDPE ranging from −2.3% to −22.3% and MDAPE ranging from 18.5% to 29%, even for obese patients [50–52]. For alfentanil, various compartmental PK models were published in the early 1980s, but did not use a true population modeling approach. The original datasets from these studies were subsequently used to develop a new model using population modeling (NONMEM) [28]. As this analysis did not evaluate effect-site concentration coupling, the authors reused the k_{e0} naively from a previous simultaneous PK/PD model [29]. More recently, a comparison of three different alfentanil PK models

[53] found that the model by Scott *et al.* [29] had poor performance (MDPE –35%, MDAPE 36%) compared to the one by Maitre *et al.* [28] (MDPE 12%, MDAPE 28%). In contrast, the Maitre model was reported to perform worse than the Scott model in two patient groups [54].

For fentanyl, a PK model was developed without covariates specifically for TCI use [7]. Since the model was derived from normal-weight patients and was not scaled to body weight, its application to obese patients may cause overprediction of fentanyl plasma concentrations. The accuracy of that fentanyl PK model in lean and obese patients was evaluated [55], and a correction to the simulated plasma concentration proposed, where corrected $C_p = C_p$ Shafer $\times$ (1 + (196.4 $\times$ e $^{-0.025\ \text{kg}}$ – 53.66)/100).

Remifentanil is the only opioid for which combined PK/PD models have been developed. Remifentanil PK can be described by a three-compartment model, and it has been studied in healthy volunteers and patients [25,26,56,57], obese patients [58], and those with hepatic or renal disease [59,60]. Neither renal nor hepatic insufficiency clinically alter remifentanil PK. Table 8.3 shows the most frequently used PK/PD model for remifentanil [25,26]. The performance of both sets for remifentanil were found to be clinically acceptable [61]. Combined PK/PD studies are not available for all opioids. However the times to peak effect after a bolus injection of alfentanil (1.4 min), fentanyl (3.6 min), and sufentanil (5.6 min) can be used to calculate the effect-site concentration using the t_{peak} algorithm [62].

For various other drugs such as benzodiazepines, muscle relaxants, and ketamine, multicompartment models have been created and tested. However, these drugs are not clinically available in the commercial TCI pumps.

Selecting the right target concentrations for TCI: variability

The PK/PD models cited in the previous paragraphs have all been derived from population pharmacology studies where the researchers try to identify and quantify how covariates like weight, age, gender, and height influence the dose–concentration relationship. The accuracy of the estimated drug concentration for any one individual is limited by interpatient variability, hence the applicability of the model is limited to the population studied to develop the model. Thus caution is needed when applying a PK/PD model for obese, elderly, children, diabetics, alcoholics, unless similar subjects were part of the study population from which the PK/PD model was derived. Most of the commercial implementations of TCI will therefore prevent selecting weight, height, etc. outside the range of the model's study population. Other potential causes of reduced model accuracy are errors (e.g., drug spill), excessive blood loss, or PK and/or PD drug interactions.

Accuracy of PK/PD models for highly variable populations can be improved if the model is built while exploring a wide range of possible covariates using parametric modeling, optionally nonlinear mixed-effects modeling [63,64]. An illustration of the importance of the study population range is an ongoing debate on the accuracy of the two PK/PD models for propofol, applying k_{e0} vs. t_{peak}. Since the only difference between the models is in the PD portion, only the initial moments are relevant for a difference in infused volume. After a few minutes, the plasma and effect-site compartment concentrations will have equilibrated for a constant simulated concentration, and both models will show an identical infusion pattern. The drug amount infused by both models during induction, using effect-site targeting, is illustrated in Fig. 8.5. Within the study population limits, there are small differences in infused drug amount for two parameter sets, but much greater differences for the third. Extrapolations outside the population tremendously reduce the accuracy of one, or any, of the models. An Internet initiative (www.opentci.org) has been started in an attempt to build more comprehensive models including more diverse populations.

Because of the above factors, no single regimen, concentration, or drug combination applies to all patients. Nevertheless, application of TCI often reduces intersubject variability in drug response compared with bolus dosing [65]. Some guidance can be found in the effective concentrations at which 50% and 95% of patients have the desired clinical effect (Table 8.4). As with all drug administration in anesthesia, clinical judgment is always required, and target concentration should be titrated according to patient clinical responses.

Closed-loop drug administration

Open-loop controlled drug administration applies PK/PD models based on the typical subject to estimate a drug concentration at certain locations in the body, without actually measuring these concentrations. The resulting inaccuracy of absolute concentration requires the clinician to manually titrate the dose regimen or target concentration based on observations of the desired therapeutic effect. The clinical benefits of a tight titration require high clinical expertise or a labor-intensive process and may divert the clinician's attention from critical actions, resulting in a suboptimal therapy or even threatening the patient's safety. Applying closed-loop drug administration techniques has the potential to optimize this process of dose titration.

The application of closed-loop systems for drug administration is complex and requires a perfect balance for all the basic components of such a system: (1) a controlled variable representative of the targeted therapeutic effect, (2) a clinically relevant set-point or target value for this variable, (3) a control actuator (in this case, the infusion pump driving the drug), (4) a system (in this case a patient), and (5) an accurate, stable control algorithm [68].

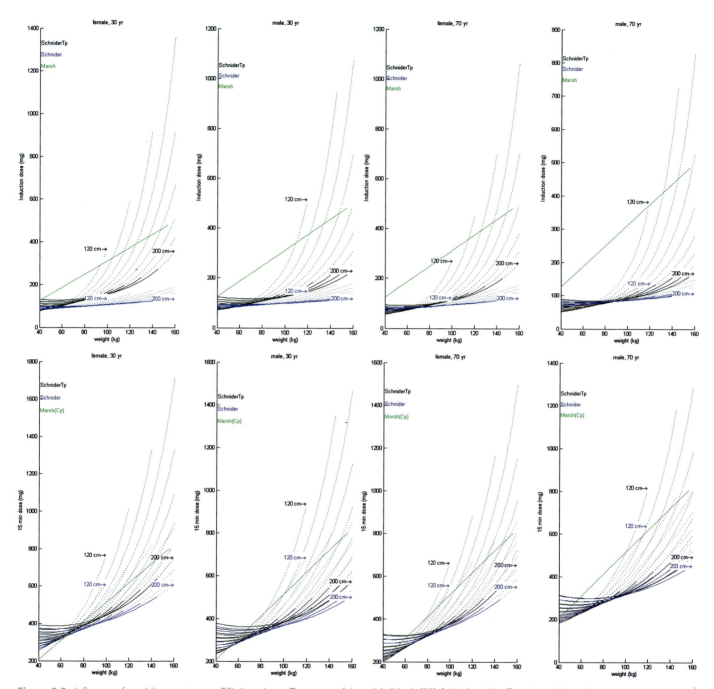

Figure 8.5. Influence of model parameters on TCI drug doses. Three propofol models (Marsh [20], Schnider with effect site calculated using a $k_{e0} = 0.456$ min^{-1} [14,15], and Schnider with effect site calculated using a $t_{peak} = 1.6$ min [14,15]) targeted an effect-site concentration of 5 µg mL^{-1}. Doses are in mg kg^{-1}, based on weight. The induction dose is the initial bolus administered. The 15 min dose is the total amount given after 15 minutes. Results are given for female and male, and for 30-year-old and 70-year-old, patients. Each line represents a specific patient height. The dotted line represents the extrapolation of the model outside the limit imposed by the maximum lean body mass (at the same time outside the study population).

The controlled variable
Pharmacokinetic closed-loop

If drug concentrations can be measured in real time, closed-loop delivery based on pharmacokinetics is possible. The clinician can select a target drug concentration and the system will adapt its delivery to attain and maintain this concentration based on concentration measurements. On-line measuring of drug concentration is not feasible for intravenous anesthetics. In contrast, inspired and end-tidal (or end-expired) concentrations of inhaled anesthetics such as isoflurane, sevoflurane, and desflurane can be measured using real-time spectroscopic

113

Table 8.4. Propofol/opioid combinations estimated to be associated with the fastest recovery from anesthesia. $C_{optimal}$ represents combinations associated with a 50% probability of a response to surgical stimuli; $C_{awakening}$ concentrations represent the estimated concentrations at which consciousness will be regained; time to awakening represents the estimated time from termination of the infusion to return of consciousness in 50% of patients. From Vuyk *et al.* [66], and modified from Absalom and Struys [67], with permission.

Infusion duration (min)		Propofol : alfentanil (μg mL^{-1} : ng mL^{-1})	Propofol : sufentanil (μg mL^{-1} : ng mL^{-1})	Propofol : remifentanil (μg mL^{-1} : ng mL^{-1})
15	$C_{optimal}$	3.25 : 99.3	3.57 : 0.17	2.57 : 4.70
	$C_{awakening}$	1.69 : 65.0	1.70 : 0.10	1.83 : 1.93
	Time to awakening (min)	8.2	9.4	5.1
60	$C_{optimal}$	3.38 : 89.7	3.34 : 0.14	2.51 : 4.78
	$C_{awakening}$	1.70 : 64.9	1.70 : 0.10	1.83 : 1.93
	Time to awakening (min)	12.2	11.9	6.1
300	$C_{optimal}$	3.40 : 88.9	3.37 : 0.14	2.51 : 4.78
	$C_{awakening}$	1.70 : 64.9	1.70 : 0.10	1.86 : 1.88
	Time to awakening (min)	16.0	15.6	6.7

methods, allowing the implementation of automated systems realizing these concentrations. The end-tidal concentration might be a reasonable surrogate for arterial blood concentration, but still shows a time lag with regard to cerebral anesthetic effects. Over the last decades, various experimental systems have been developed [69,70]. Recently, a commercial closed-circuit anesthesia ventilator (Zeus; Dräger Medical, Lübeck, Germany) was released. This machine targets the end-tidal concentrations of inhaled anesthetics and controls the fresh gas flow and sets anesthetic concentration using closed-loop technology [71].

Pharmacokinetic-dynamic closed-loop

The effectiveness of closed-loop systems for drug administration strongly depends on the reliability, monotonicity, and linearity (in contrary to on/off or saturation behavior) of the physiological signal as the indicator for the desired clinical effect. Examples of observable clinical endpoints are blood pressure [72] or neuromuscular function [73]. As "depth of hypnosis" or "level of analgesia" is not measurable, surrogate measures have to be applied as controlled variables. A clinician should be aware that a certain surrogate measure does not show 100% correlation with the desired therapeutic effect, and should back up his or her therapeutic decisions using secondary variables. Reliable closed-loop systems should integrate this common sense by applying the same secondary variables as boundaries to increase the efficacy and safety of the overall system.

The electroencephalogram (EEG), representing cortical activity, is widely accepted as a marker for depth of hypnosis. Several computerized EEG derivatives such as spectral edge frequency and median frequency have been used as controlled variables for closed-loop systems in the past [74]. More recently, the Bispectral Index (BIS) has been tested and

validated as a measure of the hypnotic component of anesthesia and has been used as the controlled variable in multiple studies. BIS has been designed using multivariate statistical analysis to combine multiple EEG features including higher-order spectra and phase correlations between spectra into a more accurate indicator. BIS values lie in the range of 0–100. BIS in the 90–100 range represents fully awake patients, while ranges around 60–70 and 40–60 indicate light and moderate hypnotic states, respectively. A BIS value below 40 indicates an excessive level of hypnosis [75]. Other EEG derivatives were designed to measure the hypnotic depth of anesthesia, but have not so far been applied in closed-loop systems. Nearly all EEG-derived parameters have the drawback that the electronics used to measure the microvolt-range signals often pick up noise from electrocoagulation or disturbances such as muscle activity. Furthermore, the actual EEG activity may be suppressed by other mechanisms induced by some volatile anesthetics, not directly related to the depth of hypnosis. One research group has tested auditory evoked potentials, more specifically the mid-latency auditory evoked potential (MLAEP) as the controlled variable for closed-loop control for propofol [76].

The development of closed-loop systems for control of analgesics (mostly opioids) still lacks an optimal measurement method. Since an adequate level of analgesia balances nociception and antinociception, an automated measurement might require a noxious stimulus to be effective. Despite a complex combined effect of both hypnotic and analgesic drugs on the hemodynamic status of the patient, most anesthesiologists rely on the autonomic and somatic changes in blood pressure, heart rate, etc. to guide their administration of perioperative opioids, supported by secondary measures such as tearing. But an automated controller for opioid control based on hemodynamic changes alone would be incapable of distinguishing between the sources of changes in blood pressure, so more complex systems are required. Recently, some preliminary reports have been published on measuring the nociception–antinociception balance by heart-rate variability, variability of the pulse plethysmography, variability in the Bispectral Index (called the composite variability index), and others [77,78].

The set-point

The set-point is the value for the controlled variable which the controller uses as its target. This target is specified by the anesthesiologist and will be approached as closely as possible during the maintenance of anesthesia; therefore an adequate individual target is essential for the accuracy of the closed-loop system. Two types of set-points can be used, based on (1) population mean data or (2) individual data measured at the start or just before the control period. The latter type could be expected to more closely correspond to clinical needs during the course of the surgical procedure.

The control algorithm

Various closed-loop strategies have been applied for drug administration. A controller classic is the proportional–integral–differential (PID) controller commonly known from general engineering [74]. A PID controller will calculate the actuator's corrective action based on a straightforward mathematical derivative of the observed error. The general formula can be written in the time domain as:

$$\mathrm{d}U/\mathrm{d}t = K_\mathrm{P} \times \mathrm{d}(err)/\mathrm{d}t + err/K_\mathrm{I} + K_\mathrm{D} \times \mathrm{d}^2(err)/\mathrm{d}^2 t \quad (8.13)$$

with err being the error between the target and the observed value, causing a response U in the actuator. The constants K_P, K_I, K_D are tuned by calculations from models of the system, by computer simulations, or derived from trials using tuning rules. For systems with a complex pharmacologic behavior, a general PID controller with U an administration rate can be slow to establish control and dangerous to use because of possible oscillations. Fine-tuning of a PID controller is difficult in this particular setting because of the complexity of the system to control (as shown in Fig. 8.1), because of interindividual pharmacologic variability, and because it is not possible to directly counteract the administration of excessive drug [79].

A better approach is to incorporate information about the dose–response into the control, by using the PID controller to set a target plasma or effect-site concentration for an underlying TCI system (Fig. 8.1: A/A′, B/B′) This approach applies the TCI system to compensate for part of the complex dose–response relationship. Even though the TCI system will only realize an approximate value for the target concentration, the dynamics of the resulting system will be of lower order [80]. PID controllers, tuned in general circumstances, may fail in situations that are different (e.g., surgical stimulation, inter-patient variability) from that for which the controller was tuned. The increasing calculation performance of computer systems may allow better control through the integration of more complex mathematical models of the overall relationship

between the drug and its effect in the human body, or by reverting to other control algorithms such as model predicted control or fuzzy logic [81,82].

The tuning of a controller does not need to be permanently fixed. In adaptive (model-based) controllers, the controller response is varied to adapt to changing circumstances. Fine-tuning of the model towards the individual patient can be done using state estimation, mixed-effects pharmacokinetic or dynamic modeling, Bayesian estimation, Kalman filtering, fuzzy logic, or other engineering techniques. Bayesian optimization [83] individualizes the PD relationship by combining individual information with the knowledge of an a-priori probability density function containing the statistical properties of the parameter to be estimated [84]. The Bayesian method starts from a standard, population-based response model providing the prior distribution of parameter values. These values are adjusted to reflect the patient's own parameters over time, based on the observed response of the individual patient under varying circumstances. Recently, this method has been used in a closed-loop system for propofol [85,86] (Fig. 8.6). The Kalman filter will apply a recursive method to calculate numbers for a given dose–response relationship for the specific patient [87]. One investigation explored how k_{e0} can be individualized on the basis of an initial bolus and estimation of time to peak effect [88]. An alternative approach of model adaptation based on fuzzy logic has been proposed [89].

Prototype examples of closed-loop drug delivery systems

Since 1950 various groups have investigated closed-loop drug delivery during anesthesia [90]. Table 8.5 shows a list of prototypes for the administration of hypnotics, analgesics, and muscle relaxants in humans based on changes in hemodynamic and cerebral drug effects. All systems were clinically tested.

Hypnotics

Lacking a better direct indicator, many closed-loop systems for hypnotics have been designed using hemodynamic feedback, as shown in Table 8.5. Early studies used the EEG median frequency as the controlled variable [103,109]. A linear two-compartment model was used to describe the drug input–concentration relation in an adaptive controller. More recently, this closed-loop system was used using EEG to study the interaction of alfentanil and propofol [126]. Each patient received a target-controlled infusion of alfentanil. Propofol was added to the alfentanil infusion by a feedback system. The set-point was the range of 1.5–2.5 Hz median frequency of the EEG. Strangely, it was concluded that the interaction between alfentanil and propofol, based on the EEG in the investigated dose range, was additive [126]. After the commercialization of the Bispectral Index derived from the EEG, closed-loop systems using BIS technology (BIS monitor; Aspect Medical, Norwood, MA, USA) were developed. Preliminary tests performed with a BIS (version 1.22)-controlled closed-loop system concluded

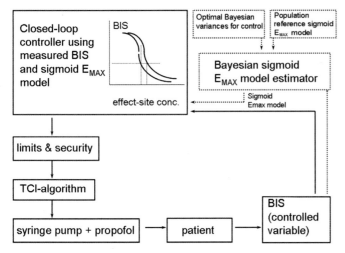

Figure 8.6. Flow chart of the closed-loop system. The straight lines represent the closed-loop control system. At each time the required effect-site concentration is calculated by the controller. This value is sent to an additional algorithm taking the safety limits into account. The result of these calculations is the required effect-site concentration sent to the TCI algorithm, which steers a pump injecting propofol to the patient. The measured BIS is used as the input of the closed-loop controller. The dotted lines represent the Bayesian sigmoid E_{MAX} model estimator. The estimator receives a-priori information from the population sigmoid E_{MAX} model, the optimal Bayesian variances for control, and the patient-measured BIS values. Reproduced with permission from De Smet et al. [85].

that the system provided intraoperative hemodynamic stability and prompt recovery from sedative-hypnotic effects of propofol [117]. The performance of a closed-loop system for administration of general anesthesia, using BIS (version 3.1) as a target for control in combination with a modified PID controller for drug administration was evaluated [116]. Anesthesia was maintained by intravenous infusion of a propofol/alfentanil mixture (via an infusion pump) or an isoflurane/nitrous-oxide-based technique (inhaled anesthetics injected in the inspiratory limb of the breathing circle). Closed-loop and manually controlled administration of anesthesia resulted in similar intraoperative conditions (cardiovascular and EEG variables) and initial recovery characteristics. The closed-loop system showed no clinical advantage over conventional, manually adjusted techniques of anesthetic administration. A similar closed-loop anesthesia system using BIS as the control variable, a PID control algorithm, and a propofol plasma-controlled TCI system as the control actuator was developed [80]. Although clinical tests showed acceptable control, the authors concluded that further studies were required to determine whether control performance could be improved by changing the gain factors or by using an effect-site-targeted TCI propofol system [127]. These researchers subsequently revised their controller algorithm, including an effect-compartment TCI in their system, which was shown to have better accuracy of control, although the PID controller might still face some stability problems [121].

Model-based adaptive control of propofol administration with BIS was previously used in a closed-loop system for sedation during spinal anesthesia and, more recently, during general anesthesia [45,115]. The latter two reports (from the same research group) describe a closed-loop control system for propofol using the BIS as the controlled variable. The implementation applied a patient-specific PD profile calculated during induction for control during surgery. More recently, the same authors further developed the adaptive part of the controller using Bayesian optimization [85].

Newer closed-loop systems have been evaluated. A new type of closed-loop control system using the BIS has been developed, and applied to the administration of inhaled isoflurane [122]. This controller uses a cascade structure, originally described by Gentilini et al. [118], which separates regulation of the PD and PK effects of isoflurane on BIS. Closed-loop control with BIS to administer isoflurane required no human intervention to maintain BIS at 50 ± 10, and performed significantly better than manual control. An indicator derived from the MLAEP, called AEPindex, has been used as the controlled variable [76], and has been used to investigate the synergistic interaction between propofol and remifentanil [128].

Opiates and muscle relaxants

There are relatively few closed-loop systems for anesthetic drug classes other than sedative-hypnotics. A model predictive controller (MPC) was designed for the control of mean arterial blood pressure during anesthesia, using alfentanil as the opiod. Opioid concentrations predicted by a PK model are used together with mean arterial pressure (MAP) by the controller algorithm to determine opioid infusion rates Many closed-loop control systems for muscle relaxants have been explored in the past, but only a few could cope with the introduction of the latest shorter-acting neuromuscular blocking drugs. Table 8.5 shows a list of various prototypes.

Future closed-loop drug delivery systems

Future development of integrated closed-loop systems for total anesthesia control are only possible if multiple input/output controllers are used to control both hypnotic and analgesic components of anesthesia [129]. The ultimate goal of the closed-loop controllers is their general acceptance in clinical practice. So far, all developed closed-loop systems have been used in well-controlled scientific trial environments. Nevertheless, closed-loop delivery systems are no longer esoteric [130]. Rather, the challenge is now to establish fully the safety, efficacy, reliability, and utility of closed-loop anesthesia for its adoption into clinical practice. However, regulatory challenges need to be solved [131].

Summary

In current clinical practice, anesthetic drugs are predominantly still administered using standard dosing guidelines and techniques, ignoring the large interindividual variability in dose–response relationships. The application of computer-controlled

Table 8.5. Closed-loop systems for hypnotics, analgesics and muscle relaxants

Reference	Drug	Controlled variable	Controller type
Bickford 1950 [90]	Thiopental	EEG	On-off
Soltero et al. 1951 [91]	Ether	EEG	P
Bellville et al. 1954 [92]	Cyclopropane	EEG	P
Kiersey et al. 1954 [79]	Thiopental	EEG	P
Bellville & Attura 1957 [93]	Cyclopropane	EEG	P
Suppan 1972 [94]	Halothane	HR	On-off/incremental
Suppan 1977 [95]	Halothane	BP	On-off/incremental
Lindkens et al. 1982 [96]	Vecuronium	NMT	PID
Rametti et al. 1985 [97]	D-Tubocurare	NMT	State estim./adaptive
Ritchie et al. 1985 [98]	Succinylcholine	NMT	PID
Rametti & Bradlow 1983 [99]	Atracurium	NMT	State estim./adaptive
Lampard et al. 1986 [100]	Atracurium	NMT	On-off
de Vries et al. 1986 [101]	Vecuronium	NMT	On-off
Schils et al. 1987 [102]	Halothane	BP + EEG	PI/model-based
Schwilden et al. 1987 [103]	Methohexital	EEG-MF	Model-based/adaptive
Webster & Cohen 1987 [104]	Atracurium	NMT	PD
Jaklitsch et al. 1987 [105]	Vecuronium	NMT	PID
Millard et al. 1988 [106]	Isoflurane	MAP	Model-based/adaptive
Monk et al. 1989 [107]	Isoflurane	MAP	Adaptive
MacLeod et al. 1989 [108]	Atracurium	NMT	PI
Schwilden et al. 1989 [109]	Propofol	EEG-MF	Model-based/adaptive
O'Hara et al. 1991 [110]	Atracurium	NMT	Miltiphase/PID
Olkkola & Schwilden 1991 [111]	Vecuronium	NMT	Model-based/adaptive
Olkkola et al. 1991 [112]	Atracurium	NMT	Model-based/adaptive
Schwilden & Stoeckel 1993 [113]	Alfentanil	EEG-MF	Model-besed/adaptive
Zbinden et al. 1995 [81]	Isoflurane	MAP	Fuzzy logic
Edwards et al. 1998 [114]	Atracurium	NMT	Fuzzy logic
Mortier et al. 1998 [115]	Propofol	EEG-BIS	Model-based, adaptive
Kenny & Mantzaridis 1999 [76]	Propofol	EEG-MLAEP	PI
Morley et al. 2000 [116]	Propofol/Isofl	EEG-BIS	PID + plasma TCI
Sakai et al. 2000 [117]	Propofol	EEG-BIS	PID
Gentilini et al. 2001 [118]	Isoflurane	EEG-BIS	Model-based, adaptive
Allen & Smith 2001 [119]	Propofol	AEP	Neuro-fuzzy
Struys et al. 2001 [45]	Propofol	EEG-BIS	Model-based, adaptive
Gentilini et al. 2002 [120]	Alfentanil	MAP	Model-based, predictive
Absalom et al. 2002 [80]	Propofol	EEG-BIS	PID + plasma TCI
Absalom & Kenny 2003 [121]	Propofol	EEG-BIS	PID + effect-site TCI
Locher et al. 2004 [122]	Isoflurane	EEG-BIS	Model-based, adaptive
Luginbühl et al. 2006 [123]	Alfentanil	MAP	Model-based,predictive
Liu et al. 2006 [124]	Propofol	EEG-BIS	PD + effect-site TCI
Puri et al. 2007 [125]	Propofol	EEG-BIS	PID
De Smet et al. 2007 [85]	Propofol	EEG-BIS	Model-based, Bayesian

EEG, electroencephalogram; MF, median frequency; MLAEP, mid-latency auditory evoked potentials; BIS, Bispectral Index; P, proportional; I, integral; D, derivative; HR, heart rate; BP, blood pressure; NMT, neuromuscular transition monitoring; MAP, mean arterial pressure; TCI, target-controlled infusion.
No animal data and no simulation data are included. This table focuses on classical hypnotics, analgesics, and NMT, and no blood-pressure controllers using inotropics are included.

continuously updated infusion rates based on mathematical models, clinical effects feedback, or, in the absence of quantifiable effects, carefully selected surrogate measures, may yield better patient-individualized dosing.

Historically conventional, open-loop drug administration targets a drug concentration or clinical effect, and uses PK/PD models based on the typical subject, to estimate a drug dose. The resulting inaccuracy of absolute concentration requires the clinician to manually titrate the dose regimen or target concentration based on observations of desired therapeutic or side effects. Achieving accurate and tightly controlled titration requires high clinical expertise or a labor-intensive process and may divert the clinician's attention away from critical actions, resulting in a suboptimal therapy or even threatening the patient's safety.

Target-controlled infusion (TCI) was developed to optimize the time course of drug effect by targeting a specific therapeutic drug concentration in a specific body compartment, mostly the plasma or the effect site. Multicompartment mammillary PK/PD models, derived from pharmacologic modeling studies, are used in TCI systems to calculate the infusion rates to achieve and maintain the target concentration as fast and accurately as possible without an overshoot in drug concentrations.

Closed-loop control takes the anesthesiologist "out of the loop." Clinicians only enter the desired clinical or surrogate effect, and a computer-based controller autonomously calculates the drug administration rate, based on the measured actual value of the controlled variable, the set-point, and, potentially, internal models of the expected dose–response relationship. The application of closed-loop systems for drug administration is complex and requires a perfect balance among all components of such a system: (1) a controlled variable representative of the targeted therapeutic effect, (2) a clinically relevant set-point or target value for this variable, (3) a control actuator (in this case, the infusion pump driving the drug), (4) a system (in this case a patient), and (5) an accurate, stable control algorithm. Applying closed-loop drug administration techniques might optimize this process of dose titration.

References

1. Kruger-Thiemer E. Continuous intravenous infusion and multicompartment accumulation. *Eur J Pharmacol* 1968; **4**: 317–24.

2. Schwilden H. A general method for calculating the dosage scheme in linear pharmacokinetics. *Eur J Clin Pharmacol* 1981; **20**: 379–86.

3. Shafer SL, Gregg KM. Algorithms to rapidly achieve and maintain stable drug concentrations at the site of drug effect with a computer-controlled infusion pump. *J Pharmacokinet Biopharm* 1992; **20**: 147–69.

4. Schüttler J, Schwilden H, Stoekel H. Pharmacokinetics as applied to total intravenous anaesthesia. Practical implications. *Anaesthesia* 1983; **38** (Suppl): 53–6.

5. Ausems ME, Stanski DR, Hug CC. An evaluation of the accuracy of pharmacokinetic data for the computer assisted infusion of alfentanil. *Br J Anaesth* 1985; **57**: 1217–25.

6. Glass PS, Jacobs JR, Smith LR, *et al.* Pharmacokinetic model-driven infusion of fentanyl: assessment of accuracy. *Anesthesiology* 1990; **73**: 1082–90.

7. Shafer SL, Varvel JR, Aziz N, Scott JC. Pharmacokinetics of fentanyl administered by computer-controlled infusion pump. *Anesthesiology* 1990; **73**: 1091–102.

8. Chaudhri S, White M, Kenny GN. Induction of anaesthesia with propofol using a target-controlled infusion system. *Anaesthesia* 1992; **47**: 551–3.

9. Glass PS, Glen JB, Kenny GN, Schüttler J, Shafer SL. Nomenclature for computer-assisted infusion devices. *Anesthesiology* 1997; **86**: 1430–1.

10. Glen JB. The development of "Diprifusor": a TCI system for propofol. *Anaesthesia* 1998; **53** (Suppl 1): 13–21.

11. Cutler DJ. Linear systems analysis in the kinetics of anaesthetic agents. *Anaesth Pharm Rev* 1994; **2**: 243–9.

12. Jacobs JR. Analytical solution to the three-compartment pharmacokinetic model. *IEEE Trans Biomed Eng* 1988; **35**: 763–5.

13. Shafer SL, Siegel LC, Cooke JE, Scott JC. Testing computer-controlled infusion pumps by simulation. *Anesthesiology* 1988; **68**: 261–6.

14. Schnider TW, Minto CF, Gambus PL, *et al.* The influence of method of administration and covariates on the pharmacokinetics of propofol in adult volunteers. *Anesthesiology* 1998; **88**: 1170–82.

15. Schnider TW, Minto CF, Shafer SL, *et al.* The influence of age on propofol pharmacodynamics. *Anesthesiology* 1999; **90**: 1502–16.

16. Struys MM, De Smet T, Depoorter B, *et al.* Comparison of plasma compartment versus two methods for effect compartment–controlled target-controlled infusion for propofol. *Anesthesiology* 2000; **92**: 399–406.

17. Van Poucke GE, Bravo LJB, Shafer SL. target controlled infusions: targeting the effect site while limiting peak plasma concentration. *IEEE Trans Biomed Eng* 2004; **51**: 1869–75.

18. Hughes MA, Glass PS, Jacobs JR. Context-sensitive half-time in multicompartment pharmacokinetic models for intravenous anesthetic drugs. *Anesthesiology* 1992; **76**: 334–41.

19. Youngs EJ, Shafer SL. Pharmacokinetic parameters relevant to recovery from opioids. *Anesthesiology* 1994; **81**: 833–42.

20. Marsh B, White M, Morton N, Kenny GN. Pharmacokinetic model driven infusion of propofol in children. *Br J Anaesth* 1991; **67**: 41–8.

21. Absalom A, Amutike D, Lal A, White M, Kenny GN. Accuracy of the "Paedfusor" in children undergoing cardiac surgery or catheterization. *Br J Anaesth* 2003; **91**: 507–13.

22. Kataria BK, Ved SA, Nicodemus HF, *et al.* The pharmacokinetics of propofol in children using three different data analysis approaches. *Anesthesiology* 1994; **80**: 104–22.

23. Absalom AR, Lee M, Menon DK, *et al.* Predictive performance of the Domino, Hijazi, and Clements models during low-dose target-controlled ketamine infusions in healthy volunteers. *Br J Anaesth* 2007; **98**: 615–23.

24. Schüttler J, Stoeckel H, Schwilden H. Pharmacokinetic and pharmacodynamic modelling of propofol ("Diprivan") in volunteers and surgical patients. *Postgrad Med J* 1985; **61**: 53–4.

25. Minto CF, Schnider TW, Shafer SL. Pharmacokinetics and pharmacodynamics of remifentanil. II. Model application. *Anesthesiology* 1997; **86**: 24–33.

26. Minto CF, Schnider TW, Egan TD, *et al.* Influence of age and gender on the pharmacokinetics and pharmacodynamics of remifentanil.

I. Model development. *Anesthesiology* 1997; **86**: 10–23.

27. Gepts E, Shafer SL, Camu F, *et al.* Linearity of pharmacokinetics and model estimation of sufentanil. *Anesthesiology* 1995; **83**: 1194–204.

28. Maitre PO, Vozeh S, Heykants J, Thomson DA, Stanski DR. Population pharmacokinetics of alfentanil: the average dose-plasma concentration relationship and interindividual variability in patients. *Anesthesiology* 1987; **66**: 3–12.

29. Scott JC, Ponganis KV, Stanski DR. EEG quantitation of narcotic effect: the comparative pharmacodynamics of fentanyl and alfentanil. *Anesthesiology* 1985; **62**: 234–41.

30. Shafer SL, Varvel JR. Pharmacokinetics, pharmacodynamics, and rational opioid selection. *Anesthesiology* 1991; **74**: 53–63.

31. Varvel JR, Donoho DL, Shafer SL. Measuring the predictive performance of computer-controlled infusion pumps. *J Pharmacokinet Biopharm* 1992; **20**: 63–94.

32. Shafer A, Doze VA, Shafer SL, White PF. Pharmacokinetics and pharmacodynamics of propofol infusions during general anesthesia. *Anesthesiology* 1988; **69**: 348–56.

33. Coetzee JF, Glen JB, Wium CA, Boshoff L. Pharmacokinetic model selection for target controlled infusions of propofol. Assessment of three parameter sets. *Anesthesiology* 1995; **82**: 1328–45.

34. Hoymork SC, Raeder J, Grimsmo B, Steen PA. Bispectral index, predicted and measured drug levels of target-controlled infusions of remifentanil and propofol during laparoscopic cholecystectomy and emergence. *Acta Anaesthesiol Scand* 2000; **44**: 1138–44.

35. Fabregas N, Rapado J, Gambus PL, *et al.* Modeling of the sedative and airway obstruction effects of propofol in patients with Parkinson disease undergoing stereotactic surgery. *Anesthesiology* 2002; **97**: 1378–86.

36. Wietasch JK, Scholz M, Zinserling J, *et al.* The performance of a target-controlled infusion of propofol in combination with remifentanil: a clinical investigation with two propofol formulations. *Anesth Analg* 2006; **102**: 430–7.

37. Struys MM, Coppens MJ, De Neve N, *et al.* Influence of Administration Rate on Propofol Plasma-Effect Site Equilibration. *Anesthesiology* 2007; **107**: 386–96.

38. Bouillon T, Shafer SL. Does size matter? *Anesthesiology* 1998; **89**: 557–60.

39. Doenicke AW, Roizen MF, Rau J, *et al.* Pharmacokinetics and pharmacodynamics of propofol in a new solvent. *Anesth Analg* 1997; **85**: 1399–403.

40. Ward DS, Norton JR, Guivarc'h PH, Litman RS, Bailey PL. Pharmacodynamics and pharmacokinetics of propofol in a medium-chain triglyceride emulsion. *Anesthesiology* 2002; **97**: 1401–8.

41. Vanluchene AL, Vereecke H, Thas O, *et al.* Spectral entropy as an electroencephalographic measure of anesthetic drug effect: a comparison with bispectral index and processed midlatency auditory evoked response. *Anesthesiology* 2004; **101**: 34–42.

42. Vanluchene AL, Struys MM, Heyse BE, Mortier EP. Spectral entropy measurement of patient responsiveness during propofol and remifentanil. A comparison with the bispectral index. *Br J Anaesth* 2004; **93**: 645–54.

43. Vereecke HE, Struys MM, Mortier EP. A comparison of bispectral index and ARX-derived auditory evoked potential index in measuring the clinical interaction between ketamine and propofol anaesthesia. *Anaesthesia* 2003; **58**: 957–61.

44. Struys MM, Vereecke H, Moerman A, *et al.* Ability of the bispectral index, autoregressive modelling with exogenous input-derived auditory evoked potentials, and predicted propofol concentrations to measure patient responsiveness during anesthesia with propofol and remifentanil. *Anesthesiology* 2003; **99**: 802–12.

45. Struys MM, De Smet T, Versichelen LF, *et al.* Comparison of closed-loop controlled administration of propofol using Bispectral Index as the controlled variable versus "standard practice" controlled administration. *Anesthesiology* 2001; **95**: 6–17.

46. Drover DR, Litalien C, Wellis V, Shafer SL, Hammer GB. Determination of the pharmacodynamic interaction of propofol and remifentanil during esophagogastroduodenoscopy in children. *Anesthesiology* 2004; **100**: 1382–6.

47. Rigouzzo A, Girault L, Louvet N, *et al.* The relationship between bispectral index and propofol during target-controlled infusion anesthesia: a comparative study between children and young adults. *Anesth Analg* 2008; **106**: 1109–16.

48. Schüttler J, Ihmsen H. Population pharmacokinetics of propofol: a multicenter study. *Anesthesiology* 2000; **92**: 727–38.

49. Cortinez LI, Delfino AE, Fuentes R, Munoz HR. Performance of the cerebral state index during increasing levels of propofol anesthesia: a comparison with the bispectral index. *Anesth Analg* 2007; **104**: 605–10.

50. Slepchenko G, Simon N, Goubaux B, *et al.* Performance of target-controlled sufentanil infusion in obese patients. *Anesthesiology* 2003; **98**: 65–73.

51. Barvais L, Heitz D, Schmartz D, *et al.* Pharmacokinetic model-driven infusion of sufentanil and midazolam during cardiac surgery: assessment of the prospective predictive accuracy and the quality of anesthesia. *J Cardiothorac Vasc Anesth* 2000; **14**: 402–8.

52. Hudson RJ, Henderson BT, Thomson IR, Moon M, Peterson MD. Pharmacokinetics of sufentanil in patients undergoing coronary artery bypass graft surgery. *J Cardiothorac Vasc Anesth* 2001; **15**: 693–9.

53. van den Nieuwenhuyzen MC, Engbers FH, Burm AG, *et al.* Computer-controlled infusion of alfentanil for postoperative analgesia. A pharmacokinetic and pharmacodynamic evaluation. *Anesthesiology* 1993; **79**: 481–92.

54. Raemer DB, Buschman A, Varvel JR, *et al.* The prospective use of population pharmacokinetics in a computer-driven infusion system for alfentanil. *Anesthesiology* 1990; **73**: 66–72.

55. Shibutani K, Inchiosa MA, Sawada K, Bairamian M. Pharmacokinetic mass of fentanyl for postoperative analgesia in lean and obese patients. *Br J Anaesth* 2005; **95**: 377–83.

56. Egan TD, Minto CF, Hermann DJ, *et al.* Remifentanil versus alfentanil: comparative pharmacokinetics and pharmacodynamics in healthy adult male volunteers. *Anesthesiology* 1996; **84**: 821–33.

57. Drover DR, Lemmens HJ. Population pharmacodynamics and pharmacokinetics of remifentanil as a supplement to nitrous oxide anesthesia for elective abdominal surgery. *Anesthesiology* 1998; **89**: 869–77.

58. Egan TD, Huizinga B, Gupta SK, *et al.* Remifentanil pharmacokinetics in obese versus lean patients. *Anesthesiology* 1998; **89**: 562–73.

59. Dershwitz M, Hoke JF, Rosow CE, *et al.* Pharmacokinetics and pharmacodynamics of remifentanil in volunteer subjects with severe liver disease. *Anesthesiology* 1996; **84**: 812–20.

60. Hoke JF, Shlugman D, Dershwitz M, *et al.* Pharmacokinetics and pharmacodynamics of remifentanil in persons with renal failure compared with healthy volunteers. *Anesthesiology* 1997; **87**: 533–41.

61. Mertens MJ, Engbers FH, Burm AG, Vuyk J. Predictive performance of computer-controlled infusion of remifentanil during propofol/remifentanil anaesthesia. *Br J Anaesth* 2003; **90**: 132–41.

62. Minto CF, Schnider TW, Gregg KM, Henthorn TK, Shafer SL. Using the time of maximum effect site concentration to combine pharmacokinetics and pharmacodynamics. *Anesthesiology* 2003; **99**: 324–33.

63. Egan TD. Remifentanil pharmacokinetics and pharmacodynamics. A preliminary appraisal. *Clin Pharmacokinet* 1995; **29**: 80–94.

64. Somma J, Donner A, Zomorodi K, *et al.* Population pharmacodynamics of midazolam administered by target controlled infusion in SICU patients after CABG surgery. *Anesthesiology* 1998; **89**: 1430–43.

65. Hu C, Horstman DJ, Shafer SL. Variability of target-controlled infusion is less than the variability after bolus injection. *Anesthesiology* 2005; **102**: 639–45.

66. Vuyk J, Mertens MJ, Olofsen E, Burm AG, Bovill JG. Propofol anesthesia and rational opioid selection: determination of optimal EC50-EC95 propofol-opioid concentrations that assure adequate anesthesia and a rapid return of consciousness. *Anesthesiology* 1997; **87**: 1549–62.

67. Absalom A, Struys MMRF. *An overview of TCI&TIVA*, 2nd edn. Gent: Academia Press, 2007.

68. O'Hara DA, Bogen DK, Noordergraaf A. The use of computers for controlling the delivery of anesthesia. *Anesthesiology* 1992; **77**: 563–81.

69. Verkaaik AP, Van Dijk G. High flow closed circuit anaesthesia. *Anaesth Intensive Care* 1994; **22**: 426–34.

70. el-Attar AM. Guided isoflurane injection in a totally closed circuit. *Anaesthesia* 1991; **46**: 1059–63.

71. Struys MM, Kalmar AF, De Baerdemaeker LE, *et al.* Time course of inhaled anaesthetic drug delivery using a new multifunctional closed-circuit anaesthesia ventilator. In vitro comparison with a classical anaesthesia machine. *Br J Anaesth* 2005; **94**: 306–17.

72. Chaudhri S, Colvin JR, Todd JG, Kenny GN. Evaluation of closed loop control of arterial pressure during hypotensive anaesthesia for local resection of intraocular melanoma. *Br J Anaesth* 1992; **69**: 607–10.

73. Claudius C, Viby-Mogensen J. Acceleromyography for use in scientific and clinical practice: a systematic review of the evidence. *Anesthesiology* 2008; **108**: 1117–40.

74. Schüttler J, Schwilden H. Closed-loop systems in clinical practice. *Current Opinion in Anesthesiology* 1997; **9**: 457–61.

75. Bruhn J, Myles PS, Sneyd R, Struys MM. Depth of anaesthesia monitoring: what's available, what's validated and what's next? *Br J Anaesth* 2006; **97**: 85–94.

76. Kenny GN, Mantzaridis H. Closed-loop control of propofol anaesthesia. *Br J Anaesth* 1999; **83**: 223–8.

77. Luginbuhl M, Ypparila-Wolters H, Rufenacht M, Petersen-Felix S, Korhonen I. Heart rate variability does not discriminate between different levels of haemodynamic responsiveness during surgical anaesthesia. *Br J Anaesth* 2007; **98**: 728–36.

78. Huiku M, Uutela K, van Gils M, *et al.* Assessment of surgical stress during general anaesthesia. *Br J Anaesth* 2007; **98**: 447–55.

79. Kiersey DK, Faulconer A, Bickford RG. Automatic electroencephalographic control of thiopental anesthesia. *Anesthesiology* 1954; **15**: 356–64.

80. Absalom AR, Sutcliffe N, Kenny GN. Closed-loop control of anesthesia using Bispectral index: performance assessment in patients undergoing major orthopedic surgery under combined general and regional anesthesia. *Anesthesiology* 2002; **96**: 67–73.

81. Zbinden AM, Feigenwinter P, Petersen-Felix S, Hacisalihzade S. Arterial pressure control with isoflurane using fuzzy logic. *Br J Anaesth* 1995; **74**: 66–72.

82. Luginbuhl M, Bieniok C, Leibundgut D, *et al.* Closed-loop control of mean arterial blood pressure during surgery with alfentanil: clinical evaluation of a novel model-based predictive controller. *Anesthesiology* 2006; **105**: 462–70.

83. Sheiner LB, Beal S, Rosenberg B, Marathe VV. Forecasting individual pharmacokinetics. *Clin Pharmacol Ther* 1979; **26**: 294–305.

84. Garraffo R, Iliadis A, Cano JP, Dellamonica P, Lapalus P. Application of Bayesian estimation for the prediction of an appropriate dosage regimen of amikacin. *J Pharm Sci* 1989; **78**: 753–7.

85. De Smet T, Struys MM, Greenwald S, Mortier EP, Shafer SL. Estimation of optimal modeling weights for a Bayesian-based closed-loop system for propofol administration using the bispectral index as a controlled variable: a simulation study. *Anesth Analg* 2007; **105**: 1629–38, table of contents.

86. De Smet T, Struys MM, Neckebroek MM, *et al.* The accuracy and clinical feasibility of a new bayesian-based

closed-loop control system for propofol administration using the bispectral index as a controlled variable. *Anesth Analg* 2008; **107**: 1200–10.

87. Sartori V, Schumacher, PM, Bouillon T, Lueginbuehl M, Morari M, eds. *On-line Estimation of Propofol Pharmacodynamic Parameters.* 27th IEEE EMBS Conference, 2005, Shangai.

88. Gentilini A, Frei CW, Glattfelder AH, Morari M, Schnider TW. Identification and targeting ploicies for computer-controlled infusion pumps. *Crit Rev Biomed Eng* 2000; **28**: 179–85.

89. Kern SE, Johnson JO, Westenskow DR. Fuzzy logic for model adaptation of a pharmacokinetic-based closed loop delivery system for pancuronium. *Artif Intell Med* 1997; **11**: 9–31.

90. Bickford R. Automatic EEEG control of general anesthesia. *Electroencephalogr Clin Neurophysiol* 1950; **2**: 93–6.

91. Soltero DE, Faulconer A, Bickford RG. The clinical application of automatic anesthesia. *Anesthesiology* 1951; **12**: 574–82.

92. Bellville JW, Artusio JF, Bulmer MW. Continuous servo motor integration of the electrical activity of the brain and its application to the control of cyclopropane anesthesia. *Electroencephalogr Clin Neurophysiol* 1954; **6**: 317–20.

93. Bellville JW, Attura GM. Servo control of general anesthesia. *Science* 1957; **126**: 827–30.

94. Suppan P. Feed-back monitoring in anaesthesia. II. Pulse rate control of halothane administration. *Br J Anaesth* 1972; **44**: 1263–71.

95. Suppan P. Feed-back monitoring in anaesthesia. IV. The indirect measurement of arterial pressure and its use for the control of halothane administration. *Br J Anaesth* 1977; **49**: 141–50.

96. Linkens DA, Asbury AJ, Rimmer SJ, Menad M. Identification and control of muscle-relaxant anaesthesia. *IEEE Proc* 1982; **129**: 136–41.

97. Rametti LB, Bradlow HS, Uys PC. Online parameter estimation and control of d-tubocurarine-induced muscle relaxation. *Med Biol Eng Comput* 1985; **23**: 556–64.

98. Ritchie G, Ebert JP, Jannett TC, Kissin I, Sheppard LC. A microcomputer based controller for neuromuscular block during surgery. *Ann Biomed Eng* 1985; **13**: 3–15.

99. Rametti LB, Bradlow HS. Online control of d-tubocurarine induced muscle relaxation: a simulation study. *Med Biol Eng Comput* 1983; **21**: 710–7.

100. Lampard DG, Brown WA, Cass NM, Ng KC. Computer-controlled muscle paralysis with atracurium in the sheep. *Anaesth Intensive Care* 1986; **14**: 7–11.

101. de Vries JW, Ros HH, Booij LH. Infusion of vecuronium controlled by a closed-loop system. *Br J Anaesth* 1986; **58**: 1100–3.

102. Schils GF, Sasse FJ, Rideout VC. Automatic control of anesthesia using two feedback variables. *Ann Biomed Eng* 1987; **15**: 19–34.

103. Schwilden H, Schüttler J, Stoeckel H. Closed-loop feedback control of methohexital anesthesia by quantitative EEG analysis in humans. *Anesthesiology* 1987; **67**: 341–7.

104. Webster NR, Cohen AT. Closed-loop administration of atracurium. Steady-state neuromuscular blockade during surgery using a computer controlled closed-loop atracurium infusion. *Anaesthesia* 1987; **42**: 1085–91.

105. Jaklitsch RR, Westenskow DR, Pace NL, Streisand JB, East KA. A comparison of computer-controlled versus manual administration of vecuronium in humans. *J Clin Monit* 1987; **3**: 269–76.

106. Millard RK, Monk CP, Prys-Roberts C. Self-tuning control of hypotension during ENT surgery using a volatile anaesthetic. *IEEE Proc* 1988; **135**: 95–105.

107. Monk CR, Millard RK, Hutton P, Prys-Roberts C. Automatic arterial pressure regulation using isoflurane: comparison with manual control. *Br J Anaesth* 1989; **63**: 22–30.

108. MacLeod AD, Asbury AJ, Gray WM, Linkens DA. Automatic control of neuromuscular block with atracurium. *Br J Anaesth* 1989; **63**: 31–5.

109. Schwilden H, Stoeckel H, Schüttler J. Closed-loop feedback control of propofol anaesthesia by quantitative EEG analysis in humans. *Br J Anaesth* 1989; **62**: 290–6.

110. O'Hara DA, Derbyshire GJ, Overdyk FJ, Bogen DK, Marshall BE. Closed-loop infusion of atracurium with four different anesthetic techniques. *Anesthesiology* 1991; **74**: 258–63.

111. Olkkola KT, Schwilden H. Adaptive closed-loop feedback control of vecuronium-induced neuromuscular relaxation. *Eur J Anaesthesiol* 1991; **8**: 7–12.

112. Olkkola KT, Schwilden H, Apffelstaedt C. Model-based adaptive closed-loop feedback control of atracurium-induced neuromuscular blockade. *Acta Anaesthesiol Scand* 1991; **35**: 420–3.

113. Schwilden H, Stoeckel H. Closed-loop feedback controlled administration of alfentanil during alfentanil-nitrous oxide anaesthesia. *Br J Anaesth* 1993; **70**: 389–93.

114. Edwards ND, Mason DG, Ross JJ. A portable self-learning fuzzy logic control system for muscle relaxation. *Anaesthesia* 1998; **53**: 136–9.

115. Mortier E, Struys M, De Smet T, Versichelen L, Rolly G. Closed-loop controlled administration of propofol using bispectral analysis. *Anaesthesia* 1998; **53**: 749–54.

116. Morley A, Derrick J, Mainland P, Lee BB, Short TG. Closed loop control of anaesthesia: an assessment of the bispectral index as the target of control. *Anaesthesia* 2000; **55**: 953–9.

117. Sakai T, Matsuki A, White PF, Giesecke AH. Use of an EEG-bispectral closed-loop delivery system for administering propofol. *Acta Anaesthesiol Scand* 2000; **44**: 1007–10.

118. Gentilini A, Rossoni-Gerosa M, Frei CW, et al. Modeling and closed-loop control of hypnosis by means of bispectral index (BIS) with isoflurane. *IEEE Trans Biomed Eng* 2001; **48**: 874–89.

119. Allen R, Smith D. Neuro-fuzzy closed-loop control of depth of anaesthesia. *Artif Intell Med* 2001; **21**: 185–91.

120. Gentilini A, Schaniel C, Morari M, et al. A new paradigm for the closed-loop intraoperative administration of analgesics in humans. *IEEE Trans Biomed Eng* 2002; **49**: 289–99.

121. Absalom AR, Kenny GN. Closed-loop control of propofol anaesthesia using bispectral index: performance assessment in patients receiving

computer-controlled propofol and manually controlled remifentanil infusions for minor surgery. *Br J Anaesth* 2003; **90**: 737–41.

122. Locher S, Stadler KS, Boehlen T, *et al.* A new closed-loop control system for isoflurane using bispectral index outperforms manual control. *Anesthesiology* 2004; **101**: 591–602.

123. Luginbuhl M, Rufenacht M, Korhonen I, *et al.* Stimulation induced variability of pulse plethysmography does not discriminate responsiveness to intubation. *Br J Anaesth* 2006; **96**: 323–9.

124. Liu N, Chazot T, Genty A, *et al.* Titration of propofol for anesthetic induction and maintenance guided by the bispectral index: closed-loop versus manual control: a prospective, randomized, multicenter study. *Anesthesiology* 2006; **104**: 686–95.

125. Puri GD, Kumar B, Aveek J. Closed-loop anaesthesia delivery system (CLADS) using bispectral index: a performance assessment study. *Anaesth Intensive Care* 2007; **35**: 357–62.

126. Schwilden H, Fechner J, Albrecht S, *et al.* Testing and modelling the interaction of alfentanil and propofol on the EEG. *Eur J Anaesthesiol* 2003; **20**: 363–72.

127. Leslie K, Absalom A, Kenny GN. Closed loop control of sedation for colonoscopy using the Bispectral Index. *Anaesthesia* 2002; **57**: 693–7.

128. Milne SE, Kenny GN, Schraag S. Propofol sparing effect of remifentanil using closed-loop anaesthesia. *Br J Anaesth* 2003; **90**: 623–9.

129. Gentilini A, Frei CW, Glattfedler AH, *et al.* Multitasked closed-loop control in anesthesia. *IEEE Eng Med Biol Mag* 2001; **20**: 39–53.

130. Glass PSA, Rampil IJ. Automated anesthesia: fact or fantasy? *Anesthesiology* 2001; **95**: 1–2.

131. Manberg PJ, Vozella CM, Kelley SD. Regulatory challenges facing closed-loop anesthetic drug infusion devices. *Clin Pharmacol Ther* 2008; **84**: 166–9.

Principles of drug action

Alternative routes of drug administration

Ola Dale

Introduction

Anesthesiologists administer drugs via a variety of routes during their everyday practice. Premedication may be given orally, intramuscularly, intravenously, or even rectally. During an operation drugs may be given intravenously, epidurally, spinally, or by inhalation. Procedural pain and pain control in the emergency treatment of injured children present additional challenges. Anesthesiologists may also be involved in control of acute and chronic cancer pain. The challenges of cancer pain control are different from those of acute care. Patients have a variety of other symptoms that may be difficult to diagnose and separate from the adverse effects of analgesics. Moreover, very high doses of opioids may be required to control pain, and many patients suffer from breakthrough pain, requiring treatment with drugs with rapid onset of effect and short duration. For these purposes alternative routes of administration, partly based on new technology, are already or will soon be available. This chapter focuses on alternative enteral and parenteral routes of drug administration. Comparative aspects related to alternative routes of administration are presented in Table 9.1.

Among the drugs commonly used in anesthetic practice, the opioids are of particular interest because of their widespread use and their capacity to be given by all routes of administration. Therefore the presentation of alternative routes will focus on opioids, although other drugs relevant to anesthetic practice will also be mentioned. Physicochemical properties determine the suitability of the opioids in this respect (Table 9.2). Taste and smell may prohibit oral and nasal transmucosal application, while local irritation/tissue toxicity affects subcutaneous and neuraxial administration. Lipid solubility and pK_a may determine the speed of transport across biological membranes, such as skin, gut epithelium, and the blood–brain barrier; it may also have pronounced effects on pharmacokinetics after neuraxial administration.

Physicochemical properties are also important from a pharmaceutical point of view. For some routes of administration the instillation volume must be low. This is very challenging, for example, in cancer pain, where the doses required

may be substantially higher than in perioperative care. Thus, for some applications it may be necessary to dissolve the opioid in small volumes, and with solvents that do not induce local irritation. It follows therefore that the potent opioids may be more favorable than the less potent ones. The development of formulations that meet these requirements can be very challenging.

Alternative routes are often used to enable drug delivery when oral bioavailability is low and/or unpredictable (e.g., parenteral fentanyl), to reduce the toxic effect of high systemic doses (e.g., neuraxial opioids), or when the nature of the pain requires rapid onset after self-administration (e.g., opioids for breakthrough cancer pain). In cancer pain, changes in the route of administration occur often, for instance from oral to a subcutaneous route. Differences in bioavailabilities between routes of administration require that drug doses must be adjusted appropriately, to avoid overdose or treatment failure.

Parenteral routes

Intramuscular administration

Intramuscular (IM) administration is a painful way of giving pain relief. However, the nonsteroidal anti-inflammatory drug (NSAID) diclofenac is often given parenterally by this route. Ketamine may also under some conditions be given by the IM route. The IM route was previously frequently used for premedication with opioids and anticholinergics. In general, IM drug administration has become far less used, and abandoned in some institutions for postoperative pain control. Time to maximum serum concentrations is about 15–20 minutes. The bioavailability is almost 100%, but time to onset of analgesia may be about 10 minutes slower than for intravenous (IV) administration, as the drug has to be absorbed from the point of injection [2]. Absorption depends on local perfusion, which may vary; hence absorption speed may depend on injection site [3]. Perfusion may be low in dehydrated and frail patients, in whom onset time and effect may be unpredictable. Safety concerns include accidental intravenous injection or accidental nerve lesions. Infections at the site of administration may also occur.

Anesthetic Pharmacology, 2nd edition, ed. Alex S. Evers, Mervyn Maze, Evan D. Kharasch. Published by Cambridge University Press. © Cambridge University Press 2011.

Both intrathecal and epidural routes deliver drug directly to spinal cord tissue. The nerve roots are also directly exposed to epidurally administered drugs. A significant difference is that the epidural drugs have to cross several barriers to reach the target, resulting in a slower onset of effect, and more drug is lost to epidural fat and cleared by epidural veins, thus requiring larger doses than for intrathecal administration. The benefit of neuraxial routes compared to systemic administration is the delivery of drugs close to the site of action. This reduces the dose compared to that for systemic administration, typically reducing systemic effects and associated potential adverse effects. In addition, clinical effects such as analgesia may be targeted to the relevant areas of the body. An

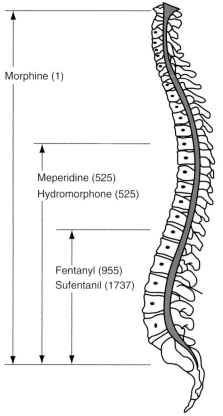

Figure 9.4. Lipid solubility and the spread of analgesia after intrathecal opioid administration in the lumbar cistern. Larger octanol:water partition coefficients (shown in parentheses) indicate greater lipid solubility. Lipophilic opioids produce more localized analgesia, while hydrophilic opioids spread rostrally and produce a broader band of analgesia. Reproduced with permission from Rathmell *et al.* [50].

important prerequisite for intrathecal and epidural dosing is that such drugs must be devoid of neurotoxicity.

The pharmacokinetics of spinally and epidurally administered drugs is complex. The key factors that determine drug behavior when given neuraxially are the physicochemical properties, especially pK_a and lipid solubility. For simplicity, the focus will be on lipid solubility of the opioids in this chapter. Host factors that determine neuraxial drug pharmacokinetics are the membrane barriers to cross, uptake to and distribution within the spinal cord, sequestration into epidural fat, and clearance of drug by spinal and epidural venous perfusion.

Morphine is the prototype hydrophilic opioid. Morphine crosses biological barriers very slowly. Epidural morphine localizes to spinal fluid, with very little sequestered into epidural fat, or into nonspecific "sites" in the spinal cord. Driven by a concentration gradient as well as by the flow of cerebrospinal fluid, morphine will slowly be distributed rostrally and exert central opioid effects (Figs. 9.4, 9.5). Thus morphine eventually exerts analgesic effects in spinal segments distant from were it was deposited. Rostral spread may cause delayed respiratory depression. Systemic clearance by venous perfusion is low for morphine. Thus the duration of effect of a single dose of morphine will be long. These characteristics results in an intrathecal to IV apparent potency ratio for morphine of at least 1 : 100 (Table 9.3) [50].

Fentanyl and sufentanil are the typical lipid-soluble opioids. Both drugs cross biological membranes rapidly. Sequestration into epidural fat is considerable, as is distribution to nonspecific "sites" in the spinal cord. Thus cerebral opioid effects of fentanyl and sufentanil via rostral spread are less likely, and their analgesic effects are more restricted to the proximity of the segmental level where they are deposited. Conversely, clearance by vascular perfusion of the cord and epidural space is far higher than for morphine, and thus the duration of effect is short compared to that of morphine. The consequence of these characteristics is that the intrathecal to IV dose ratio for fentanyl is 1 : 10, which is far lower than for morphine [50].

Epidural differs from intrathecal administration in that much larger doses are required to achieve analgesic effects. Far more drug will be sequestered to epidural fat, and far more will be cleared by epidural vascular perfusion, which is

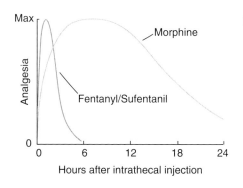

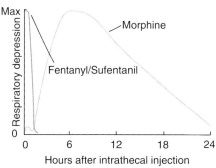

Figure 9.5. Time course of opioid effects after intrathecal administration. Lipophilic opioids (fentanyl and sufentanil) produce rapid onset of effect, while hydrophilic opioids (morphine) have a slower onset and longer duration. Analgesia results from effects at the spinal level, while respiratory depression results from rostral spread to the brainstem. Reproduced with permission from Rathmell *et al.* [50].

Table 9.3. Morphine doses relative to route

Route	Dose (mg)
Intravenous	10
Intramuscular	9
Subcutaneous	8
Oral	30
Nasal	20
Epidural	5
Spinal	0.1

especially true for fentanyl. Thus prolonged infusion of fentanyl may eventually result in systemic concentrations high enough to produce pharmacologic effects. The epidural to intravenous potency ratio for fentanyl was only 1.9 [51].

Safety

Deposition of chemical entities in the vicinity of tissue with pivotal impact on major functions, and with little regenerative capability, such as the spinal cord, requires certainty about safety. Although cauda equina syndromes are reported [49], neuraxial drug administration is generally considered safe. Any action, therapeutic or nontherapeutic, must be completely reversible, and any inflammatory or toxic effects on tissue are unacceptable. It is important to understand that a drug preparation not only contains the active pharmaceutical ingredient but may also contain excipients to facilitate drug delivery. Thus excipients such as preservatives may have unwanted effects: for instance, parabens in local anesthetic preparations are considered to provoke adverse reactions when given neuraxially. All drugs administered neuraxially must undergo the standard procedures for safety assessment as required by regulatory authorities before there is any clinical use.

Summary

Alternative routes are often used to enable drug delivery when oral bioavailability is low and/or unpredictable, or to reduce the toxic effect of high systemic doses. For analgesics specifically, alternative routes are often used when the nature of the pain requires rapid onset after self-administration. Alternative routes of drug administration include parenteral (intramuscular, subcutaneous, transdermal, and inhalation), "partial parenteral" (transmucosal), enteral (rectal), and neuraxial routes.

The benefit of alternatives to oral administration is that they allow administration of drugs to patients who cannot take oral drugs, or where oral onset of effects is too slow, or for drugs which simply cannot be given orally. Relative to intravenous administration, oral or nasal transmucosal dosing permits patient self-administration, with rapid onset of clinical effects. The transdermal route may give a continuous supply of a drug without the need for indwelling devices. The neuraxial routes may offer more profound effects with less systemic adverse effects than other routes. Physicochemical properties are important for determining the suitability of a drug for various alternative routes. The various alternative routes generally have different bioavailablities for any particular drug. Knowledge of relative and absolute bioavailabilities is important for determining equivalent doses when routes are switched. To avoid overdose or treatment failure, differences in bioavailabilities between routes of administration require that drug doses must be adjusted appropriately. Patient preference, the clinical situation, and safety are important factors for the choice of route.

References

1. Dale O. Opioid drugs via other routes. In: Davies A, ed., *Cancer-Related Breakthrough Pain.* New York, NY: Oxford University Press, 2006: 73–82.

2. Tveita T, Thoner J, Klepstad P, Jystad A, Borchgrevink PC. A controlled comparison between single doses of intravenous and intramuscular morphine with respect to analgesic effects and patient safety. *Acta Anaesthesiol Scand* 2008; **52**: 920–5.

3. Kirkpatrick T, Henderson PD, Nimmo WS. Plasma morphine concentrations after intramuscular injection into the deltoid or gluteal muscles. *Anaesthesia* 1988; **43**: 293–5.

4. Walker G, Wilcock A, Manderson C, Weller R, Crosby V. The acceptability of different routes of administration of analgesia for breakthrough pain. *Palliat Med* 2003; **17**: 219–21.

5. Stuart-Harris R, Joel SP, McDonald P, Currow D, Slevin ML. The pharmacokinetics of morphine and morphine glucuronide metabolites after subcutaneous bolus injection and subcutaneous infusion of morphine. *Br J Clin Pharmacol* 2000; **49**: 207–14.

6. Mercadante S, Radbruch L, Caraceni A, *et al.* Episodic (breakthrough) pain: consensus conference of an expert working group of the European Association for Palliative Care. *Cancer* 2002; **94**: 832–9.

7. Paix A, Coleman A, Lees J, *et al.* Subcutaneous fentanyl and sufentanil infusion substitution for morphine intolerance in cancer pain management. *Pain* 1995; **63**: 263–9.

8. Enting RH, Mucchiano C, Oldenmenger WH, *et al.* The "pain pen" for breakthrough cancer pain: a promising treatment. *J Pain Symptom Manage* 2005; **29**: 213–7.

9. Alternative routes of drug administration: advantages and disadvantages (subject review). American Academy of Pediatrics. Committee on Drugs. *Pediatrics* 1997; **100**: 143–52.

10. Evans HC, Easthope SE. Transdermal buprenorphine. *Drugs* 2003; **63**: 1999–2010.

11. Poulain P, Denier W, Douma J, *et al.* Efficacy and safety of transdermal buprenorphine: a randomized,

placebo-controlled trial in 289 patients with severe cancer pain. *J Pain Symptom Manage* 2008; **36**: 117–25.

12. Gourlay GK. Treatment of cancer pain with transdermal fentanyl. *Lancet Oncol* 2001; **2**: 165–72.

13. Varvel JR, Shafer SL, Hwang SS, Coen PA, Stanski DR. Absorption characteristics of transdermally administered fentanyl. *Anesthesiology* 1989; **70**: 928–34.

14. Rozen D, Grass GW. Perioperative and intraoperative pain and anesthetic care of the chronic pain and cancer pain patient receiving chronic opioid therapy. *Pain Pract* 2005; **5**: 18–32.

15. Rawal N, Langford RM. Current practices for postoperative pain management in Europe and the potential role of the fentanyl HCl iontophoretic transdermal system. *Eur J Anaesthesiol* 2007; **24**: 299–308.

16. Viscusi ER, Reynolds L, Chung F, Atkinson LE, Khanna S. Patient-controlled transdermal fentanyl hydrochloride vs intravenous morphine pump for postoperative pain: a randomized controlled trial. *JAMA* 2004; **291**: 1333–41.

17. Thipphawong JB, Babul N, Morishige RJ, *et al.* Analgesic efficacy of inhaled morphine in patients after bunionectomy surgery. *Anesthesiology* 2003; **99**: 693–700.

18. Farr SJ, Otulana BA. Pulmonary delivery of opioids as pain therapeutics. *Adv Drug Deliv Rev* 2006; **58**: 1076–88.

19. Dershwitz M, Walsh JL, Morishige RJ, *et al.* Pharmacokinetics and pharmacodynamics of inhaled versus intravenous morphine in healthy volunteers. *Anesthesiology* 2000; **93**: 619–28.

20. Zeppetella G. Nebulized and intranasal fentanyl in the management of cancer-related breakthrough pain. *Palliat Med* 2000; **14**: 57–8.

21. Miner JR, Kletti C, Herold M, Hubbard D, Biros MH. Randomized clinical trial of nebulized fentanyl citrate versus i.v. fentanyl citrate in children presenting to the emergency department with acute pain. *Acad Emerg Med* 2007; **14**: 895–8.

22. Lennernas B, Hedner T, Holmberg M, *et al.* Pharmacokinetics and tolerability of different doses of fentanyl following

sublingual administration of a rapidly dissolving tablet to cancer patients: a new approach to treatment of incident pain. *Br J Clin Pharmacol* 2005; **59**: 249–53.

23. Streisand JB, Varvel JR, Stanski DR, *et al.* Absorption and bioavailability of oral transmucosal fentanyl citrate. *Anesthesiology* 1991; **75**: 223–9.

24. Darwish M, Kirby M, Robertson P, Tracewell W, Jiang JG. Absolute and relative bioavailability of fentanyl buccal tablet and oral transmucosal fentanyl citrate. *J Clin Pharmacol* 2007; **47**: 343–50.

25. Streisand JB, Busch MA, Egan TD, *et al.* Dose proportionality and pharmacokinetics of oral transmucosal fentanyl citrate. *Anesthesiology* 1998; **88**: 305–9.

26. Coluzzi PH, Schwartzberg L, Conroy JD, *et al.* Breakthrough cancer pain: a randomized trial comparing oral transmucosal fentanyl citrate (OTFC) and morphine sulfate immediate release (MSIR). *Pain* 2001; **91**: 123–30.

27. Portenoy RK, Taylor D, Messina J, Tremmel L. A randomized, placebo-controlled study of fentanyl buccal tablet for breakthrough pain in opioid-treated patients with cancer. *Clin J Pain* 2006; **22**: 805–11.

28. Carr DB, Goudas LC, Denman WT, *et al.* Safety and efficacy of intranasal ketamine for the treatment of breakthrough pain in patients with chronic pain: a randomized, double-blind, placebo-controlled, crossover study. *Pain* 2004; **108**: 17–27.

29. Dale O, Hoffer C, Sheffels P, Kharasch ED. Disposition of nasal, intravenous, and oral methadone in healthy volunteers. *Clin Pharmacol Ther* 2002; **72**: 536–45.

30. Finn J, Wright J, Fong J, *et al.* A randomised crossover trial of patient controlled intranasal fentanyl and oral morphine for procedural wound care in adult patients with burns. *Burns* 2004; **30**: 262–8.

31. Borland M, Jacobs I, King B, O'Brien D. A randomized controlled trial comparing intranasal fentanyl to intravenous morphine for managing acute pain in children in the Emergency Department. *Ann Emerg Med* 49, 335–340. 2007.

32. Wolfe TR, Macfarlane TC. Intranasal midazolam therapy for pediatric status epilepticus. *Am J Emerg Med* 2006; **24**: 343–6.

33. Kerr D, Dietze P, Kelly AM. Intranasal naloxone for the treatment of suspected heroin overdose. *Addiction* 2008; **103**: 379–86.

34. Dale O, Hjortkjaer R, Kharasch ED. Nasal administration of opioids for pain management in adults. *Acta Anaesthesiol Scand* 2002; **46**: 759–70.

35. Moksnes K, Fredheim OM, Klepstad P, *et al.* Early pharmacokinetics of nasal fentanyl: is there a significant arterio-venous difference? *Eur J Clin Pharmacol* 2008; **64**: 497–502.

36. Djupesland PG, Skretting A, Windren M, Holand T. A novel concept for nasal delivery of aerosols can prevent lung inhalation. *J Aerosol Med* 2004; **17**: 249–59.

37. Kendall JM, Reeves BC, Latter VS. Multicentre randomised controlled trial of nasal diamorphine for analgesia in children and teenagers with clinical fractures. *BMJ* 2001; **322**: 261–5.

38. Fitzgibbon D, Morgan D, Dockter D, Barry C, Kharasch ED. Initial pharmacokinetic, safety and efficacy evaluation of nasal morphine gluconate for breakthrough pain in cancer patients. *Pain* 2003; **106**: 309–15.

39. Pavis H, Wilcock A, Edgecombe J, *et al.* Pilot study of nasal morphine-chitosan for the relief of breakthrough pain in patients with cancer. *J Pain Symptom Manage* 2002; **24**: 598–602.

40. Zeppetella G. An assessment of the safety, efficacy, and acceptability of intranasal fentanyl citrate in the management of cancer-related breakthrough pain: a pilot study. *J Pain Symptom Manage* 2000; **20**: 253–8.

41. Paech MJ, Lim CB, Banks SL, Rucklidge MW, Doherty DA. A new formulation of nasal fentanyl spray for postoperative analgesia: a pilot study. *Anaesthesia* 2003; **58**: 740–4.

42. Kendall JM, Latter VS. Intranasal diamorphine as an alternative to intramuscular morphine: pharmacokinetic and pharmacodynamic aspects. *Clin Pharmacokinet* 2003; **42**: 501–13.

43. Warren DE. Practical use of rectal medications in palliative care. *J Pain Symptom Manage* 1996; **11**: 378–87.

44. Ripamonti C, Zecca E, Brunelli C, *et al.* Rectal methadone in cancer patients with pain. A preliminary clinical and pharmacokinetic study. *Ann Oncol* 1995; **6**: 841–3.

45. van Hoogdalem E, de Boer AG, Breimer DD. Pharmacokinetics of rectal drug administration, Part I. General considerations and clinical applications of centrally acting drugs. *Clin Pharmacokinet* 1991; **21**: 11–26.

46. Dale O, Sheffels P, Kharasch ED. Bioavailabilities of rectal and oral methadone in healthy subjects. *Br J Clin Pharmacol* 2004; **58**: 156–62.

47. Yaksh TL, Rudy TA. Analgesia mediated by a direct spinal action of narcotics. *Science* 1976; **192**: 1357–8.

48. Walker SM, Goudas LC, Cousins MJ, Carr DB. Combination spinal analgesic chemotherapy: a systematic review. *Anesth Analg* 2002; **95**: 674–715.

49. Schug SA, Saunders D, Kurowski I, Paech MJ. Neuraxial drug administration: a review of treatment options for anaesthesia and analgesia. *CNS Drugs* 2006; **20**: 917–33.

50. Rathmell JP, Lair TR, Nauman B. The role of intrathecal drugs in the treatment of acute pain. *Anesth Analg* 2005; **101**: S30–43.

51. Polley LS, Columb MO, Naughton NN, *et al.* Effect of intravenous versus epidural fentanyl on the minimum local analgesic concentration of epidural bupivacaine in labor. *Anesthesiology* 2000; **93**: 122–8.

Principles of drug action

Principles of pharmacogenetics

Kirk Hogan

Introduction

Anesthesiology more than any other medical specialty is characterized by polypharmacy, with up to 10 drugs used for the most straightforward procedure in the healthiest patient and over 25 drugs required for the anesthetic care of very ill patients having complex surgeries. In turn, many drugs used in anesthesia have narrow or even inverted therapeutic ratios [1]. If not for the continuous vigilance of caregivers and means for chemical and mechanical support of vital signs at their immediate disposal, coma-inducing anesthetics, neuromuscular paralytic drugs, and potent analgesics at doses routinely employed in the operating room would be lethal. For these reasons, the relevance of inherited predispositions to inefficacy or toxicity was recognized very shortly after the introduction of anesthesia in the 1850s. Today, anesthesiology remains at the forefront of the translation of pharmacogenetic insights to the bedside.

Epidemiologic evidence has long established that adverse drug reactions are severe, common, and growing causes of death, disability, and resource consumption in North America and Europe [2–4]. Between 1998 and 2005, the numbers of reported adverse drug reactions and deaths arising from such reactions both increased over twofold [5]. Adverse drug reactions remain a significant problem during drug development, and approximately 4% of all newly introduced medications are withdrawn from the market due to deleterious outcomes [6]. Because the reported complications occur during treatment with approved drug doses, thereby excluding intentional or accidental overdose, errors in administration, and noncompliance, it has been suggested that 50% of mortality could be potentially preventable by a-priori genomic drug susceptibility profiling [7,8]. Remarkable advances made in biotechnology over the past two decades have surmounted many barriers to the introduction of molecular medicine into perioperative care. Based upon precise detection of DNA sequence variations at pharmacokinetic and pharmacodynamic loci, medicine is at the threshold of substantial improvements in patient safety and welfare during and after surgery. Anesthesiology is well situated to take advantage of these advances, and to enhance patient safety by rational selection of technique, drug, and dose based on individualized DNA signatures.

Pharmacogenetic concepts

The term pharmacogenomics first entered scientific discourse in the early 1990s as amplification of human DNA fragments by polymerase chain reaction (PCR) and direct DNA sequencing became robust and cost-effective [9]. Thereafter, *pharmacogenomics* came to refer generally to correlation of drug-specific traits with genome-wide DNA sequence variations, whereas *pharmacogenetics* connotes a sharper focus on traditional pedigree and population analysis of single gene effects [10]. In practice the two terms are synonymous, both implying study of the influence of genetic diversity on drug response.

Until recently, measurement of the physical manifestations of a trait (the phenotype) was considered to be relatively clear-cut, but accessing human DNA sequence variation (the genotype) was reserved for science fiction. With publication of the first "draft" human genome sequence [11], and widespread availability of low-cost, accurate molecular technologies, acquisition of genomic data is now facile, such that the assembly of reliable phenotypic databases has become the bottleneck in pharmacogenomic research. For many investigators it came as a surprise that the number of discrete human genes ranges from only 25 000 to 30 000. Each human gene, however, encodes a mean of 3–5 distinct proteins (many more for some), with limitless potential for genetic variation at each locus, and a much greater degree of human genomic variation than was previously thought to exist. DNA sequence variations, termed polymorphisms if they appear in more than 1% of the population, and mutations if in less than 1%, are staggering in frequency and in kind, ranging from single base-pair substitutions to whole gene deletions and duplications [12]. Contrary to early doctrine that most genetic changes would be deleterious, the preponderance of sequence alterations and copy number variations elicit no phenotypic effect whatsoever, for example those appearing in noncoding regions or as a redundant third base of a codon specifying an amino acid

Anesthetic Pharmacology, 2nd edition, ed. Alex S. Evers, Mervyn Maze, Evan D. Kharasch. Published by Cambridge University Press. © Cambridge University Press 2011.

[13]. Others, including single base changes, may be sufficient to kill in the presence of an environmental trigger, e.g., malignant hyperthermia.

Each nucleated human cell contains a genome composed of approximately 3 billion base pairs of DNA. Sorting through the 3 million polymorphisms unique to each human is motivated by the principle that a pharmacogenetic predictor will not change throughout life, and thus will need to be sought only once for each individual. Achieving this task is the central objective of bioinformatics, a silicon-based, web-enabled discipline that integrates clinical traits and outcomes with archived files of DNA sequence and its variations [14,15]. Virtually all of the traits in this chapter are considered to be monogenic, in which a proportion of variability in a given trait between two individuals can be traced to the presence or absence of a causal mutation in a single gene. The existence of a mono-pharmacogenetic trait is established when DNA sequence variations within one gene correlate with segregation of the larger population into smaller groups on the basis of distinct drug effects, i.e., a bimodal distribution. Hence most currently recognized pharmacogenetic traits reflect single gene defects, disclosed by the severity of their corresponding phenotypes [16]. More sophisticated bioinformatic models, enhanced computational capacity, and high-throughput genotyping are required to draw predictive correlations between drug responses and patterns of DNA sequence variations at more than one site in a gene, genes, or surrounding sequence (haplotypes) to predict susceptibilities characterized by polygenic, multifactorial inheritance.

Pharmacogenetic phenotypes

Many drugs used by anesthesiologists exhibit significant inter-individual variation in efficacy and toxicity, often in conformation to differences in drug or metabolite concentration in a given compartment (e.g., plasma or urine) for a given dose. Nonetheless, most pharmacogenetic susceptibilities go undetected in affected persons until a drug substrate for the impaired enzyme or target is administered. The search for genetic factors consonant with these observations must first address whether, in the setting of divergent responses to an identical dose, the cause is pharmacokinetic (compartment drug concentrations differ) or pharmacodynamic (response to a concentration differs). Pharmacokinetic polymorphisms that alter drug concentrations may be further subdivided into those that govern drug absorption, distribution, metabolism, or excretion (ADME). By far the most numerous and well-studied of these are polymorphisms in the genes encoding drug-metabolizing enzymes, accounting for up to 10- to 10 000-fold variations in drug activity.

Not only may detection of genotypes incommensurate with dosing regimens predict inefficacy or toxicity, but they may also warn of potential drug–drug interactions if, for example, two drugs share a mutant pathway [17]. Drug interactions are a particularly common cause of adverse reactions during the polypharmacy characteristic of perioperative management. Patients awaiting surgery may be taking any prescribed, over-the-counter, or herbal remedy, in addition to suspected and unsuspected drugs of abuse. In this context, fixed and discrete genomic data have the potential to anticipate the incidence and severity of untoward responses. For these reasons, as the number and predictive power of the pertinent genotypes expands, it will be increasingly important for anesthesiologists to acquire familiarity with the principles and practice of pharmacogenetics [18].

Pharmacogenetic genotypes

Proposed schemes to classify variations in drug response associated with specific DNA sequences are not mutually exclusive, and may be conveniently cross-referenced, i.e., by type of genetic alteration, by class or structure of encoded protein, by phylogenetic relation, by mechanism of trait inheritance, or by functional role in drug response. Because each drug interacts with numerous carrier proteins, cell-membrane transporters, metabolizing enzymes, receptors, and secondary messengers, and because most genes in outbred human populations are polymorphic, pharmacogenomic profiles will be essential to interpret variances around dose–response sample means in subpopulations defined by shared stratification of risk. Most recently, genome-wide association approaches have been introduced wherein disequilibrium between genetic variations at many thousands of loci spanning an entire genome is sought in comparison with predisposition to a trait of interest, and pharmacogenomic applications are anticipated [12]. An important constraint in the interpretation of genome-wide association data is the substantial risk for large numbers of false-positive associations that may arise from multiple comparison testing on this scale. Nevertheless, control of the genomic contribution to heterogeneity in drug response emerging from these methods will assist investigations of environmental and acquired factors by permitting exposed patients to be matched on the basis of shared genetic constitutions.

Genotype–phenotype correlations

Whether pharmacogenomic data made available in advance of surgery is of any value to the caregiver or patient (the data are "medically actionable") hinges on the extent to which the patient's genotype predicts changes in phenotype after administration of the drug in question. Accordingly, knowledge of the genotype must be *analytically valid* (the chosen DNA test method accurately detects the genotype) and *clinically valid* (the genotype correctly predicts the phenotype), and must demonstrate *clinical utility* (the genotype specifies an available step to improve patient safety and health outcomes) [19].

Analytical validity
With regard to analytical validity, the genotyping method chosen must be sufficiently flexible to discriminate a wide variety of

genetic pathologies within a shared platform to include wild-type and mutant homozygotes and heterozygotes, single nucleotide polymorphisms (SNPs) in coding regions, introns and promoters, multiple alleles at both single and multiple loci, insertions, deletions, copy-number variations, and pseudogenes. Assays capable of distinguishing these variations with greater than 99% precision, at pennies per allele, and in as short an interval as 1–2 hours are currently available. To assure appropriate use of test data, practitioners must be well-versed in the practical as well as theoretical limitations of the analysis method, including the need for standardized protocols, details of specimen handling, and control of the volume of information available from each patient.

Clinical validity

Currently, declarations of an association between a genotype and phenotype (clinical validity) often elude the level of scrutiny that would ordinarily greet news of other newly proposed, nongenetic clinical correlations. But as pharmacogenomic data inevitably flow from the laboratory bench to the operating room, it will be crucial that practitioners adopt an attitude of skepticism. The primary distinction to be made falls between a DNA polymorphism, or random sequence variation that may have no functional role but may still be inherited, and a causal mutation which either alone or in a major way contributes to the genesis of a phenotype. Morevoer, a given sequence variation may become meaningful (causal) only if it is reported and interpreted in the context of additional genetic and environmental factors acting in concert. A quantifiable clinical drug response may be causally correlated with a DNA nucleotide change on the basis of statistical, inferential, and biologic-functional lines of evidence collectively referred as functional genomics. Because each of these categoric criteria is subtle and vulnerable to error, clinicians must insist on a high degree of reproducibility and correspondence before weighing pharmacogenomic data in management decisions. Stringent standards for genetic association studies have recently been proposed [20], and a checklist of the fundamental issues of methodological quality that must be considered in the design of a pharmacogenetic trial has been provided [21]. The prospect of abundant, novel genotype–phenotype correlations for anesthetic drugs and adjuncts balances these concerns in exploiting the spectrum of inborn human diversity in drug treatment.

Clinical utility

Pharmacogenomic screening of the surgical patient will become widespread only when the capacity to detect susceptibility is matched by the ability to modulate risk at acceptable cost (clinical utility). Unless enrolled in research protocols with appropriate consent, patients must not be tested for phamacogenomic alleles in the absence of alternative interventions of proven benefit. Conversely, even if the group of genotypes accounting for a specific trait is known to be partial, and even if the causality arguments for each genotype are incompletely settled, knowledge of the positive presence of an at-risk genotype may be life-saving if a safer intervention is at hand, for example, in patients with malignant hyperthermia susceptibility.

Lack of an at-risk pharmacogenomic marker in a tested patient does not assure that there is no risk in the setting of allelic or locus heterogeneity, nor will genotyping ever substitute for vigilance and clinical judgment. However, by virtue of testing net risk may be reduced to a measurable degree. Pharmacogenomic testing of the surgical patient may thus help to unravel complex clinical responses and raise warning signals of impending trouble, but it does not guarantee freedom from complications or the promise of safety in the absence of an informed and experienced caregiver. Only by learning how patients subtly differ one from the other at the molecular level will it be possible to decrease pharmacogenetic complications with less reliance on downstream early detection and rescue when clinical warnings are issued.

Genetic pharmacokinetics

Since their presence was first suspected, it has been clear that genes encoding proteins responsible for drug ADME could not have evolved by exposure to modern pharmaceuticals. Rather, it is hypothesized that close chemical homologs expressed in ingested plants were rendered innocuous by these adaptations in our progenitors [22]. Why the genes responsible for transmission of pharmacokinetic defenses exhibit such a high degree of polymorphism is a second mystery. In part, the answer may reside in the loss of reproductive advantage of polymorphisms as environments and diets change with accumulation of neutral mutations, some of which may be deleterious in a novel environment, e.g., the operating room. Another possibility is that the extent of pharmacokinetic polymorphism reflects heterogeneity of the environments in which humans have evolved, corresponding to varying allele frequencies in groups with distinct ethnic origins. In either case, for most ADME polymorphisms, there are no phenotypes apparent on medical history or physical examination to warn caregivers ahead of a challenge with the drug itself. This lack of easily detected phenotypic markers explains the delay in recognition of genetic correlates of drug responses as clinically important phenomena, and underscores the tremendous potential for growth of knowledge now that DNA-based technologies are widely available. Polymorphisms in genes encoding proteins participating in intracellular drug metabolism (e.g., the cytochrome P450 enzymes) and drug transporters of interest to anesthesiologists are addressed elsewhere in this volume (Chapters 6 and 7), and are also the subject of recent reviews [23].

Metabolism and biotransformation

Butyrylcholinesterase deficiency

The circulating enzyme plasma cholinesterase, or butyrylcholinesterase (BChE), is responsible wholly or in part for the metabolism and elimination of a variety of anesthetic drugs sharing a vulnerable ester bond, including succinylcholine,

Table 10.1. Variants of butyrylcholinesterase

Name	Abbreviation	Mutation	Allele frequency	Description
Usual	U	—	0.85	Normal
Atypical	A	A209G	0.018	Reduced activity, dibucaine-resistant
Fluoride-resistant	F	C728T, G1169T	0.002	Reduced activity, fluoride-resistant
Silent	S	Multiple	?	No activity
H	H	G424A	?	Approximately 10% reduced concentration
J	J	A1490T	0.002	Approximately 33% reduced concentration
K	K	G1615A	0.128	Approximately 66% reduced concentration

From Levano [24], with permission.

mivacurium, cocaine, chloroprocaine, and tetracaine. Approximately 3/1000 patients are homozygous for the "atypical" mutation, in which a glycine is substituted for an aspartate in the anionic binding site of the protein (Table 10.1) [25]. The mutation abolishes electrostatic interactions essential to drug–substrate binding, thereby prolonging its duration of action. Approximately 1/100 patients of European origin are homozygous for a milder second polymorphism, the K variant, with an overall allele frequency in both homozygotes and heterozygotes of 10%, compared with a 17.5% allele frequency in Japanese populations [26]. In addition to the atypical and K-variant polymorphisms, more than 60 rare mutations have been identified, with the possibility of compound heterozygotes, i.e., a distinct predisposing mutation inherited from each parent, confirmed by direct sequencing [27,28]. A simple and accurate phenotypic test of butyrylcholinesterase activity was proposed in 1968 [29] but never became routine, attesting to anesthesiologists' general preference for safety systems dependent on early warning rather than prevention.

Screening for *BChE* polymorphisms that cause prolonged paralysis after administration of the usually short-acting muscle relaxant succinylcholine has been suggested to be one of only two indications for pharmacokinetic genetic testing suitable for clinical practice based on present-day knowledge of analytical validity, clinical validity, and clinical utility [30]. In a study of 36 patients with prolonged neuromuscular blockade after succinycholine or mivacurium, testing for the *BChE* atypical (A) variant improved diagnosis in 30% of individuals compared to biochemical tests of enzyme activity [31]. Noting the limitations of testing for a single allele in the earlier study, full-length sequencing of the four *BChE* exons, intron–exon boundaries, and the untranslated region of the *BChE* mRNA was subsequently performed [32]. Based on the more comprehensive assessment, it was demonstrated that the Kalow (K) variant causes a clinically relevant prolongation of mivacurium paralysis in heterozygotes also carrying the usual (U) allele, with a more pronounced effect when the K and A alleles are found on the same chromosome (U/AK). The most protracted

duration of effect occurs in patients who are compound homozygotes for both the K and A variant (AK/AK). In another study employing full-length sequencing of the four *BChE* exons, a high prevalence of *BChE* polymorphisms was observed in patients with a history of delayed recovery [24]. In addition to confirming a relatively high allele frequency of 0.128 for the K variant, and detection of a novel *BChE* allele (G1294T), the results underscore substantial differences in the duration of neuromuscular blockade between patients with apparently identical *BChE* genotypes. This observation, which may be caused in part by superimposition of acquired deficiencies of *BChE* (e.g., pregnancy, chronic illness, blood loss) or by undetected *BChE* allelic or locus heterogeneity, are of particular significance in view of the possible future introduction of drugs other than neuromuscular relaxants that are designed to be metabolized by the BChE pathway, e.g., the investigatory anesthetic induction and maintenance drug TD-4756 [33]. Whereas retrospective *BChE* testing of patients who may have experienced prolonged paralysis is advocated for the future safety of probands and their families [30], introduction of drugs intended for more widespread use than niche applications of succinylcholine or mivacurium may more plausibly engender routine prospective *BChE* genotyping as a companion diagnostic test.

Genetic pharmacodynamics

Drugs exert their actions through binding to specific macromolecular targets most often encoded by distinct genes. Given identical plasma concentrations, pharmacodynamic variation may originate as a result of DNA sequence changes in drug targets. Most drug targets consist of membrane receptors, enzymes, or ion channels serving as the cell's sensor elements to hormones, neurotransmitters, or other mediators, e.g., circulating cytokines. Functional genetic polymorphisms may be expressed in the effector molecules themselves, or in the intracellular second-messenger pathways activated by association of a drug ligand with its target. Of note, the targets of both inhalational and intravenous general anesthetics are remarkably free of polymorphisms conferring a change in function. Because these proteins fulfill essential cellular roles, nonsynonymous polymorphisms (those that alter the amino acid composition of a polypeptide) are apparently less well tolerated than allelic variants of genes encoding pharmacokinetic proteins. Similarly, disease-causing mutations in drug targets are more likely to produce severe or even lethal phenotypes, and thus are less widely perpetuated in a population compared with mutations that only become apparent on exposure to a drug. Variability surrounding the sample means of pharmacodynamic effects is typically large, reflecting the many molecular contributors to even the most narrowly delineated drug response. Investigations aimed at correlating interindividual differences in pharmacodynamic drug response to DNA sequence variations are further challenged by phenotypes that are much more diverse and difficult to quantify than distributions of drug and metabolite levels in corresponding body fluids.

Despite these obstacles to detection of genetic differences in pharmacodynamic effects, it is noteworthy that cognizance of the dramatic malignant hyperthermia phenotype took place only within the memory of living clinicians, and that recognition of the pharmacogenetic contribution to nitrous oxide toxicity only occurred in the past five years. The failure of pharmacodynamic syndromes to be identified with a frequency comparable to pharmacokinetic genetic predictors over the preceding three decades implies that many more of the former remain to be discovered.

Efficacy
Opioid responsivity

Multiple analgesics with distinct kinetic profiles and potencies are required in the interval before, during, and after surgery to control acute pain arising from tissue injury. Whereas interindividual differences in pain severity, and in response to drugs used for modulation of chronic and experimental pain, have been the subject of several decades of research, the perioperative setting has only recently drawn similar attention [34–36]. For example, in over 3000 patients, morphine dosage requirements for analgesia after hip replacement vary almost 40-fold [37]. Although wide interpatient variability in analgesia may arise from many acquired sources – e.g., cultural, psychological, and environmental factors, coexisting diseases, and drug interactions – recent studies suggest pharmacogenetic predictors also play an important role.

The μ-opioid receptor is a principal site of action for the endogenous ligand β-endorphin and is the target for the most commonly used exogenous opioids. More than 100 single nucleotide polymophisms (SNPs) are found in the 10 exons comprising the μ-opioid receptor gene OPRM1 [38]. Twenty of these produce amino acid changes with polymorphic frequencies greater than 1%. The most common, A118G, with an ethnicity-dependent allele frequency of 2–48%, results in an amino acid exchange at position 40 in exon 1 from asparagine to aspartate, thereby deleting a presumed N-glycosylation site in the extracellular receptor region [39]. The variant receptor protein is thought by some to express altered binding with β-endorphin compared with the more common wild-type allele, although this surmise has been contested [40,41]. Patients with chronic pain from malignant disease who are homozygous for the 118G allele require significantly higher doses of morphine to achieve pain relief than heterozygote or wild-type patients [42]. In subjects with acute, nonmalignant pain, carriers of the 118G allele have a two- to threefold decrease in opioid potency, requiring, for example, higher alfentanil concentrations to produce the same degree of antinociception [43]. Differences are also seen in the incidence of opioid-induced side effects; the same investigation reports that GG homozygotes are protected against opioid-induced respiratory depression, although this finding has been disputed for morphine (Fig. 10.1) [35].

Multiple reports suggest that carriers of the 118G allele require greater amounts of opioid for comparable levels of postoperative pain relief. However, the magnitude of the effect is often small, and the strength of the association may be weak. For example, a linear trend was observed for higher doses of morphine needed after colorectal surgery in patients with one

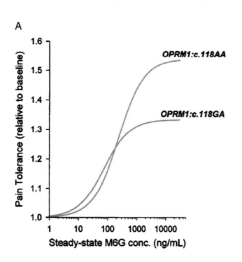
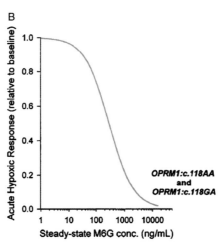

Figure 10.1. Steady-state response of morphine-6-glucuronide (M6G) concentration versus (A) pain tolerance and (B) the acute hypoxic ventilatory response. For pain tolerance, but not for respiration, a significant difference was observed between the OPRM1:c.118AA and OPRM1:c.118GA genotype, with lesser M6G efficacy in OPRM1:c.118GA heterozygotes. Reproduced with permission from Romberg et al. [35].

or two copies of the mutant allele, but the limited number of mutant GG homozygotes resulted in a study that was inadequately powered to draw firmer conclusions [44]. Correspondingly, in Taiwanese women homozygous for the 118G polymorphism, up to 18% higher doses of morphine delivered by patient-controlled analgesia were required in the first 24 hours after abdominal hysterectomy compared to women who were wild-type homozygotes [45]. Similar results were reported in a study of 147 male and female patients undergoing total knee arthroplasty at both 24 and 48 hours after surgery [46]. A difference in morphine requirement was not observed between the wild-type AA and heterozygote AG genotypes in either study, nor was A118G genotype a predictor of postoperative nausea and vomiting. In 101 patients undergoing elective laparoscopic abdominal surgery, there was no difference predicted by genotype in the amount of opioid used intraoperatively or in the postanesthesia care unit (PACU) interval [47]. In turn, no differences were observed in the average postoperative pain score between AA and AG genotypes. In this investigation, only one patient was identified as a GG homozygote, hence the investigation was also underpowered. In contrast, the AG heterozygote did confer a significant enhancement of intrathecal fentanyl analgesia for labor when compared to the wild-type AA homozygote [48,49].

In sum, the *OPRM1* A118G polymorphism apparently causes a reduced perioperative effect of opioids, and an increased opioid dosage requirement [50]. The magnitude of these associations may be drug- and response-specific, and in most reports does not appear to be large, particularly when the two-fold genetic difference is compared with 40-fold differences observed in clinical morphine requirement. In order to more clearly resolve the contribution of *OPRM1* polymorphisms to differences in postoperative pain, larger and more sophisticated trials with objective indices of pain and mood, together with genotyping at multiple loci and control of other variables known to influence analgesia, are needed [51–53].

Toxicity
Anesthetic myopathy syndrome: malignant hyperthermia

Hereditary rhabdomyolysis associated with administration of volatile anesthetic drugs and depolarizing muscle relaxants exemplifies the paradigm of a pharmacodynamic toxic response [54,55]. Currently, the Malignant Hyperthermia Association of the United States (MHAUS) is notified of about 200 probable trigger events per year, with several deaths unfortunately part of each annual report. Perhaps the most important message of recent publications addressing the syndrome known as malignant hyperthermia (MH), i.e., muscle destruction and consequent hyperkalemia, acidosis, dysrhythmia, renal failure, and disseminated intravascular coagulation after parenteral succinylcholine or inhalation of potent anesthetic vapors, is that the disorder is still fatal in a significant

proportion of patients despite early detection and appropriate management including provision of dantrolene [56]. A harrowing description of a trigger event provides ample warning that anesthetic and surgical caregivers must never let down their guard, and serves as a reminder that basic and clinical research efforts have much yet to disclose [57]. It is now well established that all volatile anesthetics, including the newer drugs sevoflurane and desflurane, are potential triggers of the syndrome, although they may not be as florid in their presentation as their predecessors [58]. Of note, an increase in temperature is often a late or inconsistent manifestation of the disorder, and recrudescence of the syndrome may occur in up to 20% of clinical reactions [59,60]. If confirmed, these observations point to the need both for earlier diagnosis based on features other than temperature (e.g., unexplained hypercarbia and dysrhythmia), and a lengthened monitoring interval and specific therapy well after a trigger arises.

For more than 30 years after its elucidation as a clinical entity [61], the syndrome was ascribed to a heterogenous inventory of underlying mechanisms including catechol excess, nonspecific membrane defects, and lipid theories. Fairhurst and colleagues, in drawing attention to the similarity between MH and toxicity of the sap of the ryana tree in Trinidadian rats, provided the first clue implicating a receptor-mediated phenomenon [62]. The observation was accorded little attention until all porcine MH triggers, and a subset of human MH events, were linked to mutations in the skeletal muscle calcium release channel, which also came to be known as the ryanodine receptor (RyR1) (Fig. 10.2) [64,65]. Currently, more than 150 *RYR1* polymorphisms have been found in patients manifesting the MH trait by clinical event or skeletal muscle contracture testing (in-vitro contracture test, or caffeine halothane contracture test), each with varying degrees of causal certainty [66]. Recently, a novel heterozygous A97G point mutation in exon 2 of *RYR1* has been identified in one patient with King–Denborough syndrome characterized by myopathy after inhalational anesthesia in the setting of multiple dysmorphic features [67]. Polymorphisms in the coding regions of *RYR1* are found in 50–70% of patients with MH, leaving 30% or more of predisposing mutations to be discovered elsewhere in *RYR1* or its surrounding genome [68]. At least five other susceptibility loci have been identified, with six mutations detected to date in the L-type calcium channel gene *CACNA1S* [55,69,70]. Mapping of predisposition to Native American myopathy, an autosomal recessive congenital disorder with muscle weakness, cleft palate, ptosis, short stature, and MH susceptibility, to chromosome 12q13.13–14.1 may point to the identification of additional candidate genes [71].

Autosomal dominant transmission is not a sine qua non of the MH diagnosis in humans. A substantial number of predisposing myopathies and conditions are recessively inherited [72,73], and de-novo mutation has been described [74]. Additionally, compound heterozygosity for *RYR1* polymorphisms is increasingly reported in patients surviving clear-cut

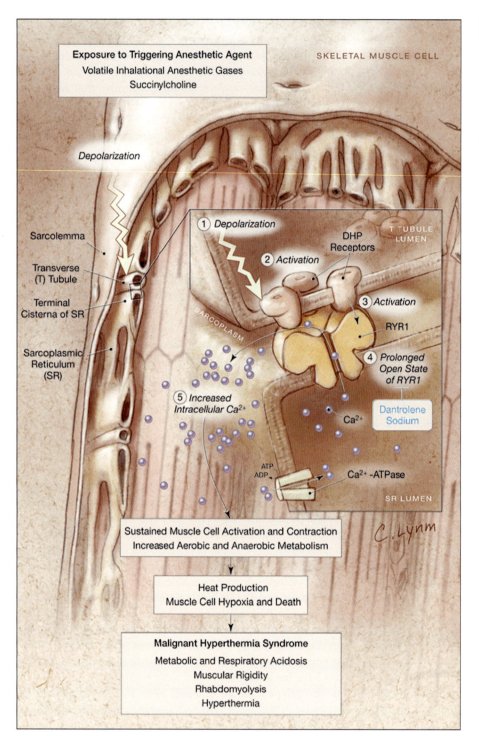

Figure 10.2. Pathophysiology of human anesthetic myopathy. Muscle-cell depolarization is sensed by the L-type calcium channel CACNA1S, also known as the dihydropyridine receptor, which signals RYR1 opening. In malignant hyperthermia, accumulation of abnormally high levels of calcium in the sarcoplasm causes uncontrolled anaerobic and aerobic metabolism and sustained muscle-cell contraction. This results in the clinical manifestations of respiratory acidosis, metabolic acidosis, muscle rigidity, and hyperthermia in some but not all patients. If the process continues, adenosine triphosphate (ATP) depletion eventually causes widespread muscle fiber hypoxia (cell death, rhabdomyolysis), which manifests clinically as hyperkalemia and myoglobinuria and an increase in creatine kinase. Dantrolene sodium binds to RYR1, causing it to favor the closed state, thereby reversing the uninhibited flow of calcium into the sarcoplasm. Reproduced with permission from Litman and Rosenberg [63].

triggers [75], and discordance between genotype and phenotype has been observed [76]. Although the incidence of clinical malignant hyperthermia varies between 1/15 000 and 1/50 000 anesthetics, the proportion of individuals in a given population with predisposing mutations may be 1/2000 or greater [77]. Based on expression of malignant hyperthermia in mice transfected with a human *RYR1* malignant-hyperthermia-associated mutation, the causality of at least one *RYR1* polymorphism in humans can no longer be considered in doubt [78,79]. However, the disproportion between the incidence of predisposing *RYR1* alleles in the general population and the apparent rarity of the full-fledged syndrome, points to additional acquired and inborn susceptibilities that have yet to be disclosed.

Although *RYR1* mutation analysis for MH susceptibility is now commercially available in the United States, genetic heterogeneity constrains the value of genetic testing [63]. While a positive test result should preclude post-hoc exposure to trigger anesthetics, a negative test result, even in a member of a family in which a known allele is segregating, cannot assure safety. In practice, an index of suspicion sufficient to motivate genetic testing is also sufficient to avoid trigger anesthetics regardless of the test result. The same line of reasoning applies to the muscle biopsy contracture testing used in the past for MH genetic counseling and research. For obvious reasons, no adequately powered sample of contracture test-negative or genotype-negative patients who have subsequently been exposed to trigger anesthetics is available. Thus, the true false-negative rate of the contracture test is unknown, and most probably is unknowable. Moreover, the thresholds distinguishing positive from negative contracture test results have been agreed upon in data from patients and family members without apparent coexisting disease. Accordingly, the value of these thresholds in the growing number of conditions that may or may not be associated with anesthetic myopathy is not known. These circumstances, coupled with limited lab-to-lab reproducibility of the contracture test [80], point to the great need for an improved malignant hyperthermia "endo-phenotype" interposed between DNA sequence variation and the clinical event, perhaps based on in-vivo contracture testing, whole muscle imaging, muscle cells grown in culture, or B-lymphocyte calcium kinetics [76]. To improve the genotype–phenotype correlation, and resolve the significant number of patients diagnosed as "MH equivocal," a number of modifications of the contracture test have been proposed, with the addition of 4-chlorochresol appearing to hold the greatest promise [81]. Although this alteration segregates many equivocal muscle bundles into either MH-susceptible or MH-normal groups, it remains premature to state whether the segregation is in fact correct (fully predictive of the clinical trigger phenotype), or to provide the precise false-equivocal rate. It is hoped that less invasive tests sufficiently sensitive to detect a single mutant *RYR1* copy may be developed in humans and model organisms, thereby sharpening phenotypic indicators for use in humans at risk. Improved phenotypic and genotypic detection is particularly desired in view of growing recognition that MH-like events may occur in susceptible patients after anesthesia, or even in the absence of exposure to trigger drugs [82–84].

As noted above, malignant hyperthermia remains fatal in a subset of young, healthy children and adults. The tragedy is compounded by an otherwise full life expectancy in the absence of exposure to trigger anesthetics. The lack of efficacy for dantrolene in up to 5% of MH patients, despite a deepening understanding of its mechanism of action, suggests that pharmacogenetic markers for this antidote itself remain to be discovered [85]. Very recently, the MHAUS has produced a comprehensive in-service kit including a DVD with mock drill and up-to-the-minute information aimed at maximizing patient safety. The kit is highly recommended, and is readily available at www.mhaus.org.

Long QT syndrome

Inherited long QT syndrome (LQTS) denotes a cardiac dysrhythmia associated with abnormal QTc-interval prolongation on the surface ECG causing syncope, torsades de pointes, ventricular fibrillation, and sudden death in patients with otherwise normal cardiac morphology. The molecular origin of LQTS can be traced to specific mutations in 70% of patients meeting clinical criteria for diagnosis of the disorder, indicating that other genetic mutations most probably exist that have yet to be identified [86]. Over 300 mutations in 10 genes are linked to LQTS, with an aggregate incidence of 1 in 2000–5000 persons [87]. Of these, 50% have mutations in *KCNQ1* (LQT1) expressing the KvLQT1 α subunit of the KvLQT1/minK channel conducting the slow (I_{ks}) current [88,89]. Up to 40% of patients have mutations in the potassium-channel gene *KCNH2* (LQT2), which encodes the hERG (human *ether-a-go-go* related gene) α subunit of the hERG/MiRP1 channel responsible for conducting the rapid component of the cardiac voltage-gated delayed rectifier K^+ current. Mutations in *KCNE1* (encoding the minK protein), *KCNE2* (encoding the MiRP1 protein), and *SCN5A* (LQT3) (encoding a cardiac sodium-channel α subunit) account for the preponderance of remaining cases. LQT1, LQT2, and LQT3 differ from one another in age at onset, the nature of triggering events (e.g., emotional or physical stress, loud noises, sleep), associated conditions (e.g., deafness), specific ECG findings (e.g., distinctive T-wave repolarization patterns), the influence of gender and pregnancy, the clinical course, and responsivity to medical interventions (Fig. 10.3) [87,90]. Therapy with β-adrenergic blockade is the mainstay for management of LQTS, with left cardiac sympathetic denervation and implantable cardioverter-defibrillators reserved for non-responders, patients with symptoms before puberty, and those with very long QTc intervals [90].

Patients who are genotypically susceptible to LQTS may have a normal QTc interval at baseline, and may first manifest torsades de pointes in the perioperative interval [91]. Many drugs commonly used in anesthetic practice interact with cardiac cation currents, causing either acquired LQTS or precipitating prolongation of the QT interval, ventricular dysrhythmia, and torsades de pointes in patients who may otherwise be presymptomatic. These include sevoflurane and isoflurane [92], atropine, glycopyrrolate [93], succinylcholine, sodium thiopental, ketamine, methadone, haloperidol, amiodarone, ketoconazole and other antimicrobial drugs, psychotropic medications, class III antiarrhythmics, sympathomimetics, depolarizing and nondepolarizing muscle relaxants [94], and local anesthetics [95–97]. Accordingly, recommendations for the anesthetic management of patients with long QT channelopathies are cautionary and generic [98]. Anesthetic drugs that do not specifically prolong the QTc interval to clinically relevant durations include propofol, nitrous oxide, vecuronium, atracurium, fentanyl, morphine, and midazolam,

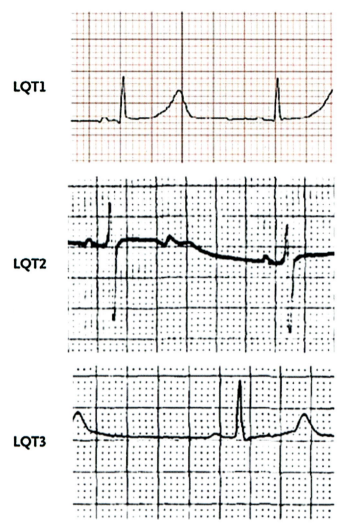

Figure 10.3. Electrocardiographic patterns in the three common forms of the long QT syndrome. LQT1 is associated with a broad T wave without a shortening of the QT interval due to exercise. LQT2 is associated with low-amplitude, often bifid, T waves. LQT3 is associated with a long isoelectric segment and a narrow-based, tall T wave. Other variants have been described. Reproduced with permission from Roden [87].

and these have been suggested as the likeliest foundation for general anesthesia [91,99]. Regional anesthesia may more effectively reduce sympathetic activity in LQTS patients than general anesthesia, and its use has been advocated in parturients with LQTS [99]. Owing to its capacity to prolong the QT interval, in 2001 the United States Food and Drug Administration (FDA) issued a "black box" warning on the use of droperidol applying broadly to the small dosages used for perioperative antiemesis [100]. To the contrary, a retrospective investigation found no incidence of torsades de pointes in over 16 000 general surgery patients exposed to droperidol in doses customarily employed for the treatment of perioperative nausea and vomiting [101]. The authors and subsequent editorialists concluded that the FDA warning is excessive and its guidelines are unlikely to improve patient safety in this setting

[102,103]. Importantly, despite the debate over the safety of droperidol in the general populations, the pharmacogenetic risk of droperidol in the known LQTS patients has not been questioned or tested.

New and emerging concepts

As noted above, a central tenet of pharmacogenomic testing has been the notion that pharmacogenetic predictors do not change throughout life, and thus need only to be sought once for each individual. Recent evidence suggests that the human genome is less genetically stable than previously considered, and that non-neoplastic, somatic genetic changes may be as significant in human drug responses as inherited germline polymorphisms (i.e., somatic mosaicism) [104,105]. The unexplained age and gender disparity in malignant hyperthermia susceptibility, with younger patients at much greater risk than older patients, could be an attractive setting in which to test this possibility. Whereas it has long been recognized that drugs alter gene expression in, for example, microsomal enzyme induction [106] and drug dependence [107], the full impact of the effects of altered expression arising from variation in small RNAs and other epigenetic mechanisms (e.g., DNA methylation and covalent modifications of histones and chromatin) on drug responses (pharmacoepigenomics) remains to be elucidated [108]. The significance of variation in gene expression at pharmacogenetic loci in explaining unexpected drug responses not traceable to environmental factors or more classical pharmacogenetics has been highlighted [109]. These and related newly identified complexities in the human genome with a bearing on pharmacogenomics are addressed with corresponding provisios in recent thought-provoking overviews [110,111].

The traits and genotypes discussed above serve to outline the general principles of pharmacogenomics in the perioperative context. Others of central interest to anesthesia caregivers are similarly well advanced – for example, the identification of alleles associated with anticoagulation [112] and responses to adrenergic agents [113–116]. A large number of perioperative events with certain pharmaocgenetic components remain that are early in their recognition and detection of causal alleles – for example, nitrous oxide toxicity (Fig. 10.4) [117–119] and postoperative nausea and vomiting [120–122]. Application of pharmacogenomic technologies and protocols to still more recently recognized conditions is compelling but awaits investigation – for example, propofol infusion syndrome [123] and postoperative cognitive dysfunction [124]. While the protein targets of general anesthetic drugs are relatively free of functional variation in humans, polymorphisms at the sites of action of regional anesthetics underlie significant interindividual differences in pain perception [125,126].

Clinical pharmacogenetic correlates of these observations remain to be explored. In each instance, interpretation of

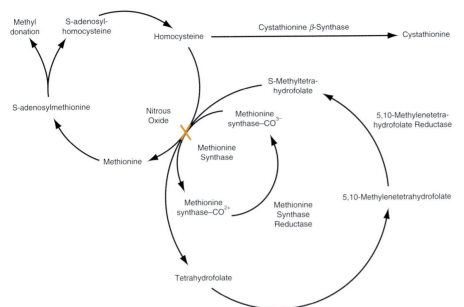

Figure 10.4. The folate and homocysteine metabolic cycles and the enzymatic site of nitrous oxide toxicity. Nitrous oxide irreversibly oxidizes the cobalt atom (Co) of vitamin B_{12}, thereby inhibiting the activity of the cobalamin-dependent enzyme methionine synthase. Methionine synthase catalyzes the remethylation of 5-methyltetrahydrofolate and homocysteine to tetrahydrofolate and methionine. Methionine, by way of its activated form, S-adenosylmethionine, is the principal substrate for methylation in most biochemical reactions, including assembly of the myelin sheath, methyl substitutions in neurotransmitters, and DNA synthesis in rapidly proliferating tissues. Pharmacogenetic susceptibility to nitrous oxide toxicity (hyperhomocysteinemia) arises from an acquired lesion of a normal protein (oxidation of methionine synthase by nitrous oxide) superimposed on an inborn lesion of a second protein, i.e., 5,10-methylenetetrahydrofolate reductase. Reproduced with permission from Selzer *et al.* [117].

pharmacogenomic data must be tempered by the background relevance of differences in gender [127–130] and ethnicity [131,132], although the molecular mechanisms for these overriding effects are unknown. However, accounting for ethnic differences in the design and analysis of pharmacogenetic investigations is fraught with methodological controversies. Guidelines toward the resolution of these matters have recently been published and are highly recommended [133,134].

During the preceding two decades, human genomics has been enabled by a series of technical leaps, first with cloning and sequencing, followed by PCR amplification of DNA fragments in vitro. With technologies adopted from silicon industries including robotics, microfluidics, microarray (i.e., "gene chip") sorting, and internet-based bioinformatics, highthroughput pharmacogenomic profiling is now feasible within clinical constraints of cost, efficiency, and precision. Before pharmaocogenomic profiling ("personalized medicine") is translated into clinical practice there is great need for large, multicenter, randomized, double-blind, well-controlled, prospective investigations to clearly demonstrate the value of prospective genotyping [135]. A model trial has been successfully completed using HLA-B genotyping to guide abacavir therapy [136], and several trials of genotype-guided warfarin dosing have been performed, showing that pharmacogenetically based dosing algorithms better predict initial and maintenance dose requirements compared with a clinical algorithm or a fixed-dose approach [137].

Risks for loss of privacy, harms from unwarranted patient labeling, and discrimination in employment or insurance coverage have drawn attention from the first conception of human genome research [138]. Today, it is acknowledged that although these risks persist, they may be tempered by

legal and technical safeguards, e.g., statutory protection of genetic information, fully informed consent, and data encryption [139,140]. For the clinician and researcher interested in tracking ethical, legal, regulatory, and social issues pertinent to pharmacogenetics, as well as up-to-the-minute syndrome and allele news, the Pharmacogenetics Research Network (www.nigms.nih.gov/pharmacogenetics), and Pharmacogenetics Knowledge Base (www.pharmgkb.org) are excellent resources [141].

Despite dogma accepted for more than a century that genetic factors are major determinants of variations in perioperative drug action between individuals and populations, technical limitations have precluded practitioners from incorporating heritable differences in drug choice and dose estimates. With the introduction of technologies able to rapidly scan DNA sequences for causal alterations, together with a composite draft of the human genome, the rate-limiting step to benefit from pharmacogenomic advances is now the availability of clinicians skilled in the recognition of drug-response outliers, and in testing novel genotype–phenotype correlations. The pharmacogenetic frontier is shifting from phase I to phase II pharmacokinetic effects, from drug metabolism to interindividual differences in pharmacodynamic responses, from monogenic to polygenic and epigenomic mechanisms, and from extreme to more subtle phenotypic correlates. As anesthetic drug administration evolves from the empiric approaches of the past to regimens customized by patient genotype, greater safety will be assured, and autonomy will be restored to the care of our most vulnerable patients including the very old, the very young, and the very sick. In the alternative, the price to be paid for ignoring genetic diversity in human drug response will grow increasingly unacceptable.

Summary

Pharmacogenetics, the study of the influence of genetic diversity on drug response, seeks to identify interindividual variation in efficacy and toxicity, often in relationship to differences in drug or metabolite concentration in a given compartment for a given dose. The genomic contribution to heterogeneity in drug response will also help delineate environmental and acquired factors that are also influencing drug responses by enabling exposed patients to be matched on the basis of shared genetic constitutions. This is an important distinction in light of recent evidence that suggests the human genome is less genetically stable than considered previously and that non-neoplastic, somatic genetic changes may be as significant in human drug responses as inherited germline polymorphisms.

Whether pharmacogenomic data made available in advance of surgery are of any value to the caregiver or patient depends on the genotype being analytically valid (the chosen DNA test method accurately detects the genotype) and clinically valid (the genotype correctly predicts the phenotype), with demonstrated clinical utility (the genotype specifies an available step to improve patient safety and health outcomes) and cost-effectiveness. Before pharmaocogenomic profiling ("personalized medicine") is translated into clinical practice there is great need for large, multicenter, randomized, double-blind, well-controlled, prospective investigations to clearly demonstrate the value of prospective genotyping.

Only by learning how patients subtly differ from one another at the molecular level will it be possible to decrease pharmacogenetic complications with less reliance on downstream early detection and rescue when adverse responses are identified. Patient safety may be enhanced by rational selection of technique, drugs, and dose based on individualized DNA signatures, and 50% of mortality could be potentially preventable by a-priori genomic drug-susceptibility profiling.

References

1. Bukaveckas BL. Adding pharmacogenetics to the clinical laboratory: narrow therapeutic index medications as a place to start. *Arch Pathol Lab Med* 2004; **128**: 1330–3.

2. Lazarou J, Pomeranz BH, Corey PN. Incidence of adverse drug reactions in hospitalized patients: a meta-analysis of prospective studies. *JAMA* 1998; **279**: 1200–5.

3. Chyka PA. How many deaths occur annually from adversed drug reactions in the United States? *Am J Med* 2000; **109**:122–30.

4. White TJ, Arakelian A, Rho JP. Counting the costs of drug-related adverse events. *Pharmacoeconomics* 1999; **15**: 445–58.

5. Moore TJ, Cohen MR, Furberg CD. Serious adverse drug reactions reported to the Food and Drug Administration, 1998–2005. *Arch Intern Med* 2007; **1667**: 1752–59.

6. Eichelbaum M, Ingelman-Sundberg M, Evans WE. Pharmacogenomics and individualized drug therapy. *Annu Rev Med* 2006; **57**: 119–37.

7. Alvan G, Bertilsson L, Dahl ML, Sjokvist F. Moving toward genetic profiling in patient care: The scope and rationale of pharmacogenetic/ecogenetic investigation. *Drug Metab Dispos* 2001; **29**: 580–5.

8. Phillips KA, Veenstra DL, Oren E, Kee JK, Sadee W. Potential role of pharmacogenomics in reducing adverse drug reactions: A systematic review. *JAMA* 2001; **286**: 2270–9.

9. Hogan K. Principles and techniques of molecular biology. In: Hemmings HC and Hopkins PM, eds., *Foundations of Anesthesia: Basic Sciences for Clinical Practice*. Philadelphia, PA: Mosby-Elsevier, 2006: 51–70.

10. Rusnak JM, Kisabeth RM, Herbert DP, McNeil DM. Pharmacogenomics: a clinician's primer on emerging technologies for improved patient care. *Mayo Clin Proc* 2001; **76**: 299–309.

11. International Human Genome Sequencing Consortium. Initial sequencing and analysis of the human genome. *Nature* 2001; **409**: 860–921.

12. Wang L, Weinschilboum RM. Pharmacogenomimcs: candidate gene identification, functional validation and mechanisms. *Hum Mol Genet* 2008; **17**: R174–9.

13. de Smith AJ, Tsalenko A, Sampas N, *et al.* Array CGH analysis of copy number variation identifies 1284 new genes variant in healthy white males: implications for association studies of complex diseases. *Hum Mol Genet* 2007; **16**: 2783–94.

14. Altman RB, Klein TE. Challenges for biomedical informatics and pharmacogenomics. *Ann Rev Pharmacol Toxicol* 2002; **42**: 113–33.

15. Ligget SB. Pharmacogenetic applications of the Human Genome project. *Nat Med* 2001; **7**: 281–3.

16. Nebert DW. Extreme discordant phenotype methodology: an intuitive approach to clinical pharmacogenetics. *Eur J Pharmacol* 2000; **41**: 107–20.

17. McLeod HL, Evans WE. Pharmacogenomics: unlocking the human genome for better drug therapy. *Annu Rev Pharmacol Toxicol* 2001; **41**: 101–21.

18. Galley HF, Mahdy A, Lowes DA. Pharmacogenetics and anesthesiologists. *Pharmacogenomics* 2005; **6**: 849–56.

19. Grossman I. Routine pharmacogenetic testing in clinical practice: dream or reality? *Pharmacogenomics* 2007; **8**: 1449–59.

20. Channock SJ, Manolio T, Boehnke M, *et al.* Replicating genotype-phenotype associations. *Nature* 2007; **447**: 655–60.

21. Jorgensen AL, Williamson PR. Methodological quality of pharmacogenetic studies: issues of concern. *Stat Med* 2008; **27**: 6547–69.

22. Kalow W. Perspectives in pharmacogenetics. *Arch Pathol Lab Med* 2001; **25**: 77–80.

23. Williams JA, Andersson T, Andersson TB, *et al.* PhRMA White Paper on ADME pharmacogenomics. *J Clin Pharmacol* 2008; **48**: 849–89.

24. Levano S, Ginz H, Siegemund M, *et al.* Genotyping the butyrylcholinesterase in patients with prolonged neuromuscular block after succinylcholine. *Anesthesiology* 2005; **102**: 531–5.

25. Levano S, Keller D, Schobinger E, Urwyler A, Girard T. Rapid and accurate detection of atypical and Kalow variants in the butyrlcholinesterase gene using denaturing high-performance liquid chromatography. *Anesth Analg* 2008; **106**: 147–51.

26. Maekawa M, Sudo K, Dey DC, *et al.* Genetic mutations of butyrylcholine esterase identified from phenotypic abnormalities in Japan. *Clin Chem* 1997; **43**: 924–9.

27. Gatke MR, Bundgaard JR, Viby-Mogensen J. Two novel mutations in the *BCHE* gene in patients with prolonged duration of action of mivacurium or succinylcholine during anaesthesia. *Pharmacogenet Genomics* 2007; **17**: 995–9.

28. Mikami LR, Wieseler S, Souza RLR, *et al.* Five new naturally occurring mutations of the BCHE gene and frequencies of 12 butyrylcholinesterase alleles in a Brazilian population. *Pharmaocogenet Genomics* 2008; **18**: 213–18.

29. Morrow AC, Motulsky AG. Rapid screening method for the common atypical pseudocholinesterase variant. *J Lab Clin Med* 1968; **71**: 350–6.

30. Gardiner SJ, Begg EJ. Pharmacogenetics, drug-metabolizing enzymes and clinical practice. *Pharmacol Rev* 2006; **58**: 521–590.

31. Cerf C, Mesguish M, Gabriel I, Amselem S, Duvaldestin P. Screening patients with prolonged neuromuscular blockade after succinylcholine and mivacurium. *Anesth Analg* 2002; **94**: 461–6.

32. Gätke M, Viby-Mogensen J, Ostergaard D, Bundgaard J. Response to mivacurium in patients carrying the k variant in the butyrylcholinesterase gene. *Anesthesiology* 2005; **102**: 503–8.

33. Kilpatrick G, Tilbrook G. Drug development in anaesthesia: industrial perspective. *Curr Opin Anaesthesiol* 2006; **19**: 385–9.

34. Belfer I, Wu T, Kingman A, *et al.* Candidate gene studies of human pain mechanisms: methods for optimizing choice of polymorphisms and sample size. *Anesthesiology* 2004; **100**: 1562–72.

35. Romberg RR, Olofsen E, Bijl H, *et al.* Polymorphism of μ-opioid receptor gene (OPRM:c118A>G) does not protect against opioid induced respiratory depression despite reduced analgesic response. *Anesthesiology* 2005; **102**: 522–30.

36. Stamer UM, Stuber F. Genetic factors in pain and its treatment. *Curr Opin Anaesthesiol* 2007; **20**: 478–84.

37. Aubrun F, Langeron O, Quesnel C, Coriat P, Riou B. Relationships between measurement of pain using visual analog scale and morphine requirements during postoperative intravenous morphine titration. *Anesthesiology* 2003; **98**: 1415–21.

38. Nagashima M, Katoh R, Sato Y, *et al.* Is there genetic polymorphism evidence for individual human sensitivity to opiates? *Curr Pain Headache Rep* 2007; **11**: 115–23.

39. Samer C, Desmeules J, Dayer P. Individualizing analgesic prescription part I: pharmacogenetics of opioid analgesics. *Per Med* 2006; **3**: 239–69.

40. Beyer A, Koch T, Schroder H, Schulz S, Hollt V. Effect of the A118G polymorphisms on binding affinity, potency and agonist-mediated endocytosis, desensitization, and resensitization of the human mu-opioid receptor. *J Neurochem* 2004; **89**: 553–60.

41. Landau R. One size does not fit all: genetic variability of the mu-opioid receptor and postoperative medicine consumption. *Anesthesiology* 2006; **105**: 235–7.

42. Klepstad P, Rakvåg T, Kaasa S, *et al.* The 118 A > G polymorphism in the human mu-opioid receptor gene may increase morphine requirements in patients with pain caused by malignant disease. *Acta Anaesthesiol Scand* 2004; **48**: 1232–9.

43. Oertel B, Schmidt R, Schneider A, Geisslinger G, Lötsch J. The mu-opioid receptor gene polymorphism 118A>G depletes alfentanil-induced analgesia and protects against respiratory depression in homozygous carriers. *Pharmacogenet Genomics* 2006; **16**: 625–36.

44. Coulbault L, Beaussier M, Verstuyft C, *et al.* Environmental and genetic factors associated with morphine response in the postoperative period. *Clin Pharmacol Ther* 2006; **79**: 316–24.

45. Chou W, Wang C, Liu P, *et al.* Human opioid receptor A118G polymorphism affects intravenous patient-controlled analgesia morphine consumption after total abdominal hysterectomy. *Anesthesiology* 2006; **105**: 334–7.

46. Chou W, Yang L, Lu H, *et al.* Association of mu-opioid receptor gene polymorphism (A118G) with variations in morphine consumption for analgesia after total knee arthroplasty. *Acta Anaesthesiol Scand* 2006; **50**: 787–92.

47. Janicki P, Schuler G, Francis D, *et al.* A genetic association study of the functional A118G polymorphism of the human mu-opioid receptor gene in patients with acute and chronic pain. *Anesth Analg* 2006; **103**: 1011–17.

48. Landau R, Kern C, Columb MO, *et al.* Genetic variability of the mu-opioid receptor influences intrathecal fentanyl requirements in laboring women. *Pain* 2008; **139**: 5–14.

49. Landau R. Pharmacogenetics and obstetric anesthesia. *Anesthesiol Clin* 2008; **26**: 183–95.

50. Sia AT, Lim Y, Lim EC, *et al.* A118G single nucleotide polymorphism of human mu-opioid receptor gene influences pain perception and patient-controlled intravenous morphine consumption after intrathecal morphine for postcesarean analgesia. *Anesthesiology* 2008; **109**: 520–6.

51. Bruehl S, Chung OY, Donahue BS, Burns JW. Anger regulation style, postoperative pain, and relationship to the A118G mu opioid receptor gene polymorphism: a preliminary study. *J Behav Med* 2006; **29**: 161–9.

52. Somogyi AA, Barratt DT, Coller JT. Pharmacogenetics of opioids. *Clin Pharmacol Ther* 2007; **81**: 429–44.

53. Campa D, Gioia A, Tomei A, Poli P, Barale R. Association of ABCB₁/MDR1 and OPRM1 gene polymorphisms with morphine pain relief. *Clin Pharmacol Ther* 2008; **83**: 559–66.

54. Hogan K. The anesthetic myopathies and malignant hyperthermias. *Curr Opin Neurol* 1998; **11**: 469–76.

55. Rosenberg H, Davis M, James D, Pollock N, Stowell K. Malignant hyperthermia. *Orphanet J Rare Dis* 2007; **2**: 21, 1–14. www.OJRD.com/content/2/1/21.

56. Larach MG, Brandom BW, Allen GC, Gronert GA, Lehman EB. Cardiac

arrests and deaths associated with malignant hyperthermia in North America from 1987 to 2006: a report from the North American Malignant Hyperthermia registry of the Malignant Hyperthermia Association of the United States. *Anesthesiology* 2008; **108**: 603–11.

57. Rosenberg H, Rothstein A. Malignant hyperthermia death holds many lessons. *Anesth Patient Saf Found Newsl* 2006; **21**: 32–4.

58. Cohen I, Kaplan R. Repeat episodes of severe muscle rigidity in a child receiving sevoflurane. *Pediatr Anesth* 2006; **16**: 1077–9.

59. Hopkins P. Recrudescence of malignant hyperthermia. *Anesthesiology* 2007; **106**: 893–4.

60. Burkman JM, Posner KL, Domino KB. Analysis of the clinical variables associated with recrudescence after malignant hyperthermia reactions. *Anesthesiology* 2007; **106**: 901–6.

61. Denborough MA. Malignant hyperthermia, 1962. *Anesthesiology* 2008; **108**: 156–7.

62. Fairhurst AS, Hamamoto V, Macri J. Modification of ryanodine toxicity by dantrolene and halothane in a model of malignant hyperthermia. *Anesthesiology* 1980; **53**: 199–204.

63. Litman R, Rosenberg H. Malignant hypterthermia: update on susceptibility testing. *JAMA* 2005; **293**: 2918–24.

64. MacLennan DH, Phillips MS. Malignant hyperthermia. *Science* 1992; **256**: 789–94.

65. Hogan K, Couch F, Powers PA, Gregg RG. A cysteine for arginine substitution (R614C) in the human skeletal muscle calcium release channel co-segregates with malignant hyperthermia. *Anesth Analg* 1992; **75**: 441–8.

66. Robinson R, Carpenter D, Shaw M, Halsall J, Hopkins P. Mutations in RYR1 in malignant hyperthermia and central core disease. *Hum Mutat* 2006; **27**: 977–89.

67. D'Arcy CE, Bjorksten A, Yiu EM, *et al.* King–Denborough syndrome caused by a novel mutation in the ryanodine receptor. *Neurology* 2008; **71**: 776–7.

68. Sambuughin N, Holley H, Muldoon S, *et al.* Screening of the entire ryanodine receptor type 1 coding region for sequence variants associated with malignant hyperthermia susceptibility in the North American population. *Anesthesiology* 2005; **102**: 515–21.

69. Hogan K, Gregg RG, Powers PA. The structure of the gene encoding the human skeletal muscle α1 subunit of the dihydropyridine-sensitive L-type calcium channel (CACNL1A3). *Genomics* 1996; **31**: 392–4.

70. Stewart SL, Hogan K, Rosenberg H, Fletcher JE. Identification of the Arg1086His mutation in the alpha subunit of the voltage-dependent calcium channel (CACNA1S) in a North American family with malignant hyperthermia. *Clin Genet* 2001; **59**: 178–84.

71. Stamm DS, Powell CM, Stajich JM, *et al.* Novel congenital myopathy locuse identified in Native American Indians at 12q13.13–14.1. *Neurology* 2008; **71**: 1764–9.

72. Zhou H, Jungbluth H, Sewry C, *et al.* Molecular mechanisms and phenotypic variation in RYR1-related congenital myopathies. *Brain* 2007; **130**: 2024–36.

73. Kossugue P, Paim J, Navarro M, *et al.* Central core disease due to recessive mutations in RYR1 gene: is it more common than described? *Muscle Nerve* 2007; **35**: 670–4.

74. Rueffert H, Olthoff D, Deutrich C. Spontaneous occurrence of disposition to malignant hyperthermia. *Anesthesiology* 2004; **100**: 731–3.

75. Anderson AA, Brown RL, Polster B, Pollock N, Stowell KM. Identification and biochemical characterization of a novel ryanodine receptor gene mutation associated with malignant hyperthermia. *Anesthesiology* 2008; **108**: 208–15.

76. Newmark J, Voelkel M, Brandom B, Wu J. Delayed onset of malignant hypothermia without creating kinase elevation in a geriatric, ryanodine receptor type 1 gene compound heterozygous patient. *Anesthesiology* 2007; **107**: 350–3.

77. Monnier N, Krivosic-Horber R, Payen J, *et al.* Presence of two different genetic traits in malignant hyperthermia families: implication for genetic analysis, diagnosis, and incidence of malignant hyperthermia. *Anesthesiology* 2002; **97**: 1067–74.

78. Yang T, Riehl J, Esteve E, *et al.* Pharmacologic and functional characterization of malignant hyperthermia in the R163C RyR1 knock-in mouse. *Anesthesiology* 2006; **105**: 1164–75.

79. Hogan K. In hot pursuit. *Anesthesiology* 2006; **105**: 1077–8.

80. Islander G, Ording H, Bendixen D, Ranklev Twetman E. Reproducibility of in vitro contracture test results in patients tested for malignant hyperthermia susceptibility. *Acta Anaesthesiol Scand* 2002; **46**: 1144–9.

81. Tegazzin V, Scutari E, Treves S, Zorzato F. Chlorocresol, an additive to commercial succinylcholine, induces contracture of human malignant hyperthermia-susceptible muscles via activation of the ryanodine receptor Ca2+ channel. *Anesthesiology* 1996; **84**: 1380–5.

82. Litman RS, Flood CD, Kaplan RF, Kim YL, Tobin JR. Postoperative malignant hyperthermia: An analysis of cases from the North American Malignant Hyperthermia Registry. *Anesthesiology* 2008; **109**: 825–9.

83. Wappler F, Fiege M, Steinfath M, *et al.* Evidence for susceptibility to malignant hyperthermia in patients with exercise-induced rhabdomyolysis. *Anesthesiology* 2001; **94**: 95–100.

84. Hopkins PM. Is there a link between malignant hyperthermia and exertional heat illness? *Br J Sports Med* 2007; **41**: 283–4.

85. Zhao X, Weisleder N, Han X, *et al.* Azumolene inhibits a component of store-operated calcium entry coupled to the skeletal muscle ryanodine receptor. *J Biol Chem* 2006; **281**: 33477–86.

86. Goldenberg I, Moss AJ. Long QT syndrome. *J Am Coll Cardiol* 2008; **24**: 2291–300.

87. Roden DM. Clinical practice. Long-QT syndrome. *N Engl J Med* 2008; **358**: 169–76.

88. Morita H, Wu J, Zipes DP. The QT syndromes: long and short. *Lancet* 2008; **372**: 750–63.

89. Boussy T, Paparella G, deAsmundis C, *et al.* Genetic basis of ventricular

arrhythmias. *Cardiol Clin* 2008; **26**: 335–53.

90. Goldenberg I, Zareba W, Moss AJ. Long QT syndrome. *Curr Probl Cardiol* 2008; **33**: 629–94.

91. Booker PD, Whyte SD, Ladusans EJ. Long QT syndrome and anaesthesia. *Br J Anaesth* 2003; **90**: 349–66.

92. Kleinsasser A, Loeckinger A, Lindner KH, *et al.* Reversing sevoflurane-associated Q-Tc prolongation by changing to propofol. *Anaesthesia* 2001; **56**: 248–50.

93. Pleym H, Bathen J, Spigset O, Gisvold SE. Ventricular fibrillation related to reversal of the neuromuscular blockade in a patient with long QT syndrome. *Acta Anaesthesiol Scand* 1999; **43**: 352–5.

94. Saarnivaara L, Klemola UM, Lindgren L. QT interval of the ECG, heart rate and arterial pressure using five non-depolarizing muscle relaxants for intubation. *Acta Anaesthesiol Scand* 1988; **32**: 623–8.

95. Siebrands CC, Binder S, Eckhoff U, *et al.* Long QT mutation *KCNQ14344V* increases local anesthetic sensitivity of the slowly activating delayed rectifier potassium current. *Anesthesiology* 2006; **105**: 511–20.

96. Vernoy K, Sicouri S, Dumaine R, *et al.* Genetic and biophysical basis for bupivacaine-induced ST segment elevation and VT/VF. Anesthesia unmasked Brugada syndrome. *Heart Rhythm* 2006; **3**: 1074–8.

97. Aersens J, Paulissemn ADC. Pharmacogenomics and acquired long QT syndrome. *Pharmacogenomics* 2005; **6**: 259–70.

98. Santambrogio L, Braschi A. Conduction abnormalities and anaesthesia. *Curr Opin Anaesthesiol* 2007; **20**: 269–73.

99. Drake E, Preston R, Douglas J. Brief review: anesthetic implications of long QT syndrome in preganancy. *Can J Anesth* 2007; **54**: 561–72.

100. Shipton E. Anaesthetics and the rate corrected interval: learning from droperidol? *Curr Opin Anaesthesiol* 2005; **18**: 419–23.

101. Nuttall GA, Eckerman KM, Jacob KA, *et al.* Does low-dose droperidol administration increase the risk of drug-induced QT prolongation and torsades de pointes in the general surgical population? *Anesthesiology* 2007; **107**: 531–6.

102. Habib AS, Gan T. PRO: the Food and Drug Administration black box warning on droperidol is not justified. *Anesth Analg* 2008; **106**: 1414–17.

103. Ludwin DB, Shafer SL. CON: the black box warning on droperidol should not be removed (but should be clarified). *Anesth Analg* 2008; **106**: 1418–20.

104. Gottlieb B, Beitel LK, Trifiro M. Somatic mosaicism and variable expressivity. *Trends Genet* 2001; **17**: 79–82.

105. Fimmel S, Kurfurst R, Bonte F, Zouboulis CC. Responsiveness to androgens and the effectiveness of antisense oligonucleotides against the androgen receptor on human epidermal keratinocytes is dependent on the age of the donor and the location of cell origin. *Horm Metab Res* 2007; **39**: 157–65.

106. Conney AH. Pharmacological implications of microsomal enzyme induction. *Pharmacol Rev* 1967; **19**: 317–66.

107. Rhodes JS, Crabbe JC. Gene expression induced by drugs of abuse. *Curr Opin Pharmacol* 2005; **5**: 26–33.

108. Dolinoy DC. Epigenetic gene regulation: early environmental exposures. *Pharmacogenomics* 2007; **8**: 5–10.

109. Kalow W. Personalized medicine: Some thoughts. *McGill J Med* 2007; **10**: 58.

110. Nebert DW, Zhang G, Vesell ES. From human genetics and genomics to pharmacogenetics and pharmacogenomics: past lessons, future directions. *Drug Metab Rev* 2008; **40**: 187–224.

111. Brockmoller J, Tzvetkov, MV. Pharmacogenetics: data, concepts and tools to improve drug discovery and drug treatment. *Eur J Clin Pharmacol* 2008; **64**: 133–57.

112. Shurin SB, Nabel EG. Pharmacogenomics: ready for prime time? *N Engl J Med* 2008; **358**: 1061–3.

113. Zaugg M, Bestmann L, Wacker J, *et al.* Adrenergic receptor genotype but not perioperative bisoprolol therapy may determine cardiovascular outcome in at-risk patients undergoing surgery with spinal block. The Swiss beta blocker in spinal anesthesia (BBSA) study: a double-blinded, placebo-controlled, multicenter trial with 1-year follow-up. *Anesthesiology* 2007; **107**: 33–44.

114. Kaymak C, Kocaba ÅŸ N, Durmaz E, Oztuna D. Beta2 adrenoceptor (ADRB2) pharmacogenetics and cardiovascular phenotypes during laryngoscopy and tracheal intubation. *Int J Toxicol* 2006; **25**: 443–9.

115. Smiley R, Blouin J, Negron M, Landau R. Beta2-adrenoceptor genotype affects vasopressor requirements during spinal anesthesia for cesarean delivery. *Anesthesiology* 2006; **104**: 644–50.

116. Talke P, Stapelfeldt C, Lobo E, *et al.* Effect of alpha2B-adrenoceptor polymorphism on peripheral vasoconstriction in healthy volunteers. *Anesthesiology* 2005; **102**: 536–42.

117. Selzer RR, Rosenblatt DS, Laxova R, Hogan K. Nitrous oxide and 5, 10-methylenetetrahydrofolate reductase deficiency. *New England Journal of Medicine* 2003; **349**: 45–50.

118. Nagele P, Zeugswetter B, Wiener C, *et al.* Influence of methylenetetrahydrofolate reductase gene polymorphisms on homocysteine concentration after nitrous oxide anesthesia. *Anesthesiology* 2008; **109**: 36–43.

119. Hogan K. Pharmacogenetics of nitrous oxide: standing at the crossroads. *Anesthesiology* 2008; **109**: 5–6.

120. Ho K, Gan T. Pharmacology, pharmacogenetics, and clinical efficacy of 5-hydroxytryptamine type 3 receptor antagonists for postoperative nausea and vomiting. *Curr Opin Anaesthesiol* 2006; **19**: 606–11.

121. Candiotti KA, Birnbach DJ, Lubarsky DA, *et al.* The impact of pharmacogenomics on postoperative nausea and vomiting: do CYP2D6 allele copy number and polymorphisms affect the success or failure of ondansetron prophylaxis? *Anesthesiology* 2005; **102**: 543–9.

122. Nielsen M, Olsen NV. Genetic polymorphisms in the cytochrome P450 system and efficacy of 5-hydroxytryptamine type-3 receptor

antagonists for postoperative nausea and vomiting. *British Journal of Anaesthesia* 2008; **101**: 441–5.

123. Corbett SM, Montoya ID, Moore FA. Propofol-related infusion syndrome in intensive care patients. *Pharmacotherapy* 2008; **28**: 250–8.

124. Monk TG, Weldon BC, Garvan CW, *et al.* Predictors of cognitive dysfunction after major noncardiac surgery. *Anesthesiology* 2008; **108**: 18–30.

125. Cox JJ, Reimann F, Nicholas AK, *et al.* An SVN9A channelopathy causes congenital inability to experience pain. *Nature* 2006; **444**: 894–8.

126. Goldberg YP, MacFarlane J, MacDonald ML, *et al.* Loss-of-function mutations in the $Na_v1.7$ gene underlie congenital indifference to pain in multiple human populations. *Clin Genet* 2007; **71**: 311–19.

127. Buchanan F, Myles P, Leslie K, *et al.* Gender and recovery after general anesthesia combined with neuromuscular blocking drugs. *Anesth Analg* 2006; **102**: 291–7.

128. Kodaka M, Suzuki T, Maeyama A, Koyama K, Miyao H. Gender differences between predicted and measured propofol C(P50) for loss of consciousness. *J Clin Anesth* 2006; **18**: 486–9.

129. Gelb MA, Gelb AW. Sex and gender in the perioperative period: wake up to reality. *Anesth Analg* 2008; **107**: 1–3.

130. Pleym H, Spigset O, Kharasch E, Dale O. Gender differences in drug effects: implications for anesthesiologists. *Acta Anaesthesiol Scand* 2003; **47**: 241–59.

131. Ezri T, Sessler D, Weisenberg M, *et al.* Association of ethnicity with the minimum alveolar concentration of sevoflurane. *Anesthesiology* 2007; **107**: 9–14.

132. Sonner J. Ethnicity can affect anesthetic requirement. *Anesthesiology* 2007; **107**: 4–5.

133. Ozdemir V, Graham JE, Godard B. Race as a variable in pharmacogenomics science: from empirical ethics to publication standards. *Pharmacogenet Genomics* 2008; **18**: 837–841.

134. Lee SS, Mountain J, Koenig B, *et al.* The ethics of characterizing difference: guiding principles on using racial categories in human genetics. *Genome Biol* 2008; **9**: 404.1– 404.4 (doi:10.1186/gb-2008-9-7-404).

135. Swen JJ, Huizinga TW, Gelderblom H, *et al.* Translating pharmacogenomics: Challenges on the road to the clinic. *PLoS Med* 2007; **4**: e209.

136. Hughes S, Huges A, Brothers C, *et al.* PREDICT-1 (CNA106030): the first powered, prospective trial of pharmacogenetic screening to reduce drug adverse events. *Pharm Stat* 2008 7: 121–9.

137. International Warfarin Pharmacogenetics Consortium, Klein TE, Altman RB, Eriksson N, *et al.* Estimation of the warfarin dose with clinical and pharmacogenetic data. *N Engl J Med* 2009; **360**: 753–64.

138. Garrison LP, Carlson RJ, Kuszler PC, *et al.* A review of public policy issues in promoting the development and commercialization of pharmacogenomic applications: challenges and implications. *Drug Metab Rev* 2008; **40**: 377–401.

139. Haga SB, Burke W. Pharmacogenetic testing: not as simple as it seems. *Genet Med* 2008; **10**: 391–5.

140. Prainsack B. What are the stakes? Genetic nondiscrimination legislation and personal genomics. *Per Med* 2008; **5**: 415–18.

141. Hernandex-Broussard T, Whirl-Carrillo M, Hebert JM, *et al.* The pharmacogenetics and pharmacogenomics knowledge base: accentuating the knowledge. *Nucleic Acids Res* 2008; **36**: 913–18.

Principles of drug action

Pharmacodynamic drug interactions in anesthesia

Talmage D. Egan and Charles F. Minto

Introduction

Understanding drug interactions is a critical part of anesthesia practice. The modern concept of "balanced anesthesia" implies the use of multiple drugs to achieve the anesthetized state. As many as a dozen drugs might be administered during a typical anesthetic, including benzodiazepines, barbiturates and other sedative-hypnotics, opioid analgesics, neuromuscular blockers, other analgesic adjuncts, antibiotics, neuromuscular blockade reversal agents, sympathomimetics, and autonomic nervous system blockers, among many others. The potential for drug interactions is therefore immense.

Anesthetic drug interactions can take several forms. Perhaps the simplest form of drug interaction in anesthesia is the **physicochemical** interaction. Physicochemical interactions occur when the physical properties of the interacting drugs are somehow incompatible; a common example of this kind of interaction in anesthesiology is the precipitation that occurs when certain neuromuscular blockers (e.g., pancuronium bromide) are injected into an intravenous line containing sodium thiopental (the precipitate is the conjugate salt of a weak acid and a weak base) [1]. A second form is the **pharmacokinetic** interaction. Pharmacokinetic interactions occur when one drug somehow alters the disposition of another drug [2]; a common example of this kind of drug interaction in anesthesiology is the increased metabolism of neuromuscular blockers observed in patients who are taking anticonvulsants chronically [3]. The final form of drug interaction is **pharmacodynamic**. Pharmacodynamic interactions occur when one drug somehow augments or reduces the effect of another drug; a common example of this kind of drug interaction in anesthesia practice is the minimum alveolar concentration (MAC) reduction that occurs for volatile anesthetics when opioids are administered as anesthetic adjuncts [4].

In anesthesiology, unlike most medical disciplines, pharmacodynamic drug interactions are frequently produced by design. Anesthesiologists take advantage of the pharmacodynamic synergy that results when two drugs with different mechanisms of action but similar therapeutic effects are combined. These synergistic combinations can be advantageous,

because the therapeutic goals of the anesthetic can often be achieved with less toxicity and faster recovery than when the individual drugs are used alone in higher doses.

In fact, except for specific, limited clinical circumstances wherein a volatile agent or propofol alone are acceptable approaches (e.g., a brief operation in a pediatric patient such as tympanostomy tubes), modern-day anesthesia is at least a two-drug process consisting of an opioid and a hypnotic agent. Opioids alone are not complete anesthetics because they cannot reliably produce unconsciousness [5,6]. Volatile anesthetics alone are inadequate unless the prestimulus hemodynamic variables are depressed to an unacceptable degree [7,8]. Modern anesthesia care is of necessity a multidrug exercise and therefore mandates that practitioners become experts in manipulating pharmacodynamic anesthetic interactions [9]. From a strictly pharmacologic perspective, anesthesiology is the practice of pharmacologic synergism using central nervous system depressants.

The goals of this chapter are threefold. First, to build the theoretical foundation for understanding the concept of pharmacodynamic synergism and to review how anesthetic drug interactions are characterized experimentally with special focus on the *isobole* concept and its three-dimensional extension, the *response surface*. Next, to review the prototypical pharmacodynamic drug interactions in anesthesiology, focusing on (1) the interaction between volatile anesthetics and opioids and (2) the interaction between propofol and opioids. Finally, to summarize the key clinical messages relating to pharmacodynamic drug interactions in anesthesia by introducing the idea of "navigating" the drug-interaction response surface as a framework for conceptualizing the pharmacology of the modern general anesthetic.

Experimental characterization of anesthetic drug interactions

Additive, synergistic, antagonistic interactions

The basic concepts of additive, synergistic, and antagonistic interactions are simple to understand. The term **additive**

Anesthetic Pharmacology, 2nd edition, ed. Alex S. Evers, Mervyn Maze, Evan D. Kharasch. Published by Cambridge University Press. © Cambridge University Press 2011.

interaction is usually used in those cases in which the combined effect of two drugs (often acting by the same mechanism) is equal to that expected by simple addition. The term **synergistic interaction** is usually used in those cases in which the combined effect of two drugs (often acting by a different mechanism) is greater than that expected by simple addition. The term **antagonistic interaction** is usually used in those cases in which the combined effect of two drugs is less than that expected by simple addition. The key concept, however, is how to define "that expected by simple addition."

Many authors define an additive interaction as one that obeys the simple effect-addition model:

$$E_{AB} = E_A + E_B \tag{11.1}$$

where the combined effect of two drugs (E_{AB}) is equal to the algebraic sum of their individual effects (E_A and E_B). Thus, the *additive* concept is often explained with reference to the simple equation $1 + 1 = 2$. With reference to this equation, the *synergy* concept is illustrated by $1 + 1 > 2$ and the *antagonism* concept by $1 + 1 < 2$. Although the basic concepts of additive, synergistic, and antagonistic interactions may be clear from this explanation, the simple effect-addition model has a major flaw. Imagine a sham experiment, in which a drug preparation is divided into two syringes, and then each syringe is treated as if it contained a different drug ("drug A" and "drug B"). In the first phase of the experiment, 1 mg of "drug A" is given. This dose causes an effect, which is 5% of the maximum response. In the second phase of the experiment, 1 mg of "drug B" is given. This dose causes an effect, which is also 5% of the maximum response. In the third phase, 1 mg of "drug A" *together with* 1 mg of "drug B" is given. What effect should be expected to observe if the interaction is additive? Will the combination cause a 10% effect, which is the algebraic sum of the individual effects (5% + 5%)? If the combination causes an effect equal to 50% of the maximum response, should it be concluded that the two drugs interact synergistically, because the effect of the combination is five times greater than expected from the algebraic sum of the individual effects? How is it possible to have a synergistic interaction when only one drug is being evaluated? Surely, by definition one drug has "no interaction" with itself! Why don't the effects just add together as described by Eq. 11.1?

The flaw with the simple effect-addition model (Eq. 11.1) is that it presupposes that the relationship between drug dose and drug effect is linear (Fig. 11.1A). It assumes that doubling the dose should double the effect. However, the hypothetical drug being investigated has a nonlinear relationship between dose and effect (Fig. 11.1B). Specifically, 1 mg causes an effect of 5% and 2 mg causes an effect of 50%. There is no synergy, because the observed effect caused by 1 mg of "drug A" combined with 1 mg of "drug B" (the same drug) is the same as the expected effect caused by a 2 mg bolus. Thus, the simple effect-addition model is only true if the dose-response relationship is linear. A more general definition of "no interaction" is required.

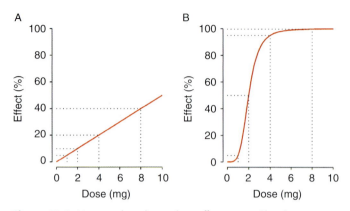

Figure 11.1. Linear and nonlinear dose–effect curves. The dose–response relationships are shown in red. Many authors define an *additive interaction* as one that obeys the simple effect addition model, where the combined effect of two drugs is equal to the algebraic sum of their individual effects (Eq. 11.1). This is only applicable if the dose–response (or concentration–response) relationship is linear (A). Often the relationship is nonlinear (B). The dotted lines represent progressive doubling of the drug dose (or concentration). In a linear relationship (A), doubling the dose will double the effect. In a nonlinear relationship (B), doubling the dose from 1 mg to 2 mg increases the effect from 5% to 50%. When the dose is doubled again, the effect increases from 50% to 95%. When the dose is doubled again, the effect only increases from 95% to 99.7%.

Isobologram

Synergism (and antagonism) can be defined as a greater (or lesser) pharmacologic effect for a two-drug combination than would be predicted for "no interaction" based on what is known about the effects of each drug individually. Thus, their definitions critically depend upon the reference model for "no interaction" [10]. We believe that the best way to obtain a clear understanding of "no interaction" is by carrying out a thought experiment based on the sham combination of one drug with itself, as described above. Knowing that syringes A and B contain the same drug, we can describe an experiment to show that "drug A" and "drug B" have "no interaction" (i.e., they are additive). Imagine syringes A and B contain 2 mg of "drug A" and 2 mg of "drug B," respectively. We perform an experiment and find that 2 mg from syringe A causes 50% effect. We perform another experiment and find that 2 mg from syringe B also causes 50% effect. Clearly, 1 mg from syringe A together with 1 mg from syringe B will also cause 50% effect, because we are still giving 2 mg of our hypothetical drug. For the same reason, 0.5 mg from syringe A together with 1.5 mg from syringe B, or 1.5 mg from syringe A together with 0.5 mg from syringe B, will also cause 50% effect. The fact that we using one or other syringe (or some combination from the two syringes) to give the same total dose makes no difference to the observed effect. This is true, whatever the shape of the dose–response relationship.

There are two important models that deserve consideration as reference standards for "no interaction" [11]. The first model is that of *Loewe additivity*, which is based on the idea that, by definition, a drug cannot interact with itself [12]. In other words, in the sham experiment in which a drug is

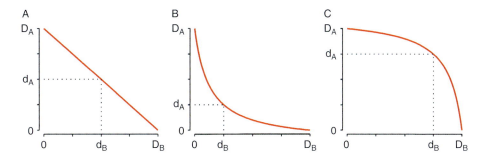

Figure 11.2. Isobolograms (shown in red) depicting (A) additivity, (B) synergy or supra-additivity, and (C) antagonism or infra-additivity. D_A and D_B are isoeffective doses of two drugs when given alone. As indicated by the dotted lines, the administration of the two drugs as the combination (d_A, d_B) results in the same effect. If D_A and D_B are the doses causing 50% effect (the D_{50}), in each case the line represents the 50% isobole. When the drugs in combination are more effective than expected (synergy), smaller amounts are needed to produce the effect, and the combination (d_A, d_B) is shifted toward the origin (B). Conversely, when the drugs in combination are less effective than expected (antagonism), greater amounts are needed to produce the effect and the combination (d_A, d_B) is shifted away from the origin [12]. The equation for the straight line in (A) is given by $y = -D_A/D_B \cdot x + D_A$, where y is d_A and x is d_B, which is the same as the equation defining Loewe additivity (Eq. 11.2).

combined with itself, the result will be Loewe additivity. The second model is *Bliss independence*, which is based on the idea of probabilistic independence, i.e., two drugs act in such a manner that neither one interferes with the other, but each contributes to a common result [13]. We prefer the Loewe additivity model as the reference for "no interaction," because it yields the intuitively correct evaluation of the sham combination of one drug with itself, whereas the Bliss independence model does not [11]. All possible combinations of "drug A" and "drug B" that cause a specified effect will be described by the equation for Loewe additivity [12]:

$$\frac{d_A}{D_A} + \frac{d_B}{D_B} = 1 \qquad (11.2)$$

where D_A is the dose of "drug A" that causes the specified effect (e.g., 50% effect), D_B is the dose of "drug B" that causes the specified effect, and (d_A, d_B) are the doses of "drug A" and "drug B" in the various combinations that also cause specified effect.

When the dose of "drug A" is plotted on the y-axis and the dose of "drug B" is plotted on the x-axis, Eq. 11.2 describes a straight line running from $D_{X,A}$ on the y-axis to $D_{X,B}$ on the x-axis. Such graphs (Fig. 11.2) are called isobolograms, and the lines on these graphs are called isoboles. Isoboles show dose combinations that result in equal effect. If the isoboles are straight lines, then the interaction is additive. If the isoboles bow towards the origin of the graph, then the interaction is synergistic. If the isoboles bow away from the origin of the graph, then the interaction is antagonistic. Although an isobole clearly shows whether an interaction is additive, synergistic, or antagonistic, it is often only determined for a single level of drug effect. For example, in the anesthesia literature, a common approach has been to determine the 50% isobole for a specific endpoint, such as preventing movement in response to an incision. Although this isobole permits a statement to be made about whether there is any evidence of synergy or antagonism, it is not possible to make inferences

about other levels of drug effect (e.g., the 95% isobole) that might be more clinically relevant. Although many different methods have been used for the analysis of drug interactions, the isobolographic method is the best validated for most applications [14].

The focus on whether drug interactions can be reduced to simple descriptors such as additive, synergistic, or antagonistic may be too simplistic. Interactions have the potential to be very complex. For example, a drug combination can be synergistic in certain regions and antagonistic in others [15]. Rather than worry about which descriptor applies, the goal should be to characterize the *response surface*. From the surface one can identify the best combination to produce the desired therapeutic effect.

Response surfaces

The name *response-surface methodology* (RSM) has been given to the statistical methodology concerned with (1) the design of studies to estimate response surfaces, (2) the actual estimation of response surfaces, and (3) the interpretation of the results. Response-surface methodology is generally employed for two principal purposes: (1) to provide a description of the response pattern *in the region of the observations studied*, and (2) to assist in finding the region where the optimal response occurs (i.e., where the response is at a maximum or a minimum).

A response surface is a mathematical equation or the graph of that equation, which relates a dependent variable (such as a drug effect) to inputs (such as two drug concentrations). Figure 11.3 shows that an isobole is obtained by making a horizontal slice through the response surface. When two agonists differ only in their potency and there is "no interaction" between the two drugs, the surface is stretched tightly between the drug A and drug B edges, and the isoboles are straight lines. Figure 11.4 shows two response surfaces (and their 50% isoboles) illustrating synergistic and antagonistic interactions between two agonists. Other interactions between full agonists, partial agonists, inverse agonists, and competitive antagonists

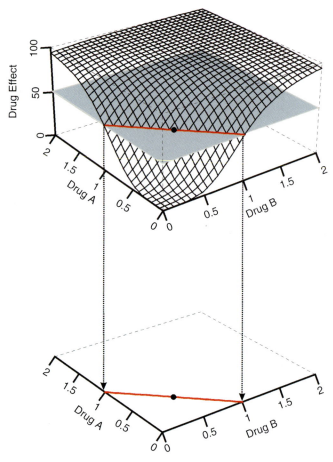

Figure 11.3. An additive response surface with a "slice" through the surface representing an isobologram at 50% of maximum drug effect. The "drug A" and "drug B" axes are labeled in units of the dose or concentration required to cause 50% of the maximum effect. The upper portion of the figure is a response surface for two agonists with "no interaction" (i.e., additive interaction). The blue horizontal plane slices the surface at the 50% effect level. The lower portion of the figure is the isobologram (shown in red) defining concentrations that result in 50% of maximum effect. The isobologram is thus a two-dimensional representation of a single slice through the three-dimensional response surface. The solid circle in both figures shows the effect resulting from 0.5 units of "drug A" combined with 0.5 units of "drug B". The study of one point on the surface will tell us whether this point shows evidence of synergism or antagonism, but tells us little about the interaction at other levels of effect (i.e., the remainder of the response surface).

can also be illustrated using response-surface models [16]. When a response surface is viewed from above, a series of equally spaced horizontal slices will appear as a series of isoboles, in the same way that contour lines drawn on a map connect points of equal height. Where the gradient of the surface is steep the contour lines will be close together, and where the gradient of the surface is shallow the contour lines will be far apart.

A large variety of experimental designs have been developed for estimating response surfaces efficiently [17]. The "ray" design studies the response (effect) for two drugs present in a number of fixed ratios. Each ratio can be considered as a single drug, which permits the analysis to be based on the same principles as that associated with single-drug experiments.

The "full factorial" design studies the response for all combinations of two drugs at a number of different doses ("fractional factorial" designs are also employed) [18–20]. When the interactions between three drugs are being investigated, the drugs should be (1) studied alone, (2) studied in three pairs, and (3) studied in the triple combination [21].

In many experimental situations unrelated to drugs and anesthesia, response surfaces are used to determine optimal response conditions. For example, a company may wish to know which combination of two variables (e.g., charge rate and temperature) maximizes the expected life of power cells [22]. However, when the two variables are two drugs, the optimum combination is sometimes more difficult to define. For example, any relatively high-dose combination of two agonists which interact synergistically will result in the maximum effect (Fig. 11.4A). However, in considering the interaction between an opioid and an hypnotic to maintain the state of general anesthesia, simply knowing that any high-dose combination works well is not particularly helpful. Determination of the optimum combination also requires considering the pharmacokinetic properties and side-effect profiles of the two drugs. The preferable combination is somewhere up on the shoulder of the surface, where the desired therapeutic effect is achieved, where the hemodynamic side effects are minimal, and where the recovery from anesthesia is predictably rapid.

A description of methods used to estimate and evaluate a fitted response surface, and of tests used to decide whether interaction effects are significant, is beyond the scope of this chapter. However, the general strategy is outlined in Table 11.1. Those seeking further information on response-surface methods can review brief [22] and full descriptions [23].

Interaction models used in anesthesia

Several investigators have modeled anesthetic drug interactions as extensions of the logistic regression model for a single drug [4,24–26]. Various models have been used in these important clinical studies, and they can be evaluated according to the characteristics of an ideal pharmacodynamic interaction model suggested in Table 11.2 [16]. In the logistic regression model for a single drug, the natural logarithm of the odds ratio (the logit) is modeled as a linear function of drug concentration (C):

$$\text{logit} = \log(\text{odds ratio}) = \log\left(\frac{P}{1-P}\right) = \beta_0 + \beta_1 \cdot \log(C) \quad (11.3)$$

where P is probability of effect, and β_0 and β_1 are estimated parameters. Alternatively, the probability of effect can be expressed as:

$$P = \frac{e^{\beta_0 + \beta_1 \cdot \log(C)}}{1 + e^{\beta_0 + \beta_1 \cdot \log(C)}} \quad (11.4)$$

If $\beta_0 = -\gamma \cdot \log(C_{50})$ and $\beta_1 = \gamma$, then Eqs. 11.3 and 11.4 are algebraically equivalent to the more intuitive and familiar sigmoid relationship:

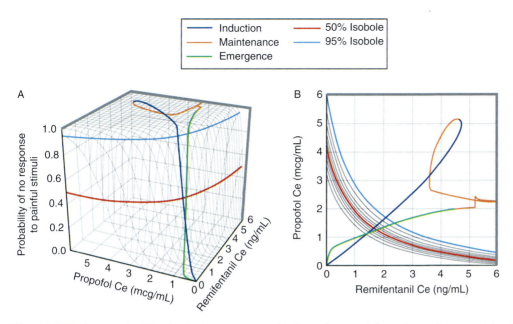

Figure 11.10. An example of "navigating the response surface" as a framework for understanding anesthesia clinical pharmacology. (A) Response surface characterizing the interaction between propofol and remifentanil for lack of response to painful stimulation. (B) Topographic view of the same response surface. Superimposed on both panels are the remifentanil and propofol effect-site concentrations that result from the simulated total intravenous anesthetic presented in Fig. 11.9. Segments of the anesthetic are color-coded to depict induction, maintenance, and emergence. See text for further explanation. Adapted with permission from Johnson and Egan [83].

pharmacokinetic simulations, the response-surface plots typically have no temporal component (i.e., time is not depicted on the plot).

Figure 11.10 illustrates several key points regarding the clinical pharmacology of the modern general anesthetic. First, it is clear that unlike most therapeutic areas in medical practice, the concentration targets are frequently changing during a typical anesthetic. The degree of the patient's central nervous system depression must be matched to the prevailing surgical stimulus. This is a dynamic process that requires frequent adjustment of the anesthetic dosage. Second, because the synergy between hypnotics and opioids is so significant, the surface is very steep. Thus, if for example anesthesia becomes inadequate at some point during an operation, moving from an isobole that predicts a 50% nonresponse rate to an isobole that predicts a 90% nonresponse rate requires only a small increase in drug concentration; when anesthesia in inadequate, often a relatively minor dosage adjustment may be sufficient to produce adequate anesthesia. The steepness of the surface is also important during emergence. Targeting concentrations that produce adequate anesthesia and yet permit rapid recovery at the end of the anesthetic necessitates staying near the steep part of the surface when formulating dosage strategy (of course, when using pharmacokinetically responsive drugs this consideration is less critical). In doing so, at the end of the anesthetic it is possible to rapidly "slide" down the steep slope of the surface to promote a rapid emergence from anesthesia.

It is important to recognize, in contrast, that the flat portion of the surface where maximal drug effect is produced also

has important clinical implications. At times during the anesthetic when "supramaximal" stimulation will occur, such as during laryngoscopy and tracheal intubation at induction of anesthesia, it is advantageous to be on the flat part of the response surface to be confident that adequate anesthesia conditions will be produced. Conversely, toward the end of the operation, targeting the flat part of the response surface (especially at excessively high concentration targets far away from the origin of the surface) is a distinct disadvantage because such a strategy will delay emergence.

Perhaps the single most important clinically relevant concept from pharmacodynamic drug-interaction response surfaces is that for any given predicted anesthetic effect, there are an infinite number of sedative–opioid target concentration pairs that will produce that same effect. Thus, a single isobolographic cut through the response surface defines a wide range of target drug concentration pairs for the sedative and the opioid that will produce the same anesthetic conditions. Choosing the best combination (e.g., high sedative/low opioid, low sedative/high opioid, etc.) is a fundamental management question that must be addressed for each anesthetic. As discussed earlier, the optimal concentration target pairs are a function of both pharmacodynamic and pharmacokinetic considerations.

Thinking about the clinical pharmacology of the modern general anesthetic in terms of response surfaces represents a new conceptual framework to guide the formulation of rational dosing strategies. The response surface is "navigated" in the sense that various points on the surface "map" are targeted at different times during the anesthetic to achieve the goals of the anesthetic (e.g., immobility, hemodynamic control, rapid emergence, good analgesia upon emergence, etc.). Rather than simply thinking about sedatives and opioids in isolation, the response-surface approach enables an in-depth, clinically relevant understanding of the tremendous synergy that results when sedatives and opioids are administered together.

Real-time visualization of response-surface models as a navigational tool

Although response-surface pharmacodynamic interaction models and traditional kinetic–dynamic models can be used to define optimal drug concentration targets and to predict the time course of drug concentration and effect for any conceivable dosage scheme, the mathematical complexity of these models has precluded their practical introduction into the operating room in real time. Thus, these models characterizing anesthetic drug behavior have primarily been used as a computer-simulation research tool to gain insight into how anesthetics can be rationally selected and administered.

Research is now being conducted to bring anesthetic pharmacology models to the operating room through automated acquisition of the drug administration scheme and real-time display of the predicted pharmacokinetics and pharmacodynamics [84,85]. Based on high-resolution pharmacokinetic-pharmacodynamic models, including a model of the synergistic pharmacodynamic interaction between sedatives (i.e., propofol and inhaled anesthetics) and opioids, this technology automatically acquires (from pumps and the anesthesia machine) the drug doses administered by the clinician and shows the drug dosing history (bolus doses, infusion rates, and expired concentrations), the predicted drug concentrations at the site of action (past, present, and future), and the predicted drug effects including sedation, analgesia, and neuromuscular blockade.

These "advisory" display systems potentially represent a significant advance compared to "passive" TCI systems, in that they include not only pharmacokinetic predictions regarding drug concentrations but also pharmacodynamic predictions regarding the likelihood of certain anesthetic effects. Response surfaces constitute the fundamental basis of these display systems; that is, the information these displays are conveying is based on response-surface, pharmacodynamic drug interaction models. Existing prototypes of these display systems actually depict three-dimensional or topographic views of response surfaces.

These display systems can perhaps best be understood as *clinical pharmacology information technology* (IT) at the point of care. In terms of the unmet need that such systems are intended to address, the basic notion is that a great deal of information regarding the behavior of anesthetic drugs exists in the form of pharmacokinetic, pharmacodynamic, and response-surface interaction models. The information

contained within these very numerous pharmacologic models is complex and is by definition mathematically oriented; much of it appears in scientific journals that are not intended for the clinician. The information initially appears in original research publications and then is interpreted and integrated into textbooks, monographs, and reviews. In total, this massive volume of mathematically based information is so large and intimidating that it is very difficult for the clinician to digest and incorporate the information into daily practice. These pharmacology display systems are meant to bring this sophisticated body of clinical pharmacology information from the scientific journals to the bedside by displaying the information in a readily understandable format in real time (i.e., clinical pharmacology IT). That clinicians cannot solve complex polyexponential equations in their heads "on the fly" to guide rational drug administration is a basic assumption of these advisory systems.

Figure 11.11 shows screen-shots of prototype displays systems currently in development. Although quite different in terms of how the information is portrayed, the two systems share in common the tabular and graphical display of predicted drug concentrations and predicted levels of drug effect, including a prediction of the synergism between hypnotics and opioids. The systems include prediction modules that allow the clinician to simulate various dosage regimens in real time and thereby rationally choose the optimal drug administration scheme to address the dynamic nature of anesthesia and surgery. For example, it is possible to simulate the decay of drug concentrations and the projected time to recovery if the drug administration were stopped five minutes into the future.

The ability to simulate various therapeutic decisions immediately before they are implemented, to explore the clinical consequences of a proposed change in therapy, is a key advance that these display systems may potentially bring to clinical care. The pharmacology display systems can be likened to the "heads-up" display systems frequently employed as a navigational aid to pilots in commercial and military aircraft. Applying the aviation analogy to anesthesia, the displays systems can potentially provide increased "situational awareness," "waypoints" to fly towards, and a smooth "glide-path" to landing.

Of course there are obvious challenges to be overcome before these display systems can be adopted into clinical practice. The utility of the systems in terms of improved clinical outcomes (e.g., faster recovery, improved analgesia on emergence, etc.) and/or user acceptance (e.g., decreased physician workload, etc.) must be satisfactorily demonstrated in clinical testing. Preliminary evidence suggests that the models displayed by these systems will perform reasonably well [87], but much work remains to be done. An additional barrier to implementation of these advisory systems is the typical clinicians' level of understanding regarding these complex models. Education and training will likely be necessary for the clinician to embrace the technology.

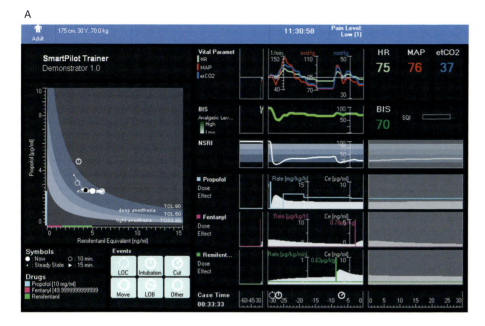

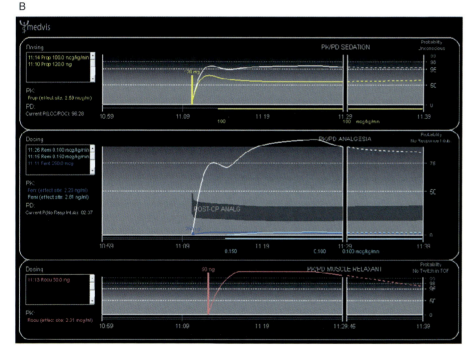

Figure 11.11. Screen-shots of two real-time clinical pharmacology advisory displays currently in development that utilize response-surface models and the concept of intelligently "navigating" the response surface. (A) The SmartPilot (Dräger, Lübeck, Germany). The two-dimensional topographic surface depicted on the left portion of the screen-shot shows the predicted effect-site concentrations of combined drugs (opioids/intravenous hypnotics or inhalation anesthetics) and the predicted anesthesia effect. Gray-shaded areas indicate different levels of anesthesia. The white point indicates the current combination of effect-site concentrations; the light gray line shows the past concentrations; the black point and arrow mark the 10- and 15-minute predictions into the future, respectively. The right portion of the screen includes simple pharmacokinetic simulations and other monitored variables. (B) The Medvis Display (Medvis, Salt Lake City, UT). The three sections of the screen depict sedation, analgesia, and neuromuscular blockade. The predicted drug effect for propofol, remifentanil, and rocuronium when administered alone are represented by the yellow, blue, and red lines, respectively. The additional drug effect resulting from synergy between propofol and remifentanil is indicated by the white lines. Drug effect is represented in terms of the probability of no response to "shake and shout" (sedation panel) and no response to laryngoscopy (analgesia panel). The drug administration history and the predicted effect-site concentrations for the individual drugs are also displayed. Adapted from Struys *et al.* [86]. Panel A was kindly provided by Peter M. Schumacher; Panel B was kindly provided by Noah Syroid.

Although it is too early to predict what role this clinical pharmacology display technology may play in future anesthesia practice, the concept is certainly an exciting area with promising potential to bring more sophisticated clinical pharmacology knowledge to the point of care. It is conceivable that in the future a real-time display of the predicted pharmacokinetics and pharmacodynamics of anesthetic drugs might be found alongside the traditional physiologic vital-sign monitors [86]. Of course the pharmacokinetic component of these systems has already been widely implemented in the form of "passive" TCI systems.

Summary

Anesthesiology is the deliberate and practical application of pharmacologic drug interactions. Anesthetic drug interactions take several forms: physicochemical, pharmacokinetic, and pharmacodynamic. Physicochemical interactions occur when the physical properties of the interacting drugs are incompatible; pharmacokinetic interactions occur when one drug alters the disposition of another drug; and pharmacodynamic interactions occur when one drug augments or reduces the effect of another drug. Beneficial drug interactions in anesthesia, often between an opioid and a hypnotic drug, aim to achieve faster recovery and diminish toxicity compared to when the individual drugs are used alone in higher doses.

Drug interactions can be represented graphically. An **isobole** shows the various combinations of doses of two drugs that result in the same degree of effect. **Additive** interactions occur when the combined effect of two drugs is equal to that expected by adding the effects of the individual drugs. Additivity often results when two drugs act by the same mechanism, and yields straight-line isoboles. **Synergistic** interactions occur when the combined effect of two drugs is greater than that expected by the sum of the effects of the individual drugs. Synergy often results when drugs act by a different mechanism, and yields a curved isobole which bows towards the origin of the graph. **Antagonism** occurs when the combined effect of two drugs is less than the sum of the effects when the drugs are given alone. Such isoboles bow away from the origin of the graph. Whereas an isobole only shows a single level of drug effect, a **response surface** depicts multiple levels of drug effect, and can be considered a family of isoboles. A response-surface graph relates a dependent variable (such as a drug effect) to inputs (such as two drug concentrations), and is used to find the region of drug effect where an optimal response occurs (i.e., where the response is at a maximum or a minimum), and the combination of drug doses which achieves that effect.

Opioid–general (volatile or sedative-hypnotic) anesthetic synergy is the pharmacologic basis of many modern anesthetic techniques because the hemodynamic depression associated with high concentrations of general anesthetics and the slow

return of spontaneous ventilation associated with high doses of opioid are both avoided. Total intravenous anesthesia with propofol and an opioid is a popular anesthetic technique internationally. Propofol–opioid interactions are characterized using the half-maximal effective concentration (EC_{50}) reduction study methodology with a clinical effect measure such as hemodynamic or movement response to surgical stimuli. Like minimum alveolar concentration (MAC) reduction studies, propofol–opioid interaction studies exhibit a general pattern irrespective of the opioid used. Opioids produce a marked reduction in the concentration of propofol required for hypnosis (and vice versa for analgesia). As the opioid concentration increases, the propofol requirement decreases asymptotically toward a non-zero minimum. The widespread availability of target-controlled infusion (TCI) technology for drugs such as propofol and intravenous opioids represents a sophisticated solution to accurately achieving specified drug concentration targets.

Perhaps the single most clinically important concept from pharmacodynamic drug interaction response surfaces is that for any given anesthetic effect there is an infinite number of sedative–opioid target concentrations pairs that will produce that same effect. Thus, a single isobolographic cut through the response surface defines a wide range of target drug concentration pairs for the sedative and the opioid that will produce the same anesthetic conditions. Choosing the best combination is a fundamental management question that must be addressed for each anesthetic, as the optimal concentration target pairs are a function of both pharmacodynamic and pharmacokinetic considerations.

References

1. Chambi D, Omoigui S. Precipitation of thiopental by some muscle relaxants. *Anesth Analg* 1995; **81**: 1112.

2. Wood M. Pharmacokinetic drug interactions in anaesthetic practice. *Clin Pharmacokinet* 1991; **21**: 285–307.

3. Alloul K, Whalley DG, Shutway F, Ebrahim Z, Varin F. Pharmacokinetic origin of carbamazepine-induced resistance to vecuronium neuromuscular blockade in anesthetized patients. *Anesthesiology* 1996; **84**: 330–9.

4. McEwan AI, Smith C, Dyar O, et al. Isoflurane minimum alveolar concentration reduction by fentanyl. *Anesthesiology* 1993; **78**: 864–9.

5. Hug CC. Does opioid "anesthesia" exist? *Anesthesiology* 1990; **73**: 1–4.

6. Wong KC. Narcotics are not expected to produce unconsciousness and amnesia. *Anesth Analg* 1983; **62**: 625–6.

7. Zbinden AM, Maggiorini M, Petersen-Felix S, et al. Anesthetic depth defined using multiple noxious stimuli during isoflurane/oxygen anesthesia. I. Motor reactions. *Anesthesiology* 1994; **80**: 253–60.

8. Zbinden AM, Petersen-Felix S, Thomson DA. Anesthetic depth defined using multiple noxious stimuli during isoflurane/oxygen anesthesia. II. Hemodynamic responses. *Anesthesiology* 1994; **80**: 261–7.

9. Kissin I. General anesthetic action: an obsolete notion? *Anesth Analg* 1993; **76**: 215–8.

10. Berenbaum MC. Criteria for analyzing interactions between biologically active agents. *Adv Cancer Res* 1981; **35**: 269–335.

11. Greco WR, Bravo G, Parsons JC. The search for synergy: a critical review from a response surface perspective. *Pharmacol Rev* 1995; **47**: 331–85.

12. Loewe S, Muischnek H. Effect of combinations: mathematical basis of problem. *Arch Exp Pathol Pharmokol* 1926; **114**: 313–26.

13. Bliss CI. The toxicity of poisons applied jointly. *Ann Appl Biol* 1939; **26**: 585–615.

14. Berenbaum MC. What is synergy? *Pharmacol Rev* 1989; **41**: 93–141.

15. Norberg L, Wahlstrom G. Anaesthetic effects of flurazepam alone and in combination with thiopental or hexobarbital evaluated with an EEG-threshold method in male rats. *Arch Int Pharmacodyn Ther* 1988; **292**: 45–57.

16. Minto CF, Schnider TW, Short TG, et al. Response surface model for anesthetic drug interactions. *Anesthesiology* 2000; **92**: 1603–16.

17. Carter WH, Wampler GL, Stablein DM. *Regression Analysis of Survival Data in Cancer Chemotherapy*. New York, NY: Marcel Dekker, 1983.

18. Kochar M, Guthrie R, Triscari J, Kassler-Taub K, Reeves RA. Matrix study of irbesartan with hydrochlorothiazide in mild-to-moderate hypertension. *Am J Hypertens* 1999; **12**: 797–805.

19. Scholze J, Zilles P, Compagnone D. Verapamil SR and trandolapril combination therapy in hypertension: a clinical trial of factorial design. German Hypertension Study Group. *Br J Clin Pharmacol* 1998; **45**: 491–5.

20. Pool JL, Cushman WC, Saini RK, Nwachuku CE, Battikha JP. Use of the factorial design and quadratic response surface models to evaluate the fosinopril and hydrochlorothiazide combination therapy in hypertension. *Am J Hypertens* 1997; **10**: 117–23.

21. Short TG, Plummer JL, Chui PT. Hypnotic and anaesthetic interactions between midazolam, propofol and alfentanil. *Br J Anaesth* 1992; **69**: 162–7.

22. Neter J, Wasserman W, Kutner MH. *Applied Linear Statistical Models*, 3rd edn. Homewood, IL: Irwin, 1990.

23. Box GEP, Draper NR. *Empirical Model-Building and Response surfaces*. New York, NY: Wiley, 1987.

24. Sebel PS, Glass PS, Fletcher JE, *et al.* Reduction of the MAC of desflurane with fentanyl. *Anesthesiology* 1992; **76**: 52–9.

25. Vuyk J, Engbers FH, Burm AG, *et al.* Pharmacodynamic interaction between propofol and alfentanil when given for induction of anesthesia. *Anesthesiology* 1996; **84**: 288–99.

26. Lang E, Kapila A, Shlugman D, *et al.* Reduction of isoflurane minimal alveolar concentration by remifentanil. *Anesthesiology* 1996; **85**: 721–8.

27. Greco WR, Park HS, Rustum YM. Application of a new approach for the quantitation of drug synergism to the combination of cis-diamminedichloroplatinum and 1-beta-D-arabinofuranosylcytosine. *Cancer Res* 1990; **50**: 5318–27.

28. Berenbaum MC. Consequences of synergy between environmental carcinogens. *Environ Res* 1985; **38**: 310–18.

29. Machado SG, Robinson GA. A direct, general approach based on isobolograms for assessing the joint action of drugs in pre-clinical experiments. *Stat Med* 1994; **13**: 2289–309.

30. Troconiz IF, Sheiner LB, Verotta D. Semiparametric models for antagonistic drug interactions. *J Appl Physiol* 1994; **76**: 2224–33.

31. Fidler M, Kern SE. Flexible interaction model for complex interactions of multiple anesthetics. *Anesthesiology* 2006; **105**: 286–96.

32. Kaminoh Y, Kamaya H, Tashiro C, Ueda I. Multi-Unit and Multi-Path system of the neural network can explain the steep dose-response of MAC. *J Anesth* 2004; **18**: 94–9.

33. Eger EI, Saidman LJ, Brandstater B. Minimum alveolar anesthetic concentration: a standard of anesthetic potency. *Anesthesiology* 1965; **26**: 756–63.

34. Rampil IJ, Lockhart SH, Zwass MS, *et al.* Clinical characteristics of desflurane in surgical patients: minimum alveolar concentration. *Anesthesiology* 1991; **74**: 429–33.

35. Stevens WD, Dolan WM, Gibbons RT, *et al.* Minimum alveolar concentrations (MAC) of isoflurande with and without nitrous oxide in patients of various ages. *Anesthesiology* 1975; **42**: 197–200.

36. Stoelting RK, Longnecker DE, Eger EI. Minimum alveolar concentrations in man on awakening from methoxyflurane, halothane, ether and fluroxene anesthesia: MAC awake. *Anesthesiology* 1970; **33**: 5–9.

37. Egan TD. Intravenous drug delivery systems: toward an intravenous "vaporizer". *J Clin Anesth* 1996; **8** (3 Suppl): 8S–14S.

38. Westmoreland CL, Sebel PS, Gropper A. Fentanyl or alfentanil decreases the minimum alveolar anesthetic concentration of isoflurane in surgical patients. *Anesth Analg* 1994; **78**: 23–8.

39. Murphy MR, Hug CC. The anesthetic potency of fentanyl in terms of its reduction of enflurane MAC. *Anesthesiology* 1982; **57**: 485–8.

40. Hall RI, Murphy MR, Hug CC. The enflurane sparing effect of sufentanil in dogs. *Anesthesiology* 1987; **67**: 518–25.

41. Hall RI, Szlam F, Hug CC. The enflurane-sparing effect of alfentanil in dogs. *Anesth Analg* 1987; **66**: 1287–91.

42. Shafer SL. Principles of pharmacokinetics and pharmacodynamics. In: Longnecker DE, Tinker JH, Morgan EG, eds. *Principles and Practice of Anesthesiology*, 2nd edn. St. Louis, MO: Mosby-Year Book, 1998: 1159–210.

43. Philbin DM, Rosow CE, Schneider RC, Koski G, D'Ambra MN. Fentanyl and sufentanil anesthesia revisited: how much is enough? *Anesthesiology* 1990; **73**: 5–11.

44. Stanski DR, Shafer SL. Quantifying anesthetic drug interaction: implications for drug dosing. *Anesthesiology* 1995; **83**: 1–5.

45. Roizen MF, Saidman LJ. Redefining anesthetic management. Goals for the anesthesiologist. *Anesthesiology* 1994; **80**: 251–2.

46. Hendrickx JF, Eger EI, Sonner JM, Shafer SL. Is synergy the rule? A review of anesthetic interactions producing hypnosis and immobility. *Anesth Analg* 2008; **107**: 494–506.

47. Harris RS, Lazar O, Johansen JW, Sebel PS. Interaction of propofol and sevoflurane on loss of consciousness and movement to skin incision during general anesthesia. *Anesthesiology* 2006; **104**: 1170–5.

48. Sebel LE, Richardson JE, Singh SP, Bell SV, Jenkins A. Additive effects of sevoflurane and propofol on gamma-aminobutyric acid receptor function. *Anesthesiology* 2006; **104**: 1176–83.

49. Egan TD. Target-controlled drug delivery: progress toward an intravenous "vaporizer" and automated anesthetic administration. *Anesthesiology* 2003; **99**: 1214–19.

50. Shafer SL, Varvel JR, Aziz N, Scott JC. Pharmacokinetics of fentanyl administered by computer-controlled infusion pump. *Anesthesiology* 1990; **73**: 1091–102.

51. Glass PS, Jacobs JR, Smith LR, *et al.* Pharmacokinetic model-driven infusion of fentanyl: assessment of accuracy. *Anesthesiology* 1990; **73**: 1082–90.

52. Shafer SL, Varvel JR. Pharmacokinetics, pharmacodynamics, and rational opioid

26. Juniper EF, Guyatt GH, Ferri PJ, *et al.* Measuring quality of life in asthma. *Am Rev Respir Dis* 1993; **147**: 832–38.

27. Ware JE, Sherbourne JD. The MOS 36-Item Short-Form Health Survey (SF-36): I. Conceptual framework and item selection. *Med Care* 1992; **30**: 473–83.

28. The EuroQol Group. EuroQol: a new facility for the measurement of health-related quality of life. *Health Policy* 1990; **16**: 199–208.

29. Torrance GW, Feeny DH, Furlong WJ, *et al.* Multiattribute utility function for a comprehensive health status classification: Health Utilities Index 2. *Med Care* 1996; **34**: 702–22.

30. Sintonen H. The 15D instrument of health-related quality of life: properties and applications. *Ann Med* 2001; **33**: 328–36.

31. Myles PS, Weitkamp B, Jones K, Melick J, Hensen S. Validity and reliability of a postoperative quality of recovery score: the QoR-40. *Br J Anaesth* 2000; **84**: 11–15.

32. Froberg DG, Kane RL. Methodology for measuring health-state preferences. II. Scaling methods. *J Clin Epidemiol* 1989; **5**: 459–71.

33. Torrance GW. Social preferences for health states: an empirical evaluation of three measurement techniques. *Socioecon Plann Sci* 1976; **10**: 129–36.

34. Tengs TO, Wallace A. One thousand health-related quality-of-life estimates. *Med Care* 2000; **38**: 583–637.

35. Rosser R, Kind P. A scale of valuations of states of illness: is there a social consensus? *Int J Epidemiol* 1978; 7: 347–58.

36. Kaplan RM, Anderson JP. The general health policy model: update and applications. *Health Serv Res* 1988; **23**: 203–35.

37. Brauer CA, Rosen AB, Greenberg D, Neumann PJ. Trends in the measurement of health utilities in published cost-utility analyses. *Value Health* 2006; **9**: 213–18.

38. Macario A, McCoy M. The pharmacy cost of delivering postoperative analgesia to patients undergoing joint replacement surgery. *J Pain* 2003; **4**: 22–8.

39. Macario A. Systematic literature review of the economics of intravenous patient-controlled analgesia. *Pharm Ther* 2005; **30**: 392–9.

40. Dexter F, Gan TJ, Naguib M, Lubarsky DA. Cost identification analysis for succinylcholine. *Anesth Analg* 2001; **92**: 693–9.

41. O'Brien B, Briggs A. Analysis of uncertainty in health care cost-effectiveness studies: an introduction to statistical issues and methods. *Stat Methods Med Res* 2002; **11**: 455–68.

42. Stinett AA, Mullahy J. Net health benefits: a new framework for the analysis of uncertainty in cost-effectiveness analysis. *Med Decis Making* 1998; **18**: S68–80.

43. Macario A, Dexter F, Lubarsky D. Meta-analysis of trials comparing postoperative recovery after anesthesia

with sevoflurane or desflurane. *Am J Health Syst Pharm* 2005; **62**: 63–8.

44. Dexter F, Macario A, Manberg PJ, Lubarsky DA. Computer simulation to determine how rapid anesthetic recovery protocols to decrease the time for emergence or increase the phase I postanesthesia care unit bypass rate affect staffing of an ambulatory surgery center. *Anesth Analg* 1999; **88**: 1053–63.

45. Macario A, Weinger M, Truong P, Lee M. Which clinical anesthesia outcomes are both common and important to avoid? The perspective of a panel of expert anesthesiologists. *Anesth Analg* 1999; **88**: 1085–91.

46. Macario A, Weinger M, Carney S, Kim A. Which clinical anesthesia outcomes are important to avoid? The perspective of patients. *Anesth Analg* 1999; **89**: 652–8.

47. Macario A, Vasanawala A. Improving quality of anesthesia care: opportunities for the new decade. *Can J Anesth* 2001; **48**: 6–11.

48. Stahl JE. Modelling methods for pharmacoeconomics and health technology assessment: an overview and guide. *Pharmacoeconomics* 2008; **26**: 131–48.

49. Wilensky GR. Developing a center for comparative effectiveness information. *Health Aff (Millwood)* 2006; **25**: w572–w585.

50. Bell CM, Urbach DR, Ray JG, *et al.* Bias in published cost effectiveness studies: systematic review. *BMJ* 2006; **332**: 699–703.

Physiologic substrates of drug action

Sleep and consciousness

George A. Mashour and Max Kelz

Introduction

Identifying the neural basis of consciousness continues to be a fundamental scientific, and philosophical, problem. Philosophers struggle with the possibility of explaining our *subjective* experience with the traditionally *objective* tools and descriptions of science [1]. Neuroscientists, however, believe that consciousness can be explained by conventional neurobiology, with a focus on the "neural correlates." The current challenge is determining the precise identity and function of these correlates, which the study of sleep and general anesthesia may help to elucidate.

Consciousness itself entails both **awareness** and **wakefulness**. Awareness denotes what we experience – the phenomenal contents of perception or what philosophers call *qualia* (e.g., the redness of a rose). Wakefulness denotes arousal or a certain requisite activity level of brain function. A persistent vegetative state is one example in which the two are dissociated: wakefulness is present in the absence of awareness (Fig. 13.1). The neural mechanisms for the phenomenal or experiential component of consciousness are thought to be primarily cortical, and may best be explored by considering anesthetic mechanism and depth. The neural mechanisms for regulating wakefulness are found primarily in subcortical structures, and are best explored through the discussion of normal sleep-cycle control. Although admittedly a simplistic framework, there are thus both "top-down" and "bottom-up" pathways to interrupt conscious processes, as occurs during general anesthesia or sleep.

Brain and cellular physiology

In the following sections we will first discuss awareness, with an emphasis on the thalamocortical system. It is important to note that "awareness" in this cognitive context denotes *only* the subjective experience of phenomena, rather than a memory of that experience. Thus it is distinct from the clinical use of the word "awareness" during general anesthesia, which includes explicit recall and which will also be discussed. Henceforth we will denote the clinical phenomenon as "awareness during general anesthesia" or "intraoperative awareness." After this

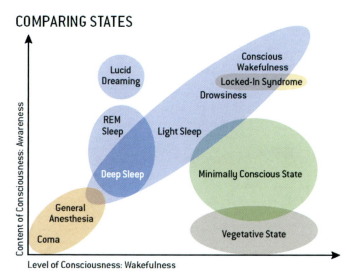

COMPARING STATES

Figure 13.1. This schematic highlights the dissociable properties of consciousness. States such as coma and general anesthesia are associated with an interruption of both wakefulness and awareness, while persistent vegetative states are associated with preserved wakefulness in the absence of awareness. Note that while the two properties of consciousness are dissociable, they are not *doubly* dissociable: it is impossible to have awareness without wakefulness, which is why there are no states of consciousness depicted at the top and far-left portion of the graph. Reproduced with permission from Laureys [2].

"top-down" discussion we will shift our focus from the cortex to the subcortical nuclei where wakefulness and sleep are regulated (a "bottom-up" approach).

Awareness

Awareness in the cognitive context

Sleep and general anesthesia share a number of common *traits* that include hypnosis (loss of consciousness), amnesia, analgesia, and even immobility [3,4]. Despite this fact and the ubiquitous clinical metaphor in anesthesiology (e.g., "You are going to sleep now, Mr. Smith" or "Time to wake up, Mrs. Jones"), general anesthesia is not the same *state* as sleep. Urethane is the only general anesthetic that has been suggested to mimic sleep in terms of EEG alternations of

Anesthetic Pharmacology, 2nd edition, ed. Alex S. Evers, Mervyn Maze, Evan D. Kharasch. Published by Cambridge University Press. © Cambridge University Press 2011.

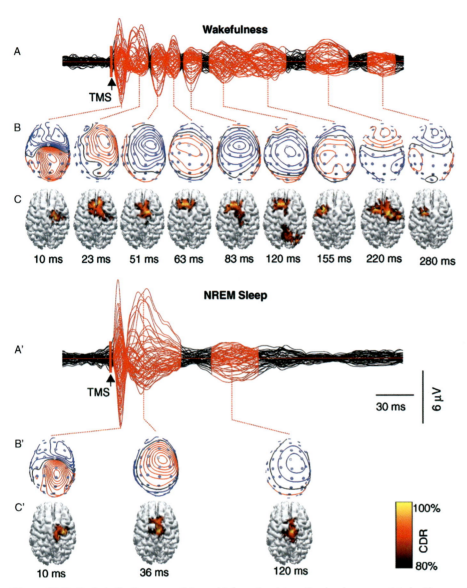

Figure 13.2. Cortical effective connectivity and information integration has been associated with normal consciousness. Accordingly, the interruption of this connectivity has been associated with general anesthesia, NREM sleep, and persistent vegetative states. This figure demonstrates how NREM sleep is associated with a diminished cortical response to a transcranial magnetic stimulus (TMS). A and A′ are averaged TMS-evoked potentials. B and B′ are contour voltage maps (red, positive; blue, negative). C and C′ show current density distribution on the cortical surface. Reproduced with permission from Massimini *et al.* [7].

"NREM"- and "REM"-like activity, as well as cholinergic and monoaminergic neuropharmacology [5]. Urethane, however, is carcinogenic and is therefore used only in nonrecovery animal experiments [6].

The common trait of unconsciousness during sleep and general anesthesia has led to the exploration of these processes for a better understanding of consciousness. There are several lines of evidence suggesting common mechanisms of sleep- and anesthetic-mediated unconsciousness. For example, it has been demonstrated that non-rapid eye movement (NREM) sleep is characterized by a loss of effective cortical connectivity, i.e., the ability of different brain structures to influence one another causally. Stimulation directed to an area of cortex (in this case, transcranial magnetic stimulation) in the awake subject

ramifies throughout the cortical mantle; during NREM sleep, however, the signal is limited and localized to the area of stimulation [7] (Fig. 13.2). Interestingly, rapid eye movement (REM) sleep is characterized by a partial return of connectivity [8]. Loss of consciousness during general anesthesia may also be associated with the interruption of such connectivity, particularly in the thalamocortical system [9,10]. Loss of consciousness due to a variety of anesthetics is associated with a dissociation of high-frequency electroencephalogram (EEG) activity throughout the cortex that is normally coordinated during consciousness [11,12]. Conversely, emergence from anesthesia is associated with a return of this integration. Thus, interrupting corticocortical and thalamocortical systems may be a common finding associated with unconsciousness during both general anesthesia and sleep. That such an interruption may be associated with unconsciousness is also supported by findings in persistent vegetative states. Loss of effective connectivity in the thalamocortical system has been identified during persistent vegetative states, while spontaneous recovery is associated with a return of such connectivity [13]. Why might the thalamocortical system be crucial for consciousness? It is thought that this system has a higher capacity to integrate information from functionally distinct cognitive modules, and that such integration is essential for the conscious representation of a multi-modal sensory experience [14,15].

Although sleep- and anesthetic-induced unconsciousness may both be associated with a lack of cortical integration, this does not necessitate that the actual *transition* to unconsciousness is mediated by the same process. The loss of consciousness at the onset of sleep is initiated by the subcortical structures regulating the sleep/wake cycle (described below). Thus, the critical process in sleep-induced unconsciousness is likely the loss of *wakefulness*. On the other hand, data from neurophysiologic recordings suggest that diminished cortical – rather than subcortical – activity is associated with the loss of consciousness induced by general anesthesia [16]. Other studies using the neurophysiologic technique of the 40 Hz auditory steady-state response concluded that there was a comparable effect of propofol on both cortical and subcortical generators of the response [17]. Further research is required to establish if anesthetic-induced unconsciousness initially results from the loss of awareness or the loss of wakefulness.

Awareness in the clinical context

We now turn to the clinical problem of awareness during general anesthesia and the assessment of anesthetic depth, both of which have been argued to play a central role in the neuroscience and philosophy of consciousness [18]. Intraoperative awareness with subsequent recall has been found to occur in approximately 1–2/1000 cases in American and European studies [19,20]. Other studies have suggested incidences that were much higher [21] and much lower [22], with prospective studies likely more reliable [23]. Victims of awareness during general anesthesia may go on to develop long-term psychological sequelae, most notably post-traumatic stress disorder (for review, see Lennmarken and Sydsjo [24]). Since subtherapeutic doses of anesthesia are associated with awareness during general anesthesia – and supratherapeutic doses have controversially been suggested to increase mortality [25] – a method of accurately assessing anesthetic depth is important.

EEG recordings were first shown to be sensitive to the effects of general anesthetics in 1937 [26]. There is no invariant "signature" common to all general anesthetics that can be detected by an unprocessed EEG [27]. As such, processed EEG monitors have been developed to aid the clinician in the evaluation of anesthetic depth. Such processing typically involves Fourier transformation, which translates a raw EEG

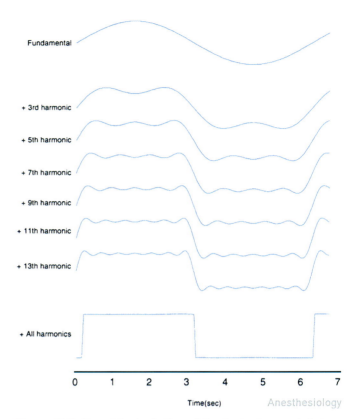

Figure 13.3. One of the implications of the Fourier theorem is that any complex waveform can be composed of, or deconstructed to, a series of simple harmonic waves. This figure demonstrates how the summation of multiple sine waves results in a square wave. The application of this theorem to EEG analysis is Fourier transformation, which is the conversion of a time domain to a frequency domain. By deconstructing the complex waveform of an EEG into its component waves, the contributions of different frequencies associated with different states of consciousness can be ascertained and interpreted. Reproduced with permission from Rampil [28].

tracing (voltage changes over time) into a frequency domain [28] (Fig. 13.3). This allows for the analysis of the contribution of each frequency to the overall EEG, which provides a "spectrum." Furthermore, waveforms of frequencies can be evaluated for their relationship to one another, which provides a "bispectrum." In addition to spectral and bispectral analysis, the presence and ratio of burst suppression is often quantified. A burst pattern, followed by quiescent EEG, is characteristic of deeper levels of anesthesia [27,29–31].

Some of the more commonly used "awareness monitors" include the Bispectral Index (BIS: Aspect Medical Systems, Norwood, MA, USA), Entropy (Datex-Ohmeda/GE Healthcare, Madison, WI, USA), Narcotrend (MonitorTechnik, Bad Bramstedt, Germany), Cerebral State Monitor/Index (Danmeter, Odense, Denmark), SEDline (Hospira, Lake Forest, IL, USA), SNAP II (Stryker, Kalamazoo, MI, USA), and the A-Line AEP (Danmeter, Odense, Denmark) monitors. We will briefly state the principles of each below [27,29–31].

- **BIS** – The BIS analyzes β power, bispectral coherence, and burst suppression. The output is a dimensionless number between 0 (isoelectric) and 100 (awake). The range for general anesthesia is considered to be 40–60. It is of interest to note that the BIS is also sensitive to natural sleep.

- **Entropy** – As anesthetic depth increases, the variability or entropy of neural function decreases. The device is based on Shannon entropy and incorporates frequency ranges of both EEG (state entropy) and EEG/EMG (response entropy).
- **Narcotrend** – This device analyzes stages and substages of anesthesia, a concept based on the EEG changes seen in sleep. The Narcotrend was based on a similar developmental process as the BIS, with a distinct algorithm.
- **Cerebral State** – This monitor calculates the α ratio and β ratio, then uses the difference between them to indicate a shift from higher to lower frequencies. Burst suppression is also analyzed.
- **SEDline** – The SEDline evolved from the Patient State Analyzer and is based on the rostrocaudal and interhemispheric loss of coherence that occurs in the anesthetized state.
- **SNAP II** – This device employs spectral analysis of low- and high-frequency components of the EEG.
- **A-Line AEP** – While the aforementioned monitors record spontaneous EEG, the stimulus–response technique of auditory-evoked potentials has also been used to assess anesthetic depth. This monitor analyzes evoked potentials in conjunction with other EEG signaling parameters.

There are numerous limitations associated with awareness monitoring. Since the BIS monitor has had the most extensive study, there is also a better understanding of its limitations [32]. For example, the BIS monitor – and EEG in general – can be activated with nitrous oxide [33,34] or ketamine [35,36], resulting in the potential for a "false positive" finding of insufficient depth. Conversely, BIS values are sensitive to nonanesthetic drugs and have been shown to decrease in patients receiving neuromuscular blockers [37,38]. This may result in the potential for a "false negative" finding of sufficient anesthetic depth. The EEG is also sensitive to physiologic changes such as hyperglycemia and hypothermia, as well as pathologic changes such as cerebral ischemia. Finally, it can be affected by electrical artifact such as cautery or warming devices.

The BIS monitor is the only device that has been studied for the prevention of intraoperative awareness. Ekman et al. showed that the use of the BIS was associated with a 0.04% incidence in awareness, compared to an incidence of 0.18% in a historical control without the BIS [39]. This represented a significant fivefold reduction in the incidence of awareness. Myles et al. conducted a prospective trial of patients at high risk for awareness (cardiac, obstetric, trauma, etc.) and found that the BIS group had significantly fewer definite awareness events (two incidents) compared to routine anesthetic care (eleven incidents) [40]. More recent data from Avidan et al. demonstrate that the BIS monitor was no more

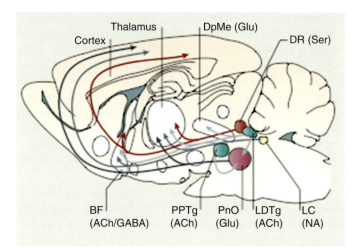

Figure 13.4. The neural substrates of wakefulness: brainstem. This sagittal cartoon illustrates that projections from the brainstem through the hypothalamus or thalamus into the cortex and forebrain form the two branches of the ascending arousal system. Cholinergic neurons in the pedunculopontine tegmentum (PPTg) and the laterodorsal tegmentum (LDTg) display dense innervation of the nonspecific intralaminar and midline nuclei and the thalamic reticular nucleus. In addition to this thalamic pathway, brainstem cholinergic neurons also project to other arousal nuclei including the deep mesencephalic reticular formation (DpMe), the pontine reticular nucleus oralis (PnO), regions of the prefrontal cortex, and magnocellular cholinergic nuclei of the basal forebrain (BF). Joining the cholinergic arousal-promoting signals are noradrenergic projections emanating from the pontine locus coeruleus (LC). LC efferent projections cause excitation through α_1- and β_1- adrenoceptors, and support arousal via an inhibitory α_2-adrenergic-receptor-mediated action upon sleep-active neurons of the basal forebrain. Midbrain serotonergic raphe nuclei (DR) send a large projection to the cortex, basal forebrain, and other arousal nuclei. Along with the LC, the DR also activates important midline and intralaminar nuclei in the thalamus. Adapted with permission from Franks [42].

successful in preventing awareness than a minimum alveolar concentration (MAC)-based protocol [41]. These data suggest that it could be the anesthetic protocol, rather than the modality itself, that is associated with a reduced incidence of awareness. Further work is required.

Wakefulness

It has been known for more than 40 years that the ascending reticular activating system in the brainstem releases excitatory neurotransmitters into the thalamus, which projects widely through cerebral cortex to promote wakefulness. Only recently has it been revealed that brainstem reticular neurons project onto the hypothalamic nuclei, which promote wakefulness by similarly releasing excitatory neurotransmitters throughout the cortex and are of key importance in regulating sleep/wake states.

The arousal-promoting circuitry of the brain is known as the ascending reticular activating system, and it consists of two branches of projections from the caudal midbrain and rostral pons area to the thalamus and hypothalamus (Fig. 13.4). The thalamic branch originates from the cholinergic pedunculopontine and laterodorsal tegmental nuclei (PPTg and LDTg

Table 13.1. EEG, EMG, and EOG characteristics of wakefulness, NREM, and REM sleep states

Sleep state	EEG	EMG	EOG
Wakefulness	Desynchronized activation (10–30 mV low voltage, 16–25 Hz fast activity) alternates with α activity (sinusoidal, 20–40 mV voltage, 8–12 Hz activity)	High or moderate, depending on degree of muscle tension	REMs abundant or scarce, depending on amount of visual scanning
NREM stage 1	Decreased α activity, little activation, mostly low-voltage, mixed-frequency activity (at 3–7 Hz)	Moderate to low	REMs absent, slow rolling eye movements
NREM stage 2	Background of low-voltage, mixed-frequency activity, bursts of distinctive 12–14 Hz sinusoidal waves ("sleep spindles") appear	Moderate to low	Eye movements rare
NREM stage 3 (SWS)	High-amplitude (> 75 mV), slow-frequency (0.5–2 Hz) δ waves appear	Moderate to low	Eye movements rare
NREM stage 4 (SWS)	Delta waves dominate the EEG trace	Moderate to low	Eye movements rare
REM	Reverts to a low-voltage, mixed-frequency pattern similar to stage 1	Small muscle twitches against virtually silent background	Bursts of prominent REMs appear

EEG, electroencephalogram; EMG, electromyogram; EOG, electro-oculogram; NREM, non-rapid eye movement; REM, rapid eye movement; SWS, slow-wave sleep.

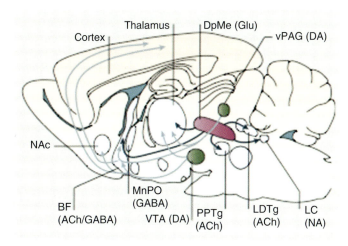

Figure 13.5. The neural substrates of wakefulness: midbrain. Glutamatergic deep mesencephalic reticular formation (DpMe) nuclei and the dopaminergic nuclei in both the ventral periaqueductal gray (vPAG) and ventral tegmental area (VTA) are the most important midbrain structures. Efferent projections from the DpMe excite thalamocortical neurons in the midline and intralaminar nuclei of the thalamus and also innervate the BF. Projections to the cholinergic PPTg and LDTg, the noradrenergic LC, and the medullary/pontine reticular formations serve to reinforce arousal-promoting excitation. vPAG neurons are wake-active, similar to other monoaminergic neurons in the LC and DR. Together with the VTA, vPAG promotes arousal by activating midline and intralaminar thalamic nuclei. Adapted with permission from Franks [42].

[43]) and projects through the paramedian midbrain reticular formation and diencephalon to the thalamus, including the intralaminar nuclei [44], thalamic relay nuclei, and the reticular nucleus. Cholinergic modulation, which is known to be crucial in activating thalamocortical neurotransmission [45], has a key role in regulating thalamic activity. The PPTg and LDTg neurons fire rapidly during both (1) wakefulness, when a low-voltage, fast cortical EEG activity is observed and (2) REM sleep, when REM and a loss of tonic muscle tone accompany a similar EEG to wakefulness. PPTg and LDTg neurons slow their activity during NREM sleep (Table 13.1).

Additionally, cortically projecting cholinergic neurons in the basal forebrain also display preferential increased firing during wakefulness (and REM sleep, but not NREM sleep), imparting a fast desynchronized EEG pattern in conjunction with brainstem ascending reticular activating inputs [46]. However, lesion and direct electrical stimulation studies suggest that unidentified, noncholinergic basal forebrain neurons may also play a role in the promotion of wakefulness [47,48].

The hypothalamic branch of the ascending arousal system originates in the caudal midbrain (Figs. 13.5, 13.6) and rostral pons and includes projections from the noradrenergic locus coeruleus (LC), serotonergic dorsal and median raphe nuclei, dopaminergic ventral periaqueductal gray (vPAG), and parabrachial nucleus and projects through the lateral hypothalamus. There it is joined by histaminergic projections from the tuberomammillary nucleus (TMN), orexin- (or hypocretin-) and melanin-concentrating, hormone-containing projections from the lateral hypothalamus, as well as cholinergic projections from the basal forebrain cholinergic nuclei. All of these pathways diffusely innervate the cortex and release neurotransmitters associated with arousal. In contrast to cholinergic arousal pathways (see earlier in this section), neurons in the monoaminergic cell groups in these pathways (i.e., from the LC, raphe nuclei, vPAG, and TMN) fire rapidly during wakefulness, very infrequently during NREM, and virtually not at all during REM sleep [49–51]. These differences in firing rates across sleep and wake states of consciousness in the

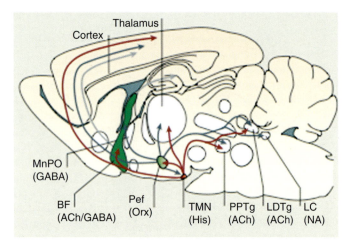

Figure 13.6. The neural substrates of wakefulness: hypothalamus and basal forebrain. Orexinergic neurons (Orx) are restricted to the dorsomedial, perifornical, and lateral hypothalamus but arborize widely throughout the entire neuraxis where they excite other arousal nuclei, thalamocortical and midline thalamic nuclei, and the cortex. A similar pattern of arousal-promoting efferent projections arises from the histaminergic neurons of the tuberomammillary nucleus (TMN) and travels through a ventral pathway to innervate BF and cortex as well as a dorsal pathway to excite the thalamus. Neurons in the BF provide a complex pattern of innervation to the limbic system and cortex. In addition to the predominantly cortical innervation of BF cholinergic neurons, these cells also target select areas of the thalamus. They provide a mainly excitatory drive through nicotinic acetylcholine receptors and muscarinic M_1 receptors. Adapted with permission from Franks [42].

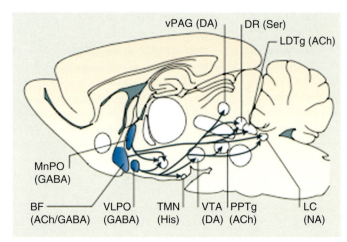

Figure 13.7. The neural substrates of sleep. The major sleep-promoting nuclei reside in the anterior hypothalamus and adjacent basal forebrain. The ventrolateral preoptic nucleus (VLPO) densely innervates and inhibits all major arousal-promoting centers via GABA and galanin. The median preoptic nucleus (MnPO) also inhibits arousal promoting nuclei such as the LC, DR, and Orx neurons, yet MnPO neurons activate the VLPO to reinforce and stabilize the sleep state. GABAergic neurons from the BF (perhaps those that are sleep-active) also provide inhibitory input to the orexinergic neurons and to the midbrain and brainstem. Adapted with permission from Franks [42].

cholinergic and monoaminergic ascending arousal systems, together with modulation by selective glutamatergic and GABAergic systems [52] (see below), are believed to modulate the generation of these different behavioral states [53].

Non-rapid eye movement (NREM) sleep

Lesion, chemical, and electrical stimulation studies have led to the recognition that sleep is an actively generated state, involving anatomically discrete supraspinal pathways in the hypothalamus and brainstem. A sleep-promoting role for the rostral hypothalamus has been recognized for 80 years [54]. Recent investigations have consistently uncovered a NREM "sleep-promoting" [55] function for neurons in preoptic anterior hypothalamus and the adjacent basal forebrain, specifically in the ventrolateral preoptic nucleus (VLPO) and median preoptic nucleus (MnPO). VLPO neurons are under inhibitory control by norepinephrine and serotonin [56,57] and discharge maximally during sleep while remaining relatively inactive during wakefulness. VLPO neurons, which form a dense cluster just lateral to the optic chiasm (the VLPO cluster, important for NREM sleep) and a diffuse population of cells extending medially and dorsally from this cluster (the extended VLPO, more important for REM sleep [58]), are defined by

three characteristics: they (1) are uniquely sleep-active (show c-Fos expression during sleep) [55]; (2) contain the colocalized (80%) inhibitory neurotransmitters γ-aminobutyric acid (GABA) and galanin across species, whereas surrounding neurons contain GABA only [59,60]; and (3) project to the arousal-promoting [61] TMN [59]. VLPO neurons also extend inhibitory projections to all of the other wake-active ascending monoaminergic, cholinergic, and orexinergic arousal-promoting sites in the brain: the noradrenergic LC, serotonergic dorsal raphe (DR), cholinergic PPTg and LDTg, and the orexinergic perifornical area (PeF) in the lateral hypothalamic area [59]; these VLPO neuronal projections inhibit their release of arousal-promoting neurotransmitters into the cortex, forebrain, and subcortical areas (Fig. 13.7).

A decrease in firing of the noradrenergic neurons in the LC of the pons releases the LC's tonic inhibition of GABAergic VLPO neurons, which are then activated and release GABA and galanin into LC, TMN, and other arousal-promoting centers [59]. At the level of the LC, this has an inhibitory effect, further decreasing firing in the LC, and therefore further decreasing norepinephrine's tonic inhibition of the VLPO neurons. At the level of the TMN, descending projections from the VLPO release GABA and galanin [59]. Inhibition of the TMN by the VLPO is believed to play a key role in causing sleep.

The inhibition of the TMN (as well as the LC, vPAG, dorsal raphe, perifornical area, and LDTg/PPTg) by GABA and galanin disinhibits VLPO neurons [62], and is believed to play a key role in causing NREM sleep. Galanin and GABA are observed in the TMN, and GABA type A (GABA$_A$) inhibitory postsynaptic potentials in the TMN region are observed when the VLPO is stimulated [63]. Discrete bilateral lesions induced by microinjection of the nonspecific excitotoxin ibotenic acid into the VLPO induce persistent insomnia in rats [64]. This may be explained by the hypothesis that GABA-mediated anesthetic drugs act by inhibiting the wake-active (c-Fos-immunoreactive during wakefulness) TMN. Discrete injections of the GABA$_A$ receptor agonist muscimol cause sedation, and at higher doses hypnosis, and potentiate the hypnotic effects of anesthetic drugs; direct injections of anesthetic drugs induce sedation, and of GABA$_A$ receptor antagonist gabazine attenuate the hypnotic effect of anesthetics [65].

Other pathways are also involved in the generation of NREM sleep. Recently, a sleep-promoting role for MnPO neurons has been recognized [66]. MnPO neurons are also sleep-active and send dense projections to the VLPO, which excite sleep-promoting VLPO neurons [56]. Moreover, most MnPO neurons appear to be GABAergic and are directly able to inhibit arousal-promoting nuclei to reinforce and stabilize sleep states [67,68]. Throughout the preoptic area that includes both VLPO and MnPO, sleep-active neurons are clustered, but still represent a minority of all cell types. Additional populations of diffusely organized neurons that display preferential activity during NREM sleep have been recognized in the magnocellular basal forebrain, where lesions that include the horizontal diagonal band may produce insomnia [69] (Fig. 13.7).

Rapid eye movement (REM) sleep

The neuronal pathways mediating REM sleep are also currently being characterized; much of what is known stems from three types of animal experiments (for review see Siegel [70]). First, transection studies have determined that the pons is sufficient to generate much of the phenomenology of REM sleep. These experiments demonstrated that when the midbrain is transected to separate the brainstem from the diencephalon and telencephalon such that the pons is connected only to midbrain and forebrain structures (and transected from the medulla and spinal cord), defining signs of REM sleep (atonia, REMs, REM-like activation of the reticular formation) are seen in rostral structures. Similarly, when the pons is connected to the medulla and spinal cord only, signs of REM sleep are observed in caudal structures and desynchronized EEG closely resembles that of wakefulness observed in rostral structures. In addition, when the junction between spinal cord and medulla is transected, rostral brain areas (medulla, pons, midbrain) show signs of REM sleep. Considered together, these findings lead to the conclusion that the pons and caudal midbrain are both necessary and sufficient to generate the basic phenomena of REM sleep.

Second, the discrete destruction of very small loci of the brainstem in an otherwise healthy brain can permanently prevent REM sleep. Discrete neuronal lesioning studies have identified a small area of the lateral pontine tegmentum corresponding to lateral portions of the pontine reticular nucleus oralis (PnO), which projects to the PPTg, and the region immediately ventral to the LC that is required for the descending components of normal REM sleep (atonia and possibly eye movements), but not the ascending components (periods of EEG desynchronization). These lesions block both the atonia of REM sleep and the expression of motor activity during REM sleep (likely by damaging areas that control locomotion). Similar lesions of the nearby noradrenergic LC, but not the PnO, do not block REM sleep, suggesting that a tiny and anatomically discrete population of neurons can recruit the massive changes in brain activity seen during REM sleep. In cats, lesions of the LDTg block REM sleep. PnO neurons modulate the atonia of REM sleep through excitatory innervation of the lower brainstem and then through projections that postsynaptically inhibit motor neurons in the spinal cord.

Third, in-vivo electrophysiology studies have localized a subpopulation of large cholinergic PPTg neurons at the mesopontine junction that are selectively active during REM sleep. These neurons project to both the thalamus (responsible for phasic pontine-geniculo-occipital wave excitation and EEG desynchronizations of REM) and the pontine reticular formation (responsible for the atonia of REM). Single-unit recording studies reveal that this subpopulation of PPTg neurons discharge at a high rate throughout REM sleep, have little or no activity during NREM sleep, and are generally silent during wakefulness (another subpopulation of PPTg/LDTg neurons are wake-active). There are three major groups of "REM-on" cells in the region encompassed by the lesions described earlier: (1) the PPTg, (2) the PnO of the pontine reticular formation, and (3) a population of glycinergic neurons in the medial medullary reticular formation. Of these, the PnO contains a subset of neurons known as the sublateral dorsal (SLD) nucleus in rodents (or as the peri-LCα or subcoeruleus in cats) that may serve as the master REM-on triggering switch [71]. While still controversial, the surprising discovery that SLD executive neurons are not cholinergic but rather glutamatergic has led to a re-examination of the role of cholinergic–monoaminergic regulation of REM sleep [52].

According to the cholinergic–monoaminergic theory, during REM sleep, noradrenergic cells of the LC and serotonergic cells of the raphe nuclei, which project to the LDTg/PPTg [72] where they are believed to inhibit cholinergic neurons, fire rapidly during wakefulness, markedly less so during NREM, and very minimally or are completely silent during REM sleep [73,74]. Thus inhibition of noradrenergic and serotonergic neurons by GABAergic inputs from the extended VLPO and caudal MnPO are thought to promote REM sleep [58,66]. Administration of physostigmine (an anticholinesterase drug that increases acetylcholine [ACh] at the synapse) precipitates REM sleep during an ongoing period of NREM sleep and enhances the phasic periods of REM sleep, whereas blocking muscarinic ACh receptors (AChRs) with a drug such as scopolamine inhibits the appearance of REM sleep and reduces phasic periods. Discrete microinjections of the cholinergic agonist carbachol into the medial pontine reticular formation (which receives projections from the PPTg) induce REM sleep in cats and rats. REM sleep can also be induced by microinjecting ACh into the PnO, and glutamate injection into the PPTg increases REM sleep. These results suggest that pontine cholinoceptive neurons (1) act on other reticular neurons to excite ascending circuits and (2) inhibit sensory and motor transmission. Noradrenergic neurons of the LC appear to act in a reciprocal manner to the cholinergic neurons, being selectively active during wakefulness (for review see Jones [75]).

It should be pointed out that a competing theory focusing upon glutamatergic–GABAergic modulation of REM sleep posits that GABAergic neurons in the deep mesencephalic reticular nucleus (DPMe) and ventrolateral part of the periaqueductal gray (vlPAG) serve as REM-off centers that tonically inhibit the SLD. Similarly, the SLD reciprocally inhibits these REM-off neurons, forming a second flip-flop switch analogous to and intertwined with the one which regulates NREM sleep [71,76]. Under the glutamatergic–GABAergic theory, vlPAG and/or DPMe GABAergic neurons are directly responsible for the inhibition of monoaminergic neurons during REM sleep. While much progress has been made in elucidating the critical neuroanatomic substrates for REM expression, further work must be done to clarify mechanisms for switching between behavioral states.

Switching between sleep and wake states

Switching between these sleep and wake states is thought to be controlled by a reciprocal relationship of mutual inhibition between the activities of sleep-promoting neurons in the VLPO and MnPO and the major monoamine areas (TMN, LC, and midbrain raphe nuclei) of the ascending reticular arousal system [53]. The VLPO and MnPO innervate the arousal system and inhibit its activity during sleep. Conversely, the nuclei of the ascending arousal system inhibit the VLPO and MnPO during wakefulness (Figs. 13.4–13.7) (see *Wakefulness* and *Non-rapid eye movement sleep*, above). Therefore when the firing rates of the VLPO and MnPO are high during sleep, they inhibit the monoaminergic arousal nuclei and thereby further disinhibit or activate their own firing. Conversely, when the monoaminergic neurons fire rapidly during wakefulness, they act to inhibit the VLPO and MnPO and disinhibit, or further activate, their own firing.

Saper and colleagues report that this reciprocal relationship tends toward two stable firing patterns (sleep or wake) and away from intermediate transition states, so that only large-scale influences such as circadian drive to sleep or a sufficient degree of sleep drive or deprivation exerts pressure on the circuit until it

reaches a critical threshold and the firing patterns reverse rapidly [53]. This functional organization evoked comparisons to the bistable circuit known to electrical engineers as a "flip-flop": when one side is firing rapidly, there is a "resistance" to "switching" such that it occurs infrequently but rapidly. When the firing of the sleep-promoting VLPO side of the circuit is weakened by ablation of the VLPO, the circuit is destabilized and animals experience insomnia plus an increased drive to sleep, which may bring the circuit balance closer to the transition state [64]. A destabilizing deficit on the waking side of this sleep switch induces the inappropriate abrupt transitions from wakefulness to sleep (particularly REM or fragments of REM sleep, such as cataplexy or the loss of muscle tone while awake) seen in the sleep disorder narcolepsy.

Saper and colleagues further hypothesized that the neurons containing orexin (also known as hypocretin) in the perifornical area of the lateral hypothalamus act as a stabilizing "finger" helping to hold the sleep switch pointing toward wakefulness and prevent switching to sleep [53]. Dysfunction of this "finger," and the consequent susceptibility to sudden and inappropriate transitions, is seen in narcolepsy, which is characterized by an orexinergic deficiency [77]. The TMN, LC, and raphe nuclei all receive input from orexinergic neurons, contain orexin receptors, and inhibit REM sleep [78] so that the inappropriate transitions into REM or fragments of REM sleep experienced with narcolepsy may be modulated by the weakening of the sleep switch reinforcement "finger." Specifically, the absence of excitatory orexin input is hypothesized to weaken the arousal system's inhibition of the extended VLPO and other REM-off clusters including the vlPAG (which modulate REM, whereas the VLPO cluster modulates NREM sleep [58]), allowing more frequent transitions into REM [53] (Fig. 13.6).

The endogenous trigger for state transitions in the absence of disease may reside within the MnPO. A subset of MnPO neurons are known to track sleep pressure, the homeostatic component of sleep that accumulates with sustained amounts of wakefulness [79]. While the exact mechanisms that trigger changes in arousal state remain unknown, the discovery of humoral factors circulating in cerebrospinal fluid capable of inducing sleep suggests potential clues. Putative somnogens include substances such as the cytokine interleukin 1β, adenosine, and prostaglandin D_2, which accumulate during wakefulness. Intracerebroventricular administration of interleukin 1β promotes sleep and is associated with activation of MnPO neurons [80]. As an inhibitory neuromodulator, adenosine promotes sleep both by inhibiting wake-promoting neurons and by depolarizing VLPO neurons. Finally, prostaglandin D_2 induces sleep when administered into the subarachnoid space along the rostral basal forebrain in close proximity to the VLPO and MnPO. Prostaglandin D_2 is known to activate VLPO neurons, possibly using adenosine as an intermediary, but whether it too also activates MnPO neurons remains unknown [81]. The endogenous clonidine-displacing substance, agmantine, is synthesized in brain, binds with high affinity to α_{2A}-adrenoceptors, and acts as a partial agonist. As such, it may possess somnogenic activity; however, to date no studies confirm this theoretical possibility.

Molecular anesthetic targets, sleep centers, and the EEG

This section discusses some of the molecular targets of anesthetics with a focus on how they relate to sleep/wake centers and the EEG. Forman and Chin have described three classes of anesthetics, which are based on molecular targets, as well as clinical and electroencephalographic effects [82]. Although a simplified framework, it is a helpful tool to consider the relationships between molecular events and macroscopic EEG changes.

Class 1

Class 1 includes intravenous drugs such as propofol, etomidate, and barbiturates, which act primarily on GABA receptors and produce unconsciousness more effectively than immobilization (Fig. 13.8). This class of drugs is associated with a decreased frequency of EEG waveforms. The direct connection between the activation of GABA$_A$ receptors and the depressed EEG is supported by the fact that GABAergic anesthetic drugs such as propofol and pentobarbital transduce their hypnotic effects via GABA$_A$ receptors in regionally discrete anatomic sites within an endogenous NREM-sleep-promoting pathway: the VLPO and TMN [65] (Fig. 13.9).

Class 2

Class 2 includes agents such as xenon, nitrous oxide, cyclopropane, and ketamine, which act primarily on N-methyl-D-aspartate (NMDA) receptors and are effective analgesics. These drugs tend to *activate* the EEG. Whereas class 1 agents acting primarily on GABA share some of the behavioral and electroencephalographic traits of NREM sleep, class 2 agents affecting NMDA share traits of REM sleep. These include an activated cortex, as well as a high propensity for dream states. Indeed, in one study a high percentage of patients who received ketamine anesthetics reported dreaming [84]. Furthermore, as discussed above, EEG-based monitors that reflect awareness primarily based on decreased waveform frequency may be relatively insensitive to the effects of NMDA antagonists because of their activating effects on the cortex. Recent data in an animal model suggest that GABAergic agents increase Fos immunoreactivity – a surrogate for metabolic activity – in the sleep-promoting VLPO region, while NMDA antagonists such as ketamine increase Fos in arousal-promoting regions such as the histaminergic TMN, dopaminergic PAG, noradrenergic LC, orexinergic hypothalamus, and the cholinergic basal forebrain [85]. It is interesting that such neurobiological interfaces of sleep and anesthesia may have implications for our approach to the clinical detection of intraoperative awareness.

Class 3

Class 3 includes the volatile anesthetics, which affect GABA and numerous other substrates, and have diverse actions. Like class 1, these drugs also are associated with a decreased frequency on EEG. In addition to effects on GABA, such actions may be related to the antagonism of the cholinergic system (Fig. 13.8). As discussed above, the cholinergic system is an important regulator of the sleep/wake cycle, promoting arousal states in both wakefulness and REM. Modulation of AChRs in critical regions may therefore contribute to anesthetic-induced unconsciousness. For example, cholinergic agonism in the central medial thalamic nucleus has been demonstrated to reverse sevoflurane-induced unconsciousness [86]. It is important to note, however, that the administration of a nicotinic antagonist, mecamylamine, in the central medial thalamic nucleus was not shown to induce anesthesia or have a MAC-sparing effect. Thus, the central medial nucleus may be an "on" switch for arousal, but not an "off" switch for anesthesia – parallel findings have been demonstrated in the orexinergic system (see below) [87]. Further evidence for the role of the cholinergic system as an "on" switch that can reverse general anesthesia comes from a rat model using cross-approximate entropy (another form of information entropy, as described above). Intracerebroventricular injection of the cholinesterase inhibitor neostigmine demonstrated behavioral and electroencephalographic signs of emergence, despite a constant concentration of isoflurane delivery [88].

Although it is clear how anesthetics affecting neurotransmitter systems such as ACh could affect consciousness by potentiating inhibition or attenuating excitation, how do we make a behavioral connection with other molecular targets such as background potassium channels? One study found that TASK-1 and TASK-3 channels mediated the change of conductance induced by halothane in thalamocortical relay neurons [89]. The thalamocortical system is characterized by 40 Hz or γ-band oscillations in the waking state, which have been associated with consciousness and cognition [90]. During NREM sleep or general anesthesia, thalamocortical activity shifts to a low frequency oscillation. It is thus possible that TASK-1 and TASK-2 play a role in that state change after administration of general anesthetics.

A new class of anesthetics?

Although not described, we might also consider a fourth class of agents that act more directly on sleep/wake centers. The α_2-agonist dexmedetomidine might be regarded as the prototypical agent, but future therapeutic agents acting on the orexin system might also fall into this class.

One of the highest densities of G-protein-coupled α_2-adrenoceptor has been detected in the LC [91], the predominant noradrenergic nucleus in the brain and an important modulator of vigilance [92]. Hypnotic and sedative effects of α_2-adrenoceptor activation have been attributed to the LC [93], which densely innervates and tonically inhibits the sleep-active

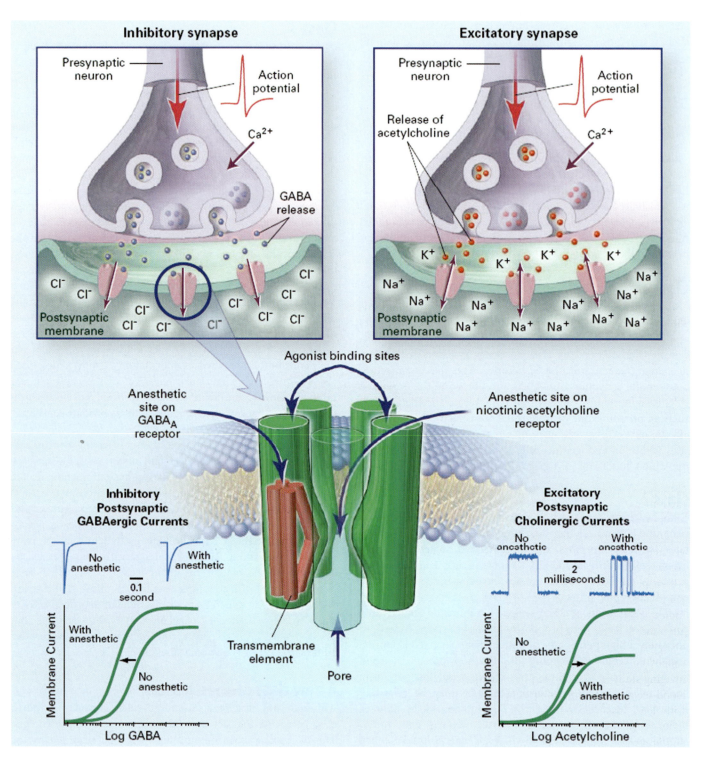

Figure 13.8. The effects of anesthetics are mediated, in part, by the potentiation of inhibitory synaptic transmission or the inhibition of excitatory transmission. This figure depicts the binding sites of anesthetics on GABA$_A$ and acetylcholine receptors, as well as the effects on postsynaptic currents. Anesthetic binding to the GABA$_A$ receptor increases the potency of the ligand, while anesthetic binding to the acetylcholine receptor decreases the potency of the ligand. Reproduced with permission from Campagna et al. [83].

VLPO during wakefulness. From an anesthetic viewpoint, hyperpolarization of noradrenergic neurons in the LC appears to be a key factor in the mechanism of action of dexmedetomidine and other α_2-adrenoceptor agonists [93,94]. Relative to its effects on the α_1-adrenoceptor, dexmedetomidine is eight times more specific for the α_2-adrenoceptor than

Awake   **NREM Sleep**

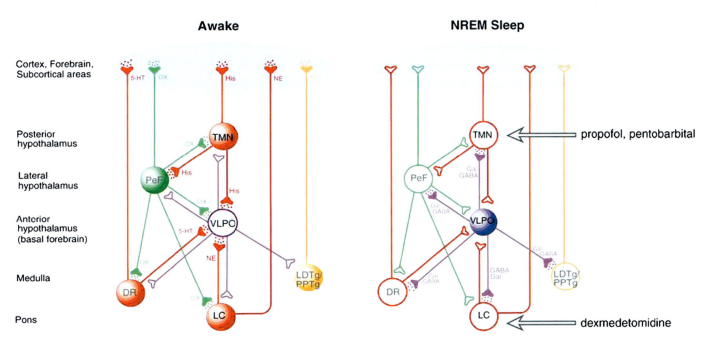

Figure 13.9. GABAergic and α₂-adrenergic anesthetic drugs converge on endogenous sleep pathways to exert their hypnotic effects. A schematic summarizing the monoaminergic (red) and cholinergic (orange) and galanin- and GABAergic (purple) neural substrates of arousal (*left*) and non-rapid eye movement (NREM) sleep (*right*). Wakefulness is promoted by the release of the arousal-promoting monoamine (red) neurotransmitters norepinephrine (NE), serotonin (5-HT), and histamine (His) in the locus coeruleus (LC), raphe nuclei, and tuberomammillary nucleus (TMN), respectively, as well as acetylcholine (ACh; orange) from the pedunculopontine and laterodorsal tegmental nuclei (PPTg and LDTg) into the forebrain and cortex. During NREM sleep, the sleep-active galanin- and GABAergic ventrolateral preoptic nucleus (VLPO; purple) inhibits the ascending arousal system to induce loss of consciousness. It is believed that the α₂-adrenergic agonist dexmedetomidine converges on this endogenous sleep circuitry at the level of the LC to exert its sedative effects, whereas putatively "GABAergic" agents such as pentobarbital and propofol converge further downstream at the level of the TMN. DR, dorsal raphe; GABA, γ-aminobutyric acid; Gal, galanin; OX, orexin; PeF, perifornical area. Adapted with permission from Nelson *et al.* [65].

clonidine, the next most selective α₂-adrenoceptor agonist (action at the α₁-adrenoceptor counteracts action at the α₂-adrenoceptor).

It is hypothesized that the decrease in firing of noradrenergic neurons in the LC results in a loss of consciousness by converging on an endogenous sleep pathway upstream of that where putatively GABAergic drugs influence these pathways [65,95] (Fig. 13.9). Qualitative observations by nursing staff indicate that dexmedetomidine induces a clinically effective sedation that is uniquely arousable (as is natural sleep), an effect not observed with any other clinically available sedatives [96]. In support of this, data from a functional magnetic resonance imaging study in healthy volunteers seemed to confirm that the blood-oxygen-level-dependent signal, which positively correlates with local brain activity, changes during dexmedetomidine-induced sedation in a manner similar to that during natural sleep and is markedly different from midazolam sedation [97]. The similarity to sleep is further supported by recent human EEG studies suggesting that dexmedetomidine sedation is associated with sleep spindles, which are thought to inhibit sensory transmission to the cortex [98]. Recent studies of clonidine sedation in humans have also revealed sleep spindles by EEG [99]. Thus, both the observed sedative "phenotype" and the underlying neurophysiologic "genotype" support α₂-agonists as inducers of a sleep-like state. The advantages of a sedative that mimics natural sleep may

perhaps best be appreciated in the critical-care setting, where many patients are sleep-deprived. One study of dexmedetomidine in medical and surgical intensive-care patients demonstrated a significant reduction in both delirium and coma states compared to the benzodiazepine lorazepam [100].

In 1998, while screening for ligands for orphan G-protein-coupled receptors, Sakurai and colleagues identified two peptides, which they named "orexin A" and "orexin B" because they promoted feeding [101]. Simultaneously, de Lecea and coworkers reported their discovery of two hypothalamus-specific mRNA coding for the same two peptides, which they termed "hypocretins" because of their sequence similarities to secretin [102]. Orexin/hypocretin knockout mice express a narcoleptic phenotype [77], canine narcolepsy is attributed to mutations in the gene for the orexin 2 receptor [103], and an absence of orexin in the hypothalamus and cerebrospinal fluid of humans with narcolepsy is observed [104].

As discussed above, orexins are involved in sleep/wake control, but they may also play a role in the neurobiology of general anesthesia. Intracerebroventricular injection of orexin A and B was found to facilitate recovery from barbiturate anesthesia in an animal model, with orexin A having a more potent effect than orexin B [105]. Conversely, the orexin antagonist SB-334867-A prolonged barbiturate anesthesia. Intracerebroventricular injection of orexin A has also been shown to activate cortical EEG and decrease burst suppression ratio during iso-flurane anesthesia [106]. Injection of orexin A and B in the basal forebrain during isoflurane anesthesia increased cortical ACh release, activated the EEG, and reduced the burst suppression ratio [107]. As with barbiturates, orexin A was more potent in its effects. The precise role of orexins in general anesthesia was not elucidated until 10 years after their discovery. Kelz et al. found that isoflurane and sevoflurane inhibited c-Fos expression in orexinergic neurons [86]. These data would suggest that anesthetics inhibit the arousal-promoting effects of the orexins, facilitating the induction of general anesthesia. Surprisingly, using a genetically modified mouse model, it was found that the absence of orexin did not alter induction, but did delay emergence. This suggests that – similar to the role of ACh in the thalamus – orexins play a role in the "on" switch for arousal, but not in an "off" switch for the induction of anesthesia.

Summary

The neural mechanisms regulating subjective awareness are thought to reside primarily in the cortex, providing a "top-down" pathway to interrupt consciousness, while those regulating wakefulness are located primarily in subcortical structures and represent "bottom-up" pathways. While there are distinctions in the EEG pattern and neuropharmacology, general anesthesia and sleep share many properties including hypnosis, amnesia, analgesia, and immobility. Both sleep and general anesthesia appear to be associated with interruption of cortical connectivity, with particular dissociation in the thalamocortical system in anesthesia and in persistent vegetative states. Failure to interrupt such cortical integration can lead to intraoperative awareness and memory, which can lead to severe psychological sequelae. Thus, accurate assessment of anesthetic depth is necessary, and several EEG-based devices are purportedly available for this purpose. However, these "awareness monitors" may be susceptible to errors arising from the activity of certain drugs, physiologic changes, pathologic changes, and electrical artifacts.

The ascending reticular activating system (RAS) projects from the caudal midbrain and rostral pons area to the thalamus and the hypothalamus. Cholinergic neurons projecting to the thalamus fire rapidly during wakefulness and rapid eye movement (REM) sleep, and more slowly during non-rapid eye movement (NREM) sleep. Monoaminergic neurons of the hypothalamic branch of the RAS fire rapidly during wakefulness, very infrequently during NREM, and generally not at all during REM sleep. Sleep is an actively generated state. NREM sleep is thought to involve neurons of the preoptic anterior hypothalamus, the ventrolateral preoptic nucleus (VLPO), and the median preoptic nucleus (MnPO). REM sleep involves activation of neurons in the pedunculopontine tegmental nucleus (PPTg), the pontine reticular nucleus oralis (PnO), and the medial medullary reticular formation. A reciprocal inhibitory mechanism is thought to mediate switching between sleep and wakefulness: VLPO and MnPO neurons have projections that inhibit the ascending arousal-promoting regions during sleep, whilst the nuclei of the ascending arousal system inhibit VLPO and MnPO neurons during wakefulness. Orexinergic neurons have been proposed to stabilize the waking state, while MnPO neurons may be involved in tracking sleep pressure.

Class 1 anesthetics act primarily on GABA receptors to produce unconsciousness that shares some traits of NREM sleep, while class 2 agents primarily act on NMDA receptors inducing analgesia and a state that in some ways resembles REM sleep. Class 3 anesthetics affect multiple systems, including GABA and cholinergic signaling. In a potential fourth class of anesthetics, α_2-adrenoceptor agonists are thought to act on the locus coeruleus, one of the sites of the monoaminergic arousal-promoting pathway, to bring about hypnotic and sedative effects. Dexmedetomidine has the highest selectivity for the α_2-adrenoceptor relative to the α_1-adrenoceptor, and produces a unique sedation with preserved arousability. Imaging and EEG studies support the similarity of this state to natural sleep. Potential future drug targets include orexin receptors. There is some evidence to suggest that orexin antagonism can delay emergence from anesthesia.

In 1899, William James wrote that "A genuine glimpse into what consciousness is would be the scientific achievement, before which all past achievements would pale." A greater understanding of states such as sleep and anesthesia – during which consciousness is effectively and reversibly suppressed – may help us achieve this glimpse. Current research in sleep and anesthesia has converged, confirming the earlier hypothesis that neural systems that have evolved to control sleep/wake states likely play a central role in the mechanism of general anesthesia [108]. Further work on this point of convergence will hopefully lead to a deeper neuroscientific understanding, enabling us to develop more sophisticated techniques of modulating and monitoring conscious and unconscious states.

References

1. Chalmers DJ. Facing up to the problem of consciousness. *J Conscious Stud* 1995; **2**: 200–19.

2. Laureys S. Eyes open, brain shut. *Sci AM* 2007; **296**(5): 84–9.

3. Lydic R, Baghdoyan HA. Sleep, anesthesiology, and the neurobiology of arousal state control. *Anesthesiology* 2005; **103**: 1268–95.

4. Tung A, Mendelson WB. Anesthesia and sleep. *Sleep Med Rev* 2004; **8**: 213–25.

5. Clement EA, Richard A, Thwaites M, *et al.* Cyclic and sleep-like spontaneous alternations of brain state under urethane anaesthesia. *PLoS ONE* 2008; **3**: e2004.

6. Koblin DD. Urethane: help or hindrance? *Anesth Analg* 2002; **94**: 241–2.

7. Massimini M, Ferrarelli F, Huber R, *et al.* Breakdown of cortical effective

connectivity during sleep. *Science* 2005; **309**: 2228–32.

8. Tononi G, Koch C. The neural correlates of consciousness: an update. *Ann N Y Acad Sci* 2008; **1124**: 239–61.

9. Alkire MT, Haier RJ, Fallon JH. Toward a unified theory of narcosis: brain imaging evidence for a thalamocortical switch as the neurophysiologic basis of anesthetic-induced unconsciousness. *Conscious Cogn* 2000; **9**: 370–86.

10. White NS, Alkire MT. Impaired thalamocortical connectivity in humans during general-anesthesia-induced unconsciousness. *Neuroimaging* 2003; **19**: 402–11.

11. John ER, Prichep LS. The anesthetic cascade: a theory of how anesthesia suppresses consciousness. *Anesthesiology* 2005; **102**: 447–71.

12. John ER, Prichep LS, Kox W, *et al.* Invariant reversible QEEG effects of anesthetics. *Conscious Cogn* 2001; **10**: 165–83.

13. Laureys S, Faymonville ME, Luxen A, *et al.* Restoration of thalamocortical connectivity after recovery from persistent vegetative state. *Lancet* 2000; **355**: 1790–1.

14. Tononi G. An information integration theory of consciousness. *BMC Neurosci* 2004; **5**: 42.

15. Tononi G, Sporns O. Measuring information integration. *BMC Neurosci* 2003; **4**: 31.

16. Velly LJ, Rey MF, Bruder NJ, *et al.* Differential dynamic of action on cortical and subcortical structures of anesthetic agents during induction of anesthesia. *Anesthesiology* 2007; **107**: 202–12.

17. Plourde G, Garcia-Asensi A, Backman S, *et al.* Attenuation of the 40-hertz auditory steady state response by propofol involves the cortical and subcortical generators. *Anesthesiology* 2008; **108**: 233–42.

18. Mashour GA, LaRock E. Inverse zombies, anesthesia awareness, ad the hard problem of uncousciousness. *Conscious Cogn* 2008; **17**:1163–8.

19. Sandin RH, Enlund G, Samuelsson P, Lennmarken C. Awareness during anaesthesia: a prospective case study. *Lancet* 2000; **355**: 707–11.

20. Sebel PS, Bowdle TA, Ghoneim MM, *et al.* The incidence of awareness during anesthesia: a multicenter United States study. *Anesth Analg* 2004; **99**: 833–9.

21. Errando CL, Sigl JC, Robles M, *et al.* Awareness with recall during general anaesthesia: a prospective observational evaluation of 4001 patients. *Br J Anaesth* 2008; **101**: 178–85.

22. Pollard RJ, Coyle JP, Gilbert RL, Beck JE. Intraoperative awareness in a regional medical system: a review of 3 years' data. *Anesthesiology* 2007; **106**: 269–74.

23. Mashour GA, Wang LYJ, Turner CR, *et al.* A retrospective study of intraoperative awareness with methodological implications. *Anesth Analg* 2009; **108**: 521–6.

24. Lennmarken C, Sydsjo G. Psychological consequences of awareness and their treatment. *Best Pract Res Clin Anaesthesiol* 2007; **21**: 357–67.

25. Monk TG, Saini V, Weldon BC, Sigl JC. Anesthetic management and one-year mortality after noncardiac surgery. *Anesth Analg* 2005; **100**: 4–10.

26. Gibbs FA, Gibbs LE, Lennox WG. Effect on the electroencephalogram of certain drugs which influence nervous activity. *Arch Intern Med* 1937; **60**: 154–66.

27. Jameson LC, Sloan TB. Using EEG to monitor anesthesia drug effects during surgery. *J Clin Monitoring Comp* 2006; **20**: 445–72.

28. Rampil IJ. A primer for EEG signal processing in anesthesia. *Anesthesiology* 1998; **89**: 980–1002.

29. Bruhn J, Myles PS, Sneyd R, Struys MM. Depth of anaesthesia monitoring: what's available, what's validated and what's next? *Br J Anaesth* 2006; **97**: 85–94.

30. Bowdle TA. Depth of anesthesia monitoring. *Anesthesiol Clin* 2006; **24**: 793–822.

31. Voss L, Sleigh J. Monitoring consciousness: the current status of EEG-based depth of anaesthesia monitors. *Best Pract Res Clin Anaesthesiol* 2007; **21**: 313–25.

32. Dahaba AA. Different conditions that could result in the bispectral index indicating an incorrect hypnotic state. *Anesth Analg* 2005; **101**: 765–73.

33. Yamamura T, Fukuda M, Takeya H, Goto Y, Furukawa K. Fast oscillatory EEG activity induced by analgesic concentrations of nitrous oxide in man. *Anesth Analg* 1981; **60**: 283–8.

34. Rampil IJ, Kim JS, Lenhardt R, Negishi C, Sessler DI. Bispectral EEG index during nitrous oxide administration. *Anesthesiology* 1998; **89**: 671–7.

35. Sakai T, Singh H, Mi WD, Kudo T, Matsuki A. The effect of ketamine on clinical endpoints of hypnosis and EEG variables during propofol infusion. *Acta Anaesthesiol Scand* 1999; **43**: 212–16.

36. Vereecke HE, Struys MM, Mortier EP. A comparison of bispectral index and ARX-derived auditory evoked potential index in measuring the clinical interaction between ketamine and propofol anaesthesia. *Anaesthesia* 2003; **58**: 957–61.

37. Messner M, Beese U, Romstock J, Dinkel M, Tschaikowsky K. The bispectral index declines during neuromuscular block in fully awake persons. *Anesth Analg* 2003; **97**: 488–91.

38. Liu N, Chazot T, Huybrechts I, Law et al. The influence of a muscle relaxant bolus on bispectral and datex-ohmeda entropy values during propofol-remifentanil induced loss of consciousness. *Anesth Analg* 2005; **101**: 1713–18.

39. Ekman A, Lindholm ML, Lennmarken C, Sandin R. Reduction in the incidence of awareness using BIS monitoring. *Acta Anaesthesiol Scand* 2004; **48**: 20–6.

40. Myles PS, Leslie K, McNeil J, Forbes A, Chan MT. Bispectral index monitoring to prevent awareness during anaesthesia: the B-Aware randomised controlled trial. *Lancet* 2004; **363**: 1757–63.

41. Avidan MS, Zhang L, Burnside BA, *et al.* Anesthesia awareness and the bispectral index. *N Engl J Med* 2008; **358**: 1097–108.

42. Franks NP. General anesthesia: from molecular targets to neuronal pathways of sleep and arousal. *Nat Rev Neurosci* 2008; **9**: 370–86.

43. Hallanger AE, Wainer BH. Ascending projections from the pedunculopontine tegmental nucleus and the adjacent mesopontine tegmentum in the rat. *J Comp Neurol* 1988; **274**: 483–515.

44. Herkenham M. Laminar organization of thalamic projections to the rat neocortex. *Science* 1980; **207**: 532–5.

45. Steriade M, McCormick DA, Sejnowski TJ. Thalamocortical oscillations in the sleeping and aroused brain. *Science* 1993; **262**: 679–85.

46. Semba K. The cholinergic basal forebrain: a critical role in cortical arousal. *Adv Exp Med Biol* 1991; **295**: 197–218.

47. Detari L. Tonic and phasic influence of basal forebrain unit activity on the cortical EEG. *Behav Brain Res* 2000; **115**: 159–70.

48. Jimenez-Capdeville ME, Dykes RW, Myasnikov AA. Differential control of cortical activity by the basal forebrain in rats: a role for both cholinergic and inhibitory influences. *J Comp Neurol* 1997; **381**: 53–67.

49. Aston-Jones G, Chiang C, Alexinsky T. Discharge of noradrenergic locus coeruleus neurons in behaving rats and monkeys suggests a role in vigilance. *Prog Brain Res* 1991; **88**: 501–20.

50. Steininger TL, Alam MN, Gong H, Szymusiak R, McGinty D. Sleep-waking discharge of neurons in the posterior lateral hypothalamus of the albino rat. *Brain Res* 1999; **840**: 138–47.

51. Lu J, Jhou TC, Saper CB. Identification of wake-active dopaminergic neurons in the ventral periaqueductal gray matter. *J Neurosci* 2006; **26**: 193–202.

52. Luppi PH, Gervasoni D, Verret L, *et al.* Paradoxical (REM) sleep genesis: the switch from an aminergic-cholinergic to a GABAergic-glutamatergic hypothesis. *J Physiol Paris* 2006; **100**: 271–83.

53. Saper CB, Chou TC, Scammell TE. The sleep switch: hypothalamic control of sleep and wakefulness. *Trends Neurosci* 2001; **24**: 726–31.

54. Von Economo C. Sleep as a problem of localization. *J Nerv Ment Dis* 1930; **71**: 248–9.

55. Sherin JE, Shiromani PJ, McCarley RW, Saper CB. Activation of ventrolateral preoptic neurons during sleep. *Science* 1996; **271**: 216–19.

56. Chou TC, Bjorkum AA, Gaus SE, *et al.* Afferents to the ventrolateral preoptic nucleus. *J Neurosci* 2002; **22**: 977–90.

57. Gallopin T, Fort P, Eggermann E, *et al.* Identification of sleep-promoting neurons in vitro. *Nature* 2000; **404**: 992–5.

58. Lu J, Bjorkum AA, Xu M, *et al.* Selective activation of the extended ventrolateral preoptic nucleus during rapid eye movement sleep. *J Neurosc* 2002; **22**: 4568–76.

59. Sherin JE, Elmquist JK, Torrealba F, Saper CB. Innervation of histaminergic tuberomammillary neurons by GABAergic and galaninergic neurons in the ventrolateral preoptic nucleus of the rat. *J Neurosc* 1998; **18**: 4705–21.

60. Gaus SE, Strecker RE, Tate BA, Parker RA, Saper CB. Ventrolateral preoptic nucleus contains sleep-active, galaninergic neurons in multiple mammalian species. *Neuroscience* 2002; **115**: 285–94.

61. Lin JS, Sakai K, Jouvet M. Evidence for histaminergic arousal mechanisms in the hypothalamus of cat. *Neuropharmacology* 1988; **27**: 111–22.

62. Steininger TL, Gong H, McGinty D, Szymusiak R. Subregional organization of preoptic area/anterior hypothalamic projections to arousal-related monoaminergic cell groups. *J Comp Neurol* 2001; **429**: 638–53.

63. Yang QZ, Hatton GI. Electrophysiology of excitatory and inhibitory afferents to rat histaminergic tuberomammillary nucleus neurons from hypothalamic and forebrain sites. *Brain Res* 1997; **773**: 162–72.

64. Lu J, Greco MA, Shiromani P, Saper CB. Effect of lesions of the ventrolateral preoptic nucleus on NREM and REM sleep. *J Neurosci* 2000; **20**: 3830–42.

65. Nelson LE, Guo TZ, Lu J, *et al.* The sedative component of anesthesia is mediated by GABA(A) receptors in an endogenous sleep pathway. *Nat Neurosci* 2002; **5**: 979–84.

66. Suntsova N, Szymusiak R, Alam MN, Guzman-Marin R, McGinty D. Sleep-waking discharge patterns of median preoptic nucleus neurons in rats. *J Physiol* 2002; **543**: 665–77.

67. Suntsova N, Guzman-Marin R, Kumar S, *et al.* The median preoptic nucleus reciprocally modulates activity of arousal-related and sleep-related neurons in the perifornical lateral hypothalamus. *J Neurosci* 2007; **27**: 1616–30.

68. Uschakov A, Gong H, McGinty D, Szymusiak R. Efferent projections from the median preoptic nucleus to sleep- and arousal-regulatory nuclei in the rat brain. *Neuroscience* 2007; **150**: 104–20.

69. Lucas EA, Sterman MB. Effect of a forebrain lesion on the polycyclic sleep-wake cycle and sleep-wake patterns in the cat. *Exp Neurol* 1975; **46**: 368–88.

70. Siegel JM. Brainstem mechanisms generating REM sleep. In: Kryger MH, Roth T, Dement WC, eds., *Principles and Practice of Sleep Medicine*, 3rd edn. Philadelphia, PA: Saunders, 2000: 112–33.

71. Lu J, Sherman D, Devor M, Saper CB. A putative flip-flop switch for control of REM sleep. *Nature* 2006; **441**: 589–94.

72. Semba K, Fibiger HC. Afferent connections of the laterodorsal and the pedunculopontine tegmental nuclei in the rat: a retro- and antero-grade transport and immunohistochemical study. *J Comp Neurol* 1992; **323**: 387–410.

73. Aston-Jones G, Bloom FE. Nonrepinephrine-containing locus coeruleus neurons in behaving rats exhibit pronounced responses to non-noxious environmental stimuli. *J Neurosci* 1981; **1**: 887–900.

74. McGinty DJ, Harper RM. Dorsal raphe neurons: depression of firing during sleep in cats. *Brain Res* 1976; **101**: 569–75.

75. Jones BE. Paradoxical sleep and its chemical/structural substrates in the brain. *Neuroscience* 1991; **40**: 637–56.

76. Saper CB, Scammell TE, Lu J. Hypothalamic regulation of sleep and circadian rhythms. *Nature* 2005; **437**: 1257–63.

77. Chemelli RM, Willie JT, Sinton CM, *et al.* Narcolepsy in orexin knockout mice: molecular genetics of sleep regulation. *Cell* 1999; **98**: 437–51.

78. Marcus JN, Aschkenasi CJ, Lee CE, *et al.* Differential expression of orexin receptors 1 and 2 in the rat brain. *J Comp Neurol* 2001; **435**: 6–25.

79. Gvilia I, Xu F, McGinty D, Szymusiak R: Homeostatic regulation of sleep: a role

for preoptic area neurons. *J Neurosci* 2006; **26**: 9426–33.

80. Baker FC, Shah S, Stewart D, *et al.* Interleukin 1beta enhances non-rapid eye movement sleep and increases c-Fos protein expression in the median preoptic nucleus of the hypothalamus. *Am J Physiol Regul Integr Comp Physiol.* 2005; **288**: R998–1005.

81. Scammell T, Gerashchenko D, Urade Y, *et al.* Activation of ventrolateral preoptic neurons by the somnogen prostaglandin D2. *Proc Nat Acad Sci U S A* 1998; **95**: 7754–9.

82. Forman SA, Chin VA. General anesthetics and molecular mechanisms of unconsciousness. *Internatl Anesthesiol Clin* 2008; **46**: 43–53.

83. Campagna JA, Miller KW, Forman SA. Mechanisms of actions of inhaled anesthetics. *N Engl J Med* 2003; **348**: 2110–24.

84. Grace RF. The effect of variable-dose diazepam on dreaming and emergence phenomena in 400 cases of ketamine–fentanyl anaesthesia. *Anaesthesia* 2003; **58**: 904–10.

85. Lu J, Nelson LE, Franks N, *et al.* Role of endogenous sleep-wake and analgesic systems in anesthesia. *J Comp Neurol* 2008; **508**: 648–62.

86. Alkire MT, McReynolds JR, Hahn EL, Trivedi AN. Thalamic microinjection of nicotine reverses sevoflurane-induced loss of righting reflex in the rat. *Anesthesiology* 2007; **107**: 264–72.

87. Kelz MB, Sun Y, Chen J, *et al.* An essential role for orexins in emergence from general anesthesia. *Proc Nat Acad Sci U S A* 2008; **105**: 1309–14.

88. Hudetz AG, Wood JD, Kampine JP. Cholinergic reversal of isoflurane anesthesia in rats as measured by cross-approximate entropy of the electroencephalogram. *Anesthesiology* 2003; **99**: 1125–31.

89. Meuth SG, Budde T, Kanyshkova T, *et al.* Contribution of TWIK-related acid-sensitive K$^+$ channel 1 (TASK1) and TASK3 channels to the control of activity modes in thalamocortical neurons. *J Neurosci* 2003; **23**: 6460–9.

90. Mashour GA. Integrating the science of consciousness and anesthesia. *Anesth Analg* 2006; **103**: 975–82.

91. MacDonald E, Scheinin M. Distribution and pharmacology of alpha 2-adrenoceptors in the central nervous system. *J Physiol Pharmacol* 1995; **46**: 241–58.

92. Aston-Jones G, Rajkowski J, Kubiak P, Alexinsky T. Locus coeruleus neurons in monkey are selectively activated by attended cues in a vigilance task. *J Neurosci* 1994; **14**: 4467–80.

93. Correa-Sales C, Rabin BC, Maze M. A hypnotic response to dexmedetomidine, an alpha 2 agonist, is mediated in the locus coeruleus in rats. *Anesthesiology* 1992; **76**: 948–52.

94. Nacif-Coelho C, Correa-Sales C, Chang LL, Maze M. Perturbation of ion channel conductance alters the hypnotic response to the alpha 2-adrenergic agonist dexmedetomidine in the locus coeruleus of the rat. *Anesthesiology* 1994; **81**: 1527–34.

95. Nelson LE, Lu J, Guo T, *et al.* The α_2-adrenoceptor agonist dexmedetomidine converges on an endogenous sleep-promoting pathway to exert its sedative effects. *Anesthesiology* 2003; **98**: 428–36.

96. Venn RM, Bradshaw CJ, Spencer R, *et al.* Preliminary UK experience of dexmedetomidine, a novel agent for postoperative sedation in the intensive care unit. *Anaesthesia* 1999; **54**: 1136–42.

97. Jones MEP, Coull MT, Egan TD, Maze M. Are subjects more easily aroused during sedation with the alpha2 agonist, dexmedetomdine? *Br J Pharmacol* 2002; **86**: 324P.

98. Huupponen E, Maksimow A, Lapinlampi P, *et al.* Electroencephalogram spindle activity during dexmedetomidine sedation and physiological sleep. *Acta Anaesthesiol Scand* 2008; **52**: 289–94.

99. Bonhomme V, Maquet P, Phillips C, *et al.* The effect of clonidine infusion on distribution of regional cerebral blood flow in volunteers. *Anesth Analg* 2008; **106**: 899–909.

100. Pandharipande PP, Pun BT, Herr DL, *et al.* Effect of sedation with dexmedetomidine vs lorazepam on acute brain dysfunction in mechanically ventilated patients: the MENDS randomized controlled trial. *JAMA* 2007; **298**: 2644–53.

101. Sakurai T, Amemiya A, Ishii M, *et al.* Orexins and orexin receptors: a family of hypothalamic neuropeptides and G protein-coupled receptors that regulate feeding behavior. *Cell* 1998; **92**: 573–85.

102. de Lecea L, Criado JR, Prospero-Garcia O, *et al.* A cortical neuropeptide with neuronal depressant and sleep-modulating properties. *Nature* 1996; **381**: 242–5.

103. Lin L, Faraco J, Li R, Kadotani H, *et al.* The sleep disorder canine narcolepsy is caused by a mutation in the hypocretin (orexin) receptor 2 gene. *Cell* 1999; **98**: 365–76.

104. Peyron C, Faraco J, Rogers W, *et al.* A mutation in a case of early onset narcolepsy and a generalized absence of hypocretin peptides in human narcoleptic brains. *Nat Med* 2000; **6**: 991–7.

105. Kushikata T, Hirota K, Yoshida H, *et al.* Orexinergic neurons and barbiturate anesthesia. *Neuroscience* 2003; **121**: 855–63.

106. Yasuda Y, Takeda A, Fukuda S, *et al.* Orexin A elicits arousal electroencephalography without sympathetic cardiovascular activation in isoflurane-anesthetized rats. *Anesth Analg* 2003; **97**: 1663–6.

107. Dong HL, Fukuda S, Murata E, Zhu Z, Higuchi T. Orexins increase cortical acetylcholine release and electroencephalographic activation through orexin-1 receptor in the rat basal forebrain during isoflurane anesthesia. *Anesthesiology* 2006; **104**: 1023–32.

108. Lydic R, Biebuyck JF. Sleep neurobiology: relevance for mechanistic studies of anaesthesia. *Br J Anaesth* 1994; **72**: 506–8.

M. B. MacIver

Introduction

Synapses form connections between neurons and provide important target sites for the actions produced by many drugs, especially those used in anesthesia. To modify activity of the nervous system – for example, during sleep, general anesthesia, or learning – requires some modification either of synapses or of neuronal excitability. Current evidence indicates that, of these two alternatives, synapses are the most important target for sleep modulators, for general anesthetics, and for memory. This chapter explores the physiology of synaptic transmission in the mammalian central nervous system (CNS). A basic knowledge of nerve cell structure is assumed, but the chapter nevertheless begins with a brief overview of the main events of synaptic transmission. A more detailed discussion of underlying processes then follows, and the chapter ends with a discussion of synaptic plasticity – i.e., the ability to alter the strength of specific synaptic connections, a necessary condition for establishing specific memories.

Since the original description of basic properties of synaptic transmission by Sherrington in the early part of the twentieth century [1], detailed mechanisms that underpin synaptic transmission have become clearer. In mammals, including humans, synapses often operate by secretion of a small quantity of a chemical (a neurotransmitter) from nerve terminals. These are known as **chemical synapses**. Some synapses operate by transmitting electrical currents to the postsynaptic cell through gap junctions between adjacent neurons. This type of synaptic transmission is known as **electrical** and these junctions neither slow action potential propagation nor exhibit the one-way transmission characteristic of chemical synapses. The importance of electrical synapses in controlling synchronized rhythmic EEG activity, and especially for synchronizing mammalian CNS inhibitory interneurons, has recently been demonstrated [2].

Systems physiology

Structure and function of electrical synapses

Gap junctions consist of specialized transmembrane proteins (connexins and/or pannexins) that form a transmembrane pore, coupling the cytoplasm of two connected cells. They allow bidirectional electrical and chemical communication between coupled cells. Electrical synapses can occur anywhere two adjacent membranes come into contact, but often involve axoaxonic coupling in pyramidal neurons, or dendrite-to-dendrite junctions in interneurons. Many inhibitory interneurons are connected by both electrical and chemical synapses to each other, thus allowing excitatory coupling via gap junctions and inhibitory coupling via chemical synapses [3].

Structure of chemical synapses

When axons reach their target cells, they form small swellings known as **synaptic boutons**. In the CNS, a single axon frequently makes contact with a number of different target neurons as it courses through the tissue. Such synapses are known as **en passant synapses**, and similar synaptic contacts also occur between autonomic nerves and their target cells. In other cases, an axon branch ends in a small swelling called a **nerve terminal**, which contacts its target cell (Fig. 14.1). The classical example of this type of synaptic contact is the neuromuscular junction (see Chapter 18). The terms *synaptic bouton* and *nerve terminal* can be used interchangeably, as their function is identical. The synaptic bouton or nerve terminal together with the underlying membrane on the target cell constitute a synapse. The nerve terminal is the presynaptic component of the synapse that is usually closely attached to the target (or postsynaptic) cell leaving only a small gap of about 20 nm between the two elements. This small gap is known as the **synaptic cleft**, which electrically isolates the presynaptic and postsynaptic cells. The synaptic boutons contain mitochondria, cytoskeletal elements, and a large number of small vesicles known as **synaptic vesicles**. Under the electron microscope these may either appear as small, round, membrane-delineated features lacking any electron-dense material in their center (as is the case for the majority of synaptic contacts in the CNS), or they may contain electron dense material of some kind. The latter are referred to as **dense-cored vesicles** and are typified by the noradrenergic nerve fibers of the sympathetic nervous system. The membrane immediately under the nerve terminal is called the

---

Anesthetic Pharmacology, 2nd edition, ed. Alex S. Evers, Mervyn Maze, Evan D. Kharasch. Published by Cambridge University Press. © Cambridge University Press 2011.

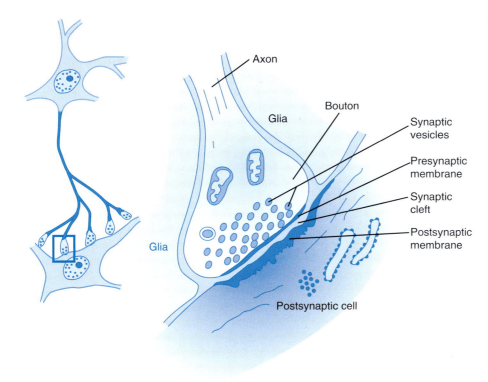

Figure 14.1. A schematic drawing of a central nervous system synapse. (*Left*) A neuron making a number of synaptic contacts with the cell body of its target cell. (*Right*) Enlargement of the area delimited by the square. The nerve terminal or bouton is shown ensheathed in glia and can be seen to possess a large number of synaptic vesicles and a number of mitochondria. The active zone is thickened, as is the postsynaptic membrane under the zone of synaptic contact. Reproduced with permission from Brodal P. [4].

postsynaptic membrane, and it often contains electron-dense material that makes it appear thicker than the plasma membrane outside the synaptic region. This is known as the postsynaptic thickening. The postsynaptic membrane contains specific receptor molecules for the neurotransmitter released by the nerve terminal.

Main stages of chemical transmission

Action potentials travel along the axon of the presynaptic neuron and invade nerve terminals, depolarizing them. This depolarization opens voltage-gated calcium channels, allowing calcium ions to enter the nerve terminal. The consequential increase in free calcium triggers the secretion of a neurotransmitter, such as acetylcholine (ACh), glutamate, or γ-aminobutyric acid (GABA), into the synaptic cleft. Neurotransmitter then diffuses across the synaptic cleft and binds to specific receptor molecules on the postsynaptic membrane. As a result, ion channels coupled to these receptors open and change the permeability of the postsynaptic membrane, modulating excitability of the postsynaptic neuron. Action potentials in the presynaptic neuron may lead to excitation or inhibition of postsynaptic cells according to the type of synaptic contact. If the transmitter directly activates an ion channel, synaptic transmission is usually both rapid and short-lived. This type of transmission is called fast synaptic transmission and is typified by the action of ACh at the neuromuscular junction. If the neurotransmitter activates a G-protein-coupled receptor, the change in the postsynaptic cell is much slower in onset and

lasts much longer. An example is the excitatory action of norepinephrine (noradrenaline) on α_1-adrenoceptors in peripheral blood vessels. The secreted neurotransmitter is removed from the synaptic cleft by diffusion, by enzymatic activity, or by uptake into the nerve terminals of surrounding glial cells. These events are summarized in Fig. 14.2. From this bare outline it is clear that synaptic transmission can be divided into two main stages: **presynaptic**, which is concerned with the mechanisms involved in controlling the secretion of the neurotransmitter, and **postsynaptic**, which is concerned with the processes that occur in the postsynaptic cell after the secreted neurotransmitter has bound to its receptor.

Chemical identity of neurotransmitters

To determine unequivocally the identity of a neurotransmitter responsible for synaptic transmission at a particular synapse is not a trivial matter. Any candidate must satisfy the following specific criteria:

(1) The substance must be synthesized and stored in the presynaptic nerve terminals, or the nerve terminals must be capable of its rapid synthesis from available precursors.
(2) The putative transmitter should be detectable in the extracellular fluid following a period of synaptic activation, and should show the same dependence on extracellular calcium as the synaptic response.
(3) Exogenous application of the putative neurotransmitter should mimic normal postsynaptic effects of activation of the synapse under consideration.

Labels: Axon, Bouton, Glia, Synaptic vesicles, Presynaptic membrane, Synaptic cleft, Postsynaptic membrane, Glia, Postsynaptic cell

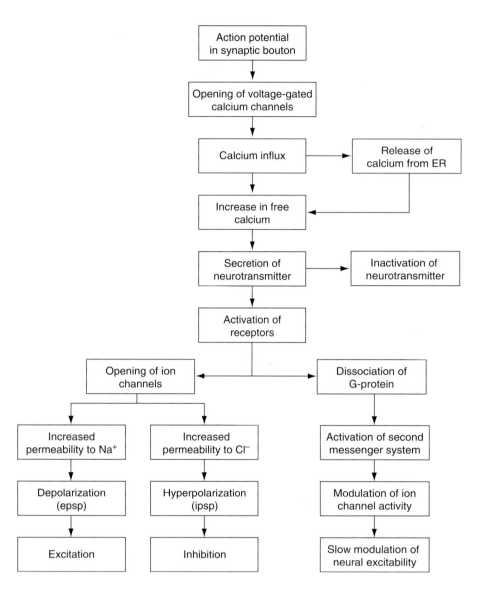

Figure 14.2. Flow chart summarizing the principal events of synaptic transmission. Postsynaptic events are summarized in the bottom half of the figure, with fast synaptic transmission on the left and slow synaptic modulation through G-protein activity on the right. ER, endoplasmic reticulum; epsp, excitatory postsynaptic potential; ipsp, inhibitory postsynaptic potential.

(4) Pharmacologic agents that modulate synaptic transmission should show similar effects on the action of the putative transmitter when it is applied artificially.

(5) There must be a means of inactivating the released neurotransmitter.

Nerve cells use a variety of neurotransmitters that can be grouped into six main classes (Table 14.1):

(1) Esters (e.g., ACh)
(2) Monoamines (e.g., norepinephrine, dopamine, and serotonin)
(3) Amino acids (e.g., glutamate and GABA)
(4) Purines (e.g., adenosine and adenosine triphosphate [ATP])
(5) Peptides (e.g., substance P and vasoactive intestinal polypeptide)
(6) Inorganic gases (e.g., nitric oxide)

At present, general anesthetics have been shown to act at multiple, agent-specific, pre- and postsynaptic sites to alter transmission at ester, monoamine, and amino acid synapses, but very little is known about actions at most types of synapses. It is likely that a better understanding of sites associated with specific anesthesia endpoints, such as loss of recall, loss of perception, loss of consciousness and blocking movement responses, will lead to safer anesthetics that target more specific neurotransmitter systems to reduce undesirable effects produced by the drugs in current use.

Dual transmission

Some nerve terminals are known to contain two different kinds of neurotransmitter. As a result, both neurotransmitters may be released when such a nerve ending is activated. This is called **cotransmission** or **dual transmission**. One

Table 14.1. Neurotransmitters and their receptors

Class of compound	Specific example	Receptor types	Physiologic role	Mechanism of action
Ester	Acetylcholine	Nicotinic	Fast excitatory synaptic transmission especially at neuromuscular junction	Activates ion channels
		Muscarinic	Both excitatory and inhibitory slow synaptic transmission depending on tissue, e.g., slowing of heart, smooth muscle relaxation in the gut	Acts via G protein
Monoamine	Norepinephrine	Various α- and β-adrenoceptors	Slow synaptic transmission in CNS and smooth muscle	Acts through G protein
	Serotonin (5-HT)	Various 5-HT receptors (e.g., 5-HT_{1A}, 5-HT_{2A}, etc.)	Slow synaptic transmission in CNS and periphery (smooth muscle and gut)	Acts through G protein
		5-HT_3	Fast excitatory synaptic transmission	Activates ion channels
	Dopamine	D_1, D_2 receptors	Slow synaptic transmission in CNS and periphery (blood vessels and gut)	Acts through G protein
Amino acid	Glutamate	AMPA	Fast excitatory synaptic transmission in CNS	Activates ion channels
		NMDA	Slow excitatory synaptic transmission in CNS	Activates ion channels
		Metabotropic	Neuromodulation	Acts through G protein
	GABA	GABA_A	Fast inhibitory synaptic transmission in CNS	Activates ion channels
		GABA_B	Slow inhibitory synaptic transmission in CNS	Acts through G protein
Purine	Adenosine	A_1 receptor	Neuromodulation	Acts through G protein
	ATP	P2X receptors	Fast excitatory synaptic transmission	Activates ion channels
		P2Y receptors	Neuromodulation	Acts through G proteins
Peptide	Substance P	NK_1	Slow excitation of smooth muscle and neurons in CNS	Acts through G protein
	Enkephalins	μ/δ-opioid	Slow synaptic signaling (reduction in excitability) Decrease in gut motility Promotes analgesia	Acts via G protein
	β-endorphin	κ-opioid	Slow synaptic signaling analgesia	Acts through G protein
Inorganic gas	Nitric oxide	Guanylate cyclase	Synaptic modulation	

AMPA, α-amino-3-hydroxy-5-methylisoxazole-4-propionic acid; ATP, adenosine triphosphate; CNS, central nervous system; GABA, γ-aminobutyric acid; GABA_A, γ-aminobutyric acid type A; GABA_B, γ-aminobutyric acid type B; NMDA, N-methyl-D-aspartate.

example of dual transmission is the parasympathetic nerves of salivary glands, which release both ACh and vasoactive intestinal polypeptide when activated. In this case, ACh acts on the acinar cells to increase secretion and vasoactive intestinal polypeptide acts on the smooth muscle of arterioles to increase local blood flow.

Cellular physiology

Storage of neurotransmitters in synaptic vesicles

Chemical analysis of nerve terminals isolated from the brain ("synaptosomes") has shown that they contain high concentrations of neurotransmitters. By careful subcellular fractionation, synaptic vesicles can be separated from other intracellular organelles of nerve terminals, and analysis of their contents has shown that vesicles contain almost all of the neurotransmitter present in terminals [5]. Thus, some form of transport mechanism must exist to concentrate neurotransmitter in the vesicles.

The mechanism responsible depends on the operation of two transporters. First, an ATP-dependent proton pump establishes a hydrogen-ion gradient between the cytoplasm and the vesicle interior, then a second transport protein exploits this proton gradient to accumulate neurotransmitter into vesicles [6]. Specific transport proteins have been characterized for vesicular uptake of ACh, catecholamines (norepinephrine and dopamine), the excitatory amino acid glutamate, and the inhibitory amino acid GABA. Vesicular transport systems permit the accumulation of high concentrations of neurotransmitter in vesicles. In cholinergic neurons, for example, the concentration of ACh in synaptic vesicles is about 0.6 M – over a thousand times more concentrated than in cytoplasm. It is unlikely that transmitter is present in free solution within the vesicle. To reduce the effective osmotic gradient across vesicle membranes, ACh is probably combined with a polyanionic matrix similar to the heparin–proteoglycan matrix of mast cells that binds histamine [7]. In addition to neurotransmitter, synaptic vesicles also contain ATP. The molar ratio of ATP/neurotransmitter varies from one neurotransmitter to another, being particularly high for catecholamines, in which the ratio is 1:3. The clear advantage of vesicular storage of transmitter lies in the ready availability of neurotransmitter for release. In view of high concentrations present in vesicles, discharge of a single vesicle in the synaptic cleft will increase extracellular concentrations of neurotransmitter to millimolar levels almost instantaneously.

Neurotransmitters secreted from synaptic vesicles are now often called classical neurotransmitters, to distinguish them from substances that are synthesized as required. An example of this latter type of transmitter is nitric oxide [8], which cannot be stored in vesicles because it rapidly diffuses through membranes.

Biochemical and molecular mechanisms underlying synaptic transmission

Mechanism of transmitter release

Secretion of neurotransmitter at a synapse is triggered by the arrival of an action potential at the nerve terminal. This process is calcium-dependent both in peripheral synapses [9] and at synapses in the CNS [10]. The entry of calcium is triggered by a depolarization-induced opening of voltage-sensitive calcium channels located in the presynaptic bouton. These presynaptic calcium channels are subdivided into N, P/Q, and R channels. Detailed analysis by Katz and colleagues of synaptic events occurring at the frog neuromuscular junction showed that neurotransmitter, in this case ACh, is spontaneously secreted at a low rate, giving rise to small random depolarizations of about 1 mV in the muscle membrane [11]. These small depolarizations are similar in time course to the main synaptic event, the endplate potential (EPP), and are called miniature endplate potentials (MEPPs). Normally, the EPP is very large and transmission between nerve and muscle is reliable. If, however, the extracellular calcium concentration in the solution is reduced and the motor nerve is stimulated with a steady train of impulses, the EPP will occasionally fail. During these conditions, the EPP fluctuates in amplitude from stimulus to stimulus in multiples of the amplitude of MEPPs. These findings led del Castillo and Katz to suggest that each MEPP is the result of secretion of a small unit of neurotransmitter or "quantum" [12].

Biochemical studies have shown that the amount of ACh in each vesicle is sufficient to account for the size of MEPPs, and synaptic vesicles quickly became the likely candidates for the origin of quanta. The idea developed that a presynaptic nerve terminal contained a large pool of vesicles from which there was a low probability that a single vesicle would be released. Depolarization by an action potential dramatically increases the chance of secreting a quantum of transmitter, and the simultaneous release of many quanta gives rise to the EPP. Thus the EPP depends on the size of individual quanta, the number of vesicles available for release (i.e., the number of release sites), and the probability of a quantum being released at a particular site.

This model of synaptic transmission is now widely accepted, and it is similar to processes occurring at CNS synapses. An important difference between the neuromuscular junction and central synapses is that nerve terminals of the CNS usually have just one release site. Because there is a finite probability that a particular release site is unable to respond to an action potential by secreting a synaptic vesicle, a CNS synapse is usually not activated by every action potential [13].

Control of vesicle secretion

Synaptic transmission depends on the nerve terminal releasing synaptic vesicles in an ordered fashion. In nerve terminals of the CNS, it is generally assumed that only one vesicle can be released per release site per action potential. The terminal itself holds many more than one vesicle, however: often close to a hundred. These vesicles must go through several steps to prepare for exocytosis. Although the number of steps and their specific nature remains unclear, they are generally grouped into three. These are known as *docking*, *priming*, and *fusion*, and all are driven by interactions between proteins found on both the plasma membrane and the vesicle membrane (which form the so-called SNARE complex).

There are three SNARE proteins, two of which, syntaxin and SNAP-25, are associated with the plasma membrane, and one, VAMP, with the vesicle membrane. The core SNARE complex also involves the ATPase NSF, its adapter protein SNAP, the Rab family of monomeric G proteins, synaptotagmin (the calcium sensor protein), synaptophysin, complexin, and VAP33. The core SNARE complex appears to represent the minimum machinery for vesicle fusion [14]. Docking reflects a linkage between the vesicle and release machinery of the plasma membrane. Priming, an ATP-dependent process, is the second step in readying a vesicle for exocytosis. This reflects a partial assembly of the SNARE complex that can then support rapid exocytosis once it is triggered [15]. Both these steps occur in advance of action potential invasion of the nerve terminal. The final step – fusion – is the exocytotic step. The vesicle moves the last few nanometers until it is in full contact with the plasma membrane, at which point the two membranes fuse together, creating an opening (the fusion pore) through which vesicle contents can diffuse out into the synaptic cleft. The trigger for vesicle fusion is thought to be binding of calcium to synaptotagmin [16].

Calcium regulation of neurosecretion

After a vesicle has been primed, it is ready to be secreted, and the step between priming and fusion with the plasma membrane is regulated by the calcium concentration in the presynaptic terminal. Several different types of calcium channels (N, P/Q, and R channels) exist in each nerve terminal. It is known that depolarization of nerve terminals leads to opening of voltage-gated calcium channels, but which of the subtypes of calcium channel are involved is known only for a few synapses. Initial studies on inhibitory postsynaptic potentials (IPSPs; see later) in spinal neurons and excitatory postsynaptic potentials (EPSPs) in hippocampal neurons suggested that N- and P-type channels mediate synaptic transmission [17]. Using synaptosomes isolated from rat brain, Turner and Dunlap showed that at least three channel types contribute to the secretion of neurotransmitter [18]. These are N, P, and a toxin-resistant channel (perhaps the R subtype described by Randall and Tsien [19]). In the hippocampus, synaptic transmission between CA3 and CA1 neurons is mediated by a combination of N-type calcium channels and Q-type channels [20]. N-type channels may even participate in the machinery for vesicle fusion discussed earlier [21]. What is striking is the absence of evidence implicating L-type and T-type channels in vesicle fusion, both of which contribute to the macroscopic calcium currents recorded from the cell body of neurons.

A major problem for the role of calcium as the trigger for exocytosis is the need for rapid on and off rates to ensure that individual action potentials control secretion in a discrete manner. Moreover, the increase in free calcium must occur in about 0.5 ms to account for the brevity of the synaptic delay at CNS synapses. The free calcium in nerve terminals must increase and decrease rapidly following invasion of nerve terminals by an action potential. Estimates made on synaptosomes suggest that free calcium in the resting nerve terminal is about 80 nM [22], but control of transmitter secretion requires that the binding site that regulates release of neurotransmitter must have a low affinity for calcium, in the micromolar region. (This requirement arises from the need to have fast on and off rates for calcium binding.) Thus the free calcium must increase more than 10-fold in about 0.5 ms. Such a large and rapid increase in intracellular calcium can occur near to open calcium channels, which suggests that these channels are associated with docked/primed vesicles [23].

The calcium dependence of vesicle fusion presents a problem, as MEPPs and their counterparts in the CNS (miniature EPSPs and IPSPs) can occur in the absence of extracellular calcium. This apparent anomaly can be explained if calcium stored within the nerve terminal can also trigger vesicle fusion. Recent experiments suggest that this is indeed the case. Discharging the internal stores of calcium with ryanodine or inhibiting the Ca^{2+} ATPase responsible for accumulating calcium into endoplasmic reticulum reduces the number of miniature synaptic events by more than 50%. Moreover, inhibition of calcium release from internal stores abolishes a form of short-term synaptic plasticity known as paired-pulse facilitation [24].

Vesicle cycling

As vesicles fuse with the plasma membrane, the surface area of a nerve terminal should increase. The surface area of a cell can be directly measured by its membrane capacitance; this was exploited by Breckenridge and Almers to follow the degranulation of mast cells, another form of vesicle fusion [25]. They found that, as predicted, capacitance increased as each granule fused with the plasma membrane. They also found that capacitance increased in discrete steps, as expected if each step represented the fusion of one vesicle. Subsequent experiments combined membrane capacitance measurements with the detection of secreted epinephrine by amperometry from chromaffin cells and showed that fusion of a single granule can be directly correlated with release of its contents [26].

The nature of the fusion pore remains a subject of debate, as does the fusion event itself. Is the pore made solely of membrane lipids (i.e., is it purely a product of two membranes coming together) or does it have a protein component? Do vesicles collapse into the plasma membrane (full fusion) or do they open a pore, stay attached for a limited time, and

Fast synaptic transmission in the central nervous system

Recordings from neurons in the CNS reveal a constant traffic of synaptic activity. The observed synaptic potentials are of varying amplitude, duration, and polarity. Those that decrease the membrane potential (depolarizing potentials) are excitatory postsynaptic potentials (EPSPs), whereas those that increase the membrane potential (hyperpolarizing potentials) are inhibitory postsynaptic potentials (IPSPs). EPSPs move the membrane potential toward the threshold for action-potential generation. Indeed, if they are large enough they will trigger an action potential. In contrast, IPSPs reduce the likelihood of an action potential occurring. Unlike action potentials, synaptic potentials sum with one another to provide a constantly changing membrane potential, and the balance between excitatory and inhibitory synapses plays an important role in determining neuronal excitability (i.e., the ease of generating an action potential).

Glutamate receptors and synaptic excitation

Fast excitatory synaptic transmission occurs when a neurotransmitter (e.g., ACh or glutamate) is released from presynaptic nerve endings and is able to bind to and open cation channels in the postsynaptic membrane. The opening of these channels causes the postsynaptic cell to depolarize for a brief time, resulting in an EPSP. A single EPSP occurring at a fast synapse reaches its peak value within 1–5 ms of the arrival of the action potential in the nerve terminal and decays to nothing over the ensuing 10–50 ms. In nerve cells, single EPSPs rarely exceed a few millivolts, although neurons may undergo large shifts in membrane potential during periods of intense excitation (Fig. 14.4A).

The membrane potential is determined by the distribution of ions across the plasma membrane and the permeability of the membrane to those ions. At rest, the membrane is much more permeable to potassium than it is to sodium and the membrane potential is therefore close to the equilibrium potential for potassium, which is about –90 mV in nerve cells. If, however, the membrane was equally permeable to both sodium and potassium, the membrane potential would be zero. Consequently, when a neurotransmitter opens a cation channel in the postsynaptic membrane, the membrane potential in the region close to the receptor approaches zero – i.e., the postsynaptic cell depolarizes. The degree of this depolarization depends on how many channels have opened.

The main excitatory neurotransmitter in the CNS is glutamate. This neurotransmitter can activate several different types of receptor. Those responsible for fast excitatory synaptic transmission are known as *ionotropic receptors* and are grouped into N-methyl-D-aspartate (NMDA) and non-NMDA types according to the agonists that activate them. These receptors are part of the same protein complex that makes up an ion channel. In addition, glutamate activates receptors linked to G proteins known as *metabotropic glutamate receptors*. The

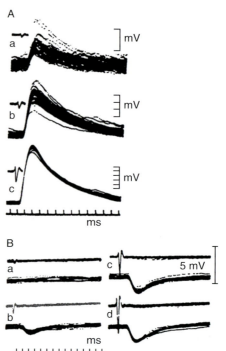

Figure 14.4. (A) Excitatory postsynaptic potentials (EPSPs) and (B) inhibitory postsynaptic potentials (IPSPs) recorded from spinal motoneurons. In each series, as the stimulus strength increases, the amplitude of the synaptic response becomes greater. Note the different voltage calibrations for the excitatory postsynaptic potential traces and the variability of the response at low stimulus strengths. Data from Eccles [41].

non-NMDA glutamate receptors are diverse in structure [42]. Those non-NMDA channels that are activated by the chemical α-amino-3-hydroxy-5-methylisoxazole-4-propionic (AMPA) are widespread in the CNS and are responsible for most fast EPSPs. These synapses can be inhibited by specific antagonists, of which 6-cyano-7-nitroquinoxaline-2,3-dione (CNQX) is the best known. When they are activated by glutamate, AMPA channels open and become permeable to small cations. This results in depolarization of the postsynaptic membrane and the generation of an EPSP. These receptor/channels rapidly inactivate so the response is of relatively short duration (10–50 ms).

NMDA receptors are activated by the agonist N-methyl-D-aspartate. Activation of NMDA receptors leads to depolarization generating an EPSP. The properties and time course of activation of NMDA receptors are, however, very different from those of the AMPA receptors. NMDA receptor channels are normally blocked by magnesium ions, but this block is relieved by depolarization. At synapses, glutamate first activates AMPA receptors and, if the resulting EPSP depolarization is sufficient, the magnesium block of NMDA receptors is relieved, resulting in the opening of NMDA channels. Inactivation of NMDA receptors is slow, so current flow through the channel is prolonged. Unlike most AMPA receptor channels, the NMDA channels are very permeable to calcium ions, and this property is important in synaptic plasticity (see below).

GABA$_A$ receptors and IPSPs

In the CNS, fast inhibitory synaptic transmission is mediated by GABA and glycine. Their receptors (GABA$_A$ and glycine receptors) are structurally related to nicotinic ACh receptors,

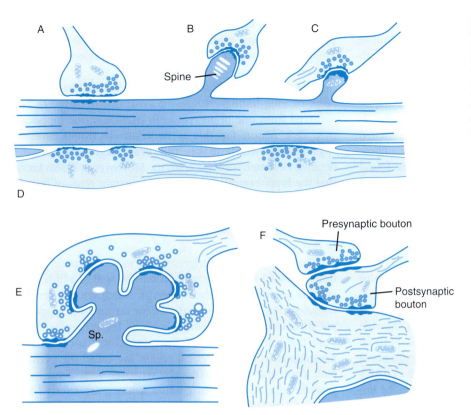

Figure 14.5. The principal kinds of synaptic contact made between neurons in the mammalian central nervous system: (A) contact between an axon terminal and the main shaft of a dendrite; (B) contact between a nerve ending and a dendritic spine; (C) en passant contact between an axon varicosity and a dendritic spine; (D) en passant boutons of an axon making contact with a dendrite; (E) a complex spine synapse; (F) an axoaxonic synapse (i.e., a synapse between two synaptic boutons).

with the important difference that the integral ion channels are permeable to chloride ions rather than to small cations. The opening of these channels causes the postsynaptic neuron to hyperpolarize, resulting in an inhibitory postsynaptic potential (IPSP; Fig. 14.4B). A single IPSP occurring at a fast synapse reaches its peak value within 1–5 ms of the arrival of the action potential in the nerve terminal. IPSPs are generally small in amplitude (about 1–5 mV). Nevertheless, they tend to last for tens of milliseconds and play an important role in determining the membrane potential and therefore the excitability of neurons. They appear to be an important target site for many general anesthetics, resulting in enhanced inhibitory transmission in the CNS [40].

Presynaptic inhibition

As illustrated in Fig. 14.5, synapses may occur between a nerve terminal and the cell body of the postsynaptic cell (axosomatic synapses), between a nerve terminal and a dendrite on the postsynaptic cell (axodendritic synapses), and between a nerve terminal and the terminal region of another axon (axoaxonic synapses). Axoaxonic synapses are generally believed to be inhibitory, and activation of an axoaxonic synapse prevents an action potential invading the nerve terminal of the postsynaptic axon. This leads to a blockade of synaptic transmission at the effected synapse. This blockade is called *presynaptic inhibition* to distinguish it from the inhibition that results from an IPSP occurring in a postsynaptic neuron (*postsynaptic inhibition*). Unlike postsynaptic inhibition, which changes the

membrane potential of the postsynaptic cell, presynaptic inhibition permits the selective blockade of a specific synaptic connection without altering the postsynaptic membrane potential.

GABA can also act on presynaptic GABA_B receptors, which are coupled to G proteins that act on calcium or potassium channels in the presynaptic terminal to reduce the influx of calcium and therefore reduce secretion of GABA, providing feedback inhibiiton. At some synapses (e.g., the varicosities of adrenergic nerve fibers), released transmitter also acts on its own presynaptic receptors to inhibit the secretion of more neurotransmitter by negative feedback.

Slow synaptic transmission

Fast synaptic transmission provides for rapid communication between neurons and, as we have seen, it depends on the direct interaction between neurotransmitter and receptor to open appropriate ion channels. In some situations, the excitability of neurons needs to be regulated over a period of seconds to minutes – for example during habituation to a constant but innocuous stimulus. This slow activation modulation of neuronal excitability is generally mediated by G-protein-coupled receptors which modulate the intracellular concentration of specific second messengers. Many neurotransmitters act on G-protein-coupled receptors (Table 14.1) to produce slow synaptic responses that are of great importance for control of such varied functions as cardiac output, the caliber of blood vessels, and secretion of hormones. Within the CNS, slow synaptic

Probably the clearest indication of the crucial nature of NMDA receptor involvement in the induction of LTP came with the demonstration that a selective NMDA receptor antagonist, AP5, blocks induction of LTP [50].

Long-term potentiation and second messengers

The high permeability of NMDA receptor/channels to Ca^{2+} gave a strong indication that an increase in intracellular Ca^{2+} was a key step in activating signaling cascades that ultimately give rise to LTP. The first demonstration of this came from Lynch *et al.*, when they showed that injecting the calcium chelator EGTA into postsynaptic cells blocks LTP induction [51]. This experiment illustrates that calcium is *necessary* for LTP induction; whether Ca^{2+} is *sufficient* to induce LTP was not, however, clear. In an attempt to address this issue, experiments were conducted with the photolabile caged Ca^{2+} compound nitr-5 [52]. On being exposed to ultraviolet light, nitr-5 liberates Ca^{2+}. By preloading CA1 cells with nitr-5, it was possible to rapidly increase intracellular Ca^{2+} by a brief flash of ultraviolet light. This approach revealed that LTP could be induced by an increase in intracellular Ca^{2+}, suggesting that Ca^{2+} is not simply *necessary* but also *sufficient* for LTP induction.

The critical role of NMDA receptors and Ca^{2+} in the induction of LTP at Schaffer collateral–CA1 cell synapses is now widely accepted. The calcium-activated processes that follow are much less well understood. Many kinase pathways have been implicated, including roles for protein kinase A, protein kinase C, protein kinase G, and tyrosine kinases. Currently, however, one pathway in particular is thought to have a pivotal role. This incorporates the Ca^{2+}/calmodulin-dependent protein kinase, CaM kinase II [49]. A number of properties of this enzyme make it an attractive candidate as the enzymatic target for increased intracellular calcium that accompanies LTP induction. First, the enzyme is found at extremely high levels within neurons, especially in the postsynaptic region of excitatory synapses. Second, the enzyme is activated by a calcium-binding protein, calmodulin, and it therefore has the capacity to sense increases in intracellular calcium. Third, the activity of this enzyme is regulated by autophosphorylation, so it remains active after calcium levels return to basal levels. This feature provides a mechanism by which a fleeting signal, the intracellular calcium rise, can be translated into a longer-lasting biochemical change, and as such may represent the "molecular switch" for LTP. Extensive experimental studies have implicated CaM kinase II in LTP. For example, the injection of selective inhibitors of CaM kinase II into individual CA1 pyramidal cells abolishes potentiation within 1 hour of the high-frequency stimulus being given. Correspondingly, injection of preactivated CaM kinase II slowly potentiates the cells into which it is added. Genetic approaches have also been used to examine the role of CaM kinase II. These experiments have included the generation of knockout animals that do not express the α isoform of CaM kinase II, the isoform found at high levels in the hippocampus. In these animals, stimuli that would normally induce LTP fail to do so. Finally, the induction of LTP produces an increase in the level of CaM kinase II in the autophosphorylated state.

Locus for the maintenance of long-term potentiation

A requirement for NMDA receptor activation, an increase in postsynaptic calcium, and a role for CaM kinase II strongly implicate the postsynaptic cell as the locus of expression for LTP. It is perhaps no surprise, therefore, that a number of models have been proposed that extend this chain of events to produce a mechanism that results in the enhancement of AMPA receptor function and thereby strengthened synaptic transmission. A number of these ideas have become firmly established as critical experimental observations have been made. These include the demonstration that CaM kinase II can phosphorylate AMPA receptors [53] and that AMPA-receptor-mediated responses are enhanced by CaM kinase II phosphorylation. The simplicity of such models adds to their appeal. There are, however, features of these models that do not adequately address all of what is known about LTP. For example, LTP lasts weeks in vivo, whereas a phosphorylation event is generally thought to be sustained for only hours. LTP is also known to be blocked by inhibitors of transcription [54] and translation [55], results consistent with the long-lasting nature of LTP. Such observations require one to look beyond post-translational phosphorylation of AMPA receptors to understand the full complement of mechanisms that underlie LTP.

Enhancement of AMPA receptor function is just one of a number of mechanisms by which synaptic transmission might be enhanced; there could also be presynaptic changes. During experimental conditions in which it was possible to monitor quantal release events, a number of investigations found that the induction of LTP was accompanied by a decrease in the number of failures of transmission [56]. This result is consistent with the idea that the probability of transmitter release increases with LTP; therefore LTP may also have a presynaptic expression mechanism. It has now become clear that that both pre- and postsynaptic loci can contribute [57].

Optical approaches for measuring presynaptic and postsynaptic components of LTP have also been used. Dyes such as FM1–43 provided a method by which the release of synaptic vesicles from the presynaptic terminal could be monitored both before and after the induction of LTP and demonstrated how the unloading of the vesicular marker dye FM1–43 was accelerated after induction of LTP. This supports the idea that maintenance of LTP has a presynaptic component. An optical approach to monitor postsynaptic responses at single synapses using entry of calcium into dendritic spines demonstrated that induction of LTP is accompanied both by an increase in the probability of transmitter release and an augmentation in the amplitude of the postsynaptic calcium transient. Thus LTP can have both a presynaptic and a postsynaptic component [58], and both components offer a number of possible sites of action for anesthetic-induced disruption, and hence, possible sites for blocking recall.

Retrograde messengers

Evidence supports the idea that LTP has a presynaptic component, yet since LTP induction is dependent on postsynaptic processes, it is necessary to consider the way in which these two loci communicate. One popular idea is that a molecule is generated by the postsynaptic cell in response to LTP induction, and this molecule diffuses in a retrograde manner across the synaptic cleft where it interacts with biochemical pathways that regulate transmitter release. There are now a number of candidate "retrograde messenger" molecules including nitric oxide, arachidonic acid, carbon monoxide, platelet-activating factor, and even the cannabinoid receptor agonist anandamide, which acts as a retrograde messenger at inhibitory synapses. Despite considerable effort, none of these molecules has been convincingly shown to be a retrograde messenger in LTP [59].

Silent synapses

A new difficulty in interpreting quantal analysis data was illustrated by the finding that NMDA and AMPA receptors are not always colocalized at a synapse. At some synapses within the CNS, NMDA receptors are found in isolation. Such synapses would be functionally inactive or "silent" at the cell resting membrane potential, as the voltage-dependent block by magnesium of the NMDA receptor would prevent current flow. To reveal the existence of such synapses, the cell membrane potential had to be experimentally manipulated (i.e., depolarized under voltage-clamp conditions) to reveal synaptically elicited currents that were not evident at the cell resting membrane potential. These currents were shown to arise from the NMDA receptor, as they are completely blocked by AP5. What has proved to be important about such synapses is that they can undergo LTP and an "unmasking" process follows the induction of LTP – i.e., AMPA receptors are thought to be inserted into the synapse, transforming it from a "silent" to an active form [60]. Evidence supporting activity-dependent trafficking of AMPA receptors came from the demonstration that the GluR1 subunit of the AMPA receptor can migrate to the cell membrane after induction of LTP [61]. The significance of these data for the debate about the relative importance of presynaptic and postsynaptic mechanisms in establishing LTP is clear. Unless it can be shown that a synaptic pathway contains no silent synapses, a decrease in the number of failures of synaptic transmission cannot be assumed to reflect a presynaptic increase in transmitter release.

Non-NMDA-dependent long-term potentiation

Although the NMDA receptor plays a critical role in the generation of potentiation at many synapses within the CNS, there are some synapses capable of showing long-lasting potentiation in which the NMDA receptor appears to play little or no role. For example, the mossy fiber synapses onto CA3 pyramidal cells show a form of LTP that is NMDA-independent. The first clear indication for this came from data obtained by Harris and Cotman showing that the NMDA receptor antagonist AP5 did not block potentiation at the mossy fiber pathway [62]. Furthermore, potentiation at these synapses does not require an increase in postsynaptic calcium. Calcium does appear to be the trigger for potentiation, because it does not occur if extracellular calcium is removed during inductive stimulation. Details of how the increase in presynaptic calcium serves to augment transmitter release are scant, although a protein kinase A second-messenger cascade has been implicated [63].

Long-term depression

The increase in synaptic strength that accompanies LTP can be *saturated* – i.e., a point is reached where a further increase in synaptic strength cannot occur. During such conditions, the encoding of new information by the brain might be compromised, and behavioural evidence exists to support this view [64]. An important feature of normal brain function might therefore include a process by which synapses can be selectively weakened. An activity-dependent mechanism able to achieve this has been described at the Schaffer collateral–CA1 cell synapses, and it is referred to as long-term depression (LTD). LTD reduces synaptic efficacy after a sustained period (10–15 minutes) of low-frequency synaptic stimulation. Experiments examining the cellular processes that underlie LTD reveal that it shares features in common with LTP: it is dependent on activation of NMDA receptors and requires calcium. The amplitude and temporal characteristics of the calcium increase are, however, different from those required to induce LTP, and it is these differences that are thought to permit the neurons to discriminate between LTP- and LTD-inducing stimuli. The biochemical processes that underlie LTD are to a degree opposite from those for LTP. For example, it has been shown that calcium-dependent phosphatases, enzymes that dephosphorylate proteins, are essential for LTD induction [65]. However, experiments exploring the mechanisms of LTD, like LTP, still have some way to go before the full complement of downstream processes and cellular targets is revealed.

Questions persist about synaptic plasticity: the locus of change that accompanies NMDA receptor-dependent LTP and LTD; the nature, or indeed existence, of the retrograde messenger(s); and the mechanisms by which LTP is maintained for periods extending to weeks. Why do different synapses have mechanistically different processes underlying the same change in efficacy? Perhaps most important of all is the question of whether the synaptic mechanisms described thus far really are processes by which the brain develops memories. Many features of these processes are highly suggestive of this possibility, and experiments comparing anesthetic effects on LTP and loss of recall in rodent models have also provided results consistent with this possibility.

Current and potential targets of drug action in synaptic transmission

Given the complexity of processes involved in synaptic transmission, there are many current and potential targets for anesthetic action [66,67]. These are exemplified nonexhaustively:

- **Synthesis of neurotransmitter** – The concentration of functional neurotransmitter can be reduced by inhibition of the rate-limiting enzymes responsible for their synthesis or by introducing a "false" substrate. Tyrosine is converted into dihydroxyphenylalanine by tyrosine hydroxylase, the rate-limiting enzyme in the synthesis of catecholamines. Competitive inhibition of this enzyme by α-methyl-para-tyrosine has been used in the treatment of pheochromocytoma. α-Methyl-dihydroxyphenylalanine (Aldomet; Merck, Whitehouse Station, NJ, USA) has been used in the treatment of hypertension through its action as a "false" neurotransmitter after it is converted to α-methyl-norepinephrine, which has almost no affinity for the α_1-adrenoceptor but relatively high affinity for the autoinhibitory α_2-adrenoceptor.
- **Storage of neurotransmitter** – Concentrating neurotransmitter into storage vesicles is an energy-dependent process. Therefore perturbations of the neuron's energy supply result in less stored neurotransmitter. The molecular pumps that concentrate neurotransmitter into vesicles could provide a useful drug target.
- **Vesicle secretion** – Vesicle secretion can be interrupted by calcium entry blockers, including specific channel toxins from conus snails, toxins acting on SNARE proteins (e.g., botox) and by a variety of anesthetics through mechanisms that appear to include presynaptic sodium, potassium, and calcium channels [66,67].
- **Vesicle cycling and endocytosis** – Currently, there are no useful therapeutic agents that target vesicle cycling and endocytosis.
- **Reuptake** – Several antidepressant agents (tricyclic antidepressants, selective serotonin reuptake inhibitors) as well as drugs of abuse (cocaine, "ecstasy") inhibit the reuptake of neurotransmitters.
- **Biotransformation of neurotransmitter** – The monoamine oxidase inhibitor class of antidepressants act by interrupting the biotransformation of neurotransmitter. These will have the effect of enhancing neurotransmission.
- **Neurotransmitter receptor agonists and antagonists** – Neurotransmitter receptors are clearly an important target for some anesthetics (e.g., as GABA receptor agonists or NMDA receptor antagonists) and adrenergic as well as acetylcholine receptors have long been important in anesthesia.

Summary

Synapses form connections between neurons and provide important target sites for many of the drugs used by anesthesiologists. There are two modes of synaptic communication between neurons: at chemical synapses one neuron secretes a chemical (neurotransmitter) which is sensed by another neuron; at electrical synapses adjacent neurons communicate by electrical signals transmitted through gap junctions. Chemical synaptic transmission can be divided into two main stages: presynaptic, which is concerned with secretion of the neurotransmitter, and postsynaptic, which is concerned with the response of of the postsynaptic neuron after the secreted neurotransmitter has bound to its receptor.

Specific neurotransmitters are responsible for synaptic transmission at a particular synapse. Neurotransmitters can be grouped into six main classes: esters, monoamines, amino acids, purines, peptides, and inorganic gases (Table 14.1). Some nerve terminals store and release two different kinds of neurotransmitters; this is called cotransmission or dual transmission.

Almost all of the neurotransmitter contained in a nerve terminal is localized in a structure referred to as a synaptic vesicle. Vesicles must go through several steps to prepare for exocytosis: docking, priming, and fusion. All are driven by interactions between plasma membrane proteins and proteins in the synaptic vesicle membrane. Docking reflects a linkage between the vesicle and the release machinery of the plasma membrane. Priming, the second step, is the partial assembly of the SNARE complex that can then support rapid exocytosis once it is triggered. Fusion is the exocytotic step during which the vesicle membrane comes in full contact with the plasma membrane and the two membranes fuse together, creating an opening (the fusion pore) through which vesicle contents can diffuse into the synaptic cleft. The step between priming and fusion with the plasma membrane is regulated by the calcium concentration in the presynaptic terminal. The fusion of the vesicular membrane with the plasma membrane increases the surface area of the secreting cell. This increase in surface area is counteracted by endocytosis, the pinching off and internalization of regions of membrane. Data linking exocytosis and endocytosis originated from electron-microscopic studies that showed evidence for vesicle fusion at sites directly opposed to postsynaptic folds, whereas membrane endocytotic budding was seen at more distant sites. There is increasing evidence that there are multiple pools of synaptic vesicles. The identification of discrete pools of releasable vesicles and reserve vesicles suggests there may be structural components within the terminal that sort vesicles, or a difference in identity (e.g., a protein marker) of vesicles.

Secretion of neurotransmitter at a synapse is triggered by the arrival of an action potential at the nerve terminal. Depolarization of the nerve terminal activates voltage-dependent calcium channels, which increases intracellular calcium concentration, triggering neurotransmitter release. The released neurotransmitters diffuse into the synaptic cleft, where they transiently achieve high local concentration, activating postsynaptic neurotransmitter receptors. Neurotransmitter concentrations in the synaptic cleft fall rapidly as a consequence of rapid enzymatic destruction, binding to sequestering proteins, reuptake into the secreting nerve terminals or into neighboring cells, and diffusion away from the synapse.

Fast excitatory synaptic transmission occurs when glutamate is released from presynaptic nerve endings and binds to and opens cation channels (glutamate receptors) in the postsynaptic membrane. The glutamate receptors responsible for fast excitatory synaptic transmission are known as ionotropic receptors and are grouped into N-methyl-D-aspartate (NMDA) and non-NMDA types according to the agonists that activate them. The non-NMDA channels are activated by the chemical α-amino-3-hydroxy-5-methylisoxazole-4-propionic acid (AMPA), are widespread in the CNS and are responsible for most fast excitatory postsynaptic potentials (EPSPs). At synapses, glutamate first activates AMPA receptors and, if the resulting EPSP depolarization is sufficient, magnesium block of NMDA receptors is relieved, resulting in the opening of NMDA channels.

In the CNS, fast inhibitory synaptic transmission is mediated by GABA and glycine. Their receptors (GABA$_A$ and glycine receptors) are permeable to chloride ions. Opening of these channels causes the postsynaptic neuron to hyperpolarize, resulting in an inhibitory postsynaptic potential. GABA$_A$ and glycine receptors are targets for many general anesthetics.

In addition to producing rapid, brief responses, chemical synapses can produce effects of greater duration. Slow modulation of neuronal excitability can be mediated by G-protein-coupled receptors which modulate the intracellular concentration of specific second messengers. Many neurotransmitters act on G-protein-coupled receptors to produce slow synaptic responses that are of great importance for control of such functions as cardiac output, the caliber of blood vessels, and secretion of hormones.

At many excitatory synapses the magnitude of synaptic response can be modulated and is said to show plasticity. Long-lasting forms of plasticity are thought to reflect the cellular basis of development, learning, and memory. Two processes, referred to as long-term potentiation (LTP) and long-term depressions (LTD), are thought to be essential early steps in synaptic plasticity. LTP has been shown to involve the activation of NMDA receptors; this occurs when a synapse receives multiple volleys of action potential leading to prolonged glutamate stimulation, postsynaptic depolarization, and the consequent release of Mg^{2+} blockade of NMDA.

The complex process of synaptic transmission is being unraveled for many mammalian systems. These processes appear to vary depending on the neurotransmitter involved, the type of synapse, and the brain region, and will require a systematic examination of anesthetic effects for each major type of neuronal pathway.

Acknowledgments

This chapter was modified from the equivalent chapter in the first edition, written by C. D. Richards, D. A. Richards, and N. J. Emptage. I thank Chris Richards for many years of leadership and guidance.

References

1. Sherrington CS. *The Integrative Action of the Nervous System*. New Haven, CT: Yale University Press, 1906.

2. Golebiewski H, Eckersdorf B, Konopacki J. Electrical coupling underlies theta rhythm in freely moving cats. *Eur J Neurosci* 2006; **24**: 1759–70.

3. Hestrin S, Galarreta M. Electrical synapses define networks of neocortical GABAergic neurons. *Trends Neurosci* 2005; **28**: 304–9.

4. Brodal P. *The Central Nervous System: Structure and Function*. New York, NY: Oxford University Press, 1992.

5. Whittaker VP, Michaelson IA, Kirkland RJA. The separation of synaptic vesicles from nerve-ending particles ('synaptosomes'). *Biochem J* 1964; **90**: 293–303.

6. Liu YJ, Edwards RH. The role of vesicular transport proteins in synaptic transmission and neural degeneration. *Ann Rev Neurosci* 1997; **20**: 125–56.

7. Rahamimoff R, Fernandez JM. Pre- and post-fusion regulation of transmitter release. *Neuron* 1997; **18**: 17–27.

8. Dawson TM, Snyder SH. Gases as biological messengers: nitric oxide and carbon monoxide in the brain. *J Neurosci* 1994; **14**: 5147–59.

9. del Castillo J, Engbak L. The nature of the neuromuscular block produced by magnesium. *J Physiol* 1954; **124**: 370–84.

10. Richards CD, Sercombe R. Calcium, magnesium and the electrical activity of guinea-pig olfactory cortex in vitro. *J Physiol* 1970; **211**: 571–84.

11. Katz B. *The Release of Neural Transmitter Substances*. Liverpool: Liverpool University Press, 1969.

12. del Castillo J, Katz B. Quantal components of the end plate potential. *J Physiol* 1954; **124**: 560–73.

13. Redman S. Quantal analysis of synaptic potentials in neurons of the central nervous system. *Physiol Rev* 1990; **70**: 165–98.

14. Weber T, Zemelman BV, McNew JA, *et al.* SNAREpins: minimal machinery for membrane fusion. *Cell* 1998; **92**: 759–72.

15. Chen YA, Scales SJ, Scheller RH. Sequential SNARE assembly underlies priming and triggering of exocytosis. *Neuron* 2001; **30**: 161–70.

16. Fernandez-Chacon R, Konigstorfer A, Gerber SH, *et al.* Synaptotagmin I functions as a calcium regulator of release probability. *Nature* 2001; **410**: 41–9.

17. Takahashi T, Momiyama A. Different types of calcium channels mediate central synaptic transmission. *Nature* 1993; **366**: 156–8.

18. Turner TJ, Dunlap K. Pharmacological characterization of presynaptic calcium channels using subsecond biochemical measurements of synaptosomal neurosecretion. *Neuropharmacology* 1995; **34**: 1469–78.

19. Randall A, Tsien RW. Pharmacological dissection of multiple types of Ca^{2+} channel currents in rat cerebellar granule neurons. *J Neurosci* 1995; **15**: 2995–3012.

20. Wheeler DB, Randall A, Tsien RW. Roles of N-type and Q-type Ca^{2+} channels in supporting hippocampal synaptic transmission. *Science* 1994; **264**: 107–11.

21. Degtiar VE, Scheller RH, Tsien RW. Syntaxin modulation of slow inactivation of N-type calcium channels. *J Neurosci* 2000; **20**: 4355–67.

22. Richards CD, Metcalfe JC, Smith GA, Hesketh TR. Free calcium levels and pH in synaptosomes during transmitter release. *Biochim Biophys Acta* 1984; **803**: 215–20.

23. Zucker RS, Fogelson AL. Relationship between transmitter release and presynaptic calcium influx when calcium enters through discrete channels. *Proc Natl Acad Sci U S A* 1986; **83**: 3032–6.

24. Emptage NJ, Reid C, Fine A. Calcium stores in hippocampal synaptic boutons mediate short-term plasticity, store operated Ca^{2+} entry and spontaneous release. *Neuron* 2001; **29**: 197–208.

25. Breckenridge LJ, Almers W. Currents through the fusion pore that forms during exocytosis of a secretory vesicle. *Nature* 1987; **328**: 814–17.

26. Chow RH, von Ruden L, Neher E. Delay in vesicle formation revealed by electrochemical monitoring of single secretory events in adrenal chromaffin cells. *Nature* 1992; **356**: 60–3.

27. Heuser JE, Reese TS. Structural changes after transmitter release at the frog neuromuscular junction. *J Cell Biol* 1981; **88**: 564–80.

28. Richards DA, Guatimosim C, Betz WJ. Two endocytic recycling routes selectively fill two vesicle pools in frog motor nerve terminals. *Neuron* 2000; **27**: 551–9.

29. Pyle JL, Kavalali ET, Choi S, Tsien RW. Visualization of synaptic activity in hippocampal slices with FM1–43 enabled by fluorescent quenching. *Neuron* 2000; **24**: 803–8.

30. Klingauf J, Kavalali ET, Tsien RW. Kinetics and regulation of fast endocytosis at hippocampal synapses. *Nature* 1998; **394**: 581–5.

31. Sankaranarayanan S, Ryan TA. Calcium accelerates endocytosis of vSNAREs at hippocampal synapses. *Nat Neurosci* 2001; **4**: 129–36.

32. He L, Wu LG. The debate on the kiss-and-run fusion at synapses. *Trends Neurosci* 2007; **30**: 447–55.

33. Schikorski T, Stevens CF. Quantitative ultrastructural analysis of hippocampal excitatory synapses. *J Neurosci* 1997; **17**: 5858–67.

34. Pieribone VA, Shupliakov O, Brodin L, *et al.* Distinct pools of synaptic vesicles in neurotransmitter release. *Nature* 1995; **375**: 493–7.

35. Eaton BA, Haugwitz M, Lau D, Moore HPH. Biogenesis of regulated exocytotic carriers in neuroendocrine cells. *J Neurosci* 2000; **20**: 7334–44.

36. Rupnik M, Kreft M, Sikdar SK, *et al.* Rapid regulated dense-core vesicle exocytosis requires the CAPS protein. *Proc Natl Acad Sci U S A* 2000; **97**: 5627–32.

37. Cole JC, Villa BR, Wilkinson RS. Disruption of actin impedes transmitter release in snake motor terminals. *J Physiol* 2000; **525**: 579–86.

38. Ryan TA. Inhibitors of myosin light chain kinase block synaptic vesicle pool mobilization during actin potential firing. *J Neurosci* 1999; **19**: 1317–23.

39. Birks R, MacIntosh FC. Acetylcholine metabolism at nerve endings. *Br Med Bull* 1957; **13**: 157–61.

40. Tanelian DL, Kosek P, Mody I, MacIver MB. The role of the $GABA_A$ receptor/chloride channel complex in anesthesia. *Anesthesiology* 1993; **78**: 757–76.

41. Eccles JC. *The Physiology of Synapses.* Berlin: Springer, 1964.

42. Hollman M, Heinemann S. Cloned glutamate receptors. *Ann Rev Neurosci* 1994; **17**: 31–108.

43. Brown DA, Adams P. Muscarinic suppression of a novel voltage-sensitive K^+ current in a vertebrate neuron. *Nature* 1980; **283**: 673–6.

44. Horn JP, Dodd J. Mono-synaptic muscarinic activation of K^+ conductance underlies the slow inhibitory postsynaptic potential in sympathetic ganglia. *Nature* 1981; **292**: 625–7.

45. North RA. Drug receptors and the inhibition of nerve cells. *Br J Pharmacol* 1989; **98**: 13–28.

46. Winegar BD, MacIver MB. Isoflurane depresses hippocampal CA1 glutamate nerve terminals without inhibiting fiber volleys. *BMC Neurosci* 2006; **7**: 5.

47. MacIver MB, Mikulec AA, Amagasu SM, Monroe FA. Volatile anesthetics depress glutamate transmission via presynaptic actions. *Anesthesiology* 1996; **85**: 823–34.

48. Bliss TV, Lømo T. Long-lasting potentiation of synaptic transmission in the dentate area of the anaesthetized rabbit following stimulation of the perforant path. *J Physiol* 1973; **232**: 331–56.

49. Lisman J, Malenka RC, Nicoll RA, Malinow R. Learning mechanisms: the case for CaM-KII. *Science* 1997; **276**: 2001–2.

50. Collingridge GL, Kehl SJ, McLennan H. Excitatory amino acids in synaptic transmission in the Schaffer collateral-commissural pathway of the rat hippocampus. *J Physiol* 1983; **334**: 33–46.

51. Lynch G, Larson J, Kelso S, *et al.* Intracellular injections of EGTA block induction of hippocampal long-term potentiation. *Nature* 1983; **305**: 719–21.

52. Malenka RC, Kauer JA, Zucker RS, Nicoll RA. Postsynaptic calcium is sufficient for potentiation of hippocampal synaptic transmission. *Science* 1988; **242**: 81–4.

53. Barria A, Derkach V, Soderling T. Identification of the CA^{2+}/ calmodulin-dependent protein kinase II regulatory phosphorylation site in the alpha-amino-3-hydroxyl-5-methyl-4-isoxazole-propionate-type glutamate receptor. *J Biol Chem* 1997; **272**: 32727–30.

54. Nguyen PV, Abel T, Kandel ER. Requirement of a critical period of transcription for induction of a late phase of LTP. *Science* 1994; **265**: 1104–7.

55. Frey U, Krug M, Reymann KG, Matthies H. Anisomycin, an inhibitor of protein synthesis, blocks late phases of LTP phenomena in the hippocampal CA1 region in vitro. *Brain Res* 1988; **452**: 57–65.

56. Stevens CF, Wang Y. Changes in reliability of synaptic function as a mechanism for plasticity. *Nature* 1994; **371**: 704–7.

57. Raymond CR. LTP forms 1, 2 and 3: different mechanisms for the 'long' in long-term potentiation. *Trends Neurosci* 2007; **30**: 167–75.

58. Zakharenko SS, Zablow L, Siegelbaum SA. Visualization of changes in presynaptic function during long-term synaptic plasticity. *Nat Neurosci* 2001; **7**: 711–17.

59. Thiagarajan TC, Lindskog M, Malgaroli A, Tsien RW. LTP and adaptation to inactivity: overlapping mechanisms and implications for metaplasticity. *Neuropharmacology* 2007; **52**: 156–75.

60. Liao D, Hessler NA, Malinow R. Activation of postsynaptically silent synapses during pairing-induced LTP in CA1 region of hippocampal slice. *Nature* 1995; **375**: 400–4.

61. Shi SH, Hayashi Y, Petralia RS, *et al.* Rapid spine delivery and redistribution of AMPA receptors after synaptic NMDA receptor activation. *Science* 1999; **284**: 1811–16.

62. Harris EW, Cotman CW. Long-term potentiation of guinea pig mossy fiber responses is not blocked by N-methyl D-aspartate antagonists. *Neurosci Lett* 1986; **70**: 132–7.

63. Weisskopf MG, Castillo PE, Zalutsky RA, Nicoll RA. Mediation of hippocampal mossy fiber long-term potentiation by cyclic AMP. *Science* 1994; **265**: 1878–82.

64. Barnes CA, Jung MW, McNaughton BL, *et al.* LTP saturation and spatial learning disruption: effects of task variables and saturation levels. *J Neurosci* 1994; **14**: 5793–806.

65. Mulkey RM, Herron CE, Malenka RC. An essential role for protein phosphatases in hippocampal long-term depression. *Science* 1993; **261**: 1051–5.

66. Pittson S, Himmel AM, MacIver MB. Multiple synaptic and membrane sites of anesthetic action in the CA1 region of rat hippocampal slices. *BMC Neurosci* 2004; **5**: 52.

67. Hemmings HC, Akabas MH, Goldstein PA, Trudell JR, Orser BA, Harrison NL. Emerging molecular mechanisms of general anesthetic action. *Trends Pharmacol Sci* 2005; **26**: 503–10.

Physiologic substrates of drug action
Memory, learning, and cognition

Robert A. Veselis

Introduction

Beyond consciousness, there is memory. Consciousness is necessary to perceive and process information from the environment, but memory allows survival in it. In fact, it may be argued that memory is a more fundamental property of nervous systems than consciousness. Consider the *Aplysia*, a sea slug with a simple nervous system whose connections are well described, often used in basic memory research. An *Aplysia* has memory – but does it have consciousness? At the other end of the spectrum from the simple memory systems found in invertebrates are those that underlie memory functions in humans. To a large extent these define us as being uniquely human – we can plan, we can project ourselves into the future, we can consciously modify our recollections [1]. Controversy surrounds whether the family pet possesses the same abilities [2]. Memory and consciousness intersect in numerous ways. From an evolutionary standpoint, the brain is likely to solve similar problems in similar ways. Thus, insights into understanding consciousness can illuminate memory function, and vice versa. Both are subserved by distributed networks of overlapping brain regions in constant, almost instantaneous communication with each other [3–5]. This form of communication is descriptively termed the "brainweb," information being transmitted by various properties emerging from the electrophysiologic interactions of large groups of neurons [6,7]. Thus, communication between brain regions is more complex than simple transmission along the axons of neurons. Simple knowledge of anatomical connections is not enough to understand memory function. Though anatomical figures are presented in this chapter, there is frequently no defined anatomical structure underlying a given memory function. Memory function is largely understood in a structure-free context, presented as taxonomies of memory systems (e.g. Fig. 15.1). Memory function in relation to the physical structure of the brain can be understood as an analog of the internet and the World Wide Web. The function of the internet, as well as memory, is dependent on what information is flowing through a given cable or deep brain tract at a particular moment, and what processes decode that information when it is received. An even better analogy for the brainweb may be wireless or satellite communications.

Though great insights into memory function can be obtained by careful study of memory function in animals, the transition to understanding human memory is multilayered in complexity. As the setting moves from human to living animal to tissue slice to synapse, this extrapolatability becomes ever more tenuous. One example is that of the process of long-term potentiation (LTP), the permanent modification of synaptic function on the basis of complex interactions between electrical signals, genes, proteins, and membranes [9]. LTP is induced in the laboratory by exogenous electrical stimulation which modifies synaptic connections in an experimental preparation of neurons [10]. Despite the suggestion that synchronous stimulation of neurons could modify synaptic connections in 1948, only recently has it been generally accepted that this is the basis of learning in animals, defined as the acquisition of new information from the environment into memory [11–13].

The functions of memory are diverse, ranging from those that are almost automatic in nature to those harnessed in creative pursuits. Such diverse functions are not subserved by a single, all-purpose system of memory. Though certain individuals argue for a grand unified system of memory, most investigators today support the concept that memory is composed of multiple, distinct systems [14]. The term *systems* does not imply anatomical structures in the brain per se. Nevertheless, a large portion of the evidence supporting distinct memory systems includes differing topographies (separate locations) of brain processes supporting different memory functions [15]. Frequently a given brain region is active in any number of distinct memory functions [16]. One way of measuring brain activity in humans is by recording the electrical activity of the brain (electroencephalogram, EEG) using electrodes that measure the electrical activity of a small portion of the brain's surface near the electrode. EEG activity is analyzed using well-described, though complex, methods that index communications between brain regions in the form of coherence or phase parameters. The response of neuronal

Anesthetic Pharmacology, 2nd edition, ed. Alex S. Evers, Mervyn Maze, Evan D. Kharasch. Published by Cambridge University Press. © Cambridge University Press 2011.

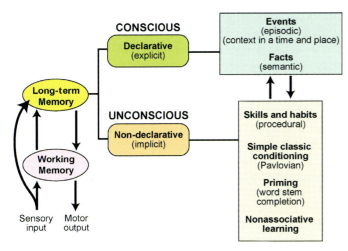

Figure 15.1. Sensory information from the environment is processed by consciousness and working memory before it is learned and becomes part of memory. Working memory also serves to organize motor output after retrieval from long-term memory. Working memory is not involved in the formation of unconscious memories. Depicted here is the most common conceptualization of the components of long-term memory (i.e., a taxonomy of memory), after Squire and Zola-Morgan [8]. Two major categories of long-term memory exist: conscious and unconscious memory. Conscious memory can be "declared" to be present, or to be true or false. The same is not true of unconscious memories. Procedural memory (skills and habits) is considered as unconscious, though it is closely related to conscious memory. The boundaries between memory systems are indistinct, and one form of memory can influence others, as shown by the arrows between the boxes on the right-hand side of the illustration. Nonassociative learning refers to habituation and sensitization. Classically, conscious memory depends on the integrity of the temporal lobes, whereas unconscious memory does not.

populations to an outside stimulus, such as a word or picture, is measured by event-related potentials (ERPs). ERPs are averaged EEG recordings time-locked to the onset of the stimulus in question. As more and more ERP responses are averaged, the common activity related to stimulus processing becomes larger, while other unrelated EEG activity is canceled out. What remains is the ERP waveform which represents activity of neuronal populations related to stimulus processing [17]. ERP waveforms that vary over different EEG electrodes define the topographical characteristics of underlying neuronal populations. Similarly, hemodynamic measures such as the blood oxygen level-dependent (BOLD) signal measured in functional magnetic resonance imaging (fMRI) accomplish similar goals. A significant portion of this chapter will be devoted to describing the nature of various memory systems, terminologies commonly used to describe these systems, and, most importantly, an understanding of the effects of drugs commonly used in anesthetic practice on memory.

Overview

As can be already appreciated, the topic of memory is vast. Memory research is a multidisciplinary effort, and to the extensive knowledge of memory function from the perspective of psychology, functional neuroimaging, electrophysiology,

receptors, cell networks, genetics, and molecular biology, the impact of pharmacologic agents on memory systems is now being added. This chapter can only provide a broad overview of current concepts, and is written with the critically interested anesthetist in mind. It is important to distinguish between temporary and permanent effects on memory function, the latter being of greater concern. Temporary amnesia is induced by all anesthetic drugs at certain concentrations, but by different mechanisms. Longer-lasting or even permanent effects on cognition and memory are different entities, represented by the states of delirium or postoperative cognitive dysfunction.

At the beginning of this chapter classic concepts and terminologies of memory function are reviewed. These are related, as best they can be, to key structures in the brain, which are the focus of much research. A simplified synthesis of memory function is then presented in which to understand the basic effects of anesthetic drugs on memory. Two major mechanisms of drug action on memory are reviewed in more detail. Sedation is contrasted with a different and more specific action of certain drugs on memory function. A particularly useful conception of memory, the SPI system, is presented. This system is useful to understand why certain drugs impair memory during consciousness, whereas at higher doses of many drugs, associated with unresponsiveness, learning of information can still occur. The parallels, or "nonparallels," between memory function in animals and humans are also considered. Much of the focus of memory research using animal models involves procedural and fear-mediated memory, whose anatomical underpinnings are well described and parallel those in humans.

Next, the mechanisms of action of drugs such as midazolam and propofol on human conscious memory are discussed. Recent research provides new insight into mechanisms of propofol's and midazolam's effects on memory, which are independent of sedation. These insights provide tantalizing prospects in the quest of relating the effects of anesthetic drugs on human memory to the vast knowledge of molecular processes of memory function. There follows a brief review of the opposing processes of consolidation and forgetting, which mold memories over time. Finally, the last major sections of the chapter provide a very brief review of changes in cognition and postoperative cognitive dysfunction, which occur in the clinical setting after surgery.

Memory in the perioperative period

A good starting point is to consider memory as being short- or long-term, unconscious or conscious (Fig. 15.1). Short-term memory is frequently equated with working memory, which is a process that holds and manipulates information for a short period of time before encoding into conscious long-term memory. The memory system that finds "where I left my keys" is long-term episodic memory, comprising the most human form of memory [18].

Episodic memory is, not surprisingly, the one most sensitive to the effects of anesthetic drugs. Memory can also be altered in the perioperative period by other, poorly defined factors. These changes in memory, not directly related to the presence of anesthetic drug, occur with delirium or another distinct cognitive state termed postoperative cognitive dysfunction (POCD). Cognition is a more general term than memory function, and includes other mental processes such as perception, attention, problem solving, mental imagery, emotion, self-awareness of one's thought processes (metacognition), and other related higher mental processes. Impaired cognition refers not only to impaired working or short-term memory, but also slowed processing abilities, disturbed perceptions about the environment, changes in mood, and so on. It is important to distinguish the acute effects of drugs on memory processes, namely amnesia for events in the operating room, and the potentially long-term changes seen in POCD. It is important to note that amnesia, POCD, and delirium are all separate entities. However, these can, and frequently do, overlap in the perioperative period. The rigorous study of the mechanisms underlying amnesia, delirium, and POCD has only begun recently. Thus it is not surprising that a detailed understanding of these entities is still lacking. An important question is whether anesthetic drugs administered in the perioperative setting only cause temporary amnesia, or whether, in combination with other factors present in the setting of surgery, there can be other, more permanent, influences on cognition.

Memory systems: fundamentals

Terminologies used to describe specific memory systems and their components are not rigorously defined. For instance, short-term memory means somewhat different things to a neuropsychologist testing a postoperative patient, a researcher using mice in a learning paradigm, and a cognitive psychologist studying event-related potentials in volunteers. Thus the descriptors of memory used in this chapter are to a greater or lesser degree nebulous. For the purposes of describing the effects of anesthetics on memory, a simple definition of memory (short or long, unconscious or conscious) becomes the starting point.

Conscious memories (closely related terms: explicit, declarative, episodic, semantic, autobiographical)

Conscious memories are those that we know we have, and that we can manipulate. For example, I remember seeing a friend last night, and I can imagine him or her wearing a particular item of clothing. I can enhance that memory, or I can actively suppress it [19]. This form of memory is referred to as *declarative* or *explicit* memory. The term declarative arises from the fact that these memories can be "declared" to be true or false,

or to have occurred at a particular time or place. Declarative memories can be divided into two broad categories, *contextual* memories and *general knowledge* memories. Contextual memories occur at a particular time and place (i.e., contextual information is a part of the memory), and are called *episodic* memories. It is this contextually rich memory remembered in a given time and place that is particularly affected by amnestic drugs [20]. Then there are memories that can be imagined (e.g., Paris in the spring), but where or when those particular memories of Paris or the meaning of spring were obtained are not known. Such knowledge of the world memories are *semantic* memories. These memories are not particularly affected by amnestic drugs. The temporal lobe is to a large extent the necessary, but not sufficient seat of those memories [21]. Distant long-term memories (e.g., first day of kindergarten) are termed *autobiographical*, as these are usually personally relevant memories (otherwise they are likely to be semantic memories) [22,23]. These are the conscious memories least affected by almost any intervention or disease, indicating that a widely distributed, robust system must support these memories.

Perception and working memory

Information from the environment must be perceived and processed before conscious memories can be formed. Many streams of sensory information are combined into a conscious image of the world called the *percept* [24]. How the brain does this is a fundamental question about consciousness, still not entirely answered [7]. Newly perceived information is held in a temporary store called *working memory* (though some refer to this as short-term memory). Information in working memory can either be transferred (encoded) into longer-term memory, or not. Memories in working memory disappear on the order of seconds, being replaced by newer information [25]. Working memory is thus of limited capacity, as demonstrated by the ability to remember and then write down a new seven-digit phone number, but not a new credit card number.

Unconscious memories (closely related terms: implicit, procedural, subliminal, priming, conditioning)

Unconscious memories are, as follows from above, memories we possess but have no conscious knowledge of. Unconscious memories are termed *implicit* or *nondeclarative* memories (they cannot be "declared" to be true or false, or whether in fact they are present). These most fascinating memories are learned unconsciously, and serve as the "workhorses" of surviving in a particular environment. Unconscious memories are formed without the involvement of working memory processes. Examples of such unconscious learning and influence include conditioning, therapeutic suggestion, emotional aversion, i.e., phobias, and subliminal advertising. The latter represents acquisition of information from a stimulus that is not consciously perceived, and is an example of a classic experiment demonstrating unconscious learning called *priming*. An item such as a word or picture is presented in such a way that no conscious memory of that item is formed, for example a picture of a face shown for a brief period of time, too short to be perceived distinctly. Within a certain period of time, reaction to a second, consciously perceived, presentation of that item is enhanced [26]. Enhanced reaction is seen in various fashions, such as faster response to that particular item, a preference for that item amongst other similar items (e.g., buying a particular brand of soft drink), or a correct completion of a partial representation of that item (e.g., a fuzzy picture that could be any face is identified as the subconsciously presented face). Relevant to anesthesia are correct completions of partial words (word stems) with words previously presented during general anesthesia [27]. This phenomenon has been demonstrated in a fairly large number of studies, with correct responses being slightly above chance guessing [28].

Procedural memory and conditioning

Similar to conscious semantic memories of world knowledge, there are unconscious memories of how to do things in the world – i.e., *procedural* memories such as playing a musical instrument. Though initially learned as conscious memories, these actions become semiautomatic and stereotypical. This explains the difficulty in, for example, playing a familiar piece of music starting at the third bar. The reader may wonder why procedural memories are "unconscious," especially as many conscious memories may surround learning a certain skill, such as driving. The reason so much learned discussion revolves around the true nature of memory is that we still do not know the true nature of memory. Indistinctness about the nature of memory comes to the fore the closer one gets to the boundaries between memory systems. Suffice it to say that conscious actions can influence unconscious memories, and vice versa. One of the biggest issues surrounding the example of word-stem completion after anesthesia mentioned above is "contamination" of experimental results by conscious influence [29]. Thus, more complex experimental paradigms have been developed to dissect out the influence of conscious from unconscious memory, such as the process dissociation procedure [30–32].

Procedural (motor) learning is mediated via the cerebellum, basal ganglia, and caudate regions of the brain (Fig. 15.2) [33,34]. A typical procedural skill used to study this form of memory is reading backwards from a mirror. Patients with damage to the basal ganglia (e.g., Huntington's disease) cannot acquire this skill, whereas patients with damage to the episodic memory system (e.g., Korsakoff's syndrome) do acquire this skill, yet have no memory of the material presented [35,36]. Procedural memory embodies Pavlovian conditioning, the classic experiment showing that dogs salivated

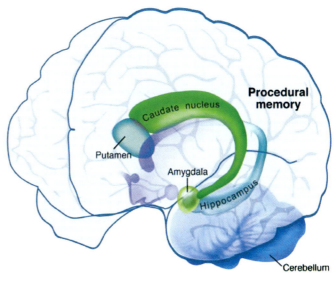

Figure 15.2. Procedural memory is mediated in different brain structures than conscious memory. Structures important in procedural memory include the cerebellum, amygdala, caudate nucleus, and putamen (basal ganglia). Procedural and conscious memory are closely related, with associated brain regions running along side by side from the medial temporal lobe to the anterior brain (Fig. 15.3). Both are influenced by the amygdala, which mediates fear and emotional influences on memory. Pavlovian and fear conditioning paradigms depend on procedural memory for learning. The amnestic effects of midazolam and propofol on this type of learning are mediated via the central nucleus of the amygdala. Whether the amnestic effect of these drugs on episodic memory in humans is also mediated in the amygdala still needs to be determined.

upon hearing a dinner bell previously learned to be associated with food. Conditioning is inherently dependent on the amygdala, the modulator of fear memory. Thus, conditioning is a "visceral" type of memory. For example, a rat quickly learns that a foot shock awaits him in an otherwise attractive environment such as a dark corridor. This type of learning, being mediated by the emotional memory system, i.e., the amygdala, demonstrates the strongest link between memory, anatomy, and animal/human behavior that exists. Emotional memories are mediated via the amygdala both in animals and humans [37]. As mentioned before, memory systems affect each other, and emotional influences on episodic memory are large and well known [38–43]. Emotionally laden episodic memories are more resistant to the amnestic effects of intravenous anesthetics [44].

Memory as a neuromechanistic process

In the past, memory was understood in terms of models of the mind, not necessarily related to brain structure. For a long time it was known that memory somehow resided in the brain, but no clear link to a specific portion of the brain was evident. That all changed in 1954 when an operation for the control of epilepsy excised a small part of the brain called the hippocampus [45]. Bilateral excision of the temporal poles resulted in the loss of the ability to form any new episodic memories. The dramatic changes in memory following the operation in this patient transformed the study of memory in humans to a

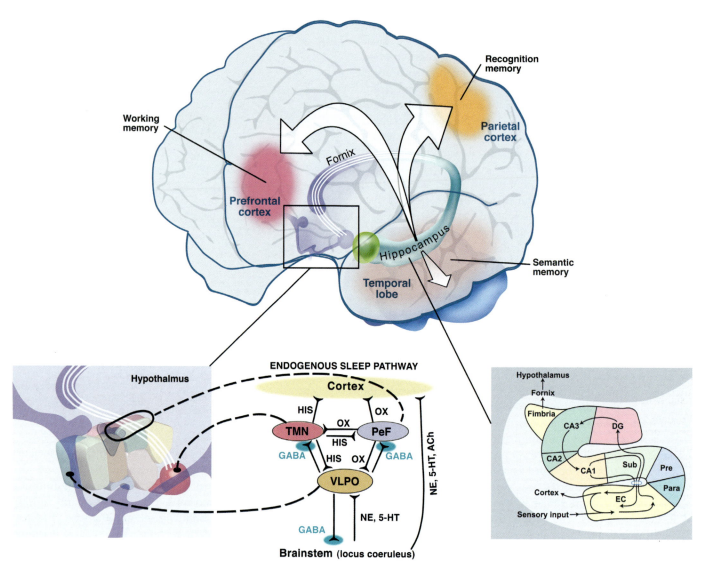

Figure 15.3. A neuromechanistic description of conscious memory in humans: conscious memory includes semantic and episodic memory. The hippocampus can be considered the seat of conscious memory, and it is located close to the amygdala, which modulates the influence of emotion and fear on episodic memory (the amygdala is located at the tip of the hippocampus: the greenish blob). The hippocampus communicates with widespread brain regions in support of episodic memory function. Working memory function is located to a large extent in the prefrontal cortex. Recognition from episodic memory involves the parietal cortex. ERP measures of recognition memory processes are shown in Fig. 15.7. A large amount of research has focused on the internal workings of the hippocampus. Input arises from close-by regions in the medial temporal lobe (entorhinal cortex, EC). Sensory input via the EC projects to the dentate gyrus (DG), the CA3 and CA1 fields of the hippocampus, and the subiculum (Sub) via the perforant pathway. The dentate gyrus projects to the CA3 field of the hippocampus via mossy fibers. CA3 neurons project to the CA1 field of the hippocampus, which in turn projects back to the subiculum. The subiculum feeds back to the EC. In the EC, superficial and deep layers are arranged to produce a recurrent loop for incoming sensory information. Some of this processed information is transferred to the hippocampus via the perforant pathways. In turn, after processing in the hippocampus, output influences information in the entorhinal reverberating circuit, which in turn repetitively activates the hippocampal formation, or is transmitted to other regions of the cerebral cortex. Pre, presubiculum; Para, parasubiculum. Based on Andersen [47] and Iijima et al. [48].

more neuromechanistic-based approach. This approach has exploded in the past decades, largely due to advanced research techniques ranging from careful study of the molecular basis of hippocampal function using genetic knockouts (animals missing a specific gene) to fMRI and ERP imaging of networks used in support of human memory function [46]. In many ways the hippocampus, and surrounding brain, can be considered as the seat of conscious memory. Quite naturally,

cellular and molecular investigations have focused on this particular brain region, as depicted in Fig. 15.3.

In this chapter, the cascade of processes put into motion after acquisition of information into memory, termed *consolidation*, is described in a simplified fashion. Two characteristics differentiate the vast number of consolidation processes; their location in the brain and the time period after learning during which they are active [49–51].

11. Hebb DO. *The Organization of Behavior: a Neuropsychological Theory*. New York, NY: Wiley, 1949.

12. Konorski J. *Conditioned Reflexes and Neuron Organization*. Cambridge: Cambridge University Press, 1948.

13. Leuner B, Falduto J, Shors TJ. Associative memory formation increases the observation of dendritic spines in the hippocampus. *J Neurosci* 2003; **23**: 659–65.

14. Tulving E, Schacter DL. Priming and human memory systems. *Science* 1990; **247**: 301–6.

15. Friedman D, Johnson R. Event-related potential (ERP) studies of memory encoding and retrieval: a selective review. *Microsc Res Tech* 2000; **51**: 6–28.

16. Cabeza R, Nyberg L. Imaging cognition II: an empirical review of 275 PET and fMRI studies. *J Cogn Neurosci* 2000; **12**: 1–47.

17. Johnson R. Event-related potential insights into the neurobiology of memory systems. In: Johnson RJ, Baron JC, eds., *Handbook of Neuropsychology*, vol 10. Amsterdam: Elsevier, 1995: 135–63.

18. Tulving E. Episodic memory: from mind to brain. *Ann Rev Psychol* 2002; **53**: 1–25.

19. Miller G. Forgetting and remembering: learning to forget. *Science* 2004; **304**: 34–6.

20. Ghoneim MM, Mewaldt SP. Benzodiazepines and human memory: a review. *Anesthesiology* 1990; **72**: 926–38.

21. Levy DA, Bayley PJ, Squire LR. The anatomy of semantic knowledge: medial vs. lateral temporal lobe. *Proc Natl Acad Sci U S A* 2004; **101**: 6710–5.

22. Burianova H, Grady CL. Common and unique neural activations in autobiographical, episodic, and semantic retrieval. *J Cogn Neurosci* 2007; **19**: 1520–34.

23. Cabeza R, St Jacques P. Functional neuroimaging of autobiographical memory. *Trends Cogn Sci* 2007; **11**: 219–27.

24. Mashour GA. Integrating the science of consciousness and anesthesia. *Anesth Analg* 2006 Oct; **103**: 975–82.

25. Lisman JE, Idiart MA. Storage of 7 +/ − 2 short-term memories in oscillatory subcycles. *Science* 1995; **267**: 1512–15.

26. Paller KA, Hutson CA, Miller BB, Boehm SG. Neural manifestations of memory with and without awareness. *Neuron* 2003; **38**: 507–16.

27. Deeprose C, Andrade J, Varma S, Edwards N. Unconscious learning during surgery with propofol anaesthesia. *Br J Anaesth* 2004; **92**: 171–7.

28. Ghoneim MM. Drugs and human memory (part 1): clinical, theoretical, and methodologic issues. *Anesthesiology* 2004; **100**: 987–1002.

29. Andrade J. Does memory priming during anesthesia matter? *Anesthesiology* 2005; **103**: 919–20.

30. Lubke GH, Kerssens C, Gershon RY, Sebel PS. Memory formation during general anesthesia for emergency cesarean sections. *Anesthesiology* 2000; **92**: 1029–34.

31. Lubke GH, Kerssens C, Phaf H, Sebel PS. Dependence of explicit and implicit memory on hypnotic state in trauma patients. *Anesthesiology* 1999; **90**: 670–80.

32. Iselin-Chaves IA, Willems SJ, Jermann FC, *et al*. Investigation of implicit memory during isoflurane anesthesia for elective surgery using the process dissociation procedure. *Anesthesiology* 2005 Nov; **103**: 925–33.

33. Ghoneim MM, Block RI, Fowles DC. No evidence of classical conditioning of electrodermal responses during anesthesia. *Anesthesiology* 1992; **76**: 682–8.

34. Ghoneim MM, El-Zahaby HM, Block RI. Classical conditioning during nitrous oxide treatment: influence of varying the interstimulus interval. *Pharmacol Biochem Behav* 1999; **62**: 449–55.

35. Cohen NJ, Squire LR. Preserved learning and retention of pattern-analyzing skill in amnesia: dissociation of knowing how and knowing that. *Science* 1980; **210**: 207–10.

36. Heindel WC, Salmon DP, Shults CW, Walicke PA, Butters N. Neuropsychological evidence for multiple implicit memory systems: a comparison of Alzheimer's, Huntington's, and Parkinson's disease patients. *J Neurosci* 1989; **9**: 582–7.

37. Cahill L, Babinsky R, Markowitsch HJ, McGaugh JL. The amygdala and emotional memory. *Nature* 1995; **377**: 295–6.

38. Cahill L, Haier RJ, Fallon J, Alkire MT, Tang C, Keator D, *et al*. Amygdala activity at encoding correlated with long-term, free recall of emotional information. *Proc Natl Acad Sci U S A* 1996; **93**: 8016–21.

39. Morris JS, Frith CD, Perrett DI, *et al*. A differential neural response in the human amygdala to fearful and happy facial expressions. *Nature* 1996; **383**: 812–15.

40. Cahill L, McGaugh JL. Mechanisms of emotional arousal and lasting declarative memory. *Trends Neurosci* 1998; **21**: 294–9.

41. Morris JS, Ohman A, Dolan RJ. Conscious and unconscious emotional learning in the human amygdala. *Nature* 1998; **393**: 467–70.

42. Kim JJ, Lee HJ, Han JS, Packard MG. Amygdala is critical for stress-induced modulation of hippocampal long-term potentiation and learning. *J Neurosci* 2001; **21**: 5222–8.

43. McGaugh JL, McIntyre CK, Power AE. Amygdala modulation of memory consolidation: interaction with other brain systems. *Neurobiol Learn Mem* 2002; **78**: 539–52.

44. Pryor KO, Veselis RA, Reinsel RA, Feshchenko VA. Enhanced visual memory effect for negative versus positive emotional content is potentiated at sub-anaesthetic concentrations of thiopental. *Br J Anaesth* 2004; **93**: 348–55.

45. Scoville WB, Milner B. Loss of recent memory after bilateral hippocampal lesions. *J Neurol Neurosurg Psychiatry* 1957; **20**: 11–21.

46. Sonner JM, Werner DF, Elsen FP, *et al*. Effect of isoflurane and other potent inhaled anesthetics on MAC, learning, and the righting reflex in mice engineered to express alpha1 GABA-A receptors unresponsive to isoflurane. *Anesthesiology* 2007; **106**: 107–13.

47. Andersen P. *The Hippocampus Book.* Oxford: Oxford University Press, 2007.

48. Iijima T, Witter MP, Ichikawa M, *et al.* Entorhinal–hippocampal interactions revealed by real-time imaging. *Science* 1996; **272**: 1176–9.

49. Abel T, Lattal KM. Molecular mechanisms of memory acquisition, consolidation and retrieval. *Vurr Opin Neurobiol* 2001; **11**: 180–7.

50. Izquierdo I, Bevilaqua LR, Rossato JI, *et al.* Different molecular cascades in different sites of the brain control memory consolidation. *Trends Neurosci* 2006; **29**: 496–505.

51. McGaugh JL. Memory: a century of consolidation. *Science* 2000; **287**: 248–51.

52. Sebel PS, Bowdle TA, Ghoneim MM, *et al.* The incidence of awareness during anesthesia: a multicenter United States study. *Anesth Analg* 2004; **99**: 833–9.

53. Veselis RA. Gone but not forgotten – or was it? *Br J Anaesth* 2004; **92**: 161–3.

54. Bullock A. *The Secret Sales Pitch: an Overview of Subliminal Advertising.* San Jose, CA: Norwich Publishers, 2004.

55. Veselis RA, Pryor KO, Reinsel RA, *et al.* Low dose propofol induced amnesia is not due to a failure of encoding: left inferior pre-frontal cortex is still active. *Anesthesiology* 2008 **109**: 213–24.

56. Veselis RA, Reinsel RA, Feshchenko VA, Johnson R. Information loss over time defines the memory defect of propofol: a comparative response with thiopental and dexmedetomidine. *Anesthesiology* 2004; **101**: 831–41.

57. Veselis RA, Reinsel RA, Feshchenko VA. Drug-induced amnesia is a separate phenomenon from sedation: electrophysiologic evidence. *Anesthesiology* 2001; **95**: 896–907.

58. Veselis RA, Reinsel RA, Feshchenko VA, Wronski M. The comparative amnestic effects of midazolam, propofol, thiopental, and fentanyl at equisedative concentrations. *Anesthesiology* 1997; **87**: 749–64.

59. Schwartz RH, Milteer R, LeBeau MA. Drug-facilitated sexual assault ("date rape"). *South Med J* 2000; **93**: 558–61.

60. Sebel PS. Memory during anesthesia: gone but not forgotten? *Anesth Analg* 1995; **81**: 668–70.

61. Schacter DL, Tulving E. *Memory Systems 1994.* Cambridge, MA: MIT Press, 1994.

62. Eichenbaum H. A cortical–hippocampal system for declarative memory. *Nat Rev Neurosci* 2000; **1**: 41–50.

63. Eichenbaum H. Hippocampus: cognitive processes and neural representations that underlie declarative memory. *Neuron* 2004; **44**: 109–20.

64. Blumenfeld RS, Ranganath C. Dorsolateral prefrontal cortex promotes long-term memory formation through its role in working memory organization. *J Neurosci* 2006; **26**: 916–25.

65. Ranganath C, Cohen MX, Brozinsky CJ. Working memory maintenance contributes to long-term memory formation: neural and behavioral evidence. *J Cogn Neurosci* 2005; **17**: 994–1010.

66. Munte S, Kobbe I, Demertzis A, Lullwitz E, Munte TF, Piepenbrock S, *et al.* Increased reading speed for stories presented during general anesthesia. *Anesthesiology* 1999; **90**: 662–9.

67. Deeprose C, Andrade J, Harrison D, Edwards N. Unconscious auditory priming during surgery with propofol and nitrous oxide anaesthesia: a replication. *Br J Anaesth* 2005; **94**: 57–62.

68. Alkire MT, Vazdarjanova A, Dickinson-Anson H, White NS, Cahill L. Lesions of the basolateral amygdala complex block propofol-induced amnesia for inhibitory avoidance learning in rats. *Anesthesiology* 2001; **95**: 708–15.

69. Dickinson-Anson H, McGaugh JL. Bicuculline administered into the amygdala after training blocks benzodiazepine-induced amnesia. *Brain Res* 1997; **752**: 197–202.

70. Alkire MT, Gruver R, Miller J, McReynolds JR, Hahn EL, Cahill L. Neuroimaging analysis of an anesthetic gas that blocks human emotional memory. *Proc Natl Acad Sci U S A* 2008; **105**: 1722–7.

71. Galinkin JL, Janiszewski D, Young CJ, *et al.* Subjective, psychomotor, cognitive, and analgesic effects of subanesthetic concentrations of sevoflurane and nitrous oxide. *Anesthesiology* 1997; **87**: 1082–8.

72. Ramani R, Qiu M, Constable RT. Sevoflurane 0.25 MAC preferentially affects higher order association areas: a functional magnetic resonance imaging study in volunteers. *Anesth Analg* 2007 Sep; **105**: 648–55.

73. Gonsowski CT, Chortkoff BS, Eger EI, Bennett HL, Weiskopf RB. Subanesthetic concentrations of desflurane and isoflurane suppress explicit and implicit learning. *Anesthesia & Analgesia* 1995; **80**: 568–72.

74. Ghoneim MM, Block RI, Dhanaraj VJ. Interaction of a subanaesthetic concentration of isoflurane with midazolam: effects on responsiveness, learning and memory. *Br J Anaesth* 1998; **80**: 581–7.

75. Nelson LE, Guo TZ, Lu J, *et al.* The sedative component of anesthesia is mediated by GABA(A) receptors in an endogenous sleep pathway. *Nat Neurosci* 2002; **5**: 979–84.

76. Nelson LE, Lu J, Guo T, *et al.* The α_2-adrenoceptor agonist dexmedetomidine converges on an endogenous sleep-promoting pathway to exert its sedative effects. *Anesthesiology* 2003; **98**: 428–36.

77. Fernandes MA, Moscovitch M. Divided attention and memory: evidence of substantial interference effects at retrieval and encoding. *J Exp Psychol Gen* 2000; **129**: 155–76.

78. Nordstrom O, Sandin R. Recall during intermittent propofol anaesthesia. *Br J Anaesth* 1996; **76**: 699–701.

79. Veselis RA, Pryor KO, Reinsel RA, Mehta M, Johnson R. Memory in the presence of Propofol or Midazolam – 30 seconds makes a difference. *Br J Anaesth* 2008; **100**: 879–80P.

80. Friedman D. ERPs during continuous recognition memory for words. *Biol Psychol* 1990; **30**: 61–87.

81. Wixted JT. A theory about why we forget what we once knew. *Curr Dir Psychol Sci* 2005; **14**: 6–9.

82. Anderson MC, Ochsner KN, Kuhl B, *et al.* Neural systems underlying the suppression of unwanted memories. *Science* 2004; **303**: 232–5.

83. Parker ES, Cahill L, McGaugh JL. A case of unusual autobiographical remembering. *Neurocase* 2006; **12**: 35–49.

84. Lynch MA. Long-term potentiation and memory. *Physiol Rev* 2004; **84**: 87–136.

85. Igaz LM, Vianna MR, Medina JH, Izquierdo I. Two time periods of hippocampal mRNA synthesis are required for memory consolidation of fear-motivated learning. *J Neurosci* 2002; **22**: 6781–9.

86. Shimizu E, Tang YP, Rampon C, Tsien JZ. NMDA receptor-dependent synaptic reinforcement as a crucial process for memory consolidation. *Science* 2000; **290**: 1170–4.

87. May A, Hajak G, Ganssbauer S, *et al.* Structural brain alterations following 5 days of intervention: dynamic aspects of neuroplasticity. *Cereb Cortex* 2007; **17**: 205–10.

88. Draganski B, Gaser C, Kempermann G, *et al.* Temporal and spatial dynamics of brain structure changes during extensive learning. *J Neurosci* 2006; **26**: 6314–17.

89. Crochet S, Fuentealba P, Cisse Y, Timofeev I, Steriade M. Synaptic plasticity in local cortical network in vivo and its modulation by the level of neuronal activity. *Cereb Cortex* 2006; **16**: 618–31.

90. Walker MP, Brakefield T, Hobson JA, Stickgold R. Dissociable stages of human memory consolidation and reconsolidation. *Nature* 2003; **425**: 616–20.

91. Dudai Y, Eisenberg M. Rites of passage of the engram: reconsolidation and the lingering consolidation hypothesis. *Neuron* 2004; **44**: 93–100.

92. Nader K. Neuroscience: re-recording human memories. *Nature* 2003; **425**: 571–2.

93. Kent C, Lamberts K. The encoding–retrieval relationship: retrieval as mental simulation. *Trends Cogn Sci* 2008; **12**: 92–8.

94. Ji D, Wilson MA. Coordinated memory replay in the visual cortex and hippocampus during sleep. *Nat Neurosci* 2007; **10**: 100–7.

95. Eichenbaum H. To sleep, perchance to integrate. *Proc Natl Acad Sci U S A* 2007; **104**: 7317–8.

96. Mölle M, Marshall L, Gais S, Born J. Learning increases human electroencephalographic coherence during subsequent slow sleep oscillations. *Proc Natl Acad Sci U S A* 2004; **101**: 13963–8.

97. Gais S, Albouy G, Boly M, Dang-Vu TT, Darsaud A, Desseilles M, *et al.* Sleep transforms the cerebral trace of declarative memories. *Proc Natl Acad Sci U S A* 2007; **104**: 18778–83.

98. Euston DR, Tatsuno M, McNaughton BL. Fast-forward playback of recent memory sequences in prefrontal cortex during sleep. *Science* 2007; **318**: 1147–50.

99. Clemens Z, Molle M, Eross L, *et al.* Temporal coupling of parahippocampal ripples, sleep spindles and slow oscillations in humans. *Brain* 2007; **130**: 2868–78.

100. Rasch BH, Born J, Gais S. Combined blockade of cholinergic receptors shifts the brain from stimulus encoding to memory consolidation. *J Cogn Neurosci* 2006, 2006; **18**: 793–802.

101. Canolty RT, Edwards E, Dalal SS, *et al.* High gamma power is phase-locked to theta oscillations in human neocortex. *Science* 2006; **313**: 1626–8.

102. Kirk IJ, Mackay JC. The role of theta-range oscillations in synchronising and integrating activity in distributed mnemonic networks. *Cortex* 2003; **39**: 993–1008.

103. Fell J, Fernandez G, Lutz MT, *et al.* Rhinal–hippocampal connectivity determines memory formation during sleep. *Brain* 2006; **129**: 108–14.

104. Fernandez G, Tendolkar I. The rhinal cortex: "gatekeeper" of the declarative memory system. *Trends Cogn Sci* 2006; **10**: 358–62.

105. Osipova D, Takashima A, Oostenveld R, *et al.* Theta and gamma oscillations predict encoding and retrieval of declarative memory. *J Neurosci* 2006; **26**: 7523–31.

106. Vertes RP. Hippocampal theta rhythm: a tag for short-term memory. *Hippocampus* 2005; **15**: 923–35.

107. Meltzer JA, Zaveri HP, Goncharova II, *et al.* Effects of working memory load on oscillatory power in human intracranial EEG. *Cereb Cortex* 2008; **18**: 1843–55.

108. Koene RA, Hasselmo ME. First-in-first-out item replacement in a model of short-term memory based on persistent spiking. *Cereb Cortex* 2007; **17**: 1766–81.

109. Lisman JE. Hippocampus, II: memory connections. *Am J Psychiatry* 2005; **162**: 239.

110. Miller GA. The magical number seven, plus or minus two: some limits on our capacity for processing information. *Psychol Rev* 1956; **63**: 81–97.

111. Montgomery SM, Buzsaki G. Gamma oscillations dynamically couple hippocampal CA3 and CA1 regions during memory task performance. *Proc Natl Acad Sci U S A* 2007; **104**: 14495–500.

112. Klimesch W, Hanslmayr S, Sauseng P, *et al.* Oscillatory EEG correlates of episodic trace decay. *Cereb Cortex* 2006; **16**: 280–90.

113. John ER, Prichep LS, Kox W, *et al.* Invariant reversible qEEG effects of anesthetics. *Conscious Cogn* 2001; **10**: 165–83.

114. Perouansky M, Hentschke H, Perkins M, Pearce RA. Amnesic concentrations of the nonimmobilizer 1,2-dichlorohexafluorocyclobutane (f6, 2n) and isoflurane alter hippocampal theta oscillations in vivo. *Anesthesiology* 2007; **106**: 1168–76.

115. O'Gorman DA, O'Connell AW, Murphy KJ, *et al.* Nefiracetam prevents propofol-induced anterograde and retrograde amnesia in the rodent without compromising quality of anesthesia. *Anesthesiology* 1998; **89**: 699–706.

116. Kozinn J, Mao L, Arora A, *et al.* Inhibition of glutamatergic activation of extracellular signal-regulated protein kinases in hippocampal neurons by the intravenous anesthetic propofol. *Anesthesiology* 2006; **105**: 1182–91.

117. Cheng VY, Martin LJ, Elliott EM, *et al.* α5GABA$_A$ receptors mediate the amnestic but not sedative-hypnotic effects of the general anesthetic etomidate. *J Neurosci* 2006; **26**: 3713–20.

118. Breitbart W, Gibson C, Tremblay A. The delirium experience: delirium recall and delirium-related distress in hospitalized patients with cancer, their spouses/caregivers, and their nurses. *Psychosomatics* 2002; **43**: 183–94.

119. Stagno D, Gibson C, Breitbart W. The delirium subtypes: a review of prevalence, phenomenology, pathophysiology, and treatment response. *Palliat Support Care* 2004; **2**: 171–9.

120. Alici-Evcimen Y, Breitbart W. An update on the use of antipsychotics in the treatment of delirium. *Palliat Support Care* 2008; **6**: 177–82.

121. Rudolph JL, Marcantonio ER, Culley DJ, *et al.* Delirium is associated with early postoperative cognitive dysfunction. *Anaesthesia* 2008; **63**: 941–7.

122. Newman S, Stygall J, Hirani S, Shaefi S, Maze M. Postoperative cognitive dysfunction after noncardiac surgery: a systematic review. *Anesthesiology* 2007; **106**: 572–90.

123. Newman MF, Kirchner JL, Phillips-Bute B, *et al.* Longitudinal assessment of neurocognitive function after coronary-artery bypass surgery. *N Engl J Med* 2001; **344**: 395–402.

124. Monk TG, Weldon BC, Garvan CW, *et al.* Predictors of cognitive dysfunction after major noncardiac surgery. *Anesthesiology* 2008; **108**: 18–30.

125. Moller JT, Cluitmans P, Rasmussen LS, *et al.* Long-term postoperative cognitive dysfunction in the elderly ISPOCD1 study. ISPOCD investigators. International Study of Post-operative Cognitive Dysfunction. *Lancet* 1998; **351**: 857–61.

126. Maze M, Todd MM. Special issue on postoperative cognitive dysfunction: selected reports from the journal-sponsored symposium. *Anesthesiology* 2007; **106**: 418–20.

127. Bedford PD. Adverse cerebral effects of anaesthesia on old people. *Lancet* 1955; **269**: 259–63.

128. Silverstein JH, Steinmetz J, Reichenberg A, Harvey PD, Rasmussen LS. Postoperative cognitive dysfunction in patients with preoperative cognitive impairment: which domains are most vulnerable? *Anesthesiology* 2007; **106**: 431–5.

129. Williams-Russo P, Sharrock NE, Mattis S, *et al.* Randomized trial of hypotensive epidural anesthesia in older adults. *Anesthesiology* 1999; **91**: 926–35.

130. Wan Y, Xu J, Ma D, *et al.* Postoperative impairment of cognitive function in rats: a possible role for cytokine-mediated inflammation in the hippocampus. *Anesthesiology* 2007; **106**: 436–43.

131. Culley DJ, Baxter MG, Yukhananov R, Crosby G. Long-term impairment of acquisition of a spatial memory task following isoflurane-nitrous oxide anesthesia in rats. *Anesthesiology* 2004; **100**: 309–14.

132. Eckenhoff RG, Johansson JS, Wei H, *et al.* Inhaled anesthetic enhancement of amyloid-beta oligomerization and cytotoxicity. *Anesthesiology* 2004; **101**: 703–9.

133. Xie Z, Dong Y, Maeda U, *et al.* The inhalation anesthetic isoflurane induces a vicious cycle of apoptosis and amyloid beta-protein accumulation. *J Neurosci* 2007; **27**: 1247–54.

134. Xie Z, Tanzi RE. Alzheimer's disease and post-operative cognitive dysfunction. *Exp Gerontol* 2006; **41**: 346–59.

Physiologic substrates of drug action
Mechanisms of pain transmission and transduction

Robert W. Gereau IV and Laura F. Cavallone

Introduction

The International Association for the Study of Pain (IASP) defines pain as "an unpleasant sensory and emotional experience associated with actual or potential tissue damage, or described in terms of such damage." Apparent from this definition is the concept that the perception of pain serves an important function – that of limiting tissue damage in the face of an injurious stimulus.

The detection of noxious stimuli (stimuli that are damaging to normal tissues) is carried out by a special subset of primary sensory neurons known as **nociceptors**. The activation of these nociceptors by peripheral stimuli is a sensory modality termed **nociception**. It is important to note that nociception can occur without eliciting the sensation of pain, and pain can be experienced in the absence of nociception. In this chapter, the organ and cellular physiology of pain and their underlying biochemical and molecular mechanisms are explained, while current and potential targets of drug action are presented in detail.

Systems physiology

Pain as a sensory system can be framed as three distinct processes:

(1) transduction
(2) transmission
(3) perception

However, anyone who has experienced even a simple ankle sprain or sunburn can also identify with a fourth process that is inherent and critical to the physiological role of this system:

(4) modulation

As mentioned above, the nociceptors are a subset of peripheral sensory neurons that are tuned for the detection of noxious stimuli. A simple "labeled line" view of the pain system would begin with **transduction** – the activation of nociceptors by a noxious stimulus. This activation generates action potentials in the nociceptor, leading to the **transmission** of this signal from the periphery to the central nervous system (CNS) via release of

neurotransmitter (glutamate and neuropeptides such as substance P) from the primary afferent onto second-order neurons in the dorsal horn of the spinal cord. Neurons in the spinal cord, either directly or through interneurons, then convey information to various areas of the nervous system that provide for the organization of reflexive withdrawal behaviors, the **perception** of pain itself, and the signals that generate learning cues for future avoidance behaviors.

Injury, disease, or experience can lead to dramatic **modulation** of pain perception. This modulation can occur in the periphery (peripheral sensitization) or within various areas of the CNS that comprise the pain neuraxis – a set of processes collectively termed *central sensitization*. In addition to the modulation of nociception produced by injury and disease, the transmission of nociceptive signals and perception of pain are subject to substantial endogenous modulation. Thus, affective state, attention, and cognitive factors can lead to substantial enhancement or suppression of nociception and/or pain perception.

In more anatomical terms, a discussion of the pain neuraxis must include a detailed understanding of at least four major components:

(1) primary afferent nociceptors
(2) spinal cord
(3) ascending pathways
(4) descending modulatory pathways

Primary afferent nociceptors

Nociceptors represent a diverse group of primary afferent sensory neurons that are variously tuned for the detection of a wide variety of potentially injurious stimuli including noxious heat, noxious pressure, tissue acidification, noxious cold, noxious chemicals, and many others.

Sensory neurons can be classified into four major categories based on the speed with which they are able to conduct action potentials (known as the conduction velocity, CV). These fiber types include the Aα fibers (CV = 80–120 m/s), Aβ fibers (30–70 m/s), Aδ fibers (5–25 m/s), and C fibers (0.6–2 m/s). The CV of an axon is impacted by the axon diameter, the extent of electrical insulation of the axon by the myelin sheath, and the

Anesthetic Pharmacology, 2nd edition, ed. Alex S. Evers, Mervyn Maze, Evan D. Kharasch. Published by Cambridge University Press. © Cambridge University Press 2011.

Table 16.1. Major types of primary sensory fibers

Type of fiber	Conduction velocity (m s^{-1})	Function of fiber
Aα	80–120	Muscle spindle afferent
		Golgi organ afferent
Aβ	30–70	G-hair, rapidly adapting innocuous mechano-sensitive
		Rapidly adapting nonhair innocuous mechano-sensitive
		Slowly adapting innocuous mechano-sensitive
Aδ	5–25	D-hair, rapidly adapting innocuous mechano-sensitive
		Slowly adapting innocuous mechano-sensitive
		Innocuous cold-sensitive
		Noxious mechano-heat-sensitive
		Noxious mechano-cold-sensitive
		Noxious mechano-sensitive
C	0.6–2	Slowly conducting innocuous mechano-sensitive
		Noxious mechano-sensitive
		Noxious mechano-cold-sensitive
		Noxious mechano-heat-sensitive
		Noxious mechano-heat-coldsensitive
		Noxious heat-sensitive "Silent" nociceptor

distance between nodes of Ranvier. Large, heavily myelinated axons conduct the fastest, while small-diameter unmyelinated axons conduct more slowly. Gasser and Erlanger showed in 1927 that fibers sensitive to innocuous stimuli include primarily the fast-conducting myelinated fibers (Aα and Aβ fibers) whereas fibers sensitive to noxious stimuli (nociceptors) were much slower-conducting, thinly myelinated or unmyelinated fibers (the Aδ and C fibers) [1]. Table 16.1 lists the various classes of primary afferent fibers, their conduction velocity, and the various functional properties of different classes of afferents.

Aα fibers originate from Golgi tendon organs or muscle spindles. Other afferent fibers originate from sensory organs or as free nerve endings in the skin, joints, or walls of various organs. These afferents are sensitive to various stimulus modalities, including thermal (heating and cooling), mechanical

(transient and/or tonic pressure), and various chemical stimuli. Fibers that respond to innocuous stimuli are generally responsive to only one stimulus type, whereas the nociceptors tend to respond to multiple noxious stimuli. This can include multiple stimulus modalities (e.g., noxious mechano-cold-heat-sensitive neurons: Table 16.1), as well as multiple chemical agents. Because of this quality, nociceptive primary afferents have been referred to as *polymodal nociceptors*. An additional group of C fibers are called *silent nociceptors*, because they do not respond to any physical stimuli under normal conditions. However, in the context of inflammation or other sensitizing conditions, these fibers can become responsive to various stimuli. These fibers may play a particularly important role in pain hypersensitivity that develops after injury. The mechanisms underlying the generation of this complexity of response properties of various primary afferents will be discussed in detail below, under *Biochemical and molecular mechanisms underlying cellular physiology*.

The spinal cord

The spinal cord is the site of the first synapses from nearly all primary afferent nociceptors. Nociceptive signals are transmitted to the CNS by synapses from nociceptor afferents onto several different populations of neurons in the dorsal horn of the spinal cord. These inputs serve to generate reflexive withdrawal responses and to transmit nociceptive signals to higher brain centers. In addition, the dorsal horn is a site of considerable descending modulation and local synaptic plasticity that can serve to inhibit or enhance pain transmission.

The organization of the spinal-cord dorsal horn includes three basic elements, as depicted in Fig. 16.1.

(1) Primary afferents synapse onto dorsal horn neurons.
(2) Dorsal-horn neurons generate two main outputs:
    (a) pathways to supraspinal sensory systems (perception, autonomic responses, affect, etc.);
    (b) pathways to motor neurons (reflex responses).
(3) Modulatory inputs from descending and propriospinal pathways influence the activity of second-order neurons in the dorsal horn, the primary afferent terminals that contact the dorsal horn, or both [2].

Considering these inputs and outputs, one can clearly see how disruption of synaptic transmission in the dorsal horn by an anesthetic drug would disconnect the upstream systems from both the external and internal environment and could contribute to immobility in the presence of noxious peripheral stimuli, both cardinal features of general anesthetics. This could occur via inhibition of excitatory transmission, enhancement of inhibitory transmission, or both, and could occur at pre- and/or postsynaptic sites. Details of sites of actions of general and local anesthetics will be discussed later in this chapter.

The subdivision of the spinal cord into 10 distinct cytoarchitectonic layers was described in the 1950s by Bror Rexed [3]. The dorsal horn, including Rexed's laminae I–VI, is rich in synaptic input from primary afferents and second-order neurons. Lamina X is also rich in nociceptive input, particularly from the viscera. Early studies of the dorsal horn posited that the different laminae subserved different classes of sensory input. Lamina IV was thought to receive inputs only from low-threshold neurons, lamina V only from nociceptors, etc. Although our knowledge of dorsal-horn circuitry is still woefully lacking, we now know that these assumptions were incorrect. Nevertheless, the great majority of sensory information regarding an animal's external and internal environment is processed at the first synapse between the primary afferent sensory neuron and a second-order neuron in the dorsal horn of the spinal cord.

Primary afferent nociceptors enter the dorsal horn of the spinal cord, where they synapse primarily in lamina I and lamina II, with additional inputs from Aδ and C fibers in

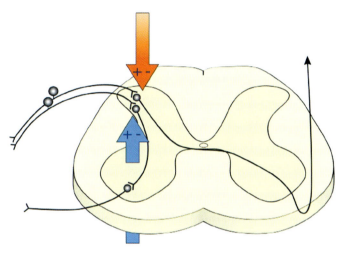

Figure 16.1. Schematic illustrating the main components of information flow through the spinal dorsal horn. Synapses between primary afferents and second-order neurons in the spinal dorsal horn are the site of information transfer from the peripheral nervous system to the central nervous system. This important center of sensory integration is influenced by propriospinal (blue) and descending supraspinal systems (orange). Integrated information is then forwarded to motor systems in the ventral horn that are involved in generation of reflex responses, and to supraspinal sites involved in pain perception.

lamina V. Aα and Aβ fibers, by contrast, synapse primarily in laminae III, IV, and V, with some inputs to lamina II. This represents a substantial oversimplification of the inputs to the dorsal horn, but serves as a useful starting point (Fig. 16.2). Recent studies have described substantial subspecialization of lamina II based on the specific subsets of nociceptors that provide input [4,5]. These studies suggest that lamina II can be divided into at least three distinct sublayers, as discussed in detail later in this chapter. Although the functional significance of this subspecialization is not fully understood, it is clear that this region of the cord, which is highly specialized for nociception, represents a functional diversity that is sure to be of substantial importance to the complexity of nociception and its modulation – both by disease states and by the actions of drugs such as anesthetics.

Ascending pathways

Neurons that project to higher centers from the cord are not uniformly distributed throughout the dorsal horn. These *projection neurons* are found in relative abundance in lamina I, are essentially absent from lamina II, and are present throughout the remainder of the dorsal horn at relatively low density [6]. Pain transmission from the spinal cord to supraspinal sites occurs predominantly via the following three pathways:

(1) The **spinothalamic tract** (STT) originates in cells within lamina I, in the deep dorsal horn (laminae IV–V) and in the intermediate zone and ventral horn (laminae VII–VIII). Lamina I neurons receive input from Aδ and C fibers, and generally convey information about pain, temperature, and itch. These cells can be nociceptive-specific, polymodal, or activated only by temperature (warming or cooling). STT neurons from laminae IV–V receive monosynaptic input from nociceptive Aδ fibers and polysynaptic input from C fibers from cutaneous, muscular, and visceral end organs. Most of these cells are called *wide dynamic range* (WDR) neurons because they respond to both innocuous and noxious stimuli.

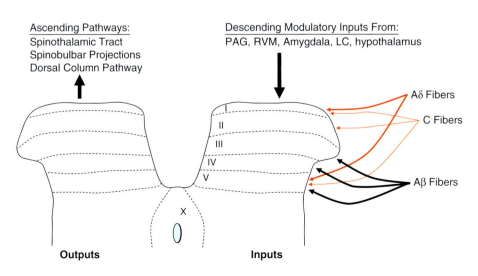

Ascending Pathways:
Spinothalamic Tract
Spinobulbar Projections
Dorsal Column Pathway

Descending Modulatory Inputs From:
PAG, RVM, Amygdala, LC, hypothalamus

Aδ Fibers
C Fibers
Aβ Fibers

Outputs

Inputs

Figure 16.2. Schematic of the spinal-cord dorsal horn, showing the approximate location of subdivisions between the laminae of Rexed (dotted lines, Rexed's laminae indicated in roman numerals). Also shown are the major sources of primary afferent input to the dorsal horn from Aδ fibers (thick red arrows), C fibers (thin red arrows), and Aβ fibers (thick black arrows), as well as the major sources of descending modulatory inputs and the major ascending output pathways from the nociceptive dorsal horn.

Laminae VII–VIII cells can respond to innocuous or noxious stimuli and have very large receptive fields which can be bilateral. Axons of the STT generally cross in spinal commissures to ascend in anterior or lateral funiculi. These fibers then synapse in several nuclei of the thalamus, most notably the posterior portion of the ventral medial nucleus and the ventrolateral, ventroposterior, and centrolateral nuclei, the ventral caudal portion of the medial dorsal nucleus, and the parafascicular nucleus.

(2) Projections from the spinal cord to the brainstem (**spinobulbar projections**) serve to provide nociceptive input to homeostatic control centers, but also serve to convey nociceptive information to forebrain regions such as the amygdala that are involved in affective components of pain. The main spinobulbar projections terminate in the parabrachial nucleus, the periaqueductal gray (PAG), the brainstem reticular formation, and the catecholamine-containing cell groups. The cells of origin for the spinobulbar projections are very similar – both in terms of location and response characteristics – to those of the cells that comprise the STT.

(3) Some nociceptive input, especially that from visceral structures, can also ascend via a specialized **dorsal column pathway**. In this system, branches of primary afferents, together with axons of postsynaptic dorsal column neurons originating in laminae IV–VI and X, ascend in the dorsal columns where they synapse with postsynaptic neurons (second or third order) in dorsal column nuclei (gracile and cuneate nuclei). The axons of these neurons then cross and ascend in the medial lemniscus to the ventral posterolateral nucleus (VPL) [7].

These pathways are shown in Fig. 16.3.

There are also several publications that suggest the presence of a spinohypothalamic tract that originates bilaterally from neurons in laminae I, V, VII, and X [8], as well as a direct projection pathway from the spinal cord to the central nucleus of the amygdala [9]. For a more detailed description of all of these ascending pain pathways, the reader is directed to an excellent treatment by Dostrovsky and Craig [10].

Beyond these first connections of the ascending pathways, functional imaging studies using PET and fMRI have identified several major sites of pain integration in the cortex. These areas include the primary and secondary somatosensory cortices (S1 and S2), the anterior cingulate cortex (ACC), and the insula. Pain-related activation of subcortical structures including the amygdala, PAG, hypothalamus, and other regions has also been reported.

Descending modulatory pathways

In 1969, a seminal paper by Reynolds demonstrated that stimulation of a midbrain site (the PAG) in the rat produced analgesia sufficient to allow pain-free surgery [11]. This finding, together with studies a few years later demonstrating the presence of an endogenous opioid system [12,13], led to decades of research that have demonstrated the presence of profoundly important descending pathways that mediate endogenous pain regulation.

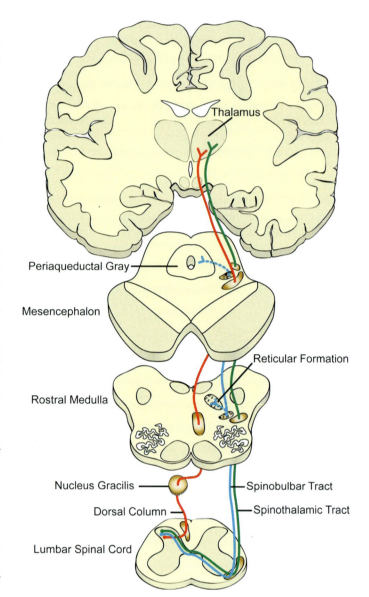

Figure 16.3. The major ascending pain pathways. This schematic drawing of the pain neuraxis shows the three main pathways by which nociceptive signals reach higher brain centers. The spinothalamic tract (*green*) carries information from the spinal dorsal horn and ascends through the anterolateral fasciculus to the thalamus. Thalamic relays will subsequently send projections to somatosensory cortex, anterior cingulate cortex and other brain centers. The dorsal column pathway (*red*) carries information primarily from visceral afferents and ascends through the dorsal column to the nucleus gracilis and nucleus cuneatus where the fibers cross and ascend through the contralateral medial lemniscus to the VPL. The spinobulbar tract (*blue*) carries nociceptive information to brainstem regions such as the periaqueductal gray and the reticular formation. Additional major projections to the parabrachial area are not shown here.

We now know that descending systems can be either antinociceptive or pronociceptive, as described below [14].

In addition to the PAG, stimulation of the rostroventromedial medulla (RVM, including both the midline nucleus raphe magnus and the adjacent reticular formation) can also elicit analgesia. These descending inhibitory systems seem to depend on serotonergic, muscarinic, and noradrenergic inputs

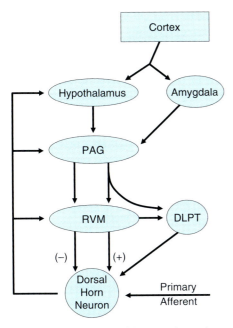

Figure 16.4. Schematic of the major descending pain modulatory circuitry. The periaqueductal gray (PAG) receives inputs from the cortex (via the hypothalamus) and amygdala, and the PAG in turn projects to the rostroventromedial medulla (RVM) and the dorsolateral pontine tegmentum (DLPT). The RVM and DLPT provide both pro- and antinociceptive descending input via the dorsolateral funiculus to the dorsal horn. Inputs to the dorsal horn from the RVM include both serotonergic and nonserotonergic fibers, while inputs from the DLPT are noradrenergic. These centers also receive ascending information from nociceptive neurons in the dorsal horn, and thus this system can function as an ascending/descending loop, with modulation of the descending input by higher centers.

to the dorsal horn. Analgesic effects of PAG stimulation are mediated via its effects on the RVM, such that inactivating the RVM prevents PAG-mediated analgesia. Various anatomical studies have led to the conclusion that the PAG and RVM are part of a larger descending pain modulatory system, as represented schematically in Fig. 16.4 [14,15]. This descending network is also involved in the analgesic actions of opioids. Thus, profound analgesia can be induced by localized injection of opioids into the PAG or RVM, as well as the amygdala.

In addition to this strong descending inhibition, early work by Zhuo and Gebhart pointed to a parallel pain-facilitating pathway originating in the RVM. Thus, stimulation in some parts of the RVM led to facilitation of the tail-flick reflex in rats – an effect that was found to be mediated by descending serotonergic fibers [16]. Subsequent studies have identified an important role for these descending facilatory inputs in maintaining pain hypersensitivity in a variety of inflammatory and neuropathic pain models. Some evidence points to a particular involvement of serotonergic descending fibers from the RVM and subsequent activation of spinal 5-HT$_3$ receptors in mediating this descending pain facilitating pathway [15]. These descending inhibitory and facilatory pathways are immensely important in modulating the overall amount of pain experienced by an organism as a result of internal and external factors.

Organ physiology

Unconscious nociceptive activity (activation of nociceptors) is at the origin of **nociceptive pain** (the term *pain* implies conscious elaboration). Nociceptive pain may originate from any tissue in the body that is innervated by nociceptors, and needs to be distinguished from **neuropathic pain**, which originates from injuries that occur within the peripheral or central nervous system.

Two distinct types of nociception exist, **somatic nociception** (superficial and deep) and **visceral nociception**, depending on the anatomical structures where the activation of peripheral nociceptors occurs, and the type and number of nociceptors that are present in that particular anatomical region.

(1) **Somatic nociception** (Table 16.2)
   Superficial (cutaneous) nociception originates from an injury to the skin or subcutaneous tissues. It produces a sharp and localized pain of short duration.
   Deep nociception originates from ligaments, tendons, bones, blood vessels, or muscles. It produces a dull, aching, poorly localized pain of longer duration.
(2) **Visceral nociception** (Table 16.3) originates from viscera and solid organs. However, not all organs are innervated by nociceptive fibers: the liver and the brain lack nociceptive innervation. Visceral pain is poorly localized and has aching or cramping qualities that may be referred to somatic structures and may have a long duration.

An important characteristic of visceral nociceptive innervation is that organs and viscera receive innervation by two systems of afferents: afferents traveling with the parasympathetic nerves (vagal and pelvic nerves) and afferents traveling with the sympathetic nerves (splanchnic nerves). It has been postulated that splanchnic innervation may be responsible for nociception, and vagal/pelvic innervation may be involved in the perception of nausea, malaise, and transmission of physiological information related to nutrient intake [17–19]. The role of this dual innervation system is not completely understood.

Cellular physiology
Primary afferents

Cell bodies of primary sensory afferents from skin, joints, muscle, plus splanchnic and pelvic visceral afferents, are located at the level of dorsal root ganglion (DRG), at the site of entrance of the dorsal root of the spinal nerves into the spinal cord, and in the trigeminal and nodose ganglia of cranial nerve V. Due to a small contribution of the cranial nerves VII, IX, and X to nociception from the external auditory meatus, the external skin of the ear, and mucous membranes of the larynx and pharynx, a small contingent of primary sensory neurons involved in nociception is also located at the level of the geniculate nucleus (VII), superior

role for this input to PKCγ interneurons in the pathophysiology of neuropathic pain.

The first synapse: spinal dorsal horn

The first synapse from primary afferent nociceptors to central dorsal horn neurons is a critical site of transmission, integration, and modulation in the pain pathway. We have a basic understanding of the location of the main primary input pathways to dorsal horn neurons as described above. The dorsal horn includes a large variety of cell types that can be classified based on response properties, morphology, neurotransmitter phenotype, and electrophysiological properties (Fig. 16.7).

Diversity of dorsal horn neurons that receive nociceptive input

Lamina I contains neurons that receive input related to pain, temperature, and itch. There are two main morphological classes of lamina I neurons: one group with dendrites that extend broadly, mostly within lamina I but some extending deeper into the dorsal horn, and a second group of smaller neurons. The dendrites of these cells can be considerably elongated along the rostrocaudal axis. These neurons can contain significant dendritic spines, although others are smooth. The functional properties of the neurons do not seem to correlate with morphological features. Many lamina I neurons are projection neurons that comprise the spinothalamic and spinobulbar pathways described above. Many of these cells are also interneurons, both excitatory and inhibitory, that contact neurons deeper in the dorsal horn [2].

As discussed above, **lamina II** includes at least three distinct sublayers in terms of types of primary afferent input. Because lamina II receives a large proportion of input from unmyelinated C fibers, this region is translucent and can be readily visualized with low-power light microscopy. This property is the source of the term *substantia gelatinosa*, referring to Rexed's lamina II. The neurons of lamina II are mostly local interneurons, both excitatory and inhibitory, making a large number of connections within lamina II but also to lamina I and others. Early studies using classical anatomical approaches suggested that there are two predominant morphologic cell types: stalked cells and islet cells. Stalked cells (possessing short stalk-like spines) have dendritic trees that form a cone-like arbor extending down through lamina II, III, and IV. The axons of these cells project superficially and synapse with lamina I neuronal dendrites. Islet cells, by contrast, have dendritic trees that extend rostrocaudally and ramify throughout lamina II. Classically, lamina II has been divided into two layers (IIo and IIi). Stalked cells are confined mostly to IIo, with islet cells mostly in IIi [26]. More recent studies, however, have identified a rich diversity of neurons in lamina II [27–29].

More recent work has led to the view that lamina II cells can be divided into four major classes based on morphology: islet cells, vertical cells (including the stalked cells described

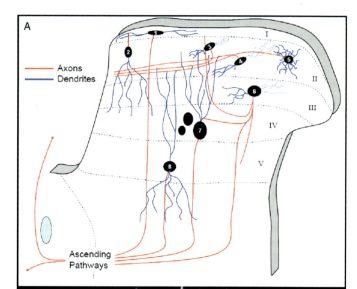

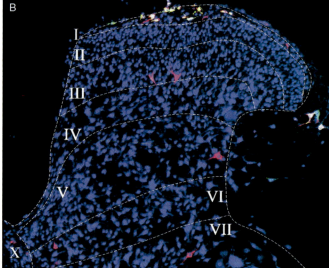

Figure 16.7. Neurons of the dorsal horn. (A) Schematic depiction of the morphology of neurons in the various laminae of the dorsal horn. In lamina I, there are multiple cell types (1), but these are relatively indistinguishable by morphology. Lamina II contains four main subtypes of cells: (2) vertical or stalked cells, (3) central cells, (4) islet cells, and (5) radial cells. Central and islet cells have dendrites that extend rostrocaudally (broken lines extending into the plane of the page). These cells have axons that are largely limited to lamina II except for vertical cells, which project to lamina I projection neurons. Lamina III neurons (6) have raustrocaudally oriented dendrites that extend through the thickness of lamina III, and the axons of these cells project throughout the dosal horn. Neurons in lamina IV and V vary in size, with some cells with large somata (7, 8). These cells have large dendritic fields that project up into superficial laminae, where they can receive primary afferent input. These cells can also be projection neurons, making up various ascending pathways. (B) Projected confocal image from a *z*-series scanned through the full thickness of a 70 µm section from L4 of the rat. The blue stain is an antibody directed against a neuronal-specific marker (NeuN) demonstrating the position of somata in the dorsal horn. The red- and green-stained neurons represent projection neurons for which axons terminate in the caudal ventrolateral medulla and parabrachial area, respectively. The rat had had a retrograde tracer (Cholera Toxin b – red) injected into the caudal ventrolateral medulla and another retrograde tracer (Fluorogold – green) in the lateral parabrachial area. Unpublished data, personal communication from Dr. Andrew Todd, University of Glasgow, with permission.

above), radial cells (with numerous dendrites radiating from the soma), and central cells (which have dendritic projections that extend rostrocaudally, though not as substantially as the islet cells) [27]. Islet cells appear to be almost entirely inhibitory interneurons, whereas the remainder of lamina II neurons have defied classification based on functional properties, with vertical, central, and radial cells all including both excitatory and inhibitory subpopulations [28]. Megumu Yoshimura's lab has demonstrated that these different classes of neurons do indeed predict the type of inputs that are typical for the various classes, however [30]. Thus, we are beginning to gain an understanding of the functional relevance of the various classes of lamina II neurons.

Neurons involved in nociception that reside deeper in the dorsal horn tend to be less specialized than those described for laminae I–II. Neurons in laminae III–V and lamina X contribute significantly in the ascending pain pathway.

In addition to the obvious distinction based on translucence of lamina II, neurons in **lamina III** can be distinguished based on their cell bodies, which are modestly larger and more widely spaced than those in lamina II. Lamina III neurons can be elongated in the rostrocaudal axis, with dendrites primarily ramifying within lamina III. Other lamina III neurons can have extremely broad dendritic trees ranging throughout laminae I–V. These cells tend to be more flattened in the rostrocaudal axis. Lamina III neurons can be projection neurons, including postsynaptic dorsal column cells, spinocervical tract cells, and others. Axons from lamina III neurons also project throughout the dorsal horn, notably to projection neurons in lamina I [2].

Neurons in **lamina IV** comprise a diverse group of cells, ranging widely in size from 8 μm to upwards of 45 μm in diameter. This variability in cell sizes, particularly the presence of very large cells, distinguishes lamina IV from lamina III. Dendrites of these neurons extend somewhat laterally and ventrally, but have prominent dorsal projections into superficial laminae. **Lamina V** can be further distinguished by the presence of many longitudinally arranged myelinated fibers, especially in the lateral region. Cell bodies of lamina V neurons are similar to those in lamina IV, but the dendritic fields radiate more widely while still possessing prominent dorsal dendrites that extend into the superficial laminae, contacting axons of central cells. These cells contribute to spinothalamic and spinocervical dorsal column pathways [2].

There is a great diversity of cell types in the dorsal horn based on morphological properties. In addition, there is great neurochemical diversity. Not only do these neurons include both excitatory (glutamatergic) and inhibitory neurons, there are multiple subtypes of each. For example, GABA is the main inhibitory transmitter in the cord, but there is also a significant population of neurons that also release glycine, which functions as an inhibitory transmitter. Neurons that release glycine appear to always corelease GABA, although the converse is not true. In addition to these fast-acting transmitters, various peptide transmitters are important contributors to dorsal horn physiology and can distinguish subsets of neurons. Notably, substance P, a neuropeptide released from the peptidergic C fibers, acts via the neurokinin 1 (NK_1) receptor in the dorsal horn. Neurons that express this NK_1 receptor are critical in the pathogenesis of chronic pain, and these neurons all appear to be excitatory, glutamatergic projection neurons [31].

Despite this level of understanding, we are only in the very early stages of understanding dorsal horn neuronal circuitry and how these cells combine to form a network that regulates information flow through the dorsal horn. As mentioned above, Yoshimura's lab has shown that lamina II neurons of differing morphologies receive different types of synaptic input [30]. Ed Perl's lab has done pioneering work utilizing paired recordings demonstrating that lamina I and II neurons organize into synaptic modules that are variously organized to transmit sensory information from Aδ and C afferent nociceptors [32]. State-of-the-art optical techniques are being used by the lab of Andrew Strassman and others who have also begun to map the various excitatory and inhibitory fields of different types of dorsal horn neurons [29]. Thus, the next few years should begin to see an emerging picture of the detailed network of neurons in the dorsal horn that subserve nociceptive transmission and modulation.

Plasticity of primary afferent inputs to the dorsal horn

Transmission at the first synapse from nociceptors onto dorsal horn neurons can be profoundly and protractedly modified by experience. Inflammation or damage to the spinal cord or peripheral nerves leads to hyperexcitability of dorsal horn neurons, known as central sensitization, which is widely thought to contribute to increased pain sensitivity. One of the main loci for central sensitization is the spinal cord dorsal horn, the first relay station for pain signals arriving from the periphery. Central sensitization involves changes in the coding of noxious signals and minimally must involve a change in synaptic strength or neuronal excitability. This type of plasticity is widespread in the nervous system. At a basic level, it involves changes in transmitter release in the presynaptic neuron and/or excitability or responsivity to transmitter in the postsynaptic neuron. Indeed, there are several examples of both of these effects associated with pain sensitization. Long-term potentiation of glutamate release from primary afferent neurons onto dorsal horn neurons in lamina I and II has been demonstrated by work from Jurgen Sandkuhler and colleagues, and work from Gereau *et al.* has demonstrated clear changes in postsynaptic excitability of dorsal horn neurons that mediate acute pain sensitization. These studies have demonstrated prominent roles for glutamate NMDA receptors and metabotropic glutamate receptors as well as NK_1 receptors in mediating central sensitization [33,34].

In addition to the changes in excitatory transmission and postsynaptic excitability described above, another key mechanism involved in pain hypersensitivity is a modulation of synaptic inhibition in the dorsal horn. Thus, either a decrease in strength of GABA/glycinergic synapses, or a loss of inhibitory interneurons in the dorsal horn, could lead to an overall increase in excitatory drive through the pain pathway, leading to enhanced pain sensation. This is a current area of extensive research and considerable disagreement in the field. However, inhibitory tone is clearly important in regulating nociceptive transmission through the cord, and indeed enhancement of this inhibition is a key mechanism of action of anesthetic drugs, as discussed later in this chapter. Furthermore, drugs that selectively enhance activity at subsets of GABA receptors are able to dramatically reduce chronic pain without side effects associated with sedation or motor impairment [35]. Thus, gaining a better understanding of the mechanisms of inhibitory transmission in the dorsal horn and how this is modulated represents an important area of current investigation into the mechanisms of analgesia and anesthesia.

Biochemical and molecular mechanisms underlying cellular physiology

There is considerable evidence now indicating that various ion channels expressed in nociceptors function as transducers of noxious mechanical, thermal, and chemical stimuli. By far the majority of noxious stimulus transduction is carried out by a group of channels belonging to the transient receptor potential (TRP) family of ion channels. These channels have been implicated in all forms of nociception, although there is significant debate as to the identity of mechanotransduction channels and noxious cold detection channels. In addition to the TRP channels, critical roles for ASIC$_3$ channels have been identified in detection of noxious chemical mediators. We will discuss each of these briefly below.

TRP channels

A subset of the very large family of TRP channels have been dubbed "thermoTRP" channels because of their activation over a wide range of temperatures. Figure 16.8 shows the varying temperature sensitivities of the six thermoTRP family members [36]. There is very convincing evidence implicating TRPV1, TRPV3, and TRPM8 in noxious heat, innocuous heat, and innocuous cold sensation, respectively. In addition, data from studies using heterologous expression systems clearly indicate that TRPV4 and TRPV2 are activated by heat in the innocuous and noxious range, respectively. To date, no genetic studies of TRPV4 or TRPV2 have been published, so in-vivo data are lacking. There are reports indicating that TRPA1 is activated by noxious cold temperatures [37], although this is still a contentious issue in the literature. Both in-vitro and

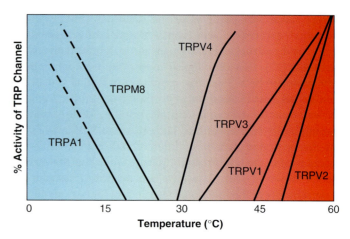

Figure 16.8. Thermo-TRP channels encode the full range of physiological temperatures. As described by Patapoutian et al. [36], there are six different TRP channels that are activated by changes in temperature. These "thermo-TRP channels" include TRPA1, M8, V1, V2, V3, and V4. As shown in the diagram, two of these (TRPM8 and TRPA1) are activated as temperatures are lowered from ambient body temperature into the innocuous and noxious cold range, respectively. TRPV4 and TRPV3 are activated by gentle warming in the innocuous range, and the activation of TRPV1 and TRPV2 occurs only as temperatures increase into the noxious range.

in-vivo studies give conflicting reports as to the role of TRPA1 in noxious cold detection [38].

ASIC channels

Tissue acidification is a major source of nociceptor activation in various conditions. Although certain TRP channels, notably TRPV1, are activated by protons, the acid-sensing ion channels (ASICs) have emerged as key mediators of proton-induced nociception. ASICs, and in particular ASIC$_3$, have been shown to be involved in a variety of pain conditions involving tissue acidification. For example, ASIC$_3$ has been indicated as an acid-sensitive receptor in the heart [39,40]. ASIC$_3$ has been shown to respond to even mild drops in pH, and these responses seem to be enhanced by the presence of lactate [41]. ASIC$_3$ knockout mice have reduced pain in a variety of acute and persistent pain tests, including a reduction in responses to mechanical stimuli [42]. However, DRG neurons from ASIC$_2$/ASIC$_3$ double-knockout mice do not have a reduction in mechanically gated channel activation, indicating at least that the mechanosensitive channels in DRG somata are not mediated by ASIC$_2$ or ASIC$_3$ [43]. Still, the significant reduction in pain behaviors in ASIC knockout mice indicate that these channels may play important roles in nociceptive transduction. Moreover, release of inflammatory mediators such as NGF and serotonin has been shown to upregulate ASIC$_3$ expression [44], so a role for ASICs in pain hypersensitivity is also a possibility.

Mechanotransduction channels

While the transduction channels described above can account for the majority of nociceptive transducers, what remains oddly elusive is the definitive identitification of the channels responsible for mechanotransduction. While several candidates have been proposed, and several have been identified in nonmammalian species, no single molecule to date has been identified in mammals that can account for a mechanotransduction channel in vivo. Nonetheless, it is clear that even in isolated DRG neurons, one can record currents, including single channel openings that are directly gated by membrane stretch [45,46]. A great deal of work is now ongoing in an attempt to identify the specific gene products that generate these mechanosensitive currents in nociceptors.

Voltage-gated channels of primary afferents

The transduction channels discussed above all serve as a mechanism for creating a generator potential that drives the sensory neuron above threshold for firing an action potential. Once this occurs, a plethora of voltage-gated sodium, calcium, and potassium channels collaborate to generate an action potential that transmits this information from the periphery to the CNS. Some voltage-gated channels are enriched or exclusively expressed in nociceptors, making them attractive targets for the development of anesthetic and/or analgesic drugs [47].

Nine sodium-channel α subunits ($Na_v1.1–1.9$) have been identified that can generate functional voltage-gated sodium channels (VGSCs) when expressed in combination with one or more β subunits. The α subunits are large proteins that contain both the voltage sensor and the pore domain of the channel. Channels formed by $Na_v1.1$, 1.2, 1.3, 1.4, 1.6, and 1.7 are sensitive to the blockade by tetrodotoxin (TTX), whereas $Na_v1.5$, $Na_v1.8$, and $Na_v1.9$ are TTX-insensitive.

Nociceptors express a rich diversity of VGSCs. Apparent from an analysis of currents that flow during an action potential in nociceptors is the predominance of TTX-resistant currents in generating nociceptor action potentials [23]. While TTX-sensitive channels contribute a relatively small amount of current, these currents are important in initiating the action potential, whereas TTX-resistant currents, mostly carried by $Na_v1.8$, result in most of the current that flows during the action potential (Fig. 16.5).

Among the VGSC subunits, particular attention has been given to $Na_v1.3$, $Na_v1.7$, $Na_v1.8$, and $Na_v1.9$ in studies of pain mechanisms. This focus arose from early studies of the distribution of these channels, their altered expression in pain models, and their biophysical properties.

$Na_v1.3$ was shown to be increased following a variety of injury models that result in persistent pain. Because the biophysical properties of $Na_v1.3$ suggest it would help to sustain high-frequency firing, the fact that it is upregulated in pain models suggested that this channel might play a key role in enhanced firing of nociceptors in persistent pain [48]. However, studies using $Na_v1.3$ knockout mice showed no phenotype in models of neuropathic pain [49]. Mixed results were obtained in various studies using antisense knockdown of $Na_v1.3$, and the role of $Na_v1.3$ in pain remains unclear [48].

A much stronger case has been made for a key role of $Na_v1.7$ in nociception. Nociceptor-specific knockout and siRNA knockdown of $Na_v1.7$ have been shown to reduce pain hypersensitivity in inflammatory (but not neuropathic) pain models in mice. More impressive is the presence of human genetic evidence for a critical role of $Na_v1.7$ in pain. Humans with mutations in the $Na_v1.7$ gene have dramatically altered pain sensitivity. For example, loss-of-function mutations in $Na_v1.7$ result in congenital insensitivity to pain [50], and gain-of-function mutations result in rare chronic pain conditions erythermalgia and paroxysmal extreme pain disorder [51,52]. All of these results strongly suggest that $Na_v1.7$ is an excellent target for the treatment of pain, and could be an important site of action for anesthetic drugs.

Results of genetic manipulation of $Na_v1.8$ have been surprisingly mixed, given the prominent role of this channel in nociceptor action potential generation and its ability to be sensitized by various inflammatory mediators [53]. Global knockout of $Na_v1.8$ does result in some modest alterations in mechanical pain [54], but these mice, as well as mice with a dual knockout of $Na_v1.8$ and $Na_v1.7$ in nociceptors, show normal neuropathic pain behaviors [55]. Results using genetic knockdown have proven more fruitful, with clear effects on neuropathic and inflammatory pain [56–58]. Taken together with the fact that a selective blocker of $Na_v1.8$ is able to reduce neuropathic pain behavior [59], it has been suggested that compensatory changes in nociceptors following genetic knockout mask the role of this channel in pain.

$Na_v1.9$ mediates a persistent TTX-resistant sodium current in sensory neurons. $Na_v1.9$ knockouts show reductions in inflammatory hyperalgesia, but no change in neuropathic pain behaviors [60,61]. $Na_v1.9$ therefore represents an attractive target for the treatment of inflammatory pain, but not neuropathic pain, based on current information [62,63].

In addition to sodium channels, voltage-gated calcium channels (VGCCs) also play an important role in shaping action potentials in nociceptors. As mentioned above, nociceptor action potentials contain a large shoulder on the falling phase. This shoulder is the result of large high-voltage-activated (HVA) calcium currents in nociceptors (Fig. 16.5) [23]. Furthermore, various mutations in the $Ca_v2.1$ gene that encodes the pore-forming $α_{1A}$ subunit of P/Q-type Ca^{2+} channels are associated with a rare hereditary form of migraine with aura termed familial hemiplegic migraine type 1 (FHM-1) [64]. There is very clear evidence for a prominent role of VGCCs in pain transmission and plasticity.

Current and potential targets of drug action

General anesthetics

Loss of consciousness, amnesia, and immobility in response to painful stimulation are considered fundamental goals of general anesthesia [65,66]. While loss of consciousness and amnesia are the result of anesthetic action in the brain, immobility in response to noxious stimulation seems to be mainly the result of anesthetic actions at the level of the spinal cord.

Both on the sensory side (dorsal horn) and on the motor side (ventral horn), several cell types and pathways have been identified as potential targets of anesthetic action to abolish movement in response to painful stimulation. The three classes of high threshold (HT), wide dynamic range (WDR), and low threshold (LT) sensory neurons have all shown depressed responses in the presence of anesthetic agents – in the noxious range of stimulation as well as in the non-noxious range. At the level of the ventral horn, excitability of motor neurons seems to be depressed by anesthetics both directly and indirectly via interneurons [67].

Effects of general anesthetics at the level of peripheral nocicepetive neurons have also been postulated and investigated [68–70]. Since the beginning of the 1990s Rampil and colleagues and Antognini and colleagues have demonstrated that immobility in response to noxious stimulation is dependent upon a direct action of the anesthetic agents at the level of the spinal cord and almost completely independent of supraspinal sites. In Rampil's studies, anesthetized rats did not display changes in minimum alveolar concentration (MAC) requirements for several hours after decerebration and after spinal-cord transection that would selectively resect descending supraspinal pathways [71]. In these two animal models, anesthetic concentration requirements to abolish movement in response to noxious stimulation did not vary compared to baseline, showing that immobility was not a consequence of supraspinal modulation.

In Antognini's studies a bypass system allowed administration of anesthetic agents selectively to the brain or the torso of anesthetized goats [72]. In these experiments, a marked increase in anesthetic requirements to suppress movement in response to noxious stimulation was observed when the brain was preferentially anesthetized with respect to the torso. This finding demonstrated that if appropriate anesthetic concentration is not reached at the level of the spinal cord, it is possible to abolish movement in response to painful stimuli only with supraclinical concentrations of anesthetic at the level of the brain. Thus, descending modulatory pathways can be engaged by anesthetics to produce these effects, but not at clinically utilized concentrations of anesthetic.

Another significant study published by Kishikawa in 1995 compared the effects of rapid eye movement (REM) sleep and propofol anesthesia on LT spinal sensory neurons [73]. During REM sleep LT neurons typically increase their response to peripheral receptive field stimulation, while motor neurons are profoundly depressed. In contrast, during propofol anesthesia, depression of LT neurons was observed. These observations of opposite effects of REM sleep and anesthesia suggest once again a separation between loss of consciousness and depression of spinal sensory neurons, which may not be mediated by descending modulation.

These studies all point to the conclusion that, besides activating descending modulatory pathways through activity at the level of the brain, general anesthetics also act directly at the level of the spinal cord, both by blocking the responses of spinal sensory neurons to noxious stimulation and by depressing excitability of spinal motor neurons [67,71,72,74–77].

Also, general anesthetics may act at other levels of the peripheral nervous system involved in sensory processing. Current research on the actions of general anesthetics on pain pathways has focused on:

- identifying **specific sites of action** for different general anesthetics within the spinal cord
- studying the effects of anesthetic agents on **nociception**
- understanding the mechanisms by which general anesthetics produce **immobility** in the face of noxious stimuli
- clarifying the relationship between nociception and immobility under general anesthesia

Recent developments in research on specific sites of action for anesthetic agents within the spinal cord have resulted in a few broadly accepted and many controversial findings. Extensive reviews discussing the contribution of various ligand- and voltage-gated channels in mediating anesthetic action at the level of the spinal cord have considered the role of opioid receptors, 5-HT$_3$, GABA$_A$, glycine, and glutamate receptors and potassium, calcium, and sodium channels [78–80]. None of these receptors or channels has been found to play a relevant role by itself, and not even any combination of actions has proven sufficient to explain the mechanism by which inhaled anesthetics produce immobility. Indeed, it is unclear whether the ability of general anesthetics to produce immobility at the level of the spinal cord results from action at a single high-affinity target or action at multiple different sites in combination [65,81].

Many anesthetic drugs have been found to exert effects on pain transduction and transmission, affecting nociception at subcortical levels. These effects may be antinociceptive and/or pronociceptive, depending on the specific properties of each single drug, the dosage and concentration of administration, and the specific site of action investigated. Particularly contradictory are the data available on the role of propofol in modulating nociception in the periphery and at the level of the spinal dorsal horn [69,70,77,82].

The relationship between the lack of motor response (immobility) to a noxious stimulus and antinociception under general anesthesia has also been extensively investigated.

In the 1960s, the development of the concept of MAC, the minimum alveolar concentration of a volatile anesthetic required to prevent movement in 50% of subjects in response to surgical noxious stimulation, represented a fundamental advance in the ability to compare clinical effects among inhaled anesthetics [83]. However, the fact that at a certain concentration of an anesthetic agent the clinical effect observed is immobility in response to painful stimulation does not imply that immobility is the consequence of a direct effect on nociception.

We know now that immobility and antinociception are to be considered separate effects, one depending only marginally upon the other [79]. Jinks and colleagues recently provided evidence to support this hypothesis, showing that the immobilizing action of isoflurane and halothane are mainly produced by action on the ventral spinal locomotor network, precisely at the level of ventrally located central pattern generators (CPG) [75,84]. Also, volatile anesthetics seem to be able to depress excitatory glutamate AMPA and NMDA currents in mouse spinal-cord motor neurons, independent of inhibitory $GABA_A$ or glycine currents [85]. Effects on $GABA_A$ and glycine receptors seem to be more relevant in explaining the mechanism of action of some intravenous anesthetic agents, such as propofol or barbiturates [79].

Table 16.4 summarizes the postulated sites of action of general anesthetics at the level of the spinal cord, the DRGs, and the peripheral nociceptors, and the relative contribution of different components of the circuitry to the effect of producing immobility and modulating nociception.

Local anesthetics

Local anesthetics (LAs) have been used for over a century to block transmission of nociceptive impulses from the periphery. The best-described mechanism of action of LAs is to block propagation of action potentials by reversibly inhibiting voltage-gated sodium channels. While this mechanism explains how LAs block impulses in peripheral nerves, it does not account for the effects of LAs administered at epidural or subarachnoid levels. At the level of the spinal cord and the DRG, LAs have been shown to act at many different sites and with distinct mechanisms that interact to produce effective clinical analgesia (Table 16.5). LAs administered at subarachnoid or epidural level have direct access to spinal dorsal horn neurons, where they act at multiple ion channels involved in the modulation of excitability and in the release of neurotransmitters. Effects mediated by pre- and postsynaptic ionotropic and metabotropic receptors have also been reported, involving interactions directly at the level of receptor proteins or with enzymes along the intracellular signaling pathways activated by these receptors [86]. The diverse mechanisms by which LAs block nociception at multiple levels suggest the possibility of developing new classes of analgesic drugs acting more selectively on the same molecular targets. A brief overview of the specific molecules and sites of action of LAs that could be of interest as targets for new selective antinociceptive drugs is provided in the following paragraphs (see Chapter 36 for additional information on local anesthetic action).

Local anesthetics and ion channels
Voltage-gated sodium channels
The most widely accepted and investigated mechanism of action of LAs is the reversible inhibition of VGSCs and resulting

block of the action potentials in excitable cells. This nonsubtype selective block of VGSCs by currently available LAs leads to restrictions in their clinical use due to limiting side effects. As previously mentioned in this chapter, VGSCs formed by α subunits $Na_v1.7$, $Na_v1.8$, $Na_v1.9$, and possibly $Na_v1.3$ are richly expressed in nociceptors and/or upregulated in pain models, suggesting that selective blockers of these channels would increase the tolerability and safety and improve analgesic efficacy in specific pain conditions: as an example, different drugs would selectively target different subunits to treat neuropathic ($Na_v1.8$) or inflammatory ($Na_v1.9$) pain conditions.

Voltage-gated potassium channels and K_{2P} channels (background or leak currents)
A considerable number of studies have demonstrated that LAs, besides exerting their effects by blocking VGSCs, also act on other types of ion channels. In particular, LAs have been shown to block voltage-gated K^+ channels and background K_{2P} channels, which have been shown to play a critical role in pain processing in the DRGs. Effects of LAs on voltage-gated K^+ channels have been investigated at the level of peripheral terminals and of the neurons in the DRG and spinal cord, and significant effects have been observed at all of these levels, with differences depending on the specific structure of each subfamily of channels and their pre- or postsynaptic location [87]. In dorsal horn neurons, LAs can equally block open and closed voltage-gated K_A channels, thus inhibiting the transient "A-type" currents. No effect has been observed at this level on sustained currents [87]. In DRG neurons, all tested LAs seem to be able to block both transient currents and sustained delayed rectifier currents [88]. The inhibition of K_{2P} channels by LAs and the consequent block of repolarization has important implications both for the clinical effect of local anesthetics and in the genesis of typical side effects of LAs such as CNS excitability and cardiac arrhythmias [89].

Voltage-gated calcium channels
Local anesthetic block of neuronal Ca^{2+} channels presents some similarities with the block of VGSCs. Lidocaine displays higher affinity for the open and inactivated channels compared to channels in the resting state. This is true for both Na^+ channels and Ca^{2+} channels [90]. An important physiological effect of local anesthetic Ca^{2+} channel blockade is the inhibition of neurotransmitter release.

VGCCs, together with VGSCs, play a determinant role in nociceptor activation and, besides being blocked by LAs, these channels are the target of clinically effective analgesic drugs used in the management of chronic pain, including gabapentin and pregabalin, which target the $\alpha_2\delta$ subunit, and ziconotide, which targets α_{1B}-containing N-type channels [63].

As a last important remark and caveat on the combined actions of LAs, in a recent review, Yanagidate and Strichartz point out that "the integrated actions of a LA agent that acts on several, physiologically coupled targets may differ from actions

Table 16.4. Postulated sites of action of general anesthetics at the level of the spinal cord, the dorsal root ganglion, and the peripheral nociceptors

Cellular targets	Molecular targets	Proposed effect
Targets of anesthetic action in the spinal cord		
Volatile anesthetics		
Ventral interneuronal network	NMDA, GABA$_A$, glycine receptors, Na$^+$ channels	Immobility
Ventral horn motor neurons	NMDA(?), AMPA receptors. (GABA$_A$, glycine rec.?)	Immobility
Dorsal horn neurons supraspinal	GABA$_A$, glycine, NMDA receptors, TREK-1 Isoflurane at 1 MAC (modulation of norepinephrine effect?) Isoflurane at subclinical concentrations: inhibition of Nicotinic receptors = inhibition of norepinephrine release	Antinociception (direct and via modulation) Immobility (indirect) Pronociception
N$_2$O		
Dorsal horn neurons	(Indirect) disinhibition of descending NE pathway (also NE effect on GABA interneurons)	Antinociception
Ventral horn motor neurons	NMDA (or non-NMDA?) glutamate receptors	Immobility
IV anesthetics (thiopental, pentobarbital, etomidate, propofol)		
Dorsal horn neurons	GABA$_A$ receptors	Antinociception
Ventral horn motor neurons	GABA$_A$ receptors	Immobility
IV anesthetics (ketamine)		
Dorsal horn neurons	NMDA receptors, K$^+$ channels (?) Nicotinic, μ-opioid receptors	Antinociception
Ventral horn motoneurons	NMDA	Immobility
Targets of anesthetic action in the DRG neurons		
N$_2$O		
	(Indirect) GABA$_A$ receptors	Antinociception
Volatile anesthetics and IV anesthetics (propofol)		
	GABA$_A$ receptors	Antinociception
Targets of anesthetic action in the periphery		
Volatile anesthetics		
Nerve endings	TRPA1 (isoflurane and desflurane)	Pronociception
IV anesthetics		
Nerve endings	NMDA receptors (propofol) TRPA1 receptors (propofol/etomidate)	Antinociception Pronociception

of the agent on the separate targets" (e.g., K$^+$ channel blockade, which by itself could result in increased excitability, acts synergistically with a concomitant Na$^+$ channel blockade in inhibiting action potentials) [86]. This consideration should be taken into account when setting out to develop new molecules that act selectively on a specific molecular target.

G-protein-coupled receptors

Of particular relevance in nociceptive pathways is the role of the following G-protein-coupled receptors: α$_1$-adrenoceptors, 5-HT$_{2A}$ receptors, group I metabotropic glutamate receptors (mGlu1 and mGlu5), M$_1$ muscarinic receptors, and NK$_1$ receptors. All of these receptors are coupled primarily via G$_q$

Table 16.5. Main targets of local anesthetic action along the sensory pathways

Spinal cord (dorsal horn neurons)

Voltage-gated K^+ channels

Two-pore-domain K^+ channels

Glutamate ionotropic receptors (AMPA + NMDA) → inhibition of ERK

G-protein-coupled receptors (G_q α subunit)

5-HT_3 receptors

DRG neurons and presynaptic terminals

Ca^{2+} channels

Two-pore-domain K^+ channels

$Na_v1.7$, $Na_v1.8$, $Na_v1.9$ $Na_v1.3$ (upregulated following injury)

5-HT_3 receptors

TRPV1 receptors

NMDA receptors

Periphery

Voltage-gated Na^+ channels

Voltage gated Ca^{2+} channels

TRPV1 receptors

5-HT_3 receptors

proteins, a class of G proteins that has been shown to be particularly sensitive to local anesthetic action in several studies [91–96]. LAs have been shown to inhibit G_q signaling in a time-dependent and reversible fashion. This inhibition occurs via an interaction of LAs with G_q proteins at the site of interaction of the G protein with the receptor [86].

In addition to the GPCR/G-protein interaction, downstream signaling molecules activated by GPCRs can also be targets of LA action. During transmission of nociceptive stimuli from the periphery, glutamate and substance P are released by the central terminals of primary sensory neurons. Of particular relevance to nociception are the identified interactions of LAs with protein kinase C (PKC), protein kinase A (PKA), and extracellular signal-regulated kinases (ERKs). Several isoforms of PKC seem to be sensitive to LAs and, as a consequence, pathways that are dependent on these enzymes are suppressed by LAs as observed in many in-vitro studies [96,97]. There is limited and somewhat controversial evidence that PKA and ERK signaling may also be inhibited by LAs [86,98].

TRPV1 channels

TRP channels are important transducers of various sensory stimuli, including many noxious stimuli. TRPV1, which is activated by noxious heat, extracellular protons, and capsaicin, is expressed in peripheral and central terminals of many

nociceptors [99,100]. LAs have been shown to interact with TRPV1 channels directly to produce inhibition, activation, sensitization, and desensitization of the channel [100,101]. Hirota *et al.* reported that lidocaine, prilocaine, and procaine were able to act as TRPV1 antagonists, suppressing capsaicin-induced calcium currents, although their site of action was not determined [101]. Activation of TRPV1 by LAs has also been described. LA activation of TRPV1 may occur by binding of the LA molecule to a site similar to the binding site for capsaicin or by interacting with a binding site on TRPV1 for phosphatidylinositol 4,5-bisphosphate (PIP_2) [4,5], which acts as an allosteric modulator of TRPV1 gating [100].

Interestingly, lidocaine at subthreshold concentrations can potentiate TRPV1 currents induced by heat or capsaicin, and lidocaine activation of the channel can be enhanced by PKC activation. Thus, in the context of inflammation or injury (many inflammatory mediators can activate PKC in nociceptors), the ability of LAs to activate TRPV1 will be enhanced. Thus, LA-mediated nociceptor activation via TRPV1 may play a significant role in neurogenic inflammation and enhancing nociceptor activation. This represents a possible mechanism of LA-induced neurotoxicity [100].

An interesting feature of TRPV1 is that the pore of these channels is able to conduct large ions. Clifford Woolf and colleagues have taken advantage of this feature, together with the selective expression of TRPV1 in nociceptors, as a novel way to deliver local anesthetics specifically to nociceptors to induce profound and specific analgesia. QX-314 is a positively charged derivative of lidocaine that lacks lipophilic properties that normally enable LAs to cross cell membranes. Thus, when QX-314 is applied externally to nerves, it is normally without effect. However, in the presence of capsaicin, which opens TRPV1 channels, QX-314 is able to gain entry to the nociceptor via the large TRPV1 pore. When applied at high enough concentrations in the presence of capsaicin, QX-314 is able to block Na^+ channels, thus blocking the generation of action potentials. Being specifically targeted to nociceptors, whose terminals selectively express TRPV1, QX-314 produces a nociceptor-specific local anesthesia, with no motor blockade or tactile deficits and limited side effects due to its selectivity for nociceptive neurons [102]. This represents a potentially exciting method for treating certain chronic pain conditions in the future.

Besides being proposed as an "entry way" for QX-314, TRPV1 channels have been targeted by agonists such as capsaicin, with the aim to desensitize the channels and produce analgesia, especially in chronic pain states [103]. More recently, a variety of increasingly selective TRPV1 antagonist molecules have been developed that have shown promising antihyperalgesic action in humans [104]. It has also been argued that TRPV1 agonists and antagonists should not be regarded as mutually exclusive treatments, but rather complementary pharmacologic approaches for pain treatment in diverse chronic pain conditions [103].

New and emerging concepts

The currently available options for treatment of acute and chronic pain states are clearly insufficient in most clinical situations. Throughout this chapter, we have mentioned several exciting concepts that could lead to novel treatments for pain. Isoform-specific sodium-channel inhibitors are one extremely promising class that we have discussed in detail. In addition, the TRPV1 agonist-assisted loading of impermeant sodium-channel blockers into nociceptors represents an exciting and novel approach to the treatment of pain. In addition to these, there are some other examples of potentially promising strategies for treating pain that bear mentioning.

Among the many different families of molecules and receptors involved in pain processing at multiple levels, nerve growth factor (NGF) and its receptor trkA (receptor tyrosine kinase A) have been identified as potential targets for a novel class of pain drugs [105]. In particular, it has been demonstrated that NGF plays a fundamental role in the generation and maintenance of pain states, that its local or systemic administration provokes long-lasting mechanical and thermal hyperalgesia [106,107], and that inhibition of NGF function is able to reduce pain and hyperalgesia in many animal models. The mechanisms by which NGF induces and maintain hyperalgesia are essentially three: (1) NGF sensitizes TRPV1 receptors by causing post-translational changes in these channels, (2) it modulates gene expression in nociceptors, and (3) it sensitizes mast cells in inflamed tissues leading to release of other pain mediators such as prostaglandins, bradykinin, and histamine. So far, inhibition of NGF activity has been attempted through diverse approaches, and research is ongoing for the development of anti-NGF monoclonal antibodies, antagonists of the NGF-TrkA binding site, and selective antagonists of trkA function [105].

Another major player in the development of chronic pain is metabotropic glutamate receptor, subtype 5 (mGlu5). Activation of mGlu5 has been demonstrated to be critical in nociceptive modulation in chronic inflammatory pain states [108] and in the development of thermal hyperalgesia in several rodent models [109,110]. Activation of mGlu5 at various points in the pain neuraxis, including the periphery, the spinal cord, and the brain, can lead to sensitization in nociceptive transmission or pain perception. In the spinal cord, activation of mGlu5 leads to central sensitization through ERK activation [111], and mGlu5 activation in the periphery induces thermal hyperalgesia by enhancing TRPV1 function in peripheral sensory neuron terminals [112]. In addition, mGlu5 expression is increased in DRG somata of A fibers following nerve injury [113]. Selective block of mGlu5 by peripheral [109], intrathecal [111,114], and systemic [108,115] administration of mGlu5 antagonists has been demonstrated to have analgesic properties in a variety of preclinical inflammatory pain models. To date, studies on mGlu5 antagonists in pain modulation have been limited to animal models, but promising molecules are available as candidates for future studies in humans. Interestingly, mGlu5 antagonists have been shown to be effective anxiolytics, both in animals and in humans. Because severe anxiety is a major comorbidity for patients with chronic pain, mGlu5 antagonists have the potential to treat both the sensory and emotional components of pain, and thus this class of drugs holds great promise as a novel strategy for the treatment of chronic pain syndromes.

Summary

The detection of noxious stimuli (stimuli that are damaging to normal tissues) is carried out by a special subset of primary sensory neurons, known as nociceptors. Pain as a sensory system can be framed in three distinct and one supplemental processes:

(1) Transduction – the activation of nociceptors by a noxious stimulus.

(2) Transmission – the nociceptor activation generates action potentials in the nociceptor, leading to the transmission of this signal from the periphery to the central nervous system via release of neurotransmitter from the primary afferent onto second-order neurons in the dorsal horn of the spinal cord. Neurons in the spinal cord, either directly or through interneurons, then convey information to various areas of the nervous system that provide for the organization of reflexive withdrawal behaviors.

(3) Perception – the perception of pain itself, and the signals that generate learning cues for future avoidance behaviors.

(4) Modulation – the affective state, attention, and cognitive factors can lead to substantial enhancement or suppression of nociception and/or pain perception.

It is important to note that nociception can occur without eliciting the sensation of pain, and pain can be experienced in the absence of nociception.

In more anatomical terms, a discussion of the pain neuraxis must include a detailed understanding of at least four major components:

(1) Primary afferent nociceptors – Nociceptors represent a diverse group of primary afferent sensory neurons that are variously tuned for the detection of a wide variety of potentially injurious stimuli including noxious heat, noxious pressure, tissue acidification, noxious cold, noxious chemicals, and many others.

(2) Spinal cord – The spinal cord is the site of the first synapses from nearly all primary afferent nociceptors. Nociceptive signals are transmitted to the CNS by synapses from nociceptor afferents onto several different populations of neurons in the dorsal horn of the spinal cord. These inputs serve to generate reflexive withdrawal responses and to transmit nociceptive signals to higher brain centers. In addition, the dorsal horn is a site of considerable descending modulation and local synaptic plasticity that can serve to inhibit or enhance pain transmission.

(3) Ascending pathways – Pain transmission from the spinal cord to supraspinal sites occurs predominantly via the following three ascending pathways: the spinothalamic tract (STT), the spinobulbar projections, and the postsynaptic dorsal column pathway.

(4) Descending modulatory pathways – Descending systems can be either anti-nociceptive or pro-nociceptive and their presence is profoundly important to mediate endogenous pain regulation.

Unconscious nociceptive activity is at the origin of nociceptive pain. Nociceptive pain may originate from any tissue in the body that is innervated by nociceptors, and needs to be distinguished from neuropathic pain, which originates from injuries that occur within the peripheral or central nervous system. Two distinct types of nociception exist: somatic nociception (superficial and deep) and visceral nociception.

Cell bodies of primary sensory afferents from skin, joints, muscle, plus splanchnic and pelvic visceral afferents, are located at the level of dorsal root ganglion (DRG), at the site of entrance of the dorsal root of the spinal nerves into the spinal cord, and in the trigeminal and nodose ganglia of cranial nerve V. All primary afferent neurons use glutamate as their principal neurotransmitter for initiating rapid responses in spinal postsynaptic neurons. The first synapse from primary afferent nociceptors to central dorsal horn neurons is a critical site of transmission, integration, and modulation in the pain pathway. The dorsal horn includes a large variety of cell types that can be classified based on response properties, morphology, neurotransmitter phenotype, and electrophysiological properties.

There is considerable evidence now indicating that various ion channels expressed in nociceptors function as transducers of noxious mechanical, thermal, and chemical stimuli. By far the majority of noxious stimulus transduction is carried out by a group of channels belonging to the transient receptor potential (TRP) family of ion channels. These channels have been implicated in all forms of nociception, although there is significant debate as to the identity of mechanotransduction channels and noxious cold detection channels. In addition to the TRP channels, critical roles for $ASIC_3$ channels have been identified in detection of noxious chemical mediators.

General anesthetics and their molecular targets in the spinal cord, the DRG and the periphery are detailed in Table 16.4, while targets of local anesthetics in the spinal cord, DRG, and peripheral nociceptors are outlined in Table 16.5.

Isoform-specific sodium-channel inhibitors are an extremely promising class of analgesic agents. In addition, the TRPV1 agonist-assisted loading of impermeant sodium-channel blockers into nociceptors represents an exciting and novel approach to the treatment of pain. Nerve growth factor (NGF) and its receptor trkA (receptor tyrosine kinase A) have been identified as potential targets for a novel class of pain drugs. Also, activation of mGlu5 has been demonstrated to be critical in nociceptive modulation in chronic inflammatory pain states and in the development of thermal hyperalgesia in several rodent models. Because severe anxiety is a major comorbidity for patients with chronic pain, mGlu5 antagonists have the potential to treat both the sensory and emotional components of pain, and thus this class of drugs holds great promise as a novel strategy for the treatment of chronic pain syndromes.

Acknowledgments
The authors wish to thank M. Morales for creating Figs. 16.1 and 16.3 and for comments on the mansucript. Work in RG's laboratory is funded by NIH grants R01NS42595, R01NS48602, and R21NS61294.

References
1. Gasser HS, Erlanger J. The role played by the sizes of the constituent fibers of a nerve-trunk in determining the form of its action potencial wave. *Am J Physiol* 1927; **80**: 522–47.

2. Willis WD, Coggeshall RE. *Sensory Mechanisms of the Spinal Cord*, 2nd edn. New York, NY: Plenum Press, 1991.

3. Rexed B. The cytoarchetectonic organization of the spinal cord in the rat. *J Comp Neurol* 1952; **96**: 415–466.

4. Neumann S, Braz JM, Skinner K, Llewellyn-Smith IJ, Basbaum AI. Innocuous, not noxious, input activates PKCgamma interneurons of the spinal dorsal horn via myelinated afferent fibers. *J Neurosci* 2008; **28**: 7936–44.

5. Zylka MJ, Rice FL, Anderson DJ. Topographically distinct epidermal nociceptive circuits revealed by axonal tracers targeted to Mrgprd. *Neuron* 2005; **45**(1): 17–25.

6. Todd AJ. Chapter 6 Anatomy and neurochemistry of the dorsal horn. *Handb Clin Neurol* 2006; **81**: 61–76.

7. Willis WD, Al-Chaer ED, Quast MJ, Westlund KN. A visceral pain pathway in the dorsal column of the spinal cord. *Proc Natl Acad Sci U S A* 1999; **96**: 7675–9.

8. Burstein R, Cliffer KD, Giesler GJ. Cells of origin of the spinohypothalamic tract in the rat. *J Comp Neurol* 1990; **291**: 329–44.

9. Burstein R, Potrebic S. Retrograde labeling of neurons in the spinal cord that project directly to the amygdala or the orbital cortex in the rat. *J Comp Neurol* 1993; **335**: 469–85.

10. Dostrovsky JO, Craig AD. Ascending projection systems. In: McMahon SB, Koltzenburg M, eds., *Wall and Melzack's Textbook of Pain*, 5th edn. Philadelphia, PA: Elsevier/Churchill Livingstone, 2005: 187–204.

11. Reynolds DV. Surgery in the rat during electrical analgesia induced by focal brain stimulation. *Science* 1969; **164**: 444–5.

12. Pert CB, Snyder SH. Opiate receptor: demonstration in nervous tissue. *Science* 1973; **179**: 1011–14.

13. Hughes J. Isolation of an endogenous compound from the brain with

pharmacological properties similar to morphine. *Brain Res* 1975; **88**: 295–308.

14. Gebhart GF. Descending modulation of pain. *Neurosci Biobehav Rev* 2004; **27**: 729–37.

15. Fields HL, Basbaum AI, Heinricher MM. Central nervous system mechanisms of pain modulation. In: McMahon SB, Koltzenburg M, eds., *Wall and Melzack's Textbook of Pain*, 5th edn. Philadelphia, PA: Elsevier/Churchill Livingstone, 2005: 125–142.

16. Gebhart GF. Can endogenous systems produce pain? *APS Journal* 1992; **1**: 79–81.

17. Andrews PL, Sanger GJ. Abdominal vagal afferent neurones: an important target for the treatment of gastrointestinal dysfunction. *Curr Opin Pharmacol* 2002; **2**: 650–6.

18. Zagon A. Does the vagus nerve mediate the sixth sense? *Trends Neurosci* 2001; **24**: 671–3.

19. Grundy D. Neuroanatomy of visceral nociception: vagal and splanchnic afferent. *Gut* 2002; **51** (Suppl 1): i2–5.

20. Loeser J, Bonica J, Butler S. *Bonica's Management of Pain*. Philadelphia, PA: Lippincott Williams & Wilkins, 2001.

21. Morgan G, Mikhail M, Murray M. *Clinical Anesthesiology*, 4th edn. New York, NY: McGraw-Hill, 2005.

22. Patestas M, LP G. *A Textbook of Neuroanatomy*. Malden, MA: Wiley-Blackwell, 2006.

23. Blair NT, Bean BP. Roles of tetrodotoxin (TTX)-sensitive Na^+ current, TTX-resistant Na^+ current, and Ca^{2+} current in the action potentials of nociceptive sensory neurons. *J Neurosci* 2002; **22**: 10277–90.

24. Snider WD, McMahon SB. Tackling pain at the source: new ideas about nociceptors. *Neuron* 1998; **20**: 629–32.

25. Lawson SN. The postnatal development of large light and small dark neurons in mouse dorsal root ganglia: a statistical analysis of cell numbers and size. *J Neurocytol* 1979; **8**: 275–94.

26. Gobel S. Golgi studies of the neurons in layer II of the dorsal horn of the medulla (trigeminal nucleus caudalis). *J Comp Neurol* 1978; **180**: 395–413.

27. Grudt TJ, Perl ER. Correlations between neuronal morphology and electrophysiological features in the rodent superficial dorsal horn. *J Physiol* 2002; **540**: 189–207.

28. Maxwell DJ, Belle MD, Cheunsuang O, Stewart A, Morris R. Morphology of inhibitory and excitatory interneurons in superficial laminae of the rat dorsal horn. *J Physiol* 2007; **584**: 521–33.

29. Kato G, Kawasaki Y, Ji RR, Strassman AM. Differential wiring of local excitatory and inhibitory synaptic inputs to islet cells in rat spinal lamina II demonstrated by laser scanning photostimulation. *J Physiol* 2007; **580**: 815–33.

30. Yasaka T, Kato G, Furue H, *et al.* Cell-type-specific excitatory and inhibitory circuits involving primary afferents in the substantia gelatinosa of the rat spinal dorsal horn in vitro. *J Physiol* 2007; **581**: 603–18.

31. Carrasquillo Y, Gereau RW. Rodent models clarify the role of cells expressing the substance P receptor in pain. *Drug Discov Today Dis Models* 2004; **1**: 107–113.

32. Lu Y, Perl ER. Modular organization of excitatory circuits between neurons of the spinal superficial dorsal horn (laminae I and II). *J Neurosci* 2005; **25**: 3900–7.

33. Hu HJ, Alter BJ, Carrasquillo Y, Qiu CS, Gereau RW. Metabotropic glutamate receptor 5 modulates nociceptive plasticity via extracellular signal-regulated kinase-Kv4.2 signaling in spinal cord dorsal horn neurons. *J Neurosci* 2007; **27**: 13181–91.

34. Sandkuhler J. Understanding LTP in pain pathways. *Mol Pain* 2007; **3**: 9.

35. Knabl J, Witschi R, Hosl K, *et al.* Reversal of pathological pain through specific spinal GABAA receptor subtypes. *Nature* 2008; **451**: 330–4.

36. Patapoutian A, Peier AM, Story GM, Viswanath V. ThermoTRP channels and beyond: mechanisms of temperature sensation. *Nat Rev Neurosci* 2003; **4**: 529–39.

37. Story GM, Peier AM, Reeve AJ, *et al.* ANKTM1, a TRP-like channel expressed in nociceptive neurons, is activated by cold temperatures. *Cell* 2003; **112**: 819–29.

38. Story GM, Gereau RW. Numbing the senses: role of TRPA1 in mechanical and cold sensation. *Neuron* 2006; **50**: 177–80.

39. Sutherland SP, Benson CJ, Adelman JP, McCleskey EW. Acid-sensing ion channel 3 matches the acid-gated current in cardiac ischemia-sensing neurons. *Proc Natl Acad Sci U S A* 2001; **98**: 711–16.

40. Cervero F, Laird JM. Understanding the signaling and transmission of visceral nociceptive events. *J Neurobiol* 2004; **61**: 45–54.

41. Immke DC, McCleskey EW. Lactate enhances the acid-sensing Na+ channel on ischemia-sensing neurons. *Nat Neurosci* 2001; **4**: 869–70.

42. Chen CC, Zimmer A, Sun WH, Hall J, Brownstein MJ. A role for ASIC3 in the modulation of high-intensity pain stimuli. *Proc Natl Acad Sci U S A* 2002; **99**: 8992–7.

43. Drew LJ, Rohrer DK, Price MP, *et al.* Acid-sensing ion channels ASIC2 and ASIC3 do not contribute to mechanically activated currents in mammalian sensory neurones. *J Physiol* 2004; **556**: 691–710.

44. Mamet J, Baron A, Lazdunski M, Voilley N. Proinflammatory mediators, stimulators of sensory neuron excitability via the expression of acid-sensing ion channels. *J Neurosci* 2002; **22**: 10662–70.

45. Cho H, Shin J, Shin CY, Lee SY, Oh U. Mechanosensitive ion channels in cultured sensory neurons of neonatal rats. *J Neurosci* 2002; **22**: 1238–47.

46. Drew LJ, Wood JN, Cesare P. Distinct mechanosensitive properties of capsaicin-sensitive and -insensitive sensory neurons. *J Neurosci* 2002; **22**: RC228.

47. McCleskey EW, Gold MS. Ion channels of nociception. *Annu Rev Physiol* 1999; **61**: 835–56.

48. Krafte DS, Bannon AW. Sodium channels and nociception: recent concepts and therapeutic opportunities. *Curr Opin Pharmacol* 2008; **8**: 50–6.

49. Nassar MA, Baker MD, Levato A, *et al.* Nerve injury induces robust allodynia and ectopic discharges in $Na_v1.3$ null mutant mice. *Mol Pain* 2006; **2**: 33.

50. Cox JJ, Reimann F, Nicholas AK, *et al.* An SCN9A channelopathy causes congenital inability to experience pain. *Nature* 2006; **444**: 894–8.

51. Fertleman CR, Baker MD, Parker KA, *et al.* SCN9A mutations in paroxysmal extreme pain disorder: allelic variants underlie distinct channel defects and phenotypes. *Neuron* 2006; **52**: 767–74.

52. Yang Y, Wang Y, Li S, *et al.* Mutations in SCN9A, encoding a sodium channel alpha subunit, in patients with primary erythermalgia. *J Med Genet* 2004; **41**: 171–4.

53. Renganathan M, Cummins TR, Waxman SG. Contribution of Na(v)1.8 sodium channels to action potential electrogenesis in DRG neurons. *J Neurophysiol* 2001; **86**: 629–40.

54. Zimmermann K, Leffler A, Babes A, *et al.* Sensory neuron sodium channel $Na_v1.8$ is essential for pain at low temperatures. *Nature* 2007; **447**: 855–8.

55. Nassar MA, Levato A, Stirling LC, Wood JN. Neuropathic pain develops normally in mice lacking both $Na_v1.7$ and $Na_v1.8$. *Mol Pain* 2005; **1**: 24.

56. Lai J, Gold MS, Kim CS, *et al.* Inhibition of neuropathic pain by decreased expression of the tetrodotoxin-resistant sodium channel, $Na_v1.8$. *Pain* 2002; **95**: 143–52.

57. Joshi SK, Mikusa JP, Hernandez G, *et al.* Involvement of the TTX-resistant sodium channel Nav 1.8 in inflammatory and neuropathic, but not post-operative, pain states. *Pain* 2006; **123**: 75–82.

58. Dong XW, Goregoaker S, Engler H, *et al.* Small interfering RNA-mediated selective knockdown of Na(V)1.8 tetrodotoxin-resistant sodium channel reverses mechanical allodynia in neuropathic rats. *Neuroscience* 2007; **146**: 812–21.

59. Jarvis MF, Honore P, Shieh CC, *et al.* A-803467, a potent and selective $Na_v1.8$ sodium channel blocker, attenuates neuropathic and inflammatory pain in the rat. *Proc Natl Acad Sci U S A* 2007; **104**: 8520–5.

60. Amaya F, Wang H, Costigan M, *et al.* The voltage-gated sodium channel Na(v)1.9 is an effector of peripheral inflammatory pain hypersensitivity. *J Neurosci* 2006; **26**: 12852–60.

61. Priest BT, Murphy BA, Lindia JA, *et al.* Contribution of the tetrodotoxin-resistant voltage-gated sodium channel $Na_v1.9$ to sensory transmission and nociceptive behavior. *Proc Natl Acad Sci U S A* 2005; **102**: 9382–7.

62. Momin A, Wood JN. Sensory neuron voltage-gated sodium channels as analgesic drug targets. *Curr Opin Neurobiol* 2008; **18**: 383–8.

63. Cao YQ. Voltage-gated calcium channels and pain. *Pain* 2006; **126**: 5–9.

64. Ophoff RA, Terwindt GM, Vergouwe MN, *et al.* Familial hemiplegic migraine and episodic ataxia type-2 are caused by mutations in the $Ca2^+$ channel gene CACNL1A4. *Cell* 1996; **87**: 543–52.

65. Grasshoff C, Antkowiak B. Effects of isoflurane and enflurane on GABAA and glycine receptors contribute equally to depressant actions on spinal ventral horn neurones in rats. *Br J Anaesth* 2006; **97**: 687–94.

66. Solt K, Forman SA. Correlating the clinical actions and molecular mechanisms of general anesthetics. *Curr Opin Anaesthesiol* 2007; **20**: 300–6.

67. Collins JG, Kendig JJ, Mason P. Anesthetic actions within the spinal cord: contributions to the state of general anesthesia. *Trends Neurosci* 1995; **18**: 549–53.

68. Antognini JF, Kien ND. Potency (minimum alveolar anesthetic concentration) of isoflurane is independent of peripheral anesthetic effects. *Anesth Analg* 1995; **81**: 69–72.

69. Sun YY, Li KC, Chen J. Evidence for peripherally antinociceptive action of propofol in rats: behavioral and spinal neuronal responses to subcutaneous bee venom. *Brain Res* 2005; **1043**: 231–5.

70. Matta JA, Cornett PM, Miyares RL, *et al.* General anesthetics activate a nociceptive ion channel to enhance pain and inflammation. *Proc Natl Acad Sci U S A* 2008; **105**: 8784–9.

71. Rampil IJ. Anesthetic potency is not altered after hypothermic spinal cord transection in rats. *Anesthesiology* 1994; **80**: 606–10.

72. Borges M, Antognini JF. Does the brain influence somatic responses to noxious stimuli during isoflurane anesthesia? *Anesthesiology* 1994; **81**: 1511–15.

73. Kishikawa K, Uchida H, Yamamori Y, Collins JG. Low-threshold neuronal activity of spinal dorsal horn neurons increases during REM sleep in cats: comparison with effects of anesthesia. *J Neurophysiol* 1995; **74**: 763–9.

74. Baars JH, Benzke M, von Dincklage F, *et al.* Presynaptic and postsynaptic effects of the anesthetics sevoflurane and nitrous oxide in the human spinal cord. *Anesthesiology* 2007; **107**: 553–62.

75. Jinks SL, Bravo M, Hayes SG. Volatile anesthetic effects on midbrain-elicited locomotion suggest that the locomotor network in the ventral spinal cord is the primary site for immobility. *Anesthesiology* 2008; **108**: 1016–24.

76. Grasshoff C, Rudolph U, Antkowiak B. Molecular and systemic mechanisms of general anaesthesia: the "multi-site and multiple mechanisms" concept. *Curr Opin Anaesthesiol* 2005; **18**: 386–91.

77. Antognini JF, Wang XW, Piercy M, Carstens E. Propofol directly depresses lumbar dorsal horn neuronal responses to noxious stimulation in goats. *Can J Anaesth* 2000; **47**: 273–9.

78. Eger EI, Koblin DD, Harris RA, *et al.* Hypothesis: inhaled anesthetics produce immobility and amnesia by different mechanisms at different sites. *Anesth Analg* 1997; **84**: 915–8.

79. Kendig JJ. In vitro networks: subcortical mechanisms of anaesthetic action. *Br J Anaesth* 2002; **89**: 91–101.

80. Sonner JM, Antognini JF, Dutton RC, *et al.* Inhaled anesthetics and immobility: mechanisms, mysteries, and minimum alveolar anesthetic concentration. *Anesth Analg* 2003; **97**: 718–40.

81. Eger EI, Raines DE, Shafer SL, Hemmings HC, Sonner JM. Is a new paradigm needed to explain how inhaled anesthetics produce immobility? *Anesth Analg* 2008; **107**: 832–48.

82. Merrill AW, Barter LS, Rudolph U, *et al.* Propofol's effects on nociceptive behavior and spinal c-fos expression after intraplantar formalin injection in mice with a mutation in the gamma-aminobutyric acid-type(A) receptor beta3 subunit. *Anesth Analg* 2006; **103**: 478–83.

83. Merkel G, Eger EI. A comparative study of halothane and halopropane anesthesia including method for determining equipotency. *Anesthesiology* 1963; **24**: 346–57.

84. Alford S, Schwartz E, Viana di Prisco G. The pharmacology of vertebrate spinal central pattern generators. *Neuroscientist* 2003; **9**: 217–28.

85. Cheng G, Kendig JJ. Enflurane directly depresses glutamate AMPA and NMDA currents in mouse spinal cord motor neurons independent of actions on GABAA or glycine receptors. *Anesthesiology* 2000; **93**: 1075–84.

86. Yanagidate F, Strichartz GR. Bupivacaine inhibits activation of neuronal spinal extracellular receptor-activated kinase through selective effects on ionotropic receptors. *Anesthesiology* 2006; **104**: 805–14.

87. Olschewski A, Hempelmann G, Vogel W, Safronov BV. Blockade of Na+ and K+ currents by local anesthetics in the dorsal horn neurons of the spinal cord. *Anesthesiology* 1998; **88**: 172–9.

88. Komai H, McDowell TS. Local anesthetic inhibition of voltage-activated potassium currents in rat dorsal root ganglion neurons. *Anesthesiology* 2001; **94**: 1089–95.

89. Kindler CH, Yost CS. Two-pore domain potassium channels: new sites of local anesthetic action and toxicity. *Reg Anesth Pain Med* 2005; **30**: 260–74.

90. Xiong Z, Strichartz GR. Inhibition by local anesthetics of Ca2+ channels in rat anterior pituitary cells. *Eur J Pharmacol* 1998; **363**: 81–90.

91. Hollmann MW, Durieux ME. Local anesthetics and the inflammatory response: a new therapeutic indication? *Anesthesiology* 2000; **93**: 858–75.

92. Hollmann MW, Herroeder S, Kurz KS, *et al.* Time-dependent inhibition of G protein-coupled receptor signaling by local anesthetics. *Anesthesiology* 2004; **100**: 852–60.

93. Hollmann MW, McIntire WE, Garrison JC, Durieux ME. Inhibition of mammalian G_q protein function by local anesthetics. *Anesthesiology* 2002; **97**: 1451–7.

94. Hollmann MW, Wieczorek KS, Berger A, Durieux ME. Local anesthetic inhibition of G protein-coupled receptor signaling by interference with Galpha(q) protein function. *Mol Pharmacol* 2001; **59**: 294–301.

95. Minami K, Uezono Y. G_q protein-coupled receptors as targets for anesthetics. *Curr Pharm Des* 2006; **12**: 1931–7.

96. Uratsuji Y, Nakanishi H, Takeyama Y, Kishimoto A, Nishizuka Y. Activation of cellular protein kinase C and mode of inhibitory action of phospholipid-interacting compounds. *Biochem Biophys Res Commun* 1985; **130**: 654–61.

97. Mikawa K, Maekawa N, Hoshina H, *et al.* Inhibitory effect of barbiturates and local anaesthetics on protein kinase C activation. *J Int Med Res* 1990; **18**: 153–60.

98. Yanagidate F, Strichartz GR. Local anesthetics. *Handb Exp Pharmacol* 2007; (**177**): 95–127.

99. Caterina MJ, Schumacher MA, Tominaga M, *et al.* The capsaicin receptor: a heat-activated ion channel in the pain pathway. *Nature* 1997; **389**: 81624.

100. Leffler A, Fischer MJ, Rehner D, *et al.* The vanilloid receptor TRPV1 is activated and sensitized by local anesthetics in rodent sensory neurons. *J Clin Invest* 2008; **118**: 763–76.

101. Hirota K, Smart D, Lambert DG. The effects of local and intravenous anesthetics on recombinant rat VR1 vanilloid receptors. *Anesth Analg* 2003; **96**: 1656–60.

102. Binshtok AM, Bean BP, Woolf CJ. Inhibition of nociceptors by TRPV1-mediated entry of impermeant sodium channel blockers. *Nature* 2007; **449**: 607–10.

103. Knotkova H, Pappagallo M, Szallasi A. Capsaicin (TRPV1 Agonist) therapy for pain relief: farewell or revival? *Clin J Pain.* 2008 Feb; **24**: 142–54.

104. Gunthorpe MJ, Chizh BA. Clinical development of TRPV1 antagonists: targeting a pivotal point in the pain pathway. *Drug Discov Today* 2009; **14**: 56–67.

105. Hefti FF, Rosenthal A, Walicke PA, *et al.* Novel class of pain drugs based on antagonism of NGF. *Trends Pharmacol Sci* 2006; **27**: 85–91.

106. Lewin GR, Rueff A, Mendell LM. Peripheral and central mechanisms of NGF-induced hyperalgesia. *Eur J Neurosci* 1994 Dec 1; **6**: 1903–12.

107. Della Seta D, de Acetis L, Aloe L, Alleva E. NGF effects on hot plate behaviors in mice. *Pharmacol Biochem Behav* 1994 Nov; **49**: 701–5.

108. Zhu CZ, Wilson SG, Mikusa JP, *et al.* Assessing the role of metabotropic glutamate receptor 5 in multiple nociceptive modalities. *Eur J Pharmacol* 2004; **506**: 107–18.

109. Bhave G, Karim F, Carlton SM, Gereau RW. Peripheral group I metabotropic glutamate receptors modulate nociception in mice. *Nat Neurosci* 2001; **4**: 417–23.

110. Lea PM, Faden AI. Metabotropic glutamate receptor subtype 5 antagonists MPEP and MTEP. *CNS Drug Rev* 2006; **12**: 149–166.

111. Karim F, Wang CC, Gereau RW. Metabotropic glutamate receptor subtypes 1 and 5 are activators of extracellular signal-regulated kinase signaling required for inflammatory pain in mice. *J Neurosci* 2001; **21**: 3771–9.

112. Hu HJ, Bhave G, Gereau RW. Prostaglandin and protein kinase A-dependent modulation of vanilloid receptor function by metabotropic glutamate receptor 5: potential mechanism for thermal hyperalgesia. *J Neurosci*, 2002; **22**: 7444–7452.

113. Hudson LJ, Bevan S, McNair K, *et al.* Metabotropic glutamate receptor 5 upregulation in A-fibers after spinal nerve injury: 2-methyl-6-(phenylethynyl)-pyridine (MPEP) reverses the induced thermal

hyperalgesia. *J Neurosci* 2002; **22**: 2660–8.

114. Walker K, Reeve A, Bowes M, *et al.* mGlu5 receptors and nociceptive function II: mGlu5 receptors functionally expressed on peripheral sensory neurones mediate inflammatory hyperalgesia. *Neuropharmacology* 2001; **40**: 10–19.

115. Montana MC, Cavallone LF, Stubbert KK, *et al.* The mGlu5 antagonist fenobam is analgesic and has improved in vivo selectivity as compared to the prototypical antagonist MPEP. *J Pharmacol Exp Ther* 2009; **330**: 834–43.

Gary R. Strichartz

Introduction

This chapter presents an analytical understanding of action potentials, what processes underly them, and how the different parameters of an excitable membrane can affect conduction velocity, refractory period, and repetitive firing.

For a complex multicellular organism to function in a coordinated way, effective communication between individual cells is of crucial importance. Communication within cells or from cell to cell involves either chemical substances (such as hormones, transmitters, or second messengers) or electrical signals (see Chapter 3). Electrical signals provide the rapid language of the nervous system, but they are also generated in almost all cells in response to a variety of stimuli.

In neurons, skeletal, cardiac, and smooth muscle, and most secretory cells action potentials are essential elements coupling stimuli to responses. Ionic currents passing through plasma membranes are the dynamic roots of action potentials. Currents through ion channels, the "conductance" elements of cell membranes, and currents originating from active transport enzymes and exchange proteins, the "electrogenic pump" elements, are the sources of electricity that determine a cell's resting potential and action potentials [1]. Such ionic channels and pumps are frequently affected by drugs used in anesthesia, either as the intended primary target, e.g., local anesthetics inhibiting Na^+ channels, or as incidental participants that contribute to therapeutic or side effects, e.g., volatile anesthetics modifying Ca^{2+} channels in cardiac membranes. Our understanding of the mechanisms of cellular excitability from the viewpoint of ion channels is therefore fundamental to an appreciation of the actions of anesthetic agents.

Importance of Ohm's law: definition of terms

Electrical phenomena occur whenever charges (Q, measured in coulombs) of opposite sign are separated or can move independently. Any net flow of charges (or a change of charge with

time, dQ/dt) is called a current (I), and is measured in amperes. In this discussion of cellular excitability, the magnitude of a current flowing between two points (e.g., from the extracellular to intracellular compartments) is determined by the **potential difference** (or "voltage," or "voltage difference") between the two points (V, measured in volts) and the resistance to current flow (R, measured in ohms), as shown in the following equation:

$$I = V/R \qquad \text{Ohm's law} \qquad (17.1a)$$

(If you are uncomfortable with electricity, try the hydraulic equivalent $F = P/R$. Here the potential difference corresponds to the pressure difference, P, and the current responds to the flow, F).

When Ohm's law is applied to biologic cell membranes, it is often easier to replace the electrical resistance by its reciprocal, the **conductance**, g, measured in reciprocal ohms, or siemens:

$$I = gV \qquad \text{Ohm's law} \qquad (17.1b)$$

For simplicity, we will assume that all resistive elements in the cell membrane behave in an "ohmic way"– i.e., their current–voltage relationship (abbreviated as I–V) is described by Eq. 17.1b: the I–V relation is linear, with a slope given by the conductance, g. This is shown graphically by the solid line in Fig. 17.1A, which represents the transmembrane current (I) measured at different transmembrane potentials (V) in a hypothetical cell. Figure 17.1B shows the experimental arrangement. Two microelectrodes are inserted into the cell (glass microelectrodes have tip diameters of 0.1–0.5 μm and can penetrate into many cells, of 10–50 μm in diameter, without apparent damage to the membrane). One electrode is connected to a voltmeter to measure the transmembrane potential. The second microelectrode is hooked up to a tunable current source (e.g., a battery of variable output), which allows us to inject current into the cell and therefore to manipulate the membrane potential. The convention used in most current literature and in this chapter (Fig. 17.1A) is that the voltage is expressed as the difference between the intracellular and the extracellular potential ($V = V_{in} - V_{out}$). At negative values of V, the cell is thought to be hyperpolarized, whereas at positive membrane potentials it is thought to be depolarized. Positive charge moving from

Anesthetic Pharmacology, 2nd edition, ed. Alex S. Evers, Mervyn Maze, Evan D. Kharasch. Published by Cambridge University Press. © Cambridge University Press 2011.

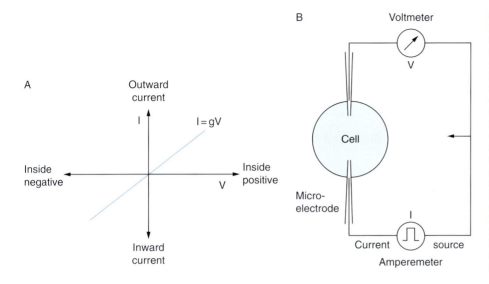

Figure 17.1. (A) Graphic representation of Ohm's law. The conventions for directions of passive current flow (I; outward and inward) in response to voltage changes (V; depolarization and hyperpolarization, respectively) are used in all contemporary electrophysiology. The conductance (g, the reciprocal of resistance) is the slope of the I versus V line. In this chapter, all ionic I–V relations are assumed to obey Ohm's law, although in reality this relationship is not usually linear because of differences in permeant ion concentration, and thus the diffusion-limited conductances, between the inside and the outside of cells. (B) Schematic diagram of the experimental arrangement for measuring a cell's electrical properties. The membrane potential difference between inside and outside the cell (V) is measured by the voltmeter coupled to one microelectrode, whereas the other microelectrode delivers current (I) across the membrane from a switchable, constant source. Both the voltmeter and the current-source electrodes are connected at their opposite pole to a ground electrode (*open triangles*) in the extracellular solution.

inside to outside is called **outward current** and represented as an upward (positive) current, whereas **inward current** is shown as a negative current deflection.

Transmembrane current is carried by ion channels

How does current actually flow through the cell membrane? Cell membranes are composed of a lipid bilayer with relatively polar regions next to the aqueous solutions and a hydrophobic layer at the center, which is practically totally impermeable to charged particles like small ions; a pure lipid bilayer presents an almost infinite resistance to ionic current flow [2]. For this reason, the presence of specialized membrane ion channels embedded in the lipid bilayer is essential for ionic currents (see Chapter 3). Each channel contains a relatively hydrophilic central pore that allows ions to cross from one side of the membrane to the other. Many different channel proteins exist, and some of them will be considered in this chapter [1]. The two most important functional properties of ion channels are: (1) their ability to discriminate between different ions (channel selectivity), and (2) that the channels fluctuate between open (conducting) and closed (nonconducting) states. This property is called channel *gating*, and its importance will become obvious when we consider the factors that control it (see below).

Channel selectivity: the Nernst equation and the resting potential

The hypothetical I–V relation shown in Fig. 17.1A does not apply to a real cell. It implies that in the absence of an externally applied current the potential difference across the membrane is

zero. In contrast, when an experimenter actually inserts a microelectrode into a resting cell, a constant ("resting") potential of –80 to –90 mV is recorded (recall that this is defined as $V_{\text{in}} - V_{\text{out}}$). What is the basis for this resting potential?

As mentioned earlier, ion channels can be selective for a particular ion. The negative resting potential in most cells is caused by the fact that the resting membrane is primarily permeable to chloride and potassium ions (i.e., Cl and K channels are almost the only channels open at rest). In particular, the membrane potential develops primarily because K^+ ions, which are 30 times more concentrated inside the cell, have diffused slightly to the outside, separating from their electrically neutralizing anions (thus leaving less positive charge inside) and forming the negative resting membrane potential.

The exact relation between concentration difference and membrane potential is given by the Nernst equation, which is described in Chapter 3.

$$V_{\text{ion}} = (RT/zF) \log_{10}([X]_{\text{o}}/[X]_{\text{i}}) \qquad (17.2)$$

V_{ion} is called the Nernst potential for ion X; it is the potential at which a membrane *specifically permeable only to ion X* would stabilize.

The extracellular and intracellular concentrations of the main inorganic ions in most cells is shown in Table 17.1. From these concentrations the Nernst potentials for the major ions can be calculated. This will show at what value of the transmembrane potential the net driving force for a particular ion will change sign, and the resulting flow of currents will change direction. At 37 °C, the constant term $RT/F \ln (10) = 61$ mV. Therefore,

$$V_{\text{Na}} = 61 \log(145/15) = +60 \text{ mV}$$

$$V_{\text{K}} = 61 \log(5/145) = -89 \text{ mV}$$

$$V_{\text{Cl}} = 61 \log(150/10) = -72 \text{ mV}$$

$$V_{\text{Ca}} = 30.5 \log(2/.0001) = +131 \text{ mV}$$

Table 17.1. Extracellular and intracellular concentrations of the main inorganic ions

Ion	Extracellular concentration	Intracellular concentration
Na$^+$	145 mM	15 mM
K$^+$	5 mM	145 mM
Cl$^-$	150 mM	10 mM
Ca^{2+}	2 mM	0.0001 mM (!!)

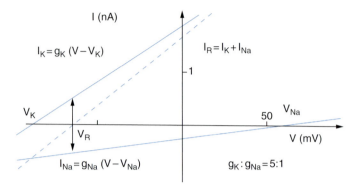

Figure 17.2. Current–voltage relations for theoretical K$^+$ and Na$^+$ currents through constant conductances in a "resting" membrane. Ohm's law now includes the Nernst potential for the permeation (V_{Na} or V_K) as an offset on the membrane potential (x-axis). The broken line represents the sum of K$^+$ and Na$^+$ currents at any membrane potential, with zero net current occurring at V_R, the resting potential. Changing the conductances g_K and g_{Na} will change the slopes of the I–V relations for the membrane and thus alter the value of V_R.

Thus the measured value of the membrane resting potential in most healthy, mature cells (–60 to –80 mV) is close to the Nernst potentials for Cl$^-$ and K$^+$ ions. It is as if the cell membrane was highly Cl- and K-selective. This is confirmed by the fact that changes in these ions' concentrations lead to predictable changes in membrane potential, whereas changes in the other ions have little effect on the resting potential.

In reality, there are multiple types of K$^+$ channels that are sensitive to a variety of intracellular and extracellular stimuli [3]. For the basic explanations in this chapter we coarsely define the K$^+$ channels that contribute to the resting conductance as *leak channels*, designated by g_l. Those K$^+$ channels that open in response to depolarization, which may include several classes, are called *voltage-gated channels*, and are generally designated in this chapter by g_K.

Notably, at the resting potential there exists a large inwardly directed electrochemical driving force for both Na$^+$ and Ca^{2+} ions. If Na$^+$ or Ca^{2+} channels, or both, were to open, this would lead to large inward currents that would depolarize the cell. Later it is shown that this is precisely the mechanism that leads to the generation of an action potential.

The balance of currents determines the potential

We can now return to our initial current–voltage relation and draw the correct relation for an open K$^+$ channel (Fig. 17.2). It will now intersect the current axis at V_K. Ohm's law still describes the I–V relation, but voltage offset (because of K$^+$ ions' asymmetric distribution) must be introduced, and Eq. 17.1b becomes:

$$I_K = g_K(V - V_K) \tag{17.3}$$

$V - V_K$ is, of course, just the electrochemical driving force at any potential V. If K$^+$ channels are the only channels open, then, as stated earlier, the membrane potential will be V_K. However, if the cell membrane also has some other measurable conductance, then V will deviate from V_K. Let us assume, for instance, that the cell also has a measurable Na$^+$ conductance, with $g_{Na}:g_K = 1:5$.

$$I_{Na} = g_{Na}(V - V_{NA})$$

I_{Na} will be zero at V_{Na} (+60 mV) and have a slope of one-fifth that of I_K (Fig. 17.2). The resting potential, V_R, in this case will settle at a value between V_{Na} and V_K, where net K efflux (I_K) is exactly balanced by net Na influx (I_{Na}). This point can easily be determined graphically from Fig. 17.2.

Since

$$I_{Na} = -I_K$$

$$g_{Na}(V_R - V_{Na}) = -g_K(V_R - V_K)$$

Rearranging terms gives:

$$V_R = V_{Na}(g_{Na})/(g_K + g_{Na}) + V_K(g_K + g_{Na}) \tag{17.4}$$

So V_R can have any value between V_{Na} and V_K. The actual value of V_R becomes a weighted average of the two Nernst potentials for Na$^+$ and K$^+$, where the weight is given by the relative conductances. In our example, with the above values for V_{Na}, V_K, and $g_{Na}:g_K$, $V_R = -64$ mV.

As expected, if $g_{Na} \gg g_K$, then $V_R = V_{Na}$

And, if $g_K \gg Ig_{Na}$, then $V_R = V_K$

Importantly, this condition of constant V_R is one of "steady state" but not of an equilibrium state. Because $V_R \neq V_{Na+}$ or V_K, there is a net driving force on both ions and a unidirectional flux for Na$^+$ and for K$^+$, even though the net current is zero.

V will only stay constant as long as the ionic gradients do not change. If there was no independently operating, active transport system (see later) to maintain the ionic gradients, they would indeed run down. Thus, although flux of ions through channels is a passive process, the energy-requiring process of active transport is necessary to maintain the gradients that drive ions through channels. In the absence of such energy, provided by cellular metabolism, gradients would collapse and cells would die.

Variable conductances: the generation of the action potential

When excitable cells are depolarized from their resting potential beyond a certain level (*threshold*), they respond with a relatively large, stereotyped potential change, the **action potential**. It is the action potential propagating away from the site of origin that constitutes impulse conduction in nerve, muscle, and heart. We will deal with impulse conduction later; in this section, we will just consider the ionic basis for the generation of the action potential. Figure 17.3 shows the typical configuration of a nerve action potential. An initial depolarization from the resting potential leads to a rapid depolarization, called the

upstroke of the action potential. After the upstroke, the action potential peaks at a positive value, about +30 mV, and then repolarizes. In many cells repolarization is followed by an "undershoot" (after-hyperpolarization) of the membrane potential, which returns to its resting value a few milliseconds after the end of the action potential.

We have seen that the resting membrane potential is determined by the relative conductances of the ion channels in the cell membrane. Fifty years ago, Hodgkin and Huxley concluded that the nerve action potential is generated by rapid conductance changes of Na^+ and K^+ channels. From Eq. 17.4 it is clear that in the presence of Na^+ and K^+ channels [4–6] the membrane potential can swing between $V_K = -90$ mV and $V_{Na} = +60$ mV. At rest, total g_K (primarily from g_l) $>> g_{Na}$, and V is just slightly more positive than V_K. Upstroke and peak of the action potential are the result of a massive increase of g_{Na}, such that at the peak of the action potential the membrane potential approaches V_{Na} because now $g_{Na} >>> g_K + g_l$. Repolarization occurs because g_{Na} returns to its resting low level and voltage-dependent g_K increases. The resulting after-hyperpolarization marks the closest agreement between V and V_K, because at this time total $g_K + g_l >>> g_{Na}$. As g_K declines, total K^+ conductance returns to its resting level, g_l, and V depolarizes to the resting level. The time courses of the changes in g_{Na} and g_K underlying the generation of the nerve action potential are also shown in Fig. 17.3.

Channel gating underlies variable conductance

As mentioned earlier, ion channels fluctuate between open and closed states, a process called channel gating. It is possible to measure the openings and closings of a single channel molecule directly using a method called "patch clamp." Figure 17.4 shows such a recording from a tiny "patch" of membrane, which contains just one K^+ channel. Current traces are shown at –20 and +20 mV. Current amplitudes are the same for every opening at one potential, but differ between these two potentials (because the electrochemical driving force differs). The other important difference between the two current traces is that the *channel is open more often at the positive potential* [7]. The fraction of time a channel spends in the open state is called the *open probability*, P_o (P_o ranges between 0 and 1).

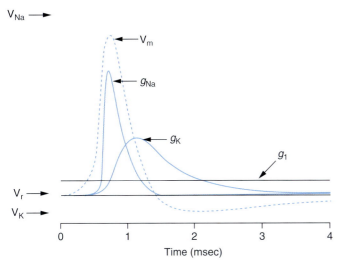

Figure 17.3. Conductance and potential changes during action potential (AP) propagation in a squid axon. The resting potential, V_r, is primarily dependent on the potential-independent and K^+-selective "leak conductance," g_l. Sodium conductance (g_{Na}) activated by depolarization, allows an inward Na^+ current that drives the rapidly depolarizing phase of the action potential, whereas the voltage-dependent potassium conductance (g_K) develops more slowly and, together with g_l, provides an outward K^+ current that reverses the AP and then hyperpolarizes the membrane for approximately 5 ms. Modified from Hodgkin and Huxley [6].

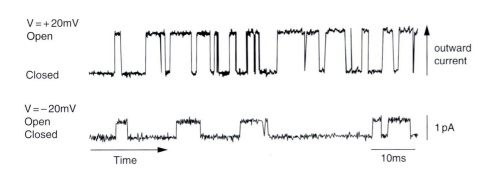

Figure 17.4. Records of a single K^+ channel showing discrete openings at two different membrane potentials. In the depolarized condition, at +20 mV, the open channel currents are larger ($V_m - V_K$ is greater) and the average closed times are briefer than in the hyperpolarized condition (–20 mV). This shows that the channel opens more frequently during the depolarized condition, but stays open for about the same time at either voltage. The average probability that the channel will be open (P_o) is $t_o/(t_o + t_c)$, where t_o is the mean open time and t_c is the mean closed time.

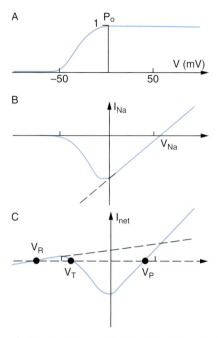

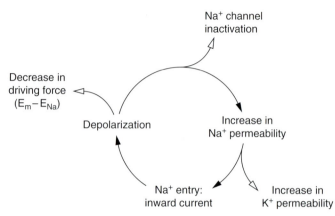

Figure 17.5. Voltage-dependent activation of Na$^+$ current. (A) The mean probability of a Na$^+$ channel reaching the open state in response to a rapid depolarization is graphed as a sigmoidal curve. Few openings occur in response to many identical depolarizations negative to −50 mV; maximum openness is reached at about 0 mV and an open probability of 50% occurs near −20 mV for this prototypical Na$^+$ channel. For a large ensemble of channels (a typical sensory neuron soma, for example, might contain 10^4 Na$^+$ channels), the fraction of all channels that open in response to one single depolarization would also equal P_o. (B) The product of voltage-dependent P_o and the I–V relation for an open channel (see I_{Na} line in Fig. 17.2) demonstrates the voltage-dependent activation of Na$^+$ current in an excitable cell. (C) The sum of the voltage-dependent Na$^+$ current in (B) and the outward K$^+$ currents (see Fig. 17.2) reveals three points where net ionic current equals zero, the resting potential (V_R), the threshold potential (V_T), and the peak of the action potential (V_P). Note that V_R is near to (but less negative than) V_K and that V_P is near to (but less positive than) V_{Na}.

Figure 17.6. Factors that drive depolarization and repolarization of the action potential. Factors in the circle, and connected by *solid arrows*, drive the rising phase. An initial depolarization is the stimulus that opens Na$^+$ channels, increasing Na$^+$ conductance and leading to the inward Na$^+$ current that can further depolarize the membrane. Factors outside the circle (*open arrows*) decrease the depolarizing tendency. Inactivation of Na$^+$ channels limits the increase in Na$^+$ conductance, the opening of K$^+$ channels produces an outward current that opposes inward Na$^+$ current, and the lessening of the force driving on Na$^+$ influx, V_m − V_{Na}, directly reduces that current. During the initial, rising phase of the action potential, the factors in the circle dominate, and during the falling, repolarizing phase, the factors outside the circle are more important.

P_o is voltage-dependent for many ion channels. **The voltage-dependent change in P_o of Na$^+$ and K$^+$ channels underlies the conductance changes that produce the action potential.** The voltage dependence of P_o for Na$^+$ channels is shown in Fig. 17.5A, while Fig. 17.5B shows the voltage dependence of the Na$^+$ current where we have now scaled the maximum conductance, g_{max} (conductance of an *open* Na$^+$ channel), with P_o to obtain $I_{Na} = g_{max} P_o$ (V − V_{Na}). Finally, Fig. 17.5C shows the *net* membrane current as the sum of the Na$^+$ channel properties and the conductance of the resting membrane (mainly g_l channels: see Fig. 17.2). The net ionic membrane current has an "N-shaped" form with three intersects of the zero-current axis. Figure 17.5C is examined in greater detail later in the descriptions of the threshold for action potential generation. Here, let us just consider the strikingly different effects of an increase in the Na$^+$ or K$^+$ conductance on membrane depolarization (Fig. 17.6).

A depolarization that activates only K$^+$ channels generates an outward current that **repolarizes** the membrane

and thus terminates itself (negative feedback), whereas a depolarization that activates Na$^+$ channels generates an inward current that, if sufficiently large, depolarizes the membrane and thus becomes **regenerative** through positive feedback between depolarization and further opening of Na$^+$ channels. This positive feedback leads to the explosive upstroke of the action potential, after the threshold is reached.

The last property of Na$^+$ channels necessary for the understanding of the action potential is **inactivation** [5]. The voltage-dependent increase of the opening probability of Na$^+$ channels is not maintained in time, but rapidly decays. When the membrane is depolarized rapidly but then held at positive potential, Na$^+$ channels open first but then enter a nonconducting "inactivated" state. The term *inactivated* means that as long as a Na$^+$ channel is in that state, it cannot be opened again by a subsequent or larger depolarization. The return of Na$^+$ channels from the inactivated to the resting (closed) state after repolarization largely determines the so-called **refractory period** – i.e., the minimal time required before the cell can be excited again to fire the next action potential. In nerve and muscle cells, this refractory period is short (a few milliseconds), but it is greatly prolonged (up to hundreds of milliseconds) in heart cells. Inactivation of Na$^+$ channels helps terminate the action potential. Reversal of inactivation requires membrane repolarization. Thus maintained depolarizations tend to drive Na$^+$ channels into the inactivated state and therefore render a cell inexcitable. (Large depolarizations will lead to inactivation after Na$^+$ channel opening, but smaller depolarizations, e.g., to −60 mV, can inactivate channels without their passage through the open state [8]. The relative number of resting versus inactivated Na^+ channels decreases steeply between –80 and –40 mV, and therefore steady depolarizations in this potential range will greatly reduce the excitability of a cell. An example of such a clinically important situation is that of elevated serum potassium levels. Of anesthetic relevance is the mechanism of inhibition of Na^+ channels by local anesthetic or class I antiarrhythmic drugs, which bind with relatively high affinity to inactivated channels and thereby stabilize this nonconducting state of the channel, reducing excitability even further [9].

Active ion pumps maintain ion gradients

To this point we have assumed that the ion gradients are not changed by the fluxes carried through ion channels during action potentials. Indeed, only a tiny fraction of the ions present on either side needs to cross the membrane to generate the required electrical signals. Nevertheless, particularly during maintained repetitive activity or prolonged (e.g., cardiac) depolarizations, the net gain in intracellular Na^+ and the loss of intracellular K^+ must be compensated. This is accomplished with a membrane transport protein called the Na^+ pump, or the Na^+/K^+ ATPase. This protein is an enzyme that transports Na^+ and K^+ ions *actively, against their electrochemical gradient*. This coupled Na^+ extrusion and K^+ uptake (three Na^+ ions are extruded for two K^+ ions taken up) requires energy, which the Na^+ pump obtains through hydrolysis of adenosine triphosphate (ATP) to adenosine diphosphate (ADP) and inorganic phosphate [10]. The Na^+ pump is present in all animal cells and has been estimated to consume as much as 60% of the basal metabolic energy. The steep chemical Na^+ gradient that the Na^+ pump creates and maintains is analogous to the energy stored in a battery. This battery is not only used for the generation of inward Na^+ current, but also at least partially provides the energy for the regulation of intracellular Ca^{2+} and protons through Na^+/Ca^{2+} and Na^+/H^+ exchangers, and it fuels the Na^+-coupled uptake of molecules such as glucose and amino acids.

Although the Na^+ pump is the most abundant active ion transporter in the plasma membrane, other ion pumps (e.g., Ca^{2+} pump) are also present and help maintain the ionic transmembrane gradients. Subcellular membranes with transport requirements differing widely from the plasma membrane also have different sets of passive (channels) and active (pumps) ion transport proteins. Examples include the membrane of the sarcoplasmic reticulum in muscle, with its very high density of Ca^{2+} pumps and Ca^{2+} release channels [11], and mitochondrial membranes with the proton pumps that form an essential part of the energy transduction mechanism.

Ion channels are formed by transmembrane proteins

All ion channels are composed of proteins that reside within the membrane and provide a pathway for ion permeation. Voltage-gated cation channels, such as the Na^+ and K^+ channels involved in the action potential, contain charged intramembrane segments that respond to the changing electrical force of a depolarization in ways that ultimately lead to channel opening and inactivation (Fig. 17.1). Rapid inactivation of the Na^+ channel requires the movement of the cytoplasmic loop that connects homologous domains III and IV [12]. Many loci on Na^+ channels can be phosphorylated by selective kinases, providing a dynamic modulation of chemical gating by second-messenger systems, activated by receptors for neurotransmitters, hormones, and ionic stimuli [13].

Although most rapid physiologic functions of voltage-gated ion channels result from activity of the α subunits, associated β subunits are important for the stability of channels in the membrane, anchoring them to cytoskeletal elements, or to extracellular basement membranes, or to both [14].

The nerve impulse: integrating the membrane properties

Previously we have discussed the conductive (resistance) properties of membranes through which ionic current flows. Now we introduce another electric element of membranes, the **capacitance**. Capacitance is simply the capability of an insulator to separate electric charge. The capacitance of the cell membrane resides specifically in the hydrophobic bilayer, which insulates the extracellular from the intracellular aqueous phase (Fig. 17.7). Capacitance (C, in farads [F]) is defined as

$$C = Q/V \qquad (17.5)$$

where Q is the amount of charge separated and V is the voltage difference across the capacitor. The physical properties of a membrane that determine its capacitance are the dielectric constant, ε, the membrane area, A, and the membrane thickness, d.

$$C = \varepsilon A/4\pi d \qquad (17.6)$$

The membrane capacitance is *proportional to the membrane area and inversely proportional to the membrane thickness*. All mammalian cell plasma membranes have about the same thickness and dielectric constant, and thus a specific membrane capacitance per area of 1 μF cm^{-2}.

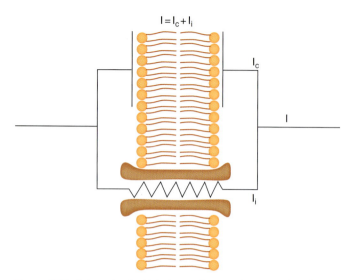

$I = I_c + I_i$

Figure 17.7. Schematic of a biologic membrane and its equivalent electrical circuit, showing the pure identity of the lipid bilayer insulator with membrane capacitance, and of the ion channel with conductance (resistance). In reality, this identity is not so segregated; bilayers have weak conductance and channels have some capacitance properties.

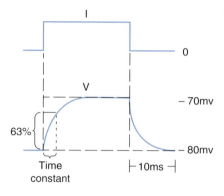

Figure 17.8. Passive response of a simple membrane. A capacitor and resistor arranged in parallel, as in the equivalent circuit of Fig. 17.7, will show a slow change in potential (V) in response to the sudden application of a constant current (I). The change of V follows exponential kinetics with a membrane time constant (the time to reach I/e or 63% of complete change, in seconds) that is the product of membrane resistance (in ohms) and membrane capacitance (in farads).

Cell capacitance and metabolic cost of an action potential

The capacitance property of a membrane determines the metabolic "cost" of an action potential, because from Eq. 17.5 it becomes clear that the greater the capacitance, the more charge must be moved to generate the voltage of an action potential. The charge is supplied by an ionic current, and the greater the current, the more energy must be expended by the Na^+/K^+ ATPase to restore the ion gradients. Because the specific capacitance of a lipid bilayer is ~1 μF cm^{-2}, one can calculate the number of Na^+ ions that must enter a cell to produce the typical depolarization of 100 mV associated with the action potential upstroke. For a spherical cell (e.g., a nerve cell body) with a diameter of 20 μm, the increase is about 8×10^{-6} Na^+ ions per action potential. In the same cell, at $[Na^+]_i = 15$ mM, the total Na^+ content is about 4×10^{10} Na^+ ions. Therefore, each action potential will increase $[Na^+]_i$ by approximately 0.05%, an increase that is not measurable chemically. After prolonged activity (i.e., hundreds of action potentials), the change in $[Na^+]_i$ will reach detectable levels and active pumping will be required to maintain the transmembrane gradient.

The relative change in ion concentration produced by each action potential varies with the surface-to-volume ratio of a cell. Because in our example we have chosen a spherical cell (minimal surface/volume ratio), the relative Na^+ accumulation can be greater in cells of different geometries. Indeed, in small cylindrical axons of nonmyelinated C fibers, with diameters 1 μm or less, as few as 5–10 action potentials can more than double $[Na^+]_i$ and stimulate the Na^+ pump, leading to an electrogenic outward pump current that, because of the high membrane resistance of such small axons, strongly hyperpolarizes the C fibers for many seconds after repetitive activity, the so-called *post-tetanic hyperpolarization* [15].

Cell capacitance and the membrane reaction time

Membranes cannot instantly change their voltages in response to sudden current changes. This is illustrated in Fig. 17.8, where we use the experimental arrangement to look at the response to a constant current pulse injected by a microelectrode. This experimental arrangement is simple but qualitatively quite similar to the physiologic situation in which currents are produced in a cell by synaptic or sensory input.

Even though in Fig. 17.8 the current applied across the membrane changes almost instantaneously, the voltage increases slowly to its new steady-state value. To understand this, we must represent the membrane by its two electric components (Fig. 17.7): the bilayer capacitance and the ionic conductance. The slow increase of the membrane potential is caused by the fact that all of the initial current flows into the capacitance. Before we can get current to flow through the conductive element (e.g., a K^+ channel in the resting membrane), we must develop a voltage across it, which requires charging the membrane capacitance.

The speed of the voltage response is expressed by the rate of change of V, i.e., by dV/dt.

From Eq. 17.5 and the definition of current ($I = dQ/dt$), we obtain

$$dV/dt_1 = 1/C_m(dQ/dt) = I_c/C_m \quad (17.7)$$

where dV/dt_1 is the initial rate of potential change, when all current flow is into the membrane's capacitance, C_m (i.e., membrane current = capacitate current). As time passes, dV/dt declines because as soon as a transmembrane voltage develops, ionic current (I_i) starts flowing through the conductance, decreasing I_c. Eventually the capacitance is fully charged, capacitate current decreases to zero ($I_c = dV/dt = 0$), and V reaches a value that is just given by the ohmic drop (Ohm's law: $V = RI$) across the resistance of the membrane. The time course of the voltage change in response to a sudden current change is exponential. For a typical membrane, the time it takes to reach 63% ("time constant") of the final steady value is about 5 ms.

The important conclusion is that because of their electrical capacitance, excitable cells take a significant time to respond to stimuli. This represents a limitation on the speed of neuronal signaling. However, it also permits closely spaced, brief stimuli to be additive; if the membrane response to the first stimulus is not yet over by the time the second stimulus is delivered, then the second response will be added on the remainder of the first one. Therefore input on the same cell membrane from more than one synapse can lead to summation, even if the inputs are separated by 5–10 ms.

Subthreshold responses are not propagated

Voltage responses such as those shown in Fig. 17.8 are called subthreshold, local, or passive responses. When they occur through synaptic or sensory input they are called excitatory postsynaptic potentials if they depolarize, or inhibitory postsynaptic potentials if they hyperpolarize the membrane. These *subthreshold responses are conducted with decrement* – i.e., their amplitude gets smaller with increasing distance from the point of origin. The reason for the decremental conduction is given (1) by the *I–V* relation of the membrane around the resting potential, and (2) by the resistive properties of cytoplasm and cell membrane. We have already examined the *I–V* relation of a nerve membrane in detail (Fig. 17.5). Let's take a closer look now at the region around the resting potential (Fig. 17.9). We can see that small depolarizations will give rise to outward current (through K^+ channels), which will hyperpolarize the membrane as soon as the depolarizing stimulus stops. Thus depolarization in that region of the *I–V* produces current that antagonizes and reverses the depolarization. The only depolarizing current available for spatial spread is the one generated locally by the synaptic or sensory input in real life, or the current-injecting microelectrode in our experiment. The inward current density will therefore be highest at the site of current injection and will decay rapidly with distance. The most tractable case is that of a cable (e.g., an axon) with uniform cytoplasmic and membrane resistance [16]. In this case, injection of current at a particular point along the axon will lead to a voltage that decays exponentially with increasing distance from the point of current injection. This is shown in Fig. 17.10. The distance at which the voltage difference has decayed to l/e is called λ, or the "space constant."

The space constant for this so-called electrotonic spread of a subthreshold depolarization depends entirely on the values of the cytoplasmic resistance and the membrane resistance. As shown schematically in Fig. 17.10, current at any point along the axon can either continue to flow axially (thereby spreading the potential difference spatially) or escape through the surface

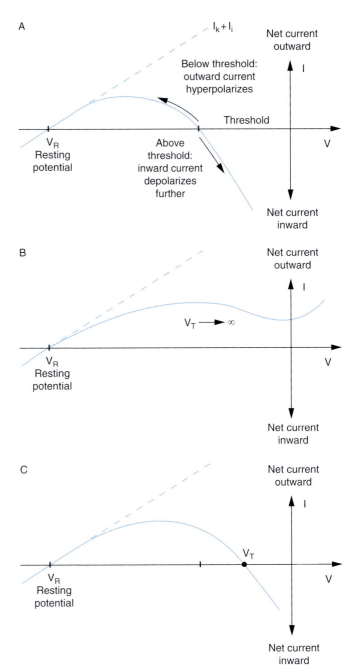

Figure 17.9. The current–voltage relationship around threshold for an excitable membrane. (A) Stimulation by an external source depolarizes the resting membrane, resulting in ionic membrane currents that reverse from outward to inward at a "threshold" potential of V_T, with a negative slope. Crossing this point on the current–voltage relation results in the "unstable" situation shown in Fig. 17.6, the regenerative feedback cycle that marks the upstroke of the action potential. In contrast, passing through the zero current point at the resting potential, V_R, on a positively sloped *I–V* relation is a "stable" condition because the resulting currents lead the potential back to rather than away from V_R. (B) Shortly after an action potential (AP) the Na^+ channels are more inactivated and the (voltage-gated) K^+ channels more activated than they are at rest. The resulting net current–voltage relations at this time yield no point of instability to induce another AP; the membrane is in the *absolute refractory period*; $V_T = \infty$. (C) Later after an AP the Na^+ channels are less inactivated and the K^+ (g_K) channels are less activated than in (B). Although the threshold is larger than at rest, a second AP can still be stimulated; the membrane is in the *relative refractory period*.

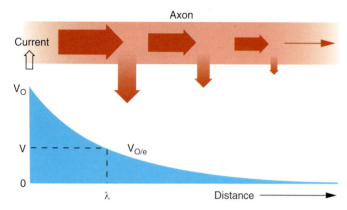

Figure 17.10. Current spread along a cylindric cell process. The passive spread of current away from its source (depolarizing or hyperpolarizing) is determined by the resistance to flow inside the cell (cytoplasmic) and the resistance to flow out from the cell (membrane). As the current density crossing the membrane decreases at increasing distance from the source (*left edge*), the (ohmic) voltage change caused by that current also decreases.

membrane. Both increased cytoplasmic resistance and decreased membrane resistance will favor current escape across the membrane and therefore shorten the distance over which the electrotonic potential spreads (shorter space constant). The cytoplasmic resistance is primarily influenced by the axon diameter. The resistance per unit length decreases with the cross-sectional area and thus with the square of the axon diameter. The resistance of the membrane close to the resting potential is determined primarily by the density of conducting channels (mainly K^+ channels, some Cl^- channels).

Typical values of space constants vary from 100 µm to several millimeters. As expected, particularly long space constants are achieved in nature by:

- **Large axon diameters** – The axial resistance decreases with the first power of the diameter. Therefore the space constant increases with the square root of the axon diameter. Squid giant axons have diameters of larger than 0.5 mm and space constants of 5 mm; very fine mammalian fibers may have space constants of 100 µm.
- **Very high membrane resistance** – Some axonal membranes have very high resistances. An example is the axon of the barnacle photoreceptor. The high membrane resistance gives this axon a space constant of 1–2 cm despite its diameter of only about 20 µm. Distal dendrites of vertebrate neurons also have high membrane resistance, favoring the spread of postsynaptic currents to a zone of summation/integration.
- **Adding outside insulation** – Myelin layers increase the effective membrane resistance in internodal regions of myelinated axons and therefore increase the space constant. Furthermore, the multiple wrapping of membranes around the axons of myelinated nerves constitutes a stack of many capacitors in a sequential configuration, a circumstance that greatly reduces the capacitance of the myelinated

axon's internodal region. As a result, much less charge is required for the passive membrane depolarization of the internode, and depolarization occurs much more rapidly than it would in an unmyelinated axon of the same diameter [17].

Propagation of the action potential

Unlike electrotonic potentials, action potentials are conducted *without decrement*. Thus as synaptic or sensory input (or spontaneous pacemaker depolarization) reaches the firing threshold, an action potential originates and then travels at constant amplitude along the entire excitable membrane of the cell. Action potentials are the "units" of information transfer along the axons of nerve fibers, and they also spread excitation in skeletal, cardiac, and smooth muscle. Even though there is considerable diversity between action potentials in different cells and different tissues, some of the fundamental properties of action-potential initiation and propagation can be generalized [6].

Let us further investigate the **threshold** for action potential initiation. We return to the I–V relation near threshold, and now include the voltage-dependent I_K as well as the leak and capacitate currents shown in Fig. 17.9. The initial positive slope of the I–V relation from these outward, passive responses flattens with progressive depolarization and turns negative as we start activating Na^+ channels. The threshold, V_T, is marked by the point where the I–V curve crosses the zero-current axis on its negative slope. The voltage range between the resting potential and this point is that of the electrotonic response, which corresponds to "subthreshold" depolarizations. Beyond this voltage range, more positive than the threshold potential, the net membrane current is now inward, which will depolarize the cell further; and it is this positive feedback between depolarization and further activation of inward current (see earlier) that produces the rapid upstroke of the action potential.

The presence of a threshold for the action potential explains why action-potential excitation is referred to as "all or nothing." An observer with a microelectrode in an axon 5 cm downstream from the site of the excitatory input can only observe either of two things: if the input reaches threshold locally, a full-blown action potential after the appropriate conduction delay will be seen, whereas if the input does not reach threshold, the observer will not see any voltage change at all (the electrotonic subthreshold response will not spread that far from the site of origin). "All or nothing" also means that once threshold is reached, a stereotyped action potential is fired that is essentially independent of the strength of the initiating stimulus. This, of course, contrasts sharply with the electrotonic response, which is a graded function of the excitatory input.

Dynamic nature of threshold

Threshold is a *condition of an excitable membrane*, not some absolute value of the membrane potential. Threshold is defined as that condition for which depolarization just produces a net inward current (Fig. 17.9A); dynamic changes in voltage-gated channels make important contributions to the threshold. The most obvious of these changes is the inactivation process of Na^+ channels: after an action potential some fraction of Na^+ channels are inactivated, effectively reducing the amount of the Na^+ current that can be generated by a stimulating depolarization. This effect shifts the threshold potential to more depolarized values; to infinity if no net inward current can be generated ($I_{Na} < I_{out}$), as in the *absolute refractory period* (Fig. 17.9B), and to values larger than that from rest, in the *relative refractory period* (Fig. 17.9C). Similarly, the shape of the stimulus will affect the threshold potential. Rapid, large depolarizations open Na^+ channels faster than their early inactivation or the slower opening of voltage-gated K^+ channels; slower-developing depolarizations permit Na^+ inactivation to occur to a greater degree and K^+ channel activation to generate more of an outward current, both factors elevating the threshold and in some cases temporarily abolishing excitability. An apparent contradiction thus occurs, as small, persistent membrane depolarizations can actually be inhibitory rather than excitatory for impulse generation.

Metabolic conditions (acidosis, hypercarbia), drugs, and diseases all can alter threshold behavior. Although action potentials are qualitatively "all or nothing," the conditions for the transition between these states are rarely constant.

Action potentials are conducted at the same amplitude

Propagation of the action potential without decrement occurs again because depolarization creates more depolarizing current, which gives the process its "regenerative" nature. All current flow must occur in loops, because the total charge moved must be conserved. Action-potential propagation is driven by a loop of current with four limbs, illustrated in Fig. 17.11, which include all the electrical elements in the cell membrane and cytoplasm that have been introduced in this chapter:

(1) Na^+ entry, down its electrochemical gradient, through open Na^+ channels. V_{Na} is shown here with the electrical sign for a battery, to indicate that it provides the driving force for the inward current.

(2) Now there exists a spatial (longitudinal) potential difference along the axoplasm, between the region of Na^+ influx and an adjacent region at rest. This results in longitudinal current flow along the axoplasm.

(3) The longitudinal current builds up charge on the membrane capacitance of the not-yet-active region. This membrane depolarizes.

(4) The current loop is closed by longitudinal current flow in the extracellular fluid, opposite to the direction of propagation. Current at any point in the loop must be the same as at any other point. Because the effective resistance of the extracellular space is only a fraction of the intracellular

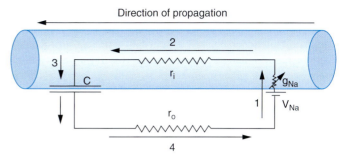

Figure 17.11. The cable properties of an axon shape the spread of depolarization during impulse propagation. In the excited region the inward Na^+ current enters the cell (process 1) where the action potential has depolarized the membrane. The difference in potential between this region and one still at rest results in longitudinal current flow inside the axon (process 2) that carries the charge to depolarize the resting membrane (mostly capacitate current for the initial depolarization; process 3). Laws of electricity require that current flow is returned to the site of original excitation along an extracellular path (process 4).

resistance, the extracellular spatial voltage differences resulting from action potential conduction are much smaller than the corresponding intracellular voltages (Ohm's law). Extracellular potentials resulting from the spatial spread of excitation can, however, be recorded, forming the basis of such widely used diagnostic techniques as the electrocardiogram, electroencephalogram, electroretinogram, and so on.

Depolarization of the not-yet-active region (limb 3 of the above loop) leads to activation of Na^+ channels in that domain. This is apparent in Fig. 17.3 as the earliest depolarization, a slow change that precedes by fractions of a millisecond the increase in g_{Na} and the corresponding rapid rise of the action potential. This region therefore becomes the new site of inward Na^+ current, and the current loop travels further downstream. Conduction will proceed unimpaired as long as the newly excited region produces at least as much depolarizing current as was needed for its own depolarization. The ratio of the charge supplied in the "forward loop" of local circuit current from an active membrane region to the charge required to bring the resting membrane to threshold is called the "margin of safety" for conduction. This ratio is 5:10 for large myelinated axons (where both parameters can be directly measured), the same or larger for small, nonmyelinated (C) axons, but substantially less for the small, myelinated (Aγ, Aδ) peripheral axons (of the motor and sensory systems, respectively).

Slowly inactivating Na^+ channels and abnormal impulse activity

Certain subtypes of Na^+ channels, including ones found exclusively in nociceptive, pain-sensing afferent nerves (e.g., $Na_v1.7$, $Na_v1.8$), do not inactivate rapidly but stay in the open, conducting state for tens of milliseconds. As a consequence, action potentials are longer in cells normally expressing these channels. Evidence shows that when the density of such channels increases, cells begin to fire repetitively in response to single brief stimuli, and that sometimes spontaneous bursts of impulses will occur, in the absence of explicit stimulation. From a clinical perspective there are two important consequences of this phenomenon. First, individuals who, often for hereditary reasons, have a surfeit of such channels in their primary nociceptors suffer from spontaneous pain. Second, such spontaneous impulse activity is exquisitely sensitive to low concentrations of Na^+ channel blockers, which may account for the therapeutic activity of micromolar lidocaine to relieve persistent, abnormal pain in many individuals.

Factors affecting conduction velocity
Membrane capacitance
A lower capacitance means less charge separation during the action potential (Eq. 17.5). Less current must flow into the capacitance and more is available for longitudinal spread. Also, the membrane can be depolarized more rapidly. The capacitance of a membrane can be decreased by making it thicker (Eq. 17.6). These principles are beautifully demonstrated in the myelinated axons (Fig. 17.12). The large reduction of the membrane capacitance through the multiple layers of myelin greatly speeds up the spread of depolarization from one node of Ranvier to the next (internodal distance = 1–2mm). This conduction is called "saltatory" (derived from Latin *saltare*, to jump). The pathophysiology of demyelinating diseases such as multiple sclerosis or Guillain–Barré syndrome is explained directly by the greatly impaired nerve conduction resulting from the loss of myelin [18].

Conductance of the resting membrane
K^+ channels tend to electrically "shunt" the depolarization induced by the inward Na^+ current. Therefore a low resting conductance favors rapid conduction, again illustrated in the myelinated axon.

Na^+ channel density
The bigger the Na^+ current, the larger the inward current in the active zone, the forward loop local current, and the conduction velocity. Local anesthetics (e.g., lidocaine) block nerve conduction by specifically binding to Na^+ channels and preventing them from opening [19]. Steady depolarization inactivates Na^+ channels, so depolarized regions of excitable tissues will conduct much more slowly. Steady depolarization beyond ~ –50 mV will completely abolish Na^+ channel-dependent conduction.

Conduction is not proportional, however, to the density of Na^+ channels [6,20], because the rapid rise of the action potential (and its brief duration) exceeds the response time for activation of Na^+ channels; only a small fraction, about 20%, of these channels actually open during one impulse. This leaves most of the channels in reserve, such that partial reduction of Na^+ channel density (e.g., by drugs, metabolic insufficiency [ischemia] or disease) to as low as 50% of

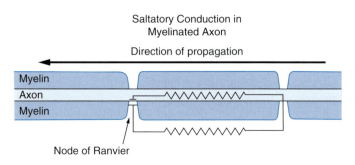

Figure 17.12. Impulse propagation in a myelinated nerve fiber. Excitation at the nonmyelinated nodes of Ranvier produces inward currents as in other excitable cells, but the heavily insulated myelinated internodes prevent ionic current from passing out through the local membrane and promote the spread of passive current much further and much faster than in a nonmyelinated axon of the same diameter. Propagation fails in demyelinated axons because of the increase of passive axonal membrane resulting from loss of myelin, loss of longitudinal current through the uninsulated internodal membrane that has no Na^+ channels, and the increase in membrane capacitance.

normal, barely affects conduction. Below that level, however, conduction deficit is easily reached and impulse failure occurs at Na^+ channel densities of 20–25% of control levels. As a result, functional losses during local anesthetic blockade are steeply dependent on dose of drug.

Axon size
Bigger axons conduct faster [21]. The increased capacitance per unit length is swamped by the decreased axial resistance, which, as noted earlier, decreases with the square of the diameter. Conduction velocity for action potentials varies greatly in nature. As expected, the fastest conduction is found in myelinated axons of large diameter (10–20 µm, speed of conduction 80–120 m s^{-1}), whereas small, nonmyelinated nerve fibers (e.g., C fibers, diameter 0.2–1.5 µm) conduct only at 0.5–2 m s^{-1}.

Whereas conduction is uniform along the entire cylindrical region of nonmyelinated axons, nonuniform behavior is evident at places where axons branch [22]. Peripheral nerves branch multiple times at their distal terminals, whether for sensory endings or skeletal muscle innervation, and sensory fibers also branch in a complex anatomy after they enter the spinal cord. For distal branches, the "summation" behavior for spatially separate terminals that converge to a common axon may present a benefit, because graded, electrotonic "generator" currents that arise from sensory transduction at spatially separated terminals will be integrated at a convergence point where the capacitance and the membrane resistance of the common, proximal axon is lower than that of the branches and, consequently, the resulting depolarization is both faster and higher. By the same reasoning, when impulses from a single axon encounter a branch point, as in the spinal cord, there may often be insufficient current from one invading impulse to raise both of the branches' membranes to threshold. Stimulation of only one branch by a single invading action potential will render it refractory, however (see earlier), so that a subsequent impulse may distribute its current to stimulate the other branch. If you imagine a train of impulses traveling along one axon toward a spread of multiple branches, you can imagine the possibilities of "activity-dependent" changes in the pattern of excitation distributed to all the nerve terminals. Add to this the dynamic responses caused by post-tetanic hyperpolarization of Na^+-loaded small branches and you will begin to appreciate the complexities of axonal firing behavior that moderate information transmission in the nervous system. In summary, although axonal conduction is characterized at its simplest by an all-or-nothing, uniformly propagated wave, at its most complex it provides a highly modulated, dynamic process for shaping information transfer in the peripheral and, likely, the central nervous system.

Summary

Ionic channels and pumps are frequently effected by drugs used in anesthesia, either as the intended primary target or as incidental participants that contribute to therapeutic or side effects. Understanding cellular excitability mechanisms from the viewpoint of ion channels is fundamental to an appreciation of the actions of anesthetic agents.

The two most important functional properties of ion channels are: (1) their ability to discriminate between different ions (channel selectivity), and (2) that the channels fluctuate between open (conducting) and closed (nonconducting) states.

At the resting potential there exists a large inwardly directed electrochemical driving force for both Na^+ and Ca^{2+} ions. If Na^+ or Ca^{2+} channels, or both, were to open, this would lead to large inward currents that would depolarize the cell. When excitable cells are depolarized from their resting potential beyond a certain level (threshold), they respond with a relatively large, stereotyped potential change, which is called the action potential. Action potentials are the "units" of information transfer along the axons of nerve fibers, and they also spread excitation in skeletal, cardiac, and smooth muscle. It is the action potential propagating away from the site of origin that constitutes impulse conduction in nerve, muscle, and heart.

When ion channels fluctuate between open and closed states, the process is called channel gating. The fraction of time a channel spends in the open state is called the open probability, P_o, and the open probability is voltage-dependent for many ion channels. The voltage-dependent change in P_o of Na^+ and K^+ channels underlies the conductance changes that produce the action potential. The voltage-dependent increase of the opening probability of Na^+ channels is not maintained, but rapidly decays. When the membrane is depolarized rapidly but then held at positive potential, Na^+ channels open first but then enter a nonconducting "inactivated" state, and as long as a Na^+ channel is in that state it cannot be opened again by a subsequent or larger depolarization. The return of Na^+ channels from the inactivated to the resting (closed) state after repolarization largely determines the refractory period. The refractory period is the minimal time required before the cell can be excited again to fire the next action potential.

Due to their electrical capacitance (the capability of an insulator to separate electric charge), excitable cells take a significant time to respond to stimuli. This represents a limitation on the speed of neuronal signaling. However, it also permits closely spaced, brief stimuli to be additive; if the membrane response to the first stimulus is not yet over by the time the second stimulus is delivered, then the second response will be added on the remainder of the first one.

References

1. Hille B. *Ionic Channels in Excitable Membranes.* Sunderland, MA: Sinauer, 1991.

2. Robertson JD. *Structure and Function of Subcellular Components.* Cambridge: Cambridge University Press, 1959.

3. Miller C. Annus mirabilis for potassium channels. *Science* 1992; **252**: 1092–6.

4. Hodgkin AL, Huxley AF. Currents carried by sodium and potassium ions through the membrane of the giant axon of Loligo. *J Physiol* 1952; **116**: 449–72.

5. Hodgkin AL, Huxley AF. The dual effect of membrane potential on sodium conductance in the giant axon of Loligo. *J Physiol* 1952; **116**: 497–506.

6. Hodgkin AL, Huxley AF. The components of membrane conductance in the giant axon of Loligo. *J Physiol* 1952; **116**: 473–96.

7. Baker OS, Larsson HP, Mannuzzu LM, Isacoff EY. Three transmembrane conformations and sequence-dependent displacement of the S4 domain in shaker K^+ channel gating. *Neuron* 1998; **20**: 1283–94.

8. Vandenberg CA, Horn R. Inactivation viewed through single sodium channels. *J Gen Physiol* 1984; **84**: 535–64.

9. Hille B. Local anesthetics: hydrophilic and hydrophobic pathways for the drug-receptor reaction. *J Gen Physiol* 1977; **69**: 497–515.

10. Glynn IM. Sodium and potassium movements in human red cells. *J Physiol* 1956; **134**: 278–310.

11. Franzini-Armstrong C, Protasi F. Ryanodine receptors of striated muscle: a complex channel capable of multiple interactions. *Physiol Rev* 1997; **77**: 699–729.

12. West JW, Patton DE, Scheuer T, *et al.* A cluster of hydrophobic amino acid residues required for fast sodium channel inactivation. *Proc Natl Acad Sci U S A* 1992; **89**: 10910–14.

13. Catterall WA. Structure and function of voltage-gated ion channels. *Annu Rev Neurosci* 1995; **64**: 493–531.

14. Isom L, De Jongh K, Patton DE, *et al.* Primary structure and functional expression of the β_1-subunit of the rat brain sodium channel. *Science* 1992; **256**: 839–42.

15. Ritchie JM, Straub RW. The hyperpolarization which follows activity in mammalian

non-myelinated nerve fibres. *J Physiol* 1957; **136**: 80–97.

16. Hodgkin AL, Rushton WAH. The electrical constants of a crustacean nerve fibre. *Proc R Soc Med* 1946; **134**: 444–79.

17. Huxley AF, Stampfli R. Evidence for saltatory conduction in peripheral myelinated nerve fibres. *J Physiol* 1949; **108**: 315–39.

18. Rasminsky M, Sears TA. Internodal conduction in undissected demyelinated nerve fibres. *J Physiol* 1972; **227**: 323–50.

19. Butterworth JF, Strichartz GR. Molecular mechanism of local anesthesia: a review. *Anesthesiology* 1990; **72**: 711–34.

20. Cohen I, Atwell D, Strichartz G. The dependence of the maximum rate of rise of the action potential upstroke on membrane properties. *Proc R Soc Lond B Biol Sci* 1981; **214**: 85–98.

21. Jack JJB, Noble D, Tsien RW. *Electric Current Flow in Excitable Cells*. London: Oxford University Press, 1975.

22. Zhou L, Chiu SY. Computer model for action potential propagation through branch point in myelinated nerves. *J Neurophysiol* 2001; **85**: 197–210.

Physiologic substrates of drug action
Neuromuscular function

Joe Henry Steinbach and Ling-Gang Wu

Introduction

The major known actions of clinically used drugs on motor function take place at the final synapse in the motor pathway: the synapse between the motor neuron and the muscle fiber. This chapter reviews the cellular structure and function of this synapse, and the role of each key molecule on synaptic transmission at this synapse. The neuromuscular junction is a highly specialized synapse, designed to enable rapid, nondecrementing and reliable transmission. Three functionally and structurally distinct parts are present: the **presynaptic terminal**, the **synaptic cleft**, and the **postsynaptic membrane**. Presynaptically, voltage-gated channels allow activity-dependent entry of Ca^{2+} ions, which results in transmitter release. The released acetylcholine (ACh) diffuses in the cleft, where it is degraded by acetylcholinesterase (AChE). Finally, ACh binds to and activates the receptors on the postsynaptic membrane to result in muscle excitation. General anesthetics may reduce transmitter release, by acting either on ion channels or on the release process. Anticholinesterases act by prolonging the time ACh persists in the cleft and so enhancing actions at the postsynaptic receptors. Neuromuscular blocking drugs inhibit the postsynaptic receptors by inhibiting binding of ACh.

Structure and function of the neuromuscular junction

Structure

The cell bodies of motor neurons are located in the ventral horn of the spinal cord or brainstem. The axon of the motor neuron innervates the muscle at a specialized region of the muscle membrane called the endplate, the neuromuscular junction (NMJ), or the neuromuscular synapse (Fig. 18.1). A myelinated axon extends from the cell body to the muscle. Inside the muscle, each axon branches to innervate between 10 and several hundred separate muscle fibers (the motor unit). At the region where the motor axon approaches the muscle fiber, the axon loses its myelin sheath and terminates on a single muscle fiber at the NMJ. The

ends of the fine branches form multiple expansions or varicosities, called synaptic boutons, from which the motor neuron releases its transmitter. Each bouton is positioned in a junctional fold, a depression in the surface of the postsynaptic muscle fiber that contains the transmitter receptors. The transmitter released by the axon terminal is ACh (see *The presynaptic terminal*), and the receptor on the muscle membrane is the nicotinic type of ACh receptor (AChR; see *The postsynaptic response*). The presynaptic and the postsynaptic membranes are separated by a synaptic cleft approximately 50 nm wide. Within the cleft is a basement membrane composed of collagen and other extracellular matrix proteins. The enzyme AChE, which rapidly hydrolyzes ACh, is anchored to the collagen fibrils of the basement membranes (see *The synaptic cleft*).

Function

The NMJ must produce very reliable and very rapid excitation of the muscle fiber in response to a presynaptic action potential. As schematically summarized in Fig. 18.2, there is minimal synaptic delay at the NMJ. The presynaptic action potential invades the axon terminal and activates voltage-dependent Ca^{2+}-selective channels. The increased intracellular Ca^{2+} concentration induces fusion of synaptic vesicles with the plasma membrane and release of the ACh into the cleft. The cleft ACh binds to postsynaptic AChR, and the channel of the receptor rapidly opens. A net inward flux of cations flows through the channels, producing a postsynaptic depolarization. This depolarization activates voltage-dependent Na^{+}-selective channels, leading to an action potential, which propagates along the muscle fiber. Finally, the action potential induces Ca^{2+} release from the sarcoplasmic reticulum that, in turn, produces muscle contraction.

The rapidity and reliability of transmission is particularly remarkable when considering that the muscle fiber is a large cell that has a low input impedance – in other words, it takes a lot of membrane current (and hence, activation of many AChRs) to excite the muscle fiber. However, it is also critical that the excitation is terminated rapidly, so that the fiber can both follow nerve activity at relatively high frequencies and so that the muscle does not show repetitive activity in response to a single presynaptic action potential.

Anesthetic Pharmacology, 2nd edition, ed. Alex S. Evers, Mervyn Maze, Evan D. Kharasch. Published by Cambridge University Press. © Cambridge University Press 2011.

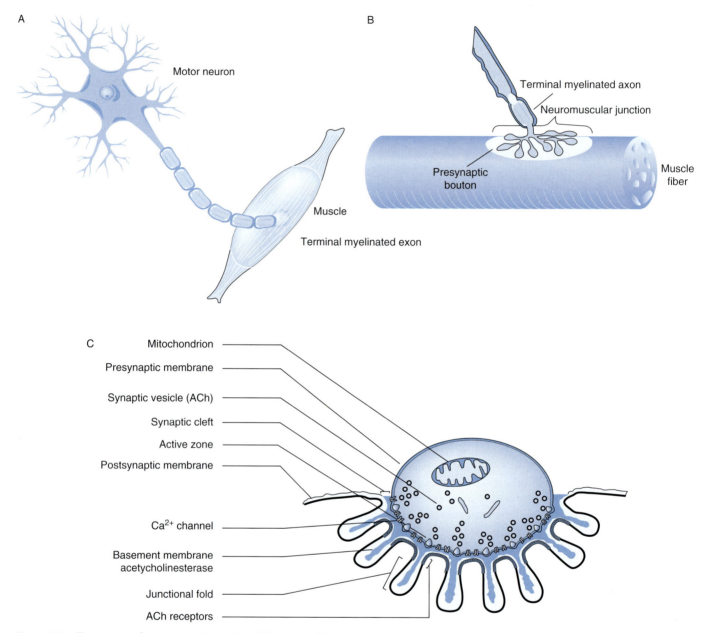

Figure 18.1. The structure of a neuromuscular junction. (A) The muscle fiber is innervated by a motor neuron whose cell body lies in the spinal cord. At the muscle, the motor axon ramifies into several fine branches. (B) Each terminal branch loses its myelin sheath and forms multiple swellings called presynaptic boutons, which are covered by a thin layer of Schwann cells. The boutons lie over a specialized region of the muscle fiber membrane, the endplate, and are separated from the muscle membrane by a 50 nm synaptic cleft. (C) Each presynaptic bouton contains mitochondria and synaptic vesicles. Synaptic vesicles are clustered around active zones, where the acetylcholine (ACh) transmitter is released. Immediately under each bouton in the endplate are several junctional folds, which contain a high density of ACh receptors at their crests. The muscle fiber is covered by a layer of connective tissue, the basement membrane (or basal lamina), consisting of collagen and glycoproteins. Both the presynaptic terminal and the muscle fiber secrete proteins into the basement membrane, including the enzyme acetylcholinesterase, which inactivates the ACh released from the presynaptic terminal by breaking it down into acetate and choline. The proteins in basement membrane also organize the synapse by aligning the presynaptic active zones with the postsynaptic junctional folds.

The presynaptic terminal: release of transmitter

Generation of an action potential

To activate voltage-gated Ca^{2+} channels, the plasma membrane of the axon and the nerve terminal use voltage-gated Na^+ and K^+ channels. An action potential is produced by rapid influx of Na^+ through Na^+ channels followed by rapid efflux of K^+ through K^+ channels [1,2] (Fig. 18.3). The Na^+ channels are responsible for depolarization or the rise of the action potential, whereas the K^+ channels are responsible for repolarization or the decay of the action potential. The half-width of a typical action potential is less than 1 millisecond, and it depolarizes the terminal by about

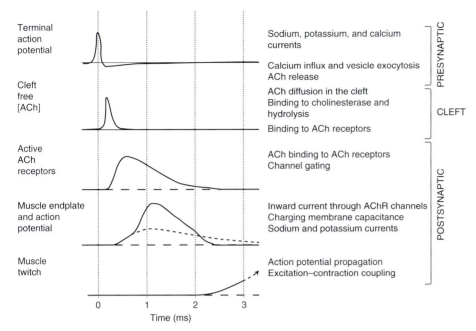

Figure 18.2. A summary of the timing of events during neuromuscular transmission, appropriate for a mammalian neuromuscular junction at 37 °C. The horizontal scale shows time (in milliseconds), starting at the peak of the action potential in the presynaptic terminal (top row). Each row shows a different phenomenon: the top shows the presynaptic action potential, the second shows the relative cleft-free acetylcholine (ACh) concentration, the third shows the relative activation of postsynaptic ACh receptors, the fourth shows the muscle membrane potential (and, *dashed line*, the endplate potential that would be observed if the action potential were blocked), while the final row shows the resulting twitch (which is mostly after the events shown). The third column lists some of the major molecules or processes that affect the time course shown. These topics are explored in greater detail in the text.

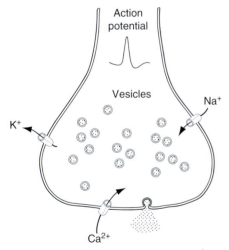

Figure 18.3. An action potential evokes Ca²⁺ influx and transmitter release. An action potential is generated by rapid Na⁺ influx, terminated by rapid K⁺ efflux. The action potential, which lasts for about 1 millisecond, activates the voltage-gated Ca²⁺ channels. The influx of Ca²⁺ through open Ca²⁺ channels triggers fusion of vesicles with the plasma membrane at the active zone. After vesicle fusion, transmitter molecules diffuse out of the fused vesicles. The dimensions are not drawn to be proportional to the real structure.

110 mV [3]. Such a brief but large depolarization activates voltage-gated Ca^{2+} channels. The amplitude and duration of the action potential determine the number of Ca^{2+} channels being opened and their opening time. Consequently, modulation of Na^+ or K^+ channels may affect the Ca^{2+} influx during an action potential and therefore alter transmitter release evoked by an action potential.

Ca^{2+} influx triggers vesicle fusion

There are many types of voltage-gated Ca^{2+} channels, including L, N, P/Q, R, and T, with specific biophysical and pharmacologic properties and different physiologic functions [4]. The distinct properties of these channel types are determined by the identity of their pore-forming subunit (termed the α_1 subunit), which is encoded by a family of related genes. Ca^{2+} channels also have associated subunits (termed α_2, β, γ, δ) that modify the properties of the channel formed by the α_1 subunits. Depending on the species, the nerve terminal of the endplate may predominantly contain P/Q or N-type Ca^{2+} channels [5–7]. The Ca^{2+} channels located in the terminal of the mammalian NMJ are P/Q-type [6,7].

There is a large inward electrochemical driving force on Ca^{2+}. The extracellular Ca^{2+} concentration is normally four orders of magnitude greater than the intracellular concentration – and therefore opening of voltage-gated Ca^{2+} channels would result in a large Ca^{2+} influx. One striking feature of transmitter release at synapses is its steep and non-linear dependence on Ca^{2+} influx – a twofold increase in Ca^{2+} influx can increase transmitter release up to 16-fold [8–11]. This relationship indicates that at some site, called the Ca^{2+} sensor, the binding of up to four or five Ca^{2+} ions is required to trigger release [12–15].

Available evidence suggests that Ca^{2+} channels are highly localized at or near active zones where transmitter release occurs [3,16–19]. Opening of these channels provides a high, local increase in Ca^{2+} concentration at the site of transmitter release during the action potential. During an action potential, the Ca^{2+} concentration at the active zone can increase 100-fold to 1000-fold (from the resting level of about 100 nM to 10–100 µM) within a few hundred microseconds [12–15]. This large and rapid Ca^{2+} transient is required for the rapid synchronous release of transmitter. The Ca^{2+} sensor responsible for transmitter release may have a relatively low affinity for Ca^{2+}, with a K_D ranging between 10 and 100 µM [13–15]. Because of the relatively low-affinity Ca^{2+} sensor, release likely takes place in a narrow region surrounding Ca^{2+} channels, where the Ca^{2+} concentration is sufficient to trigger release [20]. The requirement for a high concentration of Ca^{2+} also ensures that release will be rapidly terminated on repolarization. The delay between Ca^{2+} influx and transmitter release is extremely short (approximately 0.2 ms) [3,21,22].

Quantal transmitter release

Transmitter is released in quantal units. Fatt and Katz first observed small spontaneous postsynaptic potentials, called miniature endplate potentials (MEPPs), at the frog NMJ [23]. The size of these MEPPs is relatively fixed, about 0.5 mV. Each MEPP is caused by release of about 7000–12 000 ACh molecules from a single vesicle [24]. During an action potential, the Ca^{2+} influx triggers fusion between the synaptic vesicle membrane and the plasma membrane. A fusion pore spans these two membranes [25]. The pore rapidly dilates, and transmitter inside the vesicle rapidly diffuses across the synaptic cleft to act on its postsynaptic receptors. The opening of postsynaptic receptors generates an EPP (see *The postsynaptic response*).

In addition to acting on the postsynaptic receptors, ACh may also act on nicotinic ACh autoreceptors on motor nerve terminals, which may depolarize the nerve terminal and increase the intracellular Ca^{2+} level [26–29]. These actions may result in facilitation of ACh release during subsequent action-potential stimulation. Consequently, inhibition of presynaptic AChRs by the muscle-relaxant drug tubocurarine may block facilitation of release during a train of presynaptic firing. This mechanism, together with the well-characterized inhibitory effect of tubocurarine on the postsynaptic AChR, may contribute to muscle relaxation during administration of tubocurarine.

An action potential triggers fusion of about 300 vesicles at a frog NMJ [30]. A smaller number of released vesicles is observed in mammalian NMJs. For example, an action potential releases about 40 vesicles in rat diaphragm [31]. During an action potential, each active zone releases about one vesicle. In each active zone, tens of vesicles are attached to the plasma membrane. These vesicles are called docked vesicles. They are believed to be immediately available for release [32,33]. The number of vesicles released from each active zone during an action potential depends on the number of immediately releasable vesicles (releasable pool size) and the mean release probability of each releasable vesicle. Modulation of either of these two parameters may change the EPP size.

Cycling of synaptic vesicles

In various physiologic conditions, the motor nerve may fire (generate action potentials) repetitively. Continued repetitive firing inevitably causes depletion of the releasable pool, which results in depression of the EPP evoked by presynaptic action potentials. To maintain synaptic transmission during repetitive firing, vesicles in a pool not adjacent to the active zone plasma membrane (called the reserve pool) must move to those empty docking sites and become available for release. This process is called vesicle mobilization [34]. The rate of mobilization might be facilitated during repetitive firing, possibly mediated by an increase of the intracellular Ca^{2+} concentration [35–38].

During prolonged repetitive firing, vesicles in the reserve pool will eventually be depleted if there is no replenishment of vesicles. To continue supplying vesicles, the vesicle membrane that is fused with the plasma membrane is retrieved and recycled, generating new synaptic vesicles [39,40]. At least three forms of vesicle retrieval (endocytosis) have been hypothesized to operate at neuromuscular junctions (Fig. 18.4). The best characterized form is the full collapse of the vesicle with the plasma membrane upon exocytosis, followed by clathrin-mediated invagination and fission during endocytosis [41,42]. This form is called full-collapse fusion and retrieval. "Kiss-and-run" exocytosis and endocytosis involves fusion followed rapidly by fission without full collapse of vesicle membrane [43,44]. The original tracer experiments of Heuser and Reese also revealed that following heavy stimulation an endosome-like intracellular structure transiently appears, from which vesicles bud off [41]. Endosome-like structures are likely the result of bulk endocytosis, retrieval of a large piece of membrane directly from the plasma membrane [45–51].

Among these three forms of endocytosis, kiss-and-run fusion and retrieval might provide two advantages over other forms of fusion and retrieval. First, in principle it could allow for rapid and economical vesicle recycling. Second, its narrow fusion pore could limit the rate of transmitter discharge out of the vesicle, resulting in a slower and smaller quantal response [52,53]. Switching between kiss-and-run and full collapse fusion has been proposed as a mechanism to regulate synaptic strength [54].

Proteins involved in vesicle fusion

The molecular mechanisms that drive vesicles to cluster near synapses, to dock at active zones, to fuse with the membrane in response to Ca^{2+} influx, and to recycle have been intensively studied [55]. Proteins have been identified that are thought to (1) restrain the vesicles so as to prevent their accidental mobilization, (2) target the freed vesicles to the active zone, (3) dock the targeted vesicles at the active zone and prime them for fusion, (4) allow fusion and exocytosis, and (5) retrieve the

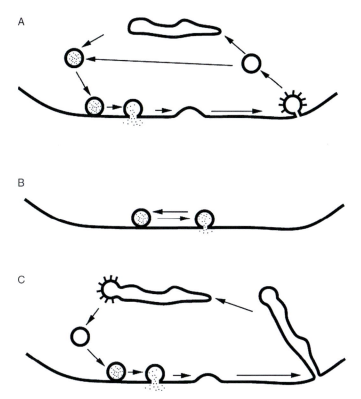

Figure 18.4. Three forms of endocytosis can be used to retrieve the vesicle membrane from the plasma membrane. (A) The vesicle can collapse fully into the plasma membrane, and then be retrieved by clathrin-mediated endocytosis. (B) The fusion pore can open transiently, then close without vesicle collapse (kiss-and-run). (C) After prolonged or massive release, vesicle membrane may be retrieved into large, endosome-like structures by bulk endocytosis.

fused membrane by endocytosis (Fig. 18.5). Synapsin I is thought to anchor vesicles that are away from active zones to a network of cytoskeletal filaments [56–58]. When the nerve terminal is depolarized and Ca^{2+} enters, synapsin is thought to become phosphorylated by Ca^{2+}/calmodulin-dependent protein kinase. Phosphorylation frees the vesicles from the cytoskeletal constraint, allowing them to move into the active zone.

The targeting of synaptic vesicles to docking sites for release is thought to be carried out by Rab3A and Rab3C, two members of a class of small proteins, related to the *ras* proto-oncogene superfamily, that bind guanosine triphosphate (GTP) and hydrolyze it to guanosine diphosphate (GDP) and inorganic phosphate [59]. Following the targeting of a vesicle to its release site, a complex set of interactions occurs between proteins in the synaptic vesicle membrane and proteins in the presynaptic membrane. Such interactions are thought to complete the docking of vesicles and to prime them so they are ready to undergo fusion in response to Ca^{2+} influx. One prominent hypothesis for this complex interaction is called the SNARE hypothesis [60,61]. According to this hypothesis, specific integral proteins in the vesicle membrane including synaptobrevin (also called VAMP) bind to specific receptor proteins in the presynaptic membrane, including syntaxin and SNAP–25.

Synaptotagmin (or p65) is an integral membrane protein of the synaptic vesicle thought to be the Ca^{2+} sensor for transmitter release [62–65]. Synaptotagmin contains two domains (the C2 domains) homologous to the regulatory region of protein kinase C. The C2 domains bind to phospholipids in a Ca^{2+}-dependent manner. This property suggests that synaptotagmin might insert into the presynaptic phospholipid bilayer in response to Ca^{2+} influx, thus serving as the Ca^{2+} sensor for exocytosis. Only a few proteins critical for transmitter release have been discussed in this chapter. There are many other vesicle proteins that may be involved in transmitter release [55]. How these proteins interact with each other and control transmitter release is currently being intensively studied. A clearer picture regarding the function of each protein in control of transmitter release may emerge in the near future.

Summary

An action potential, generated by rapid Na^+ influx and K^+ efflux, activates Ca^{2+} channels. The Ca^{2+} influx through Ca^{2+} channels triggers vesicle fusion and transmitter release. Vesicle mobilization and recycling ensures sufficient supply of vesicles for release. These processes may be the sites where anesthetics act. For example, local anesthetic drugs stop sensation by blocking conduction of nerve impulses, an effect achieved by blocking Na^+ channels [66]. Volatile anesthetics may activate K^+ channels, including two-pore potassium channels, and inhibit Ca^{2+} channels, which may contribute to their inhibitory effect on transmitter release [67–74]. Genetic evidence suggests that volatile anesthetics may modulate transmitter release by interaction with syntaxin, a membrane protein that interacts with vesicle proteins and Ca^{2+} channels [75]. Vesicle mobilization and recycling processes might also be targets for anesthetics.

The synaptic cleft: diffusion and hydrolysis

Acetylcholinesterase

The synaptic cleft provides the delimited volume in which released ACh diffuses to the AChR on the postsynaptic membrane. The major macromolecular component of the cleft, in the context of neuromuscular transmission, is AChE. AChE at the NMJ is a large complex, comprising four catalytic subunits bound to a long collagenous "tail" that serves to anchor AChE to the extracellular matrix in the cleft [76].

Physical dimensions

The synaptic cleft is about 50 nm across. The very small volume of the cleft means that the local concentrations of critical molecules can be very high. For example, there are about 2000 AChE active sites per square micrometer at the NMJ [77]. If this number is uniformly distributed through the volume of the cleft, the concentration of active sites is about 60 μM. Similarly, the density of AChR in the postsynaptic membrane is about 10 000

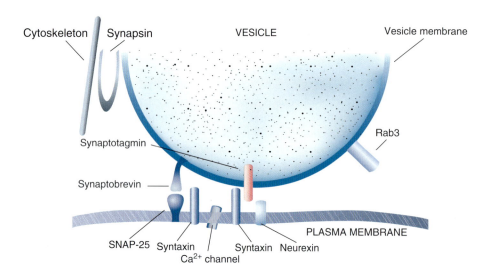

Figure 18.5. Some characterized vesicle proteins and their postulated localization and function. Synapsins are vesicle-associated proteins that are thought to mediate interaction between the synaptic vesicle and the cytoskeletal elements of the nerve terminal. The Rab proteins appear to be involved in vesicle trafficking within the cell and also in targeting of vesicles within the nerve terminal. The docking and fusion of vesicles appear to involve interactions between vesicle proteins and proteins of the nerve terminal plasma membrane: synaptobrevin (VAMP) and synaptotagmin (p65) on the vesicle membrane, and SNAP-25, syntaxins, and neurexins on the nerve terminal membrane.

per square micrometer [77], giving an averaged concentration of binding sites (two on each receptor) of about 600 μM.

The small dimensions also can result in rapid processes. Because the diffusion constant for ACh is approximately 1×10^{-5} cm^2 s^{-1}, it will take only about 1 microsecond for ACh released at the presynaptic membrane to equilibrate across the cleft. It is also true that the concentration of ACh in the cleft reaches a very high level. The estimated number of ACh molecules in a vesicle is 7000–12 000 (see *Quantal transmitter release*). When this number of molecules is rapidly released, the concentration in the cleft is likely to approach 1 mM for a brief period [77,78].

There are three basic events that a free ACh molecule can experience: it can continue to diffuse in the cleft, it can bind to cholinesterase (and be degraded), or it can bind to a postsynaptic AChR (and participate in activation). Free diffusion is important immediately after release, because the binding sites on AChE and AChR are saturated by the high local ACh concentration. However, the high concentration of sites means that the free ACh is rapidly bound and immobilized (Fig. 18.2); for example, a disk of radius 0.4 μm in the cleft contains about 10 000 binding sites on AChR and 1000 on AChE.

Muscle excitation follows after binding of ACh to the AChR, and is discussed in the next section. Binding of ACh to AChE results in cleavage of ACh to acetate and choline. This reaction is rapid, with an association rate of $\sim 2 \times 10^8$ M^{-1} s^{-1} and a dissociation constant of about 50 μM [76]. The catalytic rate for AChE is $\sim 10^4$ s^{-1}, corresponding to an average time between binding of ACh and hydrolysis of 100 microseconds. Choline is, in general, a very weak activator of the AChR and therefore the hydrolysis products are inactive. Choline, in turn, is cleared from the synaptic cleft by diffusion and by a high-affinity uptake transporter, which is located on the presynaptic nerve membrane. It should be noted, however, that at least one of the mutations of the AChR that is found in congenital myasthenic syndrome has a significantly greater likelihood of being activated by choline [79]. Accordingly, choline may serve as a long-lasting activator at the NMJ in some patients.

After the initial high concentration, there is a slow release of ACh from AChR with closed channels. Because the release is not synchronized, the concentration stays low and AChE hydrolyzes the free ACh.

Acetylcholinesterase inhibition

AChE is clearly an essential component of the NMJ. Indeed, the toxicity of anticholinesterases (including some pesticides and nerve gases) is due in part to muscle paralysis [80]. The mechanism(s) by which paralysis is produced is still somewhat controversial, and it may be that different mechanisms are relatively more important at different times after intoxication or in different species. However, all of the processes are initiated by the fact that the ACh in the cleft is not degraded. In this case, the postsynaptic receptors are exposed to high concentrations of ACh for a longer period of time. In addition, the ACh can diffuse from the synaptic cleft and reach portions of the nerve terminal axon that normally would not be exposed to ACh during neuromuscular transmission.

There are likely to be at least two postsynaptic and two presynaptic processes involved in paralysis after esterase inhibition. On the postsynaptic side, the first is prolonged depolarization of the muscle fiber in response to trains of nerve action potentials [81,82]. Prolonged depolarization initially produces multiple action potentials in the muscle fiber in response to a single nerve action potential, and can enhance the twitch. However, prolonged depolarization results in inactivation of voltage-gated Na$^+$ channels in the muscle fiber near the NMJ, and a resulting failure of action-potential generation. A second action is desensitization of the AChR [82], as a result of the continued presence of ACh (see *Receptor desensitization*).

On the presynaptic side, a common observation is the presence of repetitive action potentials in the motor axons

[83,84]. This repetitive activity reflects depolarization of the axon as a result of the activation of nicotinic receptors that are located on the terminal axon, although not immediately at the nerve terminal. Prolonged depolarization could produce Na^+ channel inactivation and failure of the action potential to invade the terminal, resulting in reduced release of ACh. The final proposed mechanism involves a second type of presynaptic nicotinic receptor that, when activated, provides a positive feedback mechanism that normally enhances release of ACh (see *Cycling of synaptic vesicles*). The prolonged presence of ACh could desensitize these receptors, which could result in a more rapid decrement in transmitter release during trains of nerve action potentials.

Longer inhibition of cholinesterase activity results in characteristic degeneration of the NMJ. The fragmentation probably results from excessive entry of Ca^{2+} into the postjunctional volume of the muscle fiber [85].

A rare congenital muscular disorder is associated with very low (or absent) AChE activity at the NMJ. Individuals with this disorder show muscle weakness and fatigability, and many die at young ages. The NMJs are smaller than usual, and show evidence of disorganization [86]. It is fascinating that the disorder does not appear to reflect a mutation in the gene encoding the AChE enzyme. Instead, all the affected individuals show mutations in the gene encoding a large extracellular molecule (collagen Q) that serves to anchor AChE in the synaptic cleft [87]. Transgenic mice have been produced with either the collagen Q gene [88] or the AChE gene [89] deleted. Both deletions result in a great increase in mortality. When the cholinesterase gene was knocked out, no animals survived past 3 weeks, whereas when the collagen Q gene was knocked out, only 50% survived after 3 weeks and only 10% lived to adulthood. That the loss of AChE activity was not immediately lethal was surprising to both groups of researchers, given the effects of acute inhibition of cholinesterase activity. Various possible compensating mechanisms may operate, including a low residual activity of either AChE or butyrylcholinesterase in the cleft [88,89].

The physiologic processes underlying interactions between neuromuscular blocking drugs and anticholinesterase drugs will be explored later (see *Neuromuscular transmission and functional consequences of drug action*).

The postsynaptic response: receptor activation, desensitization, and block

Muscle nicotinic acetylcholine receptors

Langley first postulated the idea of a "receptive substance" on the muscle fiber, localized to the site of nerve contact [90]. Subsequent physiologic studies demonstrated that the muscle response consisted of a depolarization caused by an increase in membrane conductance [91]. The channel is selective for cations over anions but relatively weakly selective among monovalent cations [92]. Divalent cations, most notably calcium ions, also are permeant through the channel [93,94]. Channel gating is dependent on membrane potential (at positive membrane potentials the channel closes more rapidly) [95,96], but the voltage dependence is weak.

The muscle nicotinic AChR is a member of an extended gene family that includes neuronal nicotinic receptors, and receptors for γ-aminobutyric acid ($GABA_A$ and $GABA_C$ receptors), glycine, and serotonin (5-HT_3 receptors) [97,98]. The neuronal nicotinic receptors in the brain play a largely presynaptic role, to modulate transmitter release [99–101]. All of the receptors in this gene family have a similar overall structure (Fig. 18.6). Each complete receptor is composed of five subunits, arranged in a donut with the gated ion channel in the middle. The nicotinic receptor at the adult NMJ is composed of two copies of the α subunit, one β subunit, one δ subunit, and one ϵ subunit. The receptor found early in fetal development and after denervation has a γ subunit replacing the ϵ subunit [102].

Each subunit of the AChR has four membrane-spanning regions (M1–M4). The pore of the ion channel is largely formed by the M2 region of each of the five subunits constituting a single receptor. The receptor has a relatively large extension into the extracellular space, with a tapering funnel leading down to the mouth of the ion channel proper [103,104]. There is a smaller extension into the cytoplasm, which interacts with the cytoplasmic proteins required to concentrate the receptors in the postsynaptic membrane [105].

The amino-terminal domains of the various subunits form the extracellular portion of the receptor and contain the binding sites for ACh. These binding sites (two on each AChR) recognize ACh and other agonists, as well as competitive antagonists. The binding sites are located at the interfaces between subunits; for the adult AChR, one binding site is located between an α subunit and the ϵ subunit, and the other between an α subunit and the δ subunit [106]. A large series of experiments has identified several regions of the α and non-α subunits which contribute to the binding site (Fig. 18.6). The crystal structure of a related ACh-binding protein suggests that the ACh binding sites are located about half of the way down the interface from the extracellular space [104]. The crystal structure also demonstrates how the protein folds bring together residues widely separated along the primary sequence of the protein to form the ACh binding site [107,108].

The second major identified pharmacologic site is located within the pore of the ion channel and is the site at which noncompetitive "channel-blocking" drugs act. These drugs are thought to enter an open channel and basically plug the hole, preventing ion movement [96].

Many of the mutations that have been found to affect the gating of the channel occur in the membrane-spanning regions. The largest number have been found in M2, but

Is the physical mechanism simple occlusion of the ion channel by the blocker, or is there a conformational change in the protein that closes the channel [96]? Do some blockers act on both closed and open channels (as has been suggested for isoflurane) [139]? Can the channel close around a noncompetitive blocker and produce a long-lived "trapped block"? Trapping has been found to occur for some drugs acting on the muscle AChR [140], but the overall importance of trapping is not known. In contrast, small molecules such as tetraethylammonium ions block the channel but the blocked channel actually closes more rapidly than usual [141].

Nondepolarizing competitive blocking drugs

The most venerable nondepolarizing blocking drug (NDB) is D-tubocurarine. Over 150 years ago, it was suggested that the paralyzing action of D-tubocurarine was caused by a block of muscle excitability, rather than an action on the nerve [142]. The greatest advance in understanding the structure of the receptor, and in understanding the interactions of drugs with the ACh binding site, came with the realization that some paralyzing snake venoms contained a toxin that bound essentially irreversibly to the AChR and prevented ACh from binding [143,144]. The use of snake α-neurotoxins as high-affinity ligands for the ACh binding sites on the AChR has been exploited to define the interactions of many drugs with these sites.

In the 1980s it was shown that there are two sites on each receptor that would bind an α-neurotoxin, and that an agonist or an NDB could occupy either of the sites. However, the two sites had different affinities for most NDBs [145]. The affinities could differ by up to 100-fold (for metocurine), or as little as 10-fold (for pancuronium) [135,145]. Subsequent biochemical work has shown that the site formed at the interface between the α and δ subunits has the lower affinity, and the α/ε (or α/γ) site has the higher affinity [106,146]. Careful comparisons of the occupancy of sites by NDBs and block of receptor activation have shown that occupancy of one or both sites results in functional block of adult receptors [135]. Accordingly, direct measurement of the inhibition of activation of AChR shows a half-blocking concentration of NDB, which is close to the affinity for the high-affinity site. It has been suggested that some NDBs might show functional synergy in block because the two sites on the AChR had opposite selectivities for some NDBs [147]. However, the data indicate that while synergy may be seen for some combinations, the basis is not likely to be due simply to site selectivity [148].

One possible complication in understanding the actions of NDBs has been the suggestion that these drugs, although they bind with high affinity, have rapid dissociation rates (possibly $> 1000 \text{ s}^{-1}$) [149]. If an NDB had an average binding time of less than 1 millisecond, then there would likely be a competitive interaction between the NDB and the high cleft ACh concentrations. This would mean that the equilibrium occupancy measurements would not be the appropriate parameters to use in understanding block of transmission. However, experiments have found that the dissociation rates from mammalian (mouse) receptors are sufficiently slow that no competition would occur during normal transmission [150,151].

The relationship between the occupancy of sites on the AChR by an NDB and block of twitch is nonlinear, as discussed in *Neuromuscular transmission and functional consequences of drug action* (see also [152]). A critical point is that block of the twitch requires occupancy of more than 90% of the ACh binding sites on the AChR, and indeed the concentrations of NDBs required to block twitch are 10 times or more greater than the concentrations necessary to block activation by 50% or to occupy half of the high-affinity binding sites [135,148].

Depolarizing blocking drugs

The depolarizing blocking drugs succinylcholine and decamethonium act as weak activators of the muscle AChR [134,153]. They produce depolarization of the muscle, can desensitize the receptor after prolonged exposure, and can also block the channel [134,153]. However, the mechanism by which they produce paralysis is still debated [154]. The same basic postsynaptic and presynaptic mechanisms have been proposed as in the case of anticholinesterases, with the exogenous depolarizing blocking drug acting as an agonist on postsynaptic or presynaptic nicotinic receptors.

Neuromuscular transmission and functional consequences of drug action

We have emphasized that during neuromuscular transmission there is a high concentration of ACh in the cleft, for a brief time. There is also a high density of binding sites, on both the AChR and AChE. Accordingly, the released ACh does not have the opportunity to diffuse any great distance, and the contents of each vesicle act only very locally. For example, the response to the exocytosis of a single vesicle produces a miniature endplate current with peak amplitude corresponding to the opening of about 1000 channels. This number of receptors is within a disk of radius less than 0.2 μm. Even though a number of quanta are released during normal transmission (about 50–100), the release sites are relatively widely separated compared with the diffusion distance, and only a small fraction of the available AChRs are involved. Accordingly, the response to the many vesicles released following an action potential can be thought of in terms of a simple summation of the response to 50 or 100 separate quantal releases [155]. Because of this, in general a reduction of transmitter release results in a proportional reduction of postsynaptic response.

A number of experimental studies and theoretic calculations have indicated that most of the ACh that is released actually is captured by AChRs (50–80%) [156–159], which occurs in a small disk of postsynaptic membrane. These considerations, and others, led to the idea that transmission occurs in a "saturated disk" – a small region of postsynaptic membrane in which most receptors bind two ACh molecules, with a relatively small annulus of partially occupied receptors [77,155,159,160]. As mentioned earlier, the ion channel opens for most receptors that have bound two molecules of ACh, but not for receptors that have bound only one, and therefore the disk of activated receptors is sharply delineated.

Transmission at the NMJ has a large safety factor: block of a twitch evoked by nerve stimulation requires a high concentration of blocking agent [161–163]. The safety factor arises from several basic mechanisms. One is that there is a nonlinear relationship between the activated conductance and the resulting membrane depolarization, so that a larger fraction of the endplate current (EPC) must be blocked to produce a similar relative reduction in endplate potential. One simple way to think about the necessary number of open channels is to compare the resting input conductance of a muscle fiber to the activatable conductance. A typical muscle fiber might have an input resistance of 500 000 ohms (or a conductance of 2×10^{-6} siemens). An adult AChR has a single-channel conductance of about 60×10^{-12} siemens; and for simplicity we will assume that the reversal potential for current through the channel is 0 mV. At steady state, to depolarize the muscle fiber from a resting potential of –70 mV to a threshold for action potential generation of –50 mV, it would be necessary to activate only about 13 000 AChRs. In contrast, there are about 50 000–100 000 AChR channels open at the peak of the evoked response (see earlier), giving a safety factor of threefold to sixfold. It is also clear that there is a large excess of AChRs available – only 0.5% to 1% of the total receptors are involved in producing a typical EPC, and only 0.1% of the receptors are required to produce an EPC that reaches threshold.

The final origin for the large safety factor arises from the properties of the "saturated disk" model for transmission. Experiments and theoretic calculations [159,164,165] have shown that the block of the evoked endplate current is not a linear function of the amount of block of the postsynaptic AChR. Instead, when only a small fraction of the receptors are blocked there is even less block of the EPC. This phenomenon arises because the released ACh can diffuse a little further to encounter an unblocked receptor; that some of the binding sites are already occupied by blocker means that ACh is then free to diffuse further and encounter more receptors. To reduce the EPC to 30% of normal, about 90% of the AChR need to be rendered inactive [152].

This last consideration is thought to underlie the ability of anticholinesterase agents to reverse the block produced by nondepolarizing blocking agents. The released ACh can diffuse further, to encounter more available AChRs, when it is not bound and hydrolyzed by AChE. It is also possible that the longer persistence of ACh in the cleft might result in more competition between ACh and blocker (depending on the dissociation rate for the blocker).

There is a possibility that the same mechanism could allow an antiesterase to reverse a block produced by desensitization of receptors by a depolarizing blocking agent. Greater diffusion of ACh could allow it to encounter a sufficient number of nondesensitized receptors to permit the re-establishment of transmission.

Summary

The axon of the motor neuron innervates the muscle at a specialized region of the muscle membrane called the endplate, the neuromuscular junction (NMJ), or the neuromuscular synapse. The NMJ must produce very reliable and very rapid excitation of the muscle fiber in response to a presynaptic action potential. At the (presynaptic) nerve terminal release of transmitter is initiated by invasion of an action potential, which depolarizes the presynaptic membrane and activates voltage-dependent Ca^{2+} channels. The resultant Ca^{2+} influx through Ca^{2+} channels triggers vesicle fusion and transmitter release. The transmitter is released in quantal units, corresponding to the neurotransmitter content of a single synaptic vesicle.

To maintain synaptic transmission during repetitive firing, the vesicle mobilization and recycling processes ensure sufficient supply of vesicles for release. Specific proteins have been identified that are involved in (1) restraining vesicles so as to prevent their accidental mobilization, (2) targeting the freed vesicles to the active zone, (3) docking the targeted vesicles at the active zone and priming them for fusion, (4) allowing fusion and exocytosis, and (5) retrieving the fused membrane by endocytosis. The precise details of acetylcholine (ACh) release and cycling at the NMJ are currently the subject of intense study.

The synaptic cleft, which is about 50 nm across, provides the delimited volume in which released ACh diffuses to the ACh receptors (AChRs) on the postsynaptic membrane. The release of ACh into the synaptic cleft results in a high synaptic concentration of ACh, which is rapidly dissipated by diffusion and by hydrolysis by acetylcholinesterase (AChE). There are three basic events that a free ACh molecule can experience: it can continue to diffuse in the cleft, it can bind to cholinesterase and be degraded, or it can bind to a postsynaptic AChR and participate in activation. ACh that binds to an AChR is slowly and asynchronously released from the channels and hydrolyzed by AChE.

An AChR is activated following the binding of two ACh molecules. An active receptor does not produce a single opening, but rather makes a "burst" of activity, which contains an average of about five openings, and the burst of activity is terminated when one ACh molecule dissociates from the receptor. An AChR can become desensitized, if ACh or another agonist is present for a long time. After approximately 1 second or longer, the receptor enters a conformation in which it binds ACh with a high affinity but is no longer able to be activated. Currently, there is no evidence that desensitization plays a role in normal transmission; however, it is possible that desensitization plays a role in some phases of neuromuscular block by depolarizing blocking drugs and anticholinesterase agents.

There are a variety of noncompetitive inhibitors of the AChR, including local anesthetics, nondepolarizing blocking agents, and even ACh itself. The primary mechanism for noncompetitive block is open-channel block, where the pharmacologic site is the actual channel, and the mechanism of action is channel occlusion. In physiologic experiments, drugs reduce the duration of channel openings by plugging the channel, thus preventing ion movement. Many cholinergic drugs are able to block channels by this mechanism. Noncompetitive blockers act only after the channel has opened, and under normal conditions the channel opens for such a brief time that the noncompetitive block cannot reach equilibrium, whereas the competitive action is established during the long periods between episodes of neuromuscular transmission.

Nondepolarizing blocking drugs (NDBs) are commonly used for skeletal muscle relaxation during anesthesia. These drugs bind to the ACh binding sites on the AChR, where they act as pharmacologic antagonists. Careful comparisons of the occupancy of sites by NDBs and block of receptor activation have shown that occupancy of one or both sites results in functional block of adult receptors. A critical point is that block of the twitch requires occupancy of more than 90% of the ACh binding sites on the AChR, and indeed the concentrations of NDBs required to block twitch are 10 times greater than the concentrations necessary to block activation by 50% or to occupy half of the high-affinity binding sites. The fact that ACh occupancy of only 10% of AChRs at the NMJ is sufficient to maintain normal transmission is referred to as a high safety factor.

The depolarizing blocking drugs succinylcholine and decamethonium also act at the ACh binding sties on the AChR, where they are weak activators (partial agonists) of the muscle AChR. They produce depolarization of the muscle, can desensitize the receptor after prolonged exposure, and can also block the channel. However, the mechanism by which they produce paralysis is still debated.

References

1. Hodgkin AL, Huxley AF. Currents carried by sodium and potassium ions through the membrane of the giant axon of loligo. *J Physiol* 1952; **116**: 449–72.

2. Hodgkin AL, Huxley AF. The components of membrane conductance in the giant axon of loligo. *J Physiol* 1952; **116**: 473–96.

3. Borst J, Sakmann B. Calcium influx and transmitter release in a fast CNS synapse. *Nature* 1996; **383**: 431–4.

4. Dunlap K, Luebke J, Turner T. Exocytotic Ca²⁺ channels in mammalian central neurons. *Trends Neurosci* 1995; **18**: 89–98.

5. Kerr L, Yoshikami D. A venom peptide with a novel presynaptic blocking action. *Nature* 1984; **308**: 282–4.

6. Uchitel O, Protti D, Sanchez V, *et al.* P-type voltage-dependent calcium channel mediates presynaptic calcium influx and transmitter release in mammalian synapses. *Proc Natl Acad Sci U S A* 1992; **89**: 3330–3.

7. Katz E, Ferro P, Weisz G, *et al.* Calcium channels involved in synaptic transmission at the mature and regenerating mouse neuromuscular junction. *J Physiol* 1996; **497**: 687–97.

8. Dodge F, Rahamimoff R. Co-operative action of calcium ions in transmitter release at the neuromuscular junction. *J Physiol* 1967; **193**: 419–32.

9. Augustine G, Charlton M, Smith S. Calcium entry and transmitter release at voltage-clamped nerve terminals of squid. *J Physiol* 1985; **369**: 163–81.

10. Landò L, Zucker R. Ca²⁺ cooperativity in neurosecretion measured using photolabile Ca²⁺ chelators. *J Neurophysiol* 1994; **72**: 825–30.

11. Wu L, Saggau P. Presynaptic calcium is increased during normal synaptic transmission and paired-pulse facilitation, but not in longterm potentiation in area CA1 of hippocampus. *J Neurosci* 1994; **14**: 645–54.

12. Llinás R, Sugimori M, Silver R. Microdomains of high calcium concentration in a presynaptic terminal. *Science* 1992; **256**: 677–9.

13. Heidelberger R, Heinemann C, Neher E, *et al.* Calcium dependence of the rate of exocytosis in a synaptic terminal. *Nature* 1994; **371**: 513–15.

14. Bollmann J, Sakmann B, Borst J. Calcium sensitivity of glutamate release in a calyx-type terminal. *Science* 2000; **289**: 953–7.

15. Schneggenburger R, Neher E. Intracellular calcium dependence of transmitter release rates at a fast central synapse. *Nature* 2000; **406**: 889–93.

16. Robitaille R, Adler E, Charlton M. Strategic location of calcium channels at transmitter release sites of frog neuromuscular synapses. *Neuron* 1990; **5**: 773–9.

17. Adler E, Augustine G, Duffy S, *et al.* Alien intracellular calcium chelators attenuate neurotransmitter release at the squid giant synapse. *J Neurosci* 1991; **11**: 1496–507.

18. Stanley E. Single calcium channels and acetylcholine release at a presynaptic nerve terminal. *Neuron* 1993; **11**: 1007–11.

19. Wu L, Westenbroek R, Borst J, *et al.* Calcium channel types with distinct presynaptic localization couple differentially to transmitter release in single calyx-type synapses. *J Neurosci* 1999; **19**: 726–36.

20. Neher E. Vesicle pools and Ca²⁺ microdomains: new tools for understanding their roles in neurotransmitter release. *Neuron* 1998; **20**: 389–99.

21. Hubbard J, Schmidt R. An electrophysiological investigation of mammalian motor nerve terminals. *J Physiol* 1963; **166**: 145–67.

22. Llinás R, Steinberg I, Walton K. Relationship between presynaptic

calcium current and postsynaptic potential in squid giant synapse. *Biophys J* 1981; **33**: 323–52.

23. Fatt P, Katz B. Spontaneous subthreshold activity at motor nerve endings. *J Physiol* 1952; **117**: 109–28.

24. Van der Kloot W. The regulation of quantal size. *Prog Neurobiol* 1991; **36**: 93–130.

25. Breckenridge L, Almers W. Currents through the fusion pore that forms during exocytosis of a secretory vesicle. *Nature* 1987; **328**: 814–17.

26. Wessler I. Control of transmitter release from the motor nerve by presynaptic nicotinic and muscarinic autoreceptors. *Trends Pharmacol Sci* 1989; **10**: 110–14.

27. Wessler I, Apel C, Garmsen M, *et al.* Effects of nicotine receptor agonists on acetylcholine release from the isolated motor nerve, small intestine and trachea of rats and guinea-pigs. *Clin Invest* 1992; **70**: 182–9.

28. Tsuneki H, Kimura I, Dezaki K, *et al.* Immunohistochemical localization of neuronal nicotinic receptor subtypes at the pre- and postjunctional sites in mouse diaphragm muscle. *Neurosci Lett* 1995; **196**: 13–16.

29. Tian L, Prior C, Dempster J, *et al.* Hexamethonium- and methyllycaconitine-induced changes in acetylcholine release from rat motor nerve terminals. *Br J Pharmacol* 1997; **122**: 1025–34.

30. Van der Kloot W, Molgó J. Quantal acetylcholine release at the vertebrate neuromuscular junction. *Physiol Rev* 1994; **74**: 899–991.

31. Glavinovic M. Voltage clamping of unparalysed cut rat diaphragm for study of transmitter release. *J Physiol* 1979; **290**: 467–80.

32. Schikorski T, Stevens C. Quantitative ultrastructural analysis of hippocampal excitatory synapses. *J Neurosci* 1997; **17**: 5858–67.

33. Schikorski T, Stevens C. Quantitative fine-structural analysis of olfactory cortical synapses. *Proc Natl Acad Sci U S A* 1999; **96**: 4107–12.

34. Zucker R. Short-term synaptic plasticity. *Annu Rev Neurosci* 1989; **12**: 13–31.

35. Kusano K, Landau E. Depression and recovery of transmission at the squid giant synapse. *J Physiol* 1975; **245**: 13–32.

36. Dittman J, Regehr W. Calcium dependence and recovery kinetics of presynaptic depression at the climbing fiber to purkinje cell synapse. *J Neurosci* 1998; **18**: 6147–62.

37. Wang L-Y, Kaczmarek L. High-frequency firing helps replenish the readily releasable pool of synaptic vesicles. *Nature* 1998; **394**: 384–8.

38. Wu L, Borst J. The reduced release probability of releasable vesicles during recovery from short-term synaptic depression. *Neuron* 1999; **23**: 821–32.

39. Heuser J, Reese T. Evidence for recycling of synaptic vesicle membrane during transmitter release at the frog neuromuscular junction. *J Cell Biol* 1973; **57**: 315–44.

40. Ceccarelli B, Hurlbut W, Mauro A. Turnover of transmitter and synaptic vesicles at the frog neuromuscular junction. *J Cell Biol* 1973; **57**: 499–524.

41. Heuser JE, Reese TS. Evidence for recycling of synaptic vesicle membrane during transmitter release at the frog neuromuscular junction. *J Cell Biol* 1973; **57**: 315–44.

42. Heuser JE. Review of electron microscopic evidence favouring vesicle exocytosis as the structural basis for quantal release during synaptic transmission. *Q J Exp Physiol* 1989; **74**: 1051–69.

43. Ceccarelli B, Hurlbut WP, Mauro A. Turnover of transmitter and synaptic vesicles at the frog neuromuscular junction. *J Cell Biol* 1973; **57**: 499–524.

44. Fesce R, Grohovaz F, Valtorta F, *et al.* Neurotransmitter release: fusion or "kiss-and-run"? *Trends Cell Biol* 1994; **4**: 1–4.

45. Wu W, Wu LG. Rapid bulk endocytosis and its kinetics of fission pore closure at a central synapse. *Proc Natl Acad Sci U S A* 2007; **104**: 10234–9.

46. Koenig JH, Ikeda K. Disappearance and reformation of synaptic vesicle membrane upon transmitter release observed under reversible blockage of membrane retrieval. *J Neurosci* 1989; **9**: 3844–60.

47. Koenig JH, Ikeda K. Synaptic vesicles have two distinct recycling pathways. *J Cell Biol* 1996; **135**: 797–808.

48. Takei K, Mundigl O, Daniell L, *et al.* The synaptic vesicle cycle: a single vesicle budding step involving clathrin and dynamin. *J Cell Biol* 1996; **133**: 1237–50.

49. Richards DA, Guatimosim C, Betz WJ. Two endocytic recycling routes selectively fill two vesicle pools in frog motor nerve terminals. *Neuron* 2000; **27**: 551–9.

50. Teng H, Wilkinson RS. Clathrin-mediated endocytosis near active zones in snake motor boutons. *J Neurosci* 2000; **20**: 7986–93.

51. Holt M, Cooke A, Wu MM, *et al.* Bulk membrane retrieval in the synaptic terminal of retinal bipolar cells. *J Neurosci* 2003; **23**: 1329–39.

52. Klyachko VA, Jackson MB. Capacitance steps and fusion pores of small and large-dense-core vesicles in nerve terminals. *Nature* 2002; **418**: 89–92.

53. He L, Wu XS, Mohan R, *et al.* Two modes of fusion pore opening revealed by cell-attached recordings at a synapse. *Nature* 2006; **444**: 102–5.

54. Choi S, Klingauf J, Tsien RW. Postfusional regulation of cleft glutamate concentration during LTP at "silent synapses". *Nat Neurosci* 2000; **3**: 330–6.

55. Fernandez-Chacon R, Sudhof T. Genetics of synaptic vesicle function: Toward the complete functional anatomy of an organelle. *Annu Rev Physiol* 1999; **61**: 753–76.

56. Rosahl T, Geppert M, Spillane D, *et al.* Short-term synaptic plasticity is altered in mice lacking synapsin I. *Cell* 1993; **75**: 661–70.

57. Rosahl T, Spillane D, Missler M, *et al.* Essential functions of synapsins I and II in synaptic vesicle regulation. *Nature* 1995; **375**: 488–93.

58. Ryan T, Li L, Chin L-S, *et al.* Synaptic vesicle recycling in synapsin I knock-out mice. *J Cell Biol* 1996; **134**: 1219–27.

59. Geppert M, Sudhof T. RAB3 and synaptotagmin: the yin and yang of synaptic membrane fusion. *Annu Rev Neurosci* 1998; **21**: 75–95.

60. Hanson P, Heuser J, Jahn R. Neurotransmitter release: four years of SNARE complexes. *Curr Opin Neurobiol* 1997; **7**: 310–15.

61. Jahn R, Sudhof T. Membrane fusion and exocytosis. *Annu Rev Biochem* 1999; **68**: 863–911.

62. Littleton J, Stern M, Schulze K, *et al.* Mutational analysis of Drosophila synaptotagmin demonstrates its essential role in Ca^{2+}-activated neurotransmitter release. *Cell* 1993; **74**: 1125–34.

63. Geppert M, Goda Y, Hammer R, *et al.* Synaptotagmin I: a major Ca^{2+} sensor for transmitter release at a central synapse. *Cell* 1994; **79**: 717–27.

64. DiAntonio A, Parfitt K, Schwarz T. Synaptic transmission persists in synaptotagmin mutants of Drosophila. *Cell* 1993; **73**: 1281–90.

65. Nonet M, Grundahl K, Meyer B, *et al.* Synaptic function is impaired but not eliminated in C. elegans mutants lacking synaptotagmin. *Cell* 1993; **73**: 1291–305.

66. Moorman J. Sodium channels. In: Yaksh C, Lynch C, Zapol W, eds., *Anesthesia: Biologic Foundations.* Philadelphia, PA: Lippincott-Raven, 1997: 145–62.

67. Franks NP, Honore E. The TREK K2P channels and their role in general anaesthesia and neuroprotection. *Trends Pharmacol Sci* 2004; **25**: 601–8.

68. Franks N, Lieb W. Volatile general anaesthetics activate a novel neuronal K^+ current. *Nature* 1988; **333**: 662–4.

69. Patel A, Honore E, Lesage F, *et al.* Inhalational anesthetics activate two-pore-domain background K^+ channels. *Nat Neurosci* 1999; **2**: 422–6.

70. Ries C, Puil E. Mechanism of anesthesia revealed by shunting actions of isoflurane on thalamocortical neurons. *J Neurophysiol* 1999; **81**: 1795–801.

71. Ries C, Puil E. Ionic mechanism of isoflurane's actions on thalamocortical neurons. *J Neurophysiol* 1999; **81**: 1802–9.

72. Takenoshita M, Steinbach J. Halothane blocks low-voltage-activated calcium current in rat sensory neurons. *J Neurosci* 1991; **11**: 1404–12.

73. Hall A, Lieb W, Franks N. Insensitivity of P-type calcium channels to inhalational and intravenous general anesthetics. *Anesthesiology* 1994; **81**: 117–23.

74. Study R. Isoflurane inhibits multiple voltage-gated calcium currents in hippocampal pyramidal neurons. *Anesthesiology* 1994; **81**: 104–16.

75. Van Swinderen B, Saifee O, Shebester L, *et al.* A neomorphic syntaxin mutation blocks volatile-anesthetic action in Caenorhabditis elegans. *Proc Natl Acad Sci U S A* 1999; **96**: 2479–84.

76. Taylor P, Radic Z. The cholinesterases: from genes to proteins. *Annu Rev Pharmacol Toxicol* 1994; **34**: 281–320.

77. Salpeter M. Vertebrate neuromuscular junctions: general morphology, molecular organization, and functional consequences. In: Salpeter M, ed., *The Vertebrate Neuromuscular Junction.* New York, NY: Liss, 1987: 1–54.

78. Steinbach J, Stevens C. Neuromuscular transmission. In: Llinas R, Precht W, eds., *Frog Neurobiology.* Berlin: Springer, 1976: 33–91.

79. Zhou M, Engel A, Auerbach A. Serum choline activates mutant acetylcholine receptors that cause slow channel congenital myasthenic syndromes. *Proc Natl Acad Sci U S A* 1999; **96**: 10466–71.

80. Karalliedde L. Organophosphorus poisoning and anaesthesia. *Anaesthesia* 1999; **54**: 1073–88.

81. Maselli R, Soliven B. Analysis of the organophosphate-induced electromyographic response to repetitive nerve stimulation: paradoxical response to edrophonium and D-tubocurarine. *Muscle Nerve* 1991; **14**: 1182–8.

82. Maselli R, Leung C. Analysis of anticholinesterase-induced neuromuscular transmission failure. *Muscle Nerve* 1993; **16**: 548–53.

83. Clark A, Hobbiger F, Terrar D. Nature of the anticholinesterase-induced repetitive response of rat and mouse striated muscle to single nerve stimuli. *J Physiol* 1984; **349**: 157–66.

84. Besser R, Vogt T, Gutmann L, *et al.* Impaired neuromuscular transmission during partial inhibition of acetylcholinesterase: the role of stimulus-induced antidromic backfiring in the generation of the decrement–increment phenomenon. *Muscle Nerve* 1992; **15**: 1072–80.

85. Leonard J, Salpeter M. Agonist-induced myopathy at the neuromuscular junction is mediated by calcium. *J Cell Biol* 1979; **82**: 811–19.

86. Ohno K, Engel A, Brengman J, *et al.* The spectrum of mutations causing end-plate acetylcholinesterase deficiency. *Ann Neurol* 2000; **47**: 162–70.

87. Engel AG, Sine SM. Current understanding of congenital myasthenic syndromes. *Curr Opin Pharmacol* 2005; **5**: 308–21.

88. Feng G, Krejci E, Molgo J, *et al.* Genetic analysis of collagen Q: roles in acetylcholinesterase and butyrylcholinesterase assembly and in synaptic structure and function. *J Cell Biol* 1999; **144**: 1349–60.

89. Xie W, Stribley J, Chatonnet A, *et al.* Postnatal developmental delay and supersensitivity to organophosphate in gene-targeted mice lacking acetylcholinesterase. *J Pharmacol Exp Ther* 2000; **293**: 896–902.

90. Langley J. Nerve endings and special excitable substances in cells. *Proc R Soc Lond B Biol Sci* 1906; **78**: 170–95.

91. Fatt P, Katz B. An analysis of the end-plate potential recorded with an intracellular electrode. *J Physiol* 1951; **115**: 320–70.

92. Takeuchi A, Takeuchi N. On the permeability of end-plate membrane during the action of transmitter. *J Physiol* 1960; **154**: 52–67.

93. Takeuchi N. Effects of calcium on the conductance change of the end-plate membrane during the action of transmitter. *J Physiol* 1963; **167**: 141–55.

94. Decker E, Dani J. Calcium permeability of the nicotinic acetylcholine receptor: the single-channel calcium influx is significant. *J Neurosci* 1990; **10**: 3413–20.

95. Magleby K, Stevens C. A quantitative description of end-plate currents. *J Physiol* 1972; **223**: 173–97.

96. Neher E, Steinbach J. Local anaesthetics transiently block currents through

single acetylcholine-receptor channels. *J Physiol* 1978; **277**: 153–76.

97. Ortells M, Lunt G. Evolutionary history of the ligand-gated ion-channel superfamily of receptors. *Trends Neurosci* 1995; **18**: 121–7.

98. Lindstrom J. The structures of neuronal nicotinic receptors. In: Clementi F, Fornasari D, Gotti C, eds., *Neuronal Nicotinic Receptors*. Berlin: Springer, 2000: 101–62.

99. Wonnacott S. Presynaptic nicotinic ACh receptors. *Trends Neurosci* 1997; **20**: 92–8.

100. Jones S, Sudweeks S, Yakel J. Nicotinic receptors in the brain: correlating physiology with function. *Trends Neurosci* 1999; **22**: 555–61.

101. Vizi E, Lendvai B. Modulatory role of presynaptic nicotinic receptors in synaptic and non-synaptic chemical communication in the central nervous system. *Brain Res Brain Res Rev* 1999; **30**: 219–35.

102. Mishina M, Takai T, Imoto K, *et al.* Molecular distinction between fetal and adult forms of muscle acetylcholine receptor. *Nature* 1986; **321**: 406–11.

103. Unwin N. Refined structure of the nicotinic acetylcholine receptor at 4A resolution. *J Mol Biol* 2005; **346**: 967–89.

104. Brejc K, van D, WJ, Klaassen R, *et al.* Crystal structure of an ACh binding protein reveals the ligand-binding domain of nicotinic receptors. *Nature* 2001; **411**: 269–76.

105. Sanes J, Lichtman J. Development of the vertebrate neuromuscular junction. *Annu Rev Neurosci* 1999; **22**: 389–442.

106. Blount P, Merlie J. Molecular basis of the two nonequivalent ligand binding sites of the muscle nicotinic acetylcholine receptor. *Neuron* 1989; **3**: 349–57.

107. Sine SM, Engel AG. Recent advances in Cys-loop receptor structure and function. *Nature* 2006; **440**: 448–55.

108. Corringer P, Le N, Changeux J. Nicotinic receptors at the amino acid level. *Annu Rev Pharmacol Toxicol* 2000; **40**: 431–58.

109. Dilger JP. The effects of general anaesthetics on ligand-gated ion channels. *Br J Anaesth* 2002; **89**: 41–51.

110. Tassonyi E, Charpantier E, Muller D, *et al.* The role of nicotinic acetylcholine receptors in the mechanisms of anesthesia. *Brain Res Bull* 2002; **57**: 133–50.

111. Akk G, Mennerick S, Steinbach JH. Actions of anesthetics on excitatory transmitter-gated channels. *Handb Exp Pharmacol* 2008; 53–84.

112. Jackson M. Kinetics of unliganded acetylcholine receptor channel gating. *Biophys J* 1986; **49**: 663–72.

113. Jackson M. Dependence of acetylcholine receptor channel kinetics on agonist concentration in cultured mouse muscle fibres. *J Physiol* 1988; **397**: 555–83.

114. Akk G, Sine S, Auerbach A. Binding sites contribute unequally to the gating of mouse nicotinic alpha-d200n acetylcholine receptors. *J Physiol* 1996; **496**: 185–96.

115. Ohno K, Wang H, Milone M, *et al.* Congenital myasthenic syndrome caused by decreased agonist binding affinity due to a mutation in the acetylcholine receptor epsilon subunit. *Neuron* 1996; **17**: 157–70.

116. Maconochie D, Steinbach J. The channel opening rate of adult- and fetal-type mouse muscle nicotinic receptors activated by acetylcholine. *J Physiol* 1998; **506**: 53–72.

117. Colquhoun D, Sakmann B. Fluctuations in the microsecond time range of the current through single acetylcholine receptor ion channels. *Nature* 1981; **294**: 464–6.

118. Katz B, Thesleff S. A study of the "desensitization" produced by acetylcholine at the motor end-plate. *J Physiol* 1957; **138**: 63–80.

119. Heidemann T, Changeux J. Structural and functional properties of the acetylcholine receptor protein in its purified and membrane-bound states. *Annu Rev Biochem* 1978; **47**: 317–57.

120. Feltz A, Trautmann A. Desensitization at the frog neuromuscular junction: a biphasic process. *J Physiol* 1982; **322**: 257–72.

121. Chesnut T. Two-component desensitization at the neuromuscular junction of the frog. *J Physiol* 1983; **336**: 229–41.

122. Paradiso K, Brehm P. Long-term desensitization of nicotinic acetylcholine receptors is regulated via protein kinase A-mediated phosphorylation. *J Neurosci* 1998; **18**: 9227–37.

123. Auerbach A, Akk G. Desensitization of mouse nicotinic acetylcholine receptor channels. *J Gen Physiol* 1998; **112**: 181–97.

124. Boyd N, Cohen J. Kinetics of binding of [3H]acetylcholine and [3H]carbamoylcholine to *Torpedo* postsynaptic membranes: slow conformational transitions of the cholinergic receptor. *Biochemistry* 1980; **19**: 5344–53.

125. Pennefather P, Quastel D. Fast desensitization of the nicotinic receptor at the mouse neuromuscular junction. *Br J Pharmacol* 1982; **77**: 395–404.

126. Magleby K, Pallotta B. A study of desensitization of acetylcholine receptors using nerve-released transmitter in the frog. *J Physiol* 1981; **316**: 225–50.

127. White B, Cohen J. Agonist-induced changes in the structure of the acetylcholine receptor M2 regions revealed by photoincorporation of an uncharged nicotinic noncompetitive antagonist. *J Biol Chem* 1992; **267**: 15770–83.

128. Leonard R, Labarca C, Charnet P, *et al.* Evidence that the M2 membrane-spanning region lines the ion channel pore of the nicotinic receptor. *Science* 1988; **242**: 1578–81.

129. Charnet P, Labarca C, Leonard R, *et al.* An open-channel blocker interacts with adjacent turns of alpha-helices in the nicotinic acetylcholine receptor. *Neuron* 1990; **4**: 87–95.

130. Sine S, Steinbach J. Agonists block currents through acetylcholine receptor channels. *Biophys J* 1984; **46**: 277–84.

131. Colquhoun D, Dreyer F, Sheridan R. The actions of tubocurarine at the frog neuromuscular junction. *J Physiol* 1979; **293**: 247–84.

132. Sine S, Steinbach J. Acetylcholine receptor activation by a site-selective ligand: nature of brief open and closed states in BC3H-1 cells. *J Physiol* 1986; **370**: 357–79.

133. Adams P, Sakmann B. Decamethonium both opens and blocks end plate channels. *Proc Natl Acad Sci U S A* 1978; **75**: 2994–8.

134. Marshall C, Ogden D, Colquhoun D. The actions of suxamethonium (succinyldicholine) as an agonist and channel blocker at the nicotinic receptor of frog muscle. *J Physiol* 1990; **428**: 155–74.

135. Fletcher G, Steinbach J. Ability of nondepolarizing neuromuscular blocking drugs to act as partial agonists at fetal and adult mouse muscle nicotinic receptors. *Mol Pharmacol* 1996; **49**: 938–47.

136. Galzi J, Revah F, Bouet F, *et al.* Allosteric transitions of the acetylcholine receptor probed at the amino acid level with a photolabile cholinergic ligand. *Proc Natl Acad Sci U S A* 1991; **88**: 5051–5.

137. Pedersen S, Sharp S, Liu W, *et al.* Structure of the noncompetitive antagonist-binding site of the Torpedo nicotinic acetylcholine receptor. [3H] meproadifen mustard reacts selectively with alpha-subunit Glu-262. *J Biol Chem* 1992; **267**: 10489–99.

138. Blanton M, Xie Y, Dangott L, *et al.* The steroid promegestone is noncompetitive antagonist of the Torpedo nicotinic acetylcholine receptor that interacts with the lipid-protein interface. *Mol Pharmacol* 1999; **55**: 269–78.

139. Dilger J, Brett R, Lesko L. Effects of isoflurane on acetylcholine receptor channels. 1. Single-channel currents. *Mol Pharmacol* 1992; **41**: 127–33.

140. Neely A, Lingle C. Trapping of an open-channel blocker at the frog neuromuscular acetylcholine channel. *Biophys J* 1986; **50**: 981–6.

141. Akk G, Steinbach JH. Activation and block of mouse muscle-type nicotinic receptors by tetraethylammonium. *J Physiol* 2003; **551**: 155–68.

142. Thomas K. *Curare: its History and Usage.* Philadelphia, PA: Lippincott, 1963.

143. Changeux JP, Kasai M, Lee CY. Use of a snake venom toxin to characterize the cholinergic receptor protein. *Proc Natl Acad Sci U S A* 1970; **67**: 1241–7.

144. Patrick J, Heinemann S, Lindstrom J, *et al.* Appearance of acetylcholine receptors during differentiation of a myogenic cell line. *Proc Natl Acad Sci U S A* 1972; **69**: 2762–6.

145. Sine S, Taylor P. Relationship between reversible antagonist occupancy and the functional capacity of the acetylcholine receptor. *J Biol Chem* 1981; **256**: 6692–9.

146. Sine S, Claudio T. Gamma- and delta-subunits regulate the affinity and the cooperativity of ligand binding to the acetylcholine receptor. *J Biol Chem* 1991; **266**: 19369–77.

147. Waud B, Waud D. Quantitative examination of the interaction of competitive neuromuscular blocking agents on the indirectly elicited muscle twitch. *Anesthesiology* 1984; **61**: 420–7.

148. Liu M, Dilger JP. Synergy between pairs of competitive antagonists at adult human muscle acetylcholine receptors. *Anesth Analg* 2008; **107**: 525–33.

149. Colquhoun D, Sheridan R. The effect of tubocurarine competition on the kinetics of agonist action on the nicotinic receptor. *Br J Pharmacol* 1982; **75**: 77–86.

150. Demazumder D, Dilger JP. The kinetics of competitive antagonism by cisatracurium of embryonic and adult nicotinic acetylcholine receptors. *Mol Pharmacol* 2001; **60**: 797–807.

151. Wenningmann I, Dilger JP. The kinetics of inhibition of nicotinic acetylcholine receptors by (+)-tubocurarine and pancuronium. *Mol Pharmacol* 2001; **60**: 790–6.

152. Lingle C, Steinbach J. Neuromuscular blocking agents. *Int Anesthesiol Clin* 1988; **26**: 288–301.

153. Liu Y, Dilger J. Decamethonium is a partial agonist at the nicotinic acetylcholine receptor. *Synapse* 1993; **13**: 57–62.

154. Feldman S, Hood J. Depolarizing neuromuscular block: a presynaptic mechanism? *Acta Anaesthesiol Scand* 1994; **38**: 535–41.

155. Hartzell H, Kuffler S, Yoshikami D. Post-synaptic potentiation: interaction between quanta of acetylcholine at the skeletal neuromuscular synapse. *J Physiol* 1975; **251**: 437–63.

156. Katz B, Miledi R. The binding of acetylcholine to receptors and its removal from the synaptic cleft. *J Physiol* 1973; **231**: 549–74.

157. Colquhoun D, Large W, Rang H. An analysis of the action of a false transmitter at the neuromuscular junction. *J Physiol* 1977; **266**: 361–5.

158. Land B, Salpeter E, Salpeter M. Acetylcholine receptor site density affects the rising phase of miniature endplate currents. *Proc Natl Acad Sci U S A* 1980; **77**: 3736–40.

159. Pennefather P, Quastel D. Relation between subsynaptic receptor blockade and response to quantal transmitter at the mouse neuromuscular junction. *J Gen Physiol* 1981; **78**: 313–44.

160. Fertuck H, Salpeter M. Quantitation of junctional and extrajunctional acetylcholine receptors by electron microscope autoradiography after ^{125}I-α-bungarotoxin binding at mouse neuromuscular junctions. *J Cell Biol* 1976; **69**: 144–58.

161. Paton W, Waud D. The margin of safety of neuromuscular transmission. *J Physiol* 1967; **191**: 59–90.

162. Waud B, Waud D. The margin of safety of neuromuscular transmission in the muscle of the diaphragm. *Anesthesiology* 1972; **37**: 417–22.

163. Waud D, Waud B. In vitro measurement of margin of safety of neuromuscular transmission. *Am J Physiol* 1975; **229**: 1632–4.

164. Albuquerque E, Barnard E, Jansson S, *et al.* Occupancy of the cholinergic receptors in relation to changes in the endplate potential. *Life Sci* 1973; **12**: 545–52.

165. Wathey J, Nass M, Lester H. Numerical reconstruction of the quantal event at nicotinic synapses. *Biophys J* 1979; **27**: 145–64.

Physiologic substrates of drug action

Vascular reactivity

Isao Tsuneyoshi, Josephine M. Garcia-Ferrer, Hung Pin Liu, and Walter A. Boyle

Introduction

The vascular system refers to the system of conduits – blood vessels – whose primary function is to deliver blood components including oxygen-carrying red cells and other essential nutrients to support the metabolic demands of the entire organism. The vascular system is also the conduit for transporting important endocrine, neurohumoral, and immunological signals to their distant targets. More recently, the pivotal role of the vascular endothelium in regulating coagulation, thrombosis, inflammation, and angiogenesis has also been appreciated. Finally, the vascular system removes cellular waste and delivers metabolic end products to the hepatic and renal systems for detoxification and removal.

The function of the vascular system is dependent on the performance of the cardiac pump – they are often referred to together as the cardiovascular system – but the role of the vascular component is far from passive. In this chapter we provide a review of vascular reactivity including both the active contraction of vascular smooth muscle (VSM), which determines systemic blood pressure and blood flow distribution, and the other important dynamic processes involving the vascular endothelium and extracellular matrix. The physiological roles of each of these elements with respect to their contribution to vascular reactivity are discussed, with an overview of the mechanisms, biochemical pathways, and molecular targets involved.

Extracellular matrix

VSM and vascular endothelial cells live within an extracellular matrix (ECM) of their own making consisting of collagen, elastin, laminin, fibronectin, vitronectin, proteoglycan, and a variety of less abundant components. The ECM proteins are particularly important as ligands for integrin receptors, a group of heterodimeric transmembrane proteins expressed in both VSM and endothelial cells [1,2]. The extracellular domains of the integrins recognize specific RGD (arginine–glycine–aspartic acid) peptide motifs of matrix components, and integrin/ECM interactions provide the organization of the vessel wall, determining the polarity and organization of the cellular elements as well as the assembly of the matrix itself [3,4]. The intracellular domains of integrins are attached to the actin cytoskeleton, providing a mechanical link between the ECM and the contractile elements [5], and thereby allowing vascular cells scattered throughout the media to function as a syncytium, even in the absence of direct cell-to-cell contact. As discussed in more detail below, ECM/cytoskeletal interactions allow changes in wall tension to be transduced to effector proteins – including the stretch-sensitive membrane ion channels and kinases involved in contraction – which are critical for development of myogenic tone. Vascular ECM collagen and von Willebrand factor (vWF) exposed by endothelial injury bind platelet GPIa/IIa and GPIb/IX, respectively, resulting in platelet activation and expression of the platelet $\alpha IIb\beta 3$ integrin (GPIIb/IIIa) receptor for fibrinogen that initiates the formation of the platelet plug. The dynamic importance of this latter vascular ECM interaction with platelets is emphasized by the remarkable efficacy of GPIIb/IIIa antagonists in treating arteriosclerotic plaque rupture and angioplasty-induced vascular injury [6]. Other important interactions of ECM with VSM and endothelial cells are discussed in the following sections.

Mutations in the genes for ECM proteins generally result in both altered matrix composition and significant vascular wall pathology [7]. Mice lacking either fibronectin or its $\alpha 5\beta 1$ integrin receptor, or collagen I or its αv integrin receptor, have severe defects in vasculogenesis and either do not survive gestation or die immediately after birth [4]. Marfan syndrome in humans appears to be caused by mutations in the gene for the matrix protein fibrillin, while Ehlers–Danlos syndrome (type IV) is associated with mutations in type III collagen found in vascular ECM [4,8]. Mutations in the elastin gene result in abnormal elastin expression and organization, and are associated with vascular thickening and subaortic stenosis [9]. Changes in matrix expression and structure also occur with aging and disease processes. For example, upregulation of both the VSM $\alpha_V\beta 3$ integrin receptor and its ECM ligand osteopontin occur in association with neointima formation in atherosclerotic vessels or following angioplasty-induced vascular

Anesthetic Pharmacology, 2nd edition, ed. Alex S. Evers, Mervyn Maze, Evan D. Kharasch. Published by Cambridge University Press. © Cambridge University Press 2011.

injury [4,10]. As discussed in the section on angiogenesis (below), proangiogenic growth factors produced in chronic inflammatory states or with tumor growth drive proliferation of endothelial cells and VSM, with production of specific ECM proteins that may contribute to the unwanted neovascularization or tissue growth in these conditions [4,10,11].

Vascular smooth muscle

VSM is the fundamental machinery of the vascular system. VSM actively contracts and relaxes to produce the changes in blood vessel diameter responsible for physiologic adjustments in blood pressure and flow. Accordingly, VSM has evolved with a complex repertoire of unique contractile proteins, ion channels, agonist receptors, and signal transduction pathways that permit VSM to carry out its specialized function [12].

VSM contractile proteins

As in cardiac and skeletal muscle, the smooth-muscle contractile apparatus is composed of actin thin filaments arranged in a hexagonal array around myosin thick filaments to form the basic contractile unit [13]. Smooth-muscle-specific α-actin is the single most abundant protein in these cells, comprising up to 70% of the total actin and 40% of cellular protein. Moreover, other than transient expression in cardiac and skeletal muscle during development, α-actin is exclusively expressed in adult smooth muscle, which contains only varying smaller amounts of smooth muscle and nonmuscle β-actin and γ-actin [14]. Globular actin monomers (G-actin) polymerize to form the actin filaments (F-actin) which are anchored at focal adhesion points on the ventral surface, as well as to more diffuse sites on the apical and nuclear membranes. These contact points are generally multiprotein structures that include actin-binding proteins and the intracellular domains of integrins. Accordingly, this complex provides a direct link between actin filaments and ECM [5].

Myosin II, the other major contractile protein expressed in VSM, is composed of two myosin heavy chains, as well as two functional and two regulatory myosin light chains. Following phosphorylation of regulatory myosin light chain (MLC), myosin heavy chains bind actin at their N-terminus, and the N-terminal myosin "head" displays ATPase ("myosin motor") activity. Actin and myosin filaments in VSM are generally oriented parallel to the long axis, resulting in a circumferential arrangement in intact vessels. Activation of these contractile proteins thus results in force generation that decreases luminal diameter as the myosin motor moves along the actin filaments [5,15].

VSM contraction mechanisms

Intracellular Ca^{2+} concentration ($[Ca^{2+}]_i$) in VSM is the major determinant of contraction. Under basal conditions, Ca^{2+} influx in VSM remains low despite a 10 000-fold concentration gradient across the sarcolemma, and $[Ca^{2+}]_i$ is maintained in the 50–100 nM range. VSM receptor agonists increase VSM $[Ca^{2+}]_i$ by receptor G-protein-coupled activation of phospholipase C (PLC), which results in inositol 1,4,5-trisphosphate

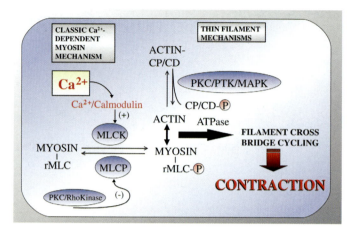

Figure 19.1. Contraction of vascular smooth muscle is dependent on the association of thin filament (actin) and thick filament (myosin) and activation of the myosin ATPase, which induces filament crossbridge cycling and force generation. The classic Ca^{2+}-dependent mechanism in smooth muscle involves activation of myosin light-chain kinase (MLCK) by Ca^{2+}/calmodulin and phosphorylation of regulatory myosin light chain (rMLC). Ca^{2+}-independent mechanisms involve inhibition of myosin light-chain phosphatase (MLCP) mediated by activation of PKC and Rho kinase. Phosphorylation of the thin-filament-associated proteins caldesmon (CD) and/or calponin (CP) by protein kinase C (PKC) or protein tyrosine kinase/mitogen-activated protein kinase (PTK/MAPK) pathways may also contribute to contraction via disinhibition of the actin–myosin interaction.

(IP_3) generation and IP_3-induced Ca^{2+} release (IICR) from intracellular stores. Stochastic Ca^{2+} release due to Ca^{2+}-induced Ca^{2+} release (CICR) also appears to be important [12,16,17].

Membrane depolarization following receptor agonists results in increased Ca^{2+} entry from the extracellular space through L-type Ca^{2+} channels, and receptor-operated Ca^{2+} channels (ROCs), Ca^{2+} release-activated channels (CRACs), and the Na^+/Ca^{2+} exchange mechanism may also contribute to Ca^{2+} influx following either agonists or mechanical stimuli (see below) [12,17].

As can be seen in Fig. 19.1, the Ca^{2+} dependence of contraction and the biochemical sequence of events leading to the formation of actin–myosin crossbridges and force development in VSM (and other smooth muscle) differs considerably from that of skeletal and cardiac muscle [18]. Rather than direct Ca^{2+} binding to thin filament proteins, activation of myosin ATPase and contraction in VSM derives its Ca^{2+} dependence from the Ca^{2+}/calmodulin-activated MLC kinase (MLCK) and MLCK-induced phosphorylation of the serine 19 residue of the 20 kDa regulatory MLC subunit [19,20].

While the central and essential role of Ca^{2+} in VSM contraction is clear, the amplitude of the contraction is not always proportional to the $[Ca^{2+}]_i$ [12]. This is most strikingly demonstrated following receptor agonists in which contraction is well maintained while $[Ca^{2+}]_i$ decreases to near baseline levels [21]. Such increases in the relative amount of contraction for a given $[Ca^{2+}]_i$ is referred to as Ca^{2+} sensitization. However, in actuality this reflects a process which is Ca^{2+}-independent, and which can be readily demonstrated in permeabilized VSM at a fixed $[Ca^{2+}]$. Recent data indicate that this phenomenon is largely explained by agonist-induced inhibition of MLC phosphatase (MLCP), the PP1A phosphatase that degrades phosphorylated MLC [22,23]. Accordingly, MLC phosphorylation levels and contraction can thereby be maintained in spite of a sharp decline in the concentration of the Ca^{2+}/calmodulin complex. Moreover, effects on MLCP activity are now recognized as the major point of convergence for the Ca^{2+}-independent contracting activities of protein kinase C (PKC) and Rho kinase (ROCK), as well as the signaling pathways involved in both myogenic contraction and endothelium-dependent relaxation (see below) [18,23–27]. Finally, as also shown in Fig. 19.1, VSM contraction may be further influenced by thin-filament mechanisms which induce contraction that is independent of either $[Ca^{2+}]_i$ or MLC phosphorylation. Phosphorylation of calponin and caldesmon by PKC or downstream protein tyrosine kinase/mitogen-activated protein kinase (PTK/MAPK) pathways, including Abelson tyrosine kinases (Abl), focal adhesion kinase (FAK), and Src family protein kinases, promote contraction by enhancing thin-filament polymerization and actin–myosin interaction [13,28]. Members of the family of small G proteins (including Rho, Cdc42, and Rac) and their associated kinases, as well as Wiskott–Aldrich syndrome protein (N-WASP), the Arp2/3 complex, profilin, cofilin, and HSP27, are also capable of modulating VSM contraction via effects on actin–myosin dynamics [13].

Ion channels involved in VSM contraction

The principal trigger for agonist-induced contraction involves Ca^{2+} release from stores via IICR and CICR channels, while sustained contraction is dependent both on the Ca^{2+} sensitization mechanism described above and on membrane depolarization and continued Ca^{2+} influx through sarcolemmal L-type (long lasting, high-voltage activated, 20–28 pS) Ca^{2+} channels (VGCCs). Membrane potential (V_m) and ion channel activity are therefore important determinants of both $[Ca^{2+}]_i$ and contraction. In relaxed VSM, membrane potential is maintained at –45 to –75 mV by voltage-dependent as well as Ca^{2+} and ATP-gated K^+ channels [19,29], and sarcolemmal and sarcoplasmic reticulum Ca^{2+} pumps and transporters maintain Ca^{2+} at sub-contracting levels [30]. Upon application of a contracting stimulus, membrane depolarization occurs with slow action potentials generated by Ca^{2+} currents through VGCCs [12]. T-type (transient, low-voltage activated, 7–15 pS) Ca^{2+} channels identified in VSM may also contribute to initial depolarization and Ca^{2+} influx. However T-type channels rapidly inactivate and remain inactivated at the depolarized potentials (–30 to 10 mV) seen in agonist-stimulated VSM [12]. Similarly, voltage-activated Na^+ channels identified in VSM may contribute to initial depolarization but they also inactivate rapidly and do not appear to contribute to sustained contraction in VSM [17]. L-type channels also inactivate with membrane depolarization, but the overlap of the activation and inactivation profiles for these channels allows for the "window currents" that are necessary to maintain Ca^{2+} entry and contraction [12].

Small GTP-binding proteins activated by agonists may also activate cation channels and inhibit K^+ channels, thereby contributing to membrane depolarization and Ca^{2+} entry through VGCCs [12]. Additionally, certain agonists such as the ATP coreleased with norepinephrine from sympathetic nerves can directly activate receptor-operated Ca^{2+} channels (ROCs). Finally, as discussed below, nonselective cation channels activated by stretch that are involved in myogenic contraction produce VSM depolarization and allow Ca^+ entry [31–33].

Gap-junction channels in VSM provide cell-to-cell electrochemical connectivity for passage of ions and small signaling molecules such as IP_3 between adjacent cells, thereby allowing for synchronized contraction or relaxation [34]. These channels are gated by intracellular stimuli, including elevations in $[Ca^{2+}]_i$ and/or phosphorylation by signaling pathways. As discussed in more detail below, endothelial-to-endothelial cell gap junctions are also important for propagating capillary endothelial cell hyperpolarization retrograde to induce relaxation of supply arteries. In addition, gap junctions between VSM and endothelial cells have been observed, potentially providing electrical coupling and a conduit for direct transfer of endothelium-dependent vasodilatory signals between cells [35,36]. The gap-junction hemi-channel is formed by the oligomerization of six connexin (Cx) protein subunits derived from a family of closely related genes, three of which, Cx37, Cx40, and Cx43, are expressed in vascular tissue [37–40].

Myogenic contraction

Myogenic contraction is a fundamental property of smooth muscle. It is manifested as a rapid and sustained contraction following increases in vascular transmural pressure, and it is independent of endothelial-cell or neural influences [41–43]. From a purely physical standpoint, myogenic contraction provides an offset to the passive dilating effect of increased transmural pressure, which would otherwise result in a reduction in vascular resistance. Accordingly, myogenic contraction is largely responsible for "autoregulation" of blood flow, the phenomenon whereby flow remains relatively constant over a range of perfusion pressures. In addition, intrinsic myogenic contraction provides for a component of vasodilatory reserve that contributes significantly to the dynamic range of blood flow responses in both directions.

As shown in Fig. 19.2, myogenic contraction is dependent on membrane depolarization and Ca^{2+} influx through voltage-dependent Ca^{2+} channels, with activation of the classic Ca^{2+}-dependent mechanisms involving MLCK phosphorylation of MLC. In addition, Ca^{2+}-independent (i.e., Ca^{2+} sensitization) mechanisms involving PKC, small G-protein-activated kinases, PTKs, as well as downstream phosphorylation of thin-filament-associated proteins such as caldesmon, also appear to be involved in myogenic contractions [41,42]. Interest in the membrane-depolarizing action of increased pressure has led to the characterization of mechanosensitive (MS) ion channels in VSM [41], including stretch-activated nonselective cation

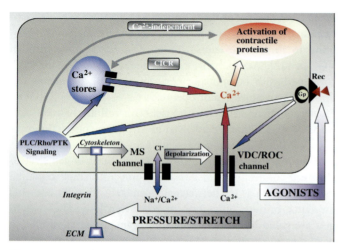

Figure 19.2. Mechanisms linking myogenic (pressure/stretch) and other G-protein (Gp) receptor (Rec) agonists to activation of contractile proteins in vascular smooth muscle cells (VSM). Integrins anchor the VSM to the extracellular matrix (ECM) and provide a physical link to VSM cytoskeleton-associated mechanosensitive (MS) channels and signaling pathways involving phospholipase C (PLC), small G proteins (e.g., Rho) kinases, and protein tyrosine kinases (PTK). Activation of MS channels results in membrane depolarization and activation of voltage-dependent calcium (VDC) channels. Receptor-operated Ca^{2+} channels (ROC) and Ca^{2+}-induced Ca^{2+} release (CICR) mechanisms also play a role.

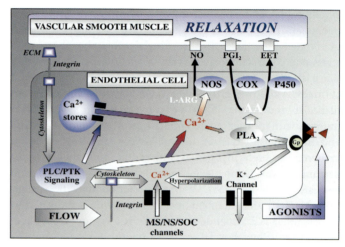

Figure 19.3. Activation of endothelium-dependent relaxation by flow is initiated by activation of mechanosensitive (MS) channels and extracellular matrix (ECM)/integrin/cytoskeleton signaling. Endothelial heterotrimeric G-protein (Gp)-coupled receptor agonists induce activation of phospholipase C (PLC) and K^+ channels, as well as activation of phospholipase A_2 (PLA$_2$). Increased release and influx of Ca^{2+} results in activation of nitric oxide synthase (NOS) and increased NO production. Vasodilatory and hyperpolarizing products of arachidonic acid (AA) metabolism are produced via the cyclooxygenase (COX) or cytochrome P450 monooxygenase (P450) pathways. EET, epoxyeicosatrienoic acids; PGI$_2$, prostacyclin; PTK, protein tyrosine kinase.

channels, which are ubiquitous in this tissue [41,44]. As shown in the model presented in Fig. 19.2, stretch is transduced directly to these channels, or to signaling pathways involved in MS ion-channel activation, by ECM interactions with VSM integrins which are "clustered" with multivalent ECM proteins at focal adhesion points. The intracellular integrin domains interact with cytoskeletal protein complexes such that the ECM/integrin/cytoskeletal complex provides a semirigid structure, analogous to the tensegrity model of R. Buckminster Fuller, from which structural deformations produced by changes in pressure are telegraphed to cytoskeleton-associated signaling proteins [41,42]. This model of "outside-in" signaling is further supported by the observations that the effector proteins, including stretch-activated channels, small G proteins, and signaling kinases involved in myogenic contraction, are anchored in cytoskeleton protein "scaffolds" linked to integrins [42,45].

Vascular endothelium

The vascular system is lined with a continuous layer of vascular endothelial cells, which provide a semipermeable barrier that regulates fluid and solute exchange [43,46].) These cells cover an estimated surface area of 3000 m^2 while having a mass less than 1 kg in the healthy adult. Small resistance vessels and capillaries represent the majority of this mass, where exposure of a relatively large endothelial surface to a small volume of blood (up to 5000 cm^2 per mL blood) facilitates the exchange of oxygen, nutrients, and metabolic products [47]. By contrast, the large conductance arteries and veins which contain most of the blood volume provide exposure to only a few square meters of endothelium (< 10 cm^2 per mL blood).

The discovery by Furchgott and Zawadzki of endothelium-derived relaxing factor (EDRF) [48] led to a major paradigm shift in our understanding of the role of the vascular endothelium in vascular reactivity. Indeed, it is now understood that endothelium-dependent vasodilation is involved in virtually every important adjustment in blood flow [49]. Moreover, altered endothelial function is now known to have a pivotal role in the changes in vascular reactivity that occur with aging as well as in a number of prevalent disease processes including hypertension, atherosclerosis, diabetes mellitus, and coronary artery disease [10,50–53] The roles of endothelial factors in the control of thrombosis and/or platelet activation, as well as in the trafficking of circulating immune cells, are also now more fully appreciated [6,54–56]. Finally, the central role of the vascular endothelium in angiogenesis – acting as both the sensor and effector for angiogenic stimuli – is now recognized, offering the potential for novel therapies to promote wound healing and tissue revascularization, as well as to prevent the unwanted angiogenesis that promotes tumor growth or chronic inflammation [57].

Endothelium-dependent relaxation

Blood flow results in elaboration of nitric oxide (NO), prostacyclin (PGI$_2$), and EDHF (epoxyeicosatrienoic acid, EET) by endothelial cells (Fig. 19.3) [58–60]. These factors produce relaxation of adjacent VSM and are important in preventing activation of platelets and the coagulation cascade, and in promoting angiogenesis. As shown in Fig. 19.3, mechanotransduction in endothelial cells leads to increases in intracellular Ca^{2+} similar to that which occurs in VSM. In contrast to VSM, however, in which downstream Ca^{2+} signaling involving MLCK activation leads to contraction (Fig. 19.1), Ca^{2+} signaling in endothelial cells activates eNOS and PLA_2, leading to release of the VSM relaxing factors shown (Fig. 19.3) [60–62].

As shown in Fig. 19.3, the extracellular domains of endothelial-cell integrins can directly detect changes in flow at the luminal surface, while perturbations in endothelial structure or diameter are telegraphed to signaling pathways via the same ECM/integrin/cytoskeletal interactions as described above for myogenic contraction [61]. Accordingly, blockade of integrin signaling with RGD peptides or β_3 integrin antibodies results in attenuation of flow-induced, endothelium-dependent vasodilation [63]. Release of endothelial relaxing factors is particularly important in metabolic autoregulation, and inhibition of endothelium-dependent relaxation results in a substantial decrease in the vasodilatory response to tissue hypoxia [64]. A working model of metabolic autoregulation involves proportional depletion of high-energy phosphate stores in relatively hypoxic tissue leading to activation of ATP-gated potassium (K_{ATP}) channels in the capillary endothelial cells. The resulting membrane hyperpolarization drives membrane potential further from the Ca^{2+} equilibration potential, Ca^{2+} influx through non-selective cation channels is thereby increased, and eNOS and PLA_2 are activated as shown (Fig. 19.3). Endothelial cell-to-cell gap junctions propagate this capillary endothelial signal upstream to the small arterioles controlling tissue blood flow, while flow-induced endothelial relaxing factor release is further propagated upstream (i.e., until the downstream requirements for oxygen are satisfied) [65,66].

Nitric oxide

Endothelium-derived relaxing factor (EDRF) is now taken to be synonymous with nitric oxide (NO), a heterodiatomic molecule synthesized from the terminal guanidino nitrogen atom(s) of L-arginine by NOS through a five-electron oxidation [48]. Three main NOS isoforms have been identified, although only the constitutive endothelial isoform, eNOS or NOS III [67] is present in vascular tissue. eNOS is activated by Ca^{2+}/calmodulin and therefore dependent on endothelial intracellular Ca^{2+} signaling. Additionally, recent evidence indicates that phospholipase-A_2 (PLA_2)-derived arachidonic acid (AA) is also essential for activation of eNOS [68]. An inducible NOS isoform (iNOS or NOS II) can also be expressed in both endothelial cells and VSM, but only after transcriptional induction by inflammatory mediators or other pathologic stimuli. Notably iNOS, unlike eNOS, once expressed in endothelial cells or VSM, is constitutively active and produces NO independent of $[Ca^{2+}]_i$. iNOS expression thereby results in vasodilation that is independent of tissue metabolism or flow [69].

Once generated in the endothelial cell, the amphophilic NO molecule rapidly crosses membranes and enters adjacent VSM cells where it is bound by the heme moiety of guanylate cyclase, activating this enzyme. The resulting increased production of cyclic guanosine $3',5'$-monophosphate (cGMP)

results in cGMP-dependent protein-kinase (PKG)-mediated VSM relaxation [70]. A number of PKG phosphorylation targets in VSM appear to be involved in the relaxing action of NO and other agonists of the cGMP/PKG pathway, including both Ca^{2+} and K^+ channels as well as the Ca^{2+} transporters and pumps involved in Ca^{2+}-activated contraction. PKG also phosphorylates the myosin recognition subunit (MYPT1) of MLCP, resulting in MLCP activation and Ca^{2+}-independent relaxation (i.e., "Ca^{2+} desensitization"). Additionally, NO may directly activate K^+ channels, producing hyperpolarization and relaxation independent of PKG [71].

Prostanoids

Activation of phospholipase A_2 (PLA_2) in endothelial cells by Ca^{2+} results in production of arachidonic acid (AA), which is the substrate for elaboration of a number of important cyclooxygenase (COX) products, most notably PGI_2 and prostaglandin E_2 (PGE_2), both of which are potent vasodilating agents. As with the NOS family of genes, there are both constitutive and inducible COX isoforms (COX-1 and COX-2, respectively), with the constitutive COX-1 being the only isoform expressed at significant levels in endothelial cells under physiological conditions [72]. Again, similar to iNOS, inflammatory stimuli may also result in increased expression of COX-2 in both endothelial and VSM cells [73]. Notably, vasoconstrictor COX products including $PGF_{2\alpha}$, PGH, and the potent constrictor TxA_2, may contribute to VSM contraction and blood flow distribution under conditions associated with increased expression of COX-2 [74].

Unlike NO, the actions of the vasodilatory prostanoids are mediated by activation of adenylate cyclase in VSM [75], resulting in increases in the intracellular concentration of cyclic adenosine $3',5'$-monophosphate (cAMP) and activation of cAMP-dependent protein kinase (protein kinase A, PKA). Interestingly, the vasorelaxing effects of cAMP in VSM also appear to be dependent on activation of PKG, which is expressed in considerably higher quantities in VSM compared to PKA. PKG thus appears to be an important point of convergence for endothelium-dependent relaxation of VSM following activation of either adenylate cyclase by PGI_2 or guanylate cyclase by NO [76,77].

Endothelium-derived hyperpolarizing factor

While both NO and PGI_2 can produce VSM hyperpolarization and relaxation, endothelium-derived hyperpolarizing factor (EDHF) activity persists in the presence of both NOS and COX inhibitors [78–80]. Although the molecular identity of EDHF in all tissues has remained unclear, PLA_2-derived AA metabolized via the cytochrome P450 monooxygenase pathway to produce epoxyeicosatrienoic acids (EETs) appears to account for the EDHF activity observed in a number of arterial preparations [78–80]. Additionally, PLA_2-derived AA metabolized via the 5'-lipoxygenase pathway, leading to the production of leukotrienes (LTA_4, LTB_4, LTC_4, and LTD_4), may also have a role in VSM hyperpolarization and relaxation in some tissues [81]. Ultimately, EDHF activity, which may arise from a number of different mediators, is related to activation of VSM K^+ channels, resulting in hyperpolarization and resistance to depolarizing agonists [82–84]. EDHF responses in some tissue are inhibited by application of the K^+ channel blockers, apamin and charybdotoxin, although coapplication appears necessary to completely block EDHF activity [84]. Notably, ATP-sensitive K^+ channels (K_{ATP}) and large-conductance Ca^{2+}-activated K^+ channels (BK_{Ca}) do not appear to play a major role in EDHF-induced hyperpolarization [85,86].

Endothelin

The vascular endothelium also may elaborate the potent VSM vasoconstrictor endothelins (ETs), a family of three closely related 21-amino-acid peptide products (ET-1, ET-2, and ET-3) of separate genes [87–89]. ETs interact with high-affinity G-protein-coupled VSM ET receptors that activate PLC, increasing VSM $[Ca^{2+}]_i$ and inducing Ca^{2+} sensitization as described above for other vasoconstricting agonists [87]. ET_A receptor has a higher affinity for ET-1, while the ET_B receptor has approximately equal affinity for all three ETs. ETs may also act as autocoids to increase endothelial NO and PGI_2 release, thereby modulating the constrictor actions of ETs [90]. Finally, while the physiological role of ETs remains unclear, their existence is of interest in a variety of conditions associated with excessive vasoconstriction. Increased ET release and ET-induced vasoconstriction and/or mitogenesis have been implicated in the pathophysiology of atherosclerosis and hypertension, as well as coronary and cerebral vasospasm [91–93]. ET-1 concentrations have also been noted to be elevated in patients with Raynaud disease, suggesting that the pathologic vasoconstriction in this condition may be related to endothelial dysregulation and excess production of ETs [94,95].)

Coagulation and inflammation

The importance of the endothelium in preventing local thrombosis and platelet aggregation has long been appreciated, and several endothelium-dependent mechanisms involved in these actions have been elucidated. Endothelium-produced NO and PGI_2 increase cyclic nucleotide concentrations in circulating platelets, thereby inhibiting platelet activation and adhesion to the vascular wall. Additionally, endothelium-derived relaxing factors attenuate the vasoconstrictor effect of platelet-produced thromboxane A_2 (TxA_2), the major COX product of activated platelets [47]. Finally, adenosine diphosphatase expressed on the endothelial cell surface hydrolyzes and neutralizes locally produced adenosine diphosphate, another potent platelet agonist [96].

Endothelial cells inhibit local activation of the coagulation cascade by a variety of mechanisms. Endothelial cells synthesize and express heparin sulfate proteoglycans, which bind and potentiate the activity of both antithrombin III (ATIII), the main inhibitor of thrombin and activated factor X, and tissue factor pathway inhibitor (TFPI), which inhibits tissue-factor-activated

factor VII complex [55,96–98]. The thrombin receptor thrombomodulin (TM), which binds and prevents thrombin from converting fibrinogen to fibrin, or activating factor V, is also expressed on the luminal surface of endothelial cells. When bound to endothelial TM, thrombin no longer activates circulating platelets, but rather activates circulating protein C, which in the presence of its cofactor protein S enzymatically inactivates factors V_a and VIII_a. Finally, the endothelium produces tissue plasminogen activator (tPA), which results in activation of the fibrinolytic system [75,96,97].

In addition to the endothelial mechanisms which prevent coagulation and platelet activation, endothelial cells synthesize and secrete important procoagulant factors including von Willebrand factor (vWF), and plasminogen activator inhibitor 1 (a tPA inhibitor) which can be vitally important under conditions involving tissue damage [96,97,99–101]. Endothelial cells elaborate a variety of adhesion molecules under such circumstances that promote coagulation as well as attachment and activation of platelets and leukocytes [6,54,55,96,102]. Involution and loss of surface proteoglycans and TM occur such that endothelial cells stimulated by thrombin (or bradykinin or histamine from leukocytes) undergo membrane translocation of Weibel–Palade bodies containing vWF and P-selectin. These in turn interact with GPIb/IX integrin receptors on platelets and leukocytes, inducing rolling along the membrane that facilitates contact with other activator molecules or exposed ECM [4,54,96,97,102–104]. ECM collagen interacts with platelet GPIa/IIa integrin, resulting in platelet activation and exposure of GPIIb/IIIa integrin, which bind one of several high-affinity GPIIb/IIIa binding sites on fibrinogen. The resulting fibrinogen–GPIIb/IIIa interaction at the endothelial surface in this circumstance is pivotal in inducing aggregation of activated platelets and formation of the provisional platelet plug [6,103]. This structure in turn serves as the assembly surface for other coagulation factors including thrombin, which catalyzes the formation of the occlusive thrombus [6,97,103].

Stimulation of endothelial cells following exposure to local or systemic inflammatory mediators, such as tumor necrosis factor α (TNFα) or interleukin 1 (IL-1), also produces a stereotypical endothelial response involving transcription and expression of endothelial-cell-specific E-selectin receptors and adhesion molecules of the immunoglobulin superfamily, including intracellular adhesion molecule 1 and 2 (ICAM-1, ICAM-2), and vascular cell adhesion molecule 1 (VCAM-1) [54,102,103]. Activated white cells expressing β_1- and β_2-integrin receptors in turn bind endothelial adhesion molecules, resulting in leukocyte diapedesis, facilitated by platelet–endothelial cell adhesion molecule 1 (PCAM-1) located at the lateral endothelial borders [54,102,103]. Thus while vascular endothelial cells play a central role in preventing thrombosis and activation of platelets and leukocytes under physiological conditions, endothelial mechanisms are equally important in inducing activation of these elements in response to injury and inflammation. Immediate platelet-activating and prothrombotic mechanisms result in containment of an injury or infection, preventing further loss of blood from the intravascular space. The second phase of the endothelial cell response involving de-novo expression of immunoglobulin superfamily receptors results in leukocyte mobilization to the site of injury or infection, which continues until the stimulus decays and the endothelial cell response subsides [54].

Under certain conditions, ongoing leukocyte-induced endothelial cell damage or apoptosis can result in a vicious cycle in which there is continued exposure of ECM and chronic inflammation [97,104]. Clinical evidence supports this concept and places the endothelium at the center of the coagulation and inflammation cascade dysregulation that occurs in both the systemic inflammatory response (SIRS) and adult respiratory distress syndromes (ARDS) [96,102,105]. This insight has further provided for the development of novel treatments directed at the procoagulation and proinflammation positive feedback loops that occur in these conditions [54]. A therapeutic trial aimed at preventing activation of prothrombotic elements and leukocytes at the endothelial surface utilizing activated protein C has resulted in promising increases in survival in patients with severe sepsis and septic shock [106]. The crosstalk between the inflammatory and coagulation cascades at the level of the vascular endothelium, including thrombin activation-mediated depletion of the counterregulatory protein C mechanism, appears to provide the basis for the benefit of this treatment in patients with septic shock [106]. In addition, activated protein C has been demonstrated to suppress both cytokine-induced activation of the NFκB pathway in circulating leukocytes and apoptotic gene expression in endothelial cells, providing another mechanism whereby the vicious cycle of endothelial damage and leukocyte activation is interrupted [107]. Such studies provide striking support for the continued pursuit of additional strategies to exploit mechanisms involved in interactions between the inflammation and coagulation cascades at the endothelial surface.

Angiogenesis

Angiogenesis, or the formation of new vessels, is first evident with proliferation of endothelial cells and the formation of de-novo endothelium-lined capillaries. It is clearly important for healing and growth [11,108,109], and intensified interest directed at understanding tumor angiogenesis has led to a number of advances, including identification of the endothelial-cell proangiogenic and antiangiogenic signaling pathways [11,108,109]. The present model indicates that tissue growth in either physiological or pathological conditions produces a state of relative tissue hypoxia that results in production of hypoxia-induced transcription factors for the vascular endothelial growth factor (VEGF) family of proteins including platelet-derived growth factor (PDGF), and angiopoietin [11,108,109]. Activation of endothelial cells by these growth factors induces secretion of matrix metalloproteinases (MMPs), which degrade

the ECM; activated endothelial cells then migrate in the interstitial space in the direction of the hypoxic stimulus [108]. Extravasation of plasma proteins from new endothelial sprouts forms a provisional fibrin-rich matrix into which the endothelial cells migrate. The endothelial cell sprouts form interconnecting vascular channels, establishing local circulation. As the hypoxic stimulus abates, endothelial cells mature and express $\alpha_V\beta_3$-integrin receptors that interact with matrix protein ligand(s) which turn off the "angiogenic switch" [2,110].

In addition to hypoxia-induced transcription factors and tissue-derived growth factors, activation of the coagulation and inflammatory cascades at the endothelial surface (described above) is an important proangiogenic stimulus involved in wound healing, as well as in the sometimes unwanted neovascularization that can occur [11]. Factors derived from activated platelets and leukocytes, including PDGF, basic fibroblast growth factor, transforming growth factor β, and TNFα, and factors expressed by activated endothelial cells, including NO, PGI_2, tPA, plasminogen activator inhibitor 1, and E-selectin, as well as thrombin and plasmin activated in the coagulation cascade, have all been demonstrated to have proangiogenic activity [11,108,109].

In addition to proangiogenic mechanisms, a number of endogenous antiangiogenic factors have also been identified and explored, particularly for their potential to control unwanted tumor angiogenesis. Endostatin and angiostatin, peptide cleavage products of vascular-specific collagen XVIII and plasminogen respectively, have been the most extensively studied, and ongoing trials are directed at determining their efficacy in treating solid tumors [11,109]. Other antiangiogenic mechanisms and strategies have included the use of anti-VEGF or anti-$\alpha_V\beta_3$ integrin antibodies, or MMP inhibitors [11,108]. Additionally, some of the unique cellular markers of dividing endothelial cells, including $\alpha_V\beta_3$-integrin and E-selectin, have been proposed as homing probes to target tumor vessels with cytotoxic or immunogenic drugs [11,110,111]. In addition to their potential as antitumor agents, such therapies may also be useful in controlling the unwanted angiogenesis that occurs in vascular malformations and diabetic retinopathy [11,108]. It has even been proposed that control of the angiogenesis necessary for adipose tissue hypertrophy could be a potential target in the treatment of morbid obesity [11].

Neurohumoral mechanisms

Sympathetic nervous system

Vascular tissue is extensively innervated by sympathetic nerves, and vascular system reactivity is strongly influenced by central nervous system control mechanisms mediated by alterations in sympathetic nerve output. Stimulation of the amygdala/hypothalamic integrative areas involved in fright, fight, flight defense reactions produces increased sympathetic nerve activity and VSM constriction resulting in increased vascular resistance and blood pressure, and decreased arterial and venous capacitance [112,113]. Stimulation of chemoreceptors in the carotid or aortic bodies by CO_2 or acidosis similarly increases sympathetic output [113]. Conversely, stimulation of baroreceptors in the carotid sinus or aortic arch elicited by elevations in blood pressure results in decreased sympathetic outflow; however, withdrawal of baroreceptor stimulation, such as occurs in hypovolemia or hypotension, is the most potent stimulus for sympathetic nervous system output [114,115].

Norepinephrine (NE) is the principal neurotransmitter released at sympathetic nerve endings, and the vasoconstrictor effect of NE is largely mediated by activation of VSM α_1-adrenoceptors. The mechanisms involve activation of PLC and increases in VSM $[Ca^{2+}]_i$ from IP_3-sensitive intracellular stores, as well as the sensitization of the contractile proteins to Ca^{2+} mediated by PKC- and Rho-kinase-induced phosphorylation of MLCP, as described above [41]. VSM α_2 receptors may also mediate vasoconstriction in some vessels via activation of Ca^{2+} channels, although presynaptic α_2-adrenoceptors inhibit NE release resulting in VSM relaxation. In endothelial cells, α_2-adrenoceptors also induce $[Ca^{2+}]_i$ increases, resulting in activation of eNOS and PLA_2 and endothelium-dependent vasodilation [116,117]. VSM β_2 receptors mediate vasodilation in coronary and skeletal muscle beds via activation of the adenylate cyclase/PKA mechanisms described above for vasodilatory prostanoids.

Sympathetic nerve terminals also contain neuropeptide Y (NPY), a 36-amino-acid protein that is capable of producing VSM contraction via G-protein-coupled receptor (GPCR) activation of the PLC/PKC/Rho-kinase pathways just as with α_1-adrenoceptors. Presynaptic NPY receptors inhibit sympathetic neurotransmitter release, similar to α_2-adrenoceptors [118]. Sympathetic nerve terminals also contain ATP, which contributes to VSM $[Ca^{2+}]_i$ increases via ROCs. Finally, purinergic receptors activated by ATP and other purines released from sympathetic nerves inhibit NE release by a presynaptic mechanism as well as by inducing endothelium-dependent vasodilator release [119–121].

Parasympathetic nervous system

In contrast to the heart and large airways, the vascular system is only sparsely innervated with parasympathetic nerves. Accordingly, the parasympathetic nervous system has comparatively little influence on vascular reactivity. As in airway smooth muscle, activation of muscarinic M_1 or M_2 receptors in VSM can induce a contractile response. However, in stark contrast to the contracting effect of acetylcholine (ACh) and other muscarinic receptor agonists on airway smooth muscle, activation of muscarinic (M_3) receptors on vascular endothelial cells predominates in the vascular system, resulting in endothelium-dependent VSM relaxation [122]. Accordingly, VSM contraction is only observed under conditions in which the endothelium is removed or damaged [123]. Again, it is

interesting that endothelial muscarinic receptors are widely distributed in the vascular system with little or no accompanying cholinergic innervation. The functional significance of the VSM and endothelial-cell muscarinic receptors in control of VSM tone thus remains unclear.

Nonadrenergic, noncholinergic nerves

Nonadrenergic, noncholinergic (NANC) mechanisms may also influence vascular reactivity. And although some actions of cotransmitters released from sympathetic or cholinergic neurons may account for effects attributed to NANC mechanisms, distinct sensory nerves are capable of releasing a variety of vasoactive substances in certain tissues, including vasoactive intestinal polypeptide (VIP), substance P, and calcitonin gene-related product (CGRP) [124]. VIP is an octapeptide structurally related to secretin and glucagon that acts via GPCRs to activate adenylate cyclase and produce vascular relaxation via a cAMP-dependent mechanism as described for β-adrenergic agonists and prostanoids [125]. Immunohistochemical studies indicate that VIP immunoreactivity may be colocalized with ACh in some parasympathetic nerves. Substance P and CGRP are generally found colocalized in sensory neurons, and are coreleased upon stimulation of the vagus or other perivascular sensory nerves of large arteries. Substance P has dual effects on vascular tissue that are analogous to those of ACh with a direct GPCR contracting effect in VSM as well as an endothelium-dependent relaxing action [126]. CGRP by contrast is a potent VSM relaxing agent, producing direct cAMP-dependent relaxation in VSM similar to that produced by VIP [127], as well as indirect relaxation related to increased endothelium-dependent vasodilator release [128]. In general, NANC mechanisms do not appear to significantly influence vascular tone under most physiological circumstances, but may potentially play a role in vasovagal responses. Substance P may also contribute to unwanted increases in vascular tone under conditions in which there is endothelial dysfunction.

Angiotensin II

Angiotensin II (AII) is an octapeptide produced by the action of angiotensin-converting enzyme on the inactive circulating form, angiotensin I, which is itself formed by the action of renin on circulating angiotensinogen. Accordingly, renin release from the renal juxtaglomerular apparatus determines AII activity, where AII is the vasoactive end product of the renin–angiotensin system that leads to efferent arteriolar constriction. Under normal physiological conditions AII levels are largely related to sodium intake and delivery to the distal tubule macula densa cells located adjacent to the glomerulus. Under conditions of organism threat or low blood pressure where there is activation of renal sympathetic nerves, significant increases in renin release and AII levels can occur that contribute both to systemic vasoconstriction and to activation of central mechanisms leading to release of arginine vasopressin (AVP) from the posterior pituitary (see below). Angiotensin II produces direct VSM constriction via specific type 1 AII (AT_1) GPCRs, with activation of the

PLC/PKC/Rho-kinase pathways and contractile apparatus as described above for other VSM agonists (Fig. 19.1). In addition, endothelial AII receptors can result in release of the potent endothelium-dependent vasoconstrictor ET-1, which can thereby contribute to AII-induced vasoconstriction. Notably, AII is also involved in regulation of plasma volume through aldosterone-regulated sodium excretion and central thirst responses, as well as in VSM cell growth, cell migration, and ECM deposition [129]. Accordingly, AT_1 receptor blockers (ARBs) are effective in blocking both the AII-induced increases in systemic resistance that occur in certain forms of hypertension and heart failure, as well as the structural and functional abnormalities of the vascular wall produced by AII in subjects with these conditions [130].

Arginine vasopressin

AVP is a neuropeptide released into the circulation from the posterior pituitary. Under most physiological conditions AVP is released in very small quantities in response to stimulation of hypothalamic osmolar sensitive cells; it then interacts with V_2 receptors to decrease free water clearance by the renal tubular cells, in its well-known role as antidiuretic hormone (ADH). However, in the presence of a perceived threat (i.e., as part of the fright, fight, flight reflex) and particularly following decreases in baroreflex input from volume and pressure sensors in the heart and great vessels, massive AVP release can occur. Moreover, AVP release under such circumstances is independent of osmolarity and results in activation of V_1 VSM receptors with significant and physiologically important AVP-induced vasoconstriction [131]. The importance of this vasopressinergic mechanism has received considerable attention in recent years, particularly in the development of vasodilatory shock, which is accompanied by exhaustion of this mechanism [132]. A number of studies using AVP replacement therapy demonstrate reversal of both the refractory hypotension and catecholamine tachyphylaxis that is present in vasodilatory shock; in further support of the physiological importance of this mechanism, a recent study indicates that AVP replacement therapy has a significant mortality benefit [133,134]. The vasoconstrictor action of AVP, mediated by interaction with VSM V_1 GPCRs, again involves PLC activation and the classic Ca^{2+}-dependent and Ca^{2+} sensitization mechanisms described above for other agonists [135]. Notably, V_1 receptors are largely absent in the renal bed, in contrast to α_1-adrenergic and AT_1 receptors. Accordingly, the role of AVP under extreme physiological conditions associated with massive AVP release may in part relate to the relative preservation of renal blood flow. In this regard, increases, not decreases, in urine output have been noted following AVP replacement therapy in vasodilatory shock [132].

Control of vascular reactivity

Vascular reactivity as it relates to VSM contraction and relaxation is regulated both by local intrinsic "autoregulatory"

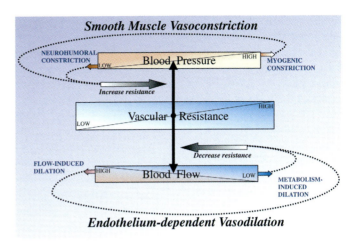

Figure 19.4. Ohm's law describes the relationships among blood pressure, vascular resistance, and blood flow. Blood pressure is directly proportional to vascular resistance and therefore increases with increases in resistance. Conversely, blood flow is inversely proportional to resistance and decreases with increases in resistance. Baseline vascular resistance, and thereby pressure and flow, are initially set by myogenic vasoconstriction which is countered by endothelium-dependent metabolism-induced and flow-induced vasodilation to meet tissue demands. During conditions in which blood pressure is low, neurohumoral constriction comes into play to increase resistance and blood pressure.

mechanisms involving myogenic contraction and by endothelium-dependent relaxation, as well as by neurohumoral factors. A model for integration of these elements is shown in Fig. 19.4. In this formulation, myogenic contraction, in response to increases in vascular transmural pressure produced by the beating heart, increases systemic resistance, thereby maintaining blood pressure. Simultaneously endothelium-dependent release of relaxing factors, in response to both tissue metabolism and blood flow, fine-tune VSM contraction so that perfusion meets tissue metabolic demands. The importance of endothelium-dependent relaxation is evident in this model (Fig. 19.4), in which elimination or dysfunction of the endothelial component can be seen to leave myogenic vasoconstriction unopposed, thereby generating a positive feedback loop leading to excessive contraction, tissue ischemia, and potentially vasospasm. During extreme physiologic conditions when blood pressure is low, or the organism otherwise perceives a threat, neurohumoral mechanisms – involving the sympathetic, renin–angiotensin, and vasopressinergic systems described above – come into play. Under such conditions, these mechanisms can have profound effects on the distribution of blood flow, primarily directed at preserving critical organ blood flow to permit the organism to survive extreme threats such as significant trauma and/or hemorrhage. Such mechanisms may thus take precedence over local endothelium-dependent mechanisms directed at matching metabolism and flow, particularly in the vessels supplying the mesenteric, muscle, and cutaneous beds, which are densely innervated by sympathetic fibers and receptor-rich with respect to both AII AT_1 and AVP V_1 GPCRs. The

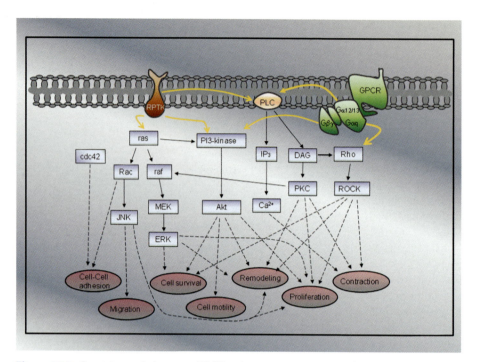

Figure 19.5. G-protein-coupled receptor (GPCR) and receptor protein tyrosine kinase (RPTK) agonists lead to activation of multiple converging and overlapping signaling pathways that result in a variety of phenotypic responses involved in vascular reactivity.

characteristic vasoconstricting response thus involves redistribution of blood flow away from the gastrointestinal tract, muscle, and skin to preserve systemic perfusion pressure and essential flow to the heart and brain. In the renal bed, sympathetic constriction may also negatively impact flow; however, juxtaglomerular apparatus and tubuloglomerular feedback mechanisms involving angiotensin-II-induced efferent arteriolar constriction, as well as the renal-bed sparing effect of vasopressin described above, preserve both glomerular filtration and critical blood flow to preserve renal tissue viability.

As shown in Fig. 19.4, neurohumoral mediator-induced vasoconstriction is integrated into the balance between myogenic constriction and endothelium-dependent relaxation such that neurohumoral mechanisms directed at organism preservation take precedence over local demands, particularly in "non-essential" beds. The endothelium-dependent mechanisms ensure that the minimum flow necessary for organ viability and the vasodilatory reserve necessary for fight and flight responses remain intact. While AVP is a known potent direct coronary constrictor [136], for example, endothelium-dependent relaxation mechanisms ensure that cardiac blood flow necessary to support cardiac and coronary vasodilatory reserve are preserved [137]. Accordingly, even under the most extreme conditions, when extrinsic vasoconstrictor mechanisms are deployed, intrinsic local control mechanisms remain essential to ensure adequate delivery of oxygen and nutrients to tissues. Finally, a number of vasodilatory compounds, including natriuretic peptides, and white-cell and platelet products such as histamine or bradykinin, can contribute to VSM tone and blood flow under certain conditions. Notably,

however, these mediators are not believed to participate in the physiological regulation of blood pressure and only appear to be important in certain pathological conditions such as systemic inflammation and allergic or anaphylactoid reactions.

The vascular system as a rich target for drug action

As the forgoing discussion has illuminated, there are a large number of potential molecular targets in the vascular system, giving rise to a multitude of pharmacologic agents that have prominent effects on vascular tone and function. The importance of these targets is further underlined by the involvement of the vascular system in virtually every important and prevalent disease state. An illustration of the complexity of the intersecting pathways in VSM and the repertoire of responses broadly included in this discussion of vascular reactivity is shown in Fig. 19.5. The responses elicited by the family of seven-transmembrane GPCRs – involved in the responses to vasoconstrictors such as NE, AVP, and AII – are shown, in which effects on contraction are mediated by activation of PLC by $G\alpha_q$ and guanine exchange factors by $G\alpha_{12/3}$ that lead to activation of small G-protein kinases, most notably ROCKs. As described earlier, ROCKs and the PKC pathways converge to produce contraction via Ca^{2+} sensitization and other Ca^{2+}-independent mechanisms. As also shown, both the PKC and ROCK pathways also converge on the signaling pathways involved in angiogenic responses involving cell proliferation and remodeling, as well as cell survival (i.e., apoptotic pathways). Similarly, receptor protein tyrosine kinases (RPTKs) such as the epidermal growth factor receptor (EGFR), as well as the $G\beta\gamma$ subunit released by GPCRs, activate the PI3K-Akt pathway, which again converges on cellular pathways involved in angiogenesis, including cell motility, and survival [15].

As Fig. 19.5 illustrates, the physiology and molecular pharmacology of the vascular system follows a pattern similar to that of other excitable tissues, with a limited number of agonists involved in diverse cellular functions which depend on the specific receptor subtypes and the coupling mechanism(s) expressed, and whether the target cell is endothelial or VSM. Sympathomimetic agonists, for example, can produce vasoconstriction or vasodilation depending on whether the GPCRs are coupled to activation of PLC or adenylate cyclase, as well as on whether α_1-, α_2-, or β_2-adrenoceptors are present on the endothelial or VSM cells, or both, in a given vessel. Notably, there is striking agonist redundancy in the vascular system, such that a number of different agonist systems converge at the level of the receptor coupling mechanisms and effector molecules to produce a similar effect on vascular reactivity. The α_1-adrenergic, V_1 vasopressin, and AT_1 angiotensin II GPCRs, as well as ET_A receptors, for example, all converge at the level of PLC, PKC, and ROCK activation, thereby all resulting in vasoconstriction and activation of other downstream processes (Fig. 19.5).

This redundancy in the actions of the various agonists in the vascular systems has additional important pharmacologic implications. First, blockade of the agonist receptor for one system generally results in compensatory increases in the activity of the other redundant system(s) such that the effects of exogenously administered agonists or antagonists are generally countered by compensatory decreases or increases in the release or activity of the other redundant systems. Accordingly, it is often difficult to ascertain which system or agonist is primarily responsible for an observed response, and multiple agents are often necessary to produce a desired effect. When attempting to block the vasoconstrictor mechanism(s) involved in the genesis of hypertension or the increased vascular resistance in heart failure, for example, it is often necessary to use multiple inhibitors to achieve the desired result. Similarly, attempts to lower blood pressure using the NO donor sodium nitroprusside (NTP) are accompanied by counterregulatory increases in sympathetic, vasopressinergic, and renin–angiotensin system activity which contribute to attenuation of NTP responsiveness, and inhibitors of all three mechanisms are thus necessary to eliminate NTP tachyphylaxis. Conversely, the redundancy in the vasoconstrictor and vasodilator mechanisms also provides additional therapeutic opportunities involving the use of multiple agents with parallel or converging mechanisms when a single agent is ineffective. The endothelium-dependent vasodilators NO and PGI_2 can be combined in the treatment of severe pulmonary hypertension owing to their different receptor mechanisms, involving guanylate and adenylate cyclase, which then converge to produce VSM relaxation [76,77].

Targeting a downstream mechanism distal to the point of convergence, at the level of the phosphodiesterase that degrades cAMP and cGMP, for example, provides another target that enhances the efficacy of NO and PGI_2 [138].

The pluripotent aspect of endogenous agonists – whereby a given agonist activates a number of receptor subtypes linked to different signaling pathways and physiological actions – is another common feature in the vascular system with important pharmacological implications. Most importantly, this allows for the development of synthetic agonists and antagonists, which are more specific for activation of a single receptor subtype than the endogenous agonists, such that a desirable pharmacological action may be emphasized and separated from one that may be less desirable. The synthetic adrenergic agonist phenylephrine (PE), for example, being a relatively specific α_1 agonist, has the advantage of allowing for exogenous vasoconstriction while avoiding the potentially deleterious β-adrenergic effects of native NE or epinephrine in patients with coronary artery disease. Similarly, specific β-adrenergic antagonists have been developed to achieve a similar degree of protection from the endogenous agonist(s). When using synthetic agonists for one receptor subtype, however, even limited agonist efficacy at the other receptor subtypes must be considered. The synthetic α_2-adrenergic agonist dexmedetomidine (DEX), for example, binds α_1 receptors with poor receptor efficacy compared to α_2 receptors, such that DEX has little undesirable effect on blood pressure. However, as a result of α_1-receptor binding, DEX competes with endogenous or exogenously administered NE, and can thereby produce undesirable hypotension in critical situations where blood pressure is dependent on endogenous sympathetic tone or exogenous adrenergic administration [139].

Finally, the opposing vasoconstricting and vasodilating actions of agonists vis-à-vis their actions on VSM versus vascular endothelial cells is another recurring theme in the vascular system. As discussed above, these opposing effects are related in large part to the fact that increases in $[Ca^{2+}]_i$, which can result from identical GPCRs and Ca^{2+} signaling pathways in the two cell types, result in activation of MLCK and contraction in VSM, while producing NOS and PLA_2 activation in endothelial cells leading to relaxation. Moreover, while the effect of a given agonist may depend on which of the two competing effects is dominant in the particular vascular bed or circumstance, the balance between VSM and endothelial function appears to be important in the physiologic product. The vasoconstricting effects of α-adrenergic agonists, for example, are significantly modulated by α-adrenergic endothelial receptors such that NE- or PE-induced vasoconstriction is markedly potentiated following removal of the endothelium. Similarly, agonists such as ACh, bradykinin, substance P, and histamine, for which endothelium-dependent vasodilation generally predominates, can produce vasoconstriction due to unopposed activation of VSM receptors when the endothelium is damaged or dysfunctional as occurs in patients with atherosclerotic disease or diabetes mellitus.

Summary

Vascular smooth muscle (VSM) contraction involves the integrated activation of a unique repertoire of membrane receptors, ion channels, transporters, signaling pathways, and messenger molecules. While these are similar to, and as complex as, those found in other excitable tissue, mechanisms distinct to smooth muscle are involved in coupling membrane receptor activation and/or depolarization to activation of contractile proteins that serve the unique functions of VSM. A complement of ion channels similar to those in skeletal and cardiac muscle produce Ca^{2+} increases that trigger contraction in VSM, for example. However, downstream signaling pathways leading to VSM contraction uniquely involve myosin light chain (MLC) phosphorylation by Ca^{2+}-activated MLC kinase (MLCK) and Ca^{2+} sensitization via inhibition of a myosin-specific phosphatase (MLCP). Indeed, these mechanisms are strikingly different than the direct Ca^{2+} binding to actin-associated proteins that produce rapid contractile protein activation and contraction in skeletal and cardiac muscle. This difference, however, serves the unique need of VSM and other smooth muscle for relatively slow and more long-lasting contractions. Similarly, while mechanosensitive channels are widely distributed in other excitable tissue, their unique interplay with the extracellular matrix (ECM)/integrin/ cytoskeletal elements leads to "myogenic" contraction in VSM and thereby provides the mechansim for autoregulation of blood flow over the physiological range of blood pressures.

The involvement of endothelial cell mechanisms in the regulation of VSM contraction, largely involving endothelial NO and PGI_2 production in response to hypoxia and flow, is another unique feature of VSM providing the link between flow and metabolism that allows for metabolic autoregulation and coupling of tissue O_2 demand with O_2 delivery. The involvement of sympathetic and other neurohumoral mediators, with their own unique complement and organ-system distribution of G-protein-coupled receptors (GPCRs) on both VSM and endothelial cells, allows for integration of metabolic demands with the survival needs of the organism under more demanding physiological conditions. Finally, the vascular system, and particularly vascular endothelial cells, participates in a number of dynamic processes involving coagulation, thrombosis, white blood cell trafficking, and angiogenesis, which are important to understanding physiological and pathological mechanisms of inflammation, healing, and tissue or tumor growth.

References

1. Hynes RO. Integrins: versatility, modulation, and signaling in cell adhesion. *Cell* 1992; **69**: 11–25.

2. Serini G, Napione L, Bussolino F. Integrins team up with tyrosine kinase receptors and plexins to control angiogenesis. *Curr Opin Hematol* 2008; **15**: 235–42.

3. Ruoslahti E. RGD and other recognition sequences for integrins. *Annu Rev Cell Dev Biol* 1996; **12**: 697–715.

4. Ruoslahti E, Engvall E. Integrins and vascular extracellular matrix assembly. *J Clin Invest* 1997; **99**: 1149–52.

5. Carpenter CL. Actin cytoskeleton and cell signaling. *Crit Care Med* 2000; **28**: N94–9.

6. Fitzgerald DJ. Vascular biology of thrombosis: the role of platelet–vessel wall adhesion. *Neurology* 2001; **57**: S1–4.

7. Pezet M, Jacob MP, Escoubet B, *et al.* Elastin haploinsufficiency induces alternative aging processes in the aorta. *Rejuvenation Res* 2008; **11**: 97–112.

8. Dietz HC, Pyeritz RE. Mutations in the human gene for fibrillin-1 (FBN1) in the Marfan syndrome and related disorders. *Hum Mol Genet* 1995; **4**: 1799–809.

9. Li DY, Faury G, Taylor DG, *et al.* Novel arterial pathology in mice and humans hemizygous for elastin. *J Clin Invest* 1998; **102**: 1783–7.

10. Ross, R. Atherosclerosis: an inflammatory disease. *N Engl J Med* 1999; **340**: 115–26.

11. Carmeliet P, Jain RK. Angiogenesis in cancer and other diseases. *Nature* 2000; **407**: 249–57.

12. Kuriyama H, Kitamura K, Itoh T, Inoue R. Physiological features of visceral smooth muscle cells, with special reference to receptors and ion channels. *Physiol Rev* 1998; **78**: 811–920.

13. Tang DD, Anfinogenova Y. Physiologic properties and regulation of the actin cytoskeleton in vascular smooth muscle. *J Cardiovasc Pharmacol Ther* 2008; **13**: 130–40.

14. Fatigati V, Murphy RA. Actin and tropomyosin variants in smooth muscles: dependence on tissue type. *J Biol Chem* 1984; **259**: 14383–8.

15. Little PJ, Ivey ME, Osman N. Endothelin-1 actions on vascular smooth muscle cell functions as a target for the prevention of atherosclerosis. *Curr Vasc Pharmacol* 2008; **6**: 195–203.

16. Berridge MJ. Inositol trisphosphate and calcium signalling. *Nature* 1993; **361**: 315–25.

17. Kuriyama H, Kitamura K, Nabata H. Pharmacological and physiological significance of ion channels and factors that modulate them in vascular tissues. *Pharmacol Rev* 1995; **47**: 387–573.

18. Savineau JP, Marthan R. Modulation of the calcium sensitivity of the smooth muscle contractile apparatus: molecular mechanisms, pharmacological and pathophysiological implications. *Fundam Clin Pharmacol* 1997; **11**: 289–99.

19. Horowitz A, Menice CB, Laporte R, Morgan KG. Mechanisms of smooth muscle contraction. *Physiol Rev* 1996; **76**: 967–1003.

20. Ikebe M, Hartshorne DJ, Elzinga M. Phosphorylation of the 20,000-dalton light chain of smooth muscle myosin by the calcium-activated, phospholipid-dependent protein kinase: phosphorylation sites and effects of phosphorylation. *J Biol Chem* 1987; **262**: 9569–73.

21. Itoh T, Kajikuri J, Kuriyama H. Characteristic features of noradrenaline-induced Ca^{2+}

mobilization and tension in arterial smooth muscle of the rabbit. *J Physiol* 1992; **457**: 297–314.

22. Kitazawa T, Gaylinn BD, Denney GH, Somlyo AP. G-protein-mediated Ca^{2+} sensitization of smooth muscle contraction through myosin light chain phosphorylation. *J Biol Chem* 1991; **266**: 1708–15.

23. Kitazawa T, Masuo M, Somlyo AP. G protein-mediated inhibition of myosin light-chain phosphatase in vascular smooth muscle. *Proc Natl Acad Sci U S A* 1991; **88**: 9307–10.

24. Gong MC, Iizuka K, Nixon G, *et al.* Role of guanine nucleotide-binding proteins – ras-family or trimeric proteins or both – in Ca^{2+} sensitization of smooth muscle. *Proc Natl Acad Sci U S A* 1996; **93**: 1340–5.

25. Hirano, K. (2007) Current topics in the regulatory mechanism underlying the Ca^{2+} sensitization of the contractile apparatus in vascular smooth muscle. *J Pharmacol Sci* 104, 109–15.

26. Noda M, Yasuda-Fukazawa C, Moriishi K, *et al.* Involvement of rho in GTP gamma S-induced enhancement of phosphorylation of 20 kDa myosin light chain in vascular smooth muscle cells: inhibition of phosphatase activity. *FEBS Lett* 1995; **367**: 246–50.

27. Somlyo AP, Somlyo AV. Signal transduction and regulation in smooth muscle. *Nature* 1994; **372**: 231–6.

28. Allen BG, Walsh MP. The biochemical basis of the regulation of smooth-muscle contraction. *Trends Biochem Sci* 1994; **19**: 362–8.

29. Nelson MT, Quayle JM. Physiological roles and properties of potassium channels in arterial smooth muscle. *Am J Physiol* 1995; **268**: C799–822.

30. O'Donnell ME, Owen NE. Regulation of ion pumps and carriers in vascular smooth muscle. *Physiol Rev* 1994; **74**: 683–721.

31. Harder DR, Madden JA, Dawson C. Hypoxic induction of Ca^{2+}-dependent action potentials in small pulmonary arteries of the cat. *J Appl Physiol* 1985; **59**: 1389–93.

32. Kirber MT, Walsh JV, Singer JJ. Stretch-activated ion channels in smooth muscle: a mechanism for the initiation of stretch-induced contraction. *Pflugers Arch* 1988; **412**: 339–45.

33. Lansman JB, Hallam TJ, Rink TJ. Single stretch-activated ion channels in vascular endothelial cells as mechanotransducers? *Nature* 1987; **325**: 811–13.

34. Christ GJ, Spray DC, el-Sabban M, Moore LK, Brink PR. Gap junctions in vascular tissues. Evaluating the role of intercellular communication in the modulation of vasomotor tone. *Circ Res* 1996; **79**: 631–46.

35. Emerson GG, Segal SS. Electrical coupling between endothelial cells and smooth muscle cells in hamster feed arteries: role in vasomotor control. *Circ Res* 2000; **87**: 474–9.

36. Sandow SL, Tare M, Coleman HA, Hill CE, Parkington HC. Involvement of myoendothelial gap junctions in the actions of endothelium-derived hyperpolarizing factor. *Circ Res* 2002; **90**: 1108–13.

37. Figueroa XF, Duling BR. Gap junctions in the control of vascular function. *Antioxid Redox Signal* 2009; **11**: 251–66.

38. Larson DM, Haudenschild CC, Beyer EC. Gap junction messenger RNA expression by vascular wall cells. *Circ Res* 1990; **66**: 1074–80.

39. Reed KE, Westphale EM, Larson DM, *et al.* Molecular cloning and functional expression of human connexin37, an endothelial cell gap junction protein. *J Clin Invest* 1993; **91**: 997–1004.

40. Hong T, Hill CE. Restricted expression of the gap junctional protein connexin 43 in the arterial system of the rat. *J Anat* 1998; **192**: 583–93.

41. Davis MJ, Hill MA. Signaling mechanisms underlying the vascular myogenic response. *Physiol Rev* 1999; **79**: 387–423.

42. Davis MJ, Wu X, Nurkiewicz TR, *et al.* Integrins and mechanotransduction of the vascular myogenic response. *Am J Physiol Heart Circ Physiol* 2001; **280**, H1427–33.

43. Vandenbroucke E, Mehta D, Minshall R, Malik AB. Regulation of endothelial junctional permeability. *Ann N Y Acad Sci* 2008; **1123**: 134–45.

44. Knot HJ, Nelson MT. Regulation of membrane potential and diameter by voltage-dependent K^+ channels in rabbit myogenic cerebral arteries. *Am J Physiol* 1995; **269**: H348–55.

45. Hall A. Rho GTPases and the actin cytoskeleton. *Science* 1998; **279**, 509–14.

46. Le Brocq M, Leslie SJ, Milliken P, Megson IL. Endothelial dysfunction: from molecular mechanisms to measurement, clinical implications, and therapeutic opportunities. *Antioxid Redox Signal* 2008; **10**: 1631–74.

47. van Hinsbergh VW. The endothelium: vascular control of haemostasis. *Eur J Obstet Gynecol Reprod Biol* 2001; **95**: 198–201.

48. Furchgott RF, Zawadzki JV. The obligatory role of endothelial cells in the relaxation of arterial smooth muscle by acetylcholine. *Nature* 1980; **288**: 373–6.

49. Alexander RW, Dzau VJ. Vascular biology: the past 50 years. *Circulation* 2000; **102**: IV112–16.

50. Cannan CR, Mathew V, Lerman A. New insight into coronary endothelial dysfunction: role of endothelin. *J Lab Clin Med* 1998; **131**: 300–5.

51. Chen YF, Oparil S. Endothelial dysfunction in the pulmonary vascular bed. *Am J Med Sci* 2000; **320**: 223–32.

52. Johnstone MT, Creager SJ, Scales KM, *et al.* Impaired endothelium-dependent vasodilation in patients with insulin-dependent diabetes mellitus. *Circulation* 1993; **88**: 2510–16.

53. Panza JA, Quyyumi AA, Brush JE, Epstein SE. Abnormal endothelium-dependent vascular relaxation in patients with essential hypertension. *N Engl J Med* 1990; **323**: 22–7.

54. Harlan JM, Winn RK. Leukocyte-endothelial interactions: clinical trials of anti-adhesion therapy. *Crit Care Med* 2002; **30**: S214–19.

55. Levi M, ten Cate H, van der Poll T. Endothelium: interface between coagulation and inflammation. *Crit Care Med* 2002; **30**: S220–4.

56. Vallet B, Wiel E. Endothelial cell dysfunction and coagulation. *Crit Care Med* 2001; **29**: S36–41.

57. Folkman J, Browder T, Palmblad J. Angiogenesis research: guidelines for translation to clinical application. *Thromb Haemost* 2001; **86**: 23–33.

58. Davies PF, Tripathi SC. Mechanical stress mechanisms and the cell.: an endothelial paradigm. *Circ Res* 1993; **72**, 239–45.

59. Bevan JA. Shear stress, the endothelium and the balance between flow-induced contraction and dilation in animals and man. *Int J Microcirc Clin Exp* 1997; **17**: 248–56.

60. Barakat AI, Davies PF. Mechanisms of shear stress transmission and transduction in endothelial cells. *Chest* 1998; **114**: 58S–63S.

61. Ali MH, Schumacker PT. Endothelial responses to mechanical stress: where is the mechanosensor? *Crit Care Med* 2002; **30**: S198–206.

62. Nerem RM, Alexander RW, Chappell DC, *et al.* The study of the influence of flow on vascular endothelial biology. *Am J Med Sci* 1998; **316**: 169–75.

63. Muller JM, Chilian WM, Davis MJ. Integrin signaling transduces shear stress-dependent vasodilation of coronary arterioles. *Circ Res* 1997; **80**: 320–26.

64. Pohl U, Busse R. Hypoxia stimulates release of endothelium-derived relaxant factor. *Am J Physiol* 1989; **256**: H1595–600.

65. Daut J, Maier-Rudolph W, von Beckerath N, *et al.* Hypoxic dilation of coronary arteries is mediated by ATP-sensitive potassium channels. *Science* 1990; **247**: 1341–4.

66. Emerson GG, Segal SS. Electrical activation of endothelium evokes vasodilation and hyperpolarization along hamster feed arteries. *Am J Physiol Heart Circ Physiol* 2001; **280**: H160–7.

67. Forstermann U, Schmidt HH, Pollock JS, *et al.* Isoforms of nitric oxide synthase: characterization and purification from different cell types. *Biochem Pharmacol* 1991; **42**: 1849–57.

68. Seegers HC, Gross RW, Boyle WA. Calcium-independent phospholipase A_2-derived arachidonic acid is essential for endothelium-dependent relaxation by acetylcholine. *J Pharmacol Exp Ther* 2002; **302**: 918–23.

69. Xie QW, Cho HJ, Calaycay J, *et al.* Cloning and characterization of inducible nitric oxide synthase from mouse macrophages. *Science* 1992; **256**: 225–8.

70. Moncada S, Palmer RM, Higgs EA. Nitric oxide: physiology, pathophysiology, and pharmacology. *Pharmacol Rev* 1991; **43**: 109–42.

71. Bolotina VM, Najibi S, Palacino JJ, Pagano PJ, Cohen RA. Nitric oxide directly activates calcium-dependent potassium channels in vascular smooth muscle. *Nature* 1994; **368**, 850–3.

72. Smith WL, Garavito RM, DeWitt DL. Prostaglandin endoperoxide H synthases (cyclooxygenases)-1 and -2. *J Biol Chem* 1996; **271**: 33157–60.

73. Wu KK. Inducible cyclooxygenase and nitric oxide synthase. *Adv Pharmacol* 1995; **33**: 179–207.

74. Selig WM, Noonan TC, Kern DF, Malik AB. Pulmonary microvascular responses to arachidonic acid in isolated perfused guinea pig lung. *J Appl Physiol* 1986; **60**: 1972–9.

75. Siegel G, Schnalke F, Stock G, Grote J. Prostacyclin, endothelium-derived relaxing factor and vasodilatation. *Adv Prostaglandin Thromboxane Leukot Res* 1989; **19**: 267–70.

76. Kawada T, Toyosato A, Islam MO, Yoshida Y, Imai S. cGMP-kinase mediates cGMP- and cAMP-induced Ca^{2+} desensitization of skinned rat artery. *Eur J Pharmacol* 1997; **323**: 75–82.

77. White RE, Kryman JP, El-Mowafy AM, Han G, Carrier GO. cAMP-dependent vasodilators cross-activate the cGMP-dependent protein kinase to stimulate BK(Ca) channel activity in coronary artery smooth muscle cells. *Circ Res* 2000; **86**: 897–905.

78. Fisslthaler B, Popp R, Kiss L, *et al.* Cytochrome P450 2C is an EDHF synthase in coronary arteries. *Nature* 1999; **401**: 493–7.

79. Hecker M, Bara AT, Bauersachs J, Busse R. Characterization of endothelium-derived hyperpolarizing factor as a cytochrome P450-derived arachidonic acid metabolite in mammals. *J Physiol* 1994; **481**: 407–14.

80. Rosolowsky M, Campbell WB. Role of PGI2 and epoxyeicosatrienoic acids in relaxation of bovine coronary arteries to arachidonic acid. *Am J Physiol* 1993; **264**: H327–35.

81. McLeod JD, Piper PJ. Effect of removing the endothelium on the vascular responses induced by leukotrienes C4 and D4 in guinea-pig isolated heart. *Eur J Pharmacol* 1992; **212**: 67–72.

82. Edwards G, Weston AH. EDHF: are there gaps in the pathway? *J Physiol* 2001; **531**: 299.

83. Khazaei M, Moien-Afshari F, Laher I. Vascular endothelial function in health and diseases. *Pathophysiology* 2008; **15**: 49–67.

84. Zygmunt PM, Hogestatt ED. Role of potassium channels in endothelium-dependent relaxation resistant to nitroarginine in the rat hepatic artery. *Br J Pharmacol* 1996; **117**: 1600–6.

85. Bryan RM, You J, Golding EM, Marrelli SP. Endothelium-derived hyperpolarizing factor: a cousin to nitric oxide and prostacyclin. *Anesthesiology* 2005; **102**: 1261–77.

86. Feletou M, Vanhoutte PM. Endothelium-dependent hyperpolarizations: past beliefs and present facts. *Ann Med* 2007; **39**: 495–516.

87. Haynes WG, Webb DJ. The endothelin family of peptides: local hormones with diverse roles in health and disease? *Clin Sci (Lond)* 1993; **84**: 485–500.

88. Inoue A, Yanagisawa M, Kimura S, *et al.* The human endothelin family: three structurally and pharmacologically distinct isopeptides predicted by three separate genes. *Proc Natl Acad Sci U S A* 1989; **86**: 2863–7.

89. Yanagisawa M, Kurihara H, Kimura S, *et al.* A novel potent vasoconstrictor peptide produced by vascular endothelial cells. *Nature* 1988; **332**: 411–15.

90. Boulanger C, Luscher TF. Release of endothelin from the porcine aorta: inhibition by endothelium-derived nitric oxide. *J Clin Invest* 1990; **85**: 587–90.

91. Best PJ, Lerman A. Endothelin in cardiovascular disease: from atherosclerosis to heart failure. *J Cardiovasc Pharmacol* 2000; **35**: S61–3.

92. Hopfner RL, Gopalakrishnan V. Endothelin: emerging role in diabetic vascular complications. *Diabetologia* 1999; **42**: 1383–94.

93. Zimmermann M, Seifert V. Endothelin and subarachnoid hemorrhage: an overview. *Neurosurgery* 1998; **43**: 863–75.

94. Stewart JT, Nisbet JA, Davies MJ. Plasma endothelin in coronary venous blood from patients with either stable or unstable angina. *Br Heart J* 1991; **66**: 7–9.

95. Zamora MR, O'Brien RF, Rutherford RB, Weil JV. Serum endothelin-1 concentrations and cold provocation in primary Raynaud's phenomenon. *Lancet* 1990; **336**, 1144–7.

96. Hack CE, Zeerleder S. The endothelium in sepsis: source of and a target for inflammation. *Crit Care Med* 2001; **29**: S21–7.

97. Aird WC. Vascular bed-specific hemostasis: role of endothelium in sepsis pathogenesis. *Crit Care Med* 2001; **29**: S28–34.

98. Marcum JA, McKenney JB, Rosenberg RD. Acceleration of thrombin-antithrombin complex formation in rat hindquarters via heparinlike molecules bound to the endothelium. *J Clin Invest* 1984; **74**: 341–50.

99. Jaffe EA, Hoyer LW, Nachman RL. Synthesis of von Willebrand factor by cultured human endothelial cells. *Proc Natl Acad Sci U S A* 1974; **71**: 1906–1909.

100. Loskutoff D.J, Edgington TE. Synthesis of a fibrinolytic activator and inhibitor by endothelial cells. *Proc Natl Acad Sci U S A* 1977; **74**: 3903–7.

101. van Mourik JA, Lawrence DA, Loskutoff DJ. Purification of an inhibitor of plasminogen activator (antiactivator) synthesized by endothelial cells. *J Biol Chem* 1984; **259**: 14914–21.

102. Zimmerman GA, Albertine KH, Carveth HJ, *et al.* Endothelial activation in ARDS. *Chest* 1999; **116**: 18S–24S.

103. Frenette PS, Wagner DD. Adhesion molecules–Part II: blood vessels and blood cells. *N Engl J Med* 1996; **335**: 43–5.

104. Van Hoozen BE, Albertson TE. Endothelial cell dysfunction: a potential new approach for the treatment of sepsis. *Crit Care Med* 1999; **27**: 2836–8.

105. Hinshaw LB. Sepsis/septic shock: participation of the microcirculation: an abbreviated review. *Crit Care Med* 1996; **24**: 1072–1078.

106. Bernard GR, Vincent JL, Laterre PF, *et al.* Efficacy and safety of recombinant human activated protein C for severe sepsis. *N Engl J Med* 2001; **344**: 699–709.

107. Joyce DE, Gelbert L, Ciaccia A, DeHoff B, Grinnell BW. Gene expression profile of antithrombotic protein c defines new mechanisms modulating inflammation and apoptosis. *J Biol Chem* 2001; **276**: 11199–203.

108. Folkman J. Angiogenesis and angiogenesis inhibition: an overview. *EXS* 1997; **79**: 1–8.

109. Griffioen AW, Barendsz-Janson AF, Mayo KH, Hillen HF. Angiogenesis, a target for tumor therapy. *J Lab Clin Med* 1998; **132**: 363–8.

110. Bischoff J. Cell adhesion and angiogenesis. *J Clin Invest* 1997; **99**: 373–6.

111. Schnitzer JE. Vascular targeting as a strategy for cancer therapy. *N Engl J Med* 1998; **339**: 472–4.

112. Anderson FL, Brown AM. Pulmonary vasoconstriction elicited by stimulation of the hypothalamic integrative area for the defense reaction. *Circ Res* 1967; **21**: 747–56.

113. Harris MC. Effects of chemoreceptor and baroreceptor stimulation on the discharge of hypothalamic supraoptic neurones in rats. *J Endocrinol* 1979; **82**: 115–25.

114. Hilz MJ, Stemper B, Neundorfer B. [Physiology and methods for studying the baroreceptor reflex]. *Fortschr Neurol Psychiatr* 2000; **68**: 37–47.

115. Kendrick JE, Matson GL, Lalley PM. Central interaction between the baroreceptor reflexes from the carotid sinus and aortic arch. *Am J Physiol* 1979; **236**: H127–33.

116. Guimaraes S, Moura D. Vascular adrenoceptors: an update. *Pharmacol Rev* 2001; **53**: 319–56.

117. Starke K, Gothert M, Kilbinger H. Modulation of neurotransmitter release by presynaptic autoreceptors. *Physiol Rev* 1989; **69**: 864–989.

118. Franco-Cereceda A, Lundberg JM, Dahlof C. Neuropeptide Y and sympathetic control of heart contractility and coronary vascular tone. *Acta Physiol Scand* 1985; **124**: 361–9.

119. Liu SF, McCormack DG, Evans TW, Barnes PJ. Characterization and distribution of P2-purinoceptor subtypes in rat pulmonary vessels. *J Pharmacol Exp Ther* 1989; **251**: 1204–10.

120. von Kugelgen I, Starke K. Noradrenaline–ATP co-transmission in the sympathetic nervous system. *Trends Pharmacol Sci* 1991; **12**: 319–24.

121. Liu SF, Crawley DE, Evans TW, Barnes PJ. Endothelium-dependent nonadrenergic, noncholinergic neural relaxation in guinea pig pulmonary artery. *J Pharmacol Exp Ther* 1992; **260**: 541–8.

122. McMahon TJ, Hood JS, Kadowitz PJ. Pulmonary vasodilator response to vagal stimulation is blocked by N omega-nitro-L-arginine methyl ester in the cat. *Circ Res* 1992; **70**: 364–9.

123. el-Kashef HA, Hofman WF, Ehrhart IC, Catravas JD. Multiple muscarinic receptor subtypes in the canine pulmonary circulation. *J Appl Physiol* 1991; **71**: 2032–43.

124. Inoue T, Kannan MS. Nonadrenergic and noncholinergic excitatory neurotransmission in rat intrapulmonary artery. *Am J Physiol* 1988; **254**: H1142–8.

125. Itoh T, Sasaguri T, Makita Y, Kanmura Y, Kuriyama H. Mechanisms of vasodilation induced by vasoactive intestinal polypeptide in rabbit mesenteric artery. *Am J Physiol* 1985; **249**: H231–40.

126. Tanaka Y, Kaneko H, Tanaka H, Shigenobu K. Pharmacologic characteristics of non-prostanoid, non-nitric oxide mediated and endothelium-dependent relaxation of guinea-pig aorta in response to substance P. *Res Commun Mol Pathol Pharmacol* 1999; **103**: 65–81.

127. McCormack DG, Mak JC, Coupe MO, Barnes PJ. Calcitonin gene-related peptide vasodilation of human pulmonary vessels. *J Appl Physiol* 1989; **67**: 1265–70.

128. Marshall I. Mechanism of vascular relaxation by the calcitonin gene-related

peptide. *Ann N Y Acad Sci* 1992; **657**: 204–15.

129. Touyz RM, Schiffrin EL. Signal transduction mechanisms mediating the physiological and pathophysiological actions of angiotensin II in vascular smooth muscle cells. *Pharmacol Rev* 2000; **52**: 639–72.

130. Schiffrin EL, Park JB, Intengan HD, Touyz RM. Correction of arterial structure and endothelial dysfunction in human essential hypertension by the angiotensin receptor antagonist losartan. *Circulation* 2000; **101**: 1653–9.

131. Laszlo FA, Laszlo F, De Wied D. Pharmacology and clinical perspectives of vasopressin antagonists. *Pharmacol Rev* 1991; **43**: 73–108.

132. Landry DW, Oliver JA. Vasopressin in septic shock. *N Engl J Med* 2008; **358**: 2736–2737.

133. Boyle WA, Leone M. Vasopressin in septic shock. *N Engl J Med* 2008; **358**: 2736.

134. Russell JA, Walley KR, Singer J, *et al.* Vasopressin versus norepinephrine infusion in patients with septic shock. *N Engl J Med* 2008; **358**: 877–87.

135. Nemenoff RA. Vasopressin signaling pathways in vascular smooth muscle. *Front Biosci* 1998; **3**: d194–207.

136. Boyle WA, Segel LD. Direct cardiac effects of vasopressin and their reversal by a vascular antagonist. *Am J Physiol* 1986; **251**: H734–41.

137. Boyle WA, Segel LD. Attenuation of vasopressin-mediated coronary constriction and myocardial depression in the hypoxic heart. *Circ Res* 1990; **66**: 710–21.

138. Ghofrani HA, Wiedemann R, Rose F, *et al.* Combination therapy with oral sildenafil and inhaled iloprost for severe pulmonary hypertension. *Ann Intern Med* 2002; **136**: 515–22.

139. Hamasaki J, Tsuneyoshi I, Katai R, *et al.* Dual α_2-adrenergic agonist and α_1-adrenergic antagonist actions of dexmedetomidine on human isolated endothelium-denuded gastroepiploic arteries. *Anesth Analg* 2002; **94**: 1434–40.

Physiologic substrates of drug action
Cardiac rhythm

Brian S. Donahue and Jeffrey R. Balser

Introduction

Cardiac arrhythmias are one of the leading causes of morbidity and mortality in the industrialized world, and remain a significant complication in the period surrounding surgery and anesthesia. At the same time, existing antiarrhythmic drug therapies are plagued by poor efficacy and specificity, as well as toxicities that include genesis of new (and sometimes lethal) cardiac arrhythmias. Fortunately, our molecular understanding of the cardiac rhythm is expanding exponentially alongside recent advances toward defining the human genome. These developments have advanced the pace of investigation aimed at defining new molecular targets for manipulating the cardiac rhythm, with the promise of new and improved antiarrhythmic therapies. This chapter follows a reductionist approach that first examines the electrophysiology of the heart as an organ and at the multicellular level and then discusses, in detail, the molecular targets that underlie the cardiac action potential in individual myocardial cells.

Systems physiology

Neural control of the heart rhythm

Our information on the neural innervation and control of cardiac rhythm derives largely from canine models, which clarify that both sympathetic efferent fibers and vagal fibers course throughout the atria and ventricles. Vagal postganglionic neurons in the atrium and the sinoatrial (SA) and atrioventricular (AV) nodes underlie the parasympathetic effects on the heart rhythm. Parasympathetic stimulation causes release of acetylcholine, which alters the rhythmic firing of the SA and AV nodal cells through two complementary mechanisms. First, through the inhibitory (guanine) regulatory protein G_i, adenylate cyclase activity is reduced, cyclic adenosine monophosphate (cAMP) concentrations decrease, and the phosphorylation of cardiac ion channels by cAMP-dependent protein kinase is attenuated. Thus the activity of L-type calcium (Ca^{2+}) channels responsible for depolarization and excitation of SA and AV nodal tissue is depressed (see *Calcium channels*, below). Second, adenosine stimulates potassium (K^+) channels (see *Cardiac*

inward rectifiers, below) that hyperpolarize the SA and AV nodal cell membranes, driving the cells further away from their firing threshold. These combined actions cause the SA node firing rate to slow, and also produce AV nodal blockade; moreover, selective vagal denervation of the atria, SA, and AV nodes reduces minute-to-minute heart-rate variability, and eliminates heart-rate baroreflex sensitivity. Notably, efferent vagal fibers that innervate the ventricular chambers travel separately, and therefore reflex-mediated autonomic changes in the SA node firing rate are not necessarily manifest in the ventricles [1].

The sympathetic nervous system stimulates both heart rate and contractility through sympathetic efferent fibers that course through the superficial epicardium of the atria and ventricles, as well as the SA and AV nodes. Catecholamines released from the sympathetic nerve terminal (or administered systemically) bind to β_1-adrenoceptors, which in turn activate stimulatory guanine regulatory proteins (G_s) that activate adenylate cyclase, increasing intracellular cAMP, and activating cAMP-dependent protein kinase. This in turn augments the activity of L-type Ca^{2+} channels in the SA and AV nodes, increasing the rate of firing by these nodal cells. At the same time, the increased Ca^{2+} channel activity in the ventricular myocytes leads to a higher intracellular Ca^{2+} concentration, with greater excitation–contraction coupling, and a positive inotropic effect.

Organ physiology

Conduction pathway

The cardiac impulse normally arises in the SA node, and passes through the atria to enter the AV node. Impulses that successfully navigate the AV node enter the specialized conduction system that includes the His bundle, the major bundle branches, and the arborizing Purkinje fiber network; this system spreads the impulse into the ventricular myocardium. Drugs or conditions that impede conduction from the SA node to (or through) the AV node prolong the interval from the P wave (which represents atrial systole) to the QRS complex (which represents ventricular systole), manifest as the PR interval on the ECG (Fig. 20.1). Conversely, conditions that prolong or modify conduction through the specialized

---

Anesthetic Pharmacology, 2nd edition, ed. Alex S. Evers, Mervyn Maze, Evan D. Kharasch. Published by Cambridge University Press. © Cambridge University Press 2011.

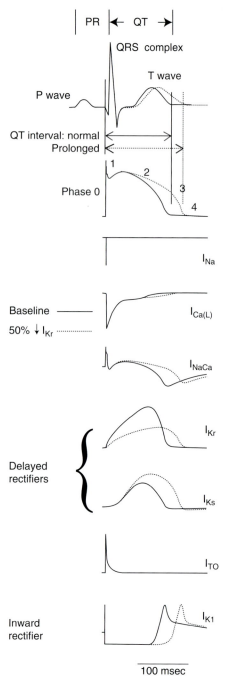

Figure 20.1. The action potential in ventricular muscle and its temporal relationship with the surface electrocardiogram. The PR interval indicates the time required for conduction of the impulse through the atrium and the atrioventricular (AV) node. The duration of the QRS complex is related to the rate of upstroke of the action potential, which partly determines the rate of impulse conduction through the ventricular myocardium. The QT interval is related to the duration of the action potential (the refractory period). The phases of the action potential are indicated, as are the major ionic currents that flow during each phase (*below*). The individual ionic currents were computed using the Luo–Rudy formalism [2]. *Solid lines* represent the baseline, and *dotted lines* represent the computation when I_{Kr} is reduced by 50%. Note that this change not only prolongs action potential duration (APD) (as expected), but also generates changes in the time course of I_{Ca-L}, I_{Ks}, and the sodium–calcium exchange current, each one of which thus also modulates the effect of reduced I_{Kr} on the APD. The amplitudes of the currents are not drawn to scale. Reproduced with permission from Roden *et al.* [3].

Table 20.1. The response of common supraventricular tachyarrhythmias to intravenous adenosine

Rhythm	Mechanism	Adenosine response
AV nodal reentry	Reentry within AV node	Termination
AV reciprocating tachycardias (orthodromic and antidromic)	Reentry involving AV node and accessory pathway (WPW)	Termination
Intra-atrial reentry	Reentry in the atrium	Transiently slows ventricular response
Atrial flutter/ fibrillation	Reentry in the atrium	Transiently slows ventricular response
Other atrial tachycardias	(1) Abnormal automaticity (2) cAMP-mediated triggered activity	(1) Transient suppression of the tachycardia (2) Termination
AV junctional rhythms	Variable	Variable
Ventricular arrhythmias	Reentry or automaticity	No response

AV, atrioventricular; cAMP, cyclic adenosine monophosphate; WPW, Wolff–Parkinson–White syndrome.
Adapted from Balser [4].

conduction system usually lengthen the QRS complex, and sometimes slur the upstroke (R wave) of this complex (see *Reentrant arrhythmias*, below).

Although the mechanistic details of each supraventricular arrhythmia are beyond the scope of this chapter, the role of the conduction system in arrhythmogenesis is nicely exemplified by the rhythm-specific action of adenosine (Table 20.1), which transiently blocks conduction within the AV node. This characteristic feature makes adenosine a choice drug for terminating supraventricular tachycardia (SVT) that originates in the AV node (or

involves the AV node in a reentrant pathway) [5]. Conversely, rhythms that originate in atrial tissue above the AV node, including atrial flutter or fibrillation, as well as paroxysmal rhythms stimulated by unopposed catecholamines, respond to adenosine only with transient slowing of the ventricular response rate, because the passage of impulses from the atrium to the ventricle through the AV node is slowed. Junctional tachycardia, common during the surgical period, arises in the specialized conduction system, and may convert to sinus rhythm in response to adenosine only if it originates very close to the AV node. Ventricular arrhythmias usually exhibit no response to adenosine, because these rhythms originate in tissues distal to the AV node.

Reentrant arrhythmias

Reentry is a mechanism that may precipitate a wide variety of supraventricular and ventricular arrhythmias, and implies the existence of a pathologic circus movement of electrical impulses around an anatomic loop or a "functional" loop generated by pathologic conductions that transiently block conduction through a segment of myocardium (e.g., ischemia). Fibrillation, in either the atrium or the ventricle, is believed to involve multiple coexistent reentrant circuits of the functional type. A classic form of anatomic reentry elicits paroxysmal supraventricular tachycardia (PSVT), and derives from reentrant circuits through abnormal accessory pathways (congenital electrical connections between the atrium and ventricle that bypass the AV node). During sinus rhythm, forward (antegrade) conduction through the accessory pathway may produce ventricular pre-excitation on the ECG (known as Wolff–Parkinson–White syndrome, WPW) with a short PR interval (<0.12 seconds), a slurred QRS upstroke (delta wave), and a wide QRS complex. The QRS complex is modified because ventricular excitation, normally facilitated by the spread of impulses through the specialized conduction system and Pürkinje network, is "bypassed" by pre-excitation through the accessory bundle.

During PSVT, when the conduction circuit is antegrade through the AV node and retrograde through the accessory bundle, the QRS complex will be narrow; however, in 5–10% of cases the conduction is antegrade through the accessory bundle, producing a wide QRS complex that may be confused with ventricular tachycardia. Normally, PSVT does not provoke a marked deterioration in hemodynamic status. However, 10–35% of patients with WPW eventually develop atrial fibrillation (AF), and an episode of PSVT sometimes precipitates AF. In this case, the rapid rate of atrial excitation (>300 impulses per minute), normally transmitted to the ventricle after considerable "filtering" by the AV nodal system, may instead be transmitted to the ventricle through the accessory bundle at a rapid rate. The danger of inducing ventricular fibrillation in this scenario is exacerbated by treatment with classic AV-nodal blocking drugs (digoxin, Ca^{2+} channel blockers, β-blockers, adenosine) because they reduce the accessory bundle refractory period. Intravenous procainamide, which slows conduction over the accessory bundle, is often the drug of choice for treating AF in this condition.

Our understanding of functional reentry and its pharmacologic termination by ion-channel current suppression is far less complete. Drugs may terminate reentry through at least two mechanisms. Agents that suppress currents responsible for initiation of the cardiac action potential, such as the sodium (Na^+) current (Fig. 20.1), may slow or block conduction in a reentrant pathway, and thus terminate an arrhythmia. Alternatively, interventions that prolong the cardiac action potential, such as potassium channel blockade (Fig. 20.1), in turn prolong the refractory period of cells in a reentrant circuit, and thus "block" impulse propagation through the circuit. In clinical trials, drugs operating through the latter mechanism have proven to be more successful in suppressing fibrillation in both the atrium [6] and the ventricle [7].

Cellular physiology

Cardiac action potential

The cardiac action potential represents the time-varying transmembrane potential of the myocardial cell during the cardiac cycle. The surface ECG can be viewed as the ensemble average of the action potentials arising from all myocardial cells, and is biased toward the activity of the left ventricle because of its greater overall mass. The effects of conditions and interventions on the ECG result from their effects on the cardiac action potential, which in turn result from their ensemble effects on any number of ionic currents (Fig. 20.1). The trajectory of the cardiac action potential is divided into five distinct phases, which reflect changes in the predominant ionic current flowing during the cardiac cycle (Fig. 20.1). The current responsible for "phase 0," the initial period of the action potential, propagates impulses through cardiac tissue. In the atria and the ventricles, the impulse is initiated by sodium current (I_{Na}) through Na^+ channels. Hence drugs that suppress Na^+ current (local anesthetic-type drugs) slow myocardial conduction and prolong the QRS complex (ventricle) and the P wave (atrium). In AV and SA nodal cells (not shown in Fig. 20.1), phase 0 is actually produced by Ca^{2+} current through L-type Ca^{2+} channels, and not through Na^+ current. Hence drugs that suppress Ca^{2+} current indirectly or directly (β-blockers and Ca^{2+} channel blockers, respectively) slow the heart rate by acting on the SA node, and also prolong the PR interval by slowing conduction through the AV node. The latter effect renders the AV node a more efficient "filter" for preventing rapid trains of atrial beats from passing into the ventricle; hence the rationale for AV nodal blockade during SVT.

The later phases of the action potential (1, 2, and 3; Fig. 20.1) inscribe repolarization. Although an electrophysiologic curiosity for years, the early "notch" of repolarization during phase 1 is induced by the transient outward current (I_{to}) and seems to be present to varying degrees in the different cell layers (greater in epicardium than in endocardium). This gradient between layers may have proarrhythmic implications during conditions that modify the Na^+ current during phase 0 (see *Layer-specific electrophysiology and arrhythmias* for detailed discussion). The long plateau (phase 2) is maintained by Ca^{2+} current and is terminated (phase 3) by a number of K^+ currents. Hence the QT interval on the ECG reflects the length of the action potential and is determined by a delicate balance between these and many other smaller inward and outward currents. Drugs that reduce Ca^{2+} current tend to abbreviate the action-potential plateau, shorten the QT, and reduce the inward movement of Ca^{2+} into the cardiac cell (hence the negative inotropic effect). Conversely, agents that block outward K^+ current prolong the action potential and the QT interval on the ECG. Notably, electrophysiologic behavior of all the voltage-gated ion channels is linked to the configuration of the cardiac action potential; hence when an intervention modifies the time-varying behavior of a single ion channel (e.g., K^+ channel blockade), the behavior of all other time-varying ionic currents is modified (Fig. 20.1). In K^+ channel blockade and QT prolongation, these complex effects on the other ionic currents may be either therapeutic or arrhythmogenic (see discussion in *Automaticity and arrhythmias*).

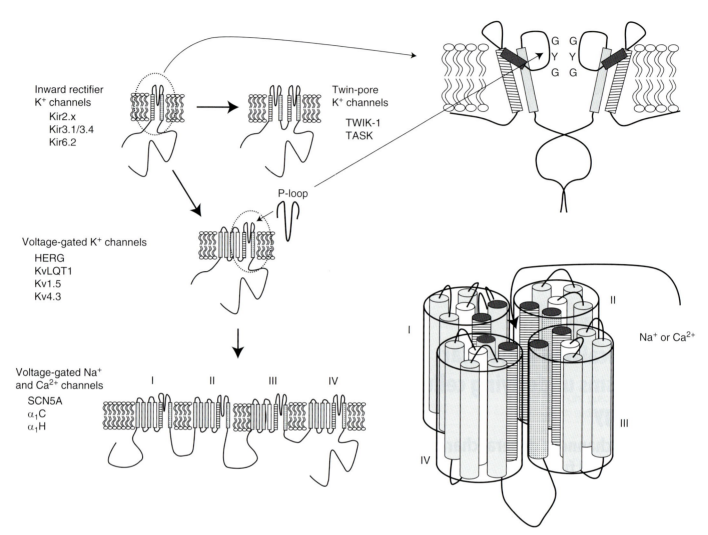

Figure 20.4. The topology of the voltage-gated ion channels in heart, presented from an "evolutionary view" of ion-channel phylogeny. The inward rectifiers include only the pore region between the two membrane-spanning segments (*shaded*), and are presumably the most primitive ion-channel structure. In this structure, a "P-loop" connecting the two transmembrane segments dips into the membrane and lines the outer pore. This P-loop structure is maintained in the voltage-gated K$^+$ channels, which also include four additional transmembrane segments (S1–S4). The S4 transmembrane segment contains positively charged amino acids that "sense" the membrane potential (*unshaded segment*) and allow voltage-dependent gating. Gene duplication of the inward rectifier structure may also have led to the "twin pore" channels (TWIK, TASK). Voltage-gated Na$^+$ and Ca^{2+} channels are assembled as four homologous domains (I—IV) that resemble the voltage-gated K$^+$ channel. In the case of Na$^+$, K$^+$, and Ca^{2+} channels, these linear amino acid sequences assemble as tetrameric three-dimensional structures with fourfold symmetry to generate ion-permeant pores (*heavy arrow*), indicated at the *bottom right* (the P-loops are omitted for clarity). Reproduced with permission from Roden *et al.* [3].

ion channels display the characteristic of inactivation gating, time-dependent entry into a nonconducting state during sustained depolarization. Inactivation provides a convenient means to terminate the flow of ionic current before the cell membrane fully repolarizes; hence the hallmark of inactivation is a slow decline of activated current during a sustained depolarization. Notably, multiple types of inactivation with varying time courses (fast, intermediate, slow) are manifest in cardiac ion channels, and a single ion channel may even enter more than one inactivated state during the cardiac cycle. Two general mechanisms of inactivation have been proposed (Fig. 20.5). The original ball-and-chain model for one type of inactivation [28], termed N-type inactivation, involves motion of a portion of the channel (often the N-terminus) to occlude the pore from inside the channel [30]. The other type of inactivation, termed C-type, usually proceeds more slowly than N-type, and involves a more complex rearrangement of residues in or near the outer pore permeation pathway (P-loops), analogous to closing the shutter on a camera [3].

Cardiac ion channels: specific features of structure and function

With the completion of the human genome project, the identification of the specific genes and gene products that comprise the cardiac ion channels is proceeding. Table 20.2 indicates the genes identified to date [3] and their various protein products.

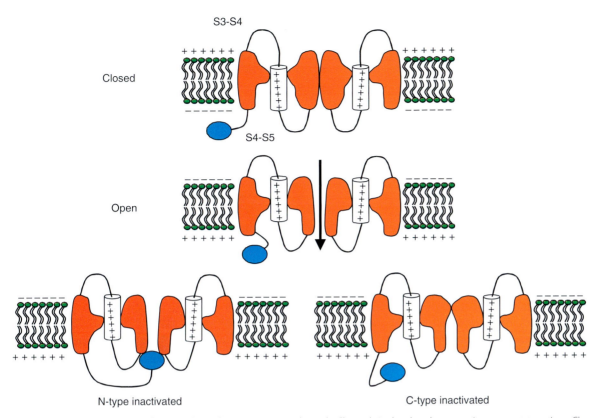

Figure 20.5. Schematic view of voltage-dependent gating in ion channels. Channels in the closed state are impermeant to cations. Channel opening (activation) involves outward movement of the voltage sensor (S4) within a water-accessible crevice in the protein complex; this outward motion initiates a protein rearrangement that opens the channel, the details of which remain undefined. Outward motion of the S4 segment also initiates channel inactivation, which again renders the channel impermeant. Two major types of inactivation are shown: N-type (ball-and-chain) involves block of the intracellular end of the pore, whereas C-type inactivation involves an outer pore rearrangement that may constrict the permeation pathway. Inactivation can occur on multiple time scales, and may be rapid or slow compared with channel opening. Reproduced with permission from Roden *et al.* [3].

Table 20.2 is organized to identify the gene products that underlie pharmacologically distinct ionic currents in heart, many of which are illustrated in Fig. 20.1. In some cases, α subunits (pore-forming) and a number of associated β subunits are listed; notably, some β subunits may be associated with multiple α subunits (e.g., minK/I_{sK}). Studies are only now clarifying the key functional manifestations of these α and β subunit interrelationships, and the details of Table 20.2 should dramatically expand in the future.

Exciting insights into the linkages between cardiac rhythm, ion-channel structure, and the genetic code have emerged from the study of monogenetic cardiac arrhythmia syndromes (Table 20.3). These include several varieties of LQTS, the idiopathic ventricular fibrillation syndromes, and genetic syndromes of conduction disease. These are discussed, with the relevant ion channels, below. Although these syndromes affect only small segments of the general population, it is clear that the mechanisms they reveal are fundamentally related to common acquired arrhythmia syndromes. For example, the inherited LQTS is a model for drug-induced QT prolongation that provokes torsades de pointes, whereas Brugada syndrome mutations may shed light on the mechanism of ischemia-induced reentry and ventricular tachycardia.

Sodium channel (I_{Na})
Structure and function
The *SCN5A* gene encodes the cardiac Na^+ channel α subunit, a 2016-amino-acid polypeptide [31]. At least two and possibly four ancillary subunits, $β_1$ through $β_4$, may interact with the cardiac Na^+ channel and regulate its function [32,33]. Recent findings indicate a direct role for β-subunit mutations in human disease (see below).

Mutation of three adjacent hydrophobic (isoleucine–phenylalanine–methionine, or IFM) residues in the cytoplasmic linker connecting domains III and IV disrupts the most rapid Na^+ channel inactivation gating process ("fast inactivation") [34]. It is thus tempting to view the III–IV linker as a "lid" that closes over the inner vestibule (an N-type inactivation mechanism), and, in this context, the IFM motif as a "latch" that holds the inactivation gate shut. Nonetheless, peptide-binding studies suggest that inactivation may not involve simple occlusive block of the inner mouth of the pore [35]; rather, the III–IV linker may bind to a site on the channel that allosterically regulates or mediates pore closure. In either scheme, a number of modulatory or "docking" sites for fast inactivation have been identified near the cytoplasmic end of the pore, including the S4–S5 linker intracellular loops and residues in the cytoplasmic portion of the S6 segment [36].

Channels that open and then rapidly inactivate can be reopened after even brief hyperpolarization that allows the channel to reassume the closed ("activatable") conformation. However, after prolonged depolarization, recovery does not occur with brief hyperpolarization, indicating the presence of other (slow) inactivated states. Several lines of evidence suggest that this may be a form of C-type inactivation (Fig. 20.5) [37].

Regulation of I_{Na}

In-vivo experiments show that chronic therapy with Na^+ channel blockers increases Na^+ channel synthesis [38]. Conversely, in experimental models of AF (where rapid rates are induced by pacing), Na^+ currents are depressed [39]. The molecular basis for regulated cardiac Na^+ channel expression during drug therapy or in arrhythmia models remains largely unexplored. The cardiac channel undergoes extensive post-translational modification, including glycosylation and phosphorylation, which modifies channel trafficking to the cell membrane, as well as channel gating function.

Phosphorylation of the Na^+ channel has complex effects on its location within the myocyte and the resulting I_{Na}. There are a number of PKA consensus sites in the I–II linker, and PKA-dependent phosphorylation of the Na^+ channel results in increased I_{Na}, probably as a result of vesicular trafficking [40]. Protein tyrosine phosphatase PTPH1 interacts with the PDZ domain binding motif at the C-terminus of the Na^+ channel, and the balance of kinase/phosphorylase activity at this locus appears to regulate channel attachment to ankyrin versus intercalated disks [41]. Ca^{2+}/calmodulin-dependent protein kinase II-dependent phosphorylation slows Na^+ channel recovery from inactivation, resulting in increased persistent current [42].

$Na_v1.5$ exhibits sensitivity to intracellular Ca^{2+} concentration ($[Ca^{2+}]_i$) in a complex manner through the dual action of an "IQ-type" calmodulin binding domain in its carboxy terminus [43,44]. This domain exhibits multiple CaM binding modes, which are influenced by Ca_i as well as an interaction with a C-terminal EF hand domain that directly binds the IQ domain at high levels of $[Ca^{2+}]_i$ [45]. In conditions where $[Ca^{2+}]_i$ is elevated, this regulatory apparatus leads to a "right shift" (depolarization) of the voltage-dependence of channel inactivation, which corresponds to destabilizing channel inactivation at the resting membrane potential, resulting in a gain-of-function effect.

Cardiac Na^+ channel dysfunction in disease

The recent advances of the Human Genome Project have enhanced our understanding of the genotype–phenotype relationships associated with ion-channel variants. Mutations in SCN5A produce a spectrum of electrophysiologic and clinical phenotypes, many with overlapping features. The foremost of these is the LQT3 variant of LQTS (Table 20.3) [46], an autosomal dominant disorder in which patients exhibit prolonged ECG QT intervals and are at risk for the polymorphic ventricular tachycardia, torsades de pointes. A common mechanism is failure of fast inactivation gating, a so-called gain of function resulting in a population of channels that exhibit recurrent openings throughout the action-potential plateau [47,48]. The small net depolarizing "pedestal" of current through these channels is sufficient to upset the balance between inward and outward currents in the action-potential plateau, and hence to prolong action-potential duration and consequently the QT interval. The first such defect to be described was a deletion of three amino acids (ΔKPQ) in the III–IV linker of the channel [47]. This finding is consistent with the prominent role of this region in normal fast inactivation [34]. The next two mutations to be described, R1644H and N1325S, are both located in cytoplasmic S4–S5 linkers (Fig. 20.4), supporting a role for these regions as docking sites for the inactivation "lid" [48,49]. Further studies have shown that mutations in other regions of the channel protein also result in defective inactivation [37].

Inherited mutations in SCN5A that cause a marked loss of I_{Na} (in contrast to LQT3 gain of function) cause the form of idiopathic ventricular fibrillation known as Brugada syndrome (Table 20.3) [10,37]. Patients with Brugada syndrome experience sudden death in the absence of any detectable heart disease (and a normal QT interval), but do display an unusual electrocardiographic feature: J-point elevation in the right precordial leads (Fig. 20.2). Some Brugada syndrome mutations result in a highly truncated and therefore nonfunctional protein, whereas others augment the inactivation gating processes (either fast or slow) to yield a loss of I_{Na}. At least one mutation, insertion of a glutamate at position 1795 in the Na^+ channel C-terminus (1795insD), produces gain-of-function defects in fast inactivation and loss-of-function defects in slow inactivation and results in both the LQT3 and Brugada syndrome phenotypes in the same carrier [50]. Thus inherited mutations have provided important insights into how structure and function in this large protein relate to arrhythmia phenotypes in the whole heart.

A third phenotype associated with Na^+ channel mutations is conduction system disease (Table 20.3) [51]. One such mutation, G514C in the I–II linker, produced a slight reduction in channel function resulting from conduction slowing that was not sufficient to elicit action-potential heterogeneities associated with LQT3 or the Brugada syndrome. Hence a small degree of loss of function is sufficient to provoke isolated cardiac conduction disease, whereas a more substantial loss of Na^+ channel function seems to provoke more lethal tachyarrhythmias.

The Brugada phenotype may also provide insight into the proarrhythmic effects of potent Na^+ channel blockade in the CAST, where investigators reported that treatment with the potent Na^+ channel blocking drugs flecainide and encainide increased mortality (likely caused by arrhythmias) in patients convalescing from acute myocardial infarction [8]. Analysis of the CAST database indicated that the group at greatest risk for an increase in drug-associated mortality was those patients at greatest risk for recurrent myocardial ischemia. Since CAST, studies have identified a reduction in Na$^+$ channel function in cardiac cells isolated from the ischemic border zone surrounding a cardiac infarct [52]. Hence the clinical observation that flecainide worsens the Brugada syndrome ECG phenotype may suggest a link between loss of Na$^+$ channel function (caused by either ischemia or genetic predisposition) and proarrhythmic susceptibility to potent Na$^+$ channel blocking drugs. Moreover, determining the extent to which DNA variants in *SCN5A* (or other ion channels) may produce little or no baseline clinical phenotype but nevertheless increase an individual patient's risk for ventricular arrhythmias on exposure to a range of stressors, including myocardial ischemia or drugs, is a critical future direction of arrhythmia research.

Recent developments in rapid DNA sequencing technology have resulted in a spectrum of rare disorders associated with variants in *SCN5A*. These epidemiologic associations are strengthened by electrophysiologic studies of the mutant channels in expression systems, verifying either gain-of-function (loss of inactivation), or loss-of-function (slower activation or shift in steady-state resting potential) physiology. Investigators have identified the role of rare Na$^+$ channel mutations in sudden cardiac death [53], familial AF [54], heart failure [55], sick sinus syndrome [56], and sudden infant death [57].

Recent evidence indicates a role for the Na$^+$ channel β subunit in human disease. Transgenic mice lacking the β$_1$-subunit gene exhibit an electrophysiologic phenotype similar to LQTS [33]. Also, in a Mexican family with congenital LQTS, researchers observed a new mutation (L179F) in the β$_4$ subunit (SCN4B) of the proband, cosegregating with the long-QT phenotype across three generations [58]. In all affected individuals, open reading frame analysis of all known LQTS genes was negative, and the SCNB4 L179F mutation was absent in 800 reference alleles. Furthermore, in HEK293 cells, coexpression of the mutant SCN4B protein with normal SCN5A channel revealed increases in the late Na$^+$ current, consistent with the current model of delayed inactivation in the etiology of LQTS.

Finally, disorders in Na$^+$ channel functioning may also arise from defects involving other myocyte elements. Dystrophin, the protein whose loss defines Duchenne muscular dystrophy, associates with the Na$^+$ channel at the PDZ domain binding motif near the C-terminus. In animal models of Duchenne muscular dystrophy, Na$^+$ channel levels and I$_{Na}$ are reduced, producing the electrophysiologic phenotype characteristic of this disorder [59].

Calcium channels (I$_{Ca}$)
Structure and function
The major Ca^{2+} channels in cardiac muscle are the L-type and T-type. The L-type Ca^{2+} channel contributes inward current to sustain the characteristically prolonged action potentials in

heart (in contrast to nerve). The calcium ions introduced into the cell act as the trigger for excitation–contraction coupling, triggering the release of myofilament-activating Ca^{2+} from sarcoplasmic reticulum stores by opening the sarcoplasmic reticulum Ca^{2+} release channel (also known as the ryanodine receptor). Whereas L-type channels are found throughout cardiac muscle, T-type channels play a role in determining automaticity, and are thus localized to SA node, AV node, atrium, and the specialized conducting system, and are thought to be absent from normal ventricle.

Calcium channels are assembled from a number of distinct α and β subunits. These include α$_{1C}$, which encodes the L-type α subunit [60], and α$_{1H}$, which encodes the T-type [61]. Two major L-type Ca^{2+} channel ancillary subunits have been identified. The β subunits are intracellular, and increase Ca^{2+} current, modify activation and inactivation gating [62], enhance prepulse facilitation, and may be involved in channel trafficking. The other major Ca^{2+} channel ancillary subunit is a large polypeptide generated by expression of a single gene, with two protein products (α$_2$ and δ subunits) that are linked by a disulfide bridge [63]. The α$_2$ protein is extracellular, whereas the δ subunit includes a single membrane-spanning segment and an extracellular domain that links to (and anchors) the α$_2$ subunit. The α$_2$δ subunit may increase cell-surface α$_1$-subunit expression. Calmodulin is now considered a subunit of the L-type Ca^{2+} channel, due to its constitutive interaction with the α$_{1C}$ subunit [64].

As mentioned earlier, a highly conserved glutamate in each of the four P-loops generates a "ring" in the pore that confers Ca^{2+} selectivity over Na$^+$. Multiple Ca^{2+} binding sites may be present within the permeation pathway, with repulsion between adjacent Ca^{2+} ions facilitating high ionic throughput [65]; indeed, Ca^{2+} channel inactivation may in part be mediated by intracellular Ca^{2+}. The intracellular Ca^{2+} sensor, while complex, involves an "EF-hand"-containing domain in the intracellular C-terminus of the channel [66], as well as two calmodulin-binding domains located nearby on the C-terminus. The mechanism involves calmodulin binding of Ca^{2+} rather than direct interaction of Ca^{2+} with the channel protein. Another unique feature of L-type Ca^{2+} channel behavior is "facilitation," whereby Ca^{2+} currents increase in size on repeated, closely coupled activating pulses. Calmodulin may also act as the Ca^{2+} sensor for facilitation; this may occur through direct binding to the Ca^{2+} channel α subunit C-terminus, or through activation of CaM kinase II.

Regulation of I$_{Ca}$
Ca^{2+} channels are heavily regulated by adrenergic pathways through the action of protein kinases. Kinase phosphorylation places the Ca^{2+} channels into distinct gating "modes:" mode 0 having rare brief openings, mode 1 showing frequent brief openings, and mode 2 being characterized by long openings that are promoted by either PKA or CaM-kinase-mediated phosphorylation [17]. Hence β-adrenergic stimulation

markedly increases I_{Ca} through the traditional G_s-related second-messenger pathway [67], causing a lengthening of action-potential duration and a positive inotropic effect in cardiac muscle.

Of the multiple consensus PKA sites in the L-type Ca^{2+} channel α_{1C} subunit, S1928 in the C-terminus appears to be functionally important [68], as do several sites on the β_2 subunit. Cardiac channel-specific A-kinase anchoring proteins appear to be crucial for mediating these PKA effects [69], which complicate studies of PKA-dependent phosphorylation in heterologous systems. While L-type Ca^{2+} channels can also be PKC-phosphorylated, the significance of this phosphorylation on cardiac rhythm is not clear. Overall, the concerted actions of protein kinases on cardiac calcium channels remains multifaceted and incompletely understood. Because myocyte calcium hemostasis is central to many important disease states, these topics constitute an area of active investigation.

Cardiac Ca^{2+} channel dysfunction in disease

Our understanding of the role of intracellular calcium in cardiac disease has advanced greatly in recent years. Alteration of normal Ca^{2+} channel functioning is central in the etiology of arrhythmias. Both L-type Ca^{2+} channels and Na^+ channels are reduced in number in atrial myocytes from animals with AF, and it is believed that these changes perpetuate the arrhythmia [39]. Calcium currents are decreased in myocytes from fibrillating atria, regardless of whether fibrillation was acute (less than 1 hour) or chronic [70,71]. Conversely, L-type Ca^{2+} channels have been implicated as a carrier of arrhythmogenic inward current. Prolongation of the action potential increases the amplitude of the intracellular Ca^{2+} transient, activating CaM kinase (and thus enhancing L-type Ca^{2+} current and other arrhythmogenic inward currents), and thereby promoting arrhythmogenic EADs and DADs (Fig. 20.3) [18]. Ca^{2+} channel blockers inhibit arrhythmogenic EADs during these conditions [72], as does CaM kinase inhibition [73].

Transient outward current (I_{to})

Structure and function

The I_{to} current (Fig. 20.1) is present in most, but not all, human ventricular epicardial and atrial cells, and is generated by a number of channels with "transient outward" gating properties that include rapid inactivation. In humans, this current regulates the level of the plateau phase of the action potential, thus indirectly affecting action-potential duration. One of the first K^+ channels cloned from human heart, $K_v1.4$, displays inactivation gating superficially typical of I_{to} in heterologous expression systems. However, human I_{to} recovers from inactivation between stimuli much more rapidly than does $K_v1.4$-mediated current [74]. By contrast, heterologous expression of $K_v4.3$ results in a transient outward current with rapid recovery from inactivation, and could thus

contribute a rapid repolarization "notch" in phase 1 (Fig. 20.1), even at rapid heart rates. $K_v4.3$ also displays drug sensitivity similar to human I_{to}, reinforcing the idea that it is a reasonable candidate for human I_{to}. There is a gradient of K_v4 subunit expression across the ventricular wall in most species, including humans, corresponding to the larger I_{to} in epicardium [75]. Whereas human endocardium does not generally display a prominent phase 1 notch during stimulation of physiologic rates, a small I_{to} with slow kinetics of recovery from inactivation can be recorded, and suggests that $K_v1.4$ may mediate I_{to} in the human endocardium (versus K_v4 in epicardium).

Numerous function-modifying subunits are present in heart and brain and modulate $K_v1.4$- and K_v4-mediated currents. Four β subunits (identified as $K_v\beta1–\beta4$) interact with the $K_v1.4$ α subunit, and have a spectrum of effects on trafficking, voltage dependence, and inactivation kinetics [76]. In addition, four additional genes have been identified which code for K_v channel-interacting proteins (KChIPs), which specifically interact with $K_v4.2$ and $K_v4.3$. KChIPs generally slow activation, accelerate inactivation, alter the gating characteristics of the channel, and promote cell-surface expression [77]. KChIPs appear to interact with K_v4 N-termini, and may act as Ca^{2+} sensors [78].

I_{to} is strongly influenced by adrenergic stimuli. The α_{1A} receptor mediates decrease in I_{to}, probably by phosphorylation by protein kinase C [79], and also decreases transcription of $K_v4.2$ and $K_v4.3$. β-Receptor activation results in increased I_{to}, but it is uncertain whether this effect can occur in the absence of α-adrenergic stimulation [80]. $K_v1.4$ and K_v4 channels contain multiple possible phosphorylation sites for PKA-, ERK-, CaM-kinase-II-, and PKG-dependent phosphorylation.

I_{to} dysfunction in disease

Action-potential shortening occurs rapidly at the onset of ischemia, too rapidly to be explained by decreases in adenosine triphosphate (ATP) stores. This may be explained by the observed decrease in I_{to}, which results in a more positive early plateau phase and more L-type Ca^{2+} channel inactivation. β-Adrenergic agonists have been shown to restore I_{to} after 24 hours. The effect of ischemia on I_{to} reduction has been consistently observed in multiple animal models but is not well understood.

Delayed rectifier K^+ currents

In contrast to I_{to}, which activates rapidly during the cardiac action potential, these K^+ currents activate after some delay (Fig. 20.1), and play a greater role in later phases of the action potential. There are three principal delayed rectifier currents (I_{Kr}, I_{Ks}, and I_{Kur}), which represent distinct gene products and are distinguishable in human heart by their kinetics of activation and deactivation, as well as their distinctive pharmacologic sensitivities.

Rapid delayed rectifier current (I_{Kr})
Structure and function

The gene *KCNH2* (*hERG*) encodes a six-membrane-spanning α subunit (hERG; Fig. 20.4) underlying the current I_{Kr} (Fig. 20.1) and is expressed abundantly in heart. In addition, hERG is associated with subunits that modify its function. The single-transmembrane domain membrane protein minK (Table 20.2) enhances expression of hERG. The minK-related gene *KCNE2* (also termed *MiRP1*) has also been implicated as a *hERG* interactor. When *MiRP1* and *hERG* are coexpressed, the unitary conductance of the hERG channel is reduced, and I_{Kr} gating and the rate of onset of drug block are both accelerated, recapitulating the experimentally observed characteristics of I_{Kr} in native myocytes [81].

Close inspection of I_{Kr} currents on membrane depolarization yields a number of unusual features. Whereas depolarization causes activation and opening of the channel, the measured current decreases markedly as depolarization potential is made more positive – i.e., the current displays striking "inward rectification." In brief, this results from an unusual C-type inactivation process (Fig. 20.5) that develops rapidly and predominates when the channel is strongly depolarized [82]. Studies have examined the time course of I_{Kr} current during a cardiac action potential, and at maintained positive potentials (such as during the action-potential plateau) inactivation is favored over channel opening, so that little outward current is generated to oppose the inward I_{Ca}. However, on sudden repolarization (i.e., phase 3 of the action potential; Fig. 20.1), I_{Kr} rapidly recovers from inactivation (before closure), and therefore a large outward current is generated that not only repolarizes the cell but also "protects" the myocyte from a spurious proarrhythmic depolarization (i.e., an EAD or DAD; Fig. 20.3) before the action potential fully terminates and the inward currents (I_{Na}, I_{Ca}) have recovered. Hence pharmacologic blockade of I_{Kr} is the most common cause of drug-induced QT prolongation with torsades de pointes.

I_{Kr} dysfunction in disease

Mutations in *KCNH2* cause the LQT2 variety of congenital LQTS (Table 20.3), just as drugs that block I_{Kr} evoke the acquired form of the disease. I_{Kr} suppression, caused by either drugs or mutations, tends to prolong the cardiac action potential with "reverse use dependence" (i.e., greatest action potential prolongation at slow rates), and patients are thus at greatest risk for torsades de pointes arrhythmias during bradycardia. A mechanism for this rate dependence may arise from the observation that the counterpart of I_{Kr}, termed I_{Ks} (see below), deactivates more slowly and incompletely at rapid heart rates. Hence I_{Ks} current accumulates at rapid heart rates and becomes larger than I_{Kr}, whereas at slow rates I_{Kr} is a relatively more important component of repolarizing current.

Hence I_{Kr} block produces marked prolongation of action potentials, and the QT interval, at slow rates or after a long diastolic interval.

hERG blockade is now widely regarded as the predominant cause of drug-induced QT prolongation [83]. Accordingly, a major challenge in drug development is early detection of compounds with hERG-blocking activity, and removal of such compounds from the development pipeline. Because hERG blockers represent a group of very diverse chemical structures, numerous methods for chemical modeling, large-scale patch clamping, in-vivo physiology, and in-silico modeling have been developed for screening candidate compounds. Although certain clinical risk factors can be identified, the development of excess QT prolongation and torsades de pointes during exposure to I_{Kr}-blocking drugs remains largely unpredictable.

Patients with inherited forms of LQTS are lifelong mutation carriers, yet have relatively rare arrhythmia events. It is postulated that risk factors, including genetic predisposition, drug exposure, hypokalemia, and so on, come together in an individual patient to culminate in torsades de pointes. Thus patients who develop excess QT prolongation on drug exposure may be viewed as having a "subclinical" genetic defect that slightly impedes repolarization, causing a reduction in "repolarization reserve." Only when repolarization reserve is sufficiently impaired (by the addition of drug therapy) does torsades de pointes occur. This hypothesis is supported by reports of patients with inherited ion-channel mutations who only present after drug challenge. Investigators have employed high-throughput genetic technology to better understand the risk associated with hERG-blocking drugs. Such approaches have heralded a new era in pharmacotherapy, with individualized drug selection [84].

These reports implicate two distinct mechanisms: first, increased sensitivity of the hERG channel complex to drug block, which has been noted primarily in patients with mutations in the MiRP1 subunit (Table 20.2), who have normal baseline ECGs but develop torsades de pointes on exposure to I_{Kr} blockers [85]; second, reduction of I_{Ks} or another repolarizing current that is well-tolerated until the superposition of I_{Kr} block [86].

Slow delayed rectifier (I_{Ks})
Structure and function

In cardiac myocytes, long depolarizing pulses also give rise to a slowly activating outward current, termed I_{Ks} for I_K slow (Fig. 20.1). Expression of *KCNQ1* (*KvLQT1*; Table 20.2), the disease gene in the LQT1 variant of inherited LQTS (Table 20.3), gives rise to rapidly activating, slowly deactivating current that does not have a readily identifiable correlate in cardiac myocytes. Conversely, coexpression of minK (the product of the gene *KCNE1*) and KvLQT1 recapitulates I_{Ks}, indicating that the coassembly of these two products produces the I_{Ks} current in cardiac myocytes [87,88]. The I_{Ks} is generated by a membrane complex consisting of four pore-forming KvLQT1 α subunits and two minK β subunits [89]. KvLQT1 retains the molecular architecture of the typical voltage-gated K^+ channel (Fig. 20.4), and accessibility data are consistent with the idea that minK resides in a crevice that is not part of the pore, but nevertheless influences movement of the mink–KvLQT1 channel complex during gating [90]. The pharmacology of KvLQT1 agonists and antagonists is modified significantly by the coexpression of minK.

Regulation of I_{Ks}

The action potential in the ventricle shortens with adrenergic stimulation, even controlling for heart rate. Because I_{Ca} increases with adrenergic stimulation (an effect that would prolong action potentials), a counterbalancing increase in outward K^+ current must also occur, and likely involves I_{Ks}. In most studies, I_{Ks} amplitude is increased by adrenergic stimulation as well as by increases in intracellular Ca^{2+} or by PKC stimulation, and a consensus PKC phosphorylation site is present in the C-terminus of human minK. In addition, studies from transgenic animals overexpressing adrenoceptors suggest possible colocalization of the *KvLQT1* and elements of the signaling pathway [91]. Coexpression of an A-kinase anchoring protein with *KvLQT1* + *minK* has been shown necessary for the I_{Ks} response to PKA stimulation [92].

I_{Ks} dysfunction in disease

Autosomal dominant mutations in *KvLQT1* or *minK* evoke (respectively) the LQT1 or LQT5 varieties of LQTS (Table 20.3). Pharmacologic I_{Ks} block tends to produce homogeneous action-potential prolongation in ventricular tissue; however, β-adrenergic agonists such as isoproterenol evoke marked heterogeneities of action-potential duration and arrhythmias. Torsades de pointes can be induced in canine hearts by the I_{Ks} blocker 293B only in the presence of isoproterenol [93]. Phosphorylation of KvLQT1 by PKA attenuates I_{Ks} block induced by quinidine, which partly explains some of the decreased potency of antiarrhythmic I_{Ks} blockers in the presence of adrenergic stimulation. This is consistent with the sensitivity of I_{Ks} to adrenergic stimulation (described earlier), and with the observation that arrhythmias in LQT1 and LQT5 patients with inherited *KvLQT1* or *minK* mutations almost always arise during periods of adrenergic stress. These findings also explain the protective effect of β-blocking drugs in patients with LQT1 or LQT5 and in the setting of increased sympathetic activity [94,95]. Examination of currents generated by heterologous expression of KvLQT1 and minK channels with inherited mutations in widely divergent areas of the protein results in a wide variety of defects that lead to a reduction in I_{Ks} current, including altered channel gating or failure of the mutant channel to traffic to the cell surface.

The rare Jervell–Lange–Nielsen (JLN) variant of LQTS (Table 20.3) associated with congenital deafness arises in children who inherit abnormal *KvLQT1* or *minK* alleles from both parents [96,97]. The *KvLQT1–minK* complex is responsible for endolymph secretion in the inner ear, and its absence in

patients with JLN results in collapse of the endolymphatic space. This situation arises through consanguinity (i.e., the child inherits alleles each encoding the same abnormal protein) or occasionally by chance (in which case the child inherits alleles that encode different abnormal proteins). Thus both parents are obligate gene carriers for LQT1 or LQT5. Although QT intervals are generally normal in these parents, it is now recognized that occasional cases of sudden unexpected death, presumably caused by LQT-related arrhythmias, can occur in the parents, an observation that has obvious implications for family screening (and preoperative assessment) of a patient with JLN [97].

Ultrarapid delayed rectifier (I_{Kur})
Structure and function

This current activates even more rapidly than I_{Kr} (hence the designation I_{Kur}, for ultrarapid), and exhibits little inactivation during sustained depolarization. Heterologous expression of the $K_v1.5$ channel subunit results in a current with gating kinetics essentially identical to I_{Kur} [98,99], and native I_{Kur} and heterologously expressed $K_v1.5$ are both sensitive to quinidine and to 4-aminopyridine, suggesting that $K_v1.5$ is the major protein substituent of I_{Kur}. $K_v1.5$ is expressed chiefly in atria, and represents the predominant delayed rectifier responsible for atrial repolarization [100].

In addition, multiple members of the $K_v\beta1$ subunit family (Table 20.2) have been cloned [101] and coexpression of $K_v\beta1.2$ with $K_v1.5$ accelerates inactivation, making the channel appear more like I_{to}. These β subunits appear to be almost exclusively cytosolic and may mediate inactivation of the $K_v1.5$ subunit through an N-type ball-and-chain mechanism (Fig. 20.5), whereby the β subunit acts as the ball [102]. The crystal structure of $K_v\beta$ has been solved and is homologous to oxido-reductase enzymes; therefore it is proposed that $K_v\beta$ subunits couple the cell redox state to K^+ channel function [26,103].

I_{Kur} regulation and dysfunction in disease

In animal models, $K_v1.5$ current is upregulated by glucocorticoids and thyroid hormone. $K_v1.5$ also contains SH3 domains that interact with tyrosine kinase, and are tyrosine-phosphorylated in human heart. In addition, $K_v1.5$ has been reported to target to lipid rafts, specific membrane regions enriched in certain subtypes of lipids (e.g., cholesterol) that may allow localization of $K_v1.5$ channels in the vicinity of signaling molecules and substrates within the cell. Moreover, adaptor proteins (ZIP1 and ZIP2) may generate a physical link between the $K_v\alpha/\beta$ complex and protein kinases [104].

Because $K_v1.5$ is abundant in human atrium but is absent from normal human ventricle, maneuvers that reduce $K_v1.5$ would be expected to prolong atrial action potentials and yet not prolong repolarization in the ventricle, thus avoiding QT prolongation and the risk for inducing torsades de pointes. Efforts to produce such a "chamber-specific" antiarrhythmic drug (targeted at AF) are ongoing, although $K_v1.5$ expression in extracardiac tissues may elicit side effects with this strategy [100,105]. Notably, in chronic AF, $K_v1.5$ mRNA and protein (like other ion currents, including I_{Ca-L} and I_{Na}) are downregulated [106], which may limit the effectiveness of this approach. Recently, a specific $K_v1.5$ and I_{to} blocking drug has shown promise in animal models of AF [107,108].

Cardiac inward rectifiers

Structure and function

These K^+ channels (I_{K1}, I_{K-ATP}, I_{K-ACh}), encoded by the *Kir* superfamily (Fig. 20.4), are notable for the absence of a charged, S4 segment (Fig. 20.5), and therefore exhibit less intrinsic voltage-dependent gating. Nonetheless, as their *inward rectifier* name implies, these K^+ channels pass inward current in preference to outward current, and are primarily operative at hyperpolarized (rather than depolarized) potentials near the cell resting potential (the potassium equilibrium potential, ~ 85 mV). Hence I_{K1} channels play a key role in clamping the myocyte resting potential. I_{K1} expression is low in nodal pacemaker cells, which explains why the diastolic potential in nodal tissue is less negative than in atrial or ventricular myocytes [109]. The inward rectification of I_{K1} results from block of outward current by intracellular constituents. For I_{K1}, Mg^{2+} alone appears sufficient [110,111], whereas for other members of this group polyamines (such as spermidine) have been implicated as further mediators of rectification [112,113].

The inward rectifier current I_{K1} likely represents expression of members of the *Kir2.x* family (Table 20.2) [114]. These channels, like the voltage-gated K^+ channels, are assembled as tetramers in the membrane, but are structurally simpler than the voltage-gated K^+ channels, consisting of only two membrane-spanning regions separated by an H5 linker region [115]. Overexpression of *Kir2.1* shortens cardiac action-potential duration and hyperpolarizes the membrane resting potential [116], whereas blockade of I_{K1} produces membrane depolarization, slows conduction velocity (by voltage-dependent Na^+ channel inactivation), and prolongs QT interval.

The acetylcholine-gated channel (I_{K-ACh}) is recapitulated in heterologous expression systems by coexpression of *Kir3.1* and *Kir3.4* (also termed *GIRK1* and *GIRK4*) [117]. Upon binding of acetylcholine to the cardiac muscarinic receptor, the βγ subunits of the receptor-associated G-protein activate I_{K-ACh} by binding directly to cytoplasmic segments of the channel [115]. This results in hyperpolarization and slowing of the nodal pacemaker cells.

The ATP-inhibited channel (K_{ATP} channel, I_{K-ATP}) can be recapitulated in vitro from coexpression of the *Kir6.2* channel with an ancillary protein, the sulfonylurea receptor (SUR2) [118]. SUR2 is a member of the ATP-binding-cassette superfamily that includes the cystic fibrosis transport regulator (CFTR). Members of this family share a common structural motif, consisting of putative 12 membrane-spanning segments and two intracellular ATP binding cassettes. Cardiac K_{ATP} channels are inhibited by physiologic concentrations of ATP. Opening of K_{ATP} channels shortens the action potential and decreases Ca^{2+} influx, protective mechanisms which preserve cellular ATP levels [119].

I_{K1} channel regulation and dysfunction in disease

In addition to maintenance of the resting membrane potential, evidence supporting a role for *Kir2.1*/I_{K1} in the terminal phase of cardiac repolarization has come from the linkage of mutations in *Kir2.1* with Andersen syndrome (Table 20.3), a neuromuscular disease whose manifestations include unusual forms of ventricular tachycardia. I_{K1} expression is downregulated in several models of cardiovascular disease, including hypertension, cardiac hypertrophy, heart failure, and cardiomyopathies [120,121], and produces prolongation of action potential, and triggered automaticity. I_{K1} expression increases in patients with chronic AF [122].

ATP-sensitive K^+ channels provide a link between the metabolic state of the cell and electrophysiologic activity. K_{ATP} channels also represent a final common pathway in ischemic and volatile-anesthetic-induced preconditioning [123,124]. Several drugs activate these channels, but are not cardiac-specific ("K^+ channel openers" such as nicorandil or pinacidil). Cardiac-specific agents, on the horizon, may be useful to protect the myocardium against the deleterious effects of ischemia (including arrhythmias). Although cardiac K_{ATP} blockers prevent action-potential shortening and ventricular fibrillation following ischemia–reperfusion, their effects on smooth muscle (vasodilation) and pancreatic β cells (hypoglycemia) limit their usefulness as antiarrhythmic agents in postinfarct settings [125]. ATP-sensitive channels are expressed not only on the cell surface, but also in mitochondria, where they may be attractive targets for cardioprotection [126].

Pacemaker current

The cardiac rhythm, a sine qua non characteristic of the heart, is generated in SA node cells by an inward current that continually depolarizes the cell toward its firing threshold during phase 4 of the action potential. Unlike other cardiac ionic currents activated by depolarization, this hyperpolarization-activated pacemaker current [127] has been termed funny (I_f) or hyperpolarization-activated (I_h). The pacemaker channel superfamily includes cyclic nucleotide binding domains in its C-terminus, and it follows that pacemaker activity is regulated in vivo by cyclic nucleotide-related (i.e., adrenergic) signaling pathways. Three members of this superfamily (*HCN1, HCN2,* and *HCN4*) have been found in mouse heart [128], and heterologous expression of these channels results in a hyperpolarization-activated current that, like I_h, displays only very weak selectivity for K^+ over Na^+ (and with a reversal potential of –35 mV). Although HCN channels display the typical six-membrane-segment spanning architecture of voltage-gated K^+ channels, the mechanisms for their unusual hyperpolarization-activated gating and lack of selectivity have not been fully determined, and might involve sequence differences in the S4 sensor and the selectivity filter regions of the pore.

In addition to pacemaker cells, I_h current can be elicited by excessive hyperpolarization in ventricular muscle cells [129], suggesting that altered regulation of this current could underlie ventricular arrhythmias during pathologic conditions. Recent studies have examined the specific pharmacology of funny channels, and drugs for altering funny-channel function are under investigation, both as research tools and as therapeutic agents [130].

Background current

In addition to currents that exhibit time- and voltage-dependent gating properties, voltage clamp studies of heart cells reveal additional currents that do not exhibit gating characteristics, known generally as "background" currents. At least three types of ion channels may underlie background currents in heart. I_{Kp} (for plateau) is a time-independent current, originally identified in guinea pig cardiomyocytes [131,132]. It has been suggested that expression of the twin-pore K^+ channel, known as TWIK1, may underlie I_{Kp} [133]. More generally, studies have identified chloride channels activated by changes in cell volume, as well as intracellular Ca^{2+} [134]. Finally, studies have shown that coexpression of *KvLQT1* with *KCNE2* (*MiRP1*) produces a background current [135], although the question of the extent of *MiRP1* expression in heart and its localization are unresolved. Moreover, whether any background currents are appropriate targets for drug therapy is unknown.

Current and potential targets of drug action

Emerging view of a common ion-channel drug receptor

The pharmacologic principles that underlie control of the cardiac rhythm (antiarrhythmic therapy) are necessarily complex, given the vast array of ion channels, receptors, and signaling pathways involved. The general principles that underlie antiarrhythmic therapy are discussed in detail in Chapter 43. This chapter focuses on the molecular mechanism whereby most antiarrhythmic compounds modulate the cardiac rhythm – i.e., suppression of ionic current through binding to voltage-gated ion channels. The ability to clone and mutagenize specific amino acid residues in channel proteins has revolutionized our approach to defining and characterizing the drug receptors and is leading toward a surprising "common view" of the mechanism whereby drugs block ion channels in multiple classes.

The first insights into the putative drug receptor in voltage-gated ion channels were provided by studies of tetraethylammonium (TEA) and the larger quaternary ammonium (QA) derivatives on delayed rectifier K^+ channels in squid axons (Fig. 20.6) [137]. These studies showed that low concentrations of QA blocked the channel from inside the cell, and that the affinity increased as the hydrophobicity (length of the QA-compound carbon tail) of the compound increased. Moreover, internal blockade by TEA suppressed outward current through the channel to a much greater degree than inward current, and increasing the inward flux of K^+ ions through the channel sped the rate of dissociation of TEA from its receptor, as if the K^+ ions "knocked off" the drug. These directional effects were best explained by a hydrophobic drug receptor that lies within the pore, in a vestibule on the internal side of a narrow selectivity "filter."

Later studies using site-specific modification of ion-channel amino acid residues satisfied these predictions and mapped the locus of the K^+ channel QA receptor to amino acid residues residing in the inner pore. Consistent with the two functional ends of QA compounds, two regions of the K^+ channel influence drug binding from inside the channel [138]. The P-loop (Fig. 20.1) primarily influences internal TEA binding, but has less effect on longer (more hydrophobic) QA derivatives. Conversely, the binding affinity of long QA derivatives is determined by the hydrophobicity of amino acid residues lining the pore in the S6 segment. The picture that emerges is a bidomain receptor, with a hydrophilic binding interaction between the charged amino head of the QA compound and the P-loop, and a hydrophobic interaction between the QA alkyl tail and hydrophobic amino acids in the S6 region (Fig. 20.6). S6 amino acid residues have been shown to be important in the binding of a number of K^+ channel blockers including 4-aminopyridine and quinidine. It has been noted that binding of the hydrophobic tail of QA derivatives to S6 residues seems to reduce the interaction of the polar amino head with the P-loop, suggesting a "tension" between binding at the two sites that might be modulated by changing the physical separation between the charged head and alkyl tail [138].

A striking parallel exists between QA binding in K^+ channels and binding of the local anesthetic class of antiarrhythmic molecules to their target, the voltage-gated Na^+ channel. These compounds contain an ionizable amino head group and a hydrophobic tail, much like the QA compounds (Fig. 20.6). An intrapore binding site for these molecules is well supported by evidence that the charged derivatives (e.g., QX–314) move deeply (50–70%) into the pore from the cytoplasmic side [139]. Specific aromatic hydrophobic residues in the S6 segments of domains I and IV line the inner pore of the channel and figure critically in block (Fig. 20.7) [140]. Analogous sites in domain IV, S6 of L-type Ca^{2+} channels, have been linked to both dihydropyridine and phenylalkylamine block of Ca^{2+} current [141,142]. At the same time, studies have shown that the polar

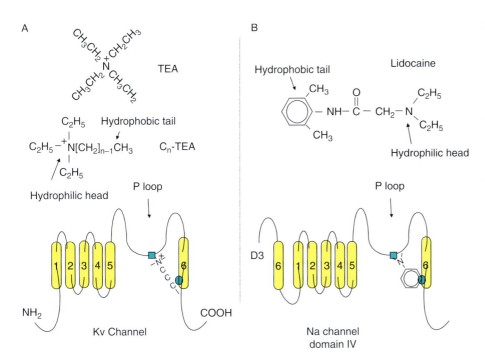

Figure 20.6. Voltage-gated K^+ and Na^+ channels have analogous bidomain drug receptor motifs. (A) The structure of tetraethylammonium (TEA) and the longer-chain TEA derivatives (Cn-TEA) are shown (*top*). Mutations in the S6 domain (*green circle*) of the Kv channel have prominent effects on the affinity of long-chain QA derivatives (*bottom*). Conversely, mutation in the P-loop (*green square*) reduces binding of TEA and short-chain QA derivatives. (B) The structure of lidocaine, a local anesthetic molecule, is shown with its hydrophobic aromatic tail and hydrophilic amino head group, separated by an amide linkage (*top*). Mutation of residues in the S6 segment of domain IV critically determines local anesthetic binding (*bottom*). In addition, residues that determine cation selectivity in the P-loops also modify local anesthetic block (see text). Reproduced with permission from Balser and George [136].

head of the compound is repelled by positively charged residues in the Na^+ channel P-region, near the selectivity filter, suggesting that this region normally restricts extracellular access to (and escape from) the intrapore binding site [143]. Notably, antiarrhythmic drug blockade of Na^+ channels increases markedly during depolarization, while the channels are mainly inactivated [144]. This "use-dependent" block may be related to gating-dependent conformational changes that secondarily increase the "affinity" of the drug receptor. For example, mutation of residues in either the III–IV linker fast inactivation gate (Fig. 20.7) or the P-loop modify the N-type and C-type Na^+ channel inactivation processes, respectively [34,146], and these modifications also markedly reduce use-dependent Na^+ channel blockade [147,148]. Moreover, recent studies suggest that drug binding to both K^+ and Na^+ channels "stabilizes" C-type inactivated conformation of the channel, and thus contributes to use-dependent current reduction partly through an allosteric mechanism [11,149].

The prominent role of the hERG channel, and the I_{Kr} channel, in the proarrhythmic effects of drugs on the cardiac rhythm warrants some additional comment. I_{Kr} channels are blocked by a myriad of drugs, both antiarrhythmics and "noncardiovascular" drugs that share the potential to produce marked QT prolongation and torsades de pointes. The recognition that hERG is "promiscuous" in its ability to be blocked by drugs from various classes has important implications for drug development; it has driven investigation into structural determinants of hERG block. Drug binding to hERG subunits occurs in the S6 region (analogous to Fig. 20.7), but is nearly irreversible, a finding that has been attributed to the channel closing during diastole with the drug trapped in its receptor within the pore [150]. In addition,

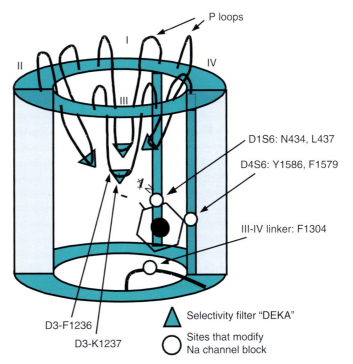

Figure 20.7. Highly schematic view of the Na^+ channel pore, lined by the four homologous domains (I–IV), with a lidocaine analog residing in the pore. The outer pore is formed by the P-loops, whereas the S6 segments line the inner pore. P-loop selectivity filter residues bridge the outer and inner pore regions (*triangles*). Residues in the selectivity filter (i.e., K1237) and the domain I and IV S6 segments interact with Na^+ channel-blocking antiarrhythmic drugs (see text). Residues in the figure are numbered according to the original sequence of the rat skeletal muscle Na^+ channel isoform [145]. D1S6 refers to domain I, S6, and so on. Adapted from Balser [36].

structural modeling, based on the sequence analogy between hERG and the KcsA K^+ channel crystal structure, reveals two unusual features of the hERG inner vestibule [151]. Most K^+ channel primary sequences include two highly conserved proline residues in the S6 segment that are predicted to "kink" the segment and limit the size of the inner vestibule. The absence of such prolines in hERG may enlarge the inner vestibule, allowing relatively bulky drugs to enter. Second, the hERG S6 sequence has two aromatic residues predicted to face the inner pore, whereas other K^+ channels have none or one (i.e., KvLQT1). Alanine mutagenesis of these residues markedly decreases drug block, suggesting that one or more of the eight aromatic residues lining the tetrameric pore can provide a high-affinity site for π-bonding interactions with aromatic groups on putative blocking drugs.

Because of the wide range of compounds capable of blocking hERG, and the possibility of lethal arrhythmias resulting from hERG blockade, regulatory agencies have now required candidate drug compounds to pass hERG screening. Even drug-induced "acquired" cardiac arrhythmias often have a genetic component, since genetic haplotypes that predispose to drug-induced arrhythmogenesis may be quite common in the population [152]. Individualized prescribing approaches may then become possible, once genetic screening methodology becomes available and cost-effective.

Summary

The normal cardiac rhythm is the result of a highly complex interplay of electrical currents generated by specific ion gradients across the myocyte membrane. Ion channels are complex transmembrane proteins which selectively permit passage of a specific ion down its concentration gradient, and can be gated by transmembrane potential or by ligand binding. Because intracellular sodium and calcium concentrations are much less than their corresponding extracellular concentrations, ion channels which are specific to these cations will produce inward currents when open, resulting in depolarization of the membrane potential from its resting baseline of –85 mV toward more positive voltage. Conversely, since intracellular potassium concentration is much greater than its extracellular concentration, potassium channels will usually produce outward currents when open, resulting in repolarization or hyperpolarization of the membrane. The resulting transmembrane potential throughout the cardiac cycle is termed the action potential, and is the result of all individual ion currents in concert. The surface ECG is the aggregate of cardiac action potentials across the entire heart.

The cardiac action potential is an essential component to cardiac pumping function because of a phenomenon whereby the action potential is converted into the contraction of the myofibrils. This is termed *excitation–contraction coupling*, and is initiated by the calcium influx at the plateau phase of the action potential.

The large number of genes comprising the existing substrate for the cardiac rhythm suggest a myriad of potential targets for antiarrhythmic therapy. However, as discussed in Chapter 43, the number of molecular targets currently exploited by existing antiarrhythmic therapies is relatively limited. Hence a major challenge is to not only expand the "arrhythmonome," genes encoding proteins that modulate cardiac excitability, but also to greatly extend our structural and functional understanding of those gene products already identified. Through an active synergy between the methods of new gene identification and the emerging technologies for high-resolution determination of protein structure and function, exciting targets for antiarrhythmic therapy are likely to be identified during the next decade. It is hoped that these new compounds will greatly improve the specificity and efficacy of antiarrhythmic therapy in both perioperative and nonsurgical settings.

Acknowledgments
Salary support was provided by the Established Investigator Award of the American Heart Association and the National Institutes of Health (R01 GM56307 and P01 HL46681).

References

1. Schwartz P, Zipes D. Autonomic modulation of cardiac arrhythmias. In: Zipes D, Jalife J, eds., *Cardiac Electrophysiology: From Cells to Bedside*, 3rd edn. Philadelphia, PA: Saunders, 2000: 300–14.

2. Luo CH, Rudy Y. A dynamic model of the cardiac ventricular action potential. II. Afterdepolarizations, triggered activity, and potentiation. *Circ Res* 1994; 74: 1097–113.

3. Roden DM, Balser JR, George AL, Anderson ME. Cardiac ion channels. *Annu Rev Physiol* 2002; 64: 431–75.

4. Balser JR. Perioperative management of arrhythmias. In: Barash PG, Fleisher LA, Prough DS, eds., *Problems in Anesthesia*. Philadelphia, PA: Lippincott-Raven, 1998: 201.

5. Engelstein ED, Lippman N, Stein KM, Lerman BB. Mechanism-specific effects of adenosine on atrial tachycardia. *Circulation* 1994; 89: 2645–54.

6. Roden DM. Ibutilide and the treatment of atrial arrhythmias. A new drug – almost unheralded – is now available to US physicians. *Circulation* 1996; 94: 1499–502.

7. Mason JW. A comparison of seven antiarrhythmic drugs in patients with ventricular tachyarrhythmias. Electrophysiologic Study versus Electrocardiographic Monitoring Investigators. *N Engl J Med* 1993; 329: 452–8.

8. Echt DS, Liebson PR, Mitchell LB, *et al.* Mortality and morbidity in patients receiving encainide, flecainide, or placebo. The Cardiac Arrhythmia Suppression Trial. *N Engl J Med* 1991; 324: 781–8.

9. Chen Q, Kirsch GE, Zhang D, *et al.* Genetic basis and molecular mechanism

for idiopathic ventricular fibrillation. *Nature* 1998; **392**: 293–6.

10. Alings M, Wilde A. "Brugada" syndrome: clinical data and suggested pathophysiological mechanism. *Circulation* 1999; **99**: 666–73.

11. Baukrowitz T, Yellen G. Use-dependent blockers and exit rate of the last ion from the multi-ion pore of a K$^+$ channel. *Science* 1996; **271**: 653–6.

12. Roden DM, Woosley RL, Primm RK. Incidence and clinical features of the quinidine-associated long QT syndrome: implications for patient care. *Am Heart J* 1986; **111**: 1088–93.

13. Priori SG, Barhanin J, Hauer RN, *et al.* Genetic and molecular basis of cardiac arrhythmias: impact on clinical management parts I and II. *Circulation* 1999; **99**: 518–28.

14. Wit A. Triggered activity. In: Podrid P, Kowey P, eds., *Cardiac Arrhythmia: Mechanisms, Diagnosis, and Management.* Baltimore, MD: Williams & Wilkins, 1995: 70–7.

15. Reuter H. Localization of beta adrenergic receptors, and effects of noradrenaline and cyclic nucleotides on action potentials, ionic currents and tension in mammalian cardiac muscle. *J Physiol* 1974; **242**: 429–51.

16. Hoch B, Meyer R, Hetzer R, Krause EG, Karczewski P. Identification and expression of delta-isoforms of the multifunctional Ca^{2+}/calmodulin-dependent protein kinase in failing and nonfailing human myocardium. *Circ Res* 1999; **84**: 713–21.

17. Dzhura I, Wu Y, Colbran RJ, Balser JR, Anderson ME. Calmodulin kinase determines calcium-dependent facilitation of L-type calcium channels. *Nat Cell Biol* 2000; **2**: 173–7.

18. Wu Y, Roden DM, Anderson ME. Calmodulin kinase inhibition prevents development of the arrhythmogenic transient inward current. *Circ Res* 1999; **84**: 906–12.

19. Yeager M. Molecular biology and structure of cardiac gap junction intercellular channels. In: Zipes D, Jalife J, eds., *Cardiac Electrophysiology: From Cells to Bedside*, 3rd edn. Philadelphia, PA: Saunders, 2000: 31–40.

20. Hamill OP, Marty A, Neher E, Sakmann B, Sigworth FJ. Improved patch-clamp techniques for high-resolution current recording from cells and cell-free membrane patches. *Pflugers Arch* 1981; **391**: 85–100.

21. Noda M, Shimizu S, Tanabe T, *et al.* Primary structure of *Electrophorus electricus* sodium channel deduced from cDNA sequence. *Nature* 1984; **312**: 121–7.

22. Hodgkin AL, Huxley AF. A quantitative description of membrane current and its application to conduction and excitation in nerve. *J Physiol* 1952; **117**: 500–44.

23. MacKinnon R, Yellen G. Mutations affecting TEA blockade and ion permeation in voltage-activated K$^+$ channels. *Science* 1990; **250**: 276–9.

24. Yellen G, Jurman ME, Abramson T, MacKinnon R. Mutations affecting internal TEA blockade identify the probable pore-forming region of a K$^+$ channel. *Science* 1991; **251**: 939–42.

25. Heinemann SH, Terlau H, Stuhmer W, Imoto K, Numa S. Calcium channel characteristics conferred on the sodium channel by single mutations. *Nature* 1992; **356**: 441–3.

26. Doyle DA, Morais Cabral J, Pfuetzner RA, *et al.* The structure of the potassium channel: molecular basis of K$^+$ conduction and selectivity. *Science* 1998; **280**: 69–77.

27. Stuhmer W, Conti F, Suzuki H, *et al.* Structural parts involved in activation and inactivation of the sodium channel. *Nature* 1989; **339**: 597–603.

28. Armstrong CM, Bezanilla F. Inactivation of the sodium channel. II. Gating current experiments. *J Gen Physiol* 1977; **70**: 567–90.

29. Yang N, George AL, Horn R. Molecular basis of charge movement in voltage-gated sodium channels. *Neuron* 1996; **16**: 113–22.

30. Hoshi T, Zagotta WN, Aldrich RW. Biophysical and molecular mechanisms of Shaker potassium channel inactivation. *Science* 1990; **250**: 533–8.

31. Gellens ME, George AL, Chen LQ, *et al.* Primary structure and functional expression of the human cardiac tetrodotoxin-insensitive voltage-dependent sodium channel. *Proc Natl Acad Sci U S A* 1992; **89**: 554–8.

32. Isom LL, De Jongh KS, Catterall WA. Auxiliary subunits of voltage-gated ion channels. *Neuron* 1994; **12**: 1183–94.

33. Meadows LS, Isom LL. Sodium channels as macromolecular complexes: implications for inherited arrhythmia syndromes. *Cardiovasc Res* 2005; **67**: 448–58.

34. West JW, Patton DE, Scheuer T, *et al.* A cluster of hydrophobic amino acid residues required for fast Na(+)-channel inactivation. *Proc Natl Acad Sci U S A* 1992; **89**: 10910–14.

35. Tang L, Kallen RG, Horn R. Role of an S4–S5 linker in sodium channel inactivation probed by mutagenesis and a peptide blocker. *J Gen Physiol* 1996; **108**: 89–104.

36. Balser JR. Structure and function of the cardiac sodium channels. *Cardiovasc Res* 1999; **42**: 327–38.

37. Balser JR. The cardiac sodium channel: gating function and molecular pharmacology. *J Mol Cell Cardiol* 2001; **33**: 599–613.

38. Taouis M, Sheldon RS, Duff HJ. Upregulation of the rat cardiac sodium channel by in vivo treatment with a class I antiarrhythmic drug. *J Clin Invest* 1991; **88**: 375–8.

39. Yue L, Melnyk P, Gaspo R, Wang Z, Nattel S. Molecular mechanisms underlying ionic remodeling in a dog model of atrial fibrillation. *Circ Res* 1999; **84**: 776–84.

40. Baba S, Dun W, Boyden PA. Can PKA activators rescue Na$^+$ channel function in epicardial border zone cells that survive in the infarcted canine heart? *Cardiovasc Res* 2004; **64**: 260–7.

41. Jespersen T, Gavillet B, van Bemmelen MX, *et al.* Cardiac sodium channel Na(v)1.5 interacts with and is regulated by the protein tyrosine phosphatase PTPH1. *Biochem Biophys Res Commun* 2006; **348**: 1455–62.

42. Wagner S, Dybkova N, Rasenack EC, *et al.* Ca^{2+}/calmodulin-dependent protein kinase II regulates cardiac Na$^+$ channels. *J Clin Invest* 2006; **116**: 3127–38.

43. Deschenes I, Neyroud N, DiSilvestre D, *et al.* Isoform-specific modulation of voltage-gated Na$^+$ channels by calmodulin. *Circ Res* 2002; **90**: E49–57.

Section 2: Physiologic substrates of drug action

44. Tan HL, Kupershmidt S, Zhang R, et al. A calcium sensor in the sodium channel modulates cardiac excitability. Nature 2002; 415: 442–7.

45. Wingo TL, Shah VN, Anderson ME, et al. An EF-hand in the sodium channel couples intracellular calcium to cardiac excitability. Nat Struct Mol Biol 2004; 11: 219–25.

46. Wang Q, Shen J, Splawski I, et al. SCN5A mutations associated with an inherited cardiac arrhythmia, long QT syndrome. Cell 1995; 80: 805–11.

47. Bennett PB, Yazawa K, Makita N, George AL. Molecular mechanism for an inherited cardiac arrhythmia. Nature 1995; 376: 683–5.

48. Dumaine R, Wang Q, Keating MT, et al. Multiple mechanisms of Na⁺ channel–linked long-QT syndrome. Circ Res 1996; 78: 916–24.

49. Wang DW, Yazawa K, George AL, Bennett PB. Characterization of human cardiac Na⁺ channel mutations in the congenital long QT syndrome. Proc Natl Acad Sci U S A 1996; 93: 13200–5.

50. Veldkamp MW, Viswanathan PC, Bezzina C, et al. Two distinct congenital arrhythmias evoked by a multidysfunctional Na(+) channel. Circ Res 2000; 86: E91–7.

51. Schott JJ, Alshinawi C, Kyndt F, et al. Cardiac conduction defects associate with mutations in SCN5A. Nat Genet 1999; 23: 20–1.

52. Pu J, Boyden PA. Alterations of Na⁺ currents in myocytes from epicardial border zone of the infarcted heart. A possible ionic mechanism for reduced excitability and postrepolarization refractoriness. Circ Res 1997; 81: 110–19.

53. Albert CM, Nam EG, Rimm EB, et al. Cardiac sodium channel gene variants and sudden cardiac death in women. Circulation 2008; 117: 16–23.

54. Ellinor PT, Nam EG, Shea MA, et al. Cardiac sodium channel mutation in atrial fibrillation. Heart Rhythm 2008; 5: 99–105.

55. Shang LL, Pfahnl AE, Sanyal S, et al. Human heart failure is associated with abnormal C-terminal splicing variants in the cardiac sodium channel. Circ Res 2007; 101: 1146–54.

56. Smits JP, Koopmann TT, Wilders R, et al. A mutation in the human cardiac sodium channel (E161K) contributes to sick sinus syndrome, conduction disease and Brugada syndrome in two families. J Mol Cell Cardiol 2005; 38: 969–81.

57. Wang DW, Desai RR, Crotti L, et al. Cardiac sodium channel dysfunction in sudden infant death syndrome. Circulation 2007; 115: 368–76.

58. Medeiros-Domingo A, Kaku T, Tester DJ, et al. SCN4B-encoded sodium channel beta4 subunit in congenital long-QT syndrome. Circulation 2007; 116: 134–42.

59. Gavillet B, Rougier JS, Domenighetti AA, et al. Cardiac sodium channel Na$_v$1.5 is regulated by a multiprotein complex composed of syntrophins and dystrophin. Circ Res 2006; 99: 407–14.

60. Schultz D, Mikala G, Yatani A, et al. Cloning, chromosomal localization, and functional expression of the alpha 1 subunit of the L-type voltage-dependent calcium channel from normal human heart. Proc Natl Acad Sci U S A 1993; 90: 6228–32.

61. Perez-Reyes E, Cribbs LL, Daud A, et al. Molecular characterization of a neuronal low-voltage-activated T-type calcium channel. Nature 1998; 391: 896–900.

62. Perez-Reyes E, Castellano A, Kim HS, et al. Cloning and expression of a cardiac/brain beta subunit of the L-type calcium channel. J Biol Chem 1992; 267: 1792–7.

63. De Jongh KS, Warner C, Catterall WA. Subunits of purified calcium channels. Alpha 2 and delta are encoded by the same gene. J Biol Chem 1990; 265: 14738–41.

64. Kim J, Ghosh S, Nunziato DA, Pitt GS. Identification of the components controlling inactivation of voltage-gated Ca²⁺ channels. Neuron 2004; 41: 745–54.

65. Hess P, Tsien RW. Mechanism of ion permeation through calcium channels. Nature 1984; 309: 453–6.

66. de Leon M, Wang Y, Jones L, et al. Essential Ca²⁺-binding motif for Ca²⁺-sensitive inactivation of L-type Ca²⁺ channels. Science 1995; 270: 1502–6.

67. Hartzell HC, Mery PF, Fischmeister R, Szabo G. Sympathetic regulation of cardiac calcium current is due exclusively to cAMP-dependent phosphorylation. Nature 1991; 351: 573–6.

68. Perets T, Blumenstein Y, Shistik E, Lotan I, Dascal N. A potential site of functional modulation by protein kinase A in the cardiac Ca²⁺ channel alpha 1C subunit. FEBS Lett 1996; 384: 189–92.

69. Gray PC, Scott JD, Catterall WA. Regulation of ion channels by cAMP-dependent protein kinase and A-kinase anchoring proteins. Curr Opin Neurobiol 1998; 8: 330–4.

70. Yue L, Feng J, Gaspo R, et al. Ionic remodeling underlying action potential changes in a canine model of atrial fibrillation. Circ Res 1997; 81: 512–25.

71. Christ T, Boknik P, Wohrl S, et al. L-type Ca2+ current downregulation in chronic human atrial fibrillation is associated with increased activity of protein phosphatases. Circulation 2004; 110: 2651–7.

72. Marban E, Robinson SW, Wier WG. Mechanisms of arrhythmogenic delayed and early afterdepolarizations in ferret ventricular muscle. J Clin Invest 1986; 78: 1185–92.

73. Mazur A, Roden DM, Anderson ME. Systemic administration of calmodulin antagonist W-7 or protein kinase A inhibitor H-8 prevents torsade de pointes in rabbits. Circulation 1999; 100: 2437–42.

74. Po S, Snyders DJ, Baker R, Tamkun MM, Bennett PB. Functional expression of an inactivating potassium channel cloned from human heart. Circ Res 1992; 71: 732–6.

75. Dixon JE, McKinnon D. Quantitative analysis of potassium channel mRNA expression in atrial and ventricular muscle of rats. Circ Res 1994; 75: 252–60.

76. Nerbonne JM, Kass RS. Physiology and molecular biology of ion channels contributing to ventricular repolarization. In: Gussack I, Antzelevitch C, eds., Cardiac Repolarization. Totowa, NJ: Humana Press, 2003: 25–62.

77. Patel SP, Campbell DL. Transient outward potassium current, "Ito",

phenotypes in the mammalian left ventricle: underlying molecular, cellular and biophysical mechanisms. *J Physiol* 2005; **569**: 7–39.

78. An WF, Bowlby MR, Betty M, *et al.* Modulation of A-type potassium channels by a family of calcium sensors. *Nature* 2000; **403**: 553–6.

79. Po SS, Wu RC, Juang GJ, Kong W, Tomaselli GF. Mechanism of alpha-adrenergic regulation of expressed hKv4.3 currents. *Am J Physiol Heart Circ Physiol* 2001; **281**: H2518–27.

80. van der Heyden MA, Wijnhoven TJ, Opthof T. Molecular aspects of adrenergic modulation of the transient outward current. *Cardiovasc Res* 2006; **71**: 430–42.

81. Abbott GW, Sesti F, Splawski I, *et al.* MiRP1 forms IKr potassium channels with HERG and is associated with cardiac arrhythmia. *Cell* 1999; **97**: 175–87.

82. Smith PL, Baukrowitz T, Yellen G. The inward rectification mechanism of the HERG cardiac potassium channel. *Nature* 1996; **379**: 833–6.

83. Thomas D, Karle CA, Kiehn J. The cardiac hERG/IKr potassium channel as pharmacological target: structure, function, regulation, and clinical applications. *Curr Pharm Des* 2006; **12**: 2271–83.

84. Vizirianakis IS. Clinical translation of genotyping and haplotyping data: implementation of in vivo pharmacology experience leading drug prescription to pharmacotyping. *Clin Pharmacokinet* 2007; **46**: 807–24.

85. Sesti F, Abbott GW, Wei J, *et al.* A common polymorphism associated with antibiotic-induced cardiac arrhythmia. *Proc Natl Acad Sci U S A* 2000; **97**: 10613–18.

86. Yang P, Wei J, Murray KT, *et al.* Frequency of ion channel mutations and polymorphisms in a large population of patients with drug-associated long QT syndrome. *Pacing Clin Electrophysiol* 2001; **24**: 579.

87. Barhanin J, Lesage F, Guillemare E, *et al.* K(V)LQT1 and lsK (minK) proteins associate to form the I(Ks) cardiac potassium current. *Nature* 1996; **384**: 78–80.

88. Sanguinetti MC, Curran ME, Zou A, *et al.* Coassembly of K(V)LQT1 and minK (IsK) proteins to form cardiac I (Ks) potassium channel. *Nature* 1996; **384**: 80–3.

89. Chen H, Kim LA, Rajan S, Xu S, Goldstein SA. Charybdotoxin binding in the I(Ks) pore demonstrates two MinK subunits in each channel complex. *Neuron* 2003; **40**: 15–23.

90. Tapper A, George AL. The KVLQT1 S6 transmembrane segment is a structural requirement for minK-mediated gating modulation. *Biophys J* 2001; **80**: 192a.

91. Dilly KW, Kurokawa J, Terrenoire C, *et al.* Overexpression of beta2-adrenergic receptors cAMP-dependent protein kinase phosphorylates and modulates slow delayed rectifier potassium channels expressed in murine heart: evidence for receptor/channel co-localization. *J Biol Chem* 2004; **279**: 40778–87.

92. Potet F, Scott JD, Mohammad-Panah R, Escande D, Baro I. AKAP proteins anchor cAMP-dependent protein kinase to KvLQT1/IsK channel complex. *Am J Physiol Heart Circ Physiol* 2001; **280**: H2038–45.

93. Shimizu W, Antzelevitch C. Cellular basis for the ECG features of the LQT1 form of the long-QT syndrome: effects of beta-adrenergic agonists and antagonists and sodium channel blockers on transmural dispersion of repolarization and torsade de pointes. *Circulation* 1998; **98**: 2314–22.

94. Kass RS, Moss AJ. Long QT syndrome: novel insights into the mechanisms of cardiac arrhythmias. *J Clin Invest* 2003; **112**: 810–15.

95. Schwartz PJ. The long QT syndrome: a clinical counterpart of hERG mutations. *Novartis Found Symp* 2005; **266**: 186–98.

96. Schulze-Bahr E, Wang Q, Wedekind H, *et al.* KCNE1 mutations cause Jervell and Lange–Nielsen syndrome. *Nat Genet* 1997; **17**: 267–8.

97. Splawski I, Timothy KW, Vincent GM, Atkinson DL, Keating MT. Molecular basis of the long-QT syndrome associated with deafness. *N Engl J Med* 1997; **336**: 1562–7.

98. Fedida D, Wible B, Wang Z, *et al.* Identity of a novel delayed rectifier current from human heart with a cloned K+ channel current. *Circ Res* 1993; **73**: 210–16.

99. Snyders DJ, Tamkun MM, Bennett PB. Arapidly activating and slowly inactivating potassium channel cloned from human heart. Functional analysis after stable mammalian cell culture expression. *J Gen Physiol* 1993; **101**: 513–43.

100. Ehrlich JR, Nattel S, Hohnloser SH. Novel anti-arrhythmic drugs for atrial fibrillation management. *Curr Vasc Pharmacol* 2007; **5**: 185–95.

101. England SK, Uebele VN, Shear H, *et al.* Characterization of a voltage-gated K+ channel beta subunit expressed in human heart. *Proc Natl Acad Sci U S A* 1995; **92**: 6309–13.

102. Wissmann R, Baukrowitz T, Kalbacher H, *et al.* NMR structure and functional characteristics of the hydrophilic N terminus of the potassium channel beta-subunit Kvbeta1.1. *J Biol Chem* 1999; **274**: 35521–5.

103. Bahring R, Milligan CJ, Vardanyan V, *et al.* Coupling of voltage-dependent potassium channel inactivation and oxidoreductase active site of Kvβ subunits. *J Biol Chem* 2001; **276**: 22923–9.

104. Gong J, Xu J, Bezanilla M, *et al.* Differential stimulation of PKC phosphorylation of potassium channels by ZIP1 and ZIP2. *Science* 1999; **285**: 1565–9.

105. Brendel J, Peukert S. Blockers of the Kv1.5 channel for the treatment of atrial arrhythmias. *Curr Med Chem Cardiovasc Hematol Agents* 2003; **1**: 273–87.

106. Van Wagoner DR, Pond AL, McCarthy PM, Trimmer JS, Nerbonne JM. Outward K+ current densities and Kv1.5 expression are reduced in chronic human atrial fibrillation. *Circ Res* 1997; **80**: 772–81.

107. de Haan S, Greiser M, Harks E, *et al.* AVE0118, blocker of the transient outward current (I_{to}) and ultrarapid delayed rectifier current (I_{Kur}), fully restores atrial contractility after cardioversion of atrial fibrillation in the goat. *Circulation* 2006; **114**: 1234–42.

108. Oros A, Volders PG, Beekman JD, van der Nagel T, Vos MA. Atrial-specific drug AVE0118 is free of torsades de pointes in anesthetized dogs with

chronic complete atrioventricular block. *Heart Rhythm* 2006; **3**: 1339–45.

109. Schram G, Pourrier M, Melnyk P, Nattel S. Differential distribution of cardiac ion channel expression as a basis for regional specialization in electrical function. *Circ Res* 2002; **90**: 939–50.

110. Matsuda H, Saigusa A, Irisawa H. Ohmic conductance through the inwardly rectifying K channel and blocking by internal Mg^{2+}. *Nature* 1987; **325**: 156–9.

111. Vandenberg CA. Inward rectification of a potassium channel in cardiac ventricular cells depends on internal magnesium ions. *Proc Natl Acad Sci U S A* 1987; **84**: 2560–4.

112. Ficker E, Taglialatela M, Wible BA, Henley CM, Brown AM. Spermine and spermidine as gating molecules for inward rectifier K^+ channels. *Science* 1994; **266**: 1068–72.

113. Lopatin AN, Makhina EN, Nichols CG. Potassium channel block by cytoplasmic polyamines as the mechanism of intrinsic rectification. *Nature* 1994; **372**: 366–9.

114. Wible BA, De Biasi M, Majumder K, Taglialatela M, Brown AM. Cloning and functional expression of an inwardly rectifying K^+ channel from human atrium. *Circ Res* 1995; **76**: 343–50.

115. Tamargo J, Caballero R, Gomez R, Valenzuela C, Delpon E. Pharmacology of cardiac potassium channels. *Cardiovasc Res* 2004; **62**: 9–33.

116. Miake J, Marban E, Nuss HB. Functional role of inward rectifier current in heart probed by Kir2.1 overexpression and dominant-negative suppression. *J Clin Invest* 2003; **111**: 1529–36.

117. Krapivinsky G, Gordon EA, Wickman K, *et al.* The G-protein-gated atrial K^+ channel IKACh is a heteromultimer of two inwardly rectifying K^+-channel proteins. *Nature* 1995; **374**: 135–41.

118. Inagaki N, Gonoi T, Clement JP, *et al.* Reconstitution of IKATP: an inward rectifier subunit plus the sulfonylurea receptor. *Science* 1995; **270**: 1166–70.

119. Gogelein H. Inhibition of cardiac ATP-dependent potassium channels by sulfonylurea drugs. *Curr Opin Investig Drugs* 2001; **2**: 72–80.

120. Nabauer M, Kaab S. Potassium channel down-regulation in heart failure. *Cardiovasc Res* 1998; **37**: 324–34.

121. Tomaselli GF, Marban E. Electrophysiological remodeling in hypertrophy and heart failure. *Cardiovasc Res* 1999; **42**: 270–83.

122. Dobrev D, Graf E, Wettwer E, *et al.* Molecular basis of downregulation of G-protein-coupled inward rectifying K (+) current (I(K,ACh) in chronic human atrial fibrillation: decrease in GIRK4 mRNA correlates with reduced I (K,ACh) and muscarinic receptor-mediated shortening of action potentials. *Circulation* 2001; **104**: 2551–7.

123. Das M, Das DK. Molecular mechanism of preconditioning. *IUBMB Life* 2008; **60**: 199–203.

124. Stadnicka A, Marinovic J, Ljubkovic M, Bienengraeber MW, Bosnjak ZJ. Volatile anesthetic-induced cardiac preconditioning. *J Anesth* 2007; **21**: 212–19.

125. Brady PA, Terzic A. The sulfonylurea controversy: more questions from the heart. *J Am Coll Cardiol* 1998; **31**: 950–6.

126. Sato T, Sasaki N, Seharaseyon J, O'Rourke B, Marban E. Selective pharmacological agents implicate mitochondrial but not sarcolemmal K (ATP) channels in ischemic cardioprotection. *Circulation* 2000; **101**: 2418–23.

127. DiFrancesco D, Borer JS. The funny current: cellular basis for the control of heart rate. *Drugs* 2007; **67** (Suppl 2): 15–24.

128. Ludwig A, Zong X, Jeglitsch M, Hofmann F, Biel M. A family of hyperpolarization-activated mammalian cation channels. *Nature* 1998; **393**: 587–91.

129. Yu H, Chang F, Cohen IS. Pacemaker current exists in ventricular myocytes. *Circ Res* 1993; **72**: 232–6.

130. Bucchi A, Barbuti A, Baruscotti M, DiFrancesco D. Heart rate reduction via selective 'funny' channel blockers. *Curr Opin Pharmacol* 2007; **7**: 208–13.

131. Backx PH, Marban E. Background potassium current active during the plateau of the action potential in guinea

pig ventricular myocytes. *Circ Res* 1993; **72**: 890–900.

132. Yue DT, Marban E. A novel cardiac potassium channel that is active and conductive at depolarized potentials. *Pflugers Arch* 1988; **413**: 127–33.

133. Lesage F, Guillemare E, Fink M, *et al.* TWIK-1, a ubiquitous human weakly inward rectifying K^+ channel with a novel structure. *EMBO J* 1996; **15**: 1004–11.

134. Hume JR, Duan D, Collier ML, Yamazaki J, Horowitz B. Anion transport in heart. *Physiol Rev* 2000; **80**: 31–81.

135. Tinel N, Diochot S, Borsotto M, Lazdunski M, Barhanin J. KCNE2 confers background current characteristics to the cardiac KCNQ1 potassium channel. *EMBO J* 2000; **19**: 6326–30.

136. Balser JR, George AL. Pharmacology of ion channels. In: Rose MR, Griggs RC, eds., *Channelopathies of the Nervous System*. Boston, MA: Butterworth-Heinemann, 2001: 23–48.

137. Armstrong CM. Ionic pores, gates, and gating currents. *Q Rev Biophys* 1975; **7**: 179.

138. Choi KL, Mossman C, Aube J, Yellen G. The internal quaternary ammonium receptor site of Shaker potassium channels. *Neuron* 1993; **10**: 533–41.

139. Strichartz GR. The inhibition of sodium currents in myelinated nerve by quaternary derivatives of lidocaine. *J Gen Physiol* 1973; **62**: 37–57.

140. Ragsdale DS, McPhee JC, Scheuer T, Catterall WA. Common molecular determinants of local anesthetic, antiarrhythmic, and anticonvulsant block of voltage-gated Na^+ channels. *Proc Natl Acad Sci U S A* 1996; **93**: 9270–5.

141. Hockerman GH, Johnson BD, Scheuer T, Catterall WA. Molecular determinants of high affinity phenylalkylamine block of L-type calcium channels. *J Biol Chem* 1995; **270**: 22119–22.

142. Schuster A, Lacinova L, Klugbauer N, *et al.* The IVS6 segment of the L-type calcium channel is critical for the action of dihydropyridines and phenylalkylamines. *EMBO J* 1996; **15**: 2365–70.

143. Sunami A, Dudley SC, Fozzard HA. Sodium channel selectivity filter regulates antiarrhythmic drug binding. *Proc Natl Acad Sci U S A* 1997; **94**: 14126–31.

144. Hille B. Local anesthetics: hydrophilic and hydrophobic pathways for the drug-receptor reaction. *J Gen Physiol* 1977; **69**: 497–515.

145. Trimmer JS, Cooperman SS, Tomiko SA, *et al.* Primary structure and functional expression of a mammalian skeletal muscle sodium channel. *Neuron* 1989; **3**: 33–49.

146. Balser JR, Nuss HB, Chiamvimonvat N, *et al.* External pore residue mediates slow inactivation in mu 1 rat skeletal muscle sodium channels. *J Physiol* 1996; **494**: 431–42.

147. Chen Z, Ong BH, Kambouris NG, *et al.* Lidocaine induces a slow inactivated state in rat skeletal muscle sodium channels. *J Physiol* 2000; **524**: 37–49.

148. Kambouris NG, Hastings LA, Stepanovic S, *et al.* Mechanistic link between lidocaine block and inactivation probed by outer pore mutations in the rat micro1 skeletal muscle sodium channel. *J Physiol* 1998; **512**: 693–705.

149. Ong BH, Tomaselli GF, Balser JR. A structural rearrangement in the sodium channel pore linked to slow inactivation and use dependence. *J Gen Physiol* 2000; **116**: 653–62.

150. Mitcheson JS, Chen J, Sanguinetti MC. Trapping of a methanesulfonanilide by closure of the HERG potassium channel activation gate. *J Gen Physiol* 2000; **115**: 229–40.

151. Mitcheson JS, Chen J, Lin M, Culberson C, Sanguinetti MC. A structural basis for drug-induced long QT syndrome. *Proc Natl Acad Sci U S A* 2000; **97**: 12329–33.

152. Roepke TK, Abbott GW. Pharmacogenetics and cardiac ion channels. *Vascul Pharmacol* 2006; **44**: 90–106.

Physiologic substrates of drug action
Myocardial performance

Pierre Foëx and Helen Higham

Introduction

The heart must be able to deliver oxygen and fuels to, and remove carbon dioxide and metabolic byproducts from, the tissues. It must also allow for the transport of hormones, vasoactive and immune substances, and a large number of metabolic mediators. Because the heart is coupled to two circulations, its performance is, to a large extent, determined by the characteristics of these circulations.

System physiology

Cardiac cycle

Before mechanical activity begins, an electrical signal is delivered by a specialized conduction system to the myocardium. This system controls the heart rate and responds to a variety of influences, notably sympathetic and parasympathetic stimulation. It provides a sequence of activation that maximizes efficient contraction and filling, while initiating the biochemical processes that underlie contraction. The conduction-system cells undergo spontaneous depolarization, thereby functioning as pacemakers. The sinoatrial node, having the fastest rate of spontaneous depolarization, provides the normal initiation of contraction.

The spread of electrical impulses through the myocardium forms, at the body surface, the signal described as the electrocardiogram (ECG). At the cellular level, electrical excitation consists of transmission of membrane depolarization followed by repolarization – the action potential that is propagated through the myocardium. The action potential arises in the sinoatrial node and spreads to the atria, causing atrial contraction. Impulses in the atrial conduction system converge on the atrioventricular node and more distally reach the His bundle. Conduction is slow in the atrioventricular node, such that there is a delay between atrial and ventricular contraction. This delay facilitates ventricular filling.

The His bundle gives rise to intraventricular fascicles, the right and left bundles, with the latter divided into left anterior and left posterior fascicles. Depolarization of the atria accounts for the P wave, while depolarization of the ventricles accounts

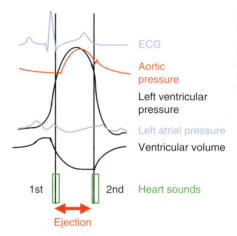

Figure 21.1. Schematic representation of the temporal relationships of electrical, mechanical, and auditory events of the cardiac cycle. ECG, electrocardiogram.

ECG

Aortic pressure

Left ventricular pressure

Left atrial pressure

Ventricular volume

1st   2nd   Heart sounds

Ejection

for the QRS complex of the ECG. Within the myocardium, the action potential spreads from myocyte to myocyte through the intercalated disks.

The mechanical cycle, conventionally, begins at end-diastole just before activation of the ventricle causes a rapid increase in intraventricular pressure (Fig. 21.1). As pressure in the ventricles exceeds atrial pressure, the atrioventricular valves close. When ventricular pressures exceed aortic and pulmonary pressures, the aortic and pulmonary valves open and ejection begins. Before ejection starts, ventricular contractions are isovolumic. During ejection, ventricular, aortic, and pulmonary artery pressures increase and decrease together. Ejection stops when aortic and pulmonary pressures exceed their respective ventricular pressures, causing the aortic and pulmonary valves to close; these events are marked by dicrotic notches. Whereas in the left ventricle there is a rapid decrease in pressure before the mitral valve opens, representing isovolumic relaxation, the low pulmonary artery pressure in respect of the right atrial pressure makes isovolumic relaxation almost nonexistent in the right ventricle [1]. Opening of the atrioventricular valves allows ventricular filling to begin. The initial rapid filling phase is followed by slow filling, and an almost complete halt (diastasis) before atrial contraction completes the ventricular filling.

Anesthetic Pharmacology, 2nd edition, ed. Alex S. Evers, Mervyn Maze, Evan D. Kharasch. Published by Cambridge University Press. © Cambridge University Press 2011.

Whereas systolic pressures between left and right ventricle differ because of differences in ventricular wall thickness and in resistance to ejection, diastolic filling pressure is only slightly greater in the left ventricle because of its thicker, less distensible, wall.

The heart attached to the circulation

Vascular systems

The heart is at the center of two series-coupled vascular circuits: the pulmonary and the systemic vascular beds. The elasticity of the larger arteries and the resistance to flow of the peripheral vessels reduce the changes in arterial and pulmonary pressures with respect to the changes in ventricular pressures.

The large arteries offer little resistance to flow, are distensible, and damp the pulsatile output of the ventricles. Their elasticity allows systolic storage and diastolic propulsion of blood flow between cardiac contractions. As blood reaches small arteries, flow is relatively steady throughout the cardiac cycle in the systemic but not in the pulmonary circulation, where it remains pulsatile. As arteries subdivide, the proportion of elastic fibers decreases and the walls become thinner. In the systemic circulation, the media of the arterioles consist predominantly of smooth muscle with a rich nerve supply. The caliber of arterioles determines the distribution of blood flow throughout the body and allows arterial pressure to be maintained within relatively narrow limits in the face of even large changes in cardiac output. In the pulmonary circulation, large changes in cardiac output are accommodated by recruitment of capillaries.

The systemic precapillary resistance vessels, consisting of small arteries and arterioles, offer the greater part of the total resistance to flow. Small changes in their diameter cause large changes in their resistance. Even though at each branching the combined cross-sectional area of the branches exceeds that of the stem, the resistance offered to flow increases because the radius of each branch is smaller than that of the stem. This is because resistance (R) is inversely proportional to the cross-sectional area of the vessel multiplied by the square of its radius:

$$R = 8\eta L/\pi r^2 \cdot r^2 \qquad (21.1)$$

where η is the fluid viscosity, L is the length of the vessel, and r is its radius.

The precapillary sphincters determine the size of the capillary exchange area by altering the number of open capillaries. The capillary exchange vessels form a dense network with a large cross-sectional area, a large surface limited by a single layer of endothelial cells, and a short length. The average dimensions of individual systemic capillaries are: radius 3 μm, length 750 μm, cross-sectional area 30 μm^2, and surface area 15 000 μm^2. At rest, 25–35% of the capillaries are open, and the effective total surface area is between 250 and 350 m^2. The pulmonary capillaries are wider (4 μm) and shorter (350 μm) than the systemic capillaries; their total effective surface area is approximately 60 m^2 at rest, increasing to 90 m^2 in heavy exercise [2,3]. The average transit time through the lung capillaries is approximately 1 second, decreasing to 0.35 s with heavy exercise.

The functional state of the greater and lesser circulations determines both the venous return to the ventricle (the preload) and the dynamic load imposed on its ejection (the afterload). The level of activity of all tissues and organs, through local regulation, determines their blood flow and the total cardiac output. As this, in turn, determines venous return, the preload of the right ventricle is a function of metabolic demands unless extraneous factors alter the size of the capacitance vessels. The pulmonary circulation passively adapts to accommodate the cardiac output with little change in pressure unless the pulmonary vasculature is diseased. Thus, in normal circumstances, the preload of the left ventricle is the same as that of the right ventricle. When metabolic demands increase, resistance to left ventricular ejection is reduced and ejection is facilitated.

Vascular resistance is the relationship between mean pressure and mean flow assuming a nonpulsatile circulation. However, pressure and flow are pulsatile, especially in the pulmonary circulation. Thus the concept of impedance, the dynamic relationship between pressure and flow, is more appropriate. Impedance includes a mean term (mean pressure and mean flow), and pulsatile terms, the impedance moduli for different harmonics of the fundamental frequency (the heart rate) [4]. In the systemic circulation, the static component of the impedance spectrum (i.e., systemic vascular resistance) is large with respect to the oscillatory components. By contrast, in the pulmonary circulation, the static term (pulmonary vascular resistance) is much smaller, and oscillatory components cannot be ignored as they contribute significantly to the load opposing right ventricular ejection.

Cardiac pump function

The effects of changes in preload on cardiac pump function have been characterized by Starling [5] and later by Sarnoff [6]. An increase in the filling of the ventricles causes a curvilinear increase in stroke volume, stroke work, and cardiac output.

Increases in contractility shift the ventricular function curve upward, whereas decreases shift it downward (Fig. 21.2). Ventricular function is also influenced by the afterload: increases and decreases in resistance shift the ventricular function curve downward and upward, respectively (Fig. 21.3). In the presence of cardiac muscle dysfunction, an increased afterload causes larger reductions of stroke volume and cardiac output than in the healthy heart.

In the healthy heart, increases in resistance cause a decrease in ejection that is limited by the presence of a homeometric mechanism: as the initial end-diastolic volume increases, the preload increases for the next contraction. This effect allows output to be relatively well maintained in the face of rising afterload, unless the heart is damaged.

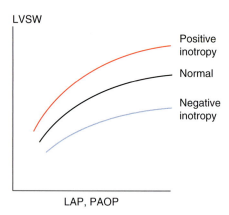

Figure 21.2. The relationship between left ventricular stroke work (LVSW) and left ventricular filling pressure, represented by left atrial pressure (LAP) and pulmonary artery occluded pressure (PAOP). Ventricular function curves are shifted upward or downward by increases/decreases in contractility.

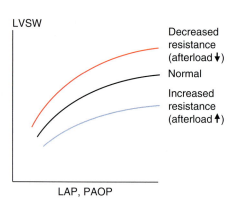

Figure 21.3. The relationship between cardiac work (stroke work) and filling pressures, as in Fig. 21.2. Ventricular function curves are shifted upward by increases and downward by reductions in vascular resistance (afterload).

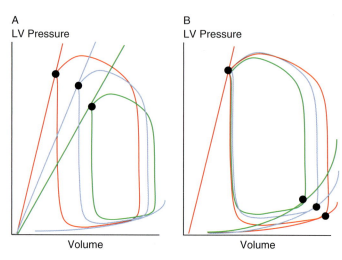

Figure 21.5. (A) Changes in contractility cause respectively an increase (positive inotropy) or a decrease (negative inotropy) of the slope of the end-systolic pressure–volume relationship (E_{max}). (B) Changes in ventricular compliance alter the shape of the end-diastolic pressure volume relationship. As a consequence, for a constant level of contractility, the width of the loop decreases (reduced compliance) or increases (increased compliance).

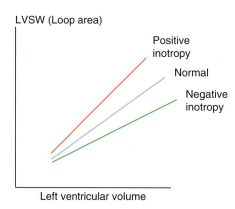

Figure 21.6. Plotting the stroke work (loop area) as a function of left ventricular volume results in straight lines, the slope of which indicates the inotropic state of the myocardium.

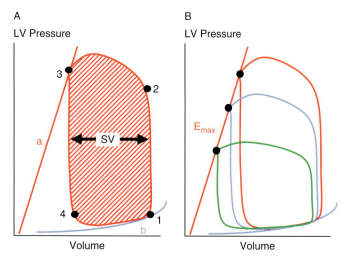

Figure 21.4. Each cardiac cycle can be represented by a pressure–volume loop. In (A), (1) denotes mitral valve closure, (2) aortic valve opening, (3) aortic valve closure, and (4) mitral valve opening. The end-systolic (a) and the end-diastolic (b) pressure–volume relationships represent the boundaries for the loops. (B) At a given inotropic state, all loops extend to the end-systolic pressure–volume relationship, also termed maximum elastance (E_{max}). SV, stroke volume.

The dynamic characteristics of the cardiac pump are best described in terms of pressure–volume relationships, represented as pressure–volume loops (Fig. 21.4A). Isovolumic contraction, ejection, isovolumic relaxation, and ventricular filling constitute the four segments of the loop and are delineated for the left ventricle, in succession, by mitral valve closure, aortic

valve opening, aortic valve closure, and mitral valve opening. The width of the pressure–volume loop represents the stroke volume and its area represents the stroke work. The *end-diastolic* pressure–volume coordinates form part of the end-diastolic pressure–volume relationship or ventricular compliance, whereas the *end-systolic* pressure–volume coordinates form part of the end-systolic pressure–volume relationship or maximum ventricular elastance (Fig. 21.4B) [7,8]. Irrespective of preload and afterload, all ventricular pressure–volume loops are bounded by these relationships unless contractility is altered resulting in a change in maximum elastance (Fig. 21.5A). Similarly, a decrease in compliance shifts the end-diastolic pressure–volume relationship upward, while an increase in compliance shifts it downward (Fig. 21.5B).

Based on the pressure–volume relationships, contractility can be represented by the preload recruitable stroke work. The area of pressure–volume loops (the stroke work) is plotted against left ventricular end-diastolic volume (Fig. 21.6); the coordinates of stroke work and end-diastolic volume form a straight line, the slope of which is an index of contractility [9]. Cardiac function is often assessed as the relationship between stroke volume and end-diastolic volume: the ejection fraction. Because the stroke volume depends on preload, afterload, contractility, and compliance, the ejection fraction is not a pure index of contractility [10].

The determinants of cardiac pump function are influenced by the activity of the autonomic nervous system. Stimulation of β_1-adrenoceptors increases contractility and heart rate, whereas β_2-adrenoceptor stimulation increases contractility and heart rate and decreases vascular tone. Stimulation of β_3-adrenoceptors decreases contractility and may play a role in the development of heart failure [11]. Stimulation of the α_1-adrenoceptors decreases venous compliance and increases systemic vascular tone.

Coronary circulation

The heart has to provide its own perfusion while supplying blood flow to the whole body. This imposes considerable metabolic demands on the heart muscle and therefore on the coronary circulation. Yet perfusion is impeded by the high extravascular compressive forces resulting from the development of wall tension during ventricular systole. Thus, oxygen extraction approaches 70% at rest [12]. Increases in myocardial oxygen consumption (mVO_2) must be met by commensurate increases in coronary blood flow, because there is little scope for an increase in extraction. Consequently, there is a linear relationship between coronary blood flow and myocardial oxygen consumption [13,14].

The large epicardial branches of the left and right coronary arteries give rise to smaller branches. These penetrate the myocardium at right angles and divide in an extensive network of small arteries and arterioles that, in turn, give rise to an extremely dense capillary network. The intercapillary distance is approximately 10–14 μm and there is one capillary for each cardiac fiber. Thus the distance between capillaries and sites of oxygen utilization is only a few micrometers. Control of subepicardial and subendocardial vessels allows the transmural distribution of blood flow to adjust oxygen supply to local demands. There are intercoronary and intracoronary collateral vessels.

The endothelium of the coronary circulation plays an important role because it is capable of releasing endothelium-dependent vasoactive substances. Shear stress, pulsatile flow, and hypoxia stimulate the production of prostacyclin, a potent coronary vasodilator [15]. Similarly, shear stress, hypoxia, and acetylcholine stimulate the constitutive nitric oxide synthase (NOS), thereby increasing the production and release of NO, resulting in cyclic guanosine monophosphate (cGMP)-mediated coronary vasodilation. Endothelium-dependent vasoconstrictors such as endothelins, thromboxane A_2, and angiotensin are also released under the influence of endogenous and exogenous substances, or stimuli, or both [16,17]. An imbalance between vasodilators and vasoconstrictors can develop in advanced coronary artery disease, especially a reduced release of NO and an increased synthesis of endothelins. The latter cause vasoconstriction and facilitate platelet adhesion, increasing the risk of thrombosis and facilitating smooth-muscle proliferation.

Regulation of myocardial perfusion

The major determinant of coronary vascular resistance is intramyocardial pressure. During systole, lateral shearing forces may completely abolish flow to certain regions of the myocardium [18]. In the wall of the left ventricle, systolic extravascular compression is so pronounced that only 20–30% of flow occurs during systole, with 70–80% during diastole. In the wall of the right ventricle, because the compressive forces are much lower than in the left ventricle, flow occurs during both systole and diastole. Because of greater metabolic requirements, subendocardial flow exceeds subepicardial flow by approximately 10% [19]. The greater degree of vasodilation at the subendocardium reduces its flow reserve and makes it more sensitive to a reduction in coronary perfusion pressure.

The coronary perfusion pressure is the difference between the upstream and downstream pressures. The former is the pressure at the aortic root during diastole, whereas the latter can be taken as the coronary sinus pressure or the left ventricular end-diastolic pressure [20]. The critical closing pressure may be a truer downstream pressure; it is derived from the pressure–flow relationship during a long diastole where flow becomes zero at a pressure that is greater than the left ventricular end-diastolic pressure [21].

The coronary flow reserve is the difference between locally regulated flow and flow when the coronary arteries are maximally dilated [22]. The coronary flow reserve varies with the coronary perfusion pressure and is reduced in the presence of coronary artery lesions.

Autoregulation of coronary blood flow

Autoregulation is the intrinsic ability of the heart to maintain constant coronary flow in the face of changing coronary perfusion pressure, as demonstrated in experimental studies where the coronary circulation is perfused independently [23]. Autoregulation may be the result of myogenic mechanisms and of changes in metabolic mediators. In the intact heart, increases in coronary perfusion pressure always result from greater systemic and left ventricular pressures, and are therefore associated with increased metabolic demands (Fig. 21.7). As metabolic demand is increasing, coronary flow must increase.

Metabolic control of myocardial blood flow

Metabolic control of coronary blood flow results from local mechanisms. Metabolic demands are the sum of basal metabolism (25–50%), wall tension (30%), external work (10–15%), activation processes (10–15%), and electrical activity (1%) [24]. The major determinants of wall tension and

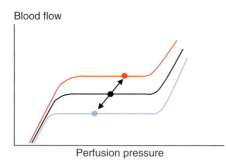

Blood flow

Perfusion pressure

Figure 21.7. The relationship between blood flow and perfusion pressure exhibits autoregulation in many tissues. In the intact heart, as metabolic requirements vary with changes in coronary perfusion pressure generated by the heart itself, coronary blood flow must be adjusted to meet the metabolic requirements.

external work are heart rate, systolic pressure, ventricular diastolic pressure, and contractility. The precise mechanisms of the coupling of blood flow and metabolic demands are not fully elucidated. They include local PO_2, PCO_2, pH, potassium and calcium concentration, osmolality, and adenosine [25]. It is postulated that a reduction in cellular oxygen partial pressure causes an increase in the synthesis and release of adenosine. Adenosine, in turn, acts on the vascular smooth muscle causing coronary vasodilation. However, adenosine does not appear to be the primary mediator of the close coupling of oxygen demand and supply. Adenosine triphosphate (ATP)-sensitive potassium channels (K_{ATP} channels), play a major role. Opening of the K_{ATP} channels results in hyperpolarization of the cell membrane. This closes the calcium channels; as cytosolic Ca^{2+} decreases, vascular smooth muscle relaxes. K_{ATP} channels are opened by receptor activation (adenosine, acetylcholine) or by metabolic factors (decreased ATP caused by hypoxia or ischemia) [26]. Blockade of K_{ATP} channels increases coronary vascular resistance and reduces coronary blood flow [27]. Other substances including prostaglandins and NO alter coronary vascular resistance, and NO plays a role in the normal control of coronary blood flow [28].

Neurogenic control of coronary blood flow

Cholinergic stimulation causes NO-mediated coronary vasodilation [29]. Adrenergic stimulation increases metabolic demands by increasing heart rate and contractility (β_1 stimulation) and arterial pressure (α_1 stimulation). This results in increases in oxygen consumption that, in turn, increase coronary blood flow because the vasoconstriction caused by α_1-adrenoceptor stimulation is overshadowed by local metabolic regulation. However, in the case of hypoperfusion, local and neurogenic regulation may compete, the latter opposing the metabolic vasodilation. Indeed, if the endothelium is damaged, α_1-mediated vasoconstriction is enhanced [30].

Redundancies in coronary vasomotor control allow for very large increases in coronary blood flow during maximum exercise. In addition, training causes an increase in resting myogenic tone that increases the scope for vasodilation and augments endothelium-dependent vasodilation throughout the coronary microcirculation mediated by increased expression of NOS [31].

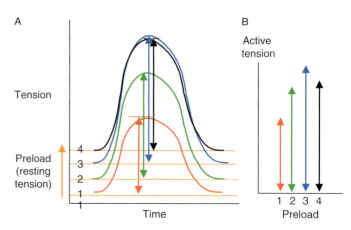

A

Tension

Preload
(resting
tension)

4
3
2
1

Time

B

Active
tension

1 2 3 4

Preload

Figure 21.8. Isometric contractions. (A) shows several contractions starting at different preloads (1–4). As can be seen in (A) and (B), increasing the preload increases the active tension up to a peak (preload 1–3), followed by a decline when preload becomes too high (preload 4).

Organ physiology

Most of the knowledge relating to cardiac mechanics derives from observations made in two experimental models: isometric and isotonic contractions.

During *isometric contractions*, from a set resting length (and its associated resting tension) representing the true preload, the muscle develops its active tension (Fig. 21.8). With increases in resting tension the active tension increases up to a maximum and then declines (Fig. 21.8). The influence of the preload on the active tension is the expression of Starling's law of the heart [5]. Studies of isolated cardiac fibers have shown that the maximum active force occurs for a sarcomere length of 2.2 μm [32]. This length is optimal for the formation of crossbridges. Below that length the overlap of actin and myosin is too extensive and fewer crossbridges are formed; alternatively, at short sarcomere lengths, actin and myosin are further apart because of an increase in interfilament lattice spacing. This results in a length dependence of Ca^{2+} sensitivity and reduced crossbridge formation [33]. Conversely, beyond the optimal length, the overlap of actin and myosin is reduced and force development is inhibited. This traditional view is now challenged as the pericellular collagen and connecting filaments within the cardiac cells confer a high resting stiffness that opposes myofibrils overstretching. The degree of actin–myosin overlap (a function of the resting length) may not be the critical factor in Starling's law of the heart [34]. Length-dependent mechanisms may increase the sensitivity of the myofilaments to Ca^{2+}.

The heart muscle is sensitive to Ca^{2+} and to a large number of hormones and drugs that increase its contractility at constant preload and rate of contraction. Positive inotropic interventions, for a given preload, increase the active force the muscle can develop; conversely, drugs with negative inotropy (halogenated anesthetics, calcium channel antagonists) decrease the active force. Inotropic interventions cause their effect through

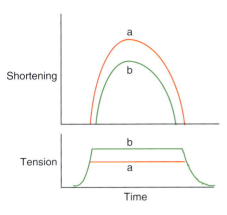

Figure 21.9. For isotonic contractions, two sets of traces show that for a lower developed tension (a, in red) there is more shortening than for a higher developed tension (b, in green).

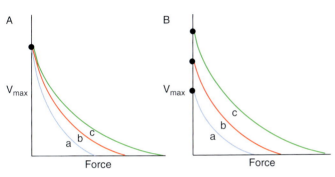

Figure 21.10. The force–velocity relationship. (A) Increases in preload (a to c) do not alter the velocity of contraction at zero force (V_{max}) as obtained by extrapolation to zero force of the velocity of shortening. (B) Increases (b to c) and decreases (b to a) in inotropy alter both V_{max} and developed force.

an increase in myoplasmic Ca^{2+} or by increasing the sensitivity of the contractile apparatus to Ca^{2+}. These effects are additive to those of increasing the preload.

During *isotonic contractions*, once enough force has developed, the muscle develops shortening at a constant load (i.e., the afterload) (Fig. 21.9). The extent of shortening and its velocity are inversely related to the afterload. Extrapolation of the velocity–force relationship to zero force yields a maximum velocity of shortening (V_{max}) that is unchanged by alterations of the preload (Fig. 21.10A). By contrast, positive inotropic interventions increase V_{max} and developed tension (Fig. 21.10B) [35,36].

In the intact heart, the maximum velocity of circumferential shortening, the maximum rate of pressure development of the ventricles, the peak power of the left ventricle, and the acceleration of the blood in the aorta relate closely to the maximum velocity of shortening. These variables are used as indices of contractility. However, they are influenced by the loading conditions of the ventricle. This is not the case for maximum elastance, which is preload- and afterload-independent.

Diastolic ventricular function

Immediately after the peak of left ventricular pressure has been reached, relaxation dominates over contraction. When the ventricular pressure becomes lower than the atrial pressure, the mitral valve opens and ventricular filling begins. Early filling is rapid but it becomes slower (diastasis), and atrial contraction may contribute as much as 25% of total ventricular filling.

Over a wide range of rates the duration of systole varies within relatively narrow limits (typically from 300 to 200 ms), but the duration of diastole decreases substantially from 500 to 125 ms as heart rate increases from 75 to 180 beats per minute. The reduced duration of diastole ultimately limits both ventricular filling and coronary perfusion.

Diastole uses approximately 15% of the energy of the cardiac cycle [37]. In hypertensive heart disease, cardiomyopathies, and myocardial ischemia, too much oxygen is used up to sustain systole and there is not enough left for effective diastole. Therfore, the diastolic characteristics of the ventricles may be affected before systolic dysfunction occurs [38].

Isovolumic relaxation can be described as an exponential function and expressed as a time constant (τ). Several equations are used for this analysis. The most frequently used is:

$$P(t) = P_o \, e^{-\nu/\tau} \tag{21.2}$$

where P is left ventricular pressure, P_o is the left ventricular pressure at peak negative dP/dt, and t is time [39].

The time constant of isovolumic relaxation (τ) depends on load, inactivation, homogeneity of relaxation in the whole ventricle, and coronary blood flow [40]. Fibers relax more quickly at high load, and this is facilitated by the diastolic engorgement of the coronary vessels that increases wall thickness, intramyocardial pressure, and diastolic load [41]. Conversely, inhomogeneity of relaxation (dyssynchrony) increases the time constant of isovolumic relaxation. Dyssynchrony is a feature of myocardial ischemia that impairs isovolumic relaxation [42].

Dissociation of the crossbridges between actin and myosin allows the sarcomeres to lengthen and the ventricles to fill. Ventricular dilation and myocardial fibrosis decrease the efficiency of filling.

The peristaltic nature of atrial contraction and the geometry of the venoatrial junctions minimize the backward transmission of pressure, especially into the pulmonary veins [43]. The Frank–Starling mechanism operates in the left atrium [44]. As a result, the contribution of atrial systole is increased in hypertrophic cardiomyopathies, in the presence of myocardial infarction, and in the elderly [45,46]. In the presence of mitral or tricuspid valve disease, large differences in rapid filling and its relationship with late filling occur. The pattern of flow through the atrioventricular valves, recorded by ultrasonography, is used to determine the severity of mitral or tricuspid lesions [47].

Ventricular compliance, or its reciprocal, ventricular stiffness, can be estimated from the relationship between pressure and volume at end-diastole and by analyzing the instantaneous relationship between pressure and volume during individual diastoles [48]. If ventricular stiffness is acutely or chronically increased, ventricular filling may be impaired such that hypo- and hypervolemia cause large changes in end-diastolic ventricular pressure and in cardiac output. With increased ventricular stiffness, hypervolemia may cause pulmonary edema, whereas hypovolemia may cause an exaggerated reduction of cardiac output.

Diastolic stiffness may be structural (ventricular hypertrophy, fibrosis) or functional (hypoxia, ischemia, altered diastolic handling of Ca^{2+}). Increased ventricular stiffness is the first manifestation of hypertrophic cardiomyopathies, hypertensive heart disease, and acute myocardial ischemia [49]. This is often reflected in a high pulmonary artery occlusion pressure (PAOP; or pulmonary capillary wedge pressure, PCWP). Episodes of regional myocardial ischemia may cause stiffening of both the ischemic and remote well-perfused myocardium, resulting in a global increase in ventricular stiffness [50].

Cellular physiology

The cardiac cell

Myocytes are branched filament-like structures 10–20 μm in diameter and 50–100 μm in length attached to one another at intercalated disks. Approximately every 2 μm in their longitudinal axis, transverse tubules (T tubules) penetrate the cells and facilitate their activation because they are regions of ion fluxes.

Cardiac cells include three systems: (1) the sarcolemmal excitation system (conduction and initiation of intracellular events responsible for contraction); (2) an intracellular excitation–contraction coupling system that converts an amplified electrical signal into a chemical signal; and (3) a contractile system within which crossbridges between actin and myosin are formed.

The basic contractile functional unit is the sarcomere, composed of two bundles of longitudinal filaments, thick and thin. The thick filaments consist of about 300 individual molecules of myosin, approximately 1.6 μm in length and 10–15 μm in width. They are placed in the center of the sarcomere's length. Each molecule of myosin has a bilobed head [51]. Half of these are oriented toward one end of the sarcomere and half toward the other. Sets of three heads are rotated about 40 degrees in relation to each other, at a distance of 14.3 μm, allowing contact with the six surrounding filaments of actin.

The thin filaments are composed of actin, tropomyosin (Tm), and troponin (Tn). The actin molecules are approximately 1 μm long; they interdigitate with the myosin filaments at one end, and they are attached to the Z-line at the other end. Actin monomers are arranged in a double helix to form the core of the thin filament [52,53]. Tm is adsorbed longitudinally along the thin filament. Troponins C, I, and T (TnC, TnI, and TnT) are adsorbed on Tm. The combined Tn-Tm complex is responsible for the ability of calcium ions to act as a switch for the initiation of crossbridge formation. Each complex is

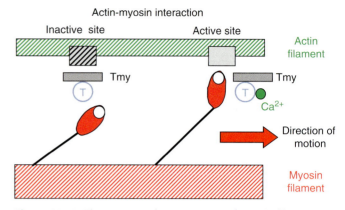

Figure 21.11. The interaction between actin and myosin filaments. As an interaction site on the actin filament becomes active, the lateral projections of myosin are elongated and the heads rotate. Tmy, tropomyosin; T, troponin.

1 μm in length and 5.7 nm in width, and they are positioned at intervals of 38 nm. TnC, the binding site for Ca^{2+}, is part of a complex that includes TnI (the inhibitory protein for the interaction of actin and myosin) and TnT, which links Tm and Tn to form the complex. Troponins are released when the myocardium is damaged. TnT and TnI are controlled by different genes in cardiac and skeletal muscle. They can be differentiated and used as markers of cardiac injury [54–56].

With activation, a change in cytosolic Ca^{2+} concentration causes calcium ions to bind to TnC and cause a rearrangement of the Tn-Tm complex with strong binding of TnI to TnC rather than to Tm. One site of Ca^{2+} binding on the TnC molecule is responsible for conformational changes in the distant region of the molecule, promoting contraction [57]. Calcium binding increases the total length of actin available for the formation of crossbridges. Calcium binding alters the position of Tm on actin and releases the inhibition of actin–myosin interaction (Fig. 21.11). The binding of Ca^{2+} to Tn causes the process of crossbridge formation to spread down the thin filament; strong binding encourages additional filament activation [58]. In addition to initiating the contractile cycle, Ca^{2+} alters the kinetics of crossbridge formation, altering the myosin ATPase activity, thereby increasing contractility [59]. During most physiologic conditions, systolic Ca^{2+} concentration does not achieve a level resulting in maximum force; this represents a contractile reserve. Once calcium is removed from the Tn-Tm complex, the active sites are blocked, the crossbridges separate, and relaxation and resting state ensue.

The mechanics of myocyte contraction are as follows: ATP supplies the energy to a process [60,61] during which there is abduction of the lateral projections of the myosin filaments with their articulated heads. This brings the heads closer to the actin filaments, thus allowing crossbridges to form at the level of new active sites on the actin molecules. Head rotation pulls on the arm and causes the actin filament to move relative to the myosin filament [62]. The formation of a crossbridge represents the consumption of one molecule of ATP. The total force developed is a function of the number of crossbridges. The rate of change of force depends on the number of crossbridges formed by unit time. Therefore both increased force development and increased rate of force development (i.e., increased contractility) contribute directly to the energy requirement of contraction.

In the absence of restraining forces, crossbridges propel the filaments at maximum speed with no force development (unloaded shortening). If an external load opposes shortening, crossbridge motion is slowed, allowing for force to be developed. At diastolic Ca^{2+} concentration, crossbridges exist in a truly detached or blocked state or a weakly attached state that does not produce force.

Myocytes are capable of rearranging the sarcomeres in response to physiologic or pathologic changes in demands. An increase in the number of sarcomeres in series increases the capacity for shortening, whereas an increase in parallel increases that for force generation.

Excitation–contraction coupling (ECC)

The excitation system consists of a transient local depolarizing inward sodium current that raises the transmembrane potential from –80 to –90 mV to slightly positive values followed by a repolarizing current. With respect to contraction, the most important component of the action potential is the slow inward Ca^{2+} current through voltage-sensitive L-type Ca^{2+} channels. Potassium efflux repolarizes the cell (timing of the various currents is displayed on Fig. 21.12). L-type Ca^{2+} channels are concentrated in the transverse tubules that are in close proximity to the sarcoplasmic reticulum (SR) membrane-associated ryanodine receptor calcium-release channels (RyRs; Fig. 21.13). The Na^+/Ca^{2+} exchanger moves calcium ions out of the cell against its concentration gradient

while using energy from the sodium gradient to move one sodium ion into the cell.

Pacemaker tissue

Pacemaker cells have the ability to depolarise spontaneously. The most important ionic current for regulating pacemaker activity in the sinoatrial node is the *funny current* (I_f), called "funny" because it has effects opposite to those of most other heart currents. I_f is a mixed Na^+/K^+ inward current activated by hyperpolarization at approximately –40 mV, and

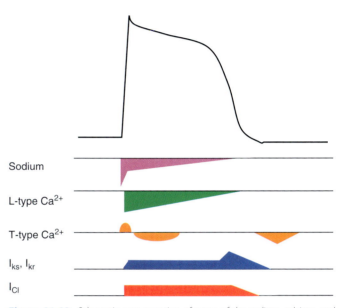

Figure 21.12. Schematic representation of some of the sodium, calcium, and potassium ion fluxes responsible for the action potential of cardiac cells. For each ion, inward fluxes are denoted by an area under the line, and outward fluxes are represented by an area above the line. Redrawn from Snyders [63].

Figure 21.13. Diagram representing channels and pumps in the vicinity of transverse tubules. (A) L-type Ca^{2+} channel; (B) sarcolemmal ryanodine receptor; (C) sarcoplasmic Ca^{2+} pump; (D) Na^+/Ca^{2+} exchange pump; (E) Ca^{2+} pump; (F) K^+ pump. The hatched area is the dyad. Modified from Katz [64].

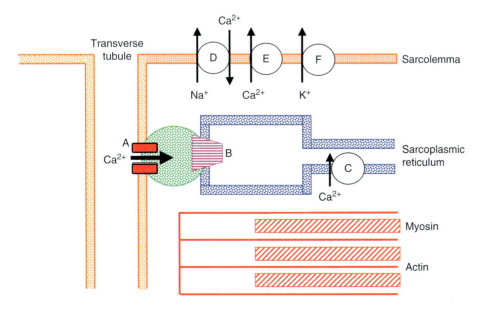

modulated by the autonomic nervous system. I_f is associated with cyclic-nucleotide-gated channels [65].

Contractile tissue

The SR encircles the contractile filaments at 1–2 μm spacing. It contains a large store of Ca^{2+} mostly bound with proteins such as calsequestrin. The action potential depolarizes the cell membrane in the region where T tubules are in close proximity to subsarcolemmal cisternae (the dyad); this opens the gate of L-type Ca^{2+} channels, allowing Ca^{2+} to cross the sarcolemma into the gap region of the dyad (Fig. 21.13). This local increase in Ca^{2+} concentration activates nearby RyRs, resulting in a triggered release of much larger amounts of Ca^{2+} from the cisternae of the SR into the cytoplasm [66,67]. As a result of this amplifying system, Ca^{2+} concentration increases from 0.1 to 1–10 μmol (peak of the Ca^{2+} transient). The interaction between L-type Ca^{2+} channels and RyRs is responsible for the high gain of graded Ca^{2+} release [68]. The steep rise in excitation–contraction coupling observed at hyperpolarized potentials is a result of increased functional coupling between L-type Ca^{2+} channels and ryanodine receptors [69].

The four monomers comprising the RyR play an important role in the dynamic of the whole receptor. This cooperativity can be affected by the binding of the FK506 binding protein. The immunophilins FKBP12 and FKBP12.6 appear to stabilize a closed state of the channel [70]. RyRs can be modulated by adrenergic stimulation via the phosphorylating action of protein kinase A (PKA). The level of cooperativity at RyRs is potentially relevant to heart failure [71].

The triggered Ca^{2+} release generates the second inward current, a component of the inward current also termed *tail current* because it is seen as a current "tail" after depolarizing pulses and is closely correlated with the contraction of the cell [72].

The increase in Ca^{2+} concentration is very transient because Ca^{2+} binds to contractile proteins and is removed both by the Na^+/Ca^{2+} exchanger and by sarcoplasmic Ca^{2+} ATPase (SERCA2) [73], a membrane-spanning protein of the SR that uses energy from ATP hydrolysis to pump Ca^{2+} back into the SR. The activity of SERCA2 is self-regulating such that its speed increases in proportion to free calcium concentration. It is also regulated by phospholamban, a key modulator of cardiac responses to adrenergic signaling [74]. As an example, β_1-adrenergic stimulation activates the cyclic adenosine monophosphate (cAMP)-dependent PKA, resulting in the phosphorylation of phospholamban. As phospholamban is phosphorylated, its inhibitory effect on SERCA2 is reduced, resulting in increased Ca^{2+} cycling and increased rate and force of contraction.

In order for relaxation to occur, Ca^{2+} concentration must return to its resting level. This involves reuptake of Ca^{2+} into the sarcoplasmic reticulum via SERCA2a, extrusion from the cell via the Na^+/Ca^{2+} exchanger (NCX1) and, to a lesser extent, the plasmalemmal Ca^{2+} ATPase (PMCA4b).

Although much of the emphasis on excitation–contraction coupling rests on Ca^{2+} channels, many other factors play an important role (Fig. 21.14). The cardiac sarcolemmal Na^+/Ca^{2+} exchange is essential for Ca^{2+} extrusion; it also contributes to a variable degree to the development of the systolic Ca^{2+} transient. Differential gene expressions of Na^+/Ca^{2+} exchange exist in cardiac disease and have implications for the excitation–contraction coupling. The Na^+/Ca^{2+} exchanger is capable of modulating SR Ca^{2+} handling, and at high expression level may interfere with the gating of the L-type Ca^{2+} current [75].

Control of contractility

Intrinsic control systems in the myocardium include the length-dependent activation and the force–frequency relation. Increases in the rate of stimulation augment the speed of contraction and relaxation and enhance the strength of contraction. This allows the stroke volume to be maintained even though less time is available for filling and emptying the ventricles. As frequency increases, there is more rapid Ca^{2+} cycling. Calcium entry increases as there is more frequent opening of L-type Ca^{2+} channels, at the same time the Ca^{2+} pump of the SR speeds up and SERCA2 activity increases.

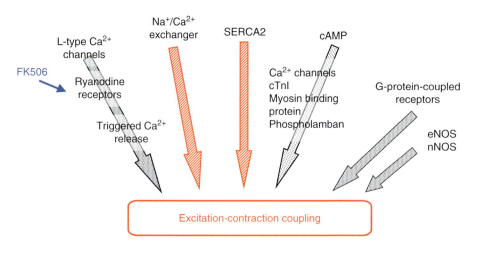

Figure 21.14. Some of the factors that determine excitation–contraction coupling, over and above the central role of calcium entry and triggered calcium release.

There are also important extrinsic control systems. cAMP is a key regulator of excitation–contraction coupling (ECC) and a mediator of the sympathetic control of the ECC through the activity of PKA. PKA phosphorylates several proteins involved in the ECC process: voltage-gated L-type Ca^{2+} channels (dihydropyridine receptors, DHPRs), sarcomeric troponin I (cTnI), myosin binding protein C (MBP-C), and phospholamban. Phosphorylation of these targets results in potentiated contraction (positive inotropy) and facilitated relaxation (lusitropy). The inotropic effect results mostly from increased Ca^{2+} currents, By contrast, the lusitropic effect is mediated by the phosphorylation of cTnI and MBP-C reducing the sensitivity of the myofilament to Ca^{2+} and speeding the dissociation of Ca^{2+} from the myofilments.

G-protein-coupled receptors other than β-adrenoceptors control metabolic enzymes and nuclear transcription factors. Such multiplicity of roles for cAMP-PKA signaling suggests that there is space-confined activity (compartmentalization) within the pathway. A family of functionally related proteins, termed A-kinase anchoring proteins (AKAP), includes more than 50 members, of which at least 13 are found in cardiac tissue. AKAP 15/180 targets PKA to the L-type Ca^{2+} channels such that the PKA-AKAP complex interacts with the α subunit of the channel. This enzyme causes rapid phosphorylation of the channel with efficient regulation in response to β-adrenergic simulation. mAKAP targets both PKA and phosphodiesterase 4D3 (PDE4D3) to RyRs. Proximity of PKA and PDE4D3 causes a two- to threefold increase in its phosphorylating activity rate. As a consequence, mAKAP-anchored PDE4D3 degrades cAMP in the vicinity of RyRs, creating a feedback loop [76].

The circulating angiotensin II peptide produces a positive inotropic effect by binding to its transmembrane G-protein-coupled receptors. A signaling cascade involves inositol 1,4,5-trisphosphate (IP_3) and protein kinase C (PKC) modulating an increase in intracellular Ca^{2+} concentration and/or increasing the sensitivity of the myofilaments to Ca^{2+}. Calcium currents, Na^+/Ca^{2+} exchange, sarcoplasmic Ca^{2+} release, Ca^{2+} transients, and contractile proteins all appear to be involved [77].

Nitric oxide (NO) also plays a role in both ECC and control of contractility [78]. NO is produced by endothelial cells and by the myocytes themselves [79]. Two isoforms of NO synthase (eNOS, nNOS) are constitutively expressed in cardiac myocytes. A third isoform, the inducible NOS (iNOS) is stimulated by inflammatory mediators.

Both eNOS and nNOS are activated by Ca^{2+} and produce NO at slower or faster rates, changing cyclically in synchrony with the heart beat. Changes in preload appear to be associated with parallel changes in intramyocardial NO concentration. Thus, NO appears to be involved in rapid autoregulatory mechanisms that modulate contraction on a beat-by-beat basis and assist in matching preload and cardiac output. As myocardial stretch causes stretch-dependent stimulation of NO

synthesis the Ca^{2+} spark rate increases and calcium waves arise from collected firing of calcium sparks [80,81]. Calcium waves, in turn, increase the developed contractile force (the Anrep effect). Stretch can also activate the Na^+/Ca^{2+} exchanger, resulting in higher intracellular Na^+, which will stimulate the entry of Ca^{2+} and put the Na^+/Ca^{2+} exchanger into reverse.

NO has been reported to alter the probability of the RyRs being in the open state. However, this does not necessarily increase the Ca^{2+} through Ca^{2+} current transient, as it will also depend upon the SR Ca^{2+} concentration. If the latter is substantially reduced, an increase in the RyR's open probability may function as a diastolic leak. NO has a negative inotropic effect mediated by cGMP possibly resulting in myofilament desensitization to calcium and a blunting of the responses to catecholamines [82]. In the failing heart, the physical association between nNOS and RyRs may decrease. Loss of nNOS-derived NO from the sarcoplasmic reticulum may result in increased free radical production [78]. This may contribute to decreased contractility in heart failure. As inflammatory cytokines enhance NOS3, through increased NO synthesis, they may depress cardiac function [83].

Myocardial metabolism

Adequate cardiac performance requires an appropriate supply of energy, as the normal myocardium utilizes approximately 6 kg of ATP daily [84]. There are three main components of cardiac metabolism: substrate utilization, oxidative phosphorylation, and ATP transfer and utilization [85].

The heart principally metabolizes free fatty acids (FFAs), which account for up to 70% of the substrate, with the remainder made up of glucose and other carbohydrates such as lactate. β-Oxidation and glycolysis, with the entry of intermediary metabolites into the Krebs cycle, are central to energy generation, as the phosphorylation of adenosine diphosphate (ADP) by the mitochondrial respiratory chain produces ATP (Fig. 21.15). The major source of energy (95%) is supplied by mitochondrial oxidative phosphorylation. For a given supply of ATP, oxidation of FFA requires 11% more oxygen than carbohydrates.

The creatine kinase energy shuttle transfers energy to the myofibril [86]. Mitochondrial creatine kinase catalyzes the transfer of the high-energy phosphate bond in ATP to creatine to form phosphocreatine and ADP. Produced by liver and kidneys, creatine is taken up in the heart by a specific transporter and two-thirds are phosphorylated into phosphocreatine in the mitochondria. It then diffuses to myofibrils, where a creatine kinase catalyzes the reformation of ATP. Finally free creatine diffuses back to the mitochondria.

Heart failure

In heart failure, substrate utilization can be reduced because of decreased substrate uptake, oxidation, or both. Fatty acid utilization is substantially decreased in advanced heart failure [87].

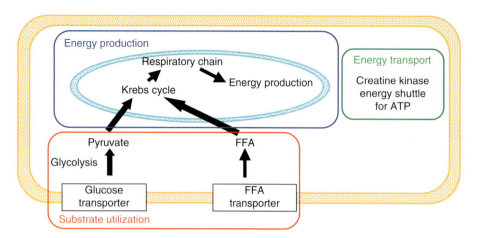

Figure 21.15. The relationships between energy substrate, production, and transfer in cardiac myocytes. Redrawn from Neubauer [85].

While glucose utilization is increased in early heart failure, it is reduced by insulin resistance in severe heart failure. Phosphocreatine and total creatine levels decrease earlier and to a greater extent than ATP. Mitochondrial creatine kinase may be reduced by 20% and myofibrillar creatine kinase by up to 50%. The loss of high-energy phosphates and creatine kinase activity reduces energy delivery to the myofibrils by up to 70% and explains the reduction in both contractility and inotropic reserve [85]. In addition, the level of uncoupling proteins may be increased, leading to generation of heat rather than ATP. This further reduces the energy available for contraction.

Several nuclear transcription factors rapidly couple gene expression with changing substrate. The peroxisome proliferator-activated receptor (PPAR) family plays an important role in fatty acid oxidation and can be altered in cardiac hypertrophy [88,89]. A nuclear-receptor coactivator, PPARγ, regulates the metabolic function of mitochondria by activating multiple genes that are responsible for fatty acid uptake and oxidation and for oxidative phosphorylation. High plasma catecholamine levels appear to reduce PPARγ through down-regulation of gene expression. This contributes to impaired oxidative phosphorylation.

Current and potential targets of drug action

The complexity of the excitation–contraction coupling is such that many mediators are involved, and new drugs could interact with these mediators and influence excitation, contraction, or coupling.

Control of arrhythmias has relied on drugs that alter sodium, calcium, and potassium fluxes and block the effects of sympathetic stimulation on the myocardium. Developments could include new compounds that have a selective effect on the funny channels. Though ivabradine has been tested for many years, there may be other compounds worthy of development.

Increasing contractility may be life-saving. However, most drugs do so by increasing the entry and triggered release of Ca^{2+}. This has two potential drawbacks: energy is needed for the reuptake of Ca^{2+} in the sarcoplasmic reticulum and for the extrusion of Ca^{2+} out of the cell, and in addition increased Ca^{2+} concentration facilitates arrhythmias. Sensitization of the troponin–tropomyosin apparatus to Ca^{2+} increases contractility. However, as Ca^{2+} concentration and Ca^{2+} fluxes are not increased there is no additional energy requirement over and above the energy required for the contractile process itself. Again, this is not new; levosimendan has been introduced, but other compounds may offer further advantages.

A different approach may be to alter substrate utilization. Partial inhibitors of fatty acid oxidation, or carnitine palmitoyl transferase 1 inhibitors, reduce fatty acid oxidation and promote glucose utilization. Trimetazidine, an inhibitor of fatty acid oxidation, has been shown to improve ventricular function in elderly patients and in patients with previous myocardial infarction and heart failure. Similarly, perhexiline or etoxomir (a carnitine palmitoyl transferase 1 inhibitor) improved left ventricular ejection fraction. Direct stimulation of oxidative phosphorylation is another possible strategy, but there is no effective stimulator available at present. Moderate stimulation of the creatine transporter may be able to reverse the decline in creatine and phosphocreatine levels. Finally, the myofibrillar efficiency of ATP utilization may be improved by calcium-sensitizing agents.

Summary

Action potentials arise in spontaneously depolarizing cells of the sinoatrial node, spreading first across the the atria via the intercalated disks between myocytes, and causing atrial contraction. Atrial contraction completes the filling of the ventricles through the atrioventricular valves. The electrical impulses converge on the atrioventricular node, and then reach the His bundle. Activation of the ventricles causes a rise in intraventricular pressure, closing the atrioventricular valves and opening the aortic and pulmonary valves, and resulting in ejection into the systemic and pulmonary circulations, respectively.

Increased oxygen demands of the myocardium are met by increased blood flow to the dense capillary beds of the coronary circulation. Perfusion is limited by extravascular compression, particularly in the left ventricular wall. Autoregulation maintains constant coronary blood flow despite changing coronary perfusion pressure, and this is mediated by local metabolic control of vascular resistance and neurogenic control mechanisms.

Cardiac function is influenced by preload, contractility, and afterload. The activity of the autonomic nervous system modifies contractility, heart rate, vascular tone, and venous compliance. A number of conditions may impair cardiac function: myocardial ischemia causes dyssynchrony and impairs isovolumic relaxation; ventricular dilation and myocardial fibrosis decrease efficiency of ventricular filling; increased ventricular stiffness can arise from structural alterations, such as hypertrophic cardiomyopathies, or functional alterations, such as myocardial ischemia.

Sarcomeres are the contractile units of myocytes, consisting of bundles of thick filaments (myosin) and thin filaments (actin, tropomyosin [Tm], and troponin [Tn]). Action potentials depolarize the cell membrane, activating voltage-sensitive L-type calcium channels in transverse tubules. The resulting local increase in Ca^{2+} concentration triggers the release of large amounts of stored Ca^{2+} from the sarcoplasmic reticulum via ryanodine receptor calcium-release channels.

Calcium binding to the Tn-Tm complex induces a conformational change, promoting ATP-dependent crossbridge formation between actin and myosin filaments, and causing contraction. Calcium not only initiates contraction, but also alters the kinetics of crossbridge formation (contractility); increased myoplasmic Ca^{2+} and increased sensitivity of the contractile apparatus to Ca^{2+} thus have a positive inotropic effect. Positive and negative inotropic effects can be mediated via a variety of drugs. The Ca^{2+} concentration increase is transient: removal is carried out by a Na^+/Ca^{2+} exchanger and the sarcoplasmic Ca^{2+} ATPase, SERCA2. Adrenergic signaling via protein kinase A (PKA) reduces phospholamban-mediated inhibition of SERCA2, resulting in increased rate and force of contraction. Other downstream targets of sympathetic stimulation and PKA for positive inotropic and lusitropic effects include voltage-gated L-type Ca^{2+} channels, sarcomeric troponin I, and myosin binding protein C. Angiotensin II binds G-protein-coupled receptors and has a positive inotropic effect. Control of excitation–contraction coupling and contractility may also be mediated by nitric oxide (NO).

To meet the demands of myocardial ATP usage, the heart metabolizes free fatty acids, glucose, and other carbohydrates. Creatine kinase catalyzes the transfer of the high-energy phosphate bond in ATP to creatine for shuttling from the mitochondria to the myofibril. In heart failure there is decreased substrate uptake or oxidation, or both. There is a reduction in creatine kinase activity and high-energy phosphates, resulting in reduced contractility and inotropic reserve. In addition to drugs which increase contractility by targeting Ca^{2+} entry and release or sensitivity of the troponin–tropomyosin apparatus to Ca^{2+}, pharmacological approaches to altering substrate utilization may be an alternative option. Arrhythmias are controlled by interventions targeting sympathetic myocardial stimulation and sodium, calcium, and potassium fluxes.

References

1. Myhre ES, Slinker BK, LeWinter MM. Absence of right ventricular isovolumic relaxation in open-chest anesthetized dogs. *Am J Physiol* 1992; **263**: H1587–90.

2. Weibel ER. Morphological basis of alveolar-capillary gas exchange. *Physiol Rev* 1973; **53**: 419–95.

3. Gil J, Bachofen H, Gehr P, Weibel ER. Alveolar volume-surface area relation in air- and saline-filled lungs fixed by vascular perfusion. *J Appl Physiol* 1979; **47**: 990–1001.

4. Noble MI. Left ventricular load, arterial impedance and their interrelationship. *Cardiovasc Res* 1979; **13**: 183–98.

5. Starling EK. *The Linacre Lecture on the Law of the Heart, Given at Cambridge 1915*. London: Longmans, 1918.

6. Sarnoff SJ, Berglund E. Ventricular function. I. Starling's law of the heart studied by means of simultaneous right and left ventricular function curves in the dog. *Circulation* 1954; **9**: 706–18.

7. Suga H. Left ventricular time-varying pressure–volume ratio in systole as an index of myocardial inotropism. *Jpn Heart J* 1971; **12**: 153–60.

8. Suga H, Sagawa K, Shoukas AA. Load independence of the instantaneous pressure–volume ratio of the canine left ventricle and effects of epinephrine and heart rate on the ratio. *Circ Res* 1973; **32**: 314–22.

9. Glower DD, Spratt JA, Snow ND, *et al.* Linearity of the Frank–Starling relationship in the intact heart: the concept of preload recruitable stroke work. *Circulation* 1985; **71**: 994–1009.

10. Robotham JL, Takata M, Berman M, Harasawa Y. Ejection fraction revisited. *Anesthesiology* 1991; **74**: 172–83.

11. Rozec B, Gauthier C. Beta3-adrenoceptors in the cardiovascular system: putative roles in human pathologies. *Pharmacol Ther* 2006; **111**: 652–73.

12. Weiss HR. Effect of coronary artery occlusion on regional arterial and venous O_2 saturation, O_2 extraction, blood flow, and O_2 consumption in the dog heart. *Circ Res* 1980; **47**: 400–7.

13. Eckenhoff JE. The physiology of the coronary circulation. *Anesthesiology* 1950; **11**: 168–77.

14. Khouri EM, Gregg DE, Rayford CR. Effect of exercise on cardiac output, left coronary flow and myocardial metabolism in the unanesthetized dog. *Circ Res* 1965; **17**: 427–37.

15. Moncada S, Vane JR. Pharmacology and endogenous roles of prostaglandin endoperoxides, thromboxane A2, and prostacyclin. *Pharmacol Rev* 1978; **30**: 293–331.

16. Rubanyi GM. Endothelium, platelets, and coronary spasm. *Coronary Artery Disease* 1990; **1**: 645–53.

17. Rubanyi GM. Endothelium-derived relaxing and contracting factors. *J Cell Biochem* 1991; **46**: 27–36.

18. Downey JM, Kirk ES. Distribution of the coronary blood flow across the canine heart wall during systole. *Circ Res* 1974; **34**: 251–7.

19. Rovai D, L'Abbate A, Lombardi M, *et al.* Nonuniformity of the transmural distribution of coronary blood flow during the cardiac cycle. In vivo documentation by contrast echocardiography. *Circulation* 1989; **79**: 179–87.

20. Klocke FJ, Mates RE, Canty JM, Ellis AK. Coronary pressure-flow relationships. Controversial issues and probable implications. *Circ Res* 1985; **56**: 310–23.

21. Bellamy RF. Diastolic coronary artery pressure–flow relations in the dog. *Circ Res* 1978; **43**: 92–101.

22. Gould KL, Lipscomb K, Hamilton GW. Physiologic basis for assessing critical coronary stenosis. Instantaneous flow response and regional distribution during coronary hyperemia as measures of coronary flow reserve. *Am J Cardiol* 1974; **33**: 87–94.

23. Marcus ML. Autoregulation in the coronary circulation. In: *The Coronary Circulation in Health and Disease.* New York, NY: McGraw-Hill, 1983: 93–112.

24. Gibbs CL, Chapman JB. Cardiac energetics. In: *Handbook of Physiology. The Cardiovascular System. The Heart.* Bethesda, MD: Amercian Physiological Society, 1979: sect. 2, vol. I, 775–804.

25. Feigl EO. Coronary physiology. *Physiol Rev* 1983; **63**: 1–205.

26. Nichols CG, Lederer WJ. Adenosine triphosphate-sensitive potassium channels in the cardiovascular system. *Am J Physiol* 1991; **261**: H1675–86.

27. Ishibashi Y, Duncker DJ, Zhang J, Bache RJ. ATP-sensitive K+ channels, adenosine, and nitric oxide-mediated mechanisms account for coronary vasodilation during exercise. *Circ Res* 1998; **82**: 346–59.

28. Feliciano L, Henning RJ. Coronary artery blood flow: physiologic and pathophysiologic regulation. *Clin Cardiol* 1999; **22**: 775–86.

29. Ludmer PL, Selwyn AP, Shook TL, *et al.* Paradoxical vasoconstriction induced by acetylcholine in atherosclerotic coronary arteries. *N Engl J Med* 1986; **315**: 1046–51.

30. Bassenge E, Heusch G. Endothelial and neuro-humoral control of coronary blood flow in health and disease. *Rev Physiol Biochem Pharmacol* 1990; **116**: 77–165.

31. Duncker DJ, Bache RJ. Regulation of coronary blood flow during exercise. *Physiol Rev* 2008; **88**: 1009–86.

32. Spiro D, Sonnenblick EH. Comparison of the ultrastructural basis of the contractile process in heart and skeletal muscle. *Circ Res* 1964; **15**: 14–37.

33. McDonald KS, Moss RL. Osmotic compression of single cardiac myocytes eliminates the reduction in Ca^{2+} sensitivity of tension at short sarcomere length. *Circ Res* 1995; **77**: 199–205.

34. Lakatta EG. Starling's law of the heart is explained by an intimate interaction of muscle length and myofilament calcium activation. *J Am Coll Cardiol* 1987; **10**: 1157–64.

35. Hill AV. Heat of shortening and dynamic constant of muscle. *Proc R Soc Lond B Biol Sci* 1938; **126**: 136–95.

36. Abbott BC, Mommaerts WF. A study of inotropic mechanisms in the papillary muscle preparation. *J Gen Physiol* 1959; **42**: 533–51.

37. Langer GA. Ion fluxes in cardiac excitation and contraction and their relation to myocardial contractility. *Physiol Rev* 1968; **48**: 708–57.

38. Van de Werf F, Boel A, Geboers J, *et al.* Diastolic properties of the left ventricle in normal adults and in patients with third heart sounds. *Circulation* 1984; **69**: 1070–8.

39. Weiss JL, Frederiksen JW, Weisfeldt ML. Hemodynamic determinants of the time-course of fall in canine left ventricular pressure. *J Clin Invest* 1976; **58**: 751–60.

40. Brutsaert DL, Rademakers FE, Sys SU. Triple control of relaxation: implications in cardiac disease. *Circulation* 1984; **69**: 190–6.

41. Brutsaert DL, Rademakers FE, Sys SU, Gillebert TC, Housmans PR. Analysis of relaxation in the evaluation of ventricular function of the heart. *Prog Cardiovasc Dis* 1985; **28**: 143–63.

42. Doyle RL, Foex P, Ryder WA, Jones LA. Differences in ischaemic dysfunction after gradual and abrupt coronary occlusion: effects on isovolumic relaxation. *Cardiovasc Res* 1987; **21**: 507–14.

43. Little WC, Downes TR. Clinical evaluation of left ventricular diastolic performance. *Prog Cardiovasc Dis* 1990; **32**: 273–90.

44. Kagawa K, Arakawa M, Miwa H, *et al.* [Left atrial function during left ventricular diastole evaluated by left atrial angiography and left ventriculography]. *J Cardiol* 1994; **24**: 317–25.

45. Arora RR, Machac J, Goldman ME, *et al.* Atrial kinetics and left ventricular diastolic filling in the healthy elderly. *J Am Coll Cardiol* 1987; **9**: 1255–60.

46. Bonow RO, Frederick TM, Bacharach SL, *et al.* Atrial systole and left ventricular filling in hypertrophic cardiomyopathy: effect of verapamil. *Am J Cardiol* 1983; **51**: 1386–91.

47. Samstad SO, Rossvoll O, Torp HG, Skjaerpe T, Hatle L. Cross-sectional early mitral flow-velocity profiles from color Doppler in patients with mitral valve disease. *Circulation* 1992; **86**: 748–55.

48. Katz AM. Influence of altered inotropy and lusitropy on ventricular pressure–volume loops. *J Am Coll Cardiol* 1988; **11**: 438–45.

49. Nonogi H, Hess OM, Bortone AS, *et al.* Left ventricular pressure–length relation during exercise-induced ischemia. *J Am Coll Cardiol* 1989; **13**: 1062–70.

50. Marsch SC, Wanigasekera VA, Ryder WA, Wong LS, Foex P. Graded myocardial ischemia is associated with a decrease in diastolic distensibility of the remote nonischemic myocardium in the anesthetized dog. *J Am Coll Cardiol* 1993; **22**: 899–906.

51. Spudich JA. How molecular motors work. *Nature* 1994; **372**: 515–18.

52. Holmes KC, Popp D, Gebhard W, Kabsch W. Atomic model of the actin filament. *Nature* 1990; **347**: 44–9.

53. Tobacman LS. Thin filament-mediated regulation of cardiac contraction. *Annu Rev Physiol* 1996; **58**: 447–81.

54. Coudrey L. The troponins. *Arch Intern Med* 1998; **158**: 1173–80.

55. Lopez-Jimenez F, Goldman L, Sacks DB, *et al.* Prognostic value of cardiac troponin T after noncardiac surgery: 6-month follow-up data. *J Am Coll Cardiol* 1997; **29**: 1241–5.

56. Metzler H, Gries M, Rehak P, *et al.* Perioperative myocardial cell injury: the role of troponins. *Br J Anaesth* 1997; **78**: 386–90.

57. Babu A, Scordilis SP, Sonnenblick EH, Gulati J. The control of myocardial contraction with skeletal fast muscle troponin C. *J Biol Chem* 1987; **262**: 5815–22.

58. Kress M, Huxley HE, Faruqi AR, Hendrix J. Structural changes during activation of frog muscle studied by time-resolved X-ray diffraction. *J Mol Biol* 1986; **188**: 325–42.

59. Brenner BM, Troy JL, Ballermann BJ. Endothelium-dependent vascular responses. Mediators and mechanisms. *J Clin Invest* 1989; **84**: 1373–8.

60. Huxley AF, Niedergerke R. Structural changes in muscle during contraction; interference microscopy of living muscle fibres. *Nature* 1954; **173**: 971–3.

61. Huxley H, Hanson J. Changes in the cross-striations of muscle during contraction and stretch and their structural interpretation. *Nature* 1954; **173**: 973–6.

62. Pollack GH, Krueger JW. Sarcomere dynamics in intact cardiac muscle. *Eur J Cardiol* 1976; **4**: 53–65.

63. Snyders DJ. Structure and function of cardiac potassium channels. *Cardiovasc Res* 1999; **42**: 377–90.

64. Katz AM. *Physiology of the Heart.* 2nd edn. New York, NY: Raven, 1992.

65. DiFrancesco D. Serious workings of the funny current. *Prog Biophys Mol Biol* 2006; **90**: 13–25.

66. Anderson K, Lai FA, Liu QY, *et al.* Structural and functional characterization of the purified cardiac ryanodine receptor-Ca^{2+} release channel complex. *J Biol Chem* 1989; **264**: 1329–35.

67. Sitsapesan R, Williams AJ. Gating of the native and purified cardiac SR Ca^{2+}-release channel with monovalent cations as permeant species. *Biophys J* 1994; **67**: 1484–94.

68. Bers DM. Cardiac excitation-contraction coupling. *Nature* 2002; **415**: 198–205.

69. Greenstein JL, Hinch R, Winslow RL. Mechanisms of excitation-contraction coupling in an integrative model of the cardiac ventricular myocyte. *Biophys J* 2006; **90**: 77–91.

70. Chelu MG, Danila CI, Gilman CP, Hamilton SL. Regulation of ryanodine receptors by FK506 binding proteins. *Trends Cardiovasc Med* 2004; **14**: 227–34.

71. Wang K, Tu Y, Rappel WJ, Levine H. Excitation-contraction coupling gain and cooperativity of the cardiac ryanodine receptor: a modeling approach. *Biophys J* 2005; **89**: 3017–25.

72. Fedida D, Noble D, Shimoni Y, Spindler AJ. Inward current related to contraction in guinea-pig ventricular myocytes. *J Physiol* 1987; **385**: 565–89.

73. Schatzmann HJ. The calcium pump of the surface membrane and of the sarcoplasmic reticulum. *Annu Rev Physiol* 1989; **51**: 473–85.

74. Koss KL, Kranias EG. Phospholamban: a prominent regulator of myocardial contractility. *Circ Res* 1996; **79**: 1059–63.

75. Reuter H, Pott C, Goldhaber JI, *et al.* Na(+)-Ca2$^+$ exchange in the regulation of cardiac excitation-contraction coupling. *Cardiovasc Res* 2005; **67**: 198–207.

76. Lissandron V, Zaccolo M. Compartmentalized cAMP/PKA signalling regulates cardiac excitation-contraction coupling. *J Muscle Res Cell Motil* 2006; **27**: 399–403.

77. Vila Petroff MG, Mattiazzi AR. Angiotensin II and cardiac excitation-contraction coupling: questions and controversies. *Heart Lung Circ* 2001; **10**: 90–8.

78. Lim G, Venetucci L, Eisner DA, Casadei B. Does nitric oxide modulate cardiac ryanodine receptor function? Implications for excitation-contraction coupling. *Cardiovasc Res* 2008; **77**: 256–64.

79. Kelly RA, Balligand JL, Smith TW. Nitric oxide and cardiac function. *Circ Res* 1996; **79**: 363–80.

80. Cheng H, Lederer MR, Lederer WJ, Cannell MB. Calcium sparks and [Ca^{2+}]i waves in cardiac myocytes. *Am J Physiol* 1996; **270**: C148–59.

81. Petroff MG, Kim SH, Pepe S, *et al.* Endogenous nitric oxide mechanisms mediate the stretch dependence of Ca^{2+} release in cardiomyocytes. *Nat Cell Biol* 2001; **3**: 867–73.

82. Kaye DM, Wiviott SD, Balligand JL, *et al.* Frequency-dependent activation of a constitutive nitric oxide synthase and regulation of contractile function in adult rat ventricular myocytes. *Circ Res* 1996; **78**: 217–24.

83. Haque R, Kan H, Finkel MS. Effects of cytokines and nitric oxide on myocardial E-C coupling. *Basic Res Cardiol* 1998; **93**: 86–94.

84. Knaapen P, Germans T, Knuuti J, *et al.* Myocardial energetics and efficiency: current status of the noninvasive approach. *Circulation* 2007; **115**: 918–27.

85. Neubauer S. The failing heart: an engine out of fuel. *N Engl J Med* 2007; **356**: 1140–51.

86. Bessman SP, Geiger PJ. Transport of energy in muscle: the phosphorylcreatine shuttle. *Science* 1981; **211**: 448–52.

87. Osorio JC, Stanley WC, Linke A, *et al.* Impaired myocardial fatty acid oxidation and reduced protein expression of retinoid X receptor-alpha in pacing-induced heart failure. *Circulation* 2002; **106**: 606–12.

88. Karbowska J, Kochan Z, Smolenski RT. Peroxisome proliferator-activated receptor alpha is downregulated in the failing human heart. *Cell Mol Biol Lett* 2003; **8**: 49–53.

89. Ashrafian H, Frenneaux MP, Opie LH. Metabolic mechanisms in heart failure. *Circulation* 2007; **116**: 434–48.

Physiologic substrates of drug action

Autonomic function

Jonathan Moss and David Glick

Introduction

The autonomic nervous system (ANS) maintains cardiovascular, gastrointestinal, and thermal homeostasis. It controls an organism's maintenance functions and its responses to homeostatic challenges. The autonomic nervous system is divided into sympathetic, parasympathetic, and enteric branches. The sympathetic nervous system responds to challenges by increasing heart rate, blood pressure, and cardiac output, dilating the bronchial tree, and shunting blood away from the viscera and toward the muscles involved in the response to the challenge. The parasympathetic nervous system acts primarily to conserve energy and to support the function of the endocrine, digestive, and urogenital systems. An additional branch of the autonomic nervous system, the enteric nervous system, has recently come into prominence.

Understanding the ANS is central to contemporary anesthetic practice for several reasons. Anesthesiologists must understand the interaction of anesthetics with the involuntary control system to avoid triggering adverse effects. Additionally, disease states may impair autonomic function and alter expected responses to surgery, anesthesia, or other stresses. Finally, the stress response itself can have both positive and negative effects that directly impact clinical care.

Systems physiology

Each branch of the autonomic nervous system exhibits a different anatomic motif, which is recapitulated on a cellular and molecular level. The underlying theme of the **sympathetic** nervous system is an **amplification** response, whereas that of the **parasympathetic** nervous system is a **discrete** and narrowly **targeted** response. The enteric nervous system is arranged nontopographically, as would be appropriate for the viscera, and relies upon the mechanism of chemical coding to differentiate between nerves subserving different functions.

Nerves are classified by the chemical transmitters they contain. Nerves that contain acetylcholine (ACh) are **cholinergic**. Nerves that contain norepinephrine (NE, noradrenaline) or epinephrine (adrenaline) are called **adrenergic**. Cholinergic

neurons may be either nicotinic or muscarinic, depending on the receptors they activate. Almost 100 years ago nicotine was found to act on ganglionic and skeletal muscle synapses, on nerve membranes, and on sensory endings. The drugs that act on those parts of the cholinergic system are called nicotinic drugs. Muscarine, a chemical isolated from mushrooms, mimics the actions of direct nerve stimulation thereby activating the parasympathetic nervous system. The enteric nervous system often contains neither NE nor ACh. Understanding nonadrenergic, noncholinergic (NANC) neurons is necessary for understanding the enteric nervous system [1].

The underlying organizational scheme of the sympathetic and parasympathetic nervous systems is given in Fig. 22.1. The largely adrenergic **sympathetic nervous system** modulates the activity of vascular and uterine smooth muscle, cardiac muscle, and glands. Aside from transmitters for a few anatomically unusual sympathetic neurons (e.g., sweat glands) the major transmitter of the sympathetic nervous system is NE. Activation of the sympathetic nervous system and the adrenal gland (which releases both NE and epinephrine) results in a robust series of coordinated activities designed to protect an organism from internal and external challenges. Sympathomimetic drugs mimic the actions of the sympathetic nervous system, and sympatholytic drugs attenuate these actions. Systemic administration of sympathomimetic drugs constricts blood vessels, which increases blood pressure, while administration of sympatholytic drugs decreases blood pressure. Epinephrine and other sympathomimetic drugs also have inotropic and chronotropic effects on cardiac muscle and are often useful when treating shock. Epinephrine decreases bronchial and uterine smooth muscle tone so it is useful as a bronchodilator and to arrest uterine contractions. The release of renin, mediated through an adrenoceptor in the kidney, potentiates many of the effects of NE.

The sympathetic nervous system originates from the spinal cord from the first thoracic through the second or third lumbar segments (Fig. 22.2). The preganglionic sympathetic neurons have cell bodies within the horns of the spinal gray matter. Nerve fibers extend from these cell bodies to three types of ganglia: the paired sympathetic ganglia, various unpaired distal plexuses, and

Anesthetic Pharmacology, 2nd edition, ed. Alex S. Evers, Mervyn Maze, Evan D. Kharasch. Published by Cambridge University Press. © Cambridge University Press 2011.

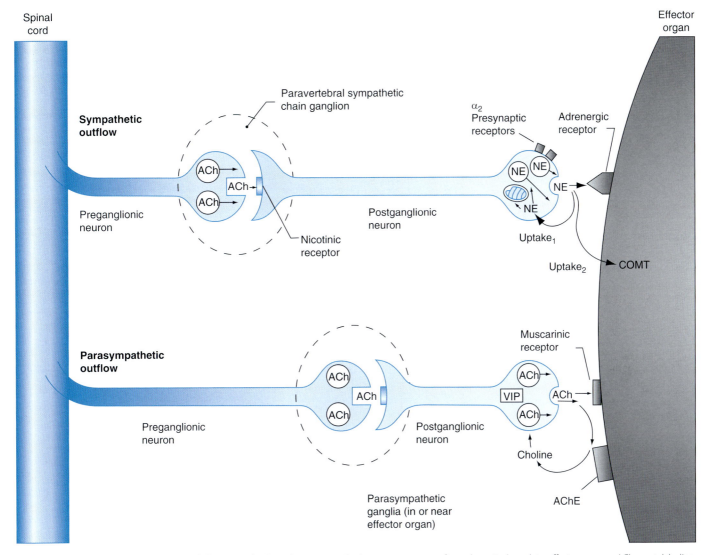

Figure 22.1. Schematic representation of the sympathetic and parasympathetic nervous systems from the spinal cord to effector organs. ACh, acetylcholine; AChE, acetylcholinesterase; COMT, catechol-O-methyltransferase; NE, norepinephrine; VIP, vasoactive intestinal polypeptide.

terminal (or collateral) ganglia near the target organ. The preganglionic fibers leave the cord within the anterior nerve roots, they join the spinal nerve trunks, and then they enter the ganglion via the white or myelinated ramus. Postsynaptic fibers reenter the spinal nerve via the gray (unmyelinated) ramus and then innervate effectors of blood vessels in the skeletal muscle and in the skin as well as the sweat glands. Sympathetic innervation to the trunk and limbs is carried by the spinal nerves.

Sympathetic preganglionic fibers are short and lie close to the central nervous system. Their distribution is diffuse and capable of amplification. In fact, at each of these ganglia there is up to 7000-fold amplification. Thus, the goal of a rapid, magnified response is served by these ganglia. Many autonomic reflexes are inhibited by supraspinal feedback, which is lost after spinal cord transection. As a result, in paraplegic patients small stimuli can evoke exaggerated sympathetic discharges. In addition to the paired ganglia, the sympathetic distribution to the head and neck

arrives via the three ganglia of the cervical sympathetic chain. Although these ganglia are fused anatomically they still demonstrate a profound ability to amplify nervous responses. The unpaired paravertabral ganglia, in the abdomen and pelvis anterior to the verebral column, include the celiac, superior mesenteric, and inferior mesenteric ganglia. The celiac ganglion, innervated by T5 to T12, innervates the spleen, liver, kidney, pancreas, small bowel, and proximal colon. Many preganglionic fibers from T5 to T12 pass through the paired paravertebral ganglia to form the splanchnic nerves. Other fibers innervate the adrenal medulla. The superior mesenteric ganglion innervates the distal colon, whereas the inferior mesenteric ganglion subserves the rectum, bladder, and genitals. The adrenal gland, which is rich in both NE and epinephrine, has its primary neuron within the organ itself.

Unlike the sympathetic nervous system, the **parasympathetic nervous system** works largely through cholinergic nerves, and its response is highly selective. The parasympathetic nervous system

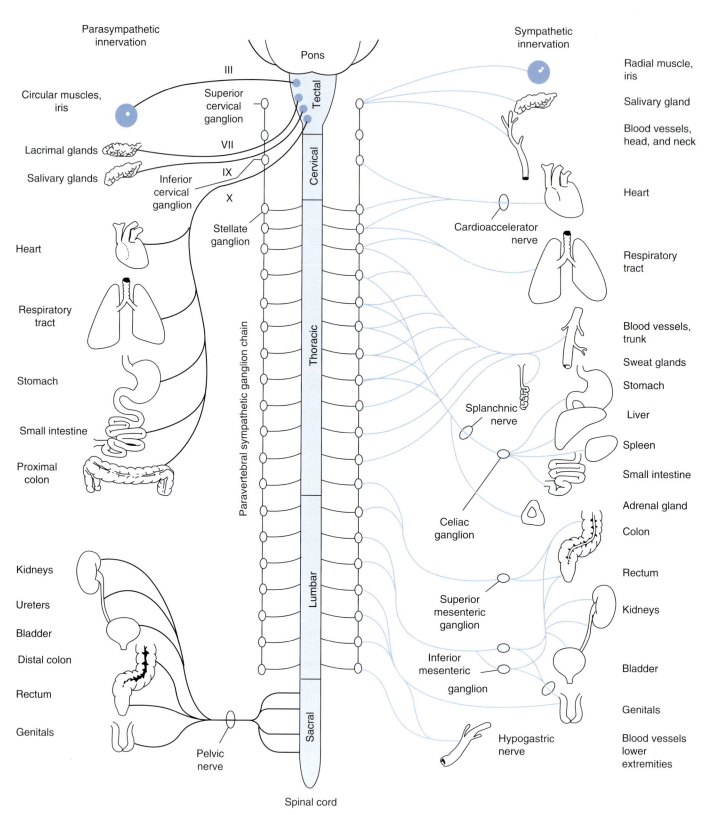

Figure 22.2. Schematic representation of the autonomic nervous system, depicting the functional innervation of peripheral effector organs and the anatomic origin of peripheral autonomic nerves from the spinal cord. Although both paravertebral sympathetic ganglia chains are presented, the sympathetic innervation to the peripheral effector organs is shown only on the right part of the figure, with the parasympathetic innervation of peripheral effector organs depicted on the left. The roman numerals on nerves originating in the tectal region of the brainstem refer to the cranial nerves that provide parasympathetic outflow to the effector organs of the head, neck, and trunk. Reproduced with permission from Ruffolo [2].

emerges from the craniosacral outflow (Fig. 22.2). The ganglia of the parasympathetic nervous system are in close proximity to, or within, the innervated organ (Fig. 22.1). Of all parasympathetic nerves, the vagus is the most important, carrying up to 75% of the efferent parasympathetic traffic. It supplies the heart, tracheo-bronchial tree, liver, spleen, kidney, and the gastrointestinal (GI) tract except for the distal colon (Fig. 22.2). The preganglionic fibers of the vagus nerve are long and its postganglionic fibers are short. This arrangement permits targeted and discrete functional responses. Usually the parasympathetic nerves synapse with a one-to-one ratio of nerve to effector cells; occasionally, as in Auerbach's plexus, there can be significant amplification.

The third branch of the autonomic nervous system is the **enteric nervous system**. An important difference between it and the other two branches of the ANS is its degree of local autonomy. This system of neurons and their supporting cells is located within the walls of the GI tract. They derive from the neural crest and migrate to the GI tract along the vagus nerve. While the gut is importantly influenced by sympathetic and parasympathetic activity, it is the enteric nervous system, through the myenteric and submucous plexi, which regulates digestive activity. Thus, digestion and peristalsis can go on after spinal cord transection or during spinal anesthesia, albeit with impaired sphincter function. Unlike the sympathetic and parasympathetic nervous systems, which have topographic representation conferring selective action, the enteric nervous system employs a pattern of chemical coding for its functional organization. The enteric nervous system is highly dependent upon the combination of amines and peptides that constitute the NANC neurons that control its function. So, while ACh is the principal excitatory trigger of the nonsphincteric portion of the enteric nervous system, causing muscle contraction, evidence has emerged that the NANC neurons, particularly the inhibitory VIP-NO (vasoactive intestinal polypeptide–nitric oxide) neurons, play an important role as well.

Organ physiology

Almost all organs are dually innervated, with sympathetic and parasympathetic inputs frequently mediating opposing effects. For example, sympathetic stimulation acts on the heart to increase rate and strength of contraction and to enhance conduction through the atrioventricular (AV) node, whereas parasympathetic stimulation tends to decrease rate and contractility and to slow conduction through the node. In nearly every instance one branch dominates and provides the "resting tone" for that organ (Table 22.1) [2]. The sympathetic nervous system is dominant in arterioles and veins while the parasympathetic nervous system dominates in the heart, GI tract, urinary tract, and salivary glands. Certain organs such as the spleen and piloerector muscles are almost exclusively innervated by the sympathetic nervous system, but this is the exception.

Administration of exogenous epinephrine activates the cardiac β_1-adrenoceptors, resulting in positive inotropic and chronotropic responses, the latter by direct action on pacemaker cells. The net result of increased heart rate and a more forceful contraction is increased cardiac output. The electrophysiologic effects of epinephrine on the pacemaker are more complex. They include increasing conduction velocity and decreasing the refractory period in the bundle of His and in Purkinje fibers, as well as activation of ectopic pacemaker cells. Premature ventricular contraction and even ventricular fibrillation can occur. While the net result of epinephrine administration is to increase blood pressure, there are important differences in regional blood flow. In blood vessels, epinephrine can act either as a vasoconstrictor or as a vasodilator depending on the relative balance of α_1 or β_2 receptors. At low doses, epinephrine causes a relaxation of vascular smooth muscle of the hepatic and mesenteric vasculature through β_2-receptor activation. In other vascular beds, particularly renal and cutaneous vessels, the α_1 receptors predominate, and epinephrine causes intense vasoconstriction.

In addition to their well-understood effects on the heart, lungs, and blood vessels, catecholamines also exert important effects by mobilizing glucose in response to hypoglycemia or stress. Overall, sympathetic nervous system stimulation increases the glycogenolysis in liver and muscle and liberates free fatty acids from adipose tissue by activation of β-adrenoceptors. In neonates, epinephrine helps maintain body temperature through exothermic breakdown of brown fat, in part by β_3 receptors. β-Receptor stimulation increases glucagon and insulin secretion while α_2 receptor activation suppresses insulin secretion and inhibits lipolysis. In the plasma, epinephrine regulates short-term changes in potassium homeostasis. Epinephrine stimulates the β_2 receptors of red cells, activating adenylate cyclase and Na^+/K^+ ATPase, driving potassium into cells. This leads to a reduction in serum potassium concentration. β-Adrenergic blockade inhibits this potassium shift [3–5].

In contrast to the amplified and diffuse discharge in the sympathetic nervous system, activation of the parasympathetic nervous system is tonic. The muscarinic effects are marked by vasodilation and decreased heart rate. The vasodilatory effects of ACh depend upon the integrity of the vascular endothelium because muscarinic receptors on the endothelium cause the release of a second messenger, nitric oxide (NO), an endothelium-derived relaxant factor [6,7]. If the endothelium is damaged, receptor activation by ACh can provoke paradoxical vasoconstriction because of the absence of NO. In the heart, ACh decreases the rate of contraction, the velocity of conduction through the sinoatrial (SA) and AV nodes, and contractility. The decrease in nodal conduction may account for the complete heart block after administration of large amounts of cholinergic agents. In the ventricle, ACh decreases automaticity and increases the fibrillation threshold. In addition, ACh can inhibit the release of NE when muscarinic receptors residing on the presynaptic terminals are stimulated. Thus, the effect of ACh on the heart results from its presynaptic inhibition of NE release from sympathetic nerve endings as well as its postsynaptic receptor-mediated

Table 22.1. Responses elicited in effector organs by stimulation of sympathetic and parasympathetic nerves

Effector organ	Adrenergic response	Receptor involved	Cholinergic response	Dominant response (A or C)
Heart				
Rate of contraction	Increase	β_1	Decrease	C
Force of contraction	Increase	β_1	Decrease	C
Blood vessels				
Arteries (most)	Vasoconstriction	α_1		A
Skeletal muscle	Vasodilation	β_2		A
Veins	Vasoconstriction	α_2		A
Bronchial tree	Bronchodilation	β_2	Bronchoconstriction	C
Splenic capsule	Contraction	α_1		A
Uterus	Contraction	α_1	Variable	A
Vas deferens	Contraction	α_1		A
Prostatic capsule	Contraction	α_1		A
Gastrointestinal tract	Relaxation	α_2	Contraction	C
Eye				
Radial muscle, iris	Contraction (mydriasis)	α_1		A
Circular muscle, iris			Contraction (miosis)	C
Ciliary muscle	Relaxation	β	Contraction (accommodation)	C
Kidney	Renin secretion	β_1		A
Urinary bladder				
Detrusor	Relaxation	β	Contraction	C
Trigone and sphincter	Contraction	α_1	Relaxation	A, C
Ureter	Contraction	α_1	Relaxation	A
Insulin release from pancreas	Decrease	α_2		A
Fat cells	Lipolysis	β_1		A
Liver glycogenolysis	Increase	α_1		A
Hair follicles, smooth muscle	Contraction (piloerection)	α_1		A
Nasal secretion			Increase	C
Salivary glands	Increase secretion	α_1	Increase secretion	C
Sweat glands	Increase secretion	α_1	Increase secretion	C

A, adrenergic; C, cholinergic.
Reproduced with permission from Ruffolo [2].

opposition of the effects of catecholamines on the myocardium. Additional effects of ACh include smooth muscle constriction (including constriction of the smooth muscle of the bronchial wall). In the GI and genitourinary tracts, there is constriction of the smooth muscle of the walls but relaxation of the sphincters. Parasympathetic input into the endocrine system causes the release of secretions from tracheobronchial, salivary, and digestive glands.

The baroreflex provides the vital link between branches of the ANS which influence cardiovascular function. The baroreflex allows the body to maintain a relatively constant blood pressure in the face of internal and external events that would otherwise push the blood pressure to extraphysiologic extremes. The baroreflex is mediated through the ANS and functions both centrally and peripherally. The central effects are predominantly controlled by the parasympathetic nervous system. High blood pressures result in increased vagal tone and a compensatory slowing of the heart rate. A decrease in blood pressure, on the other hand, leads to a decrease in vagal activity and a higher heart rate. The peripheral components of the baroreflex are tied to vascular smooth muscle tone, and it is the sympathetic nervous system that determines this component of systemic blood pressure. Low blood pressures lead to increased sympathetic outflow and increased vascular tone, while elevated blood pressure leads to reflex relaxation of the vascular smooth muscle.

Cellular physiology

NE is synthesized from tyrosine, which is actively transported into the varicosity of the preganglionic sympathetic nerve terminal. The rate-limiting step in the conversion of tyrosine to NE and epinephrine depends on the enzyme tyrosine hydroxylase. High levels of NE inhibit tyrosine hydroxylase while low levels stimulate the enzyme. In chronic stress there is evidence for induction of this enzyme [8]. Tyrosine hydroxylase is exquisitely dependent upon the presence of molecular oxygen. As a result, hypoxemia may significantly reduce NE synthesis [9].

An adrenergic response results when the nerve potential arrives at the varicosity, a fine beadlike specialization of the neuroeffector junction. Small amounts of calcium are translocated across the membrane and cause fusion of the NE-containing vesicle with the cell membrane. It is important to note that NE is not alone within the sympathetic nerve vesicle. A number of studies have documented the importance of adenosine triphosphate (ATP) and neuropeptide Y (NPY) as cotransmitters and neuromodulators [10–14].

The dominant mechanism of release is exocytosis, in which the vesicles merge with the membrane of the cell and express their contents (Fig. 22.3). The detailed mechanism by which docking and fusion occurs is incompletely understood, but appears to be a highly differentiated process in which a series of soluble binding proteins – SNAP (soluble NSF [*N*-ethylmaleimide sensitive factor] attachment proteins) and SNARE (soluble NSF receptors) – interact [15,16]. In vesicular docking and release a subpopulation of vesicles is tethered to the active zone of the prejunctional neuron. Some of these vesicles, called readily releasable vesicles, are primed for fusion in response to Ca^{2+} influx. A series of proteins called complexins are the key molecules in initiating exocytosis, possibly acting in concert with calcium sensors [17].

In the adrenal gland, NE and epinephrine are stored in and secreted from separate chromaffin cell subtypes [18]. In addition to the NE, these vesicles also contain calcium, NPY, and ATP. Depending on the nature and frequency of the stimuli received at the presynaptic nerve ending, ATP is selectively released to cause an immediate postsynaptic effect via purinoreceptors [14]. Newly synthesized or recently taken-up transmitter is preferentially incorporated into the actively recycling vesicles and is therefore the first to be released on stimulation.

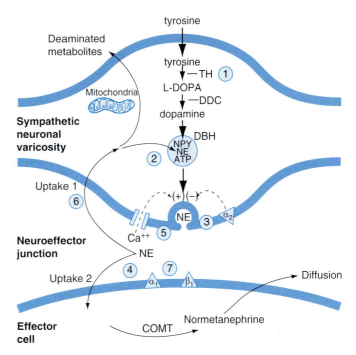

Figure 22.3. Norepinephrine synthesis, release, reuptake, and metabolism at the sympathetic postganglionic synapse. ATP, adenosine triphosphate; COMT, catechol-*O*-methyltransferase; DBH, dopamine-β-hydroxylase; DDC, dopamine decarboxylase; MAO, monoamine oxidase; NE, norepinephrine; NPY, neuropeptide Y; TH, tyrosine hydroxylase.

Thus, drugs such as ephedrine, which are taken up into the presynaptic terminal and cause vesicular fusion and NE release, initially liberate newly synthesized or newly taken-up amine.

Following nerve stimulation, NE is removed rapidly from the synaptic cleft. The reuptake into the presynaptic terminal represents the first and most important step in the inactivation of released NE. Approximately 75% of the released NE is transported into the storage vesicle for reuse. Drugs such as cocaine and tricyclic antidepressants are potent antagonists of the uptake pump and decrease the amount of NE reuptake. The transporter is extremely efficient, but it is not entirely specific. Therefore, many other clinically important amines can be taken up into the presynaptic terminal. Tyramine, contained within many foods, is such an agent. In addition, drugs which mimic NE may be taken up into the presynaptic terminal and packaged as false neurotransmitters. Ephedrine and bretylium act in this fashion.

There are important differences in the adrenergic function of the peripheral blood vessels and the heart. The heart has the highest rate of reuptake and the lowest rate of synthesis of NE. The converse is true of the blood vessels. Therefore, drugs that selectively affect reuptake have a greater effect on cardiac function, while drugs that affect biosynthesis of NE act predominantly on blood vessels.

The NE that escapes reuptake spills over into plasma. Metabolism of this plasma-borne NE occurs in the blood, liver, kidney [19], and in the lungs, where up to 25% of the NE is removed (except when pulmonary hypertension is present) [20].

The biotransformation of NE involves the mitochondrial enzyme monoamine oxidase (MAO) and the cytoplasmic enzyme catechol-O-methyltransferase (COMT). These enzymes metabolize NE and epinephrine as well as several of the sympathomimetic drugs. The end-product of metabolic inactivation of these amines is vanillylmandeic acid (VMA) which is excreted in the urine. As a result, urinary VMA levels can be used to identify patients with catecholamine-secreting tumors. COMT is present in abundance in the liver, where it metabolizes circulating catecholamines. Drug-induced inhibition of MAO is surprisingly well tolerated, but this stability belies the fact that amine metabolism is fundamentally changed. Anesthesiologists must be attuned to these changes, as they may produce life-threatening events (Chapter 40).

Release of NE in the neuroeffector junction stimulates adrenoceptors. Adrenoceptors have been classified as α_1, α_2, and β. Each class has three major subtypes (Fig. 22.4). In general, the receptors in cardiac tissue are β_1, and those acting on smooth muscle and exocrine glands are β_2. The latter can respond to NE but they are primarily stimulated by epinephrine released from the adrenal gland. Excess NE within the cleft binds to presynaptic α_2 receptors, inhibiting the release of additional NE. In clinical practice, agonists and antagonists are available for α_1, α_2, β_1, and β_2 receptors (Chapter 30). While α_1 and α_2 receptors are differentiated on the basis of their pharmacologic characteristics, it is generally true that α_1 receptors are expressed postsynaptically while α_2 receptors are expressed presynaptically in the ANS.

Cholinergic physiology

Much of our knowledge of the role of ACh in the parasympathetic nervous system is derived from studies of the neuromuscular junction, which demonstrates prototypical nicotinic transmission and is presented in detail in Chapter 18. In brief, ACh is synthesized intraneuronally from acetyl coenzyme

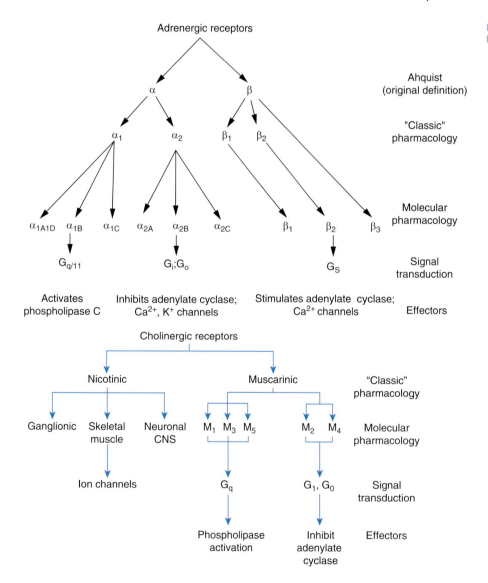

Figure 22.4. Classification of adrenergic and cholinergic receptors.

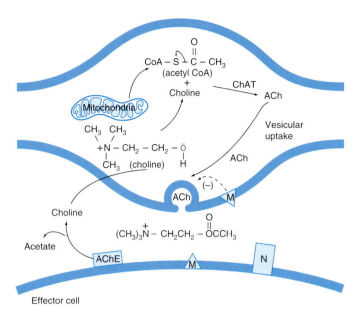

Figure 22.5. Synthesis, release, and metabolism of acetylcholine at the parasympathetic postganglionic synapse. ACh, acetylcholine; AChE, acetylcholinesterase; ChAT, choline acetyltransferase; CoA, coenzyme A; M, muscarinic; N, nicotinic.

A (CoA) and choline (Fig. 22.5). ACh coexists with vasoactive intestinal polypeptide (VIP) in parasympathetic nerves. Unlike the sympathetic system, where NPY, ATP, and NE are contained within the same vesicle, ACh and VIP are stored in separate vesicles within the presynaptic muscarinic terminal and are released differentially depending on the frequency of stimulation. VIP is thought to be released at high-frequency stimulation to augment the effects of ACh [11,21,22].

Drawing on evidence from work on the neuromuscular junction, it is believed that the presynaptic cholinergic neuron releases its contents largely by the process of exocytosis (as described above). Most of the ACh released into the neuroeffector junction is hydrolyzed by acetylcholinesterase, a membrane-bound enzyme that is present in all cholinergic synapses. This exceptionally efficient enzyme is also present in red blood cells. The acetylcholinesterase regenerates choline, most of which is taken up into the presynaptic terminal and repackaged.

Biochemical mechanisms

The biochemical and molecular mechanisms underlying both parasympathetic and sympathetic nervous function are well understood. It is at this level that most drugs exert important pharmacologic activity.

Dopamine can and does act as a neurotransmitter, particularly in the viscera and kidney. However, in most adrenergic neurons, dopamine is biotransformed by MAO or converted to NE within the dense core vesicles by dopamine β-hydroxylase. In the adrenal medulla, where the appropriate methyltransferase is present, there is a further conversion of about 85% of the NE to epinephrine.

The NE that is released into the neuroeffector junction acts on postsynaptic α- and β-adrenoceptors either alone or in concert with neuromodulators such as NPY. β-adrenoceptors were among the first receptors to be identified and characterized [23] and are one of a superfamily of receptors that have seven helices woven through the cellular membrane. The intracellular terminus can modulate the function of the β receptor and its subsequent interaction with G proteins via kinases [24]. The β receptor has mechanistic and structural similarities with muscarinic but not nicotinic receptors, primarily in the transmembrane domains. In fact, both muscarinic and β receptors are coupled via G proteins to adenylate cyclase and both can initiate the opening of ion channels. All three subtypes of β receptors (β_1, β_2, and β_3) increase cyclic adenosine monophosphate (cAMP) through adenylate cyclase and G-protein mediators, as detailed in Chapter 2.

Beta-adrenoceptors are not fixed but change significantly in response to the amount of NE present in the synaptic cleft or in plasma. Clinically, and at the cellular level, responses to many hormones and neurotransmitters wane rapidly despite continuous exposure to adrenergic agonists [25]. This phenomenon, termed desensitization, has been particularly well studied for the stimulation of cAMP levels by plasma membrane β-adrenoceptors [26]. Mechanisms postulated for desensitization include uncoupling, sequestration, and downregulation initiated by phosphorylation. The converse is also true, so β-receptor blockade increases receptor number and activity. This is why a sudden discontinuation of chronic β-adrenoceptor blockade causes rebound tachycardia and increases the incidence of myocardial infarction and ischemia [27].

The best-studied example of a change in receptor number involves chronic congestive heart failure. Traditionally, β_1 receptors were thought to be isolated to cardiac muscle and β_2 receptors were believed to be restricted to vascular and bronchial smooth muscle. The β_2 receptor population in cardiac muscle is actually quite sizeable, accounting for 15% of the β receptors in the ventricles and 30–40% in the atria [28]. These receptors may play a compensatory role in congestive heart failure. When the failing heart is depleted of catecholamines, plasma levels of catecholamines are markedly increased to maintain systemic vascular resistance. This leads to a decrease in β receptors in the heart, which explains why administration of β-agonists in this syndrome is largely ineffective. Interestingly, though β_1-receptor density is markedly decreased, β_2 density remains unchanged [29,30]. Thus, β_2 receptors account for 60% of the inotropic response in CHF [31]. Because β_3 receptors lack cytoplasmic phosphorylation sites, they are relatively refractory to desensitization, and as a result they may also play a part in the compensatory response [32].

In addition to α and β receptors there are also dopamine receptors. Although dopamine in higher doses acts on both α and β receptors, Goldberg and Rajfer demonstrated conclusively that distinct dopamine receptors exist and are physiologically important [33]. Although five dopamine receptors have been cloned only dopamine 1 (D_1) and dopamine 2 (D_2) subtypes are of physiologic importance [34]. D_1 receptors are postsynaptic and mediate vasodilation. Certain drugs such as fenoldopam act as direct D_1 agonists and are important in selective vasodilation of renal and mesenteric beds. The D_2 receptors are presynaptic and inhibit the release of NE and dopamine. Central D_2 receptors are targeted by butyrophenones.

Second messengers

Following adrenoceptor stimulation, the extracellular signal is transformed into an intracellular signal by a process known as signal transduction, in which the α_1 and β receptors are coupled to G proteins [35]. Thorough discussions of receptor–effector coupling and signal transduction via the G proteins are found elsewhere in this text (Chapter 2).

In the parasympathetic system the links between stimulus and response are different in nicotinic and muscarinic receptors. ACh receptors of the nicotinic type belong to the superfamily of ligand-gated ion channels, which includes glutamate and glycine receptors. The nicotinic receptors are heteropentameric membrane proteins that form nonselective cation channels. There are two α subunits and one each of β, ε, and δ [36]. The α subunits present the binding sites for ACh or nicotinic antagonists. When ACh occupies both α subunits, the channel opens. If only one site is occupied, the channel remains closed and there is no flow of ions or change in electrical potential. The motif of a targeted response is recapitulated in synaptic electrophysiology, as the postjunctional action of several vesicles appears to be necessary to initiate a response. Further, unlike adrenoceptors, which react instantly to changes in catecholamine levels via phosphorylation of the receptor, changes to nicotinic receptor number and function take days [37].

In contrast to the ion-gated nicotinic receptors, muscarinic receptors belong to the superfamily of G-protein-coupled receptors and are more homologous to adrenoceptors than to nicotinic receptors. Five muscarinic receptors are known. Receptors in the muscarinic series are coupled to a second-messenger system such as cyclic nucleotides or phosphoinositides that are in turn coupled to ion channels. The nature of the response is determined by the specific cation involved. The M_2 and M_3 receptors are particularly important as they have been identified in the airway smooth muscle of many species. The M_3 receptor also mediates contractile and secretory response. Muscarinic receptors exhibit different signal transduction mechanisms. Odd-numbered receptors (M_1, M_3, M_5) work predominantly through the hydrolysis of phosphoinositide and release of intracellular calcium, whereas even-numbered receptors (M_2, M_4) work primarily through the G_i proteins to inhibit adenylate cyclase [38].

Assessment of autonomic function

The increased operative risk of aged and diabetic patients with autonomic dysfunction [39] makes the diagnosis of autonomic neuropathy extremely important. Five evocative tests of cardiovascular function have been developed to evaluate autonomic function in diabetic patients [40]. The tests include heart-rate responses to the Valsalva maneuver, standing up, and deep breathing, and blood-pressure responses to standing up and sustained handgrip. The tests involving changes in heart rate measure injury to the parasympathetic system and precede changes in the measures of blood pressure, which reflect sympathetic injury (Table 22.2).

In addition to clinical tests of autonomic function, sensitive and reliable techniques for measurement of plasma NE and epinephrine have been available for three decades; however, the interpretation of such data is confounded by other influences. Plasma epinephrine levels (normally 100–400 pg mL^{-1}) reflect adrenal release but vary considerably with psychological and physical stress. Thus, although marked increases in plasma catecholamines may be significant, isolated levels of less than 1000 pg must be interpreted with caution.

Autonomic failure and hyperactivity

Failure of the ANS such as occurs in aging or diabetes can be associated with increased morbidity and mortality [41]. The common clinical manifestations of autonomic dysfunction in the elderly are orthostatic hypotension, postprandial hypotension, hypothermia, and heat stroke. These presentations are all consequences of the limited ability of elderly patients to adapt to stresses with normal, autonomic-mediated vasoconstriction and vasodilation.

The decrement in autonomic function with aging is not the result of lower neurotransmitter levels or fewer postjunctional receptors but of fewer prejunctional terminals. Clinically, there is a marked attenuation of physiologic response to β-adrenergic stimulation in the elderly. Exogenous β-adrenergic agonists have a lesser effect on heart rate, left ventricular ejection fraction, cardiac output, and vasodilation in the healthy elderly [42]. The decreased response to adrenergic stimulation in the elderly appears to be the result of decreased affinity (not number) of the β receptors for the agonist and decreases in the coupling of the G_s protein and the adenylate cyclase unit [42].

Another example of autonomic failure occurs in diabetics. Diabetic autonomic neuropathy is the most common form of autonomic neuropathy and the most extensively investigated. It occurs in 20–40% of all insulin-dependent diabetic patients. Common manifestations of diabetic autonomic neuropathy include impotence, postural hypotension, gastroparesis, diarrhea, and sweating abnormalities. When impotence or diarrhea are the sole manifestations, there is little effect on

Table 22.2. Clinical assessment of the autonomic nervous system

Clinical examination	Technique	Normal value
Parasympathetic		
HR response to Valsalva	The seated subject blows into a mouthpiece (maintaining a pressure of 40 mmHg) for 15 seconds. The Valsalva ratio is the ratio of the longest R–R interval (which comes shortly after the release) to the shortest R–R interval (which occurs during the maneuver).	Ratio of > 1.21
HR response to standing	HR is measured as the subject moves from a resting supine position to standing. Normal tachycardic response is maximal around the 15th beat following rising. A relative bradycardia follows that is most marked around the 30th beat after standing. The response to standing is expressed as the "30 : 15" ratio and is the ratio of the longest R–R interval around the 30th beat to the shortest R–R interval around the 15th beat.	Ratio of > 1.04
HR response to deep breathing	The subject takes six deep breaths in 1 minute. The maximum and minimum heart rates during each cycle are measured and the mean of the differences (maximum HR – minimum HR) during three successive breathing cycles is taken as the maximum – minimum HR.	Mean difference > 15 bpm
Sympathetic		
BP response to standing	The subject moves from resting supine to standing and the standing SBP is subtracted from the supine SBP.	Difference < 10 mmHg
BP response to sustained handgrip	The subject maintains a handgrip of 30% of maximal squeeze for up to 5 minutes. The blood pressure is measured every minute, and the initial DBP is subtracted from the DBP just prior to release.	Difference > 16 mmHg

BP, blood pressure; bpm, beats per minute; DBP, diastolic blood pressure; HR, heart rate; SBP, systolic blood pressure.

survival; however, with postural hypotension or gastroparesis 5-year mortality rates are greater than 50% [43].

The symptoms associated with diabetic autonomic neuropathy confer an increased risk during anesthesia and surgery by both direct and secondary mechanisms. Gastroparesis increases the risk of aspiration. Systemic injury to the vasa vasorum in patients with postural hypotension increases the risk of hemodynamic instability and cardiovascular collapse in the perioperative period. Even in seemingly minor surgery, diabetic autonomic neuropathy can lead to significant complications. In a series of ophthalmologic procedures requiring general anesthesia, diabetics with autonomic neuropathy had a significantly greater drop in blood pressure with induction and a greater need for vasopressors than did diabetic patients without autonomic dysfunction [44]. Furthermore, Page and Watkins reported five cases of unexpected cardiorespiratory arrest in young diabetic patients, all of whom had symptoms of autonomic neuropathy [45]. In a large prospective study of diabetic autonomic neuropathy using the five evocative clinical tests discussed above, parasympathetic dysfunction preceded sympathetic failure in 96% of the patients followed [46]. This battery of autonomic tests identifies patients with autonomic neuropathy and is highly predictive of both mortality and perioperative risk [39,43].

Sympathetic hyperactivity

While autonomic failure presents a challenge for anesthesiologists, there is increasing evidence that sympathetic overstimulation

may also increase morbidity and mortality. Surgical stress results in profound metabolic and endocrine responses. The combination of autonomic, hormonal, and catabolic changes that accompany surgery has been termed the "surgical stress response" [47]. The extent of this response depends on the preoperative condition of the patient, the magnitude of the operation, and the surgical and anesthetic techniques. The weight of current evidence suggests that treatment of the acute stress response may be of limited value, but a comprehensive anesthetic plan that focuses on attenuation of the stress response during the entire perioperative period may influence morbidity and mortality.

Three separate lines of evidence suggest that interruption of the sympathetic response to surgery markedly reduces surgical stress intra- and postoperatively and improves outcomes [48]. The use of continuous thoracic epidural infusions of local anesthetics minimized the rise in plasma catecholamines, cortisol, and glucagon and improved outcome. This improved outcome was independent of a decrease in pain perception, as patients receiving other methods of pain relief (including NSAIDs and opioids) did not exhibit similar reductions in metabolic and endocrine responses to surgery [48]. Continuation of epidural infusions well into the postoperative period was regarded as essential to improving outcome [48].

A separate line of evidence supporting the hypothesis that long-term attenuation of the stress response alters outcome comes from the pediatric literature. When neonates with complex congenital heart disease underwent cardiac surgery, those who received high-dose sufentanil infusions intraoperatively and for the first 24 hours postoperatively to reduce the stress response had lower β-endorphin, NE, epinephrine, glucagon, aldosterone and cortisol levels compared to controls [49]. The mortality rate in the high-dose opiate group was significantly lower than in the study or historical controls.

A third line of evidence which has proved to be compelling involves the results from the multicenter study of the perioperative ischemia research group [50]. Surgical patients were randomized to receive either atenolol or placebo before and after surgery (until their discharge from the hospital) and followed over 2 years. The overall mortality was significantly less in the atenolol group and persisted at the 2-year follow-up. Survival 2 years after surgery was 68% in the placebo group and 83% in the atenolol group. This powerful demonstration that β-blockade could decrease perioperative cardiac risk and improve survival outcome to 2 years led to tremendous political and administrative pressure to increase the use of β-blockers perioperatively [51]. More recent research, however, has brought the value of routine perioperative β-blockade into question, even for patients with significant cardiovascular risk factors [52–54].

Taken as a whole, these various lines of evidence are very suggestive that anesthetics or adjuvants which can interfere with the stress response in the perioperative period can markedly improve morbidity and mortality. Newer anesthetic drugs such as the α2-agonists, which can also target presynaptic receptors to block the stress response, have been shown to influence outcome in the same fashion [55].

Pharmacologic modulation of the ANS

Because of its central importance in homeostasis, the autonomic nervous system has long been studied for potential therapeutic intervention at virtually every biochemical and cellular site. A primary clinical goal has been to develop drugs that target the synthesis, storage, release, and reuptake of NE. Drugs such as methyltyrosine inhibit tyrosine hydroxylase and have been used in the management of pheochromocytomas. Carbidopa, which is derived from methyldopa but does not cross the blood–brain barrier, is used with L-dopa in Parkinson's disease to inhibit the amino acid decarboxylase enzyme. The developoment of reserpine, which prevents vesicular reuptake of NE, was the first of these important drugs.

The psychiatric community has also shown an interest in uptake inhibitors. Correlation between mood and amine availability in the synaptic cleft underlies the basis of modern psychopharmacology [56]. Cocaine and tricyclic antidepressants specifically block the NE transporter of the reuptake system. In addition, other drugs such as guanethidine or methyldopa are precursors for the elaboration of false neurotransmitters that have different selectivity for adrenoceptors

than the endogenous neurotransmitter. Guanethidine depletes NE in the presynaptic terminal, while α-methyldopa is taken up and converted to α-methylnorepinephrine, which displaces NE from the vesicle but exerts minimal biological activity.

In addition to drugs that target vesicular and synaptic uptake and release, there are many drugs that inhibit the MAO enzyme. The role of this enzyme in catabolizing monoamines (catecholamines, serotonin) has long been recognized, but it was not until the euphoria associated with the antituberculosis drug iproniazid was appreciated that highly potent and specific MAO inhibitors (MAOIs) were developed. Although still useful as antidepressants, their interactions with certain drugs (notably meperidine) and foods (those containing tyramine, such as aged cheeses and wine) has limited their use. In patients who are taking MAOIs, tyramine that is ingested is not catabolized and remains at high levels in plasma. Tyramine is then taken up by sympathetic nerve terminals as a "false transmitter" and converted to octopamine, which is biologically inactive. Thus, many patients taking MAOIs have symptoms of autonomic failure such as orthostatic hypotension. Perhaps of greater consequence, if foods high in tyramine are ingested by patients taking MAOIs, there is the potential for massive displacement of NE into the cleft and for a life-threatening hypertensive crisis.

Although virtually every component of sympathetic, and to a lesser extent parasympathetic, function has been accessed pharmacologically, the areas of most intensive interest have been receptor ligands. The appreciation that certain receptor subtypes may play unique roles in autonomic function has led to the development of superselective agonists and antagonists. This has already achieved clinical use with the introduction of dexmedetomidine, a selective α2-agonist, as a sedative–analgesic for ICU use [57]. A greater understanding of the regional distribution of receptor subtypes in the vasculature [58], brain [59,60], and spinal cord will permit their targeting by new autonomic agonist and antagonist drugs.

While the development of selective antagonists has already achieved clinical usage, there has also been renewed interest in the mechanisms of receptor regeneration and coupling. Observations that β receptors may be uncoupled from G proteins during cardiopulmonary bypass [61] suggest that the linkage between receptor and G protein may be a target. An increased understanding of the molecular mechanisms of receptor desensitization [62,63] may provide another useful target for drug development. Another approach, recognizing a possible immunologic role in entities such as cardiomyopathy [64,65], where antibodies to both β and muscarinic receptors have been identified, suggests that an immunologic strategy may be developed. The recognition of the importance of cotransmission and neuromodulation in autonomic function provides yet another potential therapeutic target [66]. Finally, the possibility of genetic strategies using adenovirus transfection to modulate autonomic function or address functionally important polymorphisms may ultimately prove to be clinically useful, as well.

There has been a recent explosion of scientific research in identifying single-nucleotide polymorphisms (SNPs) in β-adrenoceptor genes and in relating them to autonomic pathophysiology [67]. In general these studies are statistical in nature, associating the incidence of SNPs with disease entities including hypertension, asthma, congestive heart failure, and arrhythmias. However, in some instances the underlying biologic links have been more intensively explored, and therapeutic implications are beginning to emerge.

While the association between asthma susceptibility and β-adrenergic polymorphisms in the general population has not been confirmed, asthma phenotypes including severity of asthma and bronchial hyperresponsiveness have been associated with β_2-receptor polymorphisms. Most notably, changes in the coding region may alter response to short- and long-acting agonists, suggesting that there may be a different therapeutic response contingent upon the underlying genetic makeup. Similarly, there has been an increasing interest in the extent to which adrenoceptor polymorphisms play a role in hypertension, heart failure [68], sudden death, and response to β-adrenergic antagonists. While intensive studies of β-receptor polymorphisms have led to a greater understanding of important clinical syndromes such as postural tachycardia syndrome [69] and sudden death, specific changes in clinical management have lagged considerably. Nowhere has this been more evident than in heart failure, where receptor function has been studied for decades [70] but to date there has been an inability to translate pharmacogenetic insights into therapeutic recommendations [71].

Recently, however, data have emerged suggesting that differences in the underlying signaling and recovery mechanism beyond receptors may play a role in autonomic pathophysiology [72]. It has been proposed that variability in the genetics of the arrestin system, which not only participates in the regeneration of adrenergic function but also can act as a second messenger, could account for differences in therapeutic efficacy of various cardiac drugs.

So, while the ANS could fairly be called primitive (it is largely preserved across all mammalian species) its considerable complexity leaves it incompletely understood. As the understanding of the genetic determinants of autonomic activity and the functional and cellular interactions of the ANS grow, the ability to interrupt or augment various autonomic effects with greater and greater precision will increase. This, in turn, will allow for improvements in both the long-term health and the acute perioperative safety of our patients.

Summary

The autonomic nervous system (ANS) maintains cardiovascular, gastrointestinal, and thermal homeostasis. It is divided into three branches: the sympathetic, parasympathetic, and enteric nervous systems. The sympathetic nervous system acts predominantly via the neurotransmitter norepinephrine (NE),

to increase blood supply to the muscles in response to challenges. The distribution of ganglia in the sympathetic nervous system, close to the central nervous system, facilitates rapid, amplified responses. By contrast, the parasympathetic nervous system allows for discrete responses, mediated largely via muscarinic acetylcholine (ACh) receptors in the target organs. Ganglia are located close to, or within, the innervated organ, and, with a few exceptions, there is usually a one-to-one ratio of nerve to effector cells. The vagus nerve carries heavy efferent parasympathetic traffic, supplying multiple organs. The enteric nervous system is located within the walls of the GI tract. While the gut is influenced by sympathetic and parasympathetic activity, enteric nervous system autonomy allows digestive and peristaltic functions to continue independently of spinal input. The enteric nervous system employs chemical coding, rather than a topographic organization, and nonadrenergic, noncholinergic (NANC) neurons play an important role.

The enzyme tyrosine hydroxylase catalyzes the rate-limiting step in the conversion of tyrosine to NE, which is stored in vesicles (together with cotransmitters and neuromodulators) within the sympathetic nerve. Nerve potentials cause a calcium influx, which triggers exocytosis. Released NE is inactivated predominantly by reuptake from the synaptic cleft. Due to differences in reuptake and NE synthesis rates in different tissues, drugs that selectively affect reuptake have a greater effect on cardiac function, while drugs that affect biosynthesis of NE act predominantly on blood vessels. Remaining NE is metabolized in the blood, liver, kidney, and lungs. ACh is synthesized from acetyl coenzyme A (CoA) and choline, and is stored in vesicles of the presynaptic terminal. Released ACh is largely hydrolyzed by the enzyme acetylcholinesterase.

Adrenoceptors are classified as α_1, generally expressed postsynaptically; α_2, generally expressed presynaptically; β_1, generally expressed in cardiac tissue; and β_2, generally expressed in smooth muscle and exocrine glands. Adrenergic β receptors act via G proteins and adenylate cyclase. The expression levels and activity of these receptors is modulated by the level of NE present. High-dose dopamine also acts on α and β receptors, although distinct dopamine receptors do exist. Fenoldopam acts as an agonist for the D_1 dopamine receptor, mediating vasodilation of renal and mesenteric beds, while butyrophenones act on presynaptic D_2 receptors, inhibiting the release of NE and dopamine. Nicotinic ACh receptors are ligand-gated ion channels, whereas muscarinic ACh receptors are G-protein-coupled receptors linked to ion channels via cyclic nucleotide or phosphoinositide second messengers.

Sympathetic and parasympathetic innervation often mediate opposing effects within target organs and tissues, as exemplified in the cardiovascular system. In the heart, exogenous epinephrine (a sympathomimetic) has positive inotropic and chronotropic effects. The effect of epinephrine on blood vessels to cause either vasoconstriction or vasodilation is determined by the balance of α_1 and β_2 receptors. The net result of epinephrine administration is an increase in blood pressure.

ACh causes a decrease in heart rate and cardiac contractility. Muscarinic ACh receptors in undamaged vascular endothelium act via second messenger nitric oxide (NO) to cause vasodilation in response to parasympathetic stimulation. The baroreflex balances sympathetic and parasympathetic cardiovascular effects to maintain relatively constant blood pressure.

Autonomic function must be evaluated in aged and diabetic patients, due to increased operative risk of autonomic dysfunction. A battery of five evocative clinical tests of cardiovascular function is available. Autonomic dysfunction in the elderly may present as orthostatic hypotension, postprandial hypotension, hypothermia, or heat stroke. Aging is also associated with a decreased response to exogenous β-adrenergic agonists. Clinical manifestations of autonomic neuropathy in diabetics include impotence, diarrhea, sweating abnormalities, postural hypotension, and gastroparesis.

There is evidence that sympathetic overstimulation may increase morbidity and mortality, and that anesthetic plans that reduce the stress response in the perioperative period may improve outcomes.

Targets for pharmacologic modulation of the ANS include the synthesis, storage, release, and reuptake of NE. Superselective agonists and antagonists allow greater control over ANS functions, which will increase in precision as the regional distribution of receptor subtypes is further delineated. Potential new drug targets include receptor coupling to G proteins and modulation of receptor expression levels. Possible alternative approaches include immunotherapy and gene therapy. Links between single nucleotide polymorphisms (SNPs) in β-adrenoceptor genes and autonomic pathophysiology are emerging, which may have implications for clinical management of a number of diseases.

References

1. Burnstock G. Autonomic neuromuscular junctions: current developments and future directions. *J Anat* 1986; **146**: 1–30.

2. Ruffolo R. Physiology and biochemistry of the peripheral autonomic nervous system. In: Wingard LB, Brody TM, Larner J, Schwartz A, eds., *Human Pharmacology: Molecular to Clinical.* St. Louis, MO: Mosby, 1991: 77–94.

3. Kharasch ED, Bowdle TA. Hypokalemia before induction of anesthesia and prevention by beta-2 adrenoceptor antagonism. *Anesth Analg* 1991; **72**: 216–20.

4. Williams ME, Gervino EV, Rosa RM, *et al.* Catecholamine modulation of rapid potassium shifts during exercise. *N Engl J Med* 1985; **312**: 823–7.

5. Struthers AD, Reid JL. The role of adrenal medullary catecholamines in potassium homoeostasis. *Clin Sci* 1984; **66**: 377–82.

6. Furchgott RF, Zawadzki JV. The obligatory role of endothelial cells in the relaxation of arterial smooth muscle by acetylcholine. *Nature* 1980; **288**: 373–6.

7. Johns RA. EDRF/nitric oxide. The endogenous nitrovasodilator and a new cellular messenger. *Anesthesiology* 1991; **75**: 927–31.

8. Wong DL, Tank AW. Stress-induced catecholaminergic function: transcriptional and post-transcriptional control. *Stress* 2007; **10**: 121–30.

9. Rostrup M. Catecholamines, hypoxia and high altitude. *Acta Physiol Scand* 1998; **162**: 389–99.

10. Von Kügelgen I, Starke K. Noradrenaline–ATP co-transmission in the sympathetic nervous system. *Trends Pharmacol Sci* 1991; **12**: 319–24.

11. Burnstock G. Local mechanisms of blood flow control by perivascular nerves and endothelium. *J Hypertens Suppl* 1990; **8**: S95–106.

12. Jacobson KA, Trivedi BK, Churchill PC, Williams M. Novel therapeutics acting via purine receptors. *Biochem Pharmacol* 1991; **41**: 1399–410.

13. Walker P, Grouzmann E, Burnier M, Waeber B. The role of neuropeptide Y in cardiovascular regulation. *Trends Pharmacol Sci* 1991; **12**: 111–15.

14. Lincoln J, Burnstock G. Neural–endothelial interactions in control of local blood flow. In:Warren J, ed., *The Endothelium: an Introduction to Current Research.* New York, NY: Wiley-Liss, 1990: 21–32.

15. Jahn R, Sudhof TC. Membrane fusion and exocytosis. *Annu Rev Biochem* 1999; **68**: 863–911.

16. Sudhof TC. The synaptic vesicle cycle revisited. *Neuron* 2000; **28**: 317–20.

17. Reim K, Mansour M, Varoqueaux F, *et al.* Complexins regulate a late step in Ca^{2+}-dependent neurotransmitter release. *Cell* 2001; **104**: 71–81.

18. Marley PD, Livett BG. Differences between the mechanism of adrenaline and noradrenaline secretion from isolated, bovine, adrenal chromaffin cells. *Neurosci Lett* 1987; **77**: 81–6.

19. Kopin IJ, Fischer JE, Musacchio JM, Horst WD, Weise VK. "False neurochemical transmitters" and the mechanism of sympathetic blockade by monoamine oxidase inhibitors. *J Pharmacol Exp Ther* 1965; **147**: 186–93.

20. Sole MJ, Drobac M, Schwartz L, Hussain MN, Vaughan-Neil EF. The extraction of circulating catecholamines by the lungs in normal man and in patients with pulmonary hypertension. *Circulation* 1979; **60**: 160–3.

21. Bloom SR, Edwards AV. Vasoactive intestinal peptide in relation to atropine resistant vasodilatation in the submaxillary gland of the cat. *J Physiol* 1980; **300**: 41–53.

22. Lundberg JM. Evidence for coexistence of vasoactive intestinal polypeptide (VIP) and acetylcholine in neurons of cat exocrine glands: morphological, biochemical and functional studies. *Acta Physiol Scand Suppl* 1981; **496**: 1–57.

23. Lefkowitz RJ. The superfamily of heptahelical receptors. *Nat Cell Biol* 2000; **2**: E133–6.

24. Raymond JR, Hnatowich M, Lefkowitz RJ, Caron MG. Adrenergic receptors: models for regulation of signal transduction processes. *Hypertension* 1990; **15**: 119–31.

25. Insel PA. Adrenergic receptors: evolving concepts and clinical implications. *N Engl J Med* 1996; **334**: 580–5.

26. Hausdorff WP, Caron MG, Lefkowitz RJ. Turning off the signal: desensitization of β-adrenergic receptor function. *FASEB J* 1990; **4**: 2881–9.

27. Nattel S, Rangno RE, Van Loon G. Mechanism of propranolol withdrawal phenomena. *Circulation* 1979; **59**: 1158–64.

28. Vanhees L, Aubert A, Fagard R, *et al.* Influence of β1- versus β2-adrenoceptor blockade on left ventricular function in humans. *J Cardiovasc Pharmacol* 1986; **8**: 1086–91.

29. Brodde OE. The functional importance of β1 and β2 adrenoceptors in the human heart. *Am J Cardiol* 1988; **62**: 24C–29C.

30. Lefkowitz RJ, Rockman HA, Koch WJ. Catecholamines, cardiac beta-adrenergic receptors, and heart failure. *Circulation* 2000; **101**: 1634–7.

31. Opie L. Ventricular overload and heart failure. In Opie LH, ed., *The Heart: Physiology and Metabolism*, 2nd edn. New York, NY: Raven Press, 1991: 396–424.

32. Gauthier C, Langin D, Balligand JL. β3-Adrenoceptors in the cardiovascular system. *Trends Pharmacol Sci* 2000; **21**: 426–31.

33. Goldberg LI, Rajfer SI. Dopamine receptors: applications in clinical cardiology. *Circulation* 1985; **72**: 245–8.

34. Missale C, Nash SR, Robinson SW, *et al.* Dopamine receptors: from structure to function. *Physiol Rev* 1998; **78**: 189–225.

35. Linder ME, Gilman AG. G proteins. *Sci Am* 1992; **267**: 56–61, 64–5.

36. Standaert F. Donuts and holes: molecules and muscle relaxants. In Katz RL, ed., *Muscle Relaxants: Basic and Clinical Aspects*. Orlando, FL: Grune & Stratton, 1984.

37. Martyn JA, White DA, Gronert GA, *et al.* Up-and-down regulation of skeletal muscle acetylcholine receptors: effects on neuromuscular blockers. *Anesthesiology* 1992; **76**: 822–43.

38. Hosey MM. Diversity of structure, signaling and regulation within the family of muscarinic cholinergic receptors. *FASEB J* 1992; **6**: 845–52.

39. Charlson ME, MacKenzie CR, Gold JP. Preoperative autonomic function abnormalities in patients with diabetes mellitus and patients with hypertension. *J Am Coll Surg* 1994; **179**: 1–10.

40. Ewing DJ, Martyn CN, Young RJ, Clarke BF. The value of cardiovascular autonomic function tests: 10 years experience in diabetes. *Diabetes Care* 1985; **8**: 491–8.

41. Veith RC, Featherstone JA, Linares OA, Halter JB. Age differences in plasma norepinephrine kinetics in humans. *J Gerontol* 1986; **41**: 319–24.

42. Lakatta EG. Deficient neuroendocrine regulation of the cardiovascular system with advancing age in healthy humans. *Circulation* 1993; **87**: 631–6.

43. Ewing DJ, Campbell IW, Clarke BF. The natural history of diabetic autonomic neuropathy. *Q J Med* 1980; **49**: 95–108.

44. Burgos LG, Ebert TJ, Asiddao C, *et al.* Increased intraoperative cardiovascular morbidity in diabetics with autonomic neuropathy. *Anesthesiology* 1989; **70**: 591–7.

45. Page MM, Watkins PJ. Cardiorespiratory arrest and diabetic autonomic neuropathy. *Lancet* 1978; **1**: 14–16.

46. Ewing DJ, Clarke BF. Diagnosis and management of diabetic autonomic neuropathy. *Br Med J* 1982; **285**: 916–18.

47. Selye H. Forty years of stress research: principal remaining problems and misconceptions. *Can Med Assoc J* 1976; **115**: 53–6.

48. Kehlet H. Manipulation of the metabolic response in clinical practice. *World J Surg* 2000; **24**: 690–5.

49. Anand KJ, Hickey PR. Halothane–morphine compared with high-dose sufentanil for anesthesia and postoperative analgesia in neonatal cardiac surgery. *N Engl J Med* 1992; **326**: 1–9.

50. Mangano DT, Layug EL, Wallace A, Tateo I. Effect of atenolol on mortality and cardiovascular morbidity after noncardiac surgery. *N Engl J Med* 1996; **335**: 1713–20.

51. Fleisher L, Beckman JA, Brown KA, *et al.* ACC/AHA 2006 guideline update on perioperative cardiovascular evaluation for noncardiac surgery: focused update on perioperative beta-blocker therapy. *Anesth Analg* 2007; **104**: 15–26.

52. Ramsay MA, Luterman DL. Dexmedetomidine as a total intravenous anesthetic agent. *Anesthesiology* 2004; **101**: 787–90.

53. Flacke J, Bloor BC, Flacke WE, *et al.* Reduced narcotic requirement by clonidine with improved hemodynamic and adrenergic stability in patients undergoing coronary bypass surgery. *Anesthesiology* 1987; **67**: 11–19.

54. POISE Study Group. Effects of extended-release metoprolol succinate in patients undergoing non-cardiac surgery (POISE trial): a randomized controlled trial. *Lancet* 2008; **371**: 1839–47.

55. Wallace AW, Galindez D, Salahieh A, *et al.* Effect of clonidine on cardiovascular morbidity and mortality after noncardiac surgery. *Anesthesiology* 2004; **101**: 284–93.

56. Schildkraut JJ. Neuropsychopharmacology and the affective disorders. *N Engl J Med* 1969; **281**: 197–201.

57. Kamibayashi T, Maze M. Clinical uses of alpha2-adrenergic agonists. *Anesthesiology* 2000; **93**: 1345–9.

58. Rudner XL, Berkowitz DE, Booth JV, *et al.* Subtype specific regulation of human vascular alpha(1)-adrenergic receptors by vessel bed and age. *Circulation* 1999; **100**: 2336–43.

59. Lakhlani PP, MacMillan LB, Guo TZ, *et al.* Substitution of a mutant alpha2a-adrenergic receptor via "hit and run" gene targeting reveals the role of this subtype in sedative, analgesic, and anesthetic-sparing responses in vivo. *Proc Natl Acad Sci U S A* 1997; **94**: 9950–5.

60. Maze M, Fujinaga M. Alpha2 adrenoceptors in pain modulation: which subtype should be targeted to produce analgesia? *Anesthesiology* 2000; **92**: 934–6.

61. Gerhardt MA, Booth JV, Chesnut LC, *et al.* Acute myocardial beta-adrenergic receptor dysfunction after cardiopulmonary bypass in patients with cardiac valve disease. Duke Heart

Center Perioperative Desensitization Group. *Circulation* 1998; **98**: II275–81.

62. McDonald PH, Chow CW, Miller WE, *et al.* Beta-arrestin 2: a receptor-regulated MAPK scaffold for the activation of JNK3. *Science* 2000; **290**: 1574–7.

63. Bohn LM, Gainetdinov RR, Lin FT, Lefkowitz RJ, Caron MG. Mu-opioid receptor desensitization by beta-arrestin-2 determines morphine tolerance but not dependence. *Nature* 2000; **408**: 720–3.

64. Wallukat G, Muller J, Podlowski S, *et al.* Agonist-like beta-adrenoceptor antibodies in heart failure. *Am J Cardiol* 1999; **83**: 75H–79H.

65. Wallukat G, Nissen E, Morwinski R, Muller J. Autoantibodies against the beta- and muscarinic receptors in cardiomyopathy. *Herz* 2000; **25**: 261–6.

66. Sneddon P, Westfall TD, Todorov LD, *et al.* Modulation of purinergic neurotransmission. *Prog Brain Res* 1999; **120**: 11–20.

67. Yang IA, Ng T, Molenaar, Fong KM. β2-adrenoceptor polymorphisms and obstructive airway diseases: important issues of study design. *Clin Exp Pharm Phys* 2007; **34**: 1029–36.

68. Muthumala A, Drenos F, Elliott PM, Humphries SE. Role of beta adrenergic receptor polymorphisms in heart failure: systematic review and meta-analysis. *Eur J Heart Fail* 2008; **10**: 3–13.

69. Jacob G, Garland EM, Costa F, *et al.* β2-adrenoceptor genotype and function affect hemodynamic profile heterogeneity in postural tachycardia syndrome. *Hypertension* 2006; **47**: 421–7.

70. Small KM, Wagoner LE, Levin AM, Kardia SLR, Liggett SB. Synergistic polymorphisms of β1- and α2c-adrenergic receptors and the risk of congestive heart failure. *N Engl J Med* 2002; **347**: 1135–42.

71. Shin J, Johnson JA. Pharmacogenetics of β-blockers. *Pharmacotherapy* 2007; **27**: 874–87.

72. Lefkowitz RJ. Seven transmembrane receptors: something old, something new. *Acta Physiol* 2007; **190**: 9–19.

Physiologic substrates of drug action
Immunity and inflammation

Nigel R. Webster and Helen F. Galley

Introduction

The immune system in humans has evolved to provide protection against invading pathogenic organisms, foreign cells, and macromolecules. This chapter describes the basic mechanisms involved in immune responses and illustrates the particular relevance for some disease processes. The immune system comprises **innate immunity** and **acquired, or adaptive, immunity**. These systems work together in a network, with huge areas of overlap and mutual interactivity, to prevent infection. The response to pathogens is a continuum with no clear dividing line where innate responses end and adaptive immunity begins. Figure 23.1 shows how innate immune responses such as phagocytosis activate adaptive responses via antigen presentation, T-cell activation, and cytokine expression. These processes follow seamlessly.

Innate immunity

Immunity is the state of protection from infectious disease or our own altered cells, and it includes both specific and nonspecific components. Nonspecific, or innate, immunity is the inbuilt resistance to disease, consisting of four defensive barriers that offer protection through anatomical, physiological, phagocytic, and inflammatory strategies (Table 23.1). It responds in exactly the same manner to any threat, whether bacterial, viral, or parasitic.

Anatomical barriers
The skin

Intact skin prevents penetration of most pathogens. The dermis is composed of connective tissue and contains blood vessels, hair follicles, sebaceous glands, and sweat glands. The sebaceous glands produce sebum, made up of lactic acid and fatty acids, which keeps the pH of the skin at around pH 4 and inhibits bacterial growth. Bacteria which metabolize sebum live on the skin and acne treatments such as isotretotoin inhibit sebum formation. Breaks in the skin such as small cuts and insect bites are obvious routes of infection, and diseases

such as malaria and Lyme disease are spread by breaching of the skin by insect bites.

Mucous membranes

Mucous membranes are protected by saliva, tears, and mucus, which wash away organisms and also contain antiviral and antibacterial substances. In the lower respiratory and gastrointestinal tracts organisms trapped in mucus are propelled out of the body by ciliary action. Some organisms have evolved to evade this defense mechanism; for example, the influenza virus has a surface molecule that enables it to attach to cells in mucous membranes, preventing it being washed away through the action of cilia. The adherence of bacteria to mucous membranes is dependent on the interaction of protrusions on the bacteria and specific glycoproteins on mucous-membrane epithelial cells, which explains why only certain tissues are susceptible to bacterial invasion.

Physiological barriers

If an organism manages to breach the anatomical barriers, there are several physiological protection mechanisms including temperature, pH, and a variety of soluble factors (such as lysozyme, interferons [IFNs] and complement). Some species (e.g., birds) have a high body temperature which inhibits the growth of certain organisms. Gastric acidity prevents the growth of many organisms, and newborn infants are more prone to some diseases since their stomach contents are less acidic. Lysozyme, found in mucus, is an enzyme which cleaves the peptidoglycan layer of bacterial cell walls. IFNs are produced by virus-infected cells and bind to nearby cells causing a generalized antiviral state (see below).

Phagocytosis

Another important innate defense mechanism is the ingestion of pathogens by the process of phagocytosis. Phagocytes are free-living cells which can move around the body, engulfing pathogens. The so-called "professional" phagocytes are the neutrophils and macrophages, while "nonprofessional" phagocytes – which do not move around the body – include

Anesthetic Pharmacology, 2nd edition, ed. Alex S. Evers, Mervyn Maze, Evan D. Kharasch. Published by Cambridge University Press. © Cambridge University Press 2011.

endothelial cells hepatocytes and glial cells. These cells, and indeed other cells of the innate immune system, express a limited number of receptors, which recognize molecules on the surface of invading pathogens. These molecules are called pathogen-associated molecular pattern molecules (PAMPs), and they are essentially repeated sugar molecules or other nonmammalian substances such as double-stranded RNA. Receptors that recognize these overall patterns rather than specific features (e.g., specific nucleotide sequences) are known either as pattern recognition receptors (PRRs) or as PAMP receptors. They recognize families of pathogens, e.g., viruses in general, rather than specific viruses such as herpes simplex or human immune deficiency virus (HIV). The two

main types of PRRs, Toll-like receptors (TLRs) and collectins, are discussed further below.

If the PRRs expressed on phagocytes recognize unusual molecules on a pathogen, it is phagocytosed and held in an intracellular vacuole or phagosome. Proteolytic enzymes are then released to destroy the pathogen. Phagocytes also release chemoattractant molecules, or chemokines, such as interleukin 8 (IL-8), which attract other phagocytes to the site of infection. Pathogens that are too big to be phagocytosed, such as parasites, can be destroyed by mast cells or eosinophils, which release massive amounts of enzymes onto the invading pathogen from intracellular granules by a process called degranulation. Intracellular infections by viruses, for example, evade phagocytosis, and cells infected with viruses and parasites are killed by large granular lymphocytes, termed natural killer (NK) cells, and eosinophils.

Interferons

Virus-infected cells release IFNs, which interfere with viral replication and prevent infection of other cells. IFNs are the first line of defense against viruses. By inducing the expression of IFN-stimulated genes, which have antiviral functions, IFNs can block virus replication. However, viruses are able to counteract this response through mechanisms which control IFN signaling and so block the actions of IFN-stimulated gene products. Studies of influenza, hepatitis C, herpes simplex, and vaccinia viruses have revealed the importance of IFNs for the control of virus replication and pathogenesis [1].

Complement

The complement system acts together with phagocytosis and is an even more rapid way of dealing with infection. Complement is a group of serum proteins which circulate in an

Table 23.1. The innate immune response

Type of barrier	Examples	Mediators
Anatomical barriers	Skin, mucous membranes	Sebum, mucous, ciliary action
Physiological barriers	pH, temperature, soluble factors	Complement, lysozyme, interferons
Phagocytosis	Neutrophils, macrophages, natural killer cells	Phagosome, lysozyme
Inflammatory response	Vasodilation, increased capillary permeability, leukocyte margination, chemical mediators	Cytokines, acute phase proteins, histamine, kinins, complement, phagocytosis

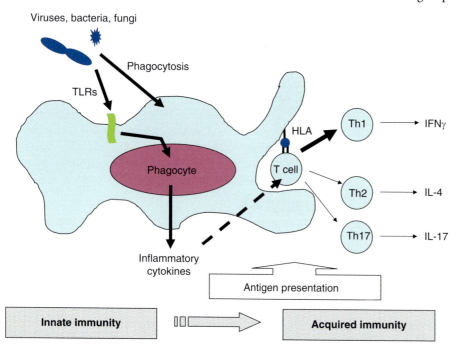

Figure 23.1. The immune system comprises innate and acquired, or adaptive, immunity. Innate immunity is the first line of defence against pathogens. The innate immune response activates adaptive immune processes through the Toll-like receptors (TLRs) and antigen presentation. Phagocytes recognize and phagocytose pathogens which promote cytokine expression and antigen presented along with human leukocyte antigens (HLA). T cells are activated and differentiated depending upon cytokine expression and antigen presentation to T helper 1 (Th1), Th2, or Th17 cells, which have roles in cellular immunity (cellular cytotoxicity), humoral or antibody-mediated immunity, and defense against extracellular pathogens respectively.

carefully
groups o
portion c
leukocyte
sion mol
(VCAM).
slow dow
adherence

Tissue
pathway.
box 1 pro
from nec
this is re
(DAMP).
promotes
migration
lia with
molecules
for adva
inflamma
leukocyte

RAGE
both as a
with extra
and drive
kinase (M
Soluble R
HMGB1.
througho
ticularly i
observed
vessels, r
other DA
peptides

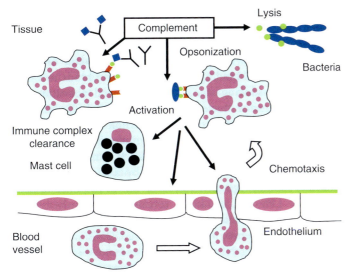

Figure 23.2. Complement has a central role in innate immunity, causing chemotaxis of phagocytes, opsonization and lysis of pathogens, and clearance of immune complexes.

inactive state. Activation converts the inactive proenzymes to active enzymes through an enzyme cascade, which results in membrane-damaging reactions, destroying pathogenic organisms and facilitating their clearance (Fig. 23.2). There are two pathways of complement activation. The classical pathway involves activation by specific immunoglobulin molecules, and the alternative pathway is activated by a variety of microorganisms and immune complexes. Each results in generation of a membrane attack complex which displaces phospholipids within cell membranes, making large holes, disrupting the membrane, and resulting in bacterial cell lysis. Complement components also amplify reactions between antigens and antibodies, attract phagocytic cells to sites of infection and promote phagocytosis, and activate B lymphocytes. Pathogens which have activated the complement cascade become coated with complement components, making them targets for phagocytosis. This is called opsonization. The complement system is nonspecific and can attack "self" cells as well as foreign cells. To prevent host-cell damage there are regulatory mechanisms which restrict complement reactions to specific targets by the release of inactivating proteins.

Acqui

The adap
diversity,
"non-self
gen, the
gen elimi
memory.

A key
the inna
increased
ecule. To
would ta
during n
ments fre
this way
molecule
genetic r
cytes call

The inflammatory response
Acute-phase response
The inflammatory response is initiated by a series of interactions involving chemical mediators, produced from the invading organisms, from damaged cells, from cells of the immune system, and from plasma enzyme systems. Among the chemical mediators released as a result of tissue damage are the acute-phase proteins, most notably the pentraxin family. C-reactive protein (CRP) is a short pentraxin produced mainly by hepatocytes in response to mediators such as IL-6. However, CRP is also produced by other cells. It binds to the C polysaccharide component

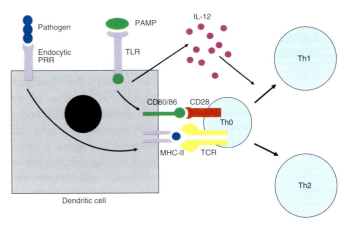

Figure 23.3. Toll-like receptors (TLRs) and other pattern recognition receptors (PRRs) sense the presence of infection through recognition of pathogen-associated molecular patterns (PAMPs). Recognition of PAMPs by TLRs expressed on antigen-presenting cells (for example dendritic cells) upregulates cell-surface expression of other molecules (e.g., CD80/CD86) and major histocompatability complex class II (MHC-II) molecules. TLRs also induce expression of cytokines, e.g., IL-12. Induction of CD80/86 on antigen-presenting cells leads to activation of T cells specific for pathogens that trigger TLR signaling, and IL-12 also contributes to the differentiation of Th cells into T helper 1 (Th1) effector cells.

found on many bacteria and fungi, activating the complement system, resulting in both complement-mediated lysis and increased phagocytosis. Pentraxin 3 is a long pentraxin produced by several cells of the innate immune system in response to PAMPs [2]. Histamine is released from mast cells, basophils, and platelets and binds to receptors on capillaries and venules, leading to increased vascular permeability and vasodilation. Kinins cause vasodilation and increased capillary permeability, and bradykinin also stimulates pain receptors in the skin.

PRRs
The PRRs or PAMP receptors mentioned above are important in the early response to pathogens by the innate immune system (Fig. 23.3). They initiate the production of phagocytosis and inflammatory responses by alerting cells to potential infection. Collectins are soluble PAMPs, and TLRs are found on the surface of cells.

Collectins are so-called because they have a collagen-like region and a lectin region. Lectins bind sugar molecules usually on the surface of bacteria. For example, mannose is found on bacteria but is not usually found on mammalian cell surfaces. The collagen domain of the collectin then interacts with effectors of the innate immune system such as phagocytes and complement. Mannose-binding lectin, ficolins, and C_{1q} are examples of collectins in the circulation, and surfactant protein A is found in the alveolar fluid in the lung [3–6]. Interestingly, the levels of mannose-binding lectin in blood are very variable in the normal population, due to genetic variations (polymorphisms) in the genes which regulate its expression. Those people who have lower levels of mannose-binding lectin have been shown to be at a higher risk of some infections than people with higher levels [7]. Children who have low levels of the Th1 phenotype, rather than generalized Th suppression. Th1 predominance is associated with cell-mediated responses, which are generally considered to be most beneficial to recovery. A shift to Th2-dominated phenotypes increases the risk for infection, for example after burn injury.

It has also been recently reported that there is an IL-23-dependent Th cell population which produces IL-17 but not IFNγ or IL-4, providing compelling evidence that the pathway that leads to generation of IL-17-producing effectors, termed the Th17 lineage, is distinct from that of the Th1 lineage, and therefore represents the third arm of the CD4 T-cell effector repertoire: Th1, Th2, and Th17 [13] (Fig. 23.6). It is thought that the Th17 lineage evolved to cope with a range of extracellular bacterial pathogens, and may be involved in autoimmune diseases, although further work will be needed to define the range of pathogens linked to Th17.

B cells and antibody

B cells are produced in the bone marrow, and through negative selection only those which are self-tolerant enter the circulation. They produce receptor though genetic recombination, but some of the receptor, unlike T cells, is actively secreted into intracellular spaces. The free B-cell receptor is called antibody or immunoglobulin. Antibody molecules consist of two identical light chains and two identical heavy chains joined by disulfide bonds. Each heavy and light chain has a variable amino acid sequence region and a constant region. The unique heavy chain constant region sequences determine the five classes or isotypes of antibody – IgM, IgG, IgA, IgD, and IgE (Table 23.3).

These isotypes vary in their function, serum concentration, and half-life. Each has a specific role. IgM is found only in blood and intercellular fluid and binds onto the surface of pathogens and stimulates the innate immune system through phagocytosis and complement activation. IgG and IgA are

found only in mammals. IgG is the most common isotype, found in most body compartments, and is the only immunoglobulin to cross the placenta. IgA is actively secreted across mucosal surfaces and so is the predominant isotype in breast milk and mucus. Neonates are very prone to infection due to their immature immune systems, and both IgG and IgA play an important role, since IgG is pumped across the placenta and IgA is secreted into breast milk. This protection for newborns probably explains why mammals need to have fewer offspring.

IgD and IgE are the least abundant isotypes. IgE mediates mast-cell degranulation and has evolved to protect against helminth infections. It binds to the surface of mast cells, and upon recognition of the parasite antigen mast-cell degranulation occurs, which causes release of mucus from the gut and stimulated gut contraction leading to worm expulsion. IgE is also involved in hypersensitivity reactions (see below).

B cells initially produce IgM but switch to production of other Ig classes after interaction with T cells. After class switching, B cells undergo somatic hypermutation to ensure production of high-affinity antibody. Any given B cell only secretes one antibody isotype. Binding of pathogens to antibodies on the cell surface of B cells leads to preferential selection of antibody-producing cells. This is termed priming, and subsequent responses are faster and amplified; this provides the basis of vaccination.

Cytokines

Regulation of immune responses depends on communication between cells by soluble molecules given the generic term cytokines, including chemokines (chemoattractant cytokines), ILs, growth factors, and IFNs. They are involved in both innate and acquired/adaptive immune responses. They are low-molecular-weight secreted proteins which regulate both the amplitude and duration of immune responses and have the properties of redundancy, pleiotrophy, synergism, and antagonism. They

Table 23.3. Characteristics of immunoglobulin isotypes

Antibody isotype	Half-life in serum	Specific effector function	Other information
IgM	5 days	Antigen receptor for naive B cells Complement activation (classical pathway)	Membrane bound
IgG	23 days	Neutralization of bacteria Facilitation of phagocytosis Complement activation (classical pathway) ADCC mediated by NK cells Inhibits B cell activation	Crosses placenta; provides neonatal passive immunity
IgA	6 days	Provides mucosal immunity	Secreted into gut lumen, respiratory tract and breast milk
IgD	3 days	Antigen receptor for naive B cells	Membrane bound, no secreted form
IgE	2 days	ADCC mediated by eosinophils Mast cell degranulation	Provides immunity against helminths Involved in hypersensitivity reactions

ADCC, antibody-dependent cellular cytotoxicity; NK, natural killer.

have a transient and tightly regulated action. Cytokines are highly active at very low concentrations, combining with small numbers of high-affinity cell-surface receptors and producing changes in the patterns of RNA and protein synthesis. They have multiple effects on growth and differentiation in a variety of cell types, with considerable overlap and redundancy between them, partially accounted for by the induction of synthesis of common proteins. Interaction may occur in a sort of network in which one cytokine induces another, through modulation of the receptor of another cytokine and through either synergism or antagonism of two cytokines acting on the same cell. Any given cytokine should not be seen specifically as a growth stimulator or inhibitor, or as having pro- or anti-inflammatory properties. Their specific actions depend on the stimulus, the cell type, and the presence of other mediators and receptors.

Interferons (IFNα, β, γ) are a family of broad-spectrum antiviral agents which also modulate the activity of other cells, particularly IL-8 and platelet activating factor (PAF) production, antibody production by B cells and activation of cytotoxic macrophages. Growth factors regulate the differentiation, proliferation, activity, and function of specific cell types. The best-known are colony stimulating factors, which cause colony formation by hematogenic progenitor cells (e.g., GM-CSF). Other examples include factors which regulate the growth of nerve cells, fibroblasts, epidermis, and hepatocytes.

In addition to the low-molecular-weight protein mediators, there are also lipid mediators of inflammation, including PAF and arachidonic acid metabolites. PAF is a labile alkyl phospholipid released from a variety of cells in the presence of antigen and leukocytes in response to immune complexes. In addition to its actions on platelets, the effects of PAF include the priming of macrophages to other inflammatory mediators and alterations of microvascular permeability. Arachidonic acid metabolites include the prostaglandins and leukotrienes, which have profound inflammatory and vascular actions, and may regulate and be regulated by other cytokines.

The biological activities of cytokines are regulated by specific cellular receptors. Often these receptors comprise multiple subunits providing phased stages of activation and biological action. For example the IL-2 receptor (IL-2R) complex consists of three subunits: IL-2Rα, IL-2Rβ, and IL-2γ. Although the IL-2Rα/β combination can bind IL-2, IL-2Rγ is also required for high-affinity binding, ligand internalization, and signaling, which all are required for maximal effect. Other cellular receptors are present in more than one type; these act alone but have different binding affinities for different forms of a cytokine protein (e.g. IL-1 receptor type I binds IL-1α better than IL-1β, and IL-1 receptor type II has more affinity for IL-1β). Binding of a cytokine to one type of receptor may result in interactions with another receptor. The two receptors for TNF, for example, use ligand passing, in which TNF binds transiently to receptor type I, with full signal transduction, but may then move on to the type II

receptor with activation of another signal for apoptosis or programmed cell killing.

Soluble cytokine receptors have been identified which compete with membrane-bound receptors, thus regulating cytokine signals. Exceptions to this are soluble receptors for IL-6 and ciliary neurotrophic factor, which act as agonists rather than antagonists. Such soluble receptors may be membrane-bound receptors, which are shed into the circulation either intact or as truncated forms (e.g., soluble TNF receptors, sTNF-R), or may begin as related precursor molecules that are enzymatically cleaved (e.g., IL-1R). Soluble receptors may appear in response to stimuli as part of a naturally occurring independent regulatory process to limit the harmful effects of a mediator (e.g., sTNF-R), but some soluble receptors have little binding activity and may represent superficial and unimportant losses of cellular receptors (e.g., the soluble form of IL-2Rα). Soluble cytokine receptors not only mediate biological activity but also control desensitization to ligands by reduced availability and decreased signaling, and by stimulating cellular mechanisms that can result in lack of activity.

The biological actions of some cytokines are also regulated by receptor antagonists. The receptor antagonist for IL-1 (IL-1ra) competes with cell receptors for IL-1, but when bound does not induce signaling. IL-1ra binds to cell receptors much more avidly than to soluble receptors, such that soluble receptors will have little effect of the inhibitory action of the receptor antagonist. The soluble receptor also inhibits activation of the pro-IL-1β precursor. The appearance of IL-1ra is independently regulated by other cytokines as part of the inflammatory process.

Immune mechanisms in disease

Hypersensitivity

Excessive inflammation caused by immune reaction is called hypersensitivity and is an important concept in the pathology of many diseases. Substances which are normally harmless such as food proteins or metal ions can cause hypersensitivity in some people. In others, harmless self-antigens which are components of normal tissues can trigger hypersensitivity through autoimmunity, and this is the basis of many manifestations of autoimmune diseases.

Hypersensitivity reactions can be classified into type I (IgE-dependent), type II (antibody-mediated cytotoxicity), type III (immune-complex-mediated hypersensitivity), and type IV (delayed-type hypersensitivity or DTH). All these reactions rely on immunological memory, via the adaptive immune system, such that prior exposure to antigen is needed for subsequent hypersensitivity reactions to occur (Table 23.4).

Type I reactions are mediated by IgE antibodies, which bind to receptors on mast cells or basophils leading to degranulation and release of mediators. The principal effects are smooth-muscle contraction and vasodilation; these can result in asthma,

Table 23.4. Description and clinical features of hypersensitivity reactions

Category	Definition	Mechanism	Time frame	Examples
Type I	Immediate hypersensitivity reaction	Mediated by IgE antibody to specific antigens, causing release of histamine from mast cells	Within 1 hour	Anaphylaxis, e.g., penicillin allergy Urticaria Angioedema Atopic allergy
Type II	Cytotoxic antibody reaction	Mediated by IgG and IgM to specific antigens	Hours	Transfusion reaction Rhesus incompatibility Goodpasture's syndrome Delayed transplant graft rejection
Type III	Immune complex reaction	Antigen–antibody complexes deposit in tissue	1–3 weeks	Systemic lupus erythematosus Rheumatoid arthritis Serum sickness
Type IV	Delayed-type hypersensitivity	Mediated by T lymphocytes to specific antigens	2–7 days	Allergic contact dermatitis (e.g., nickel allergy)

hay fever, eczema, and serious life-threatening systemic anaphylaxis. Immediate hypersensitivity reactions occur within 8 hours of secondary allergen exposure. Allergy is defined as having specific IgE antibodies to certain antigens – termed allergens – causing the clinical symptoms of allergy, which are caused by an immediate (type I) hypersensitivity reaction mediated by IgE binding to mast cells. Atopy is the state of being at high risk of allergy.

Type II hypersensitivity reactions occur when antibody reacts with antigenic markers on cell surfaces, leading to cell death through complement-mediated lysis or antibody-dependent cytotoxicity. Classic type II reactions include blood-group reactions, e.g., ABO or hemolytic (Rh) disease of the newborn, and autoimmune diseases such as Goodpasture's syndrome and myasthenia gravis.

Type III reactions are mediated by antigen–antibody or immune-complex deposition and subsequent complement activation. Deposition of immune complexes near the site of antigen entry can cause the release of lytic enzymes from accumulated neutrophils and localized tissue damage. Formation of circulating immune complexes contributes to the pathogenesis of a number of conditions, including allergies to penicillin, infectious diseases (e.g., hepatitis), and autoimmune diseases (e.g., rheumatoid arthritis).

Type IV or delayed hypersensitivity (DTH) can occur when activated Th1 cells encounter certain antigens. Tissue damage is usually limited, and DTH plays an important role in defense against intracellular pathogens and contact antigens. Development of a DTH response requires a prior sensitization period when T cells are activated and clonally expanded by antigen presented along with the required HLA molecule on an appropriate antigen-presenting cell. A further antigen contact induces an effector response, where the expanded clonal Th cell population can respond immediately by producing a variety of cytokines leading to recruitment and activation of macrophages and other nonspecific inflammatory cells.

A DTH response becomes apparent about 24 hours following secondary antigen contact, peaking at 48–72 hours. The delay occurs because of the time required for cytokines to activate and recruit macrophages. A complex and amplified interaction of many nonspecific cells occurs, with only about 5% of the participating cells being antigen-specific. Prolonged DTH responses can be damaging, ultimately leading to tissue necrosis in extreme cases. Examples of DTH are contact dermatitis against, for example, nickel. Nickel is not antigenic by itself but it acts as a hapten when it combines with host proteins in the skin; this then triggers Th1 recruitment. The next time nickel is encountered, memory T cells migrate to the exposure site and secrete IFNγ, resulting in an inflammatory response lasting several days.

Mixed hypersensitivity responses can also occur. Asthma is a prime example, where exposure to an antigen such as dog hair in a sensitized individual will produce an immediate reaction with all the characteristics of a type I reaction. However, persistent exposure will result in eosinophil recruitment with the features of a type IV reaction and Th1 cytokine involvement.

Cancer
Some tumors are many times more common in patients with defective immune systems, including lymphoma, carcinoma of the cervix, and Kaposi's sarcoma. Many of the tumors which develop in such immunodeficient patients are linked to viral infections, however – for example Epstein–Barr virus (lymphoma), human herpes virus 8 (Kaposi's sarcoma), and papilloma virus (cervical carcinoma). Hence it is not clear if the immune system is responding to the tumor itself or to oncogenic viruses.

In most cases tumors are not caused by viruses but are the result of genetic damage by environmental factors. There is some evidence that novel proteins produced by tumor cells can stimulate an immune response and such tumor cells display surface structures which are recognized as antigenic and which promote an immune response. Macrophages mediate tumor destruction by lytic enzymes and production of TNFα; NK cells recognize tumor cells by an unknown mechanism and either bind to antibody-coated tumor cells – this is called antibody-dependent cell-mediated cytotoxicity – or by secretion of a cytotoxic factor which is apparently only cytotoxic for tumor cells. Tumor-cell antigens can often elicit the generation of specific serum antibodies, which activate the complement system. Complement products can also induce chemotaxis of macrophages and neutrophils and release of toxic mediators. Ironically, antibodies to tumor cells may also enhance tumor growth, possibly by masking tumor antigens and preventing recognition by NK cells. Most cancers, however, are not associated with novel proteins that can be recognized by the immune system, although they may occasionally produce normal proteins at high levels. A cancer cell with low HLA expression may evade immune surveillance. Unlike infections, tumors do not activate a "danger signal." Boosting the immune system to recognize tumors has been used as a therapeutic strategy – for example, using drugs that bind to TLRs to create danger signals, and using antibodies to B cells to promote phagocytosis of lymphomas. Antibodies can also be conjugated to toxins such as ricin [14] or radioactive yttrium [15] with a much greater therapeutic success rate.

HIV

Human immunodeficiency virus (HIV) is a retrovirus that is the causative agent for acquired immunodeficiency syndrome (AIDS). It has a small RNA genome containing three genes encoding its viral envelope and the enzymes reverse transcriptase and protease. HIV uses its envelope to bind to CD4 molecules and chemokine receptors (CCR5 and CXCR4) on cell membranes. Once in the cell, it produces a DNA copy of its genome with its reverse transcriptase; viral DNA then integrates into the host chromosomal DNA, forming a provirus that can remain in a dormant state for varying lengths of time. Reverse transcriptase introduces mutations into the HIV genome, leading to constantly changing amino acid sequences of its three proteins. Activation of an HIV-infected CD4-positive Th cell triggers activation of the provirus, leading to destruction of the host-cell plasma membrane and cell death; this leads to severe immunodepression and infection of other cells. Since only about 0.01% of the CD4-positive Th cells are infected by HIV in an HIV-infected individual, the extensive depletion of the T-cell population implies that uninfected CD4 cells are also destroyed. Several mechanisms have been proposed for this, including complement-mediated lysis, apoptosis, or antibody-mediated cytotoxicity. Early immunological abnormalities include loss of in-vitro proliferative responses of T cells, reduced IgM synthesis, increased cytokine synthesis, and reduced DTH responses. Later abnormalities include loss of germinal centers in lymph nodes, marked decreases in T-cell numbers and functions, lack of proliferation of HIV-specific B cells, lack of anti-HIV antibodies, shift in cytokine production from Th1 to Th2 subsets, and complete absence of DTH responses.

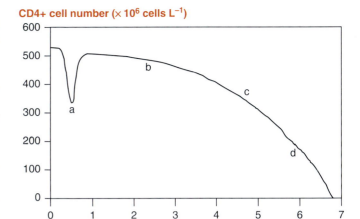

CD4+ cell number ($\times 10^6$ cells L^{-1})

Years after infection

Figure 23.7. The progress of CD-positive cell count after HIV infection. Early in infection there is little control of HIV infected cells and CD4-positive Th cells are destroyed rapidly, leading to (a) an acute dip in CD4 cell count. An asymptomatic period follows, with Tc responses to the virus leading to (b) only a gradual destruction of CD4-positive T cells. Ultimately the Tc cell response can no longer cope with the virus and the loss of CD-positive cells gradually increases to a critical point (c). As the CD4 count falls below around 400×10^6 cells L^{-1} opportunistic mild infections from pathogens such as *Candida* or herpes zoster can occur, but once the count falls below 200×10^6 cells L^{-1} more severe infections such as pneumonias are seen (d). Virus driven-tumors such Kaposi's sarcoma can also develop.

As is the case for many viruses, antibodies can provide some protection early in the infection, but cytotoxic T cells are much more important. In most cases Tc cells cannot sustain a response against established HIV infection because Tc cells are not receiving costimulation from Th cells, many of which have been destroyed. In addition, HIV mutates and is gradually able to evade immune responses. Ultimately significant damage to the immune system occurs, with ensuing opportunist infection and development of AIDS. Monitoring of CD4-positive cells is a useful means of measuring the number of surviving Th cells as an indication of immune status. Figure 23.7 shows the progress of the CD-positive cell count over several years after HIV infection, and summarizes the possible development of clinical manifestations.

Treatment of HIV is at present limited to delaying progression to AIDS. Individuals may have different rates of disease progression depending on genetic variation in HLA class I molecules and chemokine receptor expression. Cytokines are involved early in HIV infection and can affect disease progression and control of virus replication [16]. Several steps, before and after retroviral integration into host DNA in T cells, are affected by cytokines, and CCR5 and CXCR4 binding chemokines can interfere with viral entry. A polymorphism in the CCR5 chemokine receptor has been shown to be linked to a lesser probability of becoming infected with HIV after exposure and to slower disease progression, presumably due to interference with virus entry into the cells of the immune system [17].

It has been known since 1995 that HIV uses chemokine coreceptors, primarily CCR5 and CXCR4, for entry into CD4-positive T cells, providing another target for the treatment of HIV infection. Drugs which can block HIV entry include CD4 receptor inhibitors, chemokine receptor inhibitors, and inhibitors of attachment and membrane fusion. These drugs may add a further treatment for HIV-1 infection along with protease inhibitors and reverse transcription inhibitors, although to date these strategies do not seem to be effective in laboratory tests against HIV-4.

Transplantation and HLA

Transplantation is the transfer of cells, tissues, or organs from one site or person to another. Tissues that are antigenically similar or histocompatible do not elicit rejection; the reverse is termed histoincompatible. *Autologous* or *syngeneic* transplants are between different parts of the body or between identical twins, *allogeneic* transplants are between non-genetically identical members of the same species, and *xenogeneic* transplants are between different species. There will always be a rejection risk for allogeneic transplants and a very high risk for xenogeneic grafts.

The key antigens that trigger rejection are the HLA molecules. There are many antigens determining histocompatibility, but it is the HLA system which is most important. HLA genes are inherited in blocks called haplotypes. Most people do not have an identical twin who could act as a donor, but there is a 1 in 4 chance that a sibling will be HLA-identical. Both parents and half the siblings of a potential transplant recipient will share half the recipient's HLA genes. This is called haploidentical, but because only half the HLA genes are identical half are different, and an allogeneic response will occur. For these reasons a better match is often found from a large pool of nonrelated donors. Most kidneys are transplanted from brain-dead donors, and the chances of an identical HLA match are small. Potential recipients often have to wait for some time for transplantation and so may be offered a partial HLA mismatch, which has a better chance of success than a haploidentical organ from a living parent or sibling.

Stem cells are able to divide constantly; they are pluripotent and develop into many types of cells, depending on stimulus. Stem cells isolated from bone marrow can be rejected just like solid organs, and must be HLA matched as closely as possible.

Mesenchymal stem cells (MSC) originated from embryonic tissue, but multipotent cells derived from other nonembryonic and nonmarrow tissues, such as adult muscle cells or the Wharton's jelly present in the umbilical cord, as well as in the dental pulp of milk teeth, are often referred to as MSCs. The term multipotent stromal cell has therefore been proposed as a better term. Adult MSCs avoid allorecognition, interfere with dendritic cell and T cell function, and generate a local immunosuppressive microenvironment by secreting cytokines. They therefore seem to be hypoimmunogenic and suitable for allogeneic transplantation, while producing immunosuppression upon transplantation [18].

Summary

The physiological function of the immune system is to provide defense against infection, although noninfectious foreign substances and even endogenous molecules can also elicit immune responses. In addition, these protective mechanisms can also cause injury and disease themselves. A more inclusive definition of immunity is the reaction to foreign substances, including pathogens, macromolecules, proteins, and sugars, even though exposure to these may not have either pathological or physiological consequences. Immunology is the study of immunity in this broader sense and includes the cellular and molecular events and exploitation of them to treat disease.

Innate immunity provides several defensive barriers. The anatomical barriers of the skin and mucous membranes prevent pathogen entry. Physiological barriers, such as temperature, pH, and various soluble factors present a challenge to the survival and growth of many invading organisms. Effector cells of innate immunity express Toll-like receptors (TLR) and interact with collectins. These pattern recognition receptors (PRR) recognize conserved molecular patterns expressed by invading organisms, alerting the innate immune system to a potential infection. Phagocytic cells engulf and destroy pathogens. Other effector cells include mast cells, eosinophils, and natural killer (NK) cells. Interferon (IFN) signaling by virus-infected cells induces antiviral functions, blocking viral replication and preventing the spread of infection. The complement system mediates bacterial cell lysis as well as a variety of actions to aid in the recognition and clearance of invading organisms by circulating phagocytes. Inflammatory mediators are produced by pathogens, damaged cells, immune cells, and plasma enzyme systems. The inflammatory response leads to increased vascular permeability, vasodilation, and expression of adhesion molecules aiding the recruitment of leukocytes to the site of infection.

Activation of TLRs expressed by antigen-presenting cells is important in the initiation of adaptive immune responses. Adaptive immunity has the capacity to produce highly specific responses to diverse antigens, and furthermore is able to generate memory in order to produce a more rapid and intense response in the event of a second encounter. The diverse repertoire of T-cell and B-cell receptor specificities is generated by random genetic recombination during maturation. Lymphocytes bearing self-reactive receptors are eliminated during development, or are functionally suppressed, allowing the adaptive immunity to distinguish self from non-self. Recognition of specific antigen leads to clonal expansion of the specific lymphocytes. Some of these specific lymphocytes will become long-lived memory cells.

The humoral branch of adaptive immunity involves B lymphocytes and the production of antibody. Antibody binds antigen, neutralizing it or facilitating its clearance by innate effector cells. There are five different isotypes of antibody (immunoglobulins), which each perform different functions. In cell-mediated immunity, T lymphocytes recognize antigen as processed peptide fragments presented by human leukocyte antigen (HLA) molecules. Generally, phagocytosed extracellular antigen is processed and displayed on HLA class II molecules expressed by antigen-presenting cells, activating CD4-positive T helper (Th) cells, while cytoplasmic peptide antigens are displayed on HLA class I molecules for recognition by CD8-positive cytotoxic T cells. Th cells produce distinct patterns of cytokines which may enhance either cell-mediated immune functions (a Th1 cytokine profile) or humoral immunity (a Th2 cytokine profile).

Beyond its function to clear infection, the immune system can play an important role in disease. Excessive inflammation, or hypersensitivity, is important in the pathology of a number of diseases, including asthma, allergy, autoimmune diseases, and some infectious diseases such as hepatitis. There is some evidence that immune surveillance plays a role in eliminating tumor cells, and this is a basis for immunotherapeutic strategies. The human immunodeficiency virus (HIV) infects CD4-expressing Th cells, causing not only the death of the infected cell, but also extensive immune dysfunction with depletion of a large proportion of CD4-positive T cells, many of which arelikely uninfected. This results in immune suppression and subsequent opportunistic infections and acquired immunodeficiency syndrome (AIDS). Current antiretroviral drugs target reverse transcription and viral proteases; HIV binding and entry represent further potential pharmacologic targets.

The histocompatibility of donor tissues in transplantation is determined by many antigens, the highly polymorphic HLA molecules being the most important. Adult mesenchymal stem cells (MSC) promote local immunosuppression and may offer potential for avoiding rejection during allogeneic transplantation.

References

1. Unterholzner L, Bowie AG. The interplay between viruses and innate immune signaling: recent insights and therapeutic opportunities. *Biochem Pharmacol* 2008; **75**: 589–602.

2. Manfredi AA, Rovere-Querini P, Bottazzi B, Garlanda C, Mantovani A. Pentraxins, humoral innate immunity and tissue injury. *Curr Opin Immunol* 2008; **21**: 1–7.

3. Aderem A, Ulevitch RJ. Toll-like receptors in the induction of the innate immune response. *Nature* 2000; **406**: 782–7.

4. Runza VL, Schwaeble W, Männel DN. Ficolins: novel pattern recognition molecules of the innate immune response. *Immunobiology* 2008; **213**: 297–306.

5. Arancibia SA, Beltrán CJ, Aguirre IM, *et al.* Toll-like receptors are key participants in innate immune responses. *Biol Res* 2007; **40**: 97–112.

6. Kuroki Y, Takahashi M, Nishitani C. Pulmonary collectins in innate immunity of the lung. *Cell Microbiol* 2007; **9**: 1871–9.

7. Summerfield JA, Sumiya M, Levin M, *et al.* Association of mutations in mannose binding protein gene with childhood infection in consecutive hospital series. *Br Med J* 1997; **314**: 1229–36.

8. Hibberd ML, Sumiya M, Summerfield JA, *et al.* Meningoccal Research Group. Association of variants of the gene for mannose-binding lectin with susceptibility to meningococcal disease. *Lancet* 1999; **353**: 1049–53.

9. Rassa JC, Ross SR. Viruses and Toll-like receptors. *Microbes Infect* 2003; **5**: 961–96.

10. Delhalle S, Blasius R, Dicato M, Diederich M. A beginner's guide to NF-kappaB signaling pathways. *Ann N Y Acad Sci* 2004; **1030**: 1–13.

11. Cohen J. TREM-1 in sepsis. *Lancet* 2001; **358**: 776–8.

12. Carneiro LA, Magalhaes JG, Tattoli I, Philpott DJ, Travassos LH.Nod-like proteins in inflammation and disease. *J Pathol* 2008; **214**: 136–48.

13. Harrington LE, Mangan PR, Weaver CT. Expanding the effector CD4 T-cell repertoire: the Th17 lineage. *Curr Opin Immunol* 2006; **18**: 349–56.

14. Kreitman RJ. Toxin-labeled monoclonal antibodies. *Curr Pharm Biotechnol* 2001; **2**: 313–25.

15. Shimoni A, Nagler A. Radioimmunotherapy and stem-cell transplantation in the treatment of aggressive B-cell lymphoma. *Leuk Lymphoma* 2007; **48**: 2110–20.

16. Alfano M, Crotti A, Vicenzi E, Poli G. New players in cytokine control of HIV infection. *Curr HIV/AIDS Rep* 2008; **5**: 27–32.

17. Reiche EM, Bonametti AM, Voltarelli JC, Morimoto HK, Watanabe MA. Genetic polymorphisms in the chemokine and chemokine receptors: impact on clinical course and therapy of the human immunodeficiency virus type 1 infection (HIV-1). *Curr Med Chem* 2007; **14**: 1325–34.

18. Ryan JM, Barry FP, Murphy JM, Mahon BP. Mesenchymal stem cells avoid allogeneic rejection. *J Inflamm* 2005; **2**: 8.

Structure–activity relationships

Using the criteria cited above, it is becoming apparent that there are several specific classes of anesthetics, each of which shares common binding sites on specific target proteins. While a complete taxonomy of classes of anesthetics is not available, it is clear that some structurally similar anesthetics share a similar mode of action and have specific structure–activity relationships. The fact that a distinct pharmacophore has been identified for several classes of anesthetics (e.g., neurosteroids, propofol, barbiturates), but not for all anesthetics as a group, indicates that previous failures to identify anesthetic structure–activity relationships are probably a consequence of improper grouping of mechanistically unrelated groups of anesthetics and imprecise selection/definition of the endpoints used to measure potency. The structure–activity relationships for each class of anesthetics are briefly reviewed below.

The structure–activity relationships for the halogenated anesthetics are not well understood. Several recent modeling studies have been performed [15–17]. These studies all identify correlations between structure and anesthetic activity, but differ in their methodology and conclusions, with different structural importance being attributed to molecular size, shape, hydrophobicity, and electrostatic interactions. In contrast, the structure–activity relationships of anesthetic barbiturates have been known for many years [18]. Sedative activity is introduced to the barbituric acid ring by the addition of hydrophobic side chains. Increasing length and branching of the side chains increases both lipophilicity and anesthetic potency. The potency of barbiturates can also be increased by replacing the two-position oxygen with sulfur. All of the anesthetic barbiturates have asymmetric carbons, and enantiomeric pairs of barbiturates differ significantly in anesthetic potency [19].

Extensive data exist for the structure–activity relationships of propofol and etomidate. Systematic structure–activity studies by Neil Harrison's group [20,21] have shown that the anesthetic potency of various propofol analogs does not correlate well with log P, a measure of lipid solubility, but does correlate with the ability of the compounds to potentiate GABA-elicited chloride currents. This indicates that the $GABA_A$ receptor is the likely target of propofol action and that the shape and size of the analogs rather than just their hydrophobicity is important for their action at $GABA_A$ receptors. A follow-up quantitative structure–activity modeling analysis indicated that the most important determinant of anesthetic potency is the presence of a hydrogen bond donor (the phenol OH group), and that hydrophobic interactions with the two- and six-position groups on the aromatic ring are also major determinants of anesthetic potency. Studies with etomidate analogs have shown that the R and S enantiomers have a greater than 10-fold difference in potency both as modulators of $GABA_A$ receptor currents and as anesthetics [6]. The methyl group at the chiral center of etomidate appears to be essential for activity, but a variety of substituents on either of the etomidate rings produce differences in the compound's potency as modulators of $GABA_A$ receptor conformation [22].

Finally, extensive structure–activity studies have been performed on anesthetic steroids. The pharmacophore for neurosteroids acting at the $GABA_A$ receptor consists of an unsaturated steroid backbone with a hydrogen-bond accepting group in a 17β configuration and a hydrogen-bond donating hydroxyl group in a 3α configuration [23,24]. While there is a correlation between lipophilicity (log P) and neurosteroid potency, there are multiple compounds that deviate from this correlation. It appears that both lipophilicity and molecular structure (electrostatic and steric interactions) contribute to the activity of neurosteroids as anesthetics [25].

Etomidate

Etomidate is a carboxylated imidazole derivative that was found to have anesthetic properties in the 1960s. It is an

---

Box 24.1. A genetics primer

Genetics methods have become increasingly important for our understanding of anesthetic mechanisms. However, most anesthesiologists and even many anesthetic mechanism scientists are somewhat intimidated by genetic methods and terminology. In order to remedy this problem for our readers, a few basic genetic concepts and methods relevant to this chapter are presented here. First, consider the basic types of genetic approaches, forward genetics and reverse genetics. **Forward genetics**, otherwise known as classical genetics, begins with an animal that expresses an interesting phenotype (for example, resistance to isoflurane) and subsequently defines the gene or genes responsible for the trait. **Reverse genetics** begins with a gene of interest (for example, a gene encoding a $GABA_A$ receptor subunit) and modifies the gene or its expression in some way to determine the role of the gene in vivo. Simply put, forward genetics goes from phenotype to genotype, and reverse genetics from genotype to phenotype. The best example of a forward genetic approach in the anesthetic mechanism field was the screening through mutant nematodes for halothane hypersensitivity and the subsequent laborious identification of the genes by classical mapping techniques [12]. Reverse genetics can be subdivided into distinct approaches, knockouts and knockins. A **knockout** animal is one where a specific gene of interest is inactivated so that no functional gene product is produced. A **knockin** animal is one where a specific gene is altered to produce a novel gene product or a change in expression level or location. The β3(N265M) $GABA_A$ receptor subunit knockin mouse is a beautiful example that provides very strong evidence that etomidate and propofol produce immobility by potentiating β3-containing $GABA_A$ receptors [13]. Both knockout and knockin animals are generated by similar methods involving injection of DNA into pluripotent germ cells (see figure) and as such are two types of **transgenic** animals, where foreign DNA is introduced into the animal.

Box 24.1. (*cont.*)

A

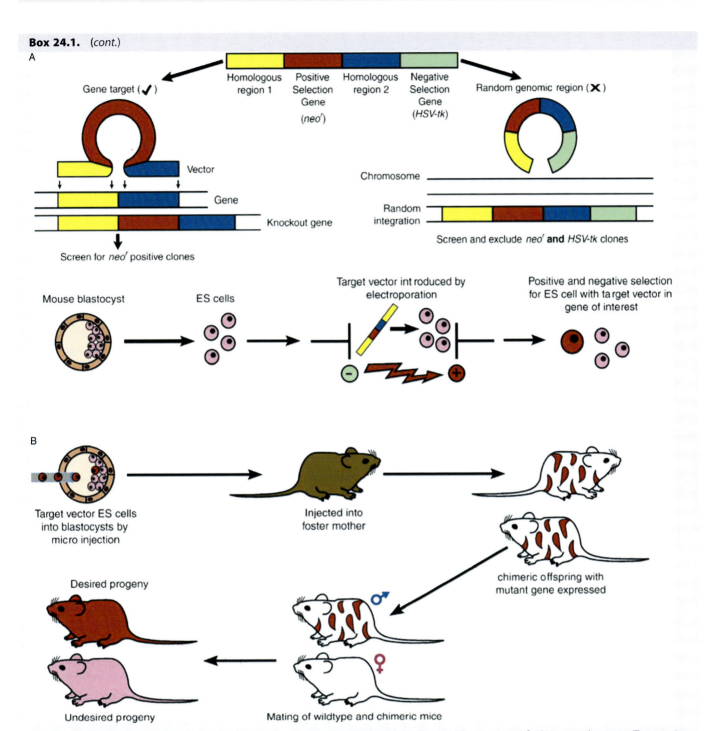

B

Making of a transgenic mouse. (A) A targeting vector is generated that has segments homologous to the native gene flanking a novel segment. The targeting vector is introduced into embryonic stem (ES) cells. ES cells that have incorporated the targeting vector into the corresponding gene by homologous recombination are selected by the presence of the positive selection gene and the absence of the negative selection gene. (B) ES cells with the targeting vector are injected into a foster mother and chimeric offspring identified. Chimeric mice are bred with wild-type mice and offspring containing the targeting vector are identified. Male and female heterozygous mice are then the founders for the transgenic strain. Adapted from Hacking [14].

efficacious hypnotic and amnestic agent, but lacks analgesic effect. The mechanism of anesthetic action of etomidate is arguably the best understood and characterized of any anesthetic. Current knowledge indicates that etomidate produces its hypnotic, amnestic and immobilizing effects via actions at the $GABA_A$ receptor. The structure and function of $GABA_A$ receptors is briefly reviewed in Box 24.2

Low concentrations of etomidate (10^{-7} – 10^{-5} M) potentiate the actions of GABA at $GABA_A$ receptors, whereas higher concentrations ($> 10^{-5}$ M) can directly activate the $GABA_A$ receptor [27–29]. Lambert and colleagues observed that the ability of etomidate to directly activate $GABA_A$ receptors is dependent on the β isoform that is present; β_2 and β_3 but not β_1 subunits support the effect of etomidate. These studies also showed that etomidate is about 10-fold more potent in potentiating the effects of GABA in β_2- than in β_1-containing receptors [30]. The realization that the actions of etomidate on $GABA_A$ receptors were subunit-specific led to studies to identify specific amino acid changes in the β_2 or β_3 subunits that could eliminate the effect of etomidate. This work resulted in the identification of a single asparganine in transmembrane spanning segment 2 (TM2) of the β_2 and β_3 subunits, which when changed to a methionine completely eliminated the ability of etomidate to either potentiate the actions of GABA or to directly activate $GABA_A$ receptors [31] (Fig. 24.3A). This asparganine is a serine in the β_1 subunit, explaining the inability of the β_1 subunit to support etomidate activity. Notably, the mutations in the β subunits did not affect the actions of pentobarbital on $GABA_A$ receptors, indicating that the critical asparganine was specific to etomidate action and might constitute part of a binding site [34]. Subsequent work has identified a methionine in the TM3 segment of the β subunits that is also essential for etomidate action [35].

Recent photolabeling studies have confirmed that etomidate binds to the β subunits of the $GABA_A$ receptor. Using azietomidate, an etomidate analog that covalently attaches to its binding site(s) on exposure to ultraviolet light (i.e., a photolabeling reagent), Li and colleagues showed that the critical methionine in TM3 (M286) of the β subunit and a methionine in TM1 (M236) of the α_1 subunit were attachment sites for azietomidate [36]. For technical reasons, they were unable to determine if the critical asparganine in TM2 of the β subunit was involved in etomidate binding. These data indicate that etomidate does directly bind to the β subunit(s) of the $GABA_A$ receptor, and suggest that etomidate may bind in a cleft between the α and β subunits (Fig. 24.3D).

To determine if the binding interaction of etomidate with the $GABA_A$ receptor is responsible for its anesthetic effect, transgenic animals were generated in which the critical asparganine in TM2 of the β_2 or β_3 subunits was changed to an amino acid (methionine) that renders the $GABA_A$ receptor insensitive to etomidate. Genetically modified mice containing an etomidate-insensitive β_2 subunit (β_2 N265S) demonstrated no change in the anesthetic actions of etomidate, as monitored by loss-of-righting reflex. The β_2-modified animals did show

reduced sedation in response to etomidate [37]. In marked contrast, genetically modified mice containing an etomidate-insensitive β_3 subunit (β_3 N265M) were completely resistant to the anesthetic effects of etomidate and propofol (as monitored by withdrawal to noxious stimulus) and were highly resistant to the effects of both drugs on loss-of-righting reflex (Fig. 24.3B,C). The response of the β_3 N265M mice to the neurosteroid alphaxalone was indistinguishable from that of wild-type animals, indicating that the β_3 mutation does not grossly alter ion channel function, but rather that it selectively interferes with the effect of etomidate [13]. These data indicate that etomidate action on $GABA_A$ receptors containing β_3 subunits is wholly responsible for its anesthetic effect. Etomidate interactions with β_2-containing $GABA_A$ receptors appear to contribute to the drug's sedative, but not anesthetic, actions.

While the preceding data provide strong evidence that the anesthetic action of etomidate is mediated by specific (β_3-containing) $GABA_A$ receptors, it is unclear if the amino acids identified constitute the actual etomidate binding site, or whether they are involved in transduction of the signal resulting from etomidate binding [32]. Additional photolabeling, modeling, and mutagenesis studies should clarify this issue.

It is clear that the β_3-containing $GABA_A$ receptors are anatomically positioned in arousal pathways in the central nervous system (CNS), appropriate locations to mediate the hypnotic effect of etomidate [38]. The amnestic effects of etomidate also appear to be mediated by $GABA_A$ receptors. Transgenic mice lacking the α_5 subunit of the $GABA_A$ receptor are resistant to the amnestic, but not the hypnotic effects of etomidate [39]. The amnestic effects of etomidate are likely mediated by $GABA_A$ receptors containing both α_5 and β_3 subunits.

The five criteria set out above to define relevant targets of anesthetic action are completely fulfilled by etomidate. (1) Its actions on $GABA_A$ receptors occur at clinically relevant concentrations, and (2) it has been shown to bind to the $GABA_A$ receptor. (3) Etomidate activates $GABA_A$ receptors, enhancing neuronal inhibition, and (4) its actions occur in critical arousal pathways in the CNS. Finally, (5) mutation of the $GABA_A$ receptor selectively eliminates the anesthetic effect of etomidate, but not of (all) other anesthetics. Unfortunately, etomidate is the only anesthetic for which the mechanism of anesthetic action is so clearly defined.

It is noteworthy that etomidate has several important non-mechanism-based effects. Unlike other anesthetics, it does not decrease blood pressure. This favorable clinical quality has been shown to be the result of etomidate acting as an agonist at α_{2B}-adrenoceptors [40]. Etomidate also has the adverse effect of suppressing adrenocortical steroid synthesis. This effect is mediated by inhibition of 11β-hydroxylase and 17α-hydroxylase, two enzymes involved in cortisol synthesis. An etomidate analog that retains its anesthetic effect, but has markedly reduced actions on cortisol synthesis, has recently been described [41].

Box 24.2. GABA_A receptors

Gamma-aminobutyric acid type A (GABA_A) receptors are the major inhibitory neurotransmitter receptors in the central nervous system. A functional GABA_A receptor is a pentamer composed of various combinations of five GABA_A subunits surrounding a central, chloride-selective, conducting pore. Eighteen mammalian GABA_A subunits have been identified by molecular cloning including 6 αs, 3 βs, 3 γs, 1 δ, 1 ϵ, 1 π, and 3 ρs. Each subunit consists of a large extracellular N-terminal domain, four transmembrane-spanning segments (TM1–TM4), and an intracellular loop between TM3 and TM4. Most GABA_A receptors are composed of 2α, 2β, and either a γ or a δ subunit. GABA binds in the extracellular domain, causing the channel to open and conduct chloride; in adult neurons this leads to hyperpolarization of the neuron and thus inhibits action-potential generation. Various anesthetics are thought to bind to the GABA_A receptor and either enhance the effects of GABA (potentiation) or directly activate the receptor in the absence of GABA. Interestingly, multiple anesthetics are thought to act through GABA_A receptors, and it appears that there are multiple distinct binding sites on the receptor for the different classes of anesthetics. It is noteworthy that GABA_A receptors are present both at the synapse and in extrasynaptic dendritic sites. At the postsynaptic membrane, activation of GABA_A receptors (generally containing a γ subunit) produces a short-lived phasic current that summates to form the inhibitory postsynaptic potential (IPSP). At extrasynaptic sites activation of GABA_A receptors (often containing a δ subunit) produces a tonic current of long duration.

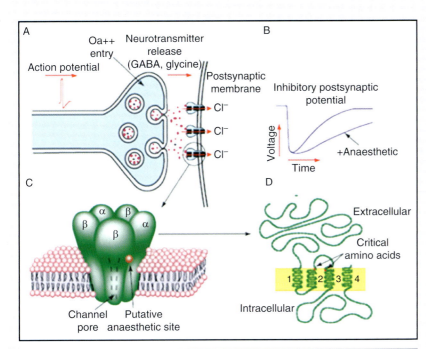

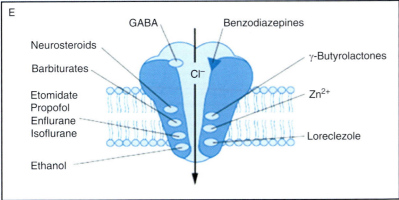

GABA_A receptors and anesthetic action. (A) GABA is released at inhibitory synapses and binds to postsynaptic GABA_A receptors. This allows chloride to enter the postsynaptic neuron. (B) The influx of chloride hyperpolarizes the neuron, generating an inhibitory postsynaptic potential (IPSP). The IPSP is enhanced by anesthetics binding to the GABA_A receptor. (C) The GABA_A receptors are pentamers of closely related subunits. (D) The membrane topology of a single subunit is illustrated. The amino acid residues thought to contribute to an isoflurane binding site are illustrated in (C) and (D) by red balls. Reproduced with permission from Franks and Lieb [26]. (E) A schematic representation of a GABA_A receptor, illustrating that in addition to binding sites for the physiologic neurotransmitter GABA, GABA_A receptors have distinct modulatory binding sites for benzodiazepines, barbiturates, neurosteroids, etomidate, propofol, and halogenated anesthetics.

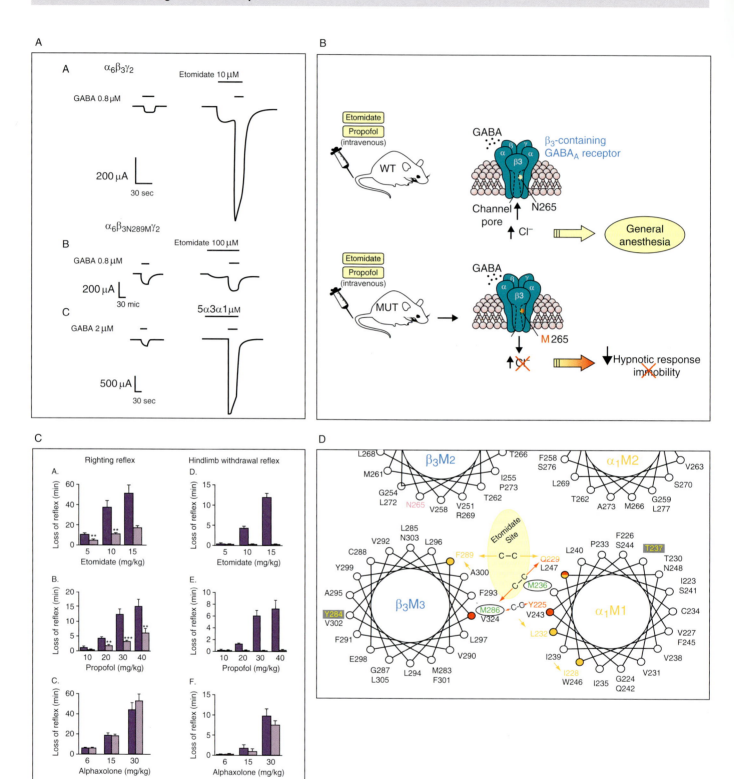

Figure 24.3. Mechanism of etomidate action. (A) Mutation of an asparagine to a methionine (N289M) in the TM2 segment of the β₃ subunit of the GABA_A receptor eliminates the ability of etomidate to activate GABA_A currents. This mutation has no effect on the ability of the neurosteroid allopregnanolone (5α3α) to enhance GABA_A currents. Reproduced with permission from Belelli et al. [31]. (B, C) Genetically modified mice with the equivalent asparagine to methionine mutation (N265M) in the β₃ subunit of the GABA_A receptor are resistant to the immobilizing and hypnotic effects of etomidate and propofol, but not the neurosteroid alphaxalone. Reproduced with permission from Jurd et al. [13]. (D) The putative binding site for etomidate as determined by photolabeling with azi-etomidate is in the interface between the TM1 segment of the α₁ subunit and the TM3 segment of the β₃ subunit. Reproduced with permission from Li et al. [33].

Propofol

Propofol is a substituted phenol that is widely used as an intravenous anesthetic, for both induction and maintenance of anesthesia. As with etomidate, the known neuropharmacologic profile of propofol suggests it to be a relatively selective modulator of the $GABA_A$ receptor. Propofol potentiates the actions of GABA to open $GABA_A$ receptors at clinical concentrations and directly activates $GABA_A$ currents at slightly higher concentrations [42]. Propofol is thought to interact primarily with β subunits of the $GABA_A$ receptor [43], but unlike etomidate shows no preference for the $β_2$ and $β_3$ subunits over the $β_1$ subunit [30]. Two specific amino acid residues have been identified as essential for potentiation of $GABA_A$ receptor function by propofol. A methionine residue (M286) in the TM3 region of the β subunit appears to be part of a propofol binding pocket, since the effect of various amino acid substitutions on propofol action varies with the bulk of the amino acid substituted at this site [44]. The same asparagine (N265) in TM2 of the $β_2$ and $β_3$ subunits that affects etomidate action is also essential to propofol effects on $GABA_A$ receptor function [31].

There are currently no direct labeling studies identifying binding sites for propofol. However, the ability of propofol to prevent etomidate photolabeling of its binding site on the $GABA_A$ receptor has been explored. These studies show that propofol partially inhibits etomidate labeling [45], suggesting that propofol and etomidate do *not* compete for a common binding site and that their binding sites are separate but allosterically linked sites on the β subunits of $GABA_A$ receptors. This is consistent with a recent molecular modeling study showing two distinct binding pockets for etomidate and propofol on the $β_2$ subunit [46].

As discussed with etomidate, genetically modified mice have been generated that have propofol-resistant $β_2$ or $β_3$ subunits (Fig. 24.3B,C). The mice with the propofol-resistant $β_3$ receptors are resistant to the anesthetic effects of propofol, demonstrating that propofol anesthesia (using the endpoints of loss of response to noxious stimulus and loss-of-righting reflex) is predominantly mediated by $β_3$-containing $GABA_A$ receptors [13]. The mice with propofol-resistant $β_2$ subunits had a reduced sedative response to propofol but a normal anesthetic response [37], indicating that $β_2$-containing receptors contribute to the sedative effect of propofol. It is important to recall that since propofol does have actions on $β_1$-containing $GABA_A$ receptors it is likely to produce a broader pattern of inhibition than etomidate. Propofol effects on $β_1$-containing $GABA_A$ receptors may contribute to its sedative action or to other behavioral components of anesthesia.

$GABA_A$ receptors meet most of the criteria for definitive identification as the molecular target of propofol. Propofol potentiates $GABA_A$ receptors at clinical concentrations, and propofol-sensitive $GABA_A$ receptors are located in arousal pathways where they could readily produce hypnosis [38]. Indeed, local injection of propofol in the tuberomammillary nucleus (TMN) of the hypothalamus, a critical nucleus in maintenance of arousal, can produce deep sedation in rats [47]. Transgenic animals with propofol-resistant $GABA_A$ receptors are resistant to the anesthetic effect of propofol, confirming the functional relevance of propofol action on $GABA_A$ receptors. The one missing criterion is definitive evidence for propofol binding to the $GABA_A$ receptor.

Propofol does have effects on other ligand-gated ion channels, including neuronal nicotinic receptors [48] and glycine receptors [49]. These interactions may contribute to other effects of propofol (e.g., analgesia, amnesia) but are clearly not sufficient for the hypnotic effects of the drug.

Barbiturates

Barbiturates have been used as intravenous anesthetic induction drugs for over 70 years. Commonly used agents include the thiobarbiturates, thiopental and thioamylal, and the oxybarbiturates, pentobarbital and methohexital. Despite their long use, the mechanisms of anesthetic action of barbiturates remain poorly defined. Anesthetic barbiturates produce effects on several kinds of ion channels at concentrations within their clinical range; these include $GABA_A$ receptors, AMPA and kainate subtypes of glutamate receptors, and neuronal nicotinic acetylcholine receptors.

Current thinking favors the $GABA_A$ receptor as an important target of barbiturate action. Barbiturates potentiate the actions of GABA at low concentration and directly activate $GABA_A$ receptors at higher concentrations [50]. There is some evidence that β subunits of the $GABA_A$ receptor are specifically involved in barbiturate action, but this work has never been pursued to completion [51,52]. There is evidence that anesthetic barbiturates do have greater effects on $GABA_A$ receptors containing δ subunits [53] and/or $α_6$ subunits [54]. This does not imply a specific interaction with the δ or $α_6$ subunit, but may indicate that extrasynaptic receptors are particularly sensitive to barbiturates, since the $α_6$ and δ subunits are preferentially expressed in extrasynaptic receptors. The actions of barbiturates on $GABA_A$ receptors have been detected in various brain regions including neocortex and thalamocortical neurons [55], indicating that barbiturate-sensitive $GABA_A$ receptors are appropriately located to be relevant targets of barbiturate action. The absence of specific identified amino acids on the $GABA_A$ receptor that are essential for barbiturate action precludes the generation of genetically modified animals that might help to define the biological relevance of barbiturate actions on $GABA_A$ receptors.

Anesthetic barbiturates also inhibit excitatory neurotransmitter receptors. Clinical concentrations of pentobarbital block both kainate and AMPA, but not NMDA-type glutamate receptors [56]. There is some evidence that the inhibitory effects of barbiturates are dependent on the specific glutamate receptor subunits expressed. For example, GluR6 homomers are more strongly inhibited by pentobarbital than are GluR3 homomers [57]. Studies examining the barbiturate sensitivity of AMPA receptors show that receptors containing the GluR2 subunit are more sensitive than other combinations of GluR1–4 subunits [58]. This enhanced sensitivity of the GluR2 site is determined by an arginine residue in the TM2 segment of the channel [59]. While there is good evidence that barbiturates can inhibit excitatory neurotransmission, the relevance of AMPA and kainate glutamate receptors as contributors to the mechanism of barbiturate anesthesia is not established.

Barbiturates also inhibit neuronal nicotinic receptors. Clinically relevant concentrations of thiopental have been shown to inhibit $\alpha_4\beta_2$ and α_7 neuronal as well as muscle-type ($\alpha\beta\gamma\delta$) nicotinic receptors. Interestingly, when the stereoisomers of thiopental were studied, neither the α_7 nor the muscle-type receptors showed stereoselectivity, but the R(+) isomer was significantly more effective than the S(−) isomer at inhibiting $\alpha_4\beta_2$ nicotinic receptors. Since the S(−) isomer is more potent than the R(+) in producing anesthesia, these data suggest that barbiturate inhibition of neuronal nicotinic receptors may not contribute to the general anesthetic properties of thiopental [60].

Based on the foregoing discussion it is clear that barbiturates can affect the function of multiple ion channels, but that none of these targets has been definitively identified as relevant to the mechanisms of barbiturate anesthesia. While GABA_A receptors remain the most likely mediator of barbiturate anesthesia, it is possible that additional targets will emerge as being important. In this regard, Puil has shown that pentobarbital induces an outward current (presumably a K^+ current) in thalamic neurons at concentrations below those required to potentiate GABA_A receptors [61].

Neurosteroids

At the current time there are no neurosteroid anesthetics in clinical use, but several neurosteroids, most notably alphaxalone (the active compound in Althesin), have been important clinical anesthetic agents in the past. Neurosteroids are an important class of compounds to consider because they are the only known endogenous anesthetics. Allopregnanolone, a neurosteroid produced in neurons and glial cells from cholesterol, is a potent anesthetic agent when administered exogenously. Its local production is thought to contribute to a variety of normal and abnormal CNS functions including anxiolysis, anticonvulsant activity, and neuroprotection [62].

In the mid 1980s neurosteroids were shown to be potent and efficacious modulators of GABA_A receptors [63]. Subsequent studies established a strong correlation between the potency of neurosteroid analogs as modulators of GABA_A receptors and their potency as anesthetics, establishing the GABA_A receptor as the likely mediator of neurosteroid anesthetic effect [64]. Neurosteroids such as alphaxalone and allopregnanolone potentiate the actions of GABA at low concentrations (10 nM – 1 μM) and directly activate GABA_A

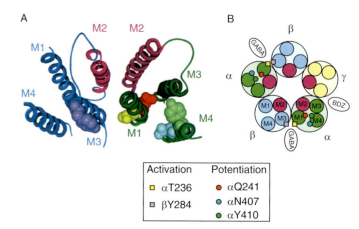

Figure 24.4. The binding sites for anesthetic neurosteroids on the GABA_A receptor. (A) Model of the juxtaposed α_1 and β_2 subunits of the GABA_A receptor (viewed from the extracellular surface) showing the amino acids identified as possible neurosteroid binding residues. (B) Schematic representation of a GABA_A receptor illustrating the locations of the neurosteroid binding site that mediates potentiation of GABA responses (red, blue, and green) and of the neurosteroid binding site that mediates direct activation of the GABA_A receptor (yellow and purple). Reproduced with permission from Hosie et al. [68].

receptor currents at higher concentrations [65]. Allopregnanolone enhances the effects of GABA on GABA_A receptors with every subunit combination that has been tested, with only modest variation in steroid potency with different α and β isoforms. The efficacy of the GABA-enhancing action of neurosteroid is significantly augmented in receptors containing a δ subunit and significantly reduced when an ε subunit is incorporated [66].

There is strong evidence that GABA_A receptors have two distinct binding sites for neurosteroids that are differentially recognized by selected neurosteroid analogs [67]. Indeed, molecular biological studies have identified amino acid residues that appear to constitute two separate binding sites: one that mediates potentiation of GABA responses and one that mediates direct activation of GABA_A currents. The potentiation site (Fig. 24.4) is composed of a cavity between the TM1 and TM4 helices of the α_1 subunit. The direct-activation site is constituted by residues from the TM1 helix of the α_1 subunit and the TM3 helix of the β_2 subunit, with the steroid binding in the cleft between the subunits [68]. These binding sites are conserved in all of the α-subunit isoforms, explaining why neurosteroids modulate all GABA_A receptors [69].

To date no data are available from animals genetically modified to have neurosteroid-resistant GABA_A receptors. It is clear that mice genetically modified to be resistant to etomidate and propofol have normal anesthetic responses to neurosteroids; this confirms that the neurosteroid binding sites are distinct and separate from etomidate or propofol binding sites on GABA_A receptors. Mice lacking the δ subunit of the GABA_A receptor are less sensitive to the anesthetic effects of alphaxalone, but not to the effects of etomidate, pentobarbital, propofol, or ketamine. This is consistent with the enhanced efficacy of neurosteroid action on δ-containing GABA$_A$ receptors and suggests a role for extrasynaptic GABA$_A$ receptors in neurosteroid anesthesia [70]. Definitive evidence for neurosteroid binding to GABA$_A$ receptors (e.g., photolabeling) is also not yet available. Overall, it appears likely that neurosteroids produce their anesthetic effects by interacting with specific binding sites on GABA$_A$ receptors, but several pieces of evidence are needed to confirm this.

Volatile anesthetics

Volatile anesthetics (VAs) have been shown to affect a large number of nervous system molecules. Consistent with this seeming lack of specificity, a prevalent hypothesis for many years has been that VAs do not bind to any particular protein target but rather alter the lipid environment in which numerous important nervous system proteins are embedded and thereby indirectly and nonspecifically disrupt neuronal signaling. However, several lines of evidence argue against a nonspecific membrane hypothesis. First, enantiomers of isoflurane have an approximately twofold difference in potency for producing anesthesia in rodents [71], whereas the lipid-perturbing effects of isoflurane are not stereoselective [5,72]. While by no means putting to rest the idea that volatile anesthetics act to alter bulk membrane properties, the observation of stereoselectivity for isoflurane is hard to reconcile with membrane theories of anesthesia. Genetics provides another strong argument for relative specificity of VA targets. In the nematode *Caenorhabditis elegans*, mutations in single genes have been isolated that make the animal's movement either hypersensitive or resistant to volatile anesthetics [73,74]. Indeed, mutations in the gene encoding the presynaptic protein syntaxin result in isoflurane sensitivities that vary over 30-fold, with one particular mutation resulting in animals fully resistant to clinical concentrations of isoflurane [73]. Large variations in anesthetic sensitivity by mutations in a single gene strongly refute hypotheses of nonspecific or highly distributed mechanisms of anesthesia. In mice, the magnitude of changes seen with mutations is smaller, but nevertheless significant differences in VA EC50s have been observed in transgenic animals. Stereospecificity and large phenotypic variability produced by single gene mutations provide strong evidence for specific and limited protein targets for VAs.

Of the proteins whose function is known to be altered by VAs, GABA$_A$ receptors are the leading candidates as relevant anesthetic targets. At concentrations within the clinical range, VAs potentiate inhibitory chloride currents through GABA$_A$ receptors by increasing the efficacy of GABA [75]. GABA$_A$ receptor potentiation produces a decrease in neuronal excitability; given the widespread and abundant expression of GABA$_A$ receptors, its potentiation is a logical mechanism of anesthesia. In support of its relevance, GABA$_A$ receptors are potentiated by isoflurane enantiomers with different potencies that match their potencies in producing anesthesia [71,76–78].

Binding of VAs to GABA$_A$ receptors has not been directly demonstrated. However, several in-vitro mutations of GABA$_A$ receptor subunits have been shown to alter the electrophysiologic effects of VAs, providing suggestive evidence for a VA binding pocket. Specifically, particular point mutations within the transmembrane domains of an α subunit of the receptor abolish VA potentiation of a GABA$_A$ receptor expressed in cultured cells [79–83]. Loss of VA potentiation was found to correlate with the calculated increase in volume of the amino acid altered by the mutation and with the molecular volume of the anesthetic (Fig. 24.5). For example, a small increase in amino acid volume abolished potentiation by isoflurane by not by halothane, a smaller molecule. A bulkier amino acid at this site abolished potentiation by both isoflurane and halothane, whereas a further reduction in free volume at a neighboring amino acid was required to block chloroform potentiation. These data can be explained by proposing a VA binding cavity of approximately 300 Å^3 formed by transmembrane domains of the α subunit of the GABA$_A$ receptor.

Genetic evidence in mouse supports a role for potentiation of the GABA$_A$ receptor in VA action [86]. Transgenic mice lacking the β_3 subunit of the GABA$_A$ receptor are significantly less sensitive to the immobilizing effects of both halothane and enflurane [87]. Likewise, a mouse in which the β_3 subunit was mutated at a site previously shown to modulate VA potentiation of the receptor β_3(N265M) was mildly but significantly resistant to immobilization by halothane and enflurane [13]. Important to the interpretation of these results is the finding, described earlier, that immobilization by etomidate and propofol is essentially abolished in the β_3(N265M) transgenic animals. This argues that potentiation of β_3-containing receptors is necessary and probably sufficient for immobilization by these intravenous anesthetics. Thus, the weak VA-resistant phenotype of these animals can not be attributed to the unimportance of β_3 subunit for mediating this behavior. Rather, it seems likely the β_3 subunit is less essential to VA immobilization. The contribution to anesthetic sensitivity of the putative anesthetic binding pocket in the transmembrane domain of the α_1 subunit was recently tested using a knockin mouse [85]. The transgenic mouse carried two mutations in the α_1 subunit, one that had been shown previously to abolish isoflurane but not halothane potentiation of the receptor and a second mutation that compensated for the effects of the first mutation on the basic properties of the channel in the absence of VAs. Thus, this mouse had relatively normal behavior and GABA$_A$ receptor physiology. Such mice were found to be mildly but significantly resistant to isoflurane but not to halothane for the loss-of-righting reflex endpoint (a measure of hypnosis) and had VA sensitivities similar to wild-type mice in immobilization and amnesia assays [85]. In summary, transgenic mouse experiments support a role for GABA$_A$ receptors in both VA immobilization and hypnosis, but the relatively weak VA-resistance phenotypes, as opposed to the strong phenotypes for etomidate and propofol, argue that VAs act on additional targets.

Glycine receptors are closely related structurally and functionally to GABA$_A$ receptors and are potentiated by VAs

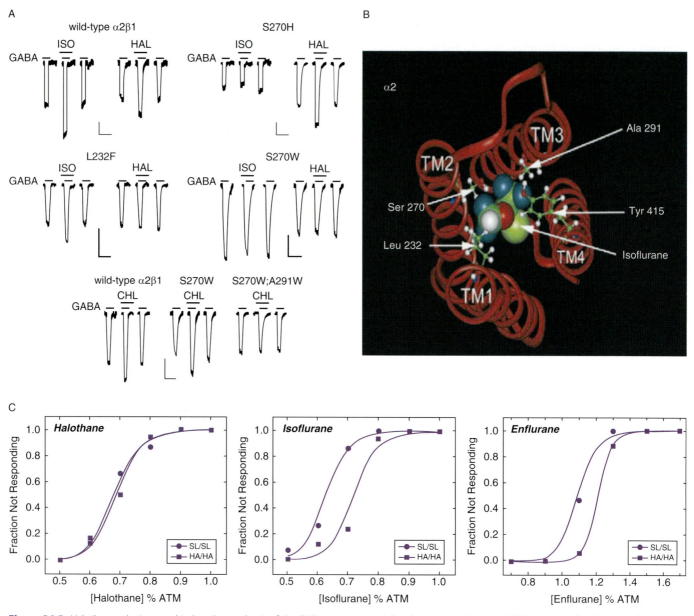

Figure 24.5. Volatile anesthetics may bind to the α subunit of the GABA$_A$ receptor and thereby promote hypnosis. (A) Expression of wild-type and mutant α$_2$ GABA$_A$ receptor subunits in heterologous cells. Mutation of serine 270 to histidine abolishes potentiation by isoflurane but not by the smaller anesthetic halothane, whereas mutation to tryptophan blocks potentiation by both anesthetics. A double mutation S270W and A291W blocks potentiation by the smallest anesthetic tested, chloroform. Reproduced with permission from Jenkins et al. [80]. (B) Molecular model of the putative anesthetic binding site based on the mutagenesis studies. Reproduced with permission from Hemmings et al. [84]. (C) Transgenic mice (designated HA) carrying the S270H mutation in the GABA$_A$ receptor α$_1$ subunit along with a compensatory mutation L277A that restores relatively normal channel properties. Consistent with the electrophysiological results, HA mice are resistant to isoflurane and enflurane but have normal halothane sensitivity. Reproduced with permission from Sonner et al. [83].

[88–90]. When activated, glycine receptors, like GABA$_A$ receptors, open a chloride-permeable channel that hyperpolarizes neurons and would generally decrease nervous system excitability. Glycine receptors are abundant in the spinal cord whereas GABA$_A$ receptors are expressed there at low levels. Thus, glycine receptors are a good candidate as a mediator of the effects of VAs on the spinal cord. Potentiation of glycine receptors has been observed with multiple VAs acting within the clinically relevant range, although sevoflurane was found to be relatively weak in this regard [88]. In-vitro mutagenesis studies are suggestive of a VA binding pocket formed by the transmembrane domains of the glycine receptor at a position similar to that proposed for the GABA$_A$ receptor [80,91,92].

Unlike the stereoselectivity of isoflurane for GABA$_A$ receptor potentiation, isoflurane enantiomers have equal potency against glycine receptors. Thus, glycine receptors are unlikely to be the target mediating the stereoselective component of the isoflurane anesthetic mechanism. Other pharmacologic tests of the role of glycine receptor potentiation have utilized intrathecal strychnine, an antagonist of the glycine receptor. Strychnine was found to increase the MAC of isoflurane in rats; however, the effect reached a plateau where MAC was maximally increased by about 40% [93]. These experiments were limited by the lack of quantification of glycine receptor antagonism by strychnine and its effect on isoflurane potentiation under these conditions. Nevertheless, the experiments do implicate an important role of the glycine receptor in MAC.

Nicotinic acetylcholine receptors (nAChRs) are structurally closely related to GABA$_A$ and glycine receptors and are modulated by VAs. However, rather than potentiation, volatile anesthetics potently inhibit nAChRs [48,94]. Indeed, MAC concentrations of isoflurane reduce currents through nAChRs expressed in vitro by at least 70% [94]; halothane and sevoflurane were found to be similarly potent and efficacious. As the precise function of nAChRs in the CNS is still poorly defined, the functional consequence of VA inhibition of these receptors is unclear. nAChRs clearly promote release of a variety of neurotransmitters, both excitatory and inhibitory [95], and are diffusely expressed in the CNS [96]. The global effect of nAChR activation is to enhance higher-order brain functions such as learning, memory, and attention [95]. nAChR antagonists impair these processes. Thus, in theory, VA inhibition of nAChRs might contribute to cognitive components of anesthesia, particularly amnesia. However, nAChRs do not appear to be important for VA immobilization, as nAChR antagonists do not alter isoflurane MAC in rats [97,98]. Moreover, "nonimmobilizer" drugs inhibit nAChRs but do not produce immobilization or hypnosis [99]. Alternatively, inhibition of nAChRs might be responsible for some of the side effects of VAs. A particularly interesting possibility is that nAChR antagonism may promote the hyperalgesia observed at subanesthetic concentrations of VAs [100]. Nicotine was shown to prevent isoflurane-induced hyperalgesia, and the nAChR antagonist mecamylamine produces a hyperalgesia that is additive with that from isoflurane [101].

Two-pore-domain potassium channels (K$_{2p}$ channels) are another likely relevant target of VAs (Box 24.3). About 20 years ago, Franks and Lieb reported that firing of a particular neuron within the nervous system of the pond snail could be silenced by VAs at concentrations within the clinically relevant range [103]. The inhibition of neuronal activity was due to activation of a potassium current of unknown identity. Other such anesthetic-activated K$^+$ currents have been found in other mollusks, yeast, and mammals [104–106]. These channels were subsequently identified as various subtypes of K$_{2p}$ channels [105–107]. K$_{2p}$ channels are an important determinant of the resting membrane potential of neurons and negatively regulate neuronal firing rate; thus, activation of K$_{2p}$ channels is a plausible mechanism to contribute to anesthesia. K$_{2p}$ channels are widely distributed in the central and peripheral nervous system and are expressed in both excitatory and inhibitory neurons, including GABAergic neurons. Thus the effect of activation of these channels on global nervous system function is difficult to predict.

Genetic experiments have shed light on the relevance of VA activation of the various K$_{2p}$ channels to anesthetic effect. The TREK-1, TASK-1, TASK-2, and TASK-3 genes have each been mutated in transgenic mice, and VA sensitivity of the mice tested. TREK-1 knockout mice are significantly resistant to several VAs (Fig. 24.6A–C). In particular, the MAC of halothane is increased by 50% (Fig. 24.6D). These mice have no gross neurological or behavioral abnormalities and have normal sensitivity to pentobarbital. Thus the halothane resistance is unlikely to be due to an indirect increase in arousability or CNS excitability that might result from deficiency of TREK-1. TASK-1 knockout mice are slightly but significantly resistant to immobilization by halothane and to the hypnotic effects of isoflurane [109]. However, TASK-1 knockout mice also show reduced sensitivity to the sedative effects of cannabinoids and dexmedetomidine; thus, the VA resistance could be due to a generalized effect on arousal. TASK-3 knockout animals have a small but significant halothane-resistant phenotype in immobilization assays whereas there is only a nonsignificant trend for isoflurane resistance [110]. TASK-3 knockout animals are also cannabinoid-resistant but are normally sensitive to other sedative and anesthetic drugs including dexmedetomidine and propofol. For TASK-2, mice with an insertion of a sequence predicted to disrupt expression of the TASK-2 gene have normal sensitivities to desflurane, halothane, and isoflurane [111]. However, whether the mutated TASK-2 gene is effectively knocked out and fails to express TASK-2 was not reported. In summary, genetic data strongly support a role of TREK-1 in VA immobilization, although the contribution to anesthesia of activation of the other K$_{2p}$ channels is unclear.

Volatile anesthetics also inhibit glutamate receptors. Inhibition of the NMDA subtype of glutamate receptor has been most extensively studied. NMDA receptors have a complex activation mechanism in which both glutamate and glycine are coagonists for opening of the channel while magnesium (Mg^{2+}) is a natural antagonist. Basal Mg^{2+} inhibition is relieved by depolarization of the neuron. This voltage-dependent disinhibition of the NMDA receptor allows it to function as a so-called coincidence detector and thereby mediate neuronal plasticity necessary for learning and memory (Box 24.4). NMDA receptor activation is also important for neuronal pattern generation and rhythmicity and thereby modulates global CNS excitability. Thus, NMDA receptor inhibition by VAs might reasonably contribute to anesthesia, particularly amnesia and unconsciousness. MAC concentrations of isoflurane reduce current through NMDA receptors by about 30%, a significant reduction [119–122]. AMPA receptors, the major glutamate receptor mediating fast excitatory synaptic transmission in the CNS, have also been found to be inhibited significantly by isoflurane, but less so than NMDA receptors

Box 24.3. Two-pore potassium channels (K$_{2p}$)

Neurons have a negative membrane potential that is essential to their electrical signaling function. This negative membrane potential is produced by so-called leak current potassium channels that are relatively voltage-independent. These K$^+$ leak channels were only recently identified as a group of structurally distinct four-transmembrane subunits with two pore-forming domains (Fig. A). Most other K$^+$ channels have only one pore domain. Although the two-pore (or tandem-pore) K$^+$ channels are relatively voltage-insensitive as a group, the opening of these channels is modulated by various factors that differ among members of the family. Lipids, protons, calcium, other second messengers, mechanical deformation of the cell membrane, and temperature have been shown to modulate the opening of one or more of the K$_{2p}$ channels. K$_{2p}$ channels not only modulate the resting potential but also regulate the action potential, neuronal automaticity, and transmitter release. K$_{2p}$ channels are composed of two subunits, usually but not necessarily identical. Thus far, 15 distinct K$_{2p}$ subunits have been identified in mammals (Fig. B). The identity of these subunits confers the basic properties to the K$_{2p}$ channels, in particular what factors modulate it, including anesthetics.

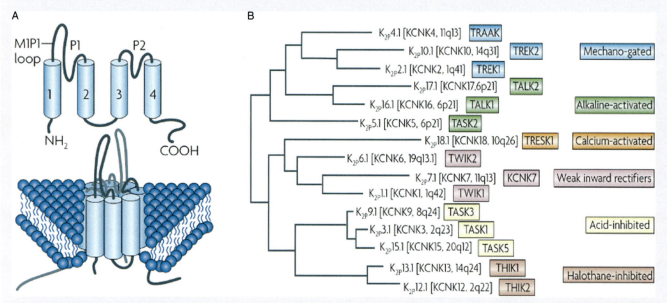

Structure of K$_{2p}$ channels. (A) K$_{2p}$ channels are composed of two subunits, usually identical, each of which has two nonidentical pore-forming domains. (B) Fifteen K$_{2p}$ subunit proteins have been identified in mammalian genomes. Subunits with similar amino acid sequence also tend to be modulated similarly and/or have similar electrophysiological properties. Adapted from Honore [102].

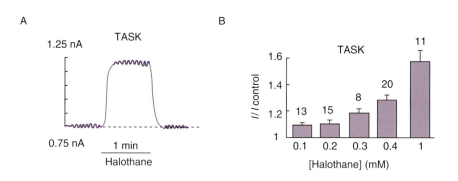

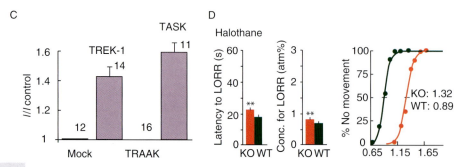

Figure 24.6. TASK-1 is activated by halothane and contributes to its hypnotic and immobilizing effects. (A) 1 mM halothane reversibly activates TASK-1 when expressed in a cell line. (B) Concentration/response curve for halothane. (C) TREK-1 and TASK-1 but not TRAAK are significantly activated by 1 mM halothane. (D) A TREK-1 knockout mouse strain is weakly resistant to the hypnotic effects of halothane and strongly resistant to immobilization by halothane. (A–C) reproduced with permission from Patel *et al.* [106]; (D) reproduced with permission from Heurteaux *et al.* [108].

Box 24.4. NMDA receptors and memory

The *N*-methyl-D-aspartate (NMDA) receptor is one of three ionotropic glutamate receptors (AMPA, kainate, NMDA). The NMDA receptor is unique among the three in that it requires glycine as well as glutamate to open its channel; however, the channel is normally blocked by magnesium (Mg^{2+}). Mg^{2+} blockade is released by membrane depolarization. Thus, the NMDA receptor is capable of serving as a detector for coincident pre- and postsynaptic activation. This property, along with the permeability of the channel to the second messenger calcium (Ca^{2+}) and prolonged channel open times, makes the NMDA receptor very well suited for regulating neuronal plasticity, which underlies learning and memory. Indeed, transgenic mice with mutations in the various subunits of the NMDA receptor were found to have markedly impaired abilities in learning and memory tasks, particular in memory acquisition [112–116]. Perhaps even more convincing is the demonstration of enhanced learning and memory in transgenic mice that overexpress the NR2B subunit of the NMDA receptor in the forebrain [117]. Thus, inhibition of NMDA receptors is a highly plausible mechanism for anesthetic-induced amnesia.

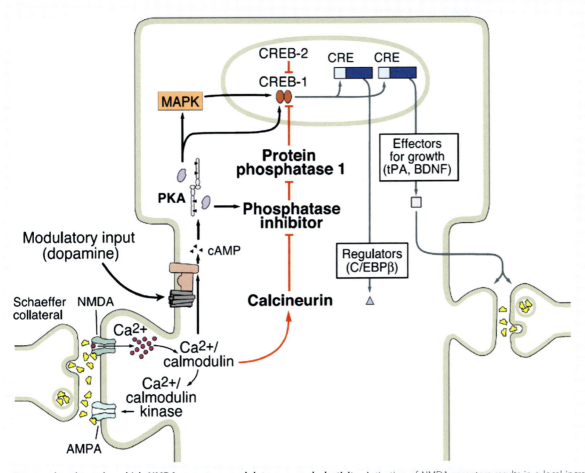

Proposed pathway by which NMDA receptors modulate neuronal plasticity. Activation of NMDA receptors results in a local increase in Ca^{2+} concentration. Ca^{2+} influx activates second-messenger pathways that ultimately alter the transcription of a variety of genes, at least in part by modulation of the transcription factor CREB-1 (cAMP response element-binding protein 1). CREB-1 binds to multiple promoters containing a sequence called the cAMP response element (CRE). CRE-containing genes promote strengthening and growth of synaptic connections. This synaptic plasticity may be a cellular basis for learning and memory. Reproduced with permission from Kandel [118].

[119]. While theoretically this level of NMDA and AMPA receptor inhibition should result in significant CNS depression, definitive genetic or pharmacologic experiments have not determined their role in anesthesia in vivo.

Volatile anesthetics have been shown to inhibit neurotransmitter release. Moreover, at clinical concentrations, VAs appear to inhibit excitatory neurotransmitter release more effectively than inhibitory [123]. Thus, the net effect should be to reduce CNS excitability – which is a plausible mechanism of anesthesia, although the mechanism of this inhibition is still a matter of investigation. Sodium (Na^+) channels have emerged as one likely target of VA inhibition of transmitter release. In studies of glutamate release from synaptosomes, which are isolated presynaptic terminals, VAs more potently

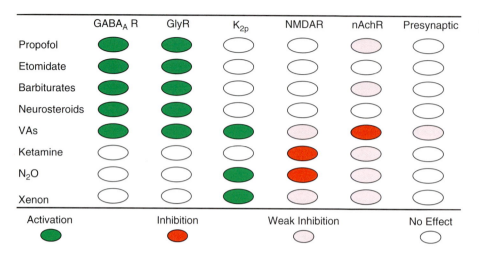

	GABA$_A$ R	GlyR	K$_{2p}$	NMDAR	nAchR	Presynaptic
Propofol	●	●	○	○	○	○
Etomidate	●	●	○	○	○	○
Barbiturates	●	●	○	○	○	○
Neurosteroids	●	●	○	○	○	○
VAs	●	●	●	○	●	○
Ketamine	○	○	○	●	○	○
N$_2$O	○	○	●	●	○	○
Xenon	○	○	●	○	○	○

Activation	Inhibition	Weak Inhibition	No Effect
●	●	○	○

Figure 24.7. Effects of anesthetics on putative targets. VAs, volatile anesthetics.

inhibit release evoked by drugs that require the function of Na$^+$ channels than by those that are Na$^+$-channel-independent [124,125]. Indeed, VAs have been shown to inhibit mammalian Na$^+$ channel currents expressed in a heterologous cell type [126]. More recently, it was shown that the amplitude of the action potential in a glutamate-releasing rat brainstem neuron is reduced by isoflurane at clinical concentrations [127]. The reduction in the action potential accounted for about two-thirds of the inhibition of glutamate release produced by isoflurane. The effect on the action potential can be explained by Na$^+$ channel inhibition, although other mechanisms are theoretically possible. The study by Wu *et al.* [127] was particularly important, because transmitter release was studied directly on native neurons in situ. Thus, it is reasonable to conclude that isoflurane and other VAs inhibit glutamate release, the major excitatory CNS neurotransmitter, at clinical concentrations in vivo. However, this study also suggested that a significant portion of VA inhibition of transmitter release was downstream of the action potential. Potential targets for this non-Na$^+$-channel-mediated presynaptic effect include TREK-1 [128,129], nicotinic acetylcholine receptors [48,94], and the transmitter release machinery itself [73,129]. A summary of the complex effects of VAs in comparison to other anesthetics is depicted in Fig. 24.7.

Ketamine

Nitrous oxide, ketamine, and xenon have similar mechanistic profiles that overlap with but are distinct from that for VAs. None of these three anesthetics significantly potentiates GABA$_A$ or glycine receptors, but all are effective inhibitors of the NMDA subtype of glutamate receptors (Box 24.4). Ketamine was the first of these anesthetics shown to be an NMDA receptor antagonist and is the best characterized [130–134]. NMDA receptors meet multiple criteria as an anesthetic target for ketamine. Ketamine inhibits NMDA receptors with an EC50 concentration of approximately 5–10 μM [135]. The average steady-state plasma concentration required for general anesthesia has been reported to be 9.3 μM, with an EC50 of 2.7 μM

[136]. Free concentrations of ketamine are estimated to be about 60% of plasma concentrations because of protein binding [137]. Assuming that plasma-free concentrations reflect those at the active site in the CNS, ketamine would significantly inhibit NMDA receptors at anesthetizing concentrations. A ketamine analog has also been shown to bind to NMDA receptors with an affinity similar to its potency against NMDA receptors [138]. Additionally, ketamine entantiomers have a selective potency against the NMDA receptor that corresponds with their potencies at producing anesthesia in intact animals [139,140]. However, the genetic evidence for a functional role of the NMDA receptor in ketamine anesthesia is limited. A genetically engineered mouse with a knocked out NR2A (ε_1) subunit of the NMDA receptor had a modestly shortened response to the hypnotic effects of a single dose of ketamine [134]. NR2A is the most abundant NR2 subunit at adult mouse cortical synapses, but other NR2 subunits can substitute for NR2A to form functional NMDA receptors. Ketamine is essentially equally potent at blocking all NR2-subtype-containing receptors [141]. Thus, the interpretation of the weakly resistant phenotype of the knockout mouse is unclear; however, one can at least conclude that the NR2A-containing NMDA receptors are necessary for normal ketamine sensitivity.

The pharmacological, biochemical, and to some degree genetic evidence implicate the NMDA receptor as an important ketamine target. However, NMDA receptor antagonism may not be the sole mechanism for ketamine anesthesia. Ketamine has also been shown to inhibit nAChRs at concentrations in the anesthetizing range [142–144]. Two reports on whether ketamine acts stereoselectively to inhibit nAChRs arrived at opposite conclusions [145,146]. Thus, it is unclear whether the criterion of stereoselectivity supports or opposes a role of nAChRs in the anesthetic mechanism of ketamine. nAChR antagonists have been tested for additivity with ketamine [147]. The assumption of this experiment is that these antagonists should reduce the concentration of ketamine required to produce anesthesia if nAChR antagonism is a relevant mechanism. None of the antagonists increased the potency or efficacy of ketamine for immobilization or hypnosis; however, one of the nAChR antagonists was shown to enhance the analgesic effect of ketamine. These experiments are difficult to interpret because of an incomplete description of the degree of antagonism of nAChRs by the combination of ketamine and the nAChR antagonists, the possibility of summation of behavioral effects through parallel mechanisms, and the possibility of other sites of action for these drugs besides nAChR. However, the experiments do suggest a role for nAChR in analgesia by ketamine. In summary, ketamine may have at least two molecular targets mediating its anesthetic action: NMDA receptors and nAChRs. More definitive genetic experiments are needed to establish their relative roles in the components of anesthesia produced by ketamine.

Nitrous oxide

Nitrous oxide (N_2O) also inhibits NMDA receptors at concentrations within the clinically relevant range [148,149]. 80% N_2O inhibits current through NMDA receptors in rat neurons by about 50% [149]. 80% N_2O corresponds to about 0.5 MAC in rats [150]. Thus, there is a close correspondence between the potency of N_2O for antagonism of the NMDA receptor current and for immobility. Genetic evidence supporting a role of NMDA receptors in N_2O anesthesia is lacking in mammals. However, in the nematode C. elegans, a null mutation in an NMDA receptor subunit fully blocks the behavioral effects of N_2O [151]. This genetic result definitively makes the molecular-to-behavioral link in C. elegans, and it shows that, at least in this animal, N_2O has only one major anesthetic target. However, in mammals N_2O may affect additional targets, one of which, like ketamine, may be the nAChR. At approximately 1/3 MAC, N_2O inhibits currents from rat nAChRs by as much as 39% [122]. Thus, N_2O and ketamine both antagonize NMDA and nACh receptors, yet these drugs produce qualitatively distinct anesthetic states, suggesting additional targets for one or both drugs. At clinically relevant concentrations, N_2O but not ketamine has been shown to enhance current through the K_{2p} channel TREK-1 [152]. As discussed for volatile anesthetics, activation of K_{2p} channels will result in decreased neuronal firing. TREK-1 is most abundant in the striatum, neocortex, and hippocampus, brain regions important for higher-order planning of movement, cognition, and short-term memory formation. Thus, activation of TREK-1 is quite plausible as a contributor to the anesthetic mechanism of N_2O. However, a more definitive answer for a role of TREK-1 in N_2O anesthesia awaits genetic evidence.

Xenon

Xenon has a pharmacological profile quite similar to N_2O. At concentrations essentially equi-MAC with N_2O, xenon significantly activates TREK-1 channels [152]. Likewise, xenon inhibits NMDA and nACh receptors at concentrations similar to those that produce anesthesia [119,122,153,154]. In addition to NMDA receptors, xenon may also act by inhibiting the AMPA subtype of glutamate receptors, although this is controversial. One set of investigators found that AMPA receptors were essentially insensitive to xenon [119] except under conditions that were thought to be nonphysiological [155]. However, another group subsequently demonstrated strong inhibition of AMPA receptors and postulated that the difference between their results and the previously published data might be explained by neuronal type differences. Thus, the role, if any, of AMPA receptors in xenon action may be limited to specific regions of the nervous system and components of anesthesia. In C. elegans, NMDA receptor mutants resistant to N_2O were found not to be resistant to xenon. Rather, a mutation in a non-NMDA receptor, structurally and functionally similar to an AMPA receptor, was resistant to xenon [156]. The conclusion that can be made from this result in the nematode is that N_2O and xenon have the potential to target different subtypes of glutamate receptors. Thus these two drugs may not have identical mechanisms.

The neuroanatomy of general anesthesia

The various targets of general anesthetics are widely distributed throughout the central and peripheral nervous systems. In theory, all components of anesthesia might be mediated by action at a single region of the nervous system. Alternatively, anesthesia could be regionally distributed, with individual components produced by anesthetic action at single specific sites in the nervous system or by action at a combination of sites. There is now very strong evidence for a distributed model, with the spinal cord mediating immobility and the sites of unconsciousness and amnesia residing within the brain.

Spinal cord

The results of several complementary experiments indicate that anesthetic action on the spinal cord produces immobility. Rampil and colleagues showed that MAC values for isoflurane are unaffected in the rat by either decerebration [157] or cervical spinal cord transection (Fig. 24.8A–C) [158]. Antognini and colleagues made clever use of the peculiar cerebral circulation of goats to administer anesthetics selectively either to the brain or to the spinal cord (Fig. 24.8D–F). They found that when isoflurane is administered only to the brain, MAC is 2.9%, whereas when it is administered to the entire animal, MAC is 1.2% [159]. Surprisingly, when isoflurane was preferentially administered to the body only, and not to the brain, isoflurane MAC was reduced to 0.8% [160]. These provocative results suggest not only that anesthetic action at the spinal cord underlies MAC, but also that anesthetic action on the brain may actually sensitize the cord to noxious stimuli. The actions of volatile anesthetics in the spinal cord may be mediated, at least in part, by direct effects on the excitability of spinal motor neurons, as the amplitude of the evoked potential F-wave

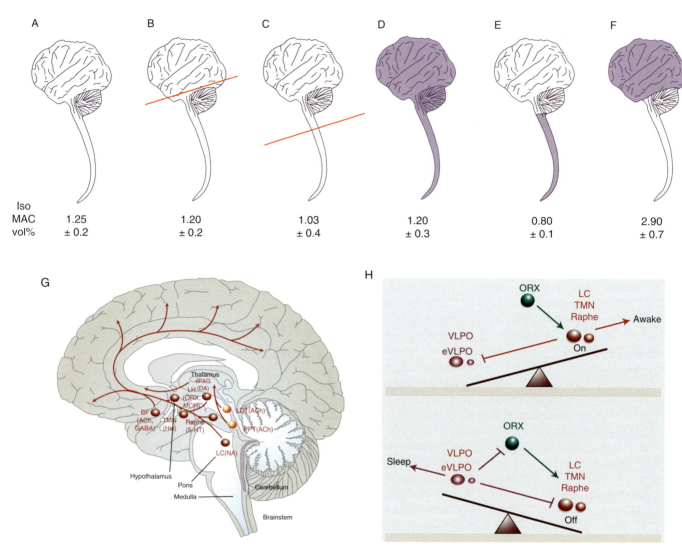

Figure 24.8. Neuroanatomical loci for MAC and hypnosis. (A–C) Decerebration or spinal cord transection at C7 level does not change MAC [157,158]. (D–F) Selective application of isoflurane (indicated by purple color) to the spinal cord results in a significant decrease in MAC for hindpaw clamp. Selective application to the forebrain results in a large increase in MAC [159–161]. (G) Brain nuclei known to control arousal. Nuclei: LDT, laterodorsal tegmental; PPT, pedunculopontine; vPAG, ventral periaqueductal gray; LH, lateral hypothalamus; LC, locus coeruleus; raphe, dorsal and median raphe; TMN, tuberomammillary; BF, basal forebrain. Neurotransmitters/modulators: NA, noradrenaline (norepinephrine); ACh, acetylcholine; 5-HT, serotonin; DA, dopamine; ORX, orexin; MCH, melanin-concentrating hormone; His, histamine; GABA, γ-aminobutyric acid. (H) A switch model for the awake or sleep state. The LC, TMN, and raphe nuclei promote wakefulness and inhibit the ventrolateral preoptic nucleus (VLPO) nuclei, which promote sleep. During wakefulness, the LC, TMN, and raphe nuclei inhibit the VLPO with reinforcement from orexinergic neurons in the LH. During sleep, the VLPO gains control and inhibits the LC/TMN/raphe nuclei and the LH. This mutually inhibitory circuit can result in rapid transitions from the awake to the sleep state and has been called a flip-flop switch. Reproduced with permission from Saper *et al.* [162].

(F-wave amplitude correlates with motor neuron excitability) is depressed by VAs [163–165]. The plausibility of the spinal cord as a locus for anesthetic immobilization is also supported by several electrophysiological studies showing inhibition of excitatory synaptic transmission in the spinal cord [166–169].

Brainstem, hypothalamic, and thalamic arousal systems

Logically, anesthetic action in the spinal cord cannot be responsible for amnesia or unconsciousness. On the other hand, the brainstem/hypothalamic/thalamic network that controls sleep and attention [170] is not only a logical site for

amnesia/unconsciousness, but it has considerable experimental support. Central to the mechanism of sleep is a set of hypothalamic nuclei that appear to form a sleep/wake switch mechanism (Fig. 24.8G,H). The ventrolateral preoptic nucleus (VLPO) in the anterior hypothalamus promotes sleep while the tuberomammillary nucleus (TMN) in the posterior hypothalamus promotes wakefulness. The VLPO and the TMN are mutually inhibitory, producing a switch-like mechanism. For example, if other modulatory sleep-promoting nuclei increase the activity of the VLPO relative to the TMN, the VLPO will ultimately shut down the output of the TMN and sleep will be favored. On the other hand, during wakefulness, the TMN is dominant and silences the VLPO. Modulatory influences on the TMN and VLPO include orexinergic neurons in the lateral hypothalamus, the circadian clock, which is directly modulated by light and contained within the hypothalamic suprachiasmatic nucleus, and multiple brainstem nuclei, in particular the locus coeruleus and dorsal raphe. Adenosine also serves as a neurohumoral factor that promotes sleep by disinhibiting the VLPO. The TMN and the VLPO are thought to promote the awake or sleep state by acting on thalamic and cortical circuits, either directly or through the reticular activating formation.

The VLPO/TMN sleep/wake switch circuit was directly implicated in anesthetic action by a set of elegant experiments from Maze, Saper, Franks, and colleagues. They showed that the application of a GABAergic antagonist directly onto the TMN diminished the efficacy of the anesthetics propofol and pentobarbital [47]. Indeed, discrete application of the GABAergic antagonist gabazine onto the TMN markedly reduced the duration of sedation produced by systemically administered propofol or pentobarbital. This effect is unlikely to be a consequence of a nonspecific increase in arousal state because systemically administered gabazine did not antagonize the potency of ketamine whereas it did antagonize propofol and pentobarbital. This result strongly implicates the VLPO/TMN sleep/wake switch as a site for the sedative action of GABAergic anesthetics such as propofol and barbiturates. (For further information on the VLPO/TMN sleep/wake circuitry, see Chapter 13.)

The reticular activating system has long been speculated to be a site of general anesthetic action on consciousness. Evidence to support this notion came from early whole-animal experiments showing that electrical stimulation of the reticular activating system could induce arousal behavior in anesthetized animals [171]. More recently, positron-emission tomography studies have shown a relatively selective effect of sevoflurane, propofol, and xenon on the thalamus and the reticular activating system [172–174]. The fact that three mechanistically distinct anesthetics all alter activity in the same brain regions is highly suggestive of a role for these brain nuclei in anesthesia. While there is evidence that the reticular formation of the brainstem is a locus for anesthetic effects, it cannot be the only anatomic site of anesthetic action for two reasons. First, as discussed above, the brainstem is not even required for anesthetics to inhibit responsiveness to noxious stimuli. Second, the reticular formation can be largely ablated without eliminating awareness [175].

The thalamus comprises a set of relay nuclei transferring somatosensory information and reticular activating system activity to the cerebral cortex. The thalamus and cortex generate positive feedback loop circuits that are thought to be necessary for consciousness. These thalamocortical/corticothalamic reentry circuits along with complex and widespread neocortical neuronal activity have been postulated to be the basis of consciousness [176]. Alkire et al. showed that regional blood flow to the thalamus is selectively reduced by VAs [174]. Subsequent studies with other anesthetics have demonstrated a similar reduction in thalamic blood flow [177]. Injection of nicotine into the thalamus results in arousal of a significant number of sevoflurane-anesthetized rats [178]. However, unlike the microinjection studies in the TMN of the hypothalamus [47], the thalamic microinjection experiments did not demonstrate specificity for subtypes of anesthetics. Thus, thalamic nicotine reversal of anesthesia may be due to a general increase in arousal and does not necessarily indicate that direct anesthetic action on the thalamus is required for anesthesia. Indeed, cortical resection ablates the electrophysiological and metabolic effects of anesthetics on the thalamus [179–181]. Thus, the effects of anesthetics on the thalamus may be secondary to other brain regions such as the cerebral cortex that have an activating influence on the thalamus.

Cerebral cortex
As discussed above, the cortex is not necessary for immobilization by VAs. However, the cerebral cortex is the major site for integration, storage, and retrieval of information. As such, it is a likely site at which anesthetics interfere with complex functions such as memory and awareness. Anesthetics clearly alter cortical electrical activity, as evidenced by the changes in surface EEG patterns recorded during anesthesia [182]. Multiple anesthetics also produce substantial depression of cortical activity as measured by changes in regional cerebral blood flow [172–174]. In particular, anesthetics have a profound effect on information transfer among cortical regions and between the cortex and subcortical nuclei [183]. However, anesthetic effects on patterns of cortical electrical activity vary widely among anesthetics, providing an initial suggestion that all anesthetics are not likely to act through identical mechanisms. More detailed in-vitro electrophysiological studies examining anesthetic effects on different cortical regions support the notion that anesthetics can differentially alter neuronal function in various cortical preparations. For example, volatile anesthetics have been shown to inhibit excitatory transmission at some synapses in the olfactory cortex [184] but not at others [185]. Similarly, whereas volatile anesthetics inhibit excitatory transmission in the dentate gyrus of the hippocampus [186], these same drugs can actually enhance excitatory transmission at other synapses in the hippocampus [187]. Anesthetics also produce a variety of effects on inhibitory transmission in the cortex. A variety of parenteral and inhalation anesthetics have been shown to enhance inhibitory transmission in olfactory cortex [184] and in the hippocampus [188]. Conversely, volatile anesthetics have also been reported to depress inhibitory transmission in hippocampus [189].

Summary
During the past several decades understanding of the mechanisms of general anesthesia has advanced on many fronts. It has become evident that nonspecific theories of anesthesia based

on perturbation of lipid membranes are incorrect and that there is not a single mechanism for all anesthetic agents (i.e., the "unitary theory of anesthesia" is incorrect). It is also abundantly clear that proteins, ion channels in particular, are the targets of anesthetic action.

It has become apparent that what we refer to as general anesthesia is actually a collection of component effects including hypnosis (unconsciousness), amnesia, immobility, attenuation of autonomic responses to noxious stimuli, and analgesia. The search for mechanisms of anesthesia needs to be restated as the search for the mechanisms through which *each* anesthetic produces *each of the components* of the anesthetic state.

Significant advances have been made in understanding how anesthetics produce loss of consciousness. It is now well established that etomidate and propofol produce unconsciousness by acting through the GABA$_A$ receptor. Binding sites for etomidate and propofol have been localized to specific β-subunit isoforms of the GABA$_A$ receptor, and genetic studies have unequivocally identified these binding sites as being responsible for the hypnotic effects of these two anesthetics. GABA$_A$ receptors have also been strongly implicated as the site of action for anesthetic neurosteroids, and two binding sites have been tentatively identified on the α subunit of the GABA$_A$ receptor.

Evidence is accumulating that halogenated volatile anesthetics are more "promiscuous" in their actions and that several molecular targets may mediate their hypnotic effect. These targets include the GABA$_A$ receptor and two-pore potassium channels. There is evidence for volatile anesthetic binding sites on each of these targets, and some genetic evidence that anesthetic actions on these targets contribute to the hypnotic effects of the VAs. Other targets that may contribute to the actions of VAs include voltage-gated sodium channels and proteins involved with presynaptic neurotransmitter release.

A third group of anesthetics, including nitrous oxide, xenon, and ketamine, have been shown to be inhibitors of NMDA-type glutamate receptors, and this effect is thought to be an important contributor to their hypnotic effect. However, the hypnotic effects of these drugs are qualitatively different from each other, and each of the drugs is likely to have additional targets that contribute to their anesthetic actions.

Finally, the science of anesthetic mechanisms is now advancing beyond identifying targets, to examining where in the nervous system each anesthetic acts and how their actions alter the complex interplay of neuronal signaling to produce the behaviors that we observe as anesthesia. Given its determining role in MAC, the spinal cord is accepted as the neuroanatomic locus for anesthetic-induced immobility. However, the site of the other components of anesthesia is unclear. The hypothalamic sleep/wake switch circuit clearly modulates hypnosis for some anesthetics and is a reasonable site of action for at least a portion of this component of anesthesia. In addition, the profound effects of anesthetics on the cerebral cortex must surely contribute to amnesia and unconsciousness – but definitive empirical support for this logical assumption is lacking.

References

1. Meyer H. Theorie der Alkoholnarkose. *Arch Exp Pathol Pharmakol* 1899; **42**: 109–18.

2. Franks NP, Lieb WR. Where do general anaesthetics act? *Nature* 1978; **274**: 339–42.

3. Franks NP, Lieb WR. Is membrane expansion relevant to anaesthesia? *Nature* 1981; **292**: 248–51.

4. Koblin DD, Chortkoff BS, Laster MJ, et al. Polyhalogenated and perfluorinated compounds that disobey the Meyer-Overton hypothesis. *Anesth Analg* 1994; **79**: 1043–8.

5. Franks NP, Lieb WR. Stereospecific effects of inhalational general anesthetic optical isomers on nerve ion channels. *Science* 1991; **254**: 427–30.

6. Tomlin SL, Jenkins A, Lieb WR, Franks NP. Stereoselective effects of etomidate optical isomers on gamma-aminobutyric acid type A receptors and animals. *Anesthesiology* 1998; **88**: 708–17.

7. Wittmer LL, Hu Y, Kalkbrenner M, et al. Enantioselectivity of steroid-induced gamma-aminobutyric acidA receptor modulation and anesthesia. *Mol Pharmacol* 1996; **50**: 1581–6.

8. Franks NP, Lieb WR. Do general anaesthetics act by competitive binding to specific receptors? *Nature* 1984; **310**: 599–601.

9. Franks NP, Jenkins A, Conti E, Lieb WR, Brick P. Structural basis for the inhibition of firefly luciferase by a general anesthetic. *Biophys J* 1998; **75**: 2205–11.

10. Forman SA, Chin VA. General anesthetics and molecular mechanisms of unconciousness. *Int Anesthesiol Clin* 2008; **46**: 43–53.

11. Wu XS, Sun JY, Evers A, Crowder M, Wu LG. Isoflurane inhibits transmitter release and the presynaptic action potential. *Anesthesiology* 2004; **100**: 663–70.

12. Humphrey JA, Hamming KS, Thacker CM, et al. A Putative cation channel and its novel regulator: cross-species conservation of effects on general anesthesia. *Curr Biol* 2007; **17**: 624–9.

13. Jurd R, Arras M, Lambert S, et al. General anesthetic actions in vivo strongly attenuated by a point mutation in the GABA(A) receptor beta3 subunit. *FASEB J* 2003; **17**: 250–2.

14. Hacking DF. "Knock, and it shall be opened": knocking out and knocking in to reveal mechanisms of disease and novel therapies. *Early Hum Dev* 2008; **84**: 821–7.

15. Sear JW. What makes a molecule an anaesthetic? Studies on the mechanisms of anaesthesia using a physicochemical approach *Br J Anaesth* 2009; **103**: 50–60.

16. Mehdipour AR, Hemmateenejad B, Miri R. QSAR studies on the anesthetic action of some polyhalogenated ethers. *Chem Biol Drug Des* 2007; **69**: 362–8.

17. Abraham MH, Acree WE, Mintz C, Payne S. Effect of anesthetic structure on inhalation anesthesia: implications

for the mechanism. *J Pharm Sci* 2008; **97**: 2373–84.

18. Dundee JW. Molecular structure–activity relationships of barbiturates. In: Halsey MJ, Millar RA, Sutton JA, eds., *Molecular Mechanism of General Anesthesia*. New York, NY: Churchill Livingstone, 1974: 16–31.

19. Andrews PR, Mark LC. Structural specificity of barbiturates and related drugs. *Anesthesiology* 1982; **57**: 314–20.

20. Krasowski MD, Jenkins A, Flood P, *et al*. General anesthetic potencies of a series of propofol analogs correlate with potency for potentiation of gamma-aminobutyric acid (GABA) current at the GABA(A) receptor but not with lipid solubility. *J Pharmacol Exp Ther* 2001; **297**: 338–51.

21. Krasowski MD, Hong X, Hopfinger AJ, Harrison NL. 4D-QSAR analysis of a set of propofol analogues: mapping binding sites for an anesthetic phenol on the GABA(A) receptor. *J Med Chem* 2002; **45**: 3210–21.

22. Atucha E, Hammerschmidt F, Zolle I, Sieghart W, Berger ML. Structure–activity relationship of etomidate derivatives at the GABA(A) receptor: comparison with binding to 11beta-hydroxylase. *Bioorg Med Chem Lett* 2009; **19**: 4284–7.

23. Veleiro AS, Burton G. Structure–activity relationships of neuroactive steroids acting on the GABA$_A$ receptor. *Curr Med Chem* 2009; **16**: 455–72.

24. Phillips GH. Structure–activity relationships in steroidal aensthetics. *J Steroid Biochem* 1975; **6**: 607–13.

25. Chisari M, Eisenmann LN, Krishnan K, *et al*. The influence of neuroactive steroid lipophilicity on GABA$_A$ receptor modulation: evidence for a low-affinity interaction. *J Neurophysiol* 2009; **102**: 1254–64.

26. Franks NP, Lieb WR. Inhibitory synapses: anaesthetics set their sites on ion channels. *Nature* 1997; **389**: 334–5.

27. Belelli D, Callachan H, Hill-Venning C, Peters JA, Lambert JJ. Interaction of positive allosteric modulators with human and Drosophila recombinant GABA receptors expressed in *Xenopus laevis* oocytes. *Br J Pharmacol* 1996; **118**: 563–76.

28. Lambert JJ, Belelli D, Hill-Venning C, Callachan H, Lambert JJ. Neurosteroid modulation of native and recombinant GABA$_A$ receptors. *Cell Mol Neurobiol* 1996; **16**: 155–74.

29. Robertson B. Actions of anaesthetics and avermectin on GABA$_A$ chloride channels in mammalian dorsal root ganglion neurones. *Br J Pharmacol* 1989; **98**: 167–76.

30. Hill-Venning C, Belelli D, Peters JA, Lambert JJ. Subunit-dependent interaction of the general anaesthetic etomidate with the gamma-aminobutyric acid type A receptor. *Br J Pharmacol* 1997; **120**: 749–56.

31. Belelli D, Lambert JJ, Peters JA, Wafford K, Whiting PJ. The interaction of the general anesthetic etomidate with the gamma-aminobutyric acid type A receptor is influenced by a single amino acid. *Proc Natl Acad Sci U S A* 1997; **94**: 11031–6.

32. Desai R, Ruesch D, Forman SA. Gamma-amino butyric acid type A receptor mutations at beta2N265 alter etomidate efficacy while preserving basal and agonist-dependent activity. *Anesthesiology* 2009; **111**: 774–84.

33. Li GD, Chiara DC, Cohen JB, Olsen RW. Neurosteroids allosterically modulate binding of the anesthetic etomidate to gamma-aminobutyric acid type A receptors. *J Biol Chem* 2009; **284**: 11771–5.

34. McGurk KA, Pistis M, Belelli D, Hope AG, Lambert JJ. The effect of a transmembrane amino acid on etomidate sensitivity of an invertebrate GABA receptor. *Br J Pharmacol* 1998; **124**: 13–20.

35. Siegwart R, Jurd R, Rudolph U. Molecular determinants for the action of general anesthetics at recombinant alpha(2)beta(3)gamma(2)gamma-aminobutyric acid(A) receptors. *J Neurochem* 2002; **80**: 140–8.

36. Li GD, Chiara DC, Sawyer GW, *et al*. Identification of a GABA$_A$ receptor anesthetic binding site at subunit interfaces by photolabeling with an etomidate analog. *J Neurosci* 2006; **26**: 11599–605.

37. Reynolds DS, Rosahl TW, Cirone J, *et al*. Sedation and anesthesia mediated by distinct GABA(A) receptor isoforms. *J Neurosci* 2003; **23**: 8608–17.

38. Zecharia AY, Nelson LE, Gent TC, *et al*. The involvement of hypothalamic sleep pathways in general anesthesia: testing the hypothesis using the GABA$_A$ receptor beta3N265M knock-in mouse. *J Neurosci* 2009; **29**: 2177–87.

39. Cheng VY, Martin LJ, Elliot EM, *et al*. Alpha5 GABA$_A$ receptors mediate the amnestic but not sedative-hypnotic effects of the general anesthetic etomidate. *J Neurosci* 2006; **26**: 3713–20.

40. Paris A, Phillipp M, Tonner PH, *et al*. Activation of alpha 2B-adrenoceptors mediates the cardiovascular effects of etomidate. *Anesthesiology* 2003; **99**: 889–95.

41. Cotten JF, Forman SA, Laha JK, *et al*. Carboetomidate: a pyrrole analog of etomidate designed not to suppress adrenocortical function. *Anesthesiology* 2010; **112**: 637–44.

42. Hales TG, Lambert JJ. The actions of propofol on inhibitory amino acid receptors of bovine adrenomedullary chromaffin cells and rodent central neurones. *Br J Pharmacol* 1991; **104**: 619–28.

43. Sanna E, Mascia MP, Klein RL, *et al*. Actions of the general anesthetic propofol on recombinant human GABA$_A$ receptors: influence of receptor subunits. *J Pharmacol Exp Ther* 1995; **274**: 353–60.

44. Krasowski MD, Nishikawa K, Nikolaeva N, Lin A, Harrison NL. Methionine 286 in transmembrane domain 3 of the GABA$_A$ receptor beta subunit controls a binding cavity for propofol and other alkylphenol general anesthetics. *Neuropharmacology* 2001; **41**: 952–64.

45. Li GD, Chiara DC, Cohen JB, Olsen RW. Numerous classes of general anesthetics inhibit etomidate binding to γ-aminobutyric acid type A (GABA$_A$) receptors. *J Biol Chem* **285**: 8615–20.

46. Campagna-Slater V, Weaver DF. Anaesthetic binding sites for etomidate and propofol on a GABA$_A$ receptor model. *Neurosci Lett* 2007; **418**: 28–33.

47. Nelson LE, Guo TZ, Lu J, *et al*. The sedative component of anesthesia is mediated by GABA(A) receptors in an endogenous sleep pathway. *Nat Neurosci* 2002; **5**: 979–84.

48. Flood P, Ramirez-Latorre J, Role L. Alpha 4 beta 2 neuronal nicotinic acetylcholine receptors in the central nervous system are inhibited by isoflurane and propofol, but alpha 7-type nicotinic acetylcholine receptors are unaffected. *Anesthesiology* 1997; **86**: 859–65.

49. Pistis M, Belelli D, Peters JA, Lambert JJ. The interaction of general anaesthetics with recombinant GABA$_A$ and glycine receptors expressed in Xenopus laevis oocytes: a comparative study. *Br J Pharmacol* 1997; **122**: 1707–19.

50. Peters JA, Kirkness EF, Callachan H, Lambert JJ, Turner AJ. Modulation of the GABA$_A$ receptor by depressant barbiturates and pregnane steroids. *Br J Pharmacol* 1988; **94**: 1257–69.

51. Cestari IN, Uchida I, Li L, Burt D, Yang J. The agonistic action of pentobarbital on GABA$_A$ beta-subunit homomeric receptors. *Neuroreport* 1996; **7**: 943–7.

52. Serafini R, Bracamontes J, Steinbach JH. Structural domains of the human GABA$_A$ receptor 3 subunit involved in the actions of pentobarbital. *J Physiol* 2000; **524** Pt 3: 649–76.

53. Feng, HJ, Bianchi MT, Macdonald RL. Pentobarbital differentially modulates alpha1beta3delta and alpha1beta3gamma2L GABA$_A$ receptor currents. *Mol Pharmacol* 2004; **66**: 988–1003.

54. Thompson SA, Whiting PJ, Wafford KA. Barbiturate interactions at the human GABA$_A$ receptor: dependence on receptor subunit combination. *Br J Pharmacol* 1996; **117**: 521–7.

55. Mathers DA, Wan X, Puil E. Barbiturate activation and modulation of GABA(A) receptors in neocortex. *Neuropharmacology* 2007; **52**: 1160–8.

56. Marszalec W, Narahashi T. Use-dependent pentobarbital block of kainate and quisqualate currents. *Brain Res* 1993; **608**: 7–15.

57. Dildy-Mayfield JE, Eger EI, Harris RA. Anesthetics produce subunit-selective actions on glutamate receptors. *J Pharmacol Exp Ther* 1996; **276**: 1058–65.

58. Taverna FA, Cameron BR, Hampson DL, Wang LY, MacDonald JF. Sensitivity of AMPA receptors to pentobarbital. *Eur J Pharmacol* 1994; **267**: R3–5.

59. Yamakura T, Sakimura K, Mishina M, Shimoji K. The sensitivity of AMPA-selective glutamate receptor channels to pentobarbital is determined by a single amino acid residue of the alpha 2 subunit. *FEBS Lett* 1995; **374**: 412–14.

60. Downie DL, Franks NP, Lieb WR. Effects of thiopental and its optical isomers on nicotinic acetylcholine receptors. *Anesthesiology* 2000; **93**: 774–83.

61. Wan X, Mathers DA, Puil E. Pentobarbital modulates intrinsic and GABA-receptor conductances in thalamocortical inhibition. *Neuroscience* 2003; **121**: 947–58.

62. Belelli D, Lambert JJ. Neurosteroids: endogenous regulators of the GABA(A) receptor. *Nat Rev Neurosci* 2005; **6**: 565–75.

63. Majewska MD, Harrison NL, Schwartz RD, Barker JL, Paul SM. Steroid hormone metabolites are barbiturate-like modulators of the GABA receptor. *Science* 1986; **232**: 1004–7.

64. Harrison NL, Majewska MD, Harrington JW, Barker JL. Structure–activity relationships for steroid interaction with the gamma-aminobutyric acid$_A$ receptor complex. *J Pharmacol Exp Ther* 1987; **241**: 346–53.

65. Callachan H, Cottrell GA, Hather NY, *et al.* Modulation of the GABA$_A$ receptor by progesterone metabolites. *Proc R Soc Lond B Biol Sci* 1987; **231**: 359–69.

66. Belelli D, Casula A, Ling A, Lambert JJ. The influence of subunit composition on the interaction of neurosteroids with GABA(A) receptors. *Neuropharmacology* 2002; **43**: 651–61.

67. Evers AS, Chen ZW, Manion BD, *et al.* A Synthetic 18-Norsteroid distinguishes between two neuroactive steroid binding sites on GABA$_A$ receptors. *J Pharmacol Exp Ther* 2010; **333**: 404–13.

68. Hosie AM, Wilkins ME, da Silva HM, Smart TG. Endogenous neurosteroids regulate GABA$_A$ receptors through two discrete transmembrane sites. *Nature* 2006; **444**: 486–9.

69. Hosie AM, Clarke L, da Silva H, Smart TG. Conserved site for neurosteroid modulation of GABA A receptors. *Neuropharmacology* 2009; **56**: 149–54.

70. Mihalek RM, Banerjee PK, Korpi ER, *et al.* Attenuated sensitivity to neuroactive steroids in gamma-aminobutyrate type A receptor delta subunit knockout mice. *Proc Natl Acad Sci U S A* 1999; **96**: 12905–10.

71. Dickinson R, White I, Lieb WR, Franks NP. Stereoselective loss of righting reflex in rats by isoflurane. *Anesthesiology* 2000; **93**: 837–43.

72. Dickinson R, Franks NP, Lieb WR. Can the stereoselective effects of the anesthetic isoflurane be accounted for by lipid solubility? *Biophys J* 1994; **66**: 2019–23.

73. van Swinderen B, Saifee O, Shebester L, *et al.* A neomorphic syntaxin mutation blocks volatile-anesthetic action in Caenorhabditis elegans. *Proc Natl Acad Sci U S A* 1999; **96**: 2479–84.

74. Kayser EB, Morgan PG, Sedensky MM. GAS-1: a mitochondrial protein controls sensitivity to volatile anesthetics in the nematode Caenorhabditis elegans. *Anesthesiology* 1999; **90**: 545–54.

75. Homanics GE, Harrison NL, Quinlan JJ, *et al.* Normal electrophysiological and behavioral responses to ethanol in mice lacking the long splice variant of the gamma2 subunit of the gamma-aminobutyrate type A receptor. *Neuropharmacology* 1999; **38**: 253–65.

76. Hall AC, Lieb WR, Franks NP. Stereoselective and non-stereoselective actions of isoflurane on the GABA$_A$ receptor. *Br J Pharmacol* 1994; **112**: 906–10.

77. Jones MV, Harrison NL. Effects of volatile anesthetics on the kinetics of inhibitory postsynaptic currents in cultured rat hippocampal neurons. *J Neurophysiol* 1993; **70**: 1339–49.

78. Moody EJ, Harris BD, Skolnick P. Stereospecific actions of the inhalation anesthetic isoflurane at the GABA$_A$ receptor complex. *Brain Res* 1993; **615**: 101–6.

79. Mihic SJ, Ye Q, Wick MJ, *et al.* Sites of alcohol and volatile anaesthetic action on GABA(A) and glycine receptors. *Nature* 1997; **389**: 385–9.

80. Krasowski MD, Harrison NL. The actions of ether, alcohol and alkane general anaesthetics on GABA$_A$ and

glycine receptors and the effects of TM2 and TM3 mutations. *Br J Pharmacol* 2000; **129**: 731–43.

81. Nishikawa K, Jenkins A, Paraskevakis I, Harrison NL. Volatile anesthetic actions on the GABA$_A$ receptors: contrasting effects of alpha 1(S270) and beta 2 (N265) point mutations. *Neuropharmacology* 2002; **42**: 337–45.

82. Koltchine VV, Finn SE, Jenkins A, *et al.* Agonist gating and isoflurane potentiation in the human gamma-aminobutyric acid type A receptor determined by the volume of a second transmembrane domain residue. *Molecular Pharmacology* 1999; **56**: 1087–93.

83. Jenkins A, Greenblatt EP, Faulkner HJ, *et al.* Evidence for a common binding cavity for three general anesthetics within the GABA$_A$ receptor. *J Neurosci* 2001; **21**: RC136.

84. Hemmings HC, Akabas MH, Goldstein PA, *et al.* Emerging molecular mechanisms of general anesthetic action. *Trends Pharmacol Sci* 2005; **26**: 503–10.

85. Sonner JM, Werner DF, Elsen FP, *et al.* Effect of isoflurane and other potent inhaled anesthetics on minimum alveolar concentration, learning, and the righting reflex in mice engineered to express alpha1 gamma-aminobutyric acid type A receptors unresponsive to isoflurane. *Anesthesiology* 2007; **106**: 107–13.

86. Rudolph U, Mohler H. Analysis of GABA$_A$ receptor function and dissection of the pharmacology of benzodiazepines and general anesthetics through mouse genetics. *Annu Rev Pharmacol Toxicol* 2004; **44**: 475.

87. Quinlan JJ, Homanics GE, Firestone LL. Anesthesia sensitivity in mice that lack the beta3 subunit of the gamma-aminobutyric acid type A receptor. *Anesthesiology* 1998; **88**: 775–80.

88. Downie DL, Hall AC, Lieb WR, Franks NP. Effects of inhalational general anaesthetics on native glycine receptors in rat medullary neurones and recombinant glycine receptors in *Xenopus* oocytes. *Br J Pharmacol* 1996; **118**: 493–502.

89. Harrison NL, Kugler JL, Jones MV, Greenblatt EP, Pritchett DB. Positive modulation of human gamma-aminobutyric acid type A and glycine receptors by the inhalation anesthetic isoflurane. *Mol Pharmacol* 1993; **44**: 628–32.

90. Wakamori M, Ikemoto Y, Akaike N. Effects of two volatile anesthetics and a volatile convulsant on the excitatory and inhibitory amino acid responses in dissociated CNS neurons of the rat. *J Neurophys* 1991; **66**: 2014–21.

91. Mihic SJ, Ye Q, Wick MJ, *et al.* Sites of alcohol and volatile anaesthetic action on GABA(A) and glycine receptors. *Nature* 1997; **389**: 385–9.

92. Yamakura T, Mihic SJ, Harris RA. Amino acid volume and hydropathy of a transmembrane site determine glycine and anesthetic sensitivity of glycine receptors. *J Biol Chem* 1999; **274**: 23006–12.

93. Zhang Y, Wu S, Eger EI, Sonner JM. Neither GABA$_A$ nor strychnine-sensitive glycine receptors are the sole mediators of MAC for isoflurane. *Anesth Analg* 2001; **92**: 123–7.

94. Violet JM, Downie DL, Nakisa RC, Lieb WR, Franks NP. Differential sensitivities of mammalian neuronal and muscle nicotinic acetylcholine receptors to general anesthetics. *Anesthesiology* 1997; **86**: 866–74.

95. Dani JA, Bertrand D. Nicotinic acetylcholine receptors and nicotinic cholinergic mechanisms of the central nervous system. *Annu Rev Pharmacol Toxicol* 2007; **47**: 699–729.

96. Gotti C, Zoli M, Clementi F. Brain nicotinic acetylcholine receptors: native subtypes and their relevance. *Trends Pharmacol Sci* 2006; **27**: 482–91.

97. Eger EI, Zhang Y, Laster M, *et al.* Acetylcholine receptors do not mediate the immobilization produced by inhaled anesthetics. *Anesth Analg* 2002; **94**: 1500–4.

98. Flood P, Sonner JM, Gong D, Coates KM. Heteromeric nicotinic inhibition by isoflurane does not mediate MAC or loss of righting reflex. *Anesthesiology* 2002; **97**: 902–5.

99. Raines DE, Claycomb RJ, Forman SA. Nonhalogenated anesthetic alkanes and perhalogenated nonimmobilizing alkanes inhibit alpha(4)beta(2) neuronal nicotinic acetylcholine receptors. *Anesth Analg* 2002; **95**: 573–7.

100. Zhang Y, Eger EI, Dutton RC, Sonner JM. Inhaled anesthetics have hyperalgesic effects at 0.1 minimum alveolar anesthetic concentration. *Anesth Analg* 2000; **91**: 462–6.

101. Flood P, Sonner JM, Gong D, Coates KM. Isoflurane hyperalgesia is modulated by nicotinic inhibition. *Anesthesiology* 2002; **97**: 192–8.

102. Honore E. *Nat Rev Neurosci* 2007; **8**: 251–61.

103. Franks N, Lieb W. Volatile general anaesthetics activate a novel K$^+$ current. *Nature* 1988; **333**: 662–4.

104. Winegar BD, Owen DF, Yost CS, Forsayeth, Mayeri E. Volatile general anesthetics produce hyperpolarization of *Aplysia* neurons by activation of a discrete population of baseline potassium channels. *Anesthesiology* 1996; **85**: 889–900.

105. Gray AT, Winegar BD, Leonoudakis DJ, Forsayeth, Yost CS. TOK1 is a volatile anesthetic stimulated K$^+$ channel. *Anesthesiology* 1998; **88**: 1076–84.

106. Patel AJ, Honoré E, Lesage F, *et al.* Inhalational anesthetics activate two-pore-domain background K$^+$ channels. *Nat Neurosci* 1999; **2**: 422–6.

107. Andres-Enguix I, Caley A, Yustos R, *et al.* Determinants of the anesthetic sensitivity of two-pore domain acid-sensitive potassium channels: molecular cloning of an anesthetic-activated potassium channel from Lymnaea stagnalis. *J Biol Chem* 2007; **282**: 20977–90.

108. Heurteaux C, Guy N, Laigle C, *et al.* TREK-1, a K$^+$ channel involved in neuroprotection and general anesthesia. *EMBO J* 2004; **23**: 2684–95.

109. Linden AM, Aller MI, Leppä E, *et al.* The in vivo contributions of TASK-1-containing channels to the actions of inhalation anesthetics, the α$_2$ adrenergic sedative dexmedetomidine, and cannabinoid agonists. *J Pharmacol Exp Ther* 2006; **317**: 615–26.

110. Linden AM, Sandu C, Aller MI, *et al.* TASK-3 knockout mice exhibit exaggerated nocturnal activity, impairments in cognitive functions, and reduced sensitivity to inhalation anesthetics. *J Pharmacol Exp Ther* 2007; **323**: 924–34.

111. Gerstin KM, Gong DH, Abdallah M, *et al.* Mutation of KCNK5 or Kir3.2 potassium channels in mice does not change minimum alveolar anesthetic concentration. *Anesth Analg* 2003; **96**: 1345–9.

112. Shimizu E, Tang YP, Rampon C, Tsien JZ. NMDA receptor-dependent synaptic reinforcement as a crucial process for memory consolidation. *Science* 2000; **290**: 1170–4.

113. Rampon C, Tang YP, Goodhouse J, *et al.* Enrichment induces structural changes and recovery from nonspatial memory deficits in CA1 NMDAR1-knockout mice. *Nat Neurosci* 2000; **3**: 238–44.

114. Nakazawa K, Sun LD, Quirk MC, *et al.* Hippocampal CA3 NMDA receptors are crucial for memory acquisition of one-time experience. *Neuron* 2003; **38**: 305–15.

115. Nakazawa K, Quirk MC, Chitwood RA, *et al.* Requirement for hippocampal CA3 NMDA receptors in associative memory recall. *Science* 2002; **297**: 211–18.

116. Tsien JZ, Huerta PT, Tonegawa S. The essential role of hippocampal CA1 NMDA receptor-dependent synaptic plasticity in spatial memory. *Cell* 1996; **87**: 1327–38.

117. Tang YP, Shimizu E, Dube GR, *et al,* Genetic enhancement of learning and memory in mice. *Nature* 1999; **401**: 63–9.

118. Kandel ER. The molecular biology of memory storage: a dialogue between genes and synapses. *Science* 2001; **294**: 1030–8.

119. de Sousa SL, Dickinson R, Lieb WR, Franks NP. Contrasting synaptic actions of the inhalational general anesthetics isoflurane and xenon. *Anesthesiology* 2000; **92**: 1055–66.

120. Hollmann MW, Liu HT, Hoenemann CW, Liu WH, Durieux ME. Modulation of NMDA receptor function by ketamine and magnesium. Part II: interactions with volatile anesthetics. *Anesth Analg* 2001; **92**: 1182–91.

121. Ogata J, Shiraishi M, Namba T, *et al.* Effects of anesthetics on mutant N-methyl-D-aspartate receptors expressed in Xenopus oocytes. *J Pharmacol Exp Ther* 2006; **318**: 434–43.

122. Yamakura T, Harris RA. Effects of gaseous anesthetics nitrous oxide and xenon on ligand-gated ion channels. Comparison with isoflurane and ethanol. *Anesthesiology* 2000; **93**: 1095–101.

123. Westphalen RI, Hemmings HC. Selective depression by general anesthetics of glutamate versus GABA release from isolated cortical nerve terminals. *J Pharmacol Exp Ther* 2003; **304**: 1188–96.

124. Lingamaneni R, Birch ML, Hemmings HC. Widespread inhibition of sodium channel-dependent glutamate release from isolated nerve terminals by isoflurane and propofol. *Anesthesiology* 2001; **95**: 1460–6.

125. Schlame M, Hemmings HC. Inhibition by volatile anesthetics of endogenous glutamate release from synaptosomes by a presynaptic mechanism. *Anesthesiology* 1995; **82**: 1406–16.

126. Rehberg B, Xiao YH, Duch DS. Central nervous system sodium channels are significantly suppressed at clinical concentrations of volatile anesthetics. *Anesthesiology* 1996; **84**: 1223–33.

127. Wu XS, Sun JY, Evers AS, Crowder M, Wu LG. Isoflurane inhibits transmitter release and the presynaptic action potential. *Anesthesiology* 2004; **100**: 663–70.

128. Westphalen RI, Krivitski M, Amarosa A, Guy N, Hemmings HC. Reduced inhibition of cortical glutamate and GABA release by halothane in mice lacking the K+ channel, TREK-1. *Br J Pharmacol* 2007; **152**: 939–45.

129. Metz LB, Dasgupta N, Liu C, Hunt SJ, Crowder CM. An evolutionarily conserved presynaptic protein is required for isoflurane sensitivity in *Caenorhabditis elegans*. *Anesthesiology* 2007; **107**: 971–82.

130. Anis NA, Berry SC, Burton NR, Lodge D. The dissociative anaesthetics, ketamine and phencyclidine, selectively reduce excitation of central mammalian neurones by N-methyl-aspartate. *Br J Pharmacol* 1983; **79**: 565–75.

131. Harrison NL, Simmonds MA. Quantitative studies on some antagonists of N-methyl D-aspartate in slices of rat cerebral cortex. *Br J Pharmacol* 1985; **84**: 381–91.

132. Thomson AM, West DC, Lodge D. An N-methylaspartate receptor-mediated synapse in rat cerebral cortex: a site of action of ketamine? *Nature* 1985; **313**: 479–81.

133. Orser BA, Pennefather PS, MacDonald JF. Multiple mechanisms of ketamine blockade of N-methyl-D-aspartate receptors. *Anesthesiology* 1997; **86**: 903–17.

134. Sato Y, Kobayashi E, Hakamata Y, *et al.* Chronopharmacological studies of ketamine in normal and NMDA ε 1 receptor knockout mice. *Br J Anaesth* 2004; **92**: 859–64.

135. MacDonald JF, Bartlett MC, Mody I, *et al.* Actions of ketamine, phencyclidine and MK-801 on NMDA receptor currents in cultured mouse hippocampal neurones. *J Physiol* 1991; **432**: 483–508.

136. Idvall J, Ahlgren I, Aronsen KR, Stenberg P. Ketamine infusions: pharmacokinetics and clinical effects. *Br J Anaesth* 1979; **51**: 1167–73.

137. Dayton PG, Stiller RL, Cook DR, Perel JM. The binding of ketamine to plasma proteins: emphasis on human plasma. *Eur J Clin Pharmacol* 1983; **24**: 825–31.

138. Keana JF, Scherz MW, Quarum M, Sonders MS, Weber E. Synthesis and characterization of a radiolabelled derivative of the phencyclidine/N-methyl-D-aspartate receptor ligand (+) MK-801 with high specific radioactivity. *Life Sci* 1988; **43**: 965–73.

139. Zeilhofer HU, Swandulla D, Geisslinger G, Brune K. Differential effects of ketamine enantiomers on NMDA receptor currents in cultured neurons. *Eur J Pharmacol* 1992; **213**: 155–8.

140. White PF, Schüttler J, Shafer A, *et al.* Comparative pharmacology of the ketamine isomers. Studies in volunteers. *Br J Anaesth* 1985; **57**: 197–203.

141. Paoletti P, Neyton J. NMDA receptor subunits: function and pharmacology. *Curr Opin Pharmacol* 2007; **7**: 39–47.

142. Furuya R, Oka K, Watanabe I, *et al.* The effects of ketamine and propofol on neuronal nicotinic acetylcholine receptors and P2x purinoceptors in PC12 cells. *Anesth Analg* 1999; **88**: 174–80.

143. Scheller M, Bufler J, Hertle I, *et al.* Ketamine blocks currents through mammalian nicotinic acetylcholine

Table 25.2. Anesthetic solubility in tissues. Note that there is considerable variability in published reports and these values should be accepted ± 10%. Blood/gas, and so tissue/blood, solubilities are especially variable: a meal may increase λ_{BG} by 15%. It is generally accepted that anesthetics obey Henry's law, i.e., the solubility coefficient is independent of partial pressure [1]

Anesthetic	Xe	N$_2$O	Desflurane	Sevoflurane	Isoflurane	Enflurane	Halothane
Saline/gas	0.093	0.46	0.22	0.34	0.54	0.73	0.86
Blood/gas (λ_{BG})	0.14	0.47	0.45	0.65	1.40	1.90	2.50
Gray matter/gas	0.14	0.50	0.61	1.02	1.84	2.24	3.76
White matter/gas	0.24	0.51	0.98	1.95	3.51	3.16	8.93
VRG/gas	0.16	0.42	0.54	1.20	2.50	3.10	4.90
Muscle/gas	0.092	0.54	0.94	2.38	4.40	3.06	9.49
Fat/gas	1.3	1.1	12	34	64	87	136
Tissue/blood solubility coefficients (λ_{TB})							
Gray matter/blood	1.1	1.1	1.4	1.6	1.3	1.2	1.5
White matter/blood	1.8	1.1	2.2	3.0	2.5	1.7	3.6
VRG/blood	1.2	0.9	1.2	1.8	1.8	1.6	2.0
Muscle/blood	0.7	1.1	2.1	3.7	3.1	1.6	3.8
Fat/blood	9.6	2.3	26.7	52.3	45.9	45.8	54.4

VRG, vessel-rich group.

pulmonary circulation initially contains no anesthetic so, in the first breath, an anesthetic partial-pressure gradient is established between alveolus and blood, driving anesthetic into the blood (uptake) and slowing the increase in anesthetic alveolar partial pressure. The greater the cardiac output and the more soluble the anesthetic in blood, the greater will be the uptake from the alveoli and the slower the increase in alveolar partial pressure, delaying the onset of anesthesia. On the other hand, if alveolar ventilation is increased then more anesthetic is brought to the alveoli, reducing the effect of uptake and accelerating the increase in alveolar anesthetic partial pressure. Historically, this was the mechanism by which the addition of carbon dioxide (CO_2) to the inspired gas mixture hastened inhalational induction with diethyl ether.

Concentration and second-gas effects

The quantity of anesthetic absorbed can be great, up to 1 liter min^{-1} for the first minute of nitrous oxide (N$_2$O) use, and this mass transfer can influence gas concentrations within the alveoli. The second-gas effect occurs when so much N$_2$O is taken out of the alveoli that the alveolar volume decreases, concentrating the remaining gases [2] and reducing expired volume. Reduced expired volume has two consequences: less volatile anesthetic is lost and less carbon dioxide is eliminated, stimulating ventilation in a spontaneously breathing patient. These effects accelerate the increase in alveolar concentration of volatile anesthetics administered with N$_2$O, but the effect is small and of doubtful clinical significance (Fig. 25.4). Indeed, there has been doubt expressed that it exists at all [3], and a recent study has suggested that it is not caused by mass transfer of N$_2$O but

by changes in regional ventilation and perfusion [4]. There is no final word on this yet. The second-gas effect will also increase the alveolar oxygen (O$_2$) concentration.

A less intuitive phenomenon is the concentration effect [5]: if N$_2$O is inhaled at a constant inspired concentration, the alveolar concentration will approach the inspired faster the greater the inspired concentration. An insight into the mechanism of this unexpected result may be gained by a simple qualitative analysis. If 1% N$_2$O is inhaled then perhaps half will be absorbed in the first breath with negligible change in lung volume, so the concentration of N$_2$O is halved. On the other hand, if 60% N$_2$O is inhaled and half absorbed, the alveolar volume would also be significantly reduced and the resulting concentration would be greater than 30%. Thus the reduction in concentration of N$_2$O due to uptake is proportionately less when a greater concentration is used (Fig. 25.4).

Distribution

Blood distributes the anesthetic around the body according to regional perfusion, and anesthetic is transferred from blood to the tissues at a rate determined by the partial-pressure gradient between arterial blood and the tissue. This transfer of anesthetic reduces its partial pressure in blood so that, on its return to the lungs, more anesthetic is again absorbed from the alveoli. It takes days to equilibrate the tissues with alveolar partial pressure, so in clinical practice uptake continues throughout anesthesia resulting in a continuing difference between inspired and alveolar anesthetic partial pressures.

The cardiac output is not distributed evenly throughout the body. Some organs are much more vascular than others,

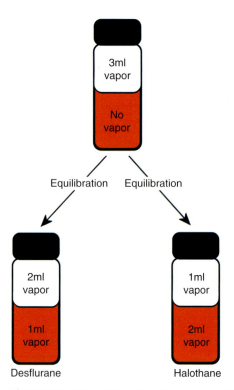

Figure 25.3. When 100 mL blood is placed in a 200 mL container and the gas space is flushed with 3% of an anesthetic before being sealed and equilibrated at 37 °C, the final concentrations are unequal between the gas and blood phases and depend upon the anesthetic, so what is actually eqilibrating? For desflurane, absorption by the blood will result in a final gas concentration of 2%: 2 mL vapor in the 100 mL gas phase and 1 mL dissolved in 100 mL blood, giving a solubility coefficient of 0.5. If 3% halothane had been used, the amounts would have been reversed: 1 mL in the gas phase, 2 mL dissolved in blood, giving a solubility coefficient of 2. In each case the partial pressure of anesthetic in blood is defined as being equal to the partial pressure in the gas phase, and it is this physical quantity that equilibrates. (Note that the values quoted are approximations.)

resulting in a greater rate of perfusion (e.g., brain gray matter 60–120 mL blood per 100 g tissue per minute, resting skeletal muscle 2 mL blood per 100 g tissue per minute). The greater the tissue perfusion, the more rapidly will anesthetic partial pressure equilibrate with blood. It is convenient to divide the body into compartments – groups of organs which are anatomically distinct but pharmacokinetically similar.

The best-perfused tissues (including brain, heart, kidney, liver, endocrine glands) are traditionally called the *vessel-rich group* [6]. They make up less than 10% of body weight but receive around 80% of the cardiac output. It is not a homogeneous group, for their perfusion varies from 20 to over 100 mL blood per 100g tissue per minute, but even the least well perfused in this group is far better perfused than the rest of the body. Muscle and skin are lean tissues and usually make up a little over 50% of the body by weight. Perfusion is very variable, depending on the physiological situation (rest or exercise, hot or cold environments), but during anesthesia they are believed to have similar perfusion of around 2 mL per 100g per minute. They can be combined into a single *muscle group*.

Anesthetics are fat-soluble drugs, so the fattier the tissue the more anesthetic it can absorb for a given partial pressure and the longer it will take longer to equilibrate with the anesthetic partial pressure in arterial blood. Therefore although *body fat* (20–30% of body weight in those of ideal body mass index, but obviously more in the obese) has a similar perfusion to muscle and skin during anesthesia, it is considered to be a separate compartment. The remaining body tissues (the *vessel-poor group*) have such a poor blood supply that their contribution to anesthetic pharmacokinetics can be ignored in the first instance.

Many find that a mathematical description of the theory is an obstacle to comprehension and prefer Mapleson's physical analog of water running between tanks [7] (Fig. 25.5).

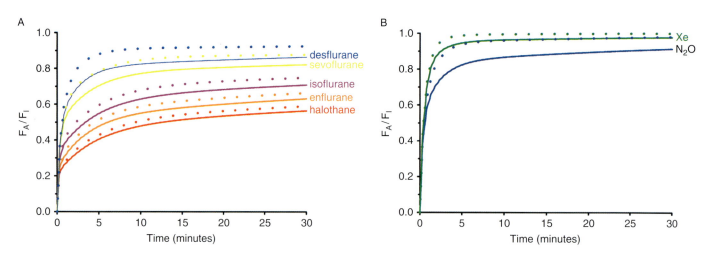

Figure 25.4. (A) The rate of rise of alveolar concentration, expressed as a fraction of the inspired concentration (F_A/F_I), for five volatile anesthetics in a simulation based on Eger's model. For each anesthetic the continuous line shows the anesthetic in an air–oxygen mixture and the dotted line shows the second-gas effect caused by anesthetic delivery in 70% nitrous oxide. The effect is greater for the less soluble agents, but it is not clinically inportant. (B) The rate of rise of alveolar concentration of nitrous oxide and xenon administered as 1% (continuous line) or 70% mixtures (dotted lines), demonstrating the concentration effect.

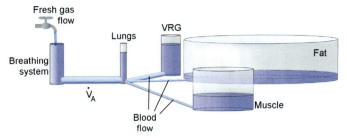

Figure 25.5. Mapleson's water analog is perhaps the most intuitive model of anesthetic uptake and distribution [7]. In this model, anesthetic is represented by water, and body compartments and the lungs are represented by containers, proportional in size to the product of the physical size of the compartment and the anesthetic solubility in it. Anesthetic partial pressure is represented by the height of the water level in the containers, for this is what determines the direction and rate of transfer between the compartments. The diameter of the pipes connecting containers represents the rate of flow of anesthetic – either the rate of alveolar ventilation or the product of the tissue perfusion and the blood/gas solubility for the anesthetic, depending upon the context. The proportions of the model differ for each anesthetic, with the model for nitrous oxide having smaller tanks and smaller pipes between them than a model for a volatile anesthetic. The behavior of this familiar physical arrangement is easily understood and exactly replicates the simple mathematical models of anesthetic uptake and distribution. In particular, it can be seen that less soluble drugs will, by draining less out of the alveolar compartment, allow the anesthetic partial pressure to be established more quickly. Mapleson adapted his water analog model to show the second-gas effect, but the modification detracts from the simplicity of the original design and is not included here. Elimination of anesthetic is simulated by allowing free drainage from the breathing-system tank.

Elimination of anesthetics

Elimination of inhaled anesthetics is almost exclusively through the lungs. Of currently available agents, only halothane undergoes enough metabolism to significantly affect its kinetics [8]. Anesthetic elimination directly from the pleural and peritoneal cavities has been measured in pigs, and it was found to be greater with more soluble anesthetics [9]. Even so, the quantities are negligible compared to elimination through the lungs and, projecting from these results to humans, loss through the skin is smaller still [10,11].

Elimination of inhaled anesthetics from the body is therefore simply the reverse process of their uptake. As blood passes through the lungs, anesthetic diffuses down the concentration gradient into the alveoli, whence it is eliminated by ventilation. Arterial blood now has a lower partial pressure of anesthetic than is present in the brain and other well-perfused tissues, and so anesthetic diffuses out of the brain into blood for elimination through the lungs. After a brief anesthetic, less well perfused and fatty tissues may still have a lower anesthetic partial pressure than arterial blood and will continue to absorb it, a phenomenon termed redistribution when applied to intravenous anesthetics. The effect will be most obvious for more fat-soluble anesthetics and will result in more rapid recovery of consciousness after a short anesthetic than might otherwise be expected, but if administration is prolonged then the depot built up in fat will delay recovery. The context-sensitive rates of elimination for different

anesthetics are predicted to increase much more for soluble anesthetics as the duration of anesthesia increases [12]. Nitrous oxide has a particularly low fat solubility and this is the reason for its rapid elimination regardless of the duration of administration. Of the volatile agents, desflurane has the smallest fat/blood solubility coefficient and so, although it is always rapidly eliminated from the body, the difference from the other anesthetics is most noticable after a long operation on an obese patient. Elimination is a slower process than uptake because the anesthetic partial-pressure gradients are smaller. The inspired concentration can be increased to "over-pressure" the alveolar space and drive anesthetic into the blood, but there is no corresponding "suction" to enhance elimination. Anesthetics can be measured in expired gas for days after surgery as they trickle out of fat depots.

In 1955 Fink described hypoxia during emergence from anesthesia as alveolar O_2 became diluted by the flood of N_2O returning from the tissues in venous blood [13]. It is the reverse of the second-gas effect seen during induction of anesthesia with N_2O, but there may be an additional effect in spontaneously breathing patients because the alveolar carbon dioxide is also diluted, leading to hypoventilation [14]. If ventilation is controlled, then an increased expired minute ventilation is observed, enhancing volatile anesthetic elimination [15]. Hypoxia due to the Fink effect is easily prevented by routine administration of supplemental O_2 when N_2O is discontinued.

Mathematics of anesthetic distribution

The theory of anesthetic distribution is based on Seymour Kety's description of the pharmacokinetics of inert gases [16]. Two assumptions are widely accepted: that the partial pressure of anesthetic in arterial blood is equal to the partial pressure in alveolar gas, of which end-expired gas provides a representative sample; and that anesthetic partial pressure equilibrates between blood and tissue during capillary transit. The first assumption was thought reasonable for many years, though later studies have reported significant end-expired to arterial gradients [17], and the second assumption is accepted almost universally.

The rate of change of anesthetic partial pressure in a tissue is proportional to the difference between the partial pressures in arterial blood and the tissue, P_a and P_T respectively:

$$dP_T/dt = k(P_a - P_T) \tag{25.1}$$

The constant of proportionality k can be derived intuitively. If the tissue is large or the anesthetic is very soluble in it, then equilibration will be slowed and k will be small. It can be convenient to think of the virtual volume of the tissue, the product of the physical volume and the solubility coefficient. For adipose tissue, the virtual volume may exceed the physical volume of the whole body by a factor of 10. If the blood flow is large then the equilibration will proceed rapidly, i.e., k will be large too, and the flow will be effectively increased if the anesthetic is more soluble in blood. Given these considerations, the simplest formula for k is $k = Q\lambda_{BG}/V\lambda_{TG}$, where Q is the absolute flow to the tissue in question, V is the tissue volume, and λ_{TG} and λ_{BG} are the tissue/gas and blood/gas solubility coefficients respectively. If care is taken with the volume units, the eventual unit is the reciprocal of time. Alternatively, Q and V can be amalgamated into q, the tissue perfusion, normally quoted in units of mL blood per 100 g tissue per minute. This must be converted to mL blood per mL tissue per minute, but that only requires a factor of 100 for acceptable accuracy. Using the blood/tissue solubility coefficient λ_{TB}, the formula for k then becomes simply $k = q/\lambda_{TB}$.

This model of anesthetic uptake into a tissue is easily extended to model uptake into the whole body by representing the body as a few homogeneous tissue compartments. The partial pressure of venous blood draining a compartment is equal to the calculated tissue partial pressure, and the mixed venous anesthetic partial pressure is calculated as a weighted sum of the venous effluents. The difference between arterial and mixed venous partial pressure allows anesthetic uptake to be calculated by Fick's principle, and it is uptake that determines the inspired/alveolar gradient. Very elaborate body models have been described [18], but Eger's original compartments are sufficient to represent uptake in a typical patient well enough for teaching purposes [6] (Fig. 25.4).

Measurements of uptake

Multicompartment models can be used to predict anesthetic uptake, but they can also be used in reverse to calculate the size and perfusion of body compartments from measurements of uptake or elimination. These measurements are not made directly, but are deduced either from measurement of inspired and expired gas volumes and anesthetic partial pressures [19], or by measurement of the amount of anesthetic added to a closed breathing system to maintain a constant end-expired anesthetic concentration, when the only loss should be from uptake by the patient [20]. The rate of uptake decreases monotonically and a function of the form $\Sigma A_i e^{-k_i t}$ can be fitted to the data by selecting appropriate values of A_i and k_i. The greater the number of exponential terms included in the sum, the better the fit (i.e., the less is the sum of all the squared differences between the measured uptake and the model) and a version of the F-test is required to confirm that additional terms in the sum are statistically justified [21]. On the assumption that the resulting sum of exponentials represents exponential uptake into tissue compartments, compartment volumes and perfusion can be calculated. The i-th compartment volume is proportional to the quotient A_i/k_i, and the perfusion is calculated for each

compartment using the expression derived above: $k = q/\lambda_{TB}$. In general the results do not match reference anatomical and physiological values very accurately. Possible reasons for the disappointing results include errors in uptake measurement, short experiments so that few data are influenced by the slower processes, and quite large confidence intervals for compartment values.

Mammillary models

It is possible to measure elimination of anesthetics in expired gas over several days but, although it is a simple matter to fit a multiexponential function to the data, redistribution between body compartments means that the model no longer predicts an exactly multiexponential washout. This prevents conclusions about the size and perfusion of compartments being drawn from the derived parameters. Mammillary analysis has been used in this situation [8]. The mammillary model has a central compartment, compartment 1, and a number of peripheral compartments which can exchange drug with the central compartment but not with other peripheral compartments. Elimination is possible from any compartment; in the model shown in Fig. 25.6, elimination was allowed through the central and vessel-rich compartments, representing the lungs and hepatic metabolism respectively.

Rather than consider the net transfer of drug between compartments 1 and 2, the analysis considers separately the

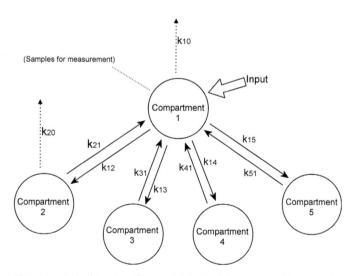

Figure 25.6. In the mammillary model the body is represented by a number of compartments. Peripheral compartments 2 to 5 exchange drug with the central compartment 1, from which samples may be drawn for measurement, but not between each other. The rate of drug transfer from any compartment is proportional to the amount of drug in that compartment, with the constant of proportionality labeled to indicate the direction of transfer (e.g., k_{31} is associated with transfer from compartment 3 to the central compartment). Elimination from the body follows a similar rule with the constant labelled k_{10}, k_{20} as appropriate. Computer modeling is typically initiated by a bolus injection of drug into the central compartment (the input), but in anesthetic studies the input is more likely to be represented by a continuous function.

amount transferred from 1 to 2, and from 2 to 1. The amount transferred out of one compartment is taken to be a fixed proportion of the total amount in that compartment, and the constant of proportionality is subscripted to indicate the transfer (e.g., k_{12} for transfer from compartment 1 to compartment 2). When drug is eliminated from the body through compartment n the constant is k_{n0}. Treating the two directions of transfer separately allows the model to cope with active uptake into compartments, but the advantage in the special case of volatile anesthetics is simply that there are sophisticated mathematical software packages readily available to handle the calculations. One disadvantage of the mammillary model is the fact that the constants do not have an obvious physical analog, and that pairs of constants k_{1i}, k_{i1} are numerically very different. In order to see the meaning in the constants, consider transfer of an inhaled anesthetic between compartments 1 and 2. Using the earlier, simple approach the net transfer is $(P_1 - P_2) \cdot k$, where P_i is the partial pressure in the i-th compartment and k depends upon solubility, compartment size, and blood flow (see above). With the mammillary approach the net transfer is the difference between the separate transfers: $A_1 \cdot k_{12} - A_2 \cdot k_{21}$, where A_i is the total amount of anesthetic in the i-th compartment. This can be rewritten in terms of partial-pressures:

$$P_1 \cdot \lambda_{\text{T1G}} \cdot V_1 \cdot k_{12} - \lambda_{\text{T2G}} \cdot V_2 \cdot k_{21} \qquad (25.2)$$

where $\lambda_{\text{T}i\text{G}}$ is the solubility coefficient of the i-th compartment and V_i is its volume. If the quantity represented by this last equation is going to be proportional to the partial-pressure difference, then it must be that

$$\lambda_{\text{T1G}} \cdot V_1 \cdot k_{12} = \lambda_{\text{T2G}} \cdot V_2 \cdot k_{21} \qquad (25.3)$$

Furthermore, each of these terms must equal the k described previously, and this links them to physiological variables.

Eger and his coworkers measured elimination of halothane, isoflurane, and desflurane following their simultaneous administration for 30 minutes. They not only fitted a multiexponential curve to their 5-day washout data, but also undertook a mammillary analysis [8]. The body was modeled as five compartments because the multiexponential analysis had supported that number. The lungs were the central compartment and the four peripheral compartments were the vessel-rich group (with a k_{20} term to allow for hepatic metabolism), the muscle group and two fat groups with differing perfusions. The smaller of these fat groups, the "fifth compartment," was thought to represent fat laid down around vascular tissue (e.g., perinephric fat), absorbing anesthetic both from its own blood supply and also by diffusion from the adjacent, well-perfused tissue which would have a high anesthetic partial pressure. There is some experimental evidence to support this idea [22], but not enough is known about regional fat perfusion to eliminate alternative explanations such as kinetically distinct core and peripheral fat compartments [23].

PBPK models

A problem common to both of the preceding analyses (multiexponential washin, mammillary washout) is that the derived parameters only define compartment volumes and perfusion when a solubility coefficient has been chosen. The coefficients are known objectively, but the choice of pairing solubility with compartment is subjective. One way around these problems is to increase the a-priori assumptions of the model. Instead of a body comprising four arbitrary compartments we can refer to standard tables to specify the size and nature of the compartments, adjusting the perfusion of the compartments to best fit the experimental data. Such physiologically based pharmacokinetic (PBPK) models have become increasingly popular in nonanesthetic pharmacokinetics and toxicology, yet although the first and most subsequent models of anesthetic uptake and distribution are physiologically based, they have rarely been given the label PBPK. PBPK models have developed independently of the anesthetic literature with just a few bridges recently built between them. They are characterized by starting with a model body comprising a number of compartments (typically 10 or more) of realistic sizes, perfusion, and partition coefficients, where known, and fitting the model predictions to measured data by adjusting one or two unknown parameters. For instance, if a drug was assumed to be metabolized in the liver but was otherwise inert, then distribution in the body and excretion through the kidneys could be included in the model using standard physiological values and the model would be tuned to the measured data by adjusting the K_m value for drug metabolism in the liver compartment.

Modern PBPK analysis has been applied retrospectively to data of anesthetic uptake and distribution with some success. Levitt found that multiple fat compartments of differing perfusion fitted the data from Eger's group [8] without the need to invoke intertissue diffusion as an explanation of those results [23]. When the Michaelis–Menten K_m and $V_{\max}$ parameters in a liver compartment were adjusted to match a PBPK model to measured data of end-expired halothane partial pressures, the derived parameters were found to be very plausible, though accurate human data are not available for exact comparison [24]. The same PBPK analysis of methoxyflurane uptake data suggested there was a marked end-expired to arterial partial-pressure gradient for this soluble anesthetic, an idea supported by direct measurement but not apparent from the mammillary analysis undertaken by the original authors.

Metabolism

Volatile anesthetics undergo metabolism to differing degrees [25]. They undergo oxidative metabolism by cytochrome P450 enzymes in the liver, kidney, and lungs, but particularly by CYP2E1, which is almost exclusively hepatic in humans [26]. There is evidence that clinical concentrations of anesthetics inhibit their own metabolism during anesthesia, but the prolonged low concentrations present in the postoperative days are metabolized much more efficiently [27]. This fact alone means that more soluble anesthetics will undergo more metabolism than those that are less soluble. Individuals who receive compounds that induce production of CYP2E1 (e.g., ethanol, isoniazid, phenobarbital) may metabolize anesthetics to a greater extent. Conversely disulfiram, an inhibitor of CYP2E1, should minimize anesthetic metabolism. Comparison of identical and nonidentical twins has shown that genetic makeup also contributes to the proportion of anesthetic metabolized [28]. Injury to the kidneys and liver from anesthetic metabolites was the stimulus to the development of the current generation of volatile anesthetics.

Methoxyflurane was abandoned from clinical use because its prolonged administration led to increasing degrees of nephrotoxicity (e.g., polyuria, hypernatremia, decrease in creatinine clearance). Enflurane can also cause a similar but milder renal injury, especially in patients whose treatment with isoniazid for tuberculosis coincidentally upregulates the metabolic pathway. Methoxyflurane-induced nephrotoxicity was associated with serum fluoride ion concentrations greater than $50\,\mu M$. Sevoflurane metabolism results in the highest serum fluoride ion levels of current anesthetics, and prolonged administration may result in serum fluoride ion concentrations greater than $100\,\mu M$. However, clinical signs of nephrotoxicity do not occur even when sevoflurane is administered for prolonged periods in low-flow breathing systems, which allow rebreathing of potentially nephrotoxic breakdown products of sevoflurane in soda lime, and subclinical injury is contentious [29,30]. One explanation for this difference between the old and the new is that the lower blood/gas partition coefficient of sevoflurane (0.65 vs. 15 for methoxyflurane) facilitates its elimination from the body after anesthesia, so the duration of exposure to $50\,\mu M$ serum fluoride ion concentration is much shorter. Additionally methoxyflurane, but very little sevoflurane, is metabolized in the kidney, exposing renal cells to greater local concentrations of fluoride [31]. Isoflurane and halothane are both associated with clinically insignificant increases in free fluoride, but desflurane is so resistant to biodegradation that there may be no measurable increase after its use.

Halothane is metabolized more than any other modern anesthetic, over 40% of amount taken up, which implies a metabolic load of several grams. It is the only modern anesthetic for which the rate of metabolism is enough to affect its pharmacokinetics, so, in spite of its greater blood and tissue solubility, its elimination (judged by the rate of reduction of alveolar concentration) is similar to that of isoflurane [8]. It is also the only anesthetic to undergo significant reductive metabolism (by the hepatic CYP2A6 and CYP3A4 cytochromes [32]), and it may be this pathway that leads to the "normal" and clinically insignificant increase in serum hepatic enzyme concentrations after anesthesia with this drug, although local hepatic hypoxia has also been put forward as an explanation. The bulk of halothane metabolism is oxidative with the formation of bromide and trifluoroacetic acid, further degradation of which may be the trigger for severe hepatic necrosis ("halothane hepatitis": see Chapter 26). Disulfiram is an inhibitor of cytochrome CYP2E1 and oral administration before surgery inhibits oxidation of halothane, so it may be a method to provide prophylaxis against halothane hepatitis [33]. Much smaller amounts of trifluoroacetic acid are generated by metabolism of the currently available fluorinated methyl-ethyl ethers, but there have been some reports of hepatitis after anesthesia with enflurane, isoflurane, and even desflurane [34]. The analog of trifluoroacetic acid in sevoflurane metabolism is hexafluoroisopropanol, and further metabolism of this compound produces relatively unreactive intermediaries. It is glucuronidated and excreted in urine with a half-life of about 20 hours [35]. The risk of severe hepatic necrosis after sevoflurane anesthesia is generally thought to be negligible.

The anesthetic gases nitrous oxide and xenon are not metabolized, and xenon seems to have minimal nonanesthetic effects in the body. Nitrous oxide, on the other hand, interferes with vital metabolic pathways and its prolonged use has been responsible for patient deaths (see Chapter 26 for details).

Special topics

Breathing systems

Just as alveolar ventilation can be a choke on the rate of rise of anesthetic concentration, so too can the fresh gas flow. As the fresh gas flow is reduced, the proportion of recycled expired gas in the inspired mixture increases. The expired gas generally contains less anesthetic than the fresh gas, so the inspired concentration will be less than has been set on a vaporizer positioned in the fresh gas flow, outside of the breathing system. This difference will be more marked when uptake is greatest, because it is uptake that reduces the expired gas concentration. For this reason, most anesthesiologists use higher fresh gas flows early in the anesthetic, reducing them later as uptake lessens. The alternative tactic to achieve an adequate inspired anesthetic concentration – very high concentrations in a low fresh gas flow – is more efficient in terms of anesthetic usage [36], but it runs a greater risk of creating unintentionally large anesthetic concentrations in the breathing system if the vaporizer setting is not reduced as uptake decreases. The water analog can be extended to include a low-flow system: instead of anesthetic entering the system by keeping the breathing-system tank filled to overflowing, an additional tank is kept filled to overflowing and a narrow pipe, the diameter representing the magnitude of the fresh gas flow, connects it to the breathing-system tank. Water can be driven into the inspired gas tank faster either by increasing the diameter of the connecting pipe or by increasing the height of the tank (analogous to increasing the fresh gas flow or increasing the vaporizer setting).

Circle systems are now used only infrequently with a vaporizer in the circle, and the interested reader is referred to a theoretical study for further information on the peculiar features of this arrangement [37].

The rubber components of the breathing system have been known to absorb anesthetics for many years, but the introduction of sevoflurane brought renewed interest in the possibility of circuit components influencing the rate of induction. Absorption into plastic and, particularly, rubber takes place with all agents in proportion to their solubility, but sevoflurane is lost into soda lime by absorption and degradation at a rate that may invalidate the measurement of uptake by injection into closed systems, though the effect is clinically unimportant [38].

The alveolar/arterial gradient

The alveolar partial pressure of anesthetic, P_A, is used as a surrogate measure of the arterial partial pressure, P_a, because it is easy to measure continuously in real time, whereas arterial sampling is invasive and intermittent, and measurement of blood partial pressure is very time-consuming. (In fact, alveolar gas is never collected and end-expired gas $P_{E'}$ is used instead, adding another step between what we can and what we want to measure; end-tidal gas is approximately 80% alveolar, 20% inspired gas during anesthesia.) Frei and colleagues found the $P_a/P_{E'}$ was 88% in ASA I patients and only 70% in ASA III patients [39]. During the first 10 minutes of inhalation the ratio was even lower, presumably because the relatively high inspired anesthetic had a greater effect on the end-expired concentration. During elimination a consistent $P_{E'}/P_a$ ratio of 80% was reported. Eger and Bahlman have suggested that the arterial anesthetic partial pressure will be within 10% of the arterial if the inspired concentration is not more than 150% of the end-expired concentration [40].

Two special clinical circumstances are worthy of mention here. During cardiopulmonary bypass the partial pressure of a volatile anesthetic in arterial blood is equal to the partial pressure in the exhaust gas of a hollow-fiber oxygenator [41], but the solid membrane used in some new oxygenators are impervious to such large molecules and the arterial partial pressure will reduce gradually during bypass as a result of redistribution within the body [42]. Secondly, in situations where it is known that the pulmonary shunt is large and oxygenation can only be maintained by a very high inspired oxygen concentration (e.g., one-lung anesthesia), it would be unwise to rely too heavily on the end-expired concentration as an index of the arterial partial pressure. The error will be less with less soluble agents because the mixed venous partial pressure will be greater, lessening the effect of the shunt.

Diffusion into gas spaces: bubbles, pneumoencephalogram, and gut

The lungs are the greatest surface area for blood–gas exchange, but diffusion will occur from blood to a gas phase wherever there is an interface. Bubbles in blood and soft tissue will enlarge as an anesthetic diffuses into them down its partial-pressure gradient, but if the gas phase is enclosed then there is the potential for pressure to develop in the closed space as diffusion is unaffected by the total pressure gradient. The rate at which pressure increases depends upon the perfusion of the surrounding tissue, the compliance of the space, and the concentration of the anesthetic. Until recently, N_2O has been the only anesthetic used in sufficient concentration for these effects to be clinically important, and most quantitative data on the rate of these pressure changes come from animal studies. Following pneumoencephalograms, cerebrospinal fluid pressure can increase threefold in 5 minutes [43]. After intraocular injection of sulfur hexafluoride, N_2O will increase pressure from 2 to 18 mmHg in 20 minutes [44]. Reports of increases in middle air pressure are variable but in the range of $1–7$ mmHg min^{-1} during the first hour of anesthesia. The concentration of N_2O within a pneumothorax increased to 50% in just 5 minutes when the lungs were ventilated with 50% N_2O in O_2 (in this instance gas transferred by diffusion from the lung surface [45]), though intestinal gas volume took 150 minutes to double in volume [46]. It can be seen that there is no safe duration of N_2O anesthesia when it is important to avoid any of these complications. The speed of the effect of N_2O on bubble size is even faster: the volume of air bubbles injected into the right atrium had tripled in volume by the time they had appeared in the pulmonary capillaries during ventilation with 80% N_2O [47]. Nitrous oxide is avoided during cardiac surgery for fear of exacerbating the adverse effects of air embolism [48]. Concerns have been expressed about these risks during xenon anesthesia, which is the only other anesthetic used at such great concentrations. Experimental work has shown that xenon does indeed diffuse into gut air and bubble emboli, but that the time course is slower and the maximum expansion less than with N_2O [49–51]. This is probably a consequence of its lesser solubility, which will reduce the quantity available locally for diffusion into the gas phase, and lesser diffusibility due to the greater bulk of the xenon atom compared to the nitrous oxide molecule.

The effects of age and pregnancy

The physiological changes of growth and senescence are not associated with much change in uptake. A faster increase in end-expired concentration of halothane in younger children compared to those over 6 years has been reported, but there is little difference between young adults and the elderly or for less soluble agents [52–54]. Similarly, young children eliminate inhaled anesthetics faster than adults [55]. In adults, age has little effect on wake-up time, though elimination is slower after 24 hours in the elderly [54].

Both cardiac output and minute ventilation are increased in pregnant women, and so the rate of rise of expired anesthetic concentrations is unchanged compared to normocapnic women [56]. The anesthetic partial pressure in umbilical venous blood appears to be independent of solubility, being approximately 70%

Table 26.1. Physicochemical properties of the potent volatile anesthetics

	Sevoflurane	Desflurane	Isoflurane	Halothane	N$_2$O
Boiling point (°C)	59	24	49	50	−88
Vapor pressure at 20 °C (mmHg)	157	669	238	243	38 770
Molecular weight (g)	200	168	184	197	44
Oil/gas partition coefficient	47	19	91	224	1.4
Blood/gas partition coefficient	0.65	0.42	1.46	2.50	0.46
Brain/blood solubility	1.7	1.3	1.6	1.9	1.1
Fat/blood solubility	47.5	27.2	44.9	51.1	2.3
Muscle/blood solubility	3.1	2.0	2.9	3.4	1.2
MAC in O$_2$, 30–60 yr (%)[a]	1.8	6.6	1.17	0.75	104
MAC in 60–70% N$_2$O (%)[a]	0.66	2.38	0.56	0.29	—
MAC in O$_2$, > 65 yr (%)[a]	1.45	5.17	1.0	0.64	—
Preservative	no	no	no	Thymol	no
Stable in moist CO$_2$ absorber	no	yes	yes	no	yes
Flammability (%) (in 70% N$_2$O/30% O$_2$)	10	17	7	4.8	—
Recovered as metabolites (%)	2–5	0.02	0.2	20	—

[a] at 37 °C and 760 mmHg.

pregnancy, severe anemia, and acute intoxication. Most of these factors also modify MAC-awake and MAC-bar. In contrast, the MAC to prevent movement to a surgical stimulus can be increased by hyperthermia, acute use of amphetamines, cocaine, or ephedrine, and by chronic alcohol consumption.

MAC decreases with age in a linear fashion, described by a model. The decreases in MAC with age are similar between anesthetics, with the exception of patients less than 1 year of age, where MAC can be lower. MAC decreases approximately 6% per decade, resulting in a 22% decrease in MAC from age 40 to age 80, and a 27% decrease in MAC from age 1 to age 40 (Fig. 26.2). MAC values are typically expressed for an intermediate age of 40–45 years, and these are: isoflurane, 1.17%; sevoflurane, 1.8%; desflurane, 6.6%; and halothane, 0.75% (Table 26.1).

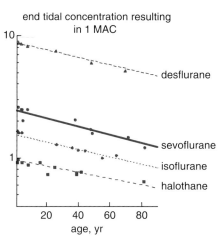

Figure 26.2. Effect of age on MAC. Regression lines are fitted to published values from separate studies. Data are from patients aged 1–80 years. Adapted from Mapleson [3].

Isoflurane

Isoflurane is a halogenated, methyl-ethyl ether that undergoes essentially no deterioration during storage for up to 5 years or on exposure to light (Fig. 26.1). It has a higher blood solubility than sevoflurane and desflurane (Table 26.1) and thus has a slower uptake and elimination, as described in Chapter 25. It maintains cardiac output and is a potent vasodilator. There were early concerns that coronary artery dilation could result in a "steal" phenomenon, where the coronary blood supply in atherosclerotic vessels is shunted to less diseased vessels from the vasodilation associated with isoflurane,

resulting in myocardial ischemia in tissue supplied by diseased vessels. Clinical use of isoflurane has not supported these concerns. A small portion of isoflurane is metabolized, and this has resulted in rare cases of immune-mediated hepatitis in sensitized individuals.

Sevoflurane

Sevoflurane is a fluorinated, methyl-isopropyl ether, with a vapor pressure slightly less than isoflurane and roughly one-fourth that of desflurane; it can be delivered in a conventional vaporizer (Fig. 26.1). Sevoflurane is less potent than isoflurane (i.e., the MAC of sevoflurane is greater than that of isoflurane), has minimal odor, no pungency, and is a potent bronchodilator. These attributes make it an excellent candidate for administration via the facemask on induction of anesthesia in both children and adults. Roughly 5% of the delivered concentration of sevoflurane is metabolized to hexafluoroisopropanol, which does not activate the immune system, and therefore immune-mediated hepatitis cannot occur. Sevoflurane can form carbon monoxide (CO) during exposure to dried carbon dioxide (CO_2) absorbents, and an exothermic reaction in dry absorbent has resulted in canister fires. Sevoflurane breaks down in the presence of CO_2 absorbers to form a vinyl halide called compound A. Compound A has been shown to be a nephrotoxin in rats at higher concentrations, but has not been associated with renal injury in controlled studies in human volunteers, patients, or renal-impaired patients. Renal injury has not been reported with clinical use.

Desflurane

Desflurane is a fluorinated, methyl-ethyl ether that differs from isoflurane by just one atom – a fluorine is substituted for a chlorine atom (Fig. 26.1). Fluorination decreases its blood and tissue solubility at the expense of potency (the MAC of desflurane is three times higher than that of sevoflurane). It also has a vapor pressure close to atmospheric pressure and must be delivered in a vaporizer modified to provide both heat and pressurization to permit a regulated concentration of desflurane as a gas. It is extremely pungent, and thus cannot be administered via the facemask in higher concentrations as it results in coughing, salivation, breath holding, and laryngospasm. Because of its pungency, when delivered in high concentrations or rapidly increasing inspired concentrations, desflurane can cause tachycardia, hypertension, and, in select cases, myocardial ischemia via activation of the sympathetic nervous system. Opioids can be used to modify this response. An extremely small portion of desflurane is metabolized, and this has been associated with a few cases of immune-mediated hepatitis in sensitized patients. In desiccated CO_2 absorbers, desflurane degrades to form CO.

Xenon

Xenon is an odorless, tasteless, inert gas that is mentioned here because of its potential to find its place in clinical practice. Similar to other noble gases, it is chemically inert and thus is not metabolized and does not harm the environment. It is difficult to obtain, limited in supply, and hence expensive. It has received considerable interest because it has many characteristics approaching those of an "ideal" inhaled anesthetic [4,5], although it can trigger malignant hyperthermia. It is nonexplosive, nonpungent, and odorless, and thus can be inhaled with ease. In addition, it does not produce significant myocardial depression [4]. Its blood/gas partition coefficient is 0.14, and unlike the other potent volatile anesthetics, xenon provides some degree of analgesia. The MAC of xenon in humans is 71%, which might prove to be a limitation. Because

of its scarcity and cost, new anesthetic systems are being developed to provide for recycling of xenon to minimize wastage when it is delivered to patients.

Halothane

Halothane has now been removed from clinical practice in most countries. It is relatively nonpungent and can be inhaled easily via facemask. It has high blood solubility, resulting in the slowest onset and offset when compared to isoflurane, sevoflurane, and desflurane as described in Chapter 25. It oxidizes spontaneously and is broken down by ultraviolet light. It is stored in amber-colored bottles with 0.01% thymol added as a preservative to prevent spontaneous oxidative decomposition (Table 26.1). It is a myocardial depressant at clinical doses, but maintains peripheral sympathetic outflow and vascular tone. It is adsorbed by contact with dry soda lime and broken down to a substance with organ toxicity in animal models. In humans, it has been associated with immune-mediated hepatitis and sensitization to epinephrine, resulting in arrhythmias. It also may cause bradycardia when used in children.

Nitrous oxide

Nitrous oxide (N_2O) was one of the first inhaled anesthetics used in the nineteenth century. It is an inorganic compound that is stable, tasteless, and odorless. At room temperature it is a gas; its boiling point is $-88.48\,^\circ C$ (Table 26.1). It is stored in cylinders and condensed to 50 atmospheres, leading to a pressure of 745 psi. This pressure is maintained in the cylinders until no liquid remains. Only cylinder weight is a reliable indicator of the volume of N_2O in storage tanks. The MAC of N_2O is 104%, and typically delivering 70% N_2O with a potent volatile anesthetic adds about 0.5 MAC to the combination. Nitrous oxide is flammable, and it should be avoided in laser surgery of the airway, as it supports combustion.

Any closed gas space in the body that contains air (i.e., nitrogen) will increase in size, pressure, or both when N_2O is administered. This is because N_2O is carried to the closed air space and diffuses from a region of high concentration outside to a region of low concentration inside the space. Nitrogen is transferred from inside to outside the space much more slowly than N_2O enters because nitrogen is much less soluble in blood and tissues (blood/gas partition coefficients at $37\,^\circ C$ of 0.46 for N_2O and 0.015 for nitrogen). The increase in volume, pressure, or both, of the air space increases with N_2O concentration and duration of exposure.

Nitrous oxide will slowly expand a closed air space in bowel obstruction. Even in patients without bowel obstruction, N_2O may delay return of normal bowel function after surgery if air is present in the bowel at the start of surgery [6]. The expansion of gas spaces in bowel by N_2O may contribute to the increased postoperative nausea and vomiting often seen after N_2O administration [7].

Untoward outcomes may arise from expansion of air spaces by N_2O, and the use of N_2O is contraindicated in these circumstances. The most rapid N_2O-induced increase in closed-air-space volume occurs with a pneumothorax. Expansion of air emboli in blood vessels by N_2O is of concern, especially air emboli in coronary vessels and in the brain. However, N_2O may be safely used in neurosurgical patients provided that it is immediately discontinued on detection of an air embolus [8]. A potential for injury also exists when N_2O increases middle ear pressure, expands intraocular gases used to treat retinal detachment, or increases pressures in air-inflated endotracheal tube cuffs to levels that cause tracheal damage [9].

Nitrous oxide is unique among the inhaled anesthetics in its ability to oxidize vitamin B_{12} and inactivate the enzyme methionine synthase, an enzyme that controls interrelations between vitamin B_{12} and folic acid metabolism. Patients given 50% N_2O for 2 hours have more than half of their hepatic methionine synthase inactivated. In almost all cases, exposure to N_2O during surgery and inactivation of methionine synthase are without clinical consequences [9]. However, severe disturbances in vitamin B_{12}/folate metabolism and marked hematologic and neurologic abnormalities may occur after N_2O exposure in individuals who abuse N_2O, in those who are critically ill, and on rare occasions in patients who have a pre-existing subclinical deficiency in vitamin B_{12}, folate, or both [9]. By disrupting vitamin B_{12} and folic acid metabolism, N_2O also increases homocysteine concentrations, and N_2O-induced increases in plasma homocysteine have been associated with increases in myocardial ischemia in patients undergoing carotid endarterectomy [10].

Delivery systems for potent inhaled anesthetics

The potent inhaled anesthetics are liquids at room temperature and atmospheric pressure. Vaporizers are closed containers where the conversion of a liquid to a vapor (vaporization) is accomplished (Fig. 26.3). Vaporization in the closed confines of a vaporizer stops when equilibrium is reached between liquid and vapor. The vapor pressure that results from molecules in the vapor phase colliding with each other and the walls of the container is unique for each of the volatile anesthetics. Thus, vaporizers are agent-specific. They are described as variable-bypass, flow-over, temperature-compensated, out-of-circuit vaporizers. Temperature compensation must be incorporated because, as an anesthetic moves from the liquid to the vapor phase, cooling occurs from the loss of heat necessary to provide energy for vaporization. The variable bypass nature of the vaporizer describes the splitting of the total fresh gas flow either into or bypassing the vaporizing chamber, the percentage of each controlled by the concentration control dial. The split portions of the fresh gas flow ultimately mix at the patient-outlet side of the vaporizer. Vaporizer output is accurate until very low fresh-gas flow rates, typically less

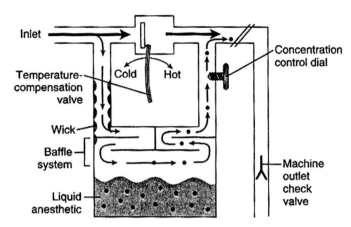

Figure 26.3. Schematic of the Tec 4 vaporizer, with temperature and pressure compensation systems. Reproduced with permission from Cole [11].

than 250 mL per minute. At these low flows, vaporizer output will fall below the dialed concentration. Desflurane requires a specially designed vaporizer because it has a vapor pressure of nearly 1 atmosphere at sea level (Fig. 26.4). At room temperature, the conventional variable-bypass vaporizer would not provide a stable and predictable concentration of desflurane. The vaporizer therefore is heated to produce gas at a pressure of approximately 2 atmospheres. When the anesthesiologist dials an increased concentration, there is a decrease in the resistance to flow of the gaseous desflurane, allowing more to be delivered to the patient. A differential pressure transducer is involved to restore the pressure in the system as desflurane is administered.

Beneficial effects of potent volatile anesthetics

Potent volatile anesthetics establish an anesthetic state of sedation and hypnosis sufficient to conduct surgical procedures. They have several beneficial effects that are extremely relevant in certain populations. For example, the patient with reactive airway disease benefits from the relaxation of bronchial smooth muscle consistently afforded by sevoflurane and halothane. The relaxation of vascular smooth muscle from volatile anesthetics benefits patients with pulmonary and systemic hypertension. Volatile anesthetics provide organ protection from ischemic injury and they favorably inhibit memory and recall.

Memory and amnesia

Low concentrations of anesthetics, typically around the MAC-awake concentration, block memory. Amnesia is less consistently produced at this concentration but more consistently achieved with a potent volatile anesthetic than with intravenous anesthetics. End-tidal gas concentrations at about 0.7 MAC may decrease the likelihood of awareness

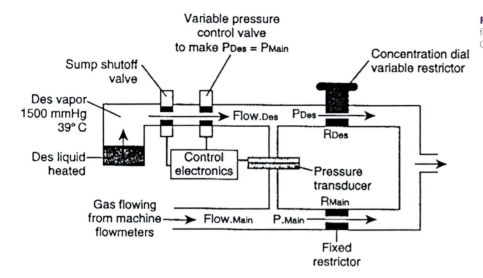

Figure 26.4. Schematic of the Tec 6 vaporizer used for desflurane. Reproduced with permission from Cole [12].

[13,14]. This effect helps achieve one of the two major goals of anesthesia: the loss of recall and the loss of movement. Nonetheless, due to variable patient sensitivities to anesthetics and the lack of 100% reliable monitors of anesthetic depth, explicit recall of intraoperative events still can occur. Anesthesia awareness can be a devastating event leading to anxiety and post-traumatic stress disorders. In a large US trial, awareness occurred at a rate of 1–2 per 1000 patients and was associated with increased ASA physical status, but was not associated with gender and age [15].

Anesthetic-mediated organ protection from ischemic injury

It is known that brief coronary occlusion to produce ischemic stress initiates a signaling cascade of intracellular events that offers 2–3 hours of protection from subsequent stress of ischemia and reperfusion. The volatile anesthetics mimic ischemic preconditioning and trigger a similar cascade of intracellular events, resulting in organ protection that lasts beyond the elimination of the anesthetic. Such protection has been reported in cardiac, neural, renal, and hepatic tissue and is discussed later in the chapter.

Adverse effects of potent volatile anesthetics

Malignant hyperthermia

Malignant hyperthermia (MH) is a clinical syndrome of acute, uncontrolled, increased skeletal muscle metabolism resulting in heightened oxygen consumption, lactate formation, heat production, and rhabdomyolysis. The hallmark findings of MH are a rapidly rising temperature, increasing by up to 1 °C every 5 minutes, increasing end-tidal CO_2, arrhythmias,

and skeletal muscle rigidity. The incidence in adults is as high as 1 in 50 000, and in children as high as 1 in 3000. MH susceptibility is inherited and is transmitted as an autosomal dominant genetic disorder with reduced penetrance and variable expression. While N_2O is considered safe in MH-susceptible patients, all of the potent volatile anesthetics serve as triggers for MH in genetically susceptible individuals [16,17]. The standard test to determine susceptibility is the caffeine-contracture test, applied to skeletal muscle biopsies. A standard muscle contraction with caffeine is not augmented by N_2O, but is augmented 3- to 11-fold with volatile anesthetics [18]. Desflurane has been associated with an unusual delayed onset of symptoms of MH in animals and humans hours after the exposure to the anesthetic gas [17,19].

Fluoride-induced nephrotoxicity

In 1971, it was determined that metabolism (biotransformation) of the volatile anesthetic methoxyflurane explained a well-described injury to renal collecting tubules [20]. This nephrotoxicity presented as a high-output renal insufficiency that was unresponsive to vasopressin and characterized by dilute polyuria, dehydration, serum hypernatremia, hyperosmolality, and an elevated blood urea nitrogen (BUN) and creatinine. An association between increased plasma fluoride concentrations and metabolism of methoxyflurane led to a "fluoride hypothesis" [21], which suggested that the nephrotoxicity was caused by metabolism of methoxyflurane to free inorganic fluoride causing renal injury. Isoflurane and desflurane are minimally metabolized, and thus fluoride-related injury should be less likely. Sevoflurane undergoes 5% metabolism, resulting in transient increases in serum fluoride concentrations, but renal concentrating defects have not been detected [22]. The lack of injury had been attributed to a short duration of the high systemic fluoride concentrations (area under the fluoride–time curve)

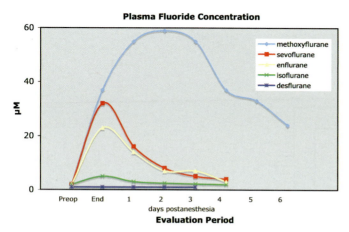

Figure 26.5. Plasma inorganic fluoride concentrations (mean ± SEM) before and after 2–4 hours of methoxyflurane, enflurane, sevoflurane, isoflurane, and desflurane anesthesia. Adapted from Njoku *et al.* [24].

and not the peak fluoride concentration (peaks above 50 μM – the toxic threshold) (Fig. 26.5) [23].

It is now known that the site of anesthetic metabolism is an important factor in toxicity, i.e., intrarenal metabolism contributes to nephrotoxicity. The renal metabolism of methoxyflurane is significantly greater than that of sevoflurane due to the multiple cytochrome P450 enzymes in the kidney responsible for metabolism of methoxyflurane (CYP2A6, CYP3A, CYP2E1) [25]. In contrast, sevoflurane is primarily metabolized by a single cytochrome, CYP2E1. Minimal intrarenal fluoride generation from sevoflurane metabolism may account for the low toxic potential. Thus, potential renal toxicity from high plasma fluoride levels following long cases and long exposures to sevoflurane are offset by the minimal amount of renal defluorination.

Other factors such as liver enzyme induction and obesity have been proven to enhance metabolism of anesthetics. The activity of hepatic cytochrome P450 enzymes is increased by a variety of drugs, including phenobarbital, phenytoin, and isoniazid [26,27]. Obesity has been shown to increase metabolism (defluorination) of isoflurane [28], but not of sevoflurane [29].

Hepatic injury

Unlike most intravenous anesthetic drugs, modern-day volatile anesthetics undergo minimal liver metabolism. Inhaled anesthetics are excreted primarily via the lungs; thus it is not surprising that today's volatile anesthetics minimally affect hepatic function. The various factors that are known to affect drug metabolism, such as age, disease, genetics, and enzyme-inducing agents, have minor effects on the excretion of the volatile anesthetics.

Nonetheless, postoperative liver dysfunction, to varying degrees, has been associated with all of the volatile anesthetics in current use [30]. Altered liver function tests have been used as an index of hepatic injury during anesthesia. The absence of changes in plasma alanine aminotransferase after sevoflurane, desflurane, or isoflurane use has been noted,

but they may not be sensitive to hepatic injury and are not uniquely specific to the liver [31,32]. Most cases of hepatic injury demonstrate lesions in the centrilobular area of the liver and, not coincidentally, this area is most susceptible to hypoxia. Therefore, a more sensitive measure of injury may be α-glutathione-S-transferase (GST), since it is distributed primarily in the centrilobular hepatocytes. In patient studies, isoflurane did not increase GST [33]. In elderly patients with no pre-existing liver disease having peripheral surgery under sevoflurane or desflurane, a brief impairment of splanchnic blood flow has been demonstrated leading to increases in GST that resolve in 24 hours [34].

There are two distinct mechanisms by which anesthetics have caused liver injury, often termed "hepatitis." One is more common and related to hepatocyte toxicity. It is relatively mild, does not require a previous exposure, and has a low morbidity. The second is associated with repeat exposure and probably represents an immune reaction to oxidatively derived metabolites of anesthetics. It has been associated with severe liver damage and fulminant hepatic failure.

Hypoxic injury to hepatocytes can be a significant contributor to postoperative hepatic injury. The liver has two blood supplies: the well-oxygenated blood from the hepatic artery and the poorly oxygenated blood from the portal vein. A beneficial attribute of the ether-based anesthetics (isoflurane, sevoflurane, and desflurane) is their ability to maintain or increase hepatic artery blood flow while decreasing (or not changing) portal vein blood flow [31,35]. In contrast, halothane causes selective hepatic artery vasoconstriction and therefore does not compensate for decreased portal vein flow [36].

Situations that decrease hepatic blood flow or increase hepatic oxygen demand make patients vulnerable to the unwanted effects of halothane. For example, surgery in the abdominal cavity, especially in the area of the liver, which might compromise hepatic blood flow, puts patients at additional risk for hepatic cell injury. Hepatic enzyme induction, which increases oxygen demand, may enhance the vulnerability of patients to the effects of volatile anesthetics. Furthermore, patients who are critically dependent upon oxygen supply for survival of remaining liver tissue, such as the cirrhotic patient, are at a higher risk for further hepatic injury during halothane anesthesia. Whether this injury can simply be explained by a direct effect of halothane during hypoxic conditions, or attributed to reductive metabolism of halothane that is enhanced under hypoxic conditions, is not entirely clear [37].

Postoperative liver dysfunction also can occur from an immune mechanism. Immune-mediated hepatitis has been associated with most of the volatile anesthetics in current use, with the exception of sevoflurane. There are many causes of postoperative jaundice and abnormal liver function tests, including viral hepatitis, coexisting liver disease (such as Gilbert's disease), blood transfusions, septicemia, drug

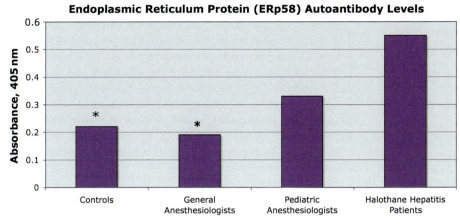

Figure 26.6. Endoplasmic reticulum protein (ERp58) autoantibody levels expressed as absorbance at 405 nm for controls ($n = 20$), general anesthesiologists ($n = 52$), pediatric anesthesiologists ($n = 105$), and halothane hepatitis patients ($n = 20$). Bars represent the median; * = statistically different from the pediatric anesthesiologist group and the halothane hepatitis patient group; $p < 0.05$. Adapted from Njoku *et al.* [51].

reactions, intra- and postoperative hypoxia and hypotension, and direct tissue trauma as a result of the surgical procedure [37]. The diagnosis of immune-mediated hepatitis is generally made based on "incomplete exclusion," defined as the appearance of liver damage within 28 days of anesthetic exposure in a person in whom other known causes of liver disease have been excluded. It is now known that oxidative metabolism of halothane, isoflurane, and desflurane, catalyzed by hepatic CYP2E1, produces a reactive intermediate, trifluoroacetic acid (TFA), which can covalently modify liver microsomal proteins. This complex can produce an immune response in some individuals that is characterized by immunoglobulin G (IgG) antibodies. A repeat exposure to an anesthetic in a sensitized individual can lead to hepatic necrosis.

Immune hypersensitivity responses are manifested by eosinophilia, fever, rash, arthralgia, and prior exposure to halothane, isoflurane, and desflurane. The possibility of a genetic susceptibility factor is suggested by case reports of immune-mediated hepatitis in closely related patients [38]. The most compelling evidence for an immune-mediated mechanism of hepatitis is the presence of circulating IgG antibodies in up to 70% of patients with the diagnosis of anesthetic-mediated hepatitis [37,39]. This antibody is not directed against the reductive metabolite of the anesthetic, but against an oxidative compound, TFA halide, which is incorporated onto the surface of the hepatocyte [40,41]. TFA proteins have been identified from the livers of rats after halothane exposure with enzyme-linked immunosorbent assays and immunoblotting techniques. These altered proteins can be seen by the immune system as non-self (neoantigens), leading to the production of antibodies. The proteins can be identified from serum samples of humans exposed to volatile anesthetics [42].

Isoflurane and desflurane are metabolized by CYP2E1 in the same manner as halothane. The expression of the neoantigens following anesthetic exposure is halothane > isoflurane > desflurane, reflecting the amount of metabolism of each of these agents [24]. Case reports have appeared in the literature linking each of these anesthetics with immune-mediated hepatitis [43–45]. If the incidence of fulminant hepatic failure after halothane is 1 in 35 000 [46], hepatic failure caused by isoflurane may be on the order of 1 in 3 500 000. Desflurane is the least metabolized of the volatile anesthetics, resulting in very small amounts of adduct, and only a few cases of hepatotoxicity from desflurane have been reported [43,47,48]. There are no reports of fulminant hepatic necrosis associated with sevoflurane in humans. Sevoflurane is not metabolized to a TFA halide; rather it is metabolized to the non-neoantigenic compound hexafluoroisopropanol [30].

Immunologic memory resulting in hepatitis has been reported 28 years after an initial halothane exposure [49]. In addition, cross-sensitivity has been reported, in which exposure to one anesthetic can sensitize a patient to a second but different anesthetic [43,50]. Autoantibodies have also been identified in 10% of healthcare workers (postanesthesia care unit nurses, nurse anesthetists, and anesthesiologists) chronically exposed to low levels of anesthetics (Fig. 26.6) [51]. This finding is intriguing, if not alarming. The newer volatile anesthetics have an extremely low potential for hepatotoxicity. The possibility of avoiding sensitization of individuals to minimize the risk of fulminant hepatic failure from a volatile anesthetic is sufficiently compelling to discourage use of the older, more metabolized anesthetics, including halothane and possibly isoflurane.

Thus, in terms of hepatocyte hypoxia, the modern volatile anesthetics have minimal adverse effects, but some have the potential to cause immune-mediated hepatitis. Volatile anesthetics might even afford protection from ischemic/hypoxic injury to cells, discussed later in the chapter.

Renal injury

Sevoflurane undergoes base catalyzed degradation in CO_2 absorbents to form a vinyl ether called compound A. The generation of compound A is augmented in low-flow or

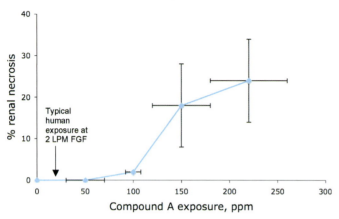

Figure 26.7. Biopsy evidence for renal cell necrosis in rat models following 3-hour exposure to (breathing of) compound A. The threshold of compound A exposure appears to be around 100 parts per million (ppm). Typical human exposure when breathing 1 MAC sevoflurane in less than 2 liters per minute (LPM) fresh gas flow (FGF) is roughly 20–30 ppm per hour, which is well below the threshold exposure to compound A in rats that causes renal cell necrosis. Adapted from Kharasch *et al.* [56].

closed-circuit breathing systems and by warm or very dry (desiccated) CO_2 absorbents [52,53]. Barium hydroxide lime produces more compound A than soda lime, and this can be attributed to slightly higher absorbent temperature during CO_2 extraction [54]. Desiccated barium hydroxide lime also has been implicated in the heat and fires associated with sevoflurane, discussed later. This absorbent has been removed from the US and European markets.

When compound A has been inhaled by rats, a threshold for renal tubular necrosis has been noted at 100 parts per million (ppm) exposure over a 3-hour period ($\sim$ 300 ppm · h) (Fig. 26.7) [56–57]. The injury appears as cell necrosis of the cortical medullary tubules in the proximal tubules [57,58]. The associated biochemical markers include increases in serum creatinine and BUN, glucosuria, and proteinuria [56,58]. In addition, increases in several enzymes derived from renal tubule cells have been noted, including urinary excretion of N-acetyl-β-D-glucosaminidase (NAG) and GST [56,58].

Renal toxicity from compound A varies by species, with the threshold greater than 612 ppm · h in pigs [59], and between 600 and 800 ppm · h in monkeys [60]. These thresholds are far above typical human exposure to compound A (Fig. 26.7). For example, in humans receiving sevoflurane in closed-circuit or low-flow delivery systems, inspired compound A concentrations averaged 8–24 ppm [61–63]. Total exposures as high as 320–400 ppm · h have had no clear effect on clinical markers of renal function [64,65]. In prospective randomized human studies, no adverse renal effects from low-flow (0.5–1.0 L min^{-1}) or closed-circuit sevoflurane anesthesia were observed based on serum creatinine and BUN concentrations, and absence of proteinuria, glucosuria, and enzymuria [62,63,66–69]. In a defining, multicenter, prospective study where patients with pre-existing renal disease were enrolled in a study designed to maximize compound A exposures, no adverse renal effects based on standard and

biochemical markers of renal injury were found [70]. The study randomized patients to sevoflurane or isoflurane, employed 1 liter per minute fresh gas flows in cases greater than 2 hours, used barium hydroxide absorbent, and employed minimal anesthetic adjuvants to maximize the dose of volatile anesthetic (and the production of compound A in the sevoflurane group). Both isoflurane and sevoflurane resulted in minor alterations in renal markers of injury, and this was consistent with other findings of nonspecific, transient proteinuria, glucosuria, and enzymuria noted after desflurane and propofol anesthesia. Desflurane and propofol do not generate compound A, making it unlikely that elevated markers of renal injury are due to sevoflurane degradation. Importantly, most countries have no gas-flow restrictions on the use of sevoflurane, and, despite an anesthesia community sensitized to potential renal concerns with sevoflurane, there has not been a single case report of renal injury after nearly 15 years of sevoflurane use in millions of patients.

One explanation for the inconsistency between the early rat studies and human studies in terms of renal injury from compound A may be related to species differences in the metabolism of compound A. The biodegradation of compound A to cysteine conjugates and the further action of a renal enzyme called β-lyase on the conjugates can result in formation of a potentially toxic thiol [55,71,72]. The cysteine conjugates can be handled in one (or both) of two ways. They can be acetylated to mercapturic acid through a detoxification pathway, which results in no organ toxicity, or acted upon by renal β-lyase to form reactive intermediates (toxification pathway) [73]. These reactive intermediates are responsible for the renal cell necrosis seen in rats. The β-lyase-dependent metabolism pathway in humans is far less extensive than the β-lyase pathway in rats (8–30 times less active) [74]. Thus, compared with rats, humans (1) receive markedly lower doses of compound A, (2) metabolize a lower fraction of compound A via the renal β-lyase pathway, and (3) have not suffered renal injury.

Hydrogen fluoride toxicity

Generic formulations of sevoflurane were introduced into the clinical market in 2006. The methods for synthesizing sevoflurane differ between manufacturers [75]. Although the active ingredient of sevoflurane from different manufacturers is chemically equivalent, the water content in the formulations differs, and this accounts for their different resistance to degradation to hydrogen fluoride when exposed to a Lewis acid (metal halides and metal oxides that are present in modern vaporizers). Adding water to the formulation inhibits the action of Lewis acids to degrade sevoflurane to hydrogen fluoride. Abbott Laboratories' formulation was changed to contain 300–400 ppm of water, based upon an early adverse experience with hydrogen fluoride formation from a low-water formulation in 1996. The generic formulation marketed by Baxter Laboratories is low in water ($\sim$ 65 ppm) and has been shown in clinical and laboratory studies to degrade to toxic and corrosive hydrogen fluoride [76]. Recent reports indicate that the Penlon Sigma Delta sevoflurane vaporizer can degrade the Baxter low-water formulation of sevoflurane resulting in etching of the site glass, corrosion of the plastic on the vaporizer, and discoloration of the anesthetic [77]. Whether these differences in formulation lead to patient safety issues remains to be determined [75,78].

Minimizing injurious effects from anesthetic degradation

Most CO_2 absorbents are strong bases and contain 13–15% water. When CO_2 absorbents become "dry" or desiccated such that the water content falls below 5%, degradation of volatile anesthetics can occur (Figs. 26.8, 26.9) [79–82]. The degradation is the result of an exothermic reaction of the anesthetics with the absorbent. The formation of carbon monoxide (CO) is related to both the anesthetic molecular structure and the presence of a strong base in the CO_2 absorbent [81]. Desflurane given through a desiccated absorbent at room temperature at just under 1 MAC can produce up to 8000 ppm of CO. This is 100 times more CO than produced under similar conditions with 2 MAC sevoflurane [82]. CO production from desflurane was nearly three times higher in desiccated barium hydroxide absorbent than in soda lime. Although desflurane produces the most CO with desiccated CO_2 absorbers, the reaction with sevoflurane produces the most heat [83]. The strong exothermic reaction has caused significant heat production, fires, and patient injuries [84–86]. Although sevoflurane is not flammable at less than 11%, formaldehyde, methanol, and formate have been identified [87], and these alone or in combination with oxygen might be flammable at high canister temperatures. In experimental settings, long exposure of 1 MAC sevoflurane to desiccated barium hydroxide resulted in canister temperatures in excess of 300 °C, which can be associated with smoldering, melting of plastic components, explosions, and fires [80]. Barium hydroxide has been removed from the US and European market.

There are newer CO_2 absorbents that do not degrade anesthetics (to either compound A or CO), and they should reduce exothermic reactions. "From a patient safety perspective, widespread adoption of a nondestructive CO_2 absorbent seems logical and would be consistent with the patient safety goals of our anesthesia society" [88]. It should be noted that the cost of these new CO_2 absorbents (Amsorb Plus and DrägerSorb Free) is higher and their absorptive capacity may be lower than that of soda lime. Nonetheless, the use of a nondestructive absorbent eliminates all of the potential complications related to anesthetic breakdown and therefore minimizes the possibility of additional costs due to any, albeit rare, complications.

Cerebral injury

Although neuroprotection from volatile anesthetics is a well-defined concept, the volatile anesthetics can cause injury in certain conditions via cerebral vasodilation and increases in

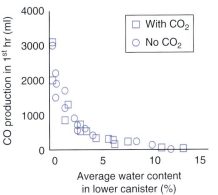

Figure 26.8. Production of carbon monoxide (CO) in the first hour resulting from desflurane breakdown in barium hydroxide lime at the specified water content. CO_2, carbon dioxide. Reproduced with permission from Woehlck *et al.* [79].

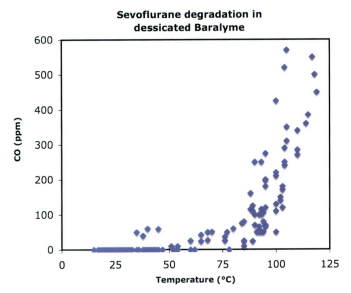

Figure 26.9. The effects of canister temperature on carbon monoxide generation during administration of sevoflurane at 2.1% through desiccated barium hydroxide lime. Reproduced with permission from Holak *et al.* [80].

intracranial pressure. A full understanding of the anesthetic effects on cerebral physiology helps prevent adverse cerebral events in clinical practice. The modern potent anesthetics, isoflurane, desflurane, and sevoflurane, all have reasonably similar effects on a wide range of parameters including cerebral metabolic rate (CMR), the electroencephalogram (EEG), cerebral blood flow (CBF), and flow–metabolism coupling. There are notable differences in effects on intracerebral pressure (ICP), cerebrospinal fluid production and resorption, CO_2 vasoreactivity, CBF autoregulation, and cerebral protection.

Cerebral metabolic rate (CMR) and EEG

All of the potent agents depress CMR to varying degrees and in a nonlinear fashion. In isoflurane-anesthetized dogs, there is a sudden decrease in $CMRO_2$ paralleling a change in the EEG from an awake to an anesthetized pattern at about 0.4–0.6 MAC [89]. For most of the potent agents, CMR is decreased only to the extent that spontaneous cortical neuronal activity (as reflected on the EEG) is decreased. Once this activity is absent (an isoelectric EEG), no further decreases in CMR are generated. (Historically, halothane was the exception. Halothane produced an isoelectric EEG at ~ 4 MAC while higher concentrations caused further decreases in $CMRO_2$.)

Isoflurane causes a larger MAC-dependent depression of CMR than halothane, and because of this greater depression in CMR it can abolish EEG activity at clinical doses that usually can be tolerated from a hemodynamic standpoint [90]. Desflurane and sevoflurane both cause decreases in CMR similar to isoflurane [91,92].

Potential for direct cerebral toxicity has been studied for sevoflurane, and compared to halothane. At normal CO_2 and blood pressure, no evidence of sevoflurane toxicity exists [93]. During sevoflurane use with extreme hyperventilation to decrease cerebral blood flow by half, brain lactate levels increase, but significantly less than with halothane. There are conflicting data as to whether sevoflurane has a proconvulsant effect [91,94,95]. High, long-lasting concentrations of sevoflurane (1.5–2.0 MAC), a sudden increase in cerebral sevoflurane concentrations, and hypocapnia can trigger EEG abnormalities that often are associated with increases in heart rate in both adults and children [96,97]. This has raised the question as to the appropriateness of sevoflurane in patients with epilepsy [98].

Cerebral blood flow (CBF), flow–metabolism coupling, and autoregulation

All of the potent volatile anesthetics increase CBF in a dose-dependent manner. Isoflurane, sevoflurane, and desflurane cause far less cerebral vasodilation than halothane at equi-MAC comparisons (Fig. 26.10). Because of this, in the past several decades halothane has been used rarely in neurosurgery. In human studies, isoflurane, sevoflurane, and desflurane, in clinically relevant doses under 1.5 MAC, produce nonsignificant changes in CBF [91,92,100,101]. The increases in CBF upon initial exposure to a volatile anesthetic can recover in several hours, despite continued exposure to the anesthetic. The mechanism of this recovery is unclear.

Increases in CBF from high concentrations of volatile anesthetics occur despite decreases in CMR. This phenomenon has been called "uncoupling," but true uncoupling of flow from metabolism may not occur. That is, as CMR is depressed by the volatile anesthetics, there still is a coupled decline in CBF opposed by a coincident direct vasodilatory effect on the cerebral blood vessels. The net effect on the cerebral vessels depends on the sum of indirect vasoconstricting and direct vasodilating influences.

Autoregulation is the intrinsic myogenic regulation of vascular tone that maintains constant organ blood flow over a range of blood pressures. Volatile anesthetics are direct vasodilators that diminish autoregulation in a dose-dependent fashion, such that at high anesthetic doses CBF is essentially

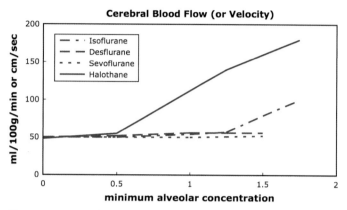

Figure 26.10. Cerebral blood flow (or velocity) measured in the presence of normocapnia and in the absence of surgical stimulation in volunteers receiving halothane or isoflurane. At light levels of anesthesia, halothane (but not isoflurane) increased cerebral blood flow. At 1.6 MAC, isoflurane also increased cerebral blood flow. Cerebral blood flow measured before and during sevoflurane and desflurane anesthesia up to 1.5 MAC showed no change. Adapted from Eger [99] and Bedforth et al. [101].

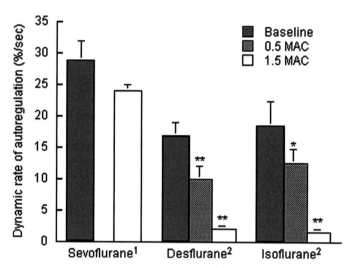

Figure 26.11. Dynamic rate of autoregulation (dRoR) during awake (or fentanyl and N_2O baseline), 0.5, and 1.5 minimum alveolar anesthetic concentration (MAC) anesthesia. Values are mean ± SE (SD for sevoflurane). * $p < 0.05$ versus baseline; ** $p < 0.001$ versus baseline and sevoflurane. Adapted from Summors et al. [102] and Strebel et al. [103].

pressure-passive. Sevoflurane preserves autoregulation up to approximately 1 MAC [91]. At 1.5 MAC, the dynamic rate of autoregulation is better preserved with sevoflurane than with isoflurane (Fig. 26.11). This may be the result of the less direct vasodilatory effect of sevoflurane, preserving the ability of the vessel to respond to changes in blood pressure at 1.5 MAC. In a separate study of dynamic autoregulation of CBF, 0.5 MAC desflurane reduced autoregulation and isoflurane did not. At 1.5 MAC, both anesthetics substantially reduced autoregulation (Fig. 26.11).

Intracerebral pressure (ICP)

For most anesthesiologists the area of greatest clinical interest is the effect of volatile anesthesia on ICP. In general, ICP will increase or decrease in proportion to changes in CBF. For perspective, halothane increases ICP to the greatest extent, reflecting its more profound effects on CBF than the other potent agents. In fact, brain protrusion during craniotomy is greater with halothane than isoflurane, consistent with the greater increase in ICP by halothane [104]. In human studies there are usually mild increases in ICP with isoflurane administration that are blocked or blunted by hyperventilation or barbiturate coadministration [105]. Like isoflurane, both sevoflurane and desflurane above 1 MAC produce mild increases in ICP, paralleling their mild increases in CBF [91,92,106,107]. One potential advantage of sevoflurane is that its lower pungency and airway irritation may lessen the risk of coughing and bucking and the associated rise in ICP as compared to desflurane or isoflurane. In fact, introduction of desflurane after propofol induction of anesthesia has led to significant increases in heart rate, mean arterial pressure, and middle cerebral artery blood flow velocity that were not noted in patients given sevoflurane [101]. This may relate to the airway irritant effects of desflurane rather than a specific alteration in neurophysiology. Several studies in both children and adults suggest that increases in ICP from desflurane are slightly greater than from either isoflurane or sevoflurane [108,109].

Cerebrospinal fluid (CSF) production and resorption

Isoflurane does not appear to alter CSF production [110], but may increase, decrease, or leave unchanged the resistance to resorption depending on dose. Sevoflurane at 1 MAC depresses CSF production up to 40% [111]. Desflurane at 1 MAC leaves CSF production unchanged or increased [108,112]. In general, anesthetic effects on ICP via changes in CSF dynamics are clinically far less important than anesthetic effects on CBF.

Cerebral blood flow response to hyper- and hypocapnia

Significant hypercapnia is associated with dramatic increases in CBF with or without volatile anesthetics. As discussed earlier, hypocapnia can blunt or abolish volatile anesthetic-induced increases in CBF depending on when the hypocapnia is produced. This vasoreactivity to CO_2 may be altered by the volatile anesthetics as compared to normal conditions. Isoflurane does not abolish hypocapnic vasoconstriction [113]. CO_2 vasoreactivity under desflurane anesthesia is normal up to 1.5 MAC [114], and CO_2 vasoreactivity for sevoflurane is preserved at 1 MAC [115].

Adverse pulmonary effects

All volatile anesthetics decrease tidal volume and increase respiratory rate such that there are only minor effects on decreasing minute ventilation. The ventilatory effects are dose-dependent, with higher concentrations of volatile anesthetics resulting in greater decreases in tidal volume and greater increases in respiratory rate, with the exception of isoflurane, which does not increase respiratory rate above 1 MAC. The net effect of a gradual decrease in minute ventilation has been associated with increasing resting P_aCO_2. The relative increases in P_aCO_2 as an index of respiratory depression with volatile anesthetics evaluated at less than 1.24 MAC are as follows: desflurane = isoflurane > sevoflurane > N_2O. The respiratory depression can be partially antagonized during surgical stimulation, where respiratory rate and tidal volume have been shown to increase, resulting in a decrease in the P_aCO_2. N_2O increases respiratory rate as much or more than the inhaled anesthetics. When N_2O is added to sevoflurane or desflurane, resting P_aCO_2 decreases relative to equi-MAC concentrations of sevoflurane or desflurane in O_2.

All of the inhaled anesthetics produce a dose-dependent depression of the ventilatory response to hypercapnia (Fig. 26.12). The threshold where respiratory drive ceases is called the apneic threshold. It is generally 4–5 mmHg below the prevailing resting P_aCO_2 in a spontaneously breathing patient. It is unrelated to the slope of the CO_2 response curves or to the level of the resting P_aCO_2. The clinical relevance of this threshold may be realized when

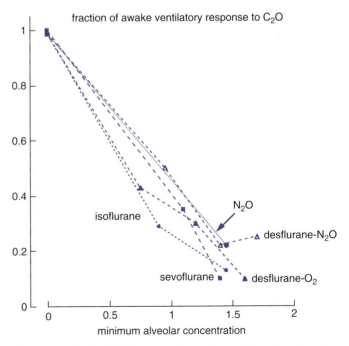

Figure 26.12. All inhaled anesthetics produce similar dose-dependent decreases in the ventilatory response to carbon dioxide. Adapted from Eger [116] and Doi and Ikeda [117].

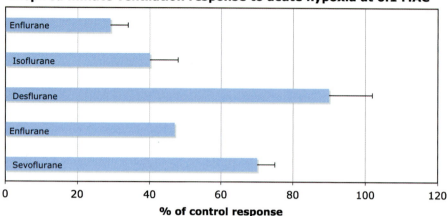

Inspired minute ventilation response to acute hypoxia at 0.1 MAC

Figure 26.13. The ventilatory responses to a decrease in end-tidal oxygen concentration during 0.1 MAC of five volatile anesthetic agents. Sevoflurane and desflurane preserved the ventilatory response better than isoflurane, enflurane, and halothane. Data are expressed as a percent of the control response (no anesthetic) to acute hypoxia; values are mean ± SD. Reproduced with permission from Sarton *et al.* [120].

assisting ventilation in an anesthetized patient who is breathing spontaneously. This only serves to lower the P_aCO_2 to approach that of the apneic threshold, therefore mandating more control of ventilation.

Inhaled anesthetics, including N_2O, also produce a dose-dependent attenuation of the ventilatory response to hypoxia [118,119]. This action appears to be dependent on the peripheral chemoreceptors. Even subanesthetic concentrations of volatile anesthetics (0.1 MAC) elicit anywhere from a 15% to a 75% depression of the ventilatory drive to hypoxia (Fig. 26.13) [121]. The mechanism of this depression still remains poorly understood. The extreme sensitivity of the hypoxic ventilation response to volatile anesthetics has important clinical implications. Residual effects of volatile anesthetics may impair the ventilatory drive of patients in the recovery room. In this regard, the short-acting anesthetics (sevoflurane and desflurane) may prove advantageous in patients who rely on hypoxic drive to set their level of ventilation, such as those in chronic respiratory failure or patients with obstructive sleep apnea.

Bronchoconstriction

Bronchoconstriction under anesthesia occurs because of direct stimulation of the laryngeal and tracheal areas, from the administration of adjuvant drugs that cause histamine release, and from noxious stimuli activating vagal afferent nerves. The reflex response to these stimuli may be enhanced in lightly anesthetized patients [122]. The responses are also enhanced in patients with known reactive airway disease, including those requiring bronchodilator therapy or those with chronic smoking histories. Airway smooth muscle extends as far distally as the terminal bronchioles and is under the influence of both parasympathetic and sympathetic nerves. The parasympathetic nerves mediate baseline airway tone and reflex bronchoconstriction via M_2 and M_3 muscarinic receptors on the airway smooth muscle, which initiate

increases in intracellular cyclic guanosine monophosphate (cGMP). Adrenoceptors also are located on bronchial smooth muscle, and the β_2-receptor subtype plays the predominant role in promoting bronchiolar muscle relaxation through an increase in intracellular cyclic adenosine monophosphate (cAMP). The volatile anesthetics relax airway smooth muscle directly by depressing smooth muscle contractility and indirectly by inhibiting the reflex neural pathways [123]. Direct effects of the volatile anesthetics partially depend on an intact bronchial epithelium, suggesting that epithelial damage or inflammation secondary to asthma may lessen their bronchodilating effect. The volatile anesthetics also may have protective effects by acting on the bronchial epithelium via a nonadrenergic, noncholinergic mechanism, possibly involving the nitric oxide pathway [124]. A study comparing patients receiving isoflurane, halothane, and sevoflurane to a control group receiving thiopental indicated that sevoflurane may have a more rapid onset of bronchodilation than isoflurane or halothane [125]. Desflurane administration shortly after thiopental induction and tracheal intubation results in a transient increase in respiratory system resistance (bronchoconstriction), and this has been attributed to a direct effect of the pungency and airway irritability of desflurane (Fig. 26.14). This effect is worsened in patients with an active smoking history [126]. Volatile anesthetics have been used effectively to treat status asthmaticus when other conventional treatments have failed [127]. Although halothane has been historically used in these situations, sevoflurane may be a better choice because of its quick onset, lack of pungency, lack of cardiovascular depression, and lower risk of cardiac arrhythmias compared to halothane.

Mucociliary function

Ciliated respiratory epithelium extends from the trachea to the terminal bronchioles. Cells and glands in the tracheobronchial tree secrete mucus that captures surface particles for transport

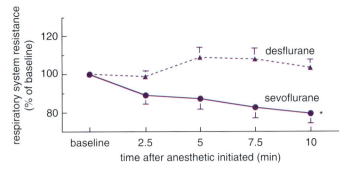

Figure 26.14. Changes in respiratory system resistance upon administering sevoflurane or desflurane to the inspired gas after intubation. Data are expressed as a percentage of the thiopental baseline recorded after tracheal intubation but prior to the administration of sevoflurane or desflurane. Airway resistance responses to sevoflurane were significantly less than to desflurane. * $p < 0.05$. Adapted from Goff et al. [126].

via ciliary action. There are a number of factors involved in diminished mucociliary function, particularly in the mechanically ventilated patient where dried, inspired gases impair ciliary movement, thicken the protective mucus, and reduce the ability of mucociliary function to transport surface particles out of the airway. Volatile anesthetics and N_2O reduce ciliary movement and alter the characteristics of mucus [128,129]. Smokers have impaired mucociliary function, and the combination of a volatile anesthetic in a smoker who is mechanically ventilated sets up a scenario for inadequate clearing of secretions, mucus plugging, atelectasis, and hypoxemia.

Pulmonary hypertension and hypoxic vasoconstriction

Although systemic vascular smooth muscle is notably affected by the volatile anesthetics, the pulmonary vascular relaxation from clinically relevant concentrations of inhaled anesthetics is minimal. The small amount of pulmonary vasodilation from volatile anesthetics is offset by anesthetic-related decreases in cardiac output, resulting in little or no change in pulmonary artery pressures and pulmonary blood flow. Even N_2O, which has little effect on cardiac output and pulmonary blood flow, has at most a small effect to increase pulmonary vascular resistance. However, pulmonary vascular constriction from N_2O may be magnified in patients with resting pulmonary hypertension [130].

Perhaps more important in terms of the effect of volatile anesthetics on pulmonary blood flow is their potential to attenuate hypoxic pulmonary vasoconstriction (HPV). During periods of hypoxemia, HPV reduces blood flow to underventilated areas of the lung, thereby diverting blood flow to areas of the lung with greater ventilation. The net effect is to improve V/Q matching, resulting in a reduced amount of venous admixture and improved arterial oxygenation. In animal models, high concentrations of all the modern inhaled anesthetics have been shown to attenuate HPV [131,132]; the situation is less clear in patient studies. This may reflect the multifactorial effects of the volatile anesthetics on the

physiologic parameters involved in pulmonary blood flow, including cardiovascular, autonomic, and humoral actions, temperature, pH, P_aCO_2, size of the hypoxic segment, and intensity of the hypoxic stimulus. Furthermore, surgical trauma can impair HPV. One-lung ventilation (OLV) serves as a human model where HPV should lessen the expected decrease in P_aO_2 and intrapulmonary shunt fraction (Q_s/Q_t). In patients undergoing thoracic surgery, clinically relevant concentrations of volatile anesthetics have had minimal effects on P_aO_2 and Q_s/Q_t when changing from two-lung ventilation to OLV [133,134]. The efficacy of HPV to decrease shunt fraction varies inversely with pulmonary blood flow and cardiac output. Isoflurane, sevoflurane, and desflurane preserve cardiac output and have minimal to modest effects on shunt fraction during OLV. Propofol appears to be no more beneficial on shunt fraction during OLV than sevoflurane [135].

Adverse circulatory effects
Hemodynamic changes
A common effect of the potent volatile anesthetics is dose-dependent reduction of arterial blood pressure. There are essentially no differences in the magnitude of blood pressure reduction at steady state, equianesthetic concentrations of the various volatile anesthetics (Fig. 26.15). Halothane decreases blood pressure via decreases in cardiac output due to a substantial depression of myocardial contractility [139]. This contrasts to the newer volatile anesthetics, desflurane, sevoflurane, and isoflurane, which are known to maintain cardiac output and lower blood pressure by decreasing regional and systemic vascular resistance [136,140].

In animal studies desflurane increases heart rate [34,141], whereas sevoflurane, in animals and humans, minimally changes heart rate (Fig. 26.15) [142,143]. Isoflurane has been associated with an increase in heart rate of 10–20% at 1 MAC. At anesthetic levels greater than 1 MAC, desflurane has been associated with an increase in heart rate equal to that of isoflurane [143]. This is generally manifest as a 10–15 beats/minute increase in heart rate. Both desflurane and, to a lesser extent, isoflurane have been associated with transient large increases in heart rate during rapid increases in the inspired concentration of either anesthetic [143,144]. The mechanism(s) underlying the transient heart rate surges is likely due to the relative pungency of these anesthetics, which stimulates airway receptors to elicit a reflex tachycardia [145]. The tachycardia can be lessened with fentanyl, alfentanil, or clonidine pretreatment [146,147].

Myocardial contractility and arrhythmias
Myocardial contractility is reduced more with halothane than with isoflurane [148]. In human studies isoflurane, sevoflurane, and desflurane have not demonstrated significant changes in echocardiographically determined indices of myocardial function. More direct measurements of myocardial contractility can be made in animals after eliminating the neural control of the heart. Under these conditions, isoflurane, desflurane, and

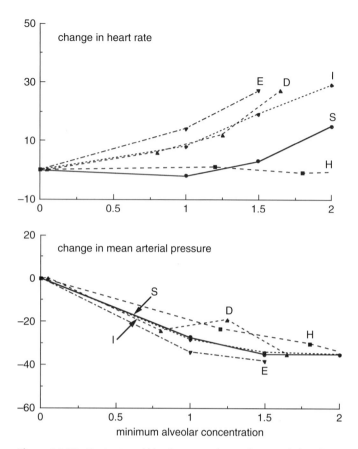

Figure 26.15. Heart rate and blood pressure changes from awake baseline in volunteers receiving general anesthesia with a potent inhaled anesthetic. Halothane and sevoflurane did not change heart rate at less than 1.5 MAC. All anesthetics caused similar decreases in blood pressure. D, desflurane; E, enflurane; H, halothane; I, isoflurane; S, sevoflurane. Adapted from Malan *et al.* [136]; Weiskopf *et al.* [137]; Calverley *et al.* [138].

sevoflurane cause a mild and similar dose-dependent depression of myocardial contractility.

In contrast to halothane, the volatile anesthetics isoflurane, sevoflurane, and desflurane do not predispose patients to ventricular arrhythmias, nor do they sensitize the heart to the arrhythmogenic effects of epinephrine. Some of the differences can be attributed to direct effects on cardiac pacemaker cells and conduction pathways [149]. Sinoatrial node discharge rate is slowed by the volatile anesthetics [150]. Conduction in the His–Purkinje system and conduction pathways in the ventricle is also prolonged by the volatile anesthetics [149]. A greater slowing by halothane than by isoflurane in the His–Purkinje system might promote dysrhythmias via a reentry phenomenon [151].

Coronary steal

The potent volatile anesthetics relax vascular smooth muscle. In the patient with ischemic heart disease, there is a mixture of normal and abnormal coronary blood vessels. Anesthetic-induced vasodilation of normal vessels might result in an effect called coronary steal: diverting blood away from diseased fixed vessels to dilated vessels. The diversion of blood from a myocardial bed with limited or inadequate perfusion to a bed with more adequate perfusion, especially one that has a remaining element of autoregulation, could result in ischemia and tissue injury. This concern was raised with the introduction of isoflurane into clinical practice. Isoflurane (like most other potent volatile anesthetics) increases coronary blood flow many times beyond that of the myocardial oxygen demand, thereby creating potential for "steal." In instrumented animal models, the pronounced coronary vasodilation produced by isoflurane was shown to cause "steal" [152], and early patient studies provided additional support [153]. However, more recent work in a chronically instrumented canine model of multivessel coronary artery obstruction has shown that neither isoflurane, sevoflurane, nor desflurane at concentrations up to 1.5 MAC resulted in abnormal collateral coronary blood flow redistribution ("steal") [154–156]. Interestingly, sevoflurane favorably increased (rather than decreased) collateral coronary blood flow in this instrumented animal model when aortic pressure was held constant by pharmacologic support of blood pressure [156].

The clinical relevance of coronary steal with isoflurane has been debated, and it is generally thought to be minimal [157,158]. Outcome studies have failed to associate the use of isoflurane in patients undergoing coronary artery bypass operations with an increased incidence of myocardial infarction or perioperative death [157,159,160]. Most studies would suggest that determinants of myocardial oxygen supply and demand, rather than the anesthetic, are of far greater importance to patient outcomes.

Ventilation mode and circulatory effects

Most of the volatile anesthetics have been studied during both controlled and spontaneous ventilation [136,161]. The process of spontaneous ventilation minimizes the increased intrathoracic pressures associated with positive-pressure ventilation. Negative intrathoracic pressure during the inspiratory phase of spontaneous ventilation augments venous return and cardiac filling and improves cardiac output and hence blood pressure. Spontaneous ventilation is associated with higher P_aCO_2, causing cerebral and systemic vascular relaxation. This contributes to an improved cardiac output via afterload reduction. Thus, spontaneous ventilation decreases systemic vascular resistance and increases heart rate, cardiac output, and stroke volume in contrast to positive-pressure ventilation. Spontaneous ventilation might improve the safety of inhaled anesthetic administration, because the concentration of a volatile anesthetic that produces cardiovascular collapse exceeds the concentration that results in apnea.

Nitrous oxide is commonly combined with potent volatile anesthetics to maintain general anesthesia. Nitrous oxide has unique cardiovascular actions. It increases sympathetic nervous system activity and vascular resistance when given in a

40% concentration [151]. Nitrous oxide combined with a volatile anesthetic results in an increased systemic vascular resistance and an improved arterial pressure with little effect on cardiac output compared to equi-MAC concentrations of a volatile anesthetic without N_2O [136,163]. These effects might not be due solely to sympathetic activation from N_2O, but may be partially attributed to a decrease in the concentration of the coadministered potent volatile anesthetic required to achieve a MAC equivalent when using N_2O.

Myocardial ischemia and cardiac outcome

Several studies have evaluated sevoflurane and desflurane to comparator anesthetics in terms of myocardial ischemia and outcome in patients with coronary artery disease undergoing either noncardiac or coronary artery bypass graft (CABG) surgery [164,165]. In both populations, sevoflurane appears to be essentially equivalent to isoflurane in terms of the incidence of myocardial ischemia and adverse cardiac outcomes. Desflurane appears to result in similar outcome effects as isoflurane in cardiac patients having CABG [166], with one exception. In a study where desflurane was given without opioids to patients with coronary artery disease requiring CABG surgery, significant ischemia mandating the use of β-blockers was noted [167]. Desflurane has not been evaluated in terms of ischemia and outcome in a patient population with coronary disease undergoing noncardiac surgery.

Adverse autonomic nervous system effects

Studies that have focused on the efferent activity of the parasympathetic and sympathetic nervous systems indicate that the volatile anesthetics depress their activity in a dose-dependent fashion [168]. The autonomic nervous system is modulated by baroreceptor reflex mechanisms. In human studies, isoflurane, sevoflurane, and desflurane reduce, in a dose-dependent fashion, arterial baroreflex modulation of vagally mediated heart-rate control [169,170]. There also is a dose-dependent depression of the reflex control of sympathetic outflow that appears to be relatively equivalent for isoflurane, sevoflurane, and desflurane. These findings may be interpreted as beneficial, as the loss of reflex responses to hypovolemia prevents the masking of the event. That is, diminished reflex vasoconstriction and tachycardia to blood loss lead to immediate hypotension, rather than masking the effect via reflex changes.

Desflurane has a unique and prominent effect on sympathetic outflow in humans, which is not apparent in animal models. With increasing steady-state concentrations of desflurane, there is a progressive increase in resting sympathetic nervous system activity and plasma norepinephrine levels [7,143,171]. Despite this increase in levels of sympathetic activity, blood pressure decreases as it does with sevoflurane and isoflurane. This raises the question as to whether desflurane has the ability to uncouple neuroeffector responses. In addition, desflurane can cause marked activation of the sympathetic nervous

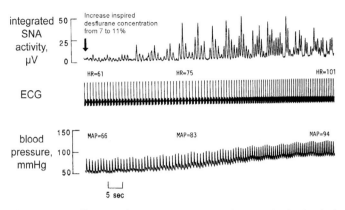

Figure 26.16. Neurocirculatory responses to an increase in the inspired concentration of desflurane in healthy, anesthetized, intubated volunteers. Within 10 seconds after increasing the desflurane concentration, large increases in peripheral sympathetic nerve activity (SNA) occur, leading to tachycardia and substantial increases in blood pressure. SNA is directed to blood vessels supplying skeletal muscles, and is recorded from a micro-needle placed into the peroneal nerve just below the knee. Adapted from Muzi et al. [172].

system when the inspired concentration is increased, especially to concentrations above 5–6% (Fig. 26.16) [7,143,171]. There is a transient surge in sympathetic outflow, leading to both hypertension and tachycardia. In addition, the endocrine axis is activated, as evidenced by 15- to 20-fold increases in plasma antidiuretic hormone and epinephrine. The hemodynamic response persists for 4–5 minutes and the endocrine response for 15–25 minutes. Adequate concentrations of opioids given prior to increasing the concentration of desflurane have been shown to attenuate these responses [135,136]. The source of the neuroendocrine activation has been actively sought, and it would appear that there are irritant receptors in both the upper and lower airways, and/or perhaps in a highly perfused tissue near the airways, that initiate the sympathetic activation [134].

Organ protection from volatile anesthetics

The potent volatile anesthetics have organ-protective effects [173–175]. Organ protection is defined as reducing tissue damage after hypoxic ischemia or toxic insult. It is now understood that lipophilic volatile anesthetics diffuse through cell membranes and alter mitochondrial electron transport leading to formation of reactive oxygen species [176]. This may be the trigger for preconditioning via protein kinase C activation of potassium (K_{ATP}) channel opening [177,178]. Numerous factors may be involved in preconditioning, including the Na^+/H^+ exchanger, the adenosine receptor (particularly α_1 and α_2 subtypes), inhibitory G proteins, protein kinase C, tyrosine kinase, and K_{ATP} channel opening. Pharmacologic blockade of these factors, e.g., with adenosine blockers, δ_1 opioids, pertussis toxin, or glibenclamide, reduces or

411

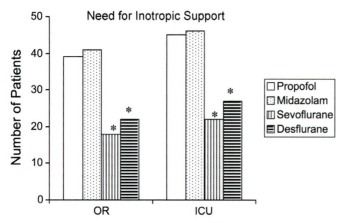

Figure 26.17. The need for inotropic support in patients undergoing coronary surgery with cardiopulmonary bypass. Significantly less support was needed in patients receiving sevoflurane and desflurane as their primary anesthetic regimen compared to propofol and midazolam groups. n = 80/group; * = statistically different from inhaled anesthetic groups. Adapted from De Hert et al. [183].

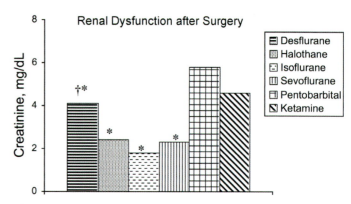

Figure 26.18. Most volatile anesthetics preserved renal function following renal ischemia–reperfusion injury in rats. The exception was desflurane. Injectable anesthetics did not preserve renal function. * = significantly different from injectable anesthetics; † = significantly different from other volatile anesthetics; p < 0.05. Adapted from Lee et al. [185].

eliminates the cardioprotective effect of ischemic or volatile anesthetic preconditioning [176,179]. Alternatively, administration of certain drugs can mimic ischemic or volatile anesthetic preconditioning. These include adenosine, opioid agonists, and K_{ATP} channel openers.

Cardioprotection

Approximately 30–40% of the cardioprotection produced by volatile anesthetics appears to be related to a reduced loading of calcium into the myocardial cells during ischemia [173]. Preconditioned hearts may tolerate ischemia for 10 minutes longer than nonconditioned hearts [180]. While these evolving data generally derive from animal models, there now is strong evidence in cardiac patients that anesthetic cardioprotection lessens myocardial damage (based on troponin levels and measures of cardiac performance) during "on and off pump" cardiac surgery [181,182]. This effect seems to be common to all current potent volatile anesthetics, and may favorably influence the need for inotropic support and ICU length of stay after coronary surgery [183] (Fig. 26.17). Sulfonylurea oral hyperglycemic drugs close K_{ATP} channels, abolishing anesthetic preconditioning. They should be discontinued 24–48 hours prior to elective surgery in high-risk patients [173]. But hyperglycemia also prevents preconditioning, so insulin therapy should be started when withholding oral agents [184].

Renal protection

Volatile anesthetics protect against renal ischemia–reperfusion (IR) injury in a rat model. When volatile anesthetics were given during or after the ischemia, there was protection based on a dramatic decrease in tubular necrosis. There also was evidence for a differential effect of the volatile anesthetics on protection from IR injury. Desflurane was less effective and showed less anti-inflammatory effects than

isoflurane and sevoflurane (Fig. 26.18). The K_{ATP} channels were not involved in the protection from renal IR injury, in contrast to protection in heart models. In addition, again in contrast to cardioprotection studies, pretreatment with a volatile anesthetic before the ischemia was not protective in the kidney [185]. The protection in the rat kidney appears to be via externalization of plasma membrane phosphatidylserine and by releasing transforming growth factor ($TGF\beta_1$), a cytokine with antinecrotic and anti-inflammatory properties [186].

Hepatic protection

The possibility that sevoflurane might lessen hepatic injury after CABG surgery was explored in a prospective randomized study of 320 patients. Postoperative biochemical markers of hepatic dysfunction were lower in the group receiving the sevoflurane-based anesthetic than in a control group receiving propofol as their primary anesthetic [187].

Cerebral protection

Brain-protective effects of volatile anesthetics have been demonstrated and attributed to the suppression of CMR. Sevoflurane, isoflurane, and desflurane have been shown to improve neurological outcome in comparison to N_2O–fentanyl after incomplete cerebral ischemia in rat models [188,189]. In piglets undergoing low-flow cardiopulmonary bypass, desflurane improved neurologic outcome compared to a fentanyl/droperidol-based anesthetic [190]. In humans, isoflurane reduced the incidence of ischemic EEG changes compared with halothane, and ischemic EEG changes occurred at a lower cerebral blood flow with isoflurane than with halothane [191,192]. Isoflurane can provide neuroprotective effects during hypoxemia or ischemia [193,194]. Desflurane has been shown to increase brain tissue PO_2 during administration, and to maintain PO_2 to a greater extent than thiopental during temporary cerebral artery occlusion during cerebrovascular surgery [195].

Summary

The pharmacodynamic effects of inhaled anesthetics are tied to their dose. Each volatile anesthetic has a unique potency, and comparisons of physiologic effects must therefore be adjusted to account for potency. To do this, the potency has been defined based on movement to a noxious stimulus. This is called the minimum alveolar concentration (MAC) and is the alveolar concentration of an anesthetic at 1 atmosphere that prevents movement in response to a surgical stimulus in 50% of patients. The most commonly administered potent volatile inhaled anesthetics for adult surgical procedures are isoflurane, sevoflurane, desflurane, and, to a lesser extent, halothane. Potent volatile anesthetics establish an anesthetic state of sedation and hypnosis sufficient to conduct surgical procedures and to effectively inhibit explicit recall. The volatile anethetics also have several major adverse effects, some of which are common to the drug class and some of which are drug-specific.

Adverse effects of potent volatile anesthetics include:

- **Malignant hyperthermia (MH)** – While nitrous oxide is considered safe in MH-susceptible patients, all of the potent volatile anesthetics serve as triggers for MH in genetically susceptible patients.
- **Injurious effects from anesthetic degradation** – Anesthetic degradation is the result of an exothermic reaction of the anesthetics with CO_2 absorbents. The use of a nondestructive absorbent eliminates all of the potential complications related to anesthetic breakdown and minimizes the possibility of complications.
- **Cerebral injury** – Although neuroprotection from volatile anesthetics is a well-defined concept, volatile anesthetics can cause injury in certain conditions via cerebral vasodilation and increases in intracranial pressure.
- **Effects on intracranial pressure** – All of the potent agents depress cerebral metabolic rate (CMR) to varying degrees and in a nonlinear fashion, and all of the potent volatile anesthetics increase cerebral blood flow (CBF), in a dose-dependent manner. The increases in CBF upon initial exposure to a volatile anesthetic can recover in several hours, despite continued exposure to the anesthetic. Intra-cerebral pressure (ICP) varies directly as a function of changes in CBF, and anesthetic-induced increases in ICP can be a dangerous in patients with an intracranial mass.
- **Hemodynamic changes** – All of the potent volatile anesthetics produce a dose-dependent decrease in blood pressure. For halothane this is predominantly due to a decrease in myocardial contractility, whereas for other agents it is the result of systemic vasodilation. Volatile anesthetics also reduce, in a dose-dependent fashion, arterial baroreflex modulation of heart rate and blood pressure.
- **Arrythmias** – Halothane can sensitize the heart to the arryhthmogenic effects of epinephrine, resulting in ventricular tachyarrhythmias. Other volatile anesthetics do not produce this effect.
- **Pulmonary effects** – All of the inhaled anesthetics produce a dose-dependent depression of the ventilatory response to hypercapnia and hypoxia.
- **Fluoride-induced nephrotoxicity** – It is now known that the site of anesthetic metabolism is an important factor in toxicity, i.e., intrarenal metabolism contributes to nephrotoxicity. This is an important mechanism of methoxyflurane nephrotoxicity.
- **Hepatic injury** – Modern-day volatile anesthetics have minimal hepatotoxic effects, but some have the potential to cause immune-mediated hepatitis.

The volatile anesthetics also provide organ protection from ischemic injury. These drugs also mimic ischemic preconditioning and trigger a similar cascade of intracellular events resulting in organ protection that lasts beyond the elimination of the anesthetic. Such protection has been reported in cardiac, neural, renal, and hepatic tissue.

- **Cardioprotection** – Approximately 30–40% of the cardioprotection produced by volatile anesthetics appears to be related to a reduced loading of calcium into the myocardial cells during ischemia. This effect seems to be common to all current potent volatile anesthetics, and may favorably influence the need for inotropic support and ICU length of stay after coronary surgery.
- **Renal protection** – When volatile anesthetics were given during or after the ischemia, there was protection based on a dramatic decrease in tubular necrosis. There was also evidence for a differential effect of the volatile anesthetics on protection from ischemia–reperfusion injury. Pretreatment with a volatile anesthetic before the ischemia was not protective in the kidney.
- **Cerebral protection** – Brain-protective effects of volatile anesthetics have been demonstrated and attributed to the suppression of cerebral metabolic rate.

References

1. Liem EB, Lin CM, Suleman MI, *et al.* Anesthetic requirement is increased in redheads. *Anesthesiology* 2004; **101**: 279–83.
2. Stekiel TA, Contney SJ, Bosnjak ZJ, *et al.* Reversal of minimum alveolar concentrations of volatile anesthetics by chromosomal substitution. *Anesthesiology* 2004; **101**: 796–8.
3. Mapleson WW. Effect of age on MAC in humans: a meta-analysis. *Br J Anaesth* 1996; **76**: 179–85.
4. Hettrick DA, Pagel PS, Kersten JR *et al.* Cardiovascular effects of xenon in isoflurane-anesthetized dogs with dilated cardiomyopathy. *Anesthesiology* 1998; **89**: 1166–73.
5. Nakata Y, Goto T, Morita S. Comparison of inhalation inductions with xenon and sevoflurane. *Acta Anaesthesiol Scand* 1997; **41**: 1157–61.
6. Scheinin B, Lindgren L, Scheinin TM. Preoperative nitrous oxide delays bowel

function after colonic surgery. *Br J Anaesth* 1990; **64**: 154–8.

7. Divatia JV, Vaidya JS, Badwe RA, *et al.* Omission of nitrous oxide during anesthesia reduces the incidence of postoperative nausea and vomiting: a meta-analysis. *Anesthesiology* 1996; **85**: 1055–62.

8. Losasso TJ, Muzzi DA, Dietz NM, *et al.* Fifty percent nitrous oxide does not increase the risk of venous air embolism in neurosurgical patients operated upon in the sitting position. *Anesthesiology* 1992; **77**: 21–30.

9. Koblin DD. Toxicity of nitrous oxide (N_2O). In: Rice SA, Fish KJ, eds., *Anesthetic Toxicity.* New York, NY: Raven Press, 1994: 135–55.

10. Badner NH, Beattie WS, Freeman D, *et al.* Nitrous oxide-induced increased homocysteine concentrations are associated with increased postoperative myocardial ischemia in patients undergoing carotid endarterectomy. *Anesth Analg* 2000; **91**: 1073–9.

11. Cole DJ, Schlunt M. *Adult Perioperative Anesthesia.* Philadelphia, PA: Elsevier Mosby, 2004: **87**.

12. Cole DJ, Schlunt M. *Adult Perioperative Anesthesia.* Philadelphia, PA: Elsevier Mosby, 2004: **88**.

13. Ghoneim MM. Awareness during anesthesia. *Anesthesiology* 2000; **92**: 597–602.

14. Gonsowski CT, Chortkoff BS, Eger EI, *et al.* Subanesthetic concentrations of desflurane and isoflurane suppress explicit and implicit learning. *Anesth Analg* 1995; **80**: 568–72.

15. Sebel PS, Bowdle TA, Ghoneim MM, *et al.* The incidence of awareness during anesthesia: a multicenter United States study. *Anesth Analg* 2004; **99**: 833–9.

16. Ducart A, Adnet P, Renaud B, *et al.* Malignant hyperthermia during sevoflurane administration. *Anesth Analg* 1995; **80**: 609–11.

17. Allen GC, Brubaker CL. Human malignant hyperthermia associated with desflurane anesthesia. *Anesth Analg* 1998; **86**: 1328–31.

18. Reed SB, Strobel GE. An in vitro model of malignant hyperthermia: differential effects of inhalation anesthetics on caffeine-induced muscle contractures. *Anesthesiology* 1978; **48**: 254–9.

19. Papadimos TJ, Almasri M, Padgett JS, Rush JE. A suspected case of delayed onset malignant hyperthermia with desflurane anesthesia. *Anesth Analg* 2004; **98**: 548–9.

20. Mazze RI, Shue GL, Jackson SH. Renal dysfunction associated with methoxyflurane anesthesia. A randomized, prospective clinical evaluation. *JAMA* 1971; **216**: 278–88.

21. Cousins MJ, Mazze RI. Methoxyflurane nephrotoxicity: a study of dose-response in man. *JAMA* 1973; **225**: 1611–16.

22. Frink EJ, Malan TP, Isner RJ, *et al.* Renal concentrating function with prolonged sevoflurane or enflurane anesthesia in volunteers. *Anesthesiology* 1994; **80**: 1019–25.

23. Mazze RI. The safety of sevoflurane in humans. *Anesthesiology* 1992; **77**: 1062–3.

24. Njoku D, Laster MJ, Gong DH, *et al.* Biotransformation of halothane, enflurane, isoflurane, and desflurane to trifluoroacetylated liver proteins: Association between protein acylation and hepatic injury. *Anesth Analg* 1997; **84**: 173–8.

25. Kharasch ED, Hankins DC, Thummel KE. Human kidney methoxyflurane and sevoflurane metabolism. Intrarenal fluoride production as a possible mechanism of methoxyflurane nephrotoxicity. *Anesthesiology* 1995; **82**: 689–99.

26. Malan TP, Kadota Y, Mata H, *et al.* Renal function after sevoflurane or enflurane anesthesia in the Fischer 344 rat. *Anesth Analg* 1993; **77**: 817–21.

27. Kharasch ED. Biotransformation of sevoflurane. *Anesth Analg* 1995; **81**: S27–38.

28. Strube PJ, Hulands GH, Halsey MJ. Serum fluoride levels in morbidly obese patients: enflurane compared with isoflurane anaesthesia. *Anaesthesia* 1987; **42**: 685–9.

29. Frink EJ, Malan TP, Brown EA, *et al.* Plasma inorganic fluoride levels with sevoflurane anesthesia in morbidly obese and nonobese patients. *Anesth Analg* 1993; **76**: 1333–7.

30. Kenna JG, Jones RM. The organ toxicity of inhaled anesthetics. *Anesth Analg* 1995; **81**: S51–66.

31. Frink EJ, Ghantous H, Malan TP, *et al.* Plasma inorganic fluoride with sevoflurane anesthesia: Correlation with indices of hepatic and renal function. *Anesth Analg* 1992; **74**: 231–5.

32. Weiskopf RB, Eger EI, Ionescu P, *et al.* Desflurane does not produce hepatic or renal injury in human volunteers. *Anesth Analg* 1992; **74**: 570–4.

33. Hussey AJ, Aldridge LM, Paul D, *et al.* Plasma glutathione-S-transferase concentration as a measure of hepatocellular integrity following a single general anaesthetic with halothane, enflurane or isoflurane. *Br J Anaesth* 1988; **60**: 130–5.

34. Suttner SW, Schmidt CC, Boldt J, *et al.* Low-flow desflurane and sevoflurane anesthesia minimally affect hepatic integrity and function in elderly patients. *Anesth Analg* 2000; **91**: 206–12.

35. Merin RG, Bernard J, Doursout M, *et al.* Comparison of the effects of isoflurane and desflurane on cardiovascular dynamics and regional blood flow in the chronically instrumented dog. *Anesthesiology* 1991; **74**: 568–74.

36. Gelman S, Fowler KC, Smith LR. Liver circulation and function during isoflurane and halothane anesthesia. *Anesthesiology* 1984; **61**: 726–30.

37. Elliott RH, Strunin L. Hepatotoxicity of volatile anaesthetics. *Br J Anaesth* 1993; **70**: 339–48.

38. Brown BR, Gandolfi AJ. Adverse effects of volatile anaesthetics. *Br J Anaesth* 1987; **59**: 14–23.

39. Kenna G, Satoh H, Christ DD, Pohl LR. Metabolic basis for drug hypersensitivity; antibodies in sera from patients with halothane hepatisis recognise liver neo-antigens that contain the tri-fluoroacetyl group derived from halothane. *J Pharmacol Exp Ther* 1988; **245**: 1103–9.

40. Kenna JG, Neuberger J, Williams R. Specific antibodies to halothane induced liver antigens in halothane associated hepatitis. *Br J Anaesth* 1987; **59**: 1286–90.

41. Kenna JG, Martin JL, Satoh H, Pohl LR. Factors affecting the expression of

trifluoroacetylated liver microsomal protein neoantigens in rats treated with halothane. *Drug Metab Dispos* 1990; **18**: 188–93.

42. Martin JL, Kenna JG, Pohl LR. Antibody assays for the detection of patients sensitised to halothane. *Anesth Analg* 1990; **2**: 154–9.

43. Martin JL, Plevak DJ, Flannery KD, *et al.* Hepatotoxicity after desflurane anesthesia. *Anesthesiology* 1995; **83**: 1125–9.

44. Stoelting RK, Blitt CD, Cohen PF, Menn RG. Hepatic dysfunction after isoflurane anesthesia. *Anesth Analg* 1987; **66**: 147–54.

45. Carrigan TW, Staughen WJ. A report of hepatic necrosis and death following isoflurane anesthesia. *Anesthesiology* 1987; **67**: 581–3.

46. Ray DC, Drummond GB. Halothane hepatitis. *Br J Anaesth* 1991; **67**: 84–99.

47. Anderson JS, Rose NR, Martin JL, *et al.* Desflurane hepatitis associated with hapten and autoantigen-specific IgG4 antibodies. *Anesth Analg* 2007; **104**: 1452–3.

48. Tung D, Yoshida EM, Wang CS, Steinbrecher UP. Severe desflurane hepatotoxicity after colon surgery in an elderly patient. *Can J Anaesth* 2005; **52**: 133–6.

49. Martin JL, Dubbink DA, Plevak DJ, *et al.* Halothane hepatitis 28 years after primary exposure. *Anesth Analg* 1992; **74**: 605–8.

50. Sigurdsen J, Hreidarsson AB, Thiodleifsson B. Enflurane hepatitis. A report of a case with a previous history of halothane hepatitis. *Acta Anaesthesiol Scand* 1985; **29**: 495–6.

51. Njoku DB, Greenberg RS, Bourdi M, *et al.* Autoantibodies associated with volatile anesthetic hepatitis found in the sera of a large cohort of pediatric anesthesiologists. *Anesth Analg* 2002; **94**: 243–9.

52. Ruzicka JA, Hidalgo JC, Tinker JH, Baker MT. Inhibition of volatile sevoflurane degradation product formation in an anesthesia circuit by a reduction in soda lime temperature. *Anesthesiology* 1994; **81**: 238–44.

53. Fang ZX, Kandel L, Laster MJ, *et al.* Factors affecting production of compound A from the interaction of sevoflurane with Baralyme and soda lime. *Anesth Analg* 1996; **82**: 775–81.

54. Frink EJ, Malan TP, Morgan SE, *et al.* Quantification of the degradation products of sevoflurane in two CO_2 absorbents during low-flow anesthesia in surgical patients. *Anesthesiology* 1992; **77**: 1064–9.

55. Kharasch ED, Thorning DT, Garton K, *et al.* Role of renal cysteine conjugate b-lyase in the mechanism of compound A nephrotoxicity in rats. *Anesthesiology* 1997; **86**: 160–71.

56. Kharasch ED, Hoffman GM, Thorning D, *et al.* Role of the renal cysteine conjugate b-lyase pathway in inhaled compound A nephrotoxicity in rats. *Anesthesiology* 1998; **88**: 1624–33.

57. Gonsowski CT, Laster MJ, Eger EI, *et al.* Toxicity of compound A in rats. Effect of a 3-hour administration. *Anesthesiology* 1994; **80**: 556–65.

58. Jin L, Baillie TA, Davis MR, Kharasch ED. Nephrotoxicity of sevoflurane compound A [fluoromethyl-2,2-difluoro-1-(trifluoromethyl)vinyl ether] in rats: Evidence for glutathione and cysteine conjugate formation and the role of renal cysteine conjugate beta-lyase. *Biochem Biophys Res Comm* 1995; **210**: 498–506.

59. Steffey EP, Laster MJ, Ionescu P, *et al.* Dehydration of baralyme increases compound A resulting from sevoflurane degradation in a standard anesthetic circuit used to anesthetize swine. *Anesth Analg* 1997; **85**: 1382–6.

60. Mazze RI, Friedman M, Delgado-Herrara L, *et al.* Renal toxicity of compound A plus sevoflurane compared with isoflurane in non-human primates. *Anesthesiology* 1998; A490.

61. Ebert TJ, Arain SR. Renal effects of low-flow anesthesia with desflurane and sevoflurane in patients. *Anesthesiology* 1999; A404.

62. Kharasch ED, Frink EJ, Zager R, *et al.* Assessment of low-flow sevoflurane and isoflurane effects on renal function using sensitive markers of tubular toxicity. *Anesthesiology* 1997; **86**: 1238–53.

63. Bito H, Ikeda K. Closed-circuit anesthesia with sevoflurane in humans. Effects on renal and hepatic function and concentrations of breakdown products with soda lime in the circuit. *Anesthesiology* 1994; **80**: 71–6.

64. Eger EI, Koblin DD, Bowland T, *et al.* Nephrotoxicity of sevoflurane versus desflurane anesthesia in volunteers. *Anesth Analg* 1997; **84**: 160–8.

65. Ebert TJ, Frink EJ, Kharasch ED. Absence of biochemical evidence for renal and hepatic dysfunction after 8 hours of 1.25 minimum alveolar concentration sevoflurane anesthesia in volunteers. *Anesthesiology* 1998; **88**: 601–10.

66. Groudine SB, Fragen RJ, Kharasch ED, *et al.* Comparison of renal function following anesthesia with low-flow sevoflurane and isoflurane. *J Clin Anesth* 1999; **11**: 201–7.

67. Bito H, Ikeda K. Renal and hepatic function in surgical patients after low-flow sevoflurane or isoflurane anesthesia. *Anesth Analg* 1996; **82**: 173–6.

68. Ebert TJ, Messana LD, Uhrich TD, Staacke TS. Absence of renal and hepatic toxicity after four hours of 1.25 minimum alveolar concentration sevoflurane anesthesia in volunteers. *Anesth Analg* 1998; **86**: 662–7.

69. Ebert TJ, Frink EJ, Kharasch ED. Absence of biochemical evidence for renal and hepatic dysfunction after 8 hours of 1.25 minimum alveolar concentration sevoflurane anesthesia in volunteers. *Anesthesiology* 1998; **88**: 601–10.

70. Conzen PF, Kharasch ED, Czerner SFA, *et al.* Low-flow sevoflurane compared with low-flow isoflurane anesthesia in patients with stable renal insufficiency. *Anesthesiology* 2002; **97**: 578–84.

71. Spracklin D, Kharasch ED. Evidence for the metabolism of fluoromethyl-1,1-difluoro-1-(trifluoromethyl)vinyl ether (Compound A), a sevoflurane degradation product, by cysteine conjugate b-lyase. *Chem Res Toxicol* 1996; **9**: 696–702.

72. Kharasch ED, Karol MD, Lanni C, Sawchuk R. Clinical sevoflurane metabolism and disposition. I. Sevoflurane and metabolite pharmacokinetics. *Anesthesiology* 1995; **82**: 1369–78.

73. Kharasch ED, Jubert C. Compound A uptake and metabolism to mercapturic acids and 3,3,3-trifluoro-2-fluoromethoxypropanoic acid during low-flow sevoflurane anesthesia. *Anesthesiology* 1999; **91**: 1267–78.

74. Iyer RA, Anders MW. Cysteine conjugate b-lyase-dependent biotransformation of the cysteine S-conjugates of the sevoflurane degradation product compound A in human, nonhuman, nonhuman primate, and rat kidney cytosol and mitochondria. *Anesthesiology* 1996; **85**: 1454–61.

75. Baker MT. Sevoflurane: are there differences in products? *Anesth Analg* 2007; **104**: 1447–51.

76. Kharasch ED, Subbarao GN, Stephens DA, *et al.* Influence of sevoflurane formulation water content on degradation to hydrogen fluoride in vaporizers. *Anesthesiology* 2007; **107**: A1591.

77. O'Neill B, Hafiz MA, De Beer DA. Corrosion of Penlon sevoflurane vaporisers. *Anaesthesia* 2007; **62**: 421.

78. Yamakage M, Hirata N, Saijo H, *et al.* Analysis of the composition of 'original' and generic sevoflurane in routine use. *Br J Anaesth* 2007; **99**: 819–23.

79. Woehlck HJ, Dunning M, Raza T, *et al.* Physical factors affecting the production of carbon monoxide from anesthetic breakdown. *Anesthesiology* 2001; **94**: 453–6.

80. Holak EJ, Mei DA, Dunning MB, *et al.* Carbon monoxide production from sevoflurane breakdown: Modeling of exposures under clinical conditions. *Anesth Analg* 2003; **96**: 757–64.

81. Baxter PJ, Garton K, Kharasch ED. Mechanistic aspects of carbon monoxide formation from volatile anesthetics. *Anesthesiology* 1998; **89**: 929–41.

82. Fang ZX, Eger EI, Laster MJ, *et al.* Carbon monoxide production from degradation of desflurane, enflurane, isoflurane, halothane, and sevoflurane by soda lime and baralyme. *Anesth Analg* 1995; **80**: 1187–93.

83. Wissing H, Kuhn I, Warnken U, Dudziak R. Carbon monoxide production from desflurane, enflurane, halothane, isoflurane and sevoflurane with dry soda lime. *Anesthesiology* 2001; **95**: 1205–12.

84. Castro BA, Freedman LA, Craig WL, Lynch C. Explosion within an anesthesia machine: Baralyme, high fresh gas flows and sevoflurane concentration. *Anesthesiology* 2004; **101**: 537–9.

85. Wu J, Previte JP, Adler E, *et al.* Spontaneous ignition, explosion, and fire with sevoflurane and barium hydroxide lime. *Anesthesiology* 2004; **101**: 534–7.

86. Fatheree RS, Leighton BL. Acute respiratory distress syndrome after an exothermic Baralyme-sevoflurane reaction. *Anesthesiology* 2004; **101**: 531–3.

87. Hanaki C, Fujii K, Morio M, Tashima T. Decomposition of sevoflurane by sodalime. *Hiroshima J Med Sci* 1987; **36**: 61–7.

88. Kharasch ED. Putting the brakes on anesthetic breakdown. *Anesthesiology* 1999; **91**: 1192–3.

89. Stullken EH, Milde JH, Michenfelder JD, Tinker JH. The non-linear responses of cerebral metabolism to low concentrations of halothane, enflurane, isoflurane and thiopental. *Anesthesiology* 1977; **46**: 28–34.

90. Smith AL, Wollman H. Cerebral blood flow and metabolism: Effects of anesthetic drugs and techniques. *Anesthesiology* 1972; **36**: 378–400.

91. Scheller MS, Nakakimura K, Fleischer JE, Zornow MH. Cerebral effects of sevoflurane in the dog: Comparison with isoflurane and enflurane. *Br J Anaesth* 1990; **65**: 388–92.

92. Lutz LJ, Milde JH, Milde LN. The cerebral functional, metabolic, and hemodynamic effects of desflurane in dogs. *Anesthesiology* 1990; **73**: 125–31.

93. Fujibayashi T, Sugiura Y, Yanagimoto M, *et al.* Brain energy metabolism and blood flow during sevoflurane and halothane anesthesia: effects of hypocapnia and blood pressure fluctuations. *Acta Anaesthesiol Scan* 1994; **38**: 413–18.

94. Osawa M, Shingu K, Murakawa M, *et al.* Effects of sevoflurane on central nervous system electrical activity in cats. *Anesth Analg* 1994; **79**: 52–7.

95. Yli-Hankala A, Vakkuri A, Särkelä M, *et al.* Epileptiform electroencephalogram during mask induction of anesthesia with sevoflurane. *Anesthesiology* 1999; **91**: 1596–603.

96. Jääskeläinen SK, Kaisti K, Suni L, *et al.* Sevoflurane is epileptogenic in healthy subjects at surgical levels of anesthesia. *Neurology* 2003; **61**: 1073–8.

97. Julliac B, Guehl D, Chopin F, *et al.* Sharp increase in cerebral sevoflurane concentration during mask induction in adults is a major risk factor of spike wave occurrence. *Anesthesiology* 2004; A–132.

98. Hisada K, Morioka T, Fukui K, *et al.* Effects of sevoflurane and isoflurane on electrocorticographic activities in patients with temporal lobe epilepsy. *J Neurosurg Anesthes* 2001; **13**: 333–7.

99. Eger El. *Isoflurane (Forane): a Compendium and Reference.* Madison, WI: Ohio Medical Products, 1985.

100. Algotsson L, Messeter K, Nordström CH, Ryding E. Cerebral blood flow and oxygen consumption during isoflurane and halothane anesthesia in man. *Acta Anaesthesiol Scand* 1988; **32**: 15–20.

101. Bedforth NM, Hardman JG, Nathanson MH. Cerebral hemodynamic response to the introduction of desflurane: A comparison with sevoflurane. *Anesth Analg* 2000; **91**: 152–5.

102. Summors AC, Gupta AK, Matta BF. Dynamic cerebral autoregulation during servoflurane anesthesia: a comparison with isoflurane. *Anesth Analg* 1999; **88**: 341–5.

103. Strebel S, Lam A, Matta B, *et al.* Dynamic and static cerebral autoregulation during isoflurane, desflurane, and propofol anesthesia. *Anesthesiology* 1995; **83**: 66–76.

104. Drummond JC, Todd MM, Toutant SM, Shapiro HM. Brain surface protrusion during enflurane, halothane, and isoflurane anesthesia in cats. *Anesthesiology* 1983; **59**: 288–93.

105. Adams RW, Cucchiara RF, Gronert GA, *et al.* Isoflurane and cerebrospinal fluid pressure in neurosurgical patients. *Anesthesiology* 1981; **54**: 97–9.

106. Talke P, Caldwell JE, Richardson CA. Sevoflurane increases lumbar

cerebrospinal fluid pressure in normocapnic patients undergoing transsphenoidal hypophysectomy. *Anesthesiology* 1999; **91**: 127–30.

107. Talke P, Caldwell J, Dodsont B, Richardson CA. Desflurane and isoflurane increases lumbar cerebrospinal fluid pressure in normocapnic patients undergoing transsphenoidal hypophysectomy. *Anesthesiology* 1996; **85**: 999–1004.

108. Muzzi DA, Losasso TJ, Dietz NM, *et al.* The effect of desflurane and isoflurane on cerebrospinal fluid pressure in humans with supratentorial mass lesions. *Anesthesiology* 1992; **76**: 720–4.

109. Sponheim S, Skraastad Ø, Helseth E, *et al.* Effects of 0.5 and 1.0 MAC isoflurane, sevoflurane and desflurane on intracranial and cerebral perfusion pressures in children. *Acta Anaesthesiol Scand* 2003; **47**: 932–8.

110. Artru AA. Isoflurane does not increase the rate of CSF production in the dog. *Anesthesiology* 1984; **60**: 193–7.

111. Sugioka S. Effects of sevoflurane on intracranial pressure and formation and absorption of cerebrospinal fluid in cats. [Japanese]. Masui. *Jpn J Anesthesiol* 1992; **41**: 1434–42.

112. Artru AA. Rate of cerebrospinal fluid formation, resistance to reabsorption of cerebrospinal fluid, brain tissue water content, and electroencephalogram during desflurane anesthesia in dogs. *J Neurosurg Anesthesiol* 1993; **5**: 178–86.

113. Drummond JC, Todd MM. The response of the feline cerebral circulation to PaCO2 during anesthesia with isoflurane and halothane and during sedation with nitrous oxide. *Anesthesiology* 1985; **62**: 268–73.

114. Lutz LJ, Milde JH, Milde LN. The response of the canine cerebral circulation to hyperventilation during anesthesia with desflurane. *Anesthesiology* 1991; **74**: 504–7.

115. Bundgaard H, von Oettingen G, Larsen KM, *et al.* Effects of sevoflurane on intracranial pressure, cerebral blood flow and cerebral metabolism. *Acta Anaesthesiol Scand* 1998; **42**: 621–7.

116. Eger EI. Desflurane. *Anesthesiol Rev* 1993; **20**: 87.

117. Doi M, Ikeda K. Respiratory effects of sevoflurane. *Anesth Analg* 1987; **66**: 241–4.

118. Yacoub O, Doell D, Kryger MH, Anthonisen NR. Depression of hypoxic ventilatory response by nitrous oxide. *Anesthesiology* 1976; **45**: 385–9.

119. Hirshman CA, McCullough RE, Cohen PJ, Weil JV. Depression of hypoxic ventilatory response by halothane, enflurane and isoflurane in dogs. *Br J Anaesth* 1977; **49**: 957–63.

120. Sarton E, Dahan A, Teppema L, *et al.* Acute pain and central nervous system arousal do not restore impaired hypoxic ventilatory response during sevoflurane sedation. *Anesthesiology* 1996; **85**: 295–303.

121. van den Elsen M, Sarton E, Teppema L, *et al.* Influence of 0.1 minimum alveolar concentration of sevoflurane, desflurane and isoflurane on dynamic ventilatory response to hypercapnia in humans. *Br J Anaesth* 1998; **80**: 174–82.

122. Hirshman CA, Bergman NA. Factors influencing intrapulmonary airway calibre during anaesthesia. *Br J Anaesth* 1990; **65**: 30–42.

123. Hirshman CA, Edelstein G, Peetz S, *et al.* Mechanism of action of inhalational anesthesia on airways. *Anesthesiology* 1982; **56**: 107–11.

124. Lindeman KS, Baker SG, Hirshman CA. Interaction between halothane and the nonadrenergic, noncholinergic inhibitory system in porcine trachealis muscle. *Anesthesiology* 1994; **81**: 641–8.

125. Rooke GA, Choi JH, Bishop MJ. The effect of isoflurane, halothane, sevoflurane, and thiopental/nitrous oxide on respiratory system resistance after tracheal intubation. *Anesthesiology* 1997; **86**: 1294–9.

126. Goff MJ, Arain SR, Ficke DJ, *et al.* Absence of bronchodilation during desflurane anesthesia: a comparison to sevoflurane and thiopental. *Anesthesiology* 2000; **93**: 404–8.

127. Mori N, Nagata H, Ohta S, Suzuki M. Prolonged sevoflurane inhalation was not nephrotoxic in two patients with refractory status asthmaticus. *Anesth Analg* 1996; **83**: 189–91.

128. Forbes AR, Horrigan RW. Mucociliary flow in the trachea during anesthesia with enflurane, ether, nitrous oxide, and morphine. *Anesthesiology* 1977; **46**: 319–21.

129. Forbes AR. Halothane depresses mucociliary flow in the trachea. *Anesthesiology* 1976; **45**: 59–63.

130. Reiz S. Nitrous oxide augments the systemic and coronary haemodynamic effects of isoflurane in patients with ischaemic heart disease. *Acta Anaesthesiol Scand* 1983; **27**: 464–9.

131. Loer SA, Scheeren TW, Tarnow J. Desflurane inhibits hypoxic pulmonary vasoconstriction in isolated rabbit lungs. *Anesthesiology* 1995; **83**: 552–6.

132. Ishibe Y, Gui X, Uno H, *et al.* Effect of sevoflurane on hypoxic pulmonary vasoconstriction in the perfused rabbit lung. *Anesthesiology* 1993; **79**: 1348–53.

133. Benumof JL, Augustine SD, Gibbons JA. Halothane and isoflurane only slightly impair arterial oxygenation during one-lung ventilation in patients undergoing thoracotomy. *Anesthesiology* 1987; **67**: 910–15.

134. Pagel PS, Fu JL, Damask MC, *et al.* Desflurane and isoflurane produce similar alterations in systemic and pulmonary hemodynamics and arterial oxygenation in patients undergoing one-lung ventilation during thoracotomy. *Anesth Analg* 1998; **87**: 800–7.

135. Beck DH, Doepfmer UR, Sinemus C, *et al.* Effects of sevoflurane and propofol on pulmonary shunt fraction during one-lung ventilation for thoracic surgery. *Br J Anaesth* 2001; **86**: 38–43.

136. Malan TP, DiNardo JA, Isner RJ, *et al.* Cardiovascular effects of sevoflurane compared with those of isoflurane in volunteers. *Anesthesiology* 1995; **83**: 918–28.

137. Weiskopf RB, Cahalan MK, Eger EI, *et al.* Cardiovascular actions of desflurane in normocarbic volunteers. *Anaesth Analg* 1991; **73**: 143–56.

138. Calverley RK, Smith NT, Prys-Roberts C, Eger EI, Jones CW. Cardiovascular effects of enflurane anesthesia during controlled ventilation in man. *Anaesth Analg* 1978; **57**: 619–28.

139. Pagel PS, Kampine JP, Schmeling WT, Warltier DC. Alteration of left ventricular diastolic function by desflurane, isoflurane, and halothane in the chronically instrumented dog with

autonomic nervous system blockade. *Anesthesiology* 1991; **74**: 1103–14.

140. Eger EI. Isoflurane: a review. *Anesthesiology* 1981; **55**: 559–76.

141. Pagel PS, Kampine JP, Schmeling WT, Warltier DC. Comparison of the systemic and coronary hemodynamic actions of desflurane, isoflurane, halothane and enflurane in the chronically instrumented dog. *Anesthesiology* 1991; **74**: 539–51.

142. Bernard JM, Wouters PF, Doursout MF, *et al.* Effects of sevoflurane and isoflurane on cardiac and coronary dynamics in chronically instrumented dogs. *Anesthesiology* 1990; **72**: 659–62.

143. Ebert TJ, Muzi M. Sympathetic hyperactivity during desflurane anesthesia in healthy volunteers. A comparison with isoflurane. *Anesthesiology* 1993; **79**: 444–53.

144. Weiskopf RB, Moore MA, Eger EI, *et al.* Rapid increase in desflurane concentration is associated with greater transient cardiovascular stimulation than with rapid increase in isoflurane concentration in humans. *Anesthesiology* 1994; **80**: 1035–45.

145. Muzi M, Ebert TJ, Hope WG, Bell LB. Site(s) mediating sympathetic activation with desflurane. *Anesthesiology* 1996; **85**: 737–47.

146. Yonker-Sell AE, Muzi M, Hope WG, Ebert TJ. Alfentanil modifies the neurocirculatory responses to desflurane. *Anesth Analg* 1996; **82**: 162–6.

147. Pacentine GG, Muzi M, Ebert TJ. Effects of fentanyl on sympathetic activation associated with the administration of desflurane. *Anesthesiology* 1995; **82**: 823–31.

148. Khambatta HJ, Sonntag H, Larsen R, *et al.* Global and regional myocardial blood flow and metabolism during equipotent halothane and isoflurane anesthesia in patients with coronary artery disease. *Anesth Analg* 1988; **67**: 936–42.

149. Atlee JL, Bosnjak ZJ. Mechanisms for cardiac dysrhythmias during anesthesia. *Anesthesiology* 1990; **72**: 347–74.

150. Bosnjak ZJ, Kampine JP. Effects of halothane, enflurane, and isoflurane on the SA node. *Anesthesiology* 1983; **58**: 314–21.

151. Atlee JL, Brownlee SW, Burstrom RE. Conscious-state comparisons of the effects of inhalation anesthetics on specialized atrioventricular conduction times in dogs. *Anesthesiology* 1986; **64**: 703–10.

152. Buffington CW, Romson JL, Levine A, *et al.* Isoflurane induces coronary steal in a canine model of chronic coronary occlusion. *Anesthesiology* 1987; **66**: 280–92.

153. Reiz S, Balfors E, Sorensen MB, *et al.* Isoflurane – a powerful coronary vasodilator in patients with coronary artery disease. *Anesthesiology* 1983; **59**: 91–7.

154. Hartman JC, Pagel PS, Kampine JP, *et al.* Influence of desflurane on regional distribution of coronary blood flow in a chronically instrumented canine model of multivessel coronary artery obstruction. *Anesth Analg* 1991; **72**: 289–99.

155. Hartman JC, Kampine JP, Schmeling WT, Warltier DC. Steal-prone coronary circulation in chronically instrumented dogs: isoflurane versus adenosine. *Anesthesiology* 1991; **74**: 744–56.

156. Kersten , Brayer AP, Pagel PS, *et al.* Perfusion of ischemic myocardium during anesthesia with sevoflurane. *Anesthesiology* 1994; **81**: 995–1004.

157. Slogoff S, Keats AS, Dear WE, *et al.* Steal-prone coronary anatomy and myocardial ischemia associated with four primary anesthetic agents in humans. *Anesth Analg* 1991; **72**: 22–7.

158. Vallance P, Collier J, Moncada S. Effects of endothelium-derived nitric oxide on peripheral arteriolar tone in man. *Lancet* 1989; **2**: 997–1000.

159. O'Young J, Mastrocostopoulos G, Hilgenberg A, *et al.* Myocardial circulatory and metabolic effects of isoflurane and sufentanil during coronary artery surgery. *Anesthesiology* 1987; **66**: 653–8.

160. Tuman KJ, McCarthy RJ, Spiess BD, *et al.* Does choice of anesthetic agent significantly affect outcome after coronary artery surgery? *Anesthesiology* 1989; **70**: 189–98.

161. Weiskopf RB, Cahalan MK, Ionescu P, *et al.* Cardiovascular actions of desflurane with and without nitrous oxide during spontaneous ventilation in humans. *Anesth Analg* 1991; **73**: 165–74.

162. Ebert TJ, Kampine JP. Nitrous oxide augments sympathetic outflow: Direct evidence from human peroneal nerve recordings. *Anesth Analg* 1989; **69**: 444–9.

163. Cahalan MK, Weiskopf RB, Eger EI, *et al.* Hemodynamic effects of desflurane/nitrous oxide anesthesia in volunteers. *Anesth Analg* 1991; **73**: 157–64.

164. Ebert TJ, Kharasch ED, Rooke GA, *et al.* Myocardial ischemia and adverse cardiac outcomes in cardiac patients undergoing noncardiac surgery with sevoflurane and isoflurane. *Anesth Analg* 1997; **85**: 993–9.

165. Searle NR, Martineau RJ, Conzen P, *et al.* Comparison of sevoflurane/fentanyl and isoflurane/fentanyl during elective coronary artery bypass surgery. *Can J Anaesth* 1996; **43**: 890–9.

166. Thomson IR, Bowering JB, Hudson RJ, *et al.* A comparison of desflurane and isoflurane in patients undergoing coronary artery surgery. *Anesthesiology* 1991; **75**: 776–81.

167. Helman JD, Leung JM, Bellows WH, *et al.* The risk of myocardial ischemia in patients receiving desflurane versus sufentanil anesthesia for coronary artery bypass graft surgery. *Anesthesiology* 1992; **77**: 47–62.

168. Seagard JL, Hopp FA, Bosnjak ZJ, *et al.* Sympathetic efferent nerve activity in conscious and isoflurane-anesthetized dogs. *Anesthesiology* 1984; **61**: 266–70.

169. Muzi M, Ebert TJ. A comparison of baroreflex sensitivity during isoflurane and desflurane anesthesia in humans. *Anesthesiology* 1995; **82**: 919–25.

170. Tanaka M, Nishikawa T. Arterial baroreflex function in humans anaesthetized with sevoflurane. *Br J Anaesth* 1999; **82**: 350–4.

171. Ebert TJ, Muzi M, Lopatka CW. Neurocirculatory responses to sevoflurane in humans. A comparison to desflurane. *Anesthesiology* 1995; **83**: 88–95.

172. Muzi M, Lopatka CW, Ebert TJ. Desflurane mediated neurocirculatory

activation in humans. Effects of concentration and rate of change on responses. *Anesthesiology* 1996; **84**: 1035–42.

173. Novalija E, Fujita S, Kampine JP, Stowe DF. Sevoflurane mimics ischemic preconditioning effects on coronary flow and nitric oxide release in isolated hearts. *Anesthesiology* 1999; **91**: 701–12.

174. Kersten , Schmeling TJ, Pagel PS, et al. Isoflurane mimics ischemic preconditioning via activation of KATP channels. *Anesthesiology* 1997; **87**: 361–70.

175. Toller WG, Kersten , Pagel PS, et al. Sevoflurane reduces myocardial infarct size and decreases the time threshold for ischemic preconditioning in dogs. *Anesthesiology* 1999; **91**: 1437–46.

176. Stowe DF, Kevin LG. Cardiac preconditioning by volatile anesthetic agents: a defining role for altered mitochondrial bioenergetics. *Antioxid Redox Signal* 2004; **6**: 439–48.

177. Novalija E, Kevin LG, Camara AK, *et al.* Reactive oxygen species precede the epsilon isoform of protein kinase C in the anesthetic preconditioning signaling cascade. *Anesthesiology* 2003; **99**: 421–8.

178. Kwok WM, Martinelli AT, Fujimoto K, *et al.* Differential modulation of the cardiac adenosine triphosphate-sensitive potassium channel by isoflurane and halothane. *Anesthesiology* 2002; **97**: 50–6.

179. Riess ML, Stowe DF, Warltier DC. Cardiac pharmacolocial preconditioning with volatile anesthetics: From bench to bedside? *Am J Physiol* 2004; **286**: H1603–7.

180. Kevin LG, Katz P, Camara AK, *et al.* Anesthetic preconditioning: effects on latency to ischemic injury in isolated hearts. *Anesthesiology* 2003; **99**: 385–91.

181. De Hert SG, Turani F, Mathur S, Stowe DF. Cardioprotection with volatile anesthetics: mechanisms and clinical implications. *Anesth Analg* 2005; **100**: 1584–93.

182. Conzen PF, Fischer S, Detter C, Peter K. Sevoflurane provides greater protection of the myocardium than propofol in patients undergoing off-pump coronary artery bypass surgery. *Anesthesiology* 2003; **99**: 826–33.

183. De Hert SG, Van der Linden PJ, Cromheecke S, *et al.* Choice of primary anesthetic regimen can influence intensive care unit length of stay after coronary surgery with cardiopulmonary bypass. *Anesthesiology* 2004; **101**: 9–20.

184. Gu W, Pagel PS, Warltier DC, Kersten JR. Modifying cardiovascular risk in diabetes mellitus. *Anesthesiology* 2003; **98**: 774–9.

185. Lee HT, Ota-Setlik A, Fu Y, *et al.* Differential protective effects of volatile anesthetics against renal ischemia–reperfusion injury in vivo. *Anesthesiology* 2004; **101**: 1313–24.

186. Lee HT, Chen SW, Doetschman TC, *et al.* Sevoflurane protects against renal ischemia and reperfusion injury in mice via the transforming growth factor-beta1 pathway. *Am J Physiol Renal Physiol* 2008; **295**: F128–36.

187. Lorsomradee S, Cromheecke S, Lorsomradee S, De Hert SG. Effects of sevoflurane on biomechanical markers of hepatic and renal dysfunction after coronary artery surgery. *J Cardiothorac Vasc Anesth* 2006; **20**: 684–90.

188. Engelhard K, Werner C, Reeker W, *et al.* Desflurane and isoflurane improve neurological outcome after incomplete cerebral ischaemia in rats. *Br J Anaesth* 1999; **83**: 415–21.

189. Werner C, Möllenberg O, Kochs E, Schulte am Esch J. Sevoflurane improves neurological outcome after incomplete cerebral ischaemia in rats. *Br J Anaesth* 1995; **75**: 756–60.

190. Loepke AW, Priestley MA, Schultz SEM, *et al.* Desflurane improves neurologic outcome after low-flow cardiopulmonary bypass in newborn pigs. *Anesthesiology* 2002; **97**: 1521–7.

191. Michenfelder JD, Sundt TM, Fode N, Sharbrough FW. Isoflurane when compared to enflurane and halothane decreases the frequency of cerebral ischemia during carotid endarterectomy. *Anesthesiology* 1987; **67**: 336–40.

192. Messick JM, Casement B, Sharbrough FW, *et al.* Correlation of regional cerebral blood flow (rCBF) with EEG changes during isoflurane anesthesia for carotid endarterectomy: Critical rCBF. *Anesthesiology* 1987; **66**: 344–9.

193. Newberg LA, Michenfelder JD. Cerebral protection by isoflurane during hypoxemia or ischemia. *Anesthesiology* 1983; **59**: 29–35.

194. Newberg LA, Milde JH, Michenfelder JD. Systemic and cerebral effects of isoflurane-induced hypotension in dogs. *Anesthesiology* 1984; **60**: 541–6.

195. Hoffman WE, Charbel FT, Edelman G, Ausman JI. Thiopental and desflurane treatment for brain protection. *Neurosurgery* 1998; **43**: 1050–3.

Pharmacokinetics of intravenous anesthetics

Frédérique S. Servin and John W. Sear

Introduction

Intravenous anesthetics are used primarily for induction of general anesthesia, and some are also used for maintenance of anesthesia or for sedation. The ideal characteristics are a rapid onset and short duration of effect terminated primarily by rapid redistribution. While metabolism and/or unchanged elimination may occur, they have comparatively little if any importance in terminating anesthetic effects. This chapter will discuss the pharmacokinetics of four groups of drugs: barbiturates, propofol, ketamine, and etomidate. These intravenous anesthetics differ in their structure and physicochemical properties, but all are highly lipid-soluble and often therefore require special solvents in their formulation.

Many of the concepts of intravenous anesthetic pharmacology which are widely used today were developed as a result of research on the disposition of the intravenous induction drugs. The earliest was thiopental, and the most recent propofol. In addition, while pharmacokinetic studies of most drugs are primarily concerned with drug elimination, those of the intravenous anesthetics are concerned with the early kinetics of the onset of drug effect, as much as with elimination kinetics.

Barbiturates

Barbiturates are formed through the "interaction" of malonic acid and urea to form the barbiturate ring structure. There are four main groups of barbiturates:

(1) **Oxybarbiturates** – with hydrogen at N1 and oxygen at C2 (these have a delayed onset and prolonged duration of action).
(2) **Thiobarbiturates** – with hydrogen at N1 and sulfur at C2 (e.g., thiopental).
(3) **Methylbarbiturates** – with a methyl group at N1 and oxygen at C2 (e.g., methohexital).
(4) **Methylthiobarbiturates** – although these are very potent, they show marked excitatory effects and are not used clinically.

Thiopental

Thiopental is the oldest intravenous anesthetic drug still in use, having been introduced into clinical practice in 1934 by Lundy and Tovell [1], and then by Pratt and colleagues [2]. The evaluation of subsequent compounds for use in the induction of anesthesia has been driven by the need to find newer drugs with fewer of the perceived disadvantages of thiopental and the other barbiturates.

Structure, stereochemistry

Thiopental is a thiobarbiturate, with a sulfur atom on the C2 position of the heterocyclic ring (Fig. 27.1). It has an asymmetric carbon atom at C5, and therefore is a racemic mixture of two enantiomers. The effects of the isomers on γ-aminobutyric acid (GABA)-induced currents have been investigated in mouse fibroblast cells [3]. The degree of stereoselectivity (defined as the ratio of GABA current potentiation by the S and R isomers) was 1.8, and was constant over the range of clinically relevant concentrations. In addition, S(–) thiopental plasma concentrations are about 24% higher than those of R(+) thiopental [4]. Thus clinical effects derive primarily from S(–) thiopental. The commercially available thiopental sodium also contains a small amount (6% of total drug) of a congener, with 1-ethylpropyl side chain at C5 instead of a 1-methylbutyl side chain. The pharmacokinetic and pharmacodynamic (PK/PD) properties of the congener are similar to those of thiopental [5].

Physicochemical properties and presentation

Thiopental is a weak base (pK_a 7.45–7.6 at 25–27 °C) [6]. It is almost insoluble in aqueous medium, with an oil/water partition coefficient around 60:1 [7]. The rapid onset of hypnosis after an intravenous dose of thiopental is caused by its swift uptake across the blood–brain barrier (as a result of its high lipid solubility and a low degree of ionization at physiological pH). Thiopental is formulated as a pale yellow powder to which 6% anhydrous sodium carbonate is added in an ampoule containing an inert atmosphere of nitrogen. Although poorly soluble in water, thiopental dissolves in the alkaline solution of the sodium carbonate, where a 2.5% solution has a pH of 10.5. There is no added preservative, but the alkaline solution is bacteriostatic. This solution will cause significant tissue damage if administered accidentally outside the vein or in an artery.

Anesthetic Pharmacology, 2nd edition, ed. Alex S. Evers, Mervyn Maze, Evan D. Kharasch. Published by Cambridge University Press. © Cambridge University Press 2011.

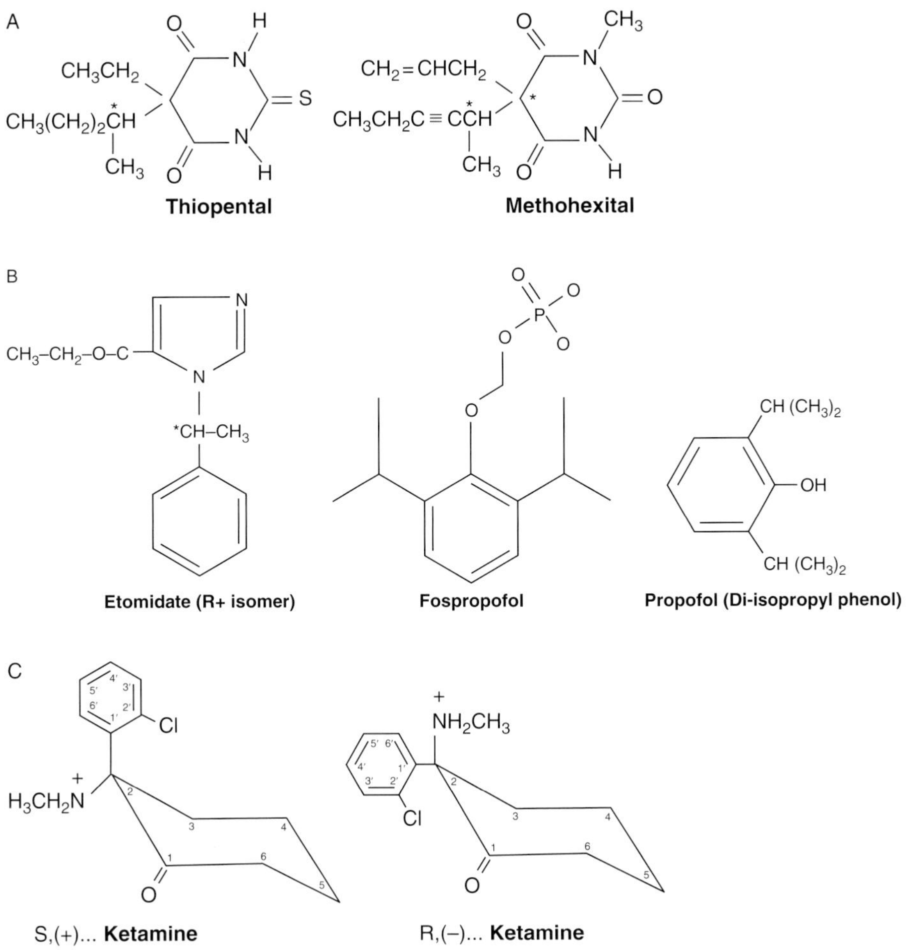

Figure 27.1. Molecular structures of thiopental, methohexital, propofol, fospropofol, ketamine and etomidate (* = chiral center).

Thiopental should not be dissolved in Ringer's lactate, since this would decrease the alkalinity of the solution and also thiopental solubility, leading to the risk of its precipitation as the free acid. The solution in water or saline is stable when kept at 4 °C for well over 7 days [8]. The usual recommended dilution for thiopental is 2.5% in the adult and 1% in children to limit the consequences of an accidental extravascular injection. When thiopental solution is administered at the same time as acidic solutions (i.e., nondepolarizing muscle relaxants), the mixture may precipitate out of solution in the intravenous tubing, resulting in an obstruction of fluid flow.

Distribution, metabolism, and excretion
Protein binding
Thiopental is extensively bound (about 80%) to plasma albumin [9]. The binding of thiopental to albumin has been described as nonlinear, with the possibility at high concentrations of a greater unbound fraction and therefore an enhanced effect [10]. Nevertheless, when systematically evaluated using an appropriate study design (i.e., early and frequent arterial blood sampling) this result could not be reproduced, and thiopental protein binding was linear over the concentration range

expected after an induction bolus dose [11]. Similarly, the simultaneous administration of drugs that might compete with thiopental for albumin binding sites did not lead to clinically significant changes in the unbound fraction [12].

Distribution
As early as 1950, the disappearance of the hypnotic effects of thiopental was related to redistribution to peripheral tissues rather than metabolism [13], and this phenomenon was more precisely described in the 1960s [14] (Fig. 27.2). After an intravenous injection, thiopental is distributed to the various tissues according to their local blood flow, tissue partition coefficients, and blood–tissue concentration gradients. The brain is initially exposed to high thiopental concentrations because of its high regional blood flow and the important lipid solubility of the drug. Blood–brain equilibration is rapid, so explaining the rapid onset of effect. Other peripheral tissues are also exposed to thiopental at an early stage, but since their volume of distribution is high and their regional blood flow is proportionally lower, thiopental concentrations increase more slowly, and continue to increase while brain concentrations have already decreased to subanesthetic concentrations. This description, which is a precursor of our

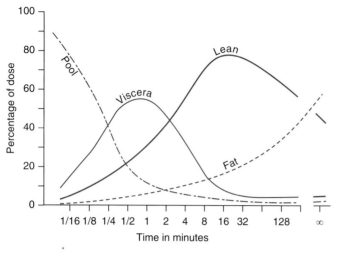

Figure 27.2. Distribution of thiopental in different body tissues at various times after its intravenous injection. Adapted from Price [14].

Table 27.1. Three-compartment mammillary model for thiopental [11,18]

Parameter	Value (mean ± SD) [13]	Population value (interindividual variability %) [16]
Rapid distribution half-life (min)	6.8 ± 2.8	
Slow distribution half-life (min)	59 ± 24	
Terminal distribution half-life (min)	719 ± 329	889
V_1 (L kg^{-1})	0.53 ± 0.18	0.079 (48%)
V_{dss} (L kg^{-1})	2.34 ± 0.75	2.73
CL (mL kg^{-1} min^{-1})	3.4 ± 0.4	3.07 (30%)

modern PK models, both compartmental and physiological, explains both how thiopental has a rapid onset and short duration of effect after a bolus dose, and how it may accumulate after an infusion.

Elimination

Thiopental is almost completely metabolized in the liver, with a very small percentage excreted unchanged in urine [13]. It is primarily oxidized by hepatic cytochrome P450 (specific isoforms responsible for metabolism have not been identified) to a carboxylic acid derivative, with a low hepatic extraction coefficient (around 15%) [11]. As a consequence, thiopental clearance is dependent on intrinsic clearance and independent of hepatic blood flow. At high thiopental concentrations, clearance is no longer linear with dose, but instead follows zero-order Michaelis–Menten elimination due to saturation of the hepatic enzymes systems that oxidize thiopental [15], the K_m for thiopental metabolism being about 30 µg m^{-1} [16]. This saturable elimination is one of the reasons for thiopental being unsuitable for the maintenance of anesthesia.

Pharmacokinetic modeling
Compartmental models

The first mammillary PK model to describe the fate of thiopental in humans [11] used a three-compartment model and a two-stage analysis in 12 young adult patients with normal weight and normal hepatic function [11]. It confirmed rapid redistribution from the central compartment (from brain to muscle), extensive metabolism, slow systemic elimination, and that hepatic metabolism contributed little to the initial rapid decline in plasma drug concentrations. A population PK analysis was subsequently performed by pooling data obtained from 64 patients recruited for various studies with different covariates (age, alcohol consumption, etc.) and administration modes (bolus, continuous infusions) [17]. Table 27.1 summarizes the

results obtained with both approaches. The main difference between the two analyses was the estimation of the initial volume of distribution, despite the use of arterial blood and early sampling (0.5 or 1 minutes after administration) in both studies. Indeed, this difficulty in characterizing initial drug distribution is a major flaw in static compartmental analysis, which considers that there is instantaneous mixing of the drug in all compartments including the central compartment.

Early mixing

Because of these difficulties in characterizing the initial (central) volume of distribution of thiopental using a traditional (three-) compartmental approach to modeling, a more precise description of thiopental early disposition was undertaken. The focus was on thiopental mixing in blood and tissues immediately after injection, which was studied by simultaneous administration of thiopental and a physiological marker which remained in the intravascular space (indocyanine green). This led to a model in which the initial volume of distribution was split into two separate compartments, one corresponding to the very rapidly circulating and central blood pools, and the other to the peripheral blood pool in rapidly equilibrating tissues [18]. Nevertheless, despite considering the role of distribution of the cardiac output in drug disposition, the limits of compartmental analysis remained in this approach, and it rapidly became obvious that some relationship with cardiac output in a quasi-physiologic model would be necessary to describe the completely non-steady-state kinetics of rapid thiopental onset [19].

Recirculatory and physiologically based pharmacokinetics

Physiologically based pharmacokinetic models (PBPK), which have a long history in the description of thiopental disposition [14], describe the time course of blood and tissue

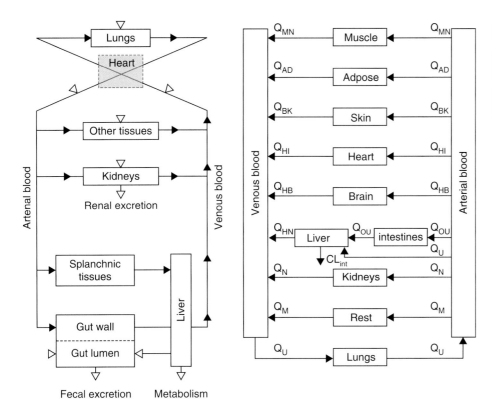

Figure 27.3. Whole-body pharmacokinetic models. Physiologically based pharmacokinetic model structure (*right*) emulates the physiological pathways of drug absorption, distribution, and elimination (*left*). The triangles show potential sites of drug administration. CL_{int}, intrinsic clearance; Q, blood flow. Reproduced with permission from Nestorov [20].

drug concentrations by considering the fraction of cardiac output distributed to each individual organ, blood–tissue distribution coefficients, and drug solubility.

Data for a PBPK model include two distinctive subsets of information:

(1) Drug-independent data based on underlying physiological processes.

(2) Drug-specific data characterizing the kinetic properties of the particular molecule under investigation. The features of a whole-body physiological model are shown in Fig. 27.3, and these can be described as a "closed circulation loop" [20]. A major concern of these models is whether or not lumping together several groups of tissues or organs into a single unit affects the accuracy of the model.

One main purpose of these models is to demonstrate the influence of pathophysiological states involving circulation (e.g., age or hypovolemia) on pharmacokinetics [21]. PBPK models are often first evaluated in animals, and then scaled up using allometric models to predict human drug disposition. Thus, the influence of cardiac output changes, either physiologically (age) or in diseases states, on thiopental dose requirements can be studied, and shown to account for a significant amount of interindividual variability in induction doses [21], but these models are unable to cope with the initial distribution of thiopental immediately after injection, which involves mixing, flow, and diffusion.

However, there are also important limitations of PBPK models: they need the input of large amounts of data (in terms of tissue drug concentrations, tissue or organ blood flows); they cannot be used to characterize drug behavior in a particular individual; nor can they input data for measured drug concentrations in either blood or tissues in the first minutes after drug dosing [22,23].

With very frequent early arterial blood sampling, recirculatory models were built which described more precisely the early fate of a drug in the vascular space [24]. Those models combined important advantages of both compartment and PBPK models. Like compartmental PK models, they can be established from blood concentrations versus time data in a variety of situations and species, and like PBPK models, they consider the influence of cardiac output and organ flows. Their main feature is to add to the traditional PK model "delay elements" which represent a kind of pharmacokinetic shunt (Fig. 27.4) [25].

This innovative description of intravenous anesthesia induction, called "front end kinetics" has direct implications in clinical practice. For example, using thiopental as a demonstration drug, and a canine model, thiopental early distribution and central volume of distribution (V_C) could be more precisely estimated, which thereby improved the initial accuracy of a thiopental target-controlled infusion (TCI) in dogs [26] The volume of the central compartment including the delay elements was about half the V_C estimated from traditional PK

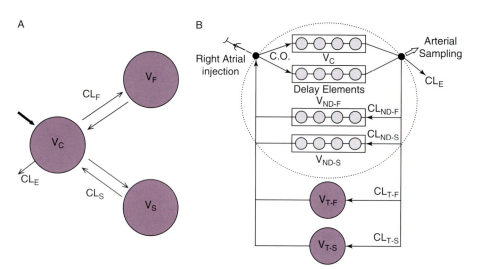

Figure 27.4. (A) Three-compartment mammillary PK model. (B) Multicompartmental recirculatory model. V_{T-F} and V_{T-S} are the fast and slow compartments of a three-compartment model, while the tank-in-series compartments (delay elements) included within the dotted circle are the expanded components of its V_C. CL_E, elimination clearance; CL_F, fast intercompartmental clearance; CL_S, slow intercompartmental clearance; V_C, central volume of distribution; V_F, fast equilibrating volume of distribution; V_S, slow equilibrating volume of distribution. Adapted from Krejcie and Avram [25] with permission of the authors and publishers of *Anesthesia and Analgesia*.

modeling with blood sampling at 1, 2, 3 minutes and all subsequent data.

The recirculatory PK model can also be adapted to compare the kinetics after rapid drug dosing by a thermally generated aerosol given in a single breath; following a 5-second intravenous injection [27]; and for drug delivery given by TCI. TCI models based on compartmental kinetic models will tend to generate plasma drug concentrations that are significantly above the target concentration until long after the infusion phase for maintenance has started [28], as overestimation of the initial volume of drug distribution will result in drug concentrations higher than the target concentration being achieved immediately after the start of the TCI infusion [29]. If recirculatory kinetics are used to control the behavior of TCI systems, the drug concentrations after the initial rapid intravenous infusion will tend to not exceed the target concentration because of the better and more accurate characterization of the initial volume of drug distribution, and hence early drug distribution.

Not only is drug disposition better characterized by physiological recirculatory models, but also the pharmacodynamics of the drugs are better delineated, as the k_{e0} (the first-order rate constant linking the central kinetic compartment and the effect site) and the EC_{50} (the drug concentration associated with a half-maximal drug effect) of the recirculatory model differ significantly from those generated by a traditional compartment model [30] and are determined with far greater precision.

Transfer to the effect site

When arterial thiopental concentrations over time after a bolus dose are compared to the time course of effect measured by the EEG, there is a delay in the onset and offset of effect compared with plasma concentrations. This delay, termed hysteresis, corresponds to the duration of all the events that occur between the movement of the drug from the arterial blood to the start of pharmacological effect [26] (Fig. 27.5). This

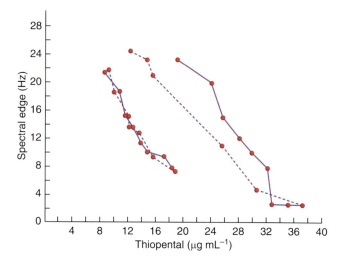

Figure 27.5. Pharmacodynamic modeling of thiopental, showing the effect of hysteresis. Venous thiopental serum concentrations vs. spectral edge hysteresis plot for two subjects. The solid line represents data during infusion of thiopental, and the dashed line represents postinfusion data. The subject to the right shows a greater degree of hysteresis. Adapted from Stanski et al. [31] with permission of the authors and publishers of *Journal of Pharmacokinetics and Biopharmaceutics*.

hysteresis can be represented by the transfer rate constant k_{e0} [31]. The k_{e0} for thiopental is around 0.58 min^{-1}, yielding a transfer half-time of 1.2 ± 0.3 minutes [26].

PK-based drug interactions

Thiopental is used only as an induction drug, and the intensity and termination of effect after a bolus dose are mainly driven by distribution processes (see above). As a consequence, few PK-based interactions have a significant impact on thiopental effect kinetics, apart from changes in cardiovascular function. Indeed, β-adrenergic blockers may modify early drug distribution through a reduction in cardiac output [32]; and volatile drugs, through their hemodynamic impact, may also modify thiopental pharmacokinetics [33,34]. However, normal sequence of drug dosing during anesthesia reduces the importance of the volatile anesthetics on the kinetics of induction drugs.

Dosage and administration

The usual dose requirements for inducing anesthesia with thiopental in an adult patient are about 5–7 mg kg^{-1}. Much of the interpatient variability may be accounted for by a simple equation: dose of thiopental (in mg) = 350 + weight (in kg) – (2 × age in years) – 50 (for female subjects) [35].

With such doses, loss of consciousness is obtained in about 1 minute and lasts 3–7 minutes. A similar duration of anesthesia may further be obtained by a second injection of about 20–25% of the initial dose (50–100 mg). Further bolus doses are not recommended because of increased risk of delayed recovery. Thiopental should not be used as a maintenance drug, due to its cumulative properties leading to delayed and unpredictable recovery.

The thiopental induction dose should be reduced in the elderly [36], mainly because hemodynamic changes in old age modify the early distribution of the drug [17,21]. However, the concentration–effect relationship seems to be little affected by ageing [17]. Neonates [37] and renal failure patients [38,39] also need reduced thiopental doses, because of decreased protein binding and therefore an increased unbound fraction of the drug. Hypovolemia and hemorrhagic shock also reduce thiopental requirements because of a preferential redistribution of blood flow to the brain [21]. In all frail patients, the appropriate induction dose should be determined by progressive titration to effect, as these elderly patients may lose consciousness with as little as 100 mg thiopental. The dose of thiopental should also be reduced where there is co-induction with benzodiazepines or an opioid drug.

Various studies examining the kinetics of the barbiturates thiopental and methohexital in the presence of renal failure, cirrhosis, alcoholism, and morbid obesity are summarized in Table 27.2 [10,11,38–43].

For the management of convulsions or treatment of increased intracranial pressure, doses of 1.5–3 mg kg^{-1} may be administered, repeated as necessary, and followed by either 25–50 mg boluses or an infusion of the barbiturate titrated against the occurrence of further fits or increased intracranial pressure (3–10 mg kg^{-1} h^{-1}). Because of altered kinetics and dynamics of thiopental, dosing adjustments may be needed in the critically ill patient with either liver or renal failure.

Methohexital

Methohexital, which was synthesized at the end of the 1950s, was designed to be a rapidly eliminated barbiturate, suitable for short-term surgery. Nevertheless, after the introduction of propofol, which had even more favorable PK properties, the use of methohexital use declined, and it is no longer available world-wide.

Structure and stereochemistry

Methohexital is an oxybarbiturate, with an oxygen substitution at position C2 of the heterocyclic ring (Fig. 27.1). It has two asymmetric carbon atoms, and thus consists of four isomers, two diastereometric pairs of enantiomers (α, β-d,l-methohexital) [44]. Because the β-enantiomers are associated with extensive motor activity, methohexital is marketed as racemic α-d,l-methohexital.

Physicochemical properties

Like thiopental, methohexital is highly lipid-soluble, with a slightly alkaline pK_a of 7.9, and therefore at physiological pH it is predominantly nonionized (75%). Methohexital is also manufactured as a sodium salt to maintain water solubility. The aqueous solution is strongly alkaline and therefore can cause the same tissue damage and precipitation with weak acids as thiopental; similarly, the aqueous solution of methohexital is bacteriostatic. It is used as a 1% solution.

Distribution, metabolism and excretion, PK modeling

Methohexital is extensively bound to serum albumin (around 80–85%) [45]. It readily crosses the placental barrier [46]. Like thiopental, methohexital is metabolized in the liver by cytochrome P450 enzymes (although the specific isoforms responsible for metabolism have not been identified). The main metabolite, 4′-hydroxymethohexital, has no pharmacologic activity. Methohexital metabolic clearance is much higher than that of thiopental, with an hepatic extraction ratio between 52% and 70% [47,48]. As a consequence, methohexital clearance depends on hepatic blood flow rather than intrinsic clearance, and the elimination half-life is shorter than that of thiopental. Methohexital pharmacokinetics are best described by a three-compartment mammillary model [48]. The main difference from thiopental is the magnitude of methohexital metabolic clearance, which reaches 700 mL min^{-1}, compared with 200–250 mL min^{-1} for thiopental [48,49]. Thus, methohexital infusions are suitable for maintenance of anesthesia [49]. Another consequence of the high clearance of methohexital, which is dependent primarily on liver blood flow, is that elimination is enhanced in the hyperkinetic state of sepsis [50,51]. There are only limited data looking at the disposition of this methoxybarbiturate in the patient with cirrhosis (Table 27.2) [52].

Methohexital was the first intravenous anesthetic drug to be implemented in a model-based closed-loop controlled anesthesia delivery system using quantitative EEG as a measure of drug effect [53,54].

Dosage and administration

The induction dose of methohexital (1.5–2.5 mg kg^{-1}) should be administered over at least 30 seconds to minimize the frequency of involuntary excitatory movements. After single-bolus dosing, the duration of loss of consciousness is similar with both thiopental and methohexital, which partly explains why methohexital as an induction drug offers few advantages over thiopental. Infusions of methohexital can be used to maintain anesthesia with either 67%

Table 27.2. Pharmacokinetics of thiopental and methohexital, and the effects of disease states and obesity (mean ± SD)

Reference	Healthy				Disease state			
	$t_{1/2}$	V_{ss}	CL_p	FF (%)	$t_{1/2}$	V_{ss}	CL_p	FF (%)
Thiopental								
Morgan [10]	690 ± 96	97.5 ± 40	150 ± 63					
Burch [11]	719 ± 329	170 ± 54	246.5 ± 29					
Ghoneim: volunteers [40]	344 ± 47	105.6 ± 0.11	242.5 ± 0.02					
Ghoneim: surgical patients [40]	308 ± 18	126.7 ± 0.38	292.1 ± 0.06					
Renal failure								
Christensen [39]	508	98.0	189	11	1069	194.2*	240	17.8*
Burch [38]	611 ± 130	144 ± 36.3	232 ± 43.5	15.7 ± 2.4	583 ± 158	216 ± 72	324 ± 79*	28.0 ± 6.5*
Cirrhosis								
Pandele [41]	529 ± 97	158.7 ± 34.5	269.1 ± 82.8	14.5 ± 3.4	714 ± 252	224 ± 121.6	340.2 ± 139	25.2 ± 3.9*
Alcoholism								
Couderc [42]	750 ± 212	199 ± 58	255 ± 62		684 ± 168	220.5 ± 139	340.2 ± 139*	
Obesity (lean 57.4 kg; obese 137.9 kg)								
Jung [43]	378	80.4 ± 26.4	198 ± 61		1671	650.9 ± 376.5*	416 ± 248*	
Methohexital								
Hudson [48]	234 ± 126	168.5 ± 53.6	835 ± 228					
Breimer [49]	96.8 ± 22.5	76.8 ± 12.9	826 ± 176					
Lange [47]			1304 ± 168					
Cirrhosis								
Duvaldestin [52]	151 ± 44	183 ± 87	2390 ± 860		204 ± 146	163 ± 97	2710 ± 1240	

$t_{1/2}$, elimination half-life (hours); V_{ss}, apparent volume of distribution at steady state (L); CL_p, plasma clearance (mL min^{-1}); FF, free fraction.
*$p < 0.05$ vs. healthy patients.

nitrous oxide or opioid supplementation, with rates between 50 and 150 μg kg^{-1} min^{-1}.

Propofol

Propofol (2,6-diisopropylphenol) is a sterically hindered phenol intravenous anesthetic first described in 1975 by ICI Pharmaceuticals. It is insoluble in water, and was first formulated in Cremophor EL (BASF) in 1977. However, because of the high incidence of adverse allergic reactions, a new

formulation was developed as a lipid emulsion in soybean oil and introduced into clinical trials in 1983 [55]. The revised propofol preparation (Diprivan) was an emulsion including 1% propofol, 10% soybean oil, and 1.2% purified egg phospholipid (emulsifier), with 2.25% of glycerol as a tonicity-adjusting agent, and sodium hydroxide to adjust the pH. This makes it appear as a highly opaque white fluid. The emulsion is isotonic and of neutral pH, and initially did not include any preservative to prevent bacterial growth. As a consequence, several clusters of infections related to Diprivan misuse were reported

[56], leading to a preservative (EDTA, sodium metabisulfite, or benzyl alcohol) being added to the initial formulation in most countries [57]. The addition of these preservatives is discussed further in Chapter 28. Even with emulsions containing a preservative to limit bacterial growth, some precautions remain mandatory. Once propofol is drawn up in a syringe from the ampoule or vial, it should be used without delay for a single patient and the remainder in the syringe discarded. Opened ampoules must not stand at room temperature. A propofol vial should never be used for several patients. Propofol emulsions are stable at room temperature and should never be frozen, and the properties of the emulsion are not modified by exposure to light [58].

Structure, stereochemistry

Propofol is an alkyl phenol, substituted with two isopropyl groups in each of the ortho positions adjacent to the hydroxyl group, and is a structural analog of vitamin E [57] (Fig. 27.1).

Physicochemical properties

At room temperature, propofol has the appearance of a slightly yellowish oil which freezes at only 19 °C. It has a neutral pH (7.4) and a pK_a of 11.0, making it 99.7% nonionized and highly lipid-soluble at physiological pH. The octanol/water partition coefficient is 6761 : 1 at a pH of 6–8.5.

Distribution, metabolism, and excretion

Propofol is extensively bound to serum albumin with a free fraction around 1.5% in the concentration range 0.5–32 µg mL^{-1} [59]. In addition, propofol avidly partitions into red blood cells. Fifty percent of blood propofol is bound to erythrocytes (of which 40% is on the red-blood-cell membranes) and 48% to serum proteins – almost exclusively to human serum albumin [59]. This high red-cell partitioning is one reason that many clinical propofol PK studies measure whole-blood propofol concentrations rather than the usual plasma concentration measurements.

After a bolus dose, propofol blood concentrations decrease rapidly due to extensive redistribution to peripheral tissues. Thus, theoretically, propofol possesses some potential for accumulation. However, at the end of administration, propofol return from the deep to the central compartment is slow, and slower than the rate of systemic elimination. As a consequence, propofol return from deep compartments cannot generate increases in blood concentration, nor persistence of a clinical effect. Propofol crosses the placental barrier [60].

The role of the lungs in the disposition and metabolism of propofol in humans has been debated. Although the pulmonary transit time of propofol was significantly longer than that of indocyanine green (22.4 vs. 2.7 seconds), there were no significant differences between pulmonary and radial arterial blood in the area under the curve (AUC) (0–60 minutes) for propofol, indicating that any propofol undergoing pulmonary uptake during the first pass is released back to the circulation by "back-diffusion" [61]. There was no pulmonary propofol

metabolism. In contrast, others found greater propofol concentrations in pulmonary artery compared with radial artery samples, and reported the formation of the metabolite 2,6-diisopropyl-1,4-quinol [62]. More recent publications support the concept of propofol trapping in the lungs followed by back-diffusion, but without significant contribution of this process to propofol clearance [63–65].

Less than 1% of administered propofol is excreted unchanged. Propofol is rapidly metabolized mainly in the liver to inactive glucuronide (by the UGT HP4 isozyme) and sulfate conjugates, and the corresponding quinol metabolites. Propofol also undergoes 4-hydroxylation by CYP2B6 to 2,6-diisopropyl-1,4-quinol, which can also undergo conjugation [66]. These metabolites are excreted via the kidneys, with 88% of the dose recoverable in the urine as hydroxylated and conjugated metabolites of propofol. The main urinary metabolite is propofol glucuronide (accounting for about 53% of an administered dose). Other metabolites are 1-(2,6-diisopropyl-1,4-quinol) glucuronide (18%); 4-(2,6-diisopropyl-1,4-quinol) glucuronide (13%) and 4-(2,6-diisopropyl-1,4-quinol) sulfate (9%). Other minor metabolites detectable in the urine include 2-(ω-propanol)-6-isopropylphenol and 2-(ω-propanol)-6-isoropyl-1,4-quinol. It is not known whether any of these metabolites have anesthetic properties. Although propofol is initially hydroxylated by CYP2B6 (which shows wide interindividual variability in human microsomal content), other cytochrome P450 isoforms with a high activity for propofol hydroxylation include CYP2C9 [66].

Although the liver has a high extraction ratio for propofol (ER $\geq$ 0.89), this cannot alone account for the total clearance of propofol being found to be greater than hepatic blood flow. Hence there is assumed to be extrahepatic metabolism (which will contribute about 40% of total propofol clearance). This has been demonstrated by the appearance of quinol and glucuronide metabolites during the anhepatic phase of liver transplant [67], and takes place mainly in the kidneys [63] and the small intestine [68].

Although the lungs do not contribute significantly to propofol clearance, tiny amounts of propofol are eliminated through the lungs. End-tidal concentrations can be measured using highly sensitive analytical methods, and may in the future be used to monitor propofol administration [69]. Propofol infusion may be associated with a green coloration of urine [70]. This phenomenon is due to metabolism of propofol, which may lead to a phenolic green chromophore that is conjugated in the liver and excreted in the urine [71].

Pharmacokinetic modeling
Compartmental analysis

The disposition of propofol can best be described by a three-compartment mammillary model. The main model characteristics are a high elimination clearance and extensive distribution to both shallow and deep peripheral compartments, with a large

Table 27.3. Main compartmental propofol pharmacokinetic models

	Gepts [73] n = 18	Marsh [74]	Schnider [75] n = 24	Schüttler [76] n = 270
V_1 (L)	16.9	$0.228 \times$ TBW [16.0]	4.27	$9.3 \times (\text{TBW}/70)^{0.71} \times (\text{age}/30)^{-0.39} \times (1 + \text{bol} \times 1.61)$ [8.31]
V_2 (L)	35	$0.472 \times$ TBW [33]	$18.9 - 0.391 \times (\text{age} - 53)$ [24]	$44.2 \times (\text{TBW}/70)^{0.61} \times (1 + \text{bol} \times 0.73)$ [44.2]
V_3 (L)	215	$2.91 \times$ TBW [204]	238	266
CL_1 (L min^{-1})	2.011	$0.027 \times$ TBW [1.899]	$1.89 + 0.0456 \times (\text{TBW} - 77) - 0.0681 \times (\text{LBM} - 59) + 0.0264 \times (\text{HT} - 177)$ [1.69]	if age $\leq$ 60 $1.44 \times (\text{TBW}/70)^{0.75}$ if age $>$ 60 $1.44 \times (\text{TBW}/70)^{0.75} - (\text{age} - 60) \times 0.045$ [1.44]
CL_2 (L min^{-1})	1.927	$0.026 \times$ TBW [1.788]	$1.29 - 0.024 \times (\text{age} - 53)$ [1.60]	$2.25 \times (\text{TBW}/70)^{0.62} \times (1 - \text{ven} \times 0.40) \times (1 + \text{bol} \times 2.02)$ [2.25]
CL_3 (L min^{-1})	0.708	$0.0096 \times$ TBW [0.669]	0.84	$0.92 \times (\text{TBW}/70)^{0.55} \times (1 - \text{bol} \times 0.48)$ [0.92]

The values in [brackets] represent the parameters for a 40-year-old, 70 kg, 175 cm male patient receiving a propofol infusion with arterial sampling.
TBW, total body weight; LBM, lean body mass; HT, height; bol, 1 for bolus data, 0 for infusion data; ven, 1 for venous samples, 0 for arterial samples.

apparent volume of distribution at steady state [72]. Several propofol compartmental models have been published. The main ones are summarized in Table 27.3, and they are typically referred to using the name of the author who reported them [73–76]. These four models differ mainly by the size of the central compartment and complexity of the model (i.e., the inclusion of significant covariates).

The Gepts model [73] was based on data from continuous constant-rate propofol infusions in 18 male adult patients of normal weight. A two-stage pharmacokinetic analysis was performed and failed to identify any covariates, possibly due to the narrow weight range in the population.

The Marsh model [74] was developed from the Gepts model, but introduced total body weight as a covariate. For a 70 kg patient, the model parameters are very similar to those published by Gepts (Table 27.3). The Marsh model was specifically designed to be used in the first commercially available TCI system, the Diprifusor [77]. The Diprifusor and other TCI delivery systems for propofol have been prospectively validated in a variety of settings [78–80], demonstrating the suitability of the March model to describe propofol PK in adult patients. The main criticism of it is the lack of covariates apart from total body weight. It is therefore not suitable to describe propofol PK in elderly patients.

The Schnider population PK model [75] was developed with data from normal-weight 26–81-year-old volunteers receiving first a bolus dose of propofol then a continuous infusion. Frequent early arterial sampling soon after dosing ensured an adequate estimate of the volume of the central compartment, which is the smallest of all propofol PK models. The Schnider model includes age and lean body mass (LBM) as significant covariates, and is therefore

recommended for use to predict concentrations in elderly patients. Unfortunately, the formula used to estimate LBM in this model [81] is obviously erroneous in the obese (leading to decreased and even a negative value of the LBM in patients with high body mass index). As a consequence, the current Schnider model is not appropriate for use in the obese patient.

The Schüttler model [76] is a population PK model derived from data pooled from five research groups, including both children and elderly patients (3–88 years old), and all of normal weight. It includes a number of significant covariates such as total body weight, age, administration mode (bolus or infusion), and site of blood sampling. Unfortunately, the presence of those two last variables, albeit very informative from a PK point of view, render it rather inconvenient for use in a TCI device. To date, two models, Marsh and Schnider, have been implemented in TCI devices. A number of pediatric models have also been established [74,76,82,83]. None of them is currently available for use in approved devices.

The main change in propofol PK in the elderly is a reduction of the fast intercompartmental clearance and as a consequence an increased early concentration for the same dose [75]. This fact can falsely be interpreted as an increased sensitivity to propofol in the elderly. Indeed, the propofol concentration–effect relationship is modified in the elderly, but only moderately so [84]. In the morbidly obese patient, propofol PK parameters are scaled to the total body weight [85], and the Marsh model is adequate in this population, as recently confirmed [80]. Propofol PK is little modified by cirrhosis of the liver [86,87], possibly because of extrahepatic metabolism pathways. In ICU patients, propofol elimination is slowed mainly by increases in unbound fraction and volumes of distribution, and alteration in effective hepatic blood flow [88,89]. During prolonged infusions, the key parameter for a stable concentration is clearance, and consequently TCI systems with models validated in anesthesia may ensure adequate control [90]. Cardiopulmonary bypass modifies propofol PK parameters, but the changes observed are moderate, and of little clinical importance [91].

The influence of old age, morbid obesity, obstructive jaundice, and liver and renal dysfunction on the disposition kinetics of propofol are shown in Table 27.4 [86–88,93–97].

Context-sensitive half-time, decrement time

In clinical anesthesia, particularly after drug infusions, the terminal half-life of multicompartmental drugs is a parameter of little value, since it is unable to describe the time course of termination of effect. This is dependent on two separate processes – distribution and elimination. Thus, a drug with a short elimination half-life will not necessarily be a short-acting drug (and vice versa), as distribution will also affect how long the dynamic effects of the drug last. For further discussion of the limitations of the elimination half-life as a descriptor of the duration of drug effect, the reader should refer to the review by Greenblatt [99].

In 1992, a new parameter was defined to describe the initial decay of drug concentrations after the end of propofol administration. The *context-sensitive half-time* was the estimated time for the plasma concentration to decrease by 50% after the end of an infusion. For propofol, context-sensitive half-time remains around 20 minutes even after 8 hours of infusion. Data simulations for thiopental, methohexital, propofol, and etomidate are shown in Fig. 27.6 [100,101]. This parameter, of great use to compare drugs or assess their cumulation potential, is of little clinical utility, since context-sensitive half-time is the same regardless of the concentration at the end of infusion, and does not relate the change in concentration to thresholds for clinical effect.

The context-sensitive half-time only describes the time for a 50% decrease in the central-compartment drug concentration. Is this always the key factor influencing recovery? A further elaboration of the concept was provided by Youngs and Shafer [102], who modeled the effects of varying infusion duration not just on the 50% decline in plasma drug concentration, but also on the 20% and 80% declines (termed the 20th, 50th, and 80th percentile *decrement times*) (Fig. 27.7). The limitations of the context-sensitive half-time have been further discussed by Schraag *et al.* [103]. Although recovery from alfentanil–propofol was faster than after sufentanil–propofol, they found that the relative decline in plasma opioid concentrations for maintenance of surgical anesthesia was greater after sufentanil than after alfentanil anesthesia (i.e., you need a greater decrease in the sufentanil concentration for extubation and discharge).

This new parameter, the decrement time, corresponds to the time from the end of infusion to a concentration value

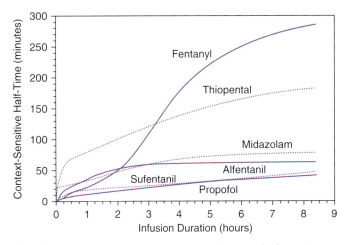

Figure 27.6. Context-sensitive half-times as a function of infusion duration for a number of anesthetic drugs. Solid and dashed line patterns are used only to permit overlapping lines to be distinguished. Adapted from Hughes *et al.* [100].

associated with 50% recovery or recovery in half of the patients [101]. The parameter includes both PK (to calculate the decrease in concentration) and PD (to define the concentration associated with 50% recovery) information, and is currently used in propofol TCI devices to estimate the recovery time.

Another index of recovery is the *mean effect time* as proposed by Bailey [104], which depends on the probability or not of whether a patient responds to a given endpoint. Whereas the 50% decrement time is the *median* recovery value for a given population of patients receiving a given drug regimen, the mean recovery index or effect time is based on the probability of an event occurring (i.e., recovery or nonrecovery) [104,105]. If there is a steep relationship between concentration and response (the γ-coefficient of the Hill equation), then the mean effect time and the 50% decrement times will be similar. For drugs with a flatter concentration–response plot, the mean effect time will be increasingly greater as the duration of drug delivery increases. The examples shown in Fig. 27.8 are for propofol and midazolam (γ-coefficients of 3.27 and 3.05, respectively) [106,107]. However, these predictors of recovery require further prospective validation to confirm their utility in providing clinically useful results.

Transfer of propofol to the effect site

Infusing propofol using PK parameters to target blood concentrations has been considered a significant improvement in propofol administration. However, the blood is not the site of propofol effect, and it rapidly appeared interesting to first describe and then target a hypothetical effect site rather than a blood concentration when using TCI systems. Thus, particular care was taken to establish propofol transfer time to the effect site, and the time course of propofol effects. Based on the

concentration was underestimated, and a nonparametric value of k_{e0} was used in the Marsh PK model without further adjustment [108]. This arose because no kinetic and dynamic indices had been determined simultaneously in the same patients. Schnider was the first to publish a PK/PD model for propofol with a transfer to the effect site described at the same time as the pharmacokinetics through an EEG parameter (semilinear canonical correlation) used as a measure of propofol hypnotic effect (PK/PD model) [84]. He also described the propofol time to peak effect, estimated as 1.6 minutes. This concept of *time to peak effect*, a physiological parameter independent from PK modeling [109], allowed the calculation of an estimate for the propofol k_{e0} to be linked to the Marsh model so that it reached the peak effect at the same time as described by Schnider [110]. The difficulty in modeling the initial phase of both PK (and hence the initial volume of drug distribution, V_C) and PD (the use of EEG monitoring with the associated computation lag time, together with the validity of the assumed sigmoid Emax model) led to discrepancies in the estimation of time to peak effect after a bolus dose or a continuous infusion [111,112].

Physiologically based PK

Similar to thiopental, propofol kinetics are influenced by cardiac output and regional blood flows, including cerebral blood flow. Consequently, the same difficulties and discrepancies already described with thiopental compartmental models have also arisen for propofol. But complex physiological models remain difficult to construct and require information on organ blood flows and tissue/blood partition coefficients not readily accessible in man, and extrapolations from animal studies may not always be appropriate. A physiologically based recirculatory model of propofol kinetics and dynamics combining information from both compartmental analysis and blood flows has been published [65]. It combines detailed descriptions of blood flows to the lungs and brain, and a more global description for flows to the rest of the body, reproducing the usual fast and slow distributions. Thus, the physiological features that are paramount to propofol induction (vascular mixing, lung kinetics and cerebral kinetics) are considered as factors that may affect drug disposition, but the global model, albeit complex, remains manageable computational analysis. So far, this model has not provided substantially new information on propofol kinetics, but the published data are in good agreement with the results of compartmental modeling [113]. The present utility of PBPK models lies in teaching and simulation, but may, in the future, lead to further clinical research and TCI improvements.

PK-based drug interactions

There is good laboratory evidence that propofol at concentrations ranging between 25 and 1000 μM in vitro inhibits drug metabolism [114–117]. More recently there have been in-vivo data indicating drug interactions with propofol leading to a reduced concomitant drug clearance. For example, propofol decreased alfentanil elimination clearance by 15%, rapid distribution clearance by 68%, slow distribution clearance by 51%, and lag time accounting for venous sampling by 62% [118]. Because mean arterial pressure and systemic vascular resistance were also significantly lowered by propofol, scaling to mean pressure improved the model. One interpretation is that the hemodynamic interaction caused by propofol may have influenced alfentanil kinetics [118], but this interpretation is at variance with the lack of liver blood flow on alfentanil clearance [119]. Propofol–remifentanil interactions have been abundantly described, and many are pharmacodynamic [120–123]. However, some interactions may be kinetic in part, through reduction in cardiac output, decreased propofol elimination, increased propofol concentrations, and hence increased propofol effect [124]. Nevertheless, in the absence of significant hemodynamic changes, remifentanil does not modify propofol PK [125].

In general, glucuronidation is a very robust metabolic pathway, and even potent inhibitors of glucuronosyltransferase are unable to significantly modify propofol clearance [126].

Administration and propofol formulations

The original propofol emulsion (Diprivan) is formulated as a 1% or 2% solution in soybean-oil emulsion [127], while generics are formulated in various lipid emulsions including a 1% solution in long-chain/medium-chain triglycerides, in cyclodextrins, in a cosolvent mixture of propylene glycol in water, as a micellar formulation, and as propofol prodrugs (see Chapter 28 for discussion of these and other investigational formulations). The use of medium- and long-chain triglycerides in the lipid carrier (MCT/LCT-propofol; B. Braun) seems associated with less discomfort on injection [128]. Owing to concern about risks associated with prolonged lipid infusions specifically in critical care patients, a 2% propofol formulation has been marketed [69]. Its pharmacological properties are similar to those of the 1% formulation [129,130].

Despite the widespread of propofol use in its current lipid formulations, some drawbacks remain and there is still room for improvement concerning emulsion stability, the need for antimicrobial drugs, hyperlipidemia, and the problem of pain on injection – which is more debatable, since the lipid vector is not painful when given alone or when used to solubilize other drugs [131]. This suggests that perhaps pain on propofol injection is due to propofol itself [132].

Effective plasma propofol concentrations in various clinical situations and populations are now well established, having been derived mainly from TCI studies. Loss of consciousness requires effect-site concentrations of 4–8 μg mL^{-1}, the absolute value depending whether or not the patient is premedicated with opioids, α_2-agonists, or benzodiazepines. During anesthesia maintenance, the concentration required depends on the intensity of surgical stimuli and coadministration of analgesics. It usually remains between 2 and 8 μg mL^{-1}. As a general rule, at the end of a propofol infusion, patients open their eyes when the predicted propofol concentration is between 0.8 and 1.5 µg mL^{-1}, depending on the residual concentrations of coadministered drugs and the physiological status of the patient. This is why, in the absence of depth-of-anesthesia monitoring, it is not recommended to target less than 2 µg mL^{-1} propofol, to avoid intraoperative awareness. When using TCI for conscious sedation, either under control by the anesthetist or in studies using patient-controlled TCI, the average effect-site concentration associated with anxiolysis and conscious sedation is 1–1.5 µg mL^{-1}. This corresponds at pseudo-steady state to a 1–3 µg kg^{-1} min^{-1} infusion rate.

Propofol analogs

The only propofol analog currently clinically approved by the US Food and Drug Administration (FDA) is a water-soluble phosphate prodrug of propofol (fospropofol; previously GPI 15715 and Aquavan; marketed as Lusedra by Eisai Pharma) [133]. The molecule is rapidly and completely cleaved by plasma alkaline phosphatase to inorganic phosphate, formaldehyde, and propofol (Fig. 27.9). It has a complex pharmacokinetic profile which requires two linked compartmental models for accurate description (one for distribution and conversion of fospropofol in propofol, and one for propofol itself [134]). Because of the need for drug cleavage, the onset of hypnotic action is delayed [98]. Fospropofol use is mainly proposed for procedural sedation.

The first fospropofol pharmacokinetic studies found unexpected propofol PK differences when compared to those obtained with lipid emulsions of Diprivan [135] (Table 27.4). One possible explanation for these is a recently discovered assay problem that may have affected the measurement of propofol-free plasma concentrations [136]. The corrected pharmacokinetics of fospropofol in humans are awaited.

Ketamine

Structure, stereochemistry

Ketamine (2-*O*-chlorophenyl-2-methylaminocyclohexanone HCl) is a phencyclidine derivative (Fig. 27.1) synthesized in 1963 [137]. Due to a chiral center in the C2 position of the molecule, it is a racemic mixture of two enantiomers, R(–)

and S(+), which exhibit different affinities to receptors and different clinical potencies. The anesthetic potency of the S(+) enantiomer is 3–4 times higher than that of the R(–) enantiomer [138]. The more potent S(+) ketamine has a better therapeutic index than the R(–) ketamine, and is commercially available as a single pharmacological entity in a number of countries. The differences between ketamine enantiomers are mainly pharmacodynamic, and concentrations of the two enantiomers in blood and brain after administration of the racemate in animals are very similar [139]. Some pharmacokinetic differences, albeit moderate, nevertheless exist (see below).

Physicochemical properties

Ketamine hydrochloride is a white crystalline salt soluble in aqueous solutions and is marketed in concentrations of 10, 50, and 100 mg ketamine base per mL. The solution is stable at room temperature, clear, and colorless. The pH values of pharmaceutical solutions range from 3.5 to 5.5. Ketamine is highly lipid-soluble, has a pK_a of 7.5, and is 44% nonionized at physiological pH.

Distribution, metabolism, and excretion

Ketamine is minimally bound to plasma proteins (12–35%) [140]. This property, in conjunction with very high lipid solubility (five times higher than thiopental) ensures an extensive distribution of the drug. A compartmental PK analysis of ketamine disposition has calculated an initial volume of distribution around 70 L, and a volume of distribution at steady state around 200 L [141,142]. Ketamine distribution is not stereospecific, and a specific active transfer across endothelial barriers seems therefore unlikely [143].

Ketamine undergoes *N*-demethylation by microsomal enzymes (cytochromes P450) to the primary metabolite norketamine, which retains about 20% of the activity of the parent drug [144]. The metabolism of ketamine is complex (Fig. 27.10) [145]. Although chiral inversion may occur during metabolism in animals (with R(–) ketamine being transformed into S(+) ketamine [146]), there is no evidence for chiral inversion of ketamine in humans in vivo. Although CYP3A4 is the principal enzyme responsible for ketamine *N*-demethylation in human liver microsomes, CYP2B6 and CYP2C9 make greater contributions to ketamine

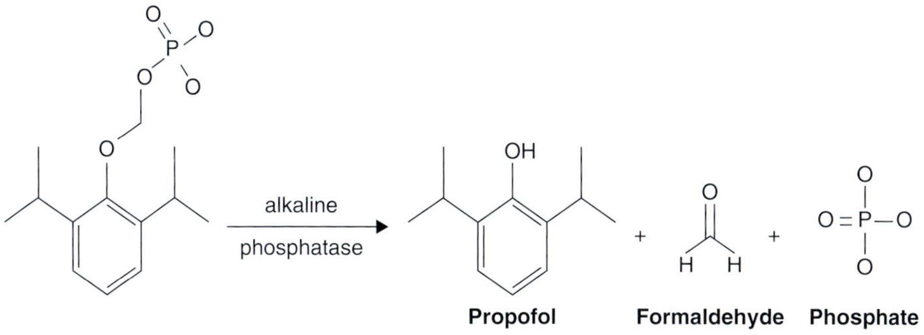

Figure 27.9. Structure of fospropofol and its proposed metabolic breakdown. Adapted from Gibiansky *et al.* [134] with permission of the authors and publishers of *Anesthesiology*.

Propofol   Formaldehyde   Phosphate

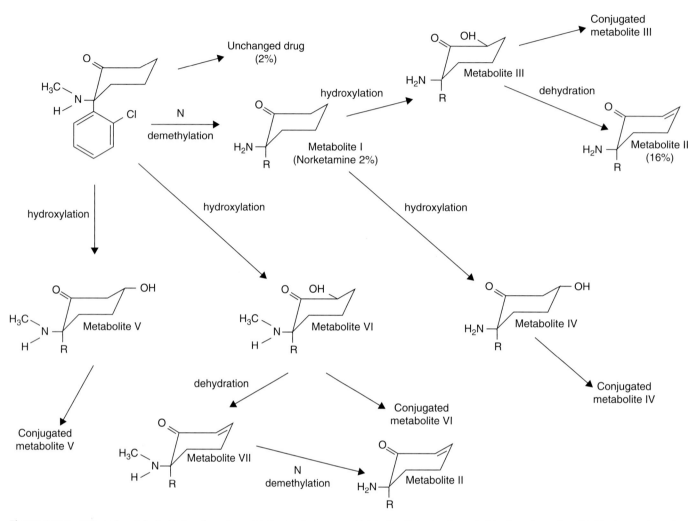

Figure 27.10. Proposed metabolic biotransformation of ketamine in humans. Metabolite III is also termed dehydronorketamine; IV, 5-hydroxynorketamine; V, 5-hydroxyketamine; VI, 6-hydroxyketamine; VII, dehydroketamine. Adapted from Lau & Domino [145].

N-demethylation at therapeutic concentrations of the drug in vivo [147,148]. Ketamine has a high metabolic clearance (1–1.6 L min^{-1}). This clearance is therefore dependent on organ blood flow and not on intrinsic metabolic capacities [142]. Ketamine and its metabolites undergo hydroxylation and conjugation prior to renal excretion, and in cases of renal failure the weak active metabolite 6-hydroxynorketamine may accumulate [149]. The main excreted metabolites are norketamine and hydroxynorketamine glucuronides, with only about 2% of a ketamine dose excreted unchanged. There is no evidence of increased concentrations of dehydronorketamine – this being an assay artifact.

The pharmacokinetics of racemic and S(+) ketamine have been compared in young male volunteers and surgical patients [140,141,150–153] (Table 27.5). The clearance of S(+) ketamine was found to be significantly higher when this isomer was administered alone than in the racemic mixture, suggesting an inhibition of S(+) clearance by the R(−) isomer [150]. In the racemic mixture, the PK parameters of both isomers were similar but not identical, with a slightly (22%) higher clearance and larger apparent volume of distribution for S(+) ketamine [150]. These findings corroborate the results of an in-vitro study on human liver microsomes in which the rate of S(+) ketamine demethylation was found to be 20% greater than that of R(−) ketamine and 10% greater than that of the racemate [154]. At clinically relevant ketamine concentrations, the rate of racemate demethylation was always less than the sum of the rates for the individual enantiomers, reflecting inhibition of metabolism of one enantiomer in the presence of the other. This interaction seems to work in two ways, R(−) inhibiting the metabolism of S(+) and vice versa, probably through competitive interaction on the same enzymes. Each ketamine enantiomer undergoes demethylation to norketamine by a high-affinity/low-capacity enzyme which accounts for 80% of ketamine metabolism at usual clinical hypnotic concentrations, and by a second low-affinity/high-capacity enzyme. S(+)-demethylation is significantly faster than R(−), hence the higher clearance.

Table 27.5. Pharmacokinetics of racemic ketamine and S(+) ketamine (mean ± SD)

Reference	$t_{1/2}$	V_{ss}	CL_p	FF (%)
Ketamine (racemic)				
White [141]	132 ± 32	203 ± 35	1130 ± 300	
Clements [153]	182 ± 25	206 ± 28	869 ± 152	
Geisslinger [152]	S 149 ± 47	230 ± 90	1340 ± 500	
(enantiomer disposition when given as racemate)				
	R 155 ± 57	211 ± 87	1150 ± 340	
Ihmsen [150]	196 ± 73	172 ± 64	1169 ± 134	
Dayton [140]				73.2 ± 4.4
Ketamine (S+)				
White [141]	158 ± 45	329 ± 77	1490 ± 110	
Geisslinger [152]	143 ± 76	199 ± 111	1150 ± 400	
Ihmsen [150]	146 ± 33	213 ± 54	2078 ± 277	
Persson [151]	80 ± 25	112 ± 33	1620 ± 300	

$t_{1/2}$, elimination half-life (hours); V_{ss}, apparent volume of distribution at steady state (L); CL_p, plasma clearance (mL min^{-1}); FF, free fraction. There are no data relating to kinetics in disease states or aging.

Table 27.6. Pharmacokinetic parameters and effective arterial concentrations of ketamine (racemic mixture) and S(+) ketamine [150]

Parameter	Racemic mixture (mean ± SD)	S(+) ketamine (mean ± SD)
CL (mL kg^{-1} min^{-1})	14.8 ± 1.7	26.3 ± 3.5
V_1 (L kg^{-1})	0.31 ± 0.05	0.41 ± 0.05
k_{12} (min^{-1})	0.096 ± 0.010	0.096 ± 0.0014
k_{21} (min^{-1})	0.023 ± 0.003	0.026 ± 0.003
k_{e0} (min^{-1})	1.03 ± 1.61	1.02 ± 0.58
Gamma	2.76 ± 0.49	1.42 ± 0.29
EC50 EEG (median frequency) (µg mL^{-1})	1.32 ± 0.57	2.08 ± 0.41
EC50 LOC (µg mL^{-1})	2.41 ± 0.90	1.11 ± 0.30
EC50 ROC (µg mL^{-1})	1.48 ± 0.46	0.75 ± 0.21
EC50 LER (µg mL^{-1})	3.68 ± 1.43	1.56 ± 0.32
EC50 RER (µg mL^{-1})	2.42 ± 0.84	1.14 ± 0.33
EC50 loss of orientation (µg mL^{-1})	1.84 ± 0.73	0.98 ± 0.34
EC50 recovery of orientation (µg mL^{-1})	1.10 ± 0.35	0.52 ± 0.16

CL, elimination clearance; V_1, initial volume of distribution; k_{12}, transfer constant from V_1 to periphery; k_{21}, transfer constant from periphery to V_1; k_{e0}, transfer constant from plasma to effect; gamma, slope of the sigmoid; EC50, concentration associated with the effect in 50% of the subjects; LOC, loss of consciousness; ROC, recovery of consciousness; LER, loss of eyelash reflex; RER, recovery of eyelash reflex.

Pharmacokinetic models, transfer to the effect site

Ketamine PK parameters from a prospective randomized crossover study of S(+) and racemic ketamine in volunteers, which also estimated ketamine transfer to the effect site, are provided in Table 27.6 [150]. The PK/PD data have been commented on to suggest that S(+) ketamine offers better titratability than the racemic mixture because of the absence of the R(−) enantiomers and hence the aforementioned metabolic enantiomeric interaction, its higher clearance, and steeper concentration–effect curve. There are, however, no substantive comparative data to support or refute this view.

Some studies suggest that norketamine may contribute to overall ketamine clinical effects. Norketamine is detected in plasma 2–3 minutes after a ketamine bolus, and peaks at about 30 minutes, but the pharmacokinetics of norketamine itself are not well characterized. Nevertheless, norketamine concentration versus time curves after a single ketamine dose, regardless of the administration route, show slower elimination than ketamine and the potential for metabolite accumulation [155]. Because of this accumulation, ketamine requirements when administered as a continuous infusion decrease over time, as the increasing norketamine concentrations in the body produce their own sedative and analgesic effects [156].

Concentration–effect relationship

The mean effective hypnotic plasma concentration (EC50) for the racemate in the presence of 67% nitrous oxide is 1.1 µg mL^{-1} (with a range 0.5–1.8 µg mL^{-1}) [157]. Table 27.6 also contains the arterial EC50s for the racemate and S(+) enantiomer for various endpoints [150]. Ketamine impairs memory at concentrations as low as 70 ng mL^{-1}, and important psychomimetic effects are seen around 500 ng mL^{-1} [158]. However, "psychedelic" effects (hallucinations, loss of the notion of time, exultation, unreal feeling) may appear at concentrations as low as 50 ng mL^{-1}, and their intensity increases linearly with concentration from 50 to 200 ng mL^{-1} [159]. Anxiety and paranoid feeling are much reduced at these higher concentrations. Bilateral nystagmus appears at concentrations around 200 ng mL^{-1}. The analgesic effect of ketamine, based on the tolerance to ischemic pain produced by tourniquet application, occurs above 100 ng mL^{-1} [153]. In another study in volunteers, the analgesic threshold was 160 ng mL^{-1} [160]. However, after oral administration, lower ketamine concentrations were associated with analgesia (40 ng mL^{-1}), due to the effects of first-pass ketamine metabolism and an enhanced contribution of the metabolite norketamine to the overall analgesia [161]. In patients suffering from hyperalgesia and allodynia after nerve damage, plasma ketamine concentrations required to reduce both hyperalgesia and allodynia need to be at least 100 ng mL^{-1} [162].

PK-based drug interactions

When a short ketamine infusion is followed by an alfentanil infusion, ketamine clearance and volumes of distribution are increased in rats. The norketamine area under the concentration–time curve is also reduced because of enhanced elimination [163]. It seems that alfentanil, through its vasodilator properties, might be able to facilitate the entrance of ketamine in the liver, the kidneys, and the gut, where most of the metabolism takes place. Conversely, ketamine has no influence on alfentanil pharmacokinetics. When taken at the same time as cocaine, ketamine may lower cocaine concentrations in rats through an increase in cocaine metabolism [164].

Another possible interaction between benzodiazepines and ketamine has been described in an ICU patient [165], but there are no definitive data to show an inhibition of ketamine N-demethylation in vivo.

Extravascular administration routes

The bioavailability of intramuscular ketamine is high (93%), with peak plasma concentrations obtained in 5 minutes. Oral ketamine effects are limited by first-pass metabolism and a low bioavailability (about 17%) [156]. In children, ketamine has been administered by both the rectal and intranasal routes. Rectal ketamine is associated with a low bioavailability (25%), in part due to first-pass metabolism, while the intranasal route is more efficient with a higher bioavailability (50%) [154]. However, intranasal dosing is not suitable for induction of anesthesia, since it requires high volumes which are in part swallowed, leading to major interindividual variability both in onset time and effect.

Dosage and administration

The recommended intravenous induction dose is 1–4.5 mg kg^{-1} (usually a dose of 2 mg kg^{-1} provides surgical anesthesia for 5–10 minutes). Maintenance of anesthesia can be achieved using a 1 mg mL^{-1} solution at a rate of 10–45 μg kg^{-1} min^{-1}. Intravenous induction doses of S(+) ketamine are 0.5–1.0 mg kg^{-1} or 2–4 mg kg^{-1} intramuscularly, with maintenance achieved by

repeated boluses of 50% of the induction dose or infusion of 0.5–3.0 mg kg^{-1} h^{-1}. For analgesia, doses of 0.1–0.25 mg kg^{-1} intravenously followed by an infusion of 0.2–1.0 mg kg^{-1} h^{-1} are needed.

Etomidate

Etomidate (R(+)-ethyl-1-(α-methyl-benzyl)-1H-imidazole-5-carboxylate) is a short-acting nonbarbiturate intravenous anesthetic drug discovered at Janssen Pharmaceutica in 1964 (Fig. 27.1).

Structures, stereochemistry

Etomidate is optically active, existing as two enantiomers. However, only the dextro (R) isomer has significant anesthetic properties (the approximate potency ratio of the enantiomers being R : S 10 : 1), and therefore etomidate has been one of the first drugs to be marketed as a single enantiomer of a racemic mixture [166].

Physicochemical properties

Etomidate has a pH of 8.1 and pK_a of 4.24. It is a base, with about 99% of the drug nonionized in the blood. The imidazole ring renders etomidate water-soluble at acidic pH and lipid-soluble at physiological pH, and hence the drug is formulated as a 2 mg mL^{-1} solution in 10 mL ampoules made up in either propylene glycol (pH solution 5.1, osmolality 4965 mOsm kg^{-1}) or in a lipid emulsion of long-chain and medium-chain triglycerides with a pH of 7.6 and osmolality of 400 mOsm kg^{-1}. This latter formulation results in significantly reduced pain on injection, myoclonus, and local thrombophlebitis, as well as less red-cell hemolysis [131,167]. Some data are currently available on a new formulation of etomidate in an aqueous solution using sulfobutyl ether-7 β-cyclodextrin (SBE-CD, Captisol) as a solubilizing agent [168]. For further discussion, see Chapter 28.

Distribution, metabolism and excretion, PK/PD modeling

Etomidate is about 75% bound to serum albumin [169]. Metabolism occurs in the liver and plasma by esterase hydrolysis to pharmacologically inactive metabolites, with only about 2% excreted unchanged in the urine [170].

Etomidate pharmacokinetics can be described by a two- or three-compartment mammillary model [171–174] with an elimination clearance in excess of 1000 mL min^{-1}, an apparent volume of distribution at steady state around 3.5–4.5 L kg^{-1}, and a terminal elimination half-life of between 1.5 and 5 hours depending on the method of dosing and the duration of blood sampling (Table 27.7). Aging reduces the central volume of distribution of etomidate, or more probably, as demonstrated with propofol, a reduced

Table 27.7. Pharmacokinetics of etomidate, and the effects of disease states (mean ± SD)

Reference		Healthy				Disease state or aging			
		$t_{1/2}$	V_{ss}	CL_p	FF (%)	$t_{1/2}$	V_{ss}	CL_p	FF (%)
Etomidate									
Van Hamme [172]		276 ± 156	339 ± 166	860 ± 230					
Schüttler [173]		68.5 ± 5.7	118.6 ± 22.5	1660 ± 271					
Fragen [174]		174 ± 66	183 ± 64	1278 ± 400					
Elderly									
Arden [171]	< 60 yrs	252 ± 58	366 ± 111	1843 ± 369					
	> 60 yrs					382 ± 186	340 ± 161	1237 ± 377	
Cirrhosis									
Bonnardot [177]		101 ± 69	226 ± 54	1539 ± 387		163 ± 93	162 ± 96	717 ± 302*	
van Beem [176]		209 ± 65	256 ± 49	889 ± 161		540 ± 150	602 ± 91	889 ± 161	
Renal failure and cirrhosis									
Carlos [178]	Healthy				24.9 ± 1.6				
	Renal failure								43.4 ± 2.9*
	Cirrhosis								44.2 ± 2.1*
Hypovolaemia									
Johnson [175] (study in swine)			53.0 ± 7.1	820 ± 90			41.3 ± 8.0	960 ± 200	

$t_{1/2}$, elimination half-life (hours); V_{ss}, apparent volume of distribution at steady state (L); CL_p, plasma clearance (mL min^{-1}); FF, free fraction.
*$p < 0.05$ vs. healthy patients.

fast intercompartmental clearance. Etomidate metabolic clearance is high, being close to liver blood flow, and therefore depends on cardiac output more than enzyme function. However, etomidate PK studies in the elderly (a population well known for reduced liver blood flow) fail to demonstrate any reduction in clearance in this population [171]. Similarly, moderate hemorrhagic shock in swine produced only minor changes in etomidate PK [175], and clearance was also unchanged in cirrhotic patients – but who have a prolonged half-life mainly through increased volumes of distribution [176,177]. The extrahepatic (plasma) clearance of etomidate may at least in part explain those discrepancies. There are significant increases in the unbound free fraction of etomidate in patients with both hepatic cirrhosis and renal failure, but there are no formal disposition studies in the latter group of patients [178]. Etomidate transfer to the effect site is rapid, with a transfer rate constant (k_{e0}) estimated round 0.43 min^{-1} (with a mean half-time for blood–brain equilibration of 1.6 min) [171].

Dosage and administration

The relationship between etomidate concentrations and hypnotic effect have been well established, with anesthetic concentrations requiring 300–500 ng mL^{-1}, and EEG burst suppression at concentrations exceeding 1 μg mL^{-1} [171]. The recommended induction dose is 0.3 mg kg^{-1}, but this is reduced in the elderly to 0.15–0.2 mg kg^{-1}. Nevertheless, since etomidate induction causes few hemodynamic effects, the clinical consequences of an overdose are minimal. In children younger than 15 years, doses up to 0.4 mg kg^{-1} may be needed. Etomidate is unsuitable for maintenance of anesthesia because it inhibits cortisol synthesis, as discussed more fully in Chapter 28.

Summary

The most commonly used intravenous induction drugs are the barbiturates thiopental and methohexital, and propofol, ketamine, and etomidate. All are characterized by rapid onset of effect due to facile brain uptake kinetics, and short duration of effect after a bolus dose. All undergo extensive hepatic biotransformation, but their duration of clinical effect is terminated by redistribution from the central vascular compartment to peripheral tissues, rather than by metabolism and systemic elimination. Pharmacokinetic drug interactions are therefore rarely a concern in the use of intravenous induction drugs.

Thiopental is the oldest of the currently used IV anesthetics, but remains an excellent induction drug. However, it is unsuitable for the maintenance of anesthesia because of slow systemic elimination and the potential for drug and metabolite accumulation. Thiopental systemic elimination is dependent on intrinsic clearance and independent of hepatic blood flow. The basic pH of its soluble form requires caution, because it causes significant tissue damage if there is inadvertent extravascular administration or if it is administered at the same time as acidic solutions (e.g., nondepolarizing muscle relaxants), and it may precipitate and obstruct intravenous tubing.

Methohexital was designed to be a rapidly eliminated barbiturate, suitable for short-duration surgery. As an induction drug, it resembles thiopental pharmacokinetically, and offers few advantages over thiopental. However, methohexital metabolic clearance is about three times greater than that of thiopental. Methohexital clearance depends more on hepatic blood flow than intrinsic clearance, and the elimination half-life is shorter than that of thiopental. Unlike thiopental, methohexital infusions are suitable for maintenance of anesthesia or longer-duration sedation.

Propofol, formulated as a lipid emulsion, is the most commonly used intravenous anesthetic, serving both as an induction drug and for maintenance of anesthesia. It is extensively metabolized, both by oxidation and by conjugation, in both the liver and extrahepatic sites. Propofol pharmacokinetics have been extensively studied to define distribution models,

in part for use in target-controlled infusion (TCI) systems. After a bolus dose, propofol blood concentrations decrease rapidly due to extensive redistribution to peripheral tissues. After prolonged administration, propofol returns slowly from peripheral compartments to the central compartment, more slowly than the rate of systemic elimination. Consequently, propofol blood concentrations decrease quickly and remain low. The result is that the context-sensitive half-time, the time for plasma concentration to decrease by 50% after the end of an infusion, remains essentially independent of the duration of drug infusion. There is interest in the development of new formulations, such as water-soluble analogs or propofol prodrugs, including the recently approved prodrug fospropofol.

Ketamine, which is variably available in certain countries as a racemate and/or the single S(+) enantiomer, is used for anesthetic induction and as an analgesic adjuvant, and may be administered as a bolus or an infusion. Ketamine is extensively metabolized, and there is evidence that some of the metabolites retain partial pharmacologic activity. Ketamine is a high-extraction drug, and systemic clearance is therefore dependent more on hepatic blood flow than on intrinsic metabolism.

Etomidate remains an unequaled induction drug in hemodynamically compromised patients, but is unsuitable for maintenance of anesthesia because it inhibits cortisol synthesis. Etomidate systemic clearance is high, approximating rates of liver blood flow, and thus it is a high-extraction drug whose clearance depends on cardiac output more than metabolism.

References

1. Lundy JS, Tovell RM. Some of the newer local and general anesthetic agents: methods of their administration. *Northwest Med* 1934; **33**: 308–11.

2. Pratt TW, Tatum AL, Hathaway HR, Waters RM. Sodium ethyl(1-methylbutyl) thiobarbiturate: Preliminary experimental and clinical study. *Am J Surg* 1936; **31**: 464.

3. Tomlin SL, Jenkins A, Lieb WR, Franks NP. Preparation of barbiturate optical isomers and their effects on GABA(A) receptors. *Anesthesiology* 1999; **90**: 1714–22.

4. Zaugg S, Caslavska J, Theurillat R, Thormann W. Characterization of the stereoselective metabolism of thiopental and its metabolite pentobarbital via analysis of their enantiomers in human plasma by capillary electrophoresis. *J Chromatogr A* 1999; **838**: 237–49.

5. Stanski DR, Burch PG, Harapat S, Richards RK. Pharmacokinetics and anesthetic potency of a thiopental isomer. *J Pharm Sci* 1983; **72**: 937–40.

6. Bush MT, Berry G, Hume A. Ultra-short-acting barbiturates as oral hypnotic agents in man. *Clin Pharmacol Ther* 1966; **7**: 373–8.

7. Mark LC, Burns JJ, Campomanes CI, *et al.* The passage of thiopental into brain. *J Pharmacol Exp Ther* 1957; **119**: 35–8.

8. Haws JL, Herman N, Clark Y, Bjoraker R, Jones D. The chemical stability and sterility of sodium thiopental after preparation. *Anesth Analg* 1998; **86**: 208–13.

9. Christensen JH, Andreasen F, Jensen EB. The binding of thiopental to human serum albumin at variable pH and temperature. *Acta Pharmacol Toxicol (Copenh)* 1983; **52**: 364–70.

10. Morgan DJ, Blackman GL, Paull JD, Wolf LJ. Pharmacokinetics and plasma binding of thiopental. I: studies in surgical patients. *Anesthesiology* 1981; **54**: 468–73.

11. Burch PG, Stanski DR. The role of metabolism and protein binding in thiopental anesthesia. *Anesthesiology* 1983; **58**: 146–52.

12. Russo H, Audran M, Bressolle F, Bres J, Maillols H. Displacement of thiopental from human serum albumin by associated drugs. *J Pharm Sci* 1993; **82**: 493–7.

13. Brodie BB, Mark LC. The fate of thiopental in man and a method for its estimation in biological material. *J Pharmacol Exp Ther* 1950; **98**: 85–96.

14. Price HL. A dynamic concept of the distribution of thiopental in the human body. *Anesthesiology* 1960; **21**: 40–5.

15. Stanski DR, Mihm FG, Rosenthal MH, Kalman SM. Pharmacokinetics of high-dose thiopental used in cerebral resuscitation. *Anesthesiology* 1980; **53**: 169–71.

16. Turcant A, Delhumeau A, Premel-Cabic A, *et al.* Thiopental pharmacokinetics under conditions of long-term infusion. *Anesthesiology* 1985; **63**: 50–4.

17. Stanski DR, Maitre PO. Population pharmacokinetics and pharmacodynamics of thiopental: the effect of age revisited. *Anesthesiology* 1990; **72**: 412–22.

18. Henthorn TK, Avram MJ, Krejcie TC. Intravascular mixing and drug distribution: the concurrent disposition of thiopental and indocyanine green. *Clin Pharmacol Ther* 1989; **45**: 56–65.

19. Hull CJ. How far can we go with compartmental models? *Anesthesiology* 1990; **72**: 399–402.

20. Nestorov I. Whole body pharmacokinetic models. *Clin Pharmacokin* 2003; **42**: 883–908

21. Wada DR, Bjorkman S, Ebling WF, *et al.* Computer simulation of the effects of alterations in blood flows and body composition on thiopental pharmacokinetics in humans. *Anesthesiology* 1997; **87**: 884–99.

22. Stanski DR. Pharmacokinetic modeling of thiopental. *Anesthesiology* 1981; **54**: 446–8.

23. Sear JW. Why not model physiologically? *Br J Anaesth* 1993; **70**: 243–245.

24. Krejcie TC, Henthorn TK, Niemann CU, *et al.* Recirculatory pharmacokinetic models of markers of blood, extracellular fluid and total body water administered concomitantly. *J Pharmacol Exp Ther* 1996; **278**: 1050–7.

25. Krejcie TC, Avram MJ. What determines anesthetic induction dose? It's the front-end kinetics, doctor! *Anesth Analg* 1999; **89**: 541–4.

26. Avram MJ, Krejcie TC. Using front-end kinetics to optimize target-controlled drug infusions. *Anesthesiology* 2003; **99**: 1078–86.

27. Avram MJ, Henthorn TK, Spyker DA, *et al.* Recirculatory pharmacokinetic model of the uptake, distribution, and bioavailability of prochlorperazine administered as a thermally generated aerosol in a single breath to dogs. *Drug Metab Dispos* 2007; **35**: 262–7.

28. Wada DR, Drover DR, Lemmens HJM. Determination of the distribution volume that can be used to calculate the intravenous loading dose. *Clin Pharmacokin* 1998; **35**: 1–7.

29. Avram MJ, Krejcie TC. Using front-end kinetics to optimise target-controlled drug infusions. *Anesthesiology* 2003; **99**: 1078–86.

30. Kuipers JA, Boer F, Olofsen E, Bovill JG, Burm AGL. Recirculatory pharmacokinetics and pharmacodynamics of rocuronium in patients: the influence of cardiac output. *Anesthesiology* 2001; **94**: 47–55.

31. Stanski DR, Hudson RJ, Homer TD, Saidman LJ, Meathe E. Pharmacodynamic modeling of thiopental anesthesia. *J Pharmacokinet Biopharm* 1984; **12**: 223–40.

32. Avram MJ, Krejcie TC, Henthorn TK, Niemann CU. Beta-adrenergic blockade affects initial drug distribution due to decreased cardiac output and altered blood flow distribution. *J Pharmacol Exp Ther* 2004; **311**: 617–24.

33. Avram MJ, Krejcie TC, Niemann CU, *et al.* Isoflurane alters the recirculatory pharmacokinetics of physiologic markers. *Anesthesiology* 2000; **92**: 1757–68.

34. Avram MJ, Krejcie TC, Niemann CU, *et al.* The effect of halothane on the recirculatory pharmacokinetics of physiologic markers. *Anesthesiology* 1997; **87**: 1381–93.

35. Avram MJ, Sanghvi R, Henthorn TK, *et al.* Determinants of thiopental induction dose requirements. *Anesth Analg* 1993; **76**: 10–17.

36. Homer TD, Stanski DR. The effect of increasing age on thiopental disposition and anesthetic requirement. *Anesthesiology* 1985; **62**: 714–24.

37. Kingston HG, Kendrick A, Sommer KM, Olsen GD, Downes H. Binding of thiopental in neonatal serum. *Anesthesiology* 1990; **72**: 428–31.

38. Burch PG, Stanski DR. Decreased protein binding and thiopental kinetics. *Clin Pharmacol Ther* 1982; **32**: 212–17.

39. Christensen JH, Andreasen F, Jansen J. Pharmacokinetics and pharmacodynamics of thiopentone in patients undergoing renal transplantation. *Acta Anaesthesiol Scand* 1983; **27**; 513–18.

40. Ghoneim MM, Van Hamme JJ. Pharmacokinetics of thiopentone; effects of enflurane and nitrous oxide anaesthesia and surgery. *Br J Anaesth* 1978; **50**; 1237–42.

41. Pandele G, Chaux F, Salvadori C *et al.* Thiopental pharmacokinetics in patients with cirrhosis. *Anesthesiology* 1983; **59**: 123–6.

42. Couderc E, Ferrier C, Haberer JP, Henzel D, Duvaldestin P. Thiopentone pharmacokinetics in patients with chronic alcoholism. *Br J Anaesth* 1984; **56**; 1393–7.

43. Jung D, Mayersohn M, Perrier D, Calkins J, Saunders R. Thiopental disposition in lean and obese patients undergoing surgery. *Anesthesiology* 1982; **56**: 269–74.

44. Brunner H. Narcotic drug methohexital: synthesis by enantioselective catalysis. *Chirality* 2001; **13**: 420–4.

45. Girard I, Ferry S. Protein binding of methohexital. Study of parameters and modulating factors using the equilibrium dialysis technique. *J Pharm Biomed Anal* 1996; **14**: 583–91.

46. Herman NL, Li AT, Van Decar TK, *et al.* Transfer of methohexital across the perfused human placenta. *J Clin Anesth* 2000; **12**: 25–30.

47. Lange H, Stephan H, Brand C, Zielmann S, Sonntag H. Hepatic disposition of methohexitone in patients undergoing coronary bypass surgery. *Br J Anaesth* 1992; **69**: 478–81.

48. Hudson RJ, Stanski DR, Burch PG. Pharmacokinetics of methohexital and thiopental in surgical patients. *Anesthesiology* 1983; **59**: 215–19.

49. Breimer DD. Pharmacokinetics of methohexitone following intravenous infusion in humans. *Br J Anaesth* 1976; **48**: 643–9.

50. Redke F, Bjorkman S. Endotoxin-induced fever increases the clearance of methohexitone in rabbits. *J Pharm Pharmacol* 1994; **46**: 887–91.

51. Redke F, Bjorkman S, Rosberg B. Pharmacokinetics and clinical experience of 20-h infusions of methohexitone in intensive care patients with postoperative pyrexia. *Br J Anaesth* 1991; **66**: 53–9.

52. Duvaldestin P, Chauvin M, Lebrault C, *et al.* Effect of upper abdominal surgery and cirrhosis upon the pharmacokinetics of methohexital. *Acta Anaesthesiol Scand* 1991; **35**; 159–63.

53. Schwilden H, Stoeckel H. Effective therapeutic infusions produced by closed-loop feedback control of methohexital administration during total intravenous anesthesia with fentanyl. *Anesthesiology* 1990; **73**: 225–9.

54. Schwilden H, Schüttler J, Stoeckel H. Closed-loop feedback control of methohexital anesthesia by quantitative EEG analysis in humans. *Anesthesiology* 1987; **67**: 341–7.

55. Cummins CG, Dixon J, Kay NH, *et al.* Dose requirements of ICI 35868 (Propofol: Diprivan) in a new formulation for induction of anaesthesia. *Anaesthesia* 1984; **39**: 1168–71.

56. Bennett SN, McNeil MM, Bland LA, *et al.* Postoperative infections traced to contamination of an intravenous anesthetic, propofol. *N Engl J Med* 1995; **333**: 147–54.

57. Baker MT, Naguib M. Propofol: the challenges of formulation. *Anesthesiology* 2005; **103**: 860–76.

58. Han J, Davis SS, Washington C. Physical properties and stability of two emulsion formulations of propofol. *Int J Pharm* 2001; **215**: 207–20.

59. Mazoit JX, Samii K. Binding of propofol to blood components: implications for pharmacokinetics and for pharmacodynamics. *Br J Clin Pharmacol* 1999; **47**: 35–42.

60. Dailland P, Cockshott ID, Lirzin JD, *et al.* Intravenous propofol during cesarean section: placental transfer, concentrations in breast milk, and neonatal effects. A preliminary study. *Anesthesiology* 1989; **71**: 827–34.

61. He YL, Ueyama H, Tashiro C, Mashimo T, Yoshiya I. Pulmonary disposition of propofol in surgical patients. *Anesthesiology* 2000; **93**: 986–91.

62. Dawidowicz AL, Fornal E, Mardarowicz M, Fijalkowska A. The role of human lungs in the biotransformation of propofol. *Anesthesiology* 2000; **93**: 992–7.

63. Hiraoka H, Yamamoto K, Miyoshi S, *et al.* Kidneys contribute to the extrahepatic clearance of propofol in humans, but not lungs and brain. *Br J Clin Pharmacol* 2005; **60**: 176–82.

64. Upton RN, Ludbrook G. A physiologically based, recirculatory model of the kinetics and dynamics of propofol in man. *Anesthesiology* 2005; **103**: 344–52.

65. Chen YZ, Zhu SM, He HL, *et al.* Do the lungs contribute to propofol elimination in patients during orthotopic liver transplantation without veno-venous bypass? *Hepatobiliary Pancreat Dis Int* 2006; **5**: 511–14.

66. Oda Y, Hamaoka N, Hiroi T, *et al.* Involvement of human liver cytochrome P4502B6 in the metabolism of propofol. *Br J Clin Pharmacol* 2001; **51**: 281–5.

67. Veroli P, O'Kelly B, Bertrand F, *et al.* Extrahepatic metabolism of propofol in man during the anhepatic phase of orthotopic liver transplantation. *Br J Anaesth* 1992; **68**: 183–6.

68. Takizawa D, Sato E, Hiraoka H, *et al.* Changes in apparent systemic clearance of propofol during transplantation of living related donor liver. *Br J Anaesth* 2005; **95**: 643–7.

69. Grossherr M, Hengstenberg A, Meier T, *et al.* Discontinuous monitoring of propofol concentrations in expired alveolar gas and in arterial and venous plasma during artificial ventilation. *Anesthesiology* 2006; **104**: 786–90.

70. Bodenham A, Culank LS, Park GR. Propofol infusion and green urine. *Lancet* 1987; **2**: 740.

71. Marik PE. Propofol: therapeutic indications and side-effects. *Curr Pharm Des* 2004; **10**: 3639–49

72. Morgan DJ, Campbell GA, Crankshaw DP. Pharmacokinetics of propofol when given by intravenous infusion. *Br J Clin Pharmacol* 1988; **30**: 144–8.

73. Gepts E, Camu F, Cockshott ID, Douglas EJ. Disposition of propofol administered as constant rate intravenous infusions in humans. *Anesth Analg* 1987; **66**: 1256–63.

74. Marsh B, White M, Morton N, Kenny GN. Pharmacokinetic model driven infusion of propofol in children. *Br J Anaesth* 1991; **67**: 41–8.

75. Schnider TW, Minto CF, Gambus PL, *et al.* The influence of method of administration and covariates on the pharmacokinetics of propofol in adult volunteers. *Anesthesiology* 1998; **88**: 1170–82.

76. Schüttler J, Ihmsen H. Population pharmacokinetics of propofol: a multicenter study. *Anesthesiology* 2000; **92**: 727–38.

77. Glen JB. The development of "Diprifusor": a TCI system for propofol. *Anaesthesia* 1998; **53**: 13–21.

78. Frolich MA, Dennis DM, Shuster JA, Melker RJ. Precision and bias of target controlled propofol infusion for sedation. *Br J Anaesth* 2005; **94**: 434–7.

79. Coetzee JF, Glen JB, Wium CA, Boshoff L. Pharmacokinetic model selection for target controlled infusions of propofol. Assessment of three parameter sets. *Anesthesiology* 1995; **82**: 1328–45.

80. Albertin A, Poli D, La Colla L, *et al.* Predictive performance of "Servin's formula" during BIS-guided propofol-remifentanil target-controlled infusion in morbidly obese patients. *Br J Anaesth* 2007; **98**: 66–75.

81. James WPT. *Research on Obesity.* London: HMSO, 1976.

82. Kataria BK, Ved SA, Nicodemus HF, *et al.* The pharmacokinetics of propofol in children using three different data analysis approaches. *Anesthesiology* 1994; **80**: 104–22.

83. Absalom A, Kenny G. "Paedfusor" pharmacokinetic data set. *Br J Anaesth* 2005; **95**: 110.

84. Schnider TW, Minto CF, Shafer SL, *et al.* The influence of age on propofol pharmacodynamics. *Anesthesiology* 1999; **90**: 1502–16.

85. Servin F, Farinotti R, Haberer JP, Desmonts JM. Propofol infusion for maintenance of anesthesia in morbidly obese patients receiving nitrous oxide. A clinical and pharmacokinetic study. *Anesthesiology* 1993; **78**: 657–65.

86. Servin F, Cockshott ID, Farinotti R, *et al.* Pharmacokinetics of propofol infusions in patients with cirrhosis. *Br J Anaesth* 1990; **65**: 177–83.

87. Servin F, Desmonts JM, Haberer JP, *et al.* Pharmacokinetics and protein

binding of propofol in patients with cirrhosis. *Anesthesiology* 1988; **69**: 887–91.

88. Albanese J, Martin C, Lacarelle B, *et al.* Pharmacokinetics of long-term propofol infusion used for sedation in ICU patients. *Anesthesiology* 1990; **73**: 214–17.

89. Barr J, Egan TD, Sandoval NF, *et al.* Propofol dosing regimens for ICU sedation based upon an integrated pharmacokinetic-pharmacodynamic model. *Anesthesiology* 2001; **95**: 324–33.

90. McMurray TJ, Johnston JR, Milligan KR, *et al.* Propofol sedation using Diprifusor target-controlled infusion in adult intensive care unit patients. *Anaesthesia* 2004; **59**: 636–41.

91. Bailey JM, Mora CT, Shafer SL. Pharmacokinetics of propofol in adult patients undergoing coronary revascularization. The Multicenter Study of Perioperative Ischemia Research Group. *Anesthesiology* 1996; **84**: 1288–97.

92. Kay NH, Sear JW, Uppington J, Cockshott ID, Douglas EJ. Disposition of propofol in patients undergoing surgery. A comparison in men and women. *Br J Anaesth* 1986; **59**: 1075–9.

93. Kirkpatrick T, Cockshott ID, Douglas EJ, Nimmo WS. Pharmacokinetics of propofol (Diprivan) in elderly patients. *Br J Anaesth* 1988; **60**: 146–50.

94. Song JC, Sun YM, Zhang MZ, *et al.* Propofol pharmacokinetics in patients with obstructive jaundice. *Current Drug Del* 2009; **6**: 317–20.

95. Kirvela M, Olkkola KT, Rosenberg PH, *et al.* Pharmacokinetics of propofol and haemodynamic changes during induction of anaesthesia in uraemic patients. *Br J Anaesth* 1992; **68**: 178–82.

96. Ickx B, Cockshott ID, Barvais L, *et al.* Propofol infusion for induction and maintenance of anaesthesia in patients with end-stage renal disease. *Br J Anaesth* 1998; **81**: 854–60.

97. Costela JL, Jimenez R, Calvo R, Suarez E, Carlos R. Serum protein binding of propofol in patients with renal failure or hepatic cirrhosis. *Acta Anaesthesiol Scand* 1996; **40**: 741–5.

98. Fechner J, Ihmsen H, Hatterscheid D, *et al.* Pharmacokinetics and clinical pharmacodynamics of the new propofol prodrug GPI 15715 in volunteers. *Anesthesiology* 2003; **99**: 303–13.

99. Greenblatt DJ. Elimination half-life of drugs: value and limitations. *Ann Rev Med* 1985; **36**: 421–7.

100. Hughes MA, Glass PS, Jacobs JR. Context-sensitive half-time in multicompartment pharmacokinetic models for intravenous anesthetic drugs. *Anesthesiology* 1992; **76**: 334–41.

101. Kharasch ED. Ketamine pharmacokinetics. In: Bowdle TA, Horita A, Kharasch ED, eds., *The Pharmacological Basis of Anesthesiology Practice: Basic Science and Clinical Applications*. New York, NY: Churchill Livingstone, 1994: 357–73.

102. Youngs EJ, Shafer SL. Pharmacokinetic parameters relevant to recovery from opioids. *Anesthesiology* 1994; **81**: 833–42.

103. Schraag S, Mohl U, Hirsch M, *et al.* Recovery from opioid anesthesia: the clinical implications of context-sensitive half-times. *Anesth Analg* 1998; **86**: 184–90.

104. Bailey JM. Technique for quantifying the duration of intravenous anesthetic effect. *Anesthesiology* 1995; **83**: 1095–103.

105. Sear JW. Recovery from anaesthesia: which is the best kinetic descriptor of a drug's recovery profile? *Anaesthesia* 1996; **51**: 997–9.

106. Wessen A, Persson P, Nilsson A, Hartvig P. Concentration-effect relationship of propofol after total intravenous anesthesia. *Anesth Analg* 1993; **77**: 1000–7.

107. Jacobs, Reves JF, Marty J, *et al.* Aging increases pharmacodynamic sensitivity to the hypnotic effects of midazolam. *Anesth Analg* 1995; **80**: 143–8.

108. White M, Schenkels MJ, Engbers FH, *et al.* Effect-site modelling of propofol using auditory evoked potentials. *Br J Anaesth* 1999; **82**: 333–9.

109. Minto CF, Schnider TW, Gregg KM, Henthorn TK, Shafer SL. Using the time of maximum effect site concentration to combine pharmacokinetics and pharmacodynamics. *Anesthesiology* 2003; **99**: 324–33.

110. Struys MM, De Smet T, Depoorter B, *et al.* Comparison of plasma compartment versus two methods for effect compartment: controlled target-controlled infusion for propofol. *Anesthesiology* 2000; **92**: 399–406.

111. Doufas AG, Bakhshandeh M, Bjorksten AR, Shafer SL, Sessler DI. Induction speed is not a determinant of propofol pharmacodynamics. *Anesthesiology* 2004; **101**: 1112–21.

112. Struys MM, Coppens MJ, De Neve N, *et al.* Influence of administration rate on propofol plasma-effect site equilibration. *Anesthesiology* 2007; **107**: 386–96.

113. Kazama T, Morita K, Ikeda T, Kurita T, Sato S. Comparison of predicted induction dose with predetermined physiologic characteristics of patients and with pharmacokinetic models incorporating those characteristics as covariates. *Anesthesiology* 2003; **98**: 299–305.

114. Baker MT, Chadam MV, Ronnenberg WC. Inhibitory effects of propofol on cytochrome P450 activities in rat hepatic microsomes. *Anesth Analg* 1993; **76**: 817–21.

115. Chen TL, Ueng TH, Chen SH, *et al.* Human cytochrome P450 mono-oxygenase system is suppressed by propofol. *Br J Anaesth* 1995; **74**: 558–62.

116. Janicki PK, James MF, Erskine WA. Propofol inhibits enzymatic degradation of alfentanil and sufentanil by isolated liver microsomes in vitro. *Br J Anaesth* 1992; **68**: 311–2.

117. Chen TL, Chen TG, Tai YT, *et al.* Propofol inhibits renal cytochrome P450 activity and enflurane defluorination in vitro in hamsters. *Can J Anaesth* 2000; **47**: 680–6.

118. Mertens MJ, Vuyk J, Olofsen E, Bovill JG, Burm AG. Propofol alters the pharmacokinetics of alfentanil in healthy male volunteers. *Anesthesiology* 2001; **94**: 949–57.

119. Henthorn TK, Avram MJ, Krejcie TC. Alfentanil clearance is independent of the polymorphic debrisoquin hydroxylase. *Anesthesiology* 1989; **71**: 635–9.

120. Johnson KB, Syroid ND, Gupta DK, *et al.* An evaluation of remifentanil propofol response surfaces for loss of responsiveness, loss of response to surrogates of painful stimuli and laryngoscopy in patients undergoing elective surgery. *Anesth Analg* 2008; **106**: 471–9.

121. Kern SE, Xie G, White JL, Egan TD. A response surface analysis of propofol–remifentanil pharmacodynamic interaction in volunteers. *Anesthesiology* 2004; **100**: 1373–81.

122. Bouillon TW, Bruhn J, Radulescu L, *et al.* Pharmacodynamic interaction between propofol and remifentanil regarding hypnosis, tolerance of laryngoscopy, bispectral index, and electroencephalographic approximate entropy. *Anesthesiology* 2004; **100**: 1353–72.

123. Mertens MJ, Olofsen E, Engbers FH, *et al.* Propofol reduces perioperative remifentanil requirements in a synergistic manner: response surface modeling of perioperative remifentanil-propofol interactions. *Anesthesiology* 2003; **99**: 347–59.

124. Ludbrook GL, Upton RN. Pharmacokinetic drug interaction between propofol and remifentanil? *Anesth Analg* 2003; **97**: 924–5.

125. Bouillon T, Bruhn J, Radu-Radulescu L, *et al.* Non-steady state analysis of the pharmacokinetic interaction between propofol and remifentanil. *Anesthesiology* 2002; **97**: 1350–62.

126. Ethell BT, Beaumont K, Rance DJ, Burchell B. Use of cloned and expressed human UDP-glucuronosyltransferases for the assessment of human drug conjugation and identification of potential drug interactions. *Drug Metab Dispos* 2001; **29**: 48–53.

127. Ward DS, Norton JR, Guivarc'h PH, Litman RS, Bailey PL. Pharmacodynamics and pharmacokinetics of propofol in a medium-chain triglyceride emulsion. *Anesthesiology* 2002; **97**: 1401–8.

128. Allford MA, Mensah JA. Discomfort on injection: a comparison between two formulations of propofol. *Eur J Anaesthesiol* 2006; **23**: 971–4.

129. Ewart MC, Yau KW, Morgan M. 2% propofol for sedation in the intensive care unit. A feasibility study. *Anaesthesia* 1992; **47**: 146–8.

130. Servin FS, Desmonts JM, Melloni C, Martinelli G. A comparison of 2% and 1% formulations of propofol for the induction and maintenance of anaesthesia in surgery of moderate duration. *Anaesthesia* 1997; **52**: 1216–21.

131. Doenicke AW, Roizen MF, Hoernecke R, Lorenz W, Ostwald P. Solvent for etomidate may cause pain and adverse effects. *Br J Anaesth* 1999; **83**: 464–6.

132. Doenicke AW, Roizen MF, Rau J, Kellermann W, Babl J. Reducing pain during propofol injection: the role of the solvent. *Anesth Analg* 1996; **82**: 472–4.

133. Silvestri GA, Vincent BD, Wahidi MM, *et al.* A phase 3, randomized, double-blind, study to assess the efficacy and safety of fospropofol disodium injection for moderate sedation in patients undergoing flexible bronchoscopy. *Chest* 2009; **135**; 41–7.

134. Gibiansky E, Struys MM, Gibiansky L, *et al.* AQUAVAN injection, a water-soluble prodrug of propofol, as a bolus injection: a phase I dose-escalation comparison with DIPRIVAN (part 1): pharmacokinetics. *Anesthesiology* 2005; **103**: 718–29.

135. Fechner J, Ihmsen H, Hatterscheid D, *et al.* Comparative pharmacokinetics and pharmacodynamics of the new propofol prodrug GPI 15715 and propofol emulsion. *Anesthesiology* 2004; **101**: 626–39.

136. Shah A, Mistry B, Gibiansky E, Gibiansky L. Fospropofol assay issues and impact on pharmacokinetic and pharmacodynamic evaluation. *Anesthesiology* 2008; **109**: 937.

137. Corssen G, Domino EF. Dissociative anesthesia: further pharmacologic studies and first clinical experience with the phencyclidine derivative CI-581. *Anesth Analg* 1966; **45**: 29–40.

138. White PF, Ham J, Way WL, Trevor AJ. Pharmacology of ketamine isomers in surgical patients. *Anesthesiology* 1980; **52**: 231–9.

139. Ryder S, Way WL, Trevor AJ. Comparative pharmacology of the optical isomers of ketamine in mice. *Eur J Pharmacol* 1978; **49**: 15–23.

140. Dayton PG, Stiller RL, Cook DR, Perel JM. The binding of ketamine to plasma proteins: emphasis on human plasma. *Eur J Clin Pharmacol* 1983; **24**: 825–31.

141. White PF, Schüttler J, Shafer A, *et al.* Comparative pharmacology of the ketamine isomers. Studies in volunteers. *Br J Anaesth* 1985; **57**: 197–203.

142. Schüttler J, Stanski DR, White PF, *et al.* Pharmacodynamic modeling of the EEG effects of ketamine and its enantiomers in man. *J Pharmacokinet Biopharm* 1987; **15**: 241–53.

143. Henthorn TK, Krejcie TC, Niemann CU, *et al.* Ketamine distribution described by a recirculatory pharmacokinetic model is not stereoselective. *Anesthesiology* 1999; **91**: 1733–43.

144. White PF, Johnston RR, Pudwill CR. Interaction of ketamine and halothane in rats. *Anesthesiology* 1975; **42**: 179–86.

145. Lau SS, Domino EF. Gas chromatography mass spectrometry assay for ketamine and its metabolites in plasma. *Biomed Mass Spectrom* 1977; **4**; 317–21.

146. Edwards SR, Mather LE. Tissue uptake of ketamine and norketamine enantiomers in the rat: indirect evidence for extrahepatic metabolic inversion. *Life Sci* 2001; **69**: 2051–66.

147. Hijazi Y, Boulieu R. Contribution of CYP3A4, CYP2B6, and CYP2C9 isoforms to N-demethylation of ketamine in human liver microsomes. *Drug Metab Dispos* 2002; **30**: 853–8.

148. Yanagihara Y, Kariya S, Ohtani M, *et al.* Involvement of CYP2B6 in n-demethylation of ketamine in human liver microsomes. *Drug Metab Dispos* 2001; **29**: 887–90.

149. Koppel C, Arndt I, Ibe K. Effects of enzyme induction, renal and cardiac function on ketamine plasma kinetics in patients with ketamine long-term analgosedation. *Eur J Drug Metab Pharmacokinet* 1990; **15**: 259–63.

150. Ihmsen H, Geisslinger G, Schüttler J. Stereoselective pharmacokinetics of ketamine: R(−)-ketamine inhibits the elimination of S(+)-ketamine. *Clin Pharmacol Ther* 2001; **70**: 431–8.

151. Persson J, Hasselstrom J, Maurset A, *et al.* Pharmacokinetics and non-analgesic effects of S- and R-ketamines in healthy volunteers with normal and reduced metabolic capacity. *Eur J Clin Pharmacol* 2002; **57**: 869–75.

152. Geisslinger G, Hering W, Thomann P, *et al.* Pharmacokinetics and pharmacodynamics of ketamine enantiomers in surgical patients using a stereoselective analytical method. *Br J Anaesth* 1993; **70**: 666–71.

153. Clements JA, Nimmo WS. Pharmacokinetics and analgesic effect of ketamine in man. *Br J Anaesth* 1981; **53**: 27–30.

154. Kharasch ED, Labroo R. Metabolism of ketamine stereoisomers by human liver microsomes. *Anesthesiology* 1992; **77**: 1201–7.

155. Malinovsky JM, Servin F, Cozian A, Lepage JY, Pinaud M. Ketamine and norketamine plasma concentrations after i.v., nasal and rectal administration in children. *Br J Anaesth* 1996; **77**: 203–7.

156. Idvall J, Ahlgren I, Aronsen KR, Stenberg P. Ketamine infusions: pharmacokinetics and clinical effects. *Br J Anaesth* 1979; **51**: 1167–73.

157. White PF, Dworsky WA, Horai Y, Trevor AJ. Comparison of continuous infusion fentanyl or ketamine versus thiopental: determining the mean effective serum concentrations for outpatient surgery. *Anesthesiology* 1983; **59**: 564–9.

158. Hartvig P, Valtysson J, Lindner KJ, *et al.* Central nervous system effects of subdissociative doses of (S)-ketamine are related to plasma and brain concentrations measured with positron emission tomography in healthy volunteers. *Clin Pharmacol Ther* 1995; **58**: 165–73.

159. Bowdle TA, Radant AD, Cowley DS *et al.* Psychedelic effects of ketamine in healthy volunteers: relationship to steady-state plasma concentrations. *Anesthesiology* 1998; **88**: 82–8.

160. Clements JA, Nimmo WS, Grant IS. Bioavailability, pharmacokinetics, and analgesic activity of ketamine in humans. *J Pharm Sci* 1982; **71**: 539–42.

161. Grant IS, Nimmo WS, Clements JA. Pharmacokinetics and analgesic effects of i.m. and oral ketamine. *Br J Anaesth* 1981; **53**: 805–10.

162. Leung A, Wallace MS, Ridgeway B, Yaksh T. Concentration-effect relationship of intravenous alfentanil and ketamine on peripheral neurosensory thresholds, allodynia and hyperalgesia of neuropathic pain. *Pain* 2001; **91**: 177–87.

163. Edwards SR, Minto CF, Mather LE. Concurrent ketamine and alfentanil administration: pharmacokinetic considerations. *Br J Anaesth* 2002; **88**: 94–100.

164. Rofael HZ, Abdel-Rahman MS. The role of ketamine on plasma cocaine pharmacokinetics in rat. *Toxicol Lett* 2002; **129**: 167–76.

165. Park GR, Manara AR, Mendel L, Bateman PE. Ketamine infusion: its use as a sedative, inotrope and bronchodilator in a critically ill patient. *Anaesthesia* 1987; **42**: 980–3.

166. Tomlins SL, Jenkins A, Lieb WR, Franks NP. Stereoselective effects of etomidate optical isomers on gamma-aminobutyric acid type A receptors and animals. *Anesthesiology* 1998; **88**: 708–17.

167. Doenicke A, Roizen MF, Hoernecke R, *et al.* Haemolysis after etomidate: comparison of propylene glycol and lipid formulations. *Br J Anaesth* 1997; **79**: 386–8.

168. McIntosh MP, Schwarting N, Rajewski RA. In vitro and in vivo evaluation of a sulfobutyl ether beta-cyclosporin enabled etomidate formulation. *J Pharm Sci* 2004; **93**: 2585–94.

169. Bright DP, Adham SD, Lemaire LC, *et al.* Identification of anesthetic binding sites on human serum albumin using a novel etomidate photolabel. *J Biol Chem* 2007; **282**: 12038–47.

170. Heykants JJ, Meuldermans WE, Michiels LJ, Lewi PJ, Janssen PA. Distribution, metabolism and excretion of etomidate, a short-acting hypnotic drug, in the rat. Comparative study of (R)-(+)-(−)-etomidate. *Arch Int Pharmacodyn Ther* 1975; **216**: 113–29.

171. Arden JR, Holley FO, Stanski DR. Increased sensitivity to etomidate in the elderly: initial distribution versus altered brain response. *Anesthesiology* 1986; **65**: 19–27.

172. Van Hamme MJ, Ghoneim MM, Ambre JJ. Pharmacokinetics of etomidate, a new intravenous anesthetic. *Anesthesiology* 1978; **49**: 274–7.

173. Schüttler J, Wilms M, Lauven PM, *et al.* Pharmacokinetische untersuchungen uber etomidat beim menschen. *Der Anaesthesist* 1980; **29**: 658–61.

174. Fragen RJ, Avrom MJ, Henthorn TK, Caldwell NJ. A pharmacokinetically designed etomidate infusion regimen for hypnosis. *Anesth Analg* 1983; **62**: 654–60.

175. Johnson KB, Egan TD, Layman J, *et al.* The influence of hemorrhagic shock on etomidate: a pharmacokinetic and pharmacodynamic analysis. *Anesth Analg* 2003; **96**: 1360–8.

176. van Beem H, Manger FW, van Boxtel C, van Bentem N. Etomidate anaesthesia in patients with cirrhosis of the liver: pharmacokinetic data. *Anaesthesia* 1983; **38**: 61–2.

177. Bonnardot JP, Levron JC, Deslauriers N, *et al.* Pharmacokinetics of continuous infusion of etomidate in cirrhosis. *Ann Fr Anesth Reanim* 1991; **10**: 443–4.

178. Carlos R, Calvo R, Erill S. Plasma protein binding of etomidate in patients with renal failure or hepatic cirrhosis. *Clin Pharmacokin* 1979; **4**: 144–8.

Essential drugs in anesthetic practice
Clinical pharmacology of intravenous anesthetics

John W. Sear

Introduction

The onset of anesthesia requires the brain drug concentration to achieve a given threshold. However, rapid achievement of this endpoint may be accompanied by significant adverse clinical effects such as hypotension, bradycardia, and respiratory depression. The greater the concentration gradient between the blood and the effect site, the greater the time needed to induce anesthesia. An overshoot in the effect-site concentration will lead to a greater incidence and severity of adverse effects. The transfer of drug from the blood to its effect site(s) is governed (in most cases) by simple diffusion. The time needed to achieve this transfer varies with the magnitude of the concentration gradient and with the individual drug's blood–brain equilibration rate constant (k_{e0}).

Conversely, the duration of drug effect from bolus administration of an intravenous hypnotic drug is terminated predominantly by drug redistribution from the blood and brain to the lean and fatty tissues of the body. This redistribution occurs by a series of different intercompartmental clearances. Bolus drug concentrations are influenced by redistribution and, to a lesser extent, by metabolic clearance. In the case of lipid-soluble hypnotic induction drugs, the sum of these clearances is dependent on the patient's cardiac output.

The kinetics of intravenous anesthetics are shown in Table 28.1, and their molecular structures in Fig. 28.1.

Barbiturates

The classification of barbiturates has been defined in Chapter 27. Present clinically used drugs are thiopental, thiamylal, and methohexital.

Thiopental

Thiopental is marketed as a pale yellow powder with added 6% anhydrous sodium carbonate in vials containing an inert atmosphere of nitrogen. Although poorly soluble in water, it dissolves in the alkaline solution of the sodium carbonate, forming a 2.5% solution with a pH of 10.5. There is no added preservative, but the alkaline solution is bacteriostatic. The alkaline thiopental is less

soluble at the pH of blood, resulting in microcrystal formation. The rapid onset of hypnosis after an intravenous dose of thiopental is caused by its uptake across the blood–brain barrier (as a result of its high lipid solubility and low degree of ionization at physiologic pH). Barbiturates are almost insoluble in aqueous, but possess weak acidic properties through their keto-enol tautomerism.

The kinetics of thiopental are shown in Table 28.1. Recovery to awakening occurs within 15–20 minutes after a 3–5 mg kg^{-1} single-bolus induction dose. At the time of awakening, only 18% of the injected dose will have undergone metabolism, compared with about 38% of a dose of methohexital and nearly 70% of propofol. The pharmacokinetics of the different intravenous induction drugs all show similar distribution half-lives, but they vary greatly in their clearance rates and the fraction of drug eliminated during the terminal elimination phase (AUCγ) (Table 28.1). As an induction drug, thiopental has a number of drawbacks. The alkalinity is extremely irritating if it is injected extravascularly or intra-arterially. It also has a low therapeutic index (median lethal dose/median effective dose [LD50/ED50] ≈ 4).

Thiopental causes a transient but significant decrease in systemic blood pressure, which is exaggerated in patients with pre-existing cardiac dysfunction (including hypertension) or hypovolemia, those receiving opioids or benzodiazepines concurrently or as premedication, and those receiving β-adrenoceptor blocking drugs or vasodilators. The effect is also more pronounced in the elderly, and when the drug is injected rapidly. Thiopental has a direct effect on the heart, reducing contractility and hence cardiac output. It also vasodilates both the arterial and venous systems, thereby decreasing venous return. Although thiopental increases pulmonary venous resistance in the rat lung, there is little evidence to indicate that the effect is of significance in humans [1,2]. Other nonhypnotic effects of thiopental include dose-related cardiorespiratory depression and an increased sensitivity to somatic pain. The side-effect profile of thiopental differs from those of other hypnotic drugs, as summarized in Table 28.2.

Population pharmacokinetic/pharmacodynamic (PK/PD) studies can be used to review the influence of different factors on thiopental elimination [3]. Although age influenced the kinetics of thiopental, it had no effect on brain responsiveness

Anesthetic Pharmacology, 2nd edition, ed. Alex S. Evers, Mervyn Maze, Evan D. Kharasch. Published by Cambridge University Press. © Cambridge University Press 2011.

Table 28.1. Disposition parameters for intravenous sedative-hypnotics used for induction of anesthesia

Drug	$t_{1/2\alpha}$ (min)	$t_{1/2\beta}$ (min)	$t_{1/2\gamma}$ (h)	CL (mL min^{-1} kg^{-1})	% AUCγ
Thiopental	2–7	42–59	5.1–11.5	2.2–3.5	0.72
Methohexital	6	2–58	1.6–3.9	8.2–12.0	0.66
Propofol	1–4	5–69	1.6–63.0	23.2–32.9	0.29
Ketamine	1–3	8–18	2.2–3.0	14.0–19.1	0.68
Etomidate	1–3	12–29	2.9–5.5	11.6–25	0.64

$t_{1/2}\alpha$, β, and γ, three half-lives for data described by a three-compartment model; CL, systemic clearance; % AUCγ, area under the curve during the terminal elimination phase as a % of the total area under the concentration–time curve (0 to infinity).

Table 28.2. Side effects of intravenous sedative-hypnotics when used for induction of anesthesia

Induction side effects	Thiopental	Methohexital	Propofol	Ketamine	Etomidate
Change in blood pressure (%)	– 8	– 8	– 17	+ 28	– 2
Change in heart rate (%)	+ 14	+ 15	+ 7	+ 33	+ 8
Induction pain (%)	0	30–50	10–30	0	40–60
Induction movement (%)	0	5	5–10	Very little	30
Induction hiccups (%)	0	30	5	Very little	20
Induction apnea (%)	6	20	40	Rare	20
Recovery restlessness (%)	10	5	5	Common	35
Recovery nausea (%)	7–10	7–10	5	Common	20
Recovery vomiting (%)	7–10	5	5	Common	20

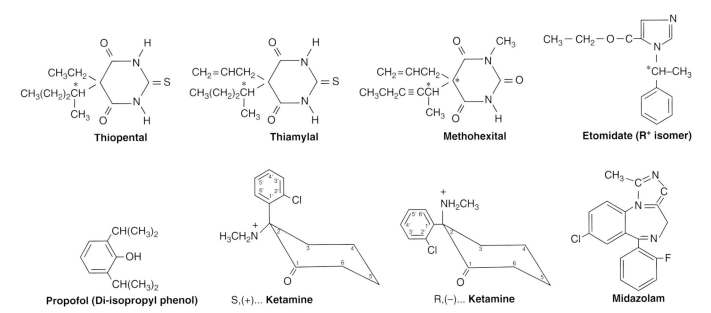

Figure 28.1. Structures of seven intravenous agents used for induction of anesthesia – thiopental; thiamylal; methohexital; etomidate; propofol; ketamine; and midazolam. Asterisks indicate chiral centers.

or pharmacodynamics when the spectral edge was used as a measure of drug effect. The induction dose requirements for thiopental will vary with patient age and weight, and, most importantly, with cardiac output. The blood–brain equilibration rate constant is $0.58 \, min^{-1}$; and the effect-compartment concentration associated with the subject dropping a syringe held at arm's length is about $17 \, \mu g \, mL^{-1}$, with a duration of effect of the induction dose (320 mg) being about 4 minutes. There are many factors that influence the kinetics and dynamics of thiopental. In the elderly patient, lower doses of thiopental are needed to cause loss of consciousness, because of a decreased rate of distribution of the barbiturate from the central compartment to the peripheral rapidly equilibrating tissues [4]. Conversely, in patients with hepatic dysfunction, the increase in the unbound drug fraction (due to decreased plasma albumin concentrations) also decreases the induction dose. Hepatic clearance of free drug is decreased, but total clearance remains unaltered.

Initial recovery from thiopental and the decline in blood (and brain) concentrations occurs mainly through redistribution. Following bolus doses and after short or low-dose infusion regimens, thiopental is eliminated by first-order kinetics and the patient promptly awakens. However, at rates in excess of $300 \, \mu g \, kg^{-1} \, min^{-1}$, thiopental concentrations increase nonlinearly as the peripheral tissue stores become saturated. Metabolism is 10–15% per hour, with the sulfur replaced by oxygen to give pentobarbital, and the side chains at the C5 position being oxidized. As well as changes in kinetics, high doses result in significant blood concentrations of the active metabolite, pentobarbital. Pentobarbital contributes to the overall hypnotic effect of thiopental, so making its effect appear to have a longer duration of action than might be expected from its kinetic profile [5]. The renal excretion of thiopental is very low (about 0.3%).

Specific clinical indications for thiopental include (1) induction of anesthesia, (2) maintenance of anesthesia by either intermittent administration or by infusion in combination with analgesics as needed, (3) anticonvulsant, and (4) sedation of and control of intracranial pressure (ICP) in the patient with head injury. The recommended induction dose is 100–150 mg over 10–15 seconds, followed by additional increments after 30–60 seconds; or a single dose of up to $4 \, mg \, kg^{-1}$. In children, doses of $2–7 \, mg \, kg^{-1}$ may be needed. For maintenance of anesthesia, thiopental infusions at rates between 150 and $300 \, \mu g \, kg^{-1} \, min^{-1}$ (with resulting plasma concentrations of $15–25 \, \mu g \, mL^{-1}$) can be used to supplement either nitrous oxide (N_2O) or as part of a total intravenous technique with opioids such as morphine, fentanyl, sufentanil, or remifentanil. In the absence of supplements, thiopental concentrations needed to abolish response to squeezing the trapezius muscle (roughly equivalent with the initial surgical incision) are about $40–50 \, \mu g \, mL^{-1}$, and the concentration needed to achieve electroencephalogram (EEG) burst suppression is about $73 \, \mu g \, mL^{-1}$ (range $42–90 \, \mu g \, mL^{-1}$) [6]. Advantages of thiopental infusions include minimal cardiovascular depression and cerebral protection during ischemic episodes. Comparable data for pentobarbital are concentrations between 25 and $35 \, \mu g \, mL^{-1}$ for effective reduction of ICP in patients with head injuries, and $25–75 \, \mu g \, mL^{-1}$ for EEG burst suppression. Use of thiobarbiturates for maintenance of anesthesia may be accompanied by prolonged recovery times. For the management of convulsions or treatment of increased ICP, doses of $1.5–3 \, mg \, kg^{-1}$ may be administered, repeated as necessary, and followed by either 25–50 mg boluses or an infusion of the barbiturate titrated against the occurrence of further seizures or ICP ($3–10 \, mg \, kg^{-1} \, h^{-1}$). Dosing adjustments may be needed in the critically ill patient with either liver or renal failure. Similar dosing strategies should be adopted with thiamylal.

Thiopental is marketed as a racemate. The S(–) enantiomer is more potent at the $GABA_A$ receptor than either the racemate or the R(+) enantiomer, although there are no stereospecific effects of thiopental on the AMPA-type glutamate receptor [7]. When the EEG effects of the two enantiomers were examined in the rat, there were differences in the potencies of the racemate, R(+), and S(–) thiopental [8]. When given by bolus or infusion to human subjects, there are some subtle effects on the kinetics of the two enantiomers; however, the 20–30% differences in the clearance and steady-state volume of distribution of the enantiomers could be accounted for by the stereoselective differences in plasma protein drug binding [5,9,10].

Thiamylal

This is another thiobarbiturate with clinical properties similar to thiopental. It is formulated as a racemic mixture, with the potency of the S(–) enantiomer twice that of the R(+) isomer. There are some kinetic differences between these enantiomers, but they are thought to have little clinical relevance [11–13]. The plasma protein binding of the R(+) and S(–) isomer are 82.5% and 88.3%, respectively. The elimination half-life of the R(+) enantiomer is 20.2 hours, the apparent volume of distribution is $3.66 \, L \, kg^{-1}$, and clearance is $0.27 \, L \, kg^{-1} \, h^{-1}$; the corresponding values for the S(–) enantiomer are 24.1 hours, $2.60 \, L \, kg^{-1}$, and $0.15 \, L \, kg^{-1} \, h^{-1}$. The barbiturate in vitro shows greater metabolism by cytochrome P450 (CYP) 2C9 than by CYP2E1 and CYP3A4, with the metabolism of the R enantiomer being greater than that of the S enantiomer. Thiamylal is formulated as an injectable 2% solution made up before use in distilled water. The powder is contained in 1, 2, and 10 g vials. The induction dose of $3–5 \, mg \, kg^{-1}$ causes less respiratory depression than an equipotent dose of thiopental.

Methohexital

Methohexital contains two asymmetric carbon atoms, and the barbiturate therefore exists as four stereoisomers. The β-l-enantiomer is the most potent, and is 4–5 times more active than the α-l-enantiomer. Because the β pair causes excessive motor activity, the drug is formulated as the α-d,l pair. Methohexital has a more appropriate kinetic profile for both induction and maintenance of intravenous anesthesia (elimination half-life of 420–460 minutes, clearance of 700–800 mL min^{-1}) when compared with thiopental. Its main metabolite, 4-OH methohexital, has no pharmacologic activity.

In healthy volunteers, venous concentrations of 3–4 µg mL^{-1} result in sleep and 10–12 µg mL^{-1} cause EEG burst suppression [14]. Based on dose–response studies, the median dose for induction of anesthesia is 1.0–1.5 mg kg^{-1}. The median infusion rate as a supplement to 67% N$_2$O is 50–65 µg kg^{-1} per minute (plasma concentrations 2–5 µg mL^{-1}), and infusion rates of 100–150 µg kg^{-1} per minute are required in the absence of N$_2$O.

Methohexital infusions depress blood pressure and cardiac output, as well as reducing baroreflex sensitivity with a resetting of the response to allow a more rapid heart rate at lower arterial pressures than when awake. Side effects include excitatory movements, pain on injection, and predisposition to convulsions. Although epileptiform activity has been recorded by EEG, clinical seizures are rare. Methohexital also causes pain if injected into arteries, but unlike thiopental this does not normally lead to thrombosis. The combination of methohexital/N$_2$O in opioid-premedicated patients may lead to significant respiratory depression, but there are no untoward effects of methohexital on liver, renal, or adrenal function. The effects of methohexital are additive with those of other CNS depressants (including ethanol and antihistamines), and administration of the drug should be avoided in patients receiving coumarin-like anticoagulants (because of the possibility of drug–drug binding interaction).

Methohexital, like thiopental, can be used both for induction of anesthesia and, by continuous infusion, for maintenance of anesthesia. It is supplied in vials containing 100 or 500 mg, which is reconstituted as a 1% solution. The usual induction dose is 1.0–1.5 mg kg^{-1}. Infusions of methohexital up to 100 µg kg^{-1} min^{-1} can be used to maintain anesthesia with either 67% N$_2$O or opioid supplementation.

Adverse effects of barbiturates

The barbiturates have a number of absolute contraindications to their use, including porphyria. Although not all types of porphyria are adversely affected by thiopental, any suspicion of the disease should be a contraindication to the barbiturates. Known susceptible types include acute intermittent porphyria, variegate porphyria, and hereditary coproporphyria. Other contraindications include proven allergy to thiopental or other barbiturates, and all patients with airway or potential airway obstruction. In addition, methohexital should be avoided in individuals with a history of epilepsy (because there is a risk that it might elicit psychomotor seizures). In patients with marked hypovolemia, including severe blood loss, cardiovascular collapse, severe uremia, in patients with a history of severe asthma, and in all patients with severe cardiac disease (e.g., ischemic heart disease, malignant or untreated severe hypertension), barbiturates should be either avoided or administered in reduced dosage.

Propofol

Propofol (2,6-diisopropylphenol) is a sterically hindered alkyl phenol first studied in 1977, when it was formulated in Cremophor EL (BASF) (Fig. 28.1). After reports of adverse allergic reactions, however, it was reformulated as an aqueous emulsion containing soybean oil and egg phosphatide (Intralipid). Propofol has a neutral pH (7.4) and a pK_a of 11.0, making it 99.7% nonionized and highly lipid-soluble. Propofol has a therapeutic index comparable to thiopental (3.4 vs. 3.9), but recovery to consciousness in both animals and humans is faster after propofol. This difference in recovery becomes more exaggerated when repeated bolus doses or infusions are administered.

Propofol has a long elimination half-life (up to 45 or more hours), a high apparent volume of distribution (1000–3940 L), and a systemic clearance between 1.0 and 1.8 L min^{-1}. Plasma protein binding is greater than 96%. Population kinetic studies of propofol have been defined using data from seven studies containing 270 patients and healthy volunteers [15]. Weight was a significant covariate for elimination clearance, the two intercompartmental clearances of the three-compartment model, and the volumes of the central and two peripheral compartments. When venous data are used, there is a decreased elimination clearance compared with arterial values.

Because of wide variability in the therapeutic drug concentration window (related to age and type of surgery) and intersubject kinetics, propofol dosing is best titrated to effect. This is easily achieved, as it has a short blood–brain equilibration time (k_{e0}) of 0.24 min^{-1}. Drug dosing can be by bolus, continuous infusion, or more recently by target-controlled infusions based on a population-kinetic model. Anesthesia requires propofol concentrations of 4–6 µg mL^{-1} when used with either N$_2$O or an opioid infusion, with recovery occurring at concentrations of about 1.0 µg mL^{-1}; higher concentrations are needed if propofol is infused alone (12–16 µg mL^{-1}).

Induction of anesthesia with propofol is smooth and associated with a low incidence of excitatory side effects. However, occasional epileptiform seizures have been reported during recovery (see later). Closing of the eyes is delayed after propofol compared with thiopental, and this may result in a relative overdosing with the drug; thus the better endpoint for induction is loss of verbal contact. Although a dose of 1.5–2.5 mg kg^{-1} is recommended as the induction dose for anesthesia, the dose of propofol is variable and depends on many factors including the initial volume of distribution and cardiac output. Using stepwise multiple linear regression modeling, four factors were found to be independently associated with the size of the induction dose: age, lean body mass, central blood volume, and liver blood flow [16]. When the dynamics of propofol are related to age, there are three functions that correlate linearly: blood–brain equilibration rate constant and time to peak effect, the steepness of the concentration–response relationships for EEG activation and depression, and the effect-site concentration associated with 50% of peak EEG activation [17].

The hemodynamic effects of induction doses of propofol are similar to those of the thiobarbiturates, but there are also accompanying decreases in systemic vascular resistance. The combination of a vagotonic effect and a decrease in vascular resistance produces significant decreases in blood pressure when used in the hypovolemic patient or the patient receiving other vagotonic drugs (e.g., opioids) [18]. Another difference between propofol and barbiturates is that the normal barore-flex increase in heart rate for a decreased blood pressure is not seen for propofol. Propofol causes a resetting of the baroreflex, with slower heart rates seen for a given arterial blood pressure when compared with awake values [19].

The ventilatory effects of induction doses of propofol are similar to those of most other hypnotic drugs – significant decreases in tidal and minute volumes, coupled with episodes of apnea greater than 30 seconds. Comparative studies show the duration of apnea after propofol to be greater than those following either eltanolone or thiopental [20]. All induction drugs decreased the ribcage and abdominal components of ventilation to a similar amount. When given by continuous infusion, propofol causes a 50% reduction in the ventilatory response to carbon dioxide, as well as in the acute ventilatory response to isocapnic hypoxia [21,22].

Propofol–drug interactions

There is evidence that propofol at clinical concentrations inhibits drug metabolism both in vitro and in vivo [23–27]. In-vitro studies show inhibition of hepatic microsomal hydroxylation and dealkylation reactions at propofol concentrations between 25 and 1000 µM [23–25]. The magnitude of inhibition varied from 30% to 71%, with the greatest effect on reactions mediated by rat CYP2B1. The wide range of rat isozymes that are inhibited (CYPs 1A1 and 2A1, as well as 2B1) suggests there may be a kinetic basis for many drug–drug interactions. Further studies showed that clinical concentrations of propofol inhibit renal mono-oxygenase (as assessed using aniline and benzo(α)pyrene) and defluorinase activities [27].

Clinical data also indicate interactions with propofol leading to a reduced drug clearance. During propofol infusions, there is decreased clearance of high-extraction (flow-dependent) and low-extraction (capacity-limited) drugs due to dose-related reductions in liver blood flow and decreases in the hepatic extraction ratio [26,28]. This may be relevant during anesthesia, where coadministered drugs during propofol infusions may show reductions in their total-body clearance. One simulation study suggested that these changes will not be seen at propofol infusion rates in the clinical range, because the kinetics of propofol were linear with regard to infusion rate at those concentrations [29]. Other data do not support this view [26]. Clinical interactions between propofol and opioids such as alfentanil and remifentanil are discussed further in Chapter 27 [30,31].

In clinical studies, combinations of two hypnotics administered to achieve loss of response to verbal command have been shown to be synergistic rather than directly additive [32]. The same approach has been further used in the technique of "co-induction." There is also increasing evidence that opioids and hypnotic drugs are similarly synergistic. For example, when used for anesthetic induction, $3 \, mg \, kg^{-1}$ propofol produced no greater hemodynanic response than a dose of $2 \, mg \, kg^{-1}$, and the addition of $2 \, \mu g \, kg^{-1}$ fentanyl blunted the responses to intubation [33]. To achieve the optimum efficacy from such combinations, the two effect-site (or biophase) drug concentrations need to peak at the same time. When a combination of hypnotic–opioid–benzodiazepine is used, there are significant reductions in dose requirements of all three, but no more synergism than can be expected from the various combinations of pairs of the drugs [34].

Propofol also interacts with α_2-agonists. Dexmedetomidine ($3 \, ng \, kg^{-1} \, min^{-1}$, producing a median plasma concentration of $0.2 \, ng \, mL^{-1}$) reduced the propofol ED50 infusion rate and EC50 blood concentration for loss of consciousness from 5.8 to $3.4 \, mg \, kg^{-1} \, h^{-1}$ and from 2.3 to $1.7 \, \mu g \, mL^{-1}$, respectively, although these differences were not statistically significant and there was no significant shift in the dose–response curve [35]. This study was originally designed with a higher infusion rate of dexmedetomidine, but during the pilot phase the highest rate was associated with a number of significant side effects (two cases of sinus arrest and one case of severe postural hypotension persisting for 24 hours after anesthesia). Sinus arrest has also been observed in other studies involving propofol and vagotonic drugs, both in patients and in healthy volunteers. It is therefore appropriate to pretreat patients (especially those younger than 40 years) with an anticholinergic drug. The final dexmedetomidine dose rate used in the study ($3 \, ng \, kg^{-1} \, min^{-1}$) blunted the responses to intubation and surgical incision, and blood pressure and heart rate remained stable during surgery and into the recovery period. In a separate study, the porpofol EC50 concentration for loss of motor response to electrical stimulation was $6.6 \, \mu g \, mL^{-1}$, but when dexmedetomidine was infused to a concentration of $0.66 \, ng \, mL^{-1}$, the propofol EC50 was decreased to $3.9 \, \mu g \, mL^{-1}$ [36]. Similar reductions were seen for the EC50 values for the clinical endpoint of the ability to retain hold of a syringe.

Nonhypnotic effects
Mood-altering, antiemetic, and antipruritic effects

Subhypnotic doses of propofol administered by a patient-controlled analgesia (PCA) system (10 mg with a 1- to 5-minute lockout) have been shown to exert sedative and anxiolytic effects in anxious patients presenting for ambulatory surgery [37,38]. Several authors have suggested a postoperative antiemetic effect of propofol (in both hypnotic and subhypnotic doses), although the site of this action remains uncertain [39]. Propofol is also effective in the prevention of nausea and emesis after cisplatin chemotherapy [39]. Subhypnotic doses of propofol (10–20 mg intravenously) are equally effective compared with naloxone in relieving pruritus caused by both epidural and spinally administered opioids [40,41] and in the treatment of pruritus caused by cholestasis [42].

Central nervous system effects

In-vitro studies demonstrate a direct vasodilating effect of propofol caused by calcium channel blockade. In-vivo studies show a decrease in mean arterial pressure and cerebral blood flow, intracranial pressure, and cerebral metabolic rate following an induction dose of the hypnotic, but there is no further decrease in cerebral blood flow or other variables when anesthesia is maintained with an infusion of 3–6 mg kg^{-1} h^{-1}. Propofol does not affect cerebrovascular autoregulation to carbon dioxide [43] and the slope of the cerebral blood flow–carbon dioxide response curve is similar to that measured in awake subjects and during anesthesia with other intravenous drugs. Evidence for a protective effect of propofol in humans and animals is controversial, although high doses of propofol have been used to afford protection during cerebral aneurysm surgery in patients requiring cardiopulmonary bypass and deep hypothermic arrest, as well as in patients undergoing nonpulsatile cardiopulmonary bypass for cardiac surgery [44,45]. Low infusion rates of propofol cause increased beta activity on the EEG, and loss of consciousness causes increased theta activity, whereas burst suppression occurs at blood concentrations greater than 6 μg mL^{-1} [46]. At these EEG suppression levels, propofol causes significant reductions in cerebral blood flow, oxygen delivery, and metabolic rate, although cerebral autoregulation remains unaltered. These changes are in contrast to the volatile anesthetics. There are many reports of opisthotonos, hyperreflexia, and hypertonus, involuntary movements, choreoathetosis, and seizure-like activity associated with propofol [47]. However, the drug has variable effect on the EEG in patients with epilepsy (some show increased spike activity, others show decreased EEG activity). Data from the UK's Committee on Safety of Medicines (CSM) from the early 1990s indicate an incidence of convulsions in association with propofol of about 1 in 47 000, with many cases seen as the drug concentration in the body is decreasing, and delayed reactions occurring in about a third of cases (www.mhra.gov.uk).

Cardiorespiratory effects

The effects of bolus doses and infusions of propofol on the cardiac and respiratory systems are similar to those of other groups of drugs in this section, excluding ketamine. After propofol administration, rare cardiac events include severe bradycardia, sinus arrest, heart block, and asystole, especially in association with the coadministration of other vagotonic drugs. Induction doses of propofol (2–3 mg kg^{-1}) also depress pharyngeal reflexes and allow satisfactory jaw tone for both insertion of the laryngeal mask and endotracheal intubation [48].

Effects on the hepatic and renal system

Bolus doses of propofol have no effect on renal or portal venous blood flows [49], and infusions of propofol in humans cause no significant changes in liver blood flow or liver function tests [50,51]. However, as mentioned previously, dose-related changes in liver blood flow have been reported in dogs during graded infusions to supraclinical concentrations [26].

Adverse effects

During the past decade, the side-effect profile of propofol has become complex. There are several case reports of allergic reactions to the drug (see below) and reports of convulsions after drug administration, although propofol also has anticonvulsant properties [18].

Adverse properties of propofol include pain on injection (especially when given into small veins and to children), hypotension, and bradycardia (which are exaggerated in the presence of other vagotonic drugs such as opioids and hypovolemia), and apnea in up to 40% patients after induction. Attempts at decreasing the pain (which varies in incidence between 30% and 70%) include pretreatment with lidocaine, fentanyl, or alfentanil, or aseptically mixing propofol with 20 mg lidocaine immediately before dosing, although the latter can destabilize the soybean emulsion. A systematic review of techniques aimed at preventing pain on injection showed intravenous administration of 40 mg lidocaine with a tourniquet 30–120 seconds before the propofol to be the best option, with a number needed to treat (NNT) of 1.6 [52]. More recently it has been shown that addition of long-chain triglyceride to propofol (Diprivan; AstraZeneca) will reduce the incidence of severe pain from about 70% to 0% [53]. The mechanism behind this result is thought to be a decrease in propofol concentration in the aqueous phase secondary to the increase in the fat content. However, this change in aqueous drug concentration does not seem to influence the kinetics or dynamics of propofol [54]. In a double-blind comparison, there was less pain with the long-chain triglyceride/medium-chain triglyceride emulsion compared with the Intralipid (Kabivitrum) emulsion [55], but there were no kinetic or dynamic differences between propofol formulations [56]. The addition of small amounts of lidocaine to propofol when given for induction may reduce the incidence of pain on injection [57]; however, addition of more than 20 mg lidocaine to 200 mg propofol and not injecting the drug immediately can cause modifications of the physicochemical nature of the emulsion [58,59].

The aqueous emulsion does not contain any preservative and is therefore a good bacterial growth medium. The etiologic factors of multiple outbreaks of postoperative infection were examined in 1996 [60]. The cause was not surgical, but rather the repeated use of propofol during nonsterile conditions during the preparation and filling of syringes and the multiuse of single-dose drug vials. A separate study demonstrated that propofol will support bacterial growth of Corpus albicans when inoculated onto agar plates [61]. Once propofol is drawn up in the syringe from the ampoule, it should be used immediately, for a single patient, and the remainder in the syringe should be discarded. Opened ampoules must not stand at room temperature. Once dispensed, a propofol syringe should be used within a few hours. Consequently, formulations of propofol containing EDTA or metabisulfite were introduced in the United States in an attempt to decrease bacterial growth. However, metabisulfite has been reported to support lipid peroxidation of the propofol emulsion.

Profound metabolic acidosis has been reported when the metabisulfite formulation of propofol was used for sedation in the adult ICU, and termed *propofol infusion syndrome* (PIS). This is partly caused by the prolonged administration (usually >48 hours) of propofol at high doses ($>4\,mg\,kg^{-1}\,h^{-1}$), resulting in a dyslipidemia from the long-chain triglycerides of the Intralipid solvent. In one such case, propofol was infused over 48 hours in an adult patient after neurosurgery. The peak serum lactate concentration reached 15 mM and was associated with cardiovascular collapse and death [62]. This situation was similar to that reported after use of the hypnotic for sedation in children [63]. The etiology of this metabolic derangement and death remains uncertain, but it may relate to propofol acting in a dose-dependent manner to antagonize myocardial β-adrenoceptor activity. Furthermore, hyperlipidema is recognized as a cause of disturbances of acyl-carnitine metabolism leading to uncoupling of oxidative phosphorylation and impaired fatty acid oxidation [64].

Because of the heterogeneity of the reported cases, and a paucity of good cardiovascular and metabolic monitoring data, it is difficult to argue for a single causal factor. Rather the clinical features (metabolic acidosis, refractory cardiac failure, bradycardia, lipidemia, and evidence of muscle cell damage) are those commonly seen in the critically ill patient and may be attributed to factors such as impairment of the microcirculation, the sympathetic neuropathy of critical illness, and septic cardiomyopathy. A recent analysis of 1139 patients with suspected propofol infusion syndrome quotes a 30% fatality [65]. Death was more likely if patients were 18 years of age or younger, if they were receiving or had received a vasopressor, and if they had some or all of the clinical features listed above. To date, there are no instances of the syndrome being reported in patients (adults or children) receiving high-dose, prolonged propofol infusions for anesthesia.

There are two absolute contraindications to the use of propofol: patients with a known hypersensitivity to propofol or related compounds and patients with disorders of fat metabolism.

Administration and dosage

Propofol can be used both in the operating room and in the ICU. In the former, propofol is administered intravenously for both induction of anesthesia and maintenance by intermittent bolus dosing or continuous infusion. Propofol is also widely used for sedation by continuous infusion, both as a supplement to regional anesthetic techniques for endoscopic procedures and in the ICU. There are reports of the drug being administered by patient control (that is, the patients themselves titrate the amount of hypnotic they receive to produce sedation).

Propofol is formulated as 1% or 2% solutions in oil emulsion (20 and 50 mL) and as a 50 mL vial for use in target-controlled infusion anesthesia and a 1% solution in long- and medium-chain triglycerides. The recommended induction dose is $1.5–2.5\,mg\,kg^{-1}$ at 20–40 mg per 10 seconds. The dose should be reduced in the patient older than 55 years. Propofol may also be used for induction of anesthesia in children older than 1 month. Maintenance of anesthesia can be achieved using 25–50 mg bolus doses or an infusion of $4–12\,mg\,kg^{-1}\,h^{-1}$ (for children older than 3 years, rates of $9–15\,mg\,kg^{-1}\,h^{-1}$ may be needed). In some countries, the use of target-controlled infusions for induction and maintenance of anesthesia is approved only for adults.

In the ICU, initial doses of propofol of about $0.3–2\,mg\,kg^{-1}$ followed by 25–50 mg boluses may be used to institute sedation for controlled ventilation. In the agitated patient, doses of up to $10\,mg\,kg^{-1}\,h^{-1}$ may be needed. The average maximum dose per day should not exceed $15\,mg\,kg^{-1}\,h^{-1}$, and the use of propofol for ICU sedation is not currently recommended in patients younger than 17 years. However, clinical trials in this area are ongoing.

Ketamine

Ketamine (2-O-chlorophenyl-2-methylaminocyclohexanone HCl) is a phencyclidine derivative formulated as a racemic mixture (Fig. 28.1). The two stereoisomers R(−) and S(+) have different anesthetic potencies (1:3–4) but similar kinetics. Ketamine is water-soluble and can be used as 1%, 5%, and 10% solutions.

Following intravenous ketamine induction doses of 1–2 mg kg^{-1}, there is rapid loss of consciousness, but recovery is slower (1–15 minutes) and less complete compared with other intravenous induction drugs.

There are limited disposition and concentration-effect data for continuous infusions of ketamine (see Chapter 27). The hypnotic and analgesic thresholds are 1.5–2.5 μg mL^{-1} and approximately 200 ng mL^{-1}, respectively. As sole drug, infusion rates of 60–80 μg kg^{-1} per minute provide clinical anesthesia.

Ketamine in vitro is a myocardial depressant, but in vivo, in contrast to other intravenous induction drugs, it causes an increase in blood pressure, heart rate, contractility, cardiac output, and systemic vascular resistance. However, these are indirect effects – as a result of an increased centrally mediated sympathetic tone and increased catecholamine release from the adrenal medulla. In the critically ill or injured patient, induction with ketamine can result in a decrease in blood pressure and cardiac output because of the direct negatively inotropic effects of both ketamine and its active metabolite, norketamine. The positive inotropic and chronotropic cardiovascular effects increase myocardial oxygen demand, so there may be circumstances in the patient with coronary artery disease where induction with ketamine results in the development of myocardial ischemia. Respiratory effects of ketamine differ from those of other intravenous induction drugs. There is no evidence of ketamine causing ventilatory depression in the healthy patient or the patient with chronic airway disease. Ketamine will also cause bronchodilation [66].

Ketamine has advantages over propofol and etomidate in being water-soluble as well as producing profound analgesia at subanesthetic doses. However, although it lacks the cardiorespiratory depressive properties of other intravenous drugs, its usefulness has been limited by the high incidence of disturbing emergence reactions (in up to 30% of patients). Compared with other induction drugs, ketamine increases the pulse rate, blood pressure, and intracranial pressure. Salivation is increased, but this can be attenuated by administration of antimuscarinic drugs such as atropine or glycopyrrolate. There is an association with a high risk of postoperative nausea and vomiting. Ketamine also causes postoperative dreaming and hallucinations. These may be attenuated by benzodiazepine or α_2-agonist premedication, although these classes of drugs prolong the elimination half-life and increase the duration of effect. Present data suggest that ketamine may also be safe for use in the management of patients susceptible to malignant hyperthermia.

Ketamine was originally marketed as a racemate. Separation of the enantiomers of ketamine has allowed clinicians to examine their relative potencies, side effects, and other pharmacologic effects. The emergence reactions referred to above are thought to be caused by the high affinity of the R(–) enantiomer for the sigma opioid receptor. The hypnotically active S(+) enantiomer is now available for use in mainland Europe (see below).

In vivo, S(+) ketamine is about twice as potent as the racemate and four times more potent than the R(–) enantiomer in terms of anesthesia, and it is associated with faster recovery. An initial study of the S(+) isomer in healthy volunteers demonstrated that ketamine doses needed for anesthesia 6 minutes in duration were 275, 140, and 429 mg for racemic, S(+), and R(–) ketamine, respectively, with recovery more rapid after the individual enantiomers [66]. This relates closely to subsequent studies showing inhibition of the metabolism of S(+) ketamine by the R(–) isomer [67]. Ketamine concentrations at time of regaining consciousness and orientation were consistent with an S : R potency ratio of 4 : 1, whereas the ratio for impairment of psychomotor function was between 3 : 1 and 5 : 1. At equipotent doses, S(+) ketamine produces longer hypnosis than the R(–) isomer, with the racemate being intermediate. However, cardiovascular stimulation and psychotomimetic effects are seen with both stereoisomers.

Crossover studies in healthy volunteers have shown that the hemodynamic and metabolic responses of the racemate and S(+) ketamine are comparable [68,69]. However, there was improved recovery with the single enantiomer. S(+) ketamine causes decreased locomotor activity, but equipotent analgesia. In studies examining the effects of racemic ketamine and the S(+) isomer on the EEG spectrum, both increased fast beta activity (21–30 Hz) with an accompanying reduction in delta power [70]. Using the IC50 for reduction of the EEG median frequency as the index of potency, the S(+) ketamine concentration was $0.8\,\mu g\;mL^{-1}$, compared with 1.8 and $2.0\,\mu g\;mL^{-1}$ for the R(–) and racemic preparations [71]. On the basis of an assumed equipotency ratio of S(+) ketamine-to-racemate of 1 : 2, Geisslinger et al. compared the kinetics and dynamics of the enantiomers of ketamine in 50 surgical patients [72]. There were no significant kinetic differences between S(+) ketamine alone and the enantiomers in the racemic mixture. However, the R(–) enantiomer showed a lower clearance and smaller apparent volumes of distribution compared with the S(+) enantiomer when administered as one component of the racemate, although there were no differences in the clearance rates of the S(+) and R(–) isomers when given as the racemate. The concentration–effect relationship for S(+) ketamine therefore lies to the left of that for the racemate and has a steeper curve.

Ketamine can cause considerable side effects. The incidence of emergence reactions is about 37%, 15%, and 5%, respectively, after R(–), racemic, and S(+) ketamine, with comparable incidences of dreaming with all three treatment groups [73]. Ketamine significantly increases blood cortisol, catecholamines, and glucose concentrations [74]; similar increases occurred with the S(+) enantiomer in surgical patients when used for elective lower limb orthopedic surgery, although the increases in circulating plasma epinephrine concentrations were greater after the racemate [75]. There are no apparent differences between the enantiomers and racemate in their hemodynamic effects.

One other important aspect of ketamine pharmacology is its ability to regulate intracellular calcium levels and inducible nitric oxide synthase activity after hypoxic insults (i.e., a neuroprotectant effect). Cell culture experiments showed that the S(+) enantiomer had a greater protective potential than the racemate, and was associated with a greater reoutgrowth of axonal neurites and an increased expression of growth-associated proteins [76,77]. R(–) ketamine is ineffective as a neuroprotectant. Use of racemic ketamine or S(+) ketamine is considered by some to be contraindicated in patients with increased ICP or intraocular pressure, and in patients with severe cardiac diseases such as arterial hypertension, ischemic, or valvular heart disease. There is also a relative contraindication to its use in patients with psychotic disorders.

Indications for use of ketamine include (1) induction of anesthesia, (2) maintenance of anesthesia, (3) sedation by use as a continuous infusion, and (4) analgesia (intraoperatively or after surgery) as a continuous infusion. Racemic ketamine is supplied in 10, 50, and 100 mg mL^{-1} strengths. The recommended induction dose is 1–4.5 mg kg^{-1} (usually a dose of 2 mg kg^{-1} provides surgical anesthesia for 5–10 minutes). Maintenance of anesthesia can be achieved using a 1 mg mL^{-1} solution at a rate of 10–45 μg kg^{-1} per minute. Anesthesia may also be achieved with intramuscular ketamine in a dose of range 6.5–13.0 mg kg^{-1} (a dose of 10 mg kg^{-1} provides 12–25 minutes for diagnostic procedures and manipulations). S(+) ketamine is supplied in 5 and 25 mg mL^{-1} strengths (5 and 20 mL vials for the 5 mg mL^{-1} strength, 2 and 10 mL vials for the 25 mg mL^{-1} strength). Induction doses of 0.5–1.0 mg kg^{-1} intravenously and 2–4 mg kg^{-1} intramuscularly are recommended. The recommended induction dose is 0.5–1.0 mg kg^{-1} intravenously or 2–4 mg kg^{-1} intramuscularly. Maintenance can be achieved by repeated boluses of 50% of the induction dose or infusion of 0.5–3.0 mg kg^{-1} h^{-1}. For analgesia, doses of 0.1–0.25 mg kg^{-1} intravenously followed by an infusion of 0.2–1.0 mg kg^{-1} h^{-1} are recommended.

Etomidate

Etomidate is a carboxylated imidazole that is unstable in water, and is currently solubilized in either 33% propylene glycol or as an emulsion (Fig. 28.1). The normal induction dose ranges from 0.2 to 0.4 mg kg^{-1}, providing hypnosis for between 5 and 15 minutes with only minimal alterations in cardiovascular parameters in healthy patients, and those with valvular or ischemic heart disease. Little is known about the interaction of etomidate with opiates or other hypnotics when used to induce loss of consciousness. Etomidate alone does little to obtund the sympathetic responses to laryngoscopy and intubation, and for a smooth hemodynamic profile, combination with an opiate or benzodiazepine is advised [78]. The action of etomidate is potentiated by the coadministration of other sedative and centrally acting drugs. Etomidate has many ideal properties (cardiostability; reduction of cerebral blood flow, cerebral metabolic rate, and ICP; no release of histamine and a low rate of allergic reactions), and it offers advantages during induction of anesthesia in patients with poor cardiac reserve and hypovolemia. Etomidate has less ventilatory depressant effect following induction of anesthesia than either thiopental or propofol, but the induction dose is still likely to result in transient apnea. However, the ventilatory depressant effects are not exaggerated in patients with chronic obstructive pulmonary disease (COPD) and there is no inhibition of the hypoxic pulmonary vasoconstrictor reflex.

Etomidate is associated with a high incidence of nausea and vomiting, pain on injection, and thrombophlebitis (up to 30% by the third postoperative day), especially if administered into the small veins of the hand, excitatory movements, and myoclonia. These excitatory movements and myoclonia can be reduced in both incidence and severity using a pretreatment regimen of a 0.03 mg kg^{-1} etomidate

dose [79]. However, there are also reports of etomidate causing convulsions in unpremedicated patients [80]. Studies suggest that the thrombophlebitis may be caused by the propylene glycol solvent. Recovery may be more uncomfortable after etomidate than for some other drugs because of increased restlessness, nausea, and vomiting [81].

Etomidate has an imidazole moiety that binds to and inhibits a number of isoenzymes of cytochrome P450. Etomidate causes dose-related reversible inhibition of adrenal steroidogenesis by interaction with mitochondrial P450 (affecting 11β-, 17α-, and 18-hydroxylases, and 20,22-lyase). This inhibition is seen after an induction dose, where the peak time to suppression of the normal plasma cortisol response to surgical stress occurs at about 4 hours after initial exposure [82]. This effect is probably not clinically significant, as there are no data to suggest that a single induction dose has long-term effects in surgical patients. However, a recent review suggests that even a single dose of etomidate may be hazardous in patients developing or with established septic shock [83]. In contrast, another study reports no harm when infusions of etomidate are given during cardiac surgery, concluding that the stress of major surgery can overcome the inhibitory effects of etomidate on cortisol synthesis [84]. Etomidate infusions in intensive care unit (ICU) patients caused significant adrenal suppression, reduced cortisol synthesis, and increased mortality [85]. There are few data exploring patient outcome when etomidate is administered by infusion for anesthesia for prolonged periods of time, with the only substantive outcome data relating to use in the ICU [85].

An emulsion formulation of etomidate was introduced in Europe, showing no change in pharmacodynamic properties, but a decreased incidence of pain on injection, myoclonus, and local thrombophlebitis, compared with the standard formulation [86,87]. An additional advantage of emulsion formulation is lower osmolality and higher pH (400 mOsm kg^{-1} and pH 7.6, compared with 4965 mOsm kg^{-1} and pH 5.1 for the propylene glycol formation), which causes less red-cell hemolysis [88]. Studies of healthy volunteers comparing the two formulations show the emulsion to be associated with both a decreased incidence of pain on injection and fewer venous sequelae [89]. A second reformulation of etomidate has 2-hydroxypropyl-β-cyclodextrin as the solvent [90], again causing a lower incidence of myoclonus and pain (17% vs. 92% and 8% vs. 58%), thrombophlebitis (0% vs. 42%), and no hemolysis. There were no alterations in the kinetics or dynamics of this etomidate formulation.

Although it is widely believed that use of etomidate is associated with an increased incidence of postoperative nausea and vomiting, this was not supported by a comparative study in which Etomidate-Lipuro and propofol were used for induction of anesthesia to supplement isoflurane/fentanyl in air in patients undergoing orthopedic procedures [91]. There were no differences in rates of nausea or in the intensity of any nausea during the early postoperative period to 24 hours.

However, the rates of vomiting among female patients after etomidate were greater (26.8% vs. 10%).

Etomidate can be used for induction of anesthesia, especially in patients with cardiovascular disease, as well as in patients with known drug hypersensitivity or atopy. Because of the effects on adrenal steroidogenesis, etomidate is no longer recommended for maintenance of anesthesia by repeat dosing or continuous infusion. Single bolus doses of etomidate (5–20 mg) may be used in the ICU for control of acute increases in ICP. Etomidate is formulated as a 2 mg mL^{-1} solution in propylene glycol or long- and medium-chain triglycerides (Etomidate-Lipuro). The recommended induction dose is 0.3 mg kg^{-1}, but this is reduced in the elderly to 0.15–0.2 mg kg^{-1}. In children younger than 15 years, doses up to 0.39 mg kg^{-1} may be needed. Use of etomidate is contraindicated in patients with acute porphyria, in patients with evidence or suggestion of depressed adrenocortical activity, and in patients with a known sensitivity to etomidate.

Midazolam

Midazolam, in contrast to other injectable benzodiazepines such as diazepam and lorazepam, is water-soluble as a result of the substituted imidazole ring structure (Fig. 28.1). The imidazole nitrogen has a pK_a of 6.2, thus being protonated and water-soluble when buffered in a solution at pH 3–4. At pH 7.4, $> 90\%$ of the midazolam exists in an unprotonated lipid-soluble form. The proposal that water solubility is due to ring opening is probably incorrect, as all benzodiazepines undergo ring opening at low pH. At pH 2, 75% of the midazolam molecules are in an open-ring configuration, while this decreases to about 9% at pH4. As midazolam is maintained at a pH of 3–4 in the vial, ring opening will account for only a small part of its water solubility at that pH, and none at physiologic pH. Hydroxylation of the methyl group in the imidazole ring decreases but does not eliminate the pharmacological activity of midazolam, and is a major route of drug clearance. This method of metabolism makes midazolam short-acting compared with other benzodiazepines.

An induction dose of midazolam (0.3 mg kg^{-1}) will cause a rapid loss of consciousness, but recovery will be slower than after equipotent doses of thiopental or propofol. In subhypnotic doses, midazolam produces amnesia for events following drug dosing (i.e., anterograde amnesia). Midazolam also has effects as an anxiolytic, as well as a low risk for producing nausea and vomiting. The myocardial depressant effects of midazolam are less than those of both thiopental and propofol when the drugs are used for induction of anesthesia. Midazolam also produces some venodilation, leading to a decrease in venous return, but unlike thiopental, midazolam has little effect on myocardial contractility. In anesthetic doses, midazolam causes a dose-dependent decrease in hypoxic ventilatory drive. Subhypnotic doses (in the absence of opioids) rarely cause apnea, but hypnotic doses produce a frequency of apnea similar to that seen with thiopental. There is marked synergy in depressing ventilatory drive between benzodiazepines and either opiates or ethanol, and in patients with COPD there is a greater sensitivity to the ventilatory depressant effects of midazolam. Midazolam has effects on cerebral metabolic rate (CMRO$_2$) and ICP similar to those of thiopental, but less in magnitude. It is an excellent anticonvulsant, but even at high doses the benzodiazepines do not cause burst suppression of the EEG or an isoelectric tracing. Hence they will not offer neuroprotection.

Case reports to date suggest that midazolam is safe to use in patients with a susceptibility to malignant hyperthermia. However, the drug should be used with caution in patients with acute intermittent porphyria, hereditary coproporphyria, and variegate porphyria. There are no substantiated hypersensitivity responses to midazolam.

Midazolam can be used for sedation in the operating room, endoscopy suite, and ICU. In the operating room, propofol is administered intravenously for both induction and maintenance of anesthesia by intermittent bolus dosing or continuous infusion. There are reports of the drug being administered by patient control. Midazolam is formulated as 10 mg in either 2 mL or 5 mL ampoules. The recommended induction dose for anesthesia is 0.1–0.3 mg kg^{-1} given slowly until loss of the eyelid reflex, response to commands, and voluntary movements. The dose should be reduced in the patient older than 55 years. The drug may also be used for induction of anesthesia in children older than 7 years. For intravenous sedation, incremental doses of 2 mg are administered over 30 seconds; if sedation is not achieved in 2 minutes, quarter incremental doses should be given. Reduced doses should be used in the elderly. Maintenance doses of 0.03–0.2 mg kg^{-1} h^{-1} by continuous infusion can be used for sedation in the ICU, with the dose being reduced in the hypovolemic, vasoconstricted, or hypothermic patient. When given in combination with an opioid, low doses (0.01–0.1 mg kg^{-1} h^{-1}) should be used to commence sedation.

New drugs and formulations

New propofol formulations

The aim of new propofol formulations is to improve the pharmacologic profile of the drug by reducing the incidence of pain on injection; to use a less toxic lipid formulation than the Intralipid solvent which has been incriminated in the development of the propofol infusion syndrome (PIS) [64]; to achieve a faster onset of effect; and to reduce the contamination risk when the drug is given by continuous infusion. The support of bacterial growth can be obtunded by addition of benzyl alcohol, sulfite, or EDTA. The problem of pain on injection is more debatable, as the lipid solvent is not associated with pain when given alone or when used to solubilize other drugs [89], suggesting that the pain may be due to the propofol itself [92].

Some new formulations have focused on the lipid used to solubilize propofol. The Lipuro formulation is solubilized in medium-chain triglycerides rather than long-chain triglycerides. It has an identical PK/PD profile to the Diprivan formulation, but is associated with less pain on injection. This formulation is not available in the USA, however, because of the lack of EDTA in the solvent. IDD-D propofol is another formulation in medium-chain triglycerides, but prepared at a 2% concentration. The drug has a slower onset of effect than Diprivan, and has an increased incidence of pain on injection. It is unlikely therefore to find widespread clinical use.

Current propofol emulsions are manufactured such that the oil droplet size averages 0.15–0.5 μm (*fine macroemulsions*) [93]. When the droplet size is less than 0.1 μm, the emulsion is known as a *microemulsion*. Microemulsions are considered highly stable [94], much more so than the ones with bigger droplets – but they require the addition of surfactants. Aquafol (Daewon Pharmaceutical Company) is a propofol microemulsion containing 1% propofol, 8% polyethylene glycol 600 hydroxystearate (solutol HS 15; BASP Co. Ltd.) as a nonionic surfactant, and 5% Glycofural (Roche) as a cosurfactant. This formulation has been compared with Diprivan 1% in volunteers. Aquafol demonstrated similar PK and PD properties to Diprivan, and similar safety profiles [95]. However, the maximum tolerated doses of surfactant and cosurfactant used in this formulation limited its administration to a maximum of 100 mL Aquafol per day. As a consequence, the microemulsion was reformulated with another, better tolerated cosurfactant (Purified polaxamer 188; PP188) [96]. This formulation has been investigated in rats, where the kinetics were found to be nonlinear [96]. Another problem which could not be assessed in this study was the presence or not of pain on injection. This might be increased in microemulsion formulations as there may be a greater amount of free propofol in the aqueous phase [97].

Three aqueous formulations of propofol solubilized using cyclodextrans have been described [98]. These use either hydroxypropyl-γ-cyclodextrin, hydroxypropyl-β-cyclodextrin (HP-βCD), or sulfobutyl-β-cyclodextrin as the solvent. The hydroxypropyl-β-cyclodextrin formulation showed favorable physicochemical and biological properties as a water-based formulation. Early porcine studies show an equivalent PK/PD profile to Diprivan [99], but there are no studies in patients to date. However, when formulations containing large amounts of the complexing agent (20% w/v) were used, intravenous dosing of the complex of propofol–hydroxypropyl-β-cyclodextrin in rats caused immediate bradycardia of variable duration while the solvent alone had no effect [100]. Hence safety issues were highlighted which might be improved by minimizing the amount of the cyclodextrin. The sulfobutyl-β-cyclodextrin is more soluble and safer than hydroxypropyl-β-cyclodextrin, and, while many of these formulations showed improved pharmacodynamic profiles, there was often an increased duration of effect and stability problems.

Other propofol formulations use cosolvent mixtures with propofol solubilized in propylene glycol : water (1 : 1 v/v) or the prolinate ester of propofol and its water-soluble derivative dissolved in water at equimolar concentrations. Studies with the prolinate ester in rats showed the formulation to have a longer induction time and longer duration of action. A micellar formulation results in a clear solution (Cleopol), which, however, is associated with an increased incidence (89%) of severe pain on injection and with the development of venous thrombophlebitis. Its only role may be use in patients demanding a pure vegetarian induction drug! A polymeric micelle formulation is a more recent water-based formulation of propofol in a poly(N-vinyl-2-pyrrolidone) block polymer (Labopharm Inc.), in which propofol is dissolved inside micelles that are 30–60 nm in diameter [101,102]. This micellar solution is then lyophilized to form Propofol-PM (propofol polymeric micelle), which instantaneously reconstitutes to a clear solution upon addition of an aqueous medium. This formulation does not support the growth of microorganisms [101]. Micellar propofol has been examined in rats, and shown to produce anesthesia. There were no differences in propofol kinetics compared with the Diprivan formulation [102]. There are few data on its use in higher species.

Propofol analogs and prodrugs

Other approaches have also been used to overcome some of the major disadvantages of propofol, specifically cardiovascular depression and pain on injection. Para-substituted propofol analogs are water-soluble and, importantly, retain anesthetic activity. The lead compound in a series of substituted phenols was a para-amino-morpholino-derivative formulated as the hydrochloride salt [103]. This was active when given intravenously over 10 seconds in producing a burst suppression ratio of $\geq$50% in the rat at a dose of 51 μmol kg^{-1} (a similar effect was observed with 39 μmol kg^{-1} propofol). These doses produced a sleep time of about 4 minutes, with recovery at the same time that the burst-suppression ratio returned to pre-drug levels.

The physicochemical features of several propofol prodrugs have been described [104,105]. The first attempt was a propofol sodium hemisuccinate prodrug, but this was unsuitable for commercialization as a stable aqueous solution. A phosphate ester formulation was studied in mice, rats, rabbits, and pigs [105]. Metabolism by phosphatases yielded inorganic phosphate and propofol with a similar kinetic profile to the parent compound. Propofol concentrations greater than 1 μg mL^{-1} were associated with sedation in rats and pigs. The median hypnotic dose (ED50) of the propofol phosphate in mice was about 10 times that seen when using propofol alone, and there was a similar increase in median lethal dose (LD50). Other highly water-soluble derivatives of propofol, formulated as cyclic amino acid esters, have been described [106]. The anesthetic properties of the most promising of these, the prolinate,

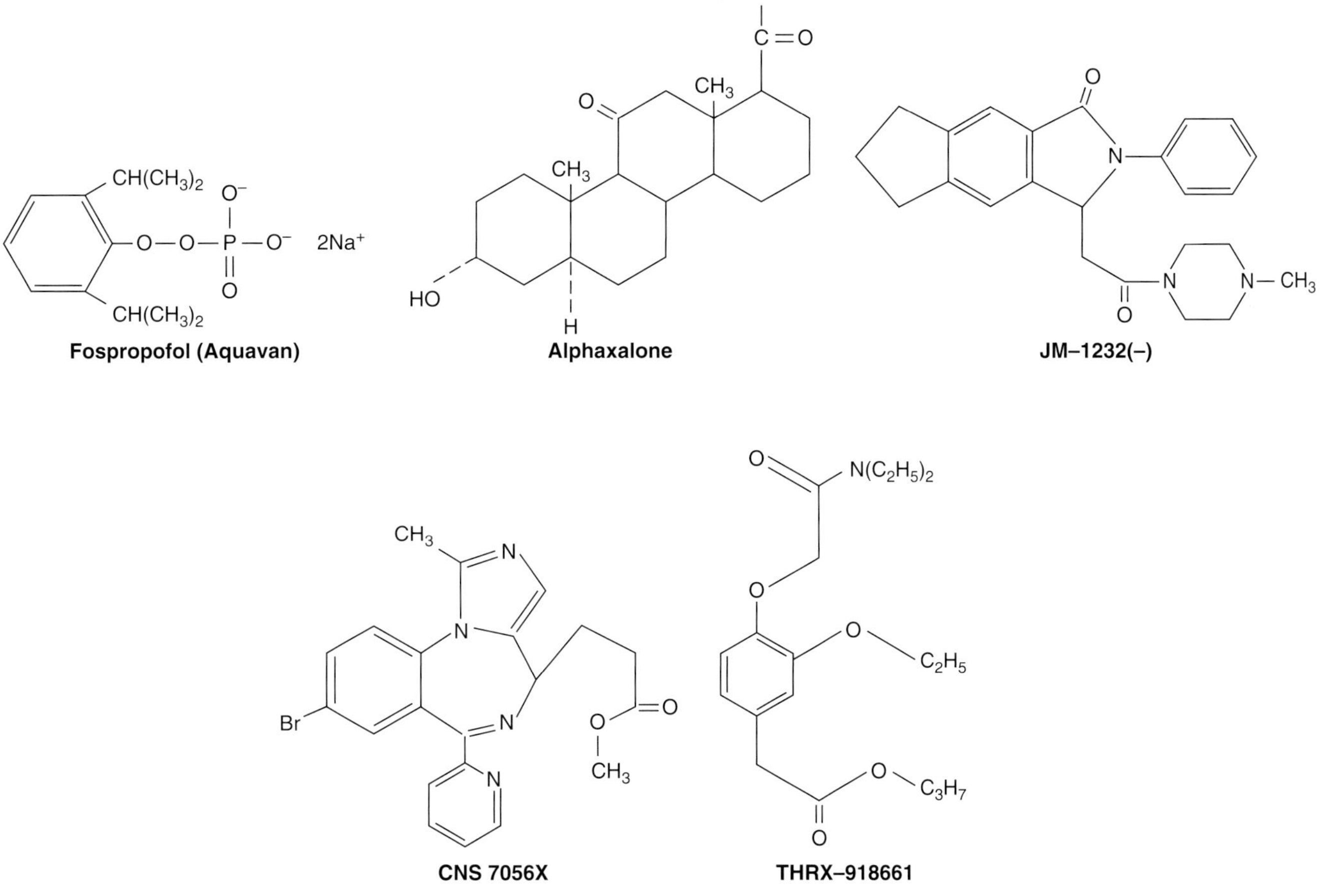

Figure 28.2. Structures of five chemical entities under evaluation as intravenous anesthetic agents – fospropofol (Aquavan); alphaxalone-CD; JM-1232(–); CNS 7056X; THRX-918661.

have been described following intraperitoneal injection in rats, and showed a faster loss of righting reflex than Diprivan.

Fospropofol (GPI-15715, Aquavan, Lusedra) is the only clinically approved propofol analog. It is a water-soluble phosphono-ester of propofol (phosphono-O-methyl-2,6-diisopropylphenol) (Fig. 28.2). It is moderately rapidly and completely broken down to propofol, inorganic phosphate, and formaldehyde by alkaline phosphatases that are widely distributed in the body. Based on the molecular weights of propofol and fospropofol, 1 mg of the latter should liberate 0.54 mg propofol. There was no reported pain on injection; two subjects reported transient and unpleasant burning sensations in the perineal region at the start of the infusion; and loss of consciousness was not achieved at the lowest dose studied. The burning sensations were accompanied by a transient increase in heart rate [107]. More recent multicenter phase 3 trials have used lower doses of fospropofol (6.5 mg kg^{-1} as compared with earlier doses of 5–14 mg kg^{-1}) to produce moderate procedural sedation, followed by subsequent titrated doses [108]. Fentanyl (50 μg) was given prior to the dose of fospropofol. Paraesthesiae occurred in about 50% of subjects, together with pruritus and perineal itching (although there was

no apparent recall of the pain or discomfort). With this dose strategy, there was rapid recovery (with a median time to full alertness of 5 minutes, and an Aldrete score >9 by 10 minutes) and improved patient outcome. In studies to date, fospropofol has been associated with a low incidence of postoperative nausea and vomiting.

In comparison with propofol, fospropofol appears to show a lower incidence of adverse effects, with only minor respiratory depression although some pain following intravenous injection. It has a slower onset of effect than propofol, and a lower maximum concentration (C_{max}) for propofol compared with the same dose of the latter when given intravenously. The metabolic products of fospropofol cause no clinically significant drug-related sedation effects. At the doses described above, 95% of subjects have a blood propofol concentration <2 μg mL^{-1}. A single dose of fospropofol has a longer duration of effect compared with the same dose of propofol. Concerns over the reliability of the assay for fospropofol have led to doubts over the published kinetics and PK/PD modeling for this drug (see Chapter 27).

Fospropofol has some apparent advantages over propofol and is associated with a lower risk of bacterial contamination as well as the absence of the infused lipid load that has been associated with organ toxicity during long-term infusions of Diprivan. Because of its slow-onset kinetics, fospropofol will probably find maximum utility for sedation in the ICU, for procedural sedation outside of the operating room, and for sedation during monitored anesthesia care or regional anesthesia per se where its slow onset is less critical. Fospropofol was approved by the US Food and Drug Administration (FDA) in December 2008 for use in monitored anesthesia care sedation in adult patients undergoing diagnostic or therapeutic procedures, and only by persons trained in the administration of general anesthesia and not involved in the conduct of the procedure.

Another prodrug of propofol, the ethyl dioxy phosphate, has been described [109]. Hydrolysis occurs in the blood by alkaline phosphatases, with a pseudo-first-order half-life of approximately 20 seconds, but without the release of formaldehyde. The bioconversion rate of this compound to propofol in the rat after intravenous dosing is faster than that of the propofol phosphate formulation.

HX0507 is another water-soluble prodrug of propofol that has been studied in mice and beagle dogs. At doses between 50 and $100\,mg\,kg^{-1}$, there were no significant differences in tail-flick latency or in counting numbers of spontaneous motor activity when it was compared with propofol $25\,mg\,kg^{-1}$ [110]. However, at the highest dose of HX0507 and with propofol, the number of mice dropping from the RotaRod was significantly greater than for controls and the low-dose groups. When examined in the beagle, $5.4\,mg\,kg^{-1}$ propofol was compared with three doses of HX0507 (30, 45, and $60\,mg\,kg^{-1}$) in animals that had previously received midazolam $0.2\,mg\,kg^{-1}$ and fentanyl $10\,\mu g\,kg^{-1}$ [111]. All three intravenous doses of HX0507 depressed respiration in a dose-dependent manner, but this depression was less than that seen following propofol. There was also dose-dependent hypotension, but there was no difference in effects between the two lower doses of HX0507 and propofol, and the decreased blood pressure was readily reversible with ephedrine.

Other new chemical entities

Steroid anesthetics

The hypnotic properties of steroid molecules were first recognised in 1927 by Cashin and Moravek [112], who induced anesthesia in cats using a colloidal suspension of cholesterol. There was no apparent relationship between the hypnotic (anesthetic) and hormonal properties of the steroids, with the most potent anesthetic steroid being pregnan-3,20-dione (pregnanedione), which is virtually devoid of endocrine activity. Over the past 80 or more years, the anesthetic properties of a large number of steroids have been assessed both in vitro and in vivo in laboratory animals and humans. One of the main problems with steroid drugs has been their lack of water

solubility [113]. Most steroids show high therapeutic indices in animals, but a variable effect in humans on the onset of hypnosis, and on the rapidity and completeness of recovery.

Althesin (a mixture of alphaxalone and alphadolone acetate; Fig. 28.2) is the only steroid anesthetic which achieved widespread clinical use, and then only in certain countries. The clinical effects of bolus doses of Althesin were similar to those of thiopental apart from more rapid recovery. It had important effects on cerebral hemodynamics, cerebral metabolism, and ICP. Induction doses of Althesin caused reductions in ICP proportional to the initial ICP, as well as decreasing the cerebrospinal fluid pressure. Given by continuous infusion, Althesin, at rates of $300\,\mu g$ total steroid per kg per hour, decreased both cerebral blood flow and cerebral metabolic rate when compared with the values in awake subjects. Althesin also reduced brain blood flow homogeneously to all cortical areas. In humans, Althesin caused only minimal effects on blood pressure, respiration, and temperature homeostasis, suggesting that its central depressive effects might be different in mechanism from those of other intravenous hypnotic drugs. Althesin had no significant effects on renal and hepatic function when given by either bolus dose or continuous infusion. It was not considered safe, however, when administered to patients with acute porphyria (both acute intermittent [Swedish] and variegate [South African] types). However, Althesin was an important drug for the maintenance of anesthesia in patients susceptible to malignant hyperthermia, and had a protective effect against arrhythmias induced by epinephrine in the cat.

Advantages of Althesin included minimal cardiovascular and respiratory depression, a low incidence of postoperative nausea and vomiting, and reduced venous sequelae. Minor side effects of Althesin for induction of anesthesia were a dose-related incidence of hiccups, coughing, laryngospasm, and involuntary muscle movements. The major adverse side effect of Althesin was allergic reactions, with an incidence of between 1/1000 and 1/18 000. The immunology of adverse reactions to Althesin was probably multietiological. Reactions on first exposure were thought to be due either to a direct nonimmunological effect on mast cells causing release of histamine and other autocoids or to alternative pathway complement activation. Reactions to repeat exposure to Althesin resulted from classical complement pathway activation, indicating an antigen–antibody interaction. This latter group of reactions generally had a more severe symptomatology and complex immunology [114–116]. There was also laboratory evidence of subclinical complement activation following both bolus doses and infusions of Althesin [117]. Whether these reactions to the Cremophor-formulated drugs such as Althesin was due to the pharmacologically active components with the Cremophor acting as an adjuvant, or to the Cremophor itself, is a matter of conjecture.

The pharmacokinetics of the Althesin steroids have been studied in humans [118]. Alphaxalone has an elimination half-life of about 30 minutes, a systemic clearance for alphaxalone of around 20 mL kg^{-1} min^{-1}, and apparent volume of distribution at steady state of 0.79 L kg^{-1}. The kinetics of alphadolone acetate in humans does not differ from that of alphaxalone. Protein binding of alphaxalone and alphadolone is mainly to albumin, but also to β-lipoproteins, with extensive plasma protein binding (96.8%) of alphaxalone [119]. Both parent steroids and the metabolite 20α-hydroxy-alphaxalone are detectable in blood after single doses and continuous infusions of Althesin [120], with alphaxalone eliminated in urine as the 20α-reduced glucuronide, and less than 1% as free drug [121].

Althesin was withdrawn from clinical use in 1984, although its use as the Cremophor EL formulation has continued in some animal species. Cremophor EL has been shown to be associated with the release of histamine on first exposure, leading to hypotension, swollen paws and ears, and occasional pulmonary edema in the cat, and severe hypotension in the dog. These effects may be avoided in the dog by using a different solvent (2-hydroxypropyl-β-cyclodextrin) as the solubilizing agent for alphaxalone alone [122] in a formulation so far registered for clinical use in dogs and cats in Australia as Alfaxan-CD RTU (Jurox Pty.). Studies in the dog showed alphaxalone-CD to have a high clearance (48–64 mL kg^{-1} min^{-1}) and an apparent volume of distribution at steady state of 2.5–3.0 L kg^{-1}. No adverse effects have been associated with injection of the steroid, although some excitation was seen during recovery at the time of awakening [123]. Repeat dosing shows no apparent accumulation in the dog. Studies in the cat confirm similar kinetics for alphaxalone; but a longer recovery profile [124].

MOC-etomidate (methoxycarbonyl-etomidate; MOC-E)

MOC-etomidate is a soft analog of etomidate presently under evaluation [125]. It has been designed to maintain the critical properties of the parent compound, but has the advantage of being rapidly broken down by esterases found in different body tissues. The aim is therefore to maintain etomidate's beneficial properties, but not to cause prolonged adrenocortical depression following bolus dose administration. The ester moiety attached to etomidate is both sterically unhindered and electronically isolated from the pi electron systems in the imidazole ring.

In *Xenopus* oocytes, MOC-E enhanced submaximal GABA-evoked GABA$_A$ receptor currents in α$_1$, β$_2$, and γ$_{2L}$ receptors, but was less potent than etomidate. MOC-E had an in-vitro metabolic half-life of 4.2 minutes in liver homogenate, compared with little effect on the breakdown of etomidate even after 40 minutes' incubation.

In tadpoles, the EC50 for loss of the righting reflex (LORR) was 8 μM (compared with 2 μM for etomidate). In the rat, the ED50s for LORR were 5.2 mg kg^{-1} for MOC-E, 1.00 mg kg^{-1} for etomidate, and 4.1 mg kg^{-1} for propofol. The decrease in mean blood pressure was similar for etomidate and MOC-E at twice the ED50 dose; but the duration of significant effect was

less (about 30 seconds) with MOC-E. After MOC-E, there was no suppression of ACTH-stimulated corticosterone production at 30 minutes after dosing, whereas there was 58% suppression by etomidate. After administering an intravenous bolus or a continuous infusion of MOC-E, adrenocortical function is predicted to recover more rapidly than after etomidate. Studies have shown that doses of etomidate needed to produce hypnosis could lead to adrenocortical suppression persisting for more than 4 days after discontinuing a prolonged infusion [22,126,127]; and even a single induction dose can cause suppression for 24 hours or more [128–130].

Whether MOC-etomidate will affect other adrenocortical enzyme systems apart from the 11β-steroid hydroxylase is unknown at present (see earlier discussion of the pharmacology of etomidate).

PF0713

PF0713 is a new induction drug presently in phase 1, human-volunteer clinical testing. The actions of PF0713 have been examined at the molecular level using rat cerebral cortex binding assays, with the greatest effect found on the chloride channel (as has been shown for propofol), and a lack of interaction with α$_2$, NMDA, PCP, benzodiazepine, or opioid receptors [131]. In a comparison with propofol on the CA1 populations of pyramidal neurons, both drugs potentiated the effects of muscimol at the GABA$_A$ receptor, suggesting that the drug acts via the picrotoxin binding site on the chloride binding channel.

PF0713 is a novel water-insoluble 2′6′dialkylphenol formulated as a 1% lipid emulsion (Fig. 28.2). When given to rats by the intravenous route, there was rapid onset of LORR, with a duration that was dose-related over the range 1.9–15.2 mg kg^{-1}. The drug appeared to be of a greater potency than propofol in this model, and the maximum tolerated dose was greater for PF0713 than propofol. However, after high doses (>7.0 mg kg^{-1}) there were suggestions of a prolonged recovery time [132].

PF0713 was administered to 24 ASA I human subjects at doses from 0.0156 to 2.0 mg kg^{-1} with no notable adverse events. At 1.0 mg kg^{-1} and 2.0 mg kg^{-1}, PF0713 produced rapid induction of general anesthesia without injection pain or agitation. The depth and duration of anesthetic effect assessed by Bispectral Index and the Richmond Agitation–Sedation Score were dose-related. Blood pressure and heart rate were adequately maintained and plasma clearance was high [133].

JM-1232(−)

JM-1232(−) is one of a series of water-soluble sedative-hypnotics presently being evaluated by the Maruishi Pharmaceutical Company [134]. The lead compound [JM-1232(−)] is an iso-indolin-1-one derivative which was shown to be active in mice (Fig. 28.2). It has a wide margin of safety – with a hypnotic ED50 of 3.1 mg kg^{-1} and LD50 of >120 mg kg^{-1} (therapeutic index >35). In-vitro binding data suggest that the compound has a high affinity for the benzodiazepine receptor, but not at the same binding site as midazolam [135]. In-vitro studies examining the effects of JM-1232(–) in a brainstem/spinal cord preparation of neonatal rats (0–4 days old) showed no effect on the C4 burst rate and amplitude at concentrations between 10 and 500 µM, but at higher concentrations there was depression of central respiratory activity which could be reversed by the addition of 100 µM flumazenil [136].

JM-1232 has recently undergone clinical evaluation. When given as a 10-minute infusion to six male volunteers, it had a rapid onset and short duration of action [137]. Doses between 0.05 and 0.8 mg kg^{-1} caused sedation, with the higher doses producing a deeper and longer reduction in the Bispectral Index. Preliminary kinetic data indicate a clearance of about 0.78 L min^{-1}, and an apparent steady-state volume of distribution of 77.3 L. Simulated context-sensitive half-times to 120 minutes infusion suggest a drug with a similar profile to propofol. Further studies in a larger population of volunteers have confirmed the drug's kinetic profile, and estimated an EC50 effect site concentration for anesthesia of 162 ng mL^{-1} (95% CI 121–203), and a $t_{1/2ke0}$ of 4.2 minutes (3.1–6.7) [138].

CNS 7056X

CNS 7056X is an ultra-short-acting benzodiazepine hypnotic drug hydrolyzed by esterases in the blood to the metabolite 7054X (Fig. 28.2). The parent compound has a very predictable offset of effect in animals with a low risk of oversedation, and is reversible by the benzodiazepine antagonist flumazenil. In vitro, CNS 7056X binds to brain benzodiazepine sites with high affinity, while the metabolite has a 300-times lower binding affinity. Neither has any affinity for other receptors, nor selectivity (just as midazolam) for specific GABA$_A$ subtypes. 7056X causes dose-dependent inhibition of neuronal firing of the substantia nigra pars reticularis. Metabolism of 7056X occurs rapidly by human, rat, mouse, and minipig liver tissue, yielding 7054X as the major metabolite. Rapid metabolism also occurs in organs other than the liver (kidney, lung, brain), but there is no metabolism by plasma in human, minipig, or dog. This metabolite profile is in keeping with CNS 7056X being a substrate for carboxylesterases rather than butyrylcholinesterase [139]. When given intravenously, 25 mg kg^{-1} midazolam and 7056X both produced immediate LORR in rats, but recovery of the righting reflex was faster with 7056X (25 vs. 10 min) [140]. The effect of 7056X is inhibited by pretreatment with flumazenil. In a kinetic and dynamic comparison with midazolam in the pig, both drugs rapidly induced sedation, but recovery was faster after 7056X [141]. Midazolam was eliminated more slowly (33 vs. 18 min half-life) and was more widely distributed (1038 vs. 440 mL kg^{-1} volume of distribution at steady state).

The first human study with CNS 7056 has recently been reported [142]. CNS 7056 was well tolerated in doses between 0.01 and 0.35 mg kg^{-1}, although episodes of hypoxia were seen with higher doses. There was no hypo- or hypertension. Plasma drug clearance was about three times that of

midazolam, and there was a linear dose–kinetic relationship. There was rapid onset of sedation (after about 1 minute with a peak at 4 minutes), and also rapid recovery (10 minutes, compared with about 40 minutes for equipotent doses of midazolam).

THRX-918661

THRX-918661 (also known as TD4756 and AZD3043) is another designer-built water-soluble drug which is a congener of the hypnotic drug propanidid, with about twice the potency (Fig. 28.2). The structure of THRX-918661 is that of an acetic acid propyl ester broken down by tissue and plasma esterases. There are no reported data on the activity of any metabolites. THRX-918661 undergoes rapid hydrolysis in vitro in whole blood of rat and guinea pig, with half-lives of 0.4 and 0.1 minutes respectively. When given intravenously to rats, doses of 5–30 mg kg^{-1} caused dose-dependent LORR and short-lived EEG suppression. After infusions ranging from 20 minutes to 5 hours, the time to recovery of the righting reflex was about 3 minutes. In contrast, the recovery from propofol anesthesia ranged between 30 and 60 minutes. Faster recovery when compared with propofol has also been demonstrated in the pig [143]. In the rat, an infusion of 2.5 mg kg^{-1} min^{-1} (in conjunction with remifentanil) maintained a surgical plane of anesthesia. After a 3-hour continuous infusion in rats, kinetic studies demonstrated there to be rapid loss of the parent compound, with none detected after about 5 minutes. Studies in the pig revealed that after a 3-hour continuous infusion clearance was about 3.4 L kg^{-1} h^{-1} and the elimination half-life 0.4 h. Recovery was faster than after propofol when given at equipotent doses [144]. However, the anesthetic appears to have a low potency, with doses for the maintenance of anesthesia in the pig being of the order of 1.5 mg kg^{-1} min^{-1}.

Melatonin

Melatonin can exert an anesthetic and antinociceptive efect in the rat [145]. In a comparison of melatonin (312 mg kg^{-1}), thiopental (23.8 mg kg^{-1}), and propofol (14.9 mg kg^{-1}) effects on the rat EEG, only relative total power, relative spectral edge 95%, and relative approximate entropy were altered by all three drugs. Of main import, all three reduced relative entropy with similar time courses for thiopental and propofol, and a slower onset and duration for melatonin [146]. No data exist, however, for dosing with intravenous melatonin or an analog in higher animals or man.

Allergic reactions to hypnotic drugs

Although the majority of allergic reactions to intravenous drugs originate from use of neuromuscular blocking drugs, there are large numbers caused by hypnotic drugs (Table 28.3). The overall incidence due to intravenous drugs is between 1/5000 and 1/20 000.

Table 28.3. Estimated incidence of adverse hypersensitivity reactions to intravenous sedative-hypnotics

Drug	Incidence
Thiopental	1/14 000 – 1/20 000
Methohexital	1/1600 – 1/7000
Propofol (Cremophor formulation; BASF)	5 in 1131
Propofol as emulsion	(estimate 1/80 000 – 1/100 000)
Ketamine	2 cases only in literature
Etomidate	10+ cases (estimate 1/50 000 – 1/450 000)
Midazolam	17 cases noted by MHRA
For comparison	
Althesin (in Cremophor)	1/400 – 1/11 000
Propanidid (in Micellophor)	1/500 – 1/17 000
Neuromuscular blocking drugs	1/5000
Penicillin	1/2500 – 1/10 000
Dextrans	1/3000
Gelatins	1/900
Hydroxyethyl starch	1/1200

Thiopental and other barbiturates

The overall incidence for barbiturates is 1/23 000 to 1/30 000, with possible cross-sensitivity between methohexital and the thiobarbiturate. The reported incidence of adverse reactions to thiopental and methohexital is about 1/14 000 and 1/7000, respectively. There have been more than 250 published cases of anaphylactic or anaphylactoid reactions to thiopental. Cutaneous and cardiovascular manifestations predominate (65% and 56%, respectively) with respiratory side effects (laryngospasm or difficulty in ventilating the patient) in about 35% of cases. There are also recorded cases of death after administration of thiopental. Many affected patients give a history of atopy, allergy, or a previous general anesthetic (presumably one of the barbiturates). Laboratory testing after a suspected reaction usually shows a significant immediate decrease in the plasma levels of IgE with no significant change in the concentration of complement proteins C_3 and C_4. In rarer cases, there is both IgE and complement involvement; complement activation probably occurs secondary to the hypotension. There are currently well-documented cases in which specific IgE antibodies to thiopental have been detected by intradermal testing [147,148].

Fifteen cases of suspected hypersensitivity to methohexital and two cases associated with thiamylal have been reported [149]. The incidence is undoubtedly low, and there have been no reported deaths. Most patients showed periorbital and facial edema with no history of allergy. One reaction presented with cutaneous signs of flushing and periorbital edema accompanied by severe hypotension. Clinical signs and laboratory tests indicate an anaphylactic response caused by a type I hypersensitivity reaction due to a possible cross-sensitivity between the two barbiturates. Data from the UK Medicines and Healthcare Products Regulatory Agency (www.mhra.gov.uk) list 85 allergic reactions to thiopental and 16 to methohexital over a 45-year period, the majority being anaphylactic.

Etomidate

The incidence of reactions to etomidate is low (about 1/450 000). There are five reports between 1978 and 1982 of possible adverse reactions to the drug [150]. Each reaction involved widespread cutaneous flushing or urticaria and the postoperative occurrence of vomiting. None of the patients showed complement activation. An additional two cases reported in 1982 also exhibited anaphylactoid responses, with signs of cyanosis, marked hypotension, and, in one case, edema [150]. Whether these were caused by etomidate is difficult to decide because the drug was administered concurrently with succinylcholine or alcuronium. Nevertheless, complement C_3 activation was shown in one of the cases. Other reactions include generalized erythema, urticaria, tachycardia and hypotension, and positive skin tests, supporting an anaphylactoid mechanism [151,152]. The first case of severe bronchospasm (leading to hypoxic cardiac arrest) and urticaria after induction of anesthesia with etomidate was reported in 1988 [153]. Complement was not activated, but the patient had an increased plasma IgE level, which was consistent with atopy. Unlike many of the other reports, a direct release of histamine or other immune mediators by the intravenous hypnotic drug seems the most likely explanation. There have been nine non-fatal allergic reactions reported to the MHRA since 1979.

Ketamine

There are only two reported allergic reactions to ketamine [154,155], one involving IgE, the other probably having a nonimmune basis.

Propofol

The incidence of reactions to propofol appears to be increasing. At least five cases of hypersensitivity were reported among the 1131 patients receiving the drug during clinical trials with a formulation made up in Cremophor EL. Reformulation of propofol as an emulsion has only resulted in 97 cases reported to date to the MHRA. These have been categorized as "allergic, anaphylactoid, or anaphylactic," with eleven associated deaths [156]. Other side effects occurring with a high incidence (and which may be related to histamine or other mediator release) include pain on injection, erythematous rashes, bronchospasm, flushing, and hypotension. When all of these hypersensitivity reactions are considered together, the overall incidence for propofol is probably between 1/80 000 and 1/100 000 administrations.

Midazolam

There have been 16 reported cases to the MHRA of suspected allergic reactions to midazolam since 1983, with two deaths.

Summary

The onset of anesthesia occurs when the concentration of drug at the brain effect site achieves a threshold value; the time to this occurring after intravenous injection will depend on the kinetics of the drug and its blood–brain equilibration time. If given as a single bolus dose, offset of effect is primarily the result of drug redistribution.

The archetypal intravenous induction drug is thiopental (a thiobarbiturate), and it is against this that all other present and newer drugs should be compared. Thiopental has a direct concentration-dependent effect on myocardial contractility, as well as causing vascular dilation of both the venous and arterial systems. It also results in a dose-dependent decrease in ventilatory drive, which is exaggerated in the elderly and patients with chronic obstructive pulmonary disease (COPD). Thiopental reduces the cerebral metabolic rate for oxygen, and by vasoconstriction of cerebral vessels it decreases intracranial pressure. Coexisting factors (such as premedication, advanced age, and concurrent diseases) will decrease drug requirements. Conversely, increased doses are needed in patients receiving anticonvulsants, if there is tolerance through chronic thiopental usage, or in cases of cross-tolerance in patients with excessive ethanol use.

Propofol is a structurally hindered phenol with central nervous system effects similar to thiopental. However, it has a greater cardiovascular depressant effect than thiopental, and also blunts the baroreflex control of heart and blood pressure, especially in conjunction with opiate drugs. Recovery from propofol is faster and more complete compared with thiopental, and patients show a low incidence of postoperative nausea and vomiting after propofol. Some studies have suggested that the drug has intrinsic antiemetic activity. One major side effect of propofol is the occurrence of pain on injection.

Ketamine is a phencyclidine derivative that causes dissociative anesthesia. When used for maintenance of anesthesia, it is difficult to monitor accurately the depth of that state. Ketamine's dynamic profile is different to that of the other intravenous anesthetics as it causes profound analgesia and salivation, increases cardiovascular parameters, has little effect on ventilatory drive, causes bronchodilation, and shows less effect on obtunding of protective airway reflexes in the anesthetized patient. Other adverse effects include postoperative psychomimetic properties, and increased intracranial pressure.

Etomidate is a carboxylated imidazole. Its central nervous system effects are similar to those of thiopental, although the drug causes a high incidence of excitatory activity. There is a lack of significant cardiovascular and ventilatory depressant effects, but etomidate inhibits 11β-steroid hydroxylation (as well as some other steroid biosynthetic enzymes), resulting in inhibition of the cortisol response to stress. There is considerable debate over whether this is relevant in surgical patients, with no study showing adverse patient outcome.

Midazolam is a water-soluble benzodiazepine which is principally a sedative with anterograde amnestic effects. It can also be used for induction of anesthesia. There is a synergy between midazolam and opioids, alcohol, and other hypnotics. COPD patients are more sensitive to its ventilatory depressant effects. It is the only marketed induction drug whose effect can be reversed – by the antagonist flumazenil.

Newer drugs are being evaluated to try and overcome the disadvantages of these compounds. Some examples include new propofol formulations and propofol prodrugs, alphaxalone in cyclodextrin, MOC-etomidate, JM-1232(–), PF0713, CNS7056X, AZD3043, and melatonin analogs.

References

1. Rich GF, Roos CM, Anderson SM, et al. Direct effects of intravenous anesthetics on pulmonary vascular resistance in the isolated rat lung. Anesth Analg 1994; 78: 961–6.

2. Todd MM, Drummond JC, U HS. The hemodynamic consequences of high-dose thiopental anesthesia. Anesth Analg 1985; 64: 681–7.

3. Stanski DR, Maitre PO. Population pharmacokinetics and pharmaco-dynamics of thiopental: The effect of age revisited. Anesthesiology 1990; 72: 412–22.

4. Avram MJ, Krejcie TC, Henthorn TK. The relationship of age to the pharmacokinetics of early drug distribution: the concurrent disposition of thiopental and indocyanine green. Anesthesiology 1990; 72: 403–11.

5. Cordato DJ, Mather LE, Gross AS, et al. Pharmacokinetics of thiopental enantiomers during and following high-dose therapy. Anesthesiology 1999; 91: 1693–702.

6. Cordata DJ, Herkes GK, Mather LE, et al. Prolonged thiopentone infusion for neurosurgical emergencies: Usefulness of therapeutic drug monitoring.

Anaesth Intensive Care 2001; 29: 339–48.

7. Tomlin SL, Jenkins A, Lieb WR, Franks NP. Preparation of barbiturate optical isomers and their effects on GABA(A) receptor. Anesthesiology 1999; 90: 1714–22.

8. Mather LE, Edwards SR, Duke CC. Electroencephalographic effects of thiopentone and its enantiomers in the rat: correlation with drug tissue distribution. Br J Pharmacol 1999; 128: 83–91.

9. Cordato DJ, Gross AS, Herkes GK, Mather LE. Pharmacokinetics of thiopentone enantiomers following intravenous injection or prolonged

infusion of rac-thiopentone. *Br J Clin Pharmacol* 1997; **43**: 355–62.

10. Nguyen KT, Stephens DP, McLeish MJ, *et al.* Pharmacokinetics of thiopental and pentobarbital enantiomers after intravenous administration of racemic thiopental. *Anesth Analg* 1996; **83**: 552–8.

11. Sueyasu M, Ikeda T, Taniyama T, *et al.* Pharmacokinetics of thiamylal enantiomers in humans. *Int J Clin Pharmacol Ther* 1997; **35**: 128–32.

12. Cook CE, Seltzman TB, Tallent CR, *et al.* Pharmacokinetics of pentobarbital enantiomers as determined by enantioselective radioimmunoassay after administration of racemate to humans and rabbits. *J Pharmacol Exp Ther* 1987; **241**: 779–85.

13. Sueyasu M, Fujito K, Shuto H, *et al.* Protein binding and the metabolism of thiamylal enantiomers in vitro. *Anesth Analg* 2000; **91**: 736–40.

14. Schwilden H, Schüttler J, Stoeckel H. Closed loop feedback control of methohexital anesthesia by quantitative EEG analysis in humans. *Anesthesiology* 1987; **67**: 341–7.

15. Schüttler J, Ihmsen H. Population pharmacokinetics of propofol: a multicenter study. *Anesthesiology* 2000; **92**: 727–38.

16. Kazama T, Ikeda K, Morita K, *et al.* Relation between initial blood distribution volume and propofol induction dose requirement. *Anesthesiology* 2001; **94**: 205–10.

17. Schnider TW, Minto CF, Shafer SL, *et al.* The influence of age on propofol pharmacodynamics. *Anesthesiology* 1999; **90**: 1502–16.

18. Bryson HM, Fulton BR, Faulds D. Propofol: An update of its use in anaesthesia and conscious sedation. *Drugs* 1995; **50**: 513–59.

19. Cullen PM, Turtle M, Prys-Roberts C, *et al.* Effect of propofol on baroreflex activity in humans. *Anesth Analg* 1987; **66**: 1115–20.

20. Spens HJ, Drummond GB. Ventilatory effects of eltanolone during induction of anaesthesia: Comparison with propofol and thiopentone. *Br J Anaesth* 1996; **77**: 194–9.

21. Nagyova B, Dorrington KL, Gill EW, *et al.* Comparison of the effects of sub-hypnotic concentrations of propofol and halothane on the acute ventilatory response to hypoxia. *Br J Anaesth* 1995; **75**: 713–18.

22. Nieuwenhuijs D, Sarton E, Teppema L, *et al.* Propofol for monitored care: Implications on hypoxic control of cardiorespiratory responses. *Anesthesiology* 2000; **92**: 46–54.

23. Janicki PK, James MFM, Erskine WAR. Propofol inhibits enzymatic degradation of alfentanil and sufentanil by isolated liver microsomes in vitro. *Br J Anaesth* 1992; **68**: 311–12.

24. Baker MT, Chadam MV, Ronnenberg WC. Inhibitory effects of propofol on cytochrome P450 activity in rat hepatic microsomes. *Anesth Analg* 1993; **76**: 817–21.

25. Chen TL, Ueng TH, Chen SH, *et al.* Human cytochrome P450 mono-oxygenase system is suppressed by propofol. *Br J Anaesth* 1995; **74**: 558–62.

26. Sear JW, Diedericks J, Foex P. Continuous infusions of propofol administered to dogs: Effects on ICG and propofol disposition. *Br J Anaesth* 1994; **72**: 451–5.

27. Chen TL, Chen TG, Tai YT, *et al.* Propofol inhibits renal cytochrome P450 activity and enflurane defluorination in vitro in hamsters. *Can J Anaesth* 2000; **47**: 680–6.

28. Coetzee JF, Glen JB, Wium CA, Boshoff L. Pharmacokinetic model selection for target controlled infusions of propofol. Assessment of three parameter sets. *Anesthesiology* 1995; **82**: 1328–45.

29. Schnider TW, Minto CF, Gambus PL, *et al.* The influence of method of administration and covariates on the pharmacokinetics of propofol in adult volunteers. *Anesthesiology* 1998; **88**: 1170–82.

30. Mertens MJ, Vuyk J, Olofsen E, *et al.* Propofol alters the pharmacokinetics of alfentanil in healthy male volunteers. *Anesthesiology* 2001; **94**: 949–57.

31. Johnson KB, Syroid ND, Gupta DK, *et al.* An evaluation of remifentanil propofol response surfaces for loss of responsiveness, loss of response to surrogates of painful stimuli and laryngoscopy in patients undergoing elective surgery. *Anesth Analg* 2008; **106**: 471–9.

32. Short TG. Pharmacodynamic interactions of anaesthetics. *Curr Opin Anaesth* 1995; **8**: 292–7.

33. Billard V, Moulla F, Bourgain JL, *et al.* Hemodynamic response to induction and intubation. Propofol/fentanyl interaction. *Anesthesiology* 1994; **81**: 1384–94.

34. Vinik HR, Bradley EL, Kissin I. Triple anesthetic combination: propofol-midazolam-alfentanil. *Anesth Analg* 1994; **78**: 354–8.

35. Peden CJ, Cloote AH, Stafford N, Prys-Roberts C. The effect of intravenous dexmedetomidine premedication on the dose requirement of propofol to induce loss of consciousness in patients receiving alfentanil. *Anaesthesia* 2001; **56**: 408–13.

36. Dutta S, Karol MD, Cohen T, *et al.* Effect of dexmedetomidine on propofol requirements in healthy subjects. *J Pharm Sci* 2001; **90**: 172–81.

37. Ure RW, Dwyer SJ, Blogg CE, White AP. Patient-controlled anxiolysis with propofol (ARS abstract). *Br J Anaesth* 1991; **67**: 657–8.

38. Rudkin GE, Osborne GA, Curtis NJ. Intra-operative patient-controlled sedation. *Anaesthesia* 1991; **46**: 90–2.

39. Borgeat A, Wilder-Smith O, Forni M, Suter PM. Adjuvant propofol enables better control of nausea and emesis secondary to chemotherapy for breast cancer. *Can J Anaesth* 1994; **41**: 1117–19.

40. Borgeat A, Wilder-Smith OHG, Salah M, *et al.* Subhypnotic doses of propofol relieve pruritus induced by epidural and intrathecal morphine. *Anesthesiology* 1992; **76**: 510–12.

41. Salah M, Borgeat A, Wilder-Smith OH, *et al.* Epidural morphine-induced pruritus: Propofol versus naloxone. *Anesth Analg* 1994; **78**: 1110–13.

42. Borgeat A, Mentha G, Savoiz D, *et al.* Prurit associe a une hepatopathie: Propofol, une nouvelle approche therapeutique? *Schweiz Med Wochenschr* 1994; **124**: 649–50.

43. Fox J, Gelb AW, Enns J, *et al.* The responsiveness of cerebral blood flow to changes in arterial carbon dioxide is

maintained during propofol-nitrous oxide in humans. *Anesthesiology* 1992; **77**: 453–6.

44. Stone JG, Young WL, Marans ZS, *et al.* Consequences of electroencephalographic suppressive doses of propofol in conjunction with deep hypothermic circulatory arrest. *Anesthesiology* 1996; **85**: 497–501.

45. Newman MF, Murkin JM, Roach G, *et al.* Cerebral physiologic effects of burst suppression doses of propofol during non-pulsatile cardiopulmonary bypass. *Anesth Analg* 1995; **81**: 452–7.

46. Illievich UM, Petricek W, Schramm W, *et al.* Electroencephalographic burst suppression by propofol infusion in humans: hemodynamic consequences. *Anesth Analg* 1993; **77**: 155–60.

47. Sear JW. Intravenous Anaesthetics. *Balliere's Clinical Anaesthesiology* 1989; **3**: 217–42.

48. McKeating K, Bali IM, Dundee JW. The effects of thiopentone and propofol on upper airway integrity. *Anaesthesia* 1988; **43**: 638–40.

49. Wouters PF, Van de Velde M, Marcus MAE, *et al.* Hemodynamic changes during induction of with eltanolone and propofol in dogs. *Anesth Analg* 1995; **81**: 125–31.

50. Sear JW, Prys-Roberts C, Dye A. Hepatic function after anaesthesia for major vascular reconstructive surgery: A comparison of four anaesthetic techniques. *Br J Anaesth* 1983; **55**: 603–9.

51. Murray JM, Trinick TR. Hepatic function and indocyanine green clearance during and after prolonged anaesthesia with propofol. *Br J Anaesth* 1992; **69**: 643–4.

52. Picard P, Tramer MR. Prevention of pain on injection with propofol: A quantitative sytematic review. *Anesth Analg* 2000; **90**: 963–9.

53. Doenicke AW, Roizen MF, Rau J, *et al.* Reducing pain during propofol injection: the role of the solvent. *Anesth Analg* 1996; **82**: 472–6.

54. Doenicke A, Roizen MF, Rau J, *et al.* Pharmacokinetics and pharmacodynamics of propofol in a new solvent. *Anesth Analg* 1997; **85**: 1399–404.

55. Rau J, Roizen MF, Doenicke AW, *et al.* Propofol in an emulsion of long- and medium-chain triglycerides: The effect on pain. *Anesth Analg* 2001; **93**: 382–4.

56. Knibbe CAJ, Aarts LPHJ, Kuks PFM, *et al.* Pharmacokinetics and pharmacodynamics of propofol 6% SAZN versus propofol 1% SAZN and Diprivan 10 for short-term sedation following coronary artery bypass surgery. *Eur J Clin Pharmacol* 2000; **56**: 89–95.

57. Gajraj NM, Nathanson MH. Preventing pain during injection of propofol: the optimal dose of lidocaine. *J Clin Anesth* 1996; **8**: 575–7.

58. Lilley EM, Isert PR, Carasso ML, Kennedy RA. The effect of the addition of lignocaine on propofol emulsion stability. *Anaesthesia* 1996; **51**: 815–18.

59. Park JW, Park ES, Chi SC, Kil HY, Lee KH. The effect of lidocaine on the globule size distribution of propofol emulsions. *Anesth Analg* 2003; **97**: 769–71.

60. Bennett SN, McNeil MM, Bland LA, *et al.* Postoperative infections traced to contamination of an intravenous anesthetic propofol. *N Engl J Med* 1995; **333**: 147–54.

61. Sosis MB, Braverman B, Villaflor E. Propofol, but not thiopental, supports the growth of Candida albicans. *Anesth Analg* 1995; **81**: 132–4.

62. Badr AE, Mychaskiw G, Eichhorn JH. Metabolic acidosis associated with a new formulation of propofol. *Anesthesiology* 2001; **94**: 536–8.

63. Matrin PH, Murthy BV, Petros AJ. Metabolic, biochemical and haemodynamic effects of infusion of propofol for long term sedation of children undergoing intensive care. *Br J Anaesth* 1997; **79**: 276–9.

64. Wysowski DK, Pollock ML. Reports of death with use of propofol (Diprivan) for nonprocedural (long-term) sedation and literature review. *Anesthesiology* 2006; **105**: 1047–51.

65. Fong JJ, Sylvia L, Ruthazer R, *et al.* Predictors of mortality in patients with suspected propofol infusion syndrome. *Crit Care Med* 2008; **36**: 2281–7.

66. White PF, Schüttler J, Shafer A, *et al.* Comparative pharmacology of the ketamine isomers. *Br J Anaesth* 1985; **57**: 197–203.

67. Kharasch ED, Labroo R. Metabolism of ketamine stereoisomers by human liver microsomes. *Anesthesiology* 1992; **77**: 1201–7.

68. Adams HA, Thiel A, Jung A, *et al.* Untersuchumgen mit S+ ketamin an probanden. Endokrine- und kreislaufreaktionen, aufwachverhalten und traumerlebnisse. *Der Anaesthesist* 1992; **41**: 588–96.

69. Albrecht S, Hering W, Schüttler J, Schwilden H. Neue intravenose anasthetika. *Der Anaesthesist* 1996; **45**: 1129–41.

70. Hering W, Geisslinger G, Kamp DH, *et al.* Changes in the EEG power spectrum after midazolam anaesthesia combined with racemic or S+ ketamine. *Acta Anaesthesiol Scand* 1994; **38**: 719–23.

71. Schüttler J, Stanski DR, White PF, *et al.* Pharmacodynamic modeling of the EEG effects of ketamine and its enantiomers in man. *J Pharmacokinet Biopharm* 1987; **15**: 241–53.

72. Geisslinger G, Hering W, Thomann P, *et al.* Pharmacokinetics and dynamics of ketamine enantiomers in surgical patients using a stereo-specific analytical method. *Br J Anaesth* 1993; **70**: 666–71.

73. White PF, Ham J, Way WL, Trevor AJ. Pharmacology of ketamine isomers in surgical patients. *Anesthesiology* 1980; **52**: 231–9.

74. Doenicke A, Angster R, Maker M, *et al.* Die wirkung von S+ ketamin auf katecholamine und cortisol im serum. *Der Anaesthesist* 1992; **41**: 597–603.

75. Adams HA, Bauer R, Gebhardt B, *et al.* TIVA mit S+ ketamin in der orthopadischen alterschirugie. *Der Anaesthesist* 1994; **43**: 92–100.

76. Pfenninger E, Himmelseher S. Neuroprotektion durch ketamin auf zellularer ebene. *Der Anaesthesist* **46**: 1997; s47–54.

77. Himmelseher S, Pfenninger E, Georgieff M. The effects of ketamine isomers on neuronal injury and regneration in rat hippocampal neurons. *Anesth Analg* 1996; **83**: 505–12.

78. Harris CE, Murray AM, Anderson JM, Grounds RM, Morgan M. Effects of thiopentone, etomidate and propofol on the haemodynamic response to trachea intubation. *Anaesthesia* 1988; **43**: 32–6.

79. Doenicke A, Roizen MF, Kugler J, *et al.* Reducing myoclonus after etomidate. *Anesthesiology* 1999; **90**: 113–19.

80. Modica PA, Tempelhoff R, White PF. Pro and anticonvulsant effects of anesthetics (Part II). *Anesth Analg* 1990; **70**: 433–44.

81. Doenicke AW, Roizen MF, Hoernecke R, Lorenz W, Ostwald P. Solvent for etomidate may cause pain and adverse effects. *Br J Anaesth* 1999; **83**: 464–6.

82. Preziosi P, Vacca M. Adrenocortical suppression and other endocrine effects of etomidate. *Life Sci* 1988; **42**: 477–89.

83. Jackson WJ. Should we use etomidate as an induction agent for endotracheal intubation in patients with septic shock? A critical appraisal. *Chest* 2005; **127**: 1031–8.

84. Crozier TA, Schlaeger M, Wuttke W, Kettler D. [TIVA with etomidate-fentanyl versus midazolam-fentanyl. The preoperative strss of coronary surgery overcomes the inhibition of corrtisol synthesus caused by etomidate-fentanyl anesthesia.] *Anaesthesist* 1994; **43**: 605–13.

85. Watt I, Ledingham IM. Mortality amonst multiple trauma patients admitted to an intensive care unit. *Anaesthesia* 1984; **39**: 973–81.

86. Vanacker B, Wiebalck A, Van Aken H, *et al.* Induktionsqualitat und nebennierenrindenfunktion: Ein klinischer vergleich von Etomidatlipuro und hypnomidate. *Der Anaesthesist* 1993; **42**: 81–9.

87. Kulka PJ, Bremer F, Schüttler J: Narkoseeinleitung mit Etomidat in Lipidemulsion. *Der Anaesthesist* 1993; **42**: 205–9.

88. Nebauer AE, Doenicke A, Hoernecke R, *et al.* Does etomidate cause haemolysis? *Br J Anaesth* 1992; **69**: 58–60.

89. Doenicke AW, Roizen MF, Hoernecke R, *et al.* Solvent for etomidate may cause pain and adverse effects. *Br J Anaesth* 1999; **83**: 464–6.

90. Doenicke A, Roizen MF, Nebauer AE, *et al.* Comparison of two formulations of etomidate, 2-hydroxypropyl-β-cyclodextrin (HPCD) and propylene glycol. *Anesth Analg* 1994; **79**: 933–9.

91. St Pierre M, Dunkel M, Rutherford A, Hering W: Does etomidate increase postoperative nausea? A double-blind controlled comparison of etomidate in lipid emulsion with propofol for balanced anaesthesia. *Eur J Anaesthesiol* 2000; **17**: 634–41.

92. Doenicke AW, Roizen MF, Rau J, Kellermann W, Babl J. Reducing pain during propofol injection: the role of the solvent. *Anesth Analg* 1996; **82**: 472–4.

93. Baker MT, Naguib M. Propofol: The challenges of formulation. *Anesthesiology* 2005; **103**: 860–76.

94. Morey TE, Modell JH, Shekhawat D, *et al.* Preparation and anesthetic properties of propofol microemulsions in rats. *Anesthesiology* 2006; **104**: 1184–90.

95. Kim KM, Choi BM, Park SW, *et al.* Pharmacokinetics and pharmacodynamics of propofol microemulsion and lipid emulsion after an intravenous bolus and variable rate infusion. *Anesthesiology* 2007; **106**; 924–34.

96. Lee EH, Lee SH, Park DY, *et al.* Physicochemical properties, pharmacokinetics, and pharmacodynamics of a reformulated microemulsion in rats. *Anesthesiology* 2008; **109**; 436–47.

97. Dubey PK, Kumar A. Pain on injection of lipid-free propofol and propofol emulsion containing medium-chain triglyceride: a comparative study. *Anesth Analg* 2005; **101**; 1060–2.

98. Trapani A, Laquintana V, Lopedota A, *et al.* Evaluation of new propofol aqueous solutions for intravenous anesthesia. *Int J Pharmaceutics* 2004; **278**; 91–8.

99. Egan TD, Kern SE, Johnson KB, Pace NL. The pharmacodynamics and pharmacodynamics of propofol in a modified cyclodextrin formulation (captisol) versus propofol on a lipid formulation (Diprivan): an encephalographic and hemodynamic study in a porcine model. *Anesth Analg* 2003; **97**; 72–9.

100. Bielen SJ, Lysko GS, Gough WB. The effect of cyclodextrin vehicle on the cardiovascular profile of propofol in rats. *Anesth Analg* 1996; **82**; 920–4.

101. Ravenelle F, Gori S, Le Garrec D, *et al.* Novel lipid and preservative-free propofol formulation: properties and pharmacodynamics. *Pharm Res* 2008; **25**; 313–19.

102. Ravenelle F, Vachon P, Rigby-Jones AE, *et al.* Anaesthetic properties of propofol polymeric micelle: a novel water soluble propofol formulation. *Br J Anaesth* 2008; **101**: 186–93.

103. Cooke A, Anderson A, Buchanan K, *et al.* water-soluble propofol analogues with intravenous anaesthetic activity. *Bioorg Med Chem Lett* 2001; **11**: 927–30.

104. Trapani G, Latrofa A, Franco M, *et al.* Water-soluble salts of aminoacid esters of the anaesthetic agent propofol. *Int J Pharmaceutics* 1998; **175**: 195–204.

105. Banaszczyk MG, Carlo AT, Millan V, *et al.* Propofol phosphate. A water-soluble propofol prodrug: in vivo evaluation. *Anesth Analg* 2002; **95**: 1285–92.

106. Altomare C, Trapani G, Latrofa A, *et al.* Highly water-soluble derivatives of the anaesthetic agent propofol: in vitro and in vivo evaluation of cyclic amino acid esters. *Europ J Pharmaceutical Sci* 2003; **20**: 17–26.

107. Gibiansky E, Struys MMRF, Gibiansky L, *et al.* AQUAVAN injection, a water-soluble prodrug of propofol, as a bolus injection: a phase I dose-escalation comparison with DIPRIVAN (part 1). *Anesthesiology* 2005; **103**: 718–29.

108. Leslie JB, Cohen LB, Silvestri G, Gan T-J. Clinical safety of fospropofol sodium sedation during diagnostic and therapeutic procedures. *Anesthesiology* 2008; **109**: A190.

109. Kumpulainen H, Jarvinen T, Mannila A, *et al.* Synthesis, in vitro and in vivo characterization of novel ethyl dioxy phosphate prodrug of propofol. *Europ J Pharmaceutical Sci* 2008; **34**: 110–17.

110. Lei L, Liu J. CNS safety of HX0507 in mice. *Anesthesiology* 2007; **107**: A1685.

111. Lei L, Liu J. Respiratory and cardiovascular safety of HX0507 in beagle dogs. *Anesthesiology* 2007; **107**: A1102.

112. Cashin MF, Moravek V. The physiological action of cholesterol. *Am J Physiol* 1927; **82**: 294–8.

113. Sear JW. ORG 21465: a new water-soluble steroid hypnotic: more of the same or something different? *Br J Anaesth* 1997; **79**: 417–19.

114. Radford SG, Lockyer JA, Simpson PJ. Immunological aspects of adverse reactions to Althesin. *Br J Anaesth* 1982; **54**: 859–63.

115. Moneret-Vautrin DA, Laxenaire MC, Viry-Babel F. Anaphylaxis caused by anti-Cremophor EL IgG STS antibodies in a case of reaction to Althesin. *Br J Anaesth* 1983; **55**: 469–71.

116. Tachon P, Descotes J, Laschi-Loquerie A, *et al.* Assessment of the allergenic potential of Althesin and its constituents. *Br J Anaesth* 1983; **55**: 715–17.

117. Simpson PJ, Radford SG, Lockyer JA, Sear JW. Some predisposing factors to hypersensitivity reactions following first exposure to Althesin. *Anaesthesia* 1985; **40**: 420–3.

118. Sear JW, Sanders RS. Intra-patient comparison of the kinetics of alphaxalone and alphadolone in man. *Eur J Anaesthesiol* 1984; **1**: 113–21.

119. Visser SAG, Smulders CJGM, Reijers BPR, *et al.* Mechanism-based pharmacokinetic-pharmacodynamic modeling of concentration-dependent hysteresis and biphasic electroencephalogram effects of alphaxalone in rats. *J Pharmacol Exp Ther* 2002; **302**: 1158–67.

120. Holly JMP, Trafford DJH, Sear JW, Makin HLJ. The in vivo metabolism of Althesin (alphaxalone + alphadolone acetate) in man. *J Pharm Pharmacol* 1981; **33**: 427–33.

121. Desmet G, Nemitz B, Biotieux JL, *et al.* Dosage de l'alphaxalone dans le serum et les urines par chromatographie gaz-liquide. *Ann Biol Clin (Paris)* 1979; **37**: 83–8.

122. Estes KS, Brewster MW, Webb AI, Bodor N. A non-surfactant formulation for alfaxalone based on an amorphous cyclodextrin: activity studies in rats and dogs. *Int J Pharmaceutics* 1990; **65**: 101.

123. Ferre PJ, Pasloske K, Whittem T, *et al.* Plasma pharmacokinetics of alphaxalone in dogs after an intravenous bolus of Alfaxan-CD RTU. *Vet Anaesth Analgesia* 2006; **33**: 229–36.

124. Whittem T, Pasloske KM, Heit MC, Ranasinghe MG. The pharmacokinetics and pharmacodynamics of alfaxalone in cats after single and multiple intravenous administration of Alfaxan at clinical and supraclinical doses. *J Vet Pharmacol Ther* 2008; **31**: 571–9.

125. Cotten JF, Husain SS, Forman SA, *et al.* Methoxycarbonyl-etomidate: a novel rapidly metabolized and ultra-short-acting etomidate analogue that does not produce prolonged adrenocortical suppression. *Anesthesiology* 2009; **111**: 240–9.

126. Ledingham IM, Watt I. Influence of sedation on mortality in critically ill multiple trauma patients. *Lancet* 1983; **1**: 1270.

127. Wagner RL, White PF, Kan PB, *et al.* Inhibition of adrenal steroidogenesis by the anesthetic etomidate. *N Engl J Med* 1984; **310**: 1415–21.

128. Absalom A, Pledger D, Kong A. Adrenocortical function in critically ill patients 24 hours after a single dose of etomidate. *Anaesthesia* 1999; **54**: 861–7.

129. den Brinker M, Hokken-Koelega AC, Hazelzet JA, *et al.* One single dose of etomidate negatively influences adrenocortical performance for at least 24 hours in children with meningococcal sepsis. *Intensive Care Med* 2007; **34**: 163–8.

130. Hildreth AN, Mejia VA, Maxwell RA, *et al.* Adrenal suppression following a single dose of etomidate for rapid sequence induction: a prospective randomized study. *J Trauma* 2008; **65**: 573–9.

131. Siegel LC, Wray J. Initial studies on the mechanism of action of PF0713, an investigational anesthetic agent. *Anesthesiology* 2008; **109**: A642.

132. Siegel LC, Pelc LR, Shaff K. Dose response of PF0713, a novel investigational intravenous anesthetic agent. *Anesthesiology* 2008; **109**: A869.

133. Siegel LC, Konstantatos A. PF0713 produced rapid infuction of general anesthesia without injection pain in a phase 1 study. *Anesthesiology* 2009; A463.

134. Kanamitsu N, Osaki T, Itsuji Y, *et al.* Novel water-soluble sedative-hypnotic agents: Isoindolin-1-one derivatives. *Chem Pharm Bull* 2007; **55**: 1682–8.

135. Yamamura Y, Uchida I, Kawatsu R, *et al.* A new benzodiazepine site agonist, JM-1232(–), as the short acting sedative-hypnotic agent. *Neuroscience* Nov. 2007, Poster 358.7/J15.

136. Kuribayashi J, Kuwana S-I, Hosokawa Y, Hatori E, Takeda J. Effect of a new sedative, JM-1232 (–) on central respiratory activity in neonatal rats. *Anesthesiology* 2008; **109**: A1767.

137. Rigby-Jones A, Ohkura T, Shimizu S, Cross M, Sneyd J. First human administration of JM1232, a novel isoindoline derivative benzodiazepine agonist. *Eur J Anaesthesiol* 2008; **25** (supplement 44): 129 (abstract 9AP2–6).

138. Rigby-Jones AE, Sneyd, , Okhura T, Tominaga H, Cross M. MR04A3 (aqueous 1.0% JM-1232 (–)) pharmacokinetics and pharmacodynamics in man. *Anesthesiology* 2009; A464.

139. Tilbrook GS, Kilpatrick GJ. CNS 7056X, an ultra-short acting benzodiazepine: in vitro metabolism. *Anesthesiology* 2006; **105**: A1611.

140. Kilpatrick GJ, McIntyre MS, Cox RF, *et al.* CNS 7056: a novel ultra-short acting benzodiazepine. *Anesthesiology* 2007; **107**: 60–6.

141. Mutter C, Rudolf G, Diemunsch PA, Tilbrook GS, Borgeat A. CNS 7056X an ultra-short acting benzodiazepine: pharmacokinetic and pharmacodynamic study in pig. *Anesthesiology* 2006; **105**: A1610.

142. Antonik LJ, Goldwater DR, Kilpatrick GJ, Tilbrook GS, Borkett KM. A phase 1 SAD study evaluating the safety, pharmacokinetics and pharmacodynamics of CNS 7056. *Anesthesiology* 2009; A1603.

143. Beattie D, Jenkins T, McCullough J *et al.* The in vivo activity of THRX-918661, a novel, pharmacokinetically responsive sedative/hypnotic agent. *Anaesthesia* 2004; **59**: 101.

144. Egan TD, Shafer SL, Jenkins TE, Beattie DT, Jaw-Tsai SS. The pharmacokinetics and pharmacodynamics of THRX-918661, a novel sedative/hypnotic agent. *Anesthesiology* 2003; **99**: A516.

145. Naguib M, Schmid PG, Baker MT. The electroencephalographic effects of iv anesthetic doses of melatonin:

comparative studies with thiopental and propofol. *Anesth Analg* 2003; **97**: 238–43.

146. Naguib M, Hammond DL, Schmid PG, *et al.* Pharmacologic effects of intravenous melatonin: comparative studies with thiopental and propofol. *Br J Anaesth* 2003; **90**: 504–7.

147. Fisher MM, Ross JD, Harle DA, Baldo B. Anaphylaxis to thiopentone: an unusual outbreak in a single hospital. *Anaesth Intensive Care* 1989; **17**: 361–5.

148. Moneret-Vautrin DA, Widmer S, Gueant J-L, *et al.* Simultaneous anaphylaxis to thiopentone and a neuromuscular blocker: A study of two cases. *Br J Anaesth* 1990; **64**: 743–5.

149. Clarke RSJ. Adverse effects of intravenously administered drugs used in anaesthetic practice. *Drugs* 1981; **22**: 26–41.

150. Watkins JA. Etomidate: an "immunologically safe" anaesthetic agent. *Anaesthesia* 1983; **38**: 34–8.

151. Krumholz W, Muller H, Gerlach H, *et al.* Ein fall von anaphylaktoider reaktion nach gabe von etomidat. *Der Anaesthesist* 1984; **33**: 161–2.

152. Sold M, Rothhammer A. Lebensbedrohliche anaphylaktoide reaktion nach etomidat. *Der Anaesthesist* 1985; **34**: 208–10.

153. Fazackerley EJ, Martin AJ, Tolhurst-Cleaver CL, Watkins J. Anaphylactoid reaction following the use of etomidate. *Anaesthesia* 1988; **43**: 953–4.

154. Mathieu A, Goudsouzian N, Snider MT. Reaction to ketamine: anaphylactoid or anaphylactic. *Br J Anaesth* 1975; **47**: 624.

155. Laxenaire MC, Moneret-Vautrin D, Vervloet D. The French experience of anaphylactoid reactions. *Int Anesthesiol Clin* 1985; **23**: 145–60.

156. Ducart AR, Watremez C, Louagie YA, *et al.* Propofol-induced anaphylactoid reaction during for cardiac surgery. *J Cardiothoracic Vasc Anesth* 2000; **14**: 200–1.

midazolam doses may be given either intravenously or intramuscularly (IM). Because of the interpatient variability in absorption and the dose–response relationship for midazolam, the use of IM midazolam should be reserved for healthy patients without IV access who receive a single IM dose of midazolam for preoperative sedation. IM midazolam must be administered 30–60 minutes in advance of the desired time to peak effect, whereas IV midazolam boluses for preoperative sedation can be administered 3–5 minutes before the start of a procedure. IV doses of midazolam for induction of anesthesia should be administered over 20–30 seconds with a peak effect occurring within 2 minutes. Patients undergoing general anesthesia who are premedicated with opioids or other sedatives should have their midazolam induction dose reduced by 25%. Subsequent doses of midazolam (approximately 25% of the induction dose) may be given intraoperatively in response to signs of lightening anesthesia. Because of the interpatient variability in the dose–response relationship for midazolam, IV midazolam boluses given for conscious sedation during procedures should be administered in divided doses and carefully titrated to the desired level of sedation for each patient, waiting at least 5 minutes between each dose.

In ICU patients receiving midazolam for continuous sedation, an IV bolus may be administered prior to the start of an infusion in order to achieve adequate levels of sedation more quickly. Boluses of midazolam should be administered in divided doses to prevent hemodynamic instability in these patients. Midazolam infusions in surgical ICU patients should be titrated frequently during the first 24–48 hours after surgery, because midazolam requirements increase initially with the resolving effects of anesthesia, then decrease with midazolam accumulation over time. Patients should be maintained at a level of sedation with midazolam that allows them to respond to simple commands without agitation. The use of a sedation scoring system to monitor depth of sedation can help to optimize the dosing of midazolam infusions in ICU patients. In addition, midazolam infusions should be temporarily suspended each day to prevent oversedation and to minimize drug accumulation. Once the patient is awake, the midazolam infusion should then be resumed at the lowest possible infusion rate to maintain the desired level of sedation. Such "sedation holidays" have been shown to hasten emergence from sedation and to improve clinical outcomes in ICU patients [59]. The concurrent use of opioid infusions for analgesia in ICU patients also significantly reduces their midazolam requirements and hastens their emergence from midazolam. ICU patients with a creatinine clearance less than 50 mL min^{-1} who receive continuous infusions of midazolam over several days may accumulate significant amounts of 1-hydroxymidazolam glucuronide, the active metabolite of midazolam, resulting in deeper levels of sedation and an even greater prolonged emergence from sedation. Alternative sedative regimens may be indicated in these patients.

Lorazepam

Table 29.5 summarizes the parenteral dosing regimens for lorazepam during a variety of clinical circumstances. Because of its slower onset of action, its longer duration of effect, and its greater potency compared with midazolam, patients require smaller and less frequent doses of lorazepam than midazolam. For every 10 years of patient age over age 60, lorazepam potency increases by about 18%, and doses should be reduced in elderly patients. Lorazepam doses should also be decreased in debilitated patients and in the presence of opioids or other preoperative sedatives, to avoid cardiorespiratory depression. Obese patients may require greater initial doses of lorazepam to achieve adequate sedation, but may exhibit delayed emergence from sedation compared with non-obese patients.

Lorazepam may be administered either intramuscularly or intravenously. When administered intravenously, lorazepam can cause venous irritation and thrombophlebitis and should be diluted with an equal volume of compatible diluent. Continuous infusions of lorazepam should be administered through central venous catheter. Because of its longer onset of effect, IM lorazepam must be administered at least 2 hours before surgery. In addition, 17% of patients experience significant pain and burning sensations with IM injections of lorazepam. For these reasons, oral administration of lorazepam may be preferable for preoperative sedation of patients. Lorazepam should not be used as a preoperative sedative in cases in which rapid emergence from anesthesia at the end of the procedure is desired. Because of its slow onset of action and its long duration of effect, lorazepam is a poor choice for the induction or maintenance of anesthesia or for use in conscious sedation.

Continuous infusions of IV lorazepam or intermittent bolus injections may be used for sedation of patients in the ICU who are intubated and mechanically ventilated. Because of its slower onset of action and its prolonged effect, lorazepam may be more difficult to titrate to a desired level of sedation compared with midazolam. As with midazolam, lorazepam infusions should be preceded by IV loading doses in awake patients to initially achieve the desired level of sedation. Lorazepam infusions should be frequently titrated over the first 24 hours to maintain optimal levels of sedation. Patients emerging from anesthesia will require less lorazepam for the first 24 hours after surgery than awake patients. Patients may still experience prolonged emergence times from sedation with lorazepam, leading to significant delays of up to several days in weaning these patients from mechanical ventilation and extubation. Strategies to minimize emergence time after discontinuation of lorazepam infusions in ICU patients include: (1) using sedation scoring systems to target the desired level of sedation with lorazepam; (2) maintaining the lightest possible level of sedation with lorazepam (i.e., the patient is still able to follow commands without being agitated); (3) using opioids together with lorazepam to minimize the amount of lorazepam required; (4) using lorazepam holidays with daily suspension of lorazepam infusions to prevent oversedation; and (5) swapping lorazepam for a shorter-acting sedative, such a propofol, 48–72 hours in advance of discontinuing sedation to allow for the lorazepam to wash out of peripheral tissues.

Diazepam

Table 29.5 summarizes the parenteral dosing regimens for diazepam for various clinical indications. Diazepam doses should be reduced in elderly or debilitated patients (especially in patients with cirrhosis) because of an increased sensitivity and longer elimination half-life for diazepam in these patients leading to oversedation and delayed emergence. Diazepam doses should also be reduced in patients receiving opioids, other sedatives, or H_2-blockers. Obese patients require greater initial doses of diazepam but may experience prolonged sedation with diazepam.

Diazepam may be given either intramuscularly or intravenously. IV diazepam should be administered through a central venous catheter to avoid venous irritation and thrombophlebitis resulting from the benzyl alcohol additive. As a preoperative sedative, IV diazepam may be administered within 3–5 minutes of the start of the procedure, compared with 15–30 minutes beforehand for IM dosing. Although the rapid onset of IV diazepam makes it a good induction drug, delayed emergence from anesthesia limit its use to ICU patients who are to remain intubated after anesthesia. Diazepam is administered intermittently, either orally or IV, for sedation of ICU patients. Diazepam dosing in these patients may need to be decreased over time as diazepam and desmethyldiazepam accumulation in peripheral tissues occurs. Emergence from sedation with diazepam in ICU patients may be hastened by switching from diazepam to a shorter-acting sedative, such as propofol, several days in advance of discontinuing sedation altogether. Diazepam should not be used for sedation of ICU patients with end-stage liver disease, because these patients may experience prolonged sedation caused by the decreased clearance of both diazepam and desmethyldiazepam.

The experimental benzodiazepine site ligand L-838,417, which is a partial agonist at α_2-, α_3-, and α_5-subunit-containing $GABA_A$ receptors and an antagonist at α_1-containing $GABA_A$ receptors, and which has anxiolytic but not sedative properties in rats [8], elicits antinociceptive actions in this species, and it is notable that over a 9-day treatment period tolerance did not develop, in contrast to morphine [60]. Novel benzodiazepine site ligands might thus be useful in the treatment of chronic pain.

Summary

Benzodiazepines act on $GABA_A$ receptors to enhance fast inhibitory neurotransmission, and are used to treat sleep disorders, anxiety disorders, status epilepticus, and muscle tension. There are separate binding sites on most $GABA_A$ receptors for benzodiazepines and the neurotransmitter GABA. In the presence of benzodiazepines, more receptors are recruited for activation by GABA. The presence of a finite number of receptors available for occupation by the neurotransmitter gives rise to a physiologic maximum of GABA-induced inhibition, which cannot be exceeded even in the presence of benzodiazepines. This is thought to result in the low toxicity and clinical safety of these drugs. Benzodiazepines also prolong the decay of the GABA response. Novel benzodiazepine site ligands might be useful in the treatment of chronic pain.

Benzodiazepines bind multiple $GABA_A$ receptor subtypes. Molecular genetic approaches have been used to delineate subtype-specific functions. Evidence indicates that the α_1-receptor subunit is involved in sedative effects and anterograde amnesia, but not hypnotic activity, while anticonvulsant effects likely rely on the combined action of several receptor subtypes. Anxiolytic and myorelaxant activity are thought to be predominantly mediated by α_2-containing $GABA_A$ receptors.

Midazolam, lorazepam, and diazepam are the most commonly used benzodiazepines for perioperative sedation. Differences in their receptor binding affinities, lipid solubilities, and pharmacokinetics give rise to differences in the onset, duration, and offset of effects with these drugs. Factors such as duration of drug administration, total dose of drug administered, patient age, weight, and liver disease have varying effects on the pharmacokinetics of each drug. Pharmacodynamic differences between the benzodiazepines should also be considered when selecting appropriate sedatives.

Benzodiazepines can suppress the hypoxic drive, causing respiratory depression. This adverse effect is amplified in the presence of opioids and other sedatives, and in patients with chronic obstructive pulmonary disease. Benzodiazepines may also cause cardiovascular depression, amplified by the presence of opioids, other sedatives, or hemodynamic instability. Adverse effects may be reversed with the benzodiazepine antagonist flumazenil, although this should be avoided in patients taking benzodiazepines long-term, because of the risk of withdrawal seizures.

Dosing regimens should take into consideration age, liver disease or other condition rendering a patient high-risk for surgery, usage of opioids, other sedatives or H_2-blockers, and obesity. Other factors include drug accumulation and the desired time for emergence from sedation, which may influence the choice of benzodiazepine. The route of administration impacts the time to peak effect, and the possibility of adverse reactions. In general, patients may receive either single oral doses or IV bolus injections for short-term sedation during a surgical procedure, or repeated IV boluses or continuous infusions for postoperative sedation in the intensive care unit. Various strategies may hasten emergence from sedation with certain benzodiazepines, such as "sedation holidays," which involve temporary suspension of infusions each day to minimize drug accumulation; maintaining an appropriate level of sedation using sedation scoring systems; and substituting long-acting sedatives for short-acting sedatives in advance of discontinuation.

References

1. Mody I, De Koninck Y, Otis TS, Soltesz I. Bridging the cleft at GABA synapses in the brain. *Trends Neurosci* 1994; **17**: 517–25.

2. Hajos N, Nusser Z, Rancz EA, Freund TF, Mody I. Cell type- and synapse-specific variability in synaptic GABA$_A$ receptor occupancy. *Eur J Neurosci* 2000; **12**: 810–18.

3. Haefely W, Martin JR, Schoch P. Novel anxiolytics that act as partial agonists at benzodiazepine receptors. *Trends Pharmacol Sci* 1990; **11**: 452–6.

4. Wieland HA, Luddens H, Seeburg PH. A single histidine in GABA$_A$ receptors is essential for benzodiazepine agonist binding. *J Biol Chem* 1992; **267**: 1426–9.

5. Kleingoor C, Wieland HA, Korpi ER, Seeburg PH, Kettenmann H. Current potentiation by diazepam but not GABA sensitivity is determined by a single histidine residue. *Neuroreport* 1993; **4**: 187–90.

6. Benson JA, Low K, Keist R, Mohler H, Rudolph U. Pharmacology of recombinant gamma-aminobutyric acid$_A$ receptors rendered diazepam-insensitive by point-mutated alpha-subunits. *FEBS Lett* 1998; **431**: 400–4.

7. Rudolph U, Crestani F, Benke D, *et al.* Benzodiazepine actions mediated by specific gamma-aminobutyric acid(A) receptor subtypes. *Nature* 1999; **401**: 796–800.

8. McKernan RM, Rosahl TW, Reynolds DS, *et al.* Sedative but not anxiolytic properties of benzodiazepines are mediated by the GABA(A) receptor alpha1 subtype. *Nat Neurosci* 2000; **3**: 587–92.

9. Zeller A, Crestani F, Camenisch I, *et al.* Cortical glutamatergic neurons mediate the motor sedative action of diazepam. *Mol Pharmacol* 2008; **73**: 282–91.

10. Low K, Crestani F, Keist R, *et al.* Molecular and neuronal substrate for the selective attenuation of anxiety. *Science* 2000; **290**: 131–4.

11. Crestani F, Keist R, Fritschy JM, *et al.* Trace fear conditioning involves hippocampal alpha5 GABA(A) receptors. *Proc Natl Acad Sci U S A* 2002; **99**: 8980–5.

12. Fradley RL, Guscott MR, Bull S, *et al.* Differential contribution of GABA(A) receptor subtypes to the anticonvulsant efficacy of benzodiazepine site ligands. *J Psychopharmacol* 2007; **21**: 384–91.

13. Crestani F, Low K, Keist R, *et al.* Molecular targets for the myorelaxant action of diazepam. *Mol Pharmacol* 2001; **59**: 442–5.

14. Tobler I, Kopp C, Deboer T, Rudolph U. Diazepam-induced changes in sleep: role of the alpha 1 GABA(A) receptor subtype. *Proc Natl Acad Sci U S A* 2001; **98**: 6464–9.

15. Kopp C, Rudolph U, Low K, Tobler I. Modulation of rhythmic brain activity by diazepam: GABA(A) receptor subtype and state specificity. *Proc Natl Acad Sci U S A* 2004; **101**: 3674–9.

16. Moschitto LJ, Greenblatt DJ. Concentration-independent plasma protein binding of benzodiazepines. *J Pharm Pharmacol* 1983; **35**: 179–80.

17. Arendt RM, Greenblatt DJ, Garland WA. Quantitation by gas chromatography of the 1- and 4-hydroxy metabolites of midazolam in human plasma. *Pharmacology* 1984; **29**: 158–64.

18. Vree TB, Baars AM, Booij LH, Driessen JJ. Simultaneous determination and pharmacokinetics of midazolam and its hydroxymetabolites in plasma and urine of man and dog by means of high-performance liquid chromatography. *Arzneimittelforschung* 1981; **31**: 2215–9.

19. Mandema JW, Tuk B, van Steveninck AL, *et al.* Pharmacokinetic-pharmacodynamic modeling of the central nervous system effects of midazolam and its main metabolite alpha-hydroxymidazolam in healthy volunteers. *Clin Pharmacol Ther* 1992; **51**: 715–28.

20. Barr J, Zomorodi K, Bertaccini EJ, Shafer SL, Geller E. A double-blind, randomized comparison of i.v. lorazepam versus midazolam for sedation of ICU patients via a pharmacologic model. *Anesthesiology* 2001; **95**: 286–98.

21. Bauer TM, Ritz R, Haberthur C, *et al.* Prolonged sedation due to accumulation of conjugated metabolites of midazolam. *Lancet* 1995; **346**: 145–7.

22. Greenblatt DJ, Schillings RT, Kyriakopoulos AA, *et al.* Clinical pharmacokinetics of lorazepam. I. Absorption and disposition of oral 14C-lorazepam. *Clin Pharmacol Ther* 1976; **20**: 329–41.

23. van der Bijl P, Roelofse JA, Joubert JJ, van Zyl JF. Comparison of various physiologic and psychomotor parameters in patients sedated with intravenous lorazepam, diazepam, or midazolam during oral surgery. *J Oral Maxillofac Surg* 1991; **49**: 672–8.

24. Herman RJ, Wilkinson GR. Disposition of diazepam in young and elderly subjects after acute and chronic dosing. *Br J Clin Pharmacol* 1996; **42**: 147–55.

25. Greenblatt DJ, Abernethy DR, Locniskar A, *et al.* Effect of age, gender, and obesity on midazolam kinetics. *Anesthesiology* 1984; **61**: 27–35.

26. Greenblatt DJ, Abernethy DR, Morse DS, Harmatz JS, Shader RI. Clinical importance of the interaction of diazepam and cimetidine. *N Engl J Med* 1984; **310**: 1639–43.

27. MacGilchrist AJ, Birnie GG, Cook A, *et al.* Pharmacokinetics and pharmacodynamics of intravenous midazolam in patients with severe alcoholic cirrhosis. *Gut* 1986; **27**: 190–5.

28. Hase I, Oda Y, Tanaka K, *et al.* I.v. fentanyl decreases the clearance of midazolam. *Br J Anaesth* 1997; **79**: 740–3.

29. Maitre PO, Funk B, Crevoisier C, Ha HR. Pharmacokinetics of midazolam in patients recovering from cardiac surgery. *Eur J Clin Pharmacol* 1989; **37**: 161–6.

30. Zomorodi K, Donner A, Somma J, *et al.* Population pharmacokinetics of midazolam administered by target controlled infusion for sedation following coronary artery bypass grafting. *Anesthesiology* 1998; **89**: 1418–29.

31. Oldenhof H, de Jong M, Steenhoek A, Janknegt R. Clinical pharmacokinetics of midazolam in intensive care patients, a wide interpatient variability? *Clin Pharmacol Ther* 1988; **43**: 263–9.

32. Hung OR, Dyck JB, Varvel J, Shafer SL, Stanski DR. Comparative absorption kinetics of intramuscular midazolam

and diazepam. *Can J Anaesth* 1996; **43**: 450–5.

33. Depoortere H, Zivkovic B, Lloyd KG, *et al.* Zolpidem, a novel nonbenzodiazepine hypnotic. I. Neuropharmacological and behavioral effect. *J Pharmacol Exp Ther* 1986; **237**: 649–58.

34. Mohler H, Okada T. Benzodiazepine receptor: demonstration in the central nervous system. *Science* 1977; **198**: 849–51.

35. Greenblatt DJ, Shader RI, Franke K, *et al.* Pharmacokinetics and bioavailability of intravenous, intramuscular, and oral lorazepam in humans. *J Pharm Sci* 1979; **68**: 57–63.

36. Kraus JW, Desmond PV, Marshall JP, *et al.* Effects of aging and liver disease on disposition of lorazepam. *Clin Pharmacol Ther* 1978; **24**: 411–19.

37. Ameer B, Greenblatt DJ. Lorazepam: a review of its clinical pharmacological properties and therapeutic uses. *Drugs* 1981; **21**: 162–200.

38. Reves JG, Fragen RJ, Vinik HR, Greenblatt DJ. Midazolam: pharmacology and uses. *Anesthesiology* 1985; **62**: 310–24.

39. Barnard ED, Skonick P, Olsen RW, *et al.* International Union of Pharmacology. XV. Subtypes of gamma-aminobutyric acid$_A$ receptors: classification on the basis of subunit structure and receptor function. *Pharmacol Rev* 1998; **2**: 291–313.

40. Klotz U, Avant GR, Hoyumpa A, Schenker S, Wilkinson GR. The effects of age and liver disease on the disposition and elimination of diazepam in adult man. *J Clin Invest* 1975; **55**: 347–59.

41. Klotz U, Reimann I. Clearance of diazepam can be impaired by its major metabolite desmethyldiazepam. *Eur J Clin Pharmacol* 1981; **21**: 161–3.

42. Mohler H, Fritschy JM, Rudolph U. A new benzodiazepine pharmacology. *J Pharmacol Exp Ther* 2001; **300**: 2–8.

43. Ochs HR, Greenblatt DJ, Kaschell HJ, *et al.* Diazepam kinetics in patients with renal insufficiency or hyperthyroidism. *Br J Clin Pharmacol* 1981; **12**: 829–32.

44. Greenblatt DJ, Sellers EM, Shader RI. Drug therapy: drug disposition in old age. *N Engl J Med* 1982; **306**: 1081–8.

45. Shapiro BA, Warren J, Egol AB, *et al.* Practice parameters for intravenous analgesia and sedation for adult patients in the intensive care unit: an executive summary. Society of Critical Care Medicine. *Crit Care Med* 1995; **23**: 1596–600.

46. Sarnquist FH, Mathers WD, Brock-Utne J, *et al.* A bioassay for a water-soluble benzodiazepine against sodium thiopental. *Anesthesiology* 1980; **52**: 149–53.

47. Crawford ME, Carl P, Andersen RS, Mikkelsen BO. Comparison between midazolam and thiopentone-based balanced anaesthesia for day-case surgery. *Br J Anaesth* 1984; **56**: 165–9.

48. Somma J, Donner A, Zomorodi K, *et al.* Population pharmacodynamics of midazolam administered by target controlled infusion in SICU patients after CABG surgery. *Anesthesiology* 1998; **89**: 1430–43.

49. Greenblatt DJ, Ehrenberg BL, Gunderman J, *et al.* Kinetic and dynamic study of intravenous lorazepam: comparison with intravenous diazepam. *J Pharmacol Exp Ther* 1989; **250**: 134–40.

50. Cole SG, Brozinsky S, Isenberg JI. Midazolam, a new more potent benzodiazepine, compared with diazepam: a randomized, double-blind study of preendoscopic sedatives. *Gastrointest Endosc* 1983; **29**: 219–22.

51. Samuelson PN, Reves JG, Kouchoukos NT, Smith LR, Dole KM. Hemodynamic responses to anesthetic induction with midazolam or diazepam in patients with ischemic heart disease. *Anesth Analg* 1981; **60**: 802–9.

52. Inomata S, Nagashima A, Itagaki F, *et al.* CYP2C19 genotype affects diazepam pharmacokinetics and emergence from general anesthesia. *Clin Pharmacol Ther* 2005; **78**: 647–55.

53. Mora CT, Torjman M, White PF. Effects of diazepam and flumazenil on sedation and hypoxic ventilatory response. *Anesth Analg* 1989; **68**: 473–8.

54. Gross JB, Zebrowski ME, Carel WD, Gardner S, Smith TC. Time course of ventilatory depression after thiopental and midazolam in normal subjects and in patients with chronic obstructive pulmonary disease. *Anesthesiology* 1983; **58**: 540–4.

55. Benson KT, Tomlinson DL, Goto H, Arakawa K. Cardiovascular effects of lorazepam during sufentanil anesthesia. *Anesth Analg* 1988; **67**: 996–8.

56. Heikkila H, Jalonen J, Arola M, Kanto J, Laaksonen V. Midazolam as adjunct to high-dose fentanyl anaesthesia for coronary artery bypass grafting operation. *Acta Anaesthesiol Scand* 1984; **28**: 683–9.

57. Ruff R, Reves JG. Hemodynamic effects of a lorazepam-fentanyl anesthetic induction for coronary artery bypass surgery. *J Cardiothorac Anesth* 1990; **4**: 314–7.

58. Spivey WH. Flumazenil and seizures: analysis of 43 cases. *Clin Ther* 1992; **14**: 292–305.

59. Kress JP, Vinayak AG, Levitt J, *et al.* Daily sedative interruption in mechanically ventilated patients at risk for coronary artery disease. *Crit Care Med* 2007; **35**: 365–71.

60. Knabl J, Witschi R, Hosl K, *et al.* Reversal of pathological pain through specific spinal GABA$_A$ receptor subtypes. *Nature* 2008; **451**: 330–4.

Robert D. Sanders and Mervyn Maze

Introduction

Sedative and amnestic drugs are used widely in procedural, perioperative, and critical care. The separation of these drugs from anesthetics is arbitrary and primarily relates to their potency for hypnotic–sedative actions and anesthetic actions. Larger doses than are used for sedative purposes may induce general anesthesia but often produce significant adverse sequelae. Dissociation between the definition of sedation and hypnosis has also been made. Hypnosis occurs at higher drug concentrations and is defined as "drug-induced impairment of the cognitive functions that are required for responding adequately to environmental stimuli." Sedation occurs at lower drug concentrations, probably by cortical effects. Electroencephalogram (EEG) differences can be derived with a shift to increased frontal beta power reflecting sedation and a delta shift signaling hypnosis and reflecting subcortical effects. However, as we will discuss, EEG effects vary between different sedative drugs.

The sedative drugs typically employed include the α_2-adrenoceptor agonists dexmedetomidine and clonidine, the benzodiazepines (notably midazolam, lorazepam, and diazepam, covered in Chapter 29), chloral hydrate, and scopolamine. While sedation can be induced with low doses of more potent inhalational or intravenous anesthetic agents, these drugs are examined thoroughly in other chapters (Chapters 25–28). Likewise opioids, used in certain settings for analgesic-based sedation, are considered elsewhere (Chapters 31–33). In this chapter we describe the pharmacology of the commonly used sedative drugs and their roles in current practice.

α_2-Adrenoceptor agonists

The prototypical α_2-adrenoceptor agonist is clonidine, which was originally developed as a nasal decongestant and then as an antihypertensive. However, sedation confounded these applications. Subsequently anesthesiologists realized that the sedative and analgesic properties (the latter considered in Chapter 35) could be used to clinical advantage, initially applying clonidine for premedication and supplementation to general anesthesia. In veterinary anesthesia, xylazine, a weak and relatively nonselective α-adrenoceptor agonist, had already been used for these purposes in veterinary anesthesia. In the early 1990s, the racemic medetomidine was introduced as a more selective α_2-agonist in veterinary anesthesia. Subsequently, its active enantiomer dexmedetomidine was developed for use as a perioperative sedative and analgesic for humans.

There are three main chemical classes of α_2-adrenoceptor agonists: the phenylethylates (such as methyldopa, guanabenz), the imidazolines (such as clonidine, dexmedetomidine, mivazerol, azepexole), and the oxaloazepines. The main α_2-adrenoceptor agonists used in anesthetic practice are the imidazolines; this is important, as these drugs also activate imidazoline receptors, which may be responsible for some of the hemodynamic side effects of these drugs, particularly hypotension [1]. Development of α_2-adrenoceptor agonists with reduced affinity for imidazoline receptors will likely expand the use of this class of drug.

Mechanism of action

There are three subtypes of α_2-adrenoceptors [2]; their physiological actions are described in Fig. 30.1. The three receptor subtypes are widely distributed, and use of genetically modified animals and specific antagonists have allowed investigators to attribute the physiological effects to one or more subtypes. Agonist action at α_{2A}-adrenoceptors mediates sedation and hypnosis, analgesia [3,4], neuroprotection [5], hyperglycemia [6], diuresis [7], and sympatholysis [8]. Alpha$_{2A}$-adrenoceptors couple to inhibitory G proteins ($G_{i/o}$; Fig. 30.2), inhibiting adenylate cyclase and activating potassium channels (such as G-protein-coupled inwardly rectifying K^+ [GIRK] channels and two-pore-domain K^+ channels) and inhibiting calcium channels; the net effect of α_{2A}-adrenoceptor activation in neurons is cellular hyperpolarization. Lakhlani and colleagues used mice expressing dysfunctional α_{2A}-adrenoceptors to show that α_2-agonist antinociception and sedation were dependent on this receptor subtype [3]. In the absence of functional α_{2A}-adrenoceptors, the drugs could not suppress voltage-gated Ca^{2+}, or activate K^+, currents

Anesthetic Pharmacology, 2nd edition, ed. Alex S. Evers, Mervyn Maze, Evan D. Kharasch. Published by Cambridge University Press. © Cambridge University Press 2011.

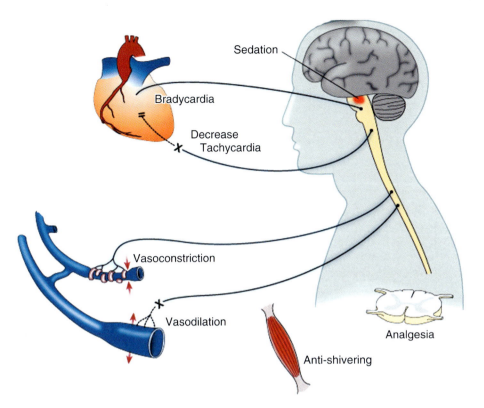

Figure 30.1. Functions mediated by α₂-adrenoceptors. The site for the sedative action is in the locus coeruleus of the brainstem, whereas the principal site for the analgesic action is probably in the spinal cord, although there are data supporting both a peripheral and a supraspinal site of action. In the heart, α₂-agonists decrease tachycardia (through block of the cardioaccelerator nerve) and produce bradycardia (through a vagomimetic action). In the peripheral vasculature, there are both a vasodilatory action (through sympatholysis) and vasoconstriction (by a direct action on the α₂-adrenoceptors on smooth-muscle cells).

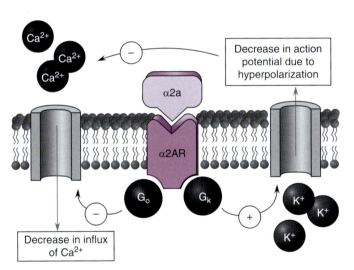

Figure 30.2. Molecular mechanism for hypnotic effect in the locus coeruleus (LC). When a selective α₂-adrenoceptor agonist binds to an α₂A-adrenoceptor in the locus coeruleus, transmembrane signaling is activated through an inwardly rectifying potassium channel allowing for a K⁺ efflux and by inhibition of voltage-gated Ca²⁺ channels. The resulting hyperpolarization decreases the firing rate in LC projections.

(Fig. 30.2). This mutation did not affect morphine analgesia but inhibited dexmedetomidine sedation and analgesia.

Stimulation of the α₂B-adrenoceptor mediates vasoconstriction [9] and probably the antishivering action [10] and the endogenous analgesic mechanism [11]. Interestingly, α₂B-adrenoceptors couple to stimulatory G proteins and thus are

an excitatory subtype, in keeping with their vasoconstrictive effects. The α₂C-adrenoceptor has been linked to learning and stress responses [12].

Preclinical pharmacology

Clonidine is a partial agonist with an α₂-adrenoceptor to α₁-adrenoceptor selectivity ratio of 220 : 1. It also shows affinity for the imidazoline receptor; the α₂-adrenoceptor : imidazoline selectivity ratio is 16 : 1. Dexmedetomidine, however, is more selective, with an α₂ : α₁-adrenoceptor ratio of 1600 : 1 and an α₂-adrenoceptor : imidazoline selectivity ratio of 32 : 1 [13]. The relative selectivity of the drugs is important, as the sedative effect of α₂-adrenoceptor agonists is antagonized by α₁-adrenoceptor activation [14], explaining why drugs that have a relatively low α₂ : α₁ affinity ratio (e.g., clonidine) have limited hypnotic effects.

The pivotal neuroanatomical locus for the sedative-hypnotic actions of α₂-agonists is the pontine noradrenergic nucleus the locus coeruleus (LC) [15–17]. Hyperpolarization of noradrenergic LC neurons also occurs in non-rapid eye movement (NREM) sleep, which involves distinct neuronal pathways, and thus dexmedetomidine appears to act by activation of, at least part of, the NREM sleep mechanism (Fig. 30.3). The sleep-promoting galanin and γ-aminobutyric acid (GABA)-containing neurons in the ventrolateral preoptic nucleus (VLPO) (in the anterior hypothalamus and basal forebrain) are under inhibitory control by norepinephrine and

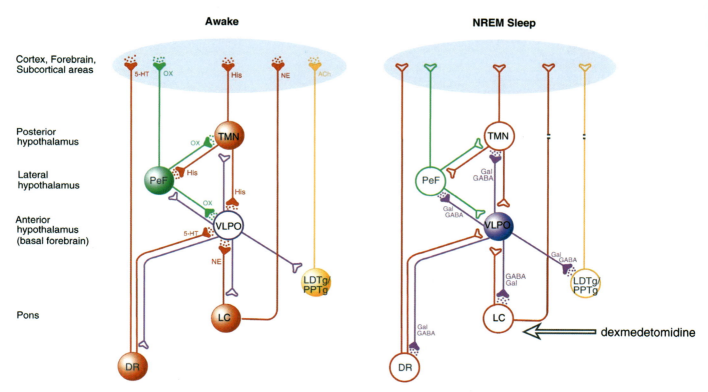

Figure 30.3. Neural substrates for sedative effect. During the hypnotic response induced by α_2-adrenoceptor agonist, a qualitatively similar pattern of neural activation is seen in rats as that observed during normal sleep; there is a decrease in the locus coeruleus (LC) and tuberomammillary nucleus (TMN) and an increase in the ventrolateral preoptic nucleus (VLPO). These changes are attenuated by a selective α_2-adrenoceptor antagonist and are not seen in mice lacking functional α_{2A}-adrenoceptors (which do not show a hypnotic response to α_2-adrenoceptor agonists). There is a hierarchical sequence of changes in which inhibition of the LC disinhibits the VLPO to release γ-aminobutyric acid (GABA) and galanin at the projections that terminate at the TMN. These inhibitory neurotransmitters inhibit firing of the TMN projections to the cortical and subcortical regions. ACh, acetylcholine; 5-HT, serotonin; His, histamine; LDTg, laterodorsal tegmental nucleus; NE, norepinephrine; NREM, non-rapid eye movement; OX, orexin; PPTg, pedunculopontine tegmental nucleus.

serotonin from the LC and raphe nucleus, respectively. Decreased noradrenergic neuron firing in the LC disinhibits inhibitory galanin and GABAergic VLPO neurons (activating them). VLPO neurons innervate the tuberomammillary nucleus (TMN), an arousal-promoting histaminergic nucleus, alongside other arousal-promoting monoaminergic, cholinergic, and orexinergic nuclei. Thus descending projections from the VLPO inhibit neurons in these arousal-promoting nuclei. Crucially, in the TMN this prevents histamine release into the cortex, forebrain, and subcortical regions, reducing arousal drive. Not only is the LC thought to be the neuroanatomical locus for the anesthetic-sparing effect of α_2-adrenoceptor agonists, it is also considered the site for the prevention or treatment of drug withdrawal syndrome after administration of opiates or cocaine.

The development of tolerance, a widespread biologic process in which responsiveness to a drug decreases with continuing drug exposure, also confounds α_2-adrenoceptor agonist sedation (like other sedatives) with tolerance to both clonidine and dexmedetomidine reported [18]. The induction of tolerance involves both N-methyl-D-aspartate-type glutamate receptors and nitric oxide synthetase [19], whereas the expression of tolerance involves the L-type Ca^{2+} channel.

While α_2-agonists are useful sedatives they are not potent amnestic drugs like other sedatives, particularly the benzodiazepines [20]. Interestingly, the α_{2A}-adrenoceptor has been implicated in playing an important role in learning and memory when activated, and this may explain their relatively weak amnestic actions [21], though it is likely that the amnestic effects are dependent on the methodology used [22].

Hemodynamic effects

Notably, α_2-adrenoceptor agonists may precipitate hypotension and bradycardia [23] by both central and peripheral mechanisms. The α_2-adrenoceptor agents exhibit no direct depressant effects on the contractile properties of the isolated myocardium [24], indicating that cardiac contractility is not affected. Depression of both spontaneous and evoked sympathetic activity in the vasomotor center of the brainstem occurs [25]. At therapeutic doses of α_2-adrenergic agonists given by oral, intravenous (slowly), or epidural routes of administration, sympatholysis is the predominant hemodynamic effect.

Alpha$_2$-adrenoceptor agonists also modulate baroreflex responses, with different effects on the tonic and phasic elements of the reflex. Clonidine produces a shift in the set-point of the baroreflex; thus, for a given arterial pressure, heart rate is lower because of a decrease in tonic activity. Conversely, changes in arterial pressure from the set-point provoke a phasic response, the amplitude of which may be even greater in the presence of α_2-adrenoceptor agonists.

As clinically used α_2-adrenoceptor agonists possess an imidazoline structure, some of the hemodynamic effects that are observed may be produced by the imidazoline I$_1$ receptors in the rostral ventrolateral medulla [1]. This would explain why hypotension produced by α_2-adrenoceptor agonists with an imidazoline structure cannot be completely reversed by the α_2-adrenoceptor antagonist yohimbine, which has a non-imidazoline structure. In contrast, idazoxan, which preferentially blocks imidazoline-preferring sites in the brainstem, completely blocks the hypotensive action of imidazole-ringed α_2-adrenoceptor agonists. A cooperative relationship between α_2-adrenoceptors and imidazoline receptors in the brainstem should also be considered as a possible mechanism for the hypotension and bradycardia that follow use of α_2-adrenoceptor agonists containing an imidazole ring in their structure [26]. Development of α_2-adrenoceptor agonists which lack affinity for imidazoline receptors would likely reduce the hypotensive effects of these drugs and might improve their safety profile.

Hypotension induced by α_2-adrenergic agonists can be reversed by vasopressors and inotropes. There appears to be an enhanced pressor response to ephedrine, phenylephrine, and dobutamine, but not to norepinephrine [27]. The responses to dopamine (which partly depends on the release of norepinephrine) and to atropine are somewhat attenuated [27].

Besides central effects, α_2-adrenergic agents produce peripheral vasoconstriction through stimulation of α_{2B}-adrenoceptors in the peripheral vasculature [9]. After rapid intravenous bolus administration of clonidine, the vasoconstrictive (α_1 and α_{2B}) effects of the drug are believed to be responsible for a transient hypertension. When the dose is slowly increased in a stepwise manner, hypotension occurs initially but is then reversed when greater concentrations are achieved, as the peripheral vasoconstrictive action overcomes the sympatholytic effect [28]. Alpha$_2$-adrenoceptor agonists have a direct vasoconstrictive effect on the coronary arteries that is partly opposed by nitric oxide, which is indirectly released by α_2-adrenoceptor agonists [29]. Interestingly, in the presence of excess nitric oxide the α_2-adrenoceptor agonists may act more as vasoconstrictors.

Overall, a reduction in myocardial oxygen demand and a decrease in coronary perfusion pressure (as a consequence of hypotension) results. On balance, myocardial energetics are usually improved; however, in some patients, hypotension may produce myocardial ischemia. In experimental studies, α_2-adrenoceptor agonists have produced anti-ischemic effects [30,31], which is also partly related to the attenuation of sympathetically mediated coronary vasoconstriction. Consequently, in patients with myocardial ischemia, α_2-adrenergic agonists have an antianginal effect [32], improve exercise tolerance, and have been shown to provide perioperative cardioprotection with a reduction in morbidity and mortality [33,34]. Importantly, abrupt discontinuation of α_2-adrenoceptor agonists after chronic administration may induce a drug withdrawal syndrome, including rebound hypertension possibly leading to myocardial ischemia.

Cerebral circulation

Activation of α_2-adrenoceptors in the cerebral vessels produces vasoconstriction [35] and reduces cerebral blood flow without influencing the metabolic rate for oxygen, indicating an uncoupling of flow and metabolic activity. Reactivity of cerebral blood flow to carbon dioxide is either preserved or modestly attenuated by dexmedetomidine [36] and clonidine [37]. Despite this, both drugs improve neurologic outcome and histopathologic lesions after cerebral ischemia in animals when the drugs are administered either before or after the start of cerebral injury [5,38]. Additionally, in animal experiments intracranial pressure did not change significantly with administration of dexmedetomidine.

Neuroprotection

Extensive preclinical evidence suggests that α_2-adrenoceptor agonists provide neuroprotection against a variety of cerebral insults [5,38]. Maier and colleagues demonstrated a neuroprotective effect even when dexmedetomidine (at a steady-state plasma concentration of 4 ng mL^{-1}) was administered post-insult, in a transient focal model of cerebral ischemia in rabbits [38]. Dexmedetomidine reduces circulating catecholamine levels but does not alter brain norepinephrine or glutamate levels. This information indicates that the neuroprotective effect may not be due to central noradrenergic mechanisms and suggests a possible direct cytoprotective mechanism of action.

Alpha$_2$-adrenoceptor agonists also show efficacy in models of perinatal asphyxia. Clonidine reduced the size of hypoxic–ischemic cortical infarcts and the mortality rate induced by unilateral carotid artery ligation compared to animals treated with the α_2-adrenoceptor antagonist yohimbine [39]. Dexmedetomidine also inhibits neuronal injury provoked by oxygen–glucose deprivation and pharmacological toxins in vitro, and in an in-vivo neonatal-asphyxia rat model, providing long-term neurocognitive protection [5]; application of an α_{2A}-adrenoceptor antagonist attenuated these effects.

It is also possible that dexmedetomidine's neuroprotective effects have already been realized clinically. In the recent MENDS study dexmedetomidine reduced the incidence of neurological dysfunction relative to lorazepam-treated controls [40].

Endocrine effects

Alpha$_2$-adrenoceptor agonists blunt the neuroendocrine stress response to surgery, with regard to cortisol, β-endorphins, arginine vasopressin, epinephrine, and norepinephrine [41], while growth hormone release is provoked by α_2-adrenoceptor agonists. These effects may alter postoperative metabolism; for example, protein catabolism is attenuated in patients administered clonidine [42]. Like most imidazoline compounds (e.g., etomidate), dexmedetomidine (at concentrations that are 100–1000 times greater than those used clinically) blocks steroidogenesis in vitro [43]. Fortunately, this does not appear to occur under clinically relevant conditions [40].

Renal effects

Alpha$_2$-adrenoceptor agonists exert a diuretic effect, as they oppose the action of arginine vasopressin (AVP) in the collecting duct of the nephron [44]. Activation of α_{2A}-adrenoceptors [7], signaling through a reduction in cyclic adenosine monophosphate (cAMP) levels and protein kinase activation, provokes reduced expression of aquaporin-2 receptors, and aquaporin-2 receptor redistribution with a consequent reduction in water and sodium transport. A second non-AVP-dependent pathway enhances osmolal clearance. While neither increasing free water clearance nor changing the solute balance of urine necessarily equates to preserved renal function in the face of a renal insult, recent animal studies have shown that α_2-adrenoceptor agonists possess renoprotective effects against hypoxic–ischemic and radiocontrast-induced injury [45,46].

Clinical pharmacology

In 1998 dexmedetomidine was licensed by the US Food and Drug Administration (FDA) as a sedative drug for use for up to 24 hours in critical care, although postmarketing evidence suggests more distinct advantages with longer periods of sedation [40]. More novel on-label indications include use for fiberoptic intubation and procedural sedation. Clonidine has been used in clinical practice for a variety of uses including the treatment of hypertension, nasal congestion, sedation, and analgesia. In 1996 the FDA licensed clonidine for the treatment of cancer pain via the epidural route, though it has been successfully employed for sedation and analgesia with administration via other routes.

It is important to note that despite their relative longevity in clinical practice (clonidine was widely introduced in the 1970s), no idiosyncratic adverse effects have been discovered, other than an extension of its pharmacologic profile (i.e., hypotension, bradycardia, xerostomia, and hypertension). As this class of drug seems to have a remarkably wide safety margin, continuing interest in these drugs as sedatives and cytoprotectives continues. Furthermore, the development of more selective drugs for the α_{2A}-adrenoceptor could further improve this safety profile.

Pharmacokinetics

Clonidine is moderately lipid-soluble and enjoys near complete bioavailability after oral administration; the peak effect occurs at 60–90 minutes, and the peak plasma concentration occurs at 1–3 hours [47]. Clonidine has a large volume of distribution (approximately 2 L kg^{-1}) and a relatively long terminal elimination half-life of 12–24 hours.

Dexmedetomidine, the dextroisomer of medetomidine, has an eight times greater affinity for α_2-adrenoceptors than does clonidine. The pharmacokinetics of dexmedetomidine were derived following intravenous administration; the distribution half-life of the drug is approximately 6 minutes, with a terminal elimination half-life of 2 hours. It is a shorter-acting, more potent agonist of α_2-adrenoceptors than clonidine with a steady-state volume of distribution of 1.33 L kg^{-1} and a clearance of 39 L h^{-1} [48]. Dexmedetomidine is highly bound ($\pm$ 94%) to albumin and α_1-glycoprotein. Metabolically it is extensively biotransformed in the liver, with the resulting methyl and glucuronide conjugates excreted by the kidneys. In vitro, dexmedetomidine weakly inhibits cytochrome P450 enzyme systems [49], and thus pharmacokinetic interactions between dexmedetomidine and other sedative/anesthetic drugs can occur.

Pharmacodynamics

Clonidine and dexmedetomidine both produce dose-dependent sedation. Nelson and colleagues suggest that α_2-adrenoceptor agonists activate the endogenous substrates for natural sleep to produce their sedative action [17], and this parallels clinical and neuroimaging evidence. Clinically, patients deeply sedated by dexmedetomidine are easily rousable to participate in clinical testing and appear calm and relaxed while breathing spontaneously [20]. Thus, mechanistic and phenotypic similarities exist between natural sleep and α_2-adrenoceptor agonist sedation. Neuroimaging research suggests that dexmedetomidine increases activity in the pulvinar nucleus of the thalamus and that this region mediates the ability of arousing stimuli to produce attention in sedated subjects [50]. At least in part, this explains why α_2-adrenoceptor agonists have only moderate amnestic effects, as patients can be easily roused to consciousness. Differences between the types of sedatives become further apparent when neuroimagining is used to compare sedation; patients sedated with dexmedetomidine or midazolam to "equivalently sedated" states show distinctive differences in the blood-oxygen-level-dependent functional magnetic resonance (BOLD fMRI) responses. Whereas there are few changes compared with placebo in the dexmedetomidine-sedated state, there are several brain regions that differ in the midazolam-sedated state from their placebo state (Fig. 30.4) [50].

EEG differences between natural sleep, sedation, and anesthesia have been recognized for many years, and therefore it is of interest that α_2-adrenoceptor agonist-induced sedation is more akin to sleep than that produced by other sedatives such as the benzodiazepines [51,52]. While further research is required into the EEG effects of α_2-adrenoceptor agonists such as dexmedetomidine, early evidence suggests that dexmedetomidine-induced sedation bears remarkable similarity to NREM sleep [52] (supported by the evidence of overlapping neurobiological substrates of action [17]).

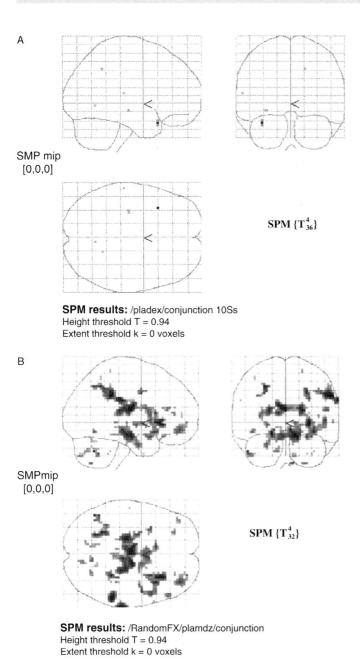

SPM {T$_{36}^{4}$}

SPM results: /pladex/conjunction 10Ss
Height threshold T = 0.94
Extent threshold k = 0 voxels

SPM {T$_{32}^{4}$}

SPM results: /RandomFX/plamdz/conjunction
Height threshold T = 0.94
Extent threshold k = 0 voxels

Figure 30.4. Functional magnetic resonance imaging (fMRI) at equisedative states produced by dexmedetomidine and midazolam in healthy volunteers. Statistical parametric mapping (SPM) projections of areas of brain, shown in sagittal, coronal, and transverse views, illustrating statistical change in activity when dexmedetomidine (A) and midazolam (B) are compared with a placebo state ($p < 0.001$). The images represent a transparent "glass brain," not a two-dimensional "slice."

Dexmedetomidine (0.2–0.7 µg kg^{-1} h^{-1}) was initally studied as a critical care sedative drug after major surgical procedures. Recent studies have successfully employed higher doses of dexmedetomidine sedation (up to 1.5 µg kg^{-1} h^{-1}) in the critical care setting with improved outcome [40]. Dexmedetomidine effectively reduces the amount of propofol or midazolam necessary to sedate intensive care

patients, but as it is relatively devoid of respiratory depressant effects it may be continued following extubation in spontaneously breathing patients [53]. Both clonidine and dexmedetomidine have been given to patients in the intensive care unit (ICU) to prevent drug withdrawal syndrome after long-term sedation with benzodiazepines and opioids or to facilitate invasive endoscopic and radiologic procedures. Furthermore, α$_2$-adrenoceptor agonists exhibit significant organ-protective effects that, in concert with their unique sedative profile, make them important drugs in critical care and perioperative sedation.

Anesthetic-sparing effects

The hypnotic actions of α$_2$-adrenoceptor agonists contribute a significant anesthetic-sparing effect, which is predominantly a pharmacodynamic mechanism, although it has been suggested that pharmacokinetic mechanisms also play a part. However, as the effect results from the action of the drugs at α$_2$-adrenoceptors and is unrelated to their imidazoline structure, it is likely that pharmacodynamic effects are of primary importance [54]. These effects have been noted at induction, maintenance, and cessation of anesthesia [55–57]. For example, premedication with clonidine (3 µg kg^{-1}) reduces the propofol and thiopental requirements for induction of anesthesia by 30–35% [57]. Clonidine (3 µg kg^{-1}) also decreases the minimum end-tidal concentration of isoflurane required for induction of burst suppression on electroencephalogram from 1.4% to 0.9% [58]. The MAC of sevoflurane required for endotracheal intubation decreased from 2.9% to 2.5% and 1.9% (35% decrease) respectively in the presence of 2 or 4 µg kg^{-1} clonidine in children. The same dose reduced the MAC of sevoflurane required for skin incision from 2.3% to 1.8% and 1.3%, respectively [59]. Doses of 0.5–5 µg kg^{-1} clonidine induce dose-dependent anesthetic-sparing effects, though higher doses become ineffective [57]. At termination of anesthesia, the MAC-awake of isoflurane (the end-tidal concentration of isoflurane corresponding to opening of the eyes on verbal command) is also reduced from 0.28% to 0.22% by clonidine administered prior to surgery [56].

Likewise, dexmedetomidine reduces the MAC of isoflurane in a dose-dependent manner [60]. However, unlike clonidine, for which the effect "plateaus" between 25% and 40% (depending on the coadministered anesthetic agent), dexmedetomidine may reduce anesthetic requirements by up to 90% [61]. This difference likely represents the increased affinity dexmedetomidine possesses for α$_2$-adrenoceptors over α$_1$-adrenoceptors. Dexmedetomidine also acts synergistically with opioids (fentanyl) to further reduce the MAC of volatile drugs. In all likelihood the analgesic properties also contribute to their anesthetic-sparing effects. While α$_2$-adrenoceptor agonists produce flaccidity and prevent opioid-induced muscle rigidity, these compounds have no clinically significant effect on the neuromuscular blocking action of muscle relaxants [62].

Amnestic effects

In a study by Ebert and colleagues a clinically relevant dexmedetomidine plasma concentration of 0.7–1.9 ng mL^{-1} produced sedation and analgesia but preserved memory (with free recall and recognition) [63]. Thus, in contrast to benzodiazepines, the amnestic properties of these drugs should be considered weak. However, in certain settings this can prove to be advantageous. Amnesia has been associated with an increased incidence of post-traumatic stress disorder in the ICU, and this lack of amnestic effect may be of use to reduce long-term neurological morbidity. Long-term follow-up of the critically ill patients sedated with dexmedetomidine may reveal this theoretical difference.

Critical care sedation

The potential implications of using sedative-hypnotic drugs that act through similar mechanisms as natural sleep to induce loss of consciousness are profound. A hypnotic that could produce the same reparative changes as natural sleep (i.e., hormone and immune function changes) might speed recovery time in an intensive care setting and counteract the effects of sleep deprivation, a common problem for patients in the ICU and for surgical patients during recovery.

Similar to NREM sleep, during dexmedetomidine sedation the arousal system appears intact. This preserved arousal state may have significant utility in the ICU; daily wake-up trials have been associated with a shortened duration of ventilation and ICU stay [64]. Therefore, the use of drugs which facilitate rousability, with the ability to revert to the sedated state when unstimulated, would appear to be a particularly attractive feature for a critical care sedative. Furthermore, increased patient rousability also facilitates neurological assessment of critically ill patients. However, another method to decrease the duration of mechanical ventilation is to reduce the incidence of delirium.

ICU-related delirium occurs in up to 80% of ICU patients and significantly increases patient mortality. Although the etiology of this condition is complex, sedation plays an important role in its genesis and also represents the most easily modifiable risk factor. A recent prospective cohort study analysed the influence of different sedative and analgesic drugs on the incidence of delirium: lorazepam is an independent risk factor for precipitating delirium; other opioid and GABAergic drugs showed a trend towards significance [65]. Understanding of the critical differences between sedation produced by α_2-adrenoceptor agonists and GABAergic drugs [17,50] provoked the MENDS (Maximizing Efficacy of target sedation and reducing Neurological DySfunction) study to evaluate the role of dexmedetomidine to reduce delirium [40].

The MENDS study enrolled 106 patients in a double-blind randomized controlled trial comparing lorazepam (maximum dose 10 mg h^{-1}) and dexmedetomidine (maximum dose 1.5 μg kg^{-1} h^{-1}) infusions (maximum duration 120 hours) with the primary outcome the incidence of delirium and coma in mechanically ventilated patients in the ICU [40]. Remarkably, patients sedated with dexmedetomidine had more days alive and free of delirium/coma (7 vs. 3, $p = 0.01$). The prevalence of coma was reduced in dexmedetomidine-treated patients (63% vs. 92%, $p < 0.001$). There was also a trend towards a lower 28-day mortality (17% vs. 27%, $p = 0.21$), though the study was not powered for this endpoint. This trial may prove to have a large impact on critical care sedation, as delirium is also an independent predictor of mortality and prolonged ICU stay. A retrospective analysis of postoperative cardiac surgery patients adds credence to these findings: the addition of dexmedetomidine to critical care sedative regimens was associated with reduced cost, length of hospital and intensive care stay, length of mechanical ventilation, and mortality (although the dexmedetomidine group was biased towards younger patients [66]).

An a-priori arranged subgroup analysis of the septic MENDS patients (39 patients admitted with sepsis, 19 in the dexmedetomidine group and 20 in the lorazepam group) revealed a fascinating effect. Baseline demographics, ICU type, and admission diagnoses of the sepsis patients were well balanced between the groups. Dexmedetomidine-treated patients had more delirium/coma-free days (8 vs. 1.5, $p = 0.002$), delirium-free days (10 vs. 7.3, $p = 0.007$), and mechanical-ventilation-free days (22.2 vs. 1.7, $p = 0.03$). The risk of dying at 28 days in dexmedetomidine patients with sepsis was reduced by 70% ($p = 0.04$) compared to lorazepam patients. Tests for interactions between treatment groups and sepsis showed that the presence of sepsis impacted the beneficial effects of dexmedetomidine for delirium/coma-free days, delirium-free days, mechanical-ventilation-free days, and 28-day mortality. It is important to note that this was a small secondary analysis, and further studies are required to evaluate this remarkable finding. Nonetheless, there is significant biological plausibility for these findings. Alpha$_2$-adrenoceptor agonists increase macrophage clearance of bacteria in vitro and thus potentiate the endogenous immune response [67]. Septic mortality also critically involves apoptotic cell death in multiple cells and tissues, and dexmedetomidine can prevent apoptotic injury in different paradigms of injury [68]. In addition to these organ-protective, including neuroprotective, effects, salubrious effects on inflammation and the unique sedative profile of α_2-adrenoceptor agonists likely contribute to the life-sparing effect of dexmedetomidine.

Anti-inflammatory effects

Activation of α_2-adrenoceptors may also modulate inflammatory cytokine signaling in many paradigms including endotoxic shock in animals [69] (compared with saline treatment) and critically ill patients [70] (compared with midazolam sedation). In these studies both IL-6 and TNFα cytokines were significantly reduced in dexmedetomidine-treated subjects. A nonsignificant reduction of the proinflammatory cytokine IL-6 was also noted in an earlier underpowered clinical study (compared with propofol) [71]. In addition, preoperative clonidine reduced TNFα levels in plasma and cerebrospinal fluid in patients undergoing peripheral revascularization procedures [72]. To what extent dexmedetomidine's modulation of central cytokine signaling contributes to its antideliriogenic, antisepsis or organ-protective properties is not known and is the subject of ongoing work. Of potential significance, when dexmedetomidine was given to animals treated with lipopolysaccharide an improvement in hemodynamic stability was noted that correlated with the observed anti-inflammatory effect [69]. In endotoxic shock, excess nitric-oxide-mediated vasodilation precipitates hypotension; in the presence of excess nitric oxide α₂-adrenoceptor agonists act to oppose this excessive vasodilation.

Hemodynamic stability

Alpha₂-adrenoceptor agonists provide hemodynamic stability, reducing "alpine anesthesia" during surgery [73] due to blunted sympathetic responses to nociceptive and surgical stimulation. Alpha₂-adrenoceptor agonists attenuate sympathetic activity during surgery and on emergence from anesthesia, and that related to administration of anesthetic drugs such as ketamine or desflurane.

Both clonidine and dexmedetomidine lead to increases in cardiac output compared to placebo under anesthesia [74], while their sympatholytic properties reduce hypertension and tachycardia during intubation of the trachea, intraoperatively, and during recovery from anesthesia [75,76]. The induced negative chronotropic effect and modest hypotension may be exacerbated in the volume-depleted patient. In clinical studies in which the double-blind study design resulted in patients receiving a "full" dose of anesthetic drugs when premedicated with clonidine or dexmedetomidine, elderly patients became particularly susceptible to hypotension and bradycardia [61]. In clinical practice, these side effects can be mitigated by appropriately decreasing the dose of coadministered anesthetic agent. Nevertheless, bradycardia may still occur in relatively young, unstimulated ASA I or II patients administered dexmedetomidine. A decrease in the incidence of shivering also reduces postoperative oxygen consumption. Thus there are multiple mechanisms through which α₂-adrenoceptor agonists may induce cardioprotection (discussed below).

Antishivering effect

Alpha₂-adrenoceptor agonists (for example, clonidine 1.5 μg kg^{-1}) prevent shivering and the subsequent increase in oxygen consumption [77]; this may contribute to their cardioprotective effects. They alter thermoregulatory control and decrease the threshold for vasoconstriction and shivering during hypothermia. Conversely, during hyperthermia, the threshold for sweating increases only slightly.

Cardioprotection

The sympatholytic properties of α₂-adrenoceptor agonists have been utilized perioperatively in both cardiac and noncardiac surgery to reduce the incidence of postoperative cardiac morbidity and mortality. A prospective, randomized, placebo-controlled trial demonstrated the efficacy of clonidine to reduce cardiac risk in noncardiac surgery patients [78]. Clonidine significantly reduced plasma epinephrine and norepinephrine levels and the incidence of perioperative myocardial ischemia. Remarkably, 30-day and 2-year mortality were reduced in the clonidine-treated group, a result comparable to the early positive β-blocker trials. Similarly, the now discontinued mivazerol reduced the incidence of intraoperative ischemia in an earlier clinical study [75]. Functionally, this cardioprotection translates to improved myocardial energetics and recovery; for example, clonidine improved recovery from myocardial stunning [79].

An earlier meta-analysis supports the findings that α₂-adrenoceptor agonists reduce perioperative cardiac mortality and ischemia [33]. This meta-analysis appears to suggest that this is a "class benefit" of α₂-adrenoceptor agonists, with the benefit probably accorded by sympatholysis, the prevention of shivering and possibly myocyte targets. Following the recent POISE study [80], in which perioperative β-blockade was associated with increased mortality, a randomized controlled trial of the protective effects of α₂-adrenoceptor agonists in this setting is urgently required. Whether improved cardiac outcomes also occur in the ICU following sedation with dexmedetomidine also awaits investigation.

Renoprotection

Consistent with preclinical evidence, a prospective double-blind randomized controlled trial of 48 cardiac surgical patients demonstrated that preoperative clonidine (4 μg kg^{-1} IV) preserved creatinine clearance on the first postoperative night [81]. Furthermore, a placebo-controlled randomized trial designed to assess postoperative pain control with dexmedetomidine treatment of thoracic surgery patients showed that dexmedetomidine-treated patients had lower serum creatinine concentrations for 7 days postoperatively [82]. While the etiology of these injuries may represent hypoperfusion, and therefore we should be cautious about extrapolating these findings to the heterogeneous syndrome of acute renal failure, these studies provide early evidence for a renoprotective effect of α₂-adrenoceptor agonists in patients.

Cerebral circulation

Despite their ability to induce vasodilation, α₂-adrenoceptor agonists decrease plasma catecholamines and do not affect intracranial pressure in patients with head injuries [83]. However, administration of clonidine in the presence of intracranial hypertension can sometimes increase intracranial pressure transiently [84], with theoretical concerns that this could aggravate cerebral ischemia because of possible decreases in perfusion pressure [84].

Gastrointestinal effects

Alpha$_2$-adrenergic agonists reduce gastrointestinal motility because of a central and peripheral action [85]. Gastric emptying is not delayed by administration of α$_2$-adrenergic agonists, but transit time is prolonged. Concurrent administration of opioids and α$_2$-agonists produces a supra-additive inhibition of gastrointestinal transit [85]. Alpha$_2$-adrenoceptor agonists do not deleteriously effect splanchnic perfusion, but appear to prevent stress-induced gastric ulcers in animals [86] and improve gut wound healing in animals, and thus they may have a specific application in anesthesia for general surgery.

Respiratory effects

Although α$_2$-adrenoceptor agonists have minimal effects on respiratory rate or tidal volume during resting ventilation, ventilatory responses to hypoxia and hypercapnia are modestly blunted in healthy volunteers and patients. The reduction in ventilatory drive can produce an obstructive upper airway ventilatory pattern.

Nevertheless, compared to opioids, clonidine exhibits little depressive effect on ventilation and does not potentiate the respiratory depressant effects of opioids [87]. Possibly through pharmacokinetic mechanisms, the simultaneous intravenous administration of clonidine and fentanyl may lead to accumulation of fentanyl that will increase the risk of respiratory depression [88]. Thus, α$_2$-adrenoceptor agonists lack the significant respiratory depression exhibited by other sedatives, and in concert with the relative rousabiliy of patients sedated with dexmedetomidine this makes it an ideal sedative to facilitate respiratory weaning in the ICU. Furthermore, the reduction in neurological dysfunction observed in the MENDS study would also improve patient cooperativity. These factors could explain why patients sedated with dexmedetomidine endured shorter periods of mechanical ventilation than lorazepam-treated patients in the recent MENDS study [40].

Dosage and administration

Premedication

Alpha$_2$-adrenoceptor agonists have distinct utility as sedative and anxiolytic premedicants. However, their amnestic effects should be considered modest and certainly inferior to those of the benzodiazepines [20]. An appropriate dose range for young healthy patients is 2–4 µg kg^{-1}; 1–2 µg kg^{-1} is more appropriate for elderly patients [89]. In children, clonidine premedication is well accepted and improves tolerance of the facemask for induction of anesthesia [90]. Likewise, dexmedetomidine has been employed at a dose of 1–4 µg kg^{-1} in this setting with effect. Other salubrious effects include analgesia and a reduction in postoperative nausea, vomiting, and agitation. The associated minimal disturbance of ventilation is no greater than that of natural sleep (in keeping with its mechanism of action). Gastrointestinal effects include xerostomia and decreased gastrointestinal transit (which is not significant for fluids). The dry mouth is rarely a problem for the patient and is useful if the airway is to be instrumented.

Anesthetic-sparing effect

The sedative qualities of qualities of α$_2$-adrenoceptor agonists can be used intraoperatively in a similar dose range to the premedicant doses. In this setting dexmedetomidine can be applied by infusion, for example during cardiopulmonary bypass [91]. Interestingly, dexmedetomidine has also been employed as the sole anesthetic in a few patients, although this is not recommended because of the risk of precipitating pulmonary or systemic hypertension.

Clinicians are sometimes loath to employ these drugs because of concerns over the hemodynamic side effects of hypotension and bradycardia. However, their prudent use leads to cardiostability and organ protection, and recognition of this means that α$_2$-adrenoceptor agonists have an expanding role in perioperative care. In certain perioperative circumstances their utility is particularly evident:

- In *drug addicts and alcoholics*, sympathetic hyperactivity is well controlled by α$_2$-adrenoceptor agonists [92], and when administered as premedication and continued after surgery, they may reduce the risk of drug withdrawal syndrome. In addition, their analgesic and opioid-sparing effects aid perioperative care in drug addicts.
- *Patients with hypertension* or *ischemic heart disease* are particularly vulnerable to marked swings in blood pressure perioperatively. Use of α$_2$-adrenoceptor agonists as premedication provides a useful way of reducing this hyperreactivity [76,78]. As with other antihypertensive medications, α$_2$-adrenoceptoragonists must not be discontinued before surgery because of the risk for a hypertensive crisis and myocardial ischemia and infarction. Several studies have demonstrated that clonidine premedication reduces the number of hypertensive episodes [55], albeit with more frequent hypotensive or bradycardic episodes. In summary, if one were to customize an "ideal" range of arterial blood pressures for surgery, patients administered α$_2$-adrenoceptor agonists would be found to spend more time within that ideal range than patients given a placebo. Furthermore, given the cardioprotective effects of this class of drugs and the recent controversy over β-blockers, use of α$_2$-adrenoceptor agonists will be of increasing importance in this group of patients [80].
- *Hypotensive anesthesa* to facilitate certain types of surgery (e.g., ear or orthopedic surgery) is aided by α$_2$-adrenoceptor agonist premedication.
- During *ophthalmic surgery*, premedication with clonidine or dexmedetomidine has the advantage of decreasing intraocular pressure and is the preferred premedicant in patients with increased intraocular pressure [89].
- In patients anesthetized with *ketamine*, and in children [90], premedication with an α$_2$-adrenoceptor agonist may prevent postanesthetic delirium.

- In the future, as the organ-protective effects of α_2-adrenoceptor agonists is further revealed, their utility to ensure perioperative organ function with long-term protection will increasingly be recognized.

Applications in critical care

Critically ill patients also stand to benefit from increased use of α_2-adrenoceptor agonists in the ICU. These drugs exhibit useful effects in many organ systems:

- *Nervous system* – α_2-adrenoceptor agonist-induced sedation is more analogous to NREM sleep than that induced by other sedatives; this may lead to salubrious effects on immune function and recovery from critical illness as patients benefit from the more natural sleep-like state. Furthermore, critically ill patients will benefit from the reduced burden of delirium, and from the putative neuroprotective effects of these drugs [40], which is associated with reduced length of ICU stay. Finally, their analgesic effects may also play an important role in ensuring patient comfort.
- *Cardiovascular system* – α_2-adrenoceptor agonists exert cardioprotective effects and promote hemodynamic stability. In part their anti-inflammatory effects may contribute in this setting.
- *Renal system* – α_2-adrenoceptor agonists possess renoprotective and diuretic actions.
- *Gastrointestinal system* – preclinical evidence suggests that these drugs may provide some gastrointestinal protection and improve wound healing.
- *Immune effects* – as shown in subgroup analysis from the MENDS study, α_2-adrenoceptor agonists may specifically improve outcomes in septic patients (though further evidence is required). This may be related to improvement in macrophage function, antiapoptotic and anti-inflammatory effects and also their unique sedative profile.

Patients may derive benefit in multiple ways from α_2-adrenoceptor agonists both in the perioperative period and in the critical care environment. While further studies are required there is accumulating evidence that we should be employing these drugs in an increasingly diverse manner, and thus it is reassuring that they are very safe when administered prudently.

Chloral hydrate

Unlike the α_2-adrenoceptor agonists, the majority of currently employed sedative drugs act, at least in part, via potentiation of GABA$_A$ receptors. Included in this important group of drugs are the benzodiazepines (Chapter 29) and chloral hydrate [93]. However, chloral hydrate exhibits no direct gating activity at GABA$_A$ receptors in the absence of GABA and acts by potentiating the action of GABA at these inotropic channels. While the subunit-dependency of chloral hydrate's effect has not been clarified, the neural networks underlying its sedative action have recently been elucidated. In a series of experiments, Lu and colleagues extended the findings of Nelson *et al.* that

Table 30.1. Effects of scopolamine

System	Effect
Central nervous system	Sedation (excitatory effects at high doses)
Cardiovascular	Tachycardia (bradycardia can occur at low doses)
Respiratory	Bronchial dilation Reduced secretions
Gastrointestinal	Reduced secretions Decreased motility
Visual	Mydriasis and cycloplegia (avoid in patients with glaucoma)

GABAergic drugs act through distinct neuronal networks to exert their sedative actions and induce some antinociceptive effect (at "anesthetic" rather than sedative concentrations) [94]. Thus, similar to propofol and pentobarbital (and in all likelihood the benzodiazepines), chloral hydrate induces hypnotic effects by actions on the VLPO (Fig. 30.4) and also activates pontine noradrenergic nuclei, thus activating descending inhibitory pathways to produce analgesia at anesthetic concentrations.

An oral dose of 40–75 mg kg^{-1} chloral hydrate produces sedative effects satisfactory for imaging studies and premedication for anesthesia [95], but it is poorly palatable. With an onset time of 20–30 minutes it is relatively slow-acting. Further, concerns over the genotoxic and carcinogenic effects have limited its chronic application. However, even in the acute setting chloral hydrate has been largely superseded by more modern sedatives.

Muscarinic antagonists

Scopolamine is an alkaloid that acts as a competitive nonselective muscarinic antagonist, thus producing both peripheral and central antimuscarinic effects. Due to blood–brain solubility, central sedative, antiemetic, and amnestic effects occur, although the sedative effects are relatively weak (Table 30.1). Peripheral parasympatholysis is useful for the reduction of gastrointestinal and bronchial secretions, smooth-muscle relaxation as well as cardiovascular effects, and therefore scopolamine is traditionally employed as a premedicant. A biphasic heart-rate response is noted, with low doses of scopolamine slowing the heart rate and higher doses increasing it dose-dependently. Doses of up to 2.8 μg kg^{-1} produce bradycardia, while at higher doses such as 8.4 μg kg^{-1} a tachycardia is observed lasting for 30 minutes and followed by a prolonged bradycardia [96].

The muscarinic cholinergic system has a well-described role in arousal and learning and memory, and therefore there is ample reason for scopolamine's utility as a sedative and an amnestic drug. Parenteral dosing of scopolamine leads to changes in EEG and cognitive performance paralleling pharmacokinetic parameters, with a dose- and time-dependent impairment of memory and attention. Following administration of scopolamine (0.4–0.8 mg SC), the drug generated a time-dependent increase in delta EEG power (1.25–4.50 Hz) and a decrease in fast alpha EEG power (9.75–12.50 Hz) for more than 8 hours [97]. Similar to the benzodiazepines, scopolamine prduces a reduction in rapid eye movement (REM) sleep. At higher doses, however, scopolamine leads to stimulation of the CNS with excitement, hallucinations, and irritability.

Scopolamine toxicity primarily relates to predictable dose-dependent anticholinergic effects including somnolence, coma, confusion, agitation, hallucinations, convulsion, visual disturbance, dry flushed skin, dry mouth, urinary retention, decreased bowel sounds, hypertension, and arrhythmias.

Dosage and administration

The use of scopolamine premedication was investigated in three groups of patients undergoing cesarean section. Scopolamine was administered intravenously (5 μg kg^{-1}), intramuscularly (10 μg kg^{-1}), or oropharyngeally (35 μg kg^{-1} in intubated patients) [98]. The patients receiving the intravenous dose were slightly sedated and lacked amnesia. However, patients in both other groups were markedly sedated and had complete amnesia up to 1.5–2 hours after the end of the anesthesia. They also reported a profound dryness of the mouth. A further study looked at male patients scheduled for minor surgery under spinal anesthesia. Patients received scopolamine (6 μg kg^{-1}) plus morphine (200 μg kg^{-1}) injected in either deltoid or gluteal muscle. The sedative effect of the drug combination was prominent and long-lasting in both groups [99]. However, because of scopolamine's significant adverse effects and its long duration of action it is rarely used now in clinical practice.

Summary

The α$_2$-adrenoceptor agonists fall into three main chemical classes: the phenylethylates, the oxaloazepines, and the imidazolines. The last, which includes clonidine, dexmedetomidine, mivazerol, and azepexole, is the chemical class predominantly used in anesthetic practice. Alpha$_2$-adrenoceptor agonists may induce a number of hemodynamic side effects. Central and peripheral sympatholytic mechanisms contribute to hypotension and bradycardia, while peripheral effects are also mediated by activation of α$_{2B}$-adrenoceptors, which induce

vasoconstriction. Binding to imidazoline receptors is thought to contribute to some of the hemodynamic side effects, and thus development of more highly selective α$_2$-adrenoceptor agonists is desirable to improve safety. Despite this, the imidazolines have a wide safety margin, with no idiosyncratic adverse effects discovered since the widespread introduction of clonidine in the 1970s.

The recent MENDS trial has highlighted some of the potential benefits of dexmedetomidine over lorazepam for critical care sedation. In mediating their sedative effects, α$_2$-adrenoceptor agonists are thought to activate neural substrates for natural sleep. It has been hypothesized that the replication of natural sleep mechanisms might bring about the reparative changes which usually accompany sleep, thus speeding recovery. Similarly, the preserved rousability and relative lack of respiratory depression associated with α$_2$-adrenoceptor agonist-mediated sedation is proposed to be beneficial in an intensive care setting, as is the possibility of reduced delirium burden. The use of α$_2$-adrenoceptor agonists as premedication can reduce anesthetic requirements, and while they have analgesic properties they are comparatively weak amnestic drugs.

There is evidence suggestive of neuroprotective and renoprotective effects for α$_2$-adrenoceptor agonists, and there is some indication that these drugs also have anti-inflammatory properties. Their sympatholytic properties can provide hemodynamic stability during surgery and recovery, and sympatholysis in combination with the prevention of shivering may provide cardioprotection.

Drugs such as chloral hydrate, which potentiates the action of GABA at GABA$_A$ receptors, and scopolamine, a competitive muscarinic antagonist, have been superseded by both benzodiazepines and α$_2$-adrenoceptor agonists, precipitating a decline in their clinical use.

Alpha$_2$-adrenoceptor agonists provide a useful and efficient solution to a number of problems encountered in the perioperative setting. As such, they deserve to be more widely used and are a useful addition to the anesthesiologist's and intensivist's armamentarium. In particular, their use in the postanesthesia care unit and critical care unit to reduce patient morbidity and mortality, as well as to improve the quality of sedation, is warranted. An evidence base for this is already established, although further research is required to elucidate the extent of these effects.

References

1. Tibiriça E, Feldman J, Mermet C, et al. An imidazoline specific mechanism for the hypotensive effect of clonidine: a study with yohimbine and idazoxan. *J Pharmacol Exp Ther* 1990; **256**: 606.

2. Bylund DB, Eikenberg DC, Hieble JP, et al. International union of pharmacology nomenclature of adrenoceptors. *Pharmacol Rev* 1994; **46**: 121–36.

3. Lakhlani PP, MacMillan LB, Guo TZ, et al. Substitution of a mutant alpha2a-adrenergic receptor via "hit and run" gene targeting reveals the role of this subtype in sedative, analgesic, and anesthetic-sparing responses in vivo.

Proc Natl Acad Sci U S A 1997; **94**: 9950–5.

4. Hunter JC, Fontana DJ, Hedley LR, et al. Assessment of the role of alpha2-adrenoceptor subtypes in the antinociceptive, sedative and hypothermic action of dexmedetomidine in transgenic mice. *Br J Pharmacol* 1997; **122**: 1339–44.

5. Ma D, Hossain M, Rajakumaraswamy N, et al. Dexmedetomidine produces its neuroprotective effect via the α$_{2A}$-adrenoceptor subtype. Eur J Pharmacol 2004; 502: 87–97.

6. Fagerholm V, Gronroos T, Marjamaki P, et al. Altered glucose homeostasis in alpha2A-adrenoceptor knockout mice. Eur J Pharmacol 2004; 505: 243–52.

7. Intengan HD, Smyth DD. Alpha-2a/d adrenoceptor subtype stimulation by guanfacine increases osmolar clearance. J Pharmacol Exp Ther 1997; 281: 48–53.

8. MacMillan LB, Hein L, Smith MS, et al. Central hypotensive effects of the alpha2a-adrenergic receptor subtype. Science 1996; 273: 801–3.

9. Link RE, Desai K, Hein L, et al. Cardiovascular regulation in mice lacking alpha 2-adrenergic receptor subtypes B and C. Science 1996; 273: 803–5.

10. Takada K, Clark DJ, Davies MF, et al. Meperidine exerts agonist activity at the alpha 2b-adrenoceptor subtype. Anesthesiology 2002; 96: 1420–6.

11. Sawamura S, Kingery WS, Davies MF, et al. Antinociceptive action of nitrous oxide is mediated by stimulation of noradrenergic neurons in the brainstem and activation of α2B adrenoceptors. J Neurosci 2000; 20: 9242–51.

12. Sallinen J, Lahdesmaki J, MacDonald E, et al. Genetic alteration of the alpha2-adrenoceptor subtype c in mice affects the development of behavioral despair and stress-induced increases in plasma corticosterone levels. Mol Psychiatry 1999; 4: 443–52.

13. Virtanen R, Savola JM, Saano V, Nyman L. Characterization of the selectivity, specificity and potency of medetomidine as an alpha 2-adrenoceptor agonist. Eur J Pharmacol 1988; 150: 9–14.

14. Guo TZ, Tinklenberg BS, Oliker R, Maze M. Central α1-adrenoreceptor stimulation functionally antagonizes the hypnotic response to dexmedetomidine and α2-adrenoreceptor agonist. Anesthesiology 1991; 75: 252–6.

15. Correa-Sales C, Rabin BC, Maze M. A hypnotic response to dexmedetomidine, an a-2 agonist, is mediated in the locus coeruleus in rats. Anesthesiology 1992; 76: 948–52.

16. Nacif-Coelho C, Correa-Sales C, Chang LL, Maze M. Perturbation of ion channel conductance alters the hypnotic response to the a2-adrenergic agonist dexmedetomidine in the locus coeruleus of the rat. Anesthesiology 1994; 81: 1527–34.

17. Nelson LE, Lu J, Guo T, et al. The alpha2-adrenoceptor agonist dexmedetomidine converges on an endogenous sleep-promoting pathway to exert its sedative effects. Anesthesiology 2003; 98: 428–36.

18. Reid K, Hayashi Y, Guo TZ, et al. Chronic administration of an alpha 2 adrenergic agonist desensitizes rats to the anesthetic effects of dexmedetomidine. Pharmacol Biochem Behav 1994; 47: 171–5.

19. Davies MF, Reid K, Guo TZ, et al. Sedative but not analgesic alpha2 agonist tolerance is blocked by NMDA receptor and nitric oxide synthase inhibitors. Anesthesiology 2001; 95: 184–91.

20. Hall JE, Uhrich TD, Barney JA, Arain SR, Ebert TJ. Sedative, amnestic, and analgesic properties of small-dose dexmedetomidine infusions. Anesth Analg 2000; 90: 699–705.

21. Wang M, Ramos BP, Paspalas CD. Alpha2A-adrenoceptors strengthen working memory networks by inhibiting cAMP-HCN channel signaling in prefrontal cortex. Cell 2007; 129: 397–410.

22. Galeotti N, Bartolini A, Gheraldini C. Alpha-2 agonist-induced memory impairment is mediated by the alpha-2A-adrenoceptor subtype. Behav Brain Res 2004; 153: 409–17.

23. Kallio A, Scheinin M, Koulu M, et al. Effects of dexmedetomidine, a selective α2-adrenoreceptor agonist, on hemodynamic control mechanisms. Clin Pharmacol Ther 1989; 46: 33–42.

24. Housmans PR. Effects of dexmedetomidine on contractility, relaxation, and intracellular calcium transients of isolated ventricular myocardium. Anesthesiology 1990; 73: 919–22.

25. Bruandet N, Rentero N, Debeer L, Quintin L. Catecholamine activation in the vasomotor center on emergence from anesthesia: the effects of α2 agonists. Anesth Analg 1998; 86: 240–5.

26. Bruban V, Estato V, Schann S, et al. Evidence for synergy between alpha(2)-adrenergic and nonadrenergic mechanisms in central blood pressure regulation. Circulation 2002; 105: 1116–21.

27. Ohata H, Iida H, Watanabe Y, Dohi S. Hemodynamic responses induced by dopamine and dobutamine in anesthetized patients premedicated with clonidine. Anesth Analg 1999; 89: 843–8.

28. Eisenach J, Detweiler D, Hood D. Hemodynamic and analgesic actions of epidurally administered clonidine. Anesthesiology 1993; 78: 277–87.

29. Coughlan MG, Lee JG, Bosnjak ZJ, et al. Direct coronary and cerebral vascular responses to dexmedetomidine: Significance of endogenous nitric oxide synthesis. Anesthesiology 1992; 77: 998–1006.

30. Roekaerts PM, Prinzen FW, Willigers HM, De Lange S. The effects of α2-adrenergic stimulation with mivazerol on myocardial blood flow and function during coronary artery stenosis in anesthetized dogs. Anesth Analg 1996; 82: 702–11.

31. Kono M, Morita S, Hayashi T, et al. The effects of intravenous clonidine on regional myocardial function in a canine model of regional myocardial ischemia. Anesth Analg 1994; 78: 1047–52.

32. Thomas MG, Quiroz AC, Rice JC, et al. Antianginal effects of clonidine. J Cardiovasc Pharmacol 1986; 8: S69–75.

33. Wijeysundera DN, Naik JS, Beattie WS. Alpha-2 adrenergic agonists to prevent perioperative cardiovascular complications: a meta-analysis. Am J Med 2003; 114: 742–52.

34. Wallace AW, Galindez D, Salahieh A, et al. Effect of clonidine on cardiovascular morbidity and mortality after noncardiac surgery. Anesthesiology 2004; 101: 284–93.

35. Ishiyama T, Dohi S, Iida H, Watanabe Y, Shimonaka H. Mechanisms of dexmedetomidine-induced cerebrovascular effects in canine in vivo experiments. Anesth Analg 1995; 81: 1208–15.

Table 31.2. Human opioid-receptor gene family

Greek name	IUPHAR name	Chromosomal location	Prefered endogenous ligands
μ-opioid receptor	MOP	6 q 24.1	β-endorphin, leu-enkephalin, met-enkephalin
δ-opioid receptor	DOP	1 p 34.3	Leu-enkephalin, met-enkephalin
κ-opioid receptor	KOP	8 q 11.2	Dynorphin
ORL1 receptor	NOP	20 q 55.18	Nociceptin

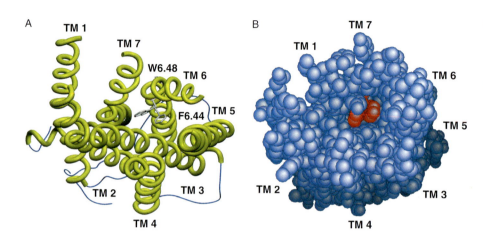

Figure 31.4. (A) Putative rhodopsin-like three-dimensional structure of an opioid receptor. (B) Top view onto the clockwise arrangement of the seven transmembrane domains (TM1–TM7) that generate a putative binding pocket for the morphine molecule (red).

from the cytoplasmic side) and form a tight helical bundle [27]. Opioid receptors interact with their ligands at several sites, extracellular as well as intramembranous. Studies on G-protein-coupled receptors indicate that while binding sites of small molecules (e.g., opium alkaloids) reside usually within the transmembrane domains, i.e., the core of the receptor protein, extracellular loops and the amino terminal are crucial for peptide recognition (e.g., opioid peptides, synthetically modified peptides).

Opioid receptor signaling

Following binding of a ligand to the opioid receptor a conformational change in the three-dimensional structure of the receptor will occur so that the ligand–receptor complex reaches a state of high affinity for intracellular $G_{\alpha}/G_{\beta\gamma}$ heterotrimeric G proteins [28]. This promotes a GDP/GTP exchange, resulting in receptor binding of the G_{α} subunit and liberation of the $G_{\beta\gamma}$ subunit. G_{α} GTP and $G_{\beta\gamma}$ target intracellular effectors including adenylate cyclases and Ca^{2+}/K^{+} ion channels, respectively (Fig. 31.5). In particular, inhibitory $G_{\alpha i/o}$ subunits show a preference for opioid receptors, resulting in reduced intracellular cAMP levels, inhibition of Ca^{2+} current, and increase in extracellular K^{+} current [28]. This will finally lead to a decrease in the neuronal excitation and to an inhibition of neurotransmitter and/or neuropetide release. Hydrolysis of

GTP to GDP returns the receptor-bound G_{α} subunit to its inactive state and subsequent dissociation. On the intracellular side of the opioid receptor the third intracellular loop and the carboxy terminal are mainly responsible for binding of the G_{α} subunit. Since there are also several putative phosphorylation sites as targets for different intracellular kinases, phosphorylation of the opioid receptor will interfere with the effective G-protein coupling of the receptor, a condition that has been described for the phenomenon of opioid tolerance (see below).

According to their ability to initiate such G-protein coupling of opioid receptors, their ligands are classified into full opioid agonists, partial agonists, antagonists, and mixed agonist-antagonists (Table 31.3). Opioid agonists elicit typical opioid effects via a reversible receptor G-protein coupling. Full opioid agonists (e.g., fentanyl, sufentanil) are highly potent and require only little receptor occupancy for maximal response. Partial opioid agonists (e.g., buprenorphine) require a higher receptor occupancy for maximal efficacy, which is usually lower than that of the full agonists.

Mechanisms of analgesic actions

A comparison of μ-opioid receptor binding and mRNA expression in the brain identified overlapping areas of high opioid receptor density as possible central sites of analgesic

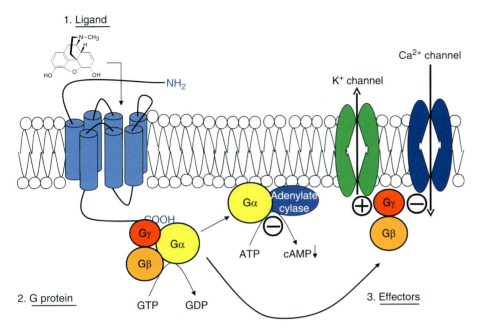

1. Ligand

NH$_2$

2. G protein

COOH

Gγ

Gα

Gβ

GTP GDP

Gα

Adenylate cyclase

ATP cAMP↓

K$^+$ channel

Ca^{2+} channel

Gγ

Gβ

3. Effectors

Figure 31.5. Mechanisms of opioid receptor-ligand-induced G-protein activation. Binding of an opioid receptor ligand such as morphine leads via a conformational change to increased receptor affinity for intracellular G proteins (i.e., Gα$_i$), which activation results in inhibition of downstream effectors such as adenylate cyclase and Ca^{2+} channels or a stimulation of K$^+$ channels. As a result, intracellular cAMP, K$^+$, and Ca^{2+} concentrations decrease, preventing neurotransmitter/neuropeptide release and excitation of the neuron.

Table 31.3. Classification of opioid ligands

Full agonists	Partial agonists	Mixed agonist-antagonists	Antagonists
Fentanyl	Buprenorphine	Pentazocine	Naloxone
Sufentanil	Tilidine	Phenazocine	Naltrexone
Remifentanil		Nalbuphine	
Alfentanil		Butorphanol	
Morphine			
Heroin			
Hydromorphone			
Levorphanol			
Codeine			
Oxycodone			
Loperamide			
Meperidine			
Methadone			

actions such as the thalamus, hypothalamus, insular cortex, amygdala, cingulate gyrus, locus coeruleus, and periaqueductal gray [29]. This was confirmed by visualization of central opioid receptors with μ-, δ-, and κ-opioid receptor-specific immuno-histochemistry [30]. More recently, functional imaging studies such as fMRI and PET scans in humans showed similar results using specific pain paradigms and radiolabeled opioid ligands (e.g., ^{11}C-carfentanil). An opioid-specific reduction in pain-induced brain activity was mainly observed in the thalamus, insula, and both anterior and posterior cingulate cortex [31–33]. More interestingly, a specific pain paradigm triggered the activation of the endogenous opioid peptide system in humans, which resulted in a competitive displacement of radiolabeled opioid ligands in the above-mentioned brain areas [34,35].

Opioid actions within the CNS are well characterized at the locus coeruleus, the periaquaeductal gray (PAG), and the ventral tegmental area, in which a high density and overlap of both opioid receptors and opioid peptides can be identified [36] (Fig. 31.6). In the PAG area administered exogenous opioids bind to opioid receptors and activate descending inhibitory pathways that project to the dorsal horn of the spinal cord to inhibit nociceptive processing [36]. These descending inhibitory pathways are also stimulated by a release of endogenous opioid peptides following certain stressful stimuli.

At the level of the spinal cord a high density of opioid-receptor binding sites has been demonstrated within the dorsal horn [37] (Fig. 31.6). Consistently, μ-, δ-, and κ-opioid receptor-specific immunohistochemistry showed distribution in laminae I and II of the spinal cord [30]. These opioid receptors are located both presynaptically on central nerve terminals of peripheral sensory neurons and postsynaptically on second-order spinal cord neurons. Interestingly, a surgical ablation of the incoming sensory neurons (i.e., rhizotomy) leads to a 50% up to 70% loss of presynaptic opioid receptor binding sites [37]. Functional studies show that intrathecal opioids inhibit the Ca^{2+} influx of incoming peripheral sensory neurons [28,38] and the subsequent spinal release of glutamate and neuropeptides such as substance P [39]. In addition, postsynaptic opioid receptors open G-protein-coupled inwardly rectifying K$^+$ (GIRK) channels and hyperpolarize the membrane [40,41]. These two mechanisms may underlie the potent

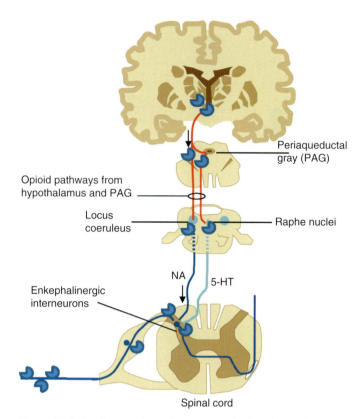

Figure 31.6. Localization of opioid receptors at the three levels of the pain pathway. A high density of opioid receptors is present in the hypothalamus, the periaqueductal gray, the locus coeruleus, the dorsal horn of the spinal cord, the dorsal root ganglia, and peripheral nerve endings of sensory neurons.

analgesic effects of intrathecally or epidurally applied opioids. The spinal cord also expresses opioid peptides, mainly enkephalin and dynorphin, which are localized in central sensory nerve terminals, inhibitory interneurons, and spinal projection neurons [30]. Under painful conditions, these endogenous opioids are presumably released and modulate incoming painful stimuli via both pre- and postsynaptic receptors. While there is clear evidence about the pain-inhibitory actions of enkephalins, the role of dynorphin seems to be more ambiguous and may depend on the state of disease [42].

Since opioid receptors were demonstrated on central nerve terminals of sensory neurons [43], it was only a matter of time before they were also discovered on peripheral nerve terminals of the same neurons [44]. Receptor protein [45,46] and mRNA [47–49] of all three opioid receptors μ, δ, and κ have been identified. Upon ligand binding, these receptors couple effectively to G proteins and lead to cAMP inhibition [50–52], which finally results in the inhibition of pain, as demonstrated in both experimental and clinical studies [53]. Under normal conditions, no endogenous opioid peptides are in the vicinity of theses peripheral opioid receptors; however, under pathological conditions such as tissue injury and inflammation, immune cells (granulocytes, macrophages, lymphocytes) migrate into subcutaneous tissue, and 30–40% of them express

endogenous opioid peptides [54]. Recent evidence shows that β-endorphin, enkephalin, and dynorphin and their respective precursors colocalize with processing enzymes in these immune cells, resulting in the vesicular accumulation of peptide end-products [55]. Trigger substances, such as CRH, initiate the Ca^{2+}-dependent release of these opioid peptides, which play a role in stress-induced analgesic effects [56,57].

Mechanisms of respiratory depression

All μ-opioid agonists in clinical use exert respiratory depression. They reduce the breathing rate, delay the expiratory time, prolong the breathing space, and promote an irregular breathing rhythm. High doses of opioids can additionally lead to continuously decreasing tidal volumes and finally to respiratory arrest without losing consciousness [58,59].

The fundamental drive to respiration is located in respiratory centers of the brainstem consisting of different groups of neuronal networks in the ventrolateral medulla. These centers do not act in isolation but are modulated by influences from different nuclei of the pons such as the nucleus tractus solitarius, the midline medullary raphe, and the locus coeruleus, known as the chemoreactive zone. All areas show a high density of opioid receptors, particularly μ and δ receptors [60]. In addition, enkephalin and opioid receptors were also identified in the glomus region of the carotid body, the main sensor for hypoxia and hypercapnia. Consistently, a central and peripheral component of the hypercapneic response to opioids can be observed, though the former contributes to it much more strongly than the latter [58,59].

Opioids reduce the responsiveness to CO_2 by elevating the end-tidal PCO_2 threshold, and attenuate the hypoxic ventilator response to a decreased PO_2. With a gradual increase in the dose of opioids, slowly developing hypercapnia maintains respiration. However, when this occurs rapidly, e.g., from an intravenous bolus, apnea occurs immediately until PCO_2 reaches a steady state which permits respiration return [61].

Because of this very complex scenario the exact mechanisms of how opioids affect the various respiratory centers involved with ventilator drive, respiratory rhythm generation, and chemoreception are still unclear. A first step towards a better understanding has been achieved with the demonstration of an antagonism of opioid-induced respiratory depression by activation of the serotonin receptor 5-HT$_{4a}$ [62]. In inspiratory neurons of the respiratory center, stimulation of the 5-HT$_{4a}$ receptor led to a reversal of the respiratory depression induced by the μ-agonist fentanyl without affecting the analgesic effect. Since both receptors colocalize on the same respiratory neuron, a reduction of intracellular cAMP by fentanyl-induced $G_{\alpha i}$ activation was counteracted by an increase in cAMP through stimulatory $G_{\alpha s}$ protein via activation of the 5-HT$_{4a}$ receptor. Unfortunately, mosapride, currently the only

5-HT$_4$ agonist available for clinical use, given as a single dose of 5 mg three times per day, was not effective [63]; other 5-HT$_{4a}$ agonists are not yet developed for clinical use.

Mechanisms of antitussive effects

In addition to the respiratory depression, opioids also suppress the coughing reflex, and this is therapeutically adopted in the use of codeine, noscapin, and dextromethorphan as antitussive drugs. This reflex is independent of the regulation of the respiratory center. The afferent arm of this reflex is represented by myelinated Aδ sensory nerve fibers (also called rapidly adapting receptors) that originate within or slightly beneath the respiratory epithelium [64]. These fibers run first in the superior laryngeal nerve and then in the vagal nerve to the nucleus tractus solitarius. The efferent arm of this reflex is represented by the motor fibers of the phrenic nerve innervating the diaphragm. There is functional and anatomical evidence of both pre- and postsynaptic opioid receptors, mainly μ- and κ-opioid receptors, within the nucleus tractus solitarius [65]. While the main antitussive effect of opioids is centrally regulated, there is increasing evidence for peripheral opioid receptors on C and Aδ nerve fibers within the tracheal and bronchial wall [66], and inhaled μ-agonists do not necessarily show antitussive effects, but seem to attenuate breathlessness and reverse reflex bronchoconstriction and mucus hypersecretion [67].

Cardiovascular mechanisms

Within the central nervous system opioids inhibit the sympathetic tone and enhance the parasympathetic tone [68]. As a consequence, hypotension, bradycardia, and sometimes even circulatory arrest may occur. The extent of these effects depends on the potency of the opioid substance and is particularly prominent following intravenous bolus injections, among other risk factors (Table 31.4). The responsible anatomical sites lie within specific areas of the brainstem such as the nucleus tractus solitarius, the dorsal vagal nucleus, the nucleus ambiguus, and the parabrachial nucleus [69,70]. In addition, opioids are known to modulate the stress response through opioid receptor-mediated actions on the hypothalamopituitary axis. The most likely anatomical location for the opioid-induced bradycardia is the nucleus ambiguus. Application of opioids in close proximity of the cardiac parasympathetic neurons of the nucleus ambiguus elicits an increase in parasympathetic cardiac activity and subsequent bradycardia [71]. Activation of postsynaptic opioid receptors of these neurons reduces inhibitory Ca^{2+} currents, which subsequently results in increased activity of cardiac parasympathetic neurons [71]. Opioid receptors are also present on endothelial cells of arterial vessels [72,73], and their activation evokes NO-mediated vasodilation [72]. While fentanyl- and sufentanil-induced hypotension is mainly due to a decrease in heart rate,

Table 31.4. Opioid-induced bradycardia: predisposing factors

Medication with β-blockers, calcium antagonists, α$_2$-adrenergic agonists

Use of muscle relaxants without parasympatholytic properties (e.g., vecuronium)

Use of muscle relaxants with parasympathetic properties (e.g., succhinylcholine)

Vagal stimuli (e.g., laryngoscopy)

High opioid dose

Fast bolus injection

remifentanil-induced hypotension is caused by both a decrease in heart rate and systemic resistance [74].

There is increasing evidence of opioid receptors expressed in the heart [68]. High abundance of δ-opioid receptors in the canine sinoatrial node and somewhat lower abundance in the atria are predominantly associated with presynaptic cholinergic nerve terminals, supporting the hypothesis hat prejunctional δ-opioid receptors regulate vagal transmission within the heart [75]. Fewer opioid receptors can also be found in cardiac myocytes, which may contribute to the cardioprotective effects of opioids in myocardial ischemia [76]. Opioid receptor stimulation resulted in a reduction in infarct size similar to that produced by ischemic preconditioning via mitochondrial ATP-sensitive K$^+$ channels [76]. Whether these results can translate into the clinical setting, however, needs to be proven.

Mechanisms of gastrointestinal effects

Opioid side effects on the gastrointestinal system are well known. In general, they reduce gastrointestinal motility, increase circular contractions, decrease gastrointestinal mucous/juice secretion, and increase fluid absorption, which finally results in constipation. In addition, they cause nausea and vomiting (Table 31.5).

Gastrointestinal motility is dependent on coordinated electrical activity of smooth muscle cells, neuronal input from the intrinsic and autonomic nervous systems, and hormonal interactions [77,78]. Opioids are known to modulate the activity of gastrointestinal sympathetic and parasympathetic neurons at the level of the myenteric and submucosal plexus. The myenteric plexus lies between the longitudinal and circular muscle layers and primarily controls the tone of the gastrointestinal wall, and the intensity and rhythm of contractions. The submucosal plexus controls local secretory and absorptive activity [77,78].

Consistent with an inhibitory effect on gut motility and fluid secretion, opioid receptors are highly abundant on neurons in the myenteric and submucus plexus, but are not

Table 31.5. Effects of opioids on the gastrointestinal tract

	Opioid actions	Consequences
Stomach	gastric motility ↓	delayed gastric emptying
	pyloric tone ↑	nausea, vomiting
	lower esophageal sphincter ↓	gastroesophageal reflux ↑
	gastric juice secretion ↓	delayed digestion
Small intestine	pancreatic and biliary secretion ↓	delayed digestion
	fluid secretion ↓	delayed transit
	propulsion ↓	delayed transit, absorption
Large intestine	propulsion ↓	bloating, distension, constipation
	circular smooth muscle contractions↑	spasm, abdominal cramps
	fluid absorption ↑	hard, dry stool
	anal sphincter tone ↑	incomplete evacuation

located on smooth muscle cells. A higher number of neurons expressing κ-receptor-like immunoreactivity were visualized in the myenteric plexus of the rat, with a small number in the submucosal plexus [79]. In contrast, numerous neurons expressing μ-receptor-like proteins were found in the submucosal plexus, with comparatively few in the myenteric plexus. However, there is also evidence for δ-opioid receptors [80,81], and different results may be related to species differences.

The exact mechanism of how opioids inhibit gastrointestinal motility via receptors in the myenteric plexus and impair fluid secretion via receptors in the submucosal plexus is still a matter of debate. A presynaptic location on parasympathetic neurons directly inhibiting the release of parasympathetic neurotransmitters [82] as well as an indirect activation of sympathetic neurons through disinhibition of serotonergic intrinsic neurons are discussed [78]. Importantly, central opioid effects leading to an activation of the sympathetic and inhibition of the parasympathetic nervous system also seem to play a role in the gastrointestinal effects of opioids. However, evidence suggests a predominantly peripheral action of opioids. Subcutaneously administered morphine inhibits intestinal transit in vagotomized animals [83], and antidiarrheal μ-opioid agonists such as loperamide and diphenoxylate, which are generally not absorbed, produce constipating effects at peripheral sites.

Because activation of opioid receptors in the gut leads to constipation, and more severely so to ileus, receptor blockade with opioid antagonists would seem to be a rational therapeutic approach. However, the challenge is to ensure that these opioid antagonists do not compromise the analgesic

efficacy, which can be prevented with a restricted passage of the blood–brain barrier. Naloxone, the classical opioid receptor antagonist, with an oral bioavailability of only 2% because of extensive first-pass metabolism, still crosses the blood–brain barrier and may reverse analgesia. Methylnaltrexone, a quarternary N-methyl derivative of the μ-receptor antagonist naltrexone, does not penetrate the blood–brain barrier and shows direct local inhibition of opioid effects in the gut [84]. A drawback is its susceptibility to demethylation to the tertiary form that then allows blood–brain barrier penetration; however, methylnaltrexone is only slightly demethylated in humans [85]. Alvimopan, a μ-receptor antagonist with a zwitterionic structure and polarity preventing blood–brain barrier penetration, shows a five-times higher μ-receptor affinity than naloxone and a 200-times higher potency of blocking peripheral than central μ-opioid receptors [86]. Orally administered alvimopan effectively blocks morphine-induced gastrointestinal inhibition without affecting analgesia [86].

Opioid-induced nausea and vomiting have a different origin. This physiological reflex to remove toxic substances from the gastrointestinal tract can be evoked either by direct stimulation of afferent neurons (vagal nerve, vestibular nerve) or by humoral substances (e.g., serotonin, dopamine, opioids) in the blood. The anatomical structure within the brain for the afferent neurons is the nucleus tractus solitarius of the vagal nerve, and for the humoral substances it is the area postrema located on the dorsal surface of the medulla oblongata (at the caudal end of the fourth ventricle). The area postrema shows excitatory chemoreceptors for different emetic substances (serotonin, histamine, dopamine). Electron microscopy also reveals μ- and δ-opioid receptors on neurons of the area postrema [87,88] that trigger emesis upon activation [89].

Finally, smooth muscle spasm induced by opioid stimulation along the gallbladder, cystic duct, and sphincter of Oddi increases intrabiliary duct pressure and triggers biliary colic [90]. This increase in intrabiliary duct pressure is particularly accentuated with a removed gall bladder and can be reversed by naloxone and atropine analogs. In the same way, opioids can cause muscle spasm in the urinary bladder, leading to urinary retention due to a decreased detrusor tone and increased sphincter tone.

Mechanisms of pruritus

The histamine-releasing properties of opioids such as codeine and morphine have been regarded for a long time as the cause of opioid-induced pruritus [91]. However, opioids such as fentanyl, sufentanil, and remifentanil are poor histamine liberators and still cause intense pruritus, particularly following intrathecal or epidural administration. Interestingly, in contrast to μ-agonists, κ-opioid agonists suppress the itch sensation. Opioid-induced pruritus seems to be mainly a central mechanism, since pruritus elicited by intravenous fentanyl, remifentanil, and morphine could be reversed by naltrexone, which enters the central nervous system, but not by methylnaltrexone, which does not penetrate the blood–brain barrier [92]. In a mouse model Kuraishi and colleagues demonstrated that intrathecal, but not intradermal, injections of morphine increased scratching of the face and trunk, suggesting that morphine-induced scratching does not occur through local histamine release but through central μ-opioid receptors [93]. The exact mechanism – whether this is a direct opioid-receptor-related effect or an indirect effect involving released mediators (e.g., serotonin, prostaglandin, dopamine) – is still unresolved.

More recently, a new explanation for opioid-induced pruritus within the central nervous system has been postulated. It is based on the fact that painful stimuli antagonize itch sensation, suggesting that pain-processing spinal neurons exert tonic inhibition to silence the distinct population of pruriceptive neurons [94]. In this regard, analgesic effects of opioids would prevent this inhibition unmasking the pruriceptive neurons to evoke the sensation of itch. Therapeutically, opioid-induced pruritus can be antagonized by naloxone and naltrexone, which unfortunately also attenuates its analgesic properties; alternatively, substances such as nalbuphine and butorphanol, which show properties of μ-opioid antagonism and κ-opioid agonism, should be considered.

Mechanisms of immunosuppression

Although there is some controversial debate about immune effects of opioids, mostly from in-vitro studies, results from opioid-receptor knockout mice strongly support an immuno-suppressive effect. Consistently, chronic use of opioids has been associated with an increased incidence of infectious diseases such as HIV and tuberculosis [94–98]. Early reports by Liebeskind and colleagues demonstrated that a single low dose of morphine (20–40 μg) injected into the lateral ventricle suppressed natural killer (NK) cell activity by activation of central opioid receptors [99]. This immunosupressive effect is dependent on the hypothalamopituitary stress axis, since serum concentrations of corticosterone were elevated and adrenalectomy attenuated the immunosupressive effect [100]. In addition, central opioid receptors seem to activate the sympathetic nervous system, since concentrations of norepinephrine in the spleen were elevated and ganglionic as well as peripheral adrenoceptor blockade diminished the immuno-suppressive effects [101,102]. The periaqueductal gray area has been identified as a brain region that has a high density of opioid receptors and that reliably responds with immuno-suppression following injections of opioids [102]. In addition to central effects, opioids exert their immunosuppressive effects via opioid receptors on various immune cells such as granulocytes, monocytes/macrophages, and lymphocytes. There is strong evidence that all opioid receptors (μ, δ, κ, and ORL1) are present on immune cells, that they couple to

$G_{\alpha i/o}$ proteins, and that they influence functional immune-cell parameters [103,104]. In addition, opioid peptides (mainly β-endorphin and enkephalin), their precursors, and required processing enzymes have been identifed in activated granulo-cytes, monocytes, and lymphocytes, suggesting a modulatory role in local inflammation [53,55]. Immunosuppressive effects are more overt following chronic opioid administration [100]. Opioids interfere with the hematopoietic cell development, resulting in atrophy of thymus and spleen and a reduced number of macrophages and B cells within the spleen. Consistently, μ-receptor knockout compared to wild-type mice lacked lymphoid organ (thymus, spleen) atrophy as well as inhibition of NK-cell activity [106]. A very impressive example of the immunosuppressive effects of opioids was demonstrated in a model of murine colon inflammation in which μ- and δ-opioid agonists resulted in a dramatic reduction of macroscopic and microscopic inflammatory signs, an almost complete reversal of immune-cell infiltration, and more importantly a significant reduction in mortality [107]. These effects are in part due to local opioid effects on immune cells, as has been shown with the use of peripherally selective opioids that profoundly diminish macroscopic and microscopic signs of arthritis [108].

Whether immunosuppressive effects of opioids are to the advantage or disadvantage of the organism is very much dependent on the context or circumstances under which opioids and the immune system interact. For example, in arthritis and autoimmune disease an immunosuppressive effect of opioids is advantageous, whereas in conditions such as HIV and drug addiction immunosuppressive effects might lead to further complications such as infections and disturbed wound healing. This becomes very clear in an experimental setting of surgery and pain that leads to enhanced regional tumor growth and an increase in widespread lung metastases [109]. In this model, effective treatment of surgical stress and pain by administration of opioids results in both a significant prevention of regional tumor growth and reduction of lung metastases [109,110].

Mechanisms of desensitization, tolerance, and physical dependence

Long-term application of opioids can result in pharmacological tolerance, i.e., a decreased effect with prolonged administration of a constant dose or increasing doses of opioids to maintain the same effect [111]. Different mechanisms underlie this phenomenon, representing cellular adaptations in response to chronic opioid -receptor activation [112] (Fig. 31.7). Early mechanisms (within seconds to minutes) occur as receptor desensitization due to receptor phosphorylation and progressively diminished receptor–G-protein coupling. Subsequent mechanisms (within minutes to 1 hour) represent receptor internalization indicating

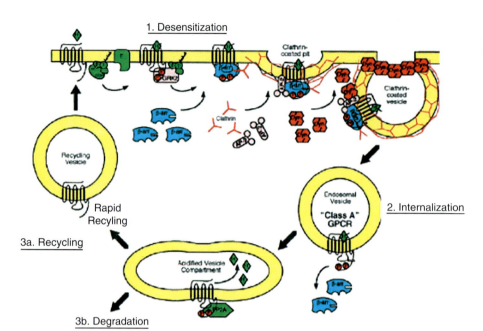

Figure 31.7. Mechanisms of opioid receptor desensitization, internalization, and recycling or degradation.

a receptor translocation from the outer cell membrane to a vesicular intracellular compartment. Late mechanisms (within minutes to several hours) show either functional recovery through recycling of the receptors to the outer cell membrane or downregulation with receptor degradation within the lysosomal compartment of the cell [113]. Even later mechanisms might occur through modulation of opioid receptor gene expression, although clear evidence is lacking [114].

Desensitization specifically refers to the loss of agonist signaling to effector systems through a functional uncoupling of receptor and effector systems. Although desensitization and internalization can occur at the same time, it has been shown that they are mediated via independent processes [115]. Homologous desensitization, in which receptor–ligand binding, G-protein-coupled receptor kinase (GRK) activation, and receptor phosphorylation eventuates, is distinguished from heterologous desensitization, which represents receptor phosphorylation through activation of other receptors, signaling cascades, and finally protein kinases such as PKC and PKA. Opioid agonist efficacy seems to be an important determinant of receptor desensitization; to wit, the highly potent etorphine induces much stronger desensitization than morphine. This is most likely due to differences in the ability to induce GRK phosphorylation of a sufficiently high fraction of opioid receptors [112].

Internalization is dependent on receptor phosphorylation of critical C-terminal residues of opioid receptors leading to an interaction with other intracellular proteins (e.g., β-arrestin) that translocate to the cell membrane and bind to the receptor. Subsequently, there is receptor clustering in clathrin-coated pits in the cell membrane and internalization of the agonist–receptor complex to interior compartments of the cell [116].

This event decreases the amount of surface receptors and ultimately leads to an attenuation of the receptor-mediated signaling transduction [117]. While full agonists (e.g., etorphine) induce rapid internalization, agonists with lower efficacy (e.g., morphine) generally show only little or no internalization [118,119]. Interestingly, when both types of agonists are applied together they support and accelerate each others' processes of internalization, most likely via binding to receptor dimer/oligomer formations [120,121]. A major player in the process of internalization appears to be β-arrestin, since β-arrestin-2 knockout mice demonstrate a significantly slower development of tolerance [122].

The internalized receptors undergo different intracellular trafficking pathways. Some can be recycled back to the cell surface, contributing to the recovery of cellular responsiveness to agonists. Alternatively, the internalized receptors can be targeted to lysosomes for degradation, resulting in a prolonged attenuation of signal transduction [123]. The internalization and intracellular trafficking of opioid receptors involve the movement of receptors between intracellular membrane vesicles [124]. Many studies have demonstrated that Rab GTPases, which belong to the small GTPases superfamily, are key regulators of the trafficking between vesicles [125]. Rab5 mediates the transport or fusion of endocytic vesicles with early endosomes. Rab4 regulates the recycling from early endosomes to the plasma membrane. Rab7 is responsible for the fusion events of late endosomes and lysosomes which finally results in receptor degradation.

There are other cellular mechanisms contributing to the development of tolerance and physical dependence. For instance, "superactivation" of the membrane-bound enzyme adenylate cyclase (AC) is suggested to occur (e.g., within the locus coeruleus) as an adaptive response to prolonged μ-opioid receptor activation [126,127]. The initial opioid-induced AC inhibition and subsequent decrease in cAMP reduces the phosphorylation state of cAMP-responsive elements (CREB) within the nucleus, initiating the adaptive increased expression of AC isoforms ("superactivation") such as ACI and ACVIII as well as PKA [127]. As a result, other receptor systems on the same cell might be activated through PKA-dependent phosphorylation, e.g., the N-methyl-D-aspartate (NMDA) receptor, leading to increased excitability of neurons that contributes to tolerance, dependence, and withdrawal. Indeed, an abrupt withdrawal of opioid tone by use of a μ-receptor antagonist unmasks the underlying enhanced AC activity and precipitates signs of withdrawal. In addition, it has been shown that NMDA receptor antagonists can reverse signs of opioid tolerance [128].

Mechanisms of opioid-associated hyperalgesia

Recently, increasing evidence shows that repeated opioid administration results not only in the development of tolerance (desensitization), but also in a pronociceptive process (sensitization) [129,130]. Collectively, both desensitization and sensitization from prolonged opioid therapy may contribute to an apparent decrease in analgesic efficacy which is often clinically not easy to differentiate. For example, postoperative patients show differences in tactile pain thresholds but not clinical pain intensity following intraoperative remifentanil [131]. Opioid-associated hyperalgesia has been well known from preclinical and clinical studies following opioid withdrawal [132]. However, recent attention has mainly focused on the observation that opioid-associated hyperalgesia also occurs during ongoing opioid treatment [133,134]. For example, patients treated with high doses of opioid infusions display overt hyperalgesia that is immediately resolved once the infusion has been stopped [129,130]. The underlying mechanisms are very similar to the above-mentioned adaptive changes during opioid therapy, i.e., immediate receptor desensitization and uncoupling, adenylate cyclase stimulation, and NMDA receptor activation [129]. This is supported by numerous experimental studies showing that both systemic and intrathecal application of opioids activate the NMDA receptor, and NMDA receptor antagonists reverse opioid-associated hyperalgesia [135].

Opioid-associated hyperalgesia should not be confused with the dose-dependent excitatory effects of morphine that are usually attributed to accumulation of morphine-3-glucuronide in plasma [136]. In addition to hyperalgesia, new pain qualities, myoclonia, and seizures can occur, indicating an accumulation of morphine-3-glucuronide. Rotating to another opioid leads to immediate improvement [137].

Summary

Endogenous opioids are inhibitory neuropeptides, released by neurons to regulate many physiological functions. While not tonically active, they are released in response to a variety of stress signals and act to maintain homeostasis in challenging conditions. Natural exogenous opioids originate from opium alkaloids of the poppy. Semisynthetic (morphine derivatives) and synthetic opioids are also available.

Three opioid G-protein-coupled receptors have been identified – μ, δ, and κ – along with a fourth which displays homology to these receptors yet fails to function similarly. Inhibitory G-protein subunits $G_{\alpha i/o}$ preferentially associate with opioid receptors, and signal transduction causes decreased cyclic adenosine monophosphate (cAMP) levels, inhibition of Ca^{2+} signaling and the activation of K^+ ion channels, ultimately attenuating neuronal excitation and preventing neurotransmitter release.

The effects of opioids on several opioid-receptor-expressing areas of the brain, such as the thalamus, hypothalamus, insular cortex, amygdala, cingulate gyrus, locus coeruleus, and periaqueductal gray, are thought to mediate analgesia. Stimulation of opioid receptors in the periaqueductal gray area activates descending pathways which inhibit nociceptive processing at the level of the dorsal horn of the spinal cord. Opioids may also act directly on opioid receptors within the dorsal horn, expressed presynaptically by the central nerve terminals of sensory neurons and postsynaptically by spinal cord neurons, perhaps providing an explanation for the potency of epidurally administered opioids. Opioid receptors are also present on peripheral nerve terminals of sensory neurons, and their activation has been shown both experimentally and clinically to inhibit pain.

Opioid receptors, particularly μ and δ, are densely expressed in respiratory centers of the brainstem and the nuclei of the pons that influence the respiratory drive, as well as in the periphery within the carotid body, which detects blood levels of O_2 and CO_2. Consequently, the μ-opioid agonists in clinical use lead to respiratory depression, and high-dose opioids can cause respiratory arrest. Opioid suppression of the coughing reflex is predominantly centrally regulated, although this is independent of opioid effects on the respiratory center. Codeine, noscapine, and dextromethorphan are used as antitussive drugs.

A further effect of opioids in the central nervous system is to inhibit sympathetic tone and enhance parasympathetic tone, with resulting hypotension, bradycardia, and possible circulatory arrest. Activation of opioid receptors on arterial endothelium results in vasodilation. The relative contributions of reduced systemic resistance and decreased heart rate to opioid-induced hypotension vary depending on the exogenous opioid administered. There is evidence of opioid receptors expressed in the heart, which are thought to regulate vagal transmission and confer a level of protection in myocardial ischemia, though these findings do not yet have clinical applications.

Opioids reduce gastrointestinal motility via receptors in the myenteric plexus, and decrease fluid secretion via receptors in the submucosal plexus. Opioids increase sympathetic activity while reducing parasympathetic activity in these regions. Although centrally mediated effects may play a role, gastrointestinal effects are thought to result predominantly from peripheral actions. Certain μ-opioid agonists that are not generally absorbed, such as loperamide and diphenoxylate, have clinical uses as antidiarrheal drugs. Use of opioid antagonists to treat morphine-induced ileus is complicated by the possibility of reversal of analgesia if the drug, or an active metabolite thereof, crosses the blood–brain barrier. Orally administered alvimopan is effective for this purpose, and does not penetrate the blood–brain barrier to affect analgesia. Activation of opioid receptors expressed in the area postrema within the brain triggers emesis. Stimulation of opioid receptors at certain peripheral sites can also cause biliary colic (reversible with naloxone and atropine analogs) and urinary retention.

There is evidence that opioid-induced pruritus is a centrally mediated mechanism. Treatment with naloxone and naltrexone attenuates analgesia; an alternative option is the use of agents which stimulate κ-opioid receptors to suppress itching while antagonizing μ-opioid receptors. Opioids are also thought to have immunosuppressive effects, mediated centrally as well as via opioid receptors on immune cells.

Chronic opioid-receptor stimulation can lead to pharmacological tolerance. Opioid tolerance occurs via multiple molecular mechanisms, including receptor desensitization, internalization, and degradation. Superactivation of adenylate cyclase and N-methyl-D-aspartate (NMDA) receptor activation may also contribute to tolerance and dependence. Similar mechanisms underlie opioid-associated hyperalgesia, which occurs during ongoing treatment as well as following withdrawal.

References

1. Dreborg S, Sundström G, Larsson TA, et al. Evolution of vertebrate opioid receptors. *Proc Natl Acad Sci U S A* 2008; **105**: 15487–92.

2. Dores RM, Lecaudé S, Bauer D, et al. Analyzing the evolution of the opioid/orphanin gene family. *Mass Spectrom Rev* 2002; **21**: 220–43.

3. Smith SM, Vale WW. The role of the hypothalamic-pituitary-adrenal axis in neuroendocrine responses to stress. *Dialogues Clin Neurosci* 2006; **8**: 383–95.

4. Archer S. Chemistry of nonpeptide opioids. In: Hertz A., ed., *Handbook of Experimental Pharmacology, Volume 104/I, Opioids I.* New York, NY: Springer, 1993.

5. Kaszor A, Matosiuk D. Non-peptide opioid receptor ligands – recent advances. Part I Agonists. *Curr Med Chem* 2002; **9**: 1567–89.

6. Hughes J, Smith TW, Kosterlitz HW, et al. Identification of two related pentapeptides from the brain with potent opiate agonist activity. *Nature* 1975; **258**: 577–80.

7. Bradbury AF, Smyth DG, Snell CR. Biosynthetic origin and receptor conformation of methionine enkephalin. *Nature* 1976; **260**: 165–6.

8. Goldstein A, Fischli W, Lowney LI, et al. Porcine pituitary dynorphin: complete amino acid sequence of the biologically active heptadecapeptide. *Proc Natl Acad Sci U S A* 1981; **78**: 7219–23.

9. Meunier JC, Mollereau C, Toll L, et al. Isolation and structure of the endogenous agonist of opioid receptor-like ORL1 receptor. *Nature* 1995; **377**: 532–5.

10. Höllt V. Opioid peptide processing processing and receptor selectivity. *Annu Rev Pharmacol Toxicol* 1986; **26**: 59–77.

11. Kieffer BL, Gavériaux-Ruff C. Exploring the opioid system by gene knockout. *Prog Neurobiol* 2002; **66**: 285–306.

12. Zadina JE, Hackler L, Ge LJ, et al. A potent and selective endogenous agonist for the mu-opiate receptor. *Nature* 1997; **386**: 499–502.

13. Fichna J, Janecka A, Costentin J. The endomorphin system and its evolving neurophysiological role. *Pharmacol Rev* 2007; **59**: 88–123.

14. Pert CB, Snyder SH. Opiate receptor: demonstration in nervous tissue. *Science* 1973; **179**: 1011–4.

15. Terenius L. Characteristics of the "receptor" for narcotic analgesics in synaptic plasma membrane fraction from rat brain. *Acta Pharmacol Toxicolog* 1973; **33**: 377–84.

16. Simon EJ, Hiller JM, Edelmand I. Stereospecific binding of the potent narcotic analgesic (3H) Etorphine to rat-brain homogenate. *Proc Natl Acad Sci U S A* 1973; **70**: 1947–9.

17. Martin WR, Eades CG, Thompson JA. The effects of morphine- and nalorphine-like drugs in the nondependent and morphine-dependent chronic spinal dog. *J Pharmacol Exp Ther* 1976; **197**: 517–32.

18. Kieffer BL, Befort K, Gaveriaux-Rull C. The delta-opioid receptor: isolation of a cDNA by expression cloning and pharmacological characterization. *Proc Natl Acad Sci U S A* 1992; **89**: 12048–52.

19. Evans CJ, Keith DE, Morrison H, et al. Cloning of a delta opioid receptor by functional expression. *Science* 1992; **258**: 1952–5.

20. Nishi M, Takeshima H, Fukuda K. cDNA cloning and pharmacological characterization of an opioid receptor with high affinities for kappa-subtype-selective ligands. *FEBS Lett* 1993; **330**: 77–80.

21. Yasuda K, Raynor K, Kong H. Cloning and functional comparison of kappa and delta opioid receptors from mouse brain. *Proc Natl Acad Sci U S A* 1993; **90**: 6736–40.

22. Wang JB, Johnson PS, Persico AM. cDNA cloning of an orphan opiate receptor gene family member and its splice variant. *FEBS Lett* 1994; **348**: 75–9.

23. Mollereaux C, Parmentier M, Mailleux P, et al. ORL1, a novel member of the opioid receptor family. Cloning,

functional expression and localization. *FEBS Lett* 1994; **341**: 33–8.

24. Bunzow JR, Saez C, Mortrud M, *et al.* Molecular cloning and tissue distribution of a putative member of the rat opioid receptor gene family that is not a mu, delta or kappa opioid receptor type. *FEBS Lett* 1994; **347**: 284–8.

25. Pasternak GW. Multiple opiate receptors: déjà vu all over again. *Neuropharmacology 47 Suppl* 2004; **1**: 312–23.

26. Sagara T, Egashira H, Okamura M, *et al.* Ligand recognition in mu opioid receptor: experimentally based modeling of mu opioid receptor binding sites and their testing by ligand docking. *Bioorg Med Chem* 1996; **4**: 2151–66.

27. Baldwin JM, Schertler GF, Unger VM. An alpha-carbon template for the transmembrane helices in the rhodopsin family of G-protein-coupled receptors. *J Mol Biol* 1997; **272**: 144–64.

28. Pan HL, Wu ZZ, Zhou HY. Modulation of pain transmission by G-protein-coupled receptors. *Pharmacol Ther* 2008; **117**: 141–61.

29. Mansour A, Fox CA, Thompson RC, *et al.* mu-Opioid receptor mRNA expression in the rat CNS: comparison to mu-receptor binding. *Brain Res* 1994; **643**: 245–65.

30. Elde R, Arvidsson U, Riedl M, *et al.* Distribution of neuropeptide receptors. New views of peptidergic neurotransmission made possible by antibodies to opioid receptors. *Ann N Y Acad Sci* 1995; **757**: 390–404.

31. Zubieta K, Smith YR, Bueller JA, *et al.* Regional mu opioid receptor regulation of sensory and affective dimensions of pain. *Science* 2001; **293**: 311–15.

32. Wise RG, Rogers R, Painter D, *et al.* Combining fMRI with a pharmacokinetic model to determine which brain areas activated by painful stimulation are specifically modulated by remifentanil. *Neuroimage* 2002; **16**: 999–1014.

33. Wagner KJ, Sprenger T, Kochs EF, *et al.* Imaging human cerebral pain modulation by dose-dependent opioid analgesia: a positron emission tomography activation study using remifentanil. *Anesthesiology* 2007; **106**: 548–56.

34. Scott DJ, Stohler CS, Koeppe RA, *et al.* Time-course of change in [11C] carfentanil and [11C]raclopride binding potential after a nonpharmacological challenge. *Synapse* 2007; **61**: 707–14.

35. Petrovic P, Kalso E, Petersson KM, *et al.* Placebo and opioid analgesia – imaging a shared neuronal network. *Science* 2002; **295**: 1737–40.

36. Fields H. State-dependent opioid control of pain. *Nat Rev Neurosci* 2004; **5**: 565–75.

37. Besson JM, Besse D, Lombard MC. Opioid peptides and pain regulation studied in animal models. *Clin Neuropharmacol* 1992; **15**: 52A–53A.

38. Taddese A, Nah SY, McCleskey EW. Selective opioid inhibition of small nociceptive neurons. *Science* 1995; **270**: 1366–9.

39. Go VL, Yaksh T. Release of substance P from the cat spinal cord. *J Physiol* 1987; **391**: 141–67.

40. Torrecilla M, Marker CL, Cintora SC, *et al.* G-protein-gated potassium channels containing Kir3.2 and Kir3.3 subunits mediate the acute inhibitory effects of opioids on locus ceruleus neurons. *J Neurosci* 2002; **22**: 4328–34.

41. Yoshimura M, North RA. Substantia gelatinosa neurones hyperpolarized in vitro by enkephalin. *Nature* 1983; **305**: 529–30.

42. Hauser KF, Aldrich JV, Anderson KJ. Pathobiology of dynorphins in trauma and disease. *Front Biosci* 2005; **10**: 216–35.

43. Simon EJ, Hiller JM. The opiate receptors. *Annu Rev Pharmacol Toxicol* 1978; **18**: 371–94.

44. Stein C, Hassan AH, Przewłocki R, *et al.* Opioids from immunocytes interact with receptors on sensory nerves to inhibit nociception in inflammation. *Proc Natl Acad Sci U S A* 1990; **87**: 5935–9.

45. Ji RR, Zhang Q, Law PY, *et al.* Expression of mu-, delta-, and kappa-opioid receptor-like immunoreactivities in rat dorsal root ganglia after carrageenan-induced inflammation. *J Neurosci* 1995; **15**: 8156–66.

46. Zhang Q, Schäfer M, Elde R, *et al.* Effects of neurotoxins and hindpaw inflammation on opioid receptor immunoreactivities in dorsal root ganglia. *Neuroscience* 1998; **85**: 281–91.

47. Schäfer M, Imai Y, Uhl GR, *et al.* Inflammation enhances peripheral mu-opioid receptor-mediated analgesia, but not mu-opioid receptor transcription in dorsal root ganglia. *Eur J Pharmacol* 1995; **279**: 165–9.

48. Puehler W, Zöllner C, Brack A, *et al.* Rapid upregulation of mu opioid receptor mRNA in dorsal root ganglia in response to peripheral inflammation depends on neuronal conduction. *Neuroscience* 2004; **129**: 473–9.

49. Puehler W, Rittner HL, Mousa SA, *et al.* Interleukin-1 beta contributes to the upregulation of kappa opioid receptor mrna in dorsal root ganglia in response to peripheral inflammation. *Neuroscience* 2006; **141**: 989–98.

50. Zöllner C, Mousa SA, Fischer O, *et al.* Chronic morphine use does not induce peripheral tolerance in a rat model of inflammatory pain. *J Clin Invest* 2008; **118**: 1065–73.

51. Zöllner C, Shaqura MA, Bopaiah CP, *et al.* Painful inflammation-induced increase in mu-opioid receptor binding and G-protein coupling in primary afferent neurons. *Mol Pharmacol* 2003; **64**: 202–10.

52. Shaqura MA, Zöllner C, Mousa SA, *et al.* Characterization of mu opioid receptor binding and G protein coupling in rat hypothalamus, spinal cord, and primary afferent neurons during inflammatory pain. *J Pharmacol Exp Ther* 2004; **308**: 712–8.

53. Stein C, Schäfer M, Machelska H. Attacking pain at its source: new perspectives on opioids. *Nat Med* 2003; **9**: 1003–8.

54. Brack A, Rittner HL, Machelska H, *et al.* Endogenous peripheral antinociception in early inflammation is not limited by the number of opioid-containing leukocytes but by opioid receptor expression. *Pain* 2004; **108**: 67–75.

55. Mousa SA, Shakibaei M, Sitte N, *et al.* Subcellular pathways of beta-endorphin synthesis, processing, and release from immunocytes in inflammatory pain. *Endocrinology* 2004; **145**: 1331–41.

56. Schäfer M, Carter L, Stein C. Interleukin 1 beta and corticotropin-releasing factor inhibit pain by releasing opioids from immune cells in inflamed tissue. *Proc Natl Acad Sci U S A* 1994; **91**: 4219–23.

57. Schäfer M, Mousa SA, Zhang Q, *et al.* Expression of corticotropin-releasing factor in inflamed tissue is required for intrinsic peripheral opioid analgesia. *Proc Natl Acad Sci U S A* 1996; **93**: 6096–100.

58. Sarton E, Teppema L, Dahan A. Sex differences in morphine-induced ventilatory depression reside within the peripheral chemoreflex loop. *Anesthesiology* 1999; **90**: 1329–38.

59. Pattinson KT. Opioids and the control of respiration. *Br J Anaesth* 2008; **100**: 747–58.

60. Winter SM, Hirrlinger J, Kirchhoff F, *et al.* Transgenic expression of fluorescent proteins in respiratory neurons. *Respir Physiol Neurobiol* 2007; **159**: 108–14.

61. Gross JB. When you breathe IN you inspire, when you DON'T breathe, you…expire: new insights regarding opioid-induced ventilatory depression. *Anesthesiology* 2003; **99**: 767–70.

62. Manzke T, Guenther U, Ponimaskin EG, *et al.* 5-HT4(a) receptors avert opioid-induced breathing depression without loss of analgesia. *Science* 2003; **301**: 226–9.

63. Lötsch J, Skarke C, Schneider A, *et al.* The 5-hydroxytryptamine 4 receptor agonist mosapride does not antagonize morphine-induced respiratory depression. *Clin Pharmacol Ther* 2005; **78**: 278–87.

64. Reynolds SM, Mackenzie AJ, Spina D, *et al.* The pharmacology of cough. *Trends Pharmacol Sci* 2004; **25**: 569–76.

65. Poole SL, Deuchars J, Lewis DI, *et al.* Subdivision-specific responses of neurons in the nucleus of the tractus solitarius to activation of mu-opioid receptors in the rat. *J Neurophysiol* 2007; **98**: 3060–71.

66. Bhargava HN, Villar VM, Cortijo J, *et al.* Binding of [3H][D-Ala2, MePhe4, Gly-ol5] enkephalin, [3H][D-Pen2, D-Pen5]enkephalin, and [3H]U-69,593 to airway and pulmonary tissues of normal and sensitized rats. *Peptides* 1997; **18**: 1603–8.

67. Jennings AL, Davies AN, Higgins JP, *et al.* A systematic review of the use of opioids in the management of dyspnoea. *Thorax* 2002; **57**: 939–44.

68. Pepe S, van den Brink OW, Lakatta EG, *et al.* Cross-talk of opioid peptide receptor and beta-adrenergic receptor signalling in the heart. *Cardiovasc Res* 2004; **63**: 414–22.

69. Moriwaki A, Wang JB, Svingos A, *et al.* Mu opiate receptor immunoreactivity in rat central nervous system. *Neurochem Res* 1996; **21**: 1315–31.

70. Ding YQ, Kaneko T, Nomura S, *et al.* Immunohistochemical localization of mu-opioid receptors in the central nervous system of the rat. *J Comp Neurol* 1996; **367**: 375–402.

71. Irnaten M, Aicher SA, Wang J, *et al.* Mu-opioid receptors are located postsynaptically and endomorphin-1 inhibits voltage-gated calcium currents in premotor cardiac parasympathetic neurons in the rat nucleus ambiguus. *Neuroscience* 2003; **116**: 573–82.

72. Stefano GB, Hartman A, Bilfinger TV, *et al.* Presence of the mu3 opiate receptor in endothelial cells. Coupling to nitric oxide production and vasodilation. *J Biol Chem* 1995; **270**: 30290–3.

73. Vidal EL, Patel NA, Wu G, *et al.* Interleukin-1 induces the expression of mu opioid receptors in endothelial cells. *Immunopharmacology* 1998; **38**: 261–6.

74. Kazmaier S, Hanekop GG, Buhre W, *et al.* Myocardial consequences of remifentanil in patients with coronary artery disease. *Br J Anaesth* 2000; **84**: 578–83.

75. Deo SH, Barlow MA, Gonzalez L, *et al.* Cholinergic location of delta-opioid receptors in canine atria and SA node. *Am J Physiol Heart Circ Physiol* 2008; **294**: H829–38.

76. Schultz JE, Hsu AK, Gross GJ. Morphine mimics the cardioprotective effect of ischemic preconditioning via a glibenclamide-sensitive mechanism in the rat heart. *Circ Res* 1996; **78**: 1100–4.

77. Kurz A, Sessler DI. Opioid-induced bowel dysfunction: pathophysiology and potential new therapies. *Drugs* 2003; **63**: 649–71.

78. De Luca A, Coupar IM. Insights into opioid action in the intestinal tract. *Pharmacol Ther* 1996; **69**: 103–15.

79. Bagnol D, Mansour A, Akil H, *et al.* Cellular localization and distribution of the cloned mu and kappa opioid receptors in rat gastrointestinal tract. *Neuroscience* 1997; **81**: 579–91.

80. Nishimura E, Buchan AM, McIntosh CH. Autoradiographic localization of mu- and delta-type opioid receptors in the gastrointestinal tract of the rat and guinea pig. *Gastroenterology* 1986; **91**: 1084–94.

81. Mihara S, North RA. Opioids increase potassium conductance in submucous neurones of guinea-pig caecum by activating delta-receptors. *Br J Pharmacol* 1986; **88**: 315–22.

82. Lord JA, Waterfield AA, Hughes J, *et al.* Endogenous opioid peptides: multiple agonists and receptors. *Nature* 1977; **267**: 495–9.

83. Stewart JJ, Weisbrodt NW, Burks TF. Central and peripheral actions of morphine on intestinal transit. *J Pharmacol Exp Ther* 1978; **205**: 547–55.

84. Yuan CS, Foss JF, Moss J. Effects of methylnaltrexone on morphine-induced inhibition of contraction in isolated guinea-pig ileum and human intestine. *Eur J Pharmacol* 1995; **276**: 107–11.

85. Kotake AN, Kuwahara SK, Burton E, *et al.* Variations in demethylation of N-methylnaltrexone in mice, rats, dogs, and humans. *Xenobiotika* 1989; **19**: 1247–54.

86. Zimmerman DM, Gidda JS, Cantrell BE, *et al.* Discovery of a potent, peripherally selective trans-3,4-dimethyl-4-(3-hydroxyphenyl) piperidine opioid antagonist for the treatment of gastrointestinal motility disorders. *J Med Chem* 1994; **37**: 2262–5.

87. Guan JL, Wang QP, Nakai Y. Electron microscopic observation of delta-opioid receptor-1 in the rat area postrema. *Peptides* 1997; **18**: 1623–8.

88. Guan JL, Wang QP, Nakai Y. Electron microscopic observation of mu-opioid receptor in the rat area postrema. *Peptides* 1999; **20**: 873–80.

89. Bhandari P, Bingham S, Andrews PL. The neuropharmacology of loperamide-induced emesis in the ferret: the role of the area postrema, vagus, opiate and 5-HT3 receptors. *Neuropharmacology* 1992; **31**: 735–42.

90. Coelho JC, Senninger N, Runkel N, *et al.* Effect of analgesic drugs on the electromyographic activity of the gastrointestinal tract and sphincter of Oddi and on biliary pressure. *Ann Surg* 1986; **204**: 53–8.

91. Ganesh A, Maxwell LG. Pathophysiology and management of opioid-induced pruritus. *Drugs* 2007; **67**: 2323–33.

92. Ko MC, Song MS, Edwards T, *et al.* The role of central mu opioid receptors in opioid-induced itch in primates. *J Pharmacol Exp Ther* 2004; **310**: 169–76.

93. Kuraishi Y, Yamaguchi T, Miyamoto T. Itch-scratch responses induced by opioids through central mu opioid receptors in mice. *J Biomed Sci* 2000; **7**: 248–52.

94. Ikoma A, Steinhoff M, Ständer S, *et al.* The neurobiology of itch. *Nat Rev Neurosci* 2006; **7**: 535–47.

95. Nath A, Hauser KF, Wojna V, *et al.* Molecular basis for interactions of HIV and drugs of abuse. *J Acquir Immune Defic Syndr* 2002; **31**: S62–9.

96. Quinn TC. The epidemiology of the acquired immunodeficiency syndrome in the 1990s. *Emerg Med Clin North Am* 1995; **13**: 1–25.

97. Chaisson RE, Keruly JC, Moore RD. Race, sex, drug use, and progression of human immunodeficiency virus disease. *N Engl J Med* 1995; **333**: 751–6.

98. Reichman LB, Felton CP, Edsall JR. Drug dependence, a possible new risk factor for tuberculosis disease. *Arch Intern Med* 1979; **139**: 337–9.

99. Shavit Y, Depaulis A, Martin FC, *et al.* Involvement of brain opiate receptors in the immune-suppressive effect of morphine. *Proc Natl Acad Sci U S A* 1986; **83**: 7114–7.

100. Bryant HU, Bernton EW, Kenner JR, *et al.* Role of adrenal cortical activation in the immunosuppressive effects of chronic morphine treatment. *Endocrinology* 1991; **128**: 3253–8.

101. Flores LR, Dretchen KL, Bayer BM. Potential role of the autonomic nervous system in the immunosuppressive effects of acute morphine administration. *Eur J Pharmacol* 1996; **318**: 437–46.

102. Hall NR, O'Grady MP, Menzies RA. Neuroimmunopharmacologic effects of drugs of abuse. *Adv Exp Med Biol* 1991; **288**: 13–23.

103. Sibinga NE, Goldstein A. Opioid peptides and opioid receptors in cells of the immune system. *Annu Rev Immunol* 1988; **6**: 219–49.

104. Bidlack JM, Khimich M, Parkhill AL, *et al.* Opioid receptors and signaling on cells from the immune system. *J Neuroimmune Pharmacol* 2006; **1**: 260–9.

105. Bryant HU, Bernton EW, Holaday JW. Morphine pellet-induced immunomodulation in mice: temporal relationships. *J Pharmacol Exp Ther* 1988; **245**: 913–20.

106. Gavériaux-Ruff C, Matthes HW, Peluso J, *et al.* Abolition of morphine-immunosuppression in mice lacking the mu-opioid receptor gene. *Proc Natl Acad Sci U S A* 1989; **95**: 6326–30.

107. Philippe D, Dubuquoy L, Groux H, *et al.* Anti-inflammatory properties of the mu opioid receptor support its use in the treatment of colon inflammation. *J Clin Invest* 2003; **111**: 1329–38.

108. Binder W, Machelska H, Mousa S, *et al.* Analgesic and antiinflammatory effects of two novel kappa-opioid peptides. *Anesthesiology* 2001; **94**: 1034–44.

109. Page GG, Ben-Eliyahu S. A role for NK cells in greater susceptibility of young rats to metastatic formation. *Dev Comp Immunol* 1999; **23**: 87–96.

110. Sasamura T, Nakamura S, Iida Y, *et al.* Morphine analgesia suppresses tumor growth and metastasis in a mouse model of cancer pain produced by orthotopic tumor inoculation. *Eur J Pharmacol* 2002; **441**: 185–91.

111. Cox BM. Mechanisms of tolerance. In: Stein C., ed., *Opioids in Pain Control.* Cambridge: Cambridge University Press, 1999.

112. Cox BM, Crowder AT. Receptor domains regulating mu opioid receptor uncoupling and internalization: relevance to opioid tolerance. *Mol Pharmacol* 2004; **65**: 492–5.

113. Bailey CP, Connor M. Opioids: cellular mechanisms of tolerance and physical dependence. *Curr Opin Pharmacol* 2005; **5**: 60–8.

114. Buzas B, Rosenberger J, Cox BM. Mu and delta opioid receptor gene expression after chronic treatment with opioid agonist. *Neuroreport* 1996; **7**: 1505–8.

115. Celver J, Xu M, Jin W, *et al.* Distinct domains of the mu-opioid receptor control uncoupling and internalization. *Mol Pharmacol* 2004; **65**: 528–37.

116. von Zastrow M, Svingos A, Haberstock-Debic H, *et al.* Regulated endocytosis of opioid receptors: cellular mechanisms and proposed roles in physiological adaptation to opiate drugs. *Curr Opin Neurobiol* 2003; **13**: 348–53.

117. Reiter E, Lefkowitz RJ. GRKs and beta-arrestins: roles in receptor silencing, trafficking and signaling. *Trends Endocrinol Metab* 2006; **17**: 159–65.

118. Alvarez VA, Arttamangkul S, Dang V, *et al.* mu-Opioid receptors: Ligand-dependent activation of potassium conductance, desensitization, and internalization. *J Neurosci* 2002; **22**: 5769–76.

119. Celver JP, Lowe J, Kovoor A, *et al.* Threonine 180 is required for G-protein-coupled receptor kinase 3- and beta-arrestin 2-mediated desensitization of the mu-opioid receptor in Xenopus oocytes. *J Biol Chem* 2001; **276**: 4894–900.

120. He L, Whistler JL. An opiate cocktail that reduces morphine tolerance and dependence. *Curr Biol* 2005; **15**: 1028–33.

121. Zöllner C, Mousa SA, Fischer O, *et al.* Chronic morphine use does not induce peripheral tolerance in a rat model of inflammatory pain. *J Clin Invest* 2008; **118**: 1065–73.

122. Bohn LM, Lefkowitz RJ, Caron MG. Differential mechanisms of morphine antinociceptive tolerance revealed in (beta)arrestin-2 knock-out mice. *J Neurosci* 2002; **22**: 10494–500.

123. Pierce KL, Premont RT, Lefkowitz RJ. Seven-transmembrane receptors. *Nat Rev Mol Cell Biol* 2002; **3**: 639–50.

124. Wang F, Chen X, Zhang X, *et al.* Phosphorylation state of mu-opioid receptor determines the alternative recycling of receptor via Rab4 or Rab11 pathway. *Mol Endocrinol* 2008; **22**: 1881–92.

125. Zerial M, McBride H. Rab proteins as membrane organizers. *Nat Rev Mol Cell Biol* 2001; **2**: 107–17.

126. Finn AK, Whistler JL. Endocytosis of the mu opioid receptor reduces tolerance and a cellular hallmark of opiate withdrawal. *Neuron* 2001; **32**: 829–39.

127. Nestler EJ. Historical review: Molecular and cellular mechanisms of opiate and cocaine addiction. *Trends Pharmacol Sci* 2004; **25**: 210–18.

128. Trujillo KA, Akil H. Inhibition of morphine tolerance and dependence by the NMDA receptor antagonist MK-801. *Science* 1991; **251**: 85–7.

129. Koppert W. Opioid-induced hyperalgesia: pathophysiology and clinical relevance. *Acute Pain* 2007; **9**: 21–34.

130. Angst MS, Clark JD. Opioid-induced hyperalgesia: a qualitative systematic review. *Anesthesiology* 2006; **104**: 570–87.

131. Wilder-Smith CH, Tassonyi E, Crul BJ, Arendt-Nielsen L. Quantitative sensory testing and human surgery: effects of analgesic management on postoperative neuroplasticity. *Anesthesiology* 2003; **98**: 1214–22.

132. Compton P, Athanasos P, Elashoff D. Withdrawal hyperalgesia after acute opioid physical dependence in nonaddicted humans: a preliminary study. *J Pain* 2003; **4**: 511–19.

133. Chu LF, Clark DJ, Angst MS. Opioid tolerance and hyperalgesia in chronic pain patients after one month of oral morphine therapy: a preliminary prospective study. *J Pain* 2006; **7**: 43–8.

134. Angst MS, Koppert W, Pahl I, *et al.* Short-term infusion of the mu-opioid agonist remifentanil in humans causes hyperalgesia during withdrawal. *Pain* 2003; **106**: 49–57.

135. Célèrier E, Laulin J, Larcher A, *et al.* Evidence for opiate-activated NMDA processes masking opiate analgesia in rats. *Brain Res* 1999; **847**: 18–25.

136. Smith MT. Neuroexcitatory effects of morphine and hydromorphone: evidence implicating the 3-glucuronide metabolites. *Clin Exp Pharmacol Physiol* 2000; **27**: 524–8.

137. Smith MT. Differences between and combinations of opioids re-visited. *Curr Opin Anaesthesiol* 2008; **21**: 596–601.

Section 3 Chapter 32
Essential drugs in anesthetic practice
Pharmacokinetics of opioids

Dhanesh K. Gupta, Tom C. Krejcie, and Michael J. Avram

Introduction

There are numerous opioids available for the treatment of opioid-responsive pain. The opioids most commonly used in the perioperative period are the μ-receptor agonists. Because of the similarity in their pharmacologic effects, the choice of appropriate opioid for each clinical setting is primarily dictated by the pharmacokinetic (PK) and pharmacodynamic (PD) properties of the drug. Thus a caregiver might administer a single intravenous dose of alfentanil if an immediate but brief burst of analgesia is needed or a single intravenous dose of morphine if analgesia of a few hours' duration is required (Fig. 32.1). Sophisticated insights into the pharmacokinetics and pharmacodynamics of many opioids achieved since the early 1980s as a result of cutting-edge research have advanced significantly not only the basis for choosing an opioid for a given clinical situation but also how it is administered to achieve the desired clinical outcome safely [3,4]. Thus, for example, understanding the importance of distributional pharmacokinetics led to the concept of context-sensitive half-time, or the time for a 50% decrease in plasma drug concentration, which depends on both drug pharmacokinetics (specifically, distribution and elimination) and its duration of administration (the context). As another example, sophisticated dosing regimens, including computer-driven target-controlled infusions (TCI), have been developed for rapid-onset, short-acting opioids that take advantage of their most desirable PK and PD properties. As a final example, we have come to understand that opioid-induced apnea may be due as much to how the opioid is administered as it is to the dose and pharmacologic properties of the drug [5].

Several advances in the formulations and mode of administration of opioids have exploited basic PK principles to make opioids safer and more effective. Sustained-release orally administered opioids and transdermal opioid delivery can provide convenient long-term administration for treating chronic moderate and severe pain, while oral transmucosal and inhalational opioid delivery provide convenient treatment of breakthrough pain.

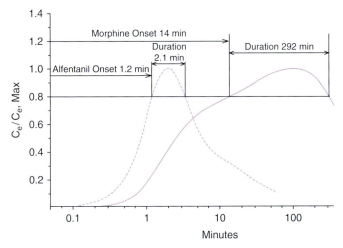

Figure 32.1. Onset and duration of opioid effect. The effect of an opioid is proportional to the concentration at the site of effect, not the plasma concentration. The effect-site concentration (C_e) is generally predicted by a combined pharmacokinetic/pharmacodynamic (PK/PD) model. In addition, drug effects may be adequate before the concentration reaches its peak in the effect compartment (biophase). Different opioids vary in their time of onset and duration of effect. This figure illustrates this concept using morphine and alfentanil as prototype opioids. Drug onset will depend on the effect being measured (e.g., incisional vs. postoperative pain, etc.), the opioid dose administered, and any pre-existing opioid concentrations. For purposes of illustrating this concept, drug onset is defined as the time from administration to the time the opioid concentration in the central nervous system (CNS) effect site reaches 80% of its maximum concentration (C_e normalized to $C_{e,max}$). Duration of effect is defined here as the time the CNS concentration remains above 80% of the maximum. The figure compares two opioids on opposite ends of the spectrum with regard to onset time and duration of effect. To highlight the differences, the time axis is logarithmic. The solid line is the CNS concentration versus time relationship for analgesia produced by intravenous morphine, based on the data from Dahan *et al.* [1]. For morphine (10 mg), the onset time of analgesia is 14 min and the duration of effect is 292 min. The dotted line depicts the effect-site concentration history for the rapid-onset synthetic opioid, alfentanil (1000 μg), with an onset time of analgesia of 1.2 min and duration of effect of 2.1 min [2]. If a larger dose was administered, the effect-site concentration would reach a therapeutic level at a lower percentage of its maximum concentration, and remain above this threshold concentration for a longer period of time. This would result in a larger dose of opioid appearing to have a more rapid onset of action and a longer duration of action. In addition, for other measures of pharmacologic effect, such as miosis or ventilatory depression, the pharmacodynamics may be different and therefore the onset and duration of effect may be different than for analgesia.

Anesthetic Pharmacology, 2nd edition, ed. Alex S. Evers, Mervyn Maze, Evan D. Kharasch. Published by Cambridge University Press. © Cambridge University Press 2011.

Rational selection and use of opioids

Although adequate anesthesia can be achieved and maintained with a potent volatile anesthetic alone, most anesthesiologists administer a combination of a hypnotic (e.g., potent volatile anesthetic, propofol, etc.) and an opioid to decrease the hemodynamic consequences of high hypnotic doses. Administering a balanced opioid–hypnotic anesthetic efficiently requires understanding the PD interactions between opioids and hypnotics (e.g., MAC reduction) to choose rational opioid target concentrations [6,7] and developing dosing strategies to achieve the desired opioid target concentration. Although PK and PD principles and data have contributed greatly to the understanding of the behavior of intravenous anesthetics and analgesics, their primary utility and ultimate purpose are to determine optimal dosing with as much mathematical precision and clinical accuracy as possible.

In most pharmacotherapeutic scenarios outside of anesthesia care, the time scales for onset of drug effect, its maintenance, and its offset are measured in days, weeks, or even years. In these cases, basic PK variables (and one-compartment models), such as total volume of distribution (V_{SS}), elimination (i.e., systemic) clearance (CL_E), and elimination half-life ($t_{1/2\beta}$) are sufficient for calculating dose regimens. In the operating room and intensive care unit, however, the temporal tolerances for onset and offset of desired drug effects are measured in minutes [8,9]. Consequently, these basic PK variables are insufficient to describe the PK behavior of drugs in the minutes to hours immediately following intravenous administration. This is particularly true of intravenously administered opioids, because distribution processes generally dominate disposition while the opioids are producing a pharmacologic response (Fig. 32.2). In addition, the clinical margin of safety of many opioids is small and two-tailed (i.e., it is possible to either underdose, resulting in inadequate analgesia, or overdose, resulting in profound ventilatory depression). Optimal dosing in these situations requires use of all the variables of a multicompartmental PK model to account for drug distribution in blood and other tissues.

It is not easy to intuit the PK behavior of a multicompartmental system by examining the kinetic variables [10]. Computer simulation is required to interpret dosing and to devise accurate new dosing regimens. In addition, there are several PK concepts that are uniquely applicable to intravenous administration of drugs with multicompartmental kinetics that must be considered when administering intravenous infusions. This section of the chapter attempts to demonstrate how PK and PD principles can be applied to the rational selection of opioids for a variety of clinical scenarios. Plasma and effect-site drug concentration versus time relationships are simulated using the PK/PD parameters for fentanyl [2,11], alfentanil [2], sufentanil [11–13], remifentanil [14], and

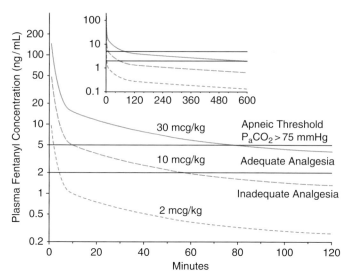

Figure 32.2. Relationship of dose to pharmacokinetic mechanism terminating drug effect. With increasing doses of an intravenous opioid, different pharmacokinetic mechanisms are primarily responsible for the decay in plasma concentrations below the lower limit of plasma concentrations associated with adequate analgesia. For small bolus doses, termination of effect is due primarily to distribution to the rapidly equilibrating compartment, whereas for larger doses termination of effect transitions from distribution to the slowly equilibrating compartment to elimination (i.e., systemic) clearance. In this figure, plasma concentration profiles are simulated for three doses of fentanyl: 2 μg kg^{-1} (long dashed line); 10 μg kg^{-1} (short dashed line); and 30 μg kg^{-1} (solid line). For the small fentanyl dose (2 μg kg^{-1}), the plasma concentration drops rapidly (i.e., within 5 min) below the lower limit of adequate analgesia, primarily because of drug distribution to the rapidly equilibrating tissues, although drug is also being taken up by the slowly equilibrating tissues and eliminated from the body. For the moderate bolus of fentanyl (10 μg kg^{-1}), the rapid-distribution phase brings the drug into the therapeutic range. However, this volume enters a state of pseudoequilibrium with the plasma (i.e., the central volume), after which decreases in plasma concentration are due to distribution into the slowly equilibrating compartment and systemic elimination. Because of the large volume of the slowly equilibrating peripheral compartment, the plasma concentration continues to decline as drug redistributes until reaching subtherapeutic levels at approximately 60 min. Finally, with a bolus of 30 μg kg^{-1} of fentanyl (e.g., "cardiac anesthetic" doses), distribution to the rapidly and slowly equilibrating volumes brings the concentrations down to levels that are still above the therapeutic window at 60 min. Systemic elimination is the predominant mechanism by which the plasma concentrations decrease into and through the therapeutic window to subanalgesic concentrations at approximately 600 min (see inset). For rapid (fast) distribution, slow distribution, and elimination half-lives of representative opioids, see Table 32.2.

morphine [1], and plasma drug concentration versus time relationships are simulated using the PK parameters for morphine [1], hydromorphone [15], and methadone [16] (Table 32.1). All simulations were performed using a fully licensed academic version of the SAAM II software system (version 1.2.1, SAAM Institute, Seattle, WA), implemented on a Windows-based PC.

Single and repeated rapid intravenous infusion (bolus) dosing of opioids

The choice of an opioid for bolus administration depends on the application. The less tolerance there is for excessive opioid effect (e.g., ventilatory depression), the more appropriate it

Table 32.1. Opioid pharmacokinetic and pharmacodynamic data

Opioid	Volume of distribution (L)[a]				Clearance (L min^{-1})[b]			$t_{1/2ke0}$[c] (min)	$t_{peak\ effect}$[d] (min)
	V_C	V_F	V_S	V_{SS}	CL_F	CL_S	CL_E		
Fentanyl [2,11]	12.7	50.3	295	358	4.83	2.27	0.62	4.7	4.2
Remifentanil [14]	7.6	9.5	4.8	21.8	1.95	0.10	2.92	0.6	1.8
Sufentanil [11–13]	18	48	482	548	4.90	1.30	1.18	3.0[e]	4.2
Alfentanil [2]	2.2	6.7	14.6	23.6	1.44	0.25	0.20	0.9	1.8
Morphine [1]	7.3	19.0	125.6	151.9	1.31	1.38	1.93	264.0	19
Hydromorphone [15]	24.4	55	243	322.4	7.2	4.4	1.66	NA	NA
Methadone [16]	76	NA	334	410	NA	8.6	0.18	NA	NA

[a] Volumes of distribution (V) for the central (V_C) and rapidly equilibrating (fast, V_F), and slowly equilibrating (V_S) compartments and the volume of distribution at steady state (V_{SS}), which is the sum of all volumes (total volume of distribution).
[b] Clearances of the rapidly equilibrating peripheral compartment (CL_F) and slowly equilibrating peripheral compartment (CL_S), and elimination (i.e., systemic) clearance (CL_E).
[c] Half-time to equilibration with the effect compartment.
[d] Time to peak effect.
[e] The effect-site drug concentration versus time relationship for a given k_{e0} is determined by the plasma drug concentration versus time relationship predicted by the pharmacokinetic model used in its estimation. Thus, k_{e0} is a rate constant developed for a specific PK/PD model that cannot be combined with other PK models to create a new PK/PD model [17]. However, to be consistent with the available literature, we have used a "hybrid" PK/PD model [11] rather than developing a new model using the model-independent pharmacodynamic parameter, time to peak effect [18].
NA, not available.

would be to choose the opioid providing the greatest margin of safety. On the other hand, when subtherapeutic opioid dosing must be avoided (e.g., inadequate analgesia for placement of Mayfield head fixation in a ruptured intracranial aneurysm), predictability is a greater concern. With six commonly used opioids from which to choose (fentanyl, the fentanyl congeners, morphine, and hydromorphone), the rational choice of the "ideal" opioid for a given clinical situation depends on integrating PK/PD principles with the tolerance for subtherapeutic and supratherapeutic dosing. Because of the lack of a combined PK/PD model for hydromorphone, we here focus mainly on fentanyl, the fentanyl congeners, and morphine.

Examination of the predicted plasma concentrations after a rapid (1 minute) intravenous infusion (bolus) of several opioids provides little insight into how to discriminate between them; within 5 minutes of administration, fentanyl, the fentanyl congeners, and morphine all have plasma concentrations less than 50% of their peak plasma concentrations (Fig. 32.3). Therefore, how does the clinician rationally choose among these opioids? Fortunately, examination of the effect-site concentration (C_e) after bolus administration of the various opioids provides the following insights (Fig. 32.4A):

(1) Remifentanil and alfentanil both produce maximum effect-site concentrations ($C_{e,max}$) most rapidly (in approximately 1.8 minutes).

(2) Remifentanil C_e decreases more rapidly than does alfentanil C_e.

(3) Fentanyl and sufentanil both achieve $C_{e,max}$ relatively rapidly (in approximately 4.2 minutes).

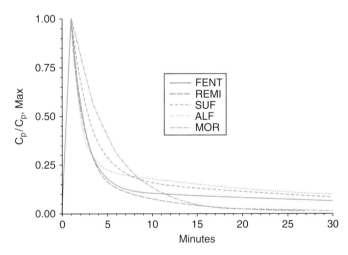

Figure 32.3. Plasma concentration profile after single bolus administration. A simulation of the normalized plasma concentration ($C_p/C_{p,max}$) profile after 1 min infusion of fentanyl (FENT), remifentanil (REMI), sufentanil (SUF), alfentanil (ALF), and morphine (MOR). After a 1 min infusion all plasma concentrations peak at the same time. The initial decreases in fentanyl, remifentanil, and alfentanil plasma concentrations overlap, whereas sufentanil and morphine plasma concentrations decrease more slowly. However, all plasma concentrations are below 25% of the peak plasma concentration by 10 min.

(4) Sufentanil C_e decreases more rapidly than does fentanyl C_e.

(5) Morphine achieves only 67% $C_{e,max}$ in the first 5 minutes, and does not achieve $C_{e,max}$ until 19 minutes – when all of the other opioids have decreased to less than 60% of their respective $C_{e,max}$.

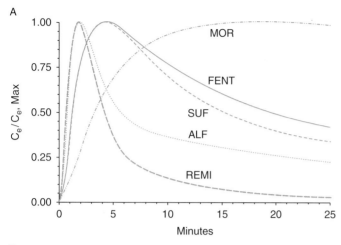

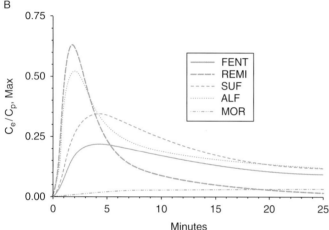

Figure 32.4. Effect-site concentration profile after single bolus administration. A simulation of the effect-site concentration (C_e) following a 1 min infusion of fentanyl (FENT), remifentanil (REMI), sufentanil (SUF), alfentanil (ALF), and morphine (MOR). (A) Effect-site concentrations are normalized to the maximum effect-site concentration ($C_e/C_{e,max}$). This clearly illustrates the similar rate of equilibration of remifentanil and alfentanil ($t_{peak\ effect}$ 1.8 min) and of sufentanil and fentanyl ($t_{peak\ effect}$ 4.2 min) and the much delayed equilibration of morphine ($t_{peak\ effect}$ 19 min). However, the effect-site concentration decreases more rapidly for remifentanil than for alfentanil, and for sufentanil than for fentanyl. (B) Effect-site concentrations are normalized to the maximum *plasma* concentration ($C_e/C_{p,max}$),. This illustrates that the rank order of efficiency of cerebral uptake of the opioids is remifentanil > alfentanil >> sufentanil > fentanyl >> morphine, despite similarities in the $t_{peak\ effect}$ of remifentanil and alfentanil, and of sufentanil and fentanyl. The effect-site concentration decreases more rapidly for remifentanil than for alfentanil, and for sufentanil than for fentanyl.

If rapidly attaining peak analgesic effect is the highest priority, then remifentanil or alfentanil are the agents of choice since both achieve $C_{e,max}$ within 90 seconds. Therefore, for short-lived, intense analgesic requirements (e.g., placement of a retro-bulbar block, placement of a Mayfield head fixation device, tracheal intubation), both of these opioids are ideal. However, because of the rapidity of equilibration with the central nervous system (CNS), boluses of either of these agents are associated with a sudden increase in the apneic threshold (discussed below) [5,19,20]. If the sudden onset of apnea cannot be tolerated, then both of these opioids are potentially dangerous.

The effect-site concentration profile normalized to the maximum plasma concentration (Fig. 32.4B) provides some additional insight that may allow differentiation between remifentanil and alfentanil. The cerebral uptake of remifentanil is more efficient than that of alfentanil; the C_e of remifentanil and alfentanil are approximately 63% and 50% of their peak plasma concentrations, respectively. Assuming that the potency ratio between alfentanil and remifentanil is constant for all PD endpoints (i.e., 50% decrease in minute ventilation, 95% probability of adequate analgesia to mild painful stimulation, 95% probability of no hemodynamic response to sternotomy, etc.) [4,14], a 26% larger dose of alfentanil would be required to achieve an effect equivalent to that produced by a unit dose of remifentanil [11]. Because of the more rapid decrease in remifentanil C_e compared to that of alfentanil, a single bolus of remifentanil may have a greater margin of safety than a single, equally efficacious bolus dose of alfentanil. In addition, because of drug accumulation, administration of subsequent bolus doses of alfentanil at 10- to 15-minute intervals will result in a sustained elevation of alfentanil C_e. In contrast, there is very little accumulation of remifentanil on repeated bolus dosing at 7- to 10-minute intervals (Fig. 32.5A). Therefore, there are significant PK advantages of remifentanil over alfentanil for single or repeated bolus dosing, if profound ventilatory depression can be tolerated.

If sudden, profound ventilatory depression is of concern, fentanyl and sufentanil, with their more gradual uptake by the CNS ($C_{e,max}$ at 4.2 minutes), are associated with a more gradual increase in the apneic threshold. While the minute ventilation decreases, there is a concomitant increase in the arterial partial pressure of CO_2, which helps prevent a sudden reduction of minute ventilation from occurring after modest doses of fentanyl and sufentanil [5,19,21,22]. Therefore, in patients who cannot tolerate a sudden onset of apnea, there is a potential safety benefit of a single bolus of fentanyl or sufentanil over remifentanil or alfentanil. However, this safety must be weighed against the slower onset of effect.

In choosing between sufentanil and fentanyl, examination of the simulated C_e profiles reveals that the relationship between sufentanil and fentanyl is similar to that between remifentanil and alfentanil. Although both sufentanil and fentanyl have similar rates of cerebral uptake ($C_{e,max}$ at 4.2 minutes), sufentanil enters the CNS more efficiently ($C_{e,max}$ 34% vs. 22% of maximum plasma concentration), and its C_e decreases more rapidly after a single bolus. Therefore, single or repeated boluses of sufentanil may have a greater margin of safety than fentanyl. In addition, if repeated boluses are required, sufentanil will accumulate less than fentanyl, thereby preserving some of the speed of recovery observed after a single bolus. However, even with 15-minute intervals between boluses, both sufentanil and fentanyl accumulate significantly with repeated boluses (Fig. 32.5B).

When choosing an opioid for bolus administration, it is necessary to determine the intensity and duration of the

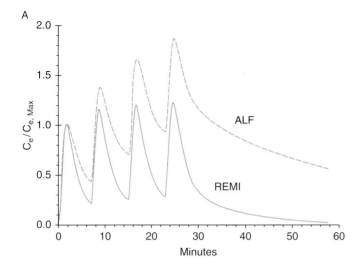

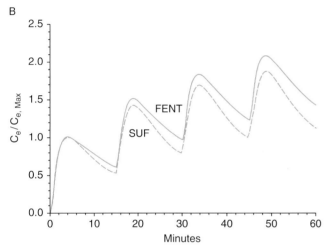

Figure 32.5. Effect-site concentration profile after repeated bolus administration. (A) Simulation of the normalized effect-site concentration ($C_e/C_{e,max\ after\ single\ dose}$) profile after repeated bolus dosing of remifentanil (REMI, *solid line*, 1 $\mu g\ kg^{-1}$ every 7 min) and alfentanil (ALF, *dashed line*, 100 $\mu g\ kg^{-1}$ every 7 min). There is approximately a 25% increase in peak effect-site concentration with each alfentanil dose, whereas all subsequent remifentanil doses only increase peak effect-site concentration 15% compared to the initial peak ($C_{e,max\ after\ single\ dose}$). In addition, the time after the last bolus dose until the alfentanil concentrations decrease below 50% is more than 30 min, while remifentanil concentrations decrease below 50% within 7 min after the last bolus dose. (B) Simulation of the normalized effect-site concentration ($C_e/C_{e,max\ after\ single\ dose}$) profile after repeated bolus dosing of fentanyl (FENT, *solid line*, 1 $\mu g\ kg^{-1}$ every 15 min) and sufentanil (SUF, *dashed line*, 0.1 $\mu g\ kg^{-1}$ every 15 min). For both opioids, there is a progressive increase (approximately 25%) in peak effect-site concentrations with each bolus dose. In addition, sufentanil concentrations decrease more rapidly after the last bolus dose than do those of fentanyl.

noxious stimulus and weigh the benefits of rapid-onset, brief-duration analgesia with profound, sudden ventilatory depression versus the benefits of slower-onset, longer-duration analgesia that allows compensation for the ventilatory depression. If inadequate analgesia is more deleterious than profound ventilatory depression, then remifentanil may be the opioid of choice (e.g., blunting the response to tracheal intubation, etc.). In contrast, if the potential danger of significant apnea outweighs the titration of one or two boluses of an opioid, then

sufentanil has significant PK/PD advantages over remifentanil. Alfentanil is a viable alternative to a single dose of remifentanil, while fentanyl is a reasonable alternative to a single bolus or repeated boluses of sufentanil.

Opioid administration by intravenous infusion

A balanced anesthetic combining a hypnotic (e.g., volatile anesthetic, propofol) and an opioid is commonly used because of the hemodynamic stability associated with opioid-based compared to hypnotic-based anesthetics. Because surgery is associated with varying levels of noxious stimulation, the dose of opioid and/or hypnotic must be adjusted to guarantee adequate amnesia, analgesia, and immobility. From the simulations presented above, it is clear that the synthetic opioids (fentanyl and its congeners) are able to attenuate patient responses to noxious stimulation rapidly (i.e., in less than 5 minutes) because of their favorable PK profile [23]. In contrast, the insoluble volatile anesthetic desflurane, with a vessel-rich group time constant of approximately 5 minutes, would require 15 minutes to reach a pseudoequilibrium between the alveoli and the vessel-rich group (brain), or the inspired concentration must be "overdosed" to achieve the desired brain concentration of desflurane in 5 minutes. Therefore, a relatively fixed dose of volatile anesthetic combined with varying doses of a short-acting opioid provides a pharmacokinetically rational method of performing a balanced anesthetic [6,7,24].

The varying opioid concentrations required with a fixed dose of hypnotic (e.g., 0.5–0.7 MAC of volatile anesthetic) for a 60-minute "idealized" procedure are shown in Fig. 32.6. With induction of anesthesia, the opioid concentration required to blunt the response to laryngoscopy and tracheal intubation is high (fentanyl dose of 7 $\mu g\ kg^{-1}$, $C_e = 6\ ng\ mL^{-1}$) for a stimulus lasting less than 5 minutes. Following intubation, there is a lack of stimulation as the patient is prepared for surgery, followed by an increase in opioid requirement with skin incision and surgical manipulation. At the end of surgery, the opioid requirement decreases, but does not completely disappear; there is a need to provide postoperative analgesia while avoiding profound ventilatory depression.

One method for providing adequate analgesia throughout a surgical procedure is to maintain a supratherapeutic opioid concentration. By maintaining an opioid effect-site concentration that provides maximal reduction of MAC and MAC$_{BAR}$ (minimum alveolar concentration that blocks autonomic response), only a modicum of the vasodilating hypnotics needs to be administered to provide adequate amnesia, immobility, and hemodynamic stability. "High-dose" opioid anesthesia was introduced by Lowenstein for morphine [25] and by Stanley for fentanyl [26]. Although opioids have minimal direct hemodynamic effects, they are profound ventilatory depressants. Therefore, high-dose opioid techniques, even with the "short-acting" agents such as alfentanil, sufentanil, and fentanyl, may require hours of postoperative mechanical ventilation.

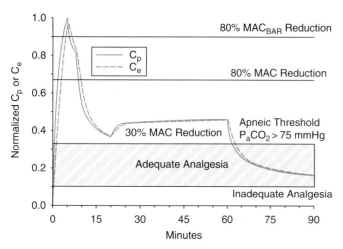

Figure 32.6. Idealized intraoperative opioid requirements. A simulation of the normalized plasma (C_p, solid line) and effect-site (C_e, dashed line) concentrations required to achieve adequate anesthesia during a "standard" balanced anesthetic with a fixed dose of hypnotic (0.5–0.6 MAC volatile anesthetic). The simulation was performed using a remifentanil PK/PD model [14] for a 1-hour surgical procedure with relatively constant surgical stimulation. The initial intense stimulation with laryngoscopy requires opioid concentrations that produce an 80% reduction in MAC$_{BAR}$ (minimum alveolar concentration that blocks autonomic response). Subsequently, for maintenance of anesthesia, the opioid requirement falls between the concentrations that produce 30–80% reduction in MAC. At the end of the procedure, the goal is to produce emergence with spontaneous ventilation with a $P_aCO_2 < 75$ mmHg and adequate analgesia for more than 30 min. (Gray shaded range of opioid concentrations.)

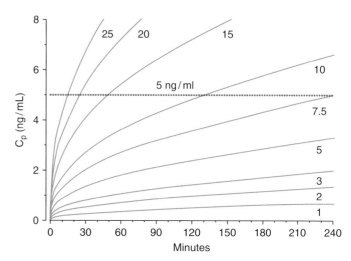

Figure 32.7. Isoconcentration nomogram for fentanyl dosing. The nomogram is based on published fentanyl PK parameters [2]. Each curved line represents the simulated plasma fentanyl concentration versus time plots that would be produced by the corresponding zero-order fentanyl infusion rate (μg kg^{-1} h^{-1}). A horizontal line is placed at the desired target plasma concentration (5 ng mL^{-1} in this example). The initial infusion (25 μg kg^{-1} h^{-1}) is continued until approximately 30 min, at which time the infusion is decreased to 20 μg kg^{-1} h^{-1}. Subsequently, the infusion will be decreased to 15, 10, and then 7.5 μg kg^{-1} h^{-1} at approximately 60, 150, and 240 min, respectively. Note that this nomogram does not give any indication of the rate of recovery after termination of the infusion.

The most efficient method for maintaining therapeutic plasma or effect-site opioid concentrations is to use a combination of boluses and varying infusion rates. If the clinician chooses to use the ultra-short-acting opioid remifentanil, then an empiric dosing strategy, based on an understanding of the PD interaction between hypnotics and remifentanil and the fact that a change in the infusion rate will equilibrate rapidly with the effect site and reach 60% of $C_{e,max}$ within 5 minutes, is sufficient to allow manual titration to effect. In contrast, to make the calculations for the various infusion rates required to maintain a target plasma concentration for the other opioids using multicompartmental PKs parameters, a clinician would need access to a basic computer and the software to perform the appropriate simulations. However, even with sophisticated PK software, this is a time-consuming process that can divert attention from the patient.

An isoconcentration nomogram is a graphical tool that was introduced in 1994 as a guide for propofol dosing [27]. It guides the clinician in the manual adjustment of an infusion pump to maintain a desired target drug concentration in the plasma. The nomogram is constructed, by calculating the plasma drug concentration versus time relationship for a variety of constant-rate infusions using the drug's multicompartmental PK parameters. As a result, the clinician has at his or her hands a graphical tool that forecasts the concentration produced by the simulated zero-order infusions. From these simulations, one can readily visualize (and estimate) the rise toward the steady-state plasma drug concentration described by the drug's PK model.

A fentanyl isoconcentration nomogram generated by simulating a range of potential fentanyl infusion rates is shown in Fig. 32.7. For best results when increasing the target concentration, a bolus equal to the product of V_c (the volume of the central compartment) and the desired *incremental* change in concentration (difference between current and newly targeted concentration) should be administered. Likewise, when a decreased concentration is desired, the best strategy is to turn off the infusion for the time predicted by the applicable context-sensitive decrement time and then resume the infusion at the rate predicted by the nomogram for the current time. The context-sensitive half-time is defined as the time required for the plasma drug concentration to decrease by 50%, where the context is the duration of the infusion [28]. Context-sensitive half-times for the common synthetic opioids fentanyl, alfentanil, sufentanil, and remifentanil are illustrated in Fig. 32.8.

Although the context-sensitive half-times are the values typically quoted for a drug (Table 32.2), the targeted decrement in opioid concentration may be more or less than 50%. Clinically relevant context-sensitive decrement times are determined by "distance" between the actual plasma concentration and the desired lower target concentration (often the threshold for ventilatory depression). This threshold, however, is not a constant value. Opioids cause ventilatory depression, changing the

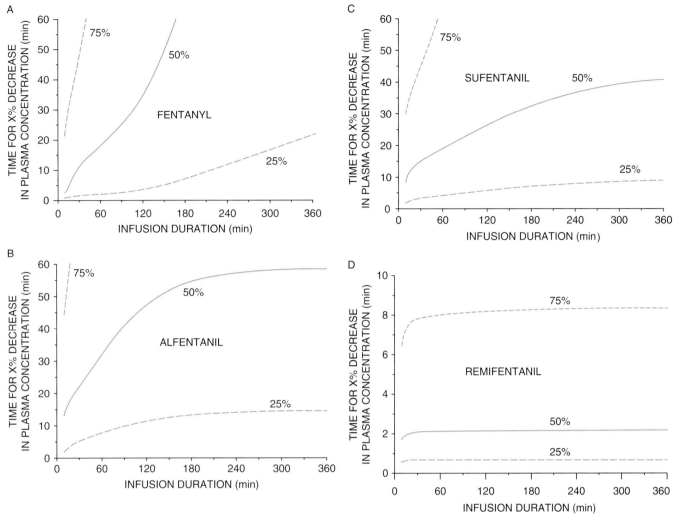

Figure 32.8. Plasma context-sensitive 25%, 50%, and 75% decrement times simulated for (A) fentanyl, (B) alfentanil, (C) sufentanil, and (D) remifentanil. For all opioids, infusions that target plasma opioid concentrations that require only a 25% decrease in concentration for emergence from anesthesia result in reasonably rapid recovery. As tissue compartments approach equilibrium with plasma, the 50% decrement time (context-sensitive half-time) approaches the elimination half-life for a drug; the context-sensitive half-time approaches, but never exceeds, the half-life. In contrast, for all of the drugs, except remifentanil, tissue drug accumulation results in a very long time until recovery if a 75% decrease in plasma concentration is needed; this value never approaches more than twice the elimination half-life of the drug. Therefore, if a high-dose opioid technique is used (e.g., tracheal surgery, laparoscopy, etc.), only remifentanil will provide a reasonable awakening time. Because remifentanil is efficiently metabolized by blood and tissue esterases, there is very little accumulation of the opioid, despite long infusions. Therefore, the context-sensitive decrement times of remifentanil are essentially independent of infusion duration but depend only on the decrease in plasma concentration required to achieve the awakening concentration.

slope and intercept of the CO_2 response curve (minute ventilation vs. end-tidal CO_2), but these changes are counteracted in the presence of pain [30]. Therefore opioid concentrations in excess of those required to provide adequate analgesia may cause some ventilatory depression. Thus the context-sensitive decrement may be 25%, 50%, 75%, or some other amount. Simulations show that the times for different percentage decreases in plasma concentration are not linear [10,11]. Therefore, if a 25% or 75% decrease in plasma concentration is required, simulations must be performed to calculate the context-sensitive 25% decrement time or context-sensitive 75% decrement time (Fig. 32.8). Examination of the 25% context-sensitive decrement times for fentanyl, alfentanil, and sufentanil

demonstrates why the typical balanced anesthetic technique (moderate hypnotic–mild/moderate opioid–relaxant) is an efficient method of achieving adequate anesthesia with an acceptably rapid awakening. In general, for procedures requiring a fairly high postoperative opioid concentration to maintain adequate analgesia, dosing schemes resulting in concentrations within 25% of the awakening analgesic concentration produce an acceptable awakening time. In contrast, in those cases where there is little postoperative opioid requirement for analgesia (e.g., employing postoperative regional analgesia, laparoscopy, etc.), excessive use of opioids will delay emergence.

Patient-controlled analgesia (PCA) regimens are often used to provide postoperative analgesia. In contrast to intraoperative

Table 32.2. Opioid pharmacokinetic half-lives

Opioid	$t_{1/2 \text{ Fast}}$ (min)	$t_{1/2 \text{ Slow}}$ (min)	$t_{1/2 \text{ Elim}}$ (min)	$t_{1/2}$ Elim (h)
Fentanyl [4]	1.0	19	475	7.9
Remifentanil [4]	0.9	6	35	0.6
Sufentanil [4]	1.4	23	562	9.4
Alfentanil [4]	0.7	13	111	1.9
Morphine [29]	1.1	8	191	3.2
Hydromorphone [15]	1.2	6	299	5.0
Methadone [16]	NA	6	2100	35

NA, not available: the pharmacokinetics of methadone were modeled with a two-compartment model.

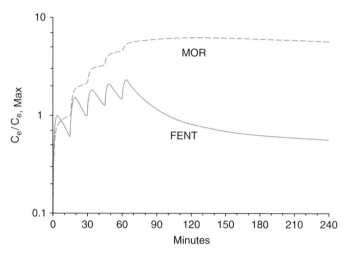

Figure 32.9. Effect-site concentration profile after repeated bolus patient-controlled analgesia (PCA) administration of fentanyl and morphine. Normalized effect-site concentration ($C_e/C_{e,\text{max after single dose}}$) profile during and after the PCA administration of five boluses of fentanyl (FENT, *solid line*, 1 µg kg^{-1} bolus every 15 min, no basal infusion) and morphine (MOR, *dashed line*, 0.02 mg kg^{-1} bolus every 15 min, no basal infusion). There is significant accumulation of morphine but only modest accumulation of fentanyl. Assuming each regimen provides equally effective analgesia at the effect-site concentration achieved with the five bolus doses at 60 min and the patient then falls asleep, the fentanyl effect-site concentration decreases over 45 min to significantly less analgesic levels, while the morphine effect-site concentrations remain elevated for at least 3 hours. Therefore, a morphine PCA has the potential for a more sustained period of analgesia without the need for rescue dosing if the patient awakens spontaneously within the first 3 hours.

opioid dosing, where excessive ventilatory depression is mainly an annoyance that may delay emergence from anesthesia, postoperative opioid dosing must provide adequate analgesia while avoiding this potentially devastating complication. Therefore, the choice of opioid to be used in the postoperative period is important.

The most commonly used opioids for PCA are morphine and fentanyl. From a PK perspective, bolus dosing of fentanyl, without a basal infusion, is an efficient method of achieving titratable analgesia (Fig. 32.9). However, once a patient achieves adequate analgesia and falls asleep, the fentanyl effect-site concentration decreases below the concentration achieved with the initial bolus within 60 minutes. Therefore, the patient who falls asleep will awaken with subtherapeutic analgesic effect-site concentrations. In contrast, while the morphine effect-site concentration takes longer to increase, it also decreases from therapeutic levels slowly. Thus, if a patient administered five doses of morphine to achieve an analgesic level (ignoring the potential contribution of the active metabolite, morphine-6-glucuronide, see below) that will allow him or her to fall asleep, the effect-site concentration would remain elevated for more than 3 hours after the last morphine dose (Fig. 32.9). This clearly illustrates the importance of understanding the plasma concentration/effect-site concentration relationship (i.e., CNS equilibration). For the rapidly equilibrating drug fentanyl, the effect-site concentration initially lags behind the plasma concentration, but with termination of an infusion (or with redistribution after a bolus), the effect-site and the plasma concentrations parallel each other closely (Fig. 32.10A). In contrast, with the slowly equilibrating morphine (and hydromorphone), the effect-site concentration lags behind the plasma concentration during administration (infusion or bolus), but it also lags in transporting drug out of the CNS. Therefore, the effect-site concentration of morphine (and hydromorphone) will remain elevated despite a relatively rapid decline in plasma concentration (Fig. 32.10B). This

simple illustration demonstrates the advantages of morphine PCA in promoting a stable analgesic level that requires minimal interval dosing while at rest. The PK/PD properties that make fentanyl useful as part of a balanced anesthetic are at odds with the requirements for efficient PCA delivery. In contrast, the PK/PD properties of morphine that make it less useful as part of a balanced anesthetic make it extremely suitable for postoperative PCA delivery.

There are some theoretical advantages of other opioids for postoperative analgesia (Fig. 32.11). Hydromorphone is associated with less nausea, one of the major opioid-related side effects that decreases patient satisfaction. In addition, plasma hydromorphone concentrations remain elevated for a long time, which may result in prolonged analgesia. However, without knowing hydromorphone PDs, it is difficult to predict the effects of a given PK profile on the effect of the drug accurately. Another opioid that may be useful in the postoperative period is methadone. With its limited elimination clearance, plasma methadone concentrations after a single bolus mimic those observed during a prolonged infusion of other drugs, making methadone appear to be an appropriate postoperative analgesic. Unfortunately a detailed PK/PD model of intravenous methadone, which could allow more accurate prediction of appropriate perioperative intravenous dosing, has not been developed.

Remifentanil has been used as an intravenous PCA opioid, especially in the obstetric population, where the minimal

A

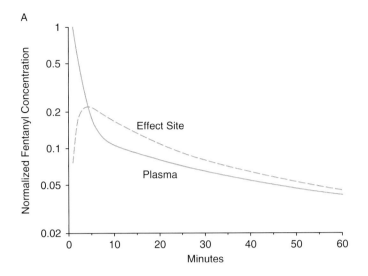

B

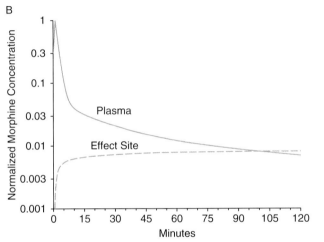

Figure 32.10. CNS uptake of fentanyl and morphine after intravenous bolus administration. Simulation of the normalized effect-site concentration (*dotted line*, $C_e/C_{p,max\ after\ single\ dose}$) and normalized plasma concentration (*solid line*, $C_p/C_{p,\ Max\ after\ single\ dose}$) profiles after a single bolus dose of (A) fentanyl and (B) morphine. The effect-site concentrations of both fentanyl and morphine initially increase, while the plasma concentrations of both drugs decrease from the moment of administration. The effect-site fentanyl concentration rapidly matches the plasma concentration, and from that point on the effect-site fentanyl concentration is higher than the plasma concentration, although the difference is small (< 25% initially, approaching < 10% at 45–60 min). In contrast, despite the continued decrease in plasma morphine concentrations, the effect-site morphine concentrations rapidly increase over the initial 8 min and then slowly increase until they surpass the plasma concentrations at approximately 105 min. The normalized effect-site morphine concentrations are less than 1% of the peak plasma concentration. Despite only achieving this low effect-site concentration, morphine is an effective and potent analgesic. This demonstrates that understanding the effect-site concentration versus time relationship for a drug with slower effect-site kinetics is more important for making accurate dosing recommendations than understanding the plasma concentration versus time relationship. In contrast, for fentanyl and other drugs with rapid effect-site kinetics, the plasma concentration versus time relationship may serve as an adequate approximation of the actual effect-site concentration versus time relationship.

effects of remifentanil on the newborn and the limited pain after delivery may make it an ideal agent [31,32]. However, in patients requiring postoperative analgesics for

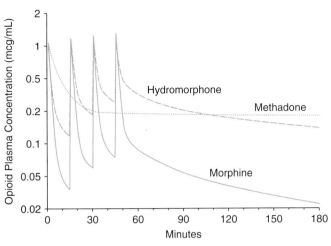

Figure 32.11. Plasma concentration profile after repeated bolus patient-controlled analgesia (PCA) administration of morphine and hydromorphone and single-dose methadone. Normalized plasma concentration ($C_p/C_{p,max\ after\ single\ dose}$) profile during and after the PCA administration of four boluses of morphine (*solid line*, 0.02 mg kg^{-1} bolus every 15 min, no basal infusion) and hydromorphone (*dashed line*, 0.0025 mg kg^{-1} bolus every 15 min, no basal infusion). There is noticeable gradual accumulation of both morphine and hydromorphone. Assuming each regimen provides equally effective analgesia at the plasma concentrations achieved with the four bolus doses at 45 min and the patient then falls asleep, the morphine plasma concentrations decrease over 45 min to significantly lower levels than those of hydromorphone. Since the morphine effect-site concentrations remain elevated for at least 3 hours (Fig. 32.9), it is tempting to assume that the hydromorphone effect-site concentrations also remain in a therapeutic range. However, without an accurate combined PK/PD model, it is impossible to predict any real PK advantage of hydromorphone over morphine for bolus PCA administration accurately. As a point of comparison, the normalized plasma concentration profile that is predicted to occur after a single intravenous bolus of 0.2 mg kg^{-1} methadone is shown (*dotted line*). The plasma methadone concentrations remain markedly elevated and decrease minimally from 30 min on. This is due to its extremely small elimination clearance and large volume of distribution. Assuming that the CNS uptake of this drug is reasonable, there may be a PK advantage of methadone over multiple PCA boluses of hydromorphone or morphine for patients with persistent pain in the perioperative period. However, without an accurate combined PK/PD model, predictions of the ideal dose or doses of methadone to administer are difficult to make.

several days, PCA with remifentanil boluses is impractical (because it requires intensive ventilatory monitoring) and inefficient (because a delay in changing the syringe will result in a loss of analgesia within 10 minutes), and it has a high potential for ventilatory complications [20]. Although achieving adequate analgesia rapidly is desirable, a slower-equilibrating opioid than remifentanil may eliminate these disadvantages.

From the previous discussion, it should be clear that the PK/PD properties of the opioids help determine their role in the perioperative pharmacopeia. As clinicians have used these opioids, they have developed regimens that take advantage of the unique properties of the ultrarapid (remifentanil and alfentanil), the short-acting (fentanyl and sufentanil), and the long-acting (morphine and hydromorphone) opioids. As new members of the μ-opioid agonist family are developed, the paradigms described in this chapter should allow the clinician to more easily extrapolate the role of these new compounds in clinical practice.

Rate of opioid administration and apnea

The useful insights into various modes of drug administration made possible by PK/PD modeling are further illustrated by the apneic effects of rapidly administering fast-onset opioids like remifentanil [19]. This was elucidated by modeling the PK and PD of both the opioid and CO_2 (the magnitude and time course of changes in minute ventilation and arterial CO_2 concentrations). The model predicts that the ventilatory effect of an opioid depends on how fast the effect-site drug concentration is achieved [5,19]. The rate of rise of the effect-site opioid concentration is influenced by the speed of drug administration (and the physicochemical properties of the drug and various drug-specific transporters at the blood–brain barrier). Thus, rapid intravenous administration of an opioid with a rapid onset of effect (e.g., remifentanil, alfentanil, sufentanil, and fentanyl) is predicted by the model to produce severe ventilatory depression or apnea. However, when the same dose of the same opioid is given by a slower intravenous infusion, minute ventilation will be decreased modestly because arterial CO_2 concentration increases gradually and stimulates continued ventilation. The same modest ventilatory decrease is predicted for the rapid administration of a slower-onset opioid like morphine. This distinction is important because elevations of arterial CO_2 are typically not detrimental to the patient but opioid-induced apnea is likely to result in hypoxemia.

Opioid metabolism

Opioids may be inactivated or activated by phase I metabolism. Many opioids, including fentanyl, alfentanil, and sufentanil, are inactivated through *N*-dealkylation by cytochrome P450 3A4 (CYP3A4) [33,34]. Methadone is inactivated via *N*-demethylation by CYP2B6 [35]. Prodrugs, such as codeine and tramadol, are bioactivated via *O*-dealkylation by CYP2D6, to morphine and *O*-desmethyltramadol, respectively [36]. Other prodrugs, such as tilidine (widely used in Germany and Belgium), are activated by *N*-demethylation [36]. Remifentanil is unique among the opioids because of its ester linkage, as a result of which it is so rapidly inactivated by nonspecific blood and tissue esterases that its effects are terminated by metabolism rather than redistribution [37]. Phase I opioid metabolites may be toxic. The best known is the meperidine metabolite normeperidine, which can have CNS excitatory effects as severe as seizures [38].

Opioids and opioid metabolites with free hydroxyl groups can undergo phase II metabolism, primarily glucuronidation by uridine diphosphate glucuronosyltransferase (UGT) 2B7, to metabolites that are readily excreted by the kidney [36]. Some of these conjugates are pharmacologically active. For example, morphine-6-glucuronide has significant μ-opioid receptor activity in vitro, although it does not cumulate enough at normal doses to have clinically significant effects in patients with normal renal function because it has poor CNS penetration due to its hydrophilicity [36]. Another phase II morphine metabolite, morphine-3-glucuronide, may or may not have antianalgesic and neuroexcitatory effects (the data are equivocal) in vivo [36].

Opioid protein binding

It is axiomatic in clinical pharmacology that the pharmacologic effect of a drug is produced by the unbound drug. Despite the numerous publications on plasma protein binding of drugs, it was not until relatively recently that the clinical relevance of protein binding was clarified [36]. Total exposure to a drug, as measured by the area under the total drug concentration versus time relationship (AUC), is independent of the protein binding of all low-extraction-ratio drugs (i.e., drugs with elimination clearances much less than clearing organ blood flow), no matter how they are administered, and of all drugs eliminated mainly by hepatic clearance when these drugs are administered orally. Therefore, there is no need to adjust dosing of these drugs for real or anticipated changes in their unbound fraction. On the other hand, changes in unbound drug exposure with changes in protein binding might be expected for high-extraction-ratio drugs (i.e., drugs with elimination clearances near clearing-organ blood flow) given intravenously, and for orally administered drugs eliminated by high-extraction-ratio extrahepatic routes. When a decrease in protein binding occurs as a result of a drug interaction, the drug must also have a low clinical margin of safety and equilibrate rapidly with its biophase for the altered protein binding to be clinically significant, because drug distribution and elimination clearance will likewise change to make up for the increased free drug fraction. According to these criteria, patients with altered protein binding caused by disease states or drug interactions are likely to have clinically significant increases in exposure to the free drug when the following drugs are administered intravenously (or by inhalation; see below): alfentanil (92% protein-bound), buprenorphine (96% protein-bound), butorphanol (80% protein-bound), fentanyl (84% protein-bound), remifentanil (92% protein-bound), and sufentanil (93% protein-bound) [39]. When the potential clinical significance of decreased protein binding of 456 drugs was evaluated, it was determined that only 25 of them might exhibit clinically significantly increased drug exposure due to decreased protein binding after nonoral administration. Nearly a quarter of these were the six opioids listed above.

Pharmacogenetics

The considerable variability in opioid dose requirements may be due to interindividual differences in PK or PD or both, which could be affected by genetically determined factors. Genetic contributions to interindividual variability in the expression and function of proteins responsible for sensitivity to pain, opioid receptors, drug transporters, and enzymes responsible for drug metabolism have been the subject of numerous studies [40], and several single nucleotide polymorphisms (SNPs) in these pathways have been identified. Although reports of their functional consequences are often conflicting or equivocal, one excellent example does illustrate the role of pharmacogenetics in opioid PK.

Codeine is a prodrug, metabolized by the highly polymorphic CYP2D6 to the more active opioid morphine [41]. One area in which there is abundant evidence that pharmacogenetics affects the opioid dose–response relationship is in the demethylation of codeine to its more potent and efficacious metabolite. Compared with "wild-type" or normal individuals (extensive metabolizers), CYP2D6 activity is reduced in 10–15% of Caucasians (intermediate metabolizers), absent in 7–10% of Caucasians (poor metabolizers), and extraordinarily high (due to gene duplications) in 1–3% of Caucasians (ultrarapid metabolizers) [41,42]. In addition, there is ethnic variability in the frequencies of these differences, as illustrated by the fact that while few Chinese are ultrarapid metabolizers (or poor metabolizers, for that matter) up to 29% of Saudi Arabians and Ethiopians are ultrarapid metabolizers [41]. Patients with absent or impaired CYP2D6 activity are unlikely to experience analgesic efficacy from codeine, while ultrarapid metabolizers may be susceptible to ventilatory depression. Similarly, coadministration of codeine with potent CYP2D6 inhibitors, such as the class IA antiarrhythmic quinidine and the selective serotonin reuptake inhibitors paroxetine and fluoxetine, even to extensive CYP2D6 metabolizers, may eliminate or decrease its analgesic efficacy due to inhibition of its metabolism to its active metabolite [43].

While dihydrocodeine, oxycodone, and hydrocodone are also metabolized by CYP2D6 to the more active opioids dihydromorphine, oxymorphone, and hydromorphone, respectively, and CYP2D6 genotype influences their metabolic conversions, the clinical implications are different than for codeine. Unlike codeine, which is inactive, dihydrocodeine, oxycodone, and hydrocodone are all active, and, the relative contribution of the active metabolites to analgesia is less than for codeine. Therefore unlike codeine, the evidence for CYP2D6 polymorphisms affecting dihydrocodeine, oxycodone, and hydrocodone analgesia is presently weak, at best [41].

At present, the importance of pharmacogenetics in determining opioid PK and PD is uncertain and remains an area of ongoing research. The possibility exists that as investigators shift their focus from SNPs to haplotypes (i.e., multiple SNPs), pharmacogenetic influences on opioid pharmacokinetics and pharmacodynamics may become clearer [40].

Drug interactions affecting opioid metabolism

Much of the evidence for the identity of the human enzymes responsible for drug metabolism and metabolic drug interactions comes from in-vitro data, extrapolations of in-vitro data, and some clinical studies. There are several examples of clinically significant metabolic drug interactions that affect opioid PK and affect both the choice of opioids and their dosing.

Fentanyl, sufentanil, and alfentanil are all metabolized (and inactivated) by CYP3A4 and CYP3A5 [33,34]. While in-vitro studies have shown that CYP3A4/5 inhibitors prevent the metabolism of all these opioids, the clinical consequences of inhibition are opioid-specific. For example, triazole antifungal agents, such as fluconazole and itraconazole, are known inhibitors of CYP3A4. While fluconazole decreased the elimination clearance of alfentanil by more than 50% [44], there was no effect of itraconazole on fentanyl elimination clearance [45]. These differences were observed because fentanyl is more efficiently metabolized by the liver than is alfentanil (i.e., it has a higher hepatic extraction ratio, which is the fraction of the drug present in the blood that is removed by the liver upon each passage), and would therefore require more extensive inhibition of metabolism to reduce its elimination clearance [46]. HIV protease inhibitors (ritonavir, lopinavir, and others) inhibit CYP3A4/5 much more strongly than most antifungals and can markedly impair opioid metabolism. Ritonavir extensively (more than 90%) inhibits the intestinal and hepatic activity of CYP3A4/5 and the metabolism of alfentanil [47]. Because of the profound inhibition, ritonavir even impaired the metabolism of fentanyl, resulting in a 67% reduction in elimination clearance [48]. Multiple dose and long-term administration of opioids (e.g., fentanyl patch) that are CYP3A4/5 substrates are best avoided in patients taking HIV protease inhibitors.

Some drug interactions speculated to occur based on in-vitro experiments have been later shown not to be clinically significant [49]. For example, CYP3A4 was the enzyme widely reported to be responsible for the metabolism of methadone, and caregivers prescribing methadone were warned by the product insert to exert extreme caution when prescribing this drug to patients taking drugs known to inhibit or induce CYP3A4. Yet recent clinical studies demonstrated that changes in CYP3A activity did not affect methadone clearance [35]. Ritonavir actually increases the elimination clearance of methadone to such an extent that withdrawal symptoms may be observed [50] despite profound inhibition of CYP3A4 [51]. Rather, it appears that CYP2B6 plays a significant role in stereoselective human methadone metabolism [35].

Not all opioids are susceptible to drug interactions, and not all opioid drug interactions are clinically significant. Remifentanil is not metabolized by hepatic cytochrome P450, but rather is metabolized by nonspecific blood and tissue esterases [37]; and there are no known drug interactions that reduce remifentanil esterase metabolism and elimination clearance. Because the effects of a single opioid (except remifentanil and methadone) dose are terminated by redistribution rather than metabolism and elimination clearance (Fig. 32.2), drug interactions affecting drug metabolism are more likely to affect multiple-dose and long-term opioid administration than they are single-dose administration.

As mentioned above, coadministration of potent CYP2D6 inhibitors, such as quinidine, paroxetine, and fluoxetine, with the orally administered opioid prodrug codeine may reduce or eliminate its analgesic efficacy because of inhibition of its metabolism to morphine [43].

Nonintravenous routes of administration

Intravenous opioid administration results in a known dose of drug entering the systemic circulation and at a known rate. Nonintravenous routes of opioid administration are distinguished from the intravenous route by differences in the rate of drug absorption into the systemic circulation (usually slower, often variable) and the proportion of the dose entering the systemic circulation (i.e., the bioavailability). Thus, many nonintravenous routes of drug administration offer the advantage of convenience over intravenous drug administration, but at a pharmacokinetic price.

Oral

Orally administered drugs are subject to first-pass elimination, or metabolism between the site of administration and the site of entry into the systemic circulation, which determines the bioavailability of the orally administered drug [52,53] (Table 32.3). Although the liver is generally considered to be the primary site of first-pass elimination, there can also be considerable intestinal metabolism. The complexity of the first-pass elimination process is well illustrated by the pharmacokinetics of orally administered alfentanil [51]. The alfentanil hepatic extraction ratio was determined to be 26%. Therefore, if orally administered alfentanil bioavailability is determined exclusively by hepatic metabolism, the predicted alfentanil bioavailability would be 74% (i.e., 1.00 – 0.26 = 0.74). However, the oral bioavailability of alfentanil was actually only 37%, because it was metabolized not only by the liver but also by the intestine, with an intestinal extraction ratio of 51%. Thus, 49% of the orally administered dose survived passage through the intestine to enter the liver, which removed

26% of that, leaving only 37% of the administered dose to enter the systemic circulation (1.00 – 0.51 = 0.49; 0.49 – (0.49* 0.26) = 0.49 – 0.12 = 0.37). This is important because each of these metabolic processes is potentially subject to inhibition by concomitantly administered drugs. Steady-state concentrations of ritonavir reduced the hepatic extraction ratio of alfentanil to 7% and the intestinal extraction ratio to zero, as a result of which the bioavailability of alfentanil was increased from 37% to 95% [51]. While not many drug interactions are as profound as this, when such an interaction occurs the results can be devastating unless the dose of the opioid is adjusted or an opioid not subject to such an interaction is substituted for the one that is.

Orally administered opioids with low oral bioavailability and narrow therapeutic window (e.g., morphine, oxycodone, and hydromorphone) generally require multiple daily doses to maintain effective plasma, and biophase, concentrations. The inconvenience of this therapeutic approach can lead to decreased patient compliance. Sustained-release dosage forms of these opioids have been developed that require less frequent dosing, resulting in improved patient compliance and better pain control.

Immediate-release morphine tablets and solutions have 30–40% oral bioavailability and produce peak plasma morphine concentrations between 30 and 90 minutes after administration [56]. Repeated dosing of the immediate-release formulation every 4–6 hours controls moderate and severe pain effectively but is inconvenient. A variety of sustained-release morphine dosage forms have been designed to prolong the time to a lower peak plasma morphine concentration while minimizing plasma morphine concentration fluctuations and maintaining the area under the drug concentration versus time relationship produced by an equivalent dose of immediate-release morphine [57]. These sustained-release morphine dosage forms have recommended dosing intervals of 12 or 24 hours, depending on the formulation. They control moderate and severe pain effectively, despite such significant differences in pharmacokinetics between formulations that they are not considered bioequivalent, so cannot be substituted directly for each other [57].

Table 32.3. Pharmacokinetics of orally administered opioids [54,55]

Opioid	F (%)	Protein binding (%)	V_{SS} (L)	CL_E (L/h)	$t_{1/2\beta}$ (hr)
Codeine	50–55	4–7	210–350	63	2.5–3.5
Meperidine	48–56	60–80	260–320	28–44	3–7
Methadone	41–99	70–90	240–330	3–12	19–58
Morphine	20–40	20–35	70–330	48–120	1.5–4.5
Tramadol	65–75	20	200–300	26–29	5–6

F, fraction of oral dose available systemically; V_{SS}, volume of distribution at steady state (total volume of distribution); CL_E, elimination (systemic) clearance; $t_{1/2\beta}$, elimination half-life, which is the time for one-half of the drug to be irreversibly eliminated from the body.

Oxycodone is available in both normal-release and controlled-release dosage forms. Normal-release oxycodone has a plasma concentration profile similar to that of intramuscular oxycodone, after adjusting for its 60% bioavailability, with monophasic absorption and peak concentrations achieved in a mean of 1 hour [58]. Controlled-release oxycodone has a biphasic absorption, with 38% of the dose absorbed with a half-life of 37 minutes and 62% absorbed with a half-life of 6.2 hours, with the resulting peak concentration achieved at an average of 3.2 hours [58]. Controlled-release oxycodone can be used to control moderate to severe chronic pain with twice-daily dosing, with normal-release oxycodone used for breakthrough pain.

Immediate-release hydromorphone has approximately 40% oral bioavailability, an onset of action in approximately 30 minutes, and a 4-hour duration of effect [59]. Like controlled-release oxycodone, controlled-release hydromorphone has biphasic absorption, with an initial peak plasma concentration at approximately 2 hours and a later peak at 18–24 hours [59].

Methadone has several pharmacokinetic properties that may make it useful for the treatment of moderate to severe chronic pain without sustained-release dosage formulation. It has a mean oral bioavailability of 85% and a mean elimination half-life of 40 hours as a result of a relatively large volume of distribution and a low elimination clearance [60]. While the time to maximum plasma methadone concentrations and maximum CNS effects (measured by its effect on pupil diameter) after oral administration of 10 mg of methadone hydrochloride was more than 2 hours, the duration of effect averaged at least 10 hours due to sustained effective concentrations resulting from its long elimination half-life [60]. However, the considerable interindividual variability in both its pharmacokinetics and its pharmacodynamics make individual methadone dose adjustment especially important [61].

An interesting exploitation of the first-pass effect for patient safety benefit is the deliberate adulteration of oral opioid dosage forms with the μ-opioid antagonist naloxone to prevent their abuse by intravenous administration [54]. Since naloxone has virtually no oral bioavailability, when it is administered orally with the opioid it does not interfere with the analgesic efficacy of the opioid. However, when it is injected intravenously with the opioid it antagonizes the effects of the opioid.

Oral transmucosal

Drug administration by the oral transmucosal (OTM) route has several potentially important advantages over administration by the traditional oral route [62]. Because of rapid absorption through the highly vascularized oral mucosa, a drug administered by the OTM route will have a shorter time to peak concentrations. In addition, especially if the drug has a high hepatic extraction ratio, a drug administered by the OTM route will have higher bioavailability because the oral mucosal blood supply does not empty into the portal circulation, thus avoiding the first-pass (i.e., presystemic) hepatic elimination. A potential disadvantage of this route is that an unknown and variable portion of the dose can be swallowed before transmucosal absorption and undergo delayed absorption and possibly significant presystemic elimination.

OTM fentanyl citrate administered by sucking on a lozenge that was consumed within 15 minutes produced average maximum arterial plasma fentanyl concentrations 22 minutes after beginning administration that were only approximately 10% of those observed after intravenous administration of the same dose to the same subjects over less than 10 minutes [63]. However, OTM fentanyl produced peak concentrations that were twice those observed after oral administration of the same dose to the same individuals in approximately one-fifth of the time. Mean bioavailability of OTM fentanyl citrate averaged 52%, while that of orally administered fentanyl averaged 32%. Therapeutic fentanyl concentrations were produced within 15 minutes of OTM administration due to OTM absorption and lasted for 1–2 hours due to delayed gastrointestinal absorption [63]. Unlike transdermal fentanyl (see below), OTM fentanyl administration does not appear to produce a drug depot, the slow absorption from which appears to prolong the elimination half-life of the drug after transdermal administration [52].

There is considerable intraindividual and interindividual variability in the bioavailability of OTM fentanyl in adults, because of variability in the amount of drug swallowed from time to time and from person to person, resulting in differences in bioavailability, time to, and magnitude of the maximum concentration. Therefore, it is not a great surprise that when OTM fentanyl was administered to children 3–12 years of age, the average maximum plasma concentration was half the dose-adjusted maximum concentration observed in adults, the times to maximum concentrations were extremely variable, and the average time more than twice that observed in adults [64]. In addition, the average bioavailability in children was only 36% [64], which was similar to that observed for orally administered (i.e., swallowed) fentanyl in adults [63], suggesting children swallowed more of the dose than did adults.

The PK/PD and physicochemical properties of some drugs do not lend themselves to OTM administration. As with transdermal delivery (see below), the low potency and low permeability of morphine make it a poor candidate for OTM delivery. In studies of OTM morphine administration, long times to maximum concentrations and low bioavailability led to the conclusion that most of the morphine was being absorbed from the gastrointestinal tract [62].

Subcutaneous

Although morphine may not have physicochemical properties that make it suitable for oral transmucosal delivery (see above) or transdermal delivery (see below), it is rapidly and completely absorbed when administered subcutaneously. Five milligrams of morphine administered subcutaneously in 0.5 mL to elderly postoperative patients produced average peak venous plasma concentrations of 87 ng mL^{-1} an average of 16 minutes after administration, although there was considerable interindividual variability [65]. Bioavailability of a subcutaneous bolus of morphine was determined to be complete [66]. Although bioavailability averaged 74% when 5 mg was infused subcutaneously in a total volume of 10 mL over 4 hours [62], continuous subcutaneous morphine administration has been reported to produce venous plasma concentrations, measured at 6-hourly intervals for 24 hours, that were not different from plasma concentrations produced by continuous intravenous administration at the same rate [67].

There are few studies of subcutaneous fentanyl administration. Subcutaneous fentanyl infusion at a median constant rate of 1200 μg per day for a minimum of 24 hours produced median plasma concentrations of 1 ng mL^{-1} [68]. If subcutaneous fentanyl has nearly complete bioavailability, as transdermal fentanyl does (see below), a steady-state concentration produced by this infusion rate would be associated with an elimination clearance of 833 mL per minute, which is consistent with that reported for this drug.

Intramuscular

The absorption of intramuscularly administered morphine is rapid and complete, like that of the subcutaneously administered drug, as described above. Average peak venous plasma morphine concentrations (56 ng mL^{-1}) were observed an average of 16 minutes after deltoid intramuscular injection of 10 mg of morphine sulfate [29]. Given an absorption half-life of less than 12 minutes and 100% bioavailability of the injected dose, at least 90% of the injected dose will be absorbed within 45 minutes after injection, during which time plasma concentrations will be relatively sustained. The time to and magnitude of peak plasma morphine concentrations after injection of 10 mg of morphine sulfate did not differ between intramuscular deltoid and subcutaneous deltoid morphine injection sites, presumably because blood flow to the skin reflects that to the underlying muscle [69].

Transdermal

Transdermal opioid administration offers a potentially convenient alternative to other (e.g., intravenous or oral) routes of administration to treat moderate to severe pain in certain clinical situations [70]. The original transdermal fentanyl delivery system, the Transdermal Therapeutic System of fentanyl (TTS-Fentanyl), has a rate-control membrane that allows fentanyl in the system reservoir to be released at a constant rate that is slower than the absorption of fentanyl into the systemic circulation after diffusion through the subcutaneous tissues. With the TTS-Fentanyl system, there was a lag time of 10–14 hours after patch application until plasma fentanyl concentrations increased to analgesic levels [71]. The plateau concentrations observed were nearly identical to those predicted for a constant intravenous fentanyl infusion at the average absorption rate from the

TTS-Fentanyl system observed beginning 4–8 hours after system placement. Based on these results, fentanyl bioavailability from the TTS-Fentanyl system was 92%. After removal of the system, there was continued absorption of fentanyl from the subcutaneous depot until it was depleted, prolonging the apparent elimination half-life.

Repeated TTS-Fentanyl dosing at 72-hour intervals achieved steady-state concentrations by the time of the second application that were maintained thereafter [72]. There was considerable interindividual variability in fentanyl concentrations. Among potential factors contributing to this interindividual variability in concentrations, such as skin thickness, body temperature, and elimination clearance, the latter was found to be the principal contributing factor [73].

The importance of an intact rate-control membrane is illustrated by the contrast of the delivery of fentanyl by the TTS with that by the fentanyl transdermal delivery system (FTDS). Fentanyl is absorbed much more rapidly from the FTDS, producing more variable and more dangerously high plateau concentrations, since only the skin controls drug absorption [74].

From these studies, it can be concluded that the PK profile of the TTS-Fentanyl system makes it suitable for treating opioid-responsive chronic pain. The TTS-Fentanyl system is available in four sizes with delivery rates of 25–100 μg per hour, determined by the surface area of the patch, for treating chronic pain [70]. However, the PK profile of the TTS-Fentanyl system does not make it suitable for safe and effective use in the treatment of postoperative pain, and therefore its use for such an indication is "absolutely contraindicated" [70].

A fentanyl HCl patient-controlled transdermal system (PCTS) has been investigated for use for postoperative patient-controlled analgesia (PCA) [75]. The PCTS delivers a fixed amount of ionized fentanyl on demand over 10 minutes using an external electrical field by a process called iontophoresis. Plasma fentanyl concentrations measured during the first hour after commencing sequential administration of two doses of PCTS fentanyl increased less rapidly than they did during and after an intravenous fentanyl infusion and, in fact, were not measurable in some subjects (the limit of quantification of the assay was 0.1 ng mL^{-1}) [76]. The bioavailability of fentanyl from the system was estimated to be nearly 100%, but only 40% of the dose was absorbed within an hour of administration and the full dose had not been absorbed until after 10 hours [77]. When subjects received two doses from the fentanyl PCTS every 4 hours for 68 hours, steady-state concentrations were observed within approximately 48 hours of beginning drug administration [78]. Unlike the TTS, there is minimal passive absorption of fentanyl from the PCTS and there is a minimal subcutaneous fentanyl depot, hence minimal continued absorption, after the device is removed [75].

Not all opioids have physicochemical properties that make them suitable for transdermal delivery. Although morphine is considered to be a poor candidate for transdermal delivery due to its low permeability through human cadaver skin and its low potency [78], morphine formulated in pluronic lecithin organogel (PLO) has been available from compounding pharmacies for topical administration to patients for whom oral opioid administration may be contraindicated. However, a randomized, double-blind, placebo-controlled, crossover study in healthy volunteers found that plasma morphine concentrations for 10 hours after application of the recommended dose (10 mg) of morphine in the PLO gel were below the limit of quantification of the assay, demonstrating morphine bioavailability from a topical gel formulation was so low it was unquantifiable [79].

Inhalational

Drugs can be delivered by inhalation to produce peak blood concentrations similar to those observed after rapid intravenous administration. Drug delivery devices have been developed that produce 1–3 μm diameter particles that deposit efficiently in the alveoli, from where they enter the systemic circulation rapidly [80,81]. These devices have the potential to deliver opioids noninvasively for the treatment of breakthrough pain because, like OTM drug delivery, the plasma concentration versus time relationships they produce match the time course of breakthrough pain, especially when combined with a steady-state concentration produced, for example, by a transdermal delivery system for the chronic pain upon which the breakthrough pain is superimposed [82].

Several studies have demonstrated the ability of aerosol delivery systems to administer morphine and fentanyl rapidly and reproducibly. Multiple sequential inhalations of morphine delivered as an aerosol from a metered dose oral inhaler (MDI) were compared with the same dose administered by a brief intravenous infusion [83]. Peak morphine concentrations were less than half those observed after intravenous administration because, on average, slightly less than half the dose was absorbed rapidly upon inhalation. Subsequent delayed absorption of the inhaled morphine increased bioavailability rapidly until 1 hour, when it averaged approximately 75%, after which it increased more slowly, until 95% of the administered dose was absorbed. Fentanyl administered to volunteers both in an aerosol from an MDI and intravenously produced similar maximum arterial plasma fentanyl concentrations at nearly the same time, possibly because the greater lipophilicity of fentanyl led to faster and more extensive initial absorption [84]. These results were in contrast to those for morphine [83]. Nonetheless, fentanyl absorption from the lung was also multiphasic, with 56% of the dose absorbed within 5 minutes of inhalation and the remainder absorbed more slowly over the next several hours. A more recent study found that fentanyl administered as a thermally generated aerosol (TGA) in a single breath produced arterial drug concentrations equivalent to those from the same dose administered as a 5-second intravenous infusion, with equivalent speed and predictably [85]. Ninety-two percent of the fentanyl dose was absorbed in three phases, with average mean transit times (MTTs) of the absorptive phases being 0.4, 1.3, and 42.3 minutes and an average of approximately 80% of the dose absorbed in the first two phases.

Intrathecal

The rate and extent of cephalad movement of morphine and fentanyl after simultaneous intrathecal administration in a slightly hypobaric (normal saline) solution at L2–3 was studied in volunteers [86]. Although there was wide interindividual variability in the initial mixing of the two opioids within the cerebrospinal fluid (CSF), within individuals the initial distribution of both drugs was very similar and, in six of eight individuals, very rapid, appearing in measurable concentrations at the sampling site up to 14 cm cephalad from the site of administration within 5 minutes. Concentrations of both drugs at the sampling site increased over 20–60 minutes after injection then stabilized or decreased slowly for the next hour, with less interindividual variability in concentration with increasing time. Thus, the differences in the rates of onset of the analgesic effect of fentanyl and morphine after intrathecal administration are due to the more rapid penetration of the lipophilic fentanyl into the tissues of the spinal cord than the hydrophilic morphine, rather than to differences in their movement through the CSF. While early ventilatory depression observed in some individuals after intrathecal fentanyl administration is due to very rapid tissue uptake of drug from the CSF during the highly variable early mixing phase, rapid clearance of fentanyl from the CSF explains the absence of late ventilatory depression after intrathecal fentanyl administration. Morphine, on the other hand, causes late ventilatory depression after intrathecal administration because its CSF concentrations remain elevated for an extended period of time due to its slow clearance from the CSF.

Epidural

The pharmacokinetics of epidural alfentanil absorption into the systemic circulation was studied using the stable isotope technique [87]. Each patient received 0.68 mg of deuterium-labeled alfentanil in 14 mL in the lumbar epidural space and a 60-minute intravenous infusion of 1 mg unlabeled alfentanil simultaneously. By measuring concentrations of labeled and unlabeled drug using mass spectrometry, disposition of alfentanil administered by the two routes was determined in the same individual at the same time, and absorption kinetics and bioavailability of epidural alfentanil characterized. Epidural alfentanil absorption was monophasic in most patients, although initial absorption rates were described as zero-order. Peak arterial plasma deuterium-labeled alfentanil concentrations averaged 8.3 ng mL^{-1}, compared with the nominal analgesic concentration of 50 ng mL^{-1} [88]. Concentrations peaked an average of 40 minutes after administration, and epidural alfentanil bioavailability was 100%, with a mean absorption time of nearly 2 hours. The slow absorption of alfentanil from the epidural space and the low plasma

breastfeeding safely. The amount of meperidine [102] and fentanyl [103] appearing in breast milk over 24 hours after administering a single dose of either opioid as part of a general anesthetic or morphine for postoperative analgesia [104] is less that 1% of the maternal dose and, therefore, unlikely to affect a healthy term infant.

The greatest concern about infant exposure to opioids through breast milk is with chronic maternal use. Although there have been few studies in opioid-taking breastfeeding mothers, there have been several in mothers on methadone maintenance programs. A representative study concluded that mothers taking medium to high doses of methadone (≥ 40 mg per day) may breastfeed safely but recommended a case-by-case assessment of the risk/benefit ratio [105].

The use of codeine by breastfeeding women has received considerable attention recently. Low codeine and morphine concentrations in breast milk and in infant plasma led to the conclusion that it was safe for nursing mothers to take 60 mg of codeine every 6 hours [106]. That perception changed with a report of an infant that died 13 days postpartum with highly elevated plasma morphine concentrations attributed to consuming milk from an ultrarapid CYP2D6 metabolizer mother who had been taking a combination of 30 mg of codeine and 500 mg of paracetamol (acetaminophen) twice a day since delivering the child [107]. This interpretation has been severely challenged [108]. A subsequent case–control study found that the mothers of 17 nursing infants experiencing CNS depression were taking 59% larger doses of codeine than the mothers of asymptomatic infants, in addition to confirming the importance of the ultrarapid CYP2D6 metabolizer genotype (in combination with UGT2B7*2/*2 genotype) in two of the 17 mothers [109]. Several conclusions from basic therapeutic principles can be drawn from the toxicity observed in the breastfeeding infants of women taking codeine, not the least of which are that toxicity is dose-related and that pharmacogenetics may play a role in determining the dose to which the infant is exposed [110].

Summary

Opioids are the foundation for the treatment of moderate to severe postoperative pain and for providing analgesia to noxious stimulation as part of a balanced anesthetic. Unfortunately, the clinical margin of safety of opioids is small. Aggressive

empiric dosing strategies that attempt to minimize inadequate analgesia due to subtherapeutic concentrations may result in supratherapeutic concentrations that produce profound ventilatory depression. The rational choice of the "ideal" opioid for a given clinical situation depends on integrating the pharmacokinetic/pharmacodynamic (PK/PD) properties of the individual opioids with the immediate and long-term analgesic needs of a patient in a given clinical situation. A clinically adequate general anesthetic state can be produced when a small, fixed dose of a volatile or an intravenous anesthetic that provides hypnosis, and amnesia is combined with a varying infusion of rapidly equilibrating opioid titrated to prevent nociceptive hemodynamic responses and reflexive movements. However, ineffective crossover from a short-duration intraoperative opioid to the long-duration opioid used to provide postoperative analgesia can result in inadequate analgesia.

Understanding the PK/PD properties of opioids should allow rational bolus and infusion regimens to be designed so that different opioids can be mixed to provide adequate analgesia throughout the perioperative period while minimizing exposure to subtherapeutic and supratherapeutic concentrations and undesired side effects.

The effects of a single dose of most opioids (with the notable exception of methadone) are usually terminated by redistribution rather than by elimination clearance. Therefore, factors affecting drug elimination are more likely to affect multiple-dose and long-term opioid administration than they are a single opioid dose. Alterations in hepatic function, and to a lesser extent renal function, and drug–drug interactions that alter opioid elimination clearance can also produce unintended supratherapeutic opioid concentrations. While the effect of a decrease in the elimination of an opioid on the plasma concentration can be easily countered by decreasing the rate of drug administration, such simple dosing regimen adjustments are not available when changes in organ function or drug–drug interactions affect the rate of conversion to active or toxic metabolites and their subsequent accumulation. In addition, genotype may affect the enteral absorption of opioids or the enterohepatic bioactivation of opioid prodrugs. Genetic contributions to interindividual variability in the expression and function of proteins responsible for sensitivity to pain, opioid receptors, drug transporters, and enzymes responsible for opioid metabolism remain an area of ongoing research.

References

1. Dahan A, Romberg R, Teppema L, *et al.* Simultaneous measurement and integrated analysis of analgesia and respiration after an intravenous morphine infusion. *Anesthesiology* 2004; **101**: 1201–9.

2. Scott JC, Stanski DR. Decreased fentanyl and alfentanil dose requirements with age. A simultaneous pharmacokinetic and pharmacodynamic evaluation. *J Pharmacol Exp Ther* 1987; **240**: 159–66.

3. Upton RN, Semple TJ, Macintyre PE. Pharmacokinetic optimization of opioid treatment in acute pain therapy. *Clin Pharmacokinet* 1997; **33**: 225–44.

4. Kern SE, Stanski DR. Pharmacokinetics and pharmacodynamics of intravenously administered anesthetic drugs: concepts and lessons for drug development. *Clin Pharmacol Ther* 2008; **84**: 153–7.

5. Gross JB. When you breathe IN you inspire, when you DON'T breathe, you ... expire. *Anesthesiology* 2003; **99**: 767–70.

6. Manyam SC, Gupta DK, Johnson KB, *et al.* Opioid-volatile anesthetic synergy:

a response surface model with remifentanil and sevoflurane as prototypes. *Anesthesiology* 2006; **105**: 267–78.

7. Vuyk J, Mertens MJ, Olofsen E, Burm AG, Bovill JG. Propofol anesthesia and rational opioid selection: determination of optimal EC50–EC95 propofol-opioid concentrations that assure adequate anesthesia and a rapid return of consciousness. *Anesthesiology* 1997; **87**: 1549–62.

8. Fisher DM. (Almost) everything you learned about pharmacokinetics was (somewhat) wrong! *Anesth Analg* 1996; **83**: 901–3.

9. Krejcie TC, Avram MJ. What determines anesthetic induction dose? It's the front-end kinetics, Doctor! *Anesth Analg* 1999; **89**: 541–4.

10. Shafer SL, Stanski DR. Improving the clinical utility of anesthetic drug pharmacokinetics. *Anesthesiology* 1992; **76**: 327–30.

11. Shafer SL, Varvel JR. Pharmacokinetics, pharmacodynamics, and rational opioid selection. *Anesthesiology* 1991; **74**: 53–63.

12. Hudson RJ, Bergstrom RG, Thomson IR, *et al.* Pharmacokinetics of sufentanil in patients undergoing abdominal aortic surgery. *Anesthesiology* 1989; **70**: 426–31.

13. Scott JC, Cooke JE, Stanski DR. Electroencephalographic quantitation of opioid effect: comparative pharmacodynamics of fentanyl and sufentanil. *Anesthesiology* 1991; **74**: 34–42.

14. Egan TD, Minto CF, Hermann DJ, *et al.* Remifentanil versus alfentanil: comparative pharmacokinetics and pharmacodynamics in healthy adult male volunteers. *Anesthesiology* 1996; **84**: 821–33.

15. Hill HF, Coda BA, Tanaka A, Schaffer R. Multiple-dose evaluation of intravenous hydromorphone pharmacokinetics in normal human subjects. *Anesth Analg* 1991; **72**: 330–6.

16. Gourlay GK, Wilson PR, Glynn CJ. Pharmacodynamics and pharmacokinetics of methadone during the perioperative period. *Anesthesiology* 1982; **57**: 458–67.

17. Gentry WB, Krejcie TC, Henthorn TK, *et al.* Effect of infusion rate on thiopental dose-response relationships. Assessment of a pharmacokinetic-pharmacodynamic model. *Anesthesiology* 1994; **81**: 316–24.

18. Minto CF, Schnider TW, Gregg KM, Henthorn TK, Shafer SL. Using the time of maximum effect site concentration to combine pharmacokinetics and pharmacodynamics. *Anesthesiology* 2003; **99**: 324–33.

19. Bouillon T, Bruhn J, Radu-Radulescu L, *et al.* A model of the ventilatory depressant potency of remifentanil in the non-steady state. *Anesthesiology* 2003; **99**: 779–87.

20. Egan TD, Kern SE, Muir KT, White J. Remifentanil by bolus injection: a safety, pharmacokinetic, pharmacodynamic, and age effect investigation in human volunteers. *Br J Anaesth* 2004; **92**: 335–43.

21. Caruso AL, Bouillon TW, Schumacher PM, Luginbuhl M, Morari M. Drug-induced respiratory depression: an integrated model of drug effects on the hypercapnic and hypoxic drive. *Conf Proc IEEE Eng Med Biol Soc* 2007; **2007**: 4259–63.

22. Mildh LH, Scheinin H, Kirvela OA. The concentration-effect relationship of the respiratory depressant effects of alfentanil and fentanyl. *Anesth Analg* 2001; **93**: 939–46.

23. Eger EI, Shafer SL. Tutorial: context-sensitive decrement times for inhaled anesthetics. *Anesth Analg* 2005; **101**: 688–96.

24. Vuyk J, Lim T, Engbers FH, *et al.* The pharmacodynamic interaction of propofol and alfentanil during lower abdominal surgery in women. *Anesthesiology* 1995; **83**: 8–22.

25. Lowenstein E, Hallowell P, Levine FH, *et al.* Cardiovascular response to large doses of intravenous morphine in man. *N Engl J Med* 1969; **281**: 1389–93.

26. Lunn JK, Stanley TH, Eisele J, Webster L, Woodward A. High dose fentanyl anesthesia for coronary artery surgery: plasma fentanyl concentrations and influence of nitrous oxide on cardiovascular responses. *Anesth Analg* 1979; **58**: 390–5.

27. Shafer SL. Towards optimal intravenous dosing strategies. *Semin Anesth* 1993; **12**: 222–34.

28. Hughes MA, Glass PS, Jacobs JR. Context-sensitive half-time in multicompartment pharmacokinetic models for intravenous anesthetic drugs. *Anesthesiology* 1992; **76**: 334–41.

29. Stanski DR, Greenblatt DJ, Lowenstein E. Kinetics of intravenous and intramuscular morphine. *Clin Pharmacol Ther* 1978; **24**: 52–9.

30. Borgbjerg FM, Nielsen K, Franks J. Experimental pain stimulates respiration and attenuates morphine-induced respiratory depression: a controlled study in human volunteers. *Pain* 1996; **64**: 123–8.

31. Kan RE, Hughes SC, Rosen MA, *et al.* Intravenous remifentanil: placental transfer, maternal and neonatal effects. *Anesthesiology* 1998; **88**: 1467–74.

32. Volikas I, Butwick A, Wilkinson C, Pleming A, Nicholson G. Maternal and neonatal side-effects of remifentanil patient-controlled analgesia in labour. *Br J Anaesth* 2005; **95**: 504–9.

33. Tateishi T, Krivoruk Y, Ueng YF, *et al.* Identification of human liver cytochrome P-450 3A4 as the enzyme responsible for fentatnyl and sufentanil delakylation. *Anesth Analg* 1996; **82**: 167–72.

34. Kharasch ED, Russell M, Mautz D, *et al.* The role of cytochrome P450 3A4 in alfentanil clearance: implications for interindividual variability in disposition and perioperative drug interactions. *Anesthesiology* 1997; **87**: 36–50.

35. Totah RA, Sheffels P, Roberts T, *et al.* Role of CYP2B6 in stereoselective human methadone metabolism. *Anesthesiology* 2008; **108**: 363–74.

36. Lötsch J. Opioid metabolites. *J Pain Symptom Manage* 2005; **29**: S10–24.

37. Egan TD. Remifentanil pharmacokinetics and pharmacodynamics. *A preliminary appraisal Clin Pharmacokinet* 1995; **29**: 80–94.

38. Kaiko RF, Foley KM, Grabinski PY, *et al.* Central nervous system excitatory effects of meperidine in cancer patients. *Ann Neurol* 1983; **13**: 180–5.

39. Benet LZ, Hoener B-A. Changes in plasma protein binding have little clinical relevance. *Clin Pharmacol Ther* 2002; **71**: 115–21.

40. Somogyi AA, Barratt DT, Coller JK. Pharmacogenetics of opioids. *Clin Pharmacol Ther* 2007; **81**: 429–44.

41. Mikus G, Weiss J. Influence of CYP2D6 genetics on opioid kinetics, metabolism, and response. *Curr Pharmacogenom* 2005; **3**: 43–52.

42. Cascorbi I. Pharmacogenetics of cytochrome P4502D6: Genetic background and clinical implication. *Eur J Clin Invest* 2003; **33**: 16–22.

43. Lurcott G. The effects of the genetic absence and inhibition of CYP2D6 on the metabolism of codeine and its derivatives, hydrocodone and oxycodone. *Anesth Prog* 1999; **45**: 154–6.

44. Palkama VJ, Isohanni MH, Neuvonen PJ, Olkkola KT. The effect of intravenous and oral fluconazole on the pharmacokinetics of intravenous alfentanil. *Anesth Analg* 1998; **87**: 190–4.

45. Palkama VJ, Neuvonen PJ, Olkkola KT. The CYP 3A4 inhibitor itraconazole has no effect on i.v. fentanyl. *Br J Anaesth Analg* 1998; **81**: 598–600.

46. Ibrahim AE, Feldman J, Karim A. Kharasch ED. Simultaneous assessment of drug interactions with low- and high-extraction opioids: Application to parecoxib effects on the pharmacokinetics and pharmacodynamics of fentanyl and alfentanil. *Anesthesiology* 2003; **98**: 853–61.

47. Kharasch ED, Bedynek PS, Walker A, Whittington D, Hoffer C. Mechanism of ritonavir changes in methadone pharmacokinetics and pharmacodynamics: II. Ritonavir effects on CYP3A and P-glycoprotein activities. *Clin Pharmacol Ther* 2008; **84**: 506–12.

48. Olkkola KT, Palkama VJ, Neuvonen PJ. Ritonavir's role in reducing fentanyl clearance and prolonging its half-life. *Anesthesiology* 1999; **91**: 681–5.

49. Lötsch, Skarke C, Tegeder I, Geisslinger G. Drug interactions with patient controlled analgesia. *Clin Pharmacokinet* 2001; **41**: 31–57.

50. Bruce RD, Altice FL, Gourevitch MN, Friedland GH. Pharmacokinetic drug interactions between opioid agonist therapy and antiretroviral medications: implications and management for clinical practice. *J Acquir Immun Defic Syndr* 2006; **41**: 563–72.

51. Kharasch E, Bedynek P, Park S, *et al.* Mechanism of ritonavir changes in methadone pharmacokinetics and pharmacodynamics: I. Evidence against CYP3A mediation of methadone clearance. *Clin Pharmacol Ther* 2008; **84**: 497–505.

52. Pond SM, Tozer TN. First-pass elimination: Basic concepts and clinical consequences. *Clin Pharmacokinet* 1984; **9**: 1–25.

53. Yam YK. Individual variation in first-pass metabolism. *Clin Pharmacokinet* 1993; **25**: 300–28.

54. Tegeder I, Lötsch J, Geisslinger G. Pharmacokinetics of opioids in liver disease. *Clin Pharmacokinet* 1999; **37**: 17–40.

55. Davies G, Kingswood C, Street M. Pharmacokinetics of opioids in renal dysfunction. *Clin Pharmacokinet* 1996; **31**: 410–22.

56. Lugo RA, Kern SE. Clinical pharmacokinetics of morphine. *J Pain Palliat Care Pharmacother* 2002; **16**: 5–18.

57. Gourlay GK. Sustained relief of chronic pain: Pharmacokinetics of sustained release morphine. *Clin Pharmacokinet* 1998; **35**: 173–90.

58. Mandema JW, Kaiko RF, Oshlack B, Reder RF, Stanski DR. Characterization and validation of a pharmacokinetic model for controlled-release oxycodone. *Br J Clin Pharmacol* 1996; **42**: 747–56.

59. Murray A, Hagen NA. Hydromorphone. *J Pain Symptom Manage* 2005; **29**: S57–66.

60. Dale O, Hoffer C, Sheffels P, Kharasch ED. Disposition of nasal, intravenous, and oral methadone in healthy volunteers. *Clin Pharmacol Ther* 2002; **72**: 536–45.

61. Eap CB, Buclin T, Baumann P. Interindividual variability of the clinical pharmacokinetics of methadone: Implications for the treatment of opioid dependence. *Clin Pharmacokinet* 2002; **41**: 1153–93.

62. Zhang H, Zhang J, Streisand JB. Oral mucosal drug delivery: Clinical pharmacokinetics and therapeutic applications. *Clin Pharmacokinet* 2002; **41**: 661–80.

63. Streisand JB, Varvel JR, Stanski DR, *et al.* Absorption and bioavailability of oral transmucosal fentanyl citrate. *Anesthesiology* 1991; **75**: 223–9.

64. Wheeler M, Birmingham PK, Dsida RM, *et al.* Uptake pharmacokinetics of the fentanyl Oralet® in children scheduled for central venous access removal: Implications for the timing of initiating painful procedures. *Paediatr Anaesth* 2002; **12**: 596–9.

65. Semple TJ, Upton RN, Macintyre PE, Runciman WB, Mather LE. Morphine blood concentrations in elderly postoperative patients following administration via an indwelling subcutaneous cannula. *Anaesthesia* 1997; **52**: 318–23.

66. Stuart-Harris R, Joel SP, McDonald P, Currow D, Slevin ML. The pharmacokinetics of morphine and morphine glucuronide metabolites after subcutaneous bolus injection and subcutaneous infusion of morphine. *Br J Clin Pharmacol* 2000; **49**: 207–14.

67. Waldmann CS, Eason JR, Rambohul E, Hanson GC. Serum morphine levels. A comparison between continuous subcutaneous infusion and continuous intravenous infusion in postoperative patients. *Anaesthesia* 1984; **39**: 768–71.

68. Miller RS, Peterson GM, Abbott F, *et al.* Plasma concentrations of fentanyl with subcutaneous infusion in palliative care patients. *Br J Clin Pharmacol* 1995; **40**: 553–6.

69. Ronald AL, Docherty D, Broom J, Chambers WA. Subarachnoid local anesthetic block does not affect morphine absorption from paired intramuscular and subcutaneous injection sites in the elderly patient. *Anesth Analg* 1993; **76**: 778–82.

70. Ground S, Radbruch L, Lehmann KA. Clinical pharmacokientics of transdermal opioids: Focus on transdermal fentanyl. *Clin Pharmacokinet* 2000; **38**: 59–89.

71. Varvel JR, Shafer SL, Hwang SS, Coen PA, Stanski DR. Absorption characteristics of transdermally

administered fentanyl. *Anesthesiology* 1989; **70**: 928–34.

72. Portenoy RK, Southam MA, Gupta SK, *et al.* Transdermal fentanyl for cancer pain: repeated dose pharmacokinetics. *Anesthesiology* 1993; **78**: 36–43.

73. Gupta SK, Southam M, Hwang SS. System functionality and physicochemical model of fentanyl transdermal system. *J Pain Symptom Manage* 1992; **7**: S17–26.

74. Fiset P, Cohane C, Browne S, Brand SC, Shafer SL. Biopharmaceutics of a new transdermal fentanyl device. *Anesthesiology* 1995; **83**: 459–69.

75. Sinatra R. The fentanyl HCl patient-controlled transdermal system (PCTS): an alternative to intravenous patient-controlled analgesia in the postoperative setting. *Clin Pharmacokinet* 2005; **44**: 1–6.

76. Sathyan G, Jaskowiak J, Evashenk M, Gupta S. Characterisation of the pharmacokinetics of the fentanyl HCl patient-controlled transdermal system (PCTS): Effect of current magnitude and multiple-day dosing and comparison with IV fentanyl administration. *Clin Pharmacokinet* 2005; **44**: 7–15.

77. Sathyan G, Zomorodi K, Gidwani S, Gupta S. The effect of dosing frequency on the pharmacokinetics of a fentanyl HCl patient-controlled transdermal system (PCTS). *Clin Pharmacokinet* 2005; **44**: 17–24.

78. Roy SD, Flynn GL. Transdermal delivery of narcotic analgesics: Comparative permeabilities of narcotic analgesics through human cadaver skin. *Pharm Res* 1989; **6**: 825–32.

79. Paice JA, Von Roenn JH, Hudgins JC, *et al.* Morphine bioavailability from a topical gel formulation in volunteers. *J Pain Symptom Manage* 2008; **35**: 314–20.

80. Labris NR, Dolovich MB. Pulmonary drug delivery. Part I: Physiological factors affecting therapeutic effectiveness of aerosolized medications. *Br J Clin Pharmacol* 2003; **56**: 588–99.

81. Patton JS, Byron PR. Inhaling medicines: Delivering drugs to the body through the lungs. *Nat Rev Drug Discov* 2007; **6**: 67–74.

82. Farr SJ, Otulana BA. Pulmonary delivery of opioids as pain therapeutics. *Adv Drug Deliv Rev* 2006; **58**: 1076–88.

83. Ward ME, Woodhouse A, Mather LE, *et al.* Morphine pharmacokinetics after pulmonary administration from a novel aerosol delivery system. *Clin Pharmacol Ther* 1997; **62**: 596–609.

84. Mather LE, Woodhouse A, Ward ME, *et al.* Pulmonary administration of aerosolised fentanyl: pharmacokinetic analysis of systemic delivery. *Br J Clin Pharmacol* 1998; **46**: 37–43.

85. Avram MJ, Henthorn TK, Spyker DA, Cassella JV. Recirculatory kinetic model of fentanyl administered as a thermally generated aerosol to volunteers. *Anesthesiology* 2008; **109**: A815.

86. Eisenach JC, Hood DM, Curry R, Shafer SL. Cephalad movement of morphine and fentanyl in humans after intrathecal injection. *Anesthesiology* 2003; **99**: 166–73.

87. Burm AGL, Haak-van der Lely F, van Kleef JW, *et al.* Pharmacokinetics of alfentanil after epidural administration: Investigation of systemic absorption kinetics with a stable isotope method. *Anesthesiology* 1994; **81**: 308–15.

88. Camu F, Debucquoy F. Alfentanil infusion for postoperative pain: A Comparison of epidural and intravenous routes. *Anesthesiology* 1991; **75**: 171–8.

89. Mather LE, Cousins MJ. The site of action of epidural fentanyl: What can be learned by studying the difference between infusion and bolus administration? The importance of history, one hopes. *Anesth Analg* 2003; **97**: 1428–38.

90. Ginosar Y, Riley ET, Angst MS. The site of action of epidural fentanyl in humans: The difference between infusion and bolus administration. *Anesth Analg* 2003; **97**: 1428–38.

91. Loper KA, Ready LB, Downey M, *et al.* Epidural and intravenous fentanyl infusions are clinically equivalent after knee surgery. *Anesth Analg* 1990; **70**: 72–5.

92. Moises EC, de Barros Duarte L, de Carvalho Cavalli R, *et al.* Pharmacokinetics and transplacental distribution of fentanyl in epidural anesthesia for normal pregnant women. *Eur J Clin Pharmacol* 2005; **61**: 517–22.

93. Ferrier C, Marty J, Bouffard Y, *et al.* Alfentanil pharmacokinetics in patients with cirrhosis. *Anesthesiology* 1985; **62**: 480–4.

94. Dershwitz M, Hoke JF, Rosow CE, *et al.* Pharmacokinetics and pharmacodynamics of remifentanil in volunteer subjects with severe liver disease. *Anesthesiology* 1996; **84**: 812–20.

95. Dean M. Opioids in renal failure and dialysis patients. *J Pain Symptom Manage* 2004; **28**: 497–504.

96. Osborne R, Joel, S, Grebenik K, Trew D, Slevin M. The pharmacokinetics of morphine and morphine glucuronides in kidney failure. *Clin Pharmacol Ther* 1993; **54**: 158–67.

97. D'Honneur G, Gilton A, Sandouk P, Scherrmann JN, Duvaldestin P. Plasma and cerebrospinal fluid concentrations of morphine and morphine glucuronides after oral morphine. The influence of renal failure. *Anesthesiology* 1994; **81**: 87–93.

98. Szeto HH, Inturrisi CE, Houde R, *et al.* Accumulation of normeperidine, an active metabolite of meperidine, an patients with renal failure of cancer. *Ann Intern Med* 1997; **86**: 738–41.

99. Syme MR, Paxton JW, Keelan JA. Drug transfer and metabolism by the human placenta. *Clin Pharmacokinet* 2004; **43**: 487–514.

100. Tomson G, Garle RI, Thalme B, *et al.* Maternal kinetics and transplacental passage of pethidine during labour. *Br J Clin Pharmacol* 1982; **13**: 653–9.

101. Nicolle E, Devillier P, Delanoy B, Durand C, Bessard G. Therapeutic monitoring of nalbuphine: Transplacental transfer and estimated pharmacokinetics in the neonate. *Eur J Clin Pharmacol* 1996; **49**: 485–9.

102. Borgatta L, Jenny RW, Gruss L, Ong C, Barad D. Clinical significance of methohexital, meperidine, and diazepam in breast milk. *J Clin Pharmacol* 1997; **37**: 186–92.

103. Nitsun M, Szokol JW, Saleh J, *et al.* Pharmacokinetics of midazolam, propofol, and fentanyl transfer to human breast milk. *Clin Pharmacol Ther* 2006; **79**: 549–57.

104. Feilberg VL, Rosenborg D, Broen Christensen C, Mogensen JV.

Excretion of morphine in human breast milk. *Acta Anaesthesiol Scand* 1989; **33**: 426–8.

105. Begg EJ, Malpas TJ, Hackett LP, Ilett KF. Distribution of R- and S-methadone into human milk during multiple, medium to high oral dosing. *Br J Clin Pharmacol.* 2001; **52**: 681–5.

106. Meny RG, Naumburg EG, Alger LS, Brill-Miller JL, Brown S. Codeine and the breastfed neonate. *J Hum Lact* 1993; **9**: 237–40.

107. Koren G, Cairns J, Chitayat D, Gaedigk A, Leeder SJ. Pharmacogentics of morphine poisoning in a breastfed neonate of a codeine prescribed mother. *Lancet* 2006; **368**: 704.

108. Bateman DN, Eddleston M, Sandilands E. Codeine and breastfeeding. *Lancet* 2008; **372**: 625.

109. Berlin CM, Paul IM, Vesell ES. Safety issues of maternal drug therapy during breastfeeding. *Clin Pharmacol Ther* 2009; **85**: 20–2.

110. Madadi P, Ross CJD, Hayden MR, *et al.* Pharmacogenetics of neonatal opioid toxicity following maternal use of codeine during breastfeeding: A cas-control study. *Clin Pharmacol Ther* 2009; **85**: 31–5.

Essential drugs in anesthetic practice
Clinical pharmacology of opioids

Carl E. Rosow and Mark Dershwitz

Introduction

Ancient writings and archeological data indicate that the Sumerians, who inhabited what is today Iraq, cultivated poppies and isolated opium from their seed capsules at the end of the third millennium BC. At first, opium may have been used as a euphoriant in religious rituals, but by the second century BC it was used medicinally. As early as the eighth century AD, Arab traders brought opium to India and China, and between the tenth and thirteenth centuries opium reached all parts of Europe [1]. Starting in the sixteenth century, manuscripts describe opium abuse in Turkey, Egypt, Germany, England, and China.

In 1806, Sertürner isolated the active ingredient in opium, naming it morphine after the god of dreams. After the invention of the hypodermic syringe and hollow needle in the 1850s, morphine began to be used for surgical procedures, for postoperative and chronic pain, and as an adjunct to general anesthetics. Because morphine had just as much potential for abuse as opium, much effort was expended in developing a safer, more efficacious, nonaddicting opioid. In 1898, heroin was synthesized and pronounced free from the liability of abuse. This was the first of many such claims for new opioids – however, no such substances currently have been introduced into clinical practice.

The first two completely synthetic opioids were meperidine (1939) and methadone (1946). N-allylnorcodeine and N-allylnormorphine (nalorphine) were the first compounds recognized to have opioid antagonist properties. Nalorphine was later found to have limited analgesic properties and was the prototype for the class of opioid agonist-antagonists. The N-allyl derivative of oxymorphone, naloxone, was introduced in 1966 as the first relatively pure competitive opioid antagonist.

Chapter 31 has already reviewed many cellular mechanisms of opioid action as well as the various opioid receptor families (μ, κ, δ, and ORL) and their ligands. Chapter 32 has reviewed the principles of opioid pharmacokinetics. This chapter will deliberately revisit portions of this material, but more briefly, and in the context of clinical application. Almost all of the clinically useful opioid agonists are alkaloids that are moderately to highly selective for the μ-opioid receptor. A few κ-type partial agonists are used clinically (see discussion of agonist-antagonist opioids), but no selective agonists are available for the other classes. Numerous subtypes have been described for each of the receptor classes, but thus far no agonist or antagonist selective for a particular opioid receptor subtype has been approved for clinical use.

Terminology

Opiates are compounds derived from opium and include morphine, codeine, and a variety of related alkaloids. The term **opioid** is broader and includes all compounds (alkaloids or peptides) that have affinity for opioid receptors. Opioid analgesics are often called **narcotics**, but the term has also been inappropriately applied to compounds producing sleep (i.e., narcosis), as well as nonopioid, abusable drugs like cocaine (the Bureau of Narcotics and Dangerous Drugs was the forerunner of today's Drug Enforcement Administration). *Opioid* is the preferred term, and *narcotic* is a descriptor best avoided by pharmacologists.

Opioid agonists

Since most of the commonly used opioid analgesics are selective for μ-opioid receptors, they produce a qualitatively similar group of pharmacodynamic (PD) effects (Table 33.1). Some opioids do produce nonspecific or non-opioid-receptor-mediated effects in normal clinical doses (Table 33.2).

The onset and duration of effect are most often the basis for selection of a particular opioid, and there is tremendous variability in the published values for most opioid pharmacokinetic (PK) parameters. Some of this variability reflects true differences between patient populations, whereas some is the result of sampling times and other technical aspects of measurement. Opioids also vary significantly in their oral bioavailability and in physical properties such as lipophilicity. Most opioids are used in both oral and parenteral formulations. Fentanyl and its congeners have low oral bioavailability, but their high lipophilicity makes them well suited for transdermal, buccal, or even nasal administration.

Anesthetic Pharmacology, 2nd edition, ed. Alex S. Evers, Mervyn Maze, Evan D. Kharasch. Published by Cambridge University Press. © Cambridge University Press 2011.

Table 33.1. Acute and chronic effects of opioids

Acute

Analgesia

Sedation

CNS stimulation/euphoria

Ventilatory depression

Cough suppression

Nausea and vomiting

Miosis

Skeletal muscle rigidity

Vasodilation

Bradycardia

Smooth muscle spasm

    Constipation

    Urinary retention

    Biliary spasm

Chronic

Tolerance

Physical dependence

Table 33.2. Opioid effects not mediated by opioid receptors

Drug	Mechanism	Effect
Morphine, meperidine, codeine	Histamine release	Flushing, vasodilation
d-Methadone	NMDA antagonism	Unknown
Meperidine	Local anesthesia	Neuronal block after intrathecal injection
Meperidine, tramadol	Block serotonin reuptake	Serotonin syndrome, interaction with MAOI
Meperidine	α_{2b}-agonist	Decrease shivering

Analgesia

Opioids are the most broadly effective analgesics available, probably a reflection of their supraspinal, spinal, and peripheral sites of action. Opioids are traditionally said to be most effective for visceral or burning pain, less effective for sharp pain (e.g., on incision), and least effective for neuropathic pain [2]. The opioid effect is selective for nociception, because touch, pressure, and other sensory modalities are generally unaffected. There is substantial disagreement about the relative contributions of spinal and supraspinal mechanisms when opioids are administered systemically [3,4] (spinal mechanisms become proportionately more important when the opioids are given by neuraxial injection). It seems likely that forebrain mechanisms play a prominent role in the production of clinical effects, because a common clinical manifestation of opioid analgesia is a change in the affective response to pain. Patients given systemic opioids will typically report that their pain is still present, but the intensity is reduced and the pain discomfort is also less. The mental clouding and dissociation from pain are often accompanied by mood elevation or even euphoria [5]. These positive mood effects may explain the relatively high patient acceptance of opioids, but they unquestionably contribute to their potential for abuse.

Opioids produce a dose- and concentration-dependent reduction in the intensity of acute pain. Many textbooks have lists of equianalgesic doses for various opioids, usually based on data from postoperative pain models. Information on relative potency is useful, but it must be emphasized that for many patients the "usual" doses can produce inadequate or excessive opioid effect. For example, a typical 100 mg intramuscular dose of meperidine is adequate for only 20% of adults with postsurgical pain [6]. The intensity of self-rated postsurgical pain decreases with increasing plasma concentrations of meperidine [7]. These data show two important characteristics of opioid analgesia: (1) for each patient, the pain scores decrease dramatically over a very small range of opioid concentrations; and (2) the threshold concentration for pain relief varies fourfold to fivefold among patients. The large interindividual variation in opioid requirement has been a consistent finding in pain studies and makes it clear why opioids need to be titrated for optimal effect.

These considerations apply equally well to the use of opioids for intraoperative pain. Because it is not possible to use subjective reports of pain during general anesthesia, opioids are commonly titrated to surrogate endpoints, such as blood pressure, heart rate, and movement. Alfentanil produces a concentration-dependent suppression of autonomic responses and movement during surgery [8] (Fig. 33.1). The data from this study were remarkably similar to those described for postoperative pain – i.e., the slope of the concentration–response curve for analgesia was steep for each patient, and the threshold concentrations among patients were highly variable.

Numerous factors contribute to interindividual variability in opioid requirement for analgesia, and this makes it difficult to isolate the effect of any one variable on clinical pain relief.

- The location and intensity of the pain stimulus is obviously important. For example, postoperative thoracotomy pain requires more opioid than pain of hernia repair. Blunting the intraoperative response to laryngoscopy requires more than blunting the response to skin incision [8].
- As with other subjective responses, a huge variety of psychological factors may affect opioid requirement. For example, previous positive or negative experiences with

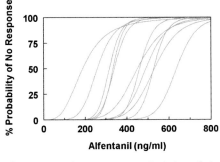

Figure 33.1. Response to manipulation of the upper abdominal viscera during general anesthesia with nitrous oxide and a variable-rate alfentanil infusion. Arterial concentrations of alfentanil were measured, and the presence or absence of response (blood pressure, heart rate, or movement) was noted. Logistic regression was used to model the probability of "analgesia" (i.e., no response) vs. alfentanil concentration for each of the 11 patients. The change from high to low probability of analgesia occurred over a small concentration range for each patient, but the threshold concentration varied considerably among patients [8].

pain relief can influence subsequent responses. It follows that a crossover study comparing analgesic versus placebo should always be randomized for the order of treatment.

- Treatment with other analgesics (cyclooxygenase inhibitors, α_2-agonists) and certain sedative-hypnotics (e.g., hydroxyzine, droperidol) can reliably potentiate opioid analgesia, and these interactions are frequently exploited for this purpose. Some CNS depressants (benzodiazepines, alcohol, barbiturates) do not have as clear an effect on analgesia, but can increase opioid adverse effects on ventilation and hemodynamics.
- Age affects opioid requirement. On average, the elderly are more sensitive to opioids, although some older patients require surprisingly high doses for adequate analgesia [9]. The age effect is partly due to PK changes (decreased clearance, decreased volumes of distribution). Simultaneous PK/PD modeling studies with fentanyl and remifentanil have also demonstrated an increase in PD sensitivity (i.e., a decrease in dose requirement) with age [10,11]. Clinicians tend to overestimate the sensitivity of elderly patients, so many of them are underdosed and have inadequate relief of pain. A recent large study of intravenous morphine for postoperative pain suggests that it may be appropriate to titrate the opioid in a similar manner for adults of all ages [12].
- Certain pathophysiologic conditions, such as hypothyroidism and pre-existing central nervous system (CNS) disease, can increase sensitivity to opioids. Patients with asthma or mild chronic obstructive pulmonary disease probably have normal sensitivity, but opioids should be used with care, because decreased cough or deep breathing can lead to inspissation of airway secretions and cause bronchospasm.
- Hepatic and renal dysfunction can lead to accumulation of both the opioid and its metabolites, but sensitivity may not change much. Two PK and PD studies demonstrated that patients with renal or hepatic failure have normal or only

slightly increased sensitivity to the ventilatory depressant effects of remifentanil when compared with healthy control subjects [13,14].
- Preliminary data suggest that sex can influence the response to opioids. There are complex sex-related differences in the ventilatory responses to a given concentration of morphine [15]. Interindividual differences in opioid sensitivity appear to be greater than differences due to sex.
- Genetic differences in drug disposition may also influence opioid requirement. As discussed in the chapter on drug metabolism, the analgesic effect of codeine is almost entirely caused by its conversion to morphine by O-demethylation. This reaction is catalyzed by CYP2D6, a cytochrome P450 enzyme that shows important genetic polymorphisms. About 10% of Caucasians [16] and most Chinese [17] are "poor metabolizers" who may have an inadequate analgesic effect from codeine. Individuals from North Africa may have multiple gene copies and show increased sensitivity to codeine [18]. There have been numerous studies of morphine's active metabolite, morphine-6-glucuronide, but little is known about the role of glucuronidation in variable responses to morphine. One study found that Colombian Indians are more sensitive than white or Latino patients to the ventilatory depressant effects of morphine [19]. Notably, Colombian Indians had less capacity to form morphine glucuronides.

Sedation

Opioids produce sedation, but, given alone, they do not generally produce hypnosis. Even very high doses of fentanyl or its analogs produce a hypnotic effect that may be brief and unreliable [20,21]. As little as 3 μg kg^{-1} alfentanil (a tiny dose that is probably subanalgesic) is sufficient to double the hypnotic potency of midazolam [22]. Opioids can also potentiate the hypnotic effect of propofol [23] and barbiturates. The κ-receptor agonist butorphanol produces a strong sedative effect and potentiates midazolam at doses lower than those used for analgesia [24].

Occasionally, opioids produce CNS excitatory effects like agitation and dysphoria, and some opioids such as meperidine and codeine are proconvulsant. Fortunately, the convulsant effect of most opioids occurs at concentrations greater than those needed for analgesia. In patients with head injury, opioids should be used with caution, if at all. They can increase intracranial pressure by causing hypercarbia, and the pupillary effects can mask changing neurologic signs. Some opioids produce a modest direct cerebral vasodilation, but this is easily overcome when ventilation is controlled [25].

Ventilatory depression

The mechanisms involved in this effect were discussed in Chapter 31. Opioids produce a dose-dependent depression of the ventilatory response to hypercapnia (technically acidosis) and hypoxia through actions on μ_2-receptors (and probably other, as yet undefined receptors) in ventilatory centers of the

other μ-receptor agonists. This cross-tolerance is often incomplete, possibly due to interaction of these drugs with multiple μ-receptor subtypes [61,62]. Tolerance develops most rapidly to opioid-induced depressant effects, such as analgesia and ventilatory depression, and very slowly to opioid-induced stimulant effects, such as constipation or miosis.

The mechanisms of tolerance to opioids may vary with the specific drug. The speed of the changes in acute tolerance suggests rapid cellular autoregulatory responses, whereas chronic tolerance appears to be a much more permanent alteration in cellular structure and function. As stated in Chapter 31, receptor phosphorylation, G-protein uncoupling, and receptor internalization (removal of receptors from the cell membrane) may all play a role. Recent research suggests that opioid tolerance also involves the activation of NMDA receptors and the production of nitric oxide. These changes may result in hyperalgesia – chronic administration of the opioid can cause increased pain that clinically manifests as a reduction in drug effect [63,64]. As a result, there have been numerous attempts to modulate tolerance to opioids by administering NMDA antagonists (dizocilpine, dextromethorphan) or nitric oxide synthase inhibitors [65,66]. Thus far, the clinical benefits of using NMDA antagonists have not been demonstrated.

Physical dependence

After sufficient doses have been administered, all opioids can induce a state of physical dependence. Discontinuation of the drug causes a stereotypical withdrawal, or abstinence, syndrome that includes restlessness, mydriasis, gooseflesh, runny nose, diarrhea, shaking chills, and drug-seeking behavior. The rate of onset of these symptoms depends on the speed of opioid elimination. Administration of an opioid antagonist can cause an immediate "precipitated" withdrawal that can sometimes be quite violent. Withdrawal symptoms can be terminated rapidly by intravenous administration of a small dose of morphine.

When a patient with known physical dependence is to be detoxified (i.e., stop taking opioids), he or she is commonly switched to administration of methadone, and the dosage is reduced slowly. The result is a mild, although protracted, withdrawal syndrome. A person dependent on heroin or methadone seeking emergency medical treatment is generally not an appropriate candidate for detoxification.

It is probable that most patients administered opioids chronically have some clinically imperceptible level of physical dependence. In most instances, withdrawal may take place without the patient or physician being aware of its occurrence. Physical dependence must be distinguished from psychological dependence or addiction, which includes compulsive drug-seeking behavior. An important concept is that drug addiction resulting from appropriate medical treatment is an unusual event [67]. Fear of addiction, however, is a common reason for inadequate pain treatment.

Use of opioids for chronic pain

The use of opioids for chronic pain is controversial. Few would deny opioids to the patient with terminal cancer, but the considerations may be different for a patient without cancer (or a cancer patient with substantial time remaining). Although many patients have received opioids chronically without apparent problems [68], it is not really known how well such opioids work, and a recent review indicates the risks may not be justified by the available data [69]. Recently, much attention has been given to the finding that neuropathic pain and centrally mediated pain are less responsive to opioids than other types of pain. Preclinical data demonstrating hyperalgesia after chronic opioid administration (see *drug tolerance*, above) suggest that chronic neuropathic pain may actually be worsened [63]. Unfortunately, a large percentage of chronic pain (both cancer and noncancer) falls into the neuropathic category.

The efficacy of opioids for low back pain and neuropathic pain has been supported (sometimes enthusiastically) by an accumulation of case reports and uncontrolled open studies [70]. Few controlled studies investigating the efficacy and side effects of opioids in these clinical settings are available [71–74]. Currently, the maximum duration of opioid treatment investigated in a double-blind, placebo-controlled study is 9 weeks [71]. All other studies have lasted a maximum of 4 weeks. These trials found a reduction in subjective pain scores, but only one study examined psychosocial features, quality of life, drug dependence, or functional status in detail [71]. No significant differences in any of the functional status parameters were detected, and there was a lack of overall patient preference for the opioid. The authors concluded that morphine may confer analgesic benefit with a low risk for addiction, but that it is unlikely to yield psychological or functional improvement [71]. Adverse opioid-induced side effects were reported in all of these investigations and led to large numbers (up to 60%) of patients withdrawing from the study.

Thus there is a lack of prospective, controlled studies examining the long-term (at least several months) administration of opioids. Future studies need to demonstrate positive outcomes, not only in subjective pain reports, but also in terms of reduced depression, functional improvement, rates of patient re-employment, and decreased use of the healthcare system.

Specific drugs

The onset or duration of effect is most often the basis for selection of a particular opioid. Many of the PK properties of opioids have been discussed generally in Chapter 32. Table 33.3 summarizes the equipotent doses and (for purpose of comparison) the approximate peak blood concentrations after an intravenous bolus dose of common opioids. Table 33.4 contains some pertinent PK and PD properties for each of the common opioid agonists. Opioids given intraoperatively during general anesthesia are almost invariably accompanied

Table 33.3. Approximately equipotent analgesic doses and peak blood concentrations for common opioids

Drug	Dose (mg)	Peak blood concentration (ng mL^{-1})	Reference
Intravenous bolus administration			
Morphine	10	1360[a,b]	[75]
Meperidine	80	1680[c,d]	[76]
Methadone	10	760[b,c]	[77]
Hydromorphone	1.5	176[c,d]	[78]
Fentanyl	0.1	3.6[a,b]	[79]
Sufentanil	0.01	0.5[a,b]	[80]
Alfentanil	0.75	320[a,b]	[10]
Remifentanil	0.1	18[a,b]	[11]
Butorphanol	2	4.0[c,d]	[81]
Nalbuphine	10	73[b,c]	[82]
Buprenorphine	0.3	34[a]	[83]
Oral administration			
Hydrocodone	24	58[c,d]	[84]
Oxycodone	24	36[c,d]	[85]
Hydromorphone	6	4.2[c,d]	[86]
Tramadol	80	247[c,d,e]	[87]

Peak concentrations are for comparative purposes only. After a bolus intravenous injection the peak concentration would be present for only a few moments. Steady-state or normal analgesic concentrations would be significantly lower.
[a]Sampled in arterial blood.
[b]Concentration simulated using the kinetic constants in the reference and a bolus dose.
[c]Sampled in venous blood.
[d]Concentration extrapolated from data in the reference.
[e]An active metabolite contributes substantially to the overall analgesic effect.

by another medication to produce hypnosis, either an inhaled anesthetic or a sedative-hypnotic drug such as propofol. Table 33.5 lists typical opioid and propofol concentrations that block the responses to various perioperative stimuli.

Opioid agonist-antagonists

The agonist-antagonist opioids are a group of synthetic and semisynthetic analgesics that are structurally related to morphine. They were developed primarily as less abusable substitutes for morphine and other pure agonists. Although that goal was achieved to some degree, these drugs have never achieved widespread popularity in medicine. They have been used primarily for moderate to severe acute pain, although in the United States buprenorphine is used only for maintenance therapy in opioid addiction. All these compounds produce some degree of competitive antagonism to morphine and the other pure agonists.

Nalorphine, the original agonist-antagonist, is no longer used clinically, but it has pharmacologic properties that illustrate the most important features of the class:

(1) A strong, but limited, analgesic effect (i.e., it is a partial agonist).
(2) A morphine antagonist effect, which depends upon the ratio of morphine to nalorphine. At very high doses of nalorphine, the agonist effects predominate.
(3) A very low potential for diversion or abuse. Administration to subjects who are physically dependent upon opioids produces a violent "precipitated withdrawal" syndrome. Former heroin addicts given nalorphine do not experience euphoria or perceive the drug as being similar to morphine.
(4) A combination of typical and atypical opioid side effects. Nalorphine produces limited ventilatory depression and gastrointestinal effects, but analgesic doses can cause severe psychotomimetic reactions.

The unusual mental effects – distressing hallucinations and dysphoria – made nalorphine clinically unacceptable as an analgesic, although it was used for many years as an opioid antagonist.

All of the modern agonist-antagonists behave as partial agonists; these drugs tend to have shallower dose–response curves and produce lower maximal effects than fentanyl or morphine [91]. This means there is a "ceiling" to the analgesic effects, but the toxic effects are limited as well. The clinically available agonist-antagonists fall into two broad categories based on their binding and intrinsic activity at μ and κ receptors:

- κ partial agonists – Pentazocine, butorphanol, and nalbuphine (and nalorphine) produce analgesia and sedation by a partial agonist effect at κ receptors. All of them act as competitive antagonists at μ receptors, and therefore reverse the effects of morphine.
- μ partial agonists – Buprenorphine binds to μ receptors with extremely high affinity but has limited efficacy. When given alone, its effects are similar to those of morphine. When given after morphine, it competes with the full agonist and causes a reduction in opioid effect. Buprenorphine is also an antagonist at κ-opioid receptors.

These drugs vary widely in their potencies, both as analgesics and as antagonists. Neither agonist versus antagonist potency nor μ versus κ interaction has proved to be a predictor of clinical utility or patient acceptance.

Analgesia

The agonist-antagonists have been shown to be effective in a variety of acute and chronic pain states. They have been given intramuscularly, orally, sublingually, intranasally, intravenously by bolus or continuous infusion, and in patient-controlled analgesia (PCA) systems. The drugs and their recommended intravenous doses are listed in Table 33.3. None of these drugs is currently approved for epidural or intrathecal use, although they have all been reported to be effective by this route.

Table 33.4. Properties of common opioid agonists

Drug	Absorption/metabolism	Clinical pharmacokinetics	Comments
Morphine	Low lipophilicity	Slow onset and offset	Pharmacology of M6G is *not* identical to parent compound
	Slow CNS penetration and rapid efflux	Poor correlation of plasma and effect-site concentration after bolus (Fig. 33.2)	Accumulation of M6G over time due to slow CNS clearance
	P-glycoprotein substrate	M3G (and possibly M6G) have excitatory effects	Greater accumulation of M6G in renal insufficiency.
	Flow-dependent clearance		Prolonged clearance with reduced liver blood flow (CHF, abdominal surgery)
	70% first-pass metabolism		
	Mainly 3-glucuronidation (M3G)		
	15% active metabolite, 6-β-glucuronide (M6G)		
	Low protein binding (albumin)		
Meperidine	Moderately lipophilic	Onset faster than morphine and shorter duration.	Toxicity with MAOI (serotonin syndrome)
	48–56% first-pass metabolism	NM has proconvulsant properties	Accumulation of NM in renal failure can lead to convulsions.
	Mainly demethylation to normeperidine (NM)		Weak antimuscarinic effect
	High protein binding (α_1-acid glycoprotein)		
Hydromorphone	Low lipophilicity	Slow onset (faster than morphine)	Commercially available in concentrated solution for PCA in tolerant patients
	62% first-pass metabolism	Duration shorter than morphine	Minimal histamine release compared to morphine
	Mainly 3-glucuronide		
	No active metabolite		
Hydrocodone	80% bioavailability	Usually administered orally every 3–6 h	Usually administered in fixed-dose combination with paracetamol
	Metabolized to hydromorphone by CYP2D6		
	Also demethylated to norhydrocodone		
Oxycodone	75% oral bioavailability	Usually administered orally every 3–6 h	Usually administered in fixed-dose combination with paracetamol
	Mainly demethylated to noroxycodone		Available in sustained-release tablets
Methadone	Lipophilic	Racemic mixture	Substantial accumulation with chronic dosing.
	80% oral bioavailability	NMDA antagonism from *d*-isomer	
	Metabolism mainly CYP2B6		
	35 h terminal half-life		
	High protein binding (α_1- acid glycoprotein)		

Table 33.4. (*cont.*)

Drug	Absorption/metabolism	Clinical pharmacokinetics	Comments
Fentanyl	Extremely lipophilic	Rapid onset (peak 3–5 min)	Efficient absorption via transdermal, intranasal, buccal routes
	60% first-pass metabolism	Short duration after bolus, but significant prolongation with repeated dosing or infusion	
	Flow-dependent hepatic clearance		
	Mainly norfentanyl (CYP3A4)		
Alfentanil	Lipophilic (less than fentanyl)	Extremely rapid effect-site equilibrium	Interaction with erythromycin
	30% first-pass metabolism	Time to peak effect 90 s	
	N-dealkylation, O-dealkylation	Short duration after bolus, but longer with repeated dosing	
	Almost all CYP3A4		
Sufentanil	Extremely lipophilic	Rapid onset	Highly selective probe for μ-receptor
	70% first-pass metabolism	Short duration after bolus, less accumulation than fentanyl	
	N-dealkylation, O-dealkylation		
Remifentanil	Hydrolyzed by nonspecific esterases in tissues, especially skeletal muscle	Rapid effect-site equilibrium ($t_{1/2ke0} = 90$ s)	Not a substrate for pseudocholinesterase
	Metabolites have minimal activity	No accumulation with prolonged infusion	Possible tachyphylaxis with infusions (see text)
	Clearance 2–3 L min^{-1}	No postoperative pain relief	
Tramadol	Hepatic metabolism (CYP2D6)	Racemic mixture	Interaction with MAOI (serotonin syndrome)
	High oral bioavailability	(+)Tramadol is weak opioid agonist	Genetic polymorphisms in metabolism.
	Both oxidative metabolism and glucuronidation	(−)Tramadol inhibits NE reuptake	
	Active O demethylated metabolite	Partially reversed by naloxone	

The agonist-antagonist opioids have been used during balanced anesthesia, but their partial agonist properties are not a particular advantage in this setting. Even extremely large doses of nalbuphine or butorphanol will not produce the intensity of analgesia one expects from fentanyl or its derivatives [92]. Compared with morphine or fentanyl, the agonist-antagonists produce more limited decreases in the requirements for potent volatile anesthetics [93].

Sedation and mood effects

The subjective effects of buprenorphine are similar to morphine throughout the dose range. The κ-type agonists have been described as producing "apathetic sedation," which may reflect the localization of κ receptors in deeper layers of the cerebral cortex [94]. Patients given pentazocine, nalbuphine, or butorphanol may experience floating and dissociation, but usually do not experience mood elevation like that seen with morphine. After analgesic doses these patients often appear extremely sedated, yet remain capable of surprisingly lucid conversation. With pentazocine, patients are increasingly likely to experience "weird" feelings, dysphoria, or even hallucinations as the dose is raised. As stated previously, these unpleasant effects may also be mediated by κ receptors. They occur less frequently with butorphanol or nalbuphine.

significant problem. These patients are highly tolerant to opioids, and residual levels of the partial agonist may antagonize other opioids for a long time. Regional anesthesia and nonopioid techniques should be used, whenever possible. If opioid treatment is required, large doses of potent opioid agonists may be needed, and advice should be sought from a specialist in addiction medicine.

Opioid antagonists

Naloxone

The first pure opioid antagonist that became available for parenteral use is naloxone, the N-allyl derivative of oxymorphone. Naloxone is a competitive antagonist at all opioid receptors, but it has greatest affinity for μ receptors. Small doses of naloxone reliably reverse or prevent the effects of pure opioid agonists and most mixed agonist-antagonists. Naloxone probably has no effect on nonopioid anesthetics, although this remains somewhat controversial [107].

Given alone, naloxone is nearly devoid of clinically demonstrable effects. In humans, extremely large doses (4 mg kg^{-1}) cause a mild increase in heart rate and systolic blood pressure, as well as slowing of EEG alpha-wave activity. Animal studies have also shown that naloxone can reduce food intake, alter sleep patterns, and improve spatial learning. In some disease states such as septic shock, large doses can have a pressor effect. This may be the result of antagonism of elevated endogenous opioid peptides [108].

Naloxone is widely distributed and rapidly achieves effective concentrations in the CNS. Plasma and brain concentrations fall precipitously because of rapid redistribution. The drug is rapidly cleared by hepatic biotransformation, mainly to the 3-glucuronide. The clearance is very high (approximately 30 mL kg^{-1} min^{-1}), which suggests that extrahepatic elimination may be occurring. The terminal half-life is 1–2 hours. The onset of antagonist effect is extremely rapid, but the duration of action is quite brief. An intravenous dose of 0.4 mg will usually antagonize morphine for less than 1 hour; increasing the dose does not increase the duration appreciably. The duration of naloxone is nearly always shorter than that of the opioids it is used to antagonize.

The presence of excessive opioid effects is a common problem in the postoperative setting. Small incremental doses of naloxone (0.04 mg in an adult, repeated every 3 minutes) can be given intravenously, usually with dramatic improvement. In many cases there is partial reversal of analgesia as well, but this can be minimized by careful dosing. Patients who receive naloxone need continued observation, and possibly repeated doses. Postoperative ventilatory compromise is frequently caused by a combination of factors, and therapy with naloxone does not eliminate the need to search for and treat conditions such as residual paralysis, bronchospasm, and airway edema.

Naloxone is used to reverse opioids in several other clinical settings:

- In the delivery suite naloxone may be used in depressed neonates whose mothers received opioids during labor. When given via an umbilical vein catheter, 0.01 mg kg^{-1} was usually sufficient [109]. Acidotic infants were slower to reverse and sometimes required a second dose.
- In the emergency department, 0.4–0.8 mg of naloxone is usually administered in cases of suspected heroin overdose. Naloxone is also useful as an aid in the differential diagnosis of coma; if a patient fails to respond to naloxone, nonopioid causes should be considered.
- Patients who receive epidural or intrathecal opioids are frequently troubled by side effects such as pruritus and urinary retention (see Chapter 9). An intravenous infusion of naloxone will prevent or reverse these side effects, but it may also produce an unacceptable reduction in analgesia [110].

Opioid reversal can sometimes have important hemodynamic consequences. Increases in systemic pressure, heart rate, and plasma levels of catecholamines can occur. This may be because of the sudden onset of pain, but these effects have been reproduced experimentally in the absence of painful stimuli [111]. There have been several case reports of fulminant pulmonary edema, dysrhythmias, and even death in young, previously healthy individuals given naloxone [112]. In one case, the dose of naloxone was only 0.1 mg [113]. The etiology of this rare, catastrophic response is not known.

Naltrexone

This is the N-cyclopropylmethyl derivative of oxymorphone. It is a relatively pure antagonist like naloxone, available in both an oral preparation and a long-acting depot formulation. The main clinical use of naltrexone is in the treatment of previously detoxified heroin addicts. When high doses are taken chronically, naltrexone will block the euphoriant effects of injected heroin and thus help to prevent relapse. It also decreases drug craving in former addicts. Naltrexone more recently has been used to maintain sobriety in alcoholics, although the mechanism of action in this indication is less clear [114].

Naltrexone is rapidly absorbed and undergoes 95% first-pass metabolism to 6-β-naltrexol. This is an active metabolite that probably accounts for most of the naltrexone activity. The metabolite accumulates during chronic treatment and has a terminal half-life of 12.9 hours, so significant antagonist effects may persist for 2–3 days after naltrexone is stopped.

In the event that a patient on naltrexone requires emergency surgery or treatment for acute pain, he or she should be managed (if possible) with regional anesthesia, nonopioid analgesics, and other nonopioid methods. If opioids are necessary, naltrexone antagonism is competitive and may be overcome with high doses of morphine or fentanyl.

Nalmefene

Nalmefene is a potent, extremely long-lasting pure antagonist. It is the 6-methylene derivative of naltrexone. The effects of repeated fentanyl injections can be blocked for more than 8 hours by 2 mg of nalmefene [115]. The long duration of nalmefene effects is probably due to its extensive distribution and long terminal half-life (9 hours).

Reversal with nalmefene can probably cause some of the undesirable autonomic activation seen with naloxone. A single dose of nalmefene should prevent recrudescence of ventilatory depression in most cases, and infusions are unlikely to be necessary. Nalmefene should be titrated carefully, because it can potentially eliminate opioid analgesia for a very long period of time.

N-Methylnaltrexone

This antagonist is a quaternary analog of naltrexone, and its permanent charge means that it will not enter the CNS and therefore will not reverse central opioid effects such as analgesia [52]. It has been approved by the US Food and Drug Administration (FDA) to be given by subcutaneous injection for the treatment of opioid-induced bowel dysfunction (OBD) in cancer patients and other chronically ill patients receiving extended treatment with opioids [116,117]. These patients often experience debilitating and painful constipation, and methylnaltrexone is useful in the significant fraction who do not respond adequately to laxatives and stool softeners. Methylnaltrexone also rapidly relieves constipation in subjects on methadone maintenance (not an approved indication), although these individuals are extremely sensitive to very small doses of the antagonist [118]. This confirms that caution should be used whenever an opioid antagonist is administered to a patient with substantial previous opioid exposure. Efficacy of an experimental oral formulation suggests that methylnaltrexone action is achieved via an effect on opioid receptors on the luminal aspect of the bowel wall [119]. The primary side effects are cramping and abdominal pain, likely related to the mode of drug action. Methylnaltrexone, like naloxone, has minimal effects on opioid-naive persons.

Other opioid gastrointestinal effects can be reversed by methylnaltrexone. In healthy volunteers given morphine, intravenous methylnaltrexone reverses depression of gastric emptying and intestinal motility, but it does not interfere with analgesia against experimental pain [50,120]. This property may prove useful in facilitating enteral nutrition in critically ill patients receiving opioids [121].

Quaternary compounds (e.g., glycopyrrolate or quaternary lidocaine) have long been useful experimental tools for pharmacologists, and methylnaltrexone has proved useful in clinical and laboratory settings as a pharmacologic "probe" to distinguish central (CNS) versus peripheral actions of opioids. For example, opioid depression of urinary function was thought to be a completely central effect, but a recent study in human volunteers showed that intravenous methylnaltrexone could reverse some of the inability to void produced by an infusion of remifentanil [56]. Recent laboratory investigations using methylnaltrexone have demonstrated that it blocks opioid effects on fundamental cellular processes such as tumor angiogenesis, vascular permeability, and cellular responses to viral and bacterial infection [52]. The clinical implications of these findings are still unknown.

Alvimopan

Alvimopan is a zwitterion and, like methylnaltrexone, is a peripherally restricted opioid receptor antagonist [122]. It is poorly absorbed after oral administration, so effective doses reverse opioid effects on gastrointestinal transit but do not cross the blood–brain barrier and do not reverse opioid analgesia [123,124]. Alvimopan has been studied and FDA-approved exclusively in an oral formulation for the treatment and prevention of postoperative ileus. Its efficacy in this case may be due to the fact that surgical insult releases endogenous opioid peptides in the bowel wall, and this accounts for some of the postoperative decrease in intestinal motility [125]. In patients undergoing bowel resection there is a high incidence of postoperative ileus, and the use of alvimopan in this specific group of patients significantly improves motility and decreases the time to hospital discharge [126,127]. In most studies, alvimopan appeared to have a low incidence of side effects, but one study of chronic dosing unexpectedly found an excess incidence of serious cardiovascular events. This has not been confirmed in other studies, but the FDA has approved the drug under a Risk Evaluation and Mitigation Strategy that limits the drug to short-term, in-hospital use.

Summary

The opioid analgesics are widely used in all facets of anesthesia practice. The common agonists are selective for μ receptors and all produce a similar group of depressant and stimulant effects. The choice of opioid is usually based upon pharmacokinetic considerations, i.e., the desired onset and duration. For example, times to onset of clinical effect after intravenous bolus are remifentanil = alfentanil < fentanyl = sufentanil << morphine. Rates of intravenous opioid elimination are remifentanil >> alfentanil > morphine > hydromorphone > sufentanil > fentanyl >> methadone. Analgesic effects increase with increasing plasma concentration, and the threshold for analgesia occurs over a very small range of concentrations. There is wide interindividual variability in the concentration needed to produce analgesia, so opioids must be titrated to effect. They are most effective in acute nociceptive pain, but any pain can probably be treated. Their use in chronic noncancer pain is not supported by many well-controlled trials. More patients are undertreated for pain than overtreated. The opioid analgesics are abusable, but the risk of addiction from appropriate medical care is low.

Opioids produce sedation, but given alone they do not generally produce hypnosis. Opioids also cause dose-dependent ventilatory depression, and doses causing analgesia will probably always produce some detectable effect on ventilatory drive. Since the analgesic and ventilatory effects of opioids occur by similar mechanisms, (1) equianalgesic doses of all opioid agonists will produce about the same effect on ventilation, and thus no drug is any more dangerous or any safer than morphine; (2) opioid antagonist reversal of ventilatory depression almost always also causes some reversal of analgesia; (3) opioid tolerance requiring increased doses for pain relief will also cause tolerance to the ventilatory depressant effects of opioids.

The agonist-antagonist opioids are used for moderate, but not severe, pain. They are mainly κ partial agonists with limited toxicity, but also limited analgesic effect. All have some antagonist effects at μ receptors. Buprenorphine is a μ-receptor partial agonist that is being used for maintenance therapy in opioid addiction. The opioid antagonists, e.g., naloxone, can immediately reverse opioid effects and cause precipitated withdrawal in patients who are physically dependent. It is very difficult to reverse undesirable opioid effects such as ventilatory depression or itching without reversing some analgesia. Two newer quaternary opioid antagonists can be used to reverse opioid constipation without antagonizing central effects such as analgesia.

References

1. Brownstein MJ. A brief history of opiates, opioid peptides, and opioid receptors. *Proc Natl Acad Sci U S A* 1993; **90**: 5391–3.

2. McQuay HJ. Pharmacological treatment of neuralgic and neuropathic pain. *Cancer Surv* 1988; **7**: 141–59.

3. Chen SR, Pan HL. Blocking mu opioid receptors in the spinal cord prevents the analgesic action from subsequent systemic opioids. *Brain Res* 2006; **1081**: 119–25.

4. Manning BH, Mayer DJ. The central nucleus of the amygdale contributes to the production of morphine antinociception in the rat tail-flick test. *J Neurosci* 1995; **15**: 8199–213.

5. Kaiko RF, Wallenstein SL, Rogers AG, *et al.* Intramuscular meptazinol and morphine in postoperative pain. *Clin Pharmacol Ther* 1985; **37**: 589–96.

6. Austin KL, Stapleton JV, Mather LE. Multiple intramuscular injections: A major source of variability in analgesic response to meperidine. *Pain* 1980; **8**: 47–62.

7. Austin KL, Stapleton JV, Mather LE. Relationship between blood meperidine concentrations and analgesic response: A preliminary report. *Anesthesiology* 1980; **53**: 460–6.

8. Ausems ME, Hug CC, Stanski DR, *et al.* Plasma concentrations of alfentanil required to supplement nitrous oxide anesthesia for general surgery. *Anesthesiology* 1986; **65**: 362–73.

9. Rooke GA, Reves JG, Rosow CE. Anesthesiology and geriatric medicine: mutual needs and opportunities. *Anesthesiology* 2002; **96**: 2–4.

10. Scott JC, Stanski DR. Decreased fentanyl and alfentanil dose requirements with age. A simultaneous pharmacokinetic and pharmacodynamic evaluation. *J Pharmacol Exp Ther* 1987; **240**: 159–66.

11. Minto CF, Schnider TW, Egan TD, *et al.* Influence of age and gender on the pharmacokinetics and pharmacodynamics of remifentanil. I. Model development. *Anesthesiology* 1997; **86**: 10–23.

12. Aubrun F, Moncel S, Langeron O, *et al.* Postoperative titration of intravenous morphine in the elderly patient. *Anesthesiology* 2002; **96**: 17–23.

13. Hoke JF, Shlugman D, Dershwitz M, *et al.* Pharmacokinetics and pharmacodynamics of remifentanil in persons with renal failure compared with healthy volunteers. *Anesthesiology* 1997; **87**: 533–41.

14. Dershwitz M, Hoke JF, Rosow CE, *et al.* Pharmacokinetics and pharmacodynamics of remifentanil in volunteer subjects with severe liver disease. *Anesthesiology* 1996; **84**: 812–20.

15. Dahan A, Sarton E, Teppema L, *et al.* Sex-related differences in the influence of morphine on ventilatory control in humans. *Anesthesiology* 1998; **88**: 903–13.

16. Eichelbaum M, Evert B. Influence of pharmacogenetics on drug disposition and response. *Clin Exp Pharmacol Physiol* 1996; **23**: 983–5.

17. Caraco Y, Sheller J, Wood AJ. Impact of ethnic origin and quinidine coadministration on codeine's disposition and pharmacokinetic effects. *J Pharmacol Exp Ther* 1999; **290**: 413–22.

18. Gasche Y, Daali Y, Fathi M, *et al.* Codeine intoxication associated with ultrarapid CYP2D6 metabolism. *N Engl J Med.* 2004; **351**: 2827–31.

19. Cepeda MS, Farrar JT, Roa JH, *et al.* Ethnicity influences morphine pharmacokinetics and pharmacodynamics. *Clin Pharmacol Ther* 2001; **70**: 351–61.

20. Bailey PL, Wilbrink J, Zwanikken P, *et al.* Anesthetic induction with fentanyl. *Anesth Analg* 1985; **64**: 48–53.

21. Silbert BS, Rosow CE, Keegan CR, *et al.* The effect of diazepam on induction of anesthesia with alfentanil. *Anesth Analg* 1986; **65**: 71–7.

22. Kissin I, Vinik HR, Castillo R, *et al.* Alfentanil potentiates midazolam-induced unconsciousness in subanalgesic doses. *Anesth Analg* 1990; **71**: 65–9.

23. Short TG, Plummer JL, Chui PT. Hypnotic and anaesthetic interactions between midazolam, propofol and alfentanil. *Br J Anaesth* 1992; **69**: 162–7.

24. Dershwitz M, Rosow CE, DiBiase PM, *et al.* Comparison of the sedative effects of butorphanol and midazolam. *Anesthesiology* 1991; **74**: 717–24.

25. Shupak RC, Harp JR. Comparison between high-dose sufentaniloxygen and high-dose fentanyl-oxygen for neuroanesthesia. *Br J Anaesth* 1985; **57**: 375–81.

26. Weil JV, McCullough RE, Kline JS, *et al.* Diminished ventilatory response to hypoxia and hypercapnia after morphine in normal man. *N Engl J Med* 1975; **292**: 1103–6.

27. Pasternak GW. Multiple opiate receptors: déjà vu all over again. *Neuropharmacol* 2004; **47**: 312–23.

28. Pattinson KTS. Opioids and the control of respiration. *Br J Anaesth* 2008; **100**: 747–58.

29. Forrest WH, Bellville JW. The effect of sleep plus morphine on the respiratory response to carbon dioxide. *Anesthesiology* 1964; **25**: 137–41.

30. Becker LD, Paulson BA, Miller RD, *et al.* Biphasic respiratory depression after fentanyl-droperidol or fentanyl alone used to supplement nitrous oxide anesthesia. *Anesthesiology* 1976; **44**: 291–6.

31. Wang SC, Glaviano VV. Locus of emetic action of morphine and hydergine in dogs. *J Pharmacol Exp Ther* 1954; **111**: 329–34.

32. Costello DJ, Borison HL. Naloxone antagonizes narcotic self-blockade of emesis in the cat. *J Pharmacol Exp Ther* 1977; **203**: 222–30.

33. Kharasch ED, Walker A, Hoffer C, Sheffels P. Sensitivity of intravenous and oral alfentanil and pupillary miosis as minimally invasive and noninvasive probes for hepatic and first-pass CYP3A activity. *J Clin Pharmacol* 2005; **45**: 1187–97.

34. Kharasch ED, Hoffer C, Whittington D. Influence of age on the pharmacokinetics and pharmacodynamics of oral transmucosal fentanyl citrate. *Anesthesiology* 2004; **101**: 738–43.

35. Benthuysen JL, Smith NT, Sanford TJ, *et al.* Physiology of alfentanil induced rigidity. *Anesthesiology* 1986; **64**: 440–6.

36. Costall B, Fortune DH, Naylor RJ. Involvement of mesolimbic and extrapyramidal nuclei in the motor depressant action of narcotic drugs. *J Pharm Pharmacol* 1978; **30**: 566–72.

37. Weinger MB, Smith NT, Blasco TA, *et al.* Brain sites mediating opiate-induced muscle rigidity in the rat: Methylnaloxonium mapping study. *Brain Res* 1991; **544**: 181–90.

38. Arandia HY, Patil VU. Glottic closure following large dose of fentanyl. *Anesthesiology* 1987; **66**: 574–5.

39. Laubie M, Schmitt H, Vincent M. Vagal bradycardia produced by microinjections of morphine-like drugs into the nucleus ambiguus in anaesthetized dogs. *Eur J Pharmacol* 1979; **59**: 287–91.

40. Urthaler F, Isobe JH, James T. Direct and vagally mediated chronotropic effects of morphine studied by selective perfusion of the sinus node of awake dogs. *Chest* 1975; **68**: 222–8.

41. Lowenstein E, Whiting DA, Bittar CA, *et al.* Local and neurally mediated effects of morphine on skeletal muscle vascular resistance. *J Pharmacol Exp Ther* 1972; **180**: 359–67.

42. Green JF, Jackman AP, Krohm KA. Mechanism of morphine-induced shifts in blood volume between extracorporeal reservoir and the systemic circulation of the dog under conditions of constant blood flow and vena caval pressures. *Circ Res* 1978; **2**: 479–86.

43. Hsu HO, Hickey RF, Forbes AR. Morphine decreases peripheral vascular resistance and increases capacitance in man. *Anesthesiology* 1979; **50**: 98–102.

44. Ebert TJ, Kortly KJ. Fentanyl-diazepam anesthesia with or without nitrous oxide does not attenuate cardiopulmonary baroreflexmediated vasoconstrictor responses to controlled hypovolemia in humans. *Anesth Analg* 1988; **67**: 548–54.

45. Ward JW, McGrath RL, Weil JV. Effects of morphine on the peripheral vascular response to sympathetic stimulation. *Am J Cardiol* 1972; **29**: 659–66.

46. Rosow CE, Moss J, Philbin DM, *et al.* Histamine release during morphine and fentanyl anesthesia. *Anesthesiology* 1982; **56**: 93–6.

47. Philbin DM, Moss J, Rosow CE, *et al.* Histamine release with intravenous narcotics: protective effects of H1 and H2 receptor antagonists. *Klin Wochenschr* 1982; **60**: 1056–9.

48. Ballantyne JC, Loach AB, Carr DB. Itching after epidural and spinal opiates. *Pain* 1988; **33**: 149–60.

49. Kurz A, Sessler DI. Opioid-induced bowel dysfunction: pathophysiology and potential new therapies. *Drugs* 2003; **63**: 649–71.

50. Murphy DB, Sutton JA, Prescott LF, *et al.* Opioid-induced delay in gastric emptying: a peripheral mechanism in humans. *Anesthesiology* 1997; **87**: 765–70.

51. Steward JJ, Weisbrodt NW, Burks TF. Central and peripheral actions of morphine on intestinal transit. *J Pharmacol Exp Ther* 1978; **205**: 547–55.

52. Moss J, Rosow C. Development of peripheral opioid antagonists: new insights into opioid effects. *Mayo Clin Proc* 2008; **83**: 1116–30.

53. Radnay PA, Duncalf D, Novakovic M, *et al.* Common bile duct pressure changes after fentanyl, morphine, meperidine, butorphanol, and naloxone. *Anesth Analg* 1984; **63**: 441–4.

54. Malinovsky JM, Le Normand L, Lepage JY, *et al.* The urodynamic effects of intravenous opioids and ketoprofen in humans. *Anesth Analg* 1998; **87**: 456–61.

55. Baldini G, Bagry H, Aprikian A, Carli F. Postoperative urinary retention: Anesthetic and perioperative considerations. *Anesthesiology* 2009; **110**: 1139–57.

56. Rosow CE, Gomery P, Chen TY, *et al.* Reversal of opioid-induced bladder dysfunction by intravenous naloxone and methylnaltrexone. *Clin Pharmacol Ther* 2007; **82**: 48–53.

57. Cicero TJ, Bell RD, Wiest WG, *et al.* Function of the male sex organs in heroin and methadone users. *N Engl J Med* 1975; **292**: 882–7.

58. Bovill JG, Sebel PS, Fiolet JW. The influence of sufentanil on endocrine and metabolic responses to cardiac anesthesia. *Anesth Analg* 1983; **62**: 391–7.

59. Rosow CE. Acute and chronic tolerance: relevance for clinical practice. In: *Problems of Drug Dependence.* Research monograph 76, National Institute on Drug Abuse. Washington, DC: US Government Printing Office, 1987: 29–34.

60. Vinik HR, Kissin I. Rapid development of tolerance to analgesia during

remifentanil infusion in humans. *Anesth Analg* 1998; **86**: 1307–11.

61. Law PY, Loh HH, Wei LN. Insights into the receptor transcription and signaling: implications in opioid tolerance and dependence. *Neuropharmacol* 2004; **47**: 300–11.

62. Pasternak GW. Multiple opiate receptors: déjà vu all over again. *Neuropharmacol* 2004; **47**: 312–23.

63. Mao J, Price DD, Mayer DJ. Mechanisms of hyperalgesia and morphine tolerance: a current view of other possible interactions. *Pain* 1995; **62**: 259–74.

64. King T, Ossipov MH, Wanderah TW, *et al.* Is paradoxical pain induced by sustained opioid exposure an underlying mechanism of opioid antinociceptive tolerance? *Neurosignals* 2005; **14**: 194–205.

65. Trujillo KA, Akil H. Inhibition of morphine tolerance and dependence by the NMDA receptor antagonist MK-801. *Science* 1991; **251**: 85–7.

66. Elliott K, Minami N, Kolesnikov YA, *et al.* The NMDA receptor antagonists, LY274614 and MK-801, and the nitric oxide synthase inhibitor, NG-nitro-L-arginine, attenuate analgesic tolerance to the mu-opioid morphine but not to kappa opioids. *Pain* 1994; **56**: 69–75.

67. Porter J, Jick H. Addiction rare in patients treated with narcotics. *N Engl J Med* 1980; **302**: 123.

68. Portenoy RK. Chronic opioid therapy in nonmalignant pain. *J Pain Symptom Manage* 1990; **5**: S46–62.

69. Chou R, Ballantyne JC, Fanciullo GJ, Fine PG, Miaskowski C. Research gaps on use of opioids for chronic noncancer pain: findings from a review of the evidence for an American Pain Society and American Academy of Pain Medicine clinical practice guideline. *J Pain* 2009; **10**: 147–59.

70. Stein C. What is wrong with opioids in chronic pain? *Curr Opin Anaesth* 2000; **13**: 557–9.

71. Moulin DE, Iezzi A, Amireh R, *et al.* Randomized trial of oral morphine for chronic non-cancer pain. *Lancet* 1996; **347**: 143–7.

72. Watson CP, Babul N. Efficacy of oxycodone in neuropathic pain: A randomized trial in postherpetic neuralgia. *Neurology* 1998; **50**: 1837–41.

73. Caldwell JR, Hale ME, Boyd RE, *et al.* Treatment of osteoarthritis pain with controlled release oxycodone or fixed combination oxycodone plus acetaminophen added to nonsteroidal antiinflammatory drugs: a double blind, randomized, multicenter, placebo controlled trial. *J Rheumatol* 1999; **26**: 862–9.

74. Peloso PM, Bellamy N, Bensen W, *et al.* Double blind randomized placebo control trial of controlled release codeine in the treatment of osteoarthritis of the hip or knee. *J Rheumatol* 2000; **27**: 764–71.

75. Dershwitz M, Walsh JL, Morishige RJ, *et al.* Pharmacokinetics and pharmacodynamics of inhaled versus intravenous morphine in healthy volunteers. *Anesthesiology* 2000; **93**: 619–28.

76. Mather LE, Meffin PJ. Clinical pharmacokinetics of pethidine. *Clin Pharmacokinet* 1978; **3**: 352–68.

77. Inturrisi CE, Colburn WA, Kaiko RF, *et al.* Pharmacokinetics and pharmacodynamics of methadone in patients with chronic pain. *Clin Pharmacol Ther* 1987; **41**: 392–401.

78. Rab PV, Ritschel WA, Coyle DE, *et al.* Pharmacokinetics of hydromorphone after intravenous, peroral and rectal administration to human subjects. *Biopharm Drug Dispos* 1988; **9**: 187–99.

79. McClain DA, Hug CC. Intravenous fentanyl kinetics. *Clin Pharmacol Ther* 1980; **28**: 106–14.

80. Hudson RJ, Bergstrom RG, Thomson IR, *et al.* Pharmacokinetics of sufentanil in patients undergoing abdominal aortic surgery. *Anesthesiology* 1989; **70**: 426–31.

81. *Package label for Stadol.* www. bedfordlabs.com/BedfordLabsWeb/products/inserts/Div-BTP-P00.pdf (accessed May 28, 2010).

82. Jaillon P, Gardin ME, Lecocq B, *et al.* Pharmacokinetics of nalbuphine in infants, young healthy volunteers, and elderly patients. *Clin Pharmacol Ther* 1989; **46**: 226–33.

83. Bullingham RE, McQuay HJ, Moore A, Bennett MR. Buprenorphine kinetics. *Clin Pharmacol Ther* 1980; **28**: 667–72.

84. *Package label for Vicodin.* www. accessdata.fda.gov/drugsatfda_docs/label/2006/088058s027lbl.pdf (accessed May 28, 2010).

85. *Package label for Roxicodone.* www. accessdata.fda.gov/drugsatfda_docs/label/2009/021011s002lbl.pdf (accessed May 28, 2010).

86. *Package label for Dilaudid.* www. accessdata.fda.gov/drugsatfda_docs/label/2007/019892s015lbl.pdf (accessed May 28, 2010).

87. *Package label for Ultram.* www.accessdata. fda.gov/drugsatfda_docs/label/2004/20281slr030,21123slr001_Ultram_lbl.pdf (accessed May 28, 2010).

88. Mertens MJ, Olofsen E, Engbers FHM, *et al.* Propofol reduces perioperative remifentanil requirements in a synergistic manner. *Anesthesiology* 2003; **99**: 347–59.

89. Vuyk J, Lim T, Engbers FH, *et al.* The pharmacodynamic interaction of propofol and alfentanil during lower abdominal surgery in women. *Anesthesiology* 1995; **83**: 8–22.

90. Kazama T, Ikeda K, Morita K. Reduction by fentanyl of the Cp50 values of propofol and hemodynamic responses to various noxious stimuli. *Anesthesiology* 1997; **87**: 213–27.

91. Rance MJ. Multiple opiate receptors: their occurrence and significance. *Clin Anaesthesiol* 1983; **1**: 183–99.

92. Stanley TH, *et al.* The cardiovascular effects of high-dose butorphanol–nitrous oxide anaesthesia before and during operation. *Can Anaesth Soc J* 1983; **30**: 337–41.

93. Murphy MR, Hug CC. The enflurane sparing effect of morphine, butorphanol and nalbuphine. *Anesthesiology* 1982; **489**: 489–92.

94. Goodman RR, Snyder SH. Autoradiographic localization of kappa opiate receptors to deep layers of the cerebral cortex may explain unique sedative and analgesic effects. *Life Sci* 1982; **31**: 1291–4.

95. Gal TJ, DiFazio CA, Moscicki J. Analgesic and respiratory depressant activity of

nalbuphine: a comparison with morphine. *Anesthesiology* 1982; **57**: 367–74.

96. Nagashima H, Karamanian A, Malovany R, *et al*. Respiratory and circulatory effects of intravenous butorphanol and morphine. *Clin Pharmacol Ther* 1976; **19**: 738–45.

97. Gal TJ. Naloxone reversal of buprenorphine induced respiratory depression. *Clin Pharmacol Ther* 1989; **45**: 66–71.

98. Yassen A, Olofsen E, van Dorp E, *et al*. Mechanism-based pharmacokinetic-pharmacodynamic modeling of the reversal of buprenorphine-induced respiratory depression by naloxone: a study in healthy volunteers. *Clin Pharmacokinet* 2007; **46**: 965–80.

99. Arguelles JE, Franatovic Y, Romo-Salas, F, *et al*. Intrabiliary pressure changes produced by narcotic drugs and inhalation anesthetics in guinea pigs. *Anesth Analg* 1979; **58**: 120–3.

100. McCammon RL, Stoelting RK, Madura JA. Effects of butorphanol nalbuphine and fentanyl on intrabiliary tract dynamics. *Anesth Analg* 1984; **63**: 139–42.

101. Tigerstedt I, Turunen M, Tammisito T, *et al*. The effect of buprenorphine and oxycodone on the intracholedochal passage pressure. *Acta Anaesth Scand* 1981; **25**: 99–102.

102. Alderman EL, Barry WH, Graham AF, *et al*. Hemodynamic effects of morphine and pentazocine differ in cardiac patients. *N Engl J Med* 1972; **27**: 623–7.

103. Popio KA, Jackson DH, Ross AM, *et al*. Hemodynamic and respiratory effects of morphine and butorphanol. *Clin Pharmacol Ther* 1978; **23**: 281–7.

104. Jaffe RS, Moldenhauer CC, Hug CC, *et al*. Nalbuphine antagonism of fentanyl-induced ventilatory depression: a randomized trial. *Anesthesiology* 1988; **68**: 254–60.

105. Preston KL, Bigelow GE, Liebson IA. Butorphanol precipitated withdrawal in opioid dependent human volunteers. *J Pharmacol Exp Ther* 1988; **246**: 441–8.

106. Fudala PJ, Bridge TP, Herbert S, *et al*. Office-based treatment of opiate addiction with a sublingual-tablet formulation of buprenorphine and naloxone. *N Engl J Med* 2003; **349**: 949–58.

107. Finck AD, Ngai SH, Berkowitz BA. Antagonism of general anesthesia by naloxone in the rat. *Anesthesiology* 1977; **46**: 241–5.

108. Bernton EW, Long JB, Holaday JW. Opioids and neuropeptides: mechanisms in circulatory shock. *Fed Proc* 1985; **44**: 290–9.

109. Clark RB, Beard AG, Barclay DL. Naloxone in the newborn infant. *Anesthiol Rev* 1975; **2**: 9–11.

110. Gueneron JP, Ecoffey C, Carli P, *et al*. Effect of naloxone infusion on analgesia and respiratory depression after epidural fentanyl. *Anesth Analg* 1988; **67**: 35–8.

111. Mills CA, Flacke JW, Miller JD, *et al*. Cardiovascular effects of fentanyl reversal by naloxone at varying arterial carbon dioxide tensions in dogs. *Anesth Analg* 1988; **67**: 730–6.

112. Andrée RA. Sudden death following naloxone administration. *Anesth Analg* 1980; **59**: 782–4.

113. Partridge L, Ward CF. Pulmonary edema following low-dose naloxone administration. *Anesthesiology* 1986; **65**: 709–10.

114. Srisurapanont M, Jarusuraisin N. Opioid antagonists for alcohol dependence. *Cochrane Database Syst Rev* 2005; (1): CD001867.

115. Gal TJ, DiFazio CA. Prolonged antagonism of opioid action with intravenous nalmefene. *Anesthesiology* 1986; **64**: 175–80.

116. Boyd TA, Yuan CS. Methylnaltrexone: investigations in treating opioid bowel dysfunction. In: Yuan CS., ed., *Handbook of Opioid Bowel Syndrome*. New York, NY: Haworth, 2005: 197–221.

117. Thomas J, Karver S, Cooney GA, *et al*. Methylnaltrexone for opioid-induced constipation in advanced illness. *N Engl J Med* 2008; **358**: 2332–43.

118. Yuan CS, Foss JF, O'Connor M, *et al*. Methylnaltrexone for reversal of constipation due to chronic methadone use: a randomized controlled trial. *JAMA* 2000; **283**: 367–72.

119. Yuan CS, Foss JF, Osinski J, *et al*. The safety and efficacy of oral methylnaltrexone in preventing morphine-induced delay in oral-cecal transit time. *Clin Pharmacol Ther* 1997; **61**: 467–75.

120. Yuan CS, Foss JF, O'Connor M, *et al*. Methylnaltrexone prevents morphine-induced delay in oral-cecal transit time without affecting analgesia: a double-blind randomized placebo-controlled trial. *Clin Pharmacol Ther* 1996; **59**: 469–75.

121. Woo M, O'Connor M, Yuan CS, Moss J. Reversal of opioid-induced gastric dysfunction in a critically ill burn patient after methylnaltrexone. *Anesth Analg* 2008; **107**: 1965–7.

122. Foss JF, Schmidt WK. Management of opioid-induced bowel dysfunction and postoperative ileus: Potential role of alvimopan In: Yuan CS., ed., *Handbook of Opioid Bowel Syndrome*. New York, NY: Haworth, 2005: 223–249.

123. Foss JF, Fisher DM, Schmidt VD. Pharmacokinetics of alvimopan and its metabolite in healthy volunteers and patiens in postoperative ileus trials. *Clin Pharmacol Ther* 2008; **83**: 770–6.

124. Liu SS, Hodgson PS, Carpenter RL, Fricke JR. ADL 8–2698, a trans- 3,4-dimethyl-4-(3-hydroxyphenyl) piperidine, prevents gastrointestinal effects of intravenous morphine without affecting analgesia. *Clin Pharmacol Ther* 2001; **69**: 66–71.

125. Taguchi A, Sharma N, Saleem RM, *et al*. Selective postoperative inhibition of gastrointestinal opioid receptors. *N Engl J Med* 2001; **345**: 935–40.

126. Wolff BG, Michelassi F, Gerkin TM, *et al*. Alvimopan, a novel, peripherally acting mu opioid antagonist. Results of a multicenter, randomized, double-blind, placebo-controlled, Phase III trial of major abdominal surgery and postoperative ileus. *Ann Surg* 2004; **240**: 728–35.

127. Delaney CP, Weese JL, Hyman NH, *et al*. Alvimopan Postoperative Ileus Study Group, phase III trial of alvimopan, a novel, peripherally acting, mu opioid antagonist for postoperative ileus after major abdominal surgery. *Dis Colon Rectum* 2005; **48**: 1114–25.

Essential drugs in anesthetic practice
Nonsteroidal anti-inflammatory drugs

Nilesh Randive and Richard M. Langford

Introduction

Nonsteroidal anti-inflammatory drugs (NSAIDs or NAIDs) may also be referred to as nonsteroidal anti-inflammatory agents/analgesics (NSAIAs) or nonsteroidal anti-inflammatory medicines (NSAIMs). Possessing analgesic, antipyretic, and anti-inflammatory effects, the term *nonsteroidal* is used to distinguish these drugs from steroids, whose broad range of effects include similar eicosanoid-depressing, anti-inflammatory action. NSAID use is ubiquitous, and their utility as nonopioid analgesics is widely exploited. Prominent members of this group of drugs are aspirin, ibuprofen, diclofenac, and naproxen, which are available over the counter in many countries. Paracetamol (acetaminophen) also has antipyretic and analgesic properties, but is not anti-inflammatory and hence not an NSAID.

NSAIDs have been used in one form or another for centuries. Extracts and preparations from plants such as the willow tree, *Salix alba*, have been used for hundreds of years for relief from pain and fever. These plants contain derivatives of salicylic acid, which were characterized as their active components in the eighteenth century and were chemically synthesized for the first time in 1860. Commercial production of salicylates began by 1874, and reports of salicylate (5–6 g per day) being able to "cure" rheumatic disorders were first published in 1876. NSAIDs are used extensively to manage pain and inflammation associated with surgical procedures, inflammatory diseases such as osteoarthritis (OA) and rheumatoid arthritis (RA), and more moderate pain associated with migraine, dysmenorrhea, myalgia, and dental pain.

The mechanism of action of NSAIDs was described in 1971. It is characterized by the inhibition of the enzyme cyclooxygenase (COX, also known as prostaglandin endoperoxide synthase) resulting in the inhibition of prostaglandin (PG) production. In the late 1980s and early 1990s, a second isoform of COX, COX-2, was identified, cloned, and sequenced. The two isoforms of COX (COX-1 and COX-2) are distinct with respect to transcriptional regulation and tissue expression patterns. COX-2 is induced by cytokines in inflammatory cells such as macrophages and monocytes, in tissue at localized sites of injury, and in the spinal cord in response to tissue damage [1–4]. In contrast, COX-1 is constitutively expressed at low levels in many tissues and is responsible for maintaining homeostatic pathways, for example in platelets [5]. COX-2 may be important in certain physiologic processes, particularly in female reproduction [6,7].

Roles of cyclooxygenase and prostaglandins in pain

Mechanism of action

Pain perception involves the processes of nociception, in which extremes of temperature, painful mechanical stimuli, and noxious chemical stimuli are detected by primary afferent (nociceptive) neurons [8,9]. The details of transmission of nociceptive signals from peripheral nociceptors to the spinal cord and higher centers are reviewed in detail in Chapters 14 and 16.

Prostaglandins (PGs) are produced during inflammation by the action of COX. They increase the sensitivity of nociceptors and nociceptive neurons to other pain-producing stimuli, such as bradykinin, histamine, and serotonin, and to mechanical, chemical, and thermal stimuli (peripheral sensitization) (Fig. 34.1). For example, pretreatment of sensory neurons in culture with prostaglandin E_2 (PGE_2) potentiates bradykinin-mediated release of substance P, which contributes to hyperalgesia [10,11].

In the early stages of peripheral sensitization, PG release leads to post-translational protein modifications in the peripheral nociceptors and in dorsal horn neurons [8–10,12]. This sensitization enhances signal transduction and transmission within nociceptive neurons [9,12]. Translational and transcriptional changes within sensory neurons create a sensitized phenotype that potentiates nociception [13,14] and results in hyperalgesia and allodynia (central sensitization) (Fig. 34.1).

Prostaglandin synthesis and action

COX oxidizes arachidonate to form the endoperoxide derivative PGG_2 [15]. A wide variety of stimuli, including cytokines, hormones, allergens, neuropeptides, mechanical and oxidative

Anesthetic Pharmacology, 2nd edition, ed. Alex S. Evers, Mervyn Maze, Evan D. Kharasch. Published by Cambridge University Press. © Cambridge University Press 2011.

Chapter 34: Nonsteroidal anti-inflammatory drugs

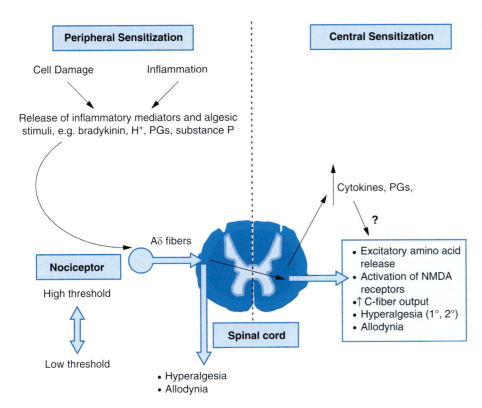

Figure 34.1. Peripheral and central sensitization to inflammatory pain. Cell damage and inflammatory stimuli in the periphery induce the release of mediators of inflammation and pain, which transmit signals through nociceptors and Aδ neurons to the central nervous system (CNS) leading to hyperalgesia and allodynia (peripheral sensitization). Peripheral sensitization, tissue injury, and inflammatory signals such as inflammatory cytokines act directly on the CNS to induce transcriptional and post-translational changes in the CNS (e.g., COX-2 upregulation) that increase pain sensitivity to mechanical, thermal, chemical, and inflammatory stimuli (central sensitization). NMDA, N-methyl-D-aspartate; PGs, prostaglandins.

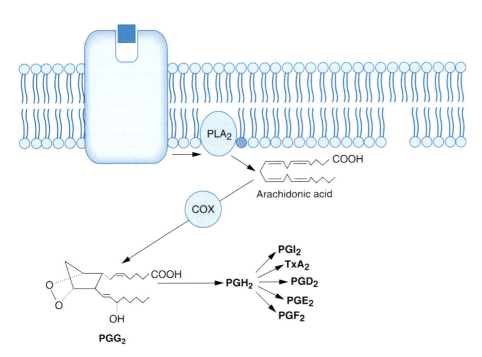

Figure 34.2. Cyclooxygenase (COX)-mediated prostaglandin (PG) production. Phospholipase A_2 (PLA_2) converts membrane phospholipids to arachidonate in response to cytokines and other extracellular stimuli, binding to membrane receptors. Arachidonate is further metabolized by COX to prostaglandin G_2 (PGG_2), the precursor for a variety of other prostaglandins including PGI_2, thromboxane A_2 (TxA_2), PGD_2, PGE_2, and $PGF_{2\alpha}$.

stress, and tissue damage activate phospholipases (PLAs) through G proteins and intracellular kinases [16]. Released arachidonate is available for oxidation by COX to the endoperoxide, PGG_2, and then to PGH_2, the unstable precursor of all PGs and thromboxane (Tx) [15]. The biologically active PGs and Tx are formed in a tissue-specific manner by PGE_2, PGD, and PGF isomerases, and by prostacyclin (PGI_2) and TxA_2 synthase (Fig. 34.2) [15].

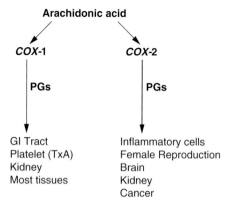

Figure 34.3. Differential expression of COX-1 and COX-2 isoenzymes in different tissues. COX-1 is constitutively expressed in most tissues including platelets and in epithelial cells of the gastric mucosa and intestine. In contrast, COX-2 is induced in response to inflammatory stimuli, including inflammatory cytokines such as interleukin 1β (IL-1β) and tumor necrosis factor α (TNFα), in inflammatory cells, in sites of inflammation and tissue damage, in the synovium of joints, in endothelial cells, and in the central nervous system. NSAIDs are nonselective inhibitors of both isoforms of COX, whereas COX-2-specific inhibitors do not inhibit COX-1 at therapeutic doses. GI, gastrointestinal; PGs, prostaglandins; TxA, thromboxane A.

Each of the PGs interacts with cognate G-protein-coupled receptors. Single receptor types have been identified for $PGF_{2\alpha}$, PGI_2, and TxA_2 (referred to as FP, IP, and TP, respectively), two subtypes of the PGD_2 (DP) receptor are known, and four distinct PGE_2 (EP) receptors have been identified [17].

COX expression and action

There are two distinct isoforms of COX (COX-1 and COX-2) associated with PG production. COX-1 and COX-2 are encoded by two genes that are differentially expressed across a variety of tissues [17,18]. COX-1 is constitutively expressed in many tissues, including lung, liver, spleen, kidney, and stomach [5]. In particular, COX-1 is expressed in platelets and in the gastric mucosa (Fig. 34.3). Nonspecific inhibition of COX-1 in these tissues by conventional NSAIDs results in reduced platelet aggregation, prolonged bleeding, damage to gastric mucosa, and gastrointestinal (GI) tract erosion and ulceration [19–22]. COX-2, the analgesic target for conventional NSAIDs and COX-2-specific inhibitors, is induced in inflamed tissues in response to mitogenic stimuli and inflammatory cytokines such as interleukin 1 (IL-1) and tumor necrosis factor α (TNFα) [1–3,5,23,24]. COX-2 is also expressed in the spinal cord and the brain [4,25–27] (Fig. 34.3), and may be involved in pain signaling and perception processes.

Peripheral COX-2 expression in response to tissue damage

The animal models of inflammation and pain have demonstrated that PGs are produced at the site of inflammation and that inhibition of their production by NSAIDs reduces swelling and nociception. A correlation between tissue damage, inflammation, and COX-2 expression has also been shown in

animal surgical models. For example, COX-2 mRNA and protein levels were increased in rat hepatocytes 3 hours after a partial hepatectomy, whereas COX-1 and PLA_2 levels were unchanged [28].

Increased production of PGs at localized sites of injury has also been demonstrated in many human surgical models. Increased PG production, particularly PGE_2, has been demonstrated in tissue surrounding surgical sites in patients who have undergone oral surgery and after major surgical procedures [29–31]. In addition, increased levels of COX-2, but not COX-1, have been demonstrated in synovial tissue and cartilage from patients with inflammatory disease such as RA and OA [32–34].

Neuronal plasticity and COX-2

Evidence in animals supports widespread induction of COX-2 in the central nervous system following peripheral tissue injury. Allodynia, artificially induced in rats by the ligation of the left lumbar L5 and L6 spinal nerves, was associated with increased expression of COX-2 protein in the dorsal spinal cord and thalamus [35]. Low basal levels of COX-2 are detectable in rat dorsal horn neurons and substantial upregulation of COX-2 mRNA and protein occurs in response to injection of carrageenan or Freund's complete adjuvant into a paw [25,26,36]. The induction of COX-2 in the spinal cord is associated with marked hyperalgesia and a substantial increase of PGE_2 in cerebrospinal fluid (CSF). Freund's complete adjuvant also leads to massive upregulation of IL-1β at the injection site and in the CSF, and also increased expression of type I IL-1β receptors [36]. IL-1β given systemically is a potent hyperalgesic agent [37]. It is postulated that the proinflammatory cytokines (interleukin 1β and 6) are responsible for transducing the signal across the blood–brain barrier and within the central nervous system (CNS). It has been proposed that PGE_2 in the CNS may thereby contribute to central sensitization to pain (hyperalgesia) [36,38]. As central inhibition of COX-2 prevents these changes in animals, there is interest in the clinical utility of NSAIDs with greater CNS penetration [38,39].

Structure of NSAIDs

NSAIDs can be classified according to their chemical structure, as shown in Table 34.1. Most NSAIDs are chiral molecules (diclofenac is a notable exception) and formulated as a racemic mixture. Typically, only a single enantiomer is pharmacologically active. For some drugs (typically profens), an isomerase enzyme exists in vivo, which converts the inactive enantiomer into the active form, although there is wide interindividual variability in this enzyme's activity. This phenomenon is likely to be responsible for the poor correlation between NSAID efficacy and plasma concentration observed in older studies, when specific analysis of the active enantiomer was not performed.

Ibuprofen and ketoprofen are now available in single active-enantiomer preparations (dexibuprofen and dexketoprofen),

Table 34.1. Classification of NSAIDs according to chemical structure

Group: chemical structure	Drug examples
Salicylates	Acetylsalicylic acid (aspirin), amoxiprin, benorylate, choline magnesium salicylate, difunisal, ethenzamide, faislamine, methyl salicylate, magnesium salicylate, salicyl salicylate, salicylamide
Arylalkanoic acids	Diclofenac, aceclofenac, acemethacin, alclofenac, bromfenac, etodolac, indomethacin, nabumetone, oxametacin, proglumetacin, sulindac, tolmentin
2-Arylpropionic acids (profens)	Ibuprofen, aminoprofen, benoxaprofen, carprofen, dexibuprofen, dexketoprofen, fenbufen, fenoprofen, flunoxaprofen, flurbiprofen, ibuproxam, indoprofen, ketoprofen, ketorolac, loxoprofen, naproxen, oxaprozin, pirprofen, suprofen, tiaprofenic acid
N-Arylanthranilic acids (fenamic acids)	Mefenamic acid, flufenamic acid, meclofenamic acid, tolfenamic acid
Pyrazolidine derivatives	Phenylbutazone, ampyrone, azapropazone, clofezone, kebuzone, metamizole, mofebutazone, oxyphenbutazone, phenazone, sulfinpyrazone
Oxicams	Piroxicam, droxicam, lornoxicam, meloxicam, tenoxicam
Sulfonamides/ sulfones	Celecoxib, lumiracoxib, valdecoxib, parecoxib, rofecoxib, etoricoxib
Sulfonanilides	Nimesulide
Others	Licofelone, omega-3 fatty acids

which purport to offer quicker onset and an improved side-effect profile. Naproxen has always been marketed as the single active enantiomer.

Nonspecific and specific COX isoform inhibition

Conventional NSAIDs are nonselective inhibitors of both COX-1 and COX-2. The anti-inflammatory activity of NSAIDs is mediated by inhibition of COX-2 [24]. Individual NSAIDs function by binding to and blocking the active site of COX, although their inhibition kinetics vary considerably. X-ray crystallography studies have advanced our understanding of the inhibitory mechanism of conventional NSAIDs and the

selectivity of COX-2-specific inhibitors [40,41]. The crystal structure of COX-1 reveals that the substrate-binding site of the enzyme is located within the catalytic domain in a pocket surrounded by three α-helices at the mouth of the channel, with charged amino acid residues at each turn in the helices [40,41]. Conventional NSAIDs bind to a charged arginine residue (Arg-120) near the active site of the enzyme, thereby blocking substrate access to amino acid residues such as tyrosine-385 that are essential for catalysis [42,43].

Differences in amino acid residues at the active sites of COX-1 and COX-2 account for the selectivity of COX-2-specific inhibitors, the most critical of which seems to be the substitution of the valine residue (Val-509) in COX-2 for isoleucine in COX-1 [44]. In the COX-2 isoform, the valine residue, with its smaller side chain, makes a side pocket adjacent to the active site accessible to COX-2-specific inhibitors [45,46]. In contrast, the COX-1 substrate channel is much narrower, because of the presence of the larger isoleucine residue, and therefore is unable to accommodate the COX-2-specific inhibitors with their bulky side chains (Fig. 34.4).

Clinical pharmacology
Nonspecific NSAIDs

Nonspecific NSAIDs are a heterogeneous class of compounds, often chemically unrelated, which share a similar therapeutic and side-effect profile [47,48]. The pharmacokinetic properties of some of the most commonly used NSAIDs are described in Table 34.2. The rates of absorption of NSAIDs are affected by a number of factors [48,49]. Consumption of NSAIDs with food often delays their absorption because of the reduction in the rate of gastric emptying. The formulation of NSAIDs affects absorption, and for most compounds soluble preparations are more rapidly absorbed [48]. However, enteric-coated tablets and sustained-release preparations have demonstrated improved bioavailability [49,50]. Absorption, peak plasma concentration, and metabolism of NSAIDs can also be significantly affected by GI pH, patient age, concomitant administration of other drugs, and the disease state of the patient [48–55]. Elimination of conventional NSAIDs is largely dependent on hepatic biotransformation and renal excretion. Therefore patients with hepatic and renal disease often demonstrate greater and more prolonged peak plasma concentrations, because rates of metabolism and elimination of the drugs are often reduced [48].

Absorption

In general, conventional NSAIDs are rapidly and well absorbed from the GI tract. Orally administered aspirin is rapidly absorbed by passive diffusion of nonionized lipophilic molecules, but it also undergoes a high degree of presystemic hydrolysis to form salicylate before absorption [49]. The

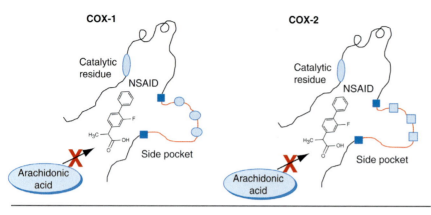

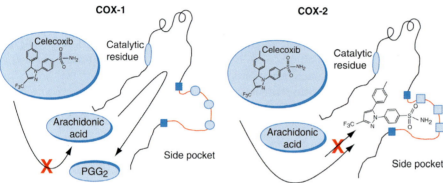

Figure 34.4. Cyclooxygenase 1 (COX-1) and COX-2 inhibition: mechanism of action. Conventional nonsteroidal anti-inflammatory drugs (NSAIDs) inhibit COX-1 and COX-2 by binding to the active site in the catalytic domain of the protein. COX-2-specific inhibitors such as celecoxib are characterized by a bulky side chain, which prohibits binding of the inhibitor in the narrow catalytic pocket of COX-1. A single amino acid change in the catalytic pocket of COX-2 exposes a side pocket that is able to accommodate the bulky side chain of COX-2-specific inhibitors.

remainder is hydrolyzed to salicylate after absorption (half-life [$t_{1/2}$] 15–20 minutes) by nonspecific esterases found in many body tissues [56]. Commercially available suppositories and soluble or enteric-coated tablet preparations of diclofenac are reported to be almost totally absorbed in the GI tract [57,58]. However, other reports suggest that diclofenac undergoes presystemic elimination, with ~ 60% of the initial dose detected in the systemic circulation unchanged.

Oral doses of ibuprofen are rapidly and almost completely absorbed (> 80%) in the GI tract [48–51]. Ibuprofen exists as two enantiomers, R(–) ibuprofen and S(+) ibuprofen. The majority of the anti-inflammatory and analgesic effects of ibuprofen have been attributed to the S enantiomer. The R enantiomer undergoes unidirectional metabolic inversion to form the S enantiomer [51]. It has been suggested that the rate of bioinversion of ibuprofen is affected by the rate of absorption. The longer ibuprofen remains in the GI tract the more likely it is that presystemic conversion will occur, thereby increasing the S:R enantiomer ratio [59]. A significant correlation between the S:R ratio and time to peak plasma concentration (T_{max}) has been observed, with a greater S:R area under the time-concentration curve (AUC) ratio in individuals with a longer T_{max}, suggesting that the absorption rate is dependent on enantiomer conversion [60]. Detection of S(+) ibuprofen after intravenous administration of R(–) ibuprofen also suggests systemic enantiomer conversion. Oral, intramuscular, and subcutaneous doses of ketorolac are rapidly absorbed, reaching

maximum concentration (C_{max}) in 30–60 minutes [54,55, 61,62]. The relative bioavailability after oral, intramuscular, and intravenous administration is 80–100%. Oral naproxen is rapidly and almost completely absorbed whether it is administered in suspension, capsule, or tablet form. Naproxen suppositories are also readily absorbed, with 94.6% bioavailability compared with tablets [52].

Paracetamol is not classified as an NSAID because it lacks anti-inflammatory activity, yet it is frequently used to treat similar conditions (i.e., acute and chronic pain). Paracetamol displays analgesic and antipyretic actions similar to aspirin and should therefore be considered in any discussion of conventional NSAIDs [63]. Oral paracetamol is rapidly absorbed from the GI tract with C_{max} reached 20–90 minutes after ingestion. Its systemic bioavailability is dose-dependent and ranges from 70% to 90%, being reduced by first-pass metabolism. Similar to NSAIDs, the absorption of paracetamol is heavily dependent on factors such as the rate of gastric emptying, pH, and formulation.

Distribution

All conventional NSAIDs are highly bound to plasma proteins, particularly albumin, limiting their distribution to extracellular spaces. As a result, volumes of distribution are often very low (< 0.2 L kg^{-1}) [48]. At therapeutic concentrations, a high proportion of NSAIDs such as salicylate (80–90%) [49], diclofenac (99%) [50,53], ibuprofen (99%) [51], ketorolac (99%)

Table 34.2. Pharmacokinetic parameters of commonly used conventional NSAIDs and COX-2-specific inhibitors

NSAID/COX-2-specific inhibitors	C_{max} (peak plasma concentration)	T_{max}	$t_{1/2}$	Clearance	Excretion
Aspirin	150–300 µg mL^{-1}				Excreted as salicylic acid or as glycine, glucuronidate conjugates
Soluble		25 min	0.25 h	39 L h^{-1}	
Tablet		4–6 h			
Diclofenac 50 mg					90% excreted within 96 h
Soluble	0.7–1.2 µg mL^{-1}	10–40 min	1–1.5 h	15.6 L h^{-1}	
Tablet	0.5–1.5 µg mL^{-1}	1.5–2 h			
Ibuprofen					70–90% excreted within 24 h
Solution 300 mg	37.9 mg mL^{-1}	1.39 h	2–2.5 h	~ 0.04–0.1 L hr^{-1} kg^{-1}	
Tablet 200–400 mg	20–30 mg mL^{-1}	~ 3 h			
Ketorolac 10 mg					91% excreted within 2 days (75% as glucuronidate conjugate, ~ 12% as para-hydroxylated form)
Intravenous	2.39 µg mL^{-1}	5 min		~ 0.01 L hr^{-1} kg^{-1}	
Intramuscular	0.6–1.44 µg mL^{-1}	20–60 min	~ 5 h	~ 0.01 L hr^{-1} kg^{-1}	
Oral (tablet)	0.7–0.9 µg mL^{-1}	1 h		~ 0.3 L hr^{-1} kg^{-1}	
Naproxen 250–500 mg	20–80 µg mL^{-1}		12–15 h	0.3 L h^{-1}	~ 80% of daily does excreted as glucuronidate conjugates
Paracetamol 0.5–2 g		20–90 min	1.9–2.5 h	~ 20–30 L h^{-1}	~ 85–95% excreted within 24 h
Celecoxib 100–200 mg	0.6–0.7 µg mL^{-1}	2–4 h	11.2–15.6 h	~ 20–40 L h^{-1}	< 2% recovered unchanged in urine
Rofecoxib 25–50 mg	207 µg mL^{-1}	2–3 h	~ 17 h	~ 7 L h^{-1}	< 1% recovered unchanged in urine
Parecoxib sodium intravenous 10–20 mg					~ 95% excreted 5–8 h
Parecoxib	2–4 µg mL^{-1}	2–3 min	15–40 min	~ 30–35 L h^{-1}	
Valdecoxib	0.1–0.4 µg mL^{-1}	1 h	5–8 h	~ 6.5–7.5 L h^{-1}	
Parecoxib sodium intramuscular 10–20 mg					~ 95% excreted 5–8 h
Parecoxib	0.4–1 µg mL^{-1}	~ 15 min	~ 0.5 h	~ 35–38 L h^{-1}	
Valdecoxib	0.13–0.27 µg mL^{-1}	~ 2.5 h	5.5–10 h	~ 6–8 L h^{-1}	

[54,55], and naproxen (99.6%) are bound to plasma protein. NSAIDs are generally distributed throughout most body tissues, including synovial fluid and CSF. Total concentrations are generally lower in the synovium and CSF than in plasma, and T_{max} is longer; but lower protein concentrations in these fluids generally lead to lower concentrations of protein-bound NSAIDs, and elimination time is longer [48]. However, unlike NSAIDs, paracetamol does not bind to plasma proteins at therapeutic doses, although approximately 15–20% of the drug is bound at concentrations associated with an overdose [63]. Therefore paracetamol is distributed throughout most tissues, and its elimination is very rapid.

healing are conflicting and difficult to interpret because of species differences in COX expression

A review of success after spinal fusion surgery revealed non-union to be greater in the ketorolac group (17%) compared with controls (4%) [89]. In another retrospective audit, long-term NSAID use was found to be more common in patients with non-union of femoral diaphysis fractures (62.5%), compared to only 13.4% of the "comparable control" group [90]. Adequately powered randomized controlled trials designed to tackle this issue are required to address the concerns regarding NSAIDs in bone healing, and to examine whether COX-1 and COX-2 blockade have different profiles.

Hepatic safety

Hepatotoxicity can occur with all NSAIDs, but appears to be more common with diclofenac and sulindac. It is more common in the first 3 months of therapy, and with increased risk in female patients, age > 50 years, with autoimmune disease, and in the presence of concomitant potentially hepatotoxic drugs [91].

Although hepatotoxicity usually resolves within 4–6 weeks of cessation of the NSAID therapy, severe acute liver failure may occur in rare cases. Cited mechanisms of diclofenac toxicity are impairment of ATP synthesis by mitochondria and production of active metabolites, particularly N,5-dihydroxydiclofenac, which causes direct cytotoxicity.

Two anti-inflammatory drugs have been restricted or withdrawn as a result of hepatic safety concerns. Nimesulide has been limited to a maximum of 15 days in some countries [92], and lumiracoxib was withdrawn following a number of spontaneous reports of serious hepatic dysfunction.

Drug–drug interactions

Nonsteroidal anti-inflammatory agents are used routinely to manage pain and inflammation, and many formulations are available in nonprescription form. Therefore the likelihood of coadministration with other drugs is high and may have implications for the absorption, pharmacokinetics, and elimination of either compound [48].

Conventional NSAIDs are associated with increased bleeding risks, including prolonged postoperative bleeding and upper GI bleeding, because of their inhibition of COX-1 [19]. It is therefore important when prescribing these drugs to consider the potential for increased bleeding risks associated with the coadministration of NSAIDs with anticoagulant agents (e.g., the coumarin derivative warfarin). Pyrazole NSAIDs, like phenylbutazone, have been shown to be particularly hazardous when coadministered with warfarin; and aspirin, at the high doses used for the treatment of severe pain (> 3 g per day), can cause increased bleeding when administered with warfarin [93–95]. COX-2-specific inhibitors, however, do not appear to have any significant interactions with anticoagulant agents [64,66]. The steady-state concentration of

warfarin is not altered by coadministration with celecoxib, and prothrombin times are not significantly affected [64,65]. Rofecoxib has shown clinically insignificant interactions with warfarin, although coadministration of the two drugs results in an 8% increase in prothrombin time in healthy subjects [66]. Coadministration of the COX-2-specific inhibitor parecoxib sodium with aspirin, administered at doses recommended for cardiovascular prophylaxis, does not appear to cause any clinically significant changes in the effects of aspirin on platelet aggregation or bleeding times [96]. Currently, there are no published data on the interaction of valdecoxib with anticoagulants.

In multimodal pain therapy, NSAIDs are frequently administered with opioid agents to enhance their analgesic potential, particularly in the treatment of postoperative pain [97].

Clinical context

Although NSAIDs have a well-established place in treating acute and chronic pain, continuing evaluation is justified regarding safety and the place of selective COX inhibitors. In chronic pain, safety concerns have driven revised prescribing strategies including the use of coxibs (European League against Rheumatism, American College of Rheumatology, NICE, and European Medicines Evaluation Agency). The voluntary worldwide withdrawal of rofecoxib in September 2004 led to widespread review of the safety of long-term NSAID and coxib usage [98,99].

By contrast, relatively little attention has been paid to the acute pain context, but it is important to separate the issues surrounding long-term use for chronic conditions from very short-term use for postoperative pain. The morphine-sparing and multimodal roles of NSAIDs are well established in acute pain management. A systematic qualitative review of 41 double-blind and randomized studies comparing paracetamol with NSAIDs concluded NSAIDs to be more effective, and that their combination conferred additional analgesic efficacy [100].

So, the question is whether coxibs confer any advantages. Clearly, in view of their cardiovascular safety profile, they are contraindicated in patients with known atherosclerotic disease and those at risk of thrombotic cardiovascular events. However, following the restrictions placed on the use of ketorolac perioperatively, the case is strengthened for a parenteral coxib drug in short-term use in an acute perioperative situation in patients with low risk of cardiovascular events. Devoid of bleeding risk, it can be administered pre- or intraoperatively, and onset prior to awakening may reduce the requirement for pain relief in the early postoperative period. A similar case holds in areas of surgery such as head and neck surgery, in which NSAIDs may traditionally be avoided. It is evident that coxibs are not as safe as initially thought, and they should be reserved for patients at low risk for thromboembolic events. Such adjunctive therapy reduces patients' opioid requirements in the range of 30–40%, with both improved pain relief and reduced opioid-associated side effects, such as nausea and vomiting.

Summary

Nonsteroidal anti-inflammatory drugs (NSAIDs) have analgesic, antipyretic, and anti-inflammatory effects that are exploited for the relief of pain and inflammation, both postoperatively and in the context of inflammatory disease, as well as for managing moderate acute pain. The NSAID group encompasses drugs with a range of chemical structures that mediate their actions via inhibition of cyclooxygenase (COX).

COX catalyzes the production of prostaglandin precursor, PGH_2, and prostaglandins act on peripheral nociceptors and nociceptive neurons, increasing their sensitivity to pain-inducing stimuli. The enzyme exists as two distinct isoforms. COX-1 is constitutively expressed in many tissues, including platelets, and in gastric mucosa. Evidence indicates that tissue inflammation in the periphery induces local expression of COX-2, as well as COX-2 expression in the central nervous system.

While the anti-inflammatory properties of the NSAIDs are mediated by inhibition of COX-2, conventional NSAIDs are nonselective COX inhibitors. The absorption, peak plasma concentration, metabolism, and elimination of NSAIDs is affected by gastrointestinal pH and rate of gastric emptying, drug formulation, patient age, drug interactions, and disease state, in particular the presence of hepatic or renal disease. Plasma protein binding results in a low volume of distribution for conventional NSAIDs, whereas paracetamol does not bind plasma proteins at therapeutic doses. COX-2-specific inhibitors (coxibs) include the orally administered drugs celecoxib and valdecoxib, and the parenterally administered parecoxib

sodium, and the kinetics of these agents are similarly affected by a number of factors.

Conventional NSAIDs and COX-2 inhibitors have been associated with increased cardiovascular risk, with the focus on long-term use. Some coxibs were withdrawn as a result of concerns. Coxibs are contraindicated for short-term use in cardiac surgical patients. There is evidence for gastrointestinal ulcer formation resulting from use of nonselective NSAIDs. Both COX-1 and COX-2 are constitutively expressed in the kidney, and transient sodium and water retention, hypertension, and edema are possible side effects occurring in the initial period of NSAID use; caution should be exercised in using NSAIDs in surgical patients with impaired renal function, perioperative dehydration, hypovolemia, or hypotension.

NSAIDs induce bronchospasm in some asthmatics, although there is some evidence that COX-2-selective blockade can be cautiously considered for use in aspirin-sensitive asthmatics. Nonselective NSAIDs may reduce platelet aggregation, and therefore the use of these drugs is discouraged in surgery where the potential for increased risk of perioperative bleeding might be particularly problematic. There have also been concerns regarding impeded bone healing with NSAID use, although further studies are required. Hepatotoxicity is a possibility with all NSAIDs, though the risk varies with specific agent, stage of therapy, sex, age, and the presence of certain disease states and other drugs. Hepatic safety concerns have led to the restriction and withdrawal of nimesulide and lumiracoxib, respectively. Coadministration of conventional NSAIDs with anticoagulant agents has the potential for increased bleeding risks, whilst coadministration of NSAIDs with opioids can improve pain relief and reduce opioid requirements.

References

1. Huang Z, Massey J. Differential regulation of cyclooxygenase-2 (COX-2) mRNA stability by interleukin-1 β (IL-1 β) and tumor necrosis factor-α (TNF- α) in human in vitro differentiated macrophages. *Biochem Pharmacol* 2000; **59**: 187–94.

2. Porreca E, Reale M, Febbo CD, *et al.* Down-regulation of cyclooxygenase-2 (COX-2) by interleukin-receptor antagonist in human monocytes. *Immunology* 1996; **89**: 424–9.

3. Kang RY, Freire-Moar, Sigal E, *et al.* Expression of cyclooxygenase-2 in human and an animal model of rheumatoid arthritis. *Br J Rheumatol* 1996; **35**: 711–18.

4. Vanegas H, Schaible HG. Prostaglandins and cyclooxygenases in the spinal cord. *Prog Neurobiol* 2001; **64**: 327–63.

5. Seibert K, Zhang Y, Leahy K, *et al.* Pharmacological and biochemical demonstration of the role of cyclooxygenase 2 in inflammation and pain. *Proc Natl Acad Sci U S A* 1994; **91**: 12013–17.

6. Matsumoto H, Ma W, Smalley W, *et al.* Diversification of cyclooxy-genase-2-derived prostaglandins in ovulation and implantation. *Biol Reprod* 2001; **64**: 1557–65.

7. Pall M, Friden B, Brännström M. Induction of delayed follicular rupture in the human by the selective COX-2 inhibitor rofecoxib: A randomized

double-blind study. *Hum Reprod* 2001; **16**: 1323–8.

8. Doubell TP, Mannion RJ, Woolf CJ. The dorsal horn: state-dependent sensory processing, plasticity and the generation of pain. In: Wall PD, Melzack R, eds., *Textbook of Pain.* Hong Kong: Churchill Livingstone, 1999.

9. Woolf CJ, Salter MW. Neuronal plasticity: increasing the gain in pain. *Science* 2000; **288**: 1765–9.

10. Vasko MR, Campbell WB, Waite KJ. Prostaglandin E2 enhances bradykinin-stimulated release of neuropeptides from rat sensory neurons in culture. *J Neurosci* 1994; **14**: 4987–97.

11. Okano K, Kuraishi Y, Satoh M. Involvement of spinal substance P and excitatory amino acids in inflammatory

hyperalgesia in rats. *Jpn J Pharmacol* 1998; **76**: 15–22.

12. Woolf CJ, Mannion RJ. Neuropathic pain: aetiology, symptoms, mechanisms, and management. *Lancet* 1999; **353**: 1959–64.

13. Mannion RJ, Costigan M, Decosterd I, *et al.* Neurotrophins: peripherally and centrally acting modulators of tactile stimulus-induced inflammatory pain hypersensitivity. *Proc Natl Acad Sci U S A* 1999; **96**: 9385–90.

14. Neumann S, Doubell TP, Leslie T, *et al.* Inflammatory pain hypersensitivity mediated by phenotypic switch in myelinated primary sensory neurons. *Nature* 1996; **384**: 360–4.

15. O'Banion MK. Cyclooxygenase-2: molecular biology, pharmacology, and neurobiology. *Crit Rev Neurobiol* 1999; **13**: 45–82.

16. Dorsam G, Taher MM, Valerie KC, *et al.* Diphenyleneiodium blocks inflammatory cytokine-induced up-regulation of group IIA phospholipase A$_2$ in rat mesangial cells. *J Pharmacol Exp Ther* 2000; **292**: 271–9.

17. Breyer R, Bagdassarian C, Myers S, *et al.* Prostanoid receptors: subtypes and signaling. *Annu Rev Pharmacol Toxicol* 2001; **41**: 661–90.

18. Kujubu DA, Fletcher BS, Varnum BC, *et al.* TIS10, a phorbol ester tumor promoter-inducible mRNA from Swiss 3T3 cells, encodes a novel prostaglandin synthase/cyclooxygenase homologue. *J Biol Chem* 1991; **266**: 12866–72.

19. Borda IT, Koff R. *NSAIDs: a Profile of Adverse Effects.* Philadelphia, PA: Hanley & Belfus, 1995.

20. Born GV, Cross MJ. The aggregation of blood platelets. *J Physiol* 1963; **168**: 178–95.

21. Gabriel SE, Jaakkimainen L, Bombardier C. Risk for serious gastrointestinal complications related to use of nonsteroidal anti-inflammatory drugs. A meta-analysis. *Ann Intern Med* 1991; **115**: 787–96.

22. Garcia Rodriguez LA, Jick H. Risk of upper gastrointestinal bleeding and perforation associated with individual non-steroidal anti-inflammatory drugs. *Lancet* 1994; **343**: 769–72.

23. Masferrer JL, Zweifel BS, Manning PT, *et al.* Selective inhibition of inducible cyclooxygenase 2 in vivo is antiinflammatory and nonulcerogenic. *Proc Natl Acad Sci U S A* 1994; **91**: 3228–32.

24. Laneuville O, Breuer DK, Dewitt DL, *et al.* Differential inhibition of human prostaglandin endoperoxide H synthases-1 and -2 by nonsteroidal anti-inflammatory drugs. *J Pharmacol Exp Ther* 1994; **271**: 927–34.

25. Hay C, de Belleroche J. Carrageenan-induced hyperalgesia is associated with increased cyclooxygenase-2 expression in spinal cord. *Neuroreport* 1997; **8**: 1249–51.

26. Hay CH, Trevethick MA, Wheeldon A, *et al.* The potential role of spinal cord cyclooxygenase-2 in the development of Freund's complete adjuvant-induced changes in hyperalgesia and allodynia. *Neuroscience* 1997; **78**: 843–50.

27. Yamagata K, Andreasson KI, Kaufmann WE, *et al.* Expression of a mitogen-inducible cyclooxygenase in brain neurons: Regulation by synaptic activity and glucocorticoids. *Neuron* 1993; **11**: 371–86.

28. Watanabe A, Nakashima S, Adachi T, *et al.* Changes in the expression of lipid-mediated signal-transducing enzymes in the rat liver after partial hepatectomy. *Surg Today* 2000; **30**: 622–30.

29. O'Brien TP, Roszkowski MT, Wolff LF, *et al.* Effect of a nonsteroidal anti-inflammatory drug on tissue levels of immunoreactive prostaglandin E2, immunoreactive leukotriene, and pain after periodontal surgery. *J Periodontol* 1996; **67**: 1307–16.

30. Power I, Cumming AD, Pugh GC. Effect of diclofenac on renal function and prostacyclin generation after surgery. *Br J Anaesth* 1992; **69**: 451–6.

31. Roszkowski MT, Swift JQ, Hargreaves KM. Effect of NSAID administration on tissue levels of immunoreactive prostaglandin E2, leukotriene B4, and (S)-flurbiprofen following extraction of impacted third molars. *Pain* 1997; **73**: 339–45.

32. Amin AR, Attur M, Patel RN, *et al.* Superinduction of cyclooxygenase-2 activity in human osteoarthritis-affected cartilage: influence of nitric oxide. *J Clin Invest* 1997; **99**: 1231–7.

33. Sano H, Hla T, Maier JA, *et al.* In vivo cyclooxygenase expression in synovial tissues of patients with rheumatoid arthritis and rats with adjuvant and streptococcal cell wall arthritis. *J Clin Invest* 1992; **89**: 97–108.

34. Siigle I, Klein T, Backman JT, *et al.* Expression of cyclooxygenase-1 and cyclooxygenase-2 in human synovial tissue: Differential elevation of cyclooxygenase in inflammatory joint disease. *Arthritis Rheum* 1998; **41**: 122–9.

35. Zhao Z, Chen SR, Eisenach JC, *et al.* Spinal cyclooxygenase-2 is involved in development of allodynia after nerve injury in rats. *Neuroscience* 2000; **97**: 743–8.

36. Samad TA, Moore KA, Sapirstein A, *et al.* Interleukin-1 beta-mediated induction of COX-2 in the CNS contributes to inflammatory pain hypersensitivity. *Nature* 2001; **410**: 471–5.

37. Ferreira SH, Lorenzetti BB, Bristow AF, *et al.* Interleukin-1β as a potent hyperalgesic agent antagonized by a tripeptide analogue. *Nature* 1988; **334**: 698–700.

38. Samad TA, Morre KA, Sapirstein A, *et al.* Interleukin-1β-mediated induction of Cox-2 in the CNS contributes to inflammatory pain hypersensitivity. *Nature* 2001; **410**: 471–5.

39. Smith CJ, Zhang Y, Koboldt CM, *et al.* Pharmacological analysis of cyclooxygenase-1 in inflammation. *Proc Natl Acad Sci U S A* 1998; **95**: 13313–18.

40. Garavito RM: The three dimensional structure of cyclooxygenases. In: Vane JR, Botting J, Botting RS, eds., *Improved Nonsteroidal Anti-Inflammatory Drugs: COX-2 Enzyme Inhibitors.* Dordrecht: Kluwer, 1996.

41. Picot D, Loll PJ, Garavito RM. The x-ray crystal structure of the membrane protein prostaglandin H2 synthase. *Nature* 1994; **367**: 243–9.

42. Loll PJ, Picot D, Ekabo O, *et al.* Synthesis and use of iodinated nonsteroidal anti-inflammatory drug analogs as crystallographic probes of the prostaglandin H2 synthase

cyclooxygenase active site. *Biochemistry* 1996; **35**: 7330–40.

43. Mancini JA, Riendeau D, Falgueyret JP, *et al.* Arginine 120 of prostaglandin G/H synthase-1 is required for the inhibition by nonsteroidal anti-inflammatory drugs containing a carboxylic acid moiety. *J Biol Chem* 1995; **270**: 29372–7.

44. Gierse JK, Koboldt CM, Walker MC, *et al.* Kinetic basis for selective inhibition of cyclo-oxygenases. *Biochem J* 1999; **339**: 607–14.

45. Kurumbail RG, Stevens AM, Gierse JK, *et al.* Structural basis for selective inhibition of cyclooxygenase-2 by anti-inflammatory agents. *Nature* 1996; **384**: 644–8.

46. Luong C, Miller A, Barnett J, *et al.* Flexibility of the NSAID binding site in the structure of human cyclooxygenase-2. *Nat Struct Biol* 1996; **3**: 927–33.

47. Fenner H. Differentiating among nonsteroidal anti-inflammatory drugs by pharmacokinetic and pharmacodynamic profiles. *Semin Arthritis Rheum* 1997; **26**: 28–33.

48. Verbeeck RK, Blackburn JL, Loewen GR. Clinical pharmacokinetics of non-steroidal anti-inflammatory drugs. *Clin Pharmacokinet* 1983; **8**: 297–331.

49. Needs CJ, Brooks PM. Clinical pharmacokinetics of the salicylates. *Clin Pharmacokinet* 1985; **10**: 164–77.

50. Brodgen RN, Heel RC, Pakes GE, *et al.* Diclofenac sodium: a review of its pharmacological properties and therapeutic use in rheumatic diseases and pain of varying origin. *Drugs* 1980; **20**: 24–48.

51. Davies NM. Clinical pharmacokinetics of ibuprofen: the first 30 years. *Clin Pharmacokinet* 1998; **34**: 101–54.

52. Davies NM, Anderson KE. Clinical pharmacokinetics of naproxen. *Clin Pharmacokinet* 1997; **32**: 268–93.

53. Davies NM, Anderson KE. Clinical pharmacokinetics of diclofenac: therapeutic insights and pitfalls. *Clin Pharmacokinet* 1997; **33**: 184–213.

54. Gillis JC, Brogden RN. Ketorolac. A reappraisal of its pharmacodynamic and pharmacokinetic properties and therapeutic use in pain management. *Drugs* 1997; **53**: 139–88.

55. Litvak KM, McEvoy GK. Ketorolac, an injectable nonnarcotic analgesic. *Clin Pharm* 1990; **9**: 921–35.

56. Rowland M, Riegleman S, Harris P, *et al.* Absorption kinetics of aspirin in man following oral administration of an aqueous solution. *J Pharmaceut Sci* 1972; **61**: 379–85.

57. Kendal M, Thornhill D, Willis J. Factors affecting the pharmacokinetics of diclofenac sodium. *Rheumatol Rehabil* 1979; **2**: 38–46.

58. Riess W, Stierlin H, Degen P, *et al.* Pharmacokinetics and metabolism of the anti-inflammatory agent Voltaren. *Scand J Rheumatol Suppl* 1978; **22**: 17–29.

59. Jamali F, Singh N, Pasutto F. Pharmacokinetics of ibuprofen enantiomers in man following oral administration of tablets with different absorption rates. *Pharm Res* 1988; **5**: 40–3.

60. Cox S, Brown M, Squires D, *et al.* Comparative human study of ibuprofen enantiomer plasma concentrations produced by two commercially available ibuprofen tablets. *Biopharm Drug Disp* 1988; **9**: 539–49.

61. Rome LH, Lands WE. Structural requirements for time-dependent inhibition of prostaglandin biosynthesis by anti-inflammatory drugs. *Proc Natl Acad Sci U S A* 1975; **72**: 4863–5.

62. Loll PJ, Picot D, Garavito RM. The structural basis of aspirin activity inferred from the crystal structure of inactivated prostaglandin H2 synthase. *Nat Struct Biol* 1995; **2**: 637–43.

63. Forrest JA, Clements JA, Prescott LF. Clinical pharmacokinetics of paracetamol. *Clin Pharmacokinet* 1982; **7**: 93–107.

64. Davies NM, McLachlan AJ, Day RO, *et al.* Clinical pharmacokinetics and pharmacodynamics of celecoxib: A selective cyclo-oxygenase-2 inhibitor. *Clin Pharmacokinet* 2000; **38**: 225–42.

65. Karim A, Tolbert D, Piergies A, *et al.* Celecoxib does not significantly alter the pharmacokinetics or hypoprothrombinemic effect of warfarin in healthy subjects. *J Clin Pharmacol* 2000; **40**: 655–63.

66. Scott LJ, Lamb HM. Rofecoxib. *Drugs* 1999; **58**: 499–505.

67. Karim A, Laurent A, Kuss M, *et al.* Single dose tolerability and pharmacokinetics of parecoxib sodium, a COX-2 specific inhibitor, following intramuscular administration. American Society of Anesthesiology Annual Congress, October 14–18, 2000, San Francisco, CA.

68. Nussmeier NA, Whelton A, Brown MT, *et al.* Safety of Parecoxib and Valdecoxib in the treatment of pain following coronary artery bypass surgery. *N Engl J Med* 2005; **352**: 1081–91.

69. Ott E, Nussmeier NA, Duke PC, *et al.* Efficacy and safety of the cyclooxygenase 2 inhibitors parecoxib and valdecoxib in patients undergoing coronary artery bypass surgery. *J Thorac Cardiovasc Surg* 2003; **125**: 1481–92.

70. Nussmeier NA, Whelton A, Brown MT, *et al.* Safety and Efficacy of the Cyclooxygenase-2 Inhibitors Parecoxib and Valdecoxib after Noncardiac Surgery. *Anesthesiology* 2006; **104**: 518–26.

71. Solomon SD, McMurray JJ, Pfeffer MA, *et al.* Cardiovascular risk associated with celecoxib in a clinical trial for colorectal adenoma prevention. *N Engl J Med* 2005; **352**: 1071–80.

72. Bresalier RS, Sandler RS, Quan H, *et al.* Cardiovascular events associated with rofecoxib in a colorectal adenoma chemoprevention trial. *N Engl J Med* 2005; **352**: 1092–102.

73. Graham DJ, Campen D, Hiu R, *et al.* Risk of acute myocardial infarction and sudden cardiac death in patients treated with cyclo-oxygenase 2 selective and non-selective non-steroidal anti-inflammatory drugs: nested case-control study. *Lancet* 2005; **365**: 475–81.

74. National Institutes of Health. Use of non-steroidal anti-inflammatory drugs suspended in large Alzheimer's disease prevention trial. Bethesda, MD: NIH, 2004.

75. Hawkey CJ. COX-2 inhibitors. *Lancet* 1999; **353**: 307–14.

76. Bombardier C, Laine I, Reicin A, *et al.* Comparison of upper gastrointestinal toxicity of rofecoxib and naproxen in patients with rheumatoid arthritis. VIGOR Study Group. *N Engl J Med* 2000; **343**: 1520–8.

77. Schnitzer TJ, Burmester GR, Mysler E, *et al.* Comparison of lumiracoxib with naproxen and ibuprofen in the Therapeutic Arthritis Research and Gastrointestinal Event Trial (TARGET), reduction in ulcer complications: randomized controlled trial. *Lancet* 2004; **364**: 665–74.

78. Farkouh ME, Kirshner H, Harrington RA, *et al.* Comparison of lumiracoxib with naproxen and ibuprofen in the Therapeutic Arthritis Research and Gastrointestinal Event Trial (TARGET), cardiovascular outcomes: randomized controlled trial. *Lancet* 2004; **364**: 675–84.

79. Komhoff M, Grone HJ, Klein T, Seyberth HW, Nusing RM. Localization of cyclooxygenase-1 and -2 in adult and fetal human kidney: implication for renal function. *Am J Physiol* 1997; **272**: F460–8.

80. Catella-Lawson F, McAdam B, Morrison BW, *et al.* Effects of specific inhibition of Cyclooxygenase-2 on sodium balance, hemodynamics and vasoactive eicosanoids. *J Pharmacol Exp Ther* 1999; **289**: 735–41.

81. Whelton A, Fort JG, Puma JA, *et al.* Cyclooxygenase-2-specific inhibitors and cardiorenal function: a randomized controlled trial of celecoxib and rofecoxib in older hypertensive osteoarthritis patients. *Am J Ther* 2001; **8**: 85–95.

82. Rossat J, Maillard M, Nussberger J, Brunner HR, Burnier M. Renal effects of selective cyclooxygenase-2 inhibition in normotensive salt-depleted subjects. *Clin Pharmacol Ther* 1999; **66**: 76–84.

83. Woessner KM, Simon RA, Stevenson DD. The safety of celecoxib in patients with aspirin-sensitive asthma. *Arthritis Rheum* 2002; **46**: 2201–6.

84. Gyllfors P, Bochenek G, Overholt J, *et al.* Biochemical and clinical evidence that aspirin-intolerant asthmatic subjects tolerate the cyclooxygenase 2-selective analgesic drug celecoxib. *J Allergy Clin Immunol* 2003; **111**: 1116–21.

85. Moiniche S, Romsing J, Dahl JB, Tramer MR. Nonsteroidal anti-inflammatory drugs and the risk of operative site bleeding after tonsillectomy: a quantitative systematic review. *Anesth Analg* 2003; **96**: 68–77.

86. Noveck RJ, Laurent A, Kuss M, Talwalker S, Hubbard RC. Parecoxib sodium does not impair platelet function in healthy elderly and non-elderly individuals. *Clin Drug Invest* 2001; **21**: 465–76.

87. Ketorolac data sheet. *ABPI Compendium* 2004.

88. Tornkvist H, Lindhom TS, Netz P, Stromberg L, Lindholm TC. Effect of ibuprofen and indomethacin on bone metabolism reflected in bone strength. *Clin Orthop* 1984; **187**: 255–9.

89. Glassman SD, Rose SM, Dimar JR, *et al.* The effect of postoperative nonsteroidal anti-inflammatory drug administration on spinal fusion. *Spine* 1998; **23**: 834–8.

90. Giannoudis PV, MacDonald DA, Matthews SJ, *et al.* Non-union of the femoral diaphysis. The influence of reaming and non-steroidal anti-inflammatory drugs. *J Bone Joint Surg Br* 2000; **82**: 655–8.

91. O'Connor N, Dargan PI, Jones AL. Hepatocellular damage from non-steroidal anti-inflammatory drugs. *Q J Med* 2003; **96**: 787–91.

92. European Medicines Agency. Press release: European Medicines Agency recommends restricted use of nimesulide-containing medicinal products. Doc. ref. EMEA/432604/2007.

93. Brouwers JR, de Smet PA. Pharmacokinetic-pharmacodynamic drug interactions with nonsteroidal anti-inflammatory drugs. *Clin Pharmacokinet* 1994; **27**: 462–85.

94. Chan TY. Adverse interactions between warfarin and nonsteroidal anti-inflammatory drugs: Mechanisms, clinical significance, and avoidance. *Ann Pharmacother* 1995; **29**: 1274–83.

95. Harder S, Thurmann P. Clinically important drug interactions with anticoagulants. An update. *Clin Pharmacokinet* 1996; **30**: 416–44.

96. Noveck RJ, Kuss M, Qian J, *et al.* Parecoxib sodium, an injectable COX-2 specific inhibitor, does not affect aspirin-mediated platelet function. American Society of Regional Anesthesia Annual Congress, May 2001, Vancouver, Canada.

97. Schug SA. Combination analgesia in 2005: a rational approach: focus on paracetamol–tramadol. *Clin Rheumatol* 2006; **25** (Suppl 1): S16–21.

98. Food and Drug Administration. FDA announces series of changes to the class of marketed non-steroidal anti-inflammatory drugs (NSAIDs). Rockville, MD: FDA, 2005.

99. European Medicines Agency. Press release: European Medicines Agency concludes action on COX-2 inhibitors EMEA Doc. ref. EMEA/207766/2005.

100. Hyllested M, Jones S, Pederson JL, Kehlet H. Comparative effect of paracetamol, NSAIDs or their combination in postoperative pain management: a qualitative review. *Br J Anaesth* 2002; **88**: 199–214.

Introduction

Physicians, whether in ancient times or in practice today, face a recurring clinical dilemma. How does one relieve a patient's pain and suffering without doing additional harm? Given the rapid advancement of the molecular neurobiology of analgesia, there has emerged a paradigm shift in analgesic treatment – away from a singular application of opioid analgesics and towards a multimodal approach utilizing drugs targeting other receptors and ion channels in the pain pathway to provide superior analgesia with fewer side effects.

NMDA antagonists: ketamine

Ketamine, introduced in the early 1960s as a dissociative anesthetic, has undergone a clinical transformation based on the observation that administration in a "low-dose" range significantly improves pain and hyperalgesia. Moreover, the analgesic effect of low-dose ketamine is without the high rate of psychomimetic effects that continues to plague ketamine's use as an intravenous anesthetic. Ketamine's benefit in multimodal analgesic therapy is most pronounced when used in the setting of the opioid-tolerant patient, refractory cancer, and neuropathic pain.

Mechanism of drug action

The analgesic action of ketamine is a consequence of its non-competitive blockade of the N-methyl-D-aspartate (NMDA) receptor expressed both in the brain (supraspinally) and in the dorsal horn of the spinal cord. Although the supraspinal action of NMDA antagonists such as ketamine has been proposed to direct analgesic effects through monoaminergic descending inhibition to the spinal cord, the action of ketamine at the level of the dorsal horn of the spinal cord has attracted considerable interest as researchers reach an understanding of how an NMDA antagonist can block sensitization/hyperalgesia produced by persistent states of inflammation and nerve injury (Fig. 35.1) [1].

Preclinical pharmacology

A key principle that has emerged to explain the analgesic action of ketamine involves blockade of NMDA-mediated neurotransmission under conditions of tissue injury (inflammation/nerve injury). Following nociceptor activation, excitatory amino acids (glutamate) are released from the central terminals of primary afferent nociceptors onto spinal neurons expressing NMDA receptors. Persistent activation of C-type nociceptors and, in turn, activation of ionotropic NMDA receptors, produce changes in neuronal plasticity at the nociceptive processing center of the spinal cord – the dorsal horn [2]. This increase in excitability of dorsal horn spinal cord neurons has been described as *central sensitization* [3]. Central sensitization encompasses several features including the spreading of pain sensitivity beyond the original site of injury (secondary hyperalgesia) as well as allodynia. Blockade of NMDA receptor function in the dorsal horn has been shown to selectively attenuate the pain, hyperalgesia, and allodynia associated with ongoing tissue injury. Importantly, the action of ketamine at the dorsal horn can block sensitization but spare the normal signaling of acute pain detection [4,5]. The notion that opioid-induced tolerance and hyperalgesia may also share a common mechanism with central sensitization has been investigated. Although the exact mechanism of opioid tolerance is not known, it is believed to include the involvement of NMDA receptors, nitric oxide pathways, and μ-opioid receptors. Importantly, ketamine was shown to reverse fentanyl- and morphine-induced tolerance/hyperalgesia in rats.

Clinical pharmacology

Ideally, use of low-dose (subanesthetic) ketamine is intended to reverse or prevent central sensitization, opioid tolerance, and hyperalgesia while improving pain control. In general, the benefit of perioperative ketamine in opioid-naive patients undergoing minor to moderately invasive operations has been limited and not generally convincing. Modest reductions in postoperative pain may not necessarily translate into improved quality of life for the patient when compared with regional techniques that have traditionally shown differences in outcome measures [6]. However, when the effect of low-dose ketamine was studied in perioperative subgroups, greater analgesic benefits were realized following major abdominal surgery and in certain types of spinal surgery [7,8].

Anesthetic Pharmacology, 2nd edition, ed. Alex S. Evers, Mervyn Maze, Evan D. Kharasch. Published by Cambridge University Press. © Cambridge University Press 2011.

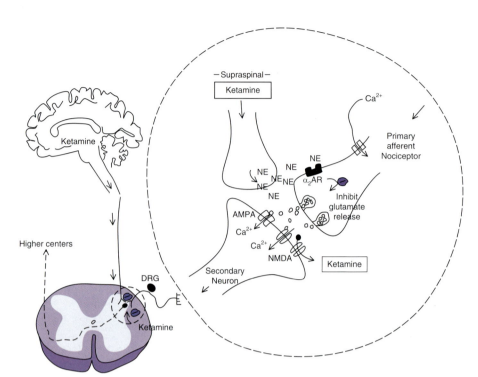

Figure 35.1. The analgesic action of ketamine involves blockade of supraspinal and spinal NMDA receptors. Supraspinal ketamine enhances descending monoaminergic inhibition at the dorsal horn of the spinal cord. Increased spinal norepinephrine (NE) acting at presynaptic α_2-adrenoceptors (α_2AR) on primary afferent nociceptors inhibits terminal depolarization and release of excitatory amino acids such as glutamate. Ketamine can also block post-synaptic NMDA receptors, decreasing nociceptive signaling and limiting the development of central sensitization under conditions of ongoing tissue injury. DRG, dorsal root ganglion.

Opioid-tolerant patients (adults and children) suffering from cancer pain or postoperative pain as a result of a malignant process have shown superior analgesia with low-dose ketamine. Escalating doses of opioids given in an attempt to manage the pain of progressive malignant diseases can drive further pain and hyperalgesia. Under these difficult clinical situations, low-dose ketamine has been show to offer dramatic improvement in pain control, and opioid dose reductions that are often greater than 50% [9].

Use of oral ketamine for pain management, especially in the opioid-tolerant patient, may have a superior analgesic effect due to the potency of its metabolite – norketamine. In practice, there is a lack of consensus on the use of ketamine as an adjunctive drug. However, adjunctive use of ketamine is generally reserved for the most refractory pain states. Wide ranges in both dose (oral dose 0.25–0.5 mg kg^{-1}) and interval (ranging from daily to every 4 hours) suggest that such off-label use should [?] be restricted to physicians experienced in pain management. The potential complications arising from the chronic use of ketamine are largely unknown, and chronic intrathecal infusions in animals produce spinal pathology [10].

Dosage and administration

Low dose – opioid sparing: 1–5 µg kg^{-1} min^{-1} intravenous/subcutaneous [9,11]

Moderate dose – analgesia: 0.1–0.3 mg kg^{-1} intravenous bolus [11]

High dose – dissociative anesthesia: 1–2 mg kg^{-1} intravenous bolus

Anticonvulsants: gabapentin, pregabalin

Gabapentin, an anticonvulsant initially introduced for the treatment of partial complex seizures, has been approved and widely used as a first-line treatment for postherpetic neuralgia (PHN). As the exclusivity of gabapentin has expired, pregabalin has been introduced and has obtained US Food and Drug Administration (FDA) approval for the treatment not only of PHN but also of diabetic polyneuropathy and fibromyalgia. In addition, gabapentin/pregabalin are being used in a widening range of off-label applications including perioperative pain management.

Mechanism of drug action

Gabapentin (a derivative of γ-aminobutyric acid, GABA) and now pregabalin (an amino acid derivative of GABA) are understood to have their analgesic action by binding and blocking a unique subunit of a voltage-gated calcium channel (VGCC) known as the $\alpha_2\delta_1$ subunit. Selective blockade of this subunit expressed in two central nervous system (CNS) regions produces antinociceptive effects through (1) enhanced descending inhibition to the dorsal horn of the spinal cord (supraspinal) and (2) inhibition of excitatory amino acid (glutamate) release from primary afferent terminals in the dorsal horn of the spinal cord (spinal) (Fig. 35.2).

Preclinical pharmacology

Under hyperalgesic conditions, gabapentin and/or pregabalin act supraspinally to reduce the release of GABA onto the locus

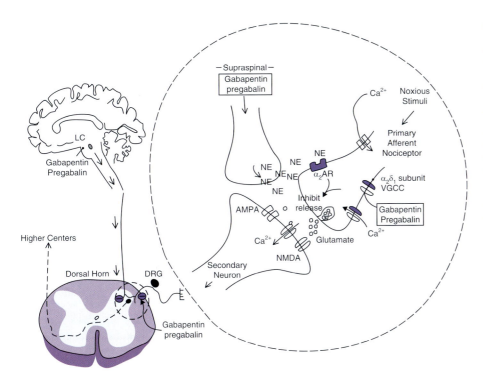

Figure 35.2. Gabapentin/pregabalin mediates analgesia through enhancing supraspinal descending inhibition and blockade of spinal Ca^{2+} channels under conditions of inflammation/nerve injury. The supraspinal action of gabapentin/pregabalin begins with the reduction of GABA released onto the locus coeruleus (LC). Subsequent loss of tonic LC inhibition enhances spinal norepinephrine (NE) release and activation of presynaptic α_2 receptors in the dorsal horn. Additionally, blockade of voltage-gated Ca^{2+} channels (VGCCs) expressing the $\alpha_2\delta_1$ subunit in nociceptors results in decreased terminal depolarization and transmitter release. Together, both supraspinal and spinal actions of gabapentin/pregabalin reduce nociceptive signaling in the spinal cord under conditions of persistent inflammation and nerve/tissue injury.

coeruleus, and this leads to the activation of the descending noradrenergic system [12]. This descending antinociceptive pathway is dependent on spinal α_2-adrenoceptor activation – presumably in the dorsal horn. Importantly, the supraspinal effect of gabapentin/pregabalin requires a hyperalgesic/neuropathic state [13].

Gabapentin/pregabalin have been shown to produce potent antinociceptive effects at the level of the spinal cord through direct binding to $\alpha_2\delta_1$ subunits of a VGCC expressed in the dorsal root ganglion (DRG) neurons (primary afferent nociceptors). Tissue and nerve injury increase $\alpha_2\delta_1$ subunit expression in the DRG and spinal cord. One consequence of this overexpression is hyperalgesia and allodynia. Under such conditions, blockade of the $\alpha_2\delta_1$ subunit with gabapentin and/or pregabalin is sufficient to reduce the excessive neurotranmitter (glutamate) release observed in the spinal cord during hyperalgesic conditions, with concurrent reduction in thermal and mechanical hyperalgesia. Evidence that the $\alpha_2\delta_1$ subunit of VGCC is the principal target site of action of pregabalin was shown by engineering of a point mutation of that subunit, resulting in a loss in pregabalin binding in the brain and spinal cord of mice [14]. Through the study of transgenic mice that constitutively overexpress the $\alpha_2\delta_1$ subunit in neuronal tissues, it was observed that the overexpressing mice had exaggerated responses to mechanical and thermal stimuli and were the most sensitive to gabapentin-induced blockade of VGCC. Moreover, radiolabeled gabapentin binding is increased in the dorsal horn region under the chronic-constriction nerve injury model. This suggests that pathophysiologic conditions

that overexpress the $\alpha_2\delta_1$ subunit provide the basis for an antihyperalgesic action of gabapentin [15].

Clinical pharmacology

Unlike opioids, neither gabapentin nor pregabalin changes the pain threshold or perception of pain at rest. However, gabapentin/pregabalin modulates the pain pathway under pathophysiologic conditions, serving as first-line drugs in the treatment of neuropathic pain. Gabapentin has been shown to be effective in the treatment of postherpetic neuralgia, a condition often refractory to commonly prescribed analgesic therapy [16]. Moreover, gabapentin monotherapy (900–3600 mg per day) was effective in pain and symptom control in patients with painful diabetic neuropathy. These initial findings are supported by later meta-analysis [17]. Although pregabalin has been approved by the FDA for the treatment of fibromyalgia, gabapentin has also been found effective in its treatment. However, gabapentin has not been effective in the treatment of postamputation/phantom-limb pain. Nevertheless, gabapentin/pregabalin may still offer a benefit to those patients who have failed other analgesic therapy. What often limits the use of gabapentin is mild/moderate sedation/altered mental status. As a consequence, a relatively small percentage of patients ever achieve a therapeutic dose range of gabapentin (2700–3600 mg per day). Gabapentin is slowly absorbed (peak 3–4 hours) and has a bioavailability of 33–66%, but pregabalin is rapidly and linearly absorbed with dose and has a higher bioavailability (90%). Both gabapentin and pregabalin are eliminated without undergoing metabolism or modification by the kidneys. Under conditions of renal failure/insufficiency, dose and interval adjustments must be made. Withdrawal syndromes associated with the acute cessation of gabapentin have been reported.

The perioperative use of gabapentin is emerging. When gabapentin (2400 mg per day) was used perioperatively in women undergoing breast surgery, there was a reduction in acute and chronic (3 and 6 months) pain [18]. Meta-analysis of 12 randomized perioperative gabapentin controlled trials with 896 patients under a variety of surgical procedures showed lower visual analog pain scores at 4 and 24 hours and a concomitant decrease in opioid requirements. One potential benefit of a reduction in either intraoperative or postoperative opioid consumption with the use of gabapentin could be a reduction in postoperative delirium [19].

Dosage and administration

Fibromyalgia: gabapentin (adult dose range 1200–2400 mg per day) oral

Postherpetic neuralgia: gabapentin (adult dose range 2700–3600 mg per day) oral

Diabetic neuropathy: gabapentin (900–3600 mg per day) oral

Preoperative gabapentin: 600–800 mg oral [20]

Perioperative gabapentin: 2400 mg per day oral [18]

Pregabalin: 300–450 mg per day oral

(Note: Gabapentin is prescribed for the treatment of pain in adults with a dose range beginning at 100–300 mg orally three times daily and slowly increased over a period of days to weeks in an attempt to avoid side effects such as sedation. Pregabalin is typically begun at 50 mg orally twice daily and increased to 150 mg twice daily within 1 week.)

Sodium channel blockers: bupivacaine, levobupivacaine, ropivacaine

Voltage-gated sodium channels (VGSCs) mediate sodium influx into cells in response to local membrane depolarization. Increases in VGSC subtype expression on primary afferent neurons (nociceptors) are linked to inflammatory and neuropathic pain [21]. Importantly, sodium currents in small-diameter (nociceptive) neurons of C and $A\delta$ fiber type are carried by members of the tetrodotoxin-resistant (TTX-R) sodium channel family (predominantly $Na_v1.8$ and $Na_v1.9$) that are differentially expressed in small-diameter pain-sensing neurons. Moreover, efforts are under way to develop a new generation of local anesthetics – sodium channel blockers that selectively block TTX-R sodium channel subtypes in sensory neurons – with the goal of obtaining an analgesic effect while sparing normal touch or motor function.

Mechanism of drug action

Local anesthetics block VGSCs through binding to a specific protein site within the aqueous pore of the sodium channel. Analgesia results when this blockade occurs on VGSCs expressed on specialized primary afferent nociceptors (C and $A\delta$ fiber-type sensory neurons). Nociceptors express predominantly TTX-R sodium channels, rather than other VGSC subtypes. There are two critical features that allow TTX-R sodium channels to play an important role in the analgesic action of local anesthetics. Firstly, TTX-R channels undergo *use-dependent* local anesthetic blockade not observed in certain TTX-sensitive channels. Secondly, in response to inflammatory/neuropathic conditions, there is an increase in TTX-R sodium channel expression that underlies the spontaneous activation of nociceptors. Therefore, the subsequent use-dependent blockade of TTX-R sodium channels transforms local anesthetics into antihyperalgesic drugs. These properties may explain why application of low-dose local anesthetics reduces the rate of action-potential firing in activated pain-sensing nociceptors while sparing TTX-sensitive channels and the function of uninjured sensory or motor neurons.

Preclinical pharmacology

It is under conditions of tissue and nerve injury that local anesthetics have their most profound analgesic effects – presumably on TTX-R channels [22]. Inflammatory mediators such as serotonin (5-HT) and prostaglandin E_2 (PGE_2) have been shown to increase TTX-R currents in dissociated sensory neurons and thereby could contribute to the development of hyperalgesia. The finding that $Na_v1.8$-null mutant mice have a significantly higher threshold for noxious mechanical stimuli as well as delayed development of inflammatory hyperalgesia further supports the importance of TTX-R sodium channels in the development of neuropathic and inflammatory pain. Although increases in TTX-sensitive channels such as $Na_v1.3$ have been observed under neuropathic pain conditions on *injured* sensory neurons, it is the concurrent increase in TTX-R channels ($Na_v1.8$) in neighboring (*uninjured*) sensory fibers that appear to drive painful sensation and hyperalgesia. Progress towards the development of a selective blocker of TTX-R sodium channel $Na_v1.8$ has been reported [23].

Clinical pharmacology

The analgesic action of local anesthetics is based on the ability to block nociceptive TTX-sensitive and TTX-resistant sodium channels at low (subanesthetic) concentrations – doses that do not block nerve conduction [24,25]. Multiple studies now show that epidural analgesia offers outcome advantages over other modes of postoperative analgesia [26]. Moreover, continuous infusion of low-dose local anesthetics adjacent to the brachial plexus or other peripheral nerves also improves postoperative outcome. The local anesthetic isomers ropivacaine and (to a degree) levobupivacaine offer a toxicity profile that is theoretically safer than bupivacaine. Nevertheless, there appears to be little difference in the analgesic action of ropivacaine, levobupivacaine, or bupivacaine when equivalent doses are compared in either epidural or peripheral nerve administration. What distinguishes these drugs clinically is their duration of action. As compared to levobupivacaine, with its longer half-life, ropivacaine is associated with a more rapid loss of segmental epidural analgesia. This is consistent with observations that low-dose thoracic epidural ropivacaine for postoperative pain management requires fentanyl ($2-4 \mu g \, mL^{-1}$) to ensure more reliable analgesia. The analgesic benefits of levobupivacaine, ropivacaine, and bupivacaine under thoracic epidural administration are indistinguishable; however, a lower profile of motor blockade has been reported with ropivacaine lumbar epidural infusion.

Dosage and administration for epidural/peripheral nerve catheter infusion

Bupivacaine: 0.0625–0.25%

Levobupivacaine – Chirocaine: pure S(–) enantiomer of bupivacaine (0.125–0.25%)

Ropivacaine – Naropin(R): pure S(–) enantiomer of ropivacaine (0.0625–0.2%)

α_2-Adrenoceptor agonists: clonidine, dexmedetomidine

Although most practitioners are familiar with the antihypertensive and sedative properties of α_2-adrenoceptor agonists, they have shown promise as analgesic drugs because of their synergistic effect with spinal opiates and efficacy in opioid-tolerant patients. Moreover, they offer an alternative analgesic strategy for patients who have failed classical opioid management for painful conditions.

Mechanism of drug action

There are two predominant mechanisms that achieve analgesia by α_2-receptor agonists, namely, activation of descending spinal inhibition and direct activation of presynaptic α_2 receptors on sensory afferent terminals in the dorsal horn [27]. One of the major descending analgesic systems in the CNS utilizes a noradrenergic system that originates in the brainstem locus coeruleus (LC) and terminates on the dorsal horn of the spinal cord. The binding of α_2-agonists in the LC, in turn, results in norepinephrine release from its descending inhibitory track onto *presynaptic* terminals of C and Aδ type primary afferent sensory neurons. The subsequent activation of presynaptic α_2 receptors by norepinephrine in the dorsal horn reduces evoked release of excitatory amino acids and neuropeptides from nociceptive neurons, resulting in an analgesic effect (Fig. 35.3) [28]. A comprehensive discussion of the general use of α_2-agonists in anesthesia can be found in Chapter 30 and elsewhere [29].

Preclincial pharmacology

Our understanding of α_2-receptor-based analgesia has matured from reports that intrathecal application of adrenergic agonists such as norepinephrine could increase nociceptive thresholds to findings that specific α_2-adrenergic agonists such as clonidine could block behavioral signs of neuropathic pain. Through the use of genetic knockout paradigms, the α_{2A} receptor subtype has emerged as a predominant target in α_2-mediated analgesia [30]. Intrathecal administration of the α_2-agonists clonidine or dexmedetomidine results in an increase in spinal levels of norepinephrine and acetylcholine, suggesting that increases in both spinal transmitters play a role in α_2-mediated spinal analgesia [31]. α_2-agonists such as clonidine can directly produce spinal analgesia, but it is their ability to synergize with morphine under nerve injury and neuropathic conditions that has emerged as a critical translational finding [32]. In addition to spinal administration, the systemic administration of α_2-agonists also recruits a descending inhibitory noradrenergic effect at the dorsal horn. Additionally, systemic administration of α_2-agonists has been shown to be effective in the treatment of an experimental neuropathic pain with a peripheral site of action.

Clinical pharmacology

Epidural/spinal clonidine has been approved for infusion in the treatment of cancer/neuropathic pain that is refractory to opioid analgesics [33]. There is no apparent cross-tolerance between clonidine and opioid analgesics at a spinal site of action. However, clonidine is not recommended for obstetric or routine perioperative pain control because of hypotension and its sequelae. Since an optimal spinal dose of clonidine has not been reported, low-dose clonidine (15 μg) administered as an adjunct to intrathecal local anesthetics may provide a successful compromise between analgesia and hypotension. Perioperative use of epidural clonidine should be reserved for the most difficult to manage and/or opioid-tolerant patient. However, such patients remain at significant risk for hypotension. The use of systemic clonidine/dexmedetomidine for the treatment of pain has been described, but evidence such as reduction in pain and postoperative opioid requirements is largely restricted to case reports and case series, with few controlled trials.

Dosage and administration

Clonidine – Duraclon: for epidural infusion up to 30 $\mu g \, h^{-1}$. Side effects: hypotension and rebound hypertension

Clonidine – Catapres: patch, TTS-1 (0.1 mg per 24 h) applied to skin every 7 days

Dexmedetomidine: 1 $\mu g \, kg^{-1}$ intravenous loading dose; 0.2–0.5 $\mu g \, kg^{-1} \, h^{-1}$ infusion

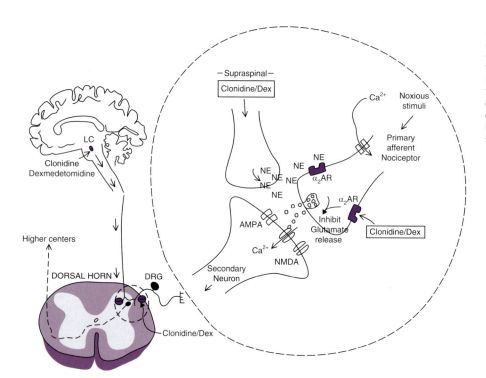

Figure 35.3. Clonidine/dexmedetomidine directs analgesia through supraspinal and spinal activation of α_2-adrenoceptors (α_2AR). Descending inhibition via norepinephrine (NE) release onto the dorsal horn is enhanced through activation of α_2 receptors on the locus coeruleus (LC). Activation of presynaptic α_2 receptors on nociceptor terminals by clonidine/dexmedetomidine together with increased spinal NE reduces glutamate release and nociceptive signaling.

Calcium channel blockers: ziconotide

Ziconotide (SNX-111), a synthetic peptide of structural similarity to the ω-conopeptide MVIIA derived from the fish-hunting snail, *Conus magus*, is approved in the United States for the treatment of chronic pain states that are intolerant to conventional therapies such as systemic analgesics or refractory to established intrathecal therapy, such as morphine. Similar approval has been established in Europe. Ziconotide represents a divergence from previous intrathecal pain therapies that have targeted opioid, α_2 receptors and/or sodium channels.

Mechanism of drug action

In contrast to established intrathecal analgesic therapies, ziconotide selectively blocks the action of neuronal N-type voltage-sensitive calcium channels in the spinal cord. N-type VGCCs are expressed presynaptically on primary afferent nociceptors in the dorsal horn of the spinal cord. Since activation of N-type VGCCs is associated with calcium influx, nerve terminal depolarization, and release of excitatory neurotransmitters (glutamate), inhibition of VGCCs in the spinal cord should result in decreased neurotransmitter release and blockade of nociceptive signaling. However, ziconotide and its analogs do not differentiate between VGCCs expressed in central versus peripheral neuronal tissues. Therefore, to achieve a more selective pharmacologic effect, a restricted administration into the

intrathecal space helps reduce unwanted systemic/peripheral effects (Fig. 35.4).

Preclinical pharmacology

VGCCs are important for the regulation of neuronal intracellular calcium concentrations, terminal depolarization, and neurotransmitter release. Therefore, suppression of calcium channel activity following inflammation/nerve injury should lead to a decrease in nociceptive excitability [34]. This approach was refined with the introduction of ziconotide, which directs a dose-dependent analgesic effect in models of inflammation and peripheral neuropathy [35]. Although these and other studies established the potent analgesic effect of intrathecal ziconotide, several studies also noted unusual motor behavior when the peptide was administered in high concentration.

Clinical pharmacology

One of the first reports of the clinical effectiveness of ziconotide came from its intrathecal use in a patient suffering from intractable brachial plexus avulsion pain. Since then, a number of studies have demonstrated improved pain control for patients who previously failed pain management strategies. However, in these same studies, the extent of adverse events associated with the clinical use of intrathecal ziconotide was revealed. In double-blind placebo-controlled randomized multicenter trials involving the treatment of refractory pain in patients with cancer or AIDS, the use of ziconotide revealed a significant improvement of pain, with 50% of patients receiving ziconotide showing improvement, compared to a 17.5%

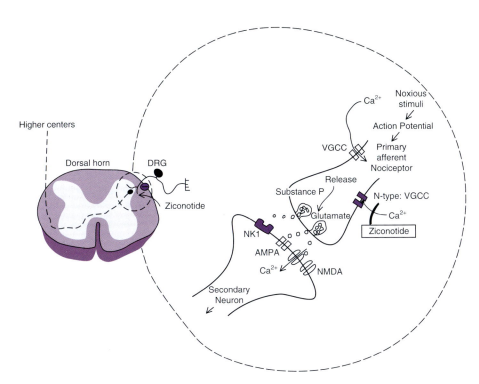

Figure 35.4. Intrathecal ziconotide binds to pre-synaptic spinal N-type Ca^{2+} channels to produce spinal analgesia. Ziconotide binds to presynaptic N-type voltage-gated Ca^{2+} channels (VGCCs) on central nociceptor terminals. Blockade of nociceptor VGCC activation results in lower evoked release of substance P and glutamate and spinal analgesia.

placebo response rate [36]. At least three randomized placebo-controlled trials have been completed supporting its analgesic action in patients with chronic pain but also revealing a narrow therapeutic window. An open-label "long-term" ziconotide trial was reported that primarily included patients receiving ziconotide for 30–90 days (some for more than 1 year) for the treatment of severe chronic pain. Importantly, the frequency of adverse events was significantly higher, with more than half (61%) of all patients discontinuing the study either temporarily or permanently because of adverse events [37]. This reflects a warning contained with the prescribing information indicating severe neurologic (confusion, mental slowing) and psychiatric disturbances (depression, anxiety) predominant among potential adverse events. Fortunately, the majority of adverse events were shown to be dose-dependent and/or reversed with either reduction or termination of ziconotide. Taken together, it is recommended to initiate ziconotide therapy at the lowest dose/rate and closely monitor the patient.

Dosage and administration

Intrathecal infusion pump: initial dose not to exceed $0.1\,\mu g\,h^{-1}$ ($2.4\,\mu g$ per day). Rate increases no greater than $0.1\,\mu g\,h^{-1}$ every 2–3 days with a maximal rate of $19.2\,\mu g$ per day at day 21.

Emerging concepts

Cannabinoids: dronabinol (Marinol)

Although the use of cannabis for its analgesic action dates back thousands of years, it has re-emerged under intense scrutiny. The activity of cannabis is believed to derive from the action of delta-9-tetrahydrocannabinol (THC) acting at G-protein-coupled receptors CB_1 and CB_2. The majority of behavioral effects of THC result from the activation of the CB_1 receptor subtype [38]. CB_1 is expressed at high levels within the brain and the dorsal horn of the spinal cord, with CB_1 residing in abundance in the superficial layers containing terminals of the primary afferent neurons responsible for nociceptive transduction ($A\delta$ and C fiber types). In contrast, the CB_2 receptor subtype appears not to be expressed in neurons but in the periphery (immune cells) and plays a role in analgesia during inflammation. The endogenous ligand for CB_1 receptors includes arachidonylethanolamide (anandamide, AEA) and is associated with analgesic activity. Although herbal preparations of cannabis contain a plethoral of compounds, oral preparations (Marinol) contain a pure isomer of THC, dronabinol (the international nonproprietary name). Use of Marinol is FDA-approved for chemotherapy-induced nausea and vomiting and AIDS-related anorexia. Although gastrointestinal absorption of dronabinol is excellent, metabolism through the enterocyte, and subsequently the liver, results in low bioavailability (~5% following oral administration, peaking 2–3 hours after ingestion). Nevertheless, modest but clinically relevant analgesic effects on central pain in patients have been reported with oral dronabinol (10 mg daily). Alternatively, clinical trials using smoked cannabis are emerging in the treatment of neuropathic pain associated with HIV [39]. Beyond the toxicity of administering these drugs through inhaled smoke, adverse events including dizziness limit their broader application. Investigation into the safe administration of cannabinoid-based analgesic drugs with a lower profile of side effects is ongoing.

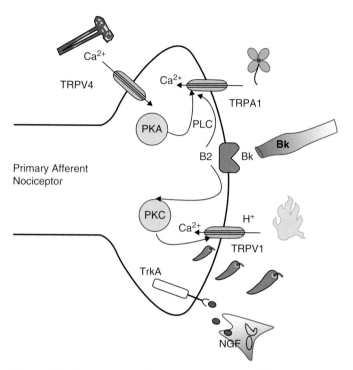

Figure 35.5. Emerging analgesic targets expressed on peripheral nociceptors. Primary afferent nociceptors are specialized primary sensory afferent neurons that detect noxious chemical, thermal, and mechanical stimuli. Certain members of the transient receptor potential (TRP) receptor superfamily are highly expressed in nociceptors and act as cellular sensors capable of detecting conditions of tissue injury. TRPV1 (capsaicin receptor) is the prototypical pain receptor/channel that is activated by multiple noxious stimuli including plant derivative, protons, heat, endogenous products of inflammation, activated protein kinase C (PKC), and bradykinin (BK) receptor activation. Through the influx of Ca^{2+} through its channel pore, nociceptive signaling is initiated. TRPA1 (activated by mustard oil) is often coexpressed with TRPV1 and is activated under inflammatory conditions mediated by activation of phospholipase C (PLC) and protein kinase A (PKA). TRPV4 can be activated by osmotic and experimental mechanical stimuli. Non-TRP channels are also known to have a profound effect on nociceptor activation and sensitization. These include the action of growth factors/neurotrophins such as nerve growth factor (NGF) acting through its high-affinity receptor-kinase TrkA.

Transient receptor potential (TRP) channels

TRP channels make up a large superfamily, some of which require both an *inflammatory mediator* and a *noxious stimulus* for activation. In general they can be considered cellular sensors, and when expressed on sensory neurons they confer specialized properties such as the detection of noxious stimuli. TRP channels functioning in this manner may serve to signal ongoing tissue injury and inflammation in addition to acute noxious stimuli. A similar mechanism may underlie mechanical hyperalgesia. Nevertheless, TRP channels likely hold an important piece of the puzzle that should one day provide a means to more effectively treat painful conditions and identify patients predisposed to the development of chronic pain (Fig. 35.5).

TRPV1 receptor antagonist-agonists

Since the cloning of the capsaicin receptor (TRPV1) in 1997 [40], our understanding of the molecular mechanisms involved in the transduction of noxious stimuli has increased

dramatically. Considerable detail has been afforded to the description of TRPV1, because it represents an archetype for a broader family of ion channels that transduce virtually all modalities of painful stimuli. In addition to TRPV1, other ion channels have been isolated and characterized that also appear to function in peripheral pain transduction (Table 35.1).

Tissue injury results in the production and release of multiple inflammatory products that have been characterized and identified to directly activate TRPV1. Anandamide, the endogenous ligand for the cannabinoid receptor (CB_1), activates rTRPV1 and is a full agonist for the human ortholog of TRPV1. Products of the lipoxygenase pathway of arachidonic acid, 12-(S)-hydroperoxyeicosatetranoic acid (12-(S)-HPETE) and leukotriene B_4 (LTB_4), have also been found to activate TRPV1 in vitro.

Therapeutic strategies targeting TRPV1

Antagonists – Given that TRPV1 is essential for the development of thermal hyperalgesia under inflammatory conditions, it has become an attractive target for the development of high-affinity antagonists. Although TRPV1 antagonists have entered phase I clinical trials, their ability to produce hyperthermia may hinder their introduction into clinical practice.

Agonists – Although initial applications of capsaicin are painful, paradoxically, repeated application of capsaicin in emollient creams has been used as a topical analgesic, producing a desensitization or destruction of nociceptive terminals. Therefore, capsaicin has the property of both exciting and inactivating capsaicin-sensitive neurons. TRPV1 is widely accepted as functional marker of an important subpopulation of sensory neurons, polymodal nociceptors, specialized primary afferent sensory neurons that are dedicated to the detection of painful stimuli. Temporary ablation of TRPV1-expressing nerve terminals by application of capsaicin produces a pronounced analgesic effect. This approach of targeting the cell population expressing TRPV1 has gained much attention with respect to the treatment of various painful conditions, including the treatment of postsurgical pain [41]. Taking a different approach, TRPV1 has been used to target nociceptors using the ion channel pore as a conduit to transport membrane-impermeable therapeutics, in this case the sodium channel blocker QX-314, to their intracellular targets [42].

TRPV4

Mechanical and thermal hyperalgesia can produce significant pain and morbidity, whether as a consequence of a surgical procedure or as the result of a chronic inflammatory process. Moreover, mechanical stimuli that initially had evoked little or no response can produce strong activation of nociceptors following exposure to inflammatory mediators. This implies that certain mechanosensitive elements remain relatively silent until costimulated with both an inflammatory event and a noxious stimulus. TRPV4 has been identified as important in the development of hyperalgesia after osmotic stimuli. It

Table 35.1. TRP ion channels active in peripheral pain transduction

Ion channel	Other names (reference)	Activation	Potential function
TRPV1	Capsaicin receptor, VR1 (*Nature* 1997; **389**; 816–24)	vanilloids (capsaicin, resiniferatoxin), heat (> 43 °C), protons, endocannabinoids, AA metabolites	chemical-thermal pain, capsaicin sensation, thermal hyperalgesia, unclear role in mechano/osmotransduction
TRPV2	VR-L1 (*Nature* 1999; **398**; 436–41)	noxious heat (> 52 °C), hypotonicity	thermal pain
TRPV3	(*Nature* 2002, **418**; 181–6) (*Nature* 2002, **418**; 186–90)	heat (30–39 °C)	warmth, thermal pain?
TRPV4	VR-OAC (*Cell* 2000; **163**; 525–35)	hypotonicity, stretch, mild hypertonicity, thermal (27–45 °C)	mechanosensation osmoregulation, nociception/pain
TRPA1	ANKTM1 (*Cell* 2003; **112**; 819–29)	mechano-stretch, cold, mustard oil, irritant anesthetics	noxious cold, inflammatory pain

appears to be highly expressed in visceral afferents and may play an important role in mediating mechanically evoked visceral pain [43]. While visceral pain (mechanical and chemical in origin) is common and often severe, it is extremely difficult to treat. The selective role for TRPV4 in visceral sensory innervation suggests that it might represent a novel target for therapeutic intervention of visceral pain arising from such conditions as inflammatory bowel disease.

TRPA1

Alongside TRPV1, TRPA1 has emerged as a general chemosensor and a key factor in sensitizing peripheral nociceptors in the setting of tissue injury and inflammation. Both receptors are activated by inflammatory mediators triggering the release of substance P and calcitonin gene-related peptide (CGRP), and promotion of neurogenic inflammation. Moreover, bradykinin, an important inflammatory mediator that has long been known to contribute to inflammatory hyperalgesia, is thought to require TRPA1 to sensitize nociceptors. Development of high-affinity antagonists to TRPA1 is ongoing, driven by its role in inflammatory pain. TRPV1 and, more importantly, TRPA1, have recently received attention with respect to their potential role in postsurgical pain. Irritant inhaled anesthetics activate TRPA1 and sensitize TRPV1 expressed on peripheral nociceptors apparently to produce a neurogenic inflammatory reaction involving the release of neuropeptides [44]. In the setting of tissue injury (e.g., surgery) leading to inflammatory sensitization of the peripheral nociceptors, the added effect of anesthetic activation of TRPA1 or sensitization of TRPV1 could potentially worsen postsurgical pain and hyperalgesia. Targeting TRPA1 and possibly TRPV1 through specific blockade may be an approach to reduce postsurgical pain.

Peptide growth factors and receptors

Nerve growth factor (NGF) is best known for its action on the developing nervous system, where it is essential for the early survival of the central and peripheral nervous system.

Increasingly, however, it has been shown to be an important link between inflammation, nerve injury, and the development of pain. For example, immunization of adult rats with NGF produces anti-NGF antibodies and subsequent hypoalgesia. Inflammation is associated with local and systemic changes. Peripheral changes include inflammatory cell migration, cytokine release, edema, erythema, pain, and hyperalgesia. Although no single factor is acting alone, there is significant evidence to support the idea that NGF has a primary role in the development of inflammatory pain and hyperalgesia through its action on nociceptors. These include the following:

(1) In experimental models of inflammation, concentrations of NGF increase within the tissue and parallel the development of behavioral signs of pain and hyperalgesia.

(2) NGF produces both early (within minutes) and delayed (hours to days) increases in pain and hyperalgesia. Antibodies and small molecules that interrupt NGF binding to its high-affinity receptor (TrkA) present another target in the treatment of inflammatory induced pain [45].

Summary

Progress in molecular neurobiology has provided alternatives to opioid analgesics. Drugs are available targeting multiple receptors and ion channels, and a multimodal approach allows for effective analgesia with fewer side effects.

Ketamine is a noncompetitive *N*-methyl-D-aspartate (NMDA) receptor antagonist which, when used in low doses, has been shown to improve pain and hyperalgesia. Ketamine is particularly beneficial for use in opioid tolerance, refractory cancer pain, and neuropathic pain. Low-dose ketamine can allow reduced opioid dose and improved pain control in opioid-tolerant cancer patients. The analgesic actions of ketamine are thought to be mediated both supraspinally and via effects at the dorsal horn of the spinal cord. Preclinical studies have shown that the action of ketamine at the dorsal horn can block central sensitization following tissue injury, whilst sparing the normal signaling of acute pain detection.

Anticonvulsant γ-aminobutyric acid (GABA) derivatives gabapentin and pregabalin selectively bind and block a unique voltage-gated calcium channel subunit, modulating pain pathways in neuropathic/hyperalgesic pain. Supraspinal effects are mediated via activation of a descending antinociceptive noradrenergic system. Gabapentin and pregabalin also act on nociceptors at the level of the spinal cord. Clinically, gabapentin and pregabalin are used in treatment of neuropathic pain, and there is emerging evidence for the use of gabapentin perioperatively to reduce opioid requirements.

Local anesthetics act via the blockade of voltage-gated sodium channels. In the setting of tissue or nerve injury, low-dose local anesthetics block sodium channels expressed on nociceptors, resulting in analgesia. Ropivacaine, bupivacaine, and levobupivacaine may be used postoperatively for epidural or peripheral nerve administration, and they differ in the duration of their effects.

Clonidine and dexmedetomidine are α_2-adrenoceptor agonists which inhibit nociception both at the level of the dorsal horn and via a descending inhibitory pathway. Spinal administration of clonidine may be used to treat opioid-refractory cancer/neuropathic pain, but because of hypotension associated with the drug its use is not recommended in routine perioperative or obstetrical pain control.

Ziconotide is a voltage-gated calcium channel blocker. Intrathecal administration aids selective inhibition of those neuronal N-type calcium channels expressed by afferent nociceptors in the dorsal horn of the spinal cord. Ziconotide may be beneficial for control of chronic pain that is refractory to conventional therapy; however, due to potential adverse events, the initiation of treatment at the lowest dose/rate with close monitoring is recommended.

Marinol is an oral preparation of dronabinol which acts on CB_1 and CB_2 cannabinoid receptors. Despite low bioavailability, oral administration has been shown to modestly improve central pain; there is evidence for the use of smoked cannabis to treat HIV-associated neuropathic pain. Use is currently limited by side effects.

Transient receptor potential (TRP) channels, such as the capsaicin receptor (TRPV1), are expressed on sensory neurons. TRPV1 and TRPA1 detect inflammatory mediators produced following tissue injury, sensitizing peripheral nociceptors. Potential therapeutic strategies targeting TRPV1 are under development, including antagonists, agonists, and the exploitation of the ion channel pore for intracellular introduction of membrane-impermeable therapeutic agents. There is also interest in the development of TRPA1 antagonists. Irritant inhaled anesthetics activate TRPA1 and sensitize TRPV1, potentially contributing to postsurgical pain. TRPV4 may represent a novel target for therapeutics aimed at treating mechanically evoked visceral pain such as occurs in inflammatory bowel disease.

There is increasing evidence that nerve growth factor (NGF) acts on nociceptors to play a role in inflammatory pain and hyperalgesia. Potential therapeutic strategies targeting NGF binding to its receptor include antibodies and small molecule inhibitors.

References

1. Nagasaka H, Nagasaka I, Sato I, et al. The effects of ketamine on the excitation and inhibition of dorsal horn WDR neuronal activity induced by bradykinin injection into the femoral artery in cats after spinal cord transection. Anesthesiology 1993; 78: 722–32.

2. Li J, Simone DA, Larson AA. Windup leads to characteristics of central sensitization. Pain 1999; 79: 75–82.

3. Woolf CJ, Costigan M. Transcriptional and posttranslational plasticity and the generation of inflammatory pain. Proc Natl Acad Sci U S A 1999; 96: 7723–30.

4. Zahn PK, Brennan TJ. Lack of effect of intrathecally administered N-methyl-D-aspartate receptor antagonists in a rat model for postoperative pain. Anesthesiology 1998; 88: 143–56.

5. Yaksh TL. Spinal systems and pain processing: development of novel analgesic drugs with mechanistically defined models. Trends Pharmacol Sci 1999; 20: 329–37.

6. Liu SS, Wu CL. The effect of analgesic technique on postoperative patient-reported outcomes including analgesia: a systematic review. Anesth Analg 2007; 105: 789–808.

7. Zakine J, Samarcq D, Lorne E, et al. Postoperative ketamine administration decreases morphine consumption in major abdominal surgery: a prospective, randomized, double-blind, controlled study. Anesth Analg 2008; 106: 1856–61.

8. Elia N, Tramer MR. Ketamine and postoperative pain: a quantitative systematic review of randomised trials. Pain 2005; 113: 61–70.

9. Eilers H, Philip LA, Bickler PE, McKay WR, Schumacher MA. The reversal of fentanyl-induced tolerance by administration of "small-dose" ketamine. Anesth Analg 2001; 93: 213–14.

10. Yaksh TL, Tozier N, Horais KA, et al. Toxicology profile of N-methyl-D-aspartate antagonists delivered by intrathecal infusion in the canine model. Anesthesiology 2008; 108: 938–49.

11. Fitzgibbon EJ, Hall P, Schroder C, Seely J, Viola R. Low dose ketamine as an analgesic adjuvant in difficult pain syndromes: a strategy for conversion from parenteral to oral ketamine. J Pain Symptom Manage 2002; 23: 165–70.

12. Hayashida K, DeGoes S, Curry R, Eisenach JC. Gabapentin activates spinal noradrenergic activity in rats and humans and reduces hypersensitivity after surgery. Anesthesiology 2007; 106: 557–62.

13. Tanabe M, Takasu K, Takeuchi Y, Ono H. Pain relief by gabapentin and pregabalin via supraspinal mechanisms after peripheral nerve injury. J Neurosci Res 2008; 86: 3258–64.

14. Field MJ, Cox PJ, Stott E, *et al.* Identification of the α2-δ-1 subunit of voltage-dependent calcium channels as a molecular target for pain mediating the analgesic actions of pregabalin. *Proc Natl Acad Sci U S A* 2006; **103**: 17537–42.

15. Li CY, Zhang XL, Matthews EA, *et al.* Calcium channel α₂δ₁ subunit mediates spinal hyperexcitability in pain modulation. *Pain* 2006; **125**: 20–34.

16. Rowbotham M, Harden N, Stacey B, Bernstein P, Magnus-Miller L. Gabapentin for the treatment of postherpetic neuralgia: a randomized controlled trial. *JAMA* 1998; **280**: 1837–42.

17. Wiffen PJ, McQuay HJ, Edwards JE, Moore RA. Gabapentin for acute and chronic pain. *Cochrane Database Syst Rev* 2005; (3): CD005452.

18. Fassoulaki A, Triga A, Melemeni A, Sarantopoulos C. Multimodal analgesia with gabapentin and local anesthetics prevents acute and chronic pain after breast surgery for cancer. *Anesth Analg* 2005; **101**: 1427–32.

19. Leung JM, Sands LP, Rico M, *et al.* Pilot clinical trial of gabapentin to decrease postoperative delirium in older patients. *Neurology* 2006; **67**: 1251–3.

20. Pandey CK, Navkar DV, Giri PJ, *et al.* Evaluation of the optimal preemptive dose of gabapentin for postoperative pain relief after lumbar diskectomy: a randomized, double-blind, placebo-controlled study. *J Neurosurg Anesthesiol* 2005; **17**: 65–8.

21. Waxman SG, Dib-Hajj S, Cummins TR, Black JA. Sodium channels and pain. *Proc Natl Acad Sci U S A* 1999; **96**: 7635–9.

22. Gold MS, Reichling DB, Shuster MJ, Levine JD. Hyperalgesic agents increase a tetrodotoxin-resistant Na+ current in nociceptors. *Proc Natl Acad Sci U S A* 1996; **93**: 1108–12.

23. Kort ME, Drizin I, Gregg RJ, *et al.* Discovery and biological evaluation of 5-aryl-2-furfuramides, potent and selective blockers of the Naᵥ1.8 sodium channel with efficacy in models of neuropathic and inflammatory pain. *J Med Chem* 2008; **51**: 407–16.

24. Devor M, Wall PD, Catalan N. Systemic lidocaine silences ectopic neuroma and DRG discharge without blocking nerve conduction. *Pain* 1992; **48**: 261–8.

25. Persaud N, Strichartz GR. Micromolar lidocaine selectively blocks propagating ectopic impulses at a distance from their site of origin. *Pain* 2002; **99**: 333–40.

26. Guay J. The benefits of adding epidural analgesia to general anesthesia: a metaanalysis. *J Anesth* 2006; **20**: 335–40.

27. Buerkle H, Yaksh TL. Pharmacological evidence for different alpha 2-adrenergic receptor sites mediating analgesia and sedation in the rat. *Br J Anaesth* 1998; **81**: 208–15.

28. Li X, Eisenach JC. alpha2A-adrenoceptor stimulation reduces capsaicin-induced glutamate release from spinal cord synaptosomes. *J Pharmacol Exp Ther* 2001; **299**: 939–44.

29. Sanders RD, Maze M. Alpha2-adrenoceptor agonists. *Curr Opin Investig Drugs* 2007; **8**: 25–33.

30. Kingery WS, Guo TZ, Davies MF, Limbird L, Maze M. The alpha(2A) adrenoceptor and the sympathetic postganglionic neuron contribute to the development of neuropathic heat hyperalgesia in mice. *Pain* 2000; **85**: 345–58.

31. Klimscha W, Tong C, Eisenach JC. Intrathecal alpha 2-adrenergic agonists stimulate acetylcholine and norepinephrine release from the spinal cord dorsal horn in sheep. An in vivo microdialysis study. *Anesthesiology* 1997; **87**: 110–16.

32. Ossipov MH, Lopez Y, Bian D, Nichols ML, Porreca F. Synergistic antinociceptive interactions of morphine and clonidine in rats with nerve-ligation injury. *Anesthesiology* 1997; **86**: 196–204.

33. Hassenbusch SJ, Gunes S, Wachsman S, Willis KD. Intrathecal clonidine in the treatment of intractable pain: a phase I/II study. *Pain Med* 2002; **3**: 85–91.

34. Malmberg AB, Yaksh TL. Voltage-sensitive calcium channels in spinal nociceptive processing: blockade of N- and P-type channels inhibits formalin-induced nociception. *J Neurosci* 1994; **14**: 4882–90.

35. Bowersox SS, Gadbois T, Singh T, *et al.* Selective N-type neuronal voltage-sensitive calcium channel blocker, SNX-111, produces spinal antinociception in rat models of acute, persistent and neuropathic pain. *J Pharmacol Exp Ther* 1996; **279**: 1243–9.

36. Staats PS, Yearwood T, Charapata SG, *et al.* Intrathecal ziconotide in the treatment of refractory pain in patients with cancer or AIDS: a randomized controlled trial. *JAMA* 2004; **291**: 63–70.

37. Wallace MS, Rauck R, Fisher R, *et al.* Intrathecal ziconotide for severe chronic pain: safety and tolerability results of an open-label, long-term trial. *Anesth Analg* 2008; **106**: 628–37.

38. Ledent C, Valverde O, Cossu G, *et al.* Unresponsiveness to cannabinoids and reduced addictive effects of opiates in CB₁ receptor knockout mice. *Science* 1999; **283**: 401–4.

39. Abrams DI, Jay CA, Shade SB, *et al.* Cannabis in painful HIV-associated sensory neuropathy: a randomized placebo-controlled trial. *Neurology* 2007; **68**: 515–21.

40. Caterina MJ, Schumacher MA, Tominaga M, *et al.* The capsaicin receptor: a heat-activated ion channel in the pain pathway. *Nature* 1997; **389**: 816–24.

41. Aasvang EK, Hansen JB, Malmstrom J, *et al.* The effect of wound instillation of a novel purified capsaicin formulation on postherniotomy pain: a double-blind, randomized, placebo-controlled study. *Anesth Analg* 2008; **107**: 282–91.

42. Binshtok AM, Bean BP, Woolf CJ. Inhibition of nociceptors by TRPV1-mediated entry of impermeant sodium channel blockers. *Nature* 2007; **449**: 607–10.

43. Brierley SM, Page AJ, Hughes PA, *et al.* Selective role for TRPV4 ion channels in visceral sensory pathways. *Gastroenterology* 2008; **134**: 2059–69.

44. Eilers H. Anesthetic activation of nociceptors: adding insult to injury? *Mol Interv* 2008; **8**: 226–9.

45. Watson JJ, Fahey MS, van den Worm E, *et al.* TrkAd5: a novel therapeutic agent for treatment of inflammatory pain and asthma. *J Pharmacol Exp Ther* 2006; **316**: 1122–9.

Francis V. Salinas and David B. Auyong

Introduction

Local anesthetics are administered to prevent or treat acute perioperative pain. They are also utilized in the diagnosis and treatment of cancer-related, chronic, and inflammatory pain disorders. The traditional mechanism of action of local anesthetics is via blockade of axonal action potential generation or propagation by prevention of voltage-gated sodium (Na^+) channel (VGSC) conductance that mediates these action potentials. Additionally, local anesthetics also interact with calcium (Ca^{2+})-signaling G-protein-coupled receptors (GPCRs), and may mediate their anti-inflammatory actions.

The clinical activity of local anesthetics is largely determined by their chemical structure and physicochemical properties. Aminoester local anesthetics are metabolized by plasma cholinesterases, and aminoamides are metabolized in the liver. The potency of local anesthetics correlates with increasing molecular weight, which confers increased lipid solubility and protein binding, both of which increase the duration of action, but slow the onset of conduction block. Local anesthetics exist in a dynamic equilibrium between the neutral lipid-soluble form (which facilitates penetration of the axonal lipid bilayer membrane to gain access to the intracellular receptor within the VGSC) and the ionized hydrophilic form (which is the active form once intracellular). The factors that govern the rate and extent of local anesthetic systemic absorption are the physicochemical properties of the local anesthetic, the total mass of drug administered, and site of injection. Epinephrine is the most widely used local anesthetic additive, and its vasoconstrictive properties prolong the duration of action of local anesthetics by decreasing vascular absorption.

Local anesthetics have the potential to cause direct toxicity of nerves, but this is a rare occurrence in clinical application. The potential systemic toxic effects of local anesthetics include methemoglobinemia (primarily due to benzocaine and the metabolite of prilocaine, *o*-toluidine), seizures, and malignant ventricular dysrhythmias with cardiovascular collapse. True allergic reactions to local anesthetics are rare, but may be associated with the metabolites of the aminoester local anesthetics or preservatives in the local anesthetic solutions.

Mechanisms of actions of local anesthetics

Functional anatomy of axons

Action potentials are the mechanism by which information is transmitted between electrically excitable cells of the central and peripheral nervous systems (see Chapter 17). VGSCs are integral membrane proteins that are responsible for initiation, propagation, and oscillation of electrical impulses in electrically excitable tissues [1] (see Chapter 3). Local anesthetics are most often administered in close proximity to nerves within the peripheral and central nervous systems. Peripheral nerves are mixed nerves containing both afferent and efferent fibers that may be myelinated or unmyelinated. Each peripheral nerve axon possesses its own cell membrane, which contains the VGSC, responsible for neural conduction. Nonmyelinated nerve fibers contain multiple axons that are simultaneously encased by a single Schwann-cell sheath. VGSCs are distributed all along the axon of nonmyelinated nerve fibers. Propagation of action potentials in nonmyelinated axons occurs when Na^+ currents enter the axoplasm generating an action potential, which then depolarizes the adjacent membrane. In contrast, myelinated nerve fibers are segmentally encased by multiple layers of myelin formed from the plasma membranes of specialized Schwann cells that wrap around a single axon. The myelin sheath may account for greater than 50% of the thickness of myelinated nerve fibers. Periodic interruptions in the myelin sheath (nodes of Ranvier) are where VGSCs are concentrated along the axons of myelinated nerve fibers. The presence of myelin significantly increases the speed of axonal conduction by electrically insulating the cell membrane from the surrounding conducting ionic medium. In myelinated axons, Na^+ currents are restricted to enter the axoplasm through the nodes of Ranvier, allowing action-potential propagation to jump from one Ranvier node to the next (saltatory conduction). In general, increasing myelination and nerve-fiber diameter are associated with

Anesthetic Pharmacology, 2nd edition, ed. Alex S. Evers, Mervyn Maze, Evan D. Kharasch. Published by Cambridge University Press. © Cambridge University Press 2011.

Table 36.1. Classification of nerve fibers

Classification	Diameter (μ)	Myelin	Conduction velocity (m s^{-1})	Location	Function
Aα	6–22	+	30–120	Efferent to muscles	Motor
Aβ	6–22	+	30–120	Afferent from skin and joints	Tactile and proprioception
Aγ	3–6	+	15–35	Efferent to muscle spindle	Muscle tone
Aδ	1–4	+	5–25	Afferent sensory nerve	Pain, cold temperature, and touch
B	< 3	+	3–15	Preganglionic sympathetic	Autonomic function
C	0.3–1.3	–	0.7–1.3	Postganglionic sympathetic	Autonomic function, warm temperature, Pain, and touch

Data from Stranding [3].

increased conduction velocity. The presence of myelin increases conduction velocity via saltatory conduction, and the increased nerve diameter increases conduction velocity via improved cable conduction properties.

The nerve fiber is the basic structural and functional unit of peripheral nerves. A typical peripheral nerve is composed of several axon bundles, or fascicles. A loose connective tissue sheath called the endoneurium, composed of nonneural glial cells, encases each axon. A second connective tissue sheath, the perineurium, composed of several alternating layers of flattened cells and collagen, encases individual fascicles. Lastly, the entire peripheral nerve, consisting of multiple fascicles, is encased in a moderately dense connective tissue sheath known as the epineurium. The presence of these multiple layers serves to protect the peripheral nerve, but also presents a significant barrier to local anesthetics reaching their intended site of action within the axonal cell membranes. For example, a rat sciatic nerve model demonstrated that only 1.6% of an administered dose of local anesthetic penetrates into the nerve to achieve a functional block [2]. A classification of peripheral nerves based on size, presence of myelin, speed of conduction, and physiological function is presented in Table 36.1.

Molecular mechanisms of local anesthetic action

Local anesthetics inhibit neuronal conduction by directly binding to and inhibiting the ability of VGSCs to conduct the inward Na$^+$ current that mediates the rapid depolarizing phase of the action potential [4]. The inhibition results from local anesthetic binding at a receptor site in the channel's inner pore, accessible from the axoplasmic opening. Binding of the local anesthetic is a dynamic process characterized by differing affinities for the receptor site based on conformational changes of the VGSC, induced by temporal changes in the membrane potential. At resting membrane potentials, VGSCs predominantly exist in a resting (closed) conformation. When a threshold depolarization is reached, VGSCs are suddenly activated (opened), allowing the inward Na$^+$ current to further depolarize the membrane potential, leading to further VGSC opening until the equilibrium potential for Na$^+$ is reached. Following activation of VGSC and initiation of the action potential, the VGSCs rapidly inactivate in order to terminate the action potential and return the membrane to its resting potential. Within a few milliseconds of activation, the VGSCs spontaneously undergo a conformational change to an inactivated state, whereupon the inward Na$^+$ current ceases. Subsequent depolarizations cannot open the VGSC from its inactivated state. The VGSC must undergo a conformational change back to the resting closed state before it is reprimed to open again. Almost simultaneously, voltage-gated K$^+$ channels are activated and open in response to depolarization, but with a slight delay and at a slower rate than the VGSCs. The inactivation of VGSCs in combination with outward K$^+$ current via the activated K$^+$ channels results in membrane repolarization to the negative resting membrane potential. During the process of repolarization, the inactivated Na$^+$ channels and activated K$^+$ channels revert to their respective resting (closed) conformations. Thus, a three-state kinetic scheme conceptually describes the changes in VGSC conformation that accounts for the changes in Na$^+$ (and K$^+$) conductance during depolarization and repolarization.

The commonly used local anesthetics are tertiary amines that exist in a dynamic equilibrium between a neutral lipid-soluble form and a hydrophilic, positively charged form, depending on pK_a and the pH of the aqueous milieu where the local anesthetic is administered. Both ionized and nonionized compounds with local anesthetic activity can inhibit VGSCs. Permanently neutral local anesthetics (e.g., the secondary amine benzocaine) freely permeate the lipid bilayer membrane and inhibit inward Na$^+$ conductance and impulse conduction, whether administered extracellularly or directly intracellularly, demonstrating that ionization is not absolutely required for local anesthetic activity. In contrast, quaternary ammonium derivatives of local anesthetics (QX-314 and QX-222), which are permanently charged and have very little membrane permeability, exhibit potent inhibition of Na^+ conductance and conduction block only when they are directly administered into the axoplasm [5]. Thus, tertiary amines must first permeate and traverse the lipid bilayer milieu in the neutral form, and having reached the axoplasm, become ionized to bind more avidly to the local anesthetic receptor within the VGSC.

In the presence of local anesthetics, VGSC activity is decreased by 30–50%, with low-frequency nerve stimulation, which is known as *tonic block*. While the neutral local anesthetic benzocaine exhibits little change in VGSC inhibition with an increased frequency of stimulation (depolarization), tertiary amines and permanently charged local anesthetic analogs exhibit increased VGSC inhibition when the axonal membrane is repetitively depolarized, known as *use-dependent (phasic) block* [6]. Increasing the frequency of stimulation increases the likelihood that VGSCs will exist in open and inactivated forms compared to the resting (closed) unstimulated state. Thus, the binding site for tertiary amine local anesthetics is thought to be located within the pore of the VGSC, and therefore not accessible when the channel is in the closed state. As a result, the terms *guarded receptor hypothesis* or *modulated receptor hypothesis* have been suggested. These theories indicate that local anesthetics bind preferentially to the VGSCs that are either open or inactivated, either because they are impeded from accessing the axoplasmic receptor site when the channel is closed ("guarded"), or because they may bind to the closed state of the channel with lower affinity (the receptor site is "modulated" by the channel conformation). More specifically, the open and inactivated conformations exhibit greater local anesthetic activity then do the closed, resting conformation. Thus, temporal changes in membrane potential influence both the VGSC conformation and affinity for local anesthetics. Local anesthetics, once bound to the channel, stabilize and prolong the duration of the inactivated state, thus inhibiting VGSC opening during further depolarization. The process of local anesthetic dissociation, which would allow the VGSC to return to its resting conformation, occurs at a much slower rate than the rapid voltage-regulated return to the resting conformation that occurs during the physiological process of repolarization.

Local anesthetic interactions with G-protein-coupled receptor systems

GPCRs are integral cell-membrane proteins that work indirectly (through an intermediary) to activate a separate membrane-associated enzyme or ion channel. The intermediaries are heterotrimeric guanosine triphosphate

(GTP)-binding complexes called G proteins, which couple membrane receptors to intracellular signaling pathways. Ca^{2+}-signaling GPCRs, which are GPCRs linked to release of Ca^{2+} from intracellular stores, have been identified as a target for local anesthetic activity [7]. More specifically, the inflammatory modulating effects of local anesthetics may result from interactions with GPCR-mediated inflammatory signaling. Inhibition of GPCRs may occur at local anesthetic concentrations that are easily reached systemically during clinical use.

The mechanisms of action of local anesthetics on GPCR signaling have been elucidated predominantly via studies in heterologous expression systems, such as *Xenopus* oocytes, where it is assumed that the enzymes that couple the GPCR to the measured endpoint are the same as those in mammalian cells expressing that particular GPCR. When expressed in *Xenopus* oocytes, Ca^{2+}-signaling GPCRs activate one of several G proteins, which in turn activate phospholipase C (PLC). Activated PLC cleaves membrane phosphatidylinositol bisphosphate (PIP_2) into inositol trisphosphate (IP_3) and diacylglycerol (DAG). IP_3 induces Ca^{2+} release via activation of a receptor channel on intracellular stores. The increase in Ca^{2+} can be measured and used as an index of GPCR activity. For almost all the local-anesthetic-sensitive GPCRs, the site of local anesthetic action can be localized to the G-protein–receptor interface. More specifically, G proteins linked to G_q α subunits have been identified as distinctively sensitive to local anesthetics, based on the known G-protein coupling of susceptible pathways [8]. This theory has been confirmed by studies where G_q was "knocked out" of a system with accompanying loss of local anesthetic sensitivity, while pathways not coupled to G_q remained unaffected.

Acute pain is often accompanied by inflammation, and certain inflammatory responses are exquisitely sensitive to local anesthetics via GPCRs. Studies on human polymorphonuclear leukocytes (PMNs) have helped to define the effects of local anesthetics on inflammation. PMNs play a crucial role in the inflammatory response, and since they do not express Na^+ channels, they are well suited to investigations on alternative sites of actions of local anesthetics. In particular, the priming of PMNs, which is the process whereby the response of PMNs to a subsequent activating stimulus is potentiated, is often crucial for their rapid and vigorous response during inflammation. This priming has been shown to be a critical component of PMN-mediated tissue injury both in vitro and in vivo. It has been shown that priming is suppressed by local anesthetic concentrations commonly observed after intravenous or epidural administration, without interfering with the activation process of PMNs [9]. These findings provide a likely explanation why local anesthetics prevent overactive inflammatory responses without impairing host defenses or suppressing normal inflammation.

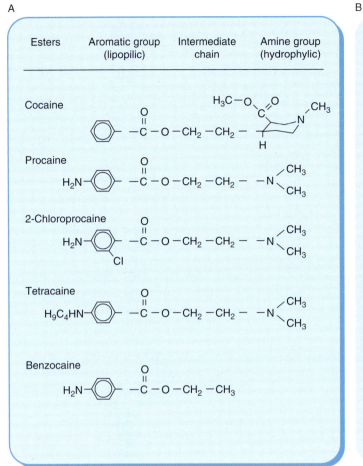

Figure 36.1. Local anesthetic structures. Clinically useful local anesthetics consist of an aromatic benzene ring linked to a hydrophilic amine group through an intermediate chain consisting of either (A) an ester or (B) an amide linkage. Benzocaine, a drug used primarily for topical anesthesia, is the only clinically useful local anesthetic lacking a tertiary amine group. Local anesthetics connected through an ester linkage are metabolized by plasma cholinesterases. Local anesthetics connected through an amide linkage are metabolized in the liver by microsomal enzymes. Adapted from Butterworth [10].

Physicochemical properties and relationships to activity and potency

The clinically useful local anesthetics consist of a lipophilic, substituted benzene ring linked to a hydrophilic amine group (tertiary or quaternary depending on pK_a and pH) through an intermediate chain consisting of either an ester or an amide linkage (Fig. 36.1). The type of linkage separates the local anesthetics into two chemically distinct classes. Plasma cholinesterase enzymes hydrolyze the aminoesters, while aminoamides undergo enzymatic biotransformation in the liver. The clinically useful aminoamide local anesthetics can be further classified based on whether the hydrophilic amino end is a straight carbon chain (e.g., lidocaine) or the amino nitrogen is within a ring structure (pipecoloxylidide, e.g., bupivacaine). The clinical activity of local anesthetics is dependent on several important physicochemical properties [11], which determine the potency, duration of action, and tendency for differential nerve block (Table 36.2).

Lipid solubility

The aromatic ring is the primary determinant of the lipophilic nature (lipid solubility) of local anesthetics. Lipid solubility correlates with the tendency of the local anesthetic to associate with and penetrate through the axonal membrane lipid bilayer and into the axoplasm, and is largely determined by the degree of alkyl substitution on either the aromatic ring or the remaining structure [13]. For example, in the mepivacaine group (N-alkylpiperidine xylidide) of the amide local anesthetics, a change from a methyl to a butyl substitution on the tertiary amino group converts mepivacaine to bupivacaine, which increases lipid solubility 26-fold. In contrast, a minor shortening of the 4-carbon butyl group of bupivacaine to a 3-carbon substitution (propyl) converts the compound to ropivacaine, which is approximately 4.5 times less lipid-soluble than bupivacaine (Fig. 36.1).

Table 36.2. Physicochemical properties of clinically used local anesthetics

Local anesthetic	pK$_a$	% Ionized (at pH 7.4)	Partition coefficient (lipid solubility)	% Protein binding
Amides				
Bupivacaine	8.1	83	3420	95
Levobupivacaine	8.1	83	3420	> 97%
Etidocaine	7.7	66	7317	94
Lidocaine	7.9	76	366	64
Mepivacaine	7.6	61	130	77
Prilocaine	7.9	76	129	55
Ropivacaine	8.1	83	775	94
Esters				
Chloroprocaine	8.7	95	810	NA
Procaine	8.9	97	100	6
Tetracaine	8.5	93	5822	94

Source: Liu [12].
NA, not available.

Lipid solubility is the primary determinant of local anesthetic potency and duration of action. The more lipophilic local anesthetics are able to permeate the axonal membranes more readily, and thus are able to bind to the VGSCs with greater affinity. Although increasing lipid solubility may hasten axonal penetration, it may also result in increased uptake and sequestration of local anesthetics by myelin and other lipid-soluble perineural compartments, which results in a net effect of a decreased onset of action. The duration of action is prolonged as the sequestration of the more lipid-soluble local anesthetics within the myelin and surrounding perineural compartments leads to decreased vascular absorption and uptake, which provides a depot for slow release of the local anesthetic. Most importantly, increased lipid solubility correlates with intrinsic local anesthetic potency. This observation may be explained by the correlation between lipid solubility and both the increased VGSC affinity and the ability to alter the VGSC conformation by directly affecting the fluidity of the axonal lipid bilayer membrane.

Protein binding

Protein binding also influences the clinical activity of local anesthetics, as only the unbound form is free to exert pharmacological activity. In general, increasing molecular weight also correlates with an increased degree of protein binding to both plasma and tissue proteins. Although the VGSC is a protein structure, it does not appear that the degree of local anesthetic protein binding correlates with increased affinity to the protein

structure of the VGSC. Studies have suggested that the binding and dissociation of local anesthetic molecules from the VGSC occurs in a matter of seconds, irrespective of the degree of protein binding [14].

Plasma protein binding more closely correlates with the degree of protein binding on the extracellular axonal membrane. It is likely that highly protein-bound local anesthetics are removed from the nerve at a decreased rate, resulting in slower uptake and absorption, which accounts for the increased duration of action. Thus, increased protein binding correlates with increased lipid solubility, which leads to increased potency and duration of action of the local anesthetic as a result of increased local anesthetic content within nerves.

Within the plasma compartment, local anesthetics are bound primarily to albumin and α$_1$-acid glycoprotein (AAG). Local anesthetics exhibit a low-affinity and high-capacity association with albumin and a high-affinity but low-capacity association with AAG. Although local anesthetics bind to AAG preferentially, binding to AAG is easily saturated with clinically relevant doses of local anesthetics [15]. Once AAG binding capacity is saturated, additional local anesthetic is bound by albumin. Because the binding capacity of albumin is very high, it can continue to bind local anesthetics at plasma concentrations that may exceed clinically desired levels. Despite the high-capacity binding of albumin, elevated plasma local anesthetic levels may increase the risk of systemic toxicity by increasing the percentage of the unbound active form. This is because the degree of protein binding is concentration-dependent and, as the transition from AAG binding to albumin binding occurs, the degree of plasma protein binding consistently decreases.

Plasma protein binding of local anesthetics is also determined by plasma pH, such that the percentage of local anesthetic that is protein-bound decreases as the pH decreases. Thus, with acidosis (as occurs with significant seizure activity secondary to CNS toxicity), the percentage of unbound active local anesthetic increases, even though the total plasma concentration may remain the same. Other clinically relevant factors also influence the degree of plasma protein binding. AAG concentrations are decreased in pregnancy and in the newborn. In contrast, AAG is increased in a variety of pathophysiological conditions such as surgery, trauma, and certain disease states (e.g., uremia), with a subsequent increase in the extent of local anesthetic binding [16].

Ionization

Local anesthetics in solution are weak bases that exist in equilibrium between the neutral lipid-soluble and the charged (protonated) hydrophilic form. The pK$_a$ (dissociation constant) of a local anesthetic is the pH at which the two forms are present in equivalent amounts. The combination of the perineural and axoplasmic pH and the pK$_a$ of a specific local anesthetic determine the percentage of each form. The primary site of action of local anesthetics appears to be on the

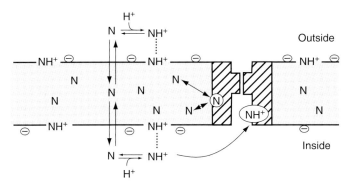

Figure 36.2. Diagram of bilayer lipid membrane of conductive tissue with Na$^+$ channel *(cross-hatching)* spanning the membrane. Clinically useful local anesthetics exist in equilibrium between the lipid-soluble neutral (N) base and the charged (NH$^+$) hydrophilic form. The neutral base (N) preferentially partitions into the lipophilic membrane interior and easily passes into the membrane. The charged hydrophilic form (NH$^+$) binds to the Na$^+$ channel at the negatively charged membrane surface. The neutral form can cause membrane expansion and closure of the Na$^+$ channel. The charged form directly inhibits the Na$^+$ channel by binding with a local anesthetic receptor. Adapted from Strichartz [18].

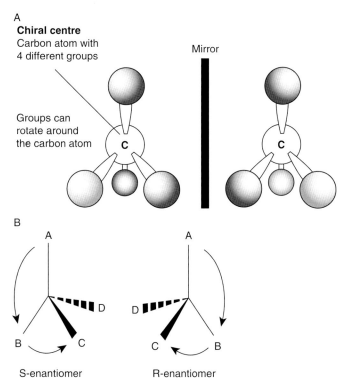

Figure 36.3. (A) Molecule with a chiral center and its enantiomers. (B) Three-dimensional projection of a pair of enantiomers that cannot be superimposed on each other. Bonds represented as solid lines are in plane, those drawn with dotted lines project away, and those represented by a wedge project toward the reader. Adapted from Burke and Henderson [19].

intracellular side of the transmembrane VGSC, and the charged form appears to be the predominantly active form within the axoplasm [17]. Thus, pK_a generally correlates with speed of onset, because penetration by the neutral lipid-soluble form across the lipid bilayer of the axonal membrane is the primary mechanism by which local anesthetics gain access to the local anesthetic binding site (Fig. 36.2). Additionally, local anesthetic uptake occuring as a result of lipophilic absorption will shift the effective pK_a downward, further favoring the neutral base form; this will have the effect of limiting diffusion of local anesthetic away from the site of administration.

The percentage of local anesthetic molecules existing in the neutral lipid-soluble form at the physiological pH of 7.4 is inversely proportional to the pK_a of the specific local anesthetic. Thus, the lower the pK_a for a given local anesthetic within a specific local tissue pH, the higher the percentage of local anesthetic that exists in the lipid-soluble form, which hastens the penetration of axonal membrane and onset of action. Sodium bicarbonate may be added to local anesthetic solutions in an attempt to raise their pH, thereby increasing the percentage of the uncharged lipid-soluble form and theoretically improving the onset of the block. In contrast, local anesthetic solutions may be less effective when administered into inflamed tissues, which may be acidic and hyperemic. The acidic milieu will result in an increased percentage of the lipid-insoluble protonated form, and the increased tissue blood flow may increase systemic absorption, further impairing the clinical activity of the administered local anesthetic.

Chirality

The majority of clinically useful local anesthetics are formulated as racemic mixtures. Racemic compounds are 1 : 1 mixtures of two types of molecules (stereoisomers) bearing identical chemical composition and binding, but with a different three-dimensional spatial orientation around an asymmetric carbon atom (Fig. 36.3). Specifically, molecules with an asymmetric carbon exist in two forms that are mirror images of each other (i.e., they exhibit "handedness" or chirality), distinguished by how they rotate light according to the orientation of the structures in three dimensions [19]. Local anesthetics exhibit a specific type of stereoisomerism termed *enantiomerism*, in which the pair of stereoisomers in three-dimensional projection cannot be superimposed on each other. A notable exception is lidocaine, which is achiral. Although enantiomers of local anesthetics have identical physicochemical properties, they exhibit potentially different clinical pharmacodynamic (e.g., potency and potential for systemic toxicity) and pharmacokinetic profiles because of differences in their interactions with the biological receptor (VGSC).

Some clinically used local anesthetics are formulated as single stereoisomers. Examples of such clinically useful local anesthetics include ropivacaine (the S-enantiomer of the bupivacaine homolog, with a propyl alkyl group rather than a butyl group) and levobupivacaine (the S-enantiomer of bupivacaine). R-enantiomers of local anesthetics appear to have greater in-vitro potency for conduction block of both neuronal and cardiac Na$^+$ channels, and thus would have the potential for greater therapeutic efficacy as well as the potential for systemic toxicity. In contrast, S-enantiomers (ropivacaine and levobupivacaine) have been shown to have equipotent clinical efficacy for neuronal conduction block, but a lower potential for systemic toxicity than either racemic mixtures or the R-enantiomer [20].

Additives to increase local anesthetic activity

Epinephrine is frequently added to local anesthetic solutions to cause vasoconstriction, and when used with larger volumes of local anesthetics (e.g., epidural and peripheral nerve blocks) it serves as a marker of intravascular injection [21]. The reported benefits of epinephrine include prolongation and increased intensity of local anesthetic block, as well as decreased systemic absorption of local anesthetic. The vasoconstrictive effects of epinephrine (and other α_1-agonists) augments local anesthetic activity via antagonism of the inherent vasodilating effects of local anesthetics [22]. Epinephrine decreases the rate of vascular absorption, thereby allowing more local anesthetics to reach the axonal membrane, which prolongs and increases the intraneural content of local anesthetics. Blood flow is decreased only briefly, and the block will persist long after the α_1-adrenergic effect on blood flow has resolved [23]. Additional analgesic effects from epinephrine may also occur through interaction with α_2-adrenoceptors in the spinal cord, which activate endogenous analgesic mechanisms via a direct pharmacodynamic mechanism [24]. The extent to which epinephrine prolongs the duration of local anesthetic block largely depends on the specific local anesthetic used and the site of administration. The most commonly used dose is 5 µg mL^{-1}, but doses as low as 1–2 µg mL^{-1} may be sufficient. The smallest effective dose should be utilized, as epinephrine in combination with local anesthetics may potentially have toxic effects on tissue, the cardiovascular system, peripheral nerves, and spinal cord [21].

Alkalinization

Alkalinization of local anesthetic solutions by the addition of sodium bicarbonate has been reported to speed the onset of conduction block. The pH of commercial local anesthetic solutions ranges from 3 to 7, and they are especially acidic if prepackaged with epinephrine. As the pK_a of commonly used local anesthetics ranges from 7.6 to 8.9 (Table 36.2), less than 3% of a commercially prepared local anesthetic exists in the lipid-soluble neutral form. Addition of sodium bicarbonate will increase the pH of the solution, which should increase the percentage of the lipid-soluble form and enhance the rate of diffusion across the nerve sheath and axonal membrane. However, local anesthetic solutions cannot be alkalinized beyond a pH of 6–8 before precipitation occurs [25], and these ranges of pH will only serve to increase the percentage of the neutral form to approximately 10%. There are conflicting data as to whether addition of sodium bicarbonate actually speeds the onset of local anesthetic block; if so, it may only decrease the latency by 5 minutes. The differences may be related to the magnitude of the pH changes and the use of local anesthetic solutions prepackaged with epinephrine. One would expect that addition of sodium bicarbonate would have its greatest impact when added to local anesthetic solutions prepackaged with epinephrine, as these solutions have a lower pH compared to epinephrine-free (plain) solutions [26]. Additionally, an animal study demonstrated that alkalinization of lidocaine actually decreased the duration of peripheral nerve block if the solution did not contain epinephrine [27]. Thus, the value of alkalinization of local anesthetics may be questioned as a clinically useful tool to improve the onset of local anesthetic block.

Opioids

Opioids are commonly added to local anesthetic solutions for spinal and epidural anesthesia as a means to increase the density and duration of the local anesthetic block. The receptor site for opioids administered in the intrathecal or epidural space is within the gray matter of substantia gelatinosa located in the dorsal horn of the spinal cord. Opioids bind to presynaptic and postsynaptic receptor sites, which selectively blocks transmission of afferent nociceptive stimuli from Aδ and C fibers [28]. Presynaptic effects include release of spinal adenosine, which seems to be an important mediator specific for spinally mediated analgesia, as well as inhibition of Ca^{2+} influx and the subsequent release of glutamate and neuropeptides (such as substance P) from primary afferent terminals [29]. Postsynaptic effects include an increase in K^+ conductance, hyperpolarizing ascending second-order projecting neurons without affecting somatosensory or motor evoked potentials [30].

Pharmacokinetics of local anesthetics

Plasma concentrations after administration of local anesthetics for neural blockade are determined by the rate of absorption from the site of injection, the rate of tissue distribution, and the rate of elimination of the specific local anesthetic drug. Patient-specific factors such as age, cardiovascular and hepatic function, and degree of plasma protein binding influence the free plasma levels of local anesthetics, which ultimately determine the potential for systemic toxicity [31].

Systemic absorption

In general, local anesthetics with decreased systemic absorption will have a greater margin of safety in clinical use. The site of injection, the total dose and physicochemical properties of the specific local anesthetic, and addition of epinephrine determine the rate and extent of systemic absorption. The relative amounts of fat and tissue perfusion surrounding

Table 36.3. Typical peak plasma levels after regional anesthesia with commonly used local anesthetics

Local anesthetic	Technique	Dose (mg)	C_{max} ($\mu g\ mL^{-1}$)	T_{max} (min)	Toxic plasma concentration ($\mu g\ mL^{-1}$)
Bupivacaine	Brachial plexus	150	1.00	20	3
	Celiac plexus	100	1.50	17	
	Epidural	150	1.26	20	
	Intercostal	140	0.90	30	
	Lumbar sympathetic	52.5	0.49	24	
	Sciatic/femoral	400	1.89	15	
Lidocaine	Brachial plexus	400	4.00	25	5
	Epidural	400	4.27	20	
	Intercostal	400	6.80	15	
Mepivacaine	Brachial plexus	500	3.68	24	5
	Epidural	500	4.95	16	
	Intercostal	500	8.06	9	
	Sciatic/femoral	500	3.59	31	
Ropivacaine	Brachial plexus	190	1.30	53	4
	Epidural	150	1.07	40	
	Intercostal	140	1.10	21	
Levobupivacaine[a]	Brachial plexus	150	0.96	43	
	Epidural	150	1.02	24	

C_{max}, peak plasma levels; T_{max}, time until C_{max}.
Sources: Liu [12] and Berrisford et al. [32].
[a]Data from [33].

the site of administration will interact with the physicochemical properties of the local anesthetic to affect the rate of systemic uptake. In general, areas with greater tissue perfusion will have more rapid and complete uptake than those with more fat, regardless of type of local anesthetic. Thus, rates of absorption generally decrease in the following order: interpleural > intercostal > caudal > epidural > brachial plexus > sciatic/femoral > subcutaneous tissue (Table 36.3). The greater the total dose of local anesthetic injected, the greater the systemic absorption and peak blood levels (C_{max}). Within the clinical range of doses used for local anesthetics, this relationship is nearly linear and is relatively unaffected by anesthetic concentration [34] and speed of injection [35]. Physicochemical properties of local anesthetics will affect systemic absorption. In general, the more potent drugs with greater lipid solubility and protein binding will result in lower systemic absorption and C_{max}. Increased binding to neural and nonneural tissue probably explains this observation. Effects of epinephrine have been previously discussed. In brief, epinephrine can counteract the inherent vasodilating characteristics of most local anesthetics. The reduction in

C_{max} with epinephrine is most effective for the less lipid-soluble, less potent, shorter-acting drugs, because increased tissue binding rather than local blood flow may be a greater determinant of absorption for the long-acting drugs.

Distribution

After systemic absorption, local anesthetics are rapidly distributed throughout all body tissues, but the relative concentration in different tissues depends on organ perfusion, partition coefficient, and plasma protein binding. The end organs of main concern for systemic toxicity are the cardiovascular system (CVS) and central nervous system (CNS), because they are considered members of the "vessel-rich group" and will have local anesthetic rapidly distributed to them. Despite the high blood perfusion, regional blood and tissue levels of local anesthetics within these organs will not initially correlate with systemic blood levels, because of hysteresis [36]. Because regional and not systemic pharmacokinetics govern subsequent pharmacodynamic effects, systemic blood levels may not correlate with effects of local anesthetics on end organs [37]. Regional pharmacokinetics of local anesthetics

anesthetics, resulting in increases in the extracellular concentration in the brain compared to administration of local anesthetics without epinephrine [69]. Thus, it appears that epinephrine may augment CNS toxicity by increasing the pharmacologically active free fraction available for transport across intracerebral neurons.

Cardiovascular toxicity

In general, significantly larger doses of local anesthetics are required to produce cardiovascular system (CVS) toxicity than CNS toxicity. Similar to CNS toxicity, the potential for CVS toxicity parallels the anesthetic potency of the drug. The more potent, more lipid-soluble drugs (bupivacaine, etidocaine, and ropivacaine) appear to have an inherently greater cardiotoxicity than the less potent drugs. In addition, the more potent drugs appear to have a different sequence of CVS toxicity compared with the less potent drugs. For example, increasing doses of lidocaine lead to hypotension, bradycardia, and hypoxia, whereas bupivacaine often results in sudden CVS collapse caused by ventricular dysrhythmias that are resistant to resuscitation [70].

The more potent local anesthetics appear to possess greater potential for direct cardiac electrophysiological toxicity. A study examining lidocaine, bupivacaine, and ropivacaine in rats has demonstrated equivalent peak effects on myocardial contractility but much greater effects on electrophysiology (prolongation of QRS) from bupivacaine and ropivacaine than from lidocaine [71]. Although all local anesthetics block the cardiac conduction system through a dose-dependent block of Na^+ channels, two features of bupivacaine's Na^+-channel-blocking abilities may enhance its cardiotoxicity. First, bupivacaine exhibits a much stronger binding affinity to resting and inactivated Na^+ channels than lidocaine [72]. Second, local anesthetics bind to Na^+ channels during systole and dissociate during diastole. Bupivacaine dissociates from Na^+ channels during cardiac diastole much more slowly than lidocaine. Indeed, bupivacaine dissociates so slowly that the duration of diastole at physiologic heart rates (60–180 beats per minute) does not allow enough time for complete recovery of Na^+ channels and bupivacaine conduction block accumulates (Fig. 36.4). In contrast, lidocaine fully dissociates from Na^+ channels during diastole and little accumulation of conduction block occurs [73]. Thus, enhanced electrophysiological effects of more potent local anesthetics on the cardiac conduction system may explain their increased potential to produce sudden CVS collapse through cardiac dysrhythmias.

CNS-mediated mechanisms may also be involved in the increased cardiotoxicity of bupivacaine. The nucleus tractus solitarius in the medulla is an important region for autonomic control of the CVS [74]. Neural activities within the nucleus tractus solitarius of rats are markedly diminished by intravenous doses of bupivacaine immediately before the development of hypotension. Furthermore, direct intracerebral injection of bupivacaine can induce sudden dysrhythmias and

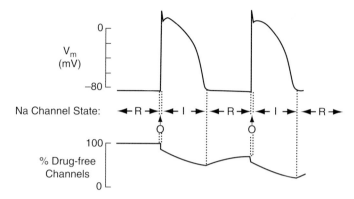

Figure 36.4. The relationship between cardiac action potential (*top*), sodium channel state (*middle*), and sodium channel block by bupivacaine (*bottom*). Sodium channels are predominantly in the resting (R) form during diastole, open (O) transiently during the upstroke of the action potential, and are in the inactive (I) form during the plateau of the action potential. Block of sodium channels by bupivacaine accumulates during the action potential (systole) with recovery occurring during diastole. Recovery of sodium channels occurs by dissociation of bupivacaine and is time-dependent. Recovery during each diastolic interval is incomplete and results in accumulation of sodium channel block with successive heart beats. Adapted from Clarkson and Hondeghem [73].

cardiovascular collapse [75]. Peripheral effects of bupivacaine on the autonomic and vasomotor systems may also augment its cardiovascular toxicity. Bupivacaine possesses potent peripheral inhibitory effects on sympathetic reflexes [76] and also has potent direct vasodilating properties that may exacerbate cardiovascular collapse [77]. The multitude of different cardiac and neural mechanisms of cardiotoxicity may in part explain the reported difficulties of resuscitation after cardiovascular collapse from bupivacaine. Once cardiovascular collapse occurs, maintenance of respiration and myocardial perfusion are vital, because hypercapnia, hypoxia, acidosis, hypothermia, hyperkalemia, hyponatremia, and myocardial ischemia will all further sensitize the heart to bupivacaine cardiotoxicity [78].

New and emerging concepts

Over three decades ago, an editorial by Albright reported a series of cases of fatal CVS toxicity associated with use of the long-acting lipophilic local anesthetics bupivacaine and etidocaine, in which there was an alarming lack of response to standard resuscitative measures in otherwise healthy patients [79]. In this editorial, Albright highlighted that the potency of bupivacaine and etidocaine correlated with their propensity to cause severe CVS toxicity, often manifested by malignant ventricular dysrhythmias, progressing to cardiovascular collapse. The treatment for severe local-anesthetic-induced CVS with bupivacaine has largely been supportive, consisting of oxygenation and ventilation with positive-pressure ventilation, in conjunction with standard advanced cardiac life support measures, including hemodynamic support with either epinephrine or vasopressin, pharmacological therapy with amiodarone, and cardioversion [58]. In spite of these aggressive efforts, bupivacaine-induced CVS toxicity may remain refractory, and cardiopulmonary bypass should be considered [80].

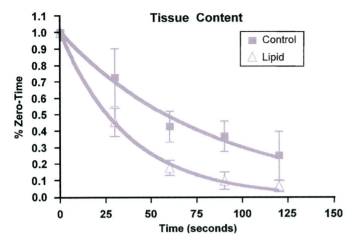

Figure 36.5. Cardiac bupivacaine content. The trends for myocardial bupivacaine content are shown during 2 minutes after a 30-second infusion of bupivacaine 500 μmol L^{-1} for control and lipid-treated hearts. Values are normalized to zero time, and error bars indicate standard deviation ($n = 5$ for both groups). Regression curves were fitted by single exponential decay functions with time constants 83 seconds ($R^2 = 0.9861$) and 37 seconds ($R^2 = 0.9978$) for control group and lipid groups respectively. Reproduced with permission from Weinberg *et al*. [83].

During a series of experiments studying the metabolic effects of bupivacaine, a group of investigators made the chance observation that pretreating rats with lipid soybean oil emulsion resulted in marked resistance to the cardiac effects of bupivacaine infusion. In a series of experiments with progressively larger animal models, lipid emulsion therapy (consisting of a bolus followed by an infusion) was administered before [81] or after [82] bupivacaine-induced cardiac arrest was established, and resulted in rapid hemodynamic recovery and uniform rescue from cardiac arrest compared to controls not given lipid emulsion. The mechanisms proposed for lipid emulsion's remarkable success included a "lipid sink" mechanism, where bupivacaine is removed from affected tissues (myocardium) by partitioning into a plasma lipid compartment created by the lipid. This hypothesis has been supported by a study clearly demonstrating that lipid emulsion not only accelerates recovery from bupivacaine toxicity, but also accelerates the removal of bupivacaine in an isolated rat heart model (Fig. 36.5) [83]. A complementary mechanism for the effectiveness of lipid emulsion is that it directly reverses bupivacaine-induced contractile dysfunction by providing an alternative source of intracellular fat content for myocardial metabolism, in the absence of normal fatty acid oxidative phosphorylation [84]. Subsequent to these animal studies, the first case of lipid emulsion in the resuscitation of severe bupivacaine-induced CVS toxicity was reported in 2006 [85]. Since then, numerous other case reports have added to the clinical evidence of the remarkable efficacy of lipid emulsion in the treatment of severe local-anesthetic-induced CVS toxicity [86–88]. The current recommended dose is 1.5 mL kg^{-1} 20% Intralipid administered as bolus, followed by a continuous infusion of 0.25 mL kg^{-1} min^{-1} continued for an hour after resumption of sinus rhythm [89]. Future areas of research include additional studies on its mechanisms of actions, as well as optimization of the treatment regimen with regards to efficacy and safety.

Summary

Action potentials are the signals through which information is transmitted between electrically excitable cells of the central and peripheral nervous systems. Local anesthetics inhibit action potentials, thus interrupting afferent (sensory) signaling from various parts of the body to the brain. Local anesthetics are most often administered in close proximity to nerves within the peripheral and central nervous systems. Multiple layers protect the peripheral nerve, thus presenting a significant barrier to local anesthetics reaching their intended site of action within the axonal cell membranes.

The traditional mechanism of action of local anesthetics is via blockade of axonal action-potential generation or propagation by prevention of the voltage-gated Na$^+$ channel (VGSC) conductances that mediate these action potentials. Additionally, local anesthetics interact with Ca^{2+} signaling and with G-protein-coupled receptors (GPCRs), which may mediate their anti-inflammatory actions.

The clinical activity of local anesthetics is dependent on several important physicochemical properties, which determine the potency, duration of action, and tendency for differential nerve block:

- The aromatic ring is the primary determinant of the lipid solubility of local anesthetics, and, in turn, lipid solubility is the primary determinant of local anesthetic potency and duration of action.
- Protein binding also influences the clinical activity of local anesthetics, as only the unbound form is free to exert pharmacological activity. In general, increasing molecular weight correlates with increased protein binding to both plasma and tissue proteins.
- The site of action of local anesthetics is on the intracellular surface of the VGSC. Local anesthetics must therefore penetrate the cell to gain access to their site of action. Only the uncharged form of the drug can penetrate the membrane. The lower the pK_a of a given local anesthetic, the greater the proportion of the drug that is unprotonated and uncharged at physiological pH. Local anesthetics with lower pK_a thus have faster onset of action.
- The majority of clinically useful local anesthetics are formulated as racemic mixtures of two enantiomers (mirror-image sterioisomers) that differ in local anesthetic potency. Several local anesthetics (ropivacaine and levobupivacaine) are marketed and administered as a single S-enantiomer. Use of a single enantiomer is thought to reduce toxicity and side effects.

Additives to increase local anesthetic activity include:

Epinephrine – Epinephrine decreases the rate of vascular absorption, thereby allowing more local anesthetics to reach the axonal membrane, which prolongs and increases the intraneural content of local anesthetics.

Alkalinization – Alkalinization of local anesthetic solutions by the addition of sodium bicarbonate has been reported to speed the onset of conduction block, but its clinical value is questionable.

Opioids – Opioids are commonly added to local anesthetic solutions for spinal and epidural anesthesia as a means of increasing the density and duration of the local anesthetic block. Opioids bind to presynaptic and postsynaptic opioid receptor sites, which selectively blocks transmission of afferent nociceptive stimuli.

Plasma concentrations after administration of local anesthetics for neural blockade are determined by the rate of absorption from the site of injection, the rate of tissue distribution, and the rate of elimination of the specific local anesthetic. Local anesthetics with decreased systemic absorption will have a greater margin of safety in clinical use. The greater the total dose of local anesthetic injected, the greater the systemic absorption and peak blood levels (C_{max}); drugs with greater lipid solubility and protein binding will result in lower systemic absorption and C_{max}. After systemic absorption, local anesthetics are rapidly distributed throughout all body tissues, but the relative concentration in different tissues depends on organ perfusion, partition coefficient, and plasma protein binding. Elimination of aminoesters is primarily dependent on hydrolysis of the ester bond by plasma cholinesterase. Aminoamides are metabolized in the liver by the cytochrome P450 enzymes CYP1A2 and CYP3A4.

The major adverse reactions to local anesthetics are allergic reactions, methemoglobinemia, cardiovascular toxicity, and central nervous system toxicity. Infusion of lipid emulsions has been shown to be highly efficacious in treating the cardiovascular toxicity of local anesthetics.

References

1. Scholz A. Mechanisms of (local) anesthetics on voltage-gated sodium and other ion channels. *Br J Anaesth* 2002; **89**: 52–61.

2. Popitz-Berger FA, Leeson S, Strichartz GR, Thalhammer JG. Relation between functional deficit and intraneural local anesthetic during peripheral nerve block. A study in the rat sciatic nerve. *Anesthesiology* 1995; **83**: 583–91.

3. Stranding S. Nervous system. In: Stranding S, Ellis H, Healy JC, *et al.*, eds., *Gray's Anatomy*, 39th edn. Edinburgh: Elsevier Churchill Livingstone, 2005.

4. Butterworth JF, Strichartz GR. Molecular mechanisms of local anesthesia: a review. *Anesthesiology* 1990; **72**: 711–34.

5. Strichartz GR. The inhibition of sodium currents in myelinated nerve by quaternary derivatives of lidocaine. *J Gen Physiol* 1973; **62**: 37–57.

6. Courtney KR, Kendig JJ, Cohen EN. The rates of interaction of local anesthetics with sodium channels in nerve. *J Pharmacol Exp Ther* 1978; **207**: 594–604.

7. Hollman MW, DiFazio CA, Duriex ME. Ca-signaling G-protein-coupled receptors: a new site of local anesthetic action? *Reg Anesth Pain Med* 2001; **26**: 565–71.

8. Hollman MW, Wieczorek KS, Berger A, Duriex ME. Local anesthetic inhibition of G protein-coupled receptor signaling by interference with Galpha(q) protein function. *Mol Pharmacol* 2001; **59**: 294–301.

9. Hollman MW, Gross A, Jelacin N, Duriex ME. Local anesthetic effects on priming and activation of human neutrophils. *Anesthesiology* 2001; **95**: 113–22.

10. Butterworth J. Mechanisms of local anesthetic action. In: Miller RA, Schwinn DA, eds., *Atlas of Anesthesia, vol. 2, Scientific Principles of Anesthesia*. Philadelphia, PA: Churchill-Livingstone, 1998: 162.

11. Strichartz GR, Sanchez V, Arthur R, Chafetz R, Martiny D. Fundamental properties of local anesthetics. II. Measuring octanol:buffer partition coefficients and pKa values of clinically used drugs. *Anesth Analg* 1990; **71**: 158–70.

12. Liu SS. Local anesthetics and analgesia. In: Ashburn MA, Rice LJ, eds., *The Management of Pain*. New York, NY: Churchill Livingstone, 1997: 141–70.

13. Courtney K, Strichartz GR. Structural elements which determine local anesthetic activity. In: Strichartz GR, ed., *Handbook of Experimental Pharmacology: Local Anesthetics*. Heidelberg: Springer-Verlag, 1987: 53.

14. Ulbricht W. Kinetics of drug action and equilibrium results at the node of Ranvier. *Physiol Rev* 1981; **61**: 785–828.

15. Denson D, Coyle D, Thompson G, Meyers J. Alpha 1-acid glycoprotein and albumin in human serum bupivacaine binding. *Clin Pharmacol Ther* 1984; **35**: 409–15.

16. Wulf H, Winckler K, Denzer D. Plasma concentrations of alpha 1-acid glycoprotein following operations and its effect on the plasma protein binding of bupivacaine. *Prog Clin Biol Res* 1989; **300**: 457–60.

17. Frazier DY, Narahashi T, Yamada M. The site of action and active form of local anesthetics. II. Experiments with quaternary compounds. *J Pharmacol Exp Ther* 1970; **171**: 45–51.

18. Strichartz GR. Neural physiology and local anesthetic action. In: Cousins MJ, Bridenbaugh PO, eds., *Neural Blockade in Clinical Anesthesia and Management of Pain*. Philadelphia, PA: Lippincott-Raven, 1998: 42.

19. Burke D, Henderson DJ. Chirality: a blueprint for the future. *Br J Anaesth* 2002; **88**: 563–76.

20. Casati A, Putzu M. Bupivacaine, levobupivacaine and ropivacaine: are they clinically different? *Best Pract Res Clin Anaesthesiol* 2005; **19**: 247–68.

21. Neal JM. Effects of epinephrine in local anesthetics on the central and peripheral nervous system: neurotoxicity and neural blood flow. *Reg Anesth Pain Med* 2003; **28**: 124–34.

22. Sinnott CJ, Cogswell LP, Johnson A, Strichartz GR. On the mechanism by which epinephrine potentiates

lidocaine's peripheral block. *Anesthesiology* 2003; **98**: 181–8.

23. Kohane DS, Lu NT, Cairns BE, Berde CB. Effects of adrenergic agonists and antagonists on tetrodotoxin-induced nerve block. *Reg Anesth Pain Med* 2001; **26**: 239–45.

24. Curatolo M, Peterson-Felix S, Arendt-Nielsen L, Zbinde AM. Epidural epinephrine and clonidine: segmental analgesia and effects on different pain modalities. *Anesthesiology* 1997; **87**: 785–94.

25. Ikuta PT, Raza SM, Durrani Z, *et al.* pH adjustment schedule for the amide local anesthetics. *Reg Anesth* 1989; **14**: 229–35.

26. Capogna G, Celleno D, Laudano D, Giunta F. Alkalinization of local anesthetics: which block, which local anesthetic? *Reg Anesth* 1995; **20**: 369–77.

27. Sinnott CJ, Garfield JM, Thalhammar JG, Strichartz GR. Addition of sodium bicarbonate to lidocaine decreases the duration of peripheral nerve block in the rat. *Anesthesiology* 2000; **93**: 1045–52.

28. Chiari A, Eisenach JC. Spinal anesthesia: mechanisms, agents, methods, and safety. *Reg Anesth Pain Med* 1998; **23**: 357–62.

29. Eisenach JC, Hood DD, Curry R, *et al.* Intrathecal but not intravenous opioids release adenosine from the spinal cord. *J Pain* 2004; **5**: 64–8.

30. Schubert A, Licina MG, Lineberry PY, Deers MA. The effect of intrathecal morphine on somatosensory evoked potentials in humans. *Anesthesiology* 1991; **75**: 401–5.

31. Rosenberg PH, Veering BT, Urmey WF. Maximum recommended dose of local anesthetics: a multifactorial concept. *Reg Anesth Pain Med* 2004; **29**: 564–75.

32. Berrisford SG, Sabanathan S, Mearns AJ, Clarke BJ, Hamdi A. Plasma concentrations of bupivacaine and its enantiomers during continuous intercostal nerve block. *Br J Anaesth* 1993; **70**: 201–4.

33. Foster RH, Markham A. Levobupivacaine: a review of its pharmacology and use as a local anesthetic. *Drugs* 2000; **59**: 551–79.

34. Morrison LM, Emanuelsson BM, McClure JH. Efficacy and kinetics of extradural ropivacaine: Comparison with bupivacaine. *Br J Anaesth* 1994; **72**: 164–9.

35. Tucker GT, Moore DC, Bridenbaugh PO, Bridenbaugh LD, Thompson GE. Systemic absorption of mepivacaine in commonly used regional block procedures. *Anesthesiology* 1972; **37**: 277–87.

36. Huang YF, Upton RN, Runciman WB. IV bolus administration of subconvulsive doses of lignocaine to conscious sheep: myocardial pharmacokinetics. *Br J Anaesth* 1993; **70**: 326–32.

37. Huang YF, Upton RN, Runciman WB. IV bolus administration of subconvulsive doses of lignocaine to conscious sheep: relationship between myocardial pharmacokinetics and pharmacodynamics. *Br J Anaesth* 1993; **70**: 556–61.

38. Denson DD. Physiology and pharmacology of local anesthetics. In: Sinatra RS, Hord AH, Ginsberg B, Preble M, eds., *Acute Pain: Mechanisms and Management*. St. Louis, MO: Mosby Year Book, 1992: 124.

39. Burm AG, van der Meer AD, van Kleef JW, Zeijlmans PW, Groen K. Pharmacokinetics of the enantiomers of bupivacaine following intravenous administration of the racemate. *Br J Clin Pharmacol* 1994; **38**: 125–9.

40. Copeland SE, Ladd LA, Gu XQ, Mather LE. The effects of general anesthesia on whole body and regional pharmacokinetics at toxic doses. *Anesth Analg* 2008; **106**: 1440–9.

41. Berkun Y, Ben-Zvi A, Levy Y, Galili D, Shalit M. Evaluation and adverse reactions to local anesthetics: experience with 236 patients. *Ann Allergy Asthma Immunol* 2003; **91**: 342–5.

42. Boren E, Teuber SS, Naguwa SM, Gershwin ME. A critical review of local anesthetic sensitivity. *Clin Rev Allergy Immunol* 2007; **32**: 119–28.

43. Lambert LA, Lambert DH, Strichartz GR. Irreversible conduction block in isolated nerve by high concentrations of local anesthetics. *Anesthesiology* 1994; **80**: 1082–93.

44. Buyukakilli B, Comelekoglu U, Tatroglu, Kanik A. Reversible conduction block in isolated sciatic nerve by high concentration of bupivacaine. *Pharmacol Res* 2003; **47**: 235–41.

45. Ravindran RS, Bond VK, Tasch MD, Gupta C, Luerssen TG. Prolonged neural blockade following regional analgesia with 2-chloroprocaine. *Anesth Analg* 1980; **59**: 447–51.

46. Reisner LS, Hochman BN, Plumer MH. Persistent neurological deficit and adhesive arachnoiditis following intrathecal 2-chloroprocaine injection. *Anesth Analg* 1980; **59**: 452–4.

47. Covino BG, Marx GF, Finster M, Zsigmond EK. Prolonged sensory/motor deficits following inadvertent spinal anesthesia. *Anesth Analg* 1980; **59**: 399–400.

48. Taniguchi M, Bollen AW, Drasner K. Sodium bisulfite: scapegoat for chloroprocaine neurotoxicity? *Anesthesiology* 2004; **100**: 85–91.

49. Casati A, Fanelli G, Danelli G, *et al.* Spinal anesthesia with lidocaine or preservative free 2-chloroprocaine for outpatient knee arthroscopy: a prospective, randomized, double blind comparison. *Anesth Analg* 2007; **104**: 959–64.

50. Yoos JR, Kopacz. Spinal 2-chloroprocaine for surgery; an initial 10-month experience. *Anesth Analg* 2005; **100**: 553–8.

51. Rigler Ml, Drasner K, Krejce TC, *et al.* Cauda equina syndrome after continuous spinal anesthesia. *Anesth Analg* 1991; **72**: 275–81.

52. Lambert DH, Hurley RJ. Cauda equina syndrome and continuous spinal anesthesia. *Anesth Analg* 1991; **72**: 817–19.

53. Pollock JE. Transient neurological symptoms: etiology, risk factors, and management. *Reg Anesth Pain Med* 2002; **27**: 581–6.

54. Pollock JE, Burkhead D, Neal JM, *et al.* Spinal nerve function in five volunteers experiencing transient neurological symptoms after lidocaine subarachnoid anesthesia. *Anesth Analg* 2000; **90**: 658–65.

55. Zaric D, Christiansen C, Pace NL, Punjasadwong Y. Transient neurological symptoms after spinal anesthesia with lidocaine versus other local anesthetics: a systematic review of randomized controlled trials. *Anesth Analg* 2005; **100**: 1811–16.

56. Moore TJ, Walsh CS, Cohen MR. Reported adverse event cases of methemoglobinemia associated with benzocaine products. *Arch Intern Med* 2004; **164**: 1192–6.

57. Vasters FG, Eberhart LHJ, Koch T, *et al.* Risk factors for prilocaine-induced methemoglobinemia following peripheral regional anesthesia. *Eur J Anaesthesiol* 2006; **23**: 760–5.

58. Salinas FV. Local anesthetic systemic toxicity. In: Atlee JL, Bucklin BA, Chaney MA, *et al.*, eds., *Complications in Anesthesia*, 2nd ed. Philadelphia, PA, Saunders Elsevier. 2007; 230–234.

59. Auroy Y, Narchi P, Messiah A, *et al.* Serious complications related to regional anesthesia; results of a prospective survey in France. *Anesthesiology* 1997; **87**: 479–86.

60. Brown DL, Ransom DM, Hall JA, *et al.* Regional anesthesia and local anesthetic-induced systemic toxicity: seizure frequency and accompanying cardiovascular changes. *Anesth Analg* 1995; **81**: 321–8.

61. Auroy Y, Benhamou D, Bargues L, *et al.* Major complications of regional anesthesia in France: the SOS regional anesthesia hotline service. *Anesthesiology* 2002; **97**: 1274–80.

62. Auroy Y, Narchi P, Messiah A, *et al.* Serious complications related to regional anesthesia: Results of a prospective survey in France. *Anesthesiology* 1997; **87**: 479–86.

63. Brown DL, Ransom DM, Hall JA, *et al.* Regional anesthesia and local anesthetic-induced systemic toxicity: Seizure frequency and accompanying cardiovascular changes. *Anesth Analg* 1995; **81**: 321–6.

64. Auroy Y, Benhamou D, Bargues L, *et al.* Major complications of regional anesthesia in France: the SOS regional anesthesia hotline service. *Anesthesiology* 2002; **97**: 1274–80.

65. Shibata M, Shingu K, Murakawa M, *et al.* Tetraphasic actions of local anesthetics on central nervous system electrical activities in cats. *Reg Anesth* 1994; **19**: 255–63.

66. Bernards CM, Carpenter RL, Rupp SM, *et al.* Effect of midazolam and diazepam premedication on central nervous and cardiovascular toxicity of bupivacaine in pigs. *Anesthesiology* 1989; **70**: 318–23.

67. Yokoyama M, Hirakawa M, Goto H. Effects of vasoconstrictive agents added to lidocaine on intravenous lidocaine-induced convulsions in rats. *Anesthesiology* 1995; **82**: 574–80.

68. Yamauchi Y, Kotania J, Ueda Y. The effects of exogenous eiphephrine on convulsive dose of lidocaine: relationship with cerebral circulation. *J Neurosurg Anesthesiol* 1998; **10**: 178–87.

69. Takahashi R, Oda Y, Tanaka K, *et al.* Epinephrine increases the extracellular lidocaine concentration in the brain: a possible mechanism for increased central nervous system toxicity. *Anesthesiology* 2006; **105**: 984–9.

70. Groban L, Deal DD, Vernon JC, James RL, Butterworth J. Cardiac resuscitation after incremental overdosage with lidocaine, bupivacaine, levobupivacaine, and ropivacaine in anesthetized dogs. *Anesth Analg* 2001; **92**: 37–43.

71. Reiz S, Haggmark S, Johansson G, Nath S. Cardiotoxicity of ropivacaine: a new amide local anesthetic agent. *Acta Anaesthesiol Scand* 1989; **33**: 93–8.

72. Guo XT, Castle NA, Chernoff DM, Strichartz GR. Comparative inhibition of voltage-gated cation channels by local anesthetics. *Ann N Y Acad Sci* 1991; **625**: 181–99.

73. Clarkson CW, Hondeghem LM. Mechanism for bupivacaine depression of cardiac conduction: fast block of sodium channels during the action potential with slow recovery from block during diastole. *Anesthesiology* 1985; **62**: 396–405.

74. Denson DD, Behbehani MM, Gregg RV. Effects of intravenously administered arrhythmogenic dose of bupivacaine at the nucleus tractus solitarius in the conscious rat. *Reg Anesth* 1990; **15**: 76–80.

75. Bernards CM, Artu AA. Hexamethonium and midazolam terminate dysrhythmias and hypertension caused by intracerebroventricular bupivacaine in rabbits. *Anesthesiology* 1991; **74**: 89–96.

76. Szocik JF, Gardener CA, Webb RC. Inhibitory effects of bupivacaine and lidocaine on adrenergic neuroeffector junctions in the rat tail artery. *Anesthesiology* 1993; **78**: 911–17.

77. Loftstrom JB. 1991 Labat lecture: the effect of local anesthetics on the peripheral vasculature. *Reg Anesth* 1992; **17**: 1–11.

78. Freysz M, Timour Q, Bertrix L, *et al.* Bupivacaine hastens the ischemia-induced decrease of the electrical ventricular fibrillation threshold. *Anesth Analg* 1995; **80**: 657–63.

79. Albright GA. Cardiac arrest following regional anesthesia with etidocaine or bupivacaine. *Anesthesiology* 1979; **51**: 285–7.

80. Soltesz EG, van Pelt F, Byrne JG. Emergent cardiopulmonary bypass for bupivacaine cardiotoxicity. *J Cardiothorac Vasc Anesth* 2003; **17**: 357–8.

81. Weinberg GL, VadeBoncouer T, Ramaraju GA, Garcia-Amaro MF, Cwik MJ. Pretreatment or resuscitation with a lipid infusion shits the dose-response to bupivacaine-induced asystole in rats. *Anesthesiology* 1998; **88**: 1071–5.

82. Weinberg GL, Ripper R, Feinstein DL, Hoffman W. Lipid emulsion infusion rescues dogs from bupivacaine-induced cardiac toxicity. *Reg Anesth Pain Med* 2003; **28**: 198–202.

83. Weinberg GL, Ripper R, Murphy P, *et al.* Lipid infusion accelerates removal of bupivacaine and recovery from bupivacaine toxicity in the isolated rat heart. *Reg Anesth Pain Med* 2006; **31**: 296–303.

84. Stehr SN, Ziegeler JC, Pexa A, *et al.* The effects of lipid infusion on myocardial function and bioenergetics in L-bupivacaine toxicity in the isolated rat heart. *Anesth Analg* 2007; **104**: 186–92.

85. Rosenblatt MA, Abel M, Fischer GW, Itzkovich CJ, Eisenkraft JB. Successful use of 20% lipid emulsion to resuscitate a patient after presumed bupivacaine-related cardiac arrest. *Anesthesiology* 2006; **105**: 217–8.

86. Ludot H, Tharin JY, Beloudah M, Mazoit JX, Malinovsky JM. Successful resuscitation after ropivacaine and lidocaine-induced ventricular arrhythmia following posterior lumbar plexus block in a child. *Anesth Analg* 2008; **106**: 1572–47.

87. Litz R, Roessel T, Heller AR, Stehr SN. Reversal of central nervous system and cardiac toxicity after local anesthetic intoxication by lipid emulsion injection. *Anesth Analg* 2008; **106**: 1575–7.

88. Warren JA, Thoma RB, Georgescu A, Shah SJ. Intravenous lipid infusion in the successful resuscitation of local anesthetic-induced cardiovascular collapse after supraclavicular brachial plexus block. *Anesth Analg* 2008; **106**: 1578–80.

89. Weinberg G. Lipid rescue resuscitation from local anaesthetic cardiac toxicity. *Toxicol Rev* 2006; **25**: 139–45.

Essential drugs in anesthetic practice
Antiepileptic and antipsychotic drugs

W. Andrew Kofke

Antiepileptic drugs

Epilepsy and uncontrolled seizures require therapy to attenuate the disabling effects of seizure and to prevent or limit seizure-induced brain damage [1]. Treatment of epilepsy should begin with monotherapy; it should be extended to include additional or alternative drugs only if monotherapy is ineffective or if unacceptable side effects arise [2].

The first generation of antiepileptic drugs (AEDs) to be used were discovered through serendipity. These drugs include phenytoin, phenobarbital, primidone, benzodiazepines, ethosuximide, carbamezepine, and valproate. Since the early 1990s a so-called second generation of AEDs has been released, including felbamate, vigabatrin, lamotrigine, gabapentin, topiramate, tiagabine, oxcarbezepine, levetiracetam, pregabalin, and zonisamide. The first-generation drugs tend to have an increased potential for interactions and adverse effects secondary to enzyme induction and/or inhibition. The newer AEDs offer advantages of decreased drug interactions, greater safety, unique mechanisms of action, and a broader spectrum of activity. However, most still have significant adverse side effects that limit efficacy [3,4].

AEDs act on diverse molecular targets, with a variety of mechanisms available to achieve antiepileptic function. These targets include specific ion channels, receptors, neurotransmitters, or neurotransmitter synthesis/breakdown systems [3]. Efficacy is generally based on the end result of modifying the excitability of neurons such that seizure activity is attenuated without disturbing normal nonepileptic neuronal activity. In general, the main mechanisms of antiepileptic activity can be categorized as:

- modulation of voltage-dependent ion channels
- enhancement of synaptic inhibition
- inhibition of synaptic excitation

The most important mechanisms of the second-generation AEDs are summarized in Fig. 37.1.

The specific FDA-approved indications for the newer drugs are summarized in Table 37.1. The table also shows the principal advantages and disadvantages that affect decision-making for each of these drugs [5,6].

Pharmacokinetics and drug interactions

AEDs as a group have varying degrees of protein binding and enzyme induction (Table 37.2) [7,8]. In general, if a drug induces the hepatic enzymes responsible for metabolism of another drug or itself then a decreased plasma concentration will arise, and, conversely, inhibition of an enzyme responsible for metabolism of another drug or itself will produce an increased plasma concentration. Other effects on free drug level may arise from competition for protein binding sites. For example, phenobarbital, phenytoin, and carbamazepine are hepatic enzyme inducers, whereas phenytoin, benzodiazepine, and valproate are highly protein-bound. This results in a bewildering array of drug and disease interactions, with significant pharmacokinetic and pharmacodynamic effects. Thus, wherever possible, safe therapy should be guided by assiduously monitoring the plasma concentration. A summary of drug interactions is shown in Table 37.3 [3,9,10]. Many other interactions with non-AED drugs occur; these are beyond the scope of this chapter, but are fully delineated in each drug's package insert or drug label.

Enzyme-inducing AEDs such as phenytoin, carbamazepine, and phenobarbital can increase the clearance and reduce the efficacy of some anticancer drugs. Use of AEDs has been associated with an increased cancer relapse rate and a decrement in survival time with some cancers [11].

Disease interactions

Evidence is conflicting regarding the neuroprotective potential of AEDs. Although neuroprotection has been reported in some animal models, this has not yet been shown in any human studies. However, some studies in both animals and humans suggest a negative influence from some first-generation AEDs. Thus it appears that AEDs should be used only cautiously or not at all in this group of patients [12]. AEDs, particularly those that are enzyme inducers, have a measurable impact on thyroid-hormone kinetics and metabolism. This usually does not have clinically significant effects except in patients with pre-existing thyroid dysfunction [13]. For AEDs that are

Anesthetic Pharmacology, 2nd edition, ed. Alex S. Evers, Mervyn Maze, Evan D. Kharasch. Published by Cambridge University Press. © Cambridge University Press 2011.

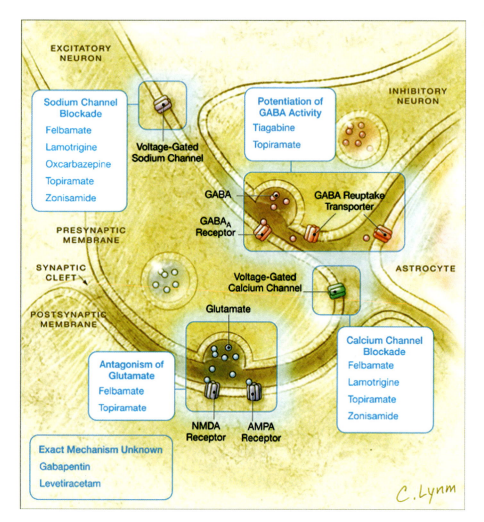

Figure 37.1. Principal mechanisms of action of the newer antiepileptic drugs include voltage-dependent ion channel blockade, enhancement of inhibitory neurotransmission, and reduction of excitatory neurotransmission. Mechanisms unique from those for traditional antiepileptic drugs include glutamate antagonism at N-methyl-D-aspartate (NMDA) receptors (felbamate) and α-amino-3-hydroxy-5-methyl-4-isoxazole propionic acid (AMPA) receptors (felbamate, topiramate) and inhibition of γ-aminobutyric acid (GABA) reuptake in neurons and astrocytes (tiagabine). Reproduced with permission from LaRoche and Helmers [4].

metabolized or eliminated by the liver or kidney, dosage adjustment is likely to be needed if one or both of these organs have significant dysfunction.

Adverse effects

Adverse effects of AEDs are usually unique to each specific drug or drug class. These include somnolence, cognitive effects, increased risk of suicide, decreased bone density with prolonged use, and pharmacokinetic/pharmacodynamic drug interactions [4]. Moreover, there has been long-standing concern regarding the use of AEDs during pregnancy [4]. Weight gain has been reported with carbamazepine, felbamate, gabapentin, pregabalin, valproate, and vigabatrin, and weight decrease with topiramate and zonixamide [13]. Common adverse effects are summarized in Table 37.4 [14,15].

With respect to potential teratogenic effects, most pregnant patients exposed to AEDs deliver normal infants. Nonetheless, fetal exposure to the first-generation AEDs has been associated with congenital anomalies. Valproate and phenobarbital are thought to have the highest risk of major malformations. Data on the teratogenicity of second-generation drugs are less clear. Notably, the metabolism of most AEDs is induced in pregnancy such that seizure control may be compromised. In addition, phenytoin, phenobarbital, primidone, and carbamazepine can cause hemorrhage in the newborn due to vitamin K deficiency [4].

AEDs have narrow therapeutic windows such that an alteration in bioavailability arising from a change in brand formulation can have serious consequences in terms of seizure control or adverse effects. For this reason the American Academy of Neurology has issued a position statement recommending that generic substitution in epilepsy be undertaken with caution, with the knowledge of both the prescribing physician and the patient. If possible, prescription refills should come from the same manufacturer [4].

A comprehensive list of AEDs can be found in Tables 37.1–37.4. Drugs more commonly encountered in the acute care context follow.

Table 37.1. Main indications, advantages, and disadvantages of new antiepileptic drugs

Drug	Main current indications in epilepsy treatment	Advantages	Disadvantages
Felbamate	Treatment of severe epilepsies, particularly Lennox–Gastaut syndrome, refractory to all other available AEDs	Broad-spectrum	Risk of aplastic anemia and liver toxicity
			CNS and gastrointestinal side effects
			Drug interactions
			Intensive safety laboratory monitoring
Gabapentin	Adjunctive treatment of refractory partial seizures, with or without secondary generalization	Rapid titration	Efficacy limited to partial epilepsies
		Good tolerability	Limited efficacy
			Multiple daily dosing
		Lack of drug interactions	Need for high doses (high cost)
		Efficacy against some comorbidities (e.g., neuropathic pain)	
Lamotrigine	Adjunctive treatment and monotherapy of partial and generalized epilepsies	Broad-spectrum	Need for slow tritration
	(may aggravate severe myoclonic epilepsy)	Good CNS tolerability	Hypersensitivity reactions
		Twice daily dosing	Vulnerability to enzyme induction and inhibition
		Efficacy against some comorbidities (e.g., bipolar depression)	
Levetiracetam	Adjunctive treatment of refractory partial seizures, with or without secondary generalization	High efficacy	Limited clinical experience
		Good tolerability, rapid titration	No data in generalized epilepsies
		No interactions	
		Twice-daily dosing	
Oxcarbazepine	Adjunctive treatment and monotherapy of partial seizures and primarily or secondarily generalized tonic-clonic seizures	Good CNS tolerability	Not broad-spectrum
		Easy titration	Interaction with oral contraceptives
		Less allergenic than carbamazepine	
		Efficacy against some comorbidities (e.g., acute mania)	Hyponatremia
Tiagabine	Adjunctive treatment of refractory partial seizures, with or without secondary generalization	Low allergenic potential	Not broad-spectrum
		No enzyme inducing effects	Need for slow titration
			Multiple daily dosing
			Inducible metabolism

Table 37.1. (*cont.*)

Drug	Main current indications in epilepsy treatment	Advantages	Disadvantages
Topiramate	Adjunctive treatment of partial and generalized epilepsies	Broad-spectrum	Need for slow titration
	(monotherapy use approved in some countries; efficacy against absence seizures has not been established)	High efficacy	CNS side effects
		Twice-daily dosing	Interactions with oral contraceptives
		Low allergenic potential	
		Efficacy against some comorbidities (e.g., binge eating disorder)	
Vigabatrin	Adjunctive treatment of partial seizures, with or without secondary generalization, refractory to all other AEDs	Easy titration	Visual field defects
	Treatment of infantile spasms	Lack of major interactions	Not broad-spectrum
		High efficacy in infantile spasms	Weight gain
Zonisamide	Adjunctive treatment of refractory partial and generalized epilepsies	Broad-spectrum	Need for slow titration
		Twice-daily dosing	CNS side effects
			Allergic reactions

Adapted from Gatti *et al.* [5] and Perucca [6].

Phenytoin

Phenytoin (5,5-diphenyl-2,4-imidazolidinedione) is a barbiturate-like drug that is effective in controlling seizure activity. It is one of the oldest AEDs, having been approved in 1953 [5,6]. Phenytoin is indicated for the control of generalized tonic–clonic (grand mal) and complex partial (psychomotor, temporal lobe) seizures and prevention and treatment of seizures occurring during or following neurosurgery [16]. Phenytoin was reported to be effective in a status epilepticus model in rats [17], a kindling model of complex partial seizures [18], and a model of topical cortical 4-aminopyridine [19]. Phenytoin was also reported to have efficacy in seizures induced by imipenum [20], pentylenetetrazole [21], electroshock [21], flurothyl [22], and opioids [23].

Pharmacokinetics

See Table 37.2 for a summary of kinetic parameters. Phenytoin undergoes hepatic degradation to inactive forms that are then renally eliminated. Alterations of hepatic enzymes affect its metabolism and kinetics [24]. Moreover, there appears to be a small subset of patients who are genetic slow metabolizers [25]. The drug is highly protein-bound and exhibits saturable pharmacokinetics [26]. The steady-state serum concentration varies nonlinearly as a function of dose. This means that with increasing dose the serum concentration increases faster for each unit increase in dose, with the opposite effect when decreasing dose (Fig. 37.2) [27]. Because of this kinetic property and its protein binding, maintaining appropriate protein-free drug levels can be problematic [26,28]. Although phenytoin has an elimination half-life of about 24 hours, it may require up to a month of continuous dosing to achieve a steady-state plasma concentration [28].

Adverse effects and interactions

Common adverse effects are summarized in Table 37.4. Most common effects include nystagmus, drowsiness, diplopia, ataxia, decreased folate levels, hyperglycemia, and cognitive effects. Hypotension and arrhythmia are associated with rapid administration. Following intravenous administration of phenytoin, severe cardiovascular reactions and fatalities have been reported with atrial and ventricular conduction depression and ventricular fibrillation [25]. Over time, gingival hyperplasia, coarsening of facial features, and hirsutism can be troublesome. It occasionally produces

Table 37.2. Pharmacokinetics of antiepileptic drugs

Drug	V_d (L kg^{-1})	Water-soluble	Protein binding (%)	Enzymatic activity	$t_{1/2}$ (h)	Elimination route (%) Renal	Liver	Maintenance dose (mg kg^{-1} d^{-1})	Normal dosing interval	Loading dose (mg kg^{-1})	Range (µg mL^{-1})
Carbamazepine	0.8	no	75	Broad-spectrum inducer	9–15	1	99	10–25	BID–TID	None	4–12
Clonazepam	3	no	85	Induces CYP2B family	20–60	<5	>90	0.03–0.3	BID	None	5–70
Ethosuximide	0.7	yes	0	None	30–60	<20	<80	15–40	OD	None	40–100
Felbamate	0.8	no	25	Induces CYP3A4, inhibits CYP2C19	13–22	50	50	15–60	BID–TID	–	30–100
Gabapentin	0.7	yes	0	None	5–7	100	0	1800–3600[a]	TID	–	4–8
Lamotrigine	1	no	55	Induces UGTs	12–62	10	90	300–500[a]	BID	–	2–4
Levetiracetam	0.5–0.7	yes	<10	None	6–8	100	0	1000–3000[a]	BID	–	20–60
Oxcarbazepine	0.8	no	40	Induces CYP3A4, UGTs, inhibits CYP2C19	9	1	99	1200–2400[a]	BID	–	5–50
Phenobarbital	0.6	yes	45	Broad-spectrum inducer	75–110	25	75	1–4	OD	18–20	10–40
Phenytoin	0.8	no	90	Broad-spectrum inducer	9–36	5	95	4–7	OD, BID	15–20	10–20
Tiagabine	1.4	no	96	None	7–9	2	98	32–56[a]	BID–QID	–	5–70
Topiramate	0.7	yes	15	Induces CYP3A4, inhibits CYP2C19	12–24	65	35	200–800[a]	BID	–	2–25
Valproate	0.2	no	90	Broad-spectrum inhibitor	6–18	2	98	10–60	BID–TID	–	50–150
Zonisamide	1.5	yes/no	40	None	63	35	65	100–600[a]	OD	–	10–40

BID, twice daily; CYP, cytochrome P450; OD, once daily; $t_{1/2}$, elimination half-life, range of therapeutic concentrations; TID, three times daily; UGT, UDP glucuronosyltransferase; V_d, volume of distribution.
[a]Maintenance dose in mg d^{-1}.
Adapted from Foldavary-Shaefer and Wyllie [7] and Lacerda et al. [8].

Table 37.3. Interactions between antiepileptic drugs

	CBZ	PHT	VPA	PB	PRD	ESM	CLB	VGA	LTG	GBP	OXC	FBM	TGB	TPM	LVT	PGB	ZNS
CBZ	↓CBZ[a]	↑↓PHT	↓VPA	0	↓PRD ↑PB	↓ESM	↓CLB ↑N-DC	0	↓LTG	0	↓OXC	↓FBM	↓TGB	↓TPM	0	0	↓ZNS
PHT	↓CBZ	—	↓VPA	↑PB	↓PRD ↑PB	↓ESM	↓CLB ↑N-DC	0	↓LTG	0	↓OXC	↓FBM	↓TGB	↓TPM	0	0	↓ZNS
VPA	↑CBZ-E	(↑)PHT, ↑fPHT	—	↑PB	↑↓PRD ↑PB	↑↓ESM	0	0	↑LTG	0	↑OXC	↑FBM	(↓)TGB	(↓)TPM	0	0	↑ZNS
PB	↓CBZ (↑)CBZ-E	↑↓PHT	↓VPA	—	?	↓ESM	↓CLB ↑N-DC	0	↓LTG	0	↓OXC	↓FBM	↓TGB	0	0	0	↓ZNS
PRD	↓CBZ (↑)CBZ-E	↑PHT	↓VPA	?	—	↓ESM	↓CLB ↑N-DC	0	↓LTG	?/0	↓OXC	↓FBM	↓TGB	0	0	0	↓ZNS
ESM	↑↓CBZ	↑↓PHT	↓VPA	↑↓PB	↑PRD ↑↓PB	—	?	?/0	?	?/0	?	?	?	?	?/0	?	?
CLB	↓CBZ	(↑)PHT	(↑)VPA	(↑)PB	(↑)PB (↑)PRD	?	—	?/0	?	?/0	0	?	?	?	?/0	?	?
VGA	0	↓PHT	0	(↓)PB	(↓)PRD	0	?	—	0	?/0	?	0	?/0	?/0	?/0	?	?
LTG	PD	0	↓VPA	0	0	0	?/0	0	↓LTG[a]	?/0	?/0	0	?/0	?/0	0	0	?
GBP	0	(↑)PHT	0	0	?/0	?/0	?/0	?/0	0/?	—	0	(↑)FBM	?/0	?/0	0	0	?
OXC	↓CBZ	↑PHT	0	↑PB	?	?	?	?	↓LTG	?	—	0	?	?	?	?	?
FBM	↓CBZ ↑CBZ-E	↑PHT	↑VPA	↑PB	?	?	?	(↑)VGA	(↑)LTG	?/0	0	—	?	?	?	?	?
TGB	0	0	(↓)VPA	?/0	?/0	?/0	?/0	?/0	?/0	?/0	?	?/0	—	?/0	?/0	0	?
TPM	0	↑PHT	(↓)VPA	0	0	?/0	?/0	?/0	?/0	?/0	?	?/0	?/0	—	?/0	0	?
LEV	0	(↑)PHT	0	0	0	?	?/0	?/0	0	0	?	?/0	?/0	?/0	—	?	?
PGB	0	0	0	0	0	?	?	?	?	?	?	?	0	0	?	—	?
ZNS	0	0	0	?	?	?	?	?	?	?	?	?	0	?	?	?	—

CBZ, carbamazepine; CBZ-E, carbamazepin-epoxid; CLB, clobazam; ESM, ethosuximide; FBM, felbamate; GBP, gabapentin; LEV, levetiracetam; LTG, lamotrigine; N-DC, N-desmethyl-clobazam; OXC, oxcarbazepine; PD, pharmacodynamic; PHT, phenytoin; fPHT, free PHT (not bound to protein); PB, phenobarbital; PGB, pregabalin; PRD, primidone; TGB, tiagabine; TPM, topiramate; VPA, valproate; VGB, vigabatrin; ZNS, zonisamide.
↓, decreased plasma level; ↑, increased plasma level; ↑↓, variable, inconsistent, or little change of plasma level; 0, no influence on plasma level; ?/0, little influence on plasma level to be expected, but not determined; ?, not determined.
[a]CBZ and LTG cause an autoinduction.
Adapted from Stefan and Feuerstein [3], Bourgeois [9], and Baumgartner and Stefan [10].

Table 37.4. Adverse effects of AEDs

AED	Adverse effect
Carbamazepine	Diplopia, nystagmus, blurred vision, ataxia, dizziness, sedation, hyponatremia
Ethosuximide	Nausea, vomiting, gastric distress, drowsiness, ataxia
Gabapentin	Weight gain, peripheral edema, behavior change
Lamotrigine	Rash, Stevens–Johnson syndrome, toxic epidermal necrolysis (especially with concomitant valproate), hypersensitivity reactions, hepatic and renal failure, disseminated intravascular coagulopathy, arthritis, tics, insomnia
Levetiracetam	Irritability, behavior change, somnolence
Oxcarbazepine	Hyponatremia, rash
Phenobarbital	Drowsiness, slurred speech, nystagmus, confusion, somnolence, ataxia, respiratory depression, coma, hypotension
Phenytoin	Vertigo, ataxia, slurred speech, nystagmus, diplopia, somnolence, stupor, coma, gingival hyperplasia, hypotension and arrhythmias (IV)
Primidone	Sedation and dizziness acutely, then similar to phenobarbital, cyrstalliuria
Tiagabine	Stupor, weakness
Topiramate	Nephrolithasis, open angle glaucoma, hypohidrosis, metabolic acidosis, weight loss, language dysfunction
Valproate	Sedation, gastric disturbance, weight gain, diarrhea, tremors, ataxia, somnolence, coma, thrombocytopenia, platelet dysfunction, hepatic failure
Zonisamide	Rash, nephrolithiasis, hypohidrosis, irritability, photosensitivity, weight loss

This is not a comprehensive list, representing only some of the more common and more serious adverse effects.
Adapted from Mattson [14] and French *et al.* [15].

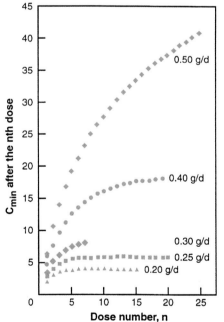

Figure 37.2. Plot of minimal phenytoin serum concentration (C_{min}) after the n-th dose. Dose rates (grams per day) are 0.50, 0.40, 0.30, 0.25, and 0.20 [28]. Reproduced with permission from Wagner [27].

Phenytoin interacts with an extensive list of drugs, with AED interactions summarized in Table 37.3. The liver is the primary site of metabolism; thus, patients with impaired liver function may show early signs of toxicity [16,25]. Phenytoin has been associated with exacerbation of porphyria [16,25]. Phenytoin is not significantly removed by hemodialysis, and supplemental dosing after hemodialysis is not required.

Fosphenytoin

Fosphenytoin sodium is a phosphate ester prodrug of phenytoin. Phenytoin is cleaved from the prodrug by phosphatases found in several tissues. Unlike phenytoin, fosphenytoin is freely soluble in aqueous solutions and was developed as a replacement for parenteral phenytoin, which is associated with many administration issues (see above) [25,29]. The indications for fosphenytoin are the same as those for phenytoin, and animal studies indicate effects equivalent to those of phenytoin [25].

Phenobarbital

First used in 1912, phenobarbital is the oldest AED in common use. Once considered a first-line drug, it is now generally considered to be a second-line therapy [30] used primarily for generalized tonic–clonic seizures [31] but also for partial seizures [32]. Absence seizures may be worsened by phenobarbital [32]. Phenobarbital's principal mechanism of action is thought to be enhancement of the inhibitory GABAergic system [33,34]. In vitro, phenobarbital enhanced postsynaptic

a morbilliform rash with a variety of other uncommon effects. It can cause soft-tissue injury with extravasation, a problem which is less likely with fosphenytoin, a prodrug of phenytoin [2,25]. Rarely, phenytoin has been associated with Stevens–Johnson syndrome and fatal hematologic/immunologic reactions [16].

GABA responses to diminish high-frequency repetitive neuronal discharges [35]. Phenobarbital has been reported to have anticonvulsant effects in a variety of animal models [19,20].

Primidone

Primidone is effective for tonic–clonic, psychomotor, and focal epileptic seizures [36]. It is thought to inactivate Na^+ channels and block rapid repetitive neuronal discharges [37]. Notably, primidone and its two metabolites phenobarbital and phenylethylmalonamide (PEMA) have anticonvulsant actions [36]. Anticonvulsant efficacy of primidone and its two metabolites has been demonstrated in electroshock and chemically induced animal seizure models [36].

Clonazepam and other benzodiazepines

Clonazepam is a benzodiazepine class drug that is used for epilepsy. Many other benzodiazepines (e.g., midazolam and lorazepam) are effective for seizures. Midazolam and lorazepam are notable for their ability to be given parenterally, and they are often used for motor seizures in the acute care context. Clonazepam is used for the alternative treatment of absence seizures, petit mal variant (Lennox–Gastaut syndrome), and akinetic and myoclonic seizures (myoclonia) resistant to therapy with other AEDs. It is generally less effective for absence seizures than ethosuximide or valproate [2,31]. It can be used alone or as an adjunct for Lennox–Gastaut syndrome [38]. The principal anticonvulsant mechanism of clonazepam is thought to be through enhancement of the inhibitory GABAergic system [33]. Clonazepam and other benzodiazepines have been reported to be efficacious in several animal models [38–40]. Notably, compated to isoflurane, ketamine, and thiopental, midazolam had the best histologic result used for two models of status epilepticus in rats [39].

Valproate

Valproate (valproic acid) is effective for monotherapy and as an adjunct in the treatment of complex partial seizures, absence seizures, and multiple seizure types that involve absence. It is a first-line drug in the treatment of absence seizures [32]. It is also effective for myoclonic, atonic, and primary generalized tonic–clonic seizures [2]. Valproate binds to the activated Na^+ channel to block rapid repetitive neuronal discharge [37]. In dissociated mouse neuron cell culture, valproate limited sustained high-frequency repetitive firing [35]. Valproate exerted anticonvulsant effects in several animal seizure models including pilocarpine [40], topical 4-aminopyridine [19,41], pentylenetetrazole [21], and flurothyl [22].

Elevation of hepatic transaminases in plasma occurs in up to 40% of patients during the first few months of therapy and is typically asymptomatic [42]. Valproate can interfere with conversion of ammonia to urea with hyperammonemia and associated lethargy. Fatal hyperammonemic encephalopathy has occurred in patients with genetic defects in urea metabolism [2]. Although serious adverse effects are uncommon, fatal liver failure has occurred. A profile of susceptibility has been established for this, with the highest risk associated with infants, AED polytherapy, mental retardation, progressive or congenital neurologic illnesses, poor nutritional status, and metabolic disorders [32].

Valproate is different from the other AEDs in that it inhibits the metabolism of drugs that are substrates for CYP2C9 and uridine diphosphate glucuronosyltransferase (UGT) and can also displace other drugs from albumin, producing an increase in unbound drug concentration [31]. It can also impair the metabolism of chemotherapeutic drugs with exacerbation of their blood dyscrasia side effects [11]. Concurrent administration with topiramate has been associated with hyperammonemia [42].

Ethosuxamide

Ethosuximide is a first-line therapy for absence (petit mal) seizures [2,32,43]. It appears to act through multiple mechanisms which include blockade of some Ca^{2+}, Na^+, and K^+ channels with a variable effect depending on brain GABA concentrations. The effects on Ca^{2+} channels are thought to be most likely responsible for its efficacy in absence seizures [44]. Microdialysis studies indicate that ethosuximide increases GABA in the ventrolateral thalamus but reduces GABA in the primary motor cortex [44]. Ethosuximide infused into various brain regions or intracerebroventricularly diminished spike and wave discharges. It was ineffective in an electroshock model of seizures [44].

Fatal blood dyscrasias, Stevens–Johnson syndrome, and systemic lupus erythematosus have been associated with ethosuxamide [2,43]. Used alone in mixed types of epilepsy, ethosuximide may increase the frequency of tonic–clonic seizures [43]. It can exacerbate porphyria, and in the presence of renal disease may lead to nephrotic syndrome. Pre-existing blood dyscrasias warrant increased vigilance for exacerbation of these problems [42].

Carbamazepine

Carbamazepine is effective for treatment of partial and secondarily generalized tonic–clonic seizures [2,45]. It is widely considered one of the drugs of choice for partial seizures, but it may make absence or myoclonic seizures worse [2,32]. Carbamazepine produces use-dependent block of Na^+ channels [7] and has been shown to be effective in rodent models of chemically and electrically induced seizure [45].

There are black-box warnings associated with carbamazepine regarding potential for aplastic anemia, agranuocytosis, thrombocytopenia, and serious dermatologic reactions that can include toxic epidermal necrolysis and Stevens–Johnson syndrome [45]. These dermatologic reactions are estimated to arise at a rate of 1–6 per 10 000 new Caucasian users with about 10-fold greater risk in patients with Chinese ancestry. In this latter group a strong association has been found with the presence of HLA-B*1502, an inherited allelic variant of the HLA-B gene. HLA-B*1502 is found almost exclusively in patients with ancestry from broad areas of Asia [45].

Oxcarbazepine

Oxcarbazepine is a keto analog of carbamazepine with many similarities to carbamazepine except for significantly less impact on hepatic microsomal enzymes and thus fewer drug interactions [3]. Oxcarbazepine is effective for monotherapy of partial seizures with or without secondary generalization [15,42,46]. Oxcarbazepine is thought to act by inhibiting voltage-dependent fast Na^+ channels. This is similar to carbamazepine's effects, but in addition oxcarbazepine also has favorable effects on K^+ and Ca^{2+} channels [3].

In-vitro electrophysiologoic studies indicate that oxcarbazepine and its active 10-monohydroxy metabolite (MHD) produce blockage of voltage-sensitive Na^+ channels. No significant interactions with brain neurotransmitters or their receptors has been observed [46]. Oxcarbazepine and MHD exhibit anticonvulsant properties in animal seizure models including electroshock and chemically induced seizures [46].

Hyponatremia and tremor can occur, and they are more common than with carbamazepine [2,46,47].

Topiramate

Topiramate is a broad-spectrum drug with minimal interactions and absence of serious side effects. Topiramate is effective as monotherapy in patients over 10 years old with partial-onset or primary generalized tonic–clonic seizures. It is also effective as an adjunct for patients over 2 years old with partial-onset seizures, primary generalized tonic–clonic seizures, or Lennox–Gestaut syndrome [2,4,48]. Several mechanisms of action have been suggested based on laboratory studies, including use-dependent Na^+ and Ca^{2+} channel blockade, potentiation of GABA, glutamate receptor antagonism, and carbonic anhydrase inhibition with resultant pH-mediated modulation of seizure [3,4,49]. Anticonvulsant activity has been demonstrated in animal electroshock, absence, and kindling models, with only weak effect in pentylenetetrazole seizure models [48].

Inhibition of carbonic anhydrase produces a metabolic acidosis and may contribute to development of nephrolithiasis [2,3,48]. There may be an increased risk of hyperammonemia in patients with inborn errors of metabolism or mitochondrial disorders [48]. Topiramate given with valproate was associated with hyperammonemia [42,48]. It has additive effects with other carbonic anhydrase-inhibiting drugs such as acetazolamide [42].

Lamotrigine

Lamotrigine, a folic acid antagonist derivative [3], was released in 1994 and is a broad-spectrum drug with minimal sedation or drug interactions [4]. Lamotrigine is effective as adjunctive therapy in adults and children over 2 years old with partial seizures or with generalized seizures associated with Lennox–Gestaut syndrome, and as monotherapy in adults with partial seizures and for juvenile myoclonic epilepsy. It is also approved as an adjunct in the therapy of primary generalized tonic–clonic seizures in patient over 2 years old. It is thought to be as effective as conventional AEDs but is better tolerated. Some reports suggest it can exacerbate myoclonus [2,14,50,51]. Lamotrigine may be effective for absence seizures, but this is a preliminary impression [32].

Lamotrigine exhibits its antiepileptic effects through Na^+ channel and to a lesser extent Ca^{2+} channel blockade [4,33,37,51]. It is an inhibitor of dihydrofolate reductase, the enzyme that catalyzes the reduction of dihydrofolate. It has been associated with reduced folate concentrations in rats. Lamotrigine was effective in electroshock and pentylenetetrazole seizure models [51], but was ineffective in some other models of status epilepticus [17].

Tiagabine

Tiagabine was FDA-approved in 1997 as an adjunct in the treatment of partial seizures in adults [3,4,14,52]. Tiagabine has a novel mechanism of action [4], enhancing the GABAergic system by inhibiting GABA uptake [33] via binding to and inhibiting the GABA transporter uptake carrier (Fig. 37.1) [3,52]. Inhibition of GABA uptake has been demonstrated in synaptosomes, neuronal cell cultures, and glial cell cultures with prolongation of GABA-mediated inhibitory postsynaptic potentials shown in rat hippocampal slices. Tiagabine inhibits pentylenetetrazole-mediated seizures [52].

There have been reports of a paradoxical effect of tiagabine to produce or exacerbate seizures or status epilepticus, particularly absence seizures [4,52]. Tiagabine is contraindicated in primary generalized seizures, because of possible induction of absence status epilepticus. There is also some concern about this with focal seizures [3].

Zonisamide

Zonisamide is a bensisoxazole with a sulfonamide side chain [3]. Zonisamide is approved for adjunctive treatment of partial seizures in adults but it appears to be effective also in infantile spasms and in myoclonic, generalized, and atypical absence seizures and possibly in other seizure types [2,3,53,54]. Zonisamide blocks Na^+ channels, reduces voltage-dependent T-type Ca^{2+} currents, and decreases glutamate-mediated excitation [3,37], thus suppressing neuronal hypersynchronization. Zonisamide binds to the GABA/benzodiazepine receptor–ionophore complex and does not appear to potentiate synaptic activity of GABA. Microdialysis studies demonstrate that it facilitates dopaminergic and serotonergic neurotransmission [54]. Studies on flurothyl seizures in rodents suggest antiepileptogenic properties of zonisamide [22]. It is also effective in other seizure models, although not effective in pentylenetetrazole seizures or in absence seizure models [3,53].

It produces an 8% increase in creatinine and blood urea nitrogen (BUN), thought to be due to an effect on glomular filtration rate, and it has been associated with kidney stones [54]. Zonisamide is a sulfonamide and should not be given to patients with known sulfa allergies.

Gabapentin

Gabapentin offers a wide margin of safety, good tolerability, and absence of significant drug interactions, but with modest efficacy. Gabapentin can be effective for mixed seizure disorders, generalized seizures, and partial seizures [2,15,47]. Gabapentin is structurally related to GABA, with many effects that may account for its efficacy. However, gabapentin does not bind to GABA receptors and is not an inhibitor of GABA uptake or degradation. It appears to have little impact on other important neurotransmitters and their receptors, although binding to voltage-activated Ca^{2+} channels has been detected. Gabapentin binds to subunits of voltage-gated Ca^{2+} channels to reduce synaptic release of neurotransmitters and decrease postsynaptic Ca^{2+} influx with diminished excitation [3]. Gabapentin exhibits anticonvulsant activity in several animal seizure models including electroshock, pentyletetrazole, and genetic epilepsy [55].

Pregabalin

Pregabalin is a GABA analog, discovered in a search for other GABA derivatives. Its pharmacologic profile is similar to that of gabapentin [53]. It is used for the adjunctive treatment of partial seizures [56]. Pregabalin is thought to be active as an anticonvulsant due to high affinity to an auxiliary subunit of voltage-gated Ca^{2+} channels, and it may alter Ca^{2+}-dependent release of several neurotransmitters [57]. Although pregabalin has little direct effect on GABA or GABA receptors, it increases the density of GABA transporter proteins and thus increases the rate of functional GABA transport while also producing a concentration-dependent increase in glutamic acid decarboxylase activity [53]. In vitro it reduces the Ca^{2+}-dependent release of several neurotransmitters [56]. Pregabalin is effective in animal seizure models [3].

Felbamate

Felbamate is a broad-spectrum AED whose release was met with much enthusiasm. Felbamate is effective for adjunctive treatment of partial seizures [32]. However, evidence of toxicity has limited its use currently. Felbamate has several mechanisms that are thought to contribute to its efficacy. These include Na^{+} and Ca^{2+} channel blockade, NMDA glutamate receptor antagonism, and AMPA glutamate receptor blockade (Fig. 37.1) [4]. Felbamate weakly binds and inhibits GABA and benzodiazepine receptors. It has antagonist effects at the strychnine-insensitive glycine recognition site of the NMDA receptor [57]. It is effective in several animal seizure models including electroshock, pentylenetetrazole, and picrotoxin [57].

Notaby, felbamate is associated with a marked increase in the incidence of aplastic anemia. Thus it should only be used when the advantages in terms of treated severe epilepsy outweigh the risk of aplastic anemia. The drug label has a black-box warning on this issue and recommends securing hematological consultation when felbamate is used [4,57]. Felbamate also confers a risk of serious hepatotoxicity, for which there is another black-box warning [4].

Levetiracetam

Levetiracetam is chemically unrelated to other AEDs, with a unique mechanism of action and high safety margin. Levetiracetam is effective as an adjunct AED for adults and children over 4 years old with partial seizures, adults and children over 6 years old with primary generalized tonic–clonic seizures, and adults and adolescents over 12 years old with myoclonic seizures [2,53,58]. The exact mechanism of action of levetiracetam is unknown but does not appear to be the result of any known interactions with inhibitory or excitatory neurotransmitters [4,53,58]. There are some data to suggest a specific interaction with synaptic proteins as a possible mechanism of action [58]. Levetiracetam has binding sites in synaptic membranes and it may alter γ-aminobutyric acid (GABA) actions through binding to neurons in specific brain nuclei such as the substantia nigra, which may be an important gateway for generalization of seizures. It is notably ineffective in electroshock and pentylenetetrazole seizure models but has shown efficacy in kindling models and models of complex partial seizures with generalization [29].

Pharmacokinetics

See Table 37.2 for a summary of kinetic parameters. Levetiracetam undergoes little hepatic metabolism, with no effect on P450 isoenzymes and no enzyme induction [3,8]. Binding to plasma protein is less than 10%, and 76% of the drug is eliminated unchanged. Plasma half-life is about 7 hours, with 95% elimination via the kidneys [3]. Dosage needs to be adjusted in patients with significant renal failure [58]. It is removed by hemodialysis, so dosing needs to be supplemented after hemodialysis [42].

Adverse effects and interactions

The most frequent adverse effects of levetiracetam are irritability, behavior change, somnolence, asthenia, headache, and infection (Table 37.4). Levetiracetam can also contribute to depression or psychosis [3,47].

Drug interactions are summarized in Table 37.3. No significant interactions with other AEDs have been reported [4]. Levetiracetam may exacerbate toxicity of carbamazepine unrelated to effects on pharmacokinetic parameters [42].

Antipsychotic drugs

The antipsychotic drugs include phenothiazines and structurally similar compounds, butyrophenones, diphenylbutylpiperidines, indolones, and other heterocyclic compounds. Apart for the treatment of psychosis, this class of drugs is used for a range of other neurologic problems including postsurgical delirium, amphetamine intoxication, paranoia, mania, affective disorders, and Alzheimer's-associated agitation [59]. Moreover, given chronically, they can also be of critical importance in maintaining control of psychosis. However, their use is

Table 37.5. Antipsychotic drugs

Typical antipsychotics		Atypical antipsychotics
Phenothiazine	*Nonphenothiazine*	
Acetophenazine	Haloperidol (butyrophenone)	Aripiprazole
Amitriptyline	Iloperidone	Clozapine
Chlorpromazine	Loxapine (tricyclic)	Fluoxetine
Fluphenazine	Molindone	Olanzapine
Meperidine	Pimozide (butyrophenone)	Paliperidone
Promethazine	Sertindole	Quetiapine
Mesoridazine	Thiothixene	Risperidone
Perphenazine	Xanomeline	Ziprasidone
Perphenazine	Zotepine	
Prochlorperazine		
Promazine		
Promethazine		
Thiethylperazine		
Thioridazine		
Trifluoperazine		

Reproduced with permission from Baldessarini and Tarazi [59].

associated with significant adverse effects. In a study evaluating the efficacy of olanzapine, perphenazine, quetiapine, risperidone, and ziprasidone in over 1000 patients, 74% of the patients discontinued their assigned medication due to perceived lack of efficacy or intolerable side effects [60].

Although there is chemical dissimilarity among the various antipsychotic drugs, there is sufficient pharmacologic similarity to allow generalizations. Among the **typical antipsychotics** the prototype for the phenothiazine–thioxanthenes is **chlorpromazine**, while **haloperidol** is the prototype for the butyrophenones and related classes of aromatic butylpiperidine-derivative drugs (Table 37.5) [59].

Atypical antipsychotic drugs are more recently developed. They are associated with a substantially lower risk of extrapyramidal effects and have varied mechanisms compared to the typical antipsychotics. The atypical antipsychotic drugs include aripiprazole, clozapine, quetiapine, ziprasidone, olanzapine, and risperidone [59,61]. These drugs have achieved widespread acceptance as preferred antipsychotic drugs [60] and, except for clozapine (the use of which is limited by severe side effects), they are deemed to be the standard of care for schizophrenia and other related psychoses [59]. In this chapter, **quetiapine** is presented as a prototype of the atypical antipsychotics.

Some antipsychotic drugs are characterized as neuroleptics, referring to the fact that they have experimental and clinical evidence of D_2 dopamine receptor antagonism that is associated with significant risk of extrapyramidal side effects and hyperprolactinemia [59].

Mechanisms of drug action

Dopamine is thought to play an integral role in the genesis of schizophrenia and both good and bad effects of treatment with antipsychotic drugs. The dopaminergic system extends to multiple brain areas, and several types of dopamine receptors have been identified and some of their effects characterized. In the limbic system, dopamine excess produces positive symptoms of schizophrenia, whereas blockade of dopamine: (1) in the mesocortical pathways produces negative symptoms of schizophrenia, (2) in mesocortical pathways causes cognitive deficits, (3) in mesolimbic areas (D_2) reduces hallucinations, (4) in nigrostriatal pathways produces extrapyramidal effects, and (5) in the tuberoinfundibular tract (D_2) leads to prolactin release [59].

The neuroleptic drugs and older phenothiazines in general are nonselective dopamine receptor antagonists. Typical antipsychotics tend to block D_2 receptors to a greater extent than D_1, and this is thought to alleviate hallucinations, delusions, and erratic behavior and speech while also contributing to the genesis of extrapyramidal symptoms [59].

In contrast, the atypical antipsychotic drugs provide a broader range of selective neurochemical effects than the typical antipsychotic drugs. These effects include, to varying extents, antiserotonergic (5-HT_{2A} and 5-HT_{1A}), antidopaminergic (D_1 and D_2), antiadrenergic, and antihistaminic (H_1) effects, with diminished anticholinergic activity. Some of the drugs interfere with serotonin (5-HT) or norepinephrine reuptake or have some 5-HT or dopaminergic agonist effects and thus also have antidepressant effects [59]. The atypical antipsychotics are further distinguished from the typical antipsychotics by properties which include a high ratio of serotonin to dopamine receptor affinity and/or D_2 receptor specificity in the limbic system. Moreover, affinity for other dopamine receptors subtypes such as D_3 and D_4 may also contribute to their therapeutic efficacy. The dual (dopamine and serotonin effects) mechanism of action of the atypical antipsychotics may contribute to their broad spectrum of efficacy [61]. The relatively lower affinity of the atypical antipsychotic drugs for D_2 receptors is thought to be one mechanism of their lower incidence of extrapyramidal effects (including tardive dyskinesia). In addition, greater occupancy at 5-HT_2 receptors relative to D_2 receptors is also a feature of atypical antipsychotic drugs and may also explain, in part, the lower propensity of these drugs to cause extrapyramidal side effects. The disparate receptor effects of the various antipsychotic drugs are summarized in Table 37.6.

Both groups of drugs to varying degrees can exhibit effects related to α_1-adrenergic antagonism and cholinergic muscarinic receptor blockade with associated symptoms derived

599

Table 37.6. Potencies of standard and experimental antipsychotic agents at neurotransmitter receptors

Receptor Drug	Dopamine D_2	Serotonin 5-HT$_2$	5-HT$_{2A}$/ D_2 ratio	Dopamine D_1	Dopamine D_4	Muscarinic cholinergic	Adrenergic α_1	Adrenergic α_2	Histamine H_1
Ziprasidone	0.42	0.42	1.0	525	32	≥1000	10	260	47
cis-Thiothixene	0.45	130	289	340	77	2500	11	200	6.0
Sertindole	0.45	0.38	0.84	28	21	≥10000	0.77	1700	500
Fluphenazine	0.80	19	24	15	9.30	2000	9	1600	21
Zotepine	1.0	0.63	0.63	84	5.80	550	3.40	960	3.40
Perphenazine	1.40	5.60	4.0	—	—	1500	10	510	—
Thioridazine	2.30	41	17.8	22	12	10	1.10	—	—
Pimozide	2.50	13	5.20	—	30	—	—	—	—
Risperidone	3.30	0.16	0.05	750	17	>10000	2.0	56	59
Aripiprazole	3.40	3.40	1.0	265	44	>10000	57	—	61
Haloperidol	4.0	36	9.0	45	10	>20000	6.20	3800	1890
Ziprasidone	4.79	0.42	0.09	339	39	≥10000	10	—	47
Mesoridazine	5.00	6.30	1.26	—	13	—	—	—	—
Sulpiride	7.40	≥1000	135	≥1000	52	≥1000	≥1000	—	—
Olanzapine	11	4	0.36	31	9.60	1.89	19	230	7.14
Chlorpromazine	19	1.40	0.07	56	12	60	0.60	750	9.10
Loxapine	71	1.69	0.02	—	12	62	28	2400	5.0
Pipamperone	93	1.20	0.01	2450	—	≥5000	66	680	≥5000
Molindone	125	5000	40	—	—	—	2500	625	>10000
Amperozide	140	20	0.14	260	—	1700	130	590	730
Quetiapine	160	294	1.84	455	1164	120	62	2500	11
Clozapine	180	1.60	0.01	38	9.6	7.50	9.0	160	2.75
Melperone	199	32	0.16	—	230	—	—	—	—
Remoxipride	275	≥10000	36	≥10000	3690	≥10000	≥10000	2900	≥10000

Data are K_i values (nM) determined by competition with radioligands for binding to the indicated receptors. Compounds are in rank order of dopamine D_2 receptor affinity; 5-HT$_{2A}$/D_2 ratio indicates relative preference for D_2 vs. 5-HT$_{2A}$ receptors. Compounds include clinically used and experimental agents. Muscarinic cholinergic receptor K_i values are pooled results obtained with radioligands that are nonselective for muscarinic receptor subtypes or that are selective for the M_1 subtype. Reproduced with permission from Baldessarini and Tarazi [59].

therefrom, including hypotension, blurred vision, xerostomia, mydriasis, nausea, adynamic ileus, urinary retention, erectile dysfunction, and constipation [59].

Pharmacokinetics

Elimination half-lives of antipsychotic drugs vary from 6 hours to 2 days, as summarized in Table 37.7.

Adverse effects

The adverse effects of the phenothiazines and butyrophenones can be problematic, with the most significant issues being extrapyramidal effects [59], some of which can be permanent [61]. Related to this are observations that antipsychotic drugs can exacerbate Parkinson's disease and inhibit the response to

antiparkinson therapy by blocking dopamine receptors in the brain [59].

Tardive dyskinesia is a particulary notable adverse effect because it is potentially irreversible, consisting of involuntary dyskinetic movements, particulary notable when perioral. The prevalence appears to highest among the elderly, especially in elderly women. The risk of developing this is thought to increase in relation to the duration of therapy, although it has also been observed after relatively brief treatment trials. There is no reliable method to predict a given patient's specific risk of developing tardive dyskinesia [62].

The atypical antipsychotic drugs have a significantly lower risk of extrapyramidal effects but still have significant potential adverse

Table 37.7. Elimination half-lives of antipsychotic drugs

Drug	Half-life (hours: average and range)
Aripiprazole	75
Chlorpromazine	24 (8–35)
Clozapine	12 (4–66)
Fluphenazine	18 (14–24)
Haloperidol	24 (12–36)[a]
Loxapine	8 (3–12)
Mesoridazine	30 (24–48)
Molindone	12 (6–24)
Olanzapine	30 (20–54)
Perphenazine	12 (8–21)
Pimozide	55 (29–111)[a]
Quetiapine	6
Risperidone	20–24[b]
Thioridazine	24 (6–40)
Thiothixene	34
Trifluoperazine	18 (14–24)[c]
Ziprasidone	7.5

[a]May have multiphasic elimination with much longer terminal half-life.
[b]Half-life of the main active metabolite (parent drug half-life ca. 3–4 hours).
[c]Estimated, assuming similarity to fluphenazine.
Sources: data from Ereshefsky (1996) and United States Pharmacopoeia (2004). Reproduced with permission from Baldessarini and Tarazi [59].

effects, which can include hypotension, seizures, weight gain, hyperglycemia, type 2 diabetes mellitus, ketoacidosis, hyperlipidemia, amongst others [59]. Atypical antipsychotic drugs in post-marketing studies were found to produce hyperglycemia and weight gain that occasionally can be so pronounced as to cause diabetic ketoacidosis, hyperosmolar and hyperglycemic states, and diabetic coma. Moreover, hyperglycemia seems to be more prevalent in patients with a family history of diabetes, in patients with African ancestry, and in obese patients. The mechanism of this effect is unclear. However the hyperglycemic propensity is not equal among these drugs. Hyperglycemia has been implicated more with olanzapine and clozapine [61].

Notably, in the above-cited study involving over 1000 patients and including both typical and atypical antipsychotics, a significant number of patients found the side effects so severe as to result in noncompliance [60]. These side effects are summarized in Table 37.8, while the neurological side effects of neuroleptic drugs and the proposed mechanism for each is summarized in Table 37.9.

Other important side effects associated with most of the antipsychotic drugs include sedation and drowsiness, decreased seizure threshold, hypotension, anticholinergic effects (constipation, nausea, xerostomia, and tachycardia), QT prolongation with concern for torsades de pointes, suicidal ideation, and elevated prolactin (variable and likely related to central D_2 antagonism). Hyperprolactinemia can cause a variety of endocrine effects that can include amenorrhea, galactorrhea, gynecomastia, and erectile dysfunction [59].

Rare but potentially lethal adverse effects

Based on data from antidepressants, there is concern that antipsychotic drugs can increase suicidality in children and adolescents. Although very unusual, neuroleptic malignant syndrome has also been associated with both typical and atypical antipsychotic drugs. The use of atypical antipsychotics for the treatment of demential psychosis in the elderly has been associated with a higher death rate [59].

Drug interactions
Phenothiazines

Phenothiazines have been associated with QT prolongation and torsades de pointes in a dose-related manner. Thus addition of phenothiazines not only to each other but to other drugs (including atypical antipsychotics) that also cause QT prolongation should be avoided if possible. Drugs which are more inclined to produce this QT-prolonging effect include thioridazine, ziprasidone, and mesoridazine. Additive adverse effects of typical and atypical antipsychotic drugs also include problems such as hypotension and central nervous system (CNS) depression [59].

Drugs which affect hepatic P450 isozymes may affect plasma concentrations of phenothiazines. Drugs that inhibit these enzymes will produce an increased plasma concentration and, conversely, drugs which induce them will produce a decreased plasma concentration of a given phenothiazine drug. For an extensive list of relevant drugs one should refer to specific drug labels or package inserts [59].

Propranolol and pindolol appear to decrease hepatic metabolism of phenothiazines, leading to up to fivefold increases in plasma concentrations. Notably, phenothiazines appear to also inhibit the metabolism of propranolol such that a positive feedback cycle may arise, possibly accounting for the marked increase in phenothiazine levels. It is not known if this interaction occurs with other hepatically metabolized β-adrenergic antagonist drugs. β-blockers with greater renal elimination, such as atenolol or nadolol, are thought to be less likely to introduce a risk of this interaction [59].

Phenothiazines can block the α-adrenergic effects of epinephrine. This can lead to a paradoxical so-called epinephrine reversal syndrome, characterized by hypotension, tachycardia, and myocardial supply/demand imbalance. There may also be a reduced response to α-adrenergic agonists such as norepinephrine and phenylephrine. Combined with clonidine and possibly other centrally acting α_2-adrenergic drugs, an additive hypotensive response may arise. Additive anticholinergic

Table 37.8. Safety and adverse effects among randomized patients receiving antipsychotic drugs

Outcome	Olanzapine (n = 336)	Quetiapine (n = 337)	Risperidone (n = 341)	Perphenazine (n = 261)*	Ziprasidone (n = 185)
Hospitalization for exacerbation of schizophrenia					
Hospitalized patients: no. (%)	38 (11)	68 (20)	51 (15)	41 (16)	33 (18)
Adverse events: no. (%)					
Any serious adverse event	32 (10)	32 (9)	33 (10)	29 (11)	19 (10)
Suicide attempt	2 (<1)	1 (<1)	2 (<1)	1 (<1)	1 (<1)
Suicidal ideation	1 (<1)	2 (<1)	4 (1)	3 (1)	2 (1)
Any moderate or severe adverse event	235 (70)	220 (65)	232 (68)	170 (65)	119 (64)
Insomnia	55 (16)	62 (18)	83 (24)	66 (25)	56 (30)
Hypersomnia, sleepiness	104 (31)	103 (31)	96 (28)	74 (28)	45 (24)
Urinary hesitancy, dry mouth, constipation	79 (24)	105 (31)	84 (25)	57 (22)	37 (20)
Decreased sex drive, arousal, ability to reach orgasm	91 (27)	69 (20)	91 (27)	64 (25)	35 (19)
Gynecomastia, galactorrhea	7 (2)	6 (2)	14 (4)	4 (2)	6 (3)
Menstrual irregularities	11 (12)	5 (6)	16 (18)	7 (11)	8 (14)
Incontinence, nocturia	18 (5)	15 (4)	25 (7)	6 (2)	10 (5)
Orthostatic faintness	31 (9)	38 (11)	37 (11)	29 (11)	24 (13)
Any moderate or severe spontaneously reported adverse event	122 (36)	113 (34)	123 (36)	79 (30)	65 (35)
Neurologic effects: no./total no. (%)					
AIMS global severity score ≥2	32/236 (14)	30/236 (13)	38/238 (16)	41/237 (17)	18/126 (14)
Barnes Akathisia Rating Scale global score ≥3	15/290 (5)	16/305 (5)	20/292 (7)	16/241 (7)	14/158 (9)
Simpson–Angus Extrapyramidal Signs Scale ≥1	23/296 (8)	12/298 (4)	23/292 (8)	15/243 (6)	6/152 (4)
Discontinuation owing to intolerability: no. (%)					
Discontinuation	62 (18)	49 (15)	34 (10)	40 (15)	28 (15)
Weight gain or metabolic effects	31 (9)	12 (4)	6 (2)	3 (1)	6 (3)
Extrapyramidal effects	8 (2)	10 (3)	11 (3)	22 (8)	7 (4)
Sedation	7 (2)	9 (3)	3 (1)	7 (3)	0
Other effects	16 (5)	18 (5)	14 (4)	8 (3)	15 (8)
Weight change from baseline to last observation					
Weight gain >7%: no./total no. (%)	92/307 (30)	49/305 (16)	42/300 (14)	29/243 (12)	12/161 (7)
Weight change (lb): mean ± SE	9.4 ± 0.9	1.1 ± 0.9	0.8 ± 0.9	−2.0 ± 1.1	−1.6 ± 1.1
Weight change (lb) per month of treatment: mean ± SE	2.0 ± 0.3	0.5 ± 0.2	0.4 ± 0.3	−0.2 ± 0.2	−0.3 ± 0.3
Change from baseline in laboratory values					
Blood glucose (mg dL^{-1}): mean ± SE	15.0 ± 2.8	6.8 ± 2.5	6.7 ± 2.0	5.2 ± 2.0	2.3 ± 3.9
Glycosylated hemoglobin (%): mean ± SE	0.41 ± 0.09	0.05 ± 0.05	0.08 ± 0.04	0.10 ± 0.06	−0.10 ± 0.14
Cholesterol (mg dL^{-1}): mean ± SE	9.7 ± 2.1	5.3 ± 2.1	−2.1 ± 1.9	0.5 ± 2.3	−9.2 ± 5.2
Triglycerides (mg dL^{-1}): mean ± SE	42.9 ± 8.4	19.2 ± 10.6	−2.6 ± 6.3	8.3 ± 11.5	−8.1 ± 9.4
Prolactin (ng dL^{-1}): mean ± SE	−6.1 ± 1.2	−9.3 ± 1.4	15.4 ± 1.5	0.4 ± 1.7	−4.5 ± 1.6
ECG findings					
Change in corrected QT interval: mean ± SE	1.2 ± 1.8	5.9 ± 1.9	0.2 ± 1.8	1.4 ± 2.0	1.3 ± 2.2
New cataracts: no./total no. (%)	3/272 (1)	1/258 (<1)	2/260 (1)	1/210 (<1)	0/142

Adapted from Lieberman *et al.* [60].

Postsynaptic physiology and pharmacology

In the healthy innervated muscle, the acetylcholine receptors (also termed *mature* acetylcholine receptors) are highly localized to the neuromuscular endplate region. The postsynaptic receptor consists of two subunits of α_1 and one each of β, δ, and ε ($2\alpha_1\beta_1\delta\varepsilon$). However, when there is deprivation of neural influence or activity, as in the fetus or after denervation, the muscle expresses *immature* or *fetal* acetylcholine receptors, in which the ε subunit is replaced by a γ subunit [8]. Thus, the subunit composition of the fetal receptor is $2\alpha_1\beta_1\delta\gamma$. These immature receptors are no longer localized to the endplate region but are inserted throughout the muscle membrane into the junctional, as well as extrajunctional, area, and they are therefore also referred to as extrajunctional receptors. This ε-to-γ switch of the acetylcholine receptor subunit has some important physiologic and metabolic consequences for the receptor itself [9–11]. The mature acetylcholine receptor is more stable metabolically, with a half-life approximating 2 weeks, whereas immature acetylcholine receptors have a metabolic half-life of around 24 hours. Immature receptors have a smaller single-channel conductance, but a 2- to 10-fold longer mean channel open time. In addition, the sensitivity and affinity to ligands differ. Agonists such as acetylcholine and succinylcholine, or its metabolite succinylmonocholine, depolarize immature receptors more easily; one-tenth to one-hundredth of normal doses of these agonists can effect depolarization [9,10]. Apart from the above-described adult and fetal acetylcholine receptors, acetylcholine receptors that contain a combination of other α subunits (α_2 to α_9) or β subunits (β_2 to β_4) have also been described [11]. These receptors are almost exclusively located in the central nervous system. Most recently, however, a homomeric receptor consisting of five α_7 subunits, previously described only in the central nervous system, has been described in muscle denervation states [11]. The clinical pharmacology of the latter receptor has not been well studied. In all of these muscle receptors, depolarization of the endplate and opening of the receptor channel occurs only when a molecule of acetylcholine binds to each of the two α_1 subunits on the receptor [8–11].

Margin of safety of neurotransmission

Approximately 10% of the total number of acetylcholine receptors at the endplate must be open for the flow of ions to increase the endplate potential from –70 mV to the threshold of –50 mV, at which a muscle action potential is initiated. The muscle action potential then runs across the muscle membrane resulting in the activation and contraction of muscle fibers. The action-potential signal is initiated by more transmitter molecules than necessary, and these molecules evoke an action-potential response greater than required. At the same time, only a small fraction of the available vesicles and receptors is used to initiate each action-potential signal. Consequently, neuromuscular transmission is said to have a substantial margin of safety or substantial reserve capacity

[12]. During the clinical administration of a neuromuscular blocker, 75% of the acetylcholine receptors must be occupied by an antagonist (neuromuscular blocker) before any effect (decrease of twitch height) is seen. After blocking the initial 75% of the receptors, the effect (twitch depression) with continued relaxant administration is relatively more rapid. This phenomenon is referred to as the "iceberg phenomenon." At least 95% receptor occupancy is necessary for complete suppression of twitch (Fig. 38.1). The percent receptor occupancy, and not the absolute number blocked, varies with dose. Therefore, concentrations reached at the neuromuscular junction vary. In other words, if the receptor number is increased, and if antagonists occupy the same percentage of receptors, the absolute number of receptors remaining unblocked is still high. In these instances, a given concentration or dose of muscle relaxant will produce a smaller effect on twitch height, provided that other factors such as acetylcholine release are unaltered. Clinically, this can be described as a resistance to antagonists (muscle relaxants).

Mechanisms of action of muscle relaxants

Muscle paralysis by muscle relaxants in a clinical setting is achieved primarily by blocking the function of the postsynaptic acetylcholine receptor. In addition to the competitive block of the acetylcholine receptor produced by nondepolarizing neuromuscular blocking drugs and the noncompetitive block by depolarizing muscle relaxants (Fig. 38.2), numerous other drugs can effect neuromuscular transmission at the receptor level.

Competitive block

Similar to acetylcholine, the nondepolarizing neuromuscular blocking drugs also bind to the α subunit of the acetylcholine receptor. They do not, however, possess any intrinsic agonist activity. That is, they do not cause a conformational change in the receptor from the closed to the open state. One molecule of nondepolarizing muscle relaxant is sufficient to occupy the receptor and prevent opening of the ion channel and consequent ion flow. Therefore, acetylcholine and the nondepolarizing muscle relaxants compete for the binding site at the receptor. Hence the term *competitive block*. The probability of binding is solely dependent on the concentration of each ligand present at the neuromuscular junction and its affinity for the receptor. Once the neuromuscular blocking drug diffuses out of the junction, the probability that acetylcholine will bind to the receptor rises and the muscle-blocking effect of the muscle relaxant diminishes.

Noncompetitive block

The neuromuscular block (paralysis) produced by the depolarizing neuromuscular blocking drugs, typified by succinylcholine, is *noncompetitive*. Succinylcholine, which is structurally two molecules of acetylcholine bound together, is a partial agonist

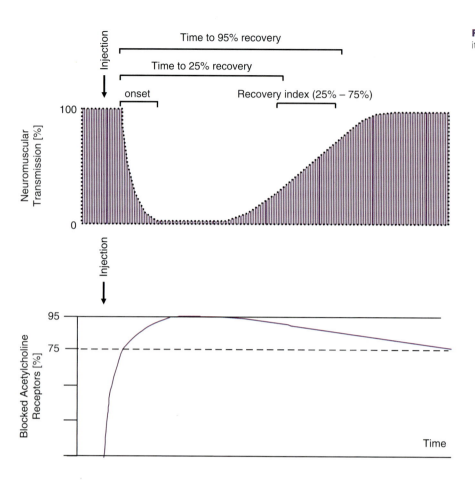

Figure 38.1. The "iceberg phenomenon" and definitions of duration of action (see text for explanation).

DRUG:	acetylcholine	succinylcholine	High or repetitive doses of succinylcholine	Benzylisoquinolones Steroid muscle relaxants
ACTION:	Agonist	Partial Agonist	Partial Antagonist	Antagonist
EFFECT:	Contraction	Non-competitve block and paralysis	Phase I-block + Phase II-block (non-competitive and competitive) with paralysis	Competitive block with paralysis

Intrinsic agonist activity

Figure 38.2. Agonistic and antagonistic interactions at the nicotinic acetylcholine receptor (nAChR).

of the acetylcholine receptor and depolarizes (opens) the ion channel. This opening requires the binding of only one molecule of succinylcholine to the α subunit. The other α subunit of the receptor can be occupied by either acetylcholine or succinylcholine. Succinylcholine cannot be hydrolyzed by acetylcholinesterase (AChE); it can therefore detach from the receptor and repeatedly bind to other acetylcholine receptors until it is cleared

from the junctional area into the plasma, where it is hydrolyzed by plasma (pseudo-)cholinesterase. Since succinylcholine is an agonist of the acetylcholine receptor, binding induces muscle fasciculation (uncoordinated mini-contractions), which occur only during the initial phase, followed by a relaxation period. Since the endplate membrane is continuously depolarized by the presence of succinylcholine, the voltage-gated sodium ion channels in the perijunctional region, which initiate the muscle action potential, are not activated after the initial depolarization. The musculature relaxes after the initial fasciculation, although the cell membrane beyond the perijunctional area is repolarized. Therefore, muscle contraction can be elicited by direct electrical stimulation of the muscle.

Phase II block

A phase II block is a complex phenomenon observed not only after high single or cumulative doses of succinylcholine, but also after normal doses of succinylcholine during lack of, or functional inefficiency of, pseudocholinesterase (the metabolizing enzyme of succinylcholine). In the latter situation, the initial phase I (depolarization) block is converted into a phase II (noncompetitive) block [13]; the decreased metabolism of succinylcholine is a relative overdose causing an increased concentration in the synaptic cleft. The exact mechanism underlying a phase II block remains unclear. It is probably due to an electrical imbalance at the junctional membrane caused by the repeated opening of the channels by succinylcholine. The junction is depolarized by the initial action of succinylcholine. Thereafter, the muscle membrane potential returns to a normal resting potential, even though the junction is still exposed to the drug. Clinically, a phase II block is characterized by a tetanic or train-of-four (TOF) fade. Usually, acetylcholinesterase inhibitors can reverse a phase II block, but they also can worsen it.

Desensitization block

The acetylcholine receptor is capable of existing in a number of conformational states. When it has been desensitized, the acetylcholine receptor cannot be activated to open its channel. It is likely that the desensitized state is a physiologic response, in which the desensitized acetylcholine receptors are in equilibrium with the sensitive receptors so as to prevent excessive muscle response to extreme neural stimulation [13]. An increase in desensitized receptors can be induced by an unphysiologically high concentration of agonist, e.g., high acetylcholine levels caused by inhibition of acetylcholinesterase enzyme, or high doses of succinylcholine after repetitive administration or decreased metabolism. Nicotine itself can also cause a desensitization of the receptor. The exact mechanism that induces a desensitization block is not fully understood. However, it is believed that it might be due to a certain acetylcholine receptor subtype that contains $\alpha_8\beta_2$ subunits instead of $\alpha_1\beta_1$. This receptor subtype is especially stimulated at high concentrations of agonists, at which the ion channel opens with a high selectivity for calcium ions. Calcium activates protein kinase C on the inside of the postjunctional membrane, which in turn phosphorylates the "normal" ($2\alpha_1\beta_1\delta\epsilon$) acetylcholine receptor, thereby desensitizing it [14].

In addition to the high levels of agonists or cholinesterase inhibitors, desensitization can also be caused by certain inhalation anesthetics, barbiturates, alcohols, local anesthetics including cocaine, phenothiazines, verapamil, or polymyxin B.

The decrease in the margin of safety, or the increase in the ability of nondepolarizing muscle relaxants to block transmission, a concomitant feature of desensitization block, is independent of the classical effect based on a competitive inhibition of acetylcholine. These effects are mediated by allosteric inhibition of receptors by binding of the drug to sites other than acetylcholine binding sites. The presence of desensitized receptors means that fewer functional receptor channels than usual are available to induce a transmembrane current. Therefore, the production of desensitized receptors decreases the efficacy or margin of safety of neuromuscular transmission. This increases the susceptibility to antagonists, i.e., nondepolarizing neuromuscular blocking drugs. If many receptors are desensitized, insufficient nondesensitized normal receptors are left to depolarize the motor endplate, and effective neuromuscular transmission will not occur.

Channel block

A noncompetitive method for blocking the physiologic opening and closing of the acetylcholine receptor channel, and thus depolarization, is by means of direct channel block. Direct channel blocking is said to occur when molecules that bind to the acetylcholine receptor change its conformation in such a way that any further binding of acetylcholine to the α subunit is prevented. Since the site of action is not located at the acetylcholine binding site, this mechanism is distinct from competitive antagonism with acetylcholine and therefore cannot be reversed by acetylcholinesterase inhibitors, which increase the concentration of acetylcholine in the synaptic cleft. Channel block is believed to play a role in some drug-induced alterations of neuromuscular function. These include antibiotics, cocaine, quinidine, piperocaine, tricyclic antidepressants, naltraxone, naloxone, and histrionicotoxin.

Muscle relaxants in high concentrations can also cause channel block [15,16]. Acetylcholine receptors are also susceptible to channel block if a profound (deep) paralysis by a nondepolarizing neuromuscular relaxant is antagonized by acetylcholinesterase inhibitors. The increased number of acetylcholine molecules displaces the muscle-relaxant molecules, and the acetylcholine competitively prevents the muscle relaxant from binding to the α subunit. The channel is, however, kept open by acetylcholine. The muscle-relaxant molecules, which are still present at a high concentration, can then enter the open channel and block the receptor for a longer duration than the original block produced by binding at the α subunit. Additionally, acetylcholinesterase inhibitors by themselves can cause a channel block.

Acetylcholinesterase enzyme

Acetylcholinesterase hydrolyzes acetylcholine to acetate and choline within 1 millisecond after its release from the presynaptic nerve terminal. By specific inhibition of acetylcholinesterase, the metabolism of acetylcholine can be prevented and

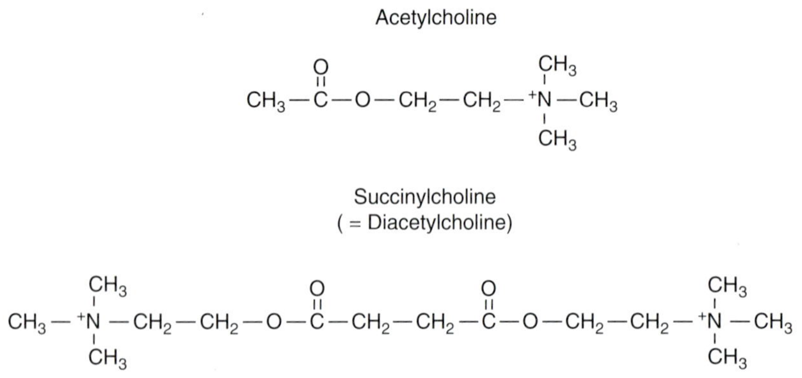

Acetylcholine

$$CH_3 - \overset{\overset{\text{O}}{\|}}{C} - O - CH_2 - CH_2 - \overset{\overset{CH_3}{|}}{\overset{+}{N}} - CH_3$$
$$\underset{|}{CH_3}$$

Succinylcholine
(= Diacetylcholine)

$$CH_3 - \overset{\overset{CH_3}{|}}{\overset{+}{N}} - CH_2 - CH_2 - O - \overset{\overset{\text{O}}{\|}}{C} - CH_2 - CH_2 - \overset{\overset{\text{O}}{\|}}{C} - O - CH_2 - CH_2 - \overset{\overset{CH_3}{|}}{\overset{+}{N}} - CH_3$$
$$\underset{CH_3}{}\qquad\qquad\qquad\qquad\qquad\qquad\qquad\qquad\qquad\qquad\qquad CH_3$$

Figure 38.3. Chemical structure of acetylcholine and succinyl-choline (diacetylcholine).

its concentration in the synaptic cleft increased. This is used to advantage in the clinical setting to reverse the effect of non-depolarizing neuromuscular blocking drugs (see Chapter 39).

Chemical structure and specific properties of muscle relaxants

Structure–activity relationship

Analogous to acetylcholine, all muscle relaxants have at least one quaternary amine group, which is involved in binding to the α subunit of the nicotinic acetylcholine receptor. Succinylcholine consists of two acetylcholine molecules bound together to form diacetylcholine (Fig. 38.3). Succinylcholine retains the depolarizing capacity of acetylcholine but is not susceptible to hydrolysis by acetylcholinesterase. Degradation is only achieved by plasma cholinesterase after succinylcholine has diffused from the synaptic cleft into the plasma. The delayed degradation of diacetylcholine (compared with acetylcholine) results in a sustained high concentration within the synaptic cleft.

Most nondepolarizing neuromuscular blocking drugs also contain two amine groups. Some, but not all, of these compounds have two quaternary amines. D-Tubocurarine, vecuronium, and rocuronium are monoquaternary at a physiological pH. The second amine group is protonated and is therefore present in an uncharged state as a tertiary amine (Fig. 38.4). The bisquaternary structure of the steriodal muscle relaxants favors the block of postganglionic muscarinic acetylcholine receptors and therefore has a vagolytic effect. The vagolytic effect is much weaker with monoquaternary drugs (e.g. vecuronium, rocuronium). The stereochemical aspects of a compound also have a role in structure–activity relationships. Muscle relaxants of the benzylisoquinoline type, including D-tubocurarine, mivacurium, and atracurium, tend to have histaminergic side effects. Some stereoisomers of atracurium have histaminergic properties, in contrast to several other isomers (e.g., cisatracurium, Fig. 38.5), which have no histaminergic side effects in clinical doses.

The affinity to the nicotinic acetylcholine receptor is important for the onset time of a muscle relaxant [17]. This

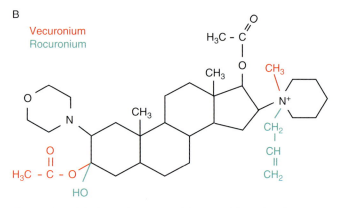

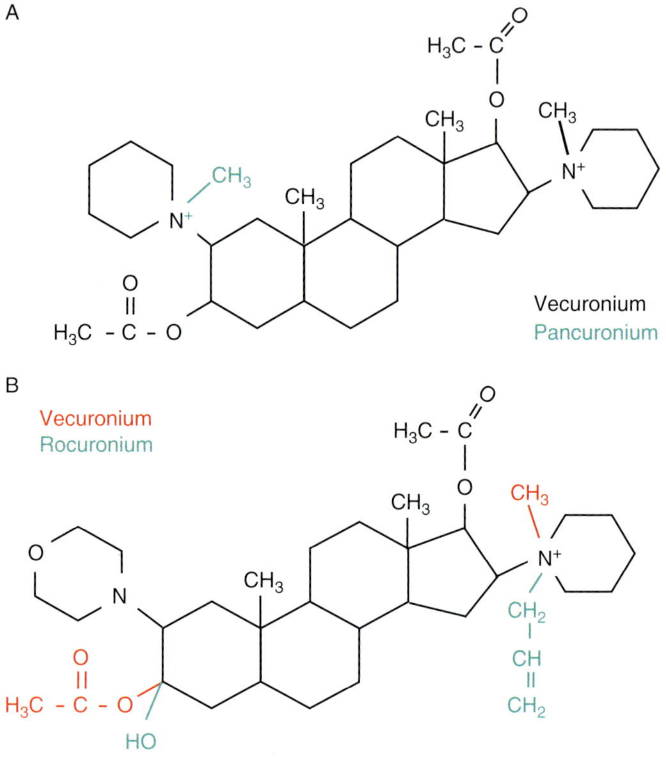

Figure 38.4. (A) Chemical structure of the steroidal muscle relaxants vecuronium and pancuronium. The bisquaternary structure of pancuronium blocks the postganglionic muscarinic acetylcholine receptors (vagolysis), unlike the monoquaternary vecuronium. (B) Chemical structure of the steroid muscle relaxants vecuronium and rocuronium. The longer aliphatic tail at the quaternary amine reduces the affinity towards the acetylcholine receptor. The hydroxyl tail at position 3 (A-ring) ensures an adequate molecular stability of rocuronium during storage in the ampullas.

principle was utilized when developing rocuronium from vecuronium (Fig. 38.4). Muscle relaxants with a lower affinity need to be administered in higher doses to achieve complete neuromuscular block. The high initial bolus dose required for this low-affinity drug, however, is associated with a higher concentration gradient between the central compartment and the neuromuscular junction, and this results in rapid diffusion of drug from the central compartment to the acetylcholine receptor, resulting in faster onset of paralysis [18].

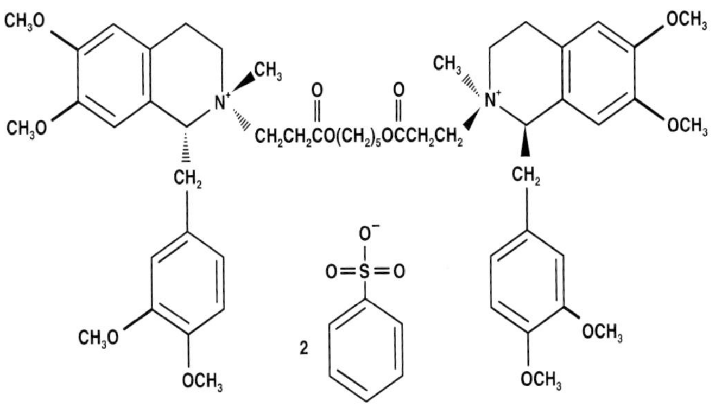

Figure 38.5. Chemical structure of cisatracurium. Cisatracurium is one of the 16 possible isomers of atracurium. The R-*cis*, R′-*cis*- conformation is approximately five times more potent than the racemate and induces almost no histamine.

Intrinsic activity at the neuromuscular nicotinic acetylcholine receptors

Molecules that bind to the nicotinic acetylcholine receptor, depending on their intrinsic activity, induce either agonistic, partial agonistic, or antagonistic activity (Fig. 38.2). The classic agonist of the acetylcholine receptor is acetylcholine: after binding of two acetylcholine molecules (one to each of the α subunits), the receptor-associated ion channel opens. Succinylcholine acts as a partial agonist: it opens the ion channel after binding to the receptor; however, it elicits only an initial depolarization with an associated muscle contraction (fasciculation). In the presence of high concentrations, succinylcholine induces a phase II block. During phase II block, repetitive stimulation will give rise to fade, simulating a nondepolarizing relaxant block. For practical purposes, nondepolarizing muscle relaxants display minimal intrinsic agonist activity (i.e., they are antagonists or competitive blockers of the acetylcholine receptor). When recording twitch responses on a mechanomyograph, however, one may observe an initial transient increase in twitch height followed by twitch depression.

Effects on acetylcholine receptors in the central and autonomic nervous system

Ganglia of the autonomic nervous system transduce either sympathetic or parasympathetic signals. In both ganglia, acetylcholine is the neurotransmitter. Succinylcholine stimulates the sympathetic as well as the parasympathetic ganglia, and additionally the postganglionic parasympathetic muscarinic receptors. Thus it is common to have increased salivary secretions and bradycardia, even in adults but more often in children, especially with repetitive doses of succinylcholine. Therapeutic doses of newer nondepolarizing neuromuscular blocking drugs have no effect on autonomic ganglia (Table 38.1). High doses of D-tubocurarine, however, can result in ganglionic block giving rise to hypotension and pupillary dilation.

Table 38.1. Effect of muscle relaxants on (a) the autonomic nervous system and (b) histamine release. The ratios provided are the quotients of the dose that has a 50% chance for producing side effects ($ED_{50}SE$) divided by the effective dose for 95% twitch depression ($ED_{95}NMB$). The higher the ratio $ED_{50}SE/ ED_{95}NMB$, the safer the drug. Values below 3 may be considered as having a low therapeutic window

	Ganglion blockade[a]	Vagolysis[a]	Histamine liberation[b]
Steroid compounds			
Pancuronium	> 100	3	none
Rocuronium	> 100	3	none
Vecuronium	> 100	20	none
Benzylisoquinolines			
Mivacurium	> 100	> 50	~ 3
Atracurium	40	16	~ 2.5
cis-Atracurium	> 50	> 50	none
Others			
Alcuronium	~ 3	~ 4	none

[a]Determined in cats.
[b]Estimated from the clinical signs of histamine liberation.

The postganglionic parasympathetic muscarinic receptors, because of their helical structure and seven transmembrane domains, have a greater similarity to adrenoceptors than to the nicotinic acetylcholine receptor and, like the adrenoceptors, they belong to the class of G-protein-coupled receptors. When succinylcholine is administered, whether or not the sympathetic or parasympathetic action in the autonomic nervous system dominates is dependent on the pre-existing dynamic equilibrium. Children, for example, often have elevated vagal tone and therefore are prone to react with bradycardia or arrhythmia during the administration of succinylcholine. To prevent this, prophylactic block of the muscarinic receptors with atropine can be attempted. Bradycardia also may be evidenced in adults when a repeat dose of succinylcholine is administered. Of the currently used nondepolarizing muscle relaxants, only pancuronium blocks muscarinic receptors in clinically relevant doses. The cardiac vagolytic effect of pancuronium is evidenced as tachycardia after injection (Table 38.1).

Effects on the carotid body

Neuronal-type nicotinic acetylcholine receptors are important in signaling of hypoxia from the peripheral chemoreceptors of the carotid body to the central nervous system. Structurally, they differ in subunit composition ($\alpha_3\beta_2$, $\alpha_3\beta_4$, $\alpha_4\beta_2$, and α_7) from muscle-type acetylcholine receptors ($\alpha_1\beta_1\delta\epsilon/\gamma$ and α_7). Inhibition of neuronal acetylcholine receptors at the carotid body by muscle relaxants reduces the acute hypoxic ventilatory response, which normally compensates for a decrease in oxygen saturation by increasing the respiratory minute volume. In clinically relevant concentrations, muscle relaxants such as atracurium and vecuronium are able to inhibit neuronal acetylcholine signaling in the carotid body, attenuating chemoreceptor responses to hypoxia [21,22].

Effects on bronchial smooth muscle

Muscarinic acetylcholine receptors belong to the family of G-protein-coupled receptors. However, they share the same ligand used by nicotinic acetylcholine receptors at the neuromuscular junction, i.e., acetylcholine. Muscarinic receptors are found not only on the postganglionic parasympathetic nerves but also on smooth muscle of the bronchi. M_2 and M_3 muscarinic receptor subtypes are present on the bronchial smooth muscle. The M_3 receptor facilitates contraction, postsynaptically. The M_2 subtype plays a role in the auto-feedback mode to inhibit or enhance the release of acetylcholine. Antagonism (block) of the M_2 receptor, which is presynaptic, enhances acetylcholine release. The released acetylcholine acts on the M_3 receptor, causing bronchoconstriction. Irritation of the airway by a foreign body, such as an endotracheal tube, can lead to parasympathetic activation and release of acetylcholine resulting in bronchoconstriction.

Since muscle relaxants are not specific to nicotinic acetylcholine receptors of the neuromuscular junction, they also are able to exert effects on muscarinic receptors. Although muscarinic-receptor control of airway tone is complicated, the net effect of neuromuscular relaxant-induced effects on airways depends on the relative block of M_2 and M_3 muscarinic receptors. Because M_3 muscarinic receptor activation is associated with initiation of airway smooth-muscle contraction, agents that are potent antagonists at the M_3 muscarinic receptor should inhibit bronchoconstriction despite the M_2 muscarinic receptor block and the increased release of acetylcholine from parasympathetic postganglionic nerves. Therefore, pancuronium, a potent M_2 antagonist, is not associated with bronchoconstriction since it is also a potent M_3 antagonist at doses in the clinical range [23]. On the other hand, rapacuronium, which was taken off the US market owing to severe bronchospasm, blocks M_2 receptors but activates M_3 receptors by allosteric binding, thereby increasing smooth-muscle tone and adding to its ability to provoke bronchospasm [24]. Vecuronium also can exert a similar muscarinic receptor activation pattern. Quite in contrast to rapacuronium, however, since the recommended intubation doses of vecuronium are 15–20 times smaller than rapacuronium, it exhibits no affinity for, or effect on, M_2 or M_3 muscarinic receptors at clinical concentrations [25]. Rocuronium also does not potentiate vagally induced bronchoconstriction; neither does cisatracurium or mivacurium [25].

Histamine release and anaphylaxis

Histamine release from mast cells can be induced either by an antigen–antibody reaction as a result of true anaphylaxis (mediated by IgE), by activation of the complement system (IgG or IgM), or by direct action of molecules on the surface of mast cells. Two types of mast cells are differentiated: mucosal (in the bronchial system and gastrointestinal tract) and serosal (vascular endothelium, skin, connective tissue) [26].

Direct effects on mast cells

In comparison to tertiary amines (e.g., morphine), the quaternary ammonium structure of muscle relaxants presents a weak histaminergic effect on mast cells. In clinical doses, succinylcholine and benzylisoquinolines (D-tubocurarine, atracurium, mivacurium) can directly liberate histamine from serosal mast cells. Clinical symptoms are erythema, rash, tachycardia, and in rare cases hypotension. The pharmacologically selective and more potent cisatracurium isoform, on the other hand, has no direct histaminergic effects [27]. Neither do any of the commonly used steroidal muscle relaxants (pancuronium, vecuronium, rocuronium). The direct effect on the surface of mast cells is subject to tachyphylaxis, meaning that slower, graduated, or repetitive administration of the drug decreases the histaminergic side effect. Prophylactic administration of histamine (H_1 and H_2) receptor blockers can suppress the clinical side effects of histamine release [28].

Anaphylactic reactions

Anaphylactic reactions to muscle relaxants are very rare, and probably are not related to other drug allergies, atopic disposition, or a sensitivity to direct mast-cell activation by individual substances. Anaphylactic reactions also have been observed at first contact with a drug, and very often crossover allergies are present. Females have a higher disposition to anaphylactic reactions with muscle relaxants (male:female ratio = 2.5:1). A causal relationship with cosmetics and cleaning chemicals, which often have quaternary ammonium structures, is speculated. Relative to the frequency with which they are used, the incidence of anaphylactic reactions after succinylcholine is approximately three times greater than after administration of nondepolarizing neuromuscular blocking drugs. The individual neuromuscular blocking drugs do not differ in their potential to elicit anaphylaxis (Table 38.1) [29].

Preclinical pharmacology and pharmacological variables of neuromuscular block

The neuromuscular blocking action of muscle relaxants is characterized by a decreased contractile response to stimulation of the respective motor nerve. Depending on the individual muscle group and blood supply, the onset, maximal effect, and duration of block following muscle relaxants differ. Usually, to determine the clinical (pharmacologic) response to a muscle relaxant, the twitch depression of a skeletal muscle (e.g., adductor pollicis) in response to its nerve stimulation is measured following incremental or single dose of the muscle relaxant. A twitch of 100% is the response in the absence of any neuromuscular block, while 0% indicates complete paralysis. Although there is tremendous variability between patients in terms of response to muscle relaxants, the compounds are characterized by determining the following pharmacologic variables as endpoints in large groups of patients (Fig. 38.1):

(1) **Potency** – The potency of a muscle relaxant is described by its *effective dose* (ED). ED_{95} and ED_{50} are the doses of muscle relaxant necessary to suppress the twitch response by 95% (5% twitch height) or 50% (50% twitch height) of baseline (100%) twitch height, respectively.

(2) **Onset** – Onset describes the interval between injection of the muscle relaxant and development of maximal neuromuscular block.

(3) **Clinical duration of action (dur25 or dur95)** – The clinical duration of action is the interval between injection of the muscle relaxant and recovery of the twitch to 25% or 95% of baseline twitch height (i.e., 75% or 5% twitch suppression). If the surgical conditions require continued relaxation, re-injection of the muscle relaxant becomes necessary at or before 25% recovery.

(4) **Recovery index** – The recovery index describes the speed of the offset of effect of a muscle relaxant, and is defined as the time taken for recovery from 25% to 75% twitch height.

(5) **Total duration of action** – The total duration of action is described by the interval between injection of the muscle relaxant and recovery of the TOF ratio to ≥ 0.9 [30].

Pharmacokinetics (distribution and elimination)

Muscle relaxants are usually administered intravenously, to ensure rapid onset, fast distribution, and predictable elimination. The desired paralytic effect after subcutaneous or intramuscular application (as with poisoned arrows in the Amazon) can only be achieved with high doses of muscle relaxants. Furthermore, the pharmacodynamics of the intramuscular nondepolarizing relaxants are unpredictable. Muscle relaxants are not absorbed through the gastrointestinal tract. Succinylcholine, however, is absorbed effectively and rapidly via the intramuscular route and therefore can be used in an emergency setting to treat laryngospasm in the absence of an intravenous line, provided there is no contraindication to its use.

Factors influencing pharmacokinetics
Volume of distribution

All muscle relaxants have a more or less positively charged quaternary ammonium group, which remains ionized independent of the pH value. The positive charge makes it almost impossible for muscle relaxants to bind to lipids. Therefore the volume of distribution (V_d) of muscle relaxants is almost exclusively in the extracellular space and consists of 0.2–0.5

$L kg^{-1}$. If muscle relaxants are administered over a prolonged period of time (> 24 hours), distribution into less perfused tissue occurs. resulting in a volume of distribution that can then increase up to 10-fold [31].

Plasma protein binding

After injection, muscle relaxants bind to plasma proteins, particularly to albumin and γ-globulins. The published values for percentage of protein binding of individual muscle relaxants are inconsistent and highly dependent on the method of determination. In the presence of inflammation, a protein called α_1-acid glycoprotein (AAG, orosomucoid), a component of α_1-globulin, increases in plasma. This protein binds to all muscle relaxants, resulting in a decreased free fraction in plasma.

Pharmacologic potency

The pharmacologic potency of a muscle relaxant is described by its affinity to the acetylcholine receptor. Many relaxants exhibit a reciprocal relationship between pharmacologic potency and onset time. If a low-affinity drug requires a high dose (e.g., higher ED_{95}) to achieve a defined twitch depression, the concentration gradient between central compartment and biophase will be high, resulting in faster delivery of the drug to the receptor. In contrast, if the drug has a high affinity for the acetylcholine receptor, it will be administered in smaller doses (lower ED_{95}) and the gradient for transfer of drug will be lower, resulting in slower onset [17,18]. Even though muscle relaxants do not all share these characteristics [18], pharmaceutical research follows this assumption when developing and synthesizing new muscle relaxants (e.g., rocuronium).

Speed of injection

Fast injection of muscle relaxant generates a high concentration gradient between the central compartment and the biophase (i.e., neuromuscular junction), and therefore expedites onset time. However, in the case of the benzylisoquinolines, especially atracurium and mivacurium, the histaminergic side effects can be associated with rapid injection [32].

Perfusion

Intravenously administered muscle relaxants must be transported via the bloodstream to their effect compartments. If the cardiac output is reduced for whatever reason, onset of the neuromuscular block is delayed [33]. Differences in regional blood flow result in different onset times in the individual muscle groups (diaphragm < laryngeal muscles < orbicular ocular muscle < adductor pollicis muscle) [34].

Obesity

At normal doses, the positive charge of the muscle relaxant prevents its absorption into fat tissue. Therefore, the body-weight-related volume of distribution ($V_d \, kg^{-1}$), and clearance in obese patients is markedly reduced compared to normal

Table 38.2. Metabolism and elimination of muscle relaxants

	Metabolism	Renal elimination	Biliary elimination
Succinylcholine	98–99% (plasma cholinesterase)	< 2% high elimination in presence of plasma cholinesterase deficiency	—
Mivacurium	95–99% (plasma cholinesterase)	< 5% (metabolites) high elimination in presence of plasma cholinesterase deficiency	—
Atracurium	70–90% (Hofmann elimination und esterases)	10–30% (laudanosine)	(laudanosine)
Cisatracurium	70–90% (Hofmann elimination and esterases)	10–30% (laudanosine)	(laudanosine)
Alcuronium	—	80–90%	10–20%
Vecuronium	30–40% (hepatic)	~ 40% (metabolites)	10–20% (metabolites)
Pancuronium	10–20% (hepatic)	60–80%	10%
Rocuronium	Minimal (hepatic)	30–40%	~ 60%

Table 38.3. Pharmacokinetic parameters of muscle relaxants at different ages

	Plasma clearance (mL kg^{-1} min^{-1})			Volume of distribution (mL kg^{-1})			Elimination half-life (min)		
	children	adults	elderly	children	adults	elderly	children	adults	elderly
Atracurium	5.1–9.1	5.0–6.2	5.4–6.5	113–210	100–140	150–190	14–20	17–23	22–23
Cisatracurium		4.1–6.5			110–180			19–25	
Mivacurium		40–120	54		120–410	290		1–3	2
Vecuronium	2.8–5.9	4.2–6.3	2.6–3.7	130–360	210–280	180–440	28–123	50–90	58–125
Rocuronium	11.4–13.5	2.2–3.5	3.4	220–300	140–220	620	38–56	70–106	137
Pancuronium	1.7	1.0–2.0	0.8–1.2	200	100–280	220–320	103	115–155	151–204

patients. The elimination half-life, however, remains almost unaltered [35].

Age

Volume of distribution for muscle relaxants is larger in children than in adults. Therefore, in children a higher dose of muscle relaxant must be injected to achieve a given concentration of relaxant. The neuromuscular junction is also more sensitive in the younger child than in the adolescent [36]. Thus the higher dose can result in prolonged duration of action. With aminosteroidal derivatives, the higher V_d of the drug can result in a prolonged duration of action and elimination [37]. The higher heart rate and cardiac index in children also shortens the onset time of neuromuscular block compared with adults. Despite the widening of the neuromuscular junction and decrease of acetylcholine receptors with aging [38,39], the sensitivity to neuromuscular blocking drugs remains unaltered [38,40,41]. However, distribution and elimination kinetics are often prolonged in the elderly. This is largely the consequence of impaired organ function, for example of heart, liver, and kidneys. Of the drugs in current use, it is usually the organ-

dependent metabolism and elimination of aminosteroidal muscle relaxants that are affected by age (Tables 38.2, 38.3).

Pregnancy

During pregnancy, the pharmacokinetics and pharmacodynamics of muscle relaxants remain virtually unaltered. However, increased potency and duration of action should be considered with the use of nondepolarizing muscle relaxants when magnesium is used as treatment for premature uterine contractions or pre-eclampsia. The ionized state of muscle relaxants minimizes the passage of drug through the blood–placenta barrier. Only after extended use, for example during prolonged mechanical ventilation with relaxants in an ICU, do muscle relaxants reach the fetus in sufficient concentrations to significantly affect muscle function [42].

Temperature

Duration of action of muscle relaxants is prolonged during hypothermia because of delayed metabolic breakdown by the organs of metabolism, as well as delayed hepatic and renal clearances [43]. In the case of atracurium and cisatracurium, it is also due to a delay in the spontaneous degradation (Hofmann elimination) [44]. The differentiation between pharmacodynamic and pharmacokinetic causes is difficult to determine during reduced body temperature. A possible exception is mivacurium, which is degraded by temperature-independent plasma cholinesterase [44,45].

Elimination and metabolism of relaxants

The neuromuscular effect of a single dose of muscle relaxant is primarily terminated by redistribution of drug from the neuromuscular junction and central compartment to the peripheral compartment. After repeated injection or continuous infusion, however, the redistribution capacity may become saturated, and the muscle relaxants and their active metabolites may be distributed back into the central compartment. In this case, neuromuscular recovery is determined primarily by the elimination of the drug.

Renal elimination

All muscle relaxants can be eliminated through the kidney, although this route may not be the primary pathway (Fig. 38.6). At physiological pH, muscle relaxants are ionized as quaternary amines. Patients with healthy renal function can eliminate muscle relaxants at a rate of approximately 1–2 mL kg^{-1} min^{-1}, which is equivalent to the normal glomerular filtration rate. Reabsorption from the tubules does not take place. Decreased renal function prolongs the elimination half-life of muscle relaxants that are excreted by the kidneys, such as pancuronium, rocuronium, and alcuronium.

Metabolism: ester hydrolysis

Succinylcholine and mivacurium are the only nondepolarizing neuromuscular blocking drugs inactivated through enzymatic cleavage by plasma cholinesterase. This inactivation takes place as long as the molecules are in the extracellular space or diffuse back into it from the synaptic cleft.

Atypical plasma cholinesterases

The incidence of individuals with heterozygous atypical plasma cholinesterase is 1/480. The duration of action of succinylcholine and mivacurium in these cases is delayed only minimally. Homozygous carriers of the atypical plasma cholinesterase (incidence 1/3200), however, can experience prolonged neuromuscular block lasting up to 3–6 hours. Numerous genotypes of plasma cholinesterase, in hetero- or homozygous form, can be differentiated: e.g., E_1^u (usual: normal form), E_1^a (atypical form: dibucaine-resistant), E_1^f (fluoride-resistant), E_1^s (silent form: no enzyme activity at all). The *dibucaine test*, introduced in 1957 by Kalow and Genest, uses the local anesthetic dibucaine to inhibit plasma cholinesterase in vitro [46]. Normal isoforms of plasma cholinesterase are more easily inhibited than the atypical isoforms. The percentage of inhibition of plasma cholinesterase is referred to as the *dibucaine number*. Normal plasma cholinesterases will be inhibited about 70% by dibucaine, whereas abnormal cholinesterases are less inhibited (Table 38.4).

Acquired cholinesterase deficiency

Different drugs can inhibit the activity of plasma cholinesterase, and thereby decrease the metabolism of succinylcholine

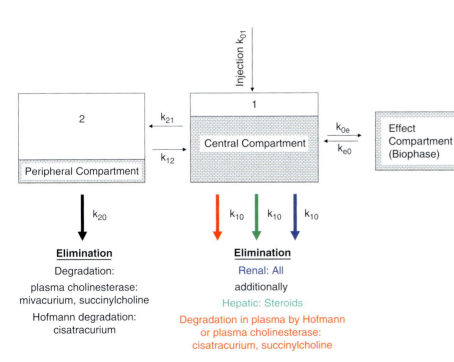

Figure 38.6. Schematic illustration of the distribution of muscle relaxants in the different compartments. The propagated model can be used to mathematically determine pharmacokinetic parameters. k_{xy} describes the redistribution constants between the different compartments.

Table 38.4. Dibucaine number, atypical plasma cholinesterase, and neuromuscular recovery after succinylcholine or mivacurium

Dibucaine number	Plasma cholinesterase	Neuromuscular recovery	Incidence
≥ 70	Normal	Normal	—
35–65	Heterozygous atypical	Minimal increase	1/480
≤ 30	Homozygous atypical	Prolonged by hours	1/3200

Table 38.5. Adverse effects of succinylcholine

Stimulation of muscarinic acetylcholine receptors of the cardiac sinoatrial node

Bradycardia

Atrioventricular node rhythm

Ventricular arrhythmia

Depolarization of the endplate

Increased intracranial pressure

Increased intraocular pressure

Increased intragastric pressure

Release of intracellular potassium

Myalgia

Masseter spasm

Trigger for malignant hyperthermia (MH)

Allergic reactions

and mivacurium. This is most obvious with the cholinesterase inhibitors neostigmine and pyridostigmine. Several other drugs, including pancuronium, antiemetic metoclopramide, echothiopate (a topical drug used to treat glaucoma), and some antiasthmatic drugs, have considerable capacity to inhibit cholinesterase. If the plasma cholinesterase activity is reduced to values around 500 IUL^{-1} (e.g., during liver failure or burn injury), the neuromuscular block induced by succinylcholine or mivacurium can be prolonged up to 2.5 times [47]. Patients with renal insufficiency, and pregnant women, may also display reduced plasma cholinesterase activity.

Metabolism: nonenzymatic decay (Hofmann elimination)

Atracurium and its isomer cisatracurium are inactivated by spontaneous temperature- and pH-dependent degradation by the so-called Hofmann elimination. They are degraded into laudanosine and monacrylate, which are inactive metabolites at the neuromuscular junction. Hofmann elimination takes place in the central and peripheral compartment and in the synaptic cleft. In addition, atracurium is degraded via ester hydrolysis into a quaternary acid and quaternary alcohol.

Metabolism: hepatic elimination

The steroidal relaxants rocuronium, pancuronium, and vecuronium are eliminated through the kidneys and the liver. Hepatic elimination of the drugs and their metabolites can be important during renal failure, but this pathway is still slightly slower than the dissipation of action due to redistribution of the drug following a single dose. Therefore, the duration of action of each repetitive injection increases, or the dose of muscle relaxant required to establish a defined neuromuscular block decreases, because the distribution volume of the drug is small. This accumulation during repetitive dosing, however, in no way compares with the accumulation of parent drug and metabolites during liver and/or kidney failure. In contrast to the benzylisoquinolines, the deacetylation by the liver of steroidal muscle relaxants in position 3 and 17 leads to metabolites, which have their own neuromuscular blocking effects and are slowly eliminated. This is of clinical relevance when these muscle relaxants are used over a long period of time (e.g., in the ICU), since the

accumulation of the metabolites can potentiate the paralysis and delay neuromuscular recovery.

Clinical pharmacology of the depolarizing relaxant succinylcholine

Succinylcholine is the only depolarizing muscle relaxant currently in clinical use, having gained international acceptance based on research by Foldes [48]. The molecular size is smaller than that of the nondepolarizing muscle relaxants. Both nitrogen atoms are quaternary, i.e., positively charged and therefore polar, water-soluble, and almost fat-insoluble. The pH of a 2% solution is around 2–3. The commercially available solutions also contain stabilizers and buffers (benzylalcohol, benzoate, and sodium chloride), which might account for some of the side effects (Table 38.5). The absolute and relative contraindications for use of succinylcholine are based on its side effects (Table 38.6). In current clinical practice, succinylcholine is used almost exclusively for rapid sequence intubation in patients with increased risk for aspiration of gastric contents, or to relieve laryngospasm.

After intravenous injection, most of the succinylcholine is immediately metabolized by the plasma cholinesterases to succinylmonocholine and choline, even before it reaches the synaptic cleft. Thus, only a fraction reaches the neuromuscular junction and it displays a depolarizing effect within 20–40 seconds. Clinically, this can be visualized within the first minute after injection as a series of muscle fasciculations, followed by complete muscle relaxation. The ED_{95} for succinylcholine is 0.3 mg kg^{-1} body weight [49]. In clinical practice,

Table 38.6. Contraindications to succinylcholine

Neuromuscular diseases

Denervation (after 2 days)

Immobilization (after 3 days)

Burns (after 2 days)

Chronic use of muscle relaxants (after 3 days)

Sepsis/severe inflammation (after 3 days)

Disposition to malignant hyperthermia

Allergy against succinylcholine

Homozygous for atypical plasma cholinesterase

to ensure fast and complete paralysis, very often 1.0 mg kg^{-1} (3 $\times$ ED$_{95}$) of succinylcholine is given. More recent studies, however, advocate a reduction in the intubating dose to 2 $\times$ ED$_{95}$ (0.6 mg kg^{-1}), which provides acceptable intubating conditions after 60 seconds, with a shortening of the duration of effect by more than 90 seconds [49]. Regardless of these dosing guidelines, in clinical situations where maximal paralyzing effect is needed quickly and good intubating conditions are mandatory, 1 mg kg^{-1} might still be a better choice. The "ideal" dose of succinylcholine therefore remains an individual decision.

Neuromuscular recovery begins after succinylcholine diffuses out of the neuromuscular junction into the extracellular space where it is enzymatically metabolized by plasma cholinesterase. Despite the development of newer nondepolarizing neuromuscular blocking drugs with faster onset times (rocuronium) or shorter duration of action (mivacurium), succinylcholine remains the only muscle relaxant that combines both properties: short onset time ($<$ 1 minute) and short duration of action (5–10 minutes). To prevent some of the unwanted side effects of succinylcholine, related to the general muscle fasciculations, the concept of *precurarization* was introduced. To achieve this effect, a small dose of nondepolarizing neuromuscular blocking drug (e.g., vecuronium 0.01 mg kg^{-1} or cisatracurium 0.01 mg kg^{-1} in an adult [50,51]), which occupies a fraction of the acetylcholine receptors, is administered before giving succinylcholine. However, since some acetylcholine receptors are blocked, the total succinylcholine dose has to be increased to achieve the same neuromuscular blocking effect. Some patients may show signs of muscle weakness (e.g., diplopia) after the precurarizing dose of the nondepolarizing relaxant. Precurarization is therefore inadvisable in patients with existing muscle weakness (e.g., myasthenia gravis). Additionally, when administering such small doses of nondepolarizing neuromuscular blocker, one has to consider that a long precurarization interval (e.g., 3–6 minutes for cisatracurium [52] owing to the small gradient between the central and effect compartment (biophase) (Fig. 38.6). The utility of administering a small dose of nondepolarizing relaxant in clinical practice has recently been questioned because of the unwanted respiratory side effects [53].

Side effects of succinylcholine on autonomic ganglia and muscarinic receptors

The effect of succinylcholine on the cardiovascular system is very diverse, since it binds to all of the cholinergic receptors of the autonomic nervous system (Table 38.5). Complete suppression of the sinoatrial node (bradycardia), idioventricular rhythm, and ventricular arrhythmias can occur as a result of stimulation of the autonomic ganglia or the vagal muscarinic receptors, especially after second and subsequent injections. These dysrhythmic effects often are observed when high vagal tone is present, which is common in pediatric patients or after vagal stimulation induced by the laryngoscopy blade. Stimulation of other parasympathetically innervated structures (dilation of cervix, stimulation of carotid body or eyeballs) can potentiate the bradycardia. High succinylcholine-induced levels of catecholamines and serum potassium can potentiate these dysrhythmias. By premedicating with atropine, bradyarrhythmias can be prevented; however, ventricular arrhythmias are not attenuated by atropine pretreatment. Additionally, a preceding injection of a small dose of succinylcholine ("self-taming") [54], or the injection of lidocaine [55] or opioids [56], cannot attenuate these unwanted cardiovascular effects, but may attenuate the side effects related to fasciculations, namely myalgia.

Effects of succinylcholine at the neuromuscular junction

By depolarizing the endplate, succinylcholine induces fasciculation (uncoordinated contraction) of all skeletal muscles and causes a variety of unwanted side effects (Table 38.5). Although a causative relationship has not yet been established, the potential to increase intragastric, intracranial, and intraocular pressures and myalgia has been attributed to the fasciculations. The relationship between fasciculations and side effects is controversial, because the precurarizing dose can weaken the intensity of the fasciculations but does not reduce the side effects overall. It is especially difficult to explain the underlying reason for elevated intracranial pressure. It has been suggested that the increase in cerebral perfusion due to an increase in afferent excitation in the context of the generalized muscle fasciculations causes the rise in intracranial pressure. Prior hyperventilation can attenuate the rise in intracranial pressure. Other studies do not confirm the rise in intracranial pressure [57]. A rise in intraocular pressure has been attributed to sustained contraction of the extraocular muscles, where each muscle fiber has multiple innervations. However, no published reports have documented further eye damage with the administration of succinylcholine in patients with open eye injury [58]. Nonetheless, this catastrophic complication influences many anesthesiologists to avoid succinylcholine [58]. The choice between succinylcholine and a nondepolarizer should therefore be weighed against the danger of aspiration of gastric contents and rise in intracranial or intraocular pressures. Inadequate paralysis by a nondepolarizing relaxant can increase intracranial and intraocular pressures from coughing or bucking during laryngoscopy.

Succinylcholine leads to a temporary small increase in serum potassium levels of approximately 0.5 mEq L^{-1} in healthy patients. Pathologic states, which lead to quantitative increases and/or qualitative changes in the acetylcholine receptor, often are associated with larger succinylcholine-induced increases in serum potassium. In certain pathologic states, the hyperkalemia can reach life-threatening levels. If a patient has a pre-existing hyperkalemia, succinylcholine is a relative contraindication. However, succinylcholine has been used in chronic renal failure patients with relatively normal potassium levels with no adverse effects [59]. The potential for hyperkalemia with succinylcholine due to denervation induced by diabetic, ischemic, and renal neuropathy should be kept in mind. The serum potassium level does not reflect the potential for increased potassium release from the muscle after succinylcholine injection. It is hoped that this dilemma will become moot as techniques for rapid intubation with other fast-onset nondepolarizing neuromuscular blocking drugs are established.

Except for the volatile anesthetics, succinylcholine is the strongest trigger of malignant hyperthermia. Masseter spasm can be associated with succinylcholine in both adults and (more frequently) in children. Although masseter muscle spasm may be an early indicator of malignant hyperthermia, it is not always predictive of malignant hyperthermia. It is not necessary to abort the anesthetic or change to a nontriggering drug when masseter spasm occurs in isolation.

Histamine release and allergic reactions following succinylcholine

Although anaphylactic reactions are rare, succinylcholine is the neuromuscular relaxant associated with their highest incidence. Should severe cardiopulmonary side effects occur after injection of succinylcholine, after excluding a hyperkalemic response, one has to consider an allergic reaction and treat the patient accordingly. Elevated serum tryptase levels will reflect the presence of an anaphylactic reaction. Postoperatively, skin testing by a dermatologist should be performed to confirm the allergen.

Clinical pharmacology of nondepolarizing neuromuscular blocking drugs

The nondepolarizing neuromuscular blocking drugs can be classified in a number of ways (Table 38.7), but it is their chemical structure that is most relevant when considering PK/PD parameters and side effects.

Standard intubation

One of the main reasons for using muscle relaxants in the context of general anesthesia is to facilitate atraumatic and/or rapid tracheal intubation. If the muscles of the oral cavity, larynx, diaphragm, and abdomen are completely relaxed that goal is achieved. In clinical practice, little emphasis is put on neuromuscular monitoring when determining the optimal time-point of intubation. Most anesthesiologists judge the time-point to be when adequate depth of anesthesia and muscle relaxation is achieved by clinical assessment. Others use the standard onset time provided by the manufacturer. Normally a $2 \times ED_{95}$ dose of a muscle relaxant is injected, and an intubation attempt is started after the standard onset time (Table 38.8). Aside from muscle relaxation, the depth of anesthesia determines the ease of intubation.

Rapid sequence induction with nondepolarizing muscle relaxants

When there is substantial risk for aspiration of gastric contents, an essential goal during induction of anesthesia is to secure the airway as rapidly as possible, usually within 60–90 seconds after loss of the protective airway reflexes. At present, succinylcholine 1 mg kg^{-1} and rocuronium 1.2 mg kg^{-1} are the only muscle relaxants with the appropriate pharmacologic characteristics to achieve this onset time. However, 1.2 mg kg^{-1} rocuronium has a prolonged duration of muscle block. This prolonged duration of action can be a serious problem if one gets into a "can't intubate, can't ventilate" situation, and it can be fatal. Many anesthesiologists are reluctant to use such high doses of rocuronium. A short-acting nondepolarizer, such as mivacurium, has a prolonged onset of action, too long for rapid sequence induction. If contraindications to succinylcholine are present (Table 38.6), alternative techniques should be used (Table 38.9).

"Priming"

Two successive injections of a nondepolarizing muscle relaxant can decrease the onset of muscle paralysis. Thus, a small subparalytic ("priming") dose is injected about 3 minutes before the full intubating dose (Table 38.9). The priming dose, by occupying a small number of receptors, decreases the margin of safety of neurotransmission and therefore speeds the onset of effect with the subsequent dose. By priming, it is possible to achieve onset times in the range of 1 minute. Just as with precurarization, some patients may show signs of muscle weakness following the priming dose, which can increase the risk for aspiration [53,60].

Increased intubating dose

By increasing the dose of nondepolarizing muscle relaxant, the onset time for paralysis can be decreased. However, the chances of unwanted cardiovascular side effects also are increased. Additionally, the time to complete neuromuscular recovery is prolonged (Table 38.9). The limitations of currently available nondepolarizing muscle relaxants for use in rapid sequence

Table 38.7. Classification of nondepolarizing muscle relaxants. Muscle relaxants can be classified according to their potency (ED_{95}), date of introduction, chemical structure, or duration of action

	ED_{95} (mg kg^{-1})	Clinical introduction	Chemical classification	Duration of action
Rocuronium	0.3	1992	Aminosteroid	Intermediate
Vecuronium	0.05–0.06	1980	Aminosteroid	Intermediate
Pancuronium	0.06–0.07	1960	Aminosteroid	Long
Mivacurium	0.08	1997	Benzylisoquinoline	Short
Atracurium	0.25	1980	Benzylisoquinoline	Intermediate
Cisatracurium	0.05	1995	Benzylisoquinoline	Intermediate
D-Tubocurarine	0.5	1942	Dibenzyl-tetrahydro-isoquinolone	Long
Alcuronium	0.2–0.25	1964	Strychnine derivative	Long

Table 38.8. Onset and duration of action after 2 × ED_{95} dose of muscle relaxant

	Onset (min)	Dur25 (min)	Duration of action until TOF ≥ 0.9 (min)	Recovery index (min)
Rocuronium	1.5–2.5	35–50	55–80	10–15
Vecuronium	2–3	30–40	50–80	10–20
Pancuronium	3.5–6	70–120	130–220	30–50
Mivacurium	2.5–4.5	15–20	25–40	5–9
Atracurium	2–3	35–50	55–80	10–15
Cisatracurium	3–6	40–55	60–90	10–15
Alcuronium	3.5–6	80–120	170–240	45–60

See Fig. 38.1 and text for definitions of onset, dur25, TOF ≥ 0.9, and recovery index.

Table 38.9. Muscle relaxants used for rapid sequence induction

	"Priming" dose (mg kg^{-1})	Intubation dose (mg kg^{-1})	Complete recovery (min)
Succinylcholine	None	0.8–1.0	5–10
Succinylcholine	Precurarization	1.5–2.0	5–10
Rocuronium	0.3	1.0–1.2	90–120
Vecuronium	0.01	0.15–0.4	90–180
Mivacurium	0.02	0.25	25–40
Atracurium	0.05	0.7–0.8	60–90
Cisatracurium	0.01	0.2–0.4	75–120

Primary goal of a rapid sequence induction is intubation within 60 seconds.

induction are (1) the relatively longer onset time for paralysis, and therefore the longer time to intubation compared with succinylcholine unless large doses of a nondepolarizing agents are given; and (2) prolonged duration of action, particularly when given in high doses to speed onset of paralysis. The latter can pose problems related to surgeries of shorter duration, and as indicated previously can result in a crisis when a "can't intubate, can't ventilate" scenario occurs. For these reasons, many anesthesiologists prefer not to use nondepolarizing muscle relaxants for rapid sequence induction. The rapid reversal of rocuronium with sugammadex does have an advantage over other drugs to produce rapid onset and offset of paralysis, particularly in "can't intubate, can't ventilate" situations.

Neuromuscular recovery from nondepolarizers

Clinical recovery from neuromuscular block is usually described by the "recovery index." By comparing the recovery index determined in one muscle (e.g., adductor pollicis) to the recovery index in another muscle (e.g., diaphragm) within the same subject, one can assess the sensitivity of different muscles groups to a drug. One also can compare the recovery index in the same muscle between individuals; however, this relationship is used mainly for studying the effect of variables, such as age, drugs, diseases, and so on.

Residual neuromuscular block (postoperative residual curarization) is a common sequela of muscle relaxant use. Approximately 30–60% of all patients who receive a muscle relaxant have residual paralysis upon leaving the operating room, depending on the length of operation [61–63]. Residual paralysis can be a serious, unrecognized, and relevant clinical problem with a potential for severe cardiorespiratory complications. Older patients are more likely to be affected [64]. The clinical consequences include hypoventilation [65–67], atelectasis, aspiration of gastric contents [60,68], lung infiltrates, pneumonia, and even death [69]. The clinical importance of monitoring neuromuscular block and its residual effects to evaluate the need for prolonged intubation or reversal of the neuromuscular block cannot be overemphasized. Simple measures such as making neuromuscular monitoring available, promoting its use, advocating the use of reversal drugs, and training that emphasizes the negative effects of postoperative residual curarization on patient outcome are highly effective tools for reducing its incidence [59–69].

Factors confounding the clinical pharmacology of muscle relaxants

Renal insufficiency

If the renal function is impaired or completely absent, there is reduced clearance (prolonged renal elimination) of relaxants. However, since the neuromuscular effect of a single injection of muscle relaxant is mainly terminated by redistribution, the reduced renal elimination rate usually does not cause prolonged recovery times after a single dose. After repetitive injections or continuous infusion, however, the decreased renal clearance of relaxants prolongs the neuromuscular effect of muscle relaxants eliminated primarily by the renal route.

The elimination (metabolic) pathways of (cis-)atracurium and mivacurium are independent of kidney function. Rocuronium can be eliminated independent of the renal function. However, even these primarily kidney-independent pathways can be impaired during concomitant diseases (Table 38.10). The activity of plasma cholinesterase is reduced in renal failure, probably related to its loss via dialysis filter membranes and as a consequence of reduced synthesis per se from uremic hepatopathy. This leads to a prolonged effect of succinylcholine [71] and mivacurium [72]. Additionally, altered fluid balances during dialysis change the V_d of the muscle relaxants, making it difficult to predict the neuromuscular blocking effect. Changes in acid–base balance as well as electrolyte status also could influence the clinical response to muscle relaxants.

Hepatic diseases

Liver failure is often associated with secondary hyperaldosteronism, which results in fluid retention and an increase in the V_d of muscle relaxants. Consequently, larger than normal doses must be administered to achieve a given paralysis. The higher dose, once administered, may stay in the central compartment for a longer time because of poor elimination by the liver. Therefore, patients with hepatobiliary diseases often have a prolonged duration of action of muscle relaxants. After a single dose, however, the elimination (clearance) times are relatively unimportant because redistribution within the compartments is the major factor determining duration of action. However, after repetitive or continuous administration of vecuronium, rocuronium, or pancuronium accumulation occurs, because the elimination of these drugs is partly dependent on hepatic function. These drugs also have metabolites that are pharmacologically active. Plasma cholinesterase activity also is decreased in liver dysfunction as a result of decreased synthesis; the ester hydrolysis of mivacurium is proportionately reduced [47,73]. The elimination times for atracurium and cisatracurium are independent of hepatic function. Since cisatracurium, compared to atracurium, is administered in lower doses owing to its higher potency, a relatively smaller amount of laudanosine is produced. The plasma protein deficiency associated with liver failure barely increases the free fraction of muscle relaxant, since the overall plasma protein binding of relaxants to albumin is relatively low.

Neuromuscular diseases

The integrity and function of pre-, intra-, and postsynaptic structures is important for development, function, and maintenance of the neuromuscular endplate. Any neuromuscular disease that influences nerve conduction or electrical activity of the muscle membrane therefore influences neuromuscular architecture and receptor function. These changes in turn affect the responses to relaxants (Fig. 38.8).

Increased expression of the acetylcholine receptor

When innervation and electrical conductivity are established between muscle and nerve, the mature receptors are localized only to the neuromuscular junction. Deprivation of the neural influences on muscle leads to an upregulation of acetylcholine receptors, as well as a spread of the receptors beyond the neuromuscular junction into the peri- and extrajunctional areas. During this time, instead of the receptor with an ε subunit ($2\alpha_1\beta_1\delta\varepsilon$) that is expressed in the normal junction, new receptors containing a γ subunit ($2\alpha_1\beta_1\delta\gamma$), also termed fetal or immature receptors, are re-expressed as seen in the fetus (see *Postsynaptic physiology and pharmacology*, above) [10,11]. The ligand sensitivity and affinity of these immature receptors are altered. Agonists such as succinylcholine depolarize immature receptors more easily, and can lead to altered and exaggerated cation fluxes. Clinically, this means that less succinylcholine is needed to open the receptor channels. Since potassium is transported from the intra- to extracellular fluid during channel opening, the upregulated acetylcholine receptors can efflux dangerously high levels of potassium into the bloodstream because of the concentration gradient. In addition α_7-acetylcholine receptors are expressed, which are depolarized not only by acetylcholine, or succinylcholine, but also by their degradation product choline [11,74]. The increased number of acetylcholine receptors and the altered receptor isoforms in the perijunctional area, on the other hand, increase the margin of safety for neuromuscular block in terms of response to muscle relaxants, leading to a resistance to nondepolarizing neuromuscular blocking drugs. Examples of conditions that induce an upregulation of acetylcholine receptors include all forms of denervation,

Table 38.10. Comparative pharmacokinetics of muscle relaxants in normal subjects versus patients with liver or kidney failure

	Plasma clearance (mL kg⁻¹ min⁻¹)			Volume of distribution (mL kg⁻¹)			Elimination half-life (min)		
	normal	kidney failure	liver failure	normal	kidney failure	liver failure	normal	kidney failure	Liver failure
Atracurium	6.8	5.5–7.0	6.5–8.0	172	140–220	200–280	21	18–25	20–25
Cisatracurium	4.3–5.3	3.8	6.6	195	161	161	22–30	25–34	24
Mivacurium	1.8	1.8	0.9	112	112	124	1–3	—	—
Vecuronium	3.0–5.3	2.5–4.5	2.4–4.3	200–510	240–470	210–250	50–110	80–150	49–98
Rocuronium	2.9	3	3	175	260	320	87	97	97
Pancuronium	1.8	0–0.9	1.1–1.5	274	210–260	310–430	132	240–1050	208–270

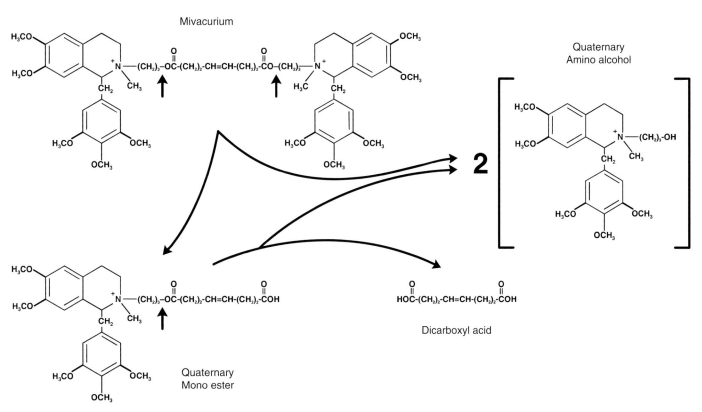

Figure 38.7. Metabolism of mivacurium by the plasma cholinesterase. The charged products are eliminated via the kidney.

immobilization, burn injury, sepsis or systemic inflammation, as well as chronic neuromuscular block (Fig. 38.8) [8,10,11,74].

Lower and upper motor neuron lesion

The potential for succinylcholine-induced hyperkalemia after a lower motor neuron lesion has been well established [75]. An increase in sensitivity to succinylcholine is already present 3–4 days after denervation and reaches a critical level after 7–8 days. Patients who demonstrate increased sensitivity to agonist (succinylcholine), due to upregulated receptors, usually also display resistance to nondepolarizing neuromuscular blocking drugs. The shorter the nerve segment distal to the lesion, the earlier the receptors become upregulated [76]. However, even a polyneuropathy in the absence of a complete transection of the nerve can cause a high potassium response to succinylcholine [77,78]. Lesions such as stroke, cerebral hemorrhage [79], head trauma [80], multiple sclerosis [81], syringomyelia, and paraplegia or quadriplegia [82] also result in upregulated acetylcholine receptors with the potential of demonstrating hypersensitivity to succinylcholine and resistance to nondepolarizing neuromuscular blocking drugs. Upper motor neuron

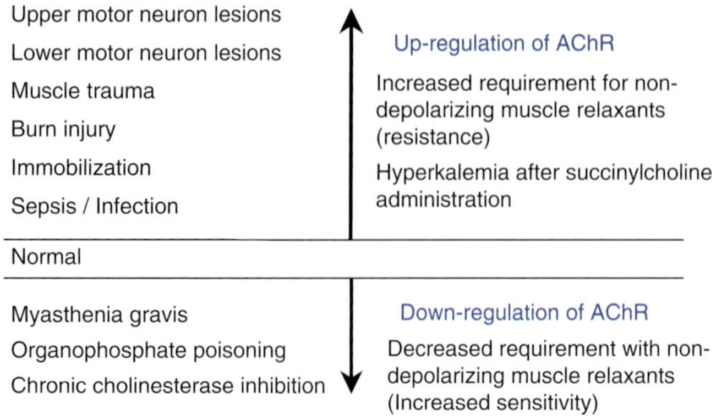

Upper motor neuron lesions
Lower motor neuron lesions
Muscle trauma
Burn injury
Immobilization
Sepsis / Infection

Normal

Myasthenia gravis
Organophosphate poisoning
Chronic cholinesterase inhibition

Up-regulation of AChR

Increased requirement for non-depolarizing muscle relaxants (resistance)

Hyperkalemia after succinylcholine administration

Down-regulation of AChR

Decreased requirement with non-depolarizing muscle relaxants (Increased sensitivity)

Figure 38.8. Conditions with altered acetylcholine receptor (AChR) expression.

lesions can lead to unilateral or bilateral changes, whereas lower motor neuron injury causes change only in the distribution of the affected nerve. The exact time period over which the receptors remain upregulated is unclear. There have been reports of increased succinylcholine sensitivity that persist for several years after the nerve injury [79]. The risk of hyperkalemia following upper or lower motor neuron injury is probably absent once the resistance to nondepolarizing muscle relaxants disappears, but no studies have defined this period. Since it is difficult to predict how a patient with neurological symptoms will react to muscle relaxants, succinylcholine should be avoided and neuromuscular function monitored when using nondepolarizing muscle relaxants.

Immobilization

The physiologic state of immobilization contrasts with denervation syndromes in that there is no direct damage to cord or nerve roots, and the muscle fibers remain innervated. However, immobilization (from isolated limbs with plaster cast to total-body immobilization as in critical illness or total-body cast) also induces an upregulation of acetylcholine receptors [83–85]. The peak effect on acetylcholine receptor regulation occurs at 14–21 days after onset of immobilization, but the duration of this change is unclear in humans [84].

Burn injury

Burn injury induces an upregulation of acetylcholine receptors in the musculature underneath the burn site, but usually not at distant muscles [86]. The iatrogenically induced immobilization of patients confined to bed, however, may cause receptor changes even in distant muscles. There is evidence that the burn injury per se leads to a direct chemical or physical denervation, since the mRNAs for γ subunits are increased, as in denervation [86]. The extent to which circulating mediators or the alterations of cell signaling pathways are involved in upregulation remains to be investigated. Burn of a single limb (8–9% body surface area) is sufficient to cause lethal

hyperkalemia following succinylcholine [87]. The prolonged administration of muscle relaxants to facilitate mechanical ventilation can accentuate the upregulation [88]. Since it takes some time to initiate the upregulation, it is safe to use succinylcholine for up to 48–72 hours after acute burn injury. Any use beyond this time should be avoided [74].

Infection and systemic inflammation

The effect of systemic infection and inflammation on the acetylcholine receptor remains controversial. There have been reports of hyperkalemia after succinylcholine administration in septic patients [89,90]. An increase in acetylcholine receptors in critically ill patients has been demonstrated; however, patients receiving intensive care treatment may have concomitant factors such as immobilization, long-term administration of muscle relaxants, and steroid treatment. Other than an increase in acetylcholine receptors, the resistance to nondepolarizing muscle relaxants also can be explained by the increased binding of relaxants to acute-phase reactant protein, AAG, which is increased in inflammatory processes. In rodents, both causes for resistance to nondepolarizing muscle relaxants have been demonstrated: inflammation alone was able to increase acetylcholine receptors as well as AAG plasma levels [91,92].

Decreased number of acetylcholine receptors
Myasthenia gravis

Myasthenia gravis is an autoimmune disease associated with a clinical picture of increasing muscle weakness and fatigue. Antibodies against the acetylcholine receptor are present in approximately 80% of the patients ("antibody-positive"). Some of the "antibody-negative" patients have antibodies against a receptor tyrosine kinase, muscle-specific kinase (MuSK), which is important for the clustering and maturation of the receptors at the neuromuscular junction [93]. It is therefore likely that "antibody-negative" patients may have antibodies against other proteins related to the neuromuscular junction. The autoantibodies to the acetylcholine receptor in myasthenic patients lead to a decrease in receptor number. Interestingly, the levels of antibodies correlate poorly with the clinical status. Symptoms of myasthenia gravis generally start with ptosis and diplopia, and proceed to bulbar paralysis. Later disease stages are marked by dysarthria, dysphagia, weakness of extremities, and weakness of respiratory muscles [94]. The therapeutic approach to myasthenia, aside from thymectomy (surgical removal of the origin of the autoantibodies), is the administration of cholinesterase inhibitors (mostly pyridostigmine). Because of the downregulation of acetylcholine receptors, patients with myasthenia are sensitive to nondepolarizing muscle relaxants. If muscle relaxants are used during clinical anesthesia, constant neuromuscular function monitoring for the duration of anesthesia is advised. Preoperative determination of the train-of-four fade can be used to predict whether or not the patient will have increased sensitivity to nondepolarizing muscle relaxants [95]. The reduced number of acetylcholine receptors, however, renders succinylcholine less capable of depolarizing the endplate effectively and raises the dose requirements of succinylcholine. For rapid sequence induction it is advisable to increase the dose of succinylcholine to 1.5–2 mg kg^{-1}. Higher doses may cause a nondepolarizing type block (see *Phase II block* and *Desensitation block*, above). The continuation of the treatment of myasthenics with cholinesterase inhibitors during the perioperative interval can cause delayed hydrolysis of succinylcholine and prolong the neuromuscular block [96]. The discontinuation of cholinesterase inhibitor therapy is, however, not recomended.

Lambert–Eaton myasthenic syndrome

Lambert–Eaton myasthenic syndrome is a paraneoplastic disease associated with small-cell carcinoma, usually of lung origin. It is an autoimmune disorder caused by the presence of antibodies directed against the PQ-type voltage-gated calcium channels [97], possibly due to a cross-reaction with the calcium channels on the carcinomatous cells [98]. More generally stated, the syndrome is caused by a prejunctional mechanism that results in the decreased quantal release of acetylcholine. The acetylcholine receptor number on the postsynaptic membrane remains normal. Clinically, patients with Lambert–Eaton syndrome display an increased sensitivity to both nondepolarizing and depolarizing muscle relaxants [99]. Again, monitoring neuromuscular function during the use of muscle relaxants will provide continuous assessment. In contrast to myasthenia gravis, repetitive (e.g., train-of-four) stimulation results in enhancement, and not fade, of twitch.

Interaction of relaxants with other drugs

Although some drugs have neuromuscular effects, because of the high margin of safety of neuromuscular transmission the effects often are seen only as a potentiation of the muscle relaxant effect. Clinically relevant interactions between these drugs and muscle relaxants can be classified into three main areas: pharmacokinetic, junctional, and muscular effects.

Pharmacokinetic interaction of relaxants with other drugs

Steroidal muscle relaxants are eliminated or metabolized by the liver to varying extents (Table 38.2). Drugs that inhibit the cytochrome P450 enzyme system (e.g., cimetidine) or reduce liver perfusion delay hepatic elimination and prolong the effect of muscle relaxants when high doses are administered [100]. Conversely, drugs that induce the cytochrome P450 system (e.g., some antiepileptic drugs) increase the rate of elimination of hepatic metabolized drugs. Thus the requirement for drugs such as vecuronium and rocuronium is increased, while that for mivacurium, which is metabolized independent of the liver [101–104], is not. Acetylcholine receptor changes and increased binding of relaxant to AAG may also play a role in the increased requirement during treatment with antiepileptic

drugs [102]. The drugs known to cause this effect are barbiturates, carbamazepine, and dilantin [101–104].

Relaxant and nonrelaxant interaction at the neuromuscular junction

Neuromuscular transmission can be influenced by drugs that act on the nerve terminal or receptor. Presynaptically, three mechanisms have been identified, all of which decrease the release of acetylcholine. First, cyclic adenosine monophosphate (cAMP) and adenosine triphosphate (ATP) are necessary to synthesize acetylcholine. Furosemide is an example of a drug that inhibits the synthesis of cAMP, thereby also decreasing presynaptic acetylcholine synthesis. Second, volatile anesthetics block presynaptic release of acetylcholine, which can be evidenced during repetitive nerve stimulation. Finally, volatile anesthetics, as well as magnesium [105,106], calcium antagonists, and aminoglycoside antibiotics [107], reduce acetylcholine release by blocking presynaptic calcium channels. Postsynaptically, numerous drugs block the α subunit of the acetylcholine receptor in a dose-dependent fashion. These include inhalational anesthetics [108], aminoglycoside antibiotics [109], quinidine [110], tricyclic antidepressants [111], ketamine [112], midazolam [113], and barbiturates [114]. Aside from binding to the α subunit, these drugs often also block the channel itself, or desensitize the acetylcholine receptor by allosteric mechanisms (see *Phase II block*, *Desensitization block*, and *Channel block*, above). It is difficult to determine, however, which of these mechanisms have the greatest effect on their ability to potentiate muscle relaxants.

Muscular effects of other drugs

Dantrolene, which inhibits calcium release and reuptake into the sarcoplasmic reticulum, is used for treatment of malignant hyperthermia. It can potentiate the effect of the nondepolarizing muscle relaxants at a muscular level without exerting an effect on neuromuscular transmission [115]. The effects of dantrolene cannot be monitored electromyographically.

Practical aspects of drug administration

Few surgical procedures mandate continuous neuromuscular paralysis. In many cases, it is unnecessary to continue the paralysis after intubation. Operations in the abdomen usually require muscle relaxation. If the depth of anesthesia is not sufficient, or if appropriate anesthetic depth cannot be achieved because of other factors (e.g., hemodynamic instability), the patient might move or cough. If the surgeon or procedure requires absolute paralysis, one can either give repetitive bolus doses of muscle relaxant or start an infusion with close monitoring of neuromuscular function. The most convenient muscle relaxants used for infusions are mivacurium or (*cis-*)

Table 38.11. Infusion rates for a continuous neuromuscular block and clinical recovery after continuous infusion

	IR$_{90}$–IR$_{95}$ (µg kg^{-1} min^{-1})	Recovery time until T1/T4 > 0.9 (min)
Mivacurium	3–15	10–20^a
Atracurium	4–12	30–70^a
Cisatracurium	0.4–4	30–70^a
Rocuronium	3–12	30–90^b

IR$_{90}$–IR$_{95}$, infusion rate for a 90–95% neuromuscular block; Recovery until T1/T4 > 0.9 (min), time from end of infusion until complete neuromuscular recovery.
^{a}Independent of infusion time.
^{b}At infusion time of up to 2 hours, significantly increased compared to single-shot injection.

atracurium, because they do not accumulate and the offset indices are constant even after repetitive injection or continuous infusion (Table 38.11) [116,117].

Differential diagnosis and therapy of residual neuromuscular block

Before reversal of residual neuromuscular block, the presence or absence of paralysis should be evaluated. The train-of-four ratio is the most common method of assessing muscle weakness, and a ratio of ≥ 0.9 is recommended for full recovery from paralysis [30,61–68]. If a nondepolarizing neuromuscular blocking drug is used, the muscle weakness beyond expected duration may be due to delayed elimination of, or increased sensitivity to, the drug. After the reversal drug has been administered, the patient should be closely monitored in the recovery room, since the half-life of the reversal drug might be shorter than that of the muscle relaxant, causing recurarization.

If succinylcholine or mivacurium was used, the underlying cause for prolonged muscle weakness could be plasma cholinesterase deficiency or atypical plasma cholinesterase. In both cases, antagonism with cholinesterase inhibitors will not be of much benefit. These patients should be mechanically ventilated until spontaneous recovery occurs, from renal elimination of the drug. This may take as long as 4–6 hours. In these instances of prolonged recovery of paralysis from succinylcholine or mivacurium, the activity of the plasma cholinesterase should be determined. If the activity of the plasma cholinesterase is reduced because of genetic factors, the patient should be advised of the results so as to avoid the same complication in future anesthetic procedures.

Use of muscle relaxants during rapid sequence induction

When inducing patients with an increased risk of aspiration of gastric contents, one of the goals is to secure the airway as early as possible. Succinylcholine continues to be the commonest drug used for this purpose. However, succinylcholine has clinically relevant side effects (Table 38.5). Myalgias

are treated either with analgesics or by reducing muscle fasciculations. The extent to which opioids are beneficial for succinylcholine-induced myalgia remains to be answered [56]. It is more common in clinical practice to treat myalgias after the fact with nonsteroidal peripheral analgesics [118]. Prevention of muscle fasciculations not only reduces the incidence of myalgias but also prevents increases in intraocular [119] and intragastric [55] pressures. The importance of increased intraocular or even intracranial pressure by succinylcholine has been questioned [57,58]. "Precurarization," by the administration of a small dose of nondepolarizing muscle relaxant preceding the administration of succinylcholine, is the most used clinical technique for reducing fasciculations. Alternative strategies include preadministration of small doses of succinylcholine ("self-taming") [54], lidocaine (100 mg) [55], or opioids [56]. In one study, 37.5% of precurarized patients had paralytic symptoms such as diplopia, heavy eyelids, difficulty with speech and swallowing. In others, signs of respiratory insufficiency were noted [53,120]. Therefore, precurarization has its own problems and side effects.

The efficacy of precurarization with nondepolarizing relaxant for reducing fasciculations is undisputed. The basis for this that is the nondepolarizing muscle relaxant has blocking effects at the pre- and postsynaptic acetylcholine receptors. Since the antagonism by nondepolarizing relaxant also affects the actual mechanism of action of succinylcholine, precurarization leads to prolonged onset time, shorter duration of action, and reduced maximal neuromuscular block by succinylcholine [121]. To overcome these effects, an increased dose of succinylcholine by approximately 25–75% is recommended (1.5–2.0 mg kg^{-1}) [122]. A higher dose of succinylcholine after precurarization and a normal dose without precurarization reveal no difference in terms of incidence of muscle fasciculations.

Succinylcholine can induce bradycardia, especially in children and particularly after the second dose. This side effect is prevented by premedication with atropine, which at the same time can cause tachycardia. Tachycardia can confound the assessment of depth of anesthesia and fluid status. Precurarization with nondepolarizing muscle relaxants does not affect the muscarinic receptors and therefore does not prevent the autonomic and cardiac effects of succinylcholine.

A systematic review published in 2008 revealed that there was no statistical difference in intubation conditions when succinylcholine 1.0 mg kg^{-1} was compared with 1.2 mg kg^{-1} rocuronium [123]. The primary drawback to administering high doses of rocuronium is the slightly prolonged onset and prolonged duration of action of approximately 2 hours versus 10 minutes after 1.0 mg kg^{-1} succinylcholine. The introduction of sugammadex (available in Europe as of September 2008), with its fast reversal of rocuronium-induced neuromuscular block, might be a real step forward in eliminating the potential hazards of succinylcholine [124–125].

Prolonged neuromuscular block in the critically ill patient

Continuous administration of neuromuscular blocking drugs in the ICU is practiced in some situations. The etiology of prolonged muscle weakness in these critically ill patients is certainly multifactorial. It is clear that extended use of muscle relaxants leads to muscle weakness. Therefore, the American College of Critical Care Medicine has published clinical practice guidelines for the prolonged use of muscle relaxants in the adult critically ill population [126]. Prolonged disruption of neuromuscular transmission by muscle relaxants can cause profound changes at the neuromuscular junction that result in aberrant responses to the future use of both depolarizing and nondepolarizing muscle relaxants. When using muscle relaxants for long periods, patients should be medicated with sedative and analgesic drugs to provide adequate amnesia and analgesia. Only after all other means have been tried without success should neuromuscular blocking drugs be added to the armamentarium. Indications for muscle relaxant therapy may include facilitation of mechanical ventilation, prevention of increase in intracranial or intrathoracic pressure during coughing and suctioning, treatment of muscle spasms (e.g., tetanus), and decrease of oxygen consumption. Other reasons for its use may include prevention of injury during seizures, or to prevent dislodgement of patient-care-related material (endotracheal tubes, arterial lines, etc.) [8].

Pancuronium or vecuronium are popular choices for relaxants in the ICU, because they are inexpensive. However, when vagolysis is contraindicated (i.e., cardiovascular disease) neuromuscular blocking drugs other than pancuronium should be used. Although the steroidal muscle relaxants may have the potential to have a more profound effect on the muscle wasting, by potentiating the effect of endogenous and exogenous steroids, this hypothesis has not been proved convincingly. In-vitro studies have documented that steroidal relaxants have no effect on enhancing the activity of nuclear steroidal receptors or the activity of steroids themselves [126]. Chemical denervation induced by muscle relaxants upregulates steroidal receptors in muscle, aggravating the steroid-induced myopathy [127]. For patients receiving neuromuscular blocking drugs and corticosteroids, therefore, every effort should be made to discontinue neuromuscular blocking drugs as soon as possible. Because of the unique organ-independent metabolism (Hofmann degradation) of atracurium and cisatracurium, these drugs are preferred in patients with significant hepatic or renal disease. If tachyphylaxis to one neuromuscular blocking drug develops, a different neuromuscular blocking drug can be tried, although cross-tolerance does exist. In general, all patients receiving neuromuscular blocking drugs for prolonged periods in the ICU should have prophylactic eye care, physical therapy, and prophylaxis for deep vein thrombosis [128].

Summary

Muscle relaxants are mostly used to facilitate endotracheal intubation and to improve operative conditions during surgery. Less commonly, muscle relaxants are used in critically ill ICU patients to facilitate mechanical ventilation, decrease oxygen consumption, and attenuate rises in intracranial or intrathoracic pressures during coughing or suctioning. Muscle relaxants are also an integral part of the pharmacologic armamentarium for sedative/hypnotic/analgesic ("balanced") anesthesia.

Muscle relaxants can be classified into depolarizing and nondepolarizing drugs. The latter, based on chemical structure, can be subdivided into steroidal and benzylisoquinoline. A depolarizing relaxant is typified by succinylcholine. Muscle paralysis by nondepolarizing relaxants is achieved primarily by blocking the function of the postsynaptic acetylcholine receptor, although these drugs also block presynaptic acetylcholine receptors. The nondepolarizers produce a competitive block by binding to the α subunit of the acetylcholine receptor, inhibiting the physiologic binding and action of the neurotransmitter acetylcholine. The neuromuscular block produced by the depolarizing relaxant is by partial agonism; succinylcholine induces paralysis by binding to the receptor, and repetitively depolarizing (opening) the ion channel until it moves out of the receptor and is degraded in the extracellular fluid by plasma (pseudo-) cholinesterase.

Muscle relaxants are administered intravenously, to ensure rapid onset, fast distribution, and predictable elimination. Muscle relaxants are not absorbed through the gastrointestinal tract. Succinylcholine, however, is rapidly absorbed via the intramuscular route and therefore can be used in an emergency situation such as laryngospasm in children who do not have intravenous access for drug administration. All muscle relaxants can be eliminated via the kidney, although this route may not be the primary pathway. The steroidal relaxants, rocuronium, pancuronium, and vecuronium, can be eliminated via the kidneys and the liver. The metabolic breakdown products of steroidal relaxants are pharmacologically active, although less potent. The benzylisoquinoline relaxants, atracurium and its isomer cisatracurium, are degraded into the inactive metabolites laudanosine and monacrylate by spontaneous, temperature- and pH-dependent, Hofmann elimination. Succinylcholine and mivacurium are inactivated through enzymatic cleavage by plasma cholinesterase. The effect of these two drugs can be prolonged in the presence of acquired or congenital pseudocholinesterase deficiency. The neuromuscular effect of a single dose of nondepolarizing muscle relaxant wanes with time primarily due to its redistribution from the neuromuscular junction and central compartment to the peripheral compartment.

Unwanted side effects of muscle relaxants can be due to histamine release (hypotension) and anaphylaxis. The bronchial and cardiovascular side effects (bronchospasm and tachycardia) of nondepolarizing relaxants, particularly the steroidal relaxants, are due to their binding to muscarinic acetylcholine receptors on the bronchi and myocardium, respectively. Succinylcholine can cause tachycardia or bradycardia by its ability to bind nicotinic receptors in the autonomic ganglia and the postsynaptic parasympathetic muscarinic receptor. It also has the potential to cause hyperkalemia and cardiac arrest when it is administered in the presence of upregulated acetylcholine receptors, as seen in denervation, burns, immobilization, sepsis and prolonged neuromuscular block. The normal acetylcholine receptor has a subunit composition of $2\alpha_1\beta_1\delta\epsilon$. In the upregulated state receptors consisting of $2\alpha_1\beta_1\delta\gamma$ and $5\alpha7$ are expressed throughout the muscle membrane. In the presence of upregulated acetylcholine receptors, there is also resistance to the neuromuscular effects of nondepolarizers.

The muscle relaxant effect of nondepolarizers can be concentration-dependently potentiated by volatile anesthetics, magnesium, aminoglycoside antibiotics, quinidine, tricyclic antidepressants, ketamine, midazolam, and barbiturates.

Myasthemia gravis is a condition in which downregulation of the acetylcholine receptors occurs due to autoantibodies against the receptor. In Lambert–Eaton myasthenic syndrome the muscle weakness is caused by decreased release of acetylcholine due to autoantibodies against the voltage-gated calcium channel present on the nerve terminal. Myasthenia gravis and Lambert–Eaton patients are more sensitive to nondepolarizing relaxants.

Neuromuscular monitoring is advocated when using muscle relaxants. A train-of-four ratio of ≥ 0.9 confirms adequate recovery from neuromuscular paralysis. In order to reverse nondepolarizer-induced neuromuscular paralysis, cholinesterase inhibitors (neostigmine, edrophonium), which increase acetylcholine levels, can be used. A steroidal muscle relaxant encapsulator, sugammadex, which rapidly reverses pancuronium-, rocuronium-, and vecuronium-induced neuromuscular block, is now available.

References

1. Bernard C. *Leçon sur les effets de substances toxiques et medicamenteuses.* Bailliere, Paris 1851: 164–190.

2. Bernard C. Etudes physiologiques sur quelques poisons americains. *Rev Deux Mondes* 1864; **53**: 164–190.

3. Griffith HR, Johnson GE. The use of curare in general anesthesia. *Anesthesiology* 1942; **3**: 418–20.

4. Mayrhofer OK. Self-experiments with succinylcholine chloride; a new ultra-short-acting muscle relaxant. *Br Med J* 1952; **1**: 1332–4.

5. Thesleff S. Succinylcholine iodide: studies on its pharmacological properties and clinical use. *Acta Physiol Scand Suppl* 1952; **27**: 1–36.

6. Bovet D. Some aspects of the relationship between chemical structure and curare-like activity. *Ann N Y Acad Sci* 1951; **54**: 407–10.

7. Baird WL, Reid AM. The neuromuscular blocking properties of a new steroid compound, pancuronium bromide: a pilot study in man. *Br J Anaesth* 1967; **39**: 775–80.

8. Martyn JAJ, Fukushima Y, Chon JY, Yang HS. Muscle relaxants in burns, trauma, and critical illness. *Int Anesthesiol Clin* 2006; **44**: 123–43.

9. Fambrough DM. Control of acetylcholine receptors in skeletal muscle. *Physiol Rev* 1979; **59**: 165–227.

10. Martyn JAJ, White DA, Gronert GA, Jaffe R, Ward JM. Up and down regulation of acetylcholine receptors: effects on neuromuscular blockers. *Anesthesiology* 1992; **76**: 822–43.

11. Martyn JAJ, Jonsson-Fagerlund M, Eriksson LI. Basic principles of neuromuscular transmission. *Anaesthesia* 2009; **64**: 1–9.

12. Paton WD, Waud DR. The margin of safety of neuromuscular transmission. *J Physiol* 1967; **191**: 59–90.

13. Lingle CJ, Steinbach JH. Neuromuscular blocking agents. *Int Anesthesiol Clin* 1988; **26**: 288–301.

14. Prince RJ, Sine SM. The ligand binding domains of the nicotinic acetylcholine receptor. In: Barrantes FJ, ed., *The Nicotinic Acetylcholine Receptor: Current Views and Future Trends.* Berlin: Springer-Verlag, 1998: 32–59.

15. Adams PR, Sakmann B. Decamethonium both opens and blocks endplate channels. *Proc Natl Acad Sci U S A* 1978; **75**: 2994–8.

16. Marshall CG, Ogden DC, Colquhoun D. The actions of suxamethonium (succinyldicholine) as an agonist and channel blocker at the nicotinic receptor of frog muscle. *J Physiol* 1990; **428**: 155–74.

17. Bowmann WC, Rodger IW, Houston J, Marshall RJ, McIndewar I. Structure: action relationships among some desacetoxy analogues of pancuronium and vecuronium in the anesthetized cat. *Anesthesiology* 1988; **69**: 57–62.

18. Kopman AF, Klewicka MM, Kopman DJ, Neuman GG. Molar potency is predictive of the speed of onset of neuromuscular block for agents of intermediate, short, and ultrashort duration. *Anesthesiology* 1999; **90**: 425–31.

19. Szenohradszky J, Trevor AJ, Bickler P, *et al.* Central nervous system effects of intrathecal muscle relaxants in rats. *Anesth Analg* 1993; **76**: 1304–9.

20. Cardone C, Szenohradszky J, Spencer Y, Bickler P. Activation of brain acetylcholine receptors by neuromuscular blocking drugs. *Anesthesiology* 1994; **80**: 1155–61.

21. Jonsson M, Kim C, Yamamoto Y, *et al.* Atracurium and vecuronium block nicotine-induced carotid body chemoreceptor responses. *Acta Anaesthesiologica Scandinavica* 2002; **46**: 488–94.

22. Jonsson M, Dabrowski M, Gurley DA, *et al.* Activation and inhibition of human muscular and neuronal nicotinic acetylcholine receptors by succinylcholine. *Anesthesiology* 2006; **104**: 724–33.

23. Hou VY, Hirshman CA, Emala CW. Neuromuscular relaxants as antagonists for M2 and M3 muscarinic receptors. *Anesthesiology* 1998; **88**: 744–50.

24. Jooste EH, Sharma A, Zhang Y, Emala CW. Rapacuronium augments acetylcholine-induced bronchoconstriction via positive allosteric interactions at the M3 muscarinic receptor. *Anesthesiology* 2005; **103**: 1195–203.

25. Jooste E, Zhang Y, Emala CW. Neuromuscular blocking agents' differential bronchoconstrictive potential in Guinea pig airways. *Anesthesiology* 2007; **106**: 763–72.

26. Lowman MA, Rees PH, Benyon RC, Church MK. Human mast cell heterogeneity: histamine release from mast cells dispersed from skin, lung, adenoids, tonsils, and colon in response to IgE-dependent and nonimmunologic stimuli. *J Allergy Clin Immunol* 1988; **81**: 590–7.

27. Lien CA, Belmont MR, Abalos A, *et al.* The cardiovascular effects and histamine-releasing properties of 51W89 in patients receiving nitrous oxide/opioid/barbiturate anesthesia. *Anesthesiology* 1995; **82**: 1131–8.

28. Scott RP, Savarese JJ, Basta SJ, *et al.* Atracurium: clinical strategies for preventing histamine release and attenuating the haemodynamic response. *Br J Anaesth* 1985; **57**: 550–3.

29. Laxenaire MC. [Epidemiology of anesthetic anaphylactoid reactions. Fourth multicenter survey (July 1994-December 1996)]. *Ann Fr Anesth Reanim* 1999; **18**: 796–809.

30. Claudius C, Viby-Mogensen J. Acceleromyography for use in scientific and clinical practice: a systematic review of the evidence. *Anesthesiology* 2008; **108**: 1117–40.

31. Waser PG, Wiederkehr H, Sin-Ren AC, Kaiser-Schonenberger E. Distribution and kinetics of 14C-vecuronium in rats and mice. *Br J Anaesth* 1987; **59**: 1044–51.

32. Savarese JJ, Ali HH, Basta SJ, *et al.* The Clinical Neuromuscular Pharmacology of Mivacurium Chloride (BW B1090U): A Short-acting Nondepolarizing Ester Neuromuscular Blocking Drug. *Anesthesiology* 1988; **68**: 723–32.

33. Iwasaki H, Igarashi M, Yamauchi M, Namiki A. The effect of cardiac output on the onset of neuromuscular block by vecuronium. *Anaesthesia* 1995; **50**: 361–2.

34. Donati F, Meistelman C, Plaud B. Vecuronium Neuromuscular Blockade at the Diaphragm, the Orbicularis Oculi, and Adductor Pollicis Muscles. *Anesthesiology* 1990; **73**: 870–5.

35. Parker CJ, Hunter JM. Relationship between volume of distribution of atracurium and body weight. *Br J Anaesth* 1993; **70**: 443–5.

36. Goudsouzian NG, Martyn JJ, Liu LM, Ali HH. The dose response effect of long-acting nondepolarizing neuromuscular blocking agents in children. *Can Anaesth Soc J* 1984; **31**: 246–50.

37. Fisher DM, Miller RD. Neuromuscular effects of vecuronium (ORG NC45) in infants and children during N2O, halothane anesthesia. *Anesthesiology* 1983; **58**: 519–23.

38. Courtney J, Steinbach JH. Age changes in neuromuscular junction morphology and acetylcholine receptor distribution on rat skeletal muscle fibres. *J Physiol* 1981; **320**: 435–47.

39. Sanes JR, Lichtman JW. Induction, assembly, maturation and maintenance of a postsynaptic apparatus. *Nat Rev Neurosci* 2001; **2**: 791–805.

40. Matteo RS, Backus WW, McDaniel DD, *et al.* Pharmacokinetics and pharmacodynamics of d-tubocurarine and metocurine in the elderly. *Anesth Analg* 1985; **64**: 23–9.

41. Yang HS, Goudsouzian NG, Cheng M, Martyn JA. The influence of the age of the rat on the neuromuscular response to mivacurium in vitro. *Paediatr Anaesth* 1996; **6**: 367–72.

42. Guay J, Grenier Y, Varin F. Clinical pharmacokinetics of neuromuscular relaxants in pregnancy. *Clin Pharmacokinet* 1998; **34**: 483.

43. Smeulers NJ, Wierda JM, van den Broek L, Gallandat Huet RC, Hennis PJ. Hypothermic cardiopulmonary bypass influences the concentration- response relationship and the biodisposition of rocuronium. *Eur J Anaesthesiol Suppl* 1995; **11**: 91–4.

44. Leslie K, Sessler DI, Bjorksten AR, Moayeri A. Mild hypothermia alters propofol pharmacokinetics and increases the duration of action of atracurium. *Anesth Analg* 1995; **80**: 1007–14.

45. Rump AF, Schierholz J, Biederbick W, *et al.* Pseudocholinesterase-activity reduction during cardiopulmonary bypass: the role of dilutional processes and pharmacological agents. *Gen Pharmacol* 1999; **32**: 65–9.

46. Kalow W, Genest K. A method for the detection of atypical forms of human serum cholinesterase: determination of dibucaine numbers. *Can J Biochem. Physiol.* 1957; **35**: 339–46.

47. Martyn JAJ, Goudsouzian NG, Chang Y, *et al.* Neuromuscular effects of mivacurium in 2- to 12-yr-old children with burn injury. *Anesthesiology* 2000; **92**: 31–7.

48. Foldes FF, Rendell-Baker L, Birch J. Causes and prevention of prolonged apnea with succinylcholine. *Anesthesia and Analgesia* 1956; **25**: 609.

49. Naguib M, Samarkandi A, Riad W, Alharby SW. Optimal dose of succinylcholine revisited. *Anesthesiology* 2003; **99**: 1045–9.

50. Engbaek J, Howardy-Hansen P, Ording H, Viby-Mogensen J. Precurarization with vecuronium and pancuronium in awake, healthy volunteers: the influence on neuromuscular transmission and pulmonary function. *Acta Anaesthesiol Scand* 1985; **29**: 117–20.

51. Joshi GP, Hailey A, Cross S, Thompson-Bell G, Whitten CC. Effects of pretreatment with cisatracurium, rocuronium, and d-tubocurarine on succinylcholine-induced fasciculations and myalgia: a comparison with placebo. *J Clin Anesth* 1999; **11**: 641–5.

52. Mencke T, Becker C, Schreiber JU, Fuchs-Buder T. A longer pretreatment interval does not improve cisatracurium precurarization. *Can J Anaesth* 2002; **49**: 640–1.

53. Han TH, Martyn JAJ. Onset and effectiveness of rocuronium for rapid onset of paralysis in patients with major burns: priming vs. large bolus. *Brit J Anaesth* 2009; **102**: 55–60.

54. Wald-Oboussier G, Lohmann C, Viell B, Doehn M. ["Self-taming": an

alternative to the prevention of succinylcholine- induced pain]. *Anaesthesist* 1987; **36**: 426–30.

55. Miller RD, Way WL. Inhibition of succinylcholine-induced increased intragastric pressure by nondepolarizing muscle relaxants and lidocaine. *Anesthesiology* 1971; **34**: 185–8.

56. Polarz H, Bohrer H, Fleischer F, *et al.* Effects of thiopentone/suxamethonium on intraocular pressure after pretreatment with alfentanil. *Eur J Clin Pharmacol* 1992; **43**: 311–3.

57. Kovarik WD, Mayberg TS, Lam AM, Mathisen TL, Winn HR. Succinylcholine does not change intracranial pressure, cerebral blood flow velocity, or the electroencephalogram in patients with neurologic injury. *Anesth Analg* 1994; **78**: 469–73.

58. Vachon CA, Warner DO, Bacon DR. Succinylcholine and the open globe: tracing the teaching. *Anesthesiology* 2003; **99**: 220–3.

59. Thapa S, Brull SJ. Succinylcholine-induced hyperkalemia in patients with renal failure: an old question revisited. *Anesth Analg* 2000; **91**: 237–41.

60. Eriksson LI, Sundman E, Olsson R, *et al.* Functional assessment of the pharynx at rest and during swallowing in partially paralyzed humans: simultaneous videomanometry and mechanomyography of awake human volunteers. *Anesthesiology* 1997; **87**: 1035–43.

61. Brull SJ, Maguib M, Miller RD. Residual neuromuscular block: rediscovering the obvious. *Anesth Analg* 2008; **107**: 11–14.

62. Hayes AH, Mirakhur RK, Breslin DS, Reid JE, McCourt KC. Postoperative residual block after intermediate-acting neuromuscular blocking drugs. *Anaesthesia* 2001; **56**: 312–18.

63. Murphy GS, Szokol JW, Marymont JH, *et al.* Residual neuromuscular blockade and critical respiratory events in the postanesthesia care unit. *Anesth Analg* 2008; **107**: 130–7.

64. Berg H, Roed J, Viby-Mogensen J, *et al.* Residual neuromuscular block is a risk factor for postoperative pulmonary complications. A prospective, randomised, and blinded study of postoperative pulmonary complications after atracurium, vecuronium and pancuronium. *Acta Anaesthesiol Scand* 1997; **41**: 1095–103.

65. Eriksson LI. The effects of residual neuromuscular blockade and volatile anesthetics on the control of ventilation. *Anesth Analg* 1999; **89**: 243–51.

66. Eriksson LI. Reduced hypoxic chemosensitivity in partially paralysed man. A new property of muscle relaxants? *Acta Anaesthesiol Scand* 1996; **40**: 520–3.

67. Eriksson LI, Sato M, Severinghaus JW. Effect of a vecuronium-induced partial neuromuscular block on hypoxic ventilatory response. *Anesthesiology* 1993; **78**: 693–9.

68. Sundman E, Witt H, Olsson R, *et al.* The incidence and mechanisms of pharyngeal and upper esophageal dysfunction in partially paralyzed humans: pharyngeal videoradiography and simultaneous manometry after atracurium. *Anesthesiology* 2000; **92**: 977–84.

69. Berg H. Is residual neuromuscular block following pancuronium a risk factor for postoperative pulmonary complications? *Acta Anaesthesiol Scand Suppl* 1997; **110**: 156–8.

70. Baillard C, Clec'h C, Catineau J, *et al.* Postoperative residual neuromuscular block: a survey of management. *Br J Anaesth* 2005; **95**: 622–6.

71. Ryan DW. Preoperative serum cholinesterase concentration in chronic renal failure. Clinical experience of suxamethonium in 81 patients undergoing renal transplant. *Br J Anaesth* 1977; **49**: 945–9.

72. Cook DR, Freeman JA, Lai AA, *et al.* Pharmacokinetics of mivacurium in normal patients and in those with hepatic or renal failure. *Br J Anaesth* 1992; **69**: 580–5.

73. Martyn JAJ, Chang Y, Goudsouzian NG, Patel SS. Pharmacodynamics of mivacurium chloride in 13- to 18-yr-old adolescents with thermal injury. *Br J Anaesth* 2002; **89**: 580–5.

74. Martyn JA, Richtsfeld M. Succinylcholine-induced hyperkalemia in acquired pathologic states: etiologic factors and molecular mechanisms. *Anesthesiology* 2006; **104**: 158–69.

75. John DA, Tobey RE, Homer LD, Rice CL. Onset of succinylcholine-induced hyperkalemia following denervation. *Anesthesiology* 1976; **45**: 294–9.

76. McArdle JJ. Molecular aspects of the trophic influence of nerve on muscle. *Prog Neurobiol* 1983; **21**: 135–98.

77. Fergusson RJ, Wright DJ, Willey RF, Crompton GK, Grant IW. Suxamethonium is dangerous in polyneuropathy. *Br Med J* 1981; **282**: 298–9.

78. Hogue CW, Itani MS, Martyn JA. Resistance to d-tubocurarine in lower motor neuron injury is related to increased acetylcholine receptors at the neuromuscular junction. *Anesthesiology* 1990; **73**: 703–9.

79. Cooperman LH. Succinylcholine-induced hyperkalemia in neuromuscular disease. *Jama* 1970; **213**: 1867–71.

80. Frankville DD, Drummond JC. Hyperkalemia after succinylcholine administration in a patient with closed head injury without paresis. *Anesthesiology* 1987; **67**: 264–6.

81. Brett RS, Schmidt JH, Gage JS, Schartel SA, Poppers PJ. Measurement of acetylcholine receptor concentration in skeletal muscle from a patient with multiple sclerosis and resistance to atracurium. *Anesthesiology* 1987; **66**: 837–9.

82. Tobey RE. Paraplegia, succinylcholine and cardiac arrest. *Anesthesiology* 1970; **32**: 359–64.

83. Ibebunjo C, Martyn JA. Fiber atrophy, but not changes in acetylcholine receptor expression, contributes to the muscle dysfunction after immobilization. *Crit Care Med* 1999; **27**: 275–85.

84. Ibebunjo C, Nosek MT, Itani MS, Martyn JA. Mechanisms for the paradoxical resistance to d-tubocurarine during immobilization-induced muscle atrophy. *J Pharmacol Exp Ther* 1997; **283**: 443–51.

85. Yanez P, Martyn JAJ. Prolonged d-tubocurarine infusion and/or immobilization cause upregulation of acetylcholine receptors and hyperkalemia to succinylcholine in rats. *Anesthesiology* 1996; **84**: 384–91.

86. Ibebunjo C, Martyn JAJ. Disparate dysfunction of skeletal muscles located near and distant from burn site in the rat. *Muscle Nerve* 2001; **24**: 1283–94.

87. Viby Mogensen J, Hanel HK, Hansen E, Graae J. Serum cholinesterase activity in burned patients. II: anaesthesia, suxamethonium and hyperkalaemia. *Acta Anaesthesiol Scand* 1975; **19**: 169–79.

88. Kim C, Hirose M, Martyn JA. d-Tubocurarine accentuates the burn-induced upregulation of nicotinic acetylcholine receptors at the muscle membrane. *Anesthesiology* 1995; **83**: 309–15.

89. Khan TZ, Khan RM. Changes in serum potassium following succinylcholine in patients with infections. *Anesth Analg* 1983; **62**: 327–31.

90. Kohlschütter B, Baur H, Roth F. Suxamethonium-induced hyperkalaemia in patients with severe intra-abdominal infections. *Br J Anaesth* 1976; **48**: 557–62.

91. Fink H, Luppa P, Mayer B, et al. Systemic inflammation leads to resistance to atracurium without increasing membrane expression of acetylcholine receptors. *Anesthesiology* 2003; **98**: 82–8.

92. Fink H, Helming M, Unterbuchner C, et al. Systemic inflammatory response syndrome increases immobility-induced neuromuscular weakness. *Crit Care Med* 2008; **36**: 910–16.

93. Hoch W, McConville J, Helms S, et al. Auto-antibodies to the receptor tyrosine kinase MuSK in patients with myasthenia gravis without acetylcholine receptor antibodies. *Nat Med* 2001; **7**: 365–8.

94. Grob D, Arsura EL, Brunner NG, Namba T. The course of myasthenia gravis and therapies affecting outcome. *Ann N Y Acad Sci* 1987; **505**: 472–99.

95. Mann R, Blobner M, Jelen-Esselborn S, Busley R, Werner C. Preanesthetic train-of-four fade predicts the atracurium requirement of myasthenia gravis patients. *Anesthesiology* 2000; **93**: 346–50.

96. Baraka A. Suxamethonium block in the myasthenic patient. Correlation with plasma cholinesterase. *Anaesthesia* 1992; **47**: 217–19.

97. Pascuzzi RM. Myasthenia gravis and Lambert-Eaton syndrome. *Ther Apher* 2002; **6**: 57–68.

98. Boonyapisit K, Kaminski HJ, Ruff RL. Disorders of neuromuscular junction ion channels. *Am J Med* 1999; **106**: 97–113.

99. Engel AG. Myasthenia gravis and myasthenic syndromes. *Ann Neurol* 1984; **16**: 519–34.

100. McCarthy G, Mirakhur RK, Elliott P, Wright J. Effect of H2-receptor antagonist pretreatment on vecuronium- and atracurium-induced neuromuscular block. *Br J Anaesth* 1991; **66**: 713–15.

101. Soriano SG, Martyn JAJ. Antiepileptic-induced resistance to neuromuscular blockers: mechanisms and clinical significance. *Clin Pharmacokinet* 2004; **43**: 71–81.

102. Kim CS, Arnold FJ, Itani MS, Martyn JA. Decreased sensitivity to metocurine during long-term phenytoin therapy may be attributable to protein binding and acetylcholine receptor changes. *Anesthesiology* 1992; **77**: 500–6.

103. Soriano SG, Kaus SJ, Sullivan LJ, Martyn JA. Onset and duration of action of rocuronium in children receiving chronic anticonvulsant therapy. *Paediatr Anaesth* 2000; **10**: 133–6.

104. Soriano SG, Sullivan LJ, Venkatakrishnan K, Greenblatt DJ, Martyn JA. Pharmacokinetics and pharmacodynamics of vecuronium in children receiving phenytoin or carbamazepine for chronic anticonvulsant therapy. *Br J Anaesth* 2001; **86**: 223–9.

105. Fuchs-Buder T, Wilder Smith OH, Borgeat A, Tassonyi E. Interaction of magnesium sulphate with vecuronium-induced neuromuscular block. *Br J Anaesth* 1995; **74**: 405–9.

106. Ghoneim MM, Long JP. The interaction between magnesium and other neuromuscular blocking agents. *Anesthesiology* 1970; **32**: 23–7.

107. Fiekers JF. Sites and mechanisms of antibiotic-induced neuromuscular block: a pharmacological analysis using quantal content, voltage clamped end-plate currents and single channel analysis. *Acta Physiol Pharmacol Ther Latinoam* 1999; **49**: 242–50.

108. Scheller M, Bufler J, Schneck H, Kochs E, Franke C. Isoflurane and sevoflurane interact with the nicotinic acetylcholine receptor channels in micromolar concentrations. *Anesthesiology* 1997; **86**: 118–27.

109. Liu M, Kato M, Hashimoto Y. Neuromuscular blocking effects of the aminoglycoside antibiotics arbekacin, astromicin, isepamicin and netilmicin on the diaphragm and limb muscles in the rabbit. *Pharmacology* 2001; **63**: 142–6.

110. Shorten GD, Crawford MW, St. Louis P. The neuromuscular effects of mivacurium chloride during propofol anesthesia in children. *Anesth Analg* 1996; **82**: 1170–5.

111. Fryer JD, Lukas RJ. Antidepressants noncompetitively inhibit nicotinic acetylcholine receptor function. *J Neurochem* 1999; **72**: 1117–24.

112. Scheller M, Bufler J, Hertle I, et al. Ketamine blocks currents through mammalian nicotinic acetylcholine receptor channels by interaction with both the open and the closed state. *Anesth Analg* 1996; **83**: 830–6.

113. Hertle I, Scheller M, Bufler J, et al. Interaction of midazolam with the nicotinic acetylcholine receptor of mouse myotubes. *Anesth Analg* 1997; **85**: 174–81.

114. Krampfl K, Schlesinger F, Dengler R, et al. Pentobarbital has curare-like effects on adult-type nicotinic acetylcholine receptor channel currents. *Anesth Analg* 2000; **90**: 970–4.

115. Driessen JJ, Wuis EW, Gielen MJ. Prolonged vecuronium neuromuscular blockade in a patient receiving orally administered dantrolene. *Anesthesiology* 1985; **62**: 523–4.

116. Ali HH, Savarese JJ, Embree PB, et al. Clinical pharmacology of mivacurium chloride (BW B1090U) infusion: comparison with vecuronium and atracurium. *Br J Anaesth* 1988; **61**: 541–6.

117. Brandom BW, Woelfel SK, Ryan Cook D, et al. Comparison of mivacurium and suxamethonium administered by bolus and infusion. *Br J Anaesth* 1989; **62**: 488–93.

118. McLoughlin C, Nesbitt GA, Howe JP. Suxamethonium induced myalgia and the effect of pre-operative administration of oral aspirin. A comparison with a standard treatment and an untreated group. *Anaesthesia* 1988; **43**: 565–7.

119. Meyers EF, Krupin T, Johnson M, Zink H. Failure of nondepolarizing neuromuscular blockers to inhibit succinylcholine-induced increased intraocular pressure, a controlled study. *Anesthesiology* 1978; **48**: 149–51.

120. Engbaek J, Viby Mogensen J. Precurarization: a hazard to the patient? *Acta Anaesthesiol Scand* 1984; **28**: 61–2.

121. Walts LF, Dillon JB. Clinical studies of the interaction between d-tubocurarine and succinylcholine. *Anesthesiology* 1969; **31**: 39–44.

122. Erkola O, Salmenpera A, Kuoppamaki R. Five non-depolarizing muscle relaxants in precurarization. *Acta Anaesthesiol Scand* 1983; **27**: 427–32.

123. Perry JJ, Lee JS, Sillberg VA, Wells GA. Rocuronium versus succinylcholine for rapid sequence induction intubation. *Cochrane Database Syst Rev* 2008; (2): CD002788.

124. Puhringer FK, Rex C, Sielenkamper AW, *et al.* Reversal of profound, high-dose rocuronium-induced neuromuscular blockade by sugammadex at two different time points: an international, multicenter, randomized, dose-finding, safety assessor-blinded, phase II trial. *Anesthesiology* 2008; **109**: 188–97.

125. Jones RK, Caldwell JE, Brull SJ, Soto RG. Reversal of profound rocuronium-induced blockade with sugammadex: a randomized comparison with neostigmine. *Anesthesiology* 2008; **109**: 816–24.

126. Yasukawa T, Kaneki M, Yasuhara S, Lee SL, Martyn JA. Steroidal nondepolarizing muscle relaxants do not simulate the effects of glucocorticoids on glucocorticoid receptor-mediated transcription in cultured skeletal muscle cells. *Anesthesiology* 2004; **100**: 1615–19.

127. DuBois DC, Almon RR. A possible role of steroids in denervation atrophy. *Muscle Nerve* 1981; **4**: 370–3.

128. Murray MJ, Cowen J, DeBlock H, *et al.* Clinical practice guidelines for sustained neuromuscular blockade in the adult critically ill patient. *Crit Care Med* 2002; **30**: 142–56.

Mohamed Naguib

Introduction

In 1942, Harold Griffith and Enid Johnson were given the opportunity of being the first to use curare (Intocostrin), the first nondepolarizing neuromuscular blocker, on some 25 patients [1]. It is important to note that Arthur Läwen, a German surgeon from Leipzig, made isolated attempts to use curare in 1912 [2].

A few years later, Dr. R. E. Pleasance, in his presidential address to the Society of Sheffield Anaesthetists on January 15, 1948, described his clinical experience using curare [3]. He stated, "one sign of ... adequate curarization is [tracheal tug] ... Under a dose of curare producing marked curarizing effects, a tracheal tug develops. As the effects of the curare wear off, this tug disappears, indicating the need for further injection of curare." Dr. Pleasance never mentioned the need for antagonizing the residual effects of curare in his patients. In fact, he stated that, during recovery, "there is no evidence that curare has any latent toxicity. It is completely and fairly rapidly eliminated." It should be noted, however, that when curarization was initially introduced, tracheal intubation was the exception to routine practice and most patients undergoing anesthesia were breathing spontaneously.

It is interesting to note that the Intocostrin package insert in 1943 stated, "When dangerous respiratory embarrassment occurs, resuscitation by ... artificial respiration may be expected to carry the patient through the paralysis. Particularly one should be certain that an airway exists. Prostigmin [neostigmine] is also a physiologic antidote; the respiratory paralysis if not too profound is removed by this drug." Nevertheless, no dosage for neostigmine was suggested at that time. It was not until 1948 that intravenous administration of neostigmine 1 mL of a 1 : 2000 dilution (0.5 mg) to treat moderate curare overdosage was suggested by E. R. Squibb & Sons. At that time, the use of neostigmine to antagonize the effects of curare on neuromuscular function was gaining momentum. In the same year, Burke and colleagues stated, in one of the early papers on the use of neostigmine for antagonism of D-tubocurarine, that "the use of neostigmine will shorten the period for the necessity of artificial respiration, but its administration should be considered as an adjuvant to treatment rather than as a substitute" [4]. The recommendation for neostigmine dosages came from Prescott and colleagues in 1946 [5]. They stated, "If prostigmin is to be effective, doses of the order of 5 mg or more must be used. Atropine 1.3 mg should also be given, to balance the parasympathomimetic action of prostigmin."

Neuromuscular junction architecture

The integrity of neuromuscular transmission is dependent on a highly orchestrated mechanism involving (1) synthesis, storage, and release of acetylcholine (ACh) from motor nerve endings (presynaptic region) at the neuromuscular junction (NMJ), (2) binding of acetylcholine to nicotinic receptors on the muscle membrane (postsynaptic region) and generation of action potentials, and (3) rapid hydrolysis of acetylcholine by the enzyme acetylcholinesterase (AChE), which is present in the synaptic cleft [6]. Many conditions, such as autoimmune or genetic defects at the presynaptic region, synaptic basal lamina, or postsynaptic structure of the neuromuscular junction, can compromise the safety margin of neuromuscular transmission and result in a diverse array of myasthenic disorders [6].

Acetylcholinesterase at the neuromuscular junction

At the neuromuscular junction, acetylcholinesterase is a type B carboxylesterase enzyme responsible for rapid hydrolysis of released acetylcholine, thereby controlling the duration of receptor activation [7]. Approximately 50% of the released acetylcholine is hydrolyzed during its diffusion across the synaptic cleft, before reaching nicotinic acetylcholine receptors (nAChR). The efficiency of acetylcholinesterase depends on its fast catalytic activity. Acetylcholinesterase has one of the highest catalytic efficiencies known. It can catalyze acetylcholine hydrolysis at a rate of 4000 molecules of acetylcholine hydrolyzed per active site per second, which is nearly the rate

Anesthetic Pharmacology, 2nd edition, ed. Alex S. Evers, Mervyn Maze, Evan D. Kharasch. Published by Cambridge University Press. © Cambridge University Press 2011.

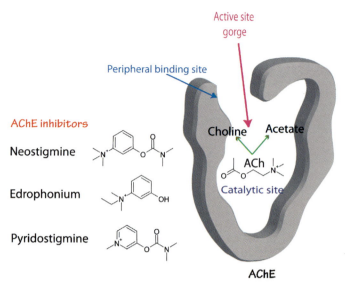

Figure 39.1. The enzyme acetylcholinesterase (AChE). The active catalytic site (lined with hydrophobic amino acid side chains) lies near the bottom of a deep and narrow cleft (gorge). Acetylcholine (ACh) must enter this cleft in the enzyme, which is blocked by a mobile ring of molecules more than 97% of the time. The entrance to the cleft opens and shuts so frequently that any ACh molecules lingering nearby have ample chances to diffuse in [9]. AChE promotes hydrolysis of ACh by forming an acetyl-AChE intermediate with the release of choline and then hydrolysis of the intermediate to release acetate. This reaction is antagonized by AChE inhibitors such as neostigmine, edrophonium, and pyridostigmine, thereby increasing the concentration of ACh.

of diffusion [7]. The active site of acetylcholinesterase lies near the bottom of a deep and narrow cleft that reaches halfway into the protein (Fig. 39.1) [8]. Acetylcholine must enter this cleft in the enzyme, which is blocked by a mobile ring of molecules more than 97% of the time. Molecular dynamics simulations showed that the entrance to the cleft opens and shuts so frequently that any acetylcholine molecules lingering nearby have ample chances to diffuse in [9]. These simulations also showed that the motions of the channel extend from the region outside the acetylcholinesterase enzyme to the active site. These fluctuations in the width of the channel are required to allow acetylcholine to move from outside into the active site. They also contribute to the selectivity of the enzyme by slowing the entrance of substrates that are larger than acetylcholine [9].

Acetylcholinesterase is highly concentrated at the neuromuscular junction but is present in a lower concentration throughout the length of muscle fibers [10]. In mammals, acetylcholinesterase is encoded by a single gene. It has been localized to chromosome 7q22 in humans [11]. Much of the acetylcholinesterase at the neuromuscular junction occurs in the asymmetric or A_{12} form, consisting of three tetramers of catalytic subunits covalently linked to a collagen-like tail. Asymmetric acetylcholinesterase is bound to the junctional basal lamina [12]. The distribution of acetylcholinesterase molecules on the synaptic basal lamina closely matches the distribution of nicotinic acetylcholine receptors [13].

Mechanisms of action of acetylcholinesterase inhibitors

Recovery from muscle relaxation induced by nondepolarizing neuromuscular blockers ultimately depends on elimination of the neuromuscular blocker from the body. Acetylcholinesterase inhibitors (e.g., neostigmine, edrophonium, and, less commonly, pyridostigmine) are used clinically to antagonize the residual effects of neuromuscular blockers and to accelerate recovery from nondepolarizing neuromuscular blockade. The acetylcholine that accumulates at the neuromuscular junction after administration of neostigmine competes with the residual molecules of the neuromuscular blocking drug for the available unoccupied nicotinic acetylcholine receptors at the neuromuscular junction. The clinical implication is that neostigmine has a ceiling effect on acetylcholinesterase. Once the inhibition of acetylcholinesterase is complete, administering additional doses of neostigmine will serve no useful purpose because the concentration of acetylcholine that can be produced at the neuromuscular junction is finite. If neostigmine is administered at a deep level of neuromuscular blockade (i.e., no response to train-of-four [TOF] stimulation), furthermore, the concentration of neuromuscular molecules will be high at the neuromuscular junction, and administration of neostigmine at this time might not be effective in antagonizing neuromuscular blockade. Indeed, administering more neostigmine at this point may in fact worsen neuromuscular recovery [14]. This points to the limitations posed by the use of neostigmine (or any other acetylcholinesterase inhibitor) in clinical practice and explains, in part, the high incidence of postoperative residual neuromuscular blockade [15].

It should be noted that the pharmacologic actions of neostigmine and edrophonium are not limited to enzyme inhibition [16,17]. Evidence suggests that the direct influences of the acetylcholinesterase inhibitors on neuromuscular transmission independent of enzyme inhibition involve at least three distinct although possibly interacting mechanisms: (1) weak agonistic action, (2) formation of desensitized receptor-complex intermediates, and (3) alteration of the conductance properties of active channels.

Clinical pharmacology of acetylcholinesterase inhibitors

Antagonism of nondepolarizing neuromuscular blockade by acetylcholinesterase inhibitors depends primarily on five factors: (1) the depth of the blockade when reversal is attempted, (2) the anticholinesterase used, (3) the dose administered, (4) the rate of spontaneous clearance of the neuromuscular blocker from plasma, and (5) the choice of anesthetic drugs and the depth of anesthesia.

Depth of neuromuscular blockade

As a general rule, it is recommended that antagonism of residual neuromuscular blockade should be attempted when there is evidence of spontaneous recovery (preferably a train-of-four [TOF] count corresponding to T1 > 25%) as detected by a conventional nerve stimulator (which requires the clinician to evaluate the evoked response visually or tactilely). Antagonism of a shallow degree of blockade is associated with faster recovery of neuromuscular function than is antagonism of deep blockade. There is, however, evidence that deep levels of neuromuscular blockade (TOF count of 0 or 1) could be antagonized by acetylcholinesterase inhibitors [18,19]. Antagonism of $1.5 \times ED_{95}$ doses of vecuronium- or rocuronium-induced neuromuscular blockade occurred at the same rate regardless of the timing of administration of $70\,\mu g\,kg^{-1}$ of neostigmine [19]. Neostigmine shortened the recovery time by approximately 40% whether it was administered at the time of 1%, 10%, or 25% of spontaneous recovery [19]. When reversing deeper levels of neuromuscular blockade, conventional monitoring of neuromuscular recovery becomes much less reliable. It should be noted, however, that both of those studies [18,19] were performed with strict protocols and the use of a quantitative neuromuscular function monitor that displays the TOF ratio (the ratio of the fourth to the first twitch height) in real time. Thus, patient safety was never compromised. In the presence of profound blockade (99% vs. 90% blockade), the dose response of reversal drugs is shifted to the right, necessitating that higher doses are required (Fig. 39.2) [20]. The magnitude of this shift is greater with either edrophonium or pyridostigmine than it is with neostigmine [20].

Anticholinesterase drugs

Edrophonium has a more rapid onset than neostigmine or pyridostigmine when used to reverse residual neuromuscular blockade [21,22]. Edrophonium $(0.5-1\,mg\,kg^{-1})$ was as effective as neostigmine $(40\,\mu g\,kg^{-1})$ in reversing moderate neuromuscular blockade (less than 90% twitch depression, corresponding to a TOF count of 1) from pancuronium, atracurium, and vecuronium [23]. Edrophonium $(1\,mg\,kg^{-1}$ but definitely not $0.5\,mg\,kg^{-1})$ was as effective as neostigmine in antagonizing deep blockade (more than 90% twitch depression) from pancuronium, atracurium, and vecuronium, but was not as effective in reversing profound (99% twitch depression) atracurium blockade (Fig. 39.2) [20,23]. Edrophonium $(1\,mg\,kg^{-1})$ was less effective than $50\,\mu g\,kg^{-1}$ of neostigmine at reversing rocuronium-induced TOF fade (Fig. 39.3A) [24]. However, this difference was not seen with cisatracurium (Fig. 39.3B), atracurium [25], or mivacurium (Fig. 39.3C) [26]. Dose–response curves for edrophonium and neostigmine are not parallel, meaning that potency ratios may differ, and may differ for single-twitch versus TOF responses, may change over time (i.e. 5 minutes vs. 10 minutes after administration)

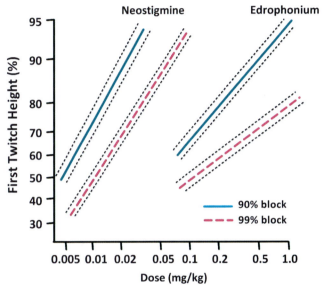

Figure 39.2. Reversal of atracurium blockade. First twitch height versus dose was measured 10 minutes after administration of neostigmine and edrophonium given at either 1% (99% block) or 10% (90% block) first twitch recovery from atracurium. Thin dashed lines represent the standard error of estimate for the mean. Reproduced with permission from Donati et al. [20].

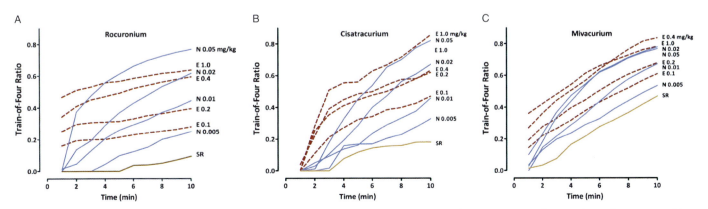

Figure 39.3. Mean train-of-four (TOF) ratio (the ratio of the fourth to the first twitch height) versus time after administration of various doses of neostigmine (N) or edrophonium (E). Antagonism of neuromuscular blockade was attempted when first twitch height had reached 10% of its control value. The neuromuscular blockers used were (A) rocuronium [24], (B) cisatracurium [25], and (C) mivacurium [26]. SR, spontaneous recovery. Reproduced with permission from Naguib et al. [24].

and may depend on the relaxant antagonized [24]. For example, 10 minutes after reversal from a rocuronium-induced blockade (at T1 = 10%), neostigmine was 27.7 times as potent as edrophonium for achieving the ED_{50} of the TOF [24]. Corresponding potency ratios for atracurium, cisatracurium, and mivacurium were 13, 11.8, and 10.4, respectively [25,26]. In general, neostigmine is recommended for reversal of more intense block.

Mixing antagonists is not advisable. Neostigmine and edrophonium do not potentiate each other; in fact, their effects in combination may not even be additive. [27]. Therefore, when inadequate reversal occurs, one should not administer a different anticholinesterase but should ensure that ventilation is supported until adequate neuromuscular function is achieved.

Anticholinesterase dose

Several studies have demonstrated that $40\,\mu g\,kg^{-1}$ of neostigmine (administered at T1 of 5–10% recovery) sufficiently antagonizes residual neuromuscular blockade, and there is no further advantage in using higher doses (e.g., $80\,\mu g\,kg^{-1}$) of neostigmine [28,29] or administering a second dose of neostigmine [18]. It is recommended that the maximal dose of neostigmine should be $70\,\mu g\,kg^{-1}$. The maximum effective dose for edrophonium appears to be $1.0\,mg\,kg^{-1}$ [23,30]. Antagonism of residual neuromuscular blockade induced by the various nondepolarizing neuromuscular blockers is similar in children and adults [31]. When neostigmine is administered to antagonize a stable level of blockade maintained by continuous infusion of vecuronium, cisatracurium, rocuronium, or mivacurium, the rate and degree of recovery are not different from those following bolus administration of each neuromuscular blocker alone [32–34].

Rate of spontaneous clearance of the neuromuscular blocker

The plasma concentrations of drugs with a short duration of action (mivacurium) decrease more rapidly than those with an intermediate (cisatracurium and rocuronium) or long duration of action (pancuronium and D-tubocurarine), and consequently the recovery of neuromuscular function is more rapid (Fig. 39.4). Following administration of an anticholinesterase, two processes contribute to recovery of neuromuscular function. The first is the antagonism induced by the effect of the anticholinesterase at the neuromuscular junction, and the second is the decrease in plasma concentration of the neuromuscular blocker due to redistribution and elimination [35,36]. Therefore, the more rapid the elimination of the neuromuscular blocker, the faster will be the recovery of adequate neuromuscular function after administration of an antagonist (Fig. 39.4). The ease and rapidity of antagonism of short- and intermediate-acting neuromuscular blockers (atracurium, vecuronium) explain the lower incidence of inadequate neuromuscular function in the postoperative period as compared with long-acting neuromuscular blockers (pancuronium)

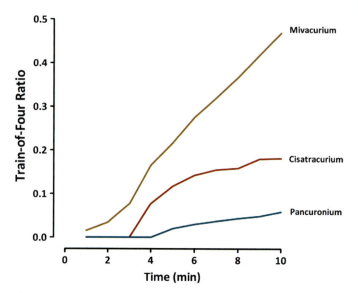

Figure 39.4. Comparative mean spontaneous recovery from neuromuscular blockade with pancuronium, cisatracurium, and mivacurium following the return to 10% first twitch height.

[37,38]. It has been erroneously suggested that routine administration of an anticholinesterase may often be omitted because spontaneous recovery from mivacurium effects is so rapid. However, this strategy may lead to inadequate recovery and postoperative weakness unless neuromuscular function is monitored quantitatively to ensure that the TOF ratio has recovered to > 0.9.

Choice of anesthetic drugs and depth of anesthesia

Volatile anesthetics potentiate the neuromuscular blocking effect of nondepolarizing neuromuscular blockers [39]. The magnitude of this potentiation depends on several factors, including the duration of anesthesia [40–42], the specific volatile anesthetic used [43], and the concentration used [44]. The rank order of potentiation is desflurane > sevoflurane > isoflurane > halothane > nitrous oxide–opioid or propofol anesthesia. Therefore, the efficacy of acetylcholinesterase inhibitors is decreased in the presence of anesthetizing concentrations of inhaled anesthetics [45,46]. For example, rocuronium reversal by neostigmine is faster under propofol than it is under sevoflurane anesthesia [46]. Reversal under isoflurane anesthesia is faster than it is under desflurane or sevoflurane [47]. Withdrawal of the volatile anesthetic at the end of surgery will speed pharmacologic reversal [48].

Other drug interactions can also prolong neuromuscular blockade. The effect of succinylcholine ($1\,mg\,kg^{-1}$) was prolonged from 11 to 35 minutes when it was given 5 minutes after administration of neostigmine (5 mg) [49]. This can be explained partly by the inhibition of butyrylcholinesterase by neostigmine. (Butyrylcholinesterase is also inhibited, to a lesser extent, by pyridostigmine.) Ninety minutes after neostigmine administration, butyrylcholinesterase activity returns to less

Table 39.1. Pharmacokinetics of neostigmine, pyridostigmine, and edrophonium in patients without and with renal failure

Cholinesterase inhibitor	Plasma clearance (mL kg^{-1} min^{-1})		Volume of distribution (mL kg^{-1})		Elimination half-life (min)	
	Normal	Kidney failure	Normal	Kidney failure	Normal	Kidney failure
Neostigmine	9.1	4.8–7.8	700	1600	77	181
Pyridostigmine	8.6	2.1–3.1	1100	1200	113	379
Edrophonium	9.5	3.9	1100	1100	110	304

Data from Cronnelly et al. [50,51] and Morris et al. [52,53].

than 50% of its baseline value. Drugs that potentiate the effects of neuromuscular blockers (e.g., aminoglycoside and tetracycline antibiotics, magnesium and calcium, local anesthetics, and antiarrhythmic drugs) would limit the efficacy of acetylcholinesterase inhibitors.

Pharmacokinetics of acetylcholinesterase inhibitors

Several factors determine the pharmacokinetics of the acetylcholinesterase inhibitors, including distribution, metabolism, and elimination (Table 39.1) [50–53]. The elimination half-life of edrophonium is similar to those of neostigmine and pyridostigmine [52] although that of pyridostigmine is somewhat longer, which likely accounts for its longer duration of effect [50,51]. Renal excretion accounts for about 50% of the elimination of neostigmine and about 75% of that of pyridostigmine and edrophonium. Renal failure decreases the plasma clearance of neostigmine, pyridostigmine, and edrophonium as much as if not more than that of the long-acting neuromuscular blockers.

Side effects of acetylcholinesterase inhibitors

Inhibition of acetylcholinesterase not only increases the concentration of acetylcholine at the neuromuscular junction (nicotinic site) but also at all other synapses that use acetylcholine as a transmitter. Despite its adverse side effects, however, neostigmine is still the anticholinesterase drug most widely used by anesthesiologists worldwide [54].

Cardiovascular side effects

Only the nicotinic effects of acetylcholinesterase inhibitors are desired. Therefore the muscarinic effects must be blocked by atropine or glycopyrrolate [55]. To minimize the muscarinic cardiovascular side effects of acetylcholinesterase inhibitors, an anticholinergic drug should be coadministered with the acetylcholinesterase inhibitor. Atropine (7–10 µg kg^{-1}) matches the onset of action and pharmacodynamic profile of the rapid-acting edrophonium (0.5–1.0 mg kg^{-1}) [55], and glycopyrrolate (7–15 µg kg^{-1}) matches the slower-acting neostigmine (40–70 µg kg^{-1}) and pyridostigmine [21,56]. In patients with pre-existing cardiac disease, glycopyrrolate may be preferable to atropine [57], and the acetylcholinesterase inhibitor and anticholinergic should be administered slowly (e.g., over 2–5 minutes).

Pulmonary and alimentary side effects

Administration of acetylcholinesterase inhibitors is associated with bronchoconstriction, increased airway resistance, increased salivation, and increased bowel motility (muscarinic effects). Anticholinergic drugs tend to reduce these effects. Findings on whether neostigmine increases the incidence of postoperative nausea and vomiting are discrepant [58]: neostigmine has been described both as having antiemetic properties [59] and as having no effect on the incidence of postoperative nausea and vomiting [60].

Monitoring of neuromuscular function

Monitoring of neuromuscular function after administration of a neuromuscular blocking drug serves at least two purposes in clinical settings. First, it allows the anesthesiologist to administer these drugs with appropriate dosing. For instance, patient movement during ophthalmologic surgery accounted for blindness in approximately 30% of patients with eye injuries [61]. No neuromuscular function monitoring was used in the patients with eye injuries who received neuromuscular blockers [61]. Second, neuromuscular monitoring ensures that the patient recovers adequately from residual effects of the neuromuscular blocker, thus guaranteeing patient safety.

In the operating room, the depth of neuromuscular blockade is typically monitored by observing the response to stimulation of any superficial neuromuscular unit. Most commonly, contraction of the adductor pollicis muscle associated with stimulation of the ulnar nerve, at either the wrist or the elbow, is monitored. In certain circumstances, the peroneal nerve or the facial nerve may be monitored. Although the centrally located muscles (such as the diaphragm and larynx) are more resistant to the effects of nondepolarizing neuromuscular blockers than are the more peripherally located muscles (such as adductor pollicis), and the EC$_{50}$ of different neuromuscular blocking drugs is 50–100% higher at the diaphragm or larynx than it is at the adductor pollicis, the neuromuscular blockade develops faster, lasts less time, and recovers more quickly in the larynx and the diaphragm than in the adductor pollicis (Fig. 39.5) [62–66]. This apparent contradiction could

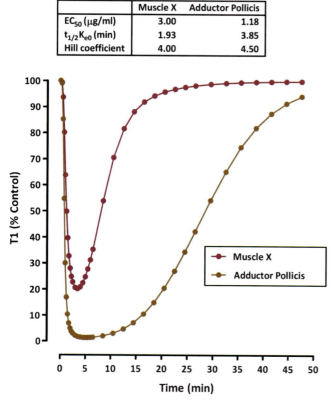

	Muscle X	Adductor Pollicis
EC_{50} (µg/ml)	3.00	1.18
$t_{1/2}K_{e0}$ (min)	1.93	3.85
Hill coefficient	4.00	4.50

Figure 39.5. Anatomical differences in neuromuscular blockade. Shown are the results from a computer simulation based on Sheiner's model [68] and data reported by Wierda *et al.* [69]. The ED_{95} of rocuronium at the adductor pollicis from this model is 0.33 mg kg^{-1}. Rocuronium 0.45 mg kg^{-1} is given as a bolus at time zero. Muscle *X* represents a muscle (such as the diaphragm or the laryngeal adductors) that is less sensitive to the effects of nondepolarizing relaxants than the adductor pollicis but has greater blood flow. In this example, the concentration of rocuronium producing 50% block (EC_{50}) of muscle *X* is 2.5 times that of the adductor pollicis, but the half-life of transport between the plasma and the effect compartment ($t_{1/2}k_{e0}$) of muscle *X* is only half as long. The rapid equilibration between plasma concentrations of rocuronium and muscle *X* results in the more rapid onset of blockade of the muscle *X* than that of the adductor pollicis. The greater EC_{50} at muscle *X* explains why this muscle recovers more quickly from neuromuscular blockade than the adductor pollicis. Lower blood concentrations of rocuronium must be achieved at the adductor pollicis than at muscle *X* before recovery begins. Reproduced with permission from Naguib and Kopman [70].

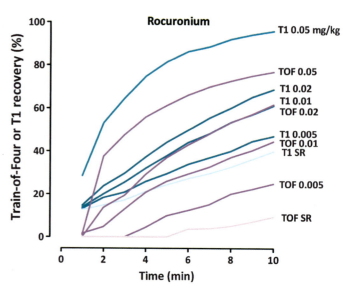

Figure 39.6. Train-of-four ratio (TOF) and first-twitch (T1) monitoring of neuromuscular blockade. Shown are mean TOF and TI versus time after administration of various doses of neostigmine. Antagonism of rocuronium-induced neuromuscular blockade was attempted when T1 height had reached 10% of its control value. SR, spontaneous recovery.

be explained by the high blood flow (greater blood flow per gram of muscle) that exists at the diaphragm and larynx, which results in rapid equilibration (i.e., shorter $t_{1/2}k_{e0}$) between plasma and the effect compartment at these central muscles [67]. The clinical implication of this is that complete recovery in the adductor pollicis implies complete recovery in the diaphragm, larynx, and other centrally located muscles.

Clinical bedside criteria for tracheal extubation (such as a 5-second head lift or the ability to generate a peak negative inspiratory force of –25 to –30 cm H_2O) are insensitive indicators of the adequacy of neuromuscular recovery [71]. A sustained 5-second head lift did not guarantee adequate reversal, since this could occur at a TOF ratio of < 0.60 [72]. It is recommended that objective monitoring (e.g., digital display of the TOF ratio in real time) be used in the clinical setting. Onset of neuromuscular blockade should be monitored with either single-twitch stimuli (T1) or TOF stimuli. Single-twitch stimulation is not a sensitive indicator of recovery, however, and does not provide any information regarding the degree of fade present (Fig. 39.6). It is important to know that the twitch response is not reduced until ~80% of the nicotinic acetylcholine receptors at the neuromuscular junction are blocked [73], and that this represents a margin of safety [74]. The response disappears completely when ≥ 90% of the receptors are blocked [73]. Greater sensitivity could be achieved with TOF stimulation; therefore, depth of the blockade during maintenance and recovery should be monitored with TOF stimulation.

Subjective (visual or tactile) evaluation of the evoked muscular response to TOF and tetanic stimulation are extremely inaccurate as estimates of fade or postoperative residual neuromuscular blockade [75,76]. Once the TOF ratio exceeds 0.40, detection of TOF fade is humanly impossible [75]. Following administration of a nondepolarizing neuromuscular blocking drug, it is essential to ensure adequate return of normal neuromuscular function to a TOF ratio of ≥ 0.9. A TOF ratio of < 0.9 in unanesthetized volunteers has been associated with difficulty in speaking and swallowing and with visual disturbances [72].

A recent meta-analysis did not demonstrate that intraoperative use of a nerve stimulator (conventional or quantitative) was associated with a reduced incidence of postoperative residual neuromuscular blockade [15]. This finding should not be interpreted as indicating that there is no clinical advantage to using an intraoperative neuromuscular function monitor, but rather that the widely cited studies are often poorly designed and inadequately detect any advantages that might be conferred by quantitative monitoring.

Perhaps the most convincing evidence that the use of an objective neuromuscular monitor (combined with a strong educational effort at the departmental level) can decrease the incidence of postoperative residual neuromuscular blockade comes from two studies by Baillard et al. [77,78]. The first was a prospective study of the incidence of postoperative residual neuromuscular blockade following administration of vecuronium in 568 consecutive patients over a 3-month period in 1995. As was customary in the authors' department, no anticholinesterase antagonists were used in this series of patients, and peripheral nerve stimulatory devices were rarely used (< 2%) intraoperatively. Postoperative residual neuromuscular blockade (indicated by an acceleromyographic TOF ratio of < 0.70) was present in 42% of patients in the postanesthesia care unit. Of 435 patients who had been extubated in the operating room, the incidence of postoperative residual neuromuscular blockade was 33% [77]. As a result of these rather alarming findings, the data on postoperative residual neuromuscular blockade were distributed to department staff acceleromyographic monitors placed in all operating rooms a short time later, and the department instituted a program of education about the use of neuromuscular monitoring and the indications for neostigmine administration. Repeat 3-month surveys of clinical practice were conducted in the years 2000 ($n = 130$), 2002 ($n = 101$), and 2004 ($n = 218$) to determine the success of the educational efforts [78]. In the 9-year interval between the initial and the 2004 survey, the use of intraoperative monitoring of neuromuscular function rose from 2% to 60%, and reversal of residual antagonism increased from 6% to 42% of cases. One other notable change was in the choice of relaxant. In 1995, all patients received vecuronium, but this drug was gradually replaced by atracurium, which was used in 99% of cases in 2004. As a result of these changes in clinical practice, the incidence of postoperative residual neuromuscular blockade (acceleromyographic TOF ratio < 0.90) decreased from 62% to < 4% [78].

Although quantitative neuromuscular function monitoring is recommended, many anesthetics are given without such monitoring. Appropriate intraoperative use of a conventional nerve stimulator may decrease (but not eliminate) the incidence of postoperative residual neuromuscular blockade [79]. If neostigmine administration is timed at a TOF count of 4, then clinically significant postoperative residual neuromuscular blockade should be rare. Quantitative monitors (such as mechanomyography, electromyography, or acceleromyography) should be seriously considered in two situations: (1) when no fade on TOF stimulation can be detected manually and the anesthesiologist is deciding not to reverse neuromuscular block, and (2) when the anesthesiologist is attempting to reverse deep nondepolarizing block (TOF count < 3) to ensure recovery of the TOF ratio to > 0.9. It is important to emphasize that even with this degree of recovery, ~80% of nicotinic acetylcholine receptors at the neuromuscular junction are still occupied by the neuromuscular blocker [73].

The problems of residual neuromuscular blockade

As indicated above, postanesthetic morbidity in the form of incomplete reversal and residual postoperative weakness is a frequent occurrence [80–82]. A 45% incidence of postoperative residual neuromuscular blockade in patients arriving in the postanesthesia care unit was reported in 2003 [81]. Patients who arrive with a TOF ratio of < 0.9 will have significant pharyngeal dysfunction that would result in a four- to fivefold increase in the risk of aspiration [83,84] and a decrease in hypoxic ventilatory drive [85].

Moreover, a 2005 survey indicated that most practitioners do not know what constitutes adequate recovery from neuromuscular blockade [86]. Although it can be argued that these problems could be attributed to (1) lack of routine use of peripheral nerve stimulators (and more importantly, the quantitative ones) or (2) the ceiling effect of the reversal drugs when administered at a deep level of neuromuscular blockade [87,88], one study found that despite both the use of nerve stimulators by clinicians with knowledge and expertise and administration of neostigmine, the incidence of critical respiratory events in the postoperative care unit remained a significant 0.8% [82]. However, the incidence of both residual neuromuscular blockade and adverse respiratory events during early recovery from anesthesia can be reduced by intraoperative use of a quantitative monitor (acceleromyography) [86].

Clearly, avoidance of critical respiratory events requires changes in clinical care. One such change could entail development of reversal drugs that act other than by acetylcholinesterase inhibition. Such drugs would interact directly with the neuromuscular blocking drugs and terminate their action at the neuromuscular junction.

Nonclassic reversal drugs

Only a few studies have explored the potential of nonclassic reversal drugs that act independently of acetylcholinesterase inhibition. One such drug, purified human plasma cholinesterase, has been shown to be effective and safe in antagonizing mivacurium-induced neuromuscular blockade [90]. Similarly, cysteine has been shown to reverse the neuromuscular blocking effects of gantacurium [91]. Sugammadex, a novel selective relaxant-binding drug, is able to reverse both shallow and profound aminosteroid-induced neuromuscular blockade, and has a unique mechanism of action (see below) that distinguishes it from cholinesterase inhibitors.

Sugammadex: a novel selective relaxant-binding drug

Chemistry

Sugammadex is a modified γ-cyclodextrin (Fig. 39.7) [92–95]. Cyclodextrins are cyclic dextrose units joined through 1–4 glycosyl bonds that are produced from starch or starch derivatives using cyclodextrin glycosyltransferase. The three natural unmodified cyclodextrins consist of 6-, 7-, and 8-cyclic oligosaccharides. They are called α-, β-, and γ-cyclodextrin, and their molecular weights are 973, 1135, and 1297, respectively. Their three-dimensional structures, which resemble a hollow, truncated cone or a doughnut, have a hydrophobic cavity and a hydrophilic exterior because of the presence of polar hydroxyl groups. Hydrophobic interactions trap the drug into the cyclodextrin cavity (the doughnut hole), resulting in formation of a water-soluble guest–host complex.

Compared with α- and β-cyclodextrins, γ-cyclodextrin exhibits more favorable properties in terms of the size of its internal cavity, water solubility, and bioavailability. This is because the α- and β-cyclodextrins have smaller lipophilic cavities (< 6.5 Å diameters) and form less stable complexes with the bulky aminosteroid neuromuscular blocker molecule (e.g., rocuronium or vecuronium; molecule width ~ 7.5 Å) than does the γ-cyclodextrin molecule, which has a larger lipophilic cavity (7.5–8.3 Å diameter) [92].

To improve the fit of the larger rigid structure of the aminosteroid neuromuscular blocker molecule within the cavity of γ-cyclodextrin, the latter was modified by adding eight side chains to extend the cavity. This modification allowed the four hydrophobic steroidal rings of rocuronium to be better accommodated within the hydrophobic cavity. Addition of negatively charged carboxyl groups at the end of each of the eight side chains served two purposes. First, the repellent forces of the negative charges keep propionic acid side chains from being disordered, thereby allowing the cavity

to remain open. Second, these negatively charged carboxyl groups enhance electrostatic binding to the positively charged quaternary nitrogen of rocuronium (Fig. 39.7) [92,93].

These modifications resulted in a compound (molecular weight of 2178), sugammadex, that is highly water-soluble with a hydrophobic cavity large enough to encapsulate steroidal neuromuscular blocking drugs, especially rocuronium [92–95]. The aqueous solution of sugammadex has a pH of approximately 7.5 and osmolality of 300–500 mOsm kg^{-1}. Sugammadex exerts its effect by forming very tight complexes at a 1 : 1 ratio with steroidal neuromuscular blocking drugs (rocuronium > vecuronium >> pancuronium) [92–95]. The intermolecular (van der Waals) forces, thermodynamic (hydrogen) bonds, and hydrophobic interactions of the sugammadex–rocuronium complex make it very tight [92]. The sugammadex–rocuronium complex has a very high association rate (an association constant of 1×10^7 M^{-1} as determined by isothermal titration calorimetry) and a very low dissociation rate. Estimates are that for every 30 million sugammadex–rocuronium complexes, only one complex dissociates.

Sugammadex is the first selective relaxant-binding drug. It exerts no effect on acetylcholinesterases or on any receptor system in the body, thus eliminating the need for anticholinergic drugs and their adverse side effects. Moreover, the unique mechanism of reversal by encapsulation is independent of the depth of neuromuscular blockade. Thus, reversal can be accomplished even during profound neuromuscular blockade.

Pharmacokinetics and metabolism

Sugammadex is biologically inactive [96–98]. When administered by itself to volunteers who had not received a neuromuscular blocking drug, doses of 0.1–8.0 mg kg^{-1} of sugammadex had a clearance rate of 120 mL per minute, an elimination half-life of 100 minutes, and a volume of distribution of 18 L [97]. Approximately 75% of the dose was eliminated through the urine. The mean percentage of the dose excreted in urine

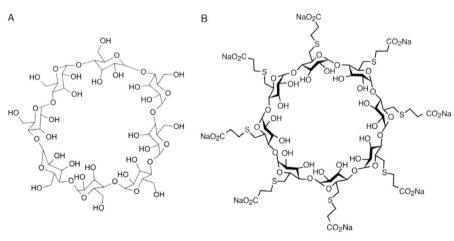

Figure 39.7. (A) γ-cyclodextrin and (B) sugammadex [6^A,6^B,6^C,6^D,6^E,6^F,6^G,6^H-octakis-S-(2-carboxyethyl)-6^A,6^B,6^C,6^D,6^E,6^F,6^G,6^H-octathio-γ-cyclodextrin octasodium salt], a modified γ-cyclodextrin.

up to 24 hours after administration varied between 59% and 80% [97]. The kinetics of sugammadex appear to be dose-dependent in that clearance increased and elimination half-life decreased when the sugammadex dose was increased from 0.15 to 1.0 mg kg^{-1} [97].

In the absence of sugammadex, rocuronium is eliminated mainly by biliary excretion ($> 75\%$) and to a lesser degree by renal excretion (10–25%). The plasma clearance of sugammadex alone is approximately three times lower than that of rocuronium alone [99]. In volunteers, the plasma clearance of rocuronium was decreased by a factor of > 2 after administration of a ≥ 2.0 mg kg^{-1} dose of sugammadex [97]. This is because the biliary route of excretion becomes unavailable for the rocuronium–sugammadex complex, and rocuronium clearance decreases to a value approaching the glomerular filtration rate (120 mL min^{-1}). As noted earlier, after administration of sugammadex, the plasma concentration of free rocuronium decreases rapidly, but the total plasma concentration of rocuronium (both free and that bound to sugammadex) increases [100].

The soluble nature of the sugammadex–rocuronium complex results in urinary excretion of the complex as the major route of elimination of rocuronium (65–97% of the administered dose is recovered in urine) [97,99]. Excretion is rapid, with approximately 70% of the administered dose excreted within 6 hours, and $> 90\%$ within 24 hours. Renal excretion of rocuronium is increased by more than 100% after administration of 4–8 mg kg^{-1} of sugammadex [99].

Sugammadex does not bind to human plasma proteins and erythrocytes to a significant extent. Metabolism of sugammadex is at most very limited, and the drug is predominantly eliminated unchanged by the kidneys. In patients with substantial renal impairment, clearance of sugammadex and rocuronium decreased by factors of 16 and 3.7, respectively, relative to that in healthy subjects, and the elimination half-

lives were increased by factors of 15 and 2.5, respectively. The effectiveness of dialysis in removing sugammadex and rocuronium from plasma was not demonstrated consistently. Therefore, sugammadex should be avoided in patients with a creatinine clearance of < 30 mL per minute.

Pharmacodynamics

Used in appropriate doses, sugammadex is capable of reversing to a TOF ratio of ≥ 0.9 within 3 minutes any depth of neuromuscular blockade induced by rocuronium or vecuronium [101]. During rocuronium- or vecuronium-induced neuromuscular blockade, intravenous administration of sugammadex results in rapid removal of free rocuronium or vecuronium molecules from the plasma. This creates a concentration gradient favoring movement of the remaining rocuronium or vecuronium molecules from the neuromuscular junction back into the plasma, where they are encapsulated by free sugammadex molecules. Those sugammadex molecules also enter the tissues and form a complex with the rocuronium or vecuronium. Therefore, the neuromuscular blockade induced by these drugs is terminated rapidly by their diffusion away from the neuromuscular junction and back into the plasma. This results in an increased total plasma concentration of rocuronium or vecuronium (both free and bound to sugammadex) [100].

The efficacy of sugammadex in antagonizing different levels of rocuronium- or vecuronium-induced neuromuscular blockade has been demonstrated in several clinical studies [99,102–108]. At appropriate doses, no recurarization has been reported in human studies. Fig. 39.8 depicts the actual course of sugammadex reversal of rocuronium-induced neuromuscular blockade at the end of surgery. This patient received 0.6 mg kg^{-1} rocuronium to facilitate tracheal intubation, which was performed when the twitch response disappeared. Complete neuromuscular blockade developed within 100 seconds (onset time). It took 43 minutes for the reappearance

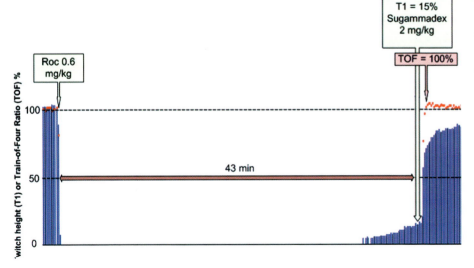

Figure 39.8. Acceleromyographic recording of the recovery of the twitch height and train-of-four (TOF) ratio after administration of 2 mg kg^{-1} of sugammadex at 15% twitch recovery from a rocuronium (Roc)-induced neuromuscular blockade. Complete neuromuscular recovery (TOF ratio of 100%) occurred 45 seconds later. Red dots depict the TOF ratio. The failure of first twitch (T1) to return to baseline height is probably a drift artifact.

of the second twitch of the TOF ratio, which was 15% of the control height. This coincided with the conclusion of the surgical procedure. Full TOF recovery occurred 45 seconds after administration of 2 mg kg^{-1} of sugammadex (Fig. 39.8). The patient was able to respond to oral commands 2 minutes after recovery of the TOF, and tracheal extubation was performed shortly thereafter. Fig. 39.9 depicts the calculated differences in the recovery duration that would be seen with 2 mg kg^{-1} of sugammadex versus 0.05 mg kg^{-1} of neostigmine.

With profound blockade induced by rocuronium or vecuronium, larger doses of sugammadex (8–16 mg kg^{-1}) are required for adequate and rapid recovery. In Fig. 39.10, the speed of recovery from 1.2 mg kg^{-1} of rocuronium followed 3 minutes later by 16 mg kg^{-1} of sugammadex is compared with the speed of spontaneous recovery from 1.0 mg kg^{-1} of succinylcholine in surgical patients [101]. The total time from administration of rocuronium until recovery of the TOF ratio to ≥ 0.9 was less than that needed for a similar degree of spontaneous recovery from the succinylcholine-induced blockade (Fig. 39.10). It should be noted, however, that all drugs behave in a dose–response manner [109]. A temporary decrease in TOF response (recurarization) was observed after reversal of muscle relaxation with an inadequate dose (0.5 mg kg^{-1}) of sugammadex administered 42 minutes after 0.9 mg kg^{-1} of rocuronium [110].

Published data indicate that if the TOF count is 2 during recovery from rocuronium-induced neuromuscular blockade, administering 2 mg kg^{-1} of sugammadex would be sufficient to produce adequate neuromuscular recovery (a TOF ratio of ≥ 0.9). Similarly, 4 mg kg^{-1} of sugammadex would be sufficient to produce adequate neuromuscular recovery from a deeper blockade at a 1–2 post-tetanic count. A still more profound blockade would require a greater dose of sugammadex, in the range of 8–16 mg kg^{-1}.

The introduction of sugammadex will allow the clinician to rapidly and fully reverse any depth of rocuronium-induced blockade, including that achieved 3 minutes after a very large dose (e.g., 1.2 mg kg^{-1}) of rocuronium. Some may erroneously argue that the use of sugammadex will render the monitoring of neuromuscular function unnecessary. This approach will definitely result not only in significant increases in the total cost of care, but also in loss of the basic understanding of

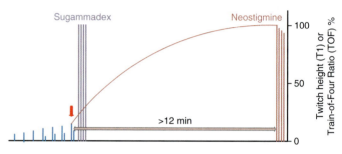

Figure 39.9. Calculated differences in the recovery course between 2 mg kg^{-1} of sugammadex and 0.05 mg kg^{-1} of neostigmine administered at a first-twitch recovery (T1) of 15% from a rocuronium-induced neuromuscular blockade (arrow). Train-of-four ratio recovery (~100%) after administration of sugammadex is prompt and complete within 2 minutes [95], compared with > 12 minutes after administration of neostigmine.

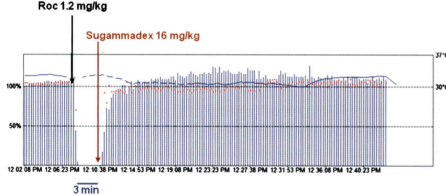

Figure 39.10. (A) Recovery of the twitch height and train-of-four (TOF) ratio after intravenous administration of 1.2 mg kg^{-1} of rocuronium, followed 3 minutes later by 16 mg kg^{-1} of sugammadex. Recovery to a first-twitch height (T1) of 90% and a TOF ratio of 0.94 occurred 110 seconds later. The onset–offset time with this sequence (i.e., the time from the end of the injection of rocuronium to a T1 recovery to 90%) was 4 minutes and 47 seconds. (B) The effects of administering 1.0 mg/kg of succinylcholine (Sch), with spontaneous recovery to a T1 of 90% occurring after 9 minutes and 23 seconds. Reproduced with permission from Naguib [101].

neuromuscular physiology and pharmacology on the part of practicing clinicians. This approach also carries the potential risk that overuse of neuromuscular blocking drugs could result in loss of the ability to discern light anesthesia, leading to increased incidence of intraoperative awareness and recall. At a minimum, routine neuromuscular monitoring with conventional nerve stimulators (those that require the clinician to evaluate the evoked response visually or tactilely) would be necessary to determine the degree of neuromuscular blockade in an anesthetized patient, and the appropriate dose of sugammadex could be administered accordingly.

Sugammadex is ineffective against succinylcholine, and against benzylisoquinoline neuromuscular blockers such as mivacurium, atracurium, and cisatracurium because it cannot form inclusion complexes with these drugs [111]. Therefore, if neuromuscular blockade must be re-established after the administration of sugammadex, one of the benzylisoquinoline neuromuscular blockers or succinylcholine should be considered. As discussed earlier, after full recovery from neuromuscular blockade, significant numbers (~80%) of nicotinic acetylcholine receptors at the neuromuscular junction are still occupied with the neuromuscular blocker [73]. Therefore, it is expected that if the neuromuscular blockade needs to be re-established after the use of sugammadex, a situation similar to "pretreatment" or "priming" will be present that would result in a delayed onset of succinylcholine effects (i.e., antagonism of depolarizing blockers) and potentiation of the effects (i.e., faster onset and prolonged duration) of benzylisoquinoline neuromuscular blockers [112–114].

Special populations

Subjects with renal impairment had a prolonged and 17-times greater exposure to sugammadex and a prolonged and four-times greater exposure to rocuronium than did subjects with normal renal function [115]. Thus, sugammadex should be avoided in patients with severe renal dysfunction (creatinine clearance rate $< 30\,\mathrm{mL\,min^{-1}}$). Recurrence of neuromuscular blockade was not observed in any patients.

Safety and tolerability

The sugammadex clinical development program included data from 30 worldwide clinical trials in 2054 subjects who received sugammadex. In all of the trial reports made available by the developer, sugammadex was compared with neostigmine (and placebo) with regard to the incidence of adverse effects. The highest sugammadex dose studied in the clinical development program was $96\,\mathrm{mg\,kg^{-1}}$ ($n = 12$ in trial 19.4.106). Sugammadex has no intrinsic pharmacologic activity and is cleared rapidly from most organs; however, it may be retained in the matrices of bone and teeth. Common adverse effects include dysgeusia, hypotension, QTc prolongation, diarrhea, headache, and polyuria [116].

Sugammadex has been approved for clinical use in several European countries. However the US Food and Drug Administration (FDA) issued a "not approvable" letter (August 2008) in response to the sugammadex new drug application, citing concerns about hypersensitivity and allergic reactions. Although the incidence of such reactions reported in all studies was < 1%, one healthy volunteer experienced a hypersensitivity reaction after his first exposure to sugammadex that resulted in discontinuation of the sugammadex infusion. The reaction was self-limiting and did not require treatment. Skin prick and intradermal tests were conducted on that volunteer, and it was concluded that he was probably hypersensitive to sugammadex. Six subjects showed signs of possible hypersensitivity to sugammadex (after the administration of $32\,\mathrm{mg\,kg^{-1}}$). Additional clinical and safety data may become available in the future and influence the FDA decisions on sugammadex.

Summary

Recovery from muscle relaxation induced by nondepolarizing neuromuscular blockers ultimately depends on elimination of the neuromuscular blocker from the body. Acetylcholinesterase inhibitors (edrophonium and more commonly neostigmine) are used clinically to antagonize the residual effects of neuromuscular blockers and to accelerate recovery from nondepolarizing neuromuscular blockade. Antagonism of nondepolarizing neuromuscular blockade by acetylcholinesterase inhibitors depends primarily on five factors: (1) the depth of the blockade when reversal is attempted, (2) the anticholinesterase used, (3) the dose administered, (4) the rate of spontaneous clearance of the neuromuscular blocker from plasma, and (5) the choice of anesthetic drugs and the depth of anesthesia. Drugs that potentiate the effects of neuromuscular blockers limit the efficacy of acetylcholinesterase inhibitors.

Inhibition of acetylcholinesterase not only increases the concentration of acetylcholine at the neuromuscular junction (nicotinic site) but also at all other synapses that use acetylcholine as a transmitter. Only the nicotinic effects of acetylcholinesterase inhibitors are desired. To minimize the muscarinic cardiovascular side effects of acetylcholinesterase inhibitors, an anticholinergic drug (atropine or glycopyrrolate) is coadministered with the acetylcholinesterase inhibitor. Administration of acetylcholinesterase inhibitors is associated with bronchoconstriction, increased airway resistance, increased salivation, and increased bowel motility (muscarinic effects). Anticholinergic drugs tend to reduce these effects.

Sugammadex is a novel reversal drug that is not an acetylcholinesterase inhibitor, and terminates action at the neuromuscular junction by interacting directly with the neuromuscular blocking drugs, specifically aminosteroids such as rocuronium and vecuronium. This eliminates the need for anticholinergic drugs and their adverse side effects. Reversal by sugammadex is independent of the depth of neuromuscular blockade, enabling reversal even during profound neuromuscular blockade.

There is a well-recognized high incidence of postoperative residual neuromuscular blockade and attendant clinical complications, and it is recommended that objective monitoring be used clinically to monitor the adequacy of reversal of neuromuscular blockade. Stimulation of the ulnar nerve, at either the wrist or the elbow, with observing contraction of the adductor pollicis, is most common. Although single-twitch monitoring is adequate for assessing onset of neuromuscular blockade, train-of-four stimulation should be used during maintenance and recovery from blockade. Objective monitoring is advantageous, since subjective (visual or tactile) evaluation of fade or postoperative residual neuromuscular blockade is inaccurate. Clinical bedside criteria for adequate antagonism of neuromuscular blockade and tracheal extubation are insensitive.

References

1. Griffith H, Johnson GE. The use of curare in general anesthesia. *Anesthesiology* 1942; **3**: 418–20.

2. Läwen A. Über die Verbindung der Lokalanästhesie mit der Narkose, über hohe Extraduralanästhesie und epidurale Injektionen anästhesierender Lösungen bei tabischen Magenkrisen. *Beitr Klin Chir* 1912; **80**: 168–80.

3. Pleasance RE. Curare. *Br J Anaesth* 1948; **21**: 2–23.

4. Burke JC, Linegar CR, Frank MN, McIntyre AR. Eserine and neostigmine antagonism of d-tubocurarine. *Anesthesiology* 1948; **9**: 251–7.

5. Prescott F, Organe G, Rothbotham S. Tubocurarine chloride as an adjunct to anaesthesia. *Lancet* 1946; **2**: 80–4.

6. Naguib M, Flood P, McArdle JJ, Brenner HR. Advances in neurobiology of the neuromuscular junction: implications for the anesthesiologist. *Anesthesiology* 2002; **96**: 202–31.

7. Rosenberry TL. Acetylcholinesterase. *Adv Enzymol Relat Areas Mol Biol* 1975; **43**: 103–218.

8. Sussman JL, Harel M, Frolow F, *et al.* Atomic structure of acetylcholinesterase from *Torpedo californica*: a prototypic acetylcholine-binding protein. *Science* 1991; **253**: 872–9.

9. Zhou HX, Wlodek ST, McCammon JA. Conformation gating as a mechanism for enzyme specificity. *Proc Natl Acad Sci U S A* 1998; **95**: 9280–3.

10. Cresnar B, Crne-Finderle N, Breskvar K, Sketelj J. Neural regulation of muscle acetylcholinesterase is exerted on the level of its mRNA. *J Neurosci Res* 1994; **38**: 294–9.

11. Ehrlich G, Viegas-Pequignot E, Ginzberg D, *et al.* Mapping the human acetylcholinesterase gene to chromosome 7q22 by fluorescent in situ hybridization coupled with selective PCR amplification from a somatic hybrid cell panel and chromosome-sorted DNA libraries. *Genomics* 1992; **13**: 1192–7.

12. McMahan UJ, Sanes JR, Marshall LM. Cholinesterase is associated with the basal lamina at the neuromuscular junction. *Nature* 1978; **271**: 172–4.

13. Hall ZW, Sanes JR. Synaptic structure and development: the neuromuscular junction. *Cell* 1993; **72**: 99–121.

14. Payne JP, Hughes R, Al Azawi S. Neuromuscular blockade by neostigmine in anaesthetized man. *Br J Anaesth* 1980; **52**: 69–76.

15. Naguib M, Kopman AF, Ensor JE. Neuromuscular monitoring and postoperative residual curarisation: a meta-analysis. *Br J Anaesth* 2007; **98**: 302–16.

16. Fiekers JF. Interactions of edrophonium, physostigmine and methanesulfonyl fluoride with the snake end-plate acetylcholine receptor-channel complex. *J Pharmacol Exp Ther* 1985; **234**: 539–49.

17. Akaike A, Ikeda SR, Brookes N, *et al.* The nature of the interactions of pyridostigmine with the nicotinic acetylcholine receptor-ionic channel complex. *Patch clamp studies. Mol Pharmacol* 1984; **25**: 102–12.

18. Magorian TT, Lynam DP, Caldwell JE, Miller RD. Can early administration of neostigmine, in single or repeated doses, alter the course of neuromuscular recovery from a vecuronium-induced neuromuscular blockade? *Anesthesiology* 1990; **73**: 410–14.

19. Bevan JC, Collins L, Fowler C, *et al.* Early and late reversal of rocuronium and vecuronium with neostigmine in adults and children. *Anesth Analg* 1999; **89**: 333–9.

20. Donati F, Smith CE, Bevan DR. Dose-response relationships for edrophonium and neostigmine as antagonists of moderate and profound atracurium blockade. *Anesth Analg* 1989; **68**: 13–19.

21. Cronnelly R, Morris RB, Miller RD. Edrophonium: duration of action and atropine requirement in humans during halothane anesthesia. *Anesthesiology* 1982; **57**: 261–6.

22. Miller RD, Van Nyhuis LS, Eger EI, Vitez TS, Way WL. Comparative times to peak effect and durations of action of neostigmine and pyridostigmine. *Anesthesiology* 1974; **41**: 27–33.

23. Rupp SM, McChristian JW, Miller RD, Taboada JA, Cronnelly R. Neostigmine and edrophonium antagonism of varying intensity neuromuscular blockade induced by atracurium, pancuronium, or vecuronium. *Anesthesiology* 1986; **64**: 711–17.

24. Naguib M, Abdulatif M, al-Ghamdi A. Dose–response relationships for edrophonium and neostigmine antagonism of rocuronium bromide (ORG 9426)-induced neuromuscular blockade. *Anesthesiology* 1993; **79**: 739–45.

25. Naguib M, Riad W. Dose–response relationships for edrophonium and neostigmine antagonism of atracurium and cisatracurium-induced neuromuscular block. *Can J Anaesth* 2000; **47**: 1074–81.

26. Naguib M, Abdulatif M, al-Ghamdi A, Hamo I, Nouheid R. Dose–response relationships for edrophonium and neostigmine antagonism of mivacurium-induced neuromuscular block. *Br J Anaesth* 1993; **71**: 709–14.

27. Naguib M, Abdulatif M. Priming with anti-cholinesterases-the effect of different combinations of anti-cholinesterases and different priming intervals. *Can J Anaesth* 1988; **35**: 47–52.

28. Jones JE, Hunter JM, Utting JE. Use of neostigmine in the antagonism of residual neuromuscular blockade produced by vecuronium. *Br J Anaesth* 1987; **59**: 1454–8.

29. Harper NJ, Wallace M, Hall IA. Optimum dose of neostigmine at two levels of atracurium-induced neuromuscular block. *Br J Anaesth* 1994; **72**: 82–5.

30. Engbaek J, Ording H, Ostergaard D, Viby-Mogensen J. Edrophonium and neostigmine for reversal of the neuromuscular blocking effect of vecuronium. *Acta Anaesthesiol Scand* 1985; **29**: 544–6.

31. Fisher DM, Cronnelly R, Sharma M, Miller RD. Clinical pharmacology of edrophonium in infants and children. *Anesthesiology* 1984; **61**: 428–33.

32. Gencarelli PJ, Miller RD. Antagonism of org NC 45 (vecuronium) and pancuronium neuromuscular blockade by neostigmine. *Br J Anaesth* 1982; **54**: 53–6.

33. Kopman AF, Kopman DJ, Ng J, Zank LM. Antagonism of profound cisatracurium and rocuronium block: the role of objective assessment of neuromuscular function. *J Clin Anesth* 2005; **17**: 30–5.

34. Lessard MR, Trepanier CA, Rouillard JF. Neostigmine requirements for reversal of neuromuscular blockade following an infusion of mivacurium. *Can J Anaesth* 1997; **44**: 836–42.

35. Beemer GH, Goonetilleke PH, Bjorksten AR. The maximum depth of an atracurium neuromuscular block antagonized by edrophonium to effect adequate recovery. *Anesthesiology* 1995; **82**: 852–8.

36. Caldwell JE, Robertson EN, Baird WL. Antagonism of vecuronium and atracurium: comparison of neostigmine and edrophonium administered at 5% twitch height recovery. *Br J Anaesth* 1987; **59**: 478–81.

37. Berg H, Roed J, Viby-Mogensen J, *et al.* Residual neuromuscular block is a risk factor for postoperative pulmonary complications. A prospective, randomised, and blinded study of postoperative pulmonary complications after atracurium, vecuronium and pancuronium. *Acta Anaesthesiol Scand* 1997; **41**: 1095–103.

38. Bevan DR, Smith CE, Donati F. Postoperative neuromuscular blockade: a comparison between atracurium, vecuronium, and pancuronium.

Anesthesiology 1988; **69**: 272–6.

39. Saitoh Y, Toyooka H, Amaha K. Recoveries of post-tetanic twitch and train-of-four responses after administration of vecuronium with different inhalation anaesthetics and neuroleptanaesthesia. *Br J Anaesth* 1993; **70**: 402–4.

40. Miller RD, Way WL, Dolan WM, Stevens WC, Eger EI. The dependence of pancuronium- and d-tubocurarine-induced neuromuscular blockades on alveolar concentrations of halothane and forane. *Anesthesiology* 1972; **37**: 573–81.

41. Miller RD, Crique M, Eger EI. Duration of halothane anesthesia and neuromuscular blockade with d-tubocurarine. *Anesthesiology* 1976; **44**: 206–10.

42. Kelly RE, Lien CA, Savarese JJ, *et al.* Depression of neuromuscular function in a patient during desflurane anesthesia. *Anesth Analg* 1993; **76**: 868–71.

43. Rupp SM, Miller RD, Gencarelli PJ. Vecuronium-induced neuromuscular blockade during enflurane, isoflurane, and halothane anesthesia in humans. *Anesthesiology* 1984; **60**: 102–5.

44. Gencarelli PJ, Miller RD, Eger EI, Newfield P. Decreasing enflurane concentrations and d-tubocurarine neuromuscular blockade. *Anesthesiology* 1982; **56**: 192–4.

45. Morita T, Tsukagoshi H, Sugaya T, *et al.* Inadequate antagonism of vecuronium-induced neuromuscular block by neostigmine during sevoflurane or isoflurane anesthesia. *Anesth Analg* 1995; **80**: 1175–80.

46. Reid JE, Breslin DS, Mirakhur RK, Hayes AH. Neostigmine antagonism of rocuronium block during anesthesia with sevoflurane, isoflurane or propofol. *Can J Anaesth* 2001; **48**: 351–5.

47. Lowry DW, Mirakhur RK, McCarthy GJ, Carroll MT, McCourt KC. Neuromuscular effects of rocuronium during sevoflurane, isoflurane, and intravenous anesthesia. *Anesth Analg* 1998; **87**: 936–40.

48. Baurain MJ, d'Hollander AA, Melot C, Dernovoi BS, Barvais L. Effects of residual concentrations of isoflurane on

the reversal of vecuronium-induced neuromuscular blockade. *Anesthesiology* 1991; **74**: 474–8.

49. Sunew KY, Hicks RG. Effects of neostigmine and pyridostigmine on duration of succinylcholine action and pseudocholinesterase activity. *Anesthesiology* 1978; **49**: 188–91.

50. Cronnelly R, Stanski DR, Miller RD, Sheiner LB, Sohn YJ. Renal function and the pharmacokinetics of neostigmine in anesthetized man. *Anesthesiology* 1979; **51**: 222–6.

51. Cronnelly R, Stanski DR, Miller RD, Sheiner LB. Pyridostigmine kinetics with and without renal function. *Clin Pharmacol Ther* 1980; **28**: 78–81.

52. Morris RB, Cronnelly R, Miller RD, Stanski DR, Fahey MR. Pharmacokinetics of edrophonium in anephric and renal transplant patients. *Br J Anaesth* 1981; **53**: 1311–14.

53. Morris RB, Cronnelly R, Miller RD, Stanski DR, Fahey MR. Pharmacokinetics of edrophonium and neostigmine when antagonizing d-tubocurarine neuromuscular blockade in man. *Anesthesiology* 1981; **54**: 399–401.

54. Suresh D, Carter JA, Whitehead JP, Goldhill DR, Flynn PJ. Cardiovascular changes at antagonism of atracurium: effects of different doses of premixed neostigmine and glycopyrronium in a ratio of 5:1. *Anaesthesia* 1991; **46**: 877–80.

55. Bowman WC. *Pharmacology of Neuromuscular Function*, 2nd edn. London: Wright, 1990.

56. Salem MG, Richardson JC, Meadows GA, Lamplugh G, Lai KM. Comparison between glycopyrrolate and atropine in a mixture with neostigmine for reversal of neuromuscular blockade. Studies in patients following open heart surgery. *Br J Anaesth* 1985; **57**: 184–7.

57. van Vlymen JM, Parlow JL. The effects of reversal of neuromuscular blockade on autonomic control in the perioperative period. *Anesth Analg* 1997; **84**: 148–54.

58. Ding Y, Fredman B, White PF. Use of mivacurium during laparoscopic surgery: effect of reversal drugs on postoperative recovery. *Anesth Analg* 1994; **78**: 450–4.

59. Boeke AJ, de Lange JJ, van Druenen B, Langemeijer JJ. Effect of antagonizing residual neuromuscular block by neostigmine and atropine on postoperative vomiting. *Br J Anaesth* 1994; **72**: 654–6.

60. Hovorka J, Korttila K, Nelskyla K, *et al.* Reversal of neuromuscular blockade with neostigmine has no effect on the incidence or severity of postoperative nausea and vomiting. *Anesth Analg* 1997; **85**: 1359–61.

61. Gild WM, Posner KL, Caplan RA, Cheney FW. Eye injuries associated with anesthesia. A closed claims analysis. *Anesthesiology* 1992; **76**: 204–8.

62. Donati F, Meistelman C, Plaud B. Vecuronium neuromuscular blockade at the adductor muscles of the larynx and adductor pollicis. *Anesthesiology* 1991; **74**: 833–7.

63. Meistelman C, Plaud B, Donati F. Rocuronium (ORG 9426) neuromuscular blockade at the adductor muscles of the larynx and adductor pollicis in humans. *Can J Anaesth* 1992; **39**: 665–9.

64. Wright PM, Caldwell JE, Miller RD. Onset and duration of rocuronium and succinylcholine at the adductor pollicis and laryngeal adductor muscles in anesthetized humans. *Anesthesiology* 1994; **81**: 1110–15.

65. Plaud B, Debaene B, Lequeau F, Meistelman C, Donati F. Mivacurium neuromuscular block at the adductor muscles of the larynx and adductor pollicis in humans. *Anesthesiology* 1996; **85**: 77–81.

66. Hemmerling TM, Schmidt J, Hanusa C, Wolf T, Schmitt H. Simultaneous determination of neuromuscular block at the larynx, diaphragm, adductor pollicis, orbicularis oculi and corrugator supercilii muscles. *Br J Anaesth* 2000; **85**: 856–60.

67. Fisher DM, Szenohradszky J, Wright PM, *et al.* Pharmacodynamic modeling of vecuronium-induced twitch depression. Rapid plasma-effect site equilibration explains faster onset at resistant laryngeal muscles than at the adductor pollicis. *Anesthesiology* 1997; **86**: 558–66.

68. Sheiner LB, Stanski DR, Vozeh S, Miller RD, Ham J. Simultaneous modeling of pharmacokinetics and pharmacodynamics: application to d-tubocurarine. *Clin Pharmacol Ther* 1979; **25**: 358–71.

69. Wierda JM, Kleef UW, Lambalk LM, Kloppenburg WD, Agoston S. The pharmacodynamics and pharmacokinetics of Org 9426, a new non-depolarizing neuromuscular blocking agent, in patients anaesthetized with nitrous oxide, halothane and fentanyl. *Can J Anaesth* 1991; **38**: 430–5.

70. Naguib M, Kopman AF. Low dose rocuronium for tracheal intubation. *Middle East J Anesthesiol* 2003; **17**: 193–204.

71. Hutton P, Burchett KR, Madden AP. Comparison of recovery after neuromuscular blockade by atracurium or pancuronium. *Br J Anaesth* 1988; **60**: 36–42.

72. Kopman AF, Yee PS, Neuman GG. Relationship of the train-of-four fade ratio to clinical signs and symptoms of residual paralysis in awake volunteers. *Anesthesiology* 1997; **86**: 765–71.

73. Waud BE, Waud DR. The relation between tetanic fade and receptor occlusion in the presence of competitive neuromuscular block. *Anesthesiology* 1971; **35**: 456–64.

74. Paton WD, Waud DR. The margin of safety of neuromuscular transmission. *J Physiol* 1967; **191**: 59–90.

75. Viby-Mogensen J, Jensen NH, Engbaek J, *et al.* Tactile and visual evaluation of the response to train-of-four nerve stimulation. *Anesthesiology* 1985; **63**: 440–3.

76. Dupuis JY, Martin R, Tetrault JP. Clinical, electrical and mechanical correlations during recovery from neuromuscular blockade with vecuronium. *Can J Anaesth* 1990; **37**: 192–6.

77. Baillard C, Gehan G, Reboul-Marty J, *et al.* Residual curarization in the recovery room after vecuronium. *Br J Anaesth* 2000; **84**: 394–5.

78. Baillard C, Clec'h C, Catineau J, *et al.* Postoperative residual neuromuscular block: a survey of management. *Br J Anaesth* 2005; **95**: 622–6.

79. Kopman AF, Ng J, Zank LM, Neuman GG, Yee PS. Residual postoperative paralysis. Pancuronium versus mivacurium, does it matter? *Anesthesiology* 1996; **85**: 1253–9.

80. Viby-Mogensen J, Jorgensen BC, Ording H. Residual curarization in the recovery room. *Anesthesiology* 1979; **50**: 539–41.

81. Debaene B, Plaud B, Dilly MP, Donati F. Residual paralysis in the PACU after a single intubating dose of nondepolarizing muscle relaxant with an intermediate duration of action. *Anesthesiology* 2003; **98**: 1042–8.

82. Murphy GS, Szokol JW, Marymont JH, *et al.* Residual neuromuscular blockade and critical respiratory events in the postanesthesia care unit. *Anesth Analg* 2008; **107**: 130–7.

83. Eriksson LI, Sundman E, Olsson R, *et al.* Functional assessment of the pharynx at rest and during swallowing in partially paralyzed humans: simultaneous videomanometry and mechanomyography of awake human volunteers. *Anesthesiology* 1997; **87**: 1035–43.

84. Sundman E, Witt H, Olsson R, *et al.* The incidence and mechanisms of pharyngeal and upper esophageal dysfunction in partially paralyzed humans: pharyngeal videoradiography and simultaneous manometry after atracurium. *Anesthesiology* 2000; **92**: 977–84.

85. Eriksson LI. The effects of residual neuromuscular blockade and volatile anesthetics on the control of ventilation. *Anesth Analg* 1999; **89**: 243–51.

86. Sorgenfrei IF, Viby-Mogensen J, Swiatek FA. [Does evidence lead to a change in clinical practice? Danish anaesthetists' and nurse anesthetists' clinical practice and knowledge of postoperative residual curarization]. *Ugeskr Laeger* 2005; **167**: 3878–82.

87. Bartkowski RR. Incomplete reversal of pancuronium neuromuscular blockade by neostigmine, pyridostigmine, and edrophonium. *Anesth Analg* 1987; **66**: 594–8.

88. Beemer GH, Bjorksten AR, Dawson PJ, *et al.* Determinants of the reversal time of competitive neuromuscular block by anticholinesterases. *Br J Anaesth* 1991; **66**: 469–75.

89. Murphy GS, Szokol JW, Marymont JH, *et al.* Intraoperative acceleromyographic

monitoring reduces the risk of residual neuromuscular blockade and adverse respiratory events in the postanesthesia care unit. *Anesthesiology* 2008; **109**: 389–98.

90. Naguib M, el-Gammal M, Daoud W, *et al.* Human plasma cholinesterase for antagonism of prolonged mivacurium-induced neuromuscular blockade. *Anesthesiology* 1995; **82**: 1288–92.

91. Belmont MR, Horochiwsky Z, Eliazo RF, Savarese JJ. Reversal of AV430A with cysteine in rhesus monkeys. *Anesthesiology* 2004: A-1180.

92. Bom A, Bradley M, Cameron K, *et al.* A novel concept of reversing neuromuscular block: chemical encapsulation of rocuronium bromide by a cyclodextrin-based synthetic host. *Angew Chem* 2002; **41**: 266–70.

93. Adam JM, Bennett DJ, Bom A, *et al.* Cyclodextrin-derived host molecules as reversal agents for the neuromuscular blocker rocuronium bromide: synthesis and structure–activity relationships. *J Med Chem* 2002; **45**: 1806–16.

94. Tarver GJ, Grove SJ, Buchanan K, *et al.* 2-O-substituted cyclodextrins as reversal agents for the neuromuscular blocker rocuronium bromide. *Bioorg Med Chem* 2002; **10**: 1819–27.

95. Cameron KS, Clark JK, Cooper A, *et al.* Modified gamma-cyclodextrins and their rocuronium complexes. *Org Lett* 2002; **4**: 3403–6.

96. Zhang MQ. Drug-specific cyclodextrins: the future of rapid neuromuscular block reversal? *Drugs Future* 2003; **28**: 347–54.

97. Gijsenbergh F, Ramael S, Houwing N, van Iersel T. First human exposure of Org 25969, a novel agent to reverse the action of rocuronium bromide. *Anesthesiology* 2005; **103**: 695–703.

98. Sorgenfrei IF, Norrild K, Larsen PB, *et al.* Reversal of rocuronium-induced neuromuscular block by the selective relaxant binding agent sugammadex: a dose-finding and safety study. *Anesthesiology* 2006; **104**: 667–74.

99. Sparr HJ, Vermeyen KM, Beaufort AM, *et al.* Early reversal of profound rocuronium-induced neuromuscular blockade by sugammadex in a randomized multicenter study: efficacy, safety, and pharmacokinetics. *Anesthesiology* 2007; **106**: 935–43.

100. Epemolu O, Bom A, Hope F, Mason R. Reversal of neuromuscular blockade and simultaneous increase in plasma rocuronium concentration after the intravenous infusion of the novel reversal agent Org 25969. *Anesthesiology* 2003; **99**: 632–7.

101. Naguib M. Sugammadex: another milestone in clinical neuromuscular pharmacology. *Anesth Analg* 2007; **104**: 575–81.

102. Shields M, Giovannelli M, Mirakhur RK, *et al.* Org 25969 (sugammadex), a selective relaxant binding agent for antagonism of prolonged rocuronium-induced neuromuscular block. *Br J Anaesth* 2006; **96**: 36–43.

103. Suy K, Morias K, Cammu G, *et al.* Effective reversal of moderate rocuronium- or vecuronium-induced neuromuscular block with sugammadex, a selective relaxant binding agent. *Anesthesiology* 2007; **106**: 283–8.

104. Groudine SB, Soto R, Lien C, Drover D, Roberts K. A randomized, dose-finding, phase II study of the selective relaxant binding drug, sugammadex, capable of safely reversing profound rocuronium-induced neuromuscular block. *Anesth Analg* 2007; **104**: 555–62.

105. de Boer HD, Driessen JJ, Marcus MA, *et al.* Reversal of rocuronium-induced (1.2 mg/kg) profound neuromuscular block by sugammadex: a multicenter, dose-finding and safety study. *Anesthesiology* 2007; **107**: 239–44.

106. Puhringer FK, Rex C, Sielenkamper AW, *et al.* Reversal of profound, high-dose rocuronium-induced neuromuscular blockade by sugammadex at two different time points: an international, multicenter, randomized, dose-finding, safety assessor-blinded, phase II trial. *Anesthesiology* 2008; **109**: 188–97.

107. Flockton EA, Mastronardi P, Hunter JM, *et al.* Reversal of rocuronium-induced neuromuscular block with sugammadex is faster than reversal of cisatracurium-induced block with neostigmine. *Br J Anaesth* 2008; **100**: 622–30.

108. Lee C, Jahr JS, Candiotti K, *et al.* Reversal of profound neuromuscular block by sugammadex administered 3 minutes after rocuronium: A comparison with spontaneous recovery from succinylcholine. Anesthesiology In press.

109. Naguib M. Sugammadex may replace best clinical practice: A misconception. *Anesth Analg* 2007; **105**: 1506–7.

110. Eleveld DJ, Kuizenga K, Proost JH, Wierda JM. A temporary decrease in twitch response during reversal of rocuronium-induced muscle relaxation with a small dose of sugammadex. *Anesth Analg* 2007; **104**: 582–4.

111. de Boer HD, van Egmond J, van de Pol F, Bom A, Booij LH. Sugammadex, a new reversal agent for neuromuscular block induced by rocuronium in the anaesthetized Rhesus monkey. *Br J Anaesth* 2006; **96**: 473–9.

112. Naguib M. Different priming techniques, including mivacurium, accelerate the onset of rocuronium. *Can J Anaesth* 1994; **41**: 902–7.

113. Naguib M, Abdulatif M, Selim M, al-Ghamdi A. Dose–response studies of the interaction between mivacurium and suxamethonium. *Br J Anaesth* 1995; **74**: 26–30.

114. Bom AH, Hope F. A higher than required dose of sugammadex prevents the creation of a situation similar to "priming". *Anesthesiology* 2007: A989.

115. Staals LM, Snoeck MM, Driessen JJ, *et al.* Multicentre, parallel-group, comparative trial evaluating the efficacy and safety of sugammadex in patients with end-stage renal failure or normal renal function. *Br J Anaesth* 2008; **101**: 492–7.

116. Naguib M, Brull SJ. Sugammadex: a novel selective relaxant binding agent. *Expert Rev Clin Pharmacol* 2009; **2**: 37–53.

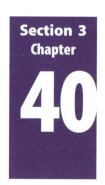

**Section 3
Chapter
40**

Essential drugs in anesthetic practice
Sympathomimetic and sympatholytic drugs

David F. Stowe and Thomas J. Ebert

Introduction

This chapter reviews only the sympathetic arm of the auto-nomic nervous system (ANS), and the hormones and drugs that stimulate or block sympathetic activity as assessed by end-organ effects. It is important for the practitioner to understand the general anatomy of the efferent sympathetic outflow from the cardiovascular center in the central nervous system (CNS) to the organs innervated via pre- and postganglionic fibers (see Chapter 22), how stimulation of baro- and chemoreceptors elicits sympathetic responses, and the nature and distribution of these responses. Knowledge of the differential effects of the two classes of adrenoceptors (α and β) and their subtypes helps us understand the effects of agonists and antagonists on these receptors. In particular, we need to differentiate the physiological effects of the most commonly used α_1- and α_2-adrenergic agonists and β_1- and β_2-adrenergic agonists. A good knowledge of the actions of the indirect-acting sympathomi-metics and their interaction with other drugs and foodstuffs is an essential part of understanding potential drug interactions and how to avoid them. Finally, a complete understanding of the most commonly prescribed α- and β-blockers, with an emphasis on their relative subtype activity, e.g., β_1 versus β_2, will assist the reader in knowledgeably selecting drugs to treat particular conditions without untoward side effects.

Sympathetic nervous system

The autonomic nervous system consists of the sympathetic and parasympathetic nervous systems that function to main-tain body homeostasis. This is achieved by integrating signals from a variety of somatic and visceral sensors to modulate organ perfusion and function. There is generally no voluntary control of the ANS, although conscious brief modulation can occur by biofeedback or during mental stress. The efferent components of the ANS are tonically active to maintain cardiac function, and visceral and vascular smooth muscle in a state of intermediate function. This permits rapid increases or decreases in efferent autonomic activity to adjust blood flow and organ activity in response to the environment.

The sympathetic nervous system (SNS) exits the spinal cord at thoracolumbar sections and has been called the "fight or flight" division. Its activation under stress (e.g., blood loss, temperature change, or exercise) increases sympathetic neural activity to the heart and other viscera, peripheral vasculature, sweat glands, ocular muscles, and piloerector muscles. Activation can affect sympathetic output in a highly differentiated manner; however, generalized activation leads to increases in cardiac output, blood glucose, pupillary dilation, and body temperature.

Basal autonomic tone

The basal "tone" of the ANS is determined by input to various regions of the lower brainstem. The primary relay or integra-tion region is called the *medullary vasomotor center*. Input into the medullary vasomotor center descends from the central autonomic network (CAN) and ascends from peripheral sensors, including the baroreceptors, chemoreceptors, and vis-ceral and somatic sensors. The CAN consists of four primary areas: the cerebral cortex, amygdala, hypothalamus, and medulla. In addition, humoral substances modulate the CAN via regions of the circumventricular organs where the blood–brain barrier is relatively deficient. Circulating substances, including angiotensin, arginine-vasopressin, and various cyto-kines, appear to cross into the CNS at the subfornical organ, in the lamina terminalis of the anterior wall of the third ventricle, and at the area postrema in the fourth ventricle. These circu-lating substances modulate reflexes initiated from peripheral receptors in blood vessels and tissues.

Medullary vasomotor center and peripheral nervous system

The medullary vasomotor center serves as the first relay station for afferent input from peripheral sensors including the baro- and chemoreceptors and gastrointestinal receptors. Ascending afferent vagal signals synapse in the nucleus tractus solitarius (NTS), found bilaterally in the dorsal medulla. The NTS relays information to higher centers of the CAN, such as the amyg-dala and hypothalamus, and also has connections with the ventrolateral medulla (VLM). From the rostral VLM, efferent

Anesthetic Pharmacology, 2nd edition, ed. Alex S. Evers, Mervyn Maze, Evan D. Kharasch. Published by Cambridge University Press. © Cambridge University Press 2011.

sympathetic outflow projects to the intermediolateral column of thoracolumbar spinal cord and increases sympathetic discharge. Neurons in the rostral VLM discharge with a rhythm linked to heart rate and can be suppressed by afferent signals from high-pressure baroreceptor discharge at peak pulse pressure. The caudal VLM interconnects with the rostral VLM and contains neurons that can suppress efferent preganglionic sympathetic activity.

The SNS disseminates and amplifies information to maintain cardiovascular homeostasis. The sympathetic nervous system consists of preganglionic *B fibers* that arise from the intermediolateral column and exit the spinal cord between the first thoracic (T1) and the third lumbar (L3) level (Fig. 40.1). They are myelinated, have a small diameter of less than 3 mm, and conduct at a speed of 2–14 m s^{-1}. Axons of these neurons leave the spinal cord in the ventral spinal roots, along with somatic neurons, then branch off in the white rami communicantes and enter the 22 paravertebral ganglia comprising the "sympathetic chain." The fine myelination of these fibers is responsible for their white appearance. The paravertebral ganglia are arranged as a bilateral vertical chain of ganglia running the length of the spinal column located anterolateral to the vertebral body. The preganglionic fibers are so named because they have not yet connected to a ganglionic cell. Likewise, postganglionic C fibers are the terminal fibers of a ganglion cell and synapse with the appropriate end organ. The preganglionic fiber has several potential destinations once it enters the "sympathetic chain": it could synapse with one or more sympathetic neurons in the ganglion it has entered; it could ascend or descend in the paravertebral chain and synapse with neurons at other levels; it could synapse in the ganglion with a postganglionic fiber that leaves the paravertebral chain via gray rami communicantes to join a somatic nerve and travel to an effector site (e.g., blood vessels). Some preganglionic fibers feed directly to peripheral ganglia before synapsing, and some make direct connections with the adrenal medulla. Because the adrenal medulla originates from neural tissue, it can be considered to be the postganglionic nerve.

Postganglionic sympathetic nerves

The postganglionic, noradrenergic, sympathetic fibers, or *C fibers*, are largely unmyelinated and have diameters ranging from 0.3 to 1.3 mm and conduction velocities of ~ 1 m s^{-1}. Like preganglionic fibers, one postganglionic fiber can synapse with a number of effector cells. Historically, activation of the SNS had been considered a "mass reflex" or total response. Current understanding is that there is selectivity of sympathetic response, although the site of differentiation or regulation of the selectivity is not known. Thus, a postganglionic fiber will synapse with only one type of end organ. In other words, one postganglionic fiber might synapse with several vascular smooth-muscle cells in blood vessels but would not simultaneously synapse with a blood vessel, a sweat gland, and a piloerector muscle. A clear example of the selectivity of the

SNS can be observed in the neural activity recorded from skin and muscle sympathetic nerves in humans [1]. The efferent sympathetic nerves to skin blood vessels, sweat glands, and piloerector muscles are generally silent during quiet resting conditions and during blood pressure fluctuation but are activated when a sudden noise is imposed or an embarrassing question is asked. In contrast, the efferent sympathetic nerves that supply skeletal-muscle blood vessels show significant tonic activity that is inversely modified by changes in blood pressure via the baroreflex. The sympathetic activity to skeletal muscle is not altered by startle maneuvers.

As one may ascertain, there is considerable dispersion in the SNS. For every one preganglionic fiber there are 20–30 postganglionic fibers. Moreover, the sympathetic terminal in a visceral organ or tissue is not a single terminal; rather it is a multiple, branched series of endings called a *terminal plexus*. A single postganglionic nerve can innervate up to 25 000 effector cells via the terminal plexus. Finally, when there is a great deal of sympathetic activity, the release of the postganglionic neurotransmitter norepinephrine (noradrenaline) may exceed the capacities of the local uptake and enzymatic breakdown systems that function to terminate its action. The excess norepinephrine (or spillover) can be dispersed by the circulatory system and can cause widespread humoral effects. The important end organs innervated by the SNS include the eyes, secretory organs (including the sweat glands), the heart, blood vessels, the adrenal medulla, the abdominal and pelvic viscera, and piloerector muscles.

Baroreflex and other neural reflexes of the sympathetic nervous system

Afferent signals from pressure sensors in the central blood vessels are integrated in the CAN, predominantly the NTS, and directly influence the ANS outflow to cardiovascular effectors. Low-pressure, cardiopulmonary baroreceptors are located primarily at the junction of the venae cavae and the right atrium, within the right atrium, and in pulmonary blood vessels (Fig. 40.2). The function of these receptors is to monitor central blood volume. For example, when the cardiopulmonary baroreceptors detect slight decreases in central venous pressure, reflex increases of peripheral sympathetic activity are initiated and blood pressure is well maintained. This reflex appears to be absent in heart transplant recipients. Arterial, or "high-pressure," baroreceptor reflexes are mediated by pressure sensors located in the arch of the aorta and in the carotid sinus (Fig. 40.2). Increased blood pressure increases afferent firing and, via CAN, stimulates increased vagal outflow and decreased sympathetic outflow, resulting in bradycardia and hypotension.

A number of other physiologic reflexes affecting ANS tonic activity have been identified. One group involves hypoxic stimulation of chemoreceptors of the aortic and carotid body exciting the SNS and increasing respiration. Another category of such reflexes involves direct stimulation of the CAN. For example, the Cushing reflex of bradycardia and hypertension

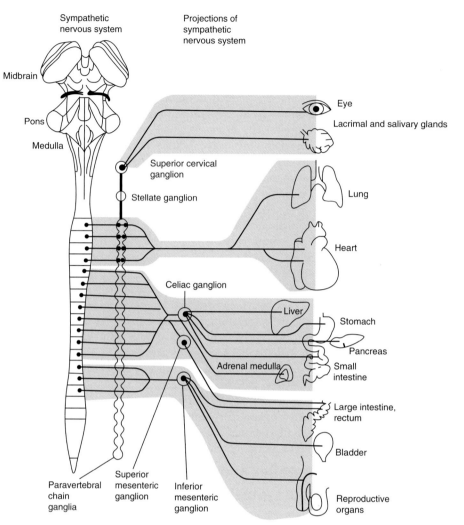

Figure 40.1. Diagramatic representation of the sympathetic nervous system and the end organs innervated by the various sympathetic nerves.

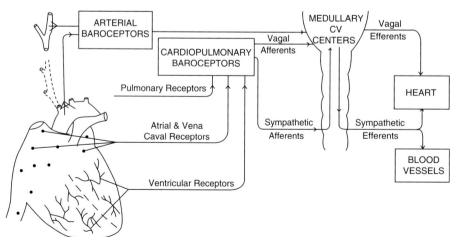

Figure 40.2. Diagramatic representation of the arterial and cardiopulmonary baroceptors and their afferent and efferent pathways.

in response to intracranial hypertension appears to be initiated by hypoxic or mechanical stimulation of the rostral VLM. Rapid changes in autonomic discharge should therefore be anticipated in states of shock, hypoxia, and from intracranial mechanical stimulation as occurs in tumor resections, brain trauma, or intracranial hemorrhage.

Anesthetics and the sympathetic nervous system

Because of the difficulty in quantifying efferent SNS activity in humans, there is a relative paucity of information relating to the direct effects of anesthetics on both basal levels of sympathetic vasoconstrictor traffic and the reflex regulation of the SNS. The technique of sympathetic microneurography permits the recording of vasoconstrictor impulses directed to blood vessels within the skeletal muscle. This technique has been applied in several studies evaluating the effects of nitrous oxide in humans [2–4]. An oxygen/nitrous oxide mixture (60%/40%) breathed by healthy volunteers induces a marked increase in sympathetic nerve traffic. Moreover, breathing nitrous oxide does not inhibit reflex sympathetic responses. Consequently, the enhanced sympathetic function permitted by adding nitrous oxide to an anesthetic regimen may, at times, provide a more ideal hemodynamic profile.

Both thiopental (thiopentone) and propofol result in near neural silence, as measured by microneurography, for a period of several minutes following their administration [5]. Part of this sympathetic silence may be related to the concomitant loss of consciousness. However, thiopental and propofol appear also to abolish the normal reflex sympathetic discharge associated with hypotension. When etomidate is infused, sympathetic outflow is well maintained despite loss of consciousness [6,7]. This maintained sympathetic activity with etomidate results in a very stable blood pressure. Etomidate also preserves reflex sympathetic discharge. In severely hypovolemic patients undergoing general anesthesia, thiopental and propofol can lead to precipitous declines in blood pressure that are mediated by reduced tonic levels of sympathetic outflow and inhibited reflex sympathetic discharge; therefore, bolus delivery of thiopental and propofol are probably contraindicated in such situations.

The volatile anesthetic desflurane has been associated with large increases in sympathetic activity and a generalized stress response when delivered at less than 1 MAC [8–11] (Fig. 40.3). The trigger for these responses is most likely irritation of airway receptors related to the high pungency and low potency of desflurane [12].

Sympathomimetic drugs

Sympathomimetic drugs produce effects similar to those produced by impulses conveyed by adrenergic postganglionic fibers of the SNS. Because these drugs resemble epinephrine (adrenaline) in physiologic action, they are also called *adrenergic* drugs.

Stimulation of postganglionic sympathetic nerve terminals, with a few exceptions, liberates norepinephrine, the major neurotransmitter at the sympathetic nerve terminal. Stimulation of the adrenal medulla releases both epinephrine and norepinephrine into the systemic circulation. Dopamine, the third naturally occurring sympathomimetic amine, serves as a neurotransmitter in multiple systems, especially in the basal ganglia of the CNS, but also in dopaminergic nerve endings and receptors elsewhere in the CNS and peripheral nervous system.

Background and history

Therapeutic use of a sympathomimetic drug was first described in China around 3000 BC [13]. The plant ma-huang was used as a diaphoretic, a circulatory stimulant, an antipyretic, and a sedative for cough. Ephedrine, the main alkaloid of ma-huang, was isolated in 1886 [14]. In 1895, adrenal extracts were described [15] and, in 1910, the phenylethanolamines were first analyzed and the term *sympathomimetic* was coined [16]. Ahlquist first subdivided adrenoceptors into two types (α and β) according to the relative potency of different sympathomimetic amines. β Receptors were later subdivided into β_1 and β_2 subtypes. This was based on the relative selectivity of β_1-agonists to stimulate the heart (positive inotropic and chronotrophic effects) and of β_2-agonists to produce bronchial and vascular dilation. Around 1939, it was proposed that epinephrine was synthesized from tyrosine in the sympathetic nerve varicosity. Discovery in the late 1950s of the second-messenger system whereby receptor stimulation by hormones leads to increased adenylate cyclase, which converts adenosine triphosphate (ATP) to cyclic adenosine monophosphate (cAMP), an activator of kinase pathways, led to a Nobel prize in 1971 to Earl Sutherland [17,18].

Mechanisms of drug action

The adrenoceptors, which play a central role in many physiologic processes, belong to the family of G-protein-coupled receptors and are subjects of intensive research [19]. Sympathomimetics produce their effects either by direct stimulation of α- and β-adrenoceptors or indirectly by displacement of norepinephrine from vesicular or extravesicular binding sites in the presynaptic adrenergic nerve terminal (see Chapter 14). The displaced norepinephrine then stimulates α- and β-adrenoceptors at the neuroeffector junction. Pretreatment with reserpine depletes presynaptic norepinephrine stores, thus allowing separation of direct and indirect sympathomimetic effects [20]. Many drugs – "mixed-acting sympathomimetics" – have both direct and indirect actions [21].

The sympathomimetic amines are derivatives of β-phenylethanolamine (Fig. 40.4). This versatile molecule allows substitutions on the benzene ring (O-dihydroxybenzene is known as catechol, thus the name *catecholamines*), on the two carbons of the ethyl side chain, resulting in enantiomers, and on the amine terminal. The subtle differences in structure produce

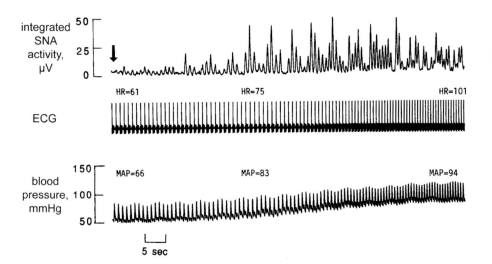

Figure 40.3. Integrated sympathetic nerve activity, heart rate, and blood pressure responses to incremental change in desflurane concentration. SNA, sympathetic nerve activity; HR, heart rate; ECG, electrocardiogram; MAP, mean arterial pressure.

not only marked differences in receptor binding and activation and metabolism of the drug but also effects on uptake mechanisms and the ratio of central to peripheral action [22]. The two-carbon distance between the benzene ring and the amine group ensures maximal sympathomimetic activity [23].

The understanding of interactions between drugs and receptors at the molecular level elucidates the significance of the subtle differences between the ligands. Computer-simulated docking arrangements to the β_2 receptor of epinephrine, ritodrine (a β_2-selective agonist), and propranolol (a β_2-antagonist) are illustrated in Fig. 40.5 [24]. The amine terminal of the agonist or antagonist forms a link with an aspartatic carboxylate group (113 on the β_2-receptor) in the third transmembrane helix of the β-adrenoceptor, and the result of this interaction affects coupling to, and activation of, adenylate cyclase by the receptor [25]. Except for phenylephrine, alkyl substitution on the amino group results in increased potency of the β_2 receptor. However, β_2-selectivity requires further substitutions on the phenylethanolamine base.

Hydrophobic substitutions on the aromatic ring and an increase in the distance between the amine group and the aromatic ring result in antagonist ligands [26]. A pouch is formed between the second and seventh transmembrane domains: in β_1 receptors a threonine is located at the base of this pocket, whereas in β_2 receptors a tyrosine residue overhangs the binding pocket [27]. Hydroxyl groups in the third and fifth position and large alkyl or aryl groups on the amino terminal contribute to β_2-receptor selectivity; the latter groups interact with the tyrosine residue in the seventh transmembrane domain [28]. Maximal α- and β-agonist activities depend on the presence of hydroxyl groups on positions 3 and 4 on the aromatic ring. Hydroxyl residues of serine 204 and 207 of the fifth transmembrane helix on the β receptor are believed to form hydrogen bonds with the catecholic hydroxyl groups [29] (Fig. 40.5). These amino acid residues not only serve as docking sites but also play an important role in regulating equilibrium dynamics between the receptor's active and inactive forms [30]. Loss of one or both hydroxyls results in dramatic reduction or complete loss of direct agonist activity.

Noncatecholamine sympathomimetics, which are missing one or both hydroxyl groups on the aromatic ring, elicit their effect by stimulating release of norepinephrine from sympathetic nerve terminals [20] (see *Indirect-acting sympathomimetics*, below). Furthermore, loss of aromatic hydroxyl groups increases the lipophilic characteristics of the compounds, allowing better penetration of the blood–brain barrier and enhancing central effects. These drugs are also resistant to metabolism by catechol-*O*-methyltransferase (COMT), which improves bioavailability and prolongs the duration of action.

Substitution at the α-carbon prevents oxidation of the compound by monoamine oxidases (MAOs), resulting in longer half-life and prolonged presence at the effector nerve terminals. This latter effect may cause prolonged presynaptic effects with sustained release of norepinephrine. One example is ephedrine, an indirect-acting sympathomimetic.

Substitution on the β-carbon increases potency on α and β receptors, but also reduces lipophilicity and lessens CNS effects. For example, β-hydroxylation of methamphetamine produces ephedrine (Fig. 40.4), which has reduced central potency but increased peripheral potency. β-Hydroxylation is necessary for storage in vesicles at the adrenergic presynaptic terminal. Substitutions at the α- and β-carbons result in stereoisomers. In general, α-carbon *d*-substitutions and β-carbon *l*-substitutions confer greater potency: *l*-epinephrine is 12 times more potent than *d*-epinephrine [31]. The coupling with an asparagine residue in the sixth transmembrane domain is responsible for the stereoselectivity of β-hydroxyl ligand binding [32].

There are now three known subtypes of each of the α_1-, α_2-, and β-adrenoceptor populations. These are $\alpha_{1A,B,C}$, $\alpha_{2A,B,C}$, and β_{1-3}. All β subtypes appear coupled to stimulation of adenylate cyclase, whereas α_2 subtypes appear coupled to inhibition of adenylate cyclase; in contrast, α_1-adrenoceptor subpopulations may couple to several effector systems (see Chapter 2).

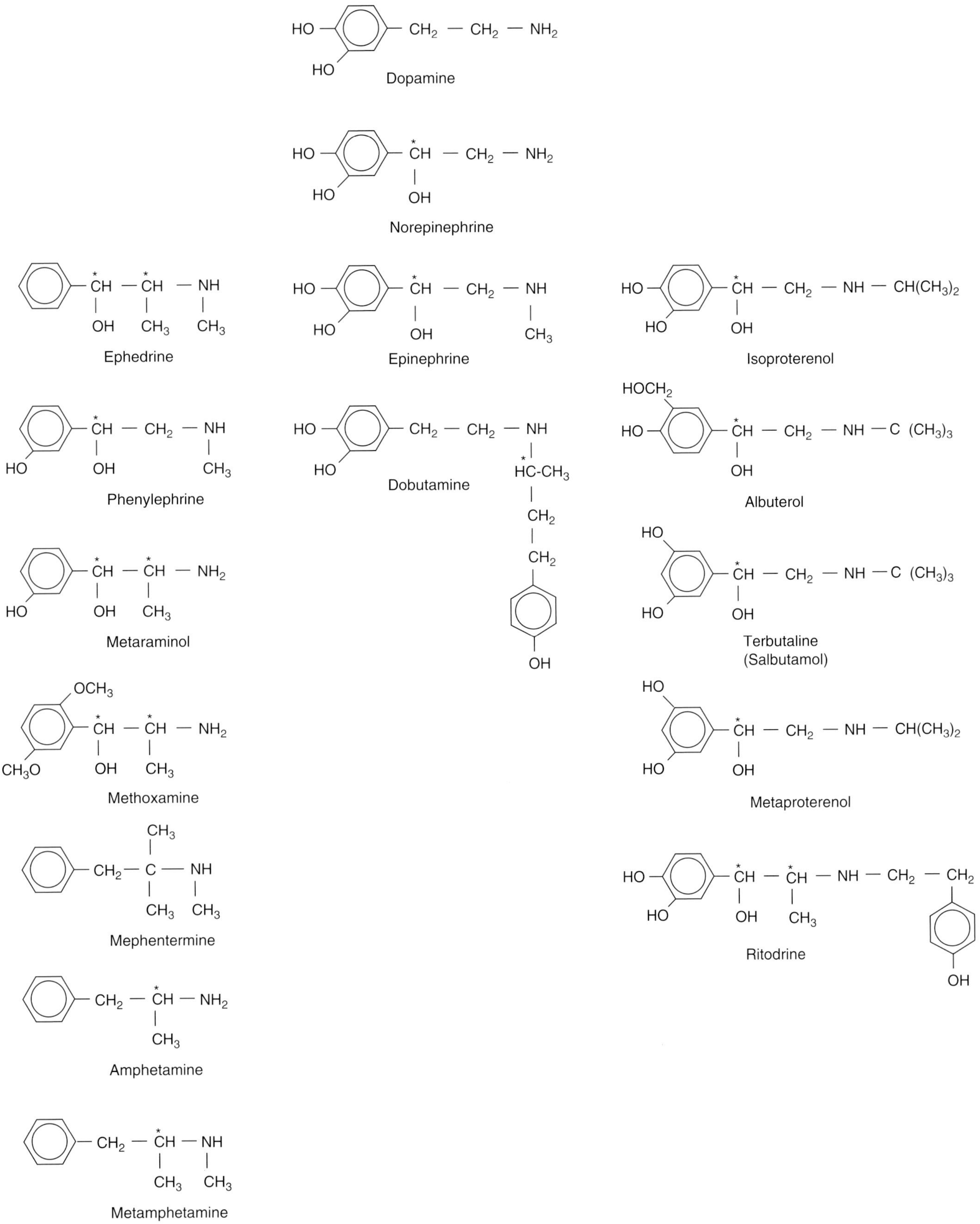

Figure 40.4. Structural formulas of phenylethanolamine sympathomimetics. (*Left*) Drugs with predominantly α-receptor agonist activity. (*Right*) β-Receptor agonists. (*Middle*) Drugs representing both receptor groups. Asterisks signal asymmetric carbons and existence of enantiomers.

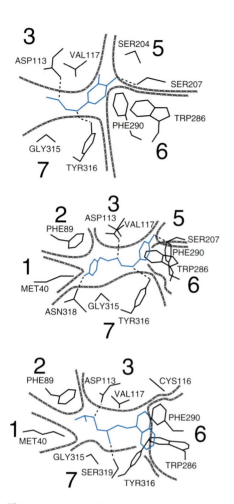

Figure 40.5. Ligand binding to the β₂ receptor. Computer-simulated models of docking of epinephrine (*top*), the β₂-agonist ritodrine (*middle*), and the nonselective β-receptor antagonist propranolol (*bottom*). The simulation presents a cross-section of the receptor, with the ligand binding site located toward the center portion. The ligands are displayed in blue. The corresponding numbers indicate the relative positions of the seven transmembrane helices. The fourth helix does not participate in the binding interaction. The amino groups of all three ligands proximate with aspartate₁₁₃ (ASP113) of the third transmembrane helix. Only the two agonists are linked with hydrogen bonds to the serine residues of the fifth helix. This interaction plays a central role in receptor activation. The tyrosine residue overhanging the binding pocket also forms links only with the agonists. Complex van der Waals interactions between hydrophobic amino acid residues and propranolol allow easy docking to the binding site. Modified from Kontoyianni *et al.* [24].

Clinical pharmacology of sympathomimetic drugs

Depending on the relative potency at the different subtypes of α and β receptors, the route of administration, and the degree of lipid solubility and biotransformation, a myriad of pharmacologic effects can be achieved by carefully selecting the drug to be used. For instance, norepinephrine has relatively little capacity to decrease bronchial resistance because the receptors in bronchial smooth muscle are largely of the β₂ subtype, whereas isoproterenol and epinephrine are both

potent bronchodilators. Blood vessels in skin express α₁ receptors, so norepinephrine and epinephrine constrict skin blood vessels but isoproterenol has little effect. The smooth muscle of vessels supplying skeletal muscle has both α₁ and β₂ receptors, so constriction or dilation of these vessels could occur with either of these drugs. But low physiological levels of epinephrine primarily activate the β₂ receptors while very high levels primarily activate the α₁ receptors. Thus a given adrenergic response depends on the receptor subtype and density in a given tissue and on the concentration of the sympathomimetic amines.

Anesthesiologists usually think of adrenergic agonists and antagonists in terms of their cardiovascular effects. But it must be remembered that the sympathomimetic drugs exert other effects on function such as tone of nonvascular smooth muscle, gland cell secretion, glycogenolysis, release of fatty acids from fat cells, secretion of insulin, renin, and pituitary hormones, and CNS effects. In the next part of this chapter, the cardiovascular and bronchiolar effects and clinical applications of the commonly used α- and β-agonists are reviewed, starting with pure agonists and ending with drugs that have multiple effects.

α₁- versus α₂-adrenoceptor agonists

Drugs that activate the α₁ receptors are located in the post-synaptic adrenergic neuron. Specific guanosine triphosphate (GTP)-binding proteins (G_{αq} proteins) interact with the α₁ receptors to activate phospholipase C to promote an increase in Ca²⁺ in smooth muscle (among other effects), which increases smooth-muscle tone. The general actions are arterial and venous vasoconstriction, decreased insulin release, and sphincter contraction.

Drugs that activate the α₂ receptors located in the presynaptic adrenergic neuron cause feedback inhibition of norepinephrine release. There are also α₂ receptors located in the postsynaptic adrenergic neuron that interact with specific GTP-binding proteins (G_{αi} proteins) to inactivate adenylate cyclase, which decreases cAMP levels and inactivates kinases, such as protein kinase A, leading to a decrease in smooth-muscle cell Ca²⁺. Overall, then, these drugs attenuate SNS activity by reducing norepinephrine release and by inactivating kinase pathways so that blood pressure and heart rate tend to be lowered. In the CNS these drugs induce sedation by a postsynaptic effect and reduce the pain threshold, as demonstrated by decreased general anesthetic and opioid requirements.

α₁-Adrenoceptor agonists
Phenylephrine

The physiologic effects of phenylephrine were first described in 1933 [33]. This drug was first used in anesthetic practice to sustain blood pressure during spinal anesthesia [34].

Phenylephrine differs from epinephrine only in lacking a hydroxy group at position 4 on the benzene ring. Phenylephrine (Fig. 40.4) is administered intravenously to counteract

Table 40.1. Recommended parenteral doses of α_1-receptor agonist drugs

Drug	IV bolus	Infusion (rate adjusted to effect)	IM/SC
Phenylephrine	40–200 µg (maximum 500 µg)	40–180 µg min^{-1}	2–5 mg IM or SC
Methoxamine	3–5 mg (1 mg min^{-1})	0.1–0.3 mg min^{-1}	10–15 mg IM
Metaraminol	0.5–5 mg	5 µg kg^{-1} min^{-1}	2–10 mg IM or SC
Mephentermine	15–30 mg	—	30–45 mg IM
Ephedrine	5–25 mg	0.5–5 mg min^{-1}	10–50 mg IM or SC

IM, intramuscular; SC, subcutaneous.

hypotension and to increase coronary and cerebral perfusion pressure. This drug is an almost pure α_1-selective agonist – only very high doses produce an effect on β receptors. Nevertheless, phenylephrine is only a partial agonist of the α_1 receptor. Because it increases vascular resistance in the skin, muscles, and renal and mesenteric vascular beds, it causes systolic and diastolic blood pressures to increase. Although a vasoconstrictor, phenylephrine has a net effect to increase coronary and cerebral blood flow due to the systemic-induced increases in cerebral and coronary (diastolic) perfusion pressures. Heart rate slows secondary to vagally mediated reflex bradycardia. Phenylephrine is probably a pulmonary arterial vasoconstrictor in humans [35], although the increases in diastolic and mean pulmonary artery blood pressures are more likely caused by translocation of the circulating blood volume from the systemic to the pulmonary capillary and venous pools. Compared with ephedrine, phenylephrine is inferior in maintaining placental blood flow during cesarean delivery under spinal anesthesia [36]. Table 40.1 shows the recommended parenteral doses for phenylephrine and other α_1-receptor agonists.

Topical phenylephrine is popular as a nasal decongestant or mydriatic. It is available in 0.25%, 0.5%, or 1% solutions for nasal decongestion and as 2.5% or 10% eye drops. However, when large doses are instilled to constrict nasal mucosa before ear, nose, and throat surgery, or to control bleeding after adenoidectomy, severe systemic effects (pulmonary edema, cardiac arrest) may occur; fatalities have been described even in American Society of Anesthesiologists (ASA) physical status I patients [37]. Inadequate management by the anesthesiologist, including deepening of inhalational anesthesia and administration of intravenous β-blocking drugs, contributed to the adverse outcome; on the contrary, no intervention to

reduce severe hypertension produced a good outcome [37]. An advisory committee for the New York State Department of Health recommended that the initial dose of phenylephrine should not exceed 0.5 mg (four drops of the 0.25% solution) in adults or 20 µg kg^{-1} in children. Mild-to-moderate hypertension should be looked for, and severe hypertension should be treated with either α_1-adrenergic antagonists, such as phentolamine or tolazoline, or direct-acting vasodilating drugs, such as hydralazine [37]. Excessive doses of phenylephrine for patients undergoing cataract surgery under general anesthesia can cause severe hypertension soon after surgery, necessitating administration of vasodilating drugs.

Methoxamine

The pharmacologic properties of methoxamine were first described in 1948 [38], and in 1950 methoxamine was used to maintain blood pressure during spinal anesthesia [39].

Although methoxamine (Fig. 40.4) has similar pharmacologic properties, but a longer duration of action than phenylephrine, large doses of methoxamine have an inhibitory effect on β receptors and may produce bradycardia [40]. In the elderly, and in those with a history of myocardial ischemia, a slow intravenous infusion of methoxamine may be superior to ephedrine in maintaining blood pressure during spinal anesthesia, because the potential for atrial tachyarrhythmias is less with methoxamine while coronary perfusion is maintained. Methoxamine has a prolonged duration of action when compared with other α_1-receptor agonists, and rebound hypertension may occur more frequently after recovery from spinal anesthesia [39]. Methoxamine is not often used to treat acute hypotension because of its long half-life. Dosage is 1–5 mg every 15 minutes to raise blood pressure.

Midodrine

Midodrine is an orally absorbed α_1-agonist used to treat autonomic failure and dialysis-related hypotension [41]; its active metabolite desglymidodrine differs from methoxamine only in lacking a methyl group. Its half-life is about 3 hours, so duration of action is 4–6 hours. This drug may be useful in treating patients with autonomic insufficiency and postural hypotension, but supine hypertension can occur.

Metaraminol, mephentermine, and the topical α_1-receptor agonists

Metaraminol (Fig. 40.4) was first used in anesthetic practice in 1954 [42]. It not only directly stimulates α_1 receptors but it also has a significant indirect effect on adrenergic terminals to stimulate release of norepinephrine; the *l*-isomer is responsible for the presynaptic effects [43]. It also has β_1 effects, and so has a positive inotropic effect on the myocardium due to the peripheral release of norepinephrine and its cotransmitters. Metaraminol is typically used to treat hypotensive states and to relieve attacks of paroxysmal atrial tachycardia. Dosage is

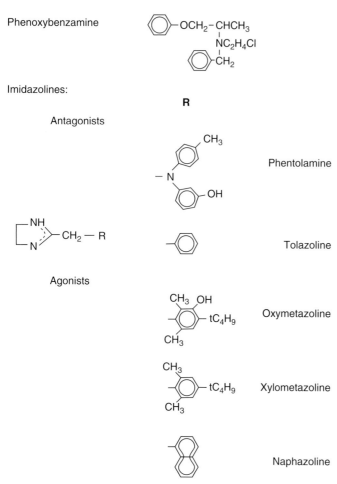

Phenoxybenzamine

Imidazolines:

Antagonists

R

Phentolamine

Tolazoline

Agonists

Oxymetazoline

Xylometazoline

Naphazoline

Figure 40.6. Structural formulas of phenoxybenzamine and the imidazoline-derivative α-receptor agonists and antagonists.

$0.1–0.5$ μg kg^{-1} min^{-1}. When discontinued after long use, metaraminol can lead to hypotension due to norepinephrine depletion.

Mephentermine (Fig. 40.4) also is a combined direct- and indirect-acting α$_1$-receptor agonist that produces a positive inotropic effect and a variable heart rate response, depending on the balance between indirect sympathetic stimulation and baroreflex-mediated inhibition of the heart. It has a prompt onset of action (5–15 minutes) and its antihypotensive effects can last for hours.

Topically active imidazoline derivatives (*naphazoline, oxymetazoline, xylometazoline,* and *tetrahydrozoline*) (Fig. 40.6) are used for the vasoconstriction of the conjunctiva and nasal mucosa. Their systemic absorption is much less than that of phenylephrine, and they are regarded as safer than phenylephrine for nasal vasoconstriction [44].

α$_2$-Adrenoceptor agonists
Clonidine

Clonidine, an imidazoline first synthesized in the 1960s, was found to produce a vasoconstrictor effect that was mediated by α-adrenoceptors. During testing clonidine also was found to cause sedation, hypotension, and bradycardia, which are not typical of α$_1$-adrenergic drugs. Clonidine is now known as a central and peripheral α$_{1,2}$-adrenergic agonist. It is used to treat drug withdrawal syndrome and has mild antihypertensive effects. Although clonidine can increase blood pressure when given intravenously, when the drug is given orally SNS activity from the brain decreases due to activation of α$_2$-adrenoceptors in the cardiovascular control centers of the CNS. The drug has a half-life of 6–24 hours.

Guanidine derivatives, α-methyldopa, and dexmedetomidine

Guanfacine and *guanabenz* are guanidine-derivative antihypertensive drugs that are structurally and functionally similar to clonidine. Guanabenz is metabolized extensively and may be safer in patients with renal failure but more problematic in those with cirrhosis [45]. Side effects of the guanidine derivatives are similar but milder than those for clonidine, and withdrawal symptoms occur less frequently [46].

α-Methyldopa produces a metabolite, α-methyl-norepinephrine, that produces a clonidine-like α$_2$-agonist effect in cardiovascular control centers that results in an antihypertensive effect due to reduced sympathetic outflow [47]. In addition, α-methyl-norepinephrine inhibits dopa-decarboxylase, and because it is resistant to breakdown by MAO it replaces norepinephrine in the storage vesicles, leading to the depletion of presynaptic norepinephrine stores. Rebound hypertension is unusual after discontinuation of the drug.

In addition to the side effects associated with the other members of this group, acquired hemolytic anemia and liver dysfunction may occur in patients taking α-methyldopa, and the drug is contraindicated in patients with cirrhosis or active liver disease. A positive direct Coombs test (formation of antibodies against red blood cells) occurs in 10–20% of patients receiving α-methyldopa therapy. Because a positive test result may delay or interfere with the cross-matching of blood for transfusion, the blood bank should be notified about this possibility as soon as possible. α-Methyldopa is used primarily to depress overall SNS activity but also can cause sedation, psychosis, and depression. It has very slow onset (4–6 hours) and very long duration of action (10–16 hours) and so is seldom used to control blood pressure. The pharmacokinetic characteristics and recommended dosing of the guanidine derivatives and α-methyldopa are presented in Table 40.2.

Dexmedetomidine is a relatively selective α$_2$- over α$_1$- (1620 : 1) adrenoceptor agonist used for continuous sedation in the intensive care setting. Presynaptic activation of these receptors hinders release of norepinephrine and postsynaptic activation of the receptors in the CNS and causes sedation and inhibition of SNS activity with a decrease in blood pressure and heart rate. Dexmedetomidine has sedative- and analgesia-sparing effects via central actions in the locus coeruleus and in

Table 40.2. Pharmacokinetic characteristics and recommended dosing of some common α_2-adrenoceptor agonist drugs

Drug	Bioavailability	Protein binding	Metabolism	Excretion	Half–life	Recommended dose
Guanfacine	~ 80%	70%	55%, liver	Renal	14 h	1–2 mg daily
Guanabenz	20–30%	10%	~ 100%, liver	Gastrointestinal, renal	3–4 h	8–32 mg daily
α-Methyldopa	8–62%	83%	Liver	Renal	1.5–2 h	1–2 g daily; max 4g[a]

[a] In children, the recommended starting daily dose is 10 mg kg^{-1} with a maximum of 65 mg kg^{-1} or 3 g, whichever is less.

the dorsal horn of the spinal cord, respectively [48,49]. Patients receiving dexmedetomidine for postsurgical pain had significantly slower early postoperative heart rates and required less than half the amount of morphine in the postanesthesia care unit (PACU) compared with a control group receiving only morphine [50]. Moreover, over half of the dexmedetomidine-treated patients had not requested additional analgesia at 1 hour into the recovery period.

There are a number of other drugs discussed elsewhere that have mild α_2-adrenergic effects in addition to their more pronounced effects on β_1, β_2, or α_1 receptors; these are dopamine, ephedrine, mephentermine, norepinephrine, and metaraminol.

β_1- versus β_2-adrenoceptor activity

Stimulation of β_1-adrenoceptors, located mostly in the heart, activates specific G proteins that stimulate adenylate cyclase to form more cAMP; this in turn activates protein kinases, which leads to increased cellular Ca^{2+}, among other effects. The net effect is an increase in heart rate and the force of myocardial contractility, and therefore an increase in cardiac output. Myocardial relaxation and diastolic filling time also increase.

Stimulation of β_2 receptors in the postsynaptic terminals activates pathways similar to those described above, resulting in decreased smooth-muscle Ca^{2+}, among other effects. The net action is peripheral arteriolar dilation in muscular, splanchnic, and renal vasculature. This leads to a reduction in vascular resistance and a decrease in diastolic blood pressure, whereas the increase or decrease of systolic blood pressure is a function of the change in cardiac output. Stimulation of β_2 receptors, also abundant in bronchial and enteric smooth muscle, leads to bronchodilation and slowing of peristalsis; it also inhibits activation of T cells [51] and release of cytokines from airway smooth-muscle cells [52]. Increased glycogenolysis in the liver is partially counterbalanced by activation of pancreatic islet cells by β receptors. Lipolysis is mediated by activation of β_3 receptors [53]. The commonly observed skeletal muscle tremor with β-agonist therapy is mediated by β_2 receptors [54].

Tables 42.2 and 42.3 (Chapter 42) furnish a list of commonly used β-adrenergic antagonists and their pharmacokinetic/pharmacodynamic profiles. Their chemical structures are shown in Figs. 40.4 and 42.7.

β_1-Adrenoceptor agonists
Isoproterenol (isoprenaline)

Isoproterenol (Fig. 40.4), the isopropyl derivative of norepinephrine, was the first synthetic β-receptor agonist in clinical use. Isoproterenol is nonselective in its β-receptor effects and has a low affinity for α receptors. Its chronotropic and dromotropic effects are caused by stimulation of β_1 and β_2 receptors [55], whereas the inotropic effect is mediated predominantly by β_1 receptors [56]. Isoproterenol lowers peripheral vascular resistance, primarily in skeletal muscle but also in renal and mesenteric vascular beds. This may result in a fall in diastolic pressure and maintained systolic pressure. This drug relaxes mostly gastrointestinal and bronchial smooth muscle and therefore can relieve bronchoconstriction.

Isoproterenol is rapidly absorbed if applied to mucous membranes but undergoes extensive metabolism by liver COMT if administered enterally. Although isoproterenol is a poor substrate of MAO, and its neuronal uptake is less than that of norepinephrine, its duration of action is brief when administered parenterally. Hence isoproterenol is administered as a continuous infusion. Current clinical indications include bradycardia caused by heart block and treatment of torsades de pointes ventricular tachycardia. Cardiac effects of isoproterenol may lead to palpitations, sinus tachycardia, and serious dysrhythmias. The use of isoproterenol as an inotropic drug has declined since the emergence of dobutamine and phosphodiesterase inhibitors. As a bronchodilator, the β_2-selective drugs have largely replaced isoproterenol. Headache, anxiety and restlessness, tremor, and skin flushes are other common side effects of isoproterenol.

β_2-Adrenoceptor agonists

Agonists that are selective for the β_2-adrenoceptors were developed to reduce the cardiovascular side effects of nonselective β-receptor agonists in the treatment of bronchial asthma. Changing the catechol ring (3,4-dihydroxybenzene) to a resorcinol ring (3,5-dihydroxybenzene) improved bioavailability, because these molecules are not methylated by COMT. Further substitutions on the amino group resulted in increased β-receptor activity and reduced α-receptor activity. This chemical change also increased the duration of action caused by decreased metabolism by MAOs [57]. These modifications led to drugs such as metaproterenol, terbutaline, and albuterol, which are not substrates for COMT. However, all currently used β_2-selective agonists are only relatively selective; they also stimulate the β_1 receptor at greater concentrations.

Further reduction in systemic side effects of β_2-adrenoceptor agonists was achieved by aerosolized administration of these drugs, as the drug reaches therapeutic concentrations in the bronchi with minimal activation of cardiac and peripheral β receptors [58]. Aerosol therapy depends on the delivery of drugs to distal airways, which in turn depends on the size of the particles, the inspiratory flow rate, tidal volume, breath-holding time, and airway diameter. Only about 10% of the aerosolized dose actually enters the lungs, although some is swallowed and ultimately absorbed. Therapeutic effects of these drugs may include suppression of release of leukotrienes and histamine from mast cells and decreased microvascular permeability.

Despite the advantages of the use of an inhalational β_2-receptor agonist, there is still an increase in the risk for arrhythmias (predominantly atrial fibrillation), necessitating hospital admission for patients with congestive heart failure [59]. Other potential adverse effects, particularly when the drug is given orally or parenterally, are skeletal muscle tremor, tachycardia, mismatching of ventilation and perfusion in the lungs, and pulmonary edema. Long-term use can lead to tolerance, bronchial hyperreactivity, and, in diabetic patients, hyperglycemia. (See Chapter 47 regarding use of β_2-selective agonists for bronchial asthma and chronic obstructive airway disease.)

Terbutaline, albuterol, and other β_2-receptor agonists

Terbutaline (Fig. 40.4) contains a resorcinol ring and therefore is not a substrate for methylation by COMT. It can be administered orally, subcutaneously, or by inhalation. It is rapidly effective by the latter two routes and effects may persist for 3–6 hours. It is used primarily long-term for obstructive pulmonary disease, and acutely for status asthmaticus, bronchospasm, and acute anaphylactic shock, where it does not have the cardiac-stimulating effects of epinephrine.

Albuterol (Fig. 40.4) is similar to terbutaline, although it is not given subcutaneously. Use of inhaled albuterol has been described in hyperkalemic familial periodic paralysis; two to four metered doses of albuterol halted the progress of both hyperkalemia and paralysis [60]. Similar emergency treatment for hyperkalemia was successful for patients in renal failure [61]. Therefore, not surprisingly, continuous infusion of β-agonists may lead to hypokalemia. There are at least seven additional inhalational β_2-receptor agonists that are marketed with actions very similar to terbutaline and albuterol but varying durations of onset and effect; these are *isoetharine, pirbuterol, bitolterol, fenoterol, formoterol, procaterol,* and *salmeterol.*

Ritodrine

The β_2-selective agonist ritodrine (Fig. 40.4) is used as a uterine relaxant to arrest premature labor [62]. Ritodrine is usually started intravenously and is continued as an oral drug if uterine contractions have stopped. Oral bioavailability is about 30%. Ritodrine is metabolized in the liver to form inactive conjugates, and about half the drug is excreted unchanged in the urine. Pulmonary edema with normal pulmonary capillary wedge pressures has been attributed to ritodrine therapy [63].

Mixed α-, β-, and dopaminergic adrenoceptor agonists

It is not surprising that some neurotransmitters have a broad effect on many types of receptors. Changing environmental conditions, such as life-threatening danger, injury, or loss of blood, may necessitate redistribution of blood from one organ to another, e.g., between splanchnic, coronary, muscle, and skin circulations, in addition to bronchodilation, an increase in blood sugar, and increases in heart rate, cardiac contractility, and peripheral vascular resistance. To engage this multiplicity of effects, natural neurotransmitters such as epinephrine and dopamine must have mixed effects on a variety of receptors. Pharmacologic biochemists have since modified natural neurotransmitters or created new molecules to selectively stimulate a receptor type or subtype for a given activity. These research and developmental advances have greatly expanded not only our knowledge of the receptor subtypes and their mechanisms of action, but also the range or treatment options.

Epinephrine (adrenaline)

Epinephrine (Fig. 40.4) is a natural catecholamine sympathetic transmitter. This hormone, secreted primarily by the adrenal medulla, has complex effects on adrenoceptors triggered in the "fight and flight" startle reaction. It has potent and rapid iontropic and chronotropic effects by β_1-adrenergic stimulation, and vasoconstrictor (precapillary resistance vessels and large veins) and vaso- and bronchodilatory effects via its α_1- and β_2-adrenoceptors. The relative effect on these receptors depends on the route of administration and the concentration of epinephrine given. When given as an intravenous bolus, the net effect on the circulation is a rapid rise in blood pressure, particularly systolic pressure. Part of the increase in blood pressure is due to the increase in cardiac contractility, but much of the increase results from increased venous return to the heart by the Starling mechanism. Epinephrine can cause a substantial redistribution of blood flow away from skin and visceral organs to skeletal muscle and the heart.

Epinephrine is not usually administered intravenously except as a cardiac stimulant (0.25–1 mg) with defibrillation after cardiac arrest, although some use epinephrine in small doses like ephedrine to increase blood pressure and heart rate. Epinephrine ($0.1–1\ \mu g\ kg^{-1}\ min^{-1}$ IV) can also be useful for inotropic support in low cardiac output states due to low heart rate and stroke volume with low to normal systemic vascular resistance. Epinephrine is efficacious for its β_2-adrenergic effects when given subcutaneously (0.1–0.5 mg) for broncho-dilation in treating acute asthma or in treating acute severe allergic reactions. Because of its broad effects, epinephrine has limited clinical uses. It is often more practical and appropriate to use adrenergic-acting drugs that have more selective effects on α and β receptors.

Norepinephrine (noradrenaline)

Norepinephrine (Fig. 40.4) is the only natural transmitter secreted by postganglionic adrenergic nerve terminals. It is the natural precursor molecule to epinephrine. Like epineph-rine, it is also a hormone released by the adrenal medulla, but in smaller amounts. Its dominant α_1 over β_2 effects make it a more effective venous and arterial vasoconstrictor than epinephrine, with lesser – but effective – positive inotropic and chronotropic actions mediated by β_1-receptor activation. Norepinephrine is equipotent to epinephrine in stimulating β_1 receptors but has relatively little effect on β_2 receptors.

Cardiovascular effects of intravenous norepinephrine infu-sion ($0.04–0.40\ \mu g\ kg^{-1}\ min^{-1}$) are an increase in both systolic and diastolic pressures, increased stroke volume, but unchanged or decreased cardiac output due to a reflex decrease in heart rate, and increased peripheral vascular resistance. Unlike epinephrine, small concentrations of norepinephrine do not cause vasodilation, or lower blood pressure, because norepinephrine only constricts vessels. Because of this effect, care must be taken to prevent necrosis from extravascular perfusion of norepinephrine and ischemic damage to organs such as kidneys and intestines with continued use.

Dopamine

Dopamine (Fig. 40.4) is the immediate metabolic precursor of norepinephrine and epinephrine. As a central neurotransmit-ter, dopamine has an important action in regulating movement, but infused dopamine does not enter the CNS. Dopamine has mixed agonist effects via dopaminergic (D) and α- and β-adrenoceptors. At low concentrations ($1–5\ \mu g\ kg^{-1}\ min^{-1}$) dopamine leads to vasodilation, especially in renal, mesenteric, and coronary beds via D_1 receptors; this effect is mediated by increasing the concentration of cAMP via activation of adeny-late cyclase. The increase in renal blood flow may be associated with increased glomerular filtration rate, Na^+ excretion, and diuresis.

At higher concentrations ($5–50\ \mu g\ kg^{-1}\ min^{-1}$) dopamine stimulates β_1-adrenoceptors directly and indirectly by release of norepinephrine from nerve terminals. Dopamine is not nearly as potent as epinephrine or norepinephrine in aug-menting cardiac contractility or heart rate at comparable concentrations. Dopamine also stimulates α_1 receptors to

increase venous return and boost blood pressure. The com-bined effect of α- and β-adrenergic stimulation is an increase in systolic pressure with minimal change in diastolic pres-sure and no change in peripheral vascular resistance at low concentrations but an increase at higher concentrations. With all sympathomimetic drugs there is increased risk of supraventricular tachycardia and ventricular tachycardia, but this is somewhat less with dopamine administration. Because dopamine is a substrate for MAO, it should be administered at a fraction of the concentrations normally used if the patient is taking a MAO inhibitor (MAOI) or tricyclic antidepressant.

An almost selective D_1-receptor agonist is fenoldopam. The $R(+)$ isomer is 200 times more potent than the $S(-)$ isomer. Fenoldopam has a small effect on α_1 receptors, but it is never-theless used primarily to treat acute malignant hypertension.

Dobutamine

The synthetic catecholamine dobutamine (Fig. 40.4) exerts its effects primarily on β_1-adrenoceptors, with lesser effects on β_2 and α_1 receptors. Dobutamine is a racemic mixture. Of the two enantiomeric forms the $(-)$ isomer is a potent agonist at α_1 receptors, whereas the $(+)$ form is a potent α_1-adrenoceptor antagonist; this effect blocks much of the α_1-agonist effects of the $(-)$ form of dobutamine. Thus compared to norepineph-rine it is not as good a vasoconstrictor. As a result of its complex effects on adrenoceptors, dobutamine has a relatively more prominent inotropic than chronotropic effect on the heart compared to isoproterenol. Because dobutamine has no effects on D_1 receptors, it does not cause renal vasodilation at lower concentrations like dopamine. Dobutamine is not as potent as epinephrine or isoproterenol in increasing heart rate and contractility. Dobutamine is used mostly as a stimulant in conducting a resting cardiac stress test and to treat acute moderate heart failure, for example after a moderate myocar-dial infarction or cardiac surgery. Intravenous dosage is $0.5–30\ \mu g\ kg^{-1}\ min^{-1}$, titrated to cardiac and vascular effects.

Indirect-acting sympathomimetics

It was long believed that sympathomimetic drugs exerted their effects by acting directly on adrenoceptors. This assumption was dispelled when it was found that chronic postganglionic denervation, or treatment with reserpine or cocaine, reduced or abolished the effects of tyramine and other catecholamines. In this case, exogenously administered norepinephrine and epinephrine caused accentuated effects. It was found that tyr-amine and other catecholamines were taken up into the adre-nergic nerve terminal where they displaced the norepinephrine from storage vesicles and across the synaptic clefts to activate the postsynaptic receptors. The depletion of catecholamines in the nerve terminals after reserpine explained the lack of effect of tyramine. In the case of cocaine, the neuronal transport of catecholamines becomes inhibited and tyramine and related amines cannot enter the adrenergic terminal. Cocaine inhibits effects of indirectly acting catecholamines but potentiates effects of directly acting catecholamines normally removed by neuronal transport.

Drugs that may have indirect effects are assessed by their actions after chronic reserpine treatment. Tyramine is almost completely an indirect-acting sympathomimetic amine, as it has little direct effect on the noradrenergic postsynaptic receptor site.

False transmitters and MAO inhibition

Monoamine oxidase is an enzyme in the cells of most tissues that catalyzes the oxidation of monoamines such as norepinephrine, serotonin (MAO-A), phenylethylamine (MAO-B), and dopamine (MAO-A,B). MAO inhibitors (MAOIs) are a class of powerful drugs (phenelzine, iproclozide, isocarboxazid, tranylcypromine, selegiline, rasagiline, moclobemide) used to treat depression and Parkinson's disease. Because of lethal dietary and drug interactions, MAOIs are generally taken only when other classes of antidepressants are unsuccessful. Dietary amines, e.g., tyramine derived from fermentation reactions in cheese, wine, and beer, can cause a hypertensive reaction in patients taking a MAOI.

Although tyrosine, and not tyramine, is the precursor to catecholamines, tyrosine can be decarboxylated to tyramine. In the presence of MAOIs, tyramine is less metabolized and competes with tyrosine in the synaptic vesicles, thereby displacing norepinephrine from the storage vesicles to provoke a hypertensive crisis. Long-term use of MAOIs may mediate the metabolism of tyramine to octopamine by β-hydroxylation, which can act as a "false transmitter" and be released like the endogenous transmitter norepinephrine. Octopamine has presynaptic agonist activity, but it is a weak postsynaptic agonist, so it tends to reduce adrenergic transmission over time.

Ephedrine

The physiologic effects of ephedrine were described in 1887 [64], but it was not until the 1920s that the drug was introduced into Western medicine [13] and clinical anesthesia. Ephedrine (Fig. 40.4) is a mixed-acting sympathomimetic: it has both direct and indirect stimulating effects on α- and β-adrenoceptors. Intravenous administration causes rapid increases in heart rate, cardiac output, and blood pressure that last 10–15 minutes; repeat doses have a decreasing effect (tachyphylaxis) [65]. Intramuscular injection has a slower rate of onset (5–10 minutes), but a longer duration of effect (35–45 minutes). Ephedrine has a half-life of 3–6 hours and is eliminated largely unchanged in the urine.

Ephedrine has a stimulatory effect on the CNS, relaxes bronchial smooth muscle, and increases trigone and sphincter muscle tone in the urinary bladder. Uterine and placental artery blood flow is not adversely affected when ephedrine is used to sustain blood pressure during spinal anesthesia for cesarean section [36], and umbilical artery vascular resistance remains unchanged [66,67]. Although ephedrine is

effective in maintaining or restoring blood pressure during spinal anesthesia when administered intravenously [68], preemptive intramuscular administration of the drug is not a reliable preventive measure [69].

Amphetamine and other central nervous system stimulants

Amphetamine and methamphetamine are powerful stimulants of the CNS in addition to their peripheral α and β actions common to indirect-acting sympathomimetics drugs. They cause the release and inhibit the reuptake of stimulatory neurotransmitters in the cortex, the motor nuclei, and the reticular activating system. Some acute consequences are wakefulness, alertness, mood elevation, a reduced sense of fatigue, increased initiative, self-confidence, euphoria, and elation. These two drugs have mild analgesic effects and may stimulate respiration obtunded by centrally acting drugs. Their peripheral indirect sympathomimetic activity leads to an acute increase in blood pressure and secondary bradycardia; large doses may cause arrhythmias [70]. Chronic use may lead to a decrease in blood pressure because d-amphetamine and d-methamphetamine are metabolized to a false neurotransmitter. Although amphetamine and methamphetamine are sometimes used to suppress appetite [71] their effect is not sustained, and tolerance and dependence often occur [72]. Amphetamine and methamphetamine are Schedule II drugs because psychological dependence often occurs with chronic use. Even though therapeutic use of has declined, their respective methylenedioxy derivatives "ice" and "ecstasy" remain popular illicit recreational drugs [73].

Repeated intoxication with amphetamine or its synthetic congeners is characterized by increasing restlessness, agitation, and irritability that progress to confusion, aggressive behavior, delirium, depression, fatigue, and paranoid delusions. Differentiation from acute schizophrenia may be difficult. Headache, shivering, palpitation and tachycardia, hypertension, and flushed or pale skin are followed by central chest pain, cardiac arrhythmias, and hypotension. Dry mouth, a metallic taste, nausea, vomiting, and abdominal cramps are the leading gastrointestinal symptoms. In fatal poisoning, convulsions, coma, and circulatory collapse are the terminal events. Gross hyperthermia, rhabdomyolysis, disseminated intravascular coagulopathy, and hepatorenal failure leading to death are most common with "ecstasy," but have also been attributed to amphetamine overdose. Treatment of acute intoxication consists of acidification of urine to enhance elimination, administration of sedatives, and control of cardiovascular side effects. Dantrolene is indicated in the event of hyperthermia [74].

Methylphenidate is a structural relative of amphetamine. It has milder CNS-stimulating activity and less effect on motor function. Methylphenidate is used to treat narcolepsy and attention-deficit hyperactivity disorder. Side effects of insomnia, anorexia, weight loss, suppression of growth, and abdominal pain have been described in children. Overdose causes symptoms similar to those of overdose with amphetamine; again, treatment is supportive.

Ergot alkaloids

Known as St. Anthony's fire in the Middle Ages, the poisoning caused by contamination of wheat or rye with the fungus *Claviceps purpurea* was characterized by mental disturbance and severe, painful peripheral vasoconstriction often leading to gangrene of the extremities.

The ergot alkaloids stimulate contraction of a variety of smooth muscles, both directly and indirectly by adrenergic and serotoninergic receptors. Contraction of vascular smooth muscle leads to coronary, cerebral, and peripheral vasoconstriction. Reflex bradycardia is commonly associated with the increase in blood pressure.

When taken orally, the alkaloids are slowly absorbed from the gut, and bioavailability is approximately 10%. The drugs are eliminated mainly in metabolized form in the bile. A number of ergot alkaloids have been isolated: *ergotamine* is used to treat migraine headaches, and *ergonovine* (also called ergometrine) is used to enhance postpartum uterine contractions.

Intravenous administration of the ergot alkaloids can produce sudden severe hypertension and should be avoided. The oral dose of ergotamine for acute migraine is 2 mg, followed by 1 mg dosages every half-hour to a maximum of 6 mg. The intramuscular dosage is 0.5 mg, repeated every half-hour to a maximum of 3 mg. Intramuscular administration of ergonovine (0.2 mg) is used to enhance postpartum uterine contractions; this dosage may be continued up to a week postpartum as an oral preparation. Contraindications to ergot alkaloids include peripheral and coronary artery disease, thyrotoxicosis, and porphyria [75].

Other sympathomimetic drugs

Pseudoephedrine and *phenylpropanolamine* are mostly commonly used as oral preparations to treat nasal congestion. They are similar to ephedrine with fewer CNS effects. Several drugs are used primarily as vasoconstrictors for local application to the nasal mucous membranes or to the eye. Examples of these are *propylhexedrine, tetrahydrozoline, oxymetazoline, naphazoline,* and *xylometazoline.*

Sympatholytic drugs

Sympatholytics (also known as *antiadrenergics*) are drugs that oppose the effects of impulses conveyed by adrenergic postganglionic fibers of the sympathetic nervous system.

Mechanisms of drug action

Sympatholytics may produce their effects in three ways: they can block α-adrenoceptors, the main result being dilation of peripheral blood vessels; they can selectively block β-adrenoceptors, the

principal pharmacologic target being the heart and vascular smooth muscle; or they can block nicotinic transmission in the sympathetic ganglia. Chapter 42 covers β-adrenoceptor antagonists. Almost all the drugs that act postsynaptically, with the exception of phenoxybenzamine, compete reversibly with agonists for the α- and β-adrenoceptors.

Clinical pharmacology of α-adrenoceptor antagonists

This class of drug, also called α-blockers, play an important role in regulating the activity of the SNS both peripherally and centrally. Blockade of α_2-adrenoceptors with selective antagonists such as yohimbine can potentiate release of norepinephrine to activate both α_1 and α_2 receptors. Antagonists to α_1-adrenoceptors such as prazosin may also stimulate release of norepinephrine but the α_1-receptor effect is blocked.

Phenoxybenzamine

Phenoxybenzamine (Fig. 40.6) is a haloalkylamine compound and an irreversible noncompetitive blocker of α-adrenoceptors. It forms a covalent link with the receptor, and recovery of receptor function requires synthesis of new receptor molecules. This sympatholytic binds to and inactivates not only α_1 and α_2 receptors, but also proteins responsible for neuronal and non-neuronal uptake of norepinephrine.

The reduction in peripheral vascular resistance is accompanied by reflex sympathetic stimulation of cardiac β_1 receptors and an increase in cardiac output. Phenoxybenzamine blocks sympathetic presynaptic inhibitory α_2 receptors in the heart and decreases elimination of myocardial norepinephrine secondary to inhibition of uptake mechanisms; these effects also contribute to the observed increase in cardiac output. Orthostatic hypotension is a characteristic of phenoxybenzamine, because baroreceptor mechanisms cannot be activated when the patient is erect [76]. Furthermore, unopposed vascular β_2-receptor stimulation may decrease vascular resistance even more.

Phenoxybenzamine is administered orally to induce hypotension. Although its half-life is approximately 18–24 hours, the duration of action depends on the cellular turnover rate of the alkylated α receptors. The major adverse effect is postural hypotension. Phenoxybenzamine remains the preferred drug for management of pheochromocytoma [77]. The unique noncompetitive nature of its α-receptor blockade prevents receptor activation by sudden catecholamine surges during surgical manipulation of the tumor. The recommended daily dose is 1–2 mg kg^{-1}. Phenoxybenzamine is also used to alleviate urinary retention caused by neurogenic bladder or benign prostatic hypertrophy [78]. The recommended dose for relief of obstruction in neurogenic bladder is 0.3–0.5 mg kg^{-1} per day in children and 10–20 mg per day in adults.

Imidazoline receptor drugs: phentolamine and tolazoline

Phentolamine and tolazoline (Fig. 40.6) are competitive non-selective α-receptor antagonists. Although these drugs have cardiovascular effects similar to those of phenoxybenzamine, α-blockade is short-lived and the effects are reversible with α-receptor agonists. Phentolamine and tolazoline can be used to treat a hypertensive crisis due to ingestion of tyramine-containing substances in patients taking MAOIs.

Tolazoline has been used to treat persistent pulmonary hypertension of the newborn [79]. Major side effects are hypotension with reflex tachycardia, arrhythmias, and pulmonary and gastrointestinal hemorrhages. Unfortunately, improved oxygenation in these newborns did not result in an improved survival rate. Since the introduction of inhaled nitric oxide, the use of tolazoline in the treatment of pulmonary hypertension has declined [80]. Tolazoline has a plasma half-life of 3–13 hours. It is excreted mainly unchanged by the kidney. The recommended dose for the treatment of persistent pulmonary hypertension of the newborn is $0.5–2$ mg kg^{-1} h^{-1} following a $0.5–2$ mg kg^{-1} loading dose administered over 10 minutes. Using a 0.5 mg load and 0.5 mg kg^{-1} h^{-1} infusion rate appears to prevent accumulation of the drug.

Piperazinyl quinazoles

Prazosin is the prototype for a family of α-adrenergic drugs that contain a piperazinyl quinazole nucleus. These drugs are given orally. Prazosin has a very high affinity for most subtypes of α$_1$-adrenoceptors. Its α$_{1B}$-receptor antagonism results in blocked constriction of arteries and veins so that there is a lowering of peripheral vascular resistance and decreased venous return to the heart. The minimal reflex response to increase heart rate may be due to a CNS effect to suppress sympathetic outflow. This antihypertensive drug is given orally (1–5 mg) and its effects last for approximately 10 hours.

Doxazosin has hemodynamic effects similar to prazosin but a duration of action about three times longer than prazosin. *Terazosin* is less potent than prazosin as an α$_1$-antagonist but has a higher bioavailability so its effects are longer. Selectivity of the α$_{1A}$ subtype over the α$_{1B}$ subtype for relaxation of bladder neck, prostate capsule, and prostatic urethra makes doxazosin, and another drug, *tamsulosin*, useful for treating benign prostatic hypertrophy with little effect on blood pressure.

Summary

Generalized activation of the sympathetic nervous system (SNS) increases cardiac output, blood glucose, pupillary dilation, and body temperature. Tonic activity maintains cardiac and smooth muscle function. The medullary vasomotor center in the brainstem relays ascending afferent signals from peripheral baroreceptors, chemoreceptors, and visceral and somatic sensors. Integration of sensory information is followed by altered efferent sympathetic signals.

Low-pressure cardiopulmonary baroreceptors monitor central blood volume, while high-pressure baroreceptors respond to blood pressure changes in the arteries. Baroreceptor signaling maintains blood pressure homeostasis via the baroreflex, which alters parasympathetic and sympathetic output. Similar physiologic reflexes generate responses to chemoreceptor signaling and intracranial hypoxic or mechanical stimulation. The effects of anesthesia on tonic sympathetic outflow and reflex sympathetic discharges vary by anesthetic drug, and should be considered in the selection of these drugs.

Sympathomimetics act either directly, by stimulation of α- and β-adrenoceptors, or indirectly, displacing norepinephrine from the presynaptic nerve terminal. The differential effects of the various sympathomimetics on adrenoceptor subtypes α$_{1A,B,C}$, α$_{2A,B,C}$, and β$_{1–3}$ allow for a degree of selective targeting. Differences in lipid solubility and biotransformation, as well as the route of administration, allow for further specificity in pharmacologic manipulation of responses.

The α$_1$-adrenoceptors generally mediate arterial and venous vasoconstriction, decreased insulin release, and sphincter contraction. Agonists include phenylephrine, methoxamine, midodrine, metaraminol, mephentermine, and topical imidazoline derivatives. Depending on their specific properties, α$_1$-receptor agonists may be selected to counteract hypotension, increase coronary and cerebral perfusion pressure, or for vasoconstriction of the nasal mucosa and conjunctiva. By contrast, α$_2$ receptors attenuate SNS activity by reducing norepinephrine release. Agonists include clonidine, guanidine derivatives, α-methyldopa, and dexmedetomidine.

The β$_1$-adrenoceptors are generally located in the heart, and they mediate positive inotropic and chronotropic effects. The β$_2$ receptors mediate bronchodilation, slowing of peristalsis, and vasodilation of muscular, splanchnic, and renal vascular beds, decreasing diastolic blood pressure. Isoproterenol is a nonselective β-adrenoceptor agonist. It has dromotropic, chronotropic, and inotropic effects, while lowering vascular resistance and relieving bronchoconstriction. Selective β$_2$-adrenoceptor agonists were developed for the treatment of bronchial asthma. Aerosolized administration aids in avoidance of cardiovascular effects mediated by β$_1$-adrenoceptors, which can also be stimulated at higher systemic concentrations. The β$_2$-adrenoceptor agonists include terbutaline, albuterol, and ritodrine.

Epinephrine, norepinephrine, and dopamine are naturally occurring sympathomimetic amines with mixed effects on multiple receptor types, such that different responses may be evoked in a variety of tissue types. Responses may be influenced by concentration and route of administration. Dobutamine is a synthetic catecholamine which has complex effects on adrenoceptors. It is used in cardiac testing and in the treatment of acute moderate heart failure.

Drugs which have an indirect effect on sympathetic activity include ephedrine, amphetamine, methamphetamine, methylphenidate, ergot alkaloids, pseudoephedrine, and phenylpropanolamine. Indirectly acting sympathomimetics have diverse clinical applications, though amphetamine, methamphetamine, and their derivatives, in particular, are associated with serious adverse effects following repeated intoxication. Despite this, derivatives of amphetamine and methamphetamine have found popularity as illegal recreational drugs. In the presence of monoamine oxidase inhibitors (MAOIs), there is an increase in tyramine-mediated displacement of norepinephrine from synaptic vesicles. Hence dietary amines can produce a hypertensive reaction in patients taking MAOIs.

Sympatholytic drugs oppose the adrenergic effects of sympathetic activity. Alpha-adrenoceptor antagonists inhibit α_1 receptors, resulting in vasodilation, or α_2 receptors, resulting in an increase in norepinephrine release. Phenoxybenzamine is an irreversible noncompetitive α-receptor antagonist used to induce hypotension. Phentolamine and tolazoline have similar cardiovascular effects, but their actions are more short-lived and the effects are reversible. Other examples of α-receptor antagonists are prazosin and doxazosin, members of the piperazinyl quinazole family of drugs. Sympatholytics may also block β-adrenoceptors or nicotinic transmission in the sympathetic ganglia.

Acknowledgements

The authors wish to thank Imre Redai, MD, and Berend Mets, MD, for their valuable and significant contributions to this chapter.

References

1. Wallin BG, Fagius J. Peripheral sympathetic neural activity in conscious humans. *Ann Rev Physiol* 1988; **50**: 565–76.

2. Ebert TJ, Kampine JP. Nitrous oxide augments sympathetic outflow: Direct evidence from human peroneal nerve recordings. *Anesth Analg* 1989; **69**: 444–9.

3. Ebert TJ. Differential effects of nitrous oxide on baroreflex control of heart rate and peripheral sympathetic nerve activity in humans. *Anesthesiology* 1990; **72**: 16–22.

4. Ebert TJ, Kotrly KJ, Kampine JP. Human muscle sympathetic efferent nerve activity is augmented by nitrous oxide. *Anesth Analg* 1989, **68**: S76.

5. Ebert TJ, Kanitz DD, Kampine JP. Inhibition of sympathetic neural outflow during thiopental anesthesia in humans. *Anesth Analg* 1990; **71**: 319–26.

6. Lopatka CW, Muzi M, Ebert TJ. The efficacy of propofol versus etomidate in reducing desflurane-mediated sympathetic activation in humans. *Anesthesiology* 1994, **81**: A136.

7. Lopatka CW, Muzi M, Ebert TJ. Propofol, but not etomidate, reduces desflurane-mediated sympathetic activation in humans. *Can J Anaesth* 1999; **46**: 342–7.

8. Ebert TJ, Muzi M. Sympathetic hyperactivity during desflurane anesthesia in healthy volunteers. A comparison with isoflurane. *Anesthesiology* 1993; **79**: 444–53.

9. Ebert TJ, Muzi M, Lopatka CW. Neurocirculatory responses to sevoflurane in humans. A comparison to desflurane. *Anesthesiology* 1995; **83**: 88–95.

10. Ebert TJ, Perez F, Uhrich TD, Deshur MA. Desflurane-mediated sympathetic activation occurs in humans despite preventing hypotension and baroreceptor unloading. *Anesthesiology* 1998; **88**: 1227–32.

11. Weiskopf RB, Eger EI, Daniel M, Noorani M. Cardiovascular stimulation induced by rapid increases in desflurane concentration in humans results from activation of tracheopulmonary and systemic receptors. *Anesthesiology* 1995; **83**: 1173–8.

12. Muzi M, Ebert TJ, Hope WG, Bell LB. Site(s) mediating sympathetic activation with desflurane. *Anesthesiology* 1996; **85**: 737–47.

13. Chen KK, Schmidt GF. The action of ephedrine, the active principle of the Chinese drug ma huang. *J Pharmacol Exp Ther* 1924; **24**: 339–57.

14. Nagai T. Ephedrin. *Pharm Zeit* 1887; **32**: 700.

15. Oliver G, Schäfer EA. The physiologic action of extract of the suprarenal capsules. *J Physiol* 1895; **18**: 230–76.

16. Barger G, Dale HH. Chemical structure and sympathomimetic action of amines. *J Physiol* 1910; **41**: 19–59.

17. Rall TW, Sutherland EW. Formation of a cyclic adenine ribonucleotide by tissue particles. *J Biol Chem* 1958; **232**: 1065–76.

18. Sutherland EW, Rall TW. Fractionation and characterization of a cyclic adenine ribonucleotide formed by tissue particles. *J Biol Chem* 1958; **232**: 1077–92.

19. Kobilka B. Adrenergic receptors as models for G protein-coupled receptors. *Annu Rev Neurosci* 1992; **15**: 87–114.

20. Burn JH, Rand MJ. The action of sympathomimetic amines in animals treated with reserpine. *J Physiol* 1958; **144**: 314–36.

21. Hoffman BB, Lefkowitz RJ. Catecholamines, sympathomimetic drugs, and adrenergic receptor antagonists. In: Hardman JG, Gilman AG, Limbird LE, eds., *Goodman and Gilman's The Pharmacological Basis of Therapeutics*, 9th edn. New York, NY: McGraw-Hill, 1996.

22. Patil PN, Miller DD, Trendelenburg U. Molecular geometry and adrenergic drug activity. *Pharmacol Rev* 1974; **26**: 323–92.

23. Bilezikian JP, Dornfeld AM, Gammon DE. Structure-binding-activity analysis of beta-adrenergic amines–I. Binding to the beta receptor and activation of adenylate cyclase. *Biochem Pharmacol* 1978; **27**: 1445–54.

24. Kontoyianni M, DeWeese C, Penzotti JE, Lybrand TP. Three-dimensional models for agonist and antagonist complexes with beta$_2$ adrenergic receptor. *J Med Chem* 1996; **39**: 4406–20.

25. Strader CD, Sigal IS, Candelore MR, *et al.* Conserved aspartic acid residues 79 and 113 of the beta-adrenergic receptor have different roles in receptor function. *J Biol Chem* 1988; **263**: 10267–71.

26. Bilezikian JP, Dornfeld AM, Gammon DE. Structure-binding-activity analysis of beta-adrenergic amines–II. Binding to the beta receptor and inhibition of adenylate cyclase. *Biochem Pharmacol* 1978; **27**: 1455–61.

27. Isogaya M, Sugimoto Y, Tanimura R, *et al.* Binding pockets of the beta(1)- and beta$_2$-adrenergic receptors for subtype-selective agonists. *Mol Pharmacol* 1999; **56**: 875–85.

28. Kurose H, Isogaya M, Kikkawa H, Nagao T. Domains of beta$_1$ and beta$_2$ adrenergic receptors to bind subtype selective agonists. *Life Sci* 1998; **62**: 1513–17.

29. Strader CD, Candelore MR, Hill WS, Sigal IS, Dixon RA. Identification of two serine residues involved in agonist activation of the beta-adrenergic receptor. *J Biol Chem* 1989; **264**: 13572–8.

30. Ambrosio C, Molinari P, Cotecchia S, Costa T. Catechol-binding serines of beta$_2$-adrenergic receptors control the equilibrium between active and inactive receptor states. *Mol Pharmacol* 2000; **57**: 198–210.

31. Cushny AR. *Biological Relations of Optically Isomeric Substances.* Baltimore, MD: Williams & Wilkins, 1926.

32. Wieland K, Zuurmond HM, Krasel C, Ijzerman AP, Lohse MJ. Involvement of Asn-293 in stereospecific agonist recognition and in activation of the beta$_2$-adrenergic receptor. *Proc Natl Acad Sci U S A* 1996; **93**: 9276–81.

33. Tainter ML, Stockton AB. Comparative actions of sympathomimetic compounds: the circulatory and local actions of the optical isomers of meta-synephrine and possible therapeutic applications. *Am J Med Sci* 1933; **185**: 832.

34. Lorhan PH, Oliverio RM. A study of the use of neosynephrine hydrochloride in spinal anesthesia in place of ephedrine for the sustaining of blood pressure. *Curr Res Anesth Analg* 1938; **17**: 44.

35. Rich S, Gubin S, Hart K. The effects of phenylephrine on right ventricular performance in patients with pulmonary hypertension. *Chest* 1990; **98**: 1102–6.

36. Alahuhta S, Rasanen J, Jouppila P, Jouppila R, Hollmen AI. Ephedrine and phenylephrine for avoiding maternal hypotension due to spinal anaesthesia for caesarean section. Effects on uteroplacental and fetal haemodynamics. *Int J Obstet Anesth* 1992; **1**: 129–34.

37. Groudine SB, Hollinger I, Jones J, DeBouno BA. New York State guidelines on the topical use of phenylephrine in the operating room. The Phenylephrine Advisory Committee. *Anesthesiology* 2000; **92**: 859–64.

38. Hjort AM, Randall LO, de Beer EJ. Pharmacology of compounds related to β-2,5-dimethoxy phenethyl amine; ethyl, isopropyl and propyl derivations. *J Pharmacol Exp Ther* 1948; **92**: 283–90.

39. King BD, Dripps RD. Use of methoxamine for maintenance of the circulation during spinal anesthesia. *Surg Gynecol Obstet* 1950; **90**: 659–65.

40. Poe MF. Use of methoxamine hydrochloride as a pressor agent during spinal analgesia. *Anesthesiology* 1952; **13**: 89–93.

41. Cruz DN. Midodrine: a selective alpha-adrenergic agonist for orthostatic hypotension and dialysis hypotension. *Expert Opin Pharmacother* 2000; **1**: 835–40.

42. Poe MF. The use of aramine as a pressor agent during spinal anesthesia. *Anesthesiology* 1954; **15**: 547.

43. Albertson NF, McKay FC, Lape HE, *et al.* The optical isomers of metaraminol. Synthesis and biological activity. *J Med Chem* 1970; **13**: 132–4.

44. Riegle EV, Gunter JB, Lusk RP, Muntz HR, Weiss KL. Comparison of vasoconstrictors for functional endoscopic sinus surgery in children. *Laryngoscope* 1992; **102**: 820–3.

45. Lasseter KC, Shapse D, Pascucci VL, Chiang ST. Pharmacokinetics of guanabenz in patients with impaired liver function. *J Cardiovasc Pharmacol* 1984; **6**: S766–70.

46. Sorkin EM, Heel RC. Guanfacine. A review of its pharmacodynamic and pharmacokinetic properties, and therapeutic efficacy in the treatment of hypertension. *Drugs* 1986; **31**: 301–36.

47. van Zwieten PA, Thoolen MJ, Timmermans PB. The hypotensive activity and side effects of methyldopa, clonidine, and guanfacine. *Hypertension* 1984; **6**: II28–33.

48. Guo TZ, Jiang JY, Buttermann AE, Maze M. Dexmedetomidine injection into the locus ceruleus produces antinociception. *Anesthesiology* 1996; **84**: 873–81.

49. Khan ZP, Ferguson CN, Jones RM. Alpha-2 and imidazoline receptor agonists. Their pharmacology and therapeutic role. *Anaesthesia* 1999; **54**: 146–65.

50. Arain SR, Ruehlow RM, Uhrich TD, Ebert TJ. Efficacy of dexmedetomidine versus morphine for post-operative analgesia following major inpatient surgery. *Anesth Analg* 2004; **98**: 153–8.

51. Paegelow I, Werner H. Influence of adrenergic agonists and antagonists on lymphokine secretion in vitro. *Int J Immunopharmacol* 1987; **9**: 761–8.

52. Hallsworth MP, Twort CH, Lee TH, Hirst SJ. beta$_2$-adrenoceptor agonists inhibit release of eosinophil-activating cytokines from human airway smooth muscle cells. *Br J Pharmacol* 2001; **132**: 729–41.

53. Arch JR, Ainsworth AT, Cawthorne MA, *et al.* Atypical beta-adrenoceptor on brown adipocytes as target for anti-obesity drugs. *Nature* 1984; **309**: 163–5.

54. Larsson S, Svedmyr N. Tremor caused by sympathomimetics is mediated by beta$_2$-adrenoreceptors. *Scand J Respir Dis* 1977; **58**: 5–10.

55. McDevitt DG. In vivo studies on the function of cardiac beta-adrenoceptors in man. *Eur Heart J* 1989; **10**: 22–8.

56. Brodde OE, Michel MC. Adrenergic and muscarinic receptors in the human heart. *Pharmacol Rev* 1999; **51**: 651–90.

57. Nelson HS. Beta adrenergic agonists. *Chest* 1982; **82**: 33S–38S.

58. Newhouse MT, Dolovich MB. Control of asthma by aerosols. *N Engl J Med* 1986; **315**: 870–4.

59. Bouvy ML, Heerdink ER, De Bruin ML, et al. Use of sympathomimetic drugs leads to increased risk of hospitalization for arrhythmias in patients with congestive heart failure. *Arch Intern Med* 2000; **160**: 2477–80.

60. Wang P, Clausen T. Treatment of attacks in hyperkalaemic familial periodic paralysis by inhalation of salbutamol. *Lancet* 1976; **1**: 221–3.

61. Brown MJ. Hypokalemia from beta$_2$-receptor stimulation by circulating epinephrine. *Am J Cardiol* 1985; **56**: 3D–9D.

62. Barden TP, Peter JB, Merkatz IR. Ritodrine hydrochloride: a betamimetic agent for use in preterm labor. I. pharmacology, clinical history, administration, side effects, and safety. *Obstet Gynecol* 1980; **56**: 1–6.

63. Wheeler AS, Patel KF, Spain J. Pulmonary edema during beta$_2$-tocolytic therapy. *Anesth Analg* 1981; **60**: 695–6.

64. Miura K. Vorläufige Mittheilung Über ephedrine, ein neues mydriaticum. *Berl Klin Wochens* 1887; **24**: 707.

65. Patil PN, Tye A, Lapidus JB. A Pharmacological study of the ephedrine isomers. *J Pharmacol Exp Ther* 1965; **148**: 158–68.

66. Lindblad A, Bernow J, Vernersson E, Marsal K. Effects of extradural anaesthesia on human fetal blood flow in utero. Comparison of three local anaesthetic solutions. *Br J Anaesth* 1987; **59**: 1265–72.

67. Räsänen J, Alahuhta S, Kangas-Saarela T, Jouppila R, Jouppila P. The effects of ephedrine and etilefrine on uterine and fetal blood flow and on fetal myocardial function during spinal anaesthesia for caesarean section. *Int J Obstet Anesth* 1991; **1**: 3–8.

68. Ferguson LK, North JP. Observations on experimental spinal anaesthesia. *Surg Gynecol Obstet* 1932; **54**: 62.

69. Dripps RD, van Deming M. An evaluation of certain drugs used to maintain blood pressure during spinal anesthesia. Comparison of ephedrine, paredrine, pitressin-ephedrine and methedrine in 2500 cases. *Surg Gynec Obstet* 1946; **83**: 312.

70. Moore KE. Toxicity and Catecholamine Releasing Actions of D- and L-Amphetamine in Isolated and Aggregated Mice. *J Pharmacol Exp Ther* 1963; **142**: 6–12.

71. Silverstone T. Appetite suppressants. A review. *Drugs* 1992; **43**: 820–36.

72. Bray GA. Use and abuse of appetite-suppressant drugs in the treatment of obesity. *Ann Intern Med* 1993; **119**: 707–13.

73. Hall AP. "Ecstasy" and the anaesthetist. *Br J Anaesth* 1997; **79**: 697–8.

74. Singarajah C, Lavies NG. An overdose of ecstasy. A role for dantrolene. *Anaesthesia* 1992; **47**: 686–7.

75. Saxena VK, De Deyn PP. Ergotamine: its use in the treatment of migraine and its complications. *Acta Neurol (Napoli)* 1992; **14**: 140–6.

76. Carruthers SG. Adverse effects of alpha 1-adrenergic blocking drugs. *Drug Saf* 1994; **11**: 12–20.

77. Kinney MA, Warner ME, vanHeerden JA, et al. Perianesthetic risks and outcomes of pheochromocytoma and paraganglioma resection. *Anesth Analg* 2000; **91**: 1118–23.

78. Caine M, Perlberg S, Meretyk S. A placebo-controlled double-blind study of the effect of phenoxybenzamine in benign prostatic obstruction. *Br J Urol* 1978; **50**: 551–4.

79. Stevenson DK, Kasting DS, Darnall RA, et al. Refractory hypoxemia associated with neonatal pulmonary disease: the use and limitations of tolazoline. *J Pediatr* 1979; **95**: 595–9.

80. Weinberger B, Weiss K, Heck DE, Laskin DL, Laskin JD. Pharmacologic therapy of persistent pulmonary hypertension of the newborn. *Pharmacol Ther* 2001; **89**: 67–79.

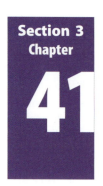

Essential drugs in anesthetic practice
Parasympathomimetic and parasympatholytic drugs

Berend Mets and Imre Redai

Parasympathomimetic drugs

Parasympathomimetics produce effects similar to those produced by stimulation of the parasympathetic nerves. These drugs preferentially stimulate postsynaptic effector muscarinic receptors. Their action is cholinergic – i.e., resembling that of acetylcholine (ACh).

Muscarinic receptors are present not only on postsynaptic visceral effectors in the periphery, but in the brain and ganglionic cells, on blood vessels, and in numerous presynaptic sites where they modulate a variety of centrally mediated functions such as locomotion, learning and memory, nociception, circadian rhythm, thermoregulation, and generation of seizure activity [1]. Acetylcholine (Fig. 41.1) is the endogenous neurotransmitter for all cholinergic receptors, both muscarinic and nicotinic. Whereas the exogenous parasympathomimetics are relatively selective for the muscarinic receptor, some nicotinic cross-reactivity may result in activation or inhibition of the nicotinic receptors.

Muscarine, pilocarpine, and arecoline (Fig. 41.2) are parasympathomimetic alkaloids derived from plants. Muscarine is an alkaloid found in some mushroom species. Pilocarpine was first isolated from the leaves of the South American shrub *Pilocarpus*. Arecoline is the alkaloid of the areca (or "betel") nut (*Areca catechu*). Betel nut is the fourth most widely used recreational drug (after nicotine, alcohol, and caffeine) and is used in masticatory mixtures by millions of people living between the east coast of Africa and the western Pacific.

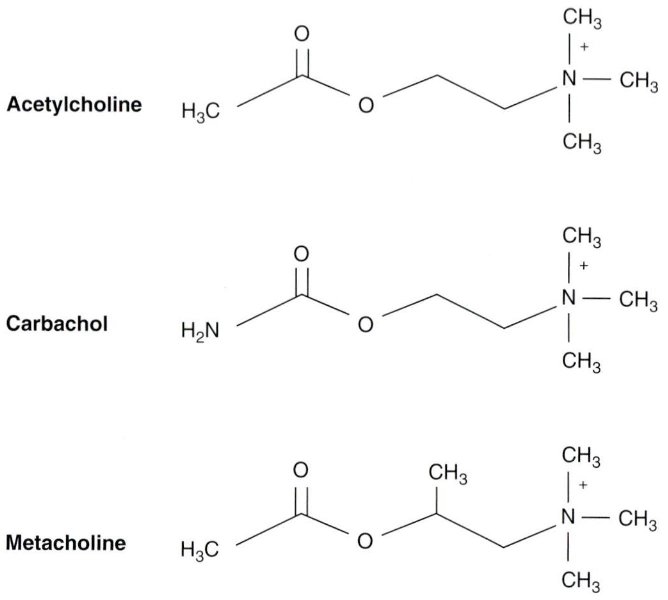

Mechanism of drug action

Five distinct muscarinic receptors have been identified and their genes have been cloned [2]. These G-protein-coupled receptors are characterized by seven highly conserved membrane-spanning domains. The receptors are divided into two subgroups: the M_1, M_3, and M_5 receptors activate G_q/G_{11} proteins leading to phospholipase C stimulation and calcium mobilization; the M_2 and M_4 receptors activate pertussis toxin-sensitive G_i/G_o proteins, which mediate inhibition of adenylate cyclase, activation of inward rectified potassium currents, and inhibition of voltage-sensitive calcium channels [3]. The structural core of the

Acetylcholine

Carbachol

Metacholine

Figure 41.1. Chemical structures of acetylcholine, metacholine, and betanechol.

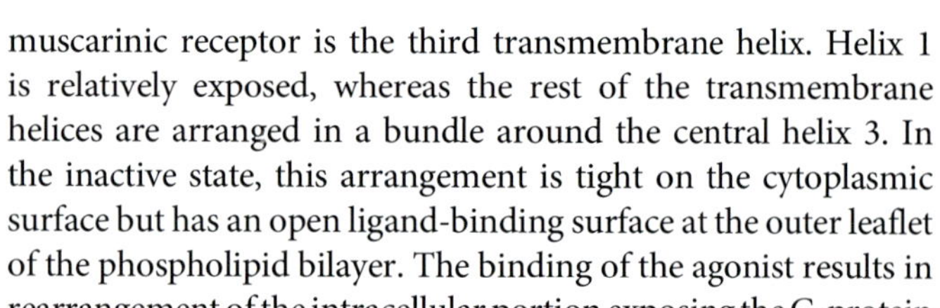

Muscarine   Pilocarpine   Arecoline

Figure 41.2. Chemical structures of muscarine, pilocarpine, and arecoline.

muscarinic receptor is the third transmembrane helix. Helix 1 is relatively exposed, whereas the rest of the transmembrane helices are arranged in a bundle around the central helix 3. In the inactive state, this arrangement is tight on the cytoplasmic surface but has an open ligand-binding surface at the outer leaflet of the phospholipid bilayer. The binding of the agonist results in rearrangement of the intracellular portion exposing the G-protein binding site [4]. The ligand binding site involves the formation

Anesthetic Pharmacology, 2nd edition, ed. Alex S. Evers, Mervyn Maze, Evan D. Kharasch. Published by Cambridge University Press. © Cambridge University Press 2011.

Table 41.1. The effects of acetylcholine and the muscarinic receptors involved [1,7,8]

Target tissue/organ	Receptor	Effect
Endothelium	M_3	Nitric oxide release, vasodilation
Vascular smooth muscle	M_2, M_3	Vasoconstriction
Cardiac conductive tissue (SA node, AV node, Purkinje fibers)	M_2	K^+ channel opening, hyperpolarization, decreased rate of spontaneous diastolic depolarization, bradycardia, slowed impulse conduction
Atrial muscle	M_2	Shortened duration of action potential
Ventricular muscle	M_2	Inhibition of cAMP-dependent activation, negative inotropy
Eye (iris, ciliary body)	M_3	Adjustment of the size of the pupil and the focal characteristics of the lens
Bronchial tree	M_3	Activation of protein kinase C, bronchoconstriction, increased mucus secretion
	M_2	Inhibition of adenylate cyclase, bronchoconstriction
Gastric mucosa	M_3, M_5	Gastric acid secretion
Gastrointestinal tract smooth muscle	M_3	Increased tone, peristaltic rate, amplitude of contractions, intestinal cramps, nausea, vomiting
	M_2	Modulation of cAMP-dependent relaxation, cramps
Gastrointestinal tract colonic mucosal cells	M_3	Increased mucus secretion, increased sodium and fluid absorption
Genitourinary tract	M_3	Increased ureteral peristalsis, contraction of detrusor muscle, relaxation of trigone and external sphincter
Lacrimal, salivary, and sweat glands	M_1, M_3	Increased lacrimation, salivation, and sweating

Table 41.1. (*cont.*)

Target tissue/organ	Receptor	Effect
Pancreatic β cells	M_3	Increased glucose-stimulated insulin secretion

Notice that while cardiac effects are predominantly associated with the M_2 receptor, in the gut, glands, and tracheobronchial tree M_3 receptors are the primary targets. In the CNS (not included) M_1 receptors appear to be the primary muscarinic targets.

of a cleft between the transmembrane domains by multiple amino acid residues. The anionic residue of aspartate 105 of the third transmembrane helix has been identified as the likely binding site for the cationic nitrogen of ACh [5]. Whereas the amino acid sequence of the muscarinic receptors is highly conservative, the large third intracellular loop, responsible for G-protein binding, displays virtually no homology among the different subtypes of muscarinic receptors [6].

Preclinical pharmacology
Acetylcholine

The pharmacological effect of ACh results from stimulation of muscarinic and nicotinic receptors. Often the effects on distant receptors combine and elicit further compensatory responses to result in a complex response in the subject. For example, in isolated heart preparations ACh reduces chronotropy, dromo-tropy, and inotropy and produces vasodilation; however in the intact animal intravenous injection of a small dose of ACh generally results in a fall in blood pressure with concomitant reflex tachycardia, and only larger doses will result in bradycardia or atrioventricular block. Furthermore, if the muscarinic effects of ACh are blocked with atropine, ACh administration will lead to an increase in blood pressure. This is the indirect result from the release of catecholamines secondary to ACh stimulating nicotinic receptors in the sympathetic ganglia and the adrenal gland [7].

The effects of ACh on tissues and organ systems and the muscarinic receptors involved [1,7,8] are detailed in Table 41.1.

Clinical pharmacology
Synthetic choline esters

Rapid hydrolysis of ACh at the neuroeffector junction and in the plasma by cholinesterases precludes systemic therapeutic application. However, a 1/100 topical preparation is available for rapid, complete miosis in ophthalmic surgery.

Muscarinic receptor activation may be achieved either by drugs resistant to cholinesterases or by blocking the degradation of endogenous ACh by cholinesterase inhibitors [9].

Cholinesterase-resistant choline esters were initially synthesized in the 1930s. Metacholine (acetyl-β-methylcholine) is resistant to hydrolysis by plasma cholinesterases and is only slowly hydrolyzed by acetylcholinesterase (AChE). It acts predominantly on the muscarinic receptors but retains mild nicotinic agonist properties. The metacholine inhalation challenge test is used in the investigation of cholinergic involvement in patients with reactive airway disease [10].

Both bethanechol and carbachol are carbamoyl ester derivatives of ACh. They are resistant to hydrolysis both by AChE and plasma cholinesterases. Bethanechol acts predominantly on muscarinic receptors, while carbachol has significant nicotinic activity, particularly in autonomic ganglia. Bethanechol and carbachol stimulate the urinary tract and the gastrointestinal tract rather selectively, and bethanechol is used in the treatment of neurogenic bladder paralysis following spinal cord injury. Bethanechol also increases lower esophageal sphincter tone and esophageal and gastric motility [11]. However, its popularity in the treatment of gastroesophageal reflux has faded with the emergence of more specific motility drugs such as metoclopramide and cisapride. The usual oral dose of bethanechol is 10–50 mg 2–4 times a day, while the subcutaneous dose is 2.5–5 mg.

Betanechol and carbachol should only be administered by the oral or subcutaneous route. When given intravenously or intramuscularly they lose their relative selectivity and the incidence and severity of side effects increases. On the other hand, oral administration of betanechol decreases the diastolic blood pressure only slightly. Muscarinic side effects are readily reversed by intravenous administration of atropine, but severe cardiovascular or bronchial side effects may need immediate treatment with epinephrine.

Cholinomimetic alkaloids

Muscarine causes diaphoresis, salivation, abdominal cramps, nausea, and severe vomiting, commonly accompanied by visual disturbances, hypotension, and bradycardia. Bronchospasm may be induced in susceptible individuals. Symptoms usually occur within 15–30 minutes after ingestion, and victims recover within 24 hours. In severe muscarine poisoning death is usually due to respiratory failure. The antidote is atropine; severe cases may need supportive ventilation. The lethal dose of muscarine in humans is 200 mg.

Whereas muscarine acts predominantly on muscarinic receptors, pilocarpine and arecoline affect both muscarinic and nicotinic receptors. Pilocarpine is currently in clinical use in the treatment of glaucoma and xerostomia. When instilled in the eye, pilocarpine causes miosis lasting several hours. A transient rise in intraocular pressure is followed by the main therapeutic effect: a prolonged fall in intraocular pressure lasting up to 8 hours. The usual concentration of pilocarpine for the treatment of open-angle glaucoma is 0.5–4%, but solutions up to 10% are also available. Oral doses of 5–10 mg four times a day are used to treat xerostomia associated with Sjögren syndrome and radiation therapy [12]. The most common side effect is diaphoresis, which is usually well tolerated. However, severe symptomatic atrioventricular block induced by pilocarpine eye drops has been documented in an elderly man [13]. Pilocarpine is also found in

several herbal preparations. Jaborandi, a South American herbal product, contains about 0.5% pilocarpine. Cevimeline, recently approved for the treatment of xerostomia associated with Sjögren syndrome, is a synthetic M_1- and M_3-receptor agonist.

Arecoline rapidly crosses the blood–brain barrier and elicits a variety of central and parasympathetic effects [14]. Although arecoline has a plasma half-life of only 1–9 minutes, holding the betel quid (the wad of the mixture used for chewing) in the buccal cavity not only bypasses first-pass hepatic metabolism but also ensures maintained alkaloid blood levels for extended periods of time. Severe and occasionally fatal cardiac dysrhythmias, myocardial infarction, acute severe asthma, and extrapyramidal symptoms have been attributed to betel nut ingestion.

Parasympatholytic drugs

Parasympatholytics are drugs that oppose the effects of the parasympathetic nervous system through anticholinergic action – i.e., they prevent ACh from acting as a neurotransmitter at muscarinic receptors.

Muscarinic receptor antagonists competitively block the binding of ACh to the muscarinic receptor and have little or no effect on the binding of ACh to the nicotinic receptor.

Several plants contain parasympatholytic alkaloids [15]. Scopolamine (hyoscine, Fig. 41.3) is found in the common Eurasian weed henbane (*Hyoscyamus niger*). It has been used as a poison since Babylonian times. In the Middle Ages henbane extract was mixed in beer to enhance the inebriating qualities. Medieval "witches" consumed and rubbed their skin with a mixture of belladonna and henbane to produce flushed skin, vivid hallucinations of flying in the air, and wild dancing.

Atropine (Fig. 41.3) is an alkaloid found in several plants, the two most common being deadly nightshade and jimsonweed. Deadly nightshade (*Atropa belladonna*) was named after Atropa, who, according to Greek mythology cuts the thread of life. The name belladonna ("pretty woman") refers to a past custom of women treating their faces with leaves of nightshade to achieve an appealing flushed complexion and dilated pupils. Deadly nightshade is a perennial plant widespread in Eurasia and the Middle East. Its poisonous qualities were long exploited, and the Roman emperor Claudius was among its victims. Legend has it that barrels of beer laced with belladonna sap saved Scotland from an invading force of Danes. Medicinal use of belladonna extracts dates back to Galen, who recommended its use for nonhealing ulcers. The use of extracts of henbane and nightshade for sedation and anesthesia was described in Avicenna's *Canon of Medicine* [16].

Jimsonweed or thorn-apple (*Datura stramonium*, meaning "thorny fruit") is a decorative but extremely poisonous plant. Originally from Asia, jimsonweed was spread all over the world by wandering gypsies. In India smoke from burned jimsonweed was used for the treatment of asthma since ancient

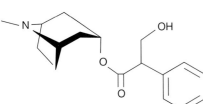

Atropine

Scopolamine

Glycopyrrolate

Figure 41.3. Chemical structures of atropine, scopolamine, and glycopyrrolate.

times. Jimsonweed was first described for medicinal purposes in the West – to treat psychosis and epilepsy – in 1762. Accidental henbane and jimsonweed poisoning still occurs, mainly in children and adolescents. Plants contain up to 0.5% alkaloid in their leaves, roots, and fruit. Prompt recognition of the poisoning is important, although in most cases (the exception being children) the outcome is not fatal.

Mechanism of drug action

Atropine, scopolamine, and their synthetic quaternary ammonium derivatives are esters of an aromatic acid containing an asymmetrical carbon atom (tropic acid or mandelic acid) and an organic base (tropine, scopine, or an N-methylated derivative of tropine) closely similar in structure. Only the l-isomers have pharmacological effect, and the intact ester link and the hydroxyl group on the acid portion are essential for the antimuscarinic action.

The structural similarity of the intramolecular arrangement around the cationic quaternary nitrogen in ACh and the organic base of the antagonists is the basis of competitive antagonism on the muscarinic receptor. The antagonists are believed to compete with ACh to form a link with the aspartate[105] residue of the third transmembrane helix. ACh binding

to the muscarinic receptor results in the receptor coupling with a G protein. This receptor–G-protein complex remains stable after the dissociation of ACh following the binding of guanosine triphosphate (GTP). Atropine was able to cause dissociation of the receptor–G-protein complex even after the agonist was removed [17]. Atropine also abolished the basal level of G-protein activation in the absence of ACh [18]. Conformational change following antagonist binding to the receptor may explain these findings. Scopolamine was shown to close inward-rectifying ACh-sensitive potassium channels, which were open at rest [19]. These findings suggest that atropine and scopolamine are in fact inverse agonists [3].

Clinical pharmacology

Atropine and scopolamine are nonselective inhibitors at the muscarinic receptor. Both are readily absorbed from the gastrointestinal tract and from mucous surfaces. Scopolamine is often administered as a transdermal patch, although it is poorly absorbed from most regions and thus the patch is applied to the postauricular area to enhance absorption. When instilled intratracheally, atropine is readily absorbed. Atropine is stable when stored in glass or plastic syringes. Pharmacokinetic characteristics of atropine, scopolamine, and glycopyrrolate are summarized in Table 41.2, and dosages are shown in Table 41.3.

Atropine

When atropine is administered intravenously a transient reduction in heart rate occurs before the onset of tachycardia [20]. This paradoxical effect was once thought to be caused by a central vagal stimulating activity of atropine. However, the effect is present with antimuscarinic drugs not crossing the blood–brain barrier. The phenomenon is best explained by the blockade of presynaptic inhibitory M_1 autoreceptors on vagus nerve terminals that usually produces negative feedback on further ACh release. Atropine-induced disinhibition leads to an increase in ACh release that initially overcomes the muscarinic blockade on sinoatrial M_2 receptors (Fig. 41.4) [21]. Although atropine increases the resting heart rate, the maximal heart rate achieved by exercise is unchanged. Atropine is also less effective at increasing the resting heart rate at the two extremes of age: in infants the resting tone is dominantly sympathetic, and in the elderly the muscarinic receptor density is reduced [22]. Complete vagal blockade requires 3 mg of intravenous atropine in a healthy adult.

Atropine shortens the functional refractory period of the atrioventricular node, which may accelerate the ventricular rate in patients with atrial flutter or fibrillation. In complete heart block the idioventricular rate may accelerate following the administration of atropine, although this response is unpredictable. Atropine has no effect on the denervated, acutely transplanted heart; parasympathetic reinnervation does occur in the long term after orthotopic heart transplantation [23]. Intravenous atropine is used to counteract the cardiodecelerator effect of vagus stimulation and is useful in preventing the parasympathomimetic effects of cholinesterase inhibitors

Table 41.2. Pharmacokinetic characteristics of atropine, scopolamine, and glycopyrrolate

Drug	Bioavailability	Protein binding	Half-life	Metabolism	Excretion
Atropine	10–25%	50%	2–4 h (terminal 12.5 h)	50–75%, liver	Renal
Scopolamine	11–48%	Variable	1.5–4.5 h (terminal 8 h)	~ 100%, liver	Renal
Glycopyrrolate	10–25%	—	0.8 h after IV 0.5–1.25 h after IM	Unchanged	Renal

IM, intramuscular; IV, intravenous.

Table 41.3. Clinical dosing, parenteral dosage forms used in anesthesia practice, and common brand names of atropine, scopolamine, glycopyrrolate, and physostigmine

Drug	Adult IV dose	Pediatric IV dose	Commercial IV dosage forms	Common brand names
Atropine	0.5–1 mg every 5 min, not to exceed a total of 3 mg or 0.04 mg kg^{-1}; may give intratracheally in 10 mL normal saline (intratracheal dose should be 2–2.5 times the IV dose)	0.02 mg kg^{-1}, minimum dose 0.1 mg, maximum single dose 0.5 mg in children and 1 mg in adolescents; may repeat at 5 min intervals to a maximum total dose of 1 mg in children or 2 mg in adolescents (Note: for intratracheal administration, give the same dose as IV diluted with normal saline to a total volume of 1–5 mL)	0.05 mg mL^{-1} (5 mL); 0.1 mg mL^{-1} (5 mL, 10 mL); 0.4 mg 0.5 mL^{-1} (0.5 mL); 0.4 mg mL^{-1} (0.5 mL, 1 mL, 20 mL); 1 mg mL^{-1} (1 mL)	Atropin Atropina Atropine Atropini sulfas Atropinsulfat
Scopolamine	0.3–0.65 mg over 2–3 minutes	6 months to 3 years: 0.1–0.15 mg 3–6 years: 0.2–0.3 mg	0.4 mg mL^{-1} (1 mL)	Scopolamine hydrobromide Hyoscine Scopamine
Glycopyrrolate	0.1 mg repeated as needed at 2–3 min intervals	0.004 mg kg^{-1}, not to exceed 0.1 mg; repeat at 2–3 min intervals as needed	0.2 mg mL^{-1} (1, 2, 5 mL)	Robinul Acpan Gastrodyn
Physostigmine	0.5–2 mg to start, repeat every 20 min until response occurs or adverse effect occurs; repeat 1–4 mg every 30–60 min as life threatening symptoms recur	0.01–0.03 mg kg^{-1} per dose; may repeat after 5–10 min to a maximum total dose of 2 mg or until response occurs or adverse cholinergic effects occur	1 mg mL^{-1} (2 mL)	Physostigmine salicylate Eserin Fisostin Anticholium

IV, intravenous.

and succinylcholine and electroconvulsive therapy. While atropine has little, if any, effect on resting vascular tone, larger doses result in cutaneous vasodilation. Vasodilation may be a compensatory response to the loss of the ability to perspire that occurs with even small doses of atropine, or a presynaptic effect on sympathetic nerves supplying the blush areas of the body. Atropine causes a marked decrease in baroreflex sensitivity and suppression of parasympathetic control mechanisms. Return to baseline functions takes 3 hours in healthy adults after a single 20 μg kg^{-1} intravenous dose [24].

Atropine does not readily penetrate the blood–brain barrier, and in the usual clinical doses of 0.5–1 mg it has negligible effect on the central nervous system (CNS). Larger doses (5–10 mg)

cause restlessness, hallucinations, and delirium. Massive intoxication leads to CNS depression and coma followed by circulatory collapse, paralysis, and respiratory failure. Elderly patients may be more vulnerable to the CNS effects of atropine than children or young adults [25].

Topical application of atropine on the conjunctiva causes mydriasis and cycloplegia. Near vision becomes blurred, and the loss of accommodation and pupillary reflexes may not fully recover for 7–12 days. These unpleasant side effects can be reversed by topical parasympathomimetics or cholinesterases. Synthetic muscarinic antagonists such as cyclopentolate and tropicamide have a much shorter duration of action and are the preferred drugs to elicit brief mydriasis and cycloplegia.

A

C

B

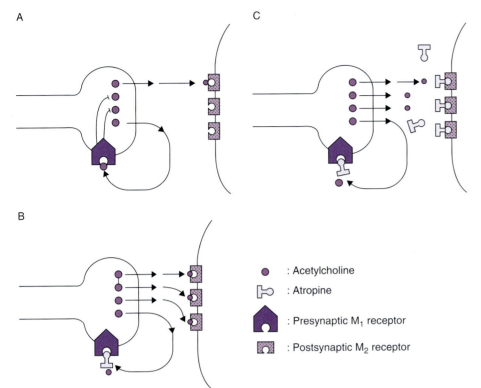

: Acetylcholine

: Atropine

: Presynaptic M_1 receptor

: Postsynaptic M_2 receptor

Figure 41.4. The heart rate response to atropine is dose-dependent [20,21]. (A) Acetylcholine (ACh) released from vagal nerve terminals interacts with effector postsynaptic M_2 receptors on sinoatrial cells and on presynaptic inhibitory M_1 receptors. (B) A small dose of atropine has little effect on M_2 receptors. On the other hand, inhibition of presynaptic M_1 receptors results in diminished feedback inhibition of ACh release. This increases release of ACh and results in bradycardia. (C) A larger dose of atropine blocks postsynaptic M_2 receptors, resulting in the classic response of tachycardia.

Large doses of atropine instilled in the eye and absorbed from the nasal mucosa or by swallowing may result in significant systemic effects. Delirium and psychosis have been reported for adults using atropine eye drops [26]. Systemic administration of atropine rarely causes ocular effects and only mildly elevates intraocular pressure. Nevertheless, in patients with narrow-angle glaucoma, sphincter constriction may lead to a sudden, dangerous rise in intraocular pressure [27]. For patients with the more common open-angle glaucoma the parenteral use of atropine and scopolamine is regarded to be safe.

Suppression of the activity of sweat glands and diminished evaporative heat loss occurs after even small doses of atropine. Administration of atropine in infants and small children with febrile disease has been associated with life-threatening hyperthermia.

Bronchial tone and bronchial secretions are partially regulated by M_3 receptors. Blockade of these receptors decreases bronchial tone [28] and thickens bronchial secretions. Although anticholinergics are most effective in alleviating bronchoconstriction from cholinergic stimulation, they also partially antagonize the effects of inflammatory mediators, suggesting a role for local or central parasympathetic reflexes in the pathophysiology of asthma and allergic airway disease. In addition, atropine has an inhibitory effect on mucociliary clearance [29] and has been used to suppress excessive bronchial secretions induced by anesthesia with ether or ketamine. Administration of atropine produces a dry mouth and difficulty in swallowing.

Atropine reduces gastric secretion of acid, mucin, and proteolytic enzymes. It also delays gastric and intestinal emptying and reduces the lower esophageal sphincter tone; this effect is not abolished by metoclopramide [30]. ACh is only one of the mediators regulating gastrointestinal tone and function, and anticholinergic drugs are only partially effective in abolishing gut motility and secretion. Atropine has no or minimal effect on the biliary sphincter mechanism and is ineffective in relieving biliary colic.

Atropine has no significant effect on the pregnant uterus. Atropine readily crosses the placenta but has no harmful effect on the fetus when used in clinically relevant doses [31].

The clinical dose of atropine is 0.5–1 mg ($20\,\mu g\,kg^{-1}$) intravenously or intramuscularly, 1–2 mg (20–$40\,\mu g\,kg^{-1}$) orally, or 2 mg ($50\,\mu g\,kg^{-1}$) intratracheally. In the past, atropine has been routinely used as a premedicant or before induction of general anesthesia. It became well recognized that perioperative use of atropine can mask the ability to monitor for important physiologic changes associated with arousal, pain, rising intracranial pressure, hypovolemia, and shock. The associated risk of arrhythmias, aspiration, and hyperthermia, postoperative sedation from central anticholinergic syndrome, as well as advances in anesthetic drugs, have all diminished the practice of routine use of atropine, in both adults and children [32,33]. Last but not least, one should remember that atropine is a parasympatholytic and has no sympathetic stimulating activity. This becomes most important during cardiopulmonary resuscitation, especially in children in the setting of severe hypoxic myocardial depression. Lives could have been saved if instead of repeat dosing of atropine patients had received epinephrine earlier in the course of resuscitation.

Scopolamine

Scopolamine readily penetrates the blood–brain barrier, and in the usual clinical doses of 0.3–0.6 mg causes drowsiness, fatigue, amnesia, dreamless (non-REM) sleep, and occasionally euphoria [34], making it a popular choice for premedication prior to surgery. However, restlessness, vertigo, hallucinations, and delirium may occur in the elderly, or in the presence of pain, even with the usual clinical doses. These adverse effects are avoidable by combining scopolamine with a benzodiazepine or an opiate.

Although scopolamine is regarded to be the most effective single drug to prevent and treat motion sickness [35], it is less effective in preventing and treating perioperative nausea and vomiting [36]. Delirium and psychosis have been reported for even transdermal use of scopolamine for motion sickness in children and the elderly [37,38]. There is a 20-fold interindividual variability in peak scopolamine concentrations after transdermal application, which may explain the adverse effects occurring in some but not all patients.

Parenteral scopolamine is likely to produce prolonged bradycardia, either as the only response or after an initial period of tachycardia [39]. Scopolamine is more potent than atropine in its effects on the eye, tracheobronchial tree, and salivary gland [35]. The drying effect on mucous membranes is better tolerated because of the associated sedation. Scopolamine inhibits bowel and bladder tone and should be avoided in patients with intestinal obstruction and obstructive uropathy. Like atropine, scopolamine readily crosses the placenta [40], but it is not considered to be teratogenic. It is safe in nursing mothers.

Adverse effects of atropine or scopolamine overdose

Accidental overdose or plant alkaloid ingestion is the most common cause of atropine or scopolamine poisoning. The diagnosis is suggested by dilated pupils, dry mucous membranes, difficulty in swallowing, dry and flushed skin, and the absence of sweating in a warm or hot patient. Usually tachycardia, blurred vision, and headache also occur. Larger doses lead to ataxia, restlessness, delirium, and coma.

The diagnosis may be confirmed by administering 1 mg physostigmine intramuscularly. If salivation, intestinal hypermotility, and sweating do not occur, anticholinergic poisoning is likely. If the poison has been ingested, gastric lavage and administration of charcoal should be initiated without delay to limit intestinal absorption of the alkaloid. Treatment consists of slow intravenous administration of physostigmine (up to 4 mg in adults, 0.5 mg in small children), which usually rapidly reverses the delirium and coma. The patient should be observed continuously, as physostigmine is metabolized more rapidly then atropine and a second dose may be needed 1–2 hours later.

If physostigmine is not available, benzodiazepines may be used to achieve sedation and control seizures. Children may need active cooling by means of alcohol sponges or immersion in cold water. Severe cases may require artificial support of ventilation.

Many drugs used in anesthesia and intensive care may cause blockade of central cholinergic transmission – the *central anticholinergic syndrome* [41]. The syndrome has the clinical characteristics of central atropine poisoning. The peripheral signs of anticholinergic overdose, such as mydriasis, are often absent immediately following general anesthesia. Although restlessness, agitation, and hallucinations may occur, motionlessness and depression rather than agitation are more often the presenting clinical features perioperatively. Central cholinergic syndrome is often mistaken for delayed recovery from the effects of anesthesia [42]. Respiratory drive may be suppressed. Differentiation of the syndrome from other causes of perioperative confusion is possible with slow intravenous administration of physostigmine (0.04 mg kg^{-1}). Treatment of the syndrome also consists of the administration of intravenous physostigmine, which may need to be repeated every 1–2 hours. It is worth mentioning that physostigmine causes nonspecific central arousal via increasing ACh and cyclic adenosine monophosphate (cAMP) levels in the CNS, which makes identification of drug-induced postoperative somnolence caused by the central anticholinergic action as opposed to a residual anesthetic effect controversial.

Glycopyrrolate (glycopyrronium bromide)

Glycopyrrolate (Fig. 41.3) is a potent quaternary antagonist of muscarinic receptors. The commercially available drug is a mixture of four stereoisomers and does not show selectivity to the individual muscarinic receptor subtypes [43].

Cardiovascular responses to glycopyrrolate are similar to those to atropine. Bradycardia may occur at lower doses, but tachycardia is usually less prominent and of shorter duration [44]. Impairment of autonomic and baroreceptor reflexes is about half the duration of that with atropine [45]. The antisialogogue effect of glycopyrrolate is pronounced and lasts up to 8 hours, which is 2–5 times longer than that of atropine [46]. Although glycopyrrolate reduces gastric volume and acidity, clinical usefulness of this effect is offset by the relaxing effect of the drug on the lower esophageal sphincter.

The usual dose of glycopyrrolate is 0.004 mg kg^{-1} as an antisialogogue or for reversal of intraoperative bradycardia. For reversal of neuromuscular blockade the recommended dose of glycopyrrolate is 0.2 mg for each 1 mg of neostigmine or 5 mg of pyridostigmine.

Other anticholinergic drugs

Several synthetic tertiary amine muscarinic receptor antagonists are in clinical use. Table 41.4 shows the pharmacokinetic characteristics and recommended dosing of these drugs.

Table 41.4. Pharmacokinetic characteristics and recommended doses of some parasympatholytic drugs

Drug	Bioavailability	Half-life	Metabolism	Elimination	Usual dose
Benztropine	NA	NA	NA	NA	1–2 mg IV or IM,[a] 0.5–6 mg PO daily
Trihexyphenidyl	Well absorbed	NA	NA	NA	1–2 mg starting dose, up to 20 mg daily
Hyoscine butylbromide	(Parenteral)	5 h	50%, liver	Renal	20 mg slow IV or IM
Oxybutinin	21%	2–2.5 h	Liver: metabolite active	Renal	10–15 mg daily (5 mg in elderly)
Propantheline	50%	1.3–2 h	95%, hydrolysis	Renal	75–120 mg daily
Tolterodine	17%[b]	2–3 h[b]	99%, liver	Renal	2–4 mg daily
Vamicamide	Well absorbed	5.5 h	20%, liver	Renal	12–36 mg daily
Pirenzepine	25%	10 h	Minimal	Renal	150 mg daily

[a]For acute dystonic reaction.
[b]In poor metabolizers (CYP2D6 deficiency) bioavailability is 65%, half-life is 10 h.
IM, intramuscular; IV, intravenous; NA, not available; PO, per os (by mouth).

Benztropine (a synthetic compound containing a tropine base and the benzohydryl portion of diphenhydramine) and trihexyphenidyl are used in the treatment of parkinsonism. These two drugs are also useful in treating extrapyramidal side effects of antidopaminergic drugs such as metoclopramide and some antipsychotic drugs. However, experimental evidence in muscarinic-receptor knockout mice suggests that selective M_4 or mixed M_1/M_4 antagonists may be more effective in Parkinson's disease, with fewer systemic side effects.

Hyoscine butylbromide is used to relieve symptoms of acute renal or biliary colic and to reduce spasm during esophagogastroduodenoscopy. Oxybutinin is recommended as the main therapy for detrusor instability or urge incontinence [48]. Propantheline is indicated as adjunctive therapy of peptic ulcer disease, gastritis, and irritable bowel syndrome. Dryness of the mouth and pupillary side effects are more common with oxybutinin. Tolterodine and vamicamide may have fewer side effects, because of tissue selectivity or accumulation in the urinary bladder. Intensive research is under way to identify receptor subtype-specific muscarinic antagonists for gastrointestinal use, and numerous compounds have been synthesized and used in laboratory research. The M_1 receptor-selective pirenzepine and telenzepine are used clinically in several countries to treat peptic ulcer. However, the role of M_1 receptors in gastric acid secretion appears to be minimal, and M_3/M_5 receptor antagonists are more likely to be effective drugs in the future. Darifenacin and solifenacin are M_3 antagonists that have preferential inhibitory action on muscarinic receptors in the gut and bladder and are approved for use in overactive bladder disease. Temiverine has not only M_3 antagonist but also calcium channel blocking activity and is awaiting FDA approval for use in patients with overactive bladder [8,48].

Alkylation of the nitrogen atom on the base of the belladonna alkaloids results in quaternary ammonium compounds. This alkylation results in poor absorption from the gut and mucous membranes, prolonged duration of action compared with that of the parent drug, increased activity on the nicotinic ACh receptors, inability to cross the blood–brain barrier, and an increased potency it the gastrointestinal tract. The N-isopropyl derivative of atropine, ipratropium bromide, is used as an inhaled bronchodilator in patients with chronic obstructive airway disease. Because ipratropium is poorly absorbed from mucous membranes of the mouth or the tracheobronchial tree, systemic side effects are minimal. Tiotropium bromide, an antagonist with a preferential slow dissociation rate from M_3 receptors [49], and revatropate, a selective M_1 and M_3 antagonist [50], may represent the first steps towards selective muscarinic antagonists in the treatment of reactive airway disease.

Summary

Parasympathomimetic and parasympatholytic drugs exert their effects on G-protein-coupled muscarinic receptors. Of the five subtypes isolated so far, M_1 and M_4 are found predominantly in the brain, M_2 is associated with cardiac tissue, and M_3 and M_5 are expressed in the lungs, gut, and glandular tissue. The naturally occurring neurotransmitter is acetylcholine (ACh). Of the three naturally occurring parasympathomimetic alkaloids, muscarine, pilocarpine, and arecoline, only pilocarpine is used in clinical practice. Accidental ingestion or intentional overdose with these alkaloids leads to characteristic symptoms of diaphoresis, salivation, abdominal cramps, nausea and vomiting, visual disturbances, hypotension, bradycardia, and bronchospasm followed by respiratory failure. Prompt treatment with atropine is important. Of the synthetic analogs, metacholine is used in inhalational challenge tests and bethanechol and carbachol are used in neurogenic bladder paralysis.

Atropine and scopolamine, two naturally occurring alkaloids, are nonselective inhibitors at the muscarinic receptor. In spite of their structural similarity their clinical effects can be quite diverse. For example, small doses of atropine may initially produce bradycardia but the usual clinical response is tachycardia. In contrast, scopolamine in large doses may elicit transient tachycardia but the usual response is bradycardia. Scopolamine also has a more pronounced sedative effect, while both drugs may cause excitation and delirium when administered in large doses. Both drugs are bronchodilators, relax the lower esophageal sphincter, and result in dry skin and mucous membranes in clinically relevant doses. In the past, atropine has been routinely used as a premedicant or before induction of general anesthesia. It became well recognized, however, that perioperative use of atropine can mask the ability to monitor for important physiologic changes associated with arousal, pain, increases in intracranial pressure, hypovolemia, and shock. Furthermore, there are associated risks of arrhythmias, aspiration, hyperthermia, and the central anticholinergic syndrome, manifesting as prolonged postoperative sedation and respiratory depression. Patients who present in the emergency room with central anticholinergic syndrome are often delirious and agitated, but the syndrome more commonly manifests itself as prolonged sedation and delayed arousal after general anesthesia. Because of this atypical presentation recognition and treatment with physostigmine is often delayed. Recognition of these risks has diminished the practice of routine use of atropine both in adults and in children.

Glycopyrrolate is a quaternary antagonist of muscarinic receptors. It does not cross the blood–brain barrier or the placenta, is less likely to cause tachycardia, and has a pronounced antisialogogue effect. It has become the parasympatholytic of choice for most anesthesiologists.

References

1. Eglen RM. Muscarinic receptor subtypes in neuronal and non-neuronal cholinergic function. *Auton and Autactoid Pharmacol* 2006; **26**: 219–33.

2. Hulme EC, Birdsall NJ, Buckley NJ. Muscarinic receptor subtypes. *Annu Rev Pharmacol Toxicol* 1990; **30**: 633–73.

3. Caulfield MP. Muscarinic receptors – characterization, coupling and function. *Pharmacol Ther* 1993; **58**: 319–79.

4. Hulme EC, Curtis CAM, Page KM, *et al.* Agonist activation of muscarinic acetylcholine receptors. *Cellular Signaling* 1993; **5**: 687–94.

5. Wess J. Molecular basis of muscarinic acetylcholine receptor function. *Trends Pharmacol Sci* 1993; **14**: 308–13.

6. Felder CC. Muscarinic acetylcholine receptors: transduction through multiple effectors. *FASEB J* 1995; **9**: 619–25.

7. Brown JH, Taylor P. Muscarinic receptor agonists and antagonists. In: Hardman JG, Gilman AG, Limbird LE, eds., *Goodman and Gilman's The Pharmacological Basis of Therapeutics.* New York, NY: McGraw-Hill, 1996.

8. Wess J, Eglen RM, Gautam D. Muscarinic acetylcholine receptors: mutant mice provide new insights for drug development. *Nat Rev Drug Discov* 2007; **6**: 721–33.

9. Cushny AR. The action of atropine, pilocarpine and physostigmine. *J Physiol* 1910; **41**: 233–45.

10. Maclagan J, Barnes PJ. Muscarinic pharmacology of the airways. *Trends Pharmacol Sci* 1989; **5**: 88–92.

11. Humphries TJ. Effects of long-term medical treatment with cimetidine and bethanechol in patients with esophagitis and Barrett's esophagus. *J Clin Gastroenterol* 1987; **9**: 28–32.

12. Nusair S, Rubinow A. The use of oral pilocarpine in xerostomia and Sjögren's syndrome. *Semin Arthritis Rheum* 1999; **28**: 360–7.

13. Littmann L, Kempler P, Rohla M, *et al.* Severe symptomatic atrioventricular block induced by pilocarpine eye drops. *Arch Intern Med* 1987; **147**: 586–7.

14. Asthana S, Greig NH, Holloway HW, *et al.* Clinical pharmacokinetics of arecoline in subjects with Alzheimer's disease. *Clin Pharmacol Ther* 1996; **60**: 276–82.

15. ThinkQuest. Poisonous plants and animals. library.thinkquest.org/C007974 (accessed June 26, 2010).

16. Aziz E, Nathan B, McKeever J. Anesthetic and analgesic practices in Avicenna's Canon of Medicine. *Am J Chinese Med* 2000; **28**: 147–51.

17. Matesic DF, Luthin GR. Atropine dissociates complexes of muscarinic acetylcholine receptor and guanine nucleotide-binding protein in heart membranes. *FEBS Letters* 1991; **284**: 184–6.

18. Hilf G, Jakobs KH. Agonist-independent inhibition of G protein activation by muscarinic acetylcholine receptor antagonists in cardiac membranes. *Eur J Pharmacol* 1992; **225**: 245–52.

19. Soejima M, Noma A. Mode of regulation of the Ach-sensitive K-channel by the muscarinic receptor in rabbit atrial cells. *Phlügers Arch* 1984; **409**: 424–31.

20. Morton HJV, Thomas ET. Effect of atropine on the heart rate. *Lancet* 1958; **2**: 1313–5.

21. Wellstein A, Pitschner HF. Complex dose-response curves of atropine in man explained by different functions of M_1- and M_2-cholinoceptors. *Naunyn-Schmiedeberg's Arch Pharmacol* 1988; **338**: 19–27.

22. Brodde OE, Konschak U, Becker K, *et al.* Cardiac muscarinic receptors decrease with age. *J Clin Invest* 1998; **101**: 471–8.

23. Überführ P, Frey AW, Reichart B. Vagal reinnervation in the long term after orthotopic heart transplantation. *J Heart Lung Transplant* 2000; **19**: 946–50.

24. Parlow JL, van Vlymen JM, Odell MJ. The duration of impairment of autonomic control after anticholinergic drug administration in humans. *Anesth Analg* 1997; **84**: 155–9.

25. Smith DS, Orkin FK, Gardner SM, *et al.* Prolonged sedation in the elderly after intraoperative atropine administration. *Anesthesiology* 1979; **51**: 348–9.

26. Kounis NG. Letter: Atropine eye-drops delirium. *Can Med Assoc J* 1974; **110**: 759.

27. Mendak JS, Minerva P, Wilson TW, *et al.* Angle closure glaucoma complicating systemic atropine use in the cardiac catheterization laboratory. *Cath Cardiovasc Diagn* 1996; **39**: 262–4.

28. Gal TJ, Suratt PM. Atropine and glycopyrrolate effects on lung mechanics in normal man. *Anesth Analg* 1981; **60**: 85–90.

29. Annis P, Landa J, Lichtiger M. Effects of atropine on velocity of tracheal mucus in anesthetized patients. *Anesthesiology* 1976; **44**: 74–7.

30. Cotton BR, Smith G. Single and combined effects of atropine and metoclopramide on the lower oesophageal sphincter pressure. *Br J Anaesth* 1981; **53**: 869–74.

31. Abboud T, Raya J, Sadri S, *et al.* Fetal and maternal cardiovascular effects of atropine and glycopyrrolate. *Anesth Analg* 1983; **62**: 426–30.

32. Leighton KM, Sanders HD. Anticholinergic premedication. *Can Anaesth Soc J* 1976; **23**: 563–6.

33. Jöhr, M. Is it time to question the routine use of anticholinergic agents in paediatric anaesthesia? *Paediatr Anaesth* 1999; **9**: 99–101.

34. Ostfeld AM, Arguete A. Central nervous system effects of hyoscine in man. *J Pharmacol Exp Ther* 1962; **137**: 133–9.

35. Renner UD, Oertel R, Kirch W. Pharmacokinetics and pharmacodynamics in clinical use of scopolamine. *Ther Drug Monit* 2005; **27**: 655–65.

36. Gibbons PA, Nicolson SC, Betts EK, *et al.* Scopolamine does not prevent postoperative emesis after pediatric eye surgery. *Anesthesiology* 1984; **61**: A435.

37. Osterholm RK, Camoriano JK. Transdermal scopolamine psychosis. *JAMA* 1982; **247**: 3081.

38. Wilkinson JA. Side effects of transdermal scopolamine. *J Emerg Med* 1987; **5**: 389–92.

39. List WF, Gravenstein JS. Effects of atropine and scopolamine on the cardiovascular system in man: II. Secondary bradycardia after scopolamine. *Anesthesiology* 1965; **26**: 299–304.

40. Kanto J, Kentala E, Kaila T, *et al.* Pharmacokinetics of scopolamine during caesarian section: relationship between serum concentration and effect. *Acta Anaesth Scan* 1989; **33**: 482–6.

41. Schnesk HJ, Ruphert J. Central anticholinergic syndrome in anaesthesia and intensive care. *Acta Anaesthesiol Belg* 1989; **40**: 219–28.

42. Brown DA, Heller F, Barkin R. Anticholinergic syndrome after anesthesia: A case report and review. *Am J Ther* 2004; **11**: 144–53.

43. Czeche S, Elgert M, Noe C, *et al.* Antimuscarinic properties of the stereoisomers of glycopyrronium bromide. *Life Sci* 1997; **60**: 1167.

44. Mirakhur RK. Intravenous administration of glycopyrronium: effects on cardiac rate and rhythm. *Anaesthesia* 1979; **34**: 458–62.

45. Ali-Melkkilä T, Kaila T, Kanto J, Iisalo E. Pharmacokinetics of i.m. glycopyrronium. *Br J Anaesth* 1990; **64**: 667–9.

46. Mirakhur RK, Dundee JW. Glycopyrrolate: pharmacology and clinical use. *Anaesthesia* 1983; **38**: 1195–204.

47. Ali-Melkkilä T, Kaila T, Kanto J, *et al.* Pharmacokinetics of glycopyrronium in parturients. *Anaesthesia* 1990; **45**: 634–7.

48. Abrams P, Andersson K-E, Buccafusco JJ, *et al.* Muscarinic receptors: their distribution and function in body systems, and the implication for treating overactive bladder. *Br J Pharmacol* 2006; **148**: 565–78.

49. Haddad EB, Mak JC, Barnes PJ. Characterization of [^{3}H]Ba 679 Br, a slowly dissociating muscarinic antagonist, in human lung: radioligand binding and autoradiographic mapping. *Mol Pharmacol* 1994; **45**: 899–907.

50. Alabaster VA. Discovery & development of selective M3 antagonists for clinical use. *Life Sci* 1997; **60**: 1053–60.

Pharmacokinetic data and recommended dosing of drugs were compiled from www.medsafe.govt.nz and www.merck.com/mmpe. Chemical structures came from Wikipedia (en.wikipedia.org).

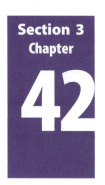

Section 3 Chapter 42

Essential drugs in anesthetic practice

Beta-blockers and other adrenoceptor antagonists

Andrew J. Patterson

Introduction

Large numbers of patients with cardiovascular disease derive benefit from the administration of adrenoceptor antagonists (blockers). For example, β-blockers decrease mortality in patients with New York Heart Association (NYHA) class II–IV congestive heart failure (CHF) [1–16] and improve outcome in high-risk vascular surgery patients during the perioperative period [17–19]. β-Blockers are also recommended for patients experiencing or having experienced myocardial infarction (MI) [20], as well as for patients with stable angina and hypertension [21,22].

Adrenoceptor blockers benefit patients in a variety of ways. Some drugs are relatively selective for one receptor subtype (such as β_1-selective antagonists). These drugs can decrease heart rate and improve myocardial oxygen balance, thereby decreasing myocardial ischemia [17,18]. In contrast, other drugs (e.g., carvedilol) appear to be most advantageous for patients with CHF through mechanisms that are not completely understood [23,24].

Adrenoceptor blockers can be classified according to the receptor(s) with which they interact. They can also be classified by the effect they have upon those receptors. Adrenoceptor blockers may be partial inverse agonists, neutral antagonists, or partial agonists that stabilize activated states of their receptor targets while inhibiting receptor interaction with full agonists [25]. Which receptor subtype these drugs interact with and the impact of this interaction upon intracellular signaling complexes appear to be the important factors that underlie their effects, both beneficial and adverse. For example, CHF patients receiving the β_1-selective partial inverse agonist metoprolol have improved outcomes [1]. In contrast, CHF patients receiving the mixed β_1/β_2/α_1 partial agonist bucindolol have worse outcomes [25,26].

The ability to inhibit adrenoceptor subtypes with a very high degree of selectivity has been elusive. Recently, the crystal structure of the human β_2-adrenoceptor in a lipid environment was elucidated while the receptor was bound to an inverse agonist [27]. This structural biology breakthrough may signal the beginning of a new era in rational drug design and the development of more effective adrenoceptor blocking drugs.

Mechanisms of drug action

Adrenoceptors mediate the primary cardiovascular effects of catecholamines in mammalian species. Both endogenous catecholamines (hormones and neurotransmitters) and exogenous catecholamines (pharmaceuticals) serve as adrenoceptor agonists. Classic pharmacology research advanced our understanding of adrenoceptors after Ahlquist first described the concept of α and β receptors more than 60 years ago [28]. During the past three decades, significant discoveries relevant to adrenoceptors have been based on advances in molecular biology and gene modification in mice.

In 1948 Ahlquist proposed that the effects of exogenously administered epinephrine were mediated by activating (α) and inhibiting (β) receptors. This classification was further modified by principal location of adrenoceptors; thus, subtypes such as α_{1A} receptors were localized to postsynaptic areas of the neuromuscular junction and were deemed excitatory, while the presynaptic variety (α_{2A} receptors) were considered autoinhibitory) [29].

As the understanding of adrenoceptor physiology accelerated during the 1980s and 1990s, researchers identified numerous roles and additional locations for α and β receptors in humans and other mammalian species. For instance, β_{1A} and β_{2A} receptors were shown to be expressed in the human sinoatrial node [30], and both receptor subtypes were shown to contribute to the capacity to increase heart rate [31,32]. It was also recognized that adrenoceptors play a role in mediating the progression of certain disease states, such as CHF [33–35]. The genes for nine distinct adrenoceptor subtypes were eventually cloned (Fig. 42.1). In addition, mutagenesis studies identified the adrenoceptor domains critical for agonist and antagonist binding, G-protein interaction, and desensitization [36–46].

Adrenoceptors are seven-transmembrane-helix receptors whose cytosolic aspects interact with signaling elements, especially G proteins. The three-dimensional structure of adrenoceptors includes pockets into which hydrophilic molecules may enter. Allosteric changes that occur within the receptors by virtue of their interactions with these hydrophilic molecules

Anesthetic Pharmacology, 2nd edition, ed. Alex S. Evers, Mervyn Maze, Evan D. Kharasch. Published by Cambridge University Press. © Cambridge University Press 2011.

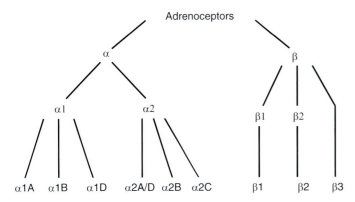

Figure 42.1. Adrenoceptors (adrenergic receptors): the genes for nine distinct adrenoceptor subtypes have now been cloned.

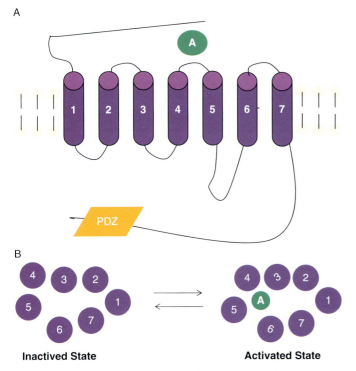

Figure 42.2. Adrenoceptor structure and activation. (A) Adrenoceptors are seven-transmembrane-helix receptors with intracellular, transmembrane, and extracellular domains. (B) The three-dimensional structures of adrenoceptors as they reside in the cellular membrane create pockets into which hydrophilic molecules (such as agonists and antagonists) can enter.

make the cytosolic elements of the receptors more or less attractive to intracellular signaling elements. Adrenoceptor agonists are molecules that induce allosteric changes and increase a receptor's affinity for intracellular signaling molecules that stimulate cellular processes (Fig. 42.2).

The mechanisms by which antagonists (such as β-blockers) act is more complicated. Conceptually, adrenoceptors are dynamic molecules that exist in a state of equilibrium between an inactivated state and numerous activated states. In the case of β-adrenoceptors, agonists stabilize activated states of the receptor and push the equilibrium toward those states. Some β-blockers stabilize the inactivated state and push the equilibrium toward that state. In contrast, other β-blockers simply serve as neutral antagonists and obstruct entry of agonists into the binding pocket without affecting a receptor's equilibrium. Still other β-blockers stabilize activated states of the receptor while obstructing access of full agonists to the receptor's binding pocket (Figs. 42.2, 42.3).

Of the nine adrenoceptor subtypes cloned, three are primary targets for commonly used antagonists: α_1, β_1, and β_2 receptors. α_1-Adrenoceptors mediate important physiologic processes such as smooth-muscle contraction and cellular hypertrophy. Consequently, α_1-antagonists include antihypertensive drugs and medications to treat benign prostatic hypertrophy [47]. β-Adrenoceptors are known to influence chronotropic and inotropic performance of the heart, pulmonary vascular tone, and peripheral vascular tone, and β-blockers are used to control heart rate and modulate the impact of hyperactive sympathetic nervous system stimulation. The remainder of this chapter will focus on these three receptor subtypes and the antagonists that act upon them.

β-Adrenoceptors and their signaling

Although the β_2-adrenoceptor was once believed to be a functional and structural duplicate of the β_1-adrenoceptor, it is now known that the two receptor subtypes differ significantly. Their genes are located on different chromosomes, the β_1 gene on chromosome 10 and the β_2 gene on chromosome 5. The receptor subtypes differ in size, with the β_1-adrenoceptor containing 423 amino acid residues while the β_2-adrenoceptor has 477 amino acids. In addition, their signaling pathways differ in ways that may help to explain some of the differences between clinically administered β-blocking drugs.

When acutely stimulated, both β_1 and β_2 subtypes enhance heart rate and contractility [48,49]. In addition, both receptor subtypes couple to stimulatory G protein (G_s). However, only β_2-adrenoceptors couple to inhibitory G protein (G_i) [50]. β_2-Adrenoceptor activation has also been shown to activate antiapoptotic signaling pathways in neonatal rat myocytes, while β_1-adrenoceptor activation in adult rat ventricular myocytes has been show to increase apoptosis [51,52]. Studies using cells from human right atrium and left ventricle have also shown that β_2-adrenoceptors couple more effectively to G_s than β_1-adrenoceptors [48,53–55].

The original concept for the consequences of activation of β_1- and β_2-adrenoceptors involves a common linear signaling pathway (Fig. 42.4). According to this paradigm, agonist binding induces conformational changes in both receptor subtypes. These conformational changes increase affinity for G_s. Interaction with either the β_1 or β_2 receptor causes G_s to disassemble into a βγ subunit and an α subunit. The α subunit activates adenylate cyclase and uses adenosine triphosphate (ATP)

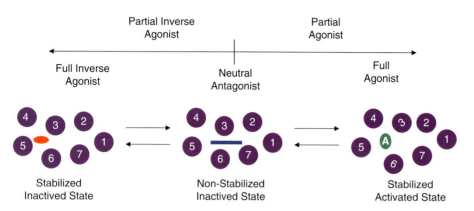

Figure 42.3. Activated and inactivated states of adrenoceptors. Each adrenoceptor exists in a dynamic equilibrium between an inactivated state and numerous activated states. Drugs that stabilize activated states and push the receptor's equilibrium toward those states are either partial or full agonists. Drugs that push the equilibrium toward the inactivated state are either full or partial inverse agonists. Drugs that simply block access to the receptor's binding pocket without affecting the state of equilibrium are neutral antagonists.

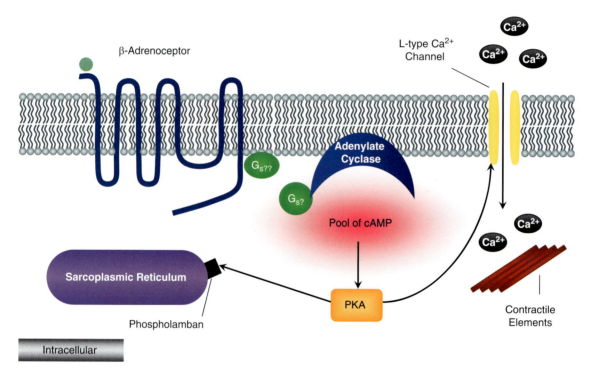

Figure 42.4. Traditional linear signaling paradigm for β-adrenoceptors. Acute activation of both β$_1$- and β$_2$-adrenoceptors increases cardiac contractility, relaxation, and heart rate. According to the traditional linear signaling paradigm, β-adrenoceptor stimulation alters calcium handling within myocytes as a consequence of protein kinase A (PKA)-mediated phosphorylation of L-type calcium channels, ryanodine receptors, and phospholamban [57,59].

to generate cyclic adenosine monophosphate (cAMP). The cAMP disinhibits protein kinase A (PKA), which in turn phosphorylates a variety of targets within the cytosol, including L-type calcium channels on the cell membrane and phospholamban and ryanodine receptors on the sarcoplasmic reticulum [56]. In cardiac myocytes, this linear signaling pathway is linked to contractile elements that enhance cardiac inotropic performance and increase contraction rate [57].

By the late 1990s evidence began to accumulate that β-adrenoceptor signaling was more complicated than a linear cascade of events. For instance, it was observed that after β$_1$-adrenoceptor stimulation, cAMP diffused throughout the cell and activated cyclic nucleotide-gated ion channels and a guanosine 5′-triphosphate (GTP) exchange factor (exchange protein-activated cAMP, EPAC). In contrast, β$_2$-adrenoceptor activation appeared to generate rises in cAMP only within specific cellular subdomains [57–59].

The linear signaling paradigm traditionally ascribed to β-adrenoceptors (Fig. 42.4) has now given way to a multidimensional schema (Fig. 42.5) in which β-adrenoceptors dynamically couple to multiple G proteins and other signaling and scaffold proteins in a temporally and spatially regulated manner. It is now recognized that the switch in coupling from G$_s$ to G$_i$ that occurs with β$_2$-adrenoceptors is a time-dependent process. Temporal regulation is also recognized as being important in the change of β$_1$-adrenoceptor signaling from PKA activation to activation of calcium/calmodulin-dependent protein kinase II (CaM kinase II) [57,59].

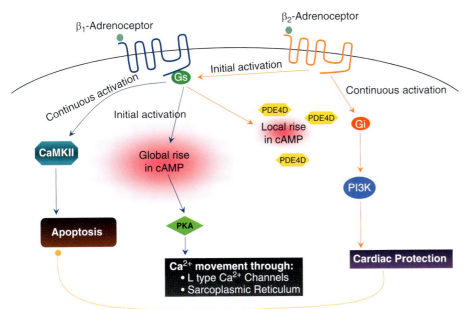

Figure 42.5. Multidimensional schema for signaling by β-adrenoceptors. Recent studies suggest that β₁- and β₂-adrenoceptor signaling involves promiscuous G-protein coupling, time-dependent changes, and G-protein-independent pathways. For example, during continuous activation, the β₂-adrenoceptor undergoes a time-dependent change in coupling from stimulatory G protein (G$_s$) to inhibitory G protein (G$_i$), which results in a phosphatidylinositol-3-kinase (PI3K)-mediated reduction in myocyte apoptosis. During continuous stimulation of the β₁-adrenoceptor, signaling changes from a protein kinase A (PKA) pathway to a calcium/calmodulin-dependent protein kinase II (CaMKII) pathway, which leads to increased myocyte apoptosis. Evidence also suggests that β₂-adrenoceptor signaling is localized to specific cellular subdomains and that phosphodiesterases (PDE) play an important role in this process [57,59].

During the past decade, in-vitro studies have elucidated several other details of the temporal and spatial regulation associated with β₁- and β₂-adrenoceptor signaling [60]. It is now appreciated that compartmentalization of cAMP allows spatially distinct pools of PKA to be differentially activated [61]. Further, by virtue of their ability to degrade cAMP, it has been shown that phosphodiesterases (PDEs) contribute to the localization of cAMP gradients within cells when β₂-adrenoceptors are stimulated [62]. Differences in cell signaling between β₁ and β₂ receptors with regard to activation of cytotoxic versus cytoprotective pathways (Fig. 42.5) explain why continuous β₁-adrenoceptor stimulation causes myocyte injury while continuous β₂-adrenoceptor stimulation does not. These differences may also help to explain why relatively β₁-selective antagonists produce favorable outcomes in humans [1,2,17,18,57,63].

The β₁- and β₂-adrenoceptor subtypes also differ in terms of the processes by which they undergo desensitization during continuous and prolonged activation. During persistent agonist activation β₁-adrenoceptors desensitize by reducing the number of available receptors on the cell surface [64]; degradation of receptors after internalization, together with a decrease in receptor mRNA, provides the mechanisms whereby the reduction persists. β₁-Adrenoceptors are desensitized when agonist-occupied receptors are phosphorylated by PKA and by G-protein-coupled receptor kinase 2 (GRK2), which is also called β-adrenergic receptor kinase 1 (βARK1) [65]. The cellular expression of GRK2 increases during continuous β₁-adrenoceptor stimulation. Following receptor phosphorylation, binding of a small protein known as β-arrestin sterically blocks G-protein activation; β-arrestin binding also directs the internalization of desensitized receptors. Studies of mice that overexpress β₁-adrenoceptors suggest that continuous β₁ stimulation leads to cardiomyocyte toxicity [66]. Studies in which the β₁/β₂-agonist

isoproterenol was administered for prolonged periods of time to β₂-adrenoceptor knockout mice also support this finding [63].

While there still is a role for β-arrestin in β₂-adrenoceptor desensitization, other aspects of the desensitization processes differ. At low agonist concentrations, β₂ receptors undergo PKA-mediated phosphorylation at serine 262 in the third intracellular loop. This process appears to depend on activation of G$_s$ by the β₂-adrenoceptor, with subsequent cAMP production and PKA activation. Under conditions of high receptor occupancy by agonist, β₂-adrenoceptors are phosphorylated by PKA at serine 262 as well as by GRKs at serines 355, 356, and 364. One such kinase is GRK2 [59,67]. GRK2 is attracted to the agonist-occupied receptor's cytosolic aspect by the G$_s$ βγ subunit, which anchors itself to the cell membrane adjacent to the receptor after separating from the G$_s$ α subunit. When bound to G$_s$ βγ, GRK2 is ideally suited to phosphorylate intracellular elements of the receptor [59]. The β₂-adrenoceptor desensitization process mediates a change in coupling of the β₂ receptor from G$_s$ to G$_i$. This process has been shown to be important for the activation of antiapoptotic pathways [52].

Several murine studies have provided evidence that the differences between β₁- and β₂-adrenoceptor activation observed in vitro are also important in vivo. Low-level transgenic overexpression (approximately fivefold) of β₁-adrenoceptors in the mouse heart has been shown to cause cardiomyopathy [66]. In contrast, 60-fold overexpression of β₂-adrenoceptors results in improved cardiac contractile force without any cardiomyopathic consequences [68]. Evidence from murine studies suggests that β₂-receptor activation actually protects the heart from prolonged β₁-receptor stimulation in vivo. For instance, mice lacking β₂-adrenoceptors (β₂-knockout) experienced significantly greater mortality and signs of more severe heart failure than wild-type controls after continuous infusion of the nonspecific β-adrenoceptor agonist isoproterenol [63]. β_2-Adrenoceptor activation has also been reported to afford cardioprotective effects in dogs [69].

α-Adrenoceptor signaling

The prototypical signaling pathway of α1 ARs involves coupling to G proteins of the $G_{q/11}$ family followed by activation of phospholipase Cβ [70–73]. The result is cleavage of phosphatidylinositol 4,5-bisphosphate (PIP_2) into inositol 1,4,5-trisphosphate (IP_3) and diacylglycerol (DAG). IP_3 promotes release of calcium ions from intracellular stores. DAG activates protein kinase C (PKC) isoforms [74,75]. Numerous other signaling molecules are now known to be activated by α_1-adrenoceptor stimulation. For example, α_1-adrenoceptors have been shown to activate pertussis-sensitive G proteins (G_i and G_o), G_s, as well as $G_{12/13}$ family G proteins. α_1-Adrenoceptors have also been shown to activate a nonheterotrimeric guanine nucleotide binding protein called G_h. Differences in signaling between α_1 subtypes, as well as between α_1 receptors in different tissues, have been demonstrated [47].

Preclinical pharmacology

In some cell types, including myocytes, it has been observed that administration of certain β-adrenoceptor blocking drugs restores responsiveness to catecholamines after β-receptor desensitization. These β-blockers lead to normalization of GRK2 activity and $G_{\alpha i}$ levels. Certain β-blockers appear to allow the intracellular signaling system to return toward a normal state despite ongoing catecholamine stimulation. In animal studies, certain β-blockers have also been shown to reverse cardiac remodeling [76,77].

Drugs such as carvedilol (and to some degree metoprolol) reverse abnormal intracellular calcium handling by promoting expression of sarcoplasmic reticulum calcium ATPase (SERCA) mRNA. They also decrease expression of detrimental β-myosin heavy-chain mRNA while increasing beneficial α-myosin heavy-chain mRNA expression [78]. Carvedilol in particular enhances secretion of atrial natriuretic peptide (ANP) [79], which inhibits the renin–angiotensin–aldosterone and sympathetic nervous systems. Celiprolol increases myocardial endothelial nitric oxide synthase (eNOS) levels and activity. Nitric oxide production has been found to be diminished during cardiac remodeling [80].

Differences in the mechanisms of action of β-blockers may explain why some drugs protect myocytes more effectively than others. β-Blockers can be classified according to which AR subtypes they antagonize (Table 42.1), as well as by whether they are inverse agonists, neutral antagonists, or partial agonists (Fig. 42.6). For example, atenolol, bisoprolol, esmolol, metoprolol, and xamoterol are relatively β_1-adrenoceptor selective antagonists, while bucindolol, carvedilol,

Table 42.1. β-blockers classified by the receptor subtypes with which they interact

β_1 blockade	β_1, β_2 blockade	β_1, β_2, α_1 blockade
Acebutolol	Carteolol	Bucindolol
Atenolol	Nadolol	Carvedilol
Betaxolol	Penbutolol	Labetalol
Bisoprolol	Pindolol	
Celiprolol	Propranolol	
Esmolol	Sotalol	
Metoprolol	Timolol	
Nebivolol		
Xamoterol		

labetalol, and propranolol are non-selective β_1/β_2-adrenoceptor blockers. Bucindolol, carvedilol, and labetalol also block α_1-adrenoceptors.

Several β-blockers actually stabilize the activated state of β-adrenoceptors, leading to coupling of the receptors to G_s. These drugs are considered partial agonists (Fig. 42.6). They block the effects of potent agonists such as epinephrine and norepinephrine while generating low-level β-adrenoceptor stimulation. Bucindolol and xamoterol are examples of partial agonists [25].

Other β-blockers are inverse agonists that stabilize the inactivated state of β-adrenoceptors. They lead to receptor upregulation rather than causing the desensitization and downregulation observed with xamoterol. Metoprolol, nebivolol, betaxolol (used in the treatment of open-angle glaucoma), and sotalol (approved for treatment of atrial fibrillation and flutter) are examples of inverse agonist β-adrenoceptor blocking drugs [25].

Many of the clinically used β-blockers are neutral antagonists that bind to β receptors without affecting their activation states. They simply block the binding of agonists. Carvedilol and propranolol are examples of neutral antagonists [25].

Based on preclinical studies, there are theoretical benefits to drugs with relatively β_1-selective properties, drugs with mixed β- and α_1-adrenoceptor blocking activity, and drugs that are partial inverse agonists. For instance, drugs such as metoprolol that preferentially block β_1-adrenoceptors may diminish detrimental myocardial remodeling while preserving the protective effects of β_2-adrenoceptor activation [81,82]. Drugs such as carvedilol that block α_1-adrenoceptors may decrease arterial vascular tone and serve as effective afterload-reducing drugs while blunting the deleterious effects of sympathetic nervous system hyperactivity. Drugs that are partial inverse agonists may diminish β-receptor desensitization while restoring functional β-receptor responsiveness.

Two β-blockers warrant further consideration. Carvedilol is a nonselective β_1/β_2 and α_1 blocking drug with a unique carbazol

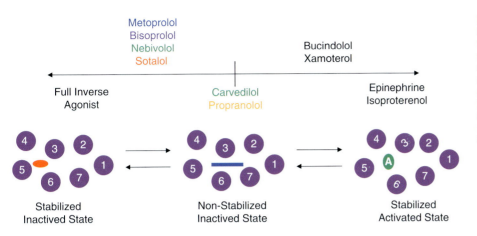

Figure 42.6. Spectrum of β-adrenoceptor blockers. Several β-blockers are inverse agonists, which stabilize the inactivated state of β-adrenoceptors. They lead to receptor upregulation rather than causing the desensitization and downregulation observed with receptor agonists. Metoprolol, bisoprolol, nebivolol, and sotalol are examples of inverse agonists. In contrast, some β-blockers are partial agonists and stabilize activated states of β-adrenoceptors, leading to coupling of the receptors to stimulatory G protein (G_s). Bucindolol and xamoterol are examples of partial agonists. Other β-blockers are neutral antagonists.

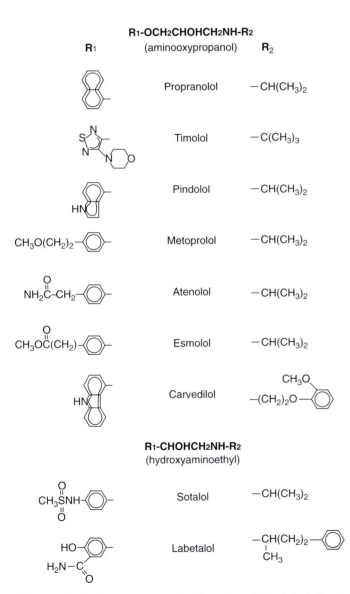

Figure 42.7. The β-receptor antagonists. The variety of side chains linking to common backbones determines the diversity of drug characteristics.

moiety. It has demonstrated greater clinical benefit than other β-blockers in the management of CHF patients and in the post-myocardial infarction (MI) setting. Carvedilol is an antioxidant with antiarrhythmic, antiapoptotic, and antiproliferative properties that affects carbohydrate and lipid metabolism [83]. Nebivolol is a highly selective β_1-adrenoceptor blocker that stimulates the vascular endothelial L-arginine/nitric oxide pathway [84]. The chemical structures of the β-blockers are shown in Fig. 42.7.

Clinical pharmacology

How β-blockers convey benefit to patients appears to vary from drug to drug. For patients with ischemic coronary artery disease, relatively β_1-selective antagonists such as atenolol and bisoprolol may improve oxygen balance by decreasing cardiac rate and contractility. They may also reduce oxygen utilization, prevent dislodging of coronary atherosclerotic plaques, and increase the threshold for ventricular fibrillation in the presence of ischemia [17,18].

For other patients, β-blockers may convey benefit by reducing detrimental myocardial remodeling. For instance, patients who suffer from CHF, patients who experience myocardial ischemia or infarction, patients who undergo cardiac surgery, and patients who endure emotional stress all demonstrate evidence of sympathetic nervous system hyperactivity. Continuous activation of β_1-adrenoceptors by catecholamines released from sympathetic nerve terminals innervating the heart (norepinephrine) and by the adrenal gland (epinephrine) can lead to the detrimental cellular and subcellular changes previously described. In humans, myocyte hypertrophy, myocyte apoptosis, reactivation of fetal gene programs, and alterations in the quantity and composition of the extracellular matrix have been shown to occur. Several β-blockers, including metoprolol and carvedilol, reduce this detrimental cardiac remodeling [85–91]. The pharmacokinetics and pharmacodynamics of the β-blockers are shown in Tables 42.2 and 42.3.

681

Table 42.2. Pharmacokinetic characteristics of some commonly used β-adrenergic antagonists

Antagonist	Absorption	First-pass metabolism	Blood level variability	Protein binding	Metabolism	Excretion	Half-life
Propranolol	~ 100%	~ 75%	High	90%	~ Full, liver	Renal	3–5 h
Pindolol	~ 100%	10–15%	Mild	40%	50%, liver	Renal	3–4 h
Oxprenolol	~ 70–90%	20–65%	High	80–90%	~ 95%, liver	Renal	1.5–4 h
Nadolol	~ 37%	Minimal	Minimal	30%	Minimal	Renal	20–24 h
Timolol	~ 100%	~ 50%	Moderate	80%	~ 80%, liver	Renal	3–5 h
Labetalol	~ 100%	~ 70%	High	50%	~ Full, liver	Renal, biliary	6–8 h PO, 5.5 h IV
Sotalol	~ 100%	~ 10%	Mild	Minimal	Minimal	Renal	7–15 h
Metoprolol	~ 100%	~ 60%	High	5–10%	~ 90%	Renal	3–4 h
Atenolol	~ 50%	<10%	Minimal	~ 3%	~ 10%	Renal	5–8 h
Acebutolol	~ 100%	~ 60%	Mild	26%	~ Full, liver	Renal, biliary	3–4 h[a]
Esmolol	IV only	NA	Minimal	50%	Erythrocyte esterase	Renal	8 min
Carvedilol	~ 100%	60–75%	Moderate	98%	Liver	Biliary	6–10 h
Celiprolol	30–70%	Minimal	Mild	30%	Minimal	Renal	4–6 h

[a] Diacetolol, the active metabolite of acebutolol, has a half-life of 8–12 hours.
IV, intravenously; NA, not available; PO, per os (by mouth).

Nonselective β$_1$/β$_2$-antagonists

Propranolol

Propranolol reduces heart rate and contractility by blocking β$_1$- and β$_2$-adrenoceptors. It is used for the control of hypertension, migraine headaches, and tremors. It is also used as an antiarrhythmic drug with quinidine-like and anesthetic-like effects on cell membranes. Propranolol can be administered orally or intravenously and is hepatically metabolized. The elimination half-life is approximately 10 hours for the sustained-release oral capsule and 4 hours for the oral nonsustained-release preparation as well as for intravenous preparations. Abrupt cessation of propranolol may cause angina exacerbation, MI, or ventricular arrhythmias [93].

Sotalol

Sotalol is an antiarrhythmic drug with Vaughan Williams class II and III properties. It causes slowing of the heart rate, increased atrioventricular (AV) node refractoriness, and reduced AV node conduction. It is administered orally and has a time to peak concentration of 2.5–4 hours. The bioavailability is 90–100%. The elimination half-life is 12 hours in adults and 9.5 hours in children. It is not metabolized. Rather, it is excreted unchanged in the urine by virtue of glomerular filtration and tubular secretion. Therefore, the elimination half-life is increased in patients with renal insufficiency. Sotalol can be removed by dialysis [93,94].

Sotalol AF is used for maintenance of sinus rhythm in patients who have experienced symptomatic atrial fibrillation or atrial flutter but are in sinus rhythm. Sotalol AF is a different medication than the non-AF preparation of sotalol and can cause life-threatening ventricular arrhythmias. In contrast, the non-AF preparation of sotalol is approved for the treatment of ventricular arrhythmias, not atrial fibrillation. Excessive dosing of both preparations of sotalol has been associated with bradycardia, hypotension, syncope, prolonged QTc interval, multifocal ventricular extrasystoles, torsades de pointes, ventricular tachycardia, ventricular fibrillation, and asystole. Like other β-blockers, sotalol can mask the symptoms of hypoglycemia. Sotalol is contraindicated in patients with baseline QT interval > 450 ms, patients with congenital or acquired long QT syndromes, patients with creatinine clearance < 40 mL min^{-1}, patients with second- and third-degree heart block, and patients with severe sinus bradycardia. Patients started on sotalol should undergo continuous cardiac monitoring for a minimum of 3 days [93,94].

Relatively β$_1$-selective antagonists

Atenolol

Atenolol is a relatively β$_1$-selective antagonist, though at higher doses it inhibits β$_2$-adrenoceptors as well. It can be administered both orally and intravenously. When administered orally, it has a bioavailability of approximately 50%, and the time to peak

Table 42.3. Pharmacodynamic characteristics and recommended dosage of some commonly used β-adrenergic antagonists

Antagonist	Receptor	Other effects	Oral dose (daily)	Intravenous dose
Propranolol	β_1, β_2	Mem stab, 5-HT$_{1C}$, 5-HT$_2$	40–320 mg	0.5–1 mg to maximum 3 mg
Pindolol	β_1, β_2	ISA, 5-HT$_{1A}$	15–45 mg	0.1–0.4 mg slowly
Oxprenolol	β_1, β_2	ISA	120–480 mg	1–2 mg slowly, maximum 5 mg
Nadolol	β_1, β_2	None	80–240 mg (maximum 320 mg)	
Timolol	β_1, β_2	None	15–45 mg (maximum 60 mg)	Ophthalmic preparation for treatment of glaucoma, 0.25–0.5 mg mL^{-1}
Labetalol	$\alpha_1, \beta_1, \beta_2$[a]	ISA	400–1200 mg	5–20 mg IV every 5–10 minutes to maximum 300 mg; infusion start at 2 mg min^{-1}
Sotalol	β_1, β_2[b]	Class III antiarrhythmic	160–320 mg (maximum 640 mg)	20–120 mg over 10 min or 1.5 mg kg^{-1} followed by 0.2–0.5 mg kg^{-1} h^{-1} (maximum 640 mg daily)
Metoprolol	β_1	None	100–400 mg	5 mg every 2 minutes to 15 mg total
Atenolol	β_1	None	50–100 mg	2.5 mg over 2.5 min every 5 min to 10 mg or 0.15 mg kg^{-1} over 20 min
Acebutolol	β_1	ISA	200–800 mg	
Esmolol	β_1	None	NA	50–100 mg bolus, 0.05–0.3 mg kg^{-1} min^{-1} infusion
Carvedilol	$\alpha_1, \beta_1, \beta_2$[c]	Mem stab, antioxidant	12.5–50 mg	
Celiprolol	β_1	Partial β_2 agonist	200–600 mg	

5-HT$_{1A}$, 5-HT$_{1C}$, 5-HT$_2$: 5-HT$_{1A}$, 5-HT$_{1C}$, 5-HT$_2$ receptor antagonism [92]; ISA, intrinsic sympathomimetic activity (partial agonist at the β_2 receptor); IV, intravenously; mem stab, membrane stabilizing effect; NA, not available.
[a] Four stereoisomers: R,R responsible for most of β activity (antagonism and ISA), S,R and S,S responsible for α_1 antagonism, R,S is inactive; β : α activity is 7 : 1 when given IV, 5 : 1 when given orally.
[b] The l-stereoisomer is responsible for the β-antagonist activity; both stereoisomers possess class III antiarrhythmic activity.
[c] The S(−) stereoisomer is responsible for the β-antagonist activity, the stereoisomers are equipotent in α_1-antagonist activity; β : α potency is 10:1. The 4′-hydroxyphenyl metabolite is a 13-times more potent β-receptor antagonist than the parent drug; two of the hydroxycarbazole metabolites are 30–80 times more potent antioxidants than the parent drug.

blood concentration is 2–4 hours. It undergoes little hepatic metabolism and is excreted by the kidney. The elimination half-life is 6–7 hours, though it can be longer in the elderly or in patients with renal insufficiency. It is FDA-approved for heart rate and blood pressure control during and after acute MI, in patients with angina, and in patients with hypertension [93].

Bisoprolol

Bisoprolol is a β_1-selective antagonist, though it can antagonize β_2-adrenoceptors at high doses. It is administered orally and has a bioavailability of about 80%. The time to peak blood concentration is 2–4 hours. It is hepatically metabolized. It is excreted renally (50%) and nonrenally with an elimination half-life of 9–12 hours. Bisoprolol is approved for the treatment of hypertension [93].

Celiprolol

Celiprolol is an investigational drug. It is a β_1-selective antagonist that causes vasodilation by stimulating peripheral β_2-adrenoceptors. It has been shown to enhance myocardial

contractility. It also appears to increase myocardial eNOS levels and activity [80]. It is orally administered, and it has been studied for the treatment of angina pectoris and hypertension. It is metabolized in the liver to a small degree. However, it is primarily excreted unmetabolized by the kidneys and to a smaller degree by the gastrointestinal tract. The elimination half-life of celiprolol is about 5.5 hours [93].

Esmolol

Esmolol is a relatively β_1-selective antagonist that is administered intravenously. It is approved for treatment of intraoperative and postoperative hypertension as well as supraventricular arrhythmias. It is metabolized in red blood cells by esterases via hydrolysis. It is excreted in the urine as an acid metabolite. Its elimination half-life is approximately 9 minutes. Esmolol is 55% protein-bound [93].

Metoprolol

Metoprolol is a relatively β_1-selective antagonist, though it blocks β_2 receptors at higher doses. It is administered either intravenously or orally. It is approved for treatment of tachycardia and hypertension in patients experiencing MI and angina pectoris. It is also approved for the treatment of CHF [95]. When administered orally, it is rapidly and completely absorbed. Only a small fraction (12%) is protein-bound. Approximately 50% of the drug is hepatically metabolized (first pass) with the metabolite excreted by the kidney with an elimination half-life of 3–7 hours [93].

Nebivolol

Nebivolol is a highly lipophilic long-acting β_1-selective antagonist that has vasodilating properties mediated by the L-arginine/nitric oxide pathway. It also inhibits reactive oxygen species [96,97]. Nebivolol is approved for the treatment of hypertension. Nebivolol is administered orally. It is metabolized via direct glucuronidation and N-dealkylation and oxidation by cytochrome P450 2D6 (CYP2D6) in the liver. Several active metabolites are produced. Excretion occurs by the fecal route and in the urine. Bioavailability and excretion characteristics vary depending on how extensively an individual metabolizes nebivolol; there is considerable variability. Bioavailability ranges from 12% (extensive metabolizers) to 96% (poor metabolizers). The elimination half-life ranges from 12 to 19 hours [93].

Mixed β_1/β_2/α_1-antagonists

Carvedilol

Carvedilol is a unique β-blocker in several ways. It antagonizes β_1-, β_2-, and α_1-adrenoceptors. It is also an antioxidant with antiarrhythmic, antiapoptotic, and antiproliferative properties that affects carbohydrate and lipid metabolism [83,93]. By virtue of its α_1-adrenoceptor blocking properties, carvedilol reduces peripheral vascular resistance. Carvedilol is administered orally and is approved for the treatment of CHF, hypertension, and impaired left ventricular dysfunction after MI. Carvedilol is hepatically metabolized via the CYP2D6 pathway that generates an active metabolite (4'-hydroxyphenyl); it is excreted in the feces after biliary elimination with an elimination half-life of 7–10 hours [93]. Carvedilol has been shown to be particularly effective for the treatment of patients with CHF, though the mechanisms by which it conveys benefit are not clear [3–7].

Labetalol

Labetalol is also a nonspecific β- and α_1-adrenoceptor blocking drug used for the treatment of hypertension in adults. It can be administered orally and intravenously; when administered orally, the time to peak concentration is considerably longer than after intravenous administration (1–2 hours, compared to several minutes). It is 50% protein-bound, and is hepatically metabolized by glucuronide conjugation and fecally and renally excreted. The elimination half-life of labetalol is 5.5 hours when administered intravenously and 6–8 hours when administered orally; both may be lengthened in elderly patients [93,98].

Looking to the future

During the next decade scientific advances may lead to pharmaceuticals that selectively inhibit detrimental elements of β-adrenoceptor signaling (such as activation of CaM kinase II) while simultaneously activating desirable signaling elements (such as phosphatidylinositol-3-kinase, PI3K). Recent breakthroughs in structural biology could lead to a better understanding of the subtle conformational changes that occur in β-adrenoceptors as they interact with various ligands (both agonists and antagonists) [27]. Revealing what these conformational states are and how they differentially affect intracellular signaling pathways could facilitate development of more targeted and effective pharmaceuticals.

Summary

Endogenous and exogenous catecholamines act via adrenoceptors to affect the cardiovascular system, and adrenoceptor blockers derive their beneficial treatment of cardiovascular disease by blocking the actions of the catecholamines on adrenoceptors. The three primary targets for commonly used antagonists are α_1-, β_1-, and β_2-adrenoceptors. α_1-Adrenoceptor antagonists counteract hypertension and cellular hypertrophy; β-antagonists are used to control heart rate and modulate sympathetic effects.

The α_1-, β_1-, and β_2-adrenoceptors are seven-transmembrane G-protein-coupled receptors that couple to multiple G proteins, as well as other signaling and scaffold proteins. In the case of the β_1- and β_2-adrenoceptors these multiple signal transduction pathways are subject to spatial and temporal regulation, which differs between the β_1-and β_2-receptor subtypes. Furthermore, there is evidence for a role of β_1-adrenoceptors in the activation of cytotoxic pathways, and for β_2-adrenoceptors in the activation of antiapoptotic pathways.

β-Blockers may be partial agonists (e.g., bucindolol and xamoterol), which result in low-level stimulation whilst blocking the effects of more potent agonists. Inverse agonists (e.g., metoprolol, nebivolol, and sotalol) stabilize the inactive state of β-adrenoceptors. Neutral antagonists (e.g., carvedilol and propranolol) simply bind to the receptor, blocking access for other agonists. Preclinical studies suggest that selectively blocking β_1-adrenoceptors may reduce myocardial remodeling, while preserving β_2-adrenoceptor-mediated protection. Continuous β_1-adrenoceptor signaling can lead to myocyte hypertrophy and apoptosis, reactivation of fetal gene programs, and changes to the extracellular matrix. Relatively selective blocking of β_1 signaling may also have a negative inotropic and chronotropic effect. Partial inverse agonists and drugs that possess both α_1- and β-adrenoceptor blocking activity may also be preferential.

Nonselective β_1- and β_2-antagonists include propranolol, which reduces heart rate and contractility. It is used to treat hypertension, migraine, tremors, and arrhythmia. Sotalol slows heart rate, increases atrioventricular (AV) node refractoriness and reduces AV node conduction. Distinct preparations are available for the maintenance of sinus rhythm following atrial fibrillation or flutter, and for the treatment of ventricular arrhythmia (Sotalol AF and non-AF, respectively).

Amongst the antagonists that are relatively selective for β_1-adrenoceptors are atenolol, which is approved for heart rate and blood pressure control in cases of myocardial infarction (MI), angina, and hypertension; bisoprolol, used to treat hypertension; and metoprolol, for treatment of congestive heart failure (CHF), as well as treatment of tachycardia and

hypertension in cases of MI and angina pectoris. These drugs also block β_2-adrenoceptors at higher doses. Esmolol is approved for treating intraoperative and postoperative hypertension and supraventricular arrhythmias. Celiprolol, an investigational drug, and nebivolol have vasodilating properties mediated via distinct pathways.

Carvedilol antagonizes α_1-, β_1-, and β_2-adrenoceptors. It is also an antioxidant with antiarrhythmic, antiapoptotic, and antiproliferative properties. It is approved for the treatment of CHF, hypertension, and impaired left ventricular dysfunction after MI. Similarly, labetalol affects mixed receptor types and is used in the treatment of hypertension.

References

1. International Steering Committee. MERTI-HF. Rationale, design, and organization of the Metoprolol CR/XL Randomized Intervention Trial in Heart Failure (MERIT-HF). *Am J Cardiol* 1997; **80**: 54J–58J.

2. CIBIS II Investigators. The Cardiac Insufficiency Bisoprolol Study II (CIBIS-II): a randomised trial. *Lancet* 1999; **353**: 9–13.

3. Packer M, Bristow MR, Cohn JN, *et al.* The effect of carvedilol on morbidity and mortality in patients with chronic heart failure. U.S. Carvedilol Heart Failure Study Group. *N Engl J Med* 1996; **334**: 1349–55.

4. Colucci WS, Packer M, Bristow MR, *et al.* Carvedilol inhibits clinical progression in patients with mild symptoms of heart failure. U.S. Carvedilol Heart Failure Study Group. *Circulation* 1996; **94**: 2800–6.

5. Packer M, Coats AJ, Fowler MB, *et al.* Effect of carvedilol on survival in severe chronic heart failure. *N Engl J Med* 2001; **344**: 1651–8.

6. Dargie HJ. Effect of carvedilol on outcome after myocardial infarction in patients with left-ventricular dysfunction: the CAPRICORN randomised trial. *Lancet* 2001; **357**: 1385–90.

7. Khand AU, Rankin AC, Martin W, *et al.* Carvedilol alone or in combination with digoxin for the management of atrial fibrillation in patients with heart failure? *J Am Coll Cardiol* 2003; **42**:1944–51.

8. Avezum A, Tsuyuki RT, Pogue J, YusufS. Beta-blocker therapy for congestive heart failure: a systematic overview and critical appraisal of the published trials. *Can J Cardiol* 1998; **14**: 1045–53.

9. Lechat P, Packer M, Chalon S, *et al.* Clinical effects of beta-adrenergic blockade in chronic heart failure: a meta-analysis of double-blind, placebo-controlled, randomized trials. *Circulation* 1998; **98**: 1184–91.

10. Doughty RN, Rodgers A, Sharpe N, MacMahon S. Effects of beta-blocker therapy on mortality in patients with heart failure. A systematic overview of randomized controlled trials. *Eur Heart J* 1997; **18**: 560–5.

11. Heidenreich PA, Lee TT, Massie BM. Effect of beta-blockade on mortality in patients with heart failure: a meta-analysis of randomized clinical trials. *J Am Coll Cardiol* 1997; **30**: 27–34.

12. Brophy JM, Joseph L, Rouleau JL. Beta-blockers in congestive heart failure: a Bayesian meta-analysis. *Ann Intern Med* 2001; **134**: 550–60.

13. Packer M, Colucci WS, Sackner-Bernstein JD, *et al.* Double-blind, placebo-controlled study of the effects of carvedilol in patients with moderate to severe heart failure. The PRECISE trial. Prospective Randomized Evaluation of Carvedilol on Symptoms and Exercise. *Circulation* 1996; **94**: 2793–9.

14. Eichhorn EJ, Heesch CM, Barnett JH, *et al.* Effect of metoprolol on myocardial function and energetics in patients with nonischemic dilated cardiomyopathy: a randomized, double-blind, placebo-controlled study. *J Am Coll Cardiol* 1994; **24**: 1310–20.

15. Waagstein F, Bristow MR, Swedberg K, *et al.* Beneficial effects of metoprolol in idiopathic dilated cardiomyopathy. Metoprolol in Dilated Cardiomyopathy (MDC) Trial Study Group. *Lancet* 1993; **342**: 1441–6.

16. Lohse MJ, Engelhardt S, Eschenhagen T. What is the role of β adrenergic signaling in heart failure? *Circ Res* 2003; **93**: 896–906.

17. Mangano DT, Layug EL, Wallace A, Tateo I. Effect of atenolol on mortality and cardiovascular morbidity after noncardiac surgery. *N Engl J Med* 1996; **335**: 1713–20.

18. Poldermans D, Boersma E, Bax JJ, *et al.* The effect of bisoprolol on perioperative mortality and myocardial infarction in high-risk patients undergoing vascular surgery. *N Engl J Med* 1999; **341**: 1789–94.

19. POISE Study Group. Effects of extended-release metoprolol succinate in patients undergoing non-cardiac surgery (POISE trial): a randomised controlled trial. *Lancet* 2008; **371**: 1839–47.

20. Braunwald E, Antman EM, Beasley JW, *et al.* ACC/AHA 2002 guideline update for the management of patients with unstable angina and non-ST-segment elevation myocardial infarction – summary article: a report of the American College of Cardiology/ American Heart Association Task Force on Practice Guidelines (Committee on the Management of Patients with Unstable Angina). *J Am Coll Cardiol* 2002; **40**: 1366–74.

21. Chobanian AV, Bakris GL, Black HR, *et al.* The seventh report of the Joint National Committee on Prevention, Detection, Evaluation, and Treatment of High Blood Pressure: the JNC 7 Report. *JAMA* 2003; **289**: 2560–72.

22. US Department of Health and Human Services, National Heart, Lung, and Blood Institute. *JNC 7 Express: the Seventh Report of the Joint National Committee on Prevention, Detection, Evaluation, and Treatment of High Blood Pressure.* Bethesda, MD: NHLBI, 2003.

23. Lowes BD, Gilbert EM, Abraham WT, *et al.* Myocardial gene expression in dilated cardiomyopathy treated with beta-blocking agents. *N Engl J Med* 2002; **346**: 1357–65.

24. Ohta Y, Watanabe K, Nakazawa M, *et al.* Carvedilol enhances atrial and brain natriuretic peptide mrna expression and release in rat heart. *J Cariovasc Pharmacol* 2000; **36**: S19–S23.

25. Engelhardt S, Grimmer Y, Fan GH, Lohse MJ. Constitutive activity of the human β1 adrenergic receptor in β1 receptor transgenic mice. *Mol Pharmacol* 2001; **60**: 712–17.

26. Bristow MR, Krause-Steinrauf H, Nuzzo R, *et al.* Effect of baseline or changes in adrenergic activity on clinical outcomes in the β Blocker Evaluation of Survival Trial. *Circulation* 2004; **110**: 1437–42.

27. Rasmussen SF, Choi HJ, Rosenbaum DM, *et al.* Crystal structure of the human β2 adrenergic g-protein-coupled receptor. *Nature* 2007; **450**: 383–8.

28. Ahlquist R. Study of adrenotropic receptors. *Am J Physiol* 1948; **153**: 586–600.

29. Hurt C, Angelotti T. Molecular insights into α 2 adrenergic receptor function: clinical implications. *Semin Anesth Perioper Med Pain* 2007; **26**: 28–34.

30. Rodefeld MD, Beau SL, Schuessler RB, Boineau JP, Saffitz JE. Beta adrenergic and muscarinic cholinergic receptor densities in the human sinoatrial node: identification of high beta 2-adrenergic receptor density. *J Cardiovasc Electrophysiol* 1996; **7**: 1039–49.

31. McDevitt DG. In vivo studies on the function of cardiac beta adrenoceptors in man. *Eur Heart J* 1989; **10**: 22–8.

32. Brodde OE. Beta 1- and Beta 2-adrenoceptors in the human heart: properties, function, and alterations in chronic heart failure. *Pharmacol Rev* 1991; **43**: 203–42.

33. Cohn JN, Levine B, Olivari MT, *et al.* Plasma norepinephrine as a guide to prognosis in patients with congestive heart failure. *N Engl J Med* 1984; **311**: 819–23.

34. Kaye DM, Lefkovits J, Jennings GL, *et al.* Adverse consequences of high sympathetic nervous activity in the failing human heart. *J Am Coll Cardiol* 1995; **26**: 1257–63.

35. Esler M, Kaye D, Lambert G, Esler D, Jennings G. Adrenergic nervous system in heart failure. *Am J Cardiol* 1997; **80**: 7L–14L.

36. Kobilka BK, Kobilka TS. Chimeric α2, β2 adrenergic receptors: delineation of domains involved in effector coupling and ligand binding specificity. *Science* 1988; **240**: 1310–16.

37. Strader CD, Sigal IS, Dixon RA. Structural basis of beta adrenergic receptor function. *Faseb J* 1989; **3**: 1825–32.

38. Strader CD, Candelore MR, Hill WS, Sigal IS, Dixon RA. Identification of two serine residues involved in agonist activation of the β adrenergic receptor. *J Biol Chem* 1989; **264**: 13572–8.

39. Green SA, Cole G, Jacinto M, Innis M, Liggett SB. A polymorphism of the human β2 adrenergic receptor within the fourth transmembrane domain alters ligand binding and functional properties of the receptor. *J Biol Chem* 1993; **268**: 23116–21.

40. Lohse MJ, Engelhardt S, Danner S, Böhm M. Mechanisms of β adrenergic receptor desensitization: from molecular biology to heart failure. *Basic Res Cardiol* 1996; **91**: 29–34.

41. Summers RJ, Kompa A, Roberts SJ. Beta-adrenoceptor subtypes and their desensitization mechanisms. *J Auton Pharmacol* 1997; **17**: 331–43.

42. Grishna G, Berlot CH. Mutations at the domain interface of Gsα impair receptor-mediated activation by altering receptor and guanine nucleotide binding. *J Biol Chem* 1998; **273**: 15053–60.

43. Broadley KJ. Review of mechanisms involved in the apparent differential desensitization of β1 and β2 adrenoreceptor-mediated functional responses. *J Auton Pharmacol* 1999; **19**: 335–45.

44. Bunemann M, Hosey MM. G protein coupled receptor kinases as modulators of G protein signaling. *J Physiol* 1999; **517**: 5–23.

45. Bunemann M, Lee KB, Pals-Rylaarsdam R, Roseberry AG, Hosey MM. Desensitization of G protein coupled receptors in the cardiovascular system. *Annu Rev Physiol* 1999; **61**: 169–92.

46. Seibold A, Williams B, Huang ZF, *et al.* Localization of the sites mediating desensitization of the β2 adrenergic receptor by the GRK pathway. *Mol Pharmacol* 2000; **58**: 1162–73.

47. Hein P, Michel MC. Signal transduction and regulation: are all α1 adrenergic receptors subtypes created equal? *Biochem Pharmacol* 2007; **73**: 1097–106.

48. Kaumann AJ, Hall JA, Murray KJ, Wells FC, Brown MJ. A comparison of the effects of adrenaline and noradrenaline on human heart: the role of beta 1 and beta 2 adrenoceptors in the stimulation of adenylate cyclase and contractile force. *Eur Heart J* 1989; **10**: 29–37.

49. Walsh DA, Van Patten SM. Multiple pathway signal transduction by the cAMP-dependent protein kinase. *Faseb J* 1994; **8**: 1227–36.

50. Xiao RP, Ji X, Lakatta EG. Functional coupling of the beta 2 adrenoceptor to pertussis toxin-sensitive G protein in cardiac myocytes. *Mol Pharmacol* 1995; **47**: 322–29.

51. Communal C, Singh K, Sawyer DB, Colucci WS. Opposing effects of beta(1) and beta(2) adrenergic receptors on cardiac myocyte apoptosis: role of pertussis toxin-sensitive G protein. *Circulation* 1999; **100**: 2210–12.

52. Chesley A, Lundberg MS, Asai T, *et al.* The beta(2)-adrenergic receptor delivers an antiapoptotic signal to cardiac myocytes through G(i)-dependent coupling to phosphatidylinositol 3'-kinase. *Circ Res* 2000; **87**: 1172–9.

53. Brodde OE, O'Hara N, Zerkowski HR, Rohm N. Human cardiac beta-adrenoceptors: both beta 1 and beta 2 adrenoceptors are functionally coupled to adenylate cyclase in right atrium. *J Cardiovasc Pharmacol* 1984; **6**: 1184–91.

54. Gille E, Lemoine H, Ehle B, Kaumann AJ. The affinity of (–)-propranolol for beta1 and beta2 adrenoceptors of human heart: differential antagonism of the positive inotropic effects and adenylate cyclase stimulation by (–)-noradrenaline and (–)-adrenaline. *Naunyn Schmiedebergs Arch Pharmacol* 1985; **331**: 60–70.

55. Bristow MR, Hershberger RE, Port JD, Minobe W, Rasmussen R. Beta 1 and beta 2 adrenergic receptor-mediated adenylate cyclase stimulation in non-failing and failing human ventricular myocardium. *Mol Pharmacol* 1989; **35**: 295–303.

56. Houslay MD, Baillie GS. β Arrestin-recruited phosphodiesterase-4 desensitizes the AKAP79/PKA-mediated switching of β2 adrenoceptors signaling to activation of ERK. *Biochem Soc Trans* 2005; **33**: 1333–6.

57. Xiao RP, Zhu W, Zheng M, *et al.* Subtype-specific α1 and β adrenoreceptor signaling in the heart. *Trends Pharmacol Sci* 2006; **27**: 330–7.

58. Richter W, Day P, Agrawal R, *et al.* Signaling from β1 and β2 adrenergic receptors is defined by differential interactions with PDE4. *EMBO J* 2008; **27**: 384–93.

59. Patterson AJ, Pearl N, Chang C. Impact of phosphodiesterase 4D on cardiac β2 adrenergic receptor signaling. *Semin Anesth Perioper Med Pain* 2007; **26**: 22–7.

60. Nikolaev VO, Bunemann M, Schmitteckert E, Lohse MJ, Engelhardt S. Cyclic AMP imaging in adult cardiac myocytes reveals far-reaching β1-adrenergic but locally confined β2-adrenergic receptor-mediated signaling. *Circ Res* 2006; **99**: 1084–91.

61. Houslay MD, Adams DR. PDE4D cAMP phosphodiesterase: modular enzymes that orchestrate signaling cross-talk, desensitization and compartmentalization. *Biochem J* 2003; **370**: 1–18.

62. Zaccolo M, Pozzan T. Discrete microdomains with high concentration of camp in stimulated rat neonatal cardiac myocytes. *Science* 2002; **295**: 1711–14.

63. Patterson AJ, Zhu W, Chow A, *et al.* Protecting the myocardium: a role for the β2 adrenergic receptor in the heart. *Crit Care Med* 2004; **32**: 1041–8.

64. Ungerer M, Bohm M, Elce JS, Schnabel P, Böhm M. Altered expression of beta-adrenergic receptor kinase and beta1 adrenergic receptors in the failing human heart. *Circulation* 1993; **87**: 454–63.

65. Hata JA, Williams ML, Koch WJ. Genetic manipulation of myocardial beta-adrenergic receptor activation and desensitization. *J Mol Cell Cardiol* 2004; **37**: 11–21.

66. Engelhardt S, Hein L, Wiesmann F, Lohse MJ. Progressive hypertrophy and heart failure in beta 1 adrenergic receptor transgenic mice. *Proc Natl Acad Sci U S A* 1999; **96**: 7059–64.

67. Vaughan DJ, Millman EE, Godines V, *et al.* Role of the G protein-coupled receptor kinase site serine cluster in β2 adrenergic receptor internalization, desensitization, and β-arrestin translocation. *J Biol Chem* 2006; **281**: 7684–92.

68. Liggett SB, Tepe NM, Lorenz JN, *et al.* Early and delayed consequences of beta (2) adrenergic receptor overexpression in mouse hearts: critical role for expression level. *Circulation* 2000; **101**: 1707–14.

69. Sosunov EA, Gainullin RZ, Moise NS, *et al.* β1 and β2 adrenergic receptor subtype effects in german shepherd dogs with inherited lethal ventricular arrhythmias. *Cardiovasc Res* 2000; **48**: 211–19.

70. Hubbard KB, Hepler JR. Cell signalling diversity of the gqα family of heterotrimeric G proteins. *Cell Signal* 2006; **18**: 135–50.

71. Offermanns S. G Proteins as transducers in transmembrane signalling. *Prog Biophys Mol Biol* 2003; **83**: 101–130.

72. Exton JH. Regulation of phosphoinositide phospholipases by hormones, neurotransmitters, and other agonists linked to G proteins. *Ann Rev Pharmacol Toxicol* 1996; **36**:481–509.

73. Wu D, Katz A, Lee CH, Simon MI. Activation of phospholipase C by α1 adrenergic receptors is mediated by the α subunits of Gq family. *J Biol Chem* 1992; **267**: 25798–802.

74. Fain JN, Garcia-Sainz JA. Role of phosphatidylinositol turnover in α1 and of adenylate cyclase inhibition in α2 effects of catecholamines. *Life Sci* 1980; **26**: 1183–94.

75. Theroux TL, Esbenshade TA, Peavy RD, Minneman KP. Coupling efficiencies of human α1 adrenergic receptor subtypes: titration of receptor density and responsiveness with inducible and repressible expression vectors. *Mol Pharmacol* 1996; **50**: 1376–87.

76. El-Armouche A, Zolk O, Rau T, Eschenhagen T. Inhibitory G-proteins and their role in desensitization of the adenylyl cyclase pathway in heart failure. *Cardiovascular Research* 2003; **60**: 478–87.

77. Brodde OE. β-adrenoceptor blocker treatment and the cardiac β-adrenoreceptor-G-protein(s)-adenylyl cyclase system in chronic heart failure. *Naunyn-Schmiedeberg's Arch Pharmacol* 2007; **374**: 361–72.

78. Lowes BD, Gilbert EM, Abraham WT, *et al.* Myocardial gene expression in dilated cardiomyopathy treated with beta-blocking agents. *N Engl J Med* 2002; **346**: 1357–65.

79. Ohta Y, Watanabe K, Nakazawa M, *et al.* Carvedilol enhances atrial and brain natriuretic peptide mRNA expression and release in rat heart. *J Cardiovasc Pharmacol* 2000; **36**: S19–S23.

80. Liao Y, Asakura M, Takashima S, *et al.* Celiprolol, A vasodilatory β blocker, inhibits pressure overload-induced cardiac hypertrophy and prevents the transition to heart failure via nitric oxide-dependent mechanisms in mice. *Circulation* 2004; **110**: 1–8.

81. Hjalmarson A, Goldstein S, Fagerberg B, *et al.* Effects of controlled-release metoprolol on total mortality, hospitalizations, and well-being in patients with heart failure: the Metoprolol CR/XL Randomized

Intervention Trial in Congestive Heart Failure (MERIT-HF). *JAMA* 2000; **283**: 1295–302.

82. Ahmet I, Krawczyk M, Zhu W, *et al.* Cardioprotective and survival benefits of long-term combined therapy with β2 adrenoreceptor (AR) agonist and β1 AR blocker in dilated cardiomyopathy postmyocardial infarction. *J Pharm Exper Therapeutics* 2008; **325**: 491–9.

83. Stroe AF, Gheorghieade M. Carvedilol: β-blockade and beyond. *Rev Cardiovasc Med* 2004; **5**: S18–S27.

84. Prisant LM. Nebivolol: pharmacologic profile of an ultraselective, vasodilatory β1 blocker. *J Clin Pharmacol* 2008; **48**: 225–39.

85. Chien KR. Stress pathways and heart failure. *Cell* 1999; **98**: 555–8.

86. Groenning BA, Nilsson JC, Sondergaard L, *et al.* Antiremodeling effects on the left ventricle during beta-blockade with metoprolol in the treatment of chronic heart failure. *J Am Coll Cardiol* 2000; **36**: 2072–80.

87. Colucci WS, Kolias TJ, Adams KF, *et al.* Metoprolol reverses left ventricular remodeling in patients with

asymptomatic systolic dysfunction: the Reversal of Ventricular Remodeling with Toprol-XL (REVERT) trial. *Circulation* 2007; **116**: 49–56.

88. Jafri SM. The effects of beta blockers on morbidity and mortality in heart failure. *Heart Fail Rev* 2004; **9**: 115–21.

89. Greenberg BH, Mehra M, Teerlink JR, *et al.* COMPARE: comparison of the effects of carvedilol CR and carvedilol IR on left ventricle ejection fraction in patients with heart failure. *Am J Cardiol* 2006; **98**: 53L–59L.

90. Chizzola PR, Goncalves de Freitas HF, Saldanha Marinho NV, *et al.* The effect of β adrenergic receptor antagonism in cardiac sympathetic neuronal remodeling in patients with heart failure. *Int J Cardiol* 2006; **106**: 29–34.

91. Udelson JE. Ventricular remodeling in heart failure and the effect of β blockade. *Am J Cardiol* 2004; **93**: 43B–48B.

92. Nishio H, Nagakura Y, Segawa T. Interactions of carteolol and other beta-

adrenoceptor blocking agents with serotonin receptor subtypes. *Arch Int Pharmacodyn Ther* 1989; **302**: 96–106.

93. Micromedex (R) Healthcare Series. *DrugPoint Summary.* Thomson Healthcare. www.thomsonhc.com (accessed June 21, 2010).

94. Lafuente-Lafuente C, Mouly S, Longas-Tejero MA, Bergmann JF. Antiarrhythmics for maintaining sinus rhythm after cardioversion of atrial fibrillation. *Cochrane Database Syst Rev* 2007; (4): CD005049.

95. Talbert RL. Pharmacokinetics and pharmacodynamics of beta blockers in heart failure. *Heart Failure Reviews* 2004; **9**: 131–7.

96. Veverka A, Nuzum DS, Jolly J. Nebivolol: a third-generation β-adrenergic blocker. *Ann Pharmacother* 2006; **40**: 1353–60.

97. Sule SS, Frishman W. Nebivolol: new therapy update. *Cardiol Rev* 2006; **14**: 259–64.

98. Pederson ME, Cockcroft JR. The vasodilatory beta-blockers. *Curr Hypertens Rep* 2007; **9**: 269–77.

Essential drugs in anesthetic practice
Antiarrhythmic drugs

Aman Mahajan and Charles W. Hogue Jr.

Introduction

Therapeutic options for patients with cardiac arrhythmias have expanded considerably in the past decade, based in part on successes with nonpharmacologic therapies such as catheter ablation treatments for patients with atrial and ventricular tachyarrhythmias [1–3]. Laboratory advances in molecular and gene-based therapeutic approaches hold promise as novel future treatments for supraventricular and ventricular arrhythmias as well as for regenerative therapies for sinoatrial (SA) node and conduction system disorders [4–9]. Nonetheless, antiarrhythmic drugs continue to have a role in the management of cardiac rhythm disorders including acute life-threatening arrhythmias, atrial fibrillation, and atrial flutter. Additionally, they are helpful in managing patients with suboptimal catheter ablation of their arrhythmia substrate and in stabilizing patients with implantable cardioverter-defibrillator devices who are receiving frequent yet appropriate shocks or cardiac pacing treatments. An appreciation of the side-effect profile of these drugs, including the negative inotropic and proarrhythmic effects, has promoted their rational clinical use and fostered development of newer, less toxic compounds [10–13]. This chapter reviews the pharmacology of antiarrhythmic drugs and their indications along with the basic principles of acute arrhythmia management.

Mechanism of drug action

The cardiac action potential (AP) is the result of balance between multiple inward and outward ionic currents, with the ionic flow through specific ion channels determining each of the five phases (Fig. 43.1) [14]. The duration of each phase of the AP varies regionally in the heart, and the specialized conduction system exhibits regional differences in ion-channel density (Fig. 43.2). This relationship between ion channels and AP phase is fundamental to understanding the cellular, antiarrhythmic, and electrocardiogram (ECG) effects of antiarrhythmic drugs. At the molecular level, antiarrhythmic drugs exert their effect on **ion channels**, **pumps** (**exchangers**), or **receptors**. Ion-specific channels exist for sodium, potassium,

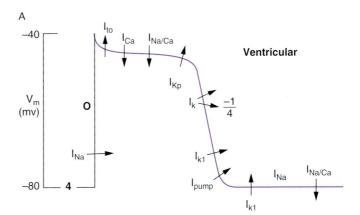

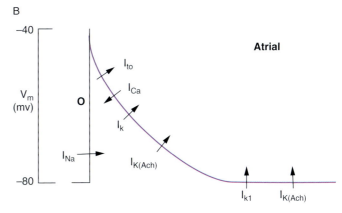

Figure 43.1. Ion channels that comprise the cardiac action potential, in (A) ventricular and (B) atrial myocardium. I_{Ca}, Ca^+ current; I_K, delayed (outwardly rectifying) K^+ current; I_{K2}, inwardly rectifying K^+ current; $I_{K(Ach)}$, acetylcholine-activated K^+ current; I_{Kp}, plateau K^+ current; I_{Na}, Na^+ current; $I_{Na/Ca}$, Na^+Ca^{2+} exchanger; I_{pump}, Na^+K^+ pump current; I_{to}, transient outward current. Redrawn from Whalley et al. [14].

calcium, and chloride. Membrane pump targets for antiarrhythmic drug therapy include the Na^+/K^+ ATPase, the Na^+/Ca^{2+} exchanger, the Na^+/H^+ exchanger, the Cl/HCO_3 exchanger, and the Na^+K^+/Cl cotransporter. Membrane receptor targets for antiarrhythmic treatments include the adrenergic β_1 and β_2 receptors, the muscarinic M_2 receptor, and the purinergic A_1 and A_2 receptors.

Anesthetic Pharmacology, 2nd edition, ed. Alex S. Evers, Mervyn Maze, Evan D. Kharasch. Published by Cambridge University Press. © Cambridge University Press 2011.

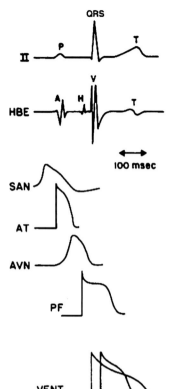

Figure 43.2. Surface ECG lead II and electrograms from locations in the heart demonstrating varying action potential characteristics resulting from different ion-channel composition and densities. The locations of the electrograms are the bundle of His (HBE), sinoatrial node (SAN), atrial tissue (AT), atrioventricular node (AVN), Purkinjie fiber (PF), and ventricular tissue (VENT).

Ion channels

Voltage- and ligand-gated ion channels are membrane-bound glycoproteins that change configuration or function in response to a stimulus (change in membrane potential or binding of ligand, respectively), thus providing a pathway of low electrical resistance across the hydrophobic lipid bilayer of the cell membrane [14,15]. Ion channels exist in **open**, **inactivated**, and **closed** states. In the open state, the channel configuration allows rapid flux of an ion along an electrochemical gradient. An activated channel usually progresses first to the inactivated state, at which time further ion conductance stops, and then to the closed state (i.e., resting state). Whereas an inactivated channel is unresponsive to a continued or new stimulus, a resting channel in the closed state can open in response to a subsequent stimulus. The resting ion channel state is more prevalent during diastole. The active state occurs during the upstroke of the AP (Fig. 43.1), and the inactivated state occurs during the plateau of repolarization. Ion channels (Na^+, Ca^{2+}) responsible for cardiac AP depolarization are predominantly in a closed state near the resting membrane potential (during diastole). The active state of Na^+ channels is seen during the upstroke of the AP with prompt inactivation of the channels that lasts throughout the plateau phase, while Ca^{2+} channels activate during the early plateau phase of the AP and become inactivated during the late repolization phase.

The net direction of ion flow through a channel is channel-specific and is referred to as **rectification**. An inward rectifying current produces a larger current when the ions are moving into the cell versus out of the cell. Ion channels that carry inward currents include the Na^+ channel (I_{Na}), Ca^{2+} channels (I_{Ca-L} and I_{Ca-T}), and the nonselective hyperpolarization Na^+ channel (I_f). Specific channel densities differ in different regions of the myocardium. For example, I_f is more prominent in pacemaker cells, and I_{Ca-T} is more dense in the SA node complex. The main outward rectifying channels are the K^+ channels, I_{K1}, I_K, with subsets I_{Kr} and I_{Ks}, and the transient outward current, I_{to}.

Two populations of channels exist in the presence of antiarrhythmic drugs: those blocked by the drug and those not blocked. In both the blocked and unblocked states, the three morphologic configurations of resting, active, and inactive channels are present. Drug association and dissociation time constants can be defined for the progression between the number of channels in each state. These rate constants in turn are affected by several factors in the cellular milieu such as hyperkalemia, hypoxia, pH changes, catecholamine release, and membrane potential. The net changes in channel blocking and state as a function of time can be described by sets of differential equations [16,17]. Antiarrhythmic drugs can be characterized in vitro based on the rate of block development and rate of recovery during repetitive stimulation. Binding kinetics of drugs to activated or inactivated channels are quantitative, but can be qualitatively described as slow, intermediate, or fast. These kinetic properties determine the overall effect of the drug on the cardiac AP and ECG.

Use-dependent block refers to drug effect on an ion channel that is more pronounced at more rapid heart rates, or after longer periods of stimulation, or both. It results when the drug affinity for open or inactivated channels exceeds the drug affinity for resting channels. **Reverse use-dependent** block, usually seen with drugs that prolong repolarization, occurs when a drug exerts a greater effect at slower heart rates. The latter is not ideal in so far as lengthening repolarization may be more desirable during tachycardia.

Specific ion channels

The cardiac I_{Na} is a transmembrane glycoprotein with multiple subunits [14]. Two gates control the flow of Na^+ ions through this channel. The m gate controls activation and the h gate controls inactivation. In the resting or closed channel configuration, the activation (m) gate is in the closed position and the inactivation (h) gate is in the open position. With membrane depolarization, the activation m gate joins the h gate in the open position, allowing the passage of Na^+ ions into the cell along their electrochemical gradient. Inward ion movement is terminated when the h gate moves to the closed position (inactivated state). The m gate then moves to the closed position (deactivation). When the h gate subsequently moves to the open position, the channel is ready to respond to the next stimulus (recovery from inactivation). Sodium channel blockers decrease the maximum upstroke velocity of phase 0 of the AP (V_{max}) and slow conduction.

Multiple K^+ channels have been identified in human cardiac tissue, and they play a primary role in repolarization of the cell membrane [14]. The voltage-gated potassium channels include I_{K1}, the inward rectifying channel; I_{to}, the transient outward current; and I_K, the delayed rectifier channel. I_K comprises the rapidly activating subtype I_{Kr} and the much more slowly activating subtype I_{Ks}. Ligand-gated potassium channels include I_{KACh}, I_{KATP}, and I_{KNa}. The different K^+ channels exhibit a diverse structural spectrum. The simplest is minK, a single polypeptide chain with a single crossing point on the cell membrane. Other K^+ channels have four subunits and multiple transmembrane helices. Potassium channel block prolongs the refractory period, increasing the effective refractory period (ERP) and AP duration, but it does not affect V_{max}. They exhibit reverse use-dependence, with decreased effectiveness in prolonging the AP at increased heart rates.

There are two extracellular and two intracellular types of Ca^{2+} channels identified in human cardiac cells [14]. L- and T-type Ca^{2+} channels are voltage-dependent plasma membrane ion channels, whereas the IP_3 receptor and the Ca^{2+} release channel (ryanodine receptor) are ligand-gated ion channels that control calcium release from the sarcoplasmic reticulum. The L-type Ca^{2+} channel, because of its close association with the ryanodine receptor, is uniquely positioned to affect both AP (by prolonging depolarization) and electromechanical coupling. Both L- and T-type Ca^{2+} channels are multiple subunit proteins; the α subunit is the target of antiarrhythmic drugs and is homologous with the voltage-dependent sodium channel.

Preclinical pharmacology

There are several classification schemes applied to antiarrhythmic drugs. The Vaughan Williams classification describes four main drug actions (Table 43.1) [18]. This classification is based on the predominant effect of the drug seen in healthy tissue. This approach is limited insofar as many of the drugs exert multiple effects and they may have active metabolites with differing mechanisms of action. Furthermore, drug effects are dependent on species, type of cardiac tissue, the presence of pathophysiologic perturbations, and other factors [19]. In 1991, the Working Group on Arrhythmias from the European Society of Cardiology proposed the Sicilian Gambit [20]. This construct emphasizes first the identification of the mechanism of the arrhythmia and its vulnerable parameter susceptible to modification, followed by identification of the target likely to affect the vulnerable parameter, and finally selection of an antiarrhythmic drug that may affect the target.

The effects of each antiarrhythmic drug on the AP and the ERP of cardiac cells are important properties that dictate clinical effect. Drugs that primarily block the inward I_{Na}

Table 43.1. Vaughan Williams classification of antiarrhythmic drugs

Class	Major electrophysiologic effect	Drugs
Ia	Block Na^+ channels leading to ↓ V_{max} and prolong AP duration, ↓ amplitude of AP, ↓ diastolic depolarization. Intermediate (< 5 s) binding kinetics	Procainamide, quinidine, disopyramide
Ib	Block Na^+ channels, shortened AP duration, no reduction in V_{max}. Fast onset/offset binding kinetics (< 500 ms)	Lidocaine, mexiletine, phenytoin, tocainide
Ic	Block Na^+ channels leading to ↓ V_{max}, slow conduction but minimal prolongation of refractoriness. Slow binding kinetics (10–20 s)	Flecainide, propafenone, moricizine
II	Blockade of β-adrenoceptor	Propranolol, atenolol, metoprolol, timolol, esmolol, etc.
III	Block K^+ channels, prolong repolarization	Amiodarone, sotalol, bretylium, azimilide, dofetilide, ibutilide
IV	Block slow Ca^{2+} channel	Verapamil, diltiazem, nifedipine, etc.

Binding kinetics refer to the rate of onset and offset of Na^+ channel blockade. AP, Action potential; V_{max}, upstroke velocity of phase 0.

current attenuate or suppress the upstroke of the AP or V_{max}. Potassium channel blockers primarily delay repolarization by prolonging the AP duration and the ERP, thus prolonging the QT interval. The net effect of a particular drug on the ECG is a combination of the electrophysiologic, pharmacodynamic, and pharmacokinetic effects (Table 43.2). The following section describes drug effects as determined in healthy human tissue.

Sodium channel blockers with intermediate binding kinetics (class Ia drugs)

Sodium channel blockers with intermediate binding kinetics include procainamide, quinidine, and disopyramide [21–24]. These drugs prolong AP duration, decrease V_{max}, decrease conduction velocity, and decrease maximum diastolic potential. The depression of V_{max} is more pronounced than the prolongation of the AP duration. They prolong atrial, His–Purkinje, and ventricular refractoriness, and thus are effective in the treatment of reentrant arrhythmias and those attributed to abnormal automaticity. These Na^+ channel blocking drugs exert little effect on cells in the SA node. Procainamide, quinidine, and disopyramide shorten the refractory period of the atrioventricular (AV) node through anticholinergic effects.

Table 43.2. Summary of the more important actions of drugs on membrane ion channels, receptors, and pumps

Drug	Channels			Ca^{2+}	K$^+$	I^f	Receptors				Pumps
	Na$^+$						α	β	M^2	P	Na$^+$/K$^+$ ATPase
	Fast	Medium	Slow								
Lidocaine	I↓										
Mexiletine	I↓										
Tocainide	↓										
Phenytoin	I↓			I↓							
Moricizine	I↑										
Procainamide		A↑			↕						
Disopyramide		A↑			↕				↓		
Quinidine		A↑			↕		↓		↓		
Propafenone		A, I↑		↓	↕			↕			
Flecainide			A↑		↓						
Encainide			A↑								
Bepridil	↓			↑	↕						
Verapamil	↓			↑					↕		
Diltiazem				↕							
Sotalol					↑			↑			
Amiodarone	↓			↓	↑		↕	↕			
Alinidine					↕	↑					
Ibutilide	*				(I$_{Kr}$)↑						
Dofetilide					(I$_{Kr}$)↑						
Azimilide					(I$_{Ks}$, I$_{Kr}$)↑						
Nadolol								↑			
Propranolol	↓							↑			
Atropine									↑		
Adenosine										*	
Digoxin									*		↑

Relative blocking potency: ↓ low; ↑ high; ↕ moderate.
* agonist; A, activated state blocker; I, inactivated state.

These effects are more pronounced during hyperkalemia in experimental tissue preparations. Procainamide has less anticholinergic properties than quinidine or disopyramide. Procainamide's major metabolite, N-acetyl procainamide (NAPA), neither suppresses the rate of phase 4 diastolic depolarization of Purkinje fibers nor affects resting membrane potential or V_{max}; however, it does prolong AP duration through K$^+$ channel blockade (class III effect) [19].

Unlike procainamide, quinidine blocks the rapid component of the K$^+$ channel, I$_{Kr}$. Quinidine has both use-dependent and reverse use-dependent effects. At slow heart rates, the K$^+$ channel is more occupied than the Na$^+$ channel and prolongation of the AP occurs, resulting in reverse use-dependence. At fast heart rates, blockage of the Na$^+$ channel predominates, consistent with use-dependent block.

Disopyramide is a racemic mixture of two stereoisomers. The S(+) isomer exhibits the electrophysiologic properties of increasing the ventricular AP duration and the QTc. The QTc prolongation by disopyramide is generally less than that seen with quinidine. The R(−) isomer shortens the AP duration and has no effect on the QT. Disopyramide's effects on I$_K$, I$_{Ca}$, and I$_{K1}$ account for prolongation of AP duration. Disopyramide, like quinidine, has anticholinergic effects and blocks the cardiac M_2 receptor. It has about one-thousandth the potency of atropine.

Sodium channel blockers with rapid binding kinetics (class Ib drugs)

This group of antiarrhythmic drugs includes lidocaine, tocainide, mexiletine, and phenytoin [21–28]. These drugs exhibit rapid association and dissociation from the Na^+ channel and preferentially block inactivated channels. These drugs slow the upstroke and prolong the duration of the AP in Purkinje fibers. They exhibit little effect on refractory periods in the SA node, atrium, or AV node.

Lidocaine suppresses abnormal automaticity in depolarized ventricular myocardium and Purkinje tissue. Modest suppression of early and delayed afterdepolarizations occurs with lidocaine. Mexiletine blocks inactivated Na^+ channels more readily than activated channels. In diseased myocardium, mexiletine administration slows conduction at the level of the AV node and His–Purkinje system. Phenytoin preferentially blocks inactivated Na^+ channels and also blocks inactivated T-type Ca^{2+} channels in ventricular myocytes. Suppression of delayed afterdepolarizations also has been described. Tocainide is a mixture of two stereoisomers; the R-isomer is electrically active. Tocainide shortens the AP duration in Purkinje fibers and ventricular myocytes. There is no effect on refractory periods in the atrium, ventricle, or specialized conduction system.

Sodium channel blockers with slow binding kinetics (class Ic drugs)

Flecainide, encainide, propafenone, and moricizine are potent Na^+ channel blockers with slow kinetics [28,29]. Flecainide is a potent depressant of V_{max}. It was developed as a fluorinated analog of procainamide, and it demonstrates tonic block of Ca^{2+} channels and Na^+ channel block. This combined effect is responsible for the minimal net effect on repolarization. Block of K^+ channels in ventricular muscle has also been described. In Purkinje tissue, both the AP duration and ERP are shortened. In ventricular tissue, the AP duration and ERP are prolonged. The AH, HV, PR, and QRS intervals are all prolonged.

Propafenone primarily blocks active and inactivated Na^+ channels. As with flecainide, I_K, I_{K1}, and I_{to} are also blocked, the latter two at supratherapeutic concentrations. Propafenone demonstrates mild block of the L-type Ca^{2+} channel. AH, HV, PR, QRS, and QT intervals are all prolonged. The ERP of the atrium, AV node, and ventricle are all prolonged. Propafenone is a weak β-adrenoceptor blocker.

Moricizine has multiple effects on the Na^+ channel. Its predominant action is to block the I_{Na}, and for that reason it is grouped with the Class I drugs in the Vaughan Williams scheme. Moricizine exhibits use-dependent properties. It slows retrograde AV nodal and His–Purkinje conduction, and has minimal effect on atrial, ventricular, and antegrade AV node refractoriness.

β-adrenoceptor blockers (class II drugs)

Beta-blockers (see Chapter 42) exhibit antiadrenergic and membrane-stabilizing effects [19,21,30,31]. The former effect results from competitive inhibition of catecholamine binding to the β receptor by the *l*-stereoisomer of the various compounds. The antiadrenergic effects decrease phase 4 depolarization, spontaneous firing, and automaticity of pacemaker cells, especially those in the AV node. As with other antiarrhythmic drugs, SA node automaticity is depressed in pre-existing SA node dysfunction. β-blockers prevent β-agonist enhancement of L-type Ca^{2+} currents. Membrane stabilization results from decreased Na^+ current that depresses V_{max} of the AP. The membrane-stabilizing effect has little clinical significance, because it occurs at concentrations 10 times greater than those necessary for β-blockade.

Class III potassium channel blockers

This group of antiarrhythmic drugs includes K^+ channel-specific drugs and those that affect multiple channels. The K^+ channel-specific drugs include azimilide, sotalol, dofetilide, and ibutilide [32–35]. These drugs prolong the ERP and increase AP duration; as such, they prolong the QT interval without other ECG effects. The pure K^+ channel blockers exhibit reverse use-dependence; the degree of block of the K^+ channel is more pronounced at slow heart rates, and there is less block at more rapid heart rates. Sotalol blocks I_{Kr}, and nonspecifically blocks $β_1$ and $β_2$ receptors. Ibutilide blocks I_{Kr} and the slow inward Na^+ channel. Dofetilide specifically targets I_{Kr}. Azimilide blocks both I_{Kr} and I_{Ks}.

Class III drugs that block multiple channels

Amiodarone is a Vaughan Williams class III drug that exert its electrophysiologic effect on multiple channels [36]. The electrophysiologic effects of amiodarone are protean. It blocks inactivated Na^+ channels in a use-dependent fashion, blocks α- and β-adrenoceptors, increases AP duration and ERP, and blocks inactivated Ca^{2+} channels. The oral form of the drug prolongs the ERP and AP duration in all cardiac tissue. In animal models, it also suppresses SA and AV node automaticity. Amiodarone blocks the slow component of the inward rectifying K^+ channel and does not exhibit reverse use-dependence. The intravenous form of amiodarone is a more potent antiadrenergic compound and Ca^{2+} channel blocker than the oral drug. There is no use-dependent block of Na^+ channels with intravenous amiodarone. The ECG demonstrates PR prolongation, QRS prolongation, and QT prolongation with chronic oral use.

Calcium channel blockers (class IV drugs)

All currently available Ca^{2+} channel antagonists (see Chapter 46) block the α subunit of the L-type Ca^{2+} channel, reducing the plateau height of the AP, slightly shortening myocardial AP, and slightly prolonging Purkinje fiber AP [37]. Verapamil and diltiazem depress the slope of diastolic depolarization of phase 0 and decrease maximum diastolic potential and the amplitude of the SA and AV nodal AP. Spontaneous sinus rate is slightly decreased and AV nodal conduction is prolonged. Heart rate may change slightly because of reflex sympathetic stimulation from systemic vasodilation (an effect attenuated with coadministration of a β-blocker). T-type Ca^{2+} channels exist in the SA node. No currently available drugs interact with T-type calcium channels. Verapamil is a racemic mixture and its d-stereoisomer exerts mild I_{Na} blocking effects.

Other antiarrhythmic drugs

Adenosine is an endogenous nucleoside whose action on cardiac ion channels is affected by catecholamine stimulation [38,39]. It directly activates the outward K^+ currents present in the SA node, atrium, and AV node (I_K, I_{Ach}, I_{Ado}), an effect similar to that of acetylcholine (or vagal stimulation). This results in a negative chronotropic and negative dromotropic response, and it also explains why adenosine can terminate some atrial arrhythmias [38]. Adenosine also decreases the inward Ca^{2+} current, the transient inward current, and the hyperpolarization current by stimulating a G protein that inhibits cyclic adenosine monophosphate (cAMP) generation. In the presence of catecholamines, adenosine also inhibits I_{Ks}.

Digoxin is a cardiac glycoside that blocks the Na^+/K^+ ATPase and exerts a positive inotropic, negative dromotropic, and negative chronotropic effect on the heart (see Chapter 44 for a discussion of inotropic effects). Intracellular Ca^{2+} is increased through the slow inward Ca^{2+} current. This in turn inhibits the Na^+/Ca^{2+} exchange. Digoxin augments vagal tone and increases the ERP of the AV node. As seen with β-blockers, SA node automaticity is depressed in underlying sick sinus syndrome. At supratherapeutic levels, digoxin increases delayed afterdepolarizations.

Magnesium is an important cellular ion involved in key enzymatic reactions, many responsible for cellular homeostasis and maintaining membrane ionic currents. Magnesium deficiency may cause intracellular potassium depletion and an increase in intracellular sodium or calcium, enhancing cellular excitability. The following tachyarrhythmias can respond favorably to magnesium therapy: intractable ventricular tachycardia and fibrillation, whether hypo- or normomagnesemic, torsades de pointes, digitalis-toxic ventricular tachyarrhythmia, multifocal atrial tachycardia. However, the role of magnesium therapy in treating acute-onset atrial fibrillation (AF), especially following cardiac surgery, is a subject of debate, with some reports showing decreased incidence of AF [40] and others suggesting little or no benefit [41].

Clinical pharmacology

Procainamide
Indications
- Life-threatening ventricular arrhythmias.
- Supraventricular arrhythmias, including the conversion of AF [23,42].

- AV reentrant tachycardia.
- Procainamide is no longer listed as treatment option in ACLS [43].

Pharmacokinetics
- Volume of distribution $\sim 2\,L\,kg^{-1}$; 20% of the drug is bound to serum proteins.
- Elimination half-life is 3–5 hours; 50–60% of elimination occurs through renal excretion; 10–30% through hepatic metabolism [19].
- Active renal tubular excretion occurs through a base-secreting pathway also used for elimination of cimetidine, ranitidine, flecainide, triamterene, and other drugs.
- Procainamide undergoes acetylation in the liver to NAPA. In "fast acetylators" $\sim 33\%$ of procainamide is converted to NAPA compared with $\sim 21\%$ in "slow acetylators" [19]. NAPA has an elimination half-life of 7–8 hours and is excreted through the kidneys.
- Serum concentrations of procainamide and NAPA need to be monitored, dosage is adjusted for patients with renal dysfunction.

Adverse effects
- Hypotension on rapid intravenous administration, negative inotropic effects, cardiac conduction abnormalities, prolonged QT interval, and polymorphic ventricular tachycardia (VT) [23].
- Anticholinergic properties can speed the conduction of atrial impulses leading to rapid ventricular response in patients with AF.
- Systemic lupus erythematosus syndrome.
- Central nervous system (CNS), gastrointestinal, and hematologic side effects have also been reported.

Quinidine
Indications
- Conversion of AF and/or maintenance of sinus rhythm.
- Life-threatening ventricular arrhythmias.
- Supraventricular arrhythmias caused by reentry.
- Conversion rate of AF with quinidine is $\sim 20\%$, but clinical trials suggests a greater mortality rate for patients receiving quinidine compared with controls [19].

Pharmacokinetics
- Eighty percent bound to serum proteins, primarily α_1-acid glycoprotein (AAG).
- Volume of distribution is 2–3 $L\,kg^{-1}$; elimination half-life is 6–8 hours in adults.
- Metabolized by cytochrome P450 (CYP) 3A4. Metabolite, 3-hydroxyquinidine, has $\sim 50\%$ of the antiarrhythmic effectiveness of the parent compound.
- Inhibits metabolism of drugs eliminated through CYP2D6 pathways, although it is not itself metabolized by the latter pathway.

However, 53% and 72% of patients administered 0.5 and 1.0 mg ibutilide, respectively, remained in sinus rhythm for at least 24 hours.

Pharmacokinetics

- Pharmacokinetics show marked interindividual variability.
- Systemic clearance is approximately equal to liver blood flow (~ 29 mL min^{-1} kg^{-1}).
- Volume of distribution is ~ 11 L kg^{-1}; little binding to plasma proteins.
- Mean elimination half-life is about 6 hours. In healthy volunteers, 82% of ibutilide was excreted in the urine, mostly as a metabolite, and 19% was recovered from the feces. There are approximately eight metabolites of ibutilide, but only the ω-hydroxy metabolites posses class III antiarrhythmic effects. The plasma concentrations of the latter are only 10% of ibutilide.

Adverse effects

- Not associated with significant hemodynamic alterations.
- Polymorphic VT with or without lengthening of the QTc interval may occur. Most events occur 40 minutes after the start of therapy, but recurrence occurs within 3 hours of the infusion. Ibutilide-related polymorphic VT is reported in up to 8% of patients, but the frequency was 1.8% when used for AF after cardiac surgery [73]. Polymorphic VT is more likely for patients with impaired LV function, history of polymorphic VT, long QT intervals, hypokalemia, or hypomagnesemia.

Dofetilide
Indications

- Conversion of AF or atrial flutter to sinus rhythm, and for the maintenance of sinus rhythm (or delay of recurrence) for patients with AF for more than 7 days who have been successfully cardioverted.
- Dofetilide is not effective for patients with paroxysmal AF. In a small study of patients with AF after cardiac surgery, conversion to sinus rhythm occurred in 36–44% of patients administered dofetilide, but this was not significantly different than with placebo (24%) [34]. In nonsurgical patients, dofetilide is more effective than placebo for converting AF to sinus rhythm [74]. After 1 year of treatment, dofetilide was more effective in maintaining sinus rhythm than placebo or sotalol.

Pharmacokinetics

- Bioavailability is greater than 90%, with peak effects occurring within 2–3 hours of ingestion.
- Plasma protein binding is 60–70%, and volume of distribution 3 L kg^{-1}.
- The terminal half-life is approximately 10 hours. Eighty percent of dofetilide is excreted unchanged in the urine, whereas 20% is in the form of inactive or minimally active

metabolites. Dofetilide is metabolized in the liver by CYP3A4 with low affinity. Renal elimination is through glomerular filtration and tubular secretion. Dosage adjustments are necessary in accordance with creatinine clearance, but not with mild or moderate hepatic impairment.
- Trimethoprim, cimetidine, prochlorperazine, and megestrol can inhibit renal clearance. Ketoconazole inhibits liver metabolism of dofetilide and increases the plasma concentrations. Verapamil, as well as the drugs listed earlier, is contraindicated in patients taking dofetilide because of the increased risk for proarrhythmia.

Adverse effects

- No decrease in inotropy or vascular resistance.
- Torsades de pointes occurs in a dose-related fashion [34,74], seen in 3.3% of patients with CHF, compared with 0.9% of patients without LV dysfunction. Proarrhythmia is most likely within 1–3 days of initiation of therapy [75].
- Dofetilide therapy is initiated in a hospital setting with continuous telemetry monitoring, with dosage guided by the QT interval and creatinine clearance.

β-Adrenoceptor blocking drugs
Indications

- Arrhythmias related to enhanced adrenergic states (e.g., thyrotoxicosis, pheochromocytoma, perioperative stress).
- Esmolol and propranolol – approved for the treatment of supraventricular arrhythmias [19]. By slowing AV conduction, β-blockers slow, terminate, or prevent recurrence of SVT involving the AV node as part of the reentrant pathway (e.g., AV nodal reentrant tachycardia [AVNRT] and orthodromic tachycardia with WPW syndrome).
- Controlling ventricular rate during AF and atrial flutter; also used for preventing these arrhythmias after cardiac surgery [76,77].
- Multifocal atrial tachycardia responds to esmolol or metoprolol [78] but is best treated with amiodarone.
- Acebutolol and propranolol – approved for frequent premature ventricular beats and VT, respectively.
- β-Blockers, particularly propranolol – effective for controlling torsades de pointes for patients with long QT intervals [79].
- Acebutolol, metoprolol, atenolol, propranolol, and timolol – approved for prevention of sudden death after myocardial infarction [19].
- Labetalol – for treating ventricular arrhythmias associated with pre-eclampsia [80].

Pharmacokinetics

- See Chapter 42 for further details of β-blockers.
- **Esmolol** – β$_1$-selective; rapidly hydrolyzed by esterases in the cytosol of red blood cells, resulting in an elimination half-life of ~ 9 minutes. Elimination kinetics are dose-independent. Approximately 2% of the drug is excreted

unchanged in the urine, whereas about 88% is recovered as the weakly active acid metabolite of esmolol.

- **Propranolol** – nonselective β-blocker; bioavailability is 25–30% because of substantial first-pass metabolism. Primarily metabolized in the liver and one metabolite (4-hydroxypropranolol) has weak β-blocking effects. Reduced hepatic blood flow from low cardiac output decreases hepatic extraction of propranolol. Although the plasma half-life is approximately 4 hours, the pharmacologic effect may persist for a longer duration.

- **Metoprolol** and **atenolol** – β$_1$-selective antagonists; available in oral and parenteral formulations. Bioavailability is approximately 50% for both. The plasma half-lives are 3–4 hours for metoprolol and 5–8 hours for atenolol. The liver extensively metabolizes metoprolol, with marked interindividual variability. Approximately 10% of the drug is excreted unchanged in the urine. Plasma concentrations of atenolol show markedly less interindividual variability than metoprolol. Atenolol is excreted mostly unchanged in the urine, and it will accumulate in patients with renal dysfunction.

Adverse effects

- Bradycardia, hypotension, myocardial depression, and bronchospasm.
- Precipitates heart failure in patients with impaired LV function, although lower doses of the drugs are well tolerated even in this group of patients for whom chronic β-blocker therapy decreased mortality rates [81].
- Cold extremities and worsening of Raynaud disease.
- Interferes with recovery from hypoglycemia in patients with diabetes, although this effect is less with β$_1$-selective compounds.
- Hypotension is more marked for patients receiving catecholamine-depleting drugs such as reserpine.
- CNS side effects include dizziness, headache, and mental status changes.
- Nausea, vomiting, abdominal cramps, and constipation; other effects such as alopecia and lupus reactions are rare.
- Upregulation of β-adrenoceptors occurs with chronic β-blocker therapy such that abrupt withdrawal may lead to tachycardia that is not tolerated by patients with coronary artery disease.

Ca^{2+} channel blocking drugs
Indications

- Verapamil and diltiazem – termination of supraventricular arrhythmias due to reentry.
- Verapamil and diltiazem – slowing the ventricular rate during AF or atrial flutter, and rarely they can convert recent-onset atrial arrhythmias to sinus rhythm.

- Verapamil and diltiazem – not generally useful for ventricular arrhythmias, although some efficacy is seen in patients with idiopathic VT [19].

Pharmacokinetics

- Verapamil undergoes considerable first-pass metabolism in the liver (bioavailability 25–30%), but it is effective in slowing ventricular rate in 30 minutes. The drug is 90% bound to plasma proteins and its half-life is 4–6 hours, with nearly 70% of the drug excreted in the kidneys. One metabolite, norverapamil, exerts clinically significant electrophysiologic effects. The bioavailability of diltiazem after oral administration is approximately 40%, and the plasma elimination half-life is 3–4.5 hours. Diltiazem is 70–80% bound to plasma proteins. Other drugs that inhibit hepatic microsomal enzymes may increase blood concentrations of diltiazem. Active metabolites of diltiazem have a much slower elimination (~20 hours). Major metabolites include desacetyldiltiazem and desmethyldiltiazem. Dosage adjustments of verapamil and diltiazem are necessary for patients with hepatic impairment.

Adverse effects

- Major effects – vasodilation leading to hypotension, light-headedness, and nausea.
- Verapamil and diltiazem also have negative inotropic effects.
- Bradycardia and transient asystole have been reported with intravenous verapamil when administered to patients with cardiac conduction abnormalities or those also receiving β-blockers.
- Peripheral edema, constipation, and rashes may occur.
- Verapamil can increase serum digoxin concentrations by 50–75% in the first week of treatment. Downward adjustments in cyclosporine dose are necessary when coadministered with diltiazem. Coadministration of oral diltiazem and carbamazepine results in increased serum levels of the latter drug.

Adenosine
Indications

- Termination of reentrant SVTs.
- Adenosine does not convert AF or atrial flutter to sinus rhythm, but helps in diagnosis by facilitating the appearance of flutter waves during transient depression of AV conduction.
- Some adrenergic-sensitive idiopathic VTs originating from the right ventricular outflow tract in patients with no structural heart disease [82,83].

Pharmacokinetics

- Adenosine has a half-life of seconds. It is taken up into most cells including the endothelium and is metabolized to inosine by adenosine deaminase.

- Dipyridamole inhibits adenosine uptake and hence potentiates the effects of adenosine. Caffeine and methylxanthines block the adenosine receptor, requiring larger doses of adenosine for clinical effect.

Adverse effects

- Because of its rapid offset, adverse effects of adenosine are short-lived, with the possible exception of patients administered dipyridamole.
- Transient asystole usually follows bolus administration.
- Rarely results in bronchospasm in patients with asthma.

Practical aspects of drug administration

Proarrhythmia refers to bradyarrhythmias or tachyarrhythmias that directly result from drugs. These complications are caused by the electrophysiologic effects of the drugs such as slowed conduction, prolonged repolarization, possibly early afterdepolarizations, and alterations in reentrant circuits, especially those resulting from dynamic interactions of existing substrate in the setting of myocardial ischemia or electrolyte disturbances. Patients particularly prone to proarrhythmic side effects include those with primary or drug-induced prolonged QT intervals, a history of VT, LV hypertrophy, myocardial ischemia, or impaired LV function [11]. For the most part, class Ic antiarrhythmic drugs are avoided in patients with structural heart disease. The use of two or more antiarrhythmic drugs is avoided when a first drug was ineffective.

In some situations, treating reversible imbalances may be sufficient for terminating arrhythmias. Examples of reversible imbalances include myocardial ischemia, hypoxemia, hypercarbia, acidosis, anemia, electrolyte abnormalities (e.g., hypokalemia, hypomagnesemia, etc.), thyrotoxicosis, hypothermia, microshock or macroshock from medical equipment and monitors, and direct mechanical irritation to the heart (e.g., central venous or pulmonary artery catheters, mediastinal drainage tubes, etc.). An exhaustive search for such factors should be initiated whenever an arrhythmia develops perioperatively.

Direct electrical cardioversion or defibrillation is used when the patient is hemodynamically unstable or the arrhythmia is associated with evidence of myocardial ischemia or CHF. Using an evidence-based approach, antiarrhythmic drugs for treating hemodynamically unstable VT or VF after failure of electrical interventions are given as class IIb (acceptable based only on fair evidence of benefit: amiodarone) or "class indeterminate" (lidocaine) in the ACLS recommendations [43]. There is no evidence that the use of any drug in these settings is associated with improved survival to hospital discharge or improved longer-term outcomes.

Polymorphic VT in the absence of pre-existing QT prolongation and associated with stable hemodynamics is treated similarly to monomorphic VT when cardioversion is not

desirable [43]. The treatment of polymorphic VT with pre-existing QT interval prolongation (torsades de pointes) should include an exhaustive search for reversible causes such as electrolyte abnormalities, medications, and ischemia. When hemodynamically stable and when cardioversion is not desirable, torsades de pointes can be treated with overdrive atrial or ventricular pacing along with β-blockers and magnesium (ACLS class indeterminate) [43].

The treatment aims for hemodynamically stable AF and atrial flutter include heart-rate control, conversion to sinus rhythm, and anticoagulation. Verapamil, diltiazem, or β-blockers can be used to slow the ventricular response in the absence of ventricular dysfunction. Digoxin is useful in the setting of LV dysfunction, but is less efficacious when there is enhanced sympathetic drive, as seen in the postoperative state. Drugs that slow AV conduction can actually precipitate fast, potentially life-threatening heart rates for patients with AF who have an accessory pathway (WPW syndrome). In these situations, antiarrhythmic drugs that slow conduction (e.g., procainamide or propafenone) are used. Drugs that are effective for treating AF or atrial flutter are given an ACLS class IIa (acceptable based on good or very good evidence) or class IIb rating (e.g., sotalol and disopyramide) [60]. The drug choice is dependent on individual risk for proarrhythmia and LV function. Left atrial thrombus is present in 13–29% of patients with AF. When atrial flutter or fibrillation have been present for more than 48 hours, anticoagulation for 3 weeks is typically recommended before pharmacologic or electrical cardioversion, but transesophageal echocardiography can be used to exclude left atrial thrombus [84].

Paroxysmal SVT usually results from a concealed accessory pathway, dual AV nodal physiology (AVNRT), or an atrial tachycardia. In the setting of stable hemodynamics, adenosine may be given. When it is successful in terminating the arrhythmia, adenosine often results in a brief period of asystole followed by sinus rhythm. Antiarrhythmic drugs such as procainamide, amiodarone, sotalol, and flecainide are considered for treating paroxysmal SVT when adenosine or AV nodal blocking drugs are unsuccessful and cardioversion is not desirable (class IIa recommendation) [43,84].

Dosage and administration

The doses of most antiarrhythmic drugs are adjusted based on therapeutic plasma concentrations. Dosing guidelines for antiarrhythmics are listed in Table 43.3.

Summary

While nonpharmacologic approaches to treating atrial and ventricular tachyarrhythmias are available, antiarrhythmic drugs still have a role in the management of cardiac rhythm disorders. There are five phases to the cardiac action potential (AP), which depend upon inward and outward ionic

Table 43.3. Dosing for Vaughan Williams class I and III drugs

Drug	Oral dose	Parenteral dose
Procainamide	500–1000 mg, then 350–1000 mg qid	1 g IV at 20 mg min^{-1} or until arrhythmia stops, hypotension develops, QRS ↑ by 50%
Quinidine	600–1000 mg, then 300–600 mg qid	
Disopyramide	300 mg, then 150–300 mg qid	
Lidocaine		1–1.5 mg kg^{-1} repeated to maximum of 300 mg, then 1–4 mg min^{-1}
Mexiletine	400–600 mg, then 50–300 mg tid or 450 mg bid	
Tocainide	400–600 mg tid or bid, then 400–600 mg tid	
Flecainide	50–100mg bid then ↑ by 50 mg daily until 400 mg daily	
Propafenone	150 mg tid ↑ to 300 mg tid over 3–4 days to maximum 900 mg daily	
Moricizine	200–300 mg tid	
Amiodarone	800–1600 mg daily for 1–3 weeks, then lowest effective dose usually 200–600 mg daily	150 mg IV over 10 min, then 1 mg min^{-1} for 6 h, then 0.5 mg min^{-1} for 18 h. Bolus may be repeated for recurrent arrhythmias
Sotalol	80 mg bid, then ↑ every 2–3 days to 80–160 mg bid	
Ibutilide		1 mg over 10 min. If < 60 kg give 0.01 mg kg^{-1}. Repeat after 10 min if needed
Dofetilide	0.125–0.5 mg bid based on creatinine clearance	
Diltiazem		0.25–0.35 mg kg^{-1} IV over 10 min, then 5–15 mg h^{-1}
Verapamil		5–10 mg IV over 2 min. May give additional 10 mg after 15–30 min
Esmolol		500 µg kg^{-1} min^{-1} IV, then ↑ in 50–100 µg kg^{-1} min^{-1} increments every 5 min until desired effect
Propranolol		1–3 mg IV at 1 mg min^{-1}. Repeat after 2 min then give effective dose every 4 hours
Metoprolol	For myocardial infarction, after IV loading, 50 mg qid for 48 h, then 100mg bid or 25–50 mg qid	1–5 mg IV
Atenolol	For myocardial infarction, after IV loading, 50 mg bid, ↑ dose to 100 mg daily; for arrhythmias, 0.3 mg kg^{-1} daily	1–5 mg IV
Acebutolol	200 mg bid ↑ until desired effect, usually 600–1200 mg daily	
Timolol	10 mg bid for myocardial infarction	

bid, 2 × daily; tid, 3 × daily; qid, 4 × daily; IV, intravenous.

currents at specific ion channels. Many antiarrhythmic drugs act to block ion channels. Use-dependent block occurs when the drug affinity for open or activated channels is greater than that for resting channels, such that effects are greater as heart rate increases or after long periods of stimulation. Antiarrhythmic drugs may be broadly divided into several classes, though the specific actions of these drugs vary both within and between classes; indications for use are drug-specific. The net effect of each drug on the ECG results from a combination of electrophysiologic, pharmacodynamic, and pharmacokinetic effects.

Sodium channel blockers generally decrease the maximum upstroke velocity of phase 0 of the AP (V_{max}), and slow conduction. Based upon their binding kinetics, these drugs are divided into three classes (Ia, Ib, and Ic). Class Ia drugs have intermediate binding kinetics and include procainamide, quinidine, and disopyramide. Class Ib drugs have rapid binding kinetics, and include lidocaine, tocainide, and mexiletine.

Class Ic have slow binding kinetics, and include flecainide, propafenone, and moricizine; the class Ic drugs are generally avoided in patients with structural heart disease.

Drugs with β-adrenoceptor blocking properties are defined as class II drugs, which act to decrease phase 4 depolarization, spontaneous firing, and automaticity of pacemaker cells. Potassium channel blockers, which include sotalol, ibutilide, and dofetilide, fall into class III. These drugs increase the effective refractory period (ERP) and AP duration without affecting V_{max}. They are reverse use-dependent, with more pronounced effects at slower heart rates. Class III also comprises drugs which act on multiple ion channel types, such as amiodarone, which also blocks α- and β-adrenoceptors.

Drugs such as verapamil and diltiazem, which act on calcium channels, fall into class IV, and may affect both AP depolarization and electromechanical coupling. Other therapeutics also exist: adenosine acts on multiple ionic currents, notably activating outward potassium currents in the sinoatrial (SA) node, atrium, and atrioventricular (AV) node; digoxin blocks the Na^+/K^+ ATPase, increasing the ERP of the AV node; magnesium therapy can be beneficial in the treatment of certain tachyarrhythmias.

Proarrhythmic side effects can occur with the use of antiarrhythmic drugs, and certain conditions render patients more susceptible to these adverse events. Some arrhythmias may be terminated by treating reversible imbalances, and factors which could contribute to these imbalances should be identified in the event of development of perioperative arrhythmias. Direct electrical cardioversion is used for arrhythmias in hemodynamically unstable patients, and those with myocardial ischemia or congestive heart failure. Where pharmacological antiarrhythmic intervention is required, choice of drug depends on multiple factors, including cause, type, and circumstances of the arrhythmia; the presence of existing QT prolongation; the presence of ventricular dysfunction in atrial fibrillation or flutter; the presence of enhanced sympathetic drive (e.g., postoperatively); response to previous therapeutic interventions; and the presence of Wolff–Parkinson–White (WPW) syndrome. Additional considerations include individual risk for proarrhythmia, potential drug interactions, and dosage adjustments necessary for some drugs in the setting of hepatic or renal dysfunction. Differing adverse effects are associated with a variety of drugs, including proarrhythmic effects, hemodynamic effects, gastrointestinal effects, pulmonary effects, and central nervous system effects.

References

1. Morady F. Radio-frequency ablation as treatment for cardiac arrhythmias. *N Engl J Med* 1999; **340**: 534–44.

2. Zeppenfeld K, Stevenson W. Ablation of ventricular tachycardia in patients with structural heart disease. *Pacing Clin Electrophysiol* 2008; **31**: 358–74.

3. Callahan T, Natale A. Catheter ablation of atrial fibrillation. *Med Clin North Am* 2008; **92**: 179–201.

4. Qu J, Barbuti A, Protas L, Cohen I, Robinson R. HNC2 overexpression in newborn and adult ventricular myocytes: distinc effects on gating and excitability. *Circ Res* 2001; **89**: E8–11.

5. Qu J, Plotnikov A, Danilo P, *et al.* Expression and function of a biological pacemaker in canine heart. *Circulation* 2003; **107**: 1106–9.

6. Plotnikov A, Sosunov E, Qu J, *et al.* A biological pacemaker implanted in the canine left bundle branc provides ventricular escape rhythms having physiologically acceptable rates. *Circulation* 2004; **109**: 506–12.

7. Kehat I, Khimovich L, Caspi O, *et al.* Electromechanical intergration of cardiomyocytes derived from human embryonic stem cells. *Nat Biotechnol* 2004; **22**: 1282–9.

8. Plotnikov A, Shlapakove I, Szabolcs M, *et al.* Xenografted adult human mesenchymal stem cells provide a platform for sustained biological pacemaker function in canine heart. *Circulation* 2007; **116**: 706–13.

9. Yankelson L, Feld Y, Bressler-Stramer T, *et al.* Cell therapy for modification of the myocardial electrophysiological substrate. *Circulation* 2008; **117**: 720–31.

10. Preliminary report: effect of encainide and flecainide on mortality in a randomized trial of arrhythmia suppression after myocardial infarction. The Cardiac Arrhythmia Suppression Trial (CAST) Investigators. *N Engl J Med* 1989; **321**: 406 –12.

11. Ben-David J, Zipes DP. Torsades de pointes and proarrhythmia. *Lancet* 1993; **341**: 1578–82.

12. Singh B, Connolly S, Crijns H, *et al.* Dronedarone afor maintenance of sinus rhythm in atrial fibrillation and flutter. *N Engl J Med* 2007; **357**: 987–99.

13. Roy D, Pratt C, Torp-Pedersen C, *et al.* Vernakalant hydrochloride for rapid conversion of atrial fibrillation. *Circulation* 2008; **117**: 1518–25.

14. Whalley DW, Wendt DJ, Grant AO. Basic concepts in cellular cardiac electrophysiology: Part I: Ion channels, membrane currents, and the action potential. *Pacin Clin Electrophysiol* 1995; **18**: 1556–74.

15. Grant AO, Whalley DW. *Mechanisms of Cardiac Arrhythmias*. Philadelphia, PA: Lippincott-Raven, 1998.

16. Hondeghem LM, Katzung BG. Time- and voltage-dependent interactions of antiarrhythmic drugs with cardiac sodium channels. *Biochim Biophys Acta* 1977; **472**: 373–98.

17. Hondeghem LM. Antiarrhythmic agents: modulated receptor applications. *Circulation* 1987; **75**: 514–20.

18. Vaughan Williams EM. A classification of antiarrhythmic actions reassessed after a decade of new drugs. *J Clin Pharmacol* 1984; **24**: 120–47.

19. Zipes DP. *Management of Cardiac Arrhythmias: Pharmacological, Electrical, and Surgical Techniques*. Philadelphia, PA: Saunders, 1997.

20. The Sicilian gambit: a new approach to the classification of antiarrhythmic drugs based on their actions on arrhythmogenic mechanisms. Task Force of the Working Group on Arrhythmias of the European

Society of Cardiology. *Circulation* 1991; **84**: 1831–51.

21. Whalley DW, Wendt DJ, Grant AO. Basic concepts in cellular cardiac electrophysiology: Part II: block of ion channels by antiarrhythmic drugs. *Pacing Clin Electrophysiol* 1995; **18**: 1686–704.

22. Grace AA, Camm AJ. Drug therapy: quinidine. *N Engl J Med* 1998; **338**: 35–45.

23. Cain ME, Josephson ME. Procainamide. In: Gould LA, ed., *Drug Treatment of Cardiac Arrhythmias*. New York, NY: Futura, 1982: 73–108.

24. Koch-Weser J. Drug therapy: disopyramide. *N Engl J Med* 1979; **300**: 957–62.

25. Manolis AS, Deering TF, Cameron J, Estes NA. Mexiletine: pharmacology and therapeutic use. *Clin Cardiol* 1990; **13**: 349–59.

26. Holmes B, Brogden RN, Heel RC, Speight TM, Avery GS. Tocainide: a review of its pharmacological properties and therapeutic efficacy. *Drugs* 1983; **26**: 93–123.

27. Roden DM, Woosley RL. Drug therapy: tocainide. *N Engl J Med* 1986; **315**: 41–5.

28. Kreeger RW, Hammill SC. New antiarrhythmic drugs: tocainide, mexiletine, flecainide, encainide, and amiodarone. *Mayo Clin Proc* 1987; **62**: 1033–50.

29. Funck-Bretano C, Kroemer HK, Lee JT, Roden DM. Drug therapy: propafenone. *N Engl J Med* 1990; **322**: 518–25.

30. Lefkowitz RJ. β-Adrenergic receptors: recognition and regulation. *N Engl J Med* 1976; **295**: 323–8.

31. Frishman WH. β-Adrenoceptor antagonists: new drugs and new indications. *N Engl J Med* 1981; **305**: 500–6.

32. Hohnloser SH, Woosley RL. Sotalol. *N Engl J Med* 1994; **331**: 31–8.

33. Karam R, Marcello S, Brooks RR, Corey AE, Moore A. Azimilide dihydrochloride: a novel antiarrhythmic agent. *Am J Cardiol* 1998; **81**: 40D–46D.

34. Frost L, Mortensen PE, Tingler J, et al. Efficacy and safety of dofetilide, a new class III antiarrhythmic agent, in acute termination of atrial fibrillation or flutter after coronary artery bypass surgery. *Int J Cardiol* 1997; **58**: 135–40.

35. Murray K. Ibutilide. *Circulation* 1998; **97**: 493–7.

36. Zipes DP, Prystowski EN, Heger JJ. Amiodarone: electrophysiologic actions, pharmacokinetics and clinical effects. *J Am Coll Cardiol* 1984; **3**: 1059–71.

37. Abernethy DR, Schwartz JB. Calcium-antagonist drugs. *N Engl J Med* 1999; **341**: 1447–57.

38. DiMarco JP, Sellers TD, Berne RM, et al. Adenosine: electrophysiologic effects and therapeutic use for terminating paroxysmal supraventricular tachycardia. *Circulation* 1983; **68**: 1254–63.

39. Belardinelli L, Linden J, Berne RM. The cardiac effects of adenosine. *Prog Cardiovasc Dis* 1989; **22**: 73–97.

40. Miller AP, Feng W, Xing D, et al. Estrogen modulates inflammatory mediator expression and neutrophil chemotaxis in injured arteries. *Circulation* 2004; **110**: 1664–9.

41. Zangrillo A, Landoni G, Sparicio D, et al. Perioperative magnesium supplementation to prevent atrial fibrillation after off-pump coronary artery surgery: a randomized controlled study. *J Cardiothorac Vasc Anesth* 2005; **19**: 723–8.

42. Madrid AH, Moro C, Marin-Huerta E, et al. Comparison of flecainide and procainamide in conversion of atrial fibrillation. *Eur Heart J* 1993; **14**: 1127–31.

43. 2005 American Heart Association guidelines for cardiopulmonary resuscitation and emergency cardiovascular care. Part 7.3: Management of symptomatic bradycardia and tachycardia. *Circulation* 2005; **112**: IV-67–77.

44. Lazzara R. Antiarrhythmic drugs and torsade de pointes. *Eur Heart J* 1993; **14**: 88–92.

45. Johnson RG, Goldberger AL, Thurer RL, et al. Lidocaine prophylaxis in coronary revascularization patients: a randomized, prospective trial. *Ann Thorac Surg* 1993; **55**: 1180–4.

46. King FG, Addetia AM, Peters SD, Peachey GO. Prophylactic lidocaine for postoperative coronary artery bypass patients, a double-blind, randomized trial. *Can J Anaesth* 1990; **37**: 363–8.

47. Hine LK, Laird N, Hewitt P, Chalmers TC. Meta-analytic evidence against prophylactic use of lidocaine in acute myocardial infarction. *Arch Intern Med* 1989; **149**: 2694–8.

48. Buchert E, Woosley RL. Clinical implications of variable antiarrhythmid drug metabolism. *Pharmacogenetics* 1992; **2**: 2–11.

49. Gill JS, Mehta D, Ward DE, Camm AJ. Efficacy of flecainide, satalol and verapamil in the treatment of right ventricular tachycardia in patients without overt cardiac abnormality. *Br Heart J* 1992; **63**: 392–7.

50. Auricchio A. Reversible protective effect of propafenone or flecainide during atrial fibrillation in patients with an accessory atrioventricular connection. *Am Heart J* 1992; **124**: 932–7.

51. Gentili C, Giordano F, Alois A, et al. Efficacy of intravenous propafenone in acute atrial fibrillation complicating open-heart surgery. *Am Heart J* 1992; **123**: 1225–8.

52. Bianconi L, Boccadamo R, Toscano S, et al. Effects of oral propafenone therapy on chronic myocardial pacing threshold. *Pacin Clin Electrophysiol* 1992; **15**: 148–54.

53. Cochrane AD, Siddins M, Rosenfeldt FL, et al. A comparison of amiodarone and digoxin for treatment of supraventricular arrhythmias after cardiac surgery. *Eur J Cardiothorac Surg* 1994; **8**: 194–8.

54. Daoud EG, Strickberger SA, Man KC, et al. Preoperative amiodarone as prophylaxis against atrial fibrillation after heart surgery. *N Engl J Med* 1997; **337**: 1785–91.

55. Guarnieri T, Nolan S, Gottlieb SO, Dudek A, Lowry DR. Intravenous amiodarone for the prevention of atrial fibrillation after open heart surgery. The Amiodarone Reduction in Coronary Heart (ARCH) trial. *J Am Coll Cardiol* 1999; **34**: 343–7.

56. Lee SH, Chang CM, Lu MD, et al. Intrevenous amiodarone for prevention of atrial fibrillation after coronary artery bypass grafting. *Ann Thorac Surg* 2000; **70**: 157–61.

57. Mitchell L, Exner D, Wyse DG, *et al.* Prophylactic oral amiodarone for the prevention of arrhythmias that begin early after revascularization, valve replacement, or repair: PAPABEAR: a randomized controlled trial. *JAMA* 2005; **294**: 3093–100.

58. Bagshaw S, Galbraith P, Mitchell L, *et al.* Prophylactic amiodarone for prevention of atrial fibrillation after cardiac surgery: a meta-analysis. *Ann Thorac Surg* 2006; **82**: 1927–37.

59. Vassallo P, Trohman R. Prescribing amiodarone: an evidence-based review of clinical indications. *J Am Med Assoc* 2007; **298**: 1312–22.

60. Fuster V, Ryden L, Cannon D, et al. ACC/AHA/ESC 2006 guidelines for the management of patients with atrial fibrillation: executive summary. *Circulation* 2006; **114**: 700–52.

61. Liberman BA, Teasdale SJ. Anesthesia and amiodarone. *Can Anaesth Soc J* 1985; **32**: 629–38.

62. Feinberg B, LaMantia K, Levy W. Amiodarone and general anesthesia: a retrospective analysis. *Anesth Analg* 1986; **65**: S49.

63. Schmid J, Rosengant T, McIntosh C, et al. Amiodarone-induced complications after cardiac operation for obstructive hypertrophic cardiomyopathy. *Ann Thorac Surg* 1989; **48**: 359–64.

64. Hohnloser SH, Klingenheben T, Singh HN. Amiodarone-associated proarrhythmic effects: a review with special reference to torsade de pointes tachycardia. *Ann Intern Med* 1994; **121**: 529–35.

65. Weinberg BA, Miles WM, Klein LS, *et al.* Five-year follow-up of 589 patients treated with amiodarone. *Am Heart J* 1993; **125**: 109–20.

66. Greenspon AJ, Kidwell GA, Hurley W, Mannion J. Amiodarone-related postoperative adult respiratory distress syndrome. *Circulation* 1991; **84**: 407–15.

67. Fitton A, Sorkin EM. Sotalol: an updated review of its pharmacological properties and therapeutic use in cardiac arrhythmias. *Drugs* 1993; **46**: 678–719.

68. Nystrom UJ, Edvardsson N, Berggren H, Pizzarelli GP, Radegran K. Oral sotalol reduces the incidence of atrial fibrillation after coronary artery bypass surgery. *J Thorac Cardiovasc Surg* 1993; **41**: 34–7.

69. Suttorp MJ, Kingma JH, Peels HO, *et al.* Effectiveness of sotalol in preventing supraventricular tachyarrhythmias shortly after coronary artery bypass grafting. *Am J Cardiol* 1991; **68**: 1163–9.

70. Campbell TJ, Gavaghan TP, Morgan JJ. Intravenous sotalol for the treatment of atrial fibrillation and flutter after cardiopulmonary bypass: comparison with disopyramide and digoxin in a randomized trial. *Br Heart J* 1985; **54**: 86–90.

71. MacNeil DJ, Davies RO, Beitchman D. Clincal safety profile of sotalol in the treatment of arrhythmias. *Am J Cardiol* 1993; **72**: 44A–50A.

72. VanderLugt JF, Mattioni T, Denker S, *et al.* Efficacy and safety of ibutilide fumarate for the conversion of atrial arrhythmias after cardiac surgery. *Circulation* 1999; **100**: 369–75.

73. Stambler BS, Wood MA, Ellenbogen KA, *et al.* Efficacy and safety of repeated intravenous doses of ibutilide for rapid conversion of atrial flutter or fibrillation. Ibutilide Repeat Dose Study Investigators. *Circulation* 1996; **94**: 1613–21.

74. Singh S, Zoble RG, Yellen L, *et al.* Efficacy and safety of oral dofetilide in converting to and maintaining sinus rhythm in patients with chronic atrial fibrillation or atrial flutter. The SAFIRE-D study. *Circulation* 2000; **102**: 2385–90.

75. Torp-Pedersen C, Moller M, Bloch-Thomsen PE, *et al.* Dofetilide in patients with congestive heart failure and left ventricular dysfunction. *N Engl J Med* 1999; **341**: 857–65.

76. Andrews TC, Reimold SC, Berlin JA, Antman EM. Prevention of supraventricular arrhythmias after coronary artery bypass surgery: a meta-analysis of randomized controlled trials. *Circulation* 1991; **84**: III236–44.

77. Kowey PR, Taylor JE, Rials SJ, Marinchak RA. Meta-analysis of the effectiveness of prophylactic drug therapy in preventing supraventricular arrhythmia early after coronary artery bypass grafting. *Am J Cardiol* 1992; **69**: 963–5.

78. Hill GA, Owens SD. Esmolol in the treatment of multifocal atrial tachycardia. *Chest* 1992; **101**: 1726–8.

79. Malfatto G, Beria G, Sala S, *et al.* Quantitative analysis of T wave abnormalities and their prognostic implications in the idiopathic long QT syndrome. *J Am Coll Cardiol* 1994; **23**: 296–301.

80. Bhorat IE, Naidoo DP, Rout CC, Moodley J. Malignant ventricular arrhythmias in eclampsia: a comparison of labetolol with dihydralazine. *Am J Obstet Gynecol* 1993; **168**: 1292–6.

81. Heidenreich PA, Lee TT, Massie BM. Effect of beta-blockade on mortality in patients with heart failure: a meta-analysis of randomized clinical trials. *J Am Coll Cardiol* 1997; **30**: 27–34.

82. Griffith MJ, Garratt CJ, Rowland E, *et al.* Effects of intravenous adenosine on verapamil-sensitive idiopathic ventricular tachycardia. *Am J Cardiol* 1994; **73**: 759–64.

83. Lerman BB. Response of nonreentrant catecholamine-mediated ventricular tachycardia in endogenous adenosine and acetylcholine: evidence for myocardial receptor-mediated effects. *Circulation* 1993; **87**: 382–90.

84. Mugge A, Kuhn H, Daniel W. The role of transesophageal echocardiography in the detection of left atrial thrombi. *Echocardiograph* 1993; **10**: 405–17.

Section 3
Chapter

44

Essential drugs in anesthetic practice
Positive inotropic drugs

Paul S. Pagel and David C. Warltier

Introduction

Heart failure occurs when the heart is unable to generate sufficient output to serve cellular metabolic requirements. Heart failure most often occurs as a result of decreases in intrinsic myocardial contractility, but abnormalities in diastolic function may also be responsible in the absence of or preceding significant impairment of systolic performance. The heart serves two major functional roles: propelling blood into the high-pressure arterial circulation during systole and collecting blood for subsequent ejection from the low-pressure venous vasculature. Thus, pathologic conditions that restrict left ventricular (LV) inflow may also produce heart failure independent of pump performance. Reductions in contractile function occur in a variety of disease states including myocardial ischemia, stunning, hibernation, infarction, pressure- or volume-overload hypertrophy, and myocyte injury produced by drugs, infectious disease, or infiltrative processes. Diastolic dysfunction may also result from these pathologic conditions or may be produced by forces outside the LV chamber (e.g., pericardial tamponade, constrictive pericarditis, ventricular interaction) that act to impair filling and compliance.

Regardless of the underlying cause, heart failure activates a series of compensatory reflexes including sympathetic nervous system stimulation, parasympathetic nervous system withdrawal, stimulation of the renin–angiotensin–aldosterone axis, and increased vasopressin release that serve to increase perfusion pressure and improve cardiac output [1]. Although these compensatory mechanisms may be adequate to maintain cardiovascular homeostasis at rest, cardiac function may subsequently decline, and clinical signs and symptoms of heart failure may ensue during periods of hemodynamic stress. This "cardiac reserve" is diminished by further reductions in contractility or exacerbations in diastolic dysfunction, and cardiac output may eventually become inadequate even during resting conditions. This progressive decline in functional reserve characterizes the well-known stages of the New York Heart Association (NYHA) classification, in which patients demonstrate significant cardiac reserve in stage I but suffer end-stage heart failure during resting conditions in stage IV.

Although activation of neural and endocrine reflexes initially maintains overall cardiovascular performance in evolving heart failure, these responses also cause adverse consequences that may eventually lead to disease progression, end-organ hypoperfusion, and death. Activation of the sympathetic nervous system and the renin–angiotensin system preserve or modestly increases arterial pressure by causing arteriolar vasoconstriction. Unfortunately, these actions also produce undesirable increases in LV afterload that further compromise already reduced LV systolic function. Aldosterone release causes retention of sodium (Na^+) and water by the kidney, but resulting increases in plasma volume combine with sympathetic nervous system-mediated reductions in venous capacitance to further exacerbate pre-existing central venous and pulmonary arterial congestion. These increases in LV afterload and preload increase LV end-systolic and end-diastolic volume and wall stress, respectively, and cause detrimental increases in myocardial oxygen consumption. The Frank–Starling mechanism that normally results in enhanced myocardial contractility, cardiac output, and stroke work in response to augmentation of LV preload is exhausted in the failing heart [2]. In fact, further reductions in LV systolic function may occur concomitant with progressive LV dilation. Lastly, increased sympathetic and decreased parasympathetic nervous system activity cause compensatory tachycardia, but this response is an energetically wasteful means of enhancing cardiac output and is especially deleterious in patients with coronary artery disease.

The search for new drugs that enhance contractility in failing myocardium has been remarkably unsuccessful [3]. The digitalis glycosides remain the only positive inotropic drugs currently available for the chronic oral treatment of heart failure, although the myofilament calcium (Ca^{2+}) sensitizer levosimendan has shown some promise in recent clinical trials [4]. Heart failure resulting from LV systolic or diastolic dysfunction appears to be most successfully treated using drugs that optimize LV loading conditions by decreasing preload (e.g., diuretics, nitrates) or afterload (e.g., angiotensin-converting enzyme inhibitors, Ca^{2+} channel blockers). Low doses of β_1-adrenoceptor antagonists have also been shown to exert beneficial effects in patients with heart failure

Anesthetic Pharmacology, 2nd edition, ed. Alex S. Evers, Mervyn Maze, Evan D. Kharasch. Published by Cambridge University Press. © Cambridge University Press 2011.

by reversing downregulation of the receptor and increasing responsiveness to endogenous catecholamines [5]. The use of these pharmacologic approaches is limited in end-stage heart failure, however, and the lack of an effective, orally administered positive inotropic drug has led to the use of procedures such as LV reduction surgery (e.g., Batista procedure) and skeletal muscle augmentation (e.g., cardiomyoplasty), which, unfortunately, are only beneficial in a small number of patients. More recently, chronic biventricular resynchronization therapy has been shown to improve functional class and quality of life in selected patients with chronic end-stage heart failure [6]. In contrast, a variety of drugs have been used successfully in the intravenous treatment of acute LV failure. Endogenous and synthetic catecholamines, phosphodiesterase 3 (PDE3) inhibitors, and new drugs such as the myofilament Ca^{2+} sensitizers are currently used or will find future use for the treatment of reduced myocardial contractility. This chapter discusses the cardiovascular pharmacology of drugs used for the treatment of acute and chronic heart failure. The use of positive inotropic drugs to enhance LV function in the cardiac surgical setting will be emphasized.

Mechanisms of drug action: an overview

Myocardial contractility is determined by several factors that affect the interaction between actin and myosin in the sarcomere. This event is dependent on the concentration of Ca^{2+} in the myoplasm and requires energy in the form of adenosine triphosphate (ATP) to occur. A transient increase in the intracellular Ca^{2+} concentration from less than 10^{-7} M to 10^{-5} M causes the cardiac myocyte to contract. Membrane depolarization causes a small amount of Ca^{2+} to enter the myocyte through voltage-regulated Ca^{2+} channels located within the sarcolemma. The total quantity of Ca^{2+} that enters the myocyte depends on the number of open channels and how long these channels remain in the open state. This small increase in intracellular Ca^{2+} concentration causes the release of stored Ca^{2+} from the cisternae of the sarcoplasmic reticulum. This process is known as Ca^{2+}-induced Ca^{2+} release and forms the basis of the "Ca^{2+} transient" measured in the experimental laboratory. Calcium-induced Ca^{2+} release from the sarcoplasmic reticulum is directly related to the quantity of and rate at which Ca^{2+} enters through sarcolemmal Ca^{2+} channels. Calcium binds to the troponin C regulatory protein of the troponin–tropomyosin complex and causes a conformational change that allows the ATP-dependent cycling of crossbridges between actin and myosin. The troponin–tropomyosin complex normally prevents the interaction of these contractile elements and inhibits contraction of the cardiac myocyte. However, the increased intracellular Ca^{2+} concentration observed after sarcolemmal depolarization permits the formation of actin–myosin crossbridges to occur. Thus, the degree of tropomyosin disinhibition, the extent of actin–myosin interaction, and the force of

contraction at constant load (i.e., inotropic state) are directly related to Ca^{2+} concentration within the myocyte.

Drugs that enhance myocardial contractility either increase the amount of Ca^{2+} for contractile activation through a variety of mechanisms or directly augment the efficacy of this ion at the contractile apparatus (Fig. 44.1). Calcium chloride and Ca^{2+} gluconate directly increase extracellular Ca^{2+} concentration and facilitate a greater influx of Ca^{2+} through sarcolemmal Ca^{2+} channels. This action leads to an increase in intracellular Ca^{2+} concentration and enhanced contractility. However, because most of the Ca^{2+} available for contractile activation is derived from the sarcoplasmic reticulum, exogenously administered Ca^{2+} may not provide a reliable, clinically evident increase in contractile function. For example, bolus doses of Ca^{2+} do not consistently increase cardiac output in patients after cardiopulmonary bypass [7], most likely because Ca^{2+} also increases LV afterload by arteriolar vasoconstriction, thereby impeding LV ejection. Cardiac glycosides (e.g., digitalis) exert positive inotropic activity by indirectly increasing intracellular Ca^{2+} concentration through reversal of the Na^+/Ca^{2+} exchanger independent of the intracellular second messenger cyclic adenosine monophosphate (cAMP). In contrast, catecholamines (e.g., epinephrine, norepinephrine) and PDE inhibitors (e.g., inamrinone, milrinone) increase Ca^{2+} concentration by positively modulating the actions of cAMP. Myofilament Ca^{2+} sensitizers (e.g., pimobendan, levosimendan) increase contractile performance by enhancing the sensitivity of the contractile proteins to Ca^{2+} without specifically affecting the intracellular concentration of this ion.

Rapid extrusion of Ca^{2+} from the myoplasm, and dissociation of Ca^{2+} from troponin C after contraction, are required for relaxation of the sarcomere to occur. Delays in this process result in incomplete myocardial relaxation and may be clinically manifested by diastolic dysfunction. Thus, simultaneous increases in the elimination of Ca^{2+} must also occur during augmentation of contractile state produced by inotropic drugs. Calcium is extruded from the myoplasm by Ca^{2+} ATPases located within the sarcolemmal membrane and the sarcoplasmic reticulum. The ATP-dependent Ca^{2+} transporter in the sarcoplasmic reticulum (SERCA) is a primary determinant of removal of Ca^{2+} from the cytosol. Calcium is also passively extruded from the myoplasm by the sarcolemmal Na^+/Ca^{2+} transporter. This ion exchanger allows Ca^{2+} to be removed from the cell in exchange for Na^+.

Pharmacology of positive inotropic drugs

Digitalis glycosides
Preclinical pharmacology
Cardiac glycosides are naturally occurring substances found in a variety of plants including foxglove (*Digitalis purpurea*). The chemical structure of digitalis glycosides contains a hydrophobic steroid nucleus and a hydrophilic unsaturated lactone

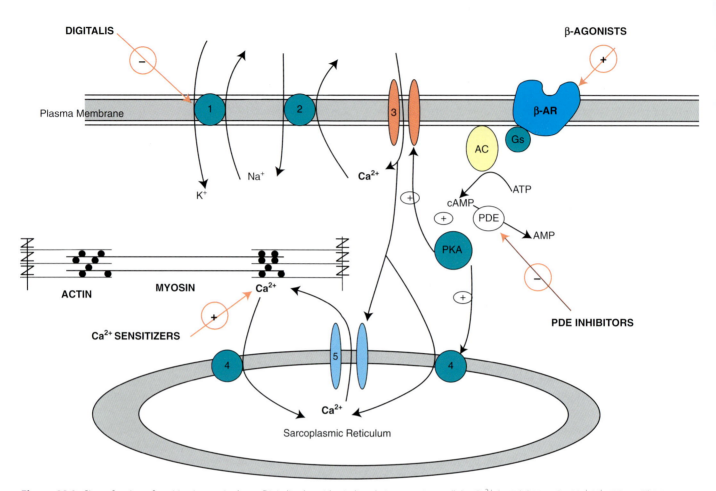

Figure 44.1. Sites of action of positive inotropic drugs. Digitalis glycosides indirectly increase intracellular Ca^{2+} by inhibiting the Na^+/K^+ ATPase. This increases intracellular Na^+, thus reducing the activity of the Na^+/Ca^{2+} exchanger. β_1-Adrenergic agonists also increase intracellular Ca^{2+}. They act by stimulating the production of cyclic adenosine monophosphate (cAMP), which activates protein kinase A (PKA). PKA in turn phosphorylates and activates both voltage-gated Ca^{2+} channels (VGCC) and the sarcoplasmic reticulum Ca^{2+} ATPase (SERCA). The increased activity of VGCC increases "trigger calcium" leading to greater activation of the Ca^{2+} release channel in sarcoplasmic reticulum. Activation of the Ca^{2+} ATPase increases Ca^{2+} uptake by sarcoplasmic reticulum, producing a positive lusitropic effect. Phosphodiesterase inhibitors increase cAMP by inhibiting its breakdown, and thus act synergistically with β_1-agonists to increase intracellular Ca^{2+}. Ca^{2+} sensitizers increase the sensitivity of the contractile apparatus to Ca^{2+} without changing intracellular Ca^{2+} concentrations. AC, adenylate cyclase; ATP, adenosine triphosphate; β_1-AR, β_1-adrenergic receptor; PDE, phosphodiesterase.

ring. Digitalis glycosides are one of only two positive inotropic drugs that are currently available for the chronic oral treatment of mild to moderate heart failure [8]. Levosimendan is available in Europe but has not been approved by the Food and Drug Administration (FDA) in the United States to date [4]. Digitalis glycosides enhance contractile function, but this positive inotropic effect is relatively minor when compared with the actions produced by other drugs used for the treatment of acute LV dysfunction. The most commonly used cardiac glycosides include digoxin and digitoxin, but a large number of related compounds also have been used clinically. Digitalis glycosides selectively and reversibly inhibit sarcolemmal Na^+/K^+ ATPase by binding to the α subunit on the extracellular surface of the enzyme complex [9]. This digitalis–sarcolemmal Na^+/K^+ ATPase binding is inhibited by increases in extracellular potassium (K^+) concentration, and, as a result, digitalis toxicity may be reversed to some degree by the administration of K^+. Conversely, digitalis toxicity is markedly

increased in the presence of hypokalemia. Inhibition of sarcolemmal Na^+/K^+ ATPase indirectly increases Ca^{2+} availability during systole, thereby augmenting myocardial contractility. The Na^+/K^+ ATPase enzyme exchanges three intracellular Na^+ ions for two extracellular K^+ ions against concentration gradients in an energy-dependent fashion. This action produces a slight increase in intracellular Na^+ concentration that, in turn, reduces extrusion of Ca^{2+} from the myoplasm by the sarcolemmal Na^+/Ca^{2+} exchanger. This additional Ca^{2+} is stored by the sarcoplasmic reticulum, providing additional Ca^{2+} for subsequent release during the next contraction. In contrast to other drugs that increase myocardial contractility, tachyphylaxis to the positive inotropic effects of digitalis glycosides does not appear to occur. The mechanism of action of digitalis glycosides is similar to that implicated for the treppe phenomenon observed in cardiac and skeletal muscle. Rapid increases in muscle stimulation or heart rate cause a lag in activity of the Na^+/K^+ ATPase, a transient increase in intracellular Na^+ concentration, and an increase in contractile force mediated by advantageous Na^+/Ca^{2+} exchange. Conversely, digitalis glycosides may simultaneously exert antiadrenergic effects in heart failure, because Na^+/K^+ ATPase has been identified as an important regulator of afferent cardiovascular baroreceptors and diminished responsiveness of these baroreceptors contributes to enhanced sympathetic nervous tone in heart failure.

Clinical pharmacology

The increase in myocardial contractility produced by digitalis glycosides occurs without change in heart rate and is associated with reductions in LV preload and afterload, LV wall tension, and myocardial oxygen consumption in the failing heart. Heart failure is characterized by a compensatory increase in sympathetic nervous system tone, and digitalis glycosides have been shown to reduce sympathetic activity by enhancing contractility and improving cardiac output. This withdrawal of sympathetic tone is accompanied by reductions in circulating and cardiac norepinephrine concentrations and reduces impedance to LV ejection. The decrease in sympathetic nervous system activity observed with digitalis glycosides is also related to the direct actions of these drugs on cardiac baroreceptors and may play an important role in reducing morbidity and mortality rates in patients with chronic congestive heart failure [8]. However, dramatic alterations in the electrophysiology of primary pacemaker cells and in the remainder of the cardiac conduction pathway may also occur as a result of digitalis-induced inhibition of the sarcolemmal Na^+/K^+ ATPase, because this enzyme is responsible for maintaining the normal resting membrane potential of the myocyte. These direct electrophysiologic effects are further complicated by indirect actions mediated by withdrawal of sympathetic and increases in parasympathetic nervous system activity. Administration of digitalis glycosides frequently leads to the development of a wide variety of arrhythmias including sinus bradycardia or arrest, atrioventricular (AV) conduction delays, and second- or third-degree heart block. Toxic levels of digitalis glycosides may paradoxically increase sympathetic nervous system tone and may precipitate the formation of malignant ventricular tachyarrhythmias. The digitalis glycosides have a low therapeutic ratio and narrow margin of safety, and mortality rates resulting from arrhythmias are directly related to the plasma concentrations of these drugs.

Digitalis glycosides are most often used during the perioperative period for the management of supraventricular tachyarrhythmias associated with a rapid ventricular response, because these drugs prolong conduction time in the AV node. Digitalis glycosides are not commonly used to increase myocardial contractility in patients with acute LV dysfunction, because of the availability of far more potent drugs with substantially less toxicity. However, digitalis glycosides continue to play an important role in the treatment of chronic congestive heart failure.

Catecholamines
Preclinical pharmacology

The cardiovascular effects of both endogenous (e.g., epinephrine, norepinephrine, dopamine) and synthetic (e.g., isoproterenol, dobutamine, dopexamine) catecholamines are mediated by activation of α- and β-adrenoceptors. These drugs mimic stimulation of the sympathetic nervous system and may be divided into those that act directly on adrenoceptors and those that act indirectly by promoting the release of norepinephrine from sympathetic nerve terminals. Catecholamines enhance myocardial contractility by activation of cardiac β_1-adrenoceptors located on the sarcolemmal surface. The β_1-adrenoceptor is coupled to the enzyme adenylate cyclase by a stimulatory guanine nucleotide-binding (G_s) protein located in the cell membrane. Adenylate cyclase converts ATP to cAMP. This second messenger binds to the regulatory subunit of protein kinase A and enhances the activity of this enzyme, resulting in the subsequent phosphorylation of sarcolemmal Ca^{2+} channels, troponin I, and phospholamban. These actions directly increase Ca^{2+} influx through voltage-dependent Ca^{2+} channels, indirectly stimulate release of Ca^{2+} from the sarcoplasmic reticulum, augment Ca^{2+} binding to the contractile apparatus, and accelerate Ca^{2+} uptake by the sarcoplasmic reticulum. Thus catecholamines exert positive inotropic effects through β_1-adrenoceptor stimulation by increasing the amount of Ca^{2+} available for contractile activation and enhancing the efficacy of Ca^{2+} at the myofilaments. Catecholamines also simultaneously accelerate myocardial relaxation (*lusitropy*) and improve diastolic function by augmenting removal of Ca^{2+} from the sarcoplasm after contraction has occurred. In addition to positive inotropic and lusitropic actions, β_1-adrenoceptor stimulation by catecholamines increases heart rate and conduction velocity (*chronotropic* and *dromotropic* effects, respectively) and may contribute to the development of supraventricular or ventricular tachyarrhythmias.

Catecholamines are used extensively to enhance myocardial contractility in the setting of acute and chronic LV dysfunction. However, the efficacy of β_1-adrenoceptor agonists in the failing heart may be influenced by the relative density and function of the β_1-adrenoceptor. This receptor is markedly downregulated and its signal transduction cascade is adversely affected in heart failure [10]. There is also strong evidence indicating that cardiopulmonary bypass and intraoperative adrenoceptor stimulation during routine surgery acutely depress β_1-adrenoceptor signaling [11]. Recognition of this phenomenon has led some investigators to advocate the use of a short-acting β_1-adrenoceptor antagonist (e.g., esmolol) during cardiopulmonary bypass to reverse downregulation of this receptor and enhance the contractile response to exogenously administered catecholamines after bypass.

Catecholamines exert a variety of pharmacologic effects in other circulatory beds, because of the widespread location and heterogenous distribution of α and β adrenoceptor subtypes. The peripheral vascular actions of catecholamines are dependent on the specific drug as a result of differences in chemical structure and selectivity for adrenoceptors. This selectivity may also be highly dose-dependent. For example, low doses of dopamine stimulate dopamine subtype 1 and 2 receptors

(D_1 and D_2) to produce arterial vasodilation, whereas progressively greater doses activate β_1- followed by α_1-adrenoceptors, thereby enhancing contractility and causing arterial vasoconstriction, respectively. α_1-Adrenoceptors are located primarily in small arterioles and veins and mediate increases in systemic vascular resistance and decreases in venous capacitance, respectively. Activation of α_1-adrenoceptors located on the sarcolemmal surface of vascular smooth-muscle cells increases the activity of phospholipase C through a G protein-mediated mechanism and leads to cleavage of cell membrane phospholipids and the production of inositol 1,4,5-trisphosphate (IP_3). This intracellular second messenger opens receptor-operated Ca^{2+} channels, stimulates Ca^{2+} release from the sarcoplasmic reticulum, and causes activation of Ca^{2+}-dependent protein kinases and phosphorylation of respective substrates. These actions increase intracellular Ca^{2+} concentration and lead to contraction of the vascular smooth muscle cell. In contrast to cutaneous blood vessels, which contain primarily α_1-adrenoceptors, skeletal muscle contains β_2-adrenoceptors, whose activation produces arteriolar vasodilation through an adenylate-cyclase-mediated mechanism.

The effects of a catecholamine on arterial pressure are determined by its actions on heart rate, myocardial contractility, arterial resistance (i.e., afterload), and venous tone (i.e., preload). For example, a pure α_1-adrenoceptor agonist produces an increase in systemic vascular resistance and a decrease in venous capacitance, actions that combine to increase arterial pressure. In contrast, a pure β-adrenoceptor agonist causes increases in heart rate, stroke volume, and cardiac output, and a decrease in systemic vascular resistance. These effects may result in a modest decline in arterial pressure. In general, catecholamines produce deleterious increases in myocardial oxygen consumption and may cause myocardial ischemia. Use of these drugs to improve LV performance in patients with coronary artery disease or congestive heart failure must be approached with caution. As a result, afterload reduction is most commonly used as an initial therapeutic approach to increase cardiac output in the pharmacologic management of acute or chronic heart failure.

Clinical pharmacology
Epinephrine
Epinephrine is an agonist of α_1-, β_1-, and β_2-adrenoceptors. An intravenous infusion of epinephrine produces an increase in mean arterial pressure characterized by selectively enhanced systolic pressure with little change in diastolic pressure. Epinephrine exerts positive chronotropic and inotropic actions by stimulation of β_1-adrenoceptors located on the cell membranes of sinoatrial node cells and cardiac myocytes, respectively. Epinephrine also increases the rate of myocardial relaxation and enhances early LV filling, thereby improving diastolic function. These combined effects result in a dramatic increase in cardiac output. For example, cardiac index increased by 0.1, 0.7, and 1.2 $L min^{-1} m^{-2}$ with the administration of epinephrine (0.01, 0.02, and 0.04 $\mu g kg^{-1} min^{-1}$, respectively) in humans [12]. The initial tachycardia observed with administration of epinephrine may be followed by a subsequent reduction in heart rate resulting from activation of baroreceptor reflexes. Epinephrine (0.01–0.03 $\mu g kg^{-1} min^{-1}$) has been shown to produce similar hemodynamic effects with less pronounced tachycardia than dobutamine (2.5–5.0 $\mu g kg^{-1} min^{-1}$) in patients after coronary artery bypass graft (CABG) surgery [13]. In fact, use of epinephrine as the primary inotropic drug for the management of LV dysfunction after cardiopulmonary bypass has been advocated by some clinicians because of the predictable increase in cardiac output observed with this endogenenous catecholamine compared with its synthetic derivatives. Such a recommendation may be especially pertinent considering recent data indicating that routine use of dobutamine in cardiac surgery adversely affects outcome [14]. Epinephrine has also been shown to increase cardiac index and oxygen delivery without affecting heart rate in patients with sepsis-induced hypotension that is unresponsive to dopamine. However, the use of epinephrine as an inotropic drug in these settings may be limited to some degree by the propensity of this catecholamine to precipitate arrhythmias. Epinephrine causes direct positive dromotropic effects, as indicated by an increase in conduction velocity and reduction of the refractory period of the AV node, His bundle, Purkinje fibers, and ventricular muscle. The increase in AV nodal conduction may produce detrimental increases in ventricular rate in patients with atrial flutter or fibrillation. The automaticity of latent pacemakers also may increase because spontaneous diastolic depolarization is accelerated. These alterations in electrophysiology caused by epinephrine may contribute to the occurrence of benign or malignant ventricular arrhythmias including premature ventricular contractions, ventricular tachycardia, and ventricular fibrillation.

Stimulation of α_1-adrenoceptors by epinephrine constricts arteriolar vascular smooth muscle located in the cutaneous, splanchnic, and renal circulations. Conversely, epinephrine-induced activation of β_2-adrenoceptors in skeletal muscle vascular beds produces vasodilation. Thus, the overall effect of epinephrine on blood flow to a specific organ depends on the relative balance of α_1- and β_2-adrenoceptors located in the vasculature. The effects of epinephrine on organ blood flow are also dose-dependent. β_2-Adrenoceptors are sensitive to lower doses of epinephrine and, as a result, peripheral vasodilation and modest reductions in arterial pressure are observed. In contrast, the effects of epinephrine on α_1-adrenoceptors predominate at greater doses. This action produces marked increases in systemic vascular resistance and arterial pressure. The intense vasoconstriction produced by high doses of epinephrine may adversely impede LV ejection by increasing afterload after cardiopulmonary bypass. Thus, greater doses of epinephrine may be used in combination with arterial vasodilators such as sodium nitroprusside to optimize contractile performance during these conditions. The venous circulation also contains a relatively high density of α_1-adrenoceptors, and venoconstriction produced by epinephrine enhances venous return. α_1-Adrenoceptors also mediate direct vasoconstriction of the pulmonary vasculature produced by epinephrine and contribute to increases in pulmonary arterial pressures. Both α_1- and β_2-adrenoceptors are located in the coronary circulation, but these receptors do not usually play a major role in determining myocardial perfusion. In contrast, epinephrine-induced increases in myocardial oxygen consumption produced by tachycardia, enhanced LV preload, augmented inotropic state, and increased afterload cause increases in coronary blood flow by metabolic autoregulation. However, during conditions of maximal coronary vasodilation, such as may be observed during myocardial ischemia, direct stimulation of α_1-adrenoceptors by epinephrine may reduce epicardial coronary artery diameter and decrease coronary blood flow.

The hemodynamic effects of epinephrine are affected by prior administration of α- or β-adrenoceptor antagonists and other vasoactive drugs. For example, the nonselective β-blocker propranolol abolishes decreases in systemic vascular resistance produced by epinephrine-induced stimulation of β_2-adrenoceptors and contributes to substantially greater peripheral vasoconstriction mediated by unopposed α_1-adrenoceptors. Clearly, the positive inotropic and chronotropic effects of epinephrine are also markedly attenuated in the presence of pre-existing β-blockade. β-Adrenoceptor antagonists competitively inhibit these adrenoceptors, and greater doses of epinephrine are required to overcome this competitive blockade. Complete pharmacologic blockade of β_1- and β_2-adrenoceptors may theoretically make the hemodynamic effects of epinephrine essentially indistinguishable from those of the pure α_1-adrenoceptor agonist phenylephrine.

Norepinephrine

Norepinephrine is the endogenous neurotransmitter released from adrenergic nerve terminals during activation of the sympathetic nervous system. Norepinephrine stimulates α_1- and β_1-adrenoceptors, but, in contrast to epinephrine, this catecholamine has little effect on β_2-adrenoceptors. These actions produce positive inotropic effects, intense vasoconstriction, increases in arterial pressure, and relative maintenance of cardiac output. In contrast to epinephrine, norepinephrine does not substantially affect heart rate because activation of baroreceptor reflexes resulting from arterial vasoconstriction usually counteracts β_1-adrenoceptor-mediated, direct, positive, chronotropic effects. Norepinephrine causes relatively greater increases in systemic vascular resistance and diastolic arterial pressure than epinephrine. Norepinephrine increases arterial pressure while simultaneously enhancing contractile state and venous return by reductions in venous capacitance, thereby augmenting stroke volume and ejection fraction. In contrast, pure α_1-adrenoceptor agonists such as phenylephrine and methoxamine further compromise cardiac output in failing myocardium and contribute to peripheral hypoperfusion despite an increase in arterial pressure.

The cardiovascular actions of norepinephrine make this catecholamine a useful drug for the treatment of refractory hypotension during severe sepsis. For example, intravenous infusions of norepinephrine (0.03–$0.90\,\mu g\,kg^{-1}$ per minute) have been shown to increase arterial pressure, LV stroke work index, cardiac index, and urine output in septic patients with hypotension that was unresponsive to volume administration, dopamine, or dobutamine. The hypertensive actions of norepinephrine may be beneficial for maintenance of coronary perfusion pressure in patients with severe coronary artery disease. The efficacy of norepinephrine in the treatment of the "low systemic vascular resistance" (also known as "vasoplegic") syndrome that is occasionally observed after cardiopulmonary bypass has also been demonstrated, although vasopressin may be more efficacious in this setting. However, although norepinephrine usually produces coronary vasodilation by indirect metabolic effects, internal mammary, gastroepiploic, or radial artery graft spasm mediated by direct α_1-adrenoceptor activation may occur in patients undergoing CABG surgery as a consequence of administration of this catecholamine. Norepinephrine may produce ventricular and supraventricular ectopy; its arrhythmogenic potential is considerably less than that of epinephrine. Thus, substitution of norepinephrine for epinephrine may be appropriate in the therapeutic management of cardiogenic shock when atrial or ventricular arrhythmias are present.

Norepinephrine-induced stimulation of pulmonary vascular α_1-adrenoceptors and simultaneous increases in venous return may increase pulmonary arterial pressures and contribute to the development of right ventricular (RV) failure. The combined use of norepinephrine administered through the left atrium and the relatively selective pulmonary vasodilator prostaglandin E_1 administered intravenously has been advocated to prevent RV dysfunction in patients with reactive pulmonary vasculature after cardiopulmonary bypass. The use of prostaglandin E_1 has been largely supplanted in favor of the inhaled highly selective pulmonary vasodilator nitric oxide, but lower doses of norepinephrine administered through the left atrium continue to be beneficial in treating LV failure associated with pulmonary hypertension, because metabolism in peripheral tissue limits the amount of norepinephrine returning to the pulmonary vasculature. When administered through the left atrium, norepinephrine enhances LV coronary perfusion by increasing diastolic arterial pressure while simultaneously increasing LV contractility. These actions lead to reductions in biventricular filling pressures and increases in cardiac output.

Norepinephrine directly reduces hepatic, skeletal muscle, splanchnic, and renal blood flow through α_1-adrenoceptor activation. However, an increase in perfusion pressure produced by norepinephrine during the treatment of profound hypotension may result in enhanced blood flow to these vascular beds. Nevertheless, decreased perfusion of renal and splanchnic beds represents a major limitation on the prolonged use of high doses of norepinephrine. Activation of renal dopamine receptors with low-dose dopamine or the selective D_1-agonist fenoldopam to counteract the deleterious actions of norepinephrine on renal blood flow may preserve renal perfusion and urine output in patients with hypotension.

Dopamine

Dopamine is an endogenous catecholamine that is the immediate biochemical precursor of norepinephrine. The pharmacology of dopamine is complex, because this drug differentially activates a variety of dopaminergic and adrenoceptor subtypes. Low doses of dopamine ($< 3\,\mu g\,kg^{-1}\,min^{-1}$) selectively stimulate D_1 receptors in and increase blood flow to renal and mesenteric vascular beds. Activation of D_2 receptors in autonomic nervous system ganglia and adrenergic nerves also reduces norepinephrine release. The combined effects of dopamine on D_1 and D_2 receptors may cause a decrease in arterial pressure during administration of lower doses of this catecholamine. Higher doses of dopamine ($3–8\,\mu g\,kg^{-1}\,min^{-1}$) appear to nonselectively stimulate both α- and β-adrenoceptors. However, dopamine activates vascular smooth muscle α_1-adrenoceptors almost exclusively, and produces arterial and venous vasoconstriction at doses exceeding $10\,\mu g\,kg^{-1}\,min^{-1}$, similar to pure α_1-agonists.

Although pedagogically useful, this traditional dose–response description of dopamine pharmacodynamics may be somewhat simplistic and may not be consistently observed even in healthy individuals [15]. In fact, a wide range of clinical responses to dopamine is more typically observed, resulting from differences in receptor regulation, the presence of drug interactions, and individual patient variability [16]. Thus, although lower doses of dopamine are frequently used for renal protection mediated through D_1 receptors, these doses may also activate α- and β-adrenoceptors that obscure the intended dopaminergic effects in some patients. Conversely, high-dose dopamine may continue to stimulate D_1 receptors despite simultaneous α_1-adrenoceptor-mediated vasoconstriction, as indicated by maintenance of renal perfusion and urine output. The renal vasodilating effects of lower doses of dopamine may be particularly useful in patients with impaired renal function or those at risk for decreases in renal perfusion associated with reduced cardiac output. Dopamine may also preserve renal perfusion during simultaneous administration of other α_1-adrenoceptor agonists that directly reduce renal blood flow. The increase in renal blood flow produced by dopamine occurs as a result of direct vasodilation of afferent and indirect vasoconstriction of efferent arterioles. These renal vascular effects enhance glomerular filtration rate, sodium excretion, and urine output. Nevertheless, a recent meta-analysis of 61 clinical trials involving 3359 patients demonstrated that although low-dose dopamine transiently increases urine output, this drug does not prevent renal dysfunction or death [17]. As a result, use of low-dose dopamine to preserve or improve renal function can no longer be recommended.

Dopamine is commonly used for inotropic support in the perioperative period. This catecholamine produces positive chronotropic, dromotropic, inotropic, and lusitropic effects by stimulation of β_1-adrenoceptors. Concomitant activation of arterial and venous α_1-adrenoceptors by greater doses of dopamine also increases LV preload and afterload. These combined effects enhance contractile performance and increase arterial pressure. However, dopamine may not be the ideal drug of choice for inotropic support in patients with elevated pulmonary arterial or LV filling pressures. For example, atrial and mean arterial pressures were greater in patients receiving dopamine than in those treated with dobutamine after cardiopulmonary bypass, despite similar levels of cardiac function. Dopamine may also produce more pronounced tachycardia than epinephrine in this clinical setting. Dopamine-induced increases in LV afterload may be reduced or eliminated by simultaneous administration of an arterial vasodilator such as sodium nitroprusside. This combined therapy (colloquially termed "dopride") preserves the positive inotropic actions of dopamine mediated through β_1-adrenoceptors and further enhances cardiac output by reducing impedance to LV ejection. Dopamine increases myocardial oxygen consumption in the normal and failing heart, impairs the functional recovery of stunned myocardium, and exacerbates injury after coronary occlusion in vivo. These data suggest that dopamine may not be the preferred drug to increase contractile function in the presence of a critical coronary artery stenosis.

Dopexamine

Dopexamine is a synthetic catecholamine that exerts activity at dopaminergic and β-adrenergic receptors. Dopexamine is structurally related to dopamine but is devoid of α-adrenoceptor activity and has a greater affinity (9.8 times) for β_2- than β_1-adrenoceptors [18]. As a result of dopamine and β_2-adrenoceptor stimulation, dopexamine acts primarily as a vasodilator. Dopexamine also enhances myocardial contractility by inhibiting presynaptic norepinephrine reuptake, whereas β_1-adrenoceptor activation does not appear to play a substantial role in the positive inotropic actions of this drug. Dopexamine has been shown to increase splanchnic and renal perfusion, reduce systemic vascular resistance, and enhance cardiac output concomitant with a baroreceptor-mediated increase in heart rate in healthy volunteers and patients with heart failure. Dopexamine ($1–4\,\mu g\,kg^{-1}\,min^{-1}$) also enhances stroke volume and cardiac output and reduces systemic and pulmonary vascular resistances in patients after cardiopulmonary bypass [19]. Dopexamine may also improve renal function and reduce the inflammatory response to cardiopulmonary bypass [20]. The use of dopexamine as a positive inotropic drug in patients with severe coronary artery disease may be limited, however, because tachycardia and increases in myocardial oxygen consumption occur at greater doses of the drug. Dopexamine may also play a role in circulatory support during sepsis, because this drug preferentially increases splanchnic and renal perfusion by activation of dopaminergic and β_2-adrenergic receptors.

Studies conducted in experimental models of and in patients with sepsis suggest that dopexamine increases cardiac output and oxygen delivery concomitant with beneficial redistribution of splanchnic blood flow. Use of dopexamine for inotropic support or reduction of LV afterload is uncommon in the United States.

Dobutamine

Dobutamine is a synthetic catecholamine composed of two stereoisomers. The (−) and (+) isomers are both β-adrenoceptor agonists, but these stereoisomers exert opposing agonist and antagonist activity, respectively, on α_1-adrenoceptors. Dobutamine produces potent β-adrenoceptor agonist stimulation with little or no effect on α_1-adrenoceptors at doses less than $5\,\mu g\,kg^{-1}\,min^{-1}$. As a result, dobutamine increases myocardial contractility and causes a modest degree of peripheral vasodilation by stimulation of cardiac β_1- and vascular smooth-muscle β_2-adrenoceptors, respectively, at these concentrations. These properties account for the reductions in LV preload and afterload and improvements in LV–arterial coupling and mechanical efficiency concomitant with enhanced contractile function observed in patients with LV dysfunction [21]. The salutary actions of dobutamine on LV–arterial matching may also account for the reductions in functional mitral insufficiency that occur with the administration of dobutamine to patients with dilated cardiomyopathy and increased LV filling pressures [22]. The (−) isomer of dobutamine stimulates the α_1-adrenoceptor at greater doses and prevents further vasodilation from occurring. As a result, LV preload, afterload, and arterial pressure are relatively maintained, whereas cardiac output is increased, and less pronounced baroreceptor reflex-mediated tachycardia may be observed. Nevertheless, dobutamine may substantially increase heart rate by direct chronotropic and dromotropic effects mediated by β_1-adrenoceptors in some patients. In fact, doses of dobutamine that enhance cardiac output and stroke volume have been shown to produce significantly greater increases in heart rate than epinephrine in patients after CABG surgery [13]. Dobutamine-induced tachycardia and enhanced myocardial contractility produce a direct increase of myocardial oxygen consumption and may cause "demand" ischemia in patients with coronary artery disease. This observation forms the basis for the use of dobutamine stress echocardiography as a diagnostic tool for the detection of functional coronary artery stenoses, because easily detected abnormalities in regional wall motion occur during these conditions [23]. Conversely, dobutamine may indirectly reduce heart rate in patients with severe heart failure if increases in cardiac output and oxygen delivery result in a simultaneous reduction of sympathetic nervous system tone, which is known to be chronically increased during these conditions. Dobutamine may also indirectly decrease myocardial oxygen consumption by reducing LV end-systolic and end-diastolic wall stress in the failing heart.

The β_2-adrenoceptor-stimulating actions of dobutamine cause modest reductions in pulmonary arterial pressure and vascular resistance. As a result, dobutamine may be used to increase cardiac output in the presence of increased pulmonary vascular resistance after cardiopulmonary bypass. In contrast, dopamine-induced, α_1-adrenoceptor-mediated vasoconstriction of pulmonary vascular smooth muscle increases pulmonary arterial pressure and results in greater LV filling pressures concomitant with augmented pulmonary venous return. Thus, dobutamine may have distinct advantages compared with dopamine in patients with heart failure and increased pulmonary arterial and LV filling pressures. However, pulmonary vasodilation produced by dobutamine may worsen ventilation/perfusion mismatch and increase pulmonary shunting. In contrast to dopamine and dopexamine, dobutamine does not exert activity at dopaminergic receptors or selectively alter renal perfusion. Nevertheless, dobutamine may indirectly enhance renal function in heart failure by augmenting cardiac output and thereby improve renal perfusion. Despite the potentially beneficial hemodynamic actions of dobutamine, administration of the drug was shown to increase mortality in patients with heart failure [24,25], and also produced adverse effects in patients during cardiac surgery [14]. As a result of these and other convincing clinical studies, many clinicians have ceased to use dobutamine for inotropic support during cardiac anesthesia.

Isoproterenol

Isoproterenol is a nonselective agonist of β-adrenoceptors. This synthetic catecholamine has a low affinity for, and consequently does not exert activity at, α-adrenoceptors. Isoproterenol reduces systemic vascular resistance by β_2-adrenoceptor-mediated arteriolar vasodilation in skeletal muscle, and to a lesser degree in renal and splanchnic vascular beds. As a result of this reduction in LV afterload, decreases in diastolic and mean arterial pressures along with relative maintenance of systolic arterial pressure are typically observed. Tachycardia produced by isoproterenol results from direct stimulation of β_1-adrenoceptors in the sinoatrial node and AV conduction system combined with activation of baroreceptor reflexes in response to decreases in arterial pressure. Isoproterenol produces dose-dependent positive inotropic effects, but clinical increases in cardiac output may be limited to some degree because tachycardia interferes with LV filling dynamics, and dilation of venous capacitance vessels occurs, further reducing LV preload. For example, isoproterenol did not significantly enhance cardiac output in patients after CABG or valve replacement surgery, in contrast to dobutamine [26]. The hemodynamic effects of isoproterenol contribute to dose-related increases in myocardial oxygen consumption concomitant with reductions in coronary perfusion pressure and diastolic filling time. As a result, myocardial ischemia or subendocardial necrosis may occur even in the absence of hemodynamically significant coronary stenoses. Thus, the use of isoproterenol may be especially detrimental in patients with severe coronary artery disease.

Isoproterenol may be used to provide sustained increases in heart rate during symptomatic bradyarrhythmias or AV conduction block before the insertion of a temporary or permanent pacemaker. However, the use of isoproterenol for these indications has been largely supplanted by transcutaneous pacing. In addition, isoproterenol increases automaticity and may precipitate supraventricular and ventricular tachyarrhythmias. Isoproterenol has been used after cardiac transplantation to increase heart rate and myocardial contractility in the denervated transplanted heart, although placement of a temporary or permanent pacemaker has replaced drug therapy in this setting as well. Finally, isoproterenol decreases pulmonary vascular resistance and may be useful in the management of RV dysfunction resulting from pulmonary hypertension, valvular or congenital heart disease, or after cardiac transplantation. However, inhaled nitric oxide therapy has essentially eliminated the use of isoproterenol for the treatment of acute RV failure as well. Thus, the current role of isoproterenol in modern clinical cardiovascular practice has become quite limited.

Ephedrine

Ephedrine is a sympathomimetic drug that exerts direct and indirect actions on adrenoceptors. This drug produces arterial and venous vasoconstriction and enhances myocardial contractility primarily by releasing norepinephrine from adrenergic nerve terminals and indirectly stimulating α_1- and β_1-adrenoceptors. Ephedrine is transported into the presynaptic terminals of adrenergic nerves and displaces norepinephrine from binding sites within and outside of the synaptic vesicles. The displaced norepinephrine is subsequently released from the presynaptic nerve terminal and stimulates postsynaptic adrenoceptors. Although the indirect effects are the predominant pharmacologic consequences of ephedrine, this drug also directly activates β_2-adrenoceptors that tend to limit the increases in arterial pressure observed with its administration. Ephedrine is frequently administered in intravenous bolus doses (e.g., 5–10 mg) to treat hypotension in the presence of bradycardia. Ephedrine causes dose-related increases in heart rate, cardiac output, and systemic vascular resistance, hemodynamic effects that are similar to those produced by epinephrine. Unlike epinephrine, however, tachyphylaxis to the hemodynamic effects of ephedrine may rapidly occur, because repetitive administration of the drug acutely depletes presynaptic norepinephrine stores. Other drugs that deplete norepinephrine from or inhibit the uptake of ephedrine into adrenergic nerves (e.g., reserpine or cocaine, respectively) will markedly reduce the cardiovascular action of this indirect-acting sympathomimetic. The pharmacology of ephedrine is further discussed in Chapter 40.

Phosphodiesterase inhibitors
Preclinical pharmacology

Phosphodiesterases (PDEs) are a group of structurally related enzymes that are responsible for a wide range of physiologic actions. The tissue distribution and subcellular isoforms of these enzymes have been intensively studied, and at least seven different subtypes that hydrolyze the second messengers cAMP or cyclic guanosine monophosphate (cGMP) have been identified. The PDE inhibitors augment the intracellular actions of cAMP and cGMP by preventing their degradation. Clinically used PDE inhibitors may demonstrate some degree of selectivity for a particular isoenzyme, but this selectivity is dose-dependent. Human cardiac and vascular smooth muscle contain the type 3 PDE isoenzyme bound to the sarcoplasmic reticulum [27], which facilitates the cleavage of cAMP to AMP. Unlike aminophylline and caffeine, which attenuate the activity of most PDE isoforms, selective inhibition of cardiac PDE3 by bypiridines (e.g., milrinone and inamrinone) or imidazoline derivatives (e.g., enoximone and piroximone) produces a series of alterations in intracellular Ca^{2+} regulation that enhance myocardial contractility independent of catecholamine release or β-adrenoceptor activation. Increases in cAMP concentration produced by these drugs augment the activity of protein kinase A and lead to the phosphorylation of the voltage-dependent Ca^{2+} channel [28] and the sarcoplasmic reticulum regulatory protein phospholamban [29]. The normal inhibition of sarcoplasmic reticular Ca^{2+} ATPases produced by phospholamban is attenuated by this cAMP-mediated phosphorylation, leading to enhanced diastolic Ca^{2+} storage in and greater systolic Ca^{2+} release from this organelle. Thus, cardiac PDE3 inhibitors not only exert positive inotropic actions by increasing the amount of Ca^{2+} available for contractile activation, but also facilitate diastolic relaxation by enhancing Ca^{2+} removal from the myoplasm. This latter positive lusitropic effect may contribute to improvements in diastolic function observed after administration of these drugs to patients with heart failure.

Clinical pharmacology

PDE3 inhibitors cause dose-dependent arterial and venous vasodilation by increasing cAMP concentration and indirectly activating cGMP-dependent protein kinase in vascular smooth muscle. In fact, the propensity of PDE3 inhibitors to enhance contractile function and simultaneously act as potent vasodilators led to use of the term *inodilator* to describe their cardiovascular effects. All PDE3 inhibitors produce more pronounced vasodilation than β-adrenoceptor agonists, including isoproterenol. Reductions in systemic and pulmonary vascular resistances enhance LV and RV ejection, respectively. The reduction in LV afterload contributes to the increases in cardiac output, LV–arterial coupling, and mechanical efficiency observed with these drugs in vivo. The relative importance of the positive inotropic effects versus the LV afterload-reducing properties of PDE3 inhibitors in augmenting cardiac output were intensely debated when these drugs were introduced into clinical practice, but it is likely that both actions contribute substantially to improvements in overall cardiovascular performance. The declines in pulmonary vascular resistance produced by PDE3 inhibitors may be especially beneficial in patients with pulmonary hypertension who are undergoing cardiac surgery [30] or heart transplantation [31]. However, the pulmonary vasodilating properties of PDE3 inhibitors may increase intrapulmonary shunt fraction and cause arterial hypoxemia. PDE3 inhibition also causes dilation of venous capacitance vessels, leading to reductions in LV and RV preload (clinically represented by pulmonary capillary occlusion and central venous pressures, respectively). The decreases in preload and afterload produced by PDE3 inhibitors may contribute to reductions in myocardial oxygen consumption observed with these drugs in patients with heart failure, despite simultaneous positive inotropic and chronotropic effects [32]. Mean arterial pressure is preserved or modestly reduced during administration of PDE3 inhibitors as long as LV preload is adequately maintained because increases in cardiac output compensate for simultaneous declines in systemic vascular resistance.

PDE3 inhibitors produce less tachycardia than catecholamines, but these drugs are arrhythmogenic because they increase intracellular cAMP and Ca^{2+} concentration [33]. The tachycardia caused by PDE3 inhibitors may be eliminated by concomitant administration of a selective β_1-adrenoceptor antagonist without adversely affecting the positive inotropic response. PDE3 inhibitors block platelet aggregation, suppress neointimal hyperplasia associated with endothelial injury, and attenuate inflammatory cytokine formation after cardiopulmonary bypass [34]. They also dilate native epicardial coronary arteries and arterial bypass conduits [35], and may produce anti-ischemic effects in patients with chronic stable angina. These data suggest that PDE3 inhibitors may exert further beneficial actions in addition to their favorable effects on LV systolic and diastolic function in patients with coronary artery disease or heart failure. Notably, the relative efficacy of PDE3 inhibitors may be reduced to some degree in the failing heart, but not to the extent observed with β-adrenoceptor agonists. This observation has been attributed to upregulation of inhibitory G proteins in heart failure and not direct structural or functional alterations in the PDE3 isoenzyme itself [27]. Nevertheless, PDE3 inhibitors remain effective positive inotropic drugs in heart failure, in contrast to the markedly attenuated actions of β-adrenoceptor agonists on contractile function in this setting [32].

PDE3 inhibitors (e.g., milrinone, enoximone, vesnarinone) are orally absorbed, and several large-scale placebo-controlled clinical trials were conducted to evaluate the efficacy of these drugs in the treatment of chronic NYHA class IV heart failure. These drugs were shown to enhance cardiac performance in this patient population, but the long-term results of these studies were discouraging, with unexpectedly high mortality as a result of malignant ventricular arrhythmias and sudden death [36]. Nevertheless, interest in PDE3 inhibitors for use in chronic heart failure has been rekindled by the use of lower doses that do not produce substantial hemodynamic effects [37] with or without simultaneous administration of β-adrenoceptor antagonists to counteract adverse electrophysiologic

side effects [38]. Despite their apparently limited applicability in the setting of chronic heart failure, PDE3 inhibitors remain a mainstay in the treatment of acute LV dysfunction, especially in the setting of cardiac surgery.

Milrinone

Milrinone is a bypiridine PDE3 inhibitor that has been used extensively during and after cardiac surgery. Milrinone is approximately 15–20 times more potent than the closely related bypiridine, inamrinone. In contrast to inamrinone, milrinone does not cause thrombocytopenia after prolonged use in cardiac surgical patients [39]. Intravenous milrinone enhances LV function and produces arterial and venous vasodilation in patients emerging from cardiopulmonary bypass [40]. Milrinone also improves the probability of successful weaning of high-risk patients from cardiopulmonary bypass [41]. The pharmacokinetics and pharmacodynamics of milrinone have been extensively studied, and a $50\,\mu g\,kg^{-1}$ loading dose was shown to be optimal compared with either 25 or $75\,\mu g\,kg^{-1}$ doses for patients separating from cardiopulmonary bypass [42]. This $50\,\mu g\,kg^{-1}$ loading dose may be used in combination with or without a $0.5\,\mu g\,kg^{-1}$ per minute infusion to increase cardiac output and oxygen delivery. A similar pharmacokinetic profile may be used to improve oxygen delivery in patients in the intensive care unit [43].

Inamrinone

Inamrinone (formerly known as amrinone) was the first clinically used bypiridine PDE3 inhibitor. Inamrinone produces cardiovascular effects that are almost identical to milrinone [40]. It increases cardiac output, reduces LV and RV filling pressures, and causes systemic and pulmonary vasodilation, while heart rate and mean arterial pressure are relatively maintained in patients with severe congestive heart failure. Inamrinone and dobutamine were shown to cause similar improvements in LV performance in patients with reduced cardiac output after CABG surgery [44]. Inamrinone and epinephrine were also equally efficacious in cardiac surgical patients with poor preoperative LV function (Fig. 44.2) [45]. Unlike milrinone, inamrinone rapidly produces clinically significant thrombocytopenia, and its use for the treatment of acute and chronic LV failure has been abandoned because of this important side effect.

Enoximone

Enoximone is a highly selective, imidazoline-derivative, PDE3 inhibitor that is used in Europe and is currently being investigated in clinical trials in the United States. The cardiovascular actions of intravenous enoximone are similar to those produced by milrinone and inamrinone. Evidence indicates that oral enoximone administered in doses that do not cause hemodynamic effects may increase functional capacity in patients with severe congestive heart failure [37]. These data suggest that enoximone may play a role in the treatment of chronic heart failure, but further study is needed to confirm this hypothesis.

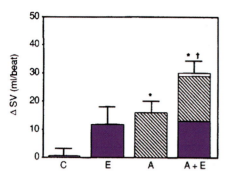

Figure 44.2. Changes in stroke volume (SV) in patients after cardiac surgery and cardiopulmonary bypass for the control (C), epinephrine (E), inamrinone (amrinone; A), and inamrinone–epinephrine (A+E) groups. The change in stroke volume for the A+E group is at least additive of the change in A and E alone (clear area). * $p < 0.05$ compared with control; † $p < 0.05$ compared to E and A alone. Reproduced from Royster et al. [46] with permission of the authors and publisher.

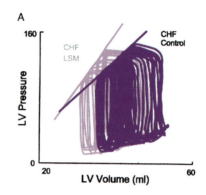

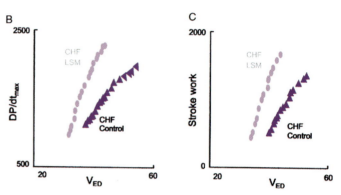

Figure 44.3. Left ventricular (LV) pressure–volume diagrams and relations determined in a conscious, chronically instrumented dog with rapid ventricular pacing-induced congestive heart failure (CHF) before and after administration of levosimendan (LSM). Treatment with LSM produced leftward shifts of (A) the LV end-systolic pressure (ESP)–end-systolic volume (ESV), (B) LV dP/dt_{max}–end-diastolic volume (V_{ED}), and (C) stroke work–end-diastolic volume relations with increased slopes. These data indicate that LSM reduces preload and increases LV contractility in the presence of CHF. Reproduced from Tachibana et al. [47] with permission of the authors and publisher.

Myofilament calcium sensitizers
Preclinical pharmacology

The myofilament Ca^{2+} sensitizers are a new class of positive inotropic vasodilating drugs that augment myocardial contractility by increasing the Ca^{2+} sensitivity of the contractile apparatus without altering intracellular Ca^{2+} concentration [4]. Myofilament Ca^{2+} sensitizers (including levosimendan, pimobendan, sulmazole, EMD 57033, and MCI-154) have received considerable attention for the treatment of acute and chronic heart failure because, unlike β_1-adrenoceptor agonists or PDE3 inhibitors, which stimulate cAMP-mediated signaling and increase intracellular Ca^{2+} concentration, these drugs do not adversely affect myocardial oxygen supply–demand relations [47], produce cardiotoxicity, or predispose to the development of arrhythmias [48]. Among the myofilament Ca^{2+} sensitizers, levosimendan has been the most extensively studied and shows the greatest promise. Levosimendan has already been approved for the treatment of acute exacerbation of chronic heart failure in several European countries following European Society of Cardiology guidelines [49]. The drug is currently undergoing phase III clinical trials in the United States (REVIVE study) to evaluate its utility for the acute or chronic management of heart failure, and has received "fast-track" status from the FDA.

The mechanisms by which myofilament Ca^{2+} sensitizers enhance inotropic state and produce vasodilation have been extensively studied [4]. Briefly, myofilament Ca^{2+} sensitizers bind to troponin C (TnC) [50] and stabilize its Ca^{2+}-bound conformation, thereby allowing unopposed interaction between actin and myosin filaments and enhancing the rate and extent of myocyte contraction [51]. These actions produce a positive inotropic effect (Fig. 44.3) [47,52]. Desensitization of the myofilaments to activator Ca^{2+} is known to occur during myocardial hypoxia, ischemia, and stunning [53], and myofilament Ca^{2+} sensitizers may be particularly useful drugs under

these conditions. A unique feature of myofilament Ca^{2+} sensitizer–TnC binding is a dependence on intracellular Ca^{2+} concentration that facilitates the interaction between TnC and Ca^{2+} during systole while simultaneously allowing Ca^{2+} to dissociate from the protein during diastole [54,55]. This Ca^{2+} dependence of TnC binding prevents deleterious abnormalities in relaxation that would otherwise be expected to occur [56]. Preservation of lusitropic function is also facilitated by the PDE-inhibiting properties of myofilament Ca^{2+} sensitizers that are observed at higher doses of these drugs. Systemic, pulmonary, and coronary vasodilation during administration of myofilament Ca^{2+} sensitizers occurs as a result of at least three distinct mechanisms. Levosimendan opens several types of K^+ channels (including voltage-dependent, ATP-sensitive, and Ca^{2+}-activated forms) in conductance and resistance vessels, actions that reduce intracellular Ca^{2+} concentration in vascular smooth muscle [57]. Interestingly, myofilament Ca^{2+} sensitizers also induce Ca^{2+} desensitization of the contractile apparatus in vascular smooth muscle that does not contain TnC, independent of intracellular Ca^{2+} concentration [58], thereby contributing to vasodilation. The PDE3-inhibiting properties of myofilament Ca^{2+} sensitizers also produce arterial and venous vasodilation. The myofilament Ca^{2+}-sensitizing characteristics of these drugs have been demonstrated convincingly in vitro [59], but the relative contribution of this Ca^{2+} sensitization to the increases in contractile state observed with these mixed myofilament Ca^{2+} sensitizer – PDE3 inhibitors remains somewhat controversial in vivo. Nevertheless, it appears likely that both mechanisms play roles in the positive inotropic effects of these drugs.

Unlike catecholamines and PDE3 inhibitors, myofilament Ca^{2+} sensitizers such as levosimendan may exert important anti-ischemic effects by virtue of ATP-sensitive K^+ (K_{ATP}) channel opening. For example, levosimendan activated sarcolemmal [60] and mitochondrial [61] K_{ATP} channels in vitro, and these channels are known to play a critical role in myocardial protection against reversible and irreversible ischemic injury. Levosimendan reduced myocardial infarct size in a canine model of ischemia and reperfusion in vivo independent of alterations in systemic hemodynamics or coronary collateral blood flow, and this beneficial action was abolished by the nonselective K_{ATP} channel antagonist glyburide [62]. Levosimendan enhanced the functional recovery of stunned myocardium after percutaneous transluminal coronary angioplasty in patients with acute myocardial ischemia [63], and was also beneficial for the treatment of cardiogenic shock resulting from stunning of border-zone myocardium during infarction [64]. Brief administration of levosimendan to patients undergoing CABG before cardiopulmonary bypass was associated with lower postoperative troponin I concentrations [65]. These latter data suggested that levosimendan may be capable of producing pharmacological preconditioning in humans, presumably as a consequence of its actions on the K_{ATP} channel.

Clinical pharmacology

Myofilament Ca^{2+} sensitizers have been shown to decrease LV filling pressure, mean arterial pressure, and pulmonary and systemic vascular resistances, and to dramatically increase cardiac output in patients with end-stage heart failure [66] and coronary artery disease [67]. Modest reductions in arterial pressure observed with these drugs are similar to those produced by pure PDE3 inhibitors, and they respond to increases in LV preload. Myofilament Ca^{2+} sensitizers also improve LV–arterial coupling and mechanical efficiency at rest and during exercise [47], while causing only minimal increases in heart rate and myocardial oxygen consumption [68].

Pimobendan

Pimobendan is a benzimidazole pyridazine derivative myofilament Ca^{2+} sensitizer that is currently used for treatment of heart failure in Japan. Pimobendan produces positive inotropic effects by increasing Ca^{2+} binding to troponin C and inhibiting PDE3. Similar to pure PDE3 inhibitors, pimobendan enhances myocardial contractility without increasing myocardial oxygen consumption, because the vasodilating properties of the drug simultaneously improve LV loading conditions in the failing heart. Pimobendan also increases myocardial blood flow and may exert antiplatelet effects that potentially improve dysfunctional microcirculation. Initial clinical trials of oral pimobendan indicated that this myofilament Ca^{2+} sensitizer increases exercise tolerance and improves quality of life in patients with heart failure [69]. However, further development of pimobendan as a chronic treatment for heart failure was halted in the United States because results of another multi-center clinical trial suggested that the drug was associated with an increase in mortality [70].

Levosimendan

Levosimendan has been shown to be clinically effacacious in patients with heart failure resulting from ischemic heart disease [71,72], dilated cardiomyopathy [72], and acute myocardial infarction [73]. Levosimendan caused dose-dependent improvements in systemic and pulmonary hemodynamics in patients with heart failure concomitant with a reduction in clinical symptoms [72], but the myofilament Ca^{2+} sensitizer did not produce hypotension, exacerbate ongoing ischemia, or contribute to mortality by increasing the incidence of arrhythmias [73]. In contrast to the findings with levosimendan, a major clinical trial of milrinone in patients with an acute exacerbation of chronic heart failure demonstrated that the pure PDE3 inhibitor did not alter in-hospital or 60-day mortality as compared to placebo, caused more frequent episodes of hypotension requiring intervention, and increased the incidence of arrhythmias compared with placebo [74]. Levosimendan also produced more favorable alterations in hemodynamics and reduced mortality in patients with low-output heart failure [25] and in those with cardiogenic shock after percutaneous coronary intervention [75] compared with dobutamine. The relative superiority of levosimendan described in these studies [25,75] may be related to the anti-inflammatory and antiapoptotic effects of the myofilament Ca^{2+} sensitizer [76]. Similar to the findings in the setting of heart failure, levosimendan has also been shown to increase cardiac performance concomitant with reductions in pulmonary capillary occlusion pressure and systemic vascular resistance in patients with normal [77] and depressed [78,79] LV function undergoing cardiac surgery with or without [80] cardiopulmonary bypass. Stroke volume was maintained to a greater extent with the combination of levosimendan and dobutamine than with milrinone and dobutamine in cardiac surgical patients with poor LV function (Fig. 44.4) [81]. These results were probably observed because levosimendan produces relatively greater reductions in systemic vascular resistance than milrinone and has a biologically active metabolite (OR-1896) with a prolonged elimination half-life [82].

Thyroid hormone

Abnormalities in thyroid hormone metabolism may occur in patients with congestive heart failure. Reversal of decreases in free triiodothyronine (T_3) concentration by administration of exogenous T_3 may enhance LV function and improve

messenger cAMP, respectively. In contrast, myofilament Ca^{2+} sensitizers (e.g., levosimendan) increase contractility by enhancing Ca^{2+} binding to the troponin C regulatory protein of the troponin–tropomyosin complex, thereby facilitating tropomyosin disinhibition and enhancing the extent and duration of actin–myosin interaction during each cardiac cycle without specifically affecting the intracellular Ca^{2+} concentration.

The development of new drugs that enhance contractile performance in patients with acute and chronic heart failure remains an important pharmacologic objective. In the treatment of chronic heart failure, options are limited. The digitalis glycosides continue to play an important role, but the currently available catecholamines and PDE3 inhibitors cannot be used, because of increased mortality rates. New drugs, such as the myofilament Ca^{2+} sensitizers, act directly on the contractile apparatus and may increase myocardial contractility without causing adverse arrhythmogenesis; one such drug, levosimendan, is available in Europe but not yet in the United States. However, catecholamines and PDE3 inhibitors remain the most common drugs used to improve contractility in cardiac surgical patients with acute LV dysfunction. A reduction in LV afterload using an arterial vasodilator should be initially considered to increase cardiac output before an inotropic drug is selected. Use of a specific positive inotropic drug is highly dependent on the hemodynamic status of each patient, and a thorough knowledge of the cardiovascular pharmacology of these drugs is required to make the most rational choice.

References

1. Packer M. The neurohormonal hypothesis: a theory to explain the mechanism of disease progression in heart failure. *J Am Coll Cardiol* 1992; **20**: 248–54.

2. Komamura K, Shannon RP, Ihara T, *et al.* Exhaustion of Frank–Starling mechanism in conscious dogs with heart failure. *Am J Physiol* 1993; **265**: H1119–H1131.

3. Armstrong PW, Moe GW. Medical advances in the treatment of congestive heart failure. *Circulation* 1993; **88**: 2941–52.

4. Toller WG, Stranz C. Levosimendan, a new inotropic and vasodilator agent. *Anesthesiology* 2006; **104**: 556–69.

5. Eichhorn EJ, Bristow MR. Practical guidelines for initiation of beta-adrenergic blockade in patients with chronic heart failure. *Am J Cardiol* 1997; **79**: 794–8.

6. Epstein AE, DiMarco JP, Ellenbogen KA, *et al.* ACC/AHA/HRS 2008 guidelines for device-based therapy of cardiac rhythm abnormalities: a report of the American College of Cardiology/American Heart Association Task Force on Practice Guidelines (Writing Committee to revise the ACC/AHA/NASPE for implantation of cardiac pacemakers and antiarrhythmia devices) developed in collaboration with the American Association for Thoracic Surgery and Society of Thoracic Surgeons. *J Am Coll Cardiol* 2008; **51**: e1–e62.

7. Royster RL, Butterworth JF, Prielipp RC, *et al.* A randomized, placebo-controlled evaluation of calcium chloride and epinephrine for inotropic support after emergence from cardiopulmonary bypass. *Anesth Analg* 1992; **74**: 3–13.

8. The effect of digoxin on mortality and morbidity in patients with heart failure. The Digitalis Investigation Group. *N Engl J Med* 1997; **336**: 525–33.

9. Hauptman PJ, Kelly RA. Digitalis. *Circulation* 1999; **99**: 1265–70.

10. Post SR, Hammond HK, Insel PA. Beta-adrenergic receptors and receptor signaling in heart failure. *Annu Rev Pharmacol Toxicol* 1999; **39**: 343–60.

11. Booth JV, Landolfo KP, Chesnut LC, *et al.* Acute depression of myocardial beta-adrenergic receptor signaling during cardiopulmonary bypass. Impairment of the adenylyl cyclase moiety. Duke Heart Center Perioperative Desensitization Group. *Anesthesiology* 1998; **89**: 602–11.

12. Leenen FH, Chan YK, Smith DL, *et al.* Epinephrine and left ventricular function in humans: effects of beta-1 vs nonselective beta blockade. *Clin Pharmacol Ther* 1988; **43**: 519–28.

13. Butterworth JF, Prielipp RC, Royster RL, *et al.* Dobutamine increases heart rate more than epinephrine in patients recovering from aortocoronary bypass surgery. *J Cardiothorac Vasc Anesth* 1992; **6**: 535–41.

14. Fellahi JL, Parienti JJ, Hanouz J, *et al.* Perioperative use of dobutamine in cardiac surgery and adverse cardiac outcome: propensity-adjusted analyses. *Anesthesiology* 2008; **108**: 979–87.

15. MacGregor DA, Smith TE, Prielipp RC, *et al.* Pharmacokinetics of dopamine in healthy male subjects. *Anesthesiology* 2000; **92**: 338–46.

16. Griffin MJ, Hines RL. Management of perioperative ventricular dysfunction. *J Cardiothorac Vasc Anesth* 2001; **15**: 90–106.

17. Friedrich JO, Adhikari N, Herridge MS, *et al.* Meta-analysis: low-dose dopamine increases urine output but does not prevent renal dysfunction or death. *Ann Intern Med* 2005; **142**: 510–24.

18. Fitton A, Benfield P. Dopexamine hydrochloride. A review of its pharmacodynamic and pharmacokinetic properties and therapeutic potential in acute cardiac insufficiency. *Drugs* 1990; **39**: 308–30.

19. MacGregor DA, Butterworth JF, Zaloga GP, *et al.* Hemodynamic and renal effects of dopexamine and dobutamine in patients with reduced cardiac output following coronary artery bypass grafting. *Chest* 1994; **106**: 835–41.

20. Berendes E, Mollhoff T, Van Aken H, *et al.* Effects of dopexamine on creatinine clearance, systemic inflammation, and splanchnic oxygenation in patients undergoing coronary artery bypass grafting. *Anesth Analg* 1997; **84**: 950–7.

21. Binkley PF, Van Fossen DB, Nunziata E, *et al.* Influence of positive inotropic therapy on pulsatile hydraulic load and ventricular-vascular coupling in congestive heart failure. *J Am Coll Cardiol* 1990; **15**: 1127–35.

22. Keren G, Laniado S, Sonnenblick EH, *et al.* Dynamics of functional mitral regurgitation during dobutamine therapy in patients with severe congestive heart failure: a Doppler echocardiograhic study. *Am Heart J* 1989; **118**: 748–54.

23. Aronson S, Dupont F, Savage R, *et al.* Changes in regional myocardial function after coronary artery bypass are predicted by intraoperative low-dose dobutamine echocardiography. *Anesthesiology* 2000; **93**: 685–92.

24. Abraham WT, Adams KF, Fonarow GC, *et al.* In-hospital mortality in patients with acute decompensated heart failure requiring intravenous vasoactive medications: an analysis from the Acute Decompensated Heart Failure National Registry (ADHERE). *J Am Coll Cardiol* 2005; **46**: 57–64.

25. Follath F, Cleland JG, Just H, *et al.* Efficacy and safety of intravenous levosimendan compared to dobutamine in severe low-output heart failure (the LIDO study): a randomised double blind trial. *Lancet* 2002; **360**: 196–202.

26. Tinker JH, Tarhan S, White RD, *et al.* Dobutamine for inotropic support during emergence from cardiopulmonary bypass. *Anesthesiology* 1976; **44**: 281–6.

27. Movsesian MA, Smith CJ, Krall J, *et al.* Sarcoplasmic reticulum-associated cyclic adenosine 5′-monophosphate phosphodiesterase activity in normal and failing human hearts. *J Clin Invest* 1991; **88**: 15–19.

28. Kajimoto K, Hagiwara N, Kasanuki H, *et al.* Contribution of phosphodiesterase isozymes to the regulation of L-type calcium current in human cardiac myocytes. *Br J Pharmacol* 1997; **121**: 1549–56.

29. Koss KL, Kranias EG. Phospholamban: a prominent regulator of myocardial contractility. *Circ Res* 1996; **79**: 1059–63.

30. Doolan LA, Jones EF, Kalman J, *et al.* A placebo-controlled trial verifying the efficacy of milrinone in weaning high-risk patients from cardiopulmonary bypass. *J Cardiothorac Vasc Anesth* 1997; **11**: 37–41.

31. Chen EP, Bittner HB, Davis RD, *et al.* Hemodynamic and inotropic effects of milrinone after heart transplantation in the setting of recipient pulmonary hypertension. *J Heart Lung Transplant* 1998; **17**: 669–78.

32. Konstam MA, Cody RJ. Short-term use of intravenous milrinone for heart failure. *Am J Cardiol* 1995; **75**: 822–6.

33. Tisdale JE, Patel R, Webb CR, *et al.* Electrophysiologic and proarrhythmic effects of intravenous inotropic agents. *Prog Cardiovasc Dis* 1995; **38**: 167–80.

34. Hayashida N, Tomoeda H, Oda T, *et al.* Inhibitory effect of milrinone on cytokine production after cardiopulmonary bypass. *Ann Thorac Surg* 1999; **68**: 1661–7.

35. Cracowski JL, Stanke-Labesque F, Chavanon O, *et al.* Vasorelaxant actions of enoximone, dobutamine, and the combination on human arterial coronary bypass grafts. *J Cardiovasc Pharmacol* 1999; **34**: 741–8.

36. Packer M, Carver JR, Rodeheffer RJ, *et al.* Effect of oral milrinone on mortality in severe chronic heart failure. The PROMISE Study Research Group. *N Engl J Med* 1991; **325**: 1468–75.

37. Lowes BD, Higginbotham M, Petrovich L, *et al.* Low dose enoximone improves exercise capacity in chronic heart failure. Enoximone Study Group. *J Am Coll Cardiol* 2000; **36**: 501–8.

38. Shakar SF, Abraham WT, Gilbert EM, *et al.* Combined oral positive inotropic and beta-blocker therapy for the treatment of refractory Class IV heart failure. *J Am Coll Cardiol* 1998; **31**: 1336–40.

39. Kikura M, Lee MK, Safon RA, *et al.* The effects of milrinone on platelets in patients undergoing cardiac surgery. *Anesth Analg* 1995; **81**: 44–8.

40. Rathmell JP, Prielipp RC, Butterworth JF, *et al.* A multicenter, randomized, blind comparison of amrinone and milrinone after elective cardiac surgery. *Anesth Analg* 1998; **86**: 683–90.

41. Feneck RO. Intravenous milrinone following cardiac surgery: II. Influence of baseline hemodynamics and patient factors on therapeutic response. The European Milrinone Multicentre Trial Group. *J Cardiothorac Vasc Anesth* 1992; **6**: 563–7.

42. Butterworth JF, Hines RL, Royster RL, *et al.* A pharmacokinetic and pharmacodynamic evaluation of milrinone in adults undergoing cardiac surgery. *Anesth Analg* 1995; **81**: 783–92.

43. Prielipp RC, MacGregor DA, Butterworth JF, *et al.* Pharmacodynamics and pharmacokinetics of milrinone administration to increase oxygen delivery in critically ill patients. *Chest* 1996; **109**: 1291–301.

44. Dupuis JY, Bondy R, Cattran C, *et al.* Amrinone and dobutamine as primary treatment of low cardiac output syndrome following coronary artery surgery: a comparison of their effects on hemodynamics and outcome. *J Cardiothorac Vasc Anesth* 1992; **6**: 542–53.

45. Butterworth JF, Royster RL, Prielipp RC, *et al.* Amrinone in cardiac surgical patients with left-ventricular dysfunction: a prospective, randomized placebo-controlled trial. *Chest* 1993; **104**: 1660–7.

46. Royster RL, Butterworth JF, Prielipp RC, *et al.* Combined inotropic effects of amrinone and epinephrine after cardiopulmonary bypass in humans. *Anesth Analg* 1993; **77**: 662–72.

47. Tachibana H, Cheng HJ, Ukai T, *et al.* Levosimendan improves LV systolic and diastolic performance at rest and during exercise after heart failure. *Am J Physiol Heart Circ Physiol* 2005; **288**: H914–22.

48. Scoote M, Williams AJ. Myocardial calcium signaling and arrhythmia pathogenesis. *Biochem Biophys Res Comm* 2004; **322**: 1286–9.

49. Nieminen MS, Bohm M, Cowie MR, *et al.* Executive summary of the guidelines on the diagnosis and treatment of acute heart failure. The Task Force on Acute Heart Failure of the European Society of Cardiology. *Eur Heart J* 2005; **26**: 384–416.

50. Haikala H, Kaivola J, Nissinen E, *et al.* Cardiac troponin C as a target for a novel calcium sensitzing drug, levosimendan. *J Mol Cell Cardiol* 1995; **27**: 1859–66.

51. Haikala H, Levijoki J, Linden IB. Troponin C-mediated calcium sensitization by levosimendan accelerates the proportional

development of isometric tension. *J Mol Cell Cardiol* 1995; **27**: 2155–65.

52. Masutani S, Cheng HJ, Hytilla-Hopponen M, *et al.* Orally available levosimendan dose-related positive inotropic and lusitropic effect in conscious chronically instrumented normal and heart failure dogs. *J Pharmacol Exp Ther* 2008; **325**: 236–47.

53. Soei LK, Sassen LMA, Fan DS, *et al.* Myofibrillar Ca^{2+} sensitization predominantly enhances function and mechanical efficiency of stunned myocardium. *Circulation* 1994; **90**: 959–69.

54. Haikala H, Nissinen E, Etemadzadeh E, *et al.* Troponin C-mediated calcium sensitization induced by levosimendan does not impair relaxation. *J Cardiovasc Pharmacol* 1995; **25**: 794–801.

55. Givertz MM, Andreou C, Conrad CH, *et al.* Direct myocardial effects of levosimendan in humans with left ventricular dysfunction: alteration of force-frequency and relaxation-frequency relationships. *Circulation* 2007; **115**: 1218–24.

56. Dernillis J, Panaretou M. Effects of levosimendan on restrictive left ventricular filling in severe heart failure: a combined hemodynamic and Doppler echocardiographic study. *Chest* 2005; **128**: 2633–9.

57. Pataricza J, Krassoi I, Hohn J, *et al.* Functional role of potassium channels in the vasodilating mechanism of levosimendan in porcine isolated coronary artery. *Cardiovasc Drugs Ther* 2003; **17**: 115–21.

58. Bowman P, Haikala H, Paul RJ. Levosimendan, a calcium sensitizer in cardiac muscle, induces relaxation in coronary smooth muscle through calcium desensitization. *J Pharmacol Exp Ther* **288**:316–325, 1999.

59. Haikala H, Linden IB. Mechanisms of action of calcium-sensitizing drugs. *J Cardiovasc Pharmacol* 1995; **26**: S10–S19.

60. Yokoshiki H, Katsube Y, Sunagawa M, *et al.* The novel calcium sensitizer levosimendan activates the ATP-sensitive K^{+} channel in rat ventricular cells. *J Pharmacol Exp Ther* 1997; **283**: 375–83.

61. Kopustinskiene DM, Pollesello P, Saris NE. Levosimendan is a mitochondrial KATP channel opener. *Eur J Pharmacol* 2001; **428**: 311–14.

62. Kersten JR, Montgomery MW, Pagel PS, *et al.* Levosimendan, a positive inotropic agent, decreases myocardial infarct size via activation of K$_{ATP}$ channels. *Anesth Analg* 2000; **90**: 5–11.

63. Sonntag S, Sundberg S, Lehtonen LA, *et al.* The calcium sensitizer levosimendan improves the function of stunned myocardium after percutaneous transluminal coronary angioplasty in acute myocardial infarction. *J Am Coll Cardiol* 2004; **43**: 2177–82.

64. Garcia-Gonzalez MJ, Dominguez-Rodriguez A, Ferrer-Hita JJ. Utility of levosimendan, a new calcium sensitizing agent, in the treatment of cardiogenic shock due to myocardial stunning in patients with ST-elevation myocardial infarction: a series of cases. *J Clin Pharmacol* 2005; **45**: 704–8.

65. Tritapepe L, De Santis V, Vitale D, *et al.* Preconditioning effects of levosimendan in coronary artery bypass grafting – a pilot study. *Br J Anaesth* 2006; **96**: 694–700.

66. Remme WJ, Wiesfeld ACP, Look MP, *et al.* Hemodynamic effects of intravenous pimobendan in patients with left ventricular dysfunction. *J Cardiovasc Pharmacol* 1989; **14**: S41–S44.

67. Thormann J, Kramer W, Schlepper M. Hemodynamic and myocardial energetic changes induced by the new cardiotonic agent, AR-L 115, in patients with coronary artery disease. *Am Heart J* 1982; **104**: 1294–302.

68. Todaka K, Wang J, Yi GH, *et al.* Effects of levosimendan on myocardial contractility and oxygen consumption. *J Pharmacol Exp Ther* 1996; **279**: 120–7.

69. Kubo SH, Gollub S, Bourge R, *et al.* Beneficial effects of pimobendan on exercise tolerance and quality of life in patients with heart failure. Results of a multicenter trial. The Pimobendan Multicenter Research Group. *Circulation* 1992; **85**: 942–9.

70. Lubsen J, Just H, Hjalmarsson AC, *et al.* Effect of pimobendan on exercise capacity in patients with heart failure: main results from the Pimobendan in Congestive Heart Failure (PICO) trial. *Heart* 1996; **76**: 223–31.

71. Nieminen MS, Akkila J, Hasenfuss G, *et al.* Hemodynamic and neurohormonal effects of continuous infusion of levosimendan in patients with congestive heart failure. *J Am Coll Cardiol* 2000; **36**: 1903–12.

72. Slawsky MT, Colucci WS, Gottlieb SS, *et al.* Acute hemodynamic and clinical effects of levosimendan in patients with severe heart failure. *Circulation* 2000; **102**: 2222–7.

73. Moiseyev VS, Poder P, Andrejevs N, *et al.* Safety and efficacy of a novel calcium sensitizer, levosimendan, in patients with left ventricular failure due to an acute myocardial infarction. A randomized, placebo-controlled, double-blind study (RUSSLAN). *Eur Heart J* 2002; **23**: 1422–32.

74. Cuffe MS, Califf RM, Adams KF, *et al.* Short-term intravenous milrinone for acute exacerbation of chronic heart failure: a controlled randomized clinical trial. Outcomes of a Prospective Trial of Intravenous Milrinone for Exacerbations of Chronic Heart Failure (OPTIME-CHF) Investigators. *JAMA* 2002; **287**: 1578–80.

75. Garcia-Gonzalez MJ, Dominguez-Rodriguez A, Ferrer-Hita JJ, *et al.* Cardiogenic shock after percutaneous coronary intervention: effects of levosimendan compared with dobutamine on haemodynamics. *Eur J Heart Fail* 2006; **8**: 723–8.

76. Adamopoulos S, Parissis JT, Iliodromitis EK, *et al.* Effects of levosimendan versus dobutamine on inflammatory and apoptotic pathways in acutely decompensated chronic heart failure. *Am J Cardiol* 2006; **98**: 102–6.

77. Lilleberg J, Nieminen MS, Akkila J, *et al.* Effects of a new calcium sensitizer, levosimendan, on haemodynamics, coronary blood flow and myocardial substrate utilization early after coronary artery bypass grafting. *Eur Heart J* 1998; **19**: 660–8.

78. Labriola C, Siro-Brigiani M, Carrata F, *et al.* Hemodynamic effects of

levosimendan in patients with low-output heart failure after cardiac surgery. *Int J Clin Pharmacol Ther* 2004; **42**: 204–11.

79. Siirila-Waris K, Suojaranta-Ylinen R, Harjola VP. Levosimendan in cardiac surgery. *J Cardiothorac Vasc Anesth* 2005; **19**: 345–9.

80. Barisin S, Husedzinovic I, Sonicki Z, *et al.* Levosimendan in off-pump coronary artery bypass: a four-times masked controlled study. *J Cardiovasc Pharmacol* 2004; **44**: 703–8.

81. De Hert SG, Lorsomradee S, Cromheecke S, *et al.* Effects of levosimendan in cardiac surgery patients with poor left ventricular function. *Anesth Analg* 2007; **104**: 766–73.

82. Kivikko M, Lehtonen L, Colucci WS. Sustained hemodynamic effects of intravenous levosimendan. *Circulation* 2003; **107**: 81–6.

83. Hamilton MA. Prevalence and clinical implications of abnormal thyroid hormone metabolism in advanced heart failure. *Ann Thorac Surg* 1993; **56**: S48–S52.

84. Jamali IN, Pagel PS, Hettrick DA, *et al.* Positive inotropic and lusitropic effects of triiodothyronine in conscious dogs with pacing-induced cardiomyopathy. *Anesthesiology* 1997; **87**: 102–9.

85. Han J, Leem C, So I, *et al.* Effects of thyroid hormone on the calcium current and isoprenaline-induced background current in rabbit ventricular myocytes. *J Mol Cell Cardiol* 1994; **26**: 925–35.

86. Ririe DG, Butterworth JF, Royster RL, *et al.* Triiodothyronine increases contractility independent of beta-adrenergic receptors or stimulation of cyclic-3',5'-adenosine monophosphate. *Anesthesiology* 1995; **82**: 1004–12.

87. Kadletz M, Mullen PG, Ding M, *et al.* Effect of triiodothyronine on postishemic myocardial function in the isolated heart. *Ann Thorac Surg* 1994; **57**: 657–62.

88. Mahaffey KW, Raya TE, Pennock GD, *et al.* Left ventricular performance and remodeling in rabbits after myocardial infarction. Effects of a thyroid hormone analogue. *Circulation* 1995; **91**: 794–801.

89. Moruzzi P, Doria E, Agostoni PG, *et al.* Usefulness of L-thyroxine to improve cardiac and exercise performance in idiopathic dilated cardiomyopathy. *Am J Cardiol* 1994; **73**: 374–8.

90. Chu SH, Huang TS, Hsu RB, *et al.* Thyroid hormone changes after cardiovascular surgery and clinical implications. *Ann Thorac Surg* 1991; **52**: 791–6.

91. Novitzky D, Cooper DK, Human PA, *et al.* Triiodothyronine therapy for heart donor and recipient. *J Heart Transplant* 1988; **7**: 370–6.

92. Dyke CM, Ding M, Abd-Elfattah AS, *et al.* Effects of triiodothyronine supplementation after myocardial ischemia. *Ann Thorac Surg* 1993; **56**: 215–22.

93. Bennett-Guerrero E, Jimenez JL, White WD, *et al.* Cardiovascular effects of intravenous triiodothyronine in patients undergoing coronary artery bypass graft surgery: a randomized, double-blind, placebo-controlled trial. Duke T_3 study group. *JAMA* 1996; **275**: 687–92.

94. Prielipp RC, MacGregor DA, Royster RL, *et al.* Dobutamine antagonizes epinephrine's biochemical and cardiotonic effects: results of an in vitro model using human lymphocytes and a clinical study in patients recovering from cardiac surgery. *Anesthesiology* 1998; **89**: 49–57.

95. Abernethy WB, Butterworth JF, Prielipp RC, *et al.* Calcium entry attenuates adenylyl cyclase activity: a possible mechanism for calcium-induced catecholamine resistance. *Chest* 1995; **107**: 1420–5.

96. McGough MF, Pagel PS, Lowe D, *et al.* Levosimendan potentiates the inotropic actions of dopamine in conscious dogs. *J Cardiovasc Pharmacol* 1996; **28**: 36–47.

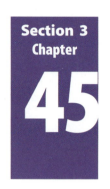

Section 3
Chapter

45

Essential drugs in anesthetic practice
Vasodilators

Roger A. Johns and Stephen Yang

Introduction

The ability to decrease vascular smooth-muscle tone and relax blood vessels is critical to many aspects of the practice of anesthesiology. In addition to controlling inappropriate hypertension, which can increase risk of stroke or cardiac ischemia, the anesthesiologist often needs to manipulate afterload and preload to improve cardiac function. In certain situations, it may be necessary to lower blood pressure below normal, such as while clipping a cerebral aneurysm or cannulating the aorta to initiate cardiopulmonary bypass. An anesthesiologist may also induce hypotension deliberately to minimize bleeding in a particular vascular bed to improve the surgical field. Thus, knowledge of the mechanisms of blood vessel contraction and relaxation, the potential sites for pharmacologic intervention, and the mechanisms and application of available drugs is essential.

Blood vessels control the flow of blood to downstream organs and its return to the heart by contracting and relaxing the surrounding vascular smooth-muscle layer. This process is critical to ensuring the delivery of oxygen and nutrients to tissues and removal of carbon dioxide and waste products. Chapter 19 discusses the physiology of blood vessels and control of vascular tone in detail. Vessel tone is determined by multiple mechanisms, including endogenous myogenic tone, neural innervation, and mediators delivered from circulating blood or released from the endothelium or the smooth muscle itself. The specific nature of these mechanisms can vary in arterial and venous circulation, depending on vessel size, and in specific organ tissue beds. To rationally approach the pharmacologic manipulation of vascular tone, an understanding of the mechanisms of vascular smooth-muscle contraction and the multiple and complex factors that modulate it is necessary.

In this chapter, we will briefly review the physiology of the vasculature, the mechanisms of vascular smooth muscle contraction, and the factors that modulate it. This will provide the basis for understanding the mechanisms of action for different vasodilator drugs. We will review the pharmacology of the different classes of vasodilators and discuss their administration in clinical practice.

Mechanisms of drug action: regulation of vascular tone and molecular basis for drug action

As described in Chapter 19, the regulation of myofilament interaction and vascular smooth-muscle contraction and tone is primarily dependent on the availability and concentration of calcium (Ca^{2+}) in the cell and regulation of the myofilaments via phosphorylation and dephosphorylation. Most vasodilator drugs ultimately act through regulation of the intracellular calcium concentration ($[Ca^{2+}]_i$), by targeting either electromechanical coupling or pharmacomechanical coupling (Fig. 45.1), or through activation of kinases.

Physiology of muscle contraction

The contractile machinery of vascular smooth muscle is composed of three elements: myosin (thick filaments), actin (thin filaments), and the regulatory proteins. Myosin is a hexamer composed of two heavy chains and two pairs of light chains (20 and 17 kDa). Actin that is involved in the contractile process is known as α-actin. The myosin and actin filaments are arranged in a diagonal pattern along the long axis of the cell; the α-actin is connected to the cytoskeleton at the dense bodies and to the cell membrane at dense plaques [2]. During contraction, the actin filaments slide along the myosin, resulting in cell shortening. This is an active process that translates chemical energy stored as adenosine triphosphate (ATP) to mechanical force. The pivotal event in smooth-muscle contraction is the increase in $[Ca^{2+}]_i$. The two major sources of Ca^{2+} are the extracellular space and the sarcoplasmic reticulum (SR). Extracellular Ca^{2+} enters the cell through voltage-gated Ca^{2+} channels (VGCC) [3]. These channels are activated by depolarization of the membrane and inactivated by repolarization and hyperpolarization. Two types of VGCC have been isolated in smooth muscle: L-type and T-type. The T-type channel has not been well described, but it is transient in nature and may be related to physically contracting smooth

Anesthetic Pharmacology, 2nd edition, ed. Alex S. Evers, Mervyn Maze, Evan D. Kharasch. Published by Cambridge University Press. © Cambridge University Press 2011.

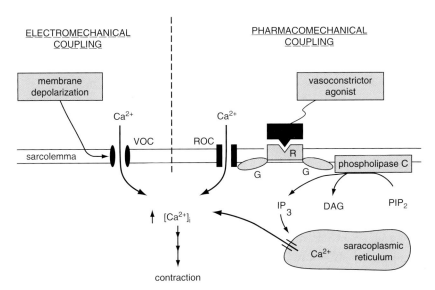

ELECTROMECHANICAL
COUPLING

PHARMACOMECHANICAL
COUPLING

Figure 45.1. Mechanisms increasing intracellular calcium ($[Ca^{2+}]_i$) in vascular smooth muscle. An increase in $[Ca^{2+}]_i$ is a critical signal in activating myosin light-chain kinase and initiating contraction of vascular smooth muscle. Ca^{2+} enters the cell through two categories of channels, voltage-operated channels (VOCs) and receptor-operated channels (ROCs). Neuronal influence leading to membrane depolarization opens VOCs and is termed electomechanical coupling. In contrast, pharmacomechanical coupling occurs at ROCs when a vaso-constrictor agonist binds to a receptor leading to extracellular Ca^{2+} entry via a ROC. Receptor coupling can also occur through activation of phospholipase C, which cleaves membrane phosphatidylinositol 4,5-bisphosphate (PIP$_2$) into diacyl-glycerol (DAG) and inositol 3-phosphate (IP$_3$). IP$_3$ initiates release of Ca^{2+} from the sarcoplasmic reticulum. Reproduced with permission from Mohrman and Heller [1].

muscle [3]. The L-type (found in vascular smooth muscle) has been extensively characterized. Its activity is enhanced by phosphorylation and is inhibited by $[Ca^{2+}]_i$ [3].

Calcium is sequestered intracellularly in the SR, which serves as the major source of Ca^{2+} that participates in muscle contraction. Ca^{2+} is released from the SR by two mechanisms. Vasoconstrictor agonists combine with receptors in the cell membrane and activate phospholipase C (PLC) through a G protein. PLC, in turn, hydrolyzes phosphatidylinositol 4,5-bisphosphate (PIP$_2$) to inositol 1,4,5-trisphosphate (IP$_3$) and diacylglycerol (DAG). The increased IP$_3$ concentration results in the activation of IP$_3$-mediated channels in the SR, which allow for the release of the sequestered Ca^{2+}. Ca^{2+} is also released from the SR in response to an increase in $[Ca^{2+}]_i$ through Ca^{2+}-dependent channels known as ryanodine receptors [4].

The increase in $[Ca^{2+}]_i$ is closely regulated through two pathways that can decrease $[Ca^{2+}]_i$: the extrusion of Ca^{2+} from the cytoplasm to the extracellular space and the resequestration of Ca^{2+} into the SR. The extrusion of Ca^{2+} is accomplished via two calcium pumps located in the cell membrane: the sodium (Na^+)/Ca^{2+} exchanger and the Ca^{2+} ATPase pump [2,3] eliminate Ca^{2+} from the cytoplasm in exchange for Na^+ and hydrogen (H^+) ions, respectively. Ca^{2+} ATPase (located in the SR membrane) activity sequesters Ca^{2+} into the SR; phospholamban is a likely regulatory protein in this process. In its unphosphorylated state, phospholamban diminishes the Ca^{2+} ATPase activity by decreasing the pump's affinity for Ca^{2+}. However, phosphorylated phospholamban dissociates from the enzyme, and the activity of the pump increases such that Ca^{2+} reuptake into the SR is enhanced. Phosphorylation of phospholamban is mediated by the activity of cyclic guanosine monophosphate (cGMP)-dependent and cyclic adenosine monophosphate (cAMP)-dependent protein kinases.

Vasodilator substances that increase cGMP (nitric oxide, atrial natriuretic peptides) or cAMP (isoproterenol, eicosanoids, catecholamines) may cause vasodilation by phosphorylating phospholamban and thus promoting the increased uptake of Ca^{2+} into the SR [5].

Troponin is not associated with smooth muscle as it is in striated muscle; rather, four Ca^{2+} ions bind to the regulatory protein calmodulin. The Ca^{2+}/calmodulin complex then binds to myosin light-chain kinase (MLCK). MLCK is a specific protein kinase that consists of a catalytic domain, a calmodulin-binding site, a putative autoinhibitory site, an actin-binding site, substrate (myosin and ATP) binding sites, and sites for phosphorylation by other protein kinases [6]. The phosphorylation sites on MLCK provide for regulation of its activity; for example, the affinity of the Ca^{2+}/calmodulin complex for MLCK is decreased by phosphorylation of its binding site. This mechanism is one by which some vasodilator drugs cause muscle relaxation (see below). Activated MLCK phosphorylates the regulatory myosin light chain at serine 19. This phosphorylation promotes the polymerization of myosin into filaments, which spontaneously bind to actin by the formation of crossbridges. The cleavage of ATP produces the energy necessary for myosin's lever action. As a result, actin slides across the myosin and causes contraction of the smooth-muscle cell. In addition to promoting myosin polymerization, phosphorylation of the regulatory light chain at serine 19 also increases the ATPase activity of the myosin heads 100-fold [7]. The mechanism by which this occurs is unclear, but it is known that two myosin heads are necessary. In in-vitro experiments, the phosphorylation of a single-headed myosin molecule is not associated with an increase in ATPase activity [8].

Phosphorylation of the regulatory light chain is a major regulatory point in vascular smooth-muscle contraction. Although the major pathway for this phosphorylation depends on free Ca^{2+}, calcium-independent pathways also exist. Guanosine triphosphate (GTP)-binding proteins can activate Rho-associated kinase (ROK) [9] and p21-activated kinase [10]. Both of these kinases are able to phosphorylate the serine 19 in the regulatory light chain, although the significance of these pathways is not clear. ROK inhibitors have been shown to decrease blood pressure [11].

Vascular smooth muscle can sustain contraction for long periods independent of the initial stimulus. That is, the contraction can be maintained despite the $[Ca^{2+}]_i$ or myosin light chain phosphorylation returning toward baseline levels [12]. One possible explanation has been termed the *latch hypothesis*. In this scenario, the regulatory light chains are phosphorylated by MLCK in response to increased $[Ca^{2+}]_i$. After the formation of the crossbridges and lever action, the myosin associates with adenosine diphosphate (ADP) and inorganic phosphorus (Pi) (MYO-ADP-Pi). Dephosphorylation of the crossbridge results in MYO-ADP; this moiety has a high affinity for actin and forms a kind of "latch." Once the latch is created, the cycling rate of the crossbridges becomes low, resulting in a prolonged contractile state [13].

Control of the contractile state
The force generated by the smooth muscle is not directly related to the $[Ca^{2+}]_i$ [4]. Several factors influence the force of contraction in response to an increase in $[Ca^{2+}]_i$. The common pathway is the activation of myosin light-chain phosphatase (MLCP). This enzyme dephosphorylates the regulatory light chains, thus decreasing the ATPase activity and lever action of the myosin heads and, ultimately, contraction. The end result is the regulation of the contractile mechanism. Several intermediaries regulate MLCP. Of particular interest is the activation of MLCP by a cGMP-dependent kinase. This enzyme promotes dephosphorylation of the regulatory light chains and decreases the contractile state [14]. MLCP is also inhibited by other kinases that promote vasoconstriction; among those are ROK and members of the protein kinase C family [3]. Inhibition of MLCP by these enzymes may be part of the cascade that maintains the prolonged contractile state that is observed.

Smooth-muscle contraction also is controlled through the activity of other regulatory proteins. One such protein is caldesmon, which is associated with the thin filaments. It has binding sites for actin, tropomyosin (a component of the thin filament), myosin, and the Ca^{2+}/calmodulin complex. In the presence of tropomyosin, caldesmon regulates the myosin-actin interaction by inhibiting the ATPase activity of the myosin head, resulting in decreased contraction [3,15]. This activity is promoted by the presence of tropomyosin and is inhibited in the presence of the Ca^{2+}/calmodulin complex.

Myogenic tone
Changes in vascular tone and diameter in response to flow is a physiologic response critical to pressure–flow autoregulation. The process by which an increase in blood in arteriolar constriction occurs as a result of an increase in intraluminal pressure (myogenic tone) dates back to 1902 when Bayliss first observed that an increase in blood flow caused a reduction in descending pressure acting on the vascular wall [16]. As pressure increases in a blood vessel, the vascular smooth muscle contracts, limiting flow. Vascular beds use this autoregulatory mechanism to keep flow relatively constant over a varying pressure range. Comparison can be made to the Frank–Starling response in cardiac muscle, in which volume stretch causes myocytes to contract, a process that involves calcium and active interaction of the actin–myosin filaments [17–18]. Although not fully understood, potential mechanisms of this response are discussed in detail in Chapter 19.

Neuronal regulation of vascular tone and electromechanical coupling
The sympathetic nervous system is the predominant neural regulator of blood vessels. Norepinephrine released from sympathetic nerves stimulates α_1-adrenoceptors in the neuroeffector junction, leading to calcium entry via receptor-operated Ca^{2+} channels. Vasoconstriction is enhanced synergistically by the simultaneous release of ATP and neuropeptide Y (Fig. 45.2) [20,21]. Molecular and electrophysiologic evidence suggests that the α_{1B}-adrenoceptor is the predominant adrenoceptor at the neuroeffector junction [22]. The α_{1A}-adrenoceptor is located outside of the neuroeffector junction and responds to circulating epinephrine and norepinephrine [21,23].

Parasympathetic nerves may induce vasodilation through release of acetylcholine (ACh) and vasoactive intestinal polypeptide (VIP). In some vascular beds, nonadrenergic, noncholinergic (NANC) neurons mediate vasodilation through the release of the vasodilator nitric oxide (NO) [22,23].

Vasoactive molecule mediators of vascular tone and pharmacomechanical coupling
Vasoactive molecules that constrict or dilate blood vessels can come from within the vascular smooth muscle itself (autocrine factors), from the endothelium (paracrine factors), or from the circulating blood (hormonal) (Fig. 45.3). Vasodilator drugs generally act on membrane receptors that lead to changes in $[Ca^{2+}]_i$ via receptor-operated channels (Fig. 45.1).

β-Adrenoceptors on smooth muscle couple via G-protein-type receptors to adenylate cyclase, which catalyzes the formation of cAMP from ATP; in turn, the cAMP activates cAMP-dependent protein kinases (PKA) [23]. Similarly, atrial natriutetic peptides couple to membrane guanylate cyclase [24], and NO [25] activates soluble guanylate cyclase, which converts GTP to cGMP to activate cGMP-dependent protein kinases (PKG). These kinases reduce Ca^{2+} availability by enhancing its movement out of the cell or into the SR. They can also affect the phosphorylation of cytoskeleton elements important to contraction (see above).

Angiotensin II is a mediator of vascular tone that is produced from angiotensin I via angiotensin-converting enzyme (ACE). It

Sympathetic Neuroeffector Mechanisms

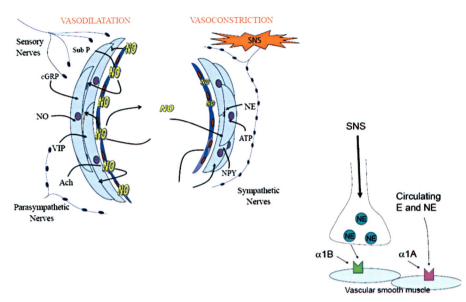

Figure 45.2. Neuronal influences on vasodilation and vasoconstriction of blood vessels. Efferent noradrenergic nerves release norepinephrine (NE) and other neuroeffectors such as neuropeptide Y (NPY) and adenosine triphosphate (ATP) which activate α_{1B}-adrenoceptors on the vascular smooth muscle at the neuroeffector junction. Circulating epinephrine (E) and NE activate α_{1A}-adrenoceptors on the vascular smooth muscle as well. Parasympathetic nerves also release neurotransmitters (e.g., acetylcholine, ACh) and vasoactive intestinal polypeptide (VIP) which can stimulate nitric oxide (NO) production leading to vasodilation. On some vessels, nonadrenergic, noncholinergic (NANC) nerve innervation directly releases NO to the vessel wall. Sensory nerves can dilate cutaneous vessels through release of neurotransmitters such as substance P (Sub P). SNS, sympathetic nervous system. Adapted with permission from Kan and Berkowitz [19].

causes vasoconstriction by acting on angiotensin-specific receptors that couple to receptor-operated Ca^{2+} channels to allow entry of Ca^{2+} into vascular smooth-muscle cells [26,27]. Similarly, endothelin [28–30], a peptide produced in the vessel wall and by circulating monocytes, can act on endothelin receptors A and B (ET_A and ET_B). Endothelin induces vessel constriction when it binds to receptors located on the smooth-muscle cell membrane. However, it can also act on ET_A receptors on the endothelium, causing production and release of NO, which activates a soluble guanylate cyclase and, as described above, leads to cGMP formation, PKG activation, and ultimately vasodilation. Influence of the endothelium on vascular tone is extremely important in vascular regulation and clinical pharmacology of vasodilators.

Importance of the endothelium in vasoactive mediator responses

Once thought to be a passive lining of blood vessels to facilitate blood flow and prevent platelet activation, over the past 25 years the endothelium has come to be recognized as a complex tissue. It has multiple functions, from mediating inflammatory responses to controlling vascular permeability, and is a critical regulator of vascular smooth-muscle tone. In addition to vasoconstrictors such as endothelin, the endothelium produces two critical vasodilators. One is prostacyclin (PGI_2), which is produced in the endothelium and acts on the smooth muscle via a

PGI_2 receptor linked to adenylate cyclase [31]. As described above, activation of adenylate cyclase catalyzes the production of cAMP from ATP. Of note, PGI_2 was the first recognized endothelium-dependent vasodilator, discovered by Moncada and Vane in 1976 [32].

The other major endothelium-dependent vasodilator is nitric oxide. The endothelium received its greatest recognition as a mediator of vasodilation in 1980, when, in a now classic experiment, Furchgott and Zawadski discovered that application of ACh caused release of an "endothelium-dependent relaxing factor (EDRF)" from the endothelium [33]. For years the vascular responses to ACh had been a puzzle to physiologists – sometimes it would cause profound vasodilation and at other times vasoconstriction. The answer was in the endothelium. These investigators took a piece of blood vessel with endothelium intact, sandwiched it against another strip of blood vessel with its endothelium removed, and mounted it to record isometric tension. When the intact "donor" vessel was sandwiched against the endothelium-denuded vessel, addition of ACh caused vasodilation; if the donor vessel with endothelium was removed, ACh caused vasoconstriction. Clearly, an endothelial-derived relaxing factor was responsible. "EDRF" was subsequently found to be NO [33]. Intensive investigation over the next two decades revealed the molecular mechanisms for the production, regulation, and actions of NO as a novel cell signaling molecule

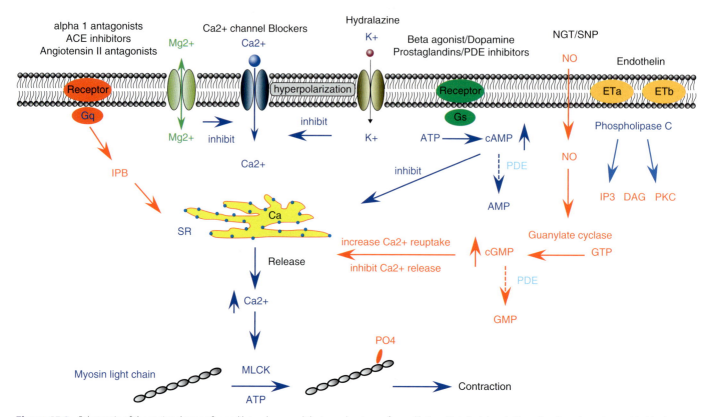

Figure 45.3. Schematic of the major classes of vasodilator drugs and their mechanisms of vasodilation. Detailed description of each pathway is provided in the text. AMP adenosine monophosphate; ATP, adenosine triphosphate; Ca^{2+}, calcium; cAMP, cyclic adenosine monophosphate; cGMP, cyclic guanosine monophosphate; DAG, diacylglycerol; ETa, endothelin receptor A; ETb, endothelin receptor B; G_q, q-type G protein; Gs, s-type G protein; GMP, guanosine monophosphate; GTP, guanosine triphosphate; IP_3, inositol trisphosphate; K^+, potassium; Mg^{2+}, magnesium; MLCK, myosin light-chain kinase; NTG, nitroglycerin; PDE, phosphodiesterase; PKC, protein kinase C; SNP, sodium nitroprusside; SR, sarcoplasmic reticulum.

(Fig. 45.4). NO is produced from L-arginine and oxygen in endothelium by endothelial NO synthase (eNOS) or inducible NO synthase (iNOS). (A third isoform, neuronal NO synthase (nNOS) is primarily localized in neural tissue.) The NO then diffuses to the vascular smooth muscle, where it binds to the heme moieties of the heterodimers of gunaylate cyclase and catalyzes the production of cGMP from GTP. In addition to the substrates L-arginine and oxygen, NOS requires calcium and tetrahydrobiopterin (BH4) as cofactors to produce NO. Regulation of arginine availability through specific arginase activity and amino acid transporters can impact NOS activity, as can availability of BH4 [34,35]. In fact, in the absence of BH4, NOS does not properly form its homodimer state and can produce damaging peroxynitrite and secondary free radicals rather than NO. Many known vascular smooth-muscle constrictors, such as adrenergic agonists and endothelin, modulate their direct contractile action on the vascular smooth muscle through simultaneous stimulation of NO production from the endothelium. Endothelial NOS can be activated by shear stress or by receptor agonists such as ACh and bradykinin. This activation causes the release of NOS from caveolae, which markedly enhances

its production of NO. iNOS is not normally present in the vasculature, but it can be induced in the endothelium or vascular smooth muscle during inflammatory processes such as sepsis or with prolonged hypoxia.

Clinical pharmacology

Nitrovasodilators

Nitrovasodilators have long been used to produce vasodilation [35], since well before it was understood that NO is an endogenous vasodilator. They release NO, which activates guanylate cyclase in the same manner as endogenous NO. NO relaxes vascular smooth muscle through both cGMP-dependent and cGMP-independent mechanisms. As noted above, NO activates guanylate cyclase to produce cGMP, which activates PKG. PKG activates MLCP, causing dephosphorylation of myosin light chains and vascular relaxation [32–34,36].

NO also activates sarco/endoplasmic reticulum Ca^{2+} ATPase (SERCA), which resides within the SR and refills intracellular Ca^{2+} stores [36]. Consequently, store-operated

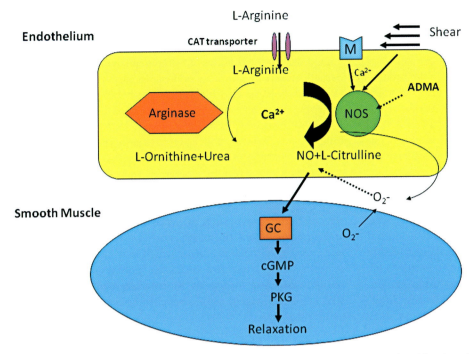

Figure 45.4. Schematic of endothelium-dependent vasodilation by nitric oxide. NO is produced from L-arginine and two molecules of oxygen (O_2^-) by the enzyme NO synthase (NOS). Activation of NOS requires binding of Ca^{2+}/calmodulin in the presence of the cofactor tetrahydrobiopterin (BH4). $[Ca^{2+}]_i$ increases in response to activation of a receptor such as the muscarinic receptor (M) or shear stress. The availability of L-arginine can be rate-limiting, and L-arginine entry to the cell is regulated by cationic amino acid (CAT) transporters and by active arginine metabolism (Arginase types I and II). NOS can also be inhibited by an analog of L-arginine, asymmetric dimethylarginine (ADMA). Once produced, NO diffuses to the smooth muscle where it avidly binds to the heme moiety of soluble guanylate cyclase (GC), catalyzing the production of cyclic GMP (cGMP) from guanosine triphosphate (GTP). cGMP, in turn, activates protein kinase G (PKG) which leads to vascular relaxation by enhancing Ca^{2+} extrusion from the cell and stimulating Ca^{2+} entry back into the sarcoplamic reticulum. It also phosphorylates phosphatases that dephosphorylate myosin light-chain kinase (MLCK).

cation channels are inhibited, and the decrease in intracellular Ca^{2+} relaxes the smooth muscle. This mechanism is predominantly cGMP-independent [36]. NO may also activate potassium (K^+) channels in the cell membrane that allow K^+ efflux from the cell. K^+ efflux leads to a decrease in membrane potential and hyperpolarization and, as a consequence, the closing of cell-membrane voltage-gated Ca^{2+} channels and vascular muscle relaxation [36–39].

Some nitrovasodilators release NO spontaneously (sodium nitroprusside) whereas others (organic nitrates such as nitroglycerin) require active reduction via intracellular sulfhydryl groups. Both nitroprusside and nitroglycerin relax arteries and veins, although low doses of nitroglycerin have a more selective action on venous circulation than on arterial circulation, making it more commonly used for reducing preload. Both drugs are commonly used intraoperatively and in the intensive care unit as continuous infusions because they have short duration of action and are easily titrated to effect. Prolonged or excessive dosing can cause methemoglobinemia, but in routine clinical use it is not usually a concern [40]. All NO donor drugs are markedly potentiated by phosphodiesterase type 5 (PDE5) inhibitors, which prevent the normal metabolism of cGMP, thus potentiating its dilating effects [41,42]. Caution must therefore be used in patients receiving sildenafil, vardenifil, or tadalafil.

Nitroglycerin and other organic nitrates induce tolerance with prolonged use, likely due to the generation of superoxide and peroxynitrite free radicals that inhibit aldehyde dehydrogenase 2. Without this enzyme, the process by which nitroglycerin and organic nitrite are biotransformed to release NO is impaired [43]. Prolonged use of sodium nitroprusside can lead to the accumulation of thiocyanate and cyanide with the potential for cyanide toxicity [44]. Cyanide toxicity can be manifest by venous hyperoxemia or metabolic acidosis. It should be treated promptly by discontinuing nitroprusside, administering sodium nitrite (5 mg kg^{-1}), and infusing thiosulfate (200 mg kg^{-1}). The sodium nitrite produces methemoglobin, which combines with the cyanide ions, from which the thiosulfate generates thiocyanate.

Drugs in the category of nitrovasodilators include isosorbide dinitrate, isosorbide mononitrate, nitroglycerin, erythrityl tetranitrate, pentaerythritol tetranitrate, and sodium nitroprusside.

Catecholamine receptor pharmacology

Catecholamines can increase or decrease smooth-muscle tone, depending on the type and density of adrenoceptors involved. Adrenoceptors are among the many G-protein-coupled receptors. The numerous subtypes of G proteins and their second-messenger systems are responsible for the diverse responses seen with receptor binding. Adding to the complexity is the presence of second-messenger isoforms with differing tissue distributions and regulatory controls [45–47].

α_1-Adrenoceptors on vascular smooth-muscle cells are linked to PLC through a G protein, G_q, resulting in the production of IP_3 and DAG with subsequent release of Ca^{2+} from the SR and smooth-muscle contraction [48]. α-Adrenoceptor antagonists competitively bind to the α_1-adrenoceptor and interfere with the ability of catecholamines to produce vasoconstriction through this mechanism. α_2-Adrenoceptors are coupled to the G_i protein complex, which is involved in inhibition of adenylate cyclase, Ca^{2+}, and K^+ channels. The net result of agonist binding to the α_2-adrenoceptor is decreased cAMP, hyperpolarization, and decreased $[Ca^{2+}]_i$. Presynaptic α_2-receptor stimulation results in decreased sympathetic output from the central nervous system (CNS), whereas agonist activity at the postsynaptic α_2 receptors in the CNS may be responsible for the sedative and analgesic properties of these drugs [49,50].

Activated β-adrenoceptors in vascular smooth muscle stimulate adenylate cyclase to produce cAMP, which in turn activates several protein kinases that interfere with vasoconstriction. One of these kinases phosphorylates the Ca^{2+} channel, inhibiting the entry of Ca^{2+} into the cell. The phosphorylation of phospholamban by another protein kinase increases the reuptake of Ca^{2+} from the cytoplasm into the SR [51]. cAMP-dependent kinases also activate MLCP [4]. This enzyme dephosphorylates the regulatory myosin light chain to promote dissociation of myosin and actin, leading to smooth-muscle relaxation.

Dopamine 1 receptors (D_1) are postsynaptic receptors that mediate vasodilation through G-protein/adenylate-cyclase coupling to produce increased cAMP and $[Ca^{2+}]_i$. Dopamine 2 receptors (D_2) are presynaptic and are coupled to the inhibitory G-protein complex that decreases cAMP levels and produces cell-membrane hyperpolarization, reducing norepinephrine release. Dopamine produces its effects in a dose-dependent manner, with predominantly D_1 receptor stimulation at lower levels, β_1 receptor stimulation at moderate doses, and α_1 receptor activity at greater concentrations. A selective D_1 receptor agonist is available for clinical use to mediate splanchnic vasodilation [52].

α_1-Adrenergic blockers

These drugs cause vascular dilation by blocking sympathetic nerve effect and circulating catecholamine actions via blockade of the α-adrenoceptor on vascular smooth muscle [53]. α-Adrenoceptors have been classified on a morphological basis as pre- and postsynaptic, and on a pharmacological basis as α_1 and α_2 subtypes. α_1 as well as α_2 receptors might be present at pre- and postsynaptic sites. In the periphery, α_1 receptors are located postsynaptically and mediate the excitatory effects of catecholamines. The α_2 receptors, on the other hand, are autoreceptors involved in the regulation of norepinephrine release. In the CNS, both α_1 and α_2 receptors exist on postsynaptic cells [45,48,49]. The α_1 receptors are located

on vascular smooth-muscle cells, whereas α_2 receptors are located both on sympathetic nerve terminals and on vascular smooth-muscle cells. Most of the α-blockers act as competitive antagonists to the binding of norepinephrine released by sympathetic nerves or produced in the adrenal glands and delivered via circulation. Some α-blockers (e.g., phenoxybenzamine) are noncompetitive and have greatly prolonged action.

Smooth-muscle (postjunctional) α_1 and α_2 receptors are linked to a G_q protein, which activates smooth-muscle contraction through the IP_3 signal transduction pathway. Prejunctional α_2 receptors located on the sympathetic nerve terminals serve as a negative feedback mechanism for norepinephrine release.

Drugs in the α_1-receptor inhibitor class include newer α_1-selective antagonists such as prazosin, terazosin, doxazosin, and timazosin and the older, nonselective drugs phentolamine and phenoxybenzamine, which will block α_2 receptors as well. These latter two drugs are potent and most commonly restricted to use in the management of hypertensive crisis associated with pheochromocytoma and similar endocrinopathies.

α_2-Adrenergic agonists

Clonidine is an α_2-adrenoceptor agonist [49,54–55]. It binds to the α_{2A} receptor in locus coeruleus neurons in the brain, inhibiting the influx of Ca^{2+} into the cell and decreasing neural activity. This results in decreased sympathetic tone, resulting in peripheral vasodilation. When administered orally, peak concentrations are reached by about 90 minutes, and duration of activity is about 6–10 hours. It takes about 2–3 days for therapeutic levels to be reached after topical application, and levels are maintained for about 8 hours. Metabolism is approximately 50% hepatic and 50% renal. The half-life is prolonged in patients with renal insufficiency. Bradycardia and orthostatic hypotension are common secondary to the decreased sympathetic tone. Rebound hypertension may occur following abrupt discontinuation of clonidine and may be severe. Sedation is a common side effect of clonidine (see Chapter 30 for a more detailed discussion); clonidine can reduce inhalational anesthetic requirements, reducing MAC by as much as 50%.

Dexmedetomidine is a highly selective α_2-adrenoceptor agonist ($\alpha_2 : \alpha_1$ selectivity ratio of 1600 : 1), which is seven times more selective than clonidine [49,54–55]. Like clonidine, dexmedetomidine decreases sympathetic tone by inhibition of Ca^{2+} influx in locus coeruleus neurons. This results in decreased heart rate and vasodilation. Dexmedetomidine also possesses hypnotic, sedative, and analgesic properties while minimally affecting respiratory drive. It is administered intravenously with an onset of action of 2–5 minutes. Elimination half-life is about 2 hours. It is primarily metabolized in the liver by direct glucuronidation and the P450 enzyme system. The dose should be reduced in patients with hepatic failure. Bradycardia and hypotension are common secondary to decreased sympathetic tone. However, if infused too rapidly during the loading dose, hypertension may result secondary to direct activation of vascular α_2-adrenoceptors. Caution must be used in hypovolemic patients. Rebound hypertension may occur after discontinuation. As with clonidine, dexmedetomidine reduces inhalational anesthetic requirements. Sedative-hypnotic and opiate requirements are also reduced by dexmedetomidine.

β_2-Adrenergic agonists

Vascular smooth-muscle cells express β_2-adrenoceptors, which are activated by catecholamines released by sympathetic adrenergic nerves. These receptors are coupled with G_s protein, which activates adenylate cyclase to stimulate the formation of cAMP from ATP. The increase in cAMP activates PKA, which phosphorylates and thereby inhibits MLCK, causing vascular smooth-muscle relaxation. Isoproterenol is the selective β-agonist most commonly used. Epinephrine at low doses can have a primary β- (versus α-) adrenergic response. Dobutamine and dopamine also can activate vascular β receptors. These drugs will induce tachycardia as a result of the chronotropic action of β receptors in the heart.

β_2-Agonists are primarily used for bronchial relaxation and are classed as short-acting (e.g., salbutamol, metaproterenol, levosabutamol, terbutaline, pirbuterol, procaterol, fenoterol, bitolterol meslate), long-acting (e.g., salmeterol, formoterol, bambuteroll, clenbuterol), and ultra long-acting (e.g., indacaterol).

Dopamine-1 agonist

Fenoldopam selectively binds to D_1 receptors, acting through G_s protein complexes to increase cAMP production, activate PKA, and thereby inhibit the cellular contractile machinery. The drug acutely decreases blood pressure and is administered through continuous infusion for the treatment of severe hypertension. It does not have D_2-receptor or β-adrenoceptor activity, but does produce reflex-mediated increases in heart rate and cardiac index [56]. Therapeutic dosages of fenoldopam increase renal blood flow, creatinine clearance, urinary flow, and excretion of sodium [57]. Fenoldopam is extensively metabolized in the liver, but in patients with liver disease plasma levels tend to be lower and clearance rates greater than in healthy volunteers, likely because of increased intrahepatic shunting and a greater volume of distribution. Although fenoldopam is given by continuous infusion, it has a relatively long duration of action (30–60 minutes); its actions can thus persist after discontinuation. Fenoldopam increases intraocular pressure and should be used with caution in patients with glaucoma or globe injury.

Renin–angiotensin pathway pharmacology
Angiotensin-converting enzyme (ACE) inhibitors

The renin–angiotensin system is critical for the regulation of arterial blood pressure and electrolyte and water balance [26,27,57–65]. Renin is produced in the kidneys and catalyzes the production of angiotensin I from angiotensinogen, a 225-amino-acid prohormone. Angiotensin-converting enzyme (ACE) then metabolizes angiotensin I to its active form, angiotensin II. Angiotensin II causes systemic vasoconstriction via angiotensin type 1 receptors, which are located on vascular smooth muscle and coupled to a G_q protein and the IP_3 signal transduction pathway. Angiotensin II also facilitates the release of norepinephrine from sympathetic adrenergic nerves and inhibits norepinephrine reuptake. It causes the release of aldosterone from the adrenal cortex and enhances renal sodium and fluid retention and stimulation of thirst, all of which lead to an increase in blood pressure. Two sites in this pathway have been pharmacologically targeted to promote vasodilation – direct inhibitors of ACE and angiotensin-receptor antagonists [26,27].

ACE is also responsible for the metabolism of bradykinin, an endogenous vasodilator. Thus ACE inhibitors, in addition to blocking the hypertensive effects of angiotensin II, also promote the vasodilatory effect of bradykinin by preventing its breakdown [26,27]. This enhanced circulating bradykinin concentration is implicated in two potential side effects of ACE inhibitors – dry cough and angioedema. Although the cough sometimes limits patient tolerance, more serious side effects such as bronchospasm and angioedema are rare [66].

In addition to their antihypertensive effects, ACE inhibitors have been shown to improve long-term outcomes in heart failure trials [59–61] and to slow renal dysfunction in diabetic nephropathy [62]. Although one might expect ACE inhibitors to be particularly effective in hypertension secondary to renal artery stenosis, a condition caused by excess renin production and activation of the angiotensin pathway, they are contraindicated because of the marked reduction in renal blood flow and risk of renal failure that ensues. A decrease in glomerular filtration rate is seen in patients treated with ACE inhibitors, and caution must be used in patients with renal impairment. Hyperkalemia can occur because of reduced production of aldosterone; therefore potassium levels should be monitored. Except for enalaprilat, all of the ACE inhibitors are administered orally. Because of its availability as an intravenous drug, enalaprilat is the only ACE inhibitor commonly used intraoperatively. Many of the ACE inhibitors are designed as prodrugs to enhance their oral bioavailability; these must undergo hepatic metabolism to the active form of the drug. Enalapril is the prodrug of the active ACE inhibitor enalaprilat, and conversion may be affected in patients with hepatic dysfunction. Captopril and lisinopril are not prodrugs. Accumulation of these ACE inhibitors occurs in renal impairment, and dose adjustment is necessary. ACE inhibitors should not be used during pregnancy. Published experience in the pediatric population is limited; although captopril and enalapril have been used with no significant adverse effects reported [63,64].

Current drugs in this class include enalapril, enaliprilat, captoprol, benazepril, fosinopril, lisinopril, moexipril, quinapril, and ramipril.

Angiotensin receptor blockers (ARBs)

Angiotensin receptor blockers (ARBs) have effects that are very similar to those of ACE inhibitors, but their pharmacologic action is through the competitive blockade of type 1 angiotensin II receptors [26,27,68]. As discussed above, these receptors are coupled to the G_q protein and IP_3 signal transduction pathway that stimulates vascular smooth muscle contraction through increases in $[Ca^{2+}]_i$. ARBs displace angiotensin II from the type 1 angiotensin receptor and produce their blood-pressure lowering effects by antagonizing angiotensin-II-induced vasoconstriction, aldosterone release, catecholamine release, arginine vasopressin release, water intake, and hypertrophic response. Unlike ACE inhibitors, ARBs do not potentiate bradykinin responses, thus avoiding the potential side effects of ACE inhibitors (cough and angioedema) that are mediated by excess bradykinin.

Current ARBs include candesartan, eprosartan, irbesartan, losartan, olmesartan, telmisartan, and valsartan, all of which are available as oral medications. No parenteral ARBs are currently available for clinical use.

Renin inhibitors

Alongside ACE inhibitors and ARBs, renin inhibitors comprise the third class of compounds that affect the renin–angiotensin–aldosterone system. Renin is responsible for converting angiotensinogen to angiotensin I, which is then converted to angiotensin II by ACE. Renin inhibitors thus prevent the formation of both angiotensin I and angiotensin II [26,27,69].

Renin inhibitors act on the juxtaglomerular cells of the kidney where renin is produced. They lead to dilation of arteries and veins by blocking angiotensin formation. They also downregulate sympathetic adrenergic activity and promote renal excretion of sodium and water as the ACE inhibitors do. Renin inhibitors do not affect kinin metabolism and, like ARBs, may produce fewer adverse effects (dry cough, angioedema) than do ACE inhibitors.

Current renin inhibitors include aliskiren and remikiren, which are available in oral form only.

Endothelin receptor antagonists

The family of endothelins (ET) consists of four closely related peptides, ET-1, ET-2, ET-3, and ET-4. They are synthesized in vascular endothelial and smooth-muscle cells, as well as in neural, renal, pulmonary, and inflammatory cells. These peptides are converted by endothelin-converting enzymes from "big endothelins" that originate from large preproendothelin peptides that are cleaved by endopeptidases. ET-1 is a 21-amino-acid peptide that has major influence on the function and structure of the vasculature, as it favors vasoconstriction and cell proliferation through activation of specific ET_A and ET_B receptors on vascular smooth-muscle cells. These receptors are coupled to a G_q protein, and receptor activation initiates a pathway to the formation of IP_3 and Ca^{2+} release from the SR [28–30,70–73].

ET-1 formation and release are stimulated by angiotensin II, arginine vasopressin, thrombin, cytokines, reactive oxygen species, and shearing forces acting on the vascular endothelium. ET-1 release is inhibited by PGI_2 and atrial natriuretic peptide as well as by NO [70–73].

Activation of ET_B receptors on endothelial cells causes vasodilation via release of NO and PGI_2, although the direct vasoconstricting actions on vascular smooth muscle are usually dominant. Additionally, ET_B receptors in the lung are a major pathway for the clearance of ET-1 from plasma. ET-receptor antagonists have been widely studied in arterial hypertension; they prevent vascular and myocardial hypertrophy. Randomized clinical trials have shown that a mixed $ET_{A/B}$-receptor antagonist effectively lowers arterial blood pressure [28–30,70–73]. Sitaxentan and ambrisentan are selective for ET_A receptors, whereas bosentan is a mixed ET_A and ET_B antagonist.

Phosphodiesterase (PDE) inhibitors

β-Agonists and NO exert much of their vasodilating action by stimulating the production of the second messengers cAMP and cGMP, respectively. The intracellular levels of cAMP and cGMP are tightly controlled both by their rate of synthesis and through their rapid hydrolysis by PDEs [40]. Cyclic AMP is primarily hydrolyzed by type 3 PDEs, whereas cGMP is specifically hydrolyzed by type 5 PDEs. Inhibition of PDEs markedly potentiates the concentration of cAMP or cGMP in the cell and the resultant vasodilation. PDEs provide a synergistic response when used in combination with a cAMP- or cGMP-stimulating agonist.

Drugs in this category include PDE3 inhibitors (milrinone, inamrinone) and PDE5 inhibitors (sildenafil, tadalafil, vardenifil).

Potassium channel openers

An important means of regulating vascular tone is through modulation of smooth-muscle cell-membrane potential. Potassium channel openers can be used to lower membrane potential and thereby alter the activity of VGCCs. Multiple K^+ channel types are present in most vascular smooth-muscle cells. Voltage-dependent K^+ (K_v) channels are activated by depolarization, may contribute to steady-state resting membrane potential, and are inhibited by certain vasoconstrictors. Calcium-activated K^+ (K_{Ca}) channels oppose the depolarization associated with intrinsic vascular tone and are activated by some endogenous vasodilators. ATP-sensitive K^+ (K_{ATP}) channels are activated by pharmacological and endogenous vasodilators. Inward rectifier K^+ (K_{ir}) channels are activated by slight changes in extracellular K^+ and may contribute to resting membrane potential [36–38,74,75].

Potassium-selective ion channels whose activity is inhibited by very small amounts of ATP have been found in a variety of cell types. Opening of the K_{ATP} channels results in cell hyperpolarization and vascular relaxation; hence, compounds that open K_{ATP} channels are vasodilators. K_{ATP} channels play an important role in the control of basal tone, autoregulation of several vascular beds, and metabolic regulation of blood flow. In the pulmonary circulation, anoxic vasodilation is in part due to activation of K_{ATP} channels [75]. The K_{ATP} channel opens when ADP levels rise and closes when ATP levels rise. It is blocked by sulfonylureas (glibenclamide, glyburide) and opened by pinacidil, cromakalim, or minoxidil.

Hydralazine is included in this class of drugs that promote the influx of potassium into vascular smooth-muscle cells, with resultant hyperpolarization and smooth-muscle relaxation [76]. It can be administered intravenously, intramuscularly, or orally and is useful in the treatment of severe hypertension, pre-eclampsia, and chronic heart failure. Onset of action may be as long as 20 minutes, even with intravenous administration, and caution must be used before re-dosing. It has a duration of action that varies from 3 to 8 hours. Metabolism is primarily hepatic by acetylation. The rate of acetylation varies among patients, with about 30% of individuals undergoing rapid acetylation and 50% slow acetylation. This rate of metabolism affects the bioavailability of the drug when it is administered orally. Rapid acetylators have lower bioavailability than slow acetylators. The acetylation rate does not appear to affect the drug concentration when it is administered intravenously. Reflex tachycardia may occur, and special care must therefore be taken if hydralazine is used in patients with coronary artery disease. Aplastic anemia and a lupus-like syndrome are associated with hydralazine use. Nonsteroidal anti-inflammatory drugs decrease the vasodilatory effect of hydralazine.

Like hydralazine, minoxidil and related drugs increase the influx of potassium into vascular smooth muscle, resulting in hyperpolarization and vasodilation [77]. Minoxidil is administered orally, has a 30-minute onset, and has a duration of approximately 24 hours. It is metabolized in the liver to minoxidil glucuronide, with an elimination half-life of about 4 hours. Reflex tachycardia is common secondary to a baroreflex response and increased sympathetic activity. Likewise, renin levels increase, leading to sodium and water retention. Minoxidil should be used in conjunction with a β-adrenergic blocker and a diuretic. Minoxidil has been associated with the development of both pulmonary edema and pericardial effusion. It also causes electrocardiographic abnormalities, particularly T-wave flattening or inversion and increased QRS amplitude. Thrombocytopenia or leukopenia may occur, and Stevens–Johnson syndrome has been associated with minoxidil use [78]. Hypertrichosis is a common side effect [79].

Ganglionic blockers

Neurotransmission within the sympathetic and parasympathetic ganglia involves the release of ACh from preganglionic efferent nerves. ACh binds to nicotinic receptors on the cell bodies of postganglionic efferent nerves. Ganglionic blockers inhibit autonomic activity by interfering with neurotransmission within autonomic ganglia. This inhibition reduces sympathetic outflow to the heart, thereby decreasing cardiac output by decreasing heart rate and contractility. Reduced sympathetic output to the vasculature decreases sympathetic vascular tone, which causes vasodilation and reduced systemic vascular resistance; the result is a reduction in arterial pressure [80]. Parasympathetic outflow is also reduced by ganglionic blockers.

Several different ganglionic blockers are available for clinical use, but only one – trimethaphan camsylate – is occasionally used in hypertensive emergencies or for producing controlled hypotension during surgery.

Magnesium

Magnesium (Mg^{2+}) may influence blood pressure by modulating vascular tone and structure through its effects on numerous biochemical reactions that control vascular contraction/dilation, growth/apoptosis, differentiation, and inflammation. Magnesium acts as a Ca^{2+} channel antagonist; it stimulates production of vasodilator prostacyclins and NO, and it alters vascular responses to vasoactive agonists [81]. Mammalian cells regulate Mg^{2+} concentration through specialized influx and efflux transport systems that have only recently been characterized. Alterations in some of these systems may contribute to hypomagnesemia and intracellular Mg^{2+} deficiency in hypertension. In particular, increased Mg^{2+} efflux through altered regulation of the vascular Na^+/Mg^{2+} exchanger and decreased Mg^{2+} influx due to defective vascular and renal TRPM6/7 expression/activity may be important.

Calcium channel blockers

The calcium channel blockers (see Chapter 46 for additional detail) bind to and inhibit calcium entry through L-type calcium channels in cardiac muscle and vascular smooth muscle as well as in cardiac nodal tissue [83–84]. Calcium channel blockers comprise three types based on their structure and relative actions on cardiac versus vascular smooth muscle: dihydropyridines, benzothiazepines, and phenylalkylamines.

The dihydropyridines act primarily on vascular smooth muscle and are used mainly to treat systemic hypertension. This class of calcium channel blockers includes amlodipine, felodipine, isradipine, nicardipine, nifedipine, nimodipine, and nitrendipine. The use of these drugs can increase cardiac output because of reflex tachycardia and decreased afterload. Nifedipine is used to prevent vasospasm of arterial conduits in coronary artery bypass surgery, while nimodipine is used to treat or prevent cerebral arterial vasospasm in patients with subarachnoid hemorrhage. Nicardipine is available in intravenous and oral preparations, whereas the others are available only in oral form. Parenteral nicardipine is usually administered by continuous infusion because of its short biologic half-life. Nicardipine does undergo relatively slow terminal elimination, and its effects can persist for several hours after discontinuation of a prolonged (e.g., > 1 day) infusion. Again, the duration of oral drugs varies depending on the type and preparation. Dose adjustments are necessary in patients with hepatic disease. Important drug interactions are possible secondary to interference with hepatic metabolism. Patients taking combinations of calcium channel blockers and ACE inhibitors or ARBs may develop marked and refractory hypotension under general anesthesia [82–84].

Diltiazem is a benzothiazepine that blocks Ca^{2+} influx in the myocardial conduction system and vascular smooth muscle. It causes mild to moderate decreases in myocardial contraction, and decreases heart rate by decreasing both the automaticity of the sinoatrial node and the rate of conduction in the atrioventricular node. It is indicated for treatment of tachyarrhythmia, angina, Raynaud syndrome, and hypertension. Diltiazem has a rapid onset when administered parenterally and may be given by intermittent bolus or continuous infusion, depending on the clinical circumstances. Diltiazem is also available in oral form, with both sustained and nonsustained preparations. It is metabolized in the liver to an active metabolite. As with other calcium channel blockers, dose reductions are necessary in patients with hepatic dysfunction, and serious drug interactions may occur.

Verapamil is a phenylalkylamine that inhibits the influx of Ca^{2+} ions in cardiac muscle, cardiac conductive tissue, and vascular smooth muscle, producing decreases in cardiac contractility, heart rate, and both coronary and peripheral vascular tone. It is used clinically in the treatment of angina, tachyarrhythmia, and hypertension. Verapamil has a rapid onset when administered intravenously, with a duration of 20–30 minutes. Oral preparations vary in their duration of action depending on their formulation (sustained vs. nonsustained). Verapamil is metabolized in the liver to norverapamil. This active metabolite has approximately 20% of the activity of the parent compound and is excreted by the kidney. Dosing adjustments are necessary in patients with renal or hepatic impairment. Because verapamil has negative inotropic and chronotropic effects, caution must be used in patients with severe left ventricular dysfunction or second- or third-degree heart block, and in those who are receiving other antiarrhythmic drugs. Verapamil may precipitate ventricular dysrhythmias in patients with Wolff–Parkinson–White syndrome. Calcium channel blockers interfere with hepatic metabolism of a number of drugs, increasing the risk for serious drug interactions. Neuromuscular blockade may be prolonged, and the doses of sedative and analgesic drugs must be reduced with concomitant administration.

Eicosanoids

Prostaglandin E_1 (PGE_1) and PGI_2 bind to specific prostanoid receptors coupled to G_s protein complexes that increase cAMP production, activate PKA, and inhibit the cellular contractile machinery to produce vasodilation [85]. Although they produce reductions in systemic vascular tone, their most common clinical uses are related to their effects on the pulmonary vasculature. PGE_1 is used in neonates with congenital heart disease to maintain ductus arteriosus patency, and PGI_2 is used predominantly for the treatment of primary pulmonary hypertension. Other important biologic effects include restoration of endothelial cell integrity, improved rheologic properties of red blood cells, decreased smooth-muscle cell proliferation, and dose-dependent inhibition of platelet aggregation, making them useful in the treatment of occlusive peripheral arterial disease. They are rapidly metabolized in the lung and require administration by continuous infusion. Desensitization occurs with prolonged exposure to PGI_2 in the treatment of primary pulmonary hypertension, making it necessary to increase doses to achieve the desired effect. These drugs may produce uterine smooth-muscle contraction and should not be used during pregnancy. Apnea occurs in approximately 10% of neonates who receive PGE_1, necessitating continuous respiratory monitoring. The potent antiplatelet effects of PGI_2 may increase bleeding risk in surgical patients or those receiving anticoagulant/antithrombotic therapy.

Calcium sensitizer (levosimendan)

Levosimendan is a calcium sensitizer and a vasodilator used in refractory heart failure. It serves to increase the cardiac myocyte sensitivity to calcium by binding to cardiac troponin C with high affinity and stabilizing the Ca^{2+}-bound conformation of the regulatory protein. It also acts as a vasodilator, primarily through opening K_{ATP} channels and inhibiting PDE, chiefly PDE3. Thus it both increases cardiac inotropicity and decreases afterload, facilitating forward blood flow and enhancing cardiac output [86–88].

Levosimendan also opens K_{ATP} channels in the cardiac mitochondria and sarcoplasmic reticulum. This activity is thought to mediate its protective effect against cardiac ischemia in a manner similar to ischemic preconditioning [87–88].

Dosage and administration

Table 45.1 lists the doses and administration of commonly used vasodilators.

New and emerging concepts

We have seen that the endothelium plays a major role in modulating vascular tone through the release of endogenous dilators such as prostacyclin and nitric oxide. Many endogenous and exogenous vasoconstrictors also modulate their contractile effect by stimulating the release of these dilators from the endothelium. So when the endothelium is injured through atherosclerosis, sepsis, or other metabolic events, the ability of vessels to dilate can become markedly impaired. To address this, many approaches are being taken to actually repair the endothelium or enhance production of endothelium dependent dilators, especially NO [89]. One approach is to increase

Table 45.1. Commonly used vasodilators: doses and routes of administration

Drugs		Doses
Nitrates	Nitroglycerin	IV: 5–200 $\mu g\ min^{-1}$, titrated to effect
		SL: 0.3–0.6 mg every 5 min
	Sodium nitroprusside	IV: start 0.25–0.3 $\mu g\ kg^{-1}\ min^{-1}$; max 10 $\mu g\ kg^{-1}\ min^{-1}$
β-Agonist	Dobutamine	IV: start 0.5–1 $\mu g\ kg^{-1}\ min^{-1}$; max 40 $\mu g\ kg^{-1}\ min^{-1}$
	Isoproterenol	IV: 0.02–0.06 mg × 1 dose, then infusion 2–20 $\mu g\ min^{-1}$
Dopamine-1 agonist	Fenoldopam	IV: start 0.025–0.3 $\mu g\ kg^{-1}\ min^{-1}$; max 1.6 $\mu g\ kg^{-1}\ min^{-1}$
Ace inhibitor	Captopril	Start 6.25–25 mg PO bid or tid; max 450 mg day^{-1}
	Enalapril	Start 2.5 mg PO daily; max 40 mg day^{-1}
	Lisinopril	Start 2.5–5 mg PO daily, max 40 mg day^{-1}
	Ramipril	Start 2.5 mg PO daily; max 10 mg day^{-1}
	Accupril	Start 10 mg PO daily; max 80 mg day^{-1}
Angiotensin II receptor antagonists	Losartan	Start 25 mg PO daily; max 100 mg day^{-1}
	Candesartan	Start 4 mg PO daily; max 32 mg day^{-1}
	Irbesartan	Start 75 mg PO daily: max 300 mg day^{-1}
	Valsartan	Start 40 mg PO daily: max 320 mg day^{-1}
	Telmisartan	Start 40 mg PO daily: max 160 mg day^{-1}
Eicosanoids	Prostaglandin E_1	IV: 0.01–0.1 $\mu g\ kg^{-1}\ min^{-1}$; max 0.4 $\mu g\ kg^{-1}\ min^{-1}$
	Prostacyclin	Administered either IV or by aerosolized inhalation device
		IV: start 2 ng $kg^{-1}\ min^{-1}$; increase by 2 ng $kg^{-1}\ min^{-1}$ every 15 min until dose-limiting side effects
Purinergic agonists	Adenosine	IV: 6 mg × 1 dose, may give 12 mg every 1–2 min × 2 doses
Calcium channel antagonists	Verapamil	IV: 2.5–10 mg per dose; max 20 mg total dose; may repeat after 15–30 min
		PO: start 40 mg tid; max 480 mg day^{-1}
	Diltiazem	Start 30 mg PO qid; max 360 mg day^{-1}
		IV: 0.25 mg kg^{-1} then 5–15 mg h^{-1}; may repeat 2nd bolus at 0.35 mg kg^{-1} after initial dose
	Nicardipine	IV: start 5 mg h^{-1}; increase to 2.5 mg h^{-1} every 5–15 min to max 15 mg h^{-1}
	Amlodipine	Start 2.5 mg PO daily; max 10 mg day^{-1}
	Felodipine	Start 2.5 mg PO daily; max 10 mg day^{-1}
	Isradipine	Start 2.5 mg PO bid; max 10 mg day^{-1}
	Nifedipine	Start 10 mg PO tid; max 180 mg day^{-1}
Phosphodiesterase inhibitors	Inamrinone	Start 0.5–1 mg kg^{-1} bolus; then 2–15 $\mu g\ kg^{-1}\ min^{-1}$
	Milrinone	Start 50 $\mu g\ kg^{-1}$ IV × 1dose, then 0.375 $\mu g\ kg^{-1}\ min^{-1}$; max 0.75 $\mu g\ kg^{-1}\ min^{-1}$
	Sildenafil	Start 25 mg PO daily; max 100 mg day^{-1}
	Tadalafil	Start 2.5 mg PO daily; max 20 mg day^{-1}
Potassium channel activators	Hydralazine	Start 10 mg PO qid; max 300 mg day^{-1}
		Alternative: 10–40 mg IM/IV every 4–6 h then switch to PO a.s.a.p.
	Minoxidil	Start 5 mg PO daily; max 100 mg PO daily

Table 45.1. (*cont.*)

Drugs		Doses
α₂-Adrenergic agonists	Clonidine	Start 0.1 mg PO bid; max 1.2 mg PO bid
		Transdermal: 0.1 mg 24 h patch; max 0.6 mg day^{-1}
	Dexmedetomidine	Loading dose: 1 mg kg^{-1} over 10 min, then 0.2–0.7 μg kg^{-1} h^{-1}
	Guanabenz	Start 2 mg PO bid; max 64 mg day^{-1}
	Guanfacine	Start 1 mg PO qhs; max 3 mg day^{-1}
	α-Methyldopa	Start 250 mg PO bid; max 3 mg day^{-1}
α₁-Adrenergic antagonists	Prazosin	Start 1 mg PO bid–tid; max 20 mg day^{-1}
	Terazosin	Start 1 mg PO Qhs; max 20 mg day^{-1}
	Doxazosin	Start 1 mg PO daily; max 16 mg day^{-1}
	Phentolamine	5 mg IM/IV bolus
Calcium sensitizer	Levosimendan	IV: 3–12 μg kg^{-1} as bolus, then infusion 0.05–0.4 μg kg^{-1} min^{-1}
Ganglionic blockers	Trimethaphan camsylate	IV: 0.3–6 mg min^{-1}
Renin inhibitors	Aliskiren	Start 150 mg PO daily
Endothelin receptor antagonist	Bosentan	Start 62.5 mg PO bid; max 250 mg day^{-1}

bid, 2 × daily; tid, 3 × daily; qid, 4 × daily; qhs, every bedtime; IM, intramuscular; IV, intravenous; PO, oral; SL, sublingual.

L-arginine availability. This is being attempted both by infusion of L-arginine and through the development of specific L-arginase inhibitors [89,90].

In the presence of severe hypoxia or high levels of free radicals, or the lack of BH4, NOS, which normally exists as a homodimer, can become "uncoupled." In its uncoupled state, NOS produces peroxynitrite (ONOO$^-$) rather than NO. Peroxynitrite then generates superoxide and hydroxyl free radicals, which can be metabolically and structurally damaging to a cell. To transform NOS back to its coupled state, approaches to increase the availability of BH4 are being developed [91,92].

It is known that statin drugs have multiple effects other than reducing serum cholesterol. Both experimental and clinical studies suggest that these drugs have vascular protective effects by improving endothelial function through both cholesterol-dependent and independent mechanisms. Reduction in endothelial NO production is used as a key marker of endothelial dysfunction. This can be due to reduced expression of eNOS, inadequate eNOS activation, or free radicals binding to and inactivating NO because of oxidative stress. Statins have been shown to significantly increase the functional NO production of endothelial cells. One mechanism by which this occurs is via the statin inhibition of Rho GTPases, preventing Rho/Rho-kinase (ROCK)-mediated changes in the actin cytoskeleton that decrease eNOS mRNA stability [93]. This leads to more eNOS production and more NO [94,95]. There are many ongoing studies using statins in the perioperative period to improve endothelial function and operative outcomes.

Stem cell therapy is also being evaluated to improve endothelial function. Intravascular delivery and engraftment of endothelial progenitor cells such as endothelial precursor cells (EPCs) is being applied to several disease processes where endothelial function is impaired, including coronary atherosclerotic disease, and peripheral vascular disease in diabetics. In some cases, these stem cells are first transfected to over-express eNOS and other vasoactive substances [96–100].

Summary

Most vasodilator drugs ultimately act through regulation of the intracellular calcium concentration ($[Ca^{2+}]_i$) in vascular smooth-muscle cells, by targeting either electromechanical or pharmacomechanical coupling, or through activation of kinases. The pivotal event in smooth-muscle contraction is the increase in $[Ca^{2+}]_i$. The two major sources of Ca^{2+} are the extracellular space and the sarcoplasmic reticulum (SR), where Ca^{2+} is sequestered intracellularly. Vasodilator substances that increase cyclic guanosine monophosphate (cGMP) or cyclic adenosine monophosphate (cAMP) may cause vasodilation by phosphorylating phospholamban and promoting the increased uptake of Ca^{2+} into the SR.

The sympathetic nervous system is the predominant neural regulator of blood vessels. Parasympathetic nerves may induce vasodilation through release of acetylcholine and vasoactive intestinal polypeptide. In some vascular beds, nonadrenergic, noncholinergic (NANC) neurons mediate vasodilation through the release of the vasodilator nitric oxide (NO). Vaso-active molecules that constrict or dilate blood vessels can come from within the vascular smooth muscle itself (autocrine factors), from the endothelium (paracrine factors), or from the circulating blood (hormonal). These drugs generally act on membrane receptors that lead to changes in $[Ca^{2+}]_i$ via receptor-operated channels.

The influence of the endothelium on vascular tone is extremely important in vascular regulation and the clinical pharmacology of vasodilators. Endothelium has multiple functions, it: (1) mediates inflammatory responses to controlling vascular permeability, (2) is a critical regulator of vascular smooth muscle tone, and (3) produces vasoconstrictors and two critical vasodilators, prostacyclin (PGI_2) and NO.

Nitrovasodilators produce vasodilation by releasing NO. Some release NO spontaneously, while others require active reduction via intracellular sulfhydryl groups. NO activates guanylate cyclase to produce cGMP, which activates cGMP-dependent protein kinases (PKG). PKG activates myosin light-chain phosphatase (MLCP), causing dephosphorylation of myosin light chains and vascular relaxation. NO also activates sarco/endoplasmic reticulum Ca^{2+} ATPase, which resides within the SR and refills intracellular Ca^{2+} stores.

Catecholamines can increase or decrease smooth-muscle tone, depending on the type and density of adrenoceptors involved. Vascular smooth-muscle cells express β_2-adrenoceptors, which activate adenylate cyclase (via G_s protein) to stimulate the formation of cAMP. The increase in cAMP activates cAMP-dependent protein kinases (PKA), which phosphorylate and thereby inhibit myosin light-chain kinase (MLCK), causing vascular smooth-muscle relaxation. Isoproterenol is the selective β-agonist most commonly used. Epinephrine at low doses can have a primary β- (versus α-) adrenergic response.

The renin–angiotensin system is critical for the regulation of arterial blood pressure and electrolyte and water balance. Two sites in the renin–angiotensin pathway have been pharmacologically targeted to promote vasodilation: direct inhibitors of angiotensin-converting enzyme (ACE) and angiotensin receptor blockers (ARBs). Renin inhibitors comprise the third class of compounds that affect the renin–angiotensin–aldosterone system.

Endothelins (peptides synthesized in vascular endothelial and smooth-muscle cells) activate endothelin (ET_A) receptors on vascular smooth-muscle cells to produce vasoconstriction. The predominant effect of endothelin antagonists is to block ET_A receptors and thus produce vasodilation.

β-Agonists and NO exert much of their vasodilating action by stimulating the production of the second messengers cAMP and cGMP, respectively. The intracellular levels of cAMP and cGMP are tightly controlled both by their rate of synthesis and through their rapid hydrolysis by phosphodiesterases (PDEs). Levels of cAMP and cGMP can be increased by using PDE inhibitors.

Potassium channel openers can be used to lower membrane potential and thereby alter the activity of voltage-dependent Ca^{2+} channels. Compounds that open ATP-sensitive K^+ channels are vasodilators. Ganglionic blockers inhibit autonomic activity by interfering with neurotransmission within autonomic ganglia. This inhibition causes vasodilation and reduced systemic vascular resistance.

Magnesium acts as a calcium channel antagonist; it also stimulates production of vasodilator prostacyclins and NO, and alters vascular responses to vasoactive agonists. Dihydropyridine-type calcium channel blockers bind to and inhibit calcium entry through L-type calcium channels in vascular smooth muscle, resulting in vasodilation.

Among the eicosanoids, prostaglandin E_1 (PGE_1) and PGI_2 bind to specific prostanoid receptors that increase cAMP production, activate PKA, and inhibit the contractile apparatus in vascular smooth muscle to produce vasodilation. PGE_1 is used in neonates with congenital heart disease to maintain ductus arteriosus patency, and PGI_2 is used predominantly for the treatment of primary pulmonary hypertension.

References

1. Mohrman DE, Heller LJ. *Cardiovascular Physiology*, 6th edn. New York, NY: McGraw-Hill, 2006 (www.accessmedicine.com).

2. Murphy R. Smooth muscle. In: Berne R, Levy M, eds., *Physiology*. St. Louis, MO: Mosby Yearbook, 1993: 309–24.

3. Horowitz A, Menice CB, Laporte R, Morgan KG. Mechanisms of smooth muscle contraction. *Physiol Rev* 1996; **76**: 967–1003.

4. Carpenter CL. Actin cytoskeleton and cell signaling. *Crit Care Med* 2000; **28**: N94–N99.

5. Tada M. Molecular structure and function of phospholamban in regulating the calcium pump from sarcoplasmic reticulum. *Ann N Y Acad Sci* 1992; **671**: 92–102.

6. Walsh MP. Calmodulin and the regulation of smooth muscle contraction. *Mol Cell Biochem* 1994; **135**: 21–41.

7. Trybus KM. Regulation of expressed truncated smooth muscle myosins: role of the essential light chain and tail length. *J Biol Chem* 1994; **269**: 20819–22.

8. Cremo CR, Sellers JR, Facemyer KC. Two heads are required for phosphorylation-dependent regulation of smooth muscle myosin. *J Biol Chem* 1995; **270**: 2171–5.

9. Van Eyk JE, Arrell DK, Foster DB, *et al.* Different molecular mechanisms for Rho family GTPase-dependent,

Ca^{2+}-independent contraction of smooth muscle. *J Biol Chem* 1998; **273**: 23433–9.

10. Chew TL, Masaracchia RA, Goeckeler ZM, Wysolmerski RB. Phosphorylation of non-muscle myosin II regulatory light chain by p21-activated kinase (gamma-PAK). *J Muscle Res Cell Motil* **19**: 839–54.

11. Uehata M, Ishizaki T, Satoh H, *et al.* Calcium sensitization of smooth muscle mediated by a Rho-associated protein kinase in hypertension. *Nature* 1997; **389**: 990–4.

12. Brophy CM. The dynamic regulation of blood vessel caliber. *J Vasc Surg* 2000; **31**: 391–5.

13. Murphy RA. What is special about smooth muscle? The significance of covalent crossbridge regulation. *FASEB J* 1994; **8**: 311–18.

14. Surks HK, Mochizuki N, Kasai Y, *et al.* Regulation of myosin phosphatase by a specific interaction with cGMP-dependent protein kinase I alpha. *Science* 1999; **286**: 1583–7.

15. Rembold CM. Regulation of contraction and relaxation in arterial smooth muscle. *Hypertension* 1992; **20**: 129–37.

16. Bayliss WM. On the local reactions ofhte arterial wall to changes of internal pressure. *J Physiol* 1902; **28**: 220–31.

17. Hill MA, Davis MJ, Meininger GA, Potocnik SJ, Murphy TV. Arteriolar myodenic signaling mechaqnisms: implications for local vascular function. *Clin Hemorheol Microcirc* 2006; **34**: 67–79.

18. Nowicki, PT, Flavahan S, Hassanian H. Redox signaling of the arteriolar myogenic response. *Circ Res* 2001; **89**: 114–16.

19. Kan R, Berkowitz D. Modulators of vascular tone: implications for new pharmacological therapies. In: Housmans PR, Nuttall GA, eds., *Advances in Cardiovascular Pharmacology*. Baltimore, MD: Lippincott Williams & Wilkins, 2008.

20. Yang XP, Chiba S. Interaction between neuropeptide YY1 receptor and alpha 1B-adrenoceptors in the neurovascular unctino of canine splenic arteries. *Eur J Pharmacol* 2003; **466**: 311–15.

21. Yang XP, Chiba S. Separate modulation of neruropeptide Y1 receptor on purinergic and on adrenergic neruoeffector transmission in canine splenic artery. *J Cardiovasc Pharmacol* 2001; **38**: S17–S20.

22. Townsend SA, Jung AS, Hoe YS. Critical role for the alpha-1B adrenergic receptor at the sympathetic neuroeffector function. *Hypertension* 2004; **44**: 776–82.

23. Welstfall TC, Westfall DP. Adrenergic agonists and antagonists. In: Bruton, LL, Lazo JP, Parker KL, eds., *Goodman and Gilman's The Pharmacologic Basis of Therapeutics*, 11th edn. New York, NY: McGraw Hill, 2006: 237–95.

24. Potter LR, Yoder AR, Flora DR, Antos LK, Dickey DM. Natriuretic peptides: their structures, receptors; hysiologic functions and therapeutic applications. *Handb Exp Pharmacol* 2009; **191**: 341–66.

25. Michell JA, Ali F, Bailey L, Moreno L, Harrington LS. Role of nitric oxide and prostacyclin as vasoactive hormones released by the endothelium. *Exp Physiol* 2008; **93**: 141–7.

26. Kumar R, Boim MA. Diversity of pathways for intracellular angiotensin II synthesis. *Curr Opin Nephrol Hypertens* 2009; **18**: 33–9.

27. Rosivall L. Intrarenal renin–angiotensin system. *Mol Cell Endocrinol* 2008; **302**: 185–92.

28. Spieker LE, Noll G, Luscher TF. Therapeutic potential for endothelin receptor antagonists in cardiovascular disorders. *Am J Cardiovasc. Drugs* 2001; **1**: 293–303.

29. Spieker LE, Noll G, Ruschitzka FT, Luscher TF. Endothelin A receptor antagonists in congestive heart failure: blocking the beast while leaving the beauty untouched? *Heart Fail Rev* 2001; **6**: 301–15.

30. Taddei S, Virdis A, Ghiadoni L, *et al.* Role of endothelin in the control of peripheral vascular tone in human hypertension. *Heart Fail Rev* 2001; **6**: 277–85.

31. Gryglewski RJ. Prostacyclin among prostanoids. *Pharmacol Rep* 2008; **60**: 3–11.

32. Moncada S, Gryglewski RJ, Bunting S, Vane JR. An enzyme isolated from the arteries transforms prostaglandin endoperoxides to an unstable substance that inhinits platelet aggregation. *Nature* 1976: **263**: 663–5.

33. Furchgott RF, Zawadski JV. The obligatory role of the endothelial cells in the relaxation of arterial smooth muscle by acetylcholine. *Nature* 1980; **288**: 373–6.

34. Palmer RM, Ferrige AG, Moncada S. Nitric oxide release accounts for the biological activity of endothelium-derived relaxing factor. *Nature* 1987; **327**: 524–6.

35. Yamamoto T, Bing RJ. Nitric oxide donors. *Proc Soc Exp Biol Med* 2000; **225**: 200–6.

36. Cohen RA, Adachi T. Nitric-oxide-induced vasodilation: regulation by physiologic s-glutathiolation and pathologic oxidation of the sarcoplasmic endoplasmic reticulum calcium ATPase. *Trends Cardiovasc Med.* 2006; **16**: 109–14.

37. Baranowska M, Kozlowska H, Korbut A, Malinowska B. [Potassium channels in blood vessels: their role in health and disease]. *Postepy Hig Med Dosw (Online)* 2007; **61**: 596–605.

38. Brayden JE. Potassium channels in vascular smooth muscle. *Clin Exp Pharmacol Physiol* 1996; **23**: 1069–76.

39. Coleman HA, Tare M, Parkington HC. Endothelial potassium channels, endothelium-dependent hyperpolarization and the regulation of vascular tone in health and disease. *Clin Exp Pharmacol Physiol* 2004; **31**: 641–9.

40. Varon J, Marik PE. Perioperative hypertension management. *Vasc Health Risk Manag* 2008; **4**: 615–27.

41. Matsumoto T, Kobayashi T, Kamata K. Phosphodiesterases in the vascular system. *J Smooth Muscle Res* 2003; **39**: 67–86.

42. Ghofrani HA, Voswinckel R, Reichenberger F, *et al.* Differences in hemodynamic and oxygenation responses to threee different phosphodiesterase-r inhibitors in patients with pulmonary arterial hypertension: a reandomized prospective study. *J Am Coll Card* 2004; **44**: 1488–96.

43. Daiber A, Mulsch A, Ink U, *et al.* The oxidative stress concept of nitrate tolerance and the antioxidant properties of hydralazine. *Am J Cardiol* 2005; **96**: 25i–36i.

44. Robin ED, McCauley R. Nitroprusside-related cyanide poisoning. Time (long past due) for urgent, effective interventions. *Chest* 1992; **102**: 1842–5.

45. Molinoff PB. Alpha- and beta-adrenergic receptor subtypes properties, distribution and regulation. *Drugs* 1984; **28**: 1–15.

46. Krupinski J, Lehman TC, Frankenfield CD, Zwaagstra JC, Watson PA. Molecular diversity in the adenylylcyclase family. Evidence for eight forms of the enzyme and cloning of type VI. *J Biol Chem* 1992; **267**: 24858–62.

47. Tang WJ, Gilman AG. Adenylyl cyclases. *Cell* 1992; **70**: 869–72.

48. Smiley RM, Kwatra MM, Schwinn DA. New developments in cardiovascular adrenergic receptor pharmacology: Molecular mechanisms and clinical relevance. *J Cardiothorac Vasc Anesth* 1998; **12**: 80–95.

49. Maze M, Tranquilli W. Alpha-2 adrenoceptor agonists: Defining the role in clinical anesthesia. *Anesthesiology* 1991; **74**: 581–605.

50. Hein TW, Kuo L. cAMP-independent dilation of coronary arterioles to adenosine: Role of nitric oxide, G proteins, and K(ATP) channels. *Circ Res* 1999; **85**: 634–42.

51. Beall AC, Kato K, Goldenring JR, Rasmussen H, Brophy CM. Cyclic nucleotide-dependent vasorelaxation is associated with the phosphorylation of a small heat shock-related protein. *J Biol Chem* 1997; **272**: 11283–7.

52. Post JB, Frishman WH. Fenoldopam: a new dopamine agonist for the treatment of hypertensive urgencies and emergencies. *J Clin Pharmacol* 1998; **38**: 2–13.

53. Stjarne L. Basic mechanisms and local modulation of nerve impulse induced secretion of neurotransmitters from individual sympathetic nerve varicosities. *Rev Physiol Biochem Pharmacol* 1998; **112**: 1–137.

54. Kamibayashi T, Maze M. Clinical uses of alpha-2 adrenergic agonists. *Anesthesiology* 2000; **93**: 1345–9.

55. Scheinin H, Virtanen R, MacDonald E, Lammintausta R, Scheinin M. Medetomidine: a novel alpha 2 adrenoceptor agonist. A review of its pharmacodynamic effects. *Prog Neuropsychopharmacol Biol Psychiatry* 1989; **13**: 635–51.

56. Gombotz H, Plaza J, Mahla E, Berger J, Metzler H. DA1-receptor stimulation by fenoldopam in the treatment of postcardiac surgical hypertension. *Acta Anaesthesiol Scand* 1998; **42**: 834–40.

57. Brogden RN, Markham A. Fenoldopam: a review of its pharmacodynamic and pharmacokinetic properties and intravenous clinical potential in the management of hypertensive urgencies and emergencies. *Drugs* 1997; **54**: 634–50.

58. Carson P, Ziesche S, Johnson G, Cohn JN. Racial differences in response to therapy for heart failure: analysis of the vasodilator-heart failure trials. Vasodilator-Heart Failure Trial Study Group. *J Card Fail* 1992; **5**: 178–87.

59. Pfeffer MA, Braunwald E, Moyé LA, *et al.* Effect of captopril on mortality and morbidity in patients with left ventricular dysfunction after myocardial infarction. Results of the survival and ventricular enlargement trial. The SAVE Investigators. *N Engl J Med* 1992; **327**: 669–77.

60. Ray S, Dargie H. Infarct-related heart failure: the choice of ACE inhibitor does not matter. *Cardiovasc Drugs Ther* 1994; **8**: 433–6.

61. Ball SG, Hall AS, Murray GD. ACE inhibition, atherosclerosis and myocardial infarction: the AIRE study in practice. Acute Infarction Ramipril Efficacy Study. *Eur Heart J* 1994; **15**: 20–25; discussion, 26–30.

62. Lewis EJ, Hunsicker LG, Bain RP, Rohde RD. The effect of angiotensin-converting-enzyme inhibition on diabetic nephropathy. The Collaborative Study Group. *N Engl J Med* 1993; **329**: 1456–62.

63. Miller K, Atkin B, Rodel PV, Walker JF. Enalapril: a well-tolerated and efficacious agent for the pediatric hypertensive patient. *J Cardiovasc Pharmacol* 1987; **10**: S154–6.

64. Pereira CM, Tam YK, Collins-Nakai RL. The pharmacokinetics of captopril in infants with congestive heart failure. *Ther Drug Monit* 1991; **13**: 209–14.

65. Crozier I, Ikram H, Awan N, *et al.* Losartan in heart failure. Hemodynamic effects and tolerability. Losartan Hemodynamic Study Group. *Circulation* 1995; **91**: 691–7.

66. Lacourciere Y, Lefebvre J. Modulation of the renin-angiotensin-aldosterone system and cough. *Can J Cardiol* 1995; **11**: 33F–39F.

67. Casas JP, Chua W, Loukogeorgakis S, *et al.* Effect of inhinitors of the renin-angiotensin system and other antihypertensive drugs on renal outcomes: systematic review and meta-analysis. *Lancet* 2005; **366**: 2026–33.

68. Lee VC, Rhew DC, Dylan M, Braunstein GD, Weingarten SR. Meta-anlaysis: angiotensin receptor blockers in chronic heart failure and high risk acute myocardial infarction. *Ann Intern Med* 2004; **141**: 693–704.

69. Anderson S, Komers R. Inhibition of the renin-angiotensin system: is more better? *Kidney Int* 2009; **75**: 12–14.

70. Dupuis J. Endothelin receptor antagonists and their developing role in cardiovascular therapeutics. *Can J Cardiol* 2000; **16**: 903–10.

71. Luscher TF, Richard V, Tschudi M, Yang ZH, Boulanger C. Endothelial control of vascular tone in large and small coronary arteries. *J Am Coll Cardiol* 1990; **15**: 519–27.

72. Rhodes CJ, Davidson A, Gibbs JS, Wharton, Wilkins MR. Therapeutic targets in pulmonary arterial hypertension. *Pharmacol Ther* 2009; **121**: 69–88

73. Barton M, Yanagisawa M. Endothelin: 20 years from discovery to therapy. *Can J Physiol Pharmacol* 2008; **86**: 485–98.

74. Misler S, Giebisch G. ATP-sensitive potassium channels in physiology, pathophysiology, and pharmacology. *Curr Opin Nephrol Hypertens* 1992; **1**: 21–33.

75. Michelakis ED, Reeve HL, Huang JM, *et al.* Potassium channel diversity in vascular smooth muscle cells. *Can J Physiol Pharmacol* 1997; **75**: 889–97.

76. Ellershaw DC, Gurne AM. Mechanisms of hydralazine induced vasodilation in rabbit aorta and pulmonary artery. *Br J Pharmacol* 2001; **134**: 621–3.

77. Devine BL, Fife R, Trust PM. Minoxidil for severe hypertension after faiolure of

other hypotensive drugs. *Br Med J* 1977; **2**: 667–9.

78. Callen EC, Church CO, Hernandez CL, Thompson ED. Stevens-Johnson syndrome associated with oral minoxidil: a case report. *J Nephrol* 2007; **20**: 91–3.

79. Rogers NI, Avram MR. Medical treatments for male and female pattern air loss. *J Am Acad Dermatol* 2008: **59**: 547–56.

80. Diedrich A, Jordan J, Tank J, *et al.* The sympathetic nervous system in hypertension: assessment by blood pressure variability and ganglionic blockade. *J Hypertens* 2003; **21**: 1677–86.

81. Guerrero-Romero F, Rodriguez-Moran M. The effect of lowering blood pressure by magnesium supplementation in diabetic hypertensive adults with low serum magnesium levels: a randomized, double-blind placebo-controlled clinical trial. *Hum Hypertens* 2009; **23**: 245–51.

82. Jamerson K, Weber MA, Bakris GL, *et al.* Benazapril plus amlodipine or hydrochlorothiazide for hypertension in high risk patients. *N Eng J Med* 2010; **375**: 1173–81.

83. Shah QA, Georgiadis A, Suri MF, Rodriguez G, Qureshi AI. Preliminary experience with intra-arterial nicardipine in patients with acute ischemic stroke. *Neurocrit Care* 2009; **7**: 53–7.

84. Sturgill MG, Seibold JR. Ratikonal use of calcium channel antagonists in Raynaud's phenomenon. *Curr Opin Rheumatol* 1999; **10**: 584–88.

85. Heinemann HO, Lee JB. Prostaglandins and blood presssure control. *Am J Med* 1976: **61**: 681–95.

86. Toller WG, Stranz C. Levosimendan, a new inotropic and vasodilator agent. *Anesthesiology* 2006; **104**: 556–69.

87. Haikala H, Levijoki, Linden JB. Troponin C-mediated calcium sensitization by levosimendan accelerates the proportional development of isometridc tension. *J Mol Cell Cardiol* 1995; **27**: 2155–65.

88. Toller W, Archan S. Levosimendan. In: Housmans PR, Nuttall GA, eds., *Advances in Cardiovascular Pharmacology*. Baltimore, MD: Lippincott Williams & Wilkins, 2008.

89. Kato GJ, Gladwin MT. Evolution of novel small-molecule therapeutics targeting sickle cell vasculopathy. *JAMA* 2008; **10**: 2638–46.

90. Berkowitz DE, White R, Li D, *et al.* Arginase reciprocally regulates nitric oxide synthase activity and contributes to endothelial dysfunction in aging vessels. *Circulation* 2003; **108**: 2000–6.

91. Alp NJ, McAteer MA, Khoo JC, *et al.* Increases in endothelial tertrahydropbiopterins synthesis by targeted transgenic GTP-cyclohydrolase I overexpression reduces endothelial dysfunction and atherosclerosis in ApoE-knockout mice. *Arterioscler Thromb Vasc Biol* 2004; **24**: 445–50.

92. Schuls E, Jansen T, Wenzel P, Daiber A, Munzel T. Nitric oxide, tetrahydrobiopterin, oxidative stress, and endothelial dysfunction in hypertension. *Antioxid Redox Signal* 2008; **10**: 1115–26.

93. Rikitake Y, Liao JK. Rho GTPases, statins, and nitric oxide. *Circ Res* 2005; **97**: 1232–5.

94. O'Driscoll G, Green D, Taylor RR. Simvastatin, an HMG-coenzyme A reductase inhibitor, improves endothelial function within 1 month. *Circulation* 1997; **95**: 1126–31.

95. Hall A. Rho GTPases and the actin cytoskeleton. *Science* 1998; **279**: 509–14.

96. Murasawa S, Asahara T. Gene modified cell transplantation for vascular regeneration. *Current Gene Therapy* 2007; **7**: 1–6.

97. Magri D, Fancher TT, Fitzgerald TN, Muto A, Dardik A. Endothelial progenitor cells: a primer for vascular surgeons. *Vascular* 2008; **6**: 384–94.

98. Melo LG, Gnecchi M, Pachori AS, *et al.* Endothelium-targeted gene and cell-based therapies for cardiovascular disease. *Arterioscler Throm Vasc Biol* 2004; **24**: 1761–74.

99. Giulati R, Lerman A, Simari RD. Therapeutic uses of autologous endothelial cells for vascular disease. *Clin Sci (London)* 2005; **109**: 27–37.

100. Theoharis S, Manunta M, Tan PH. Gene delivery to vascular endothelium using chemical vectors: implications for cardiovascular gene therapy. *Expert Opin Biol Ther* 2007; **7**: 627–43.

Essential drugs in anesthetic practice
Calcium channel blockers

W. Scott Beattie

Introduction

The role of calcium has been studied in virtually all aspects of muscular function. However, the subject is particularly important in perioperative medicine, since it controls most aspects of cardiovascular function and dysfunction, specifically including hypertension, ventricular hypertrophy, heart failure, and arrhythmia. Calcium homeostasis is critical; the influx of calcium through the calcium channel controls vascular smooth-muscle tone and hence vascular resistance [1]. In cardiac nodal tissue, Ca^{2+} channels play an important role in pacemaker currents and in phase 0 of the action potential. In skeletal muscle, calcium is important in regulating muscular contraction through effects mediated more by intracellular mechanisms outside the calcium channels.

Calcium channel blockers (CCBs) are a heterogeneous group of compounds with marked differences in chemical structure, binding sites, and tissue selectivity imparting major differences in clinical activity. Calcium channel blockers have been divided into three discrete chemical types: the **phenylalkylamines** (e.g., verapamil), the **benzothiazepines** (e.g., diltiazem), and the **dihydropyridines** (e.g., nifedipine). The pharmacologic profiles of verapamil and diltiazem are similar to one another and distinct from those of the dihydropyridines. Skeletal muscular tone and function can also be partially inhibited with dantrolene, by mechanisms other than those of the calcium channel.

Hemodynamic action of calcium channel blockers

The main feature of CCBs is vasodilation resulting in decreased vascular resistance, with concomitant increased blood flow. Nifedipine, as an example of the properties of the dihydropyridines (DHPs), has a potent vasodilating effect on both the coronary and peripheral vasculatures [2]. Diltiazem produces coronary vasodilation but is a less potent peripheral vasodilator than either nifedipine or verapamil. The coronary vasodilatory activity of verapamil is weaker than that of diltiazem or nifedipine, and its effect on the peripheral vasculature is intermediate between the two. The cardiovascular effects of the different classes of CCB are compared in Table 46.1.

All CCBs have negative inotropic properties. The newer DHPs (amlodipine) apparently possess fewer cardiac effects, but this property has not been demonstrated clinically. Verapamil is the most powerful negative inotropic CCB, and diltiazem also has a negative inotropic profile, while the DHPs have little effect on the cardiac conductive tissue. Verapamil decreases conduction in the atrioventricular (AV) node, prolonging functional recovery and thereby decreasing heart rate. The major effects of diltiazem on HR are meditated directly by the sinoatrial (SA) node. Intravenous verapamil and diltiazem are indicated for heart-rate control in patients with supraventricular tachycardia.

Clinical utility of calcium channel blockers

Hypertension

This class of drug is widely used in hypertension but has not achieved acceptance as a primary drug [3], because of early reports suggesting nifedipine causes harm. Several observational studies and individual randomized hypertensive trials had suggested that, compared with other drugs, calcium antagonists may be associated with a higher risk of coronary events, despite similar blood-pressure control. A subsequent meta-analysis, limited to short-acting dihydropyridines, suggested that CCBs were inferior to other antihypertensive drugs [3]. The sudden decrease in blood pressure was purported to increase reflex tachycardia and secondarily increase myocardial oxygen requirements. However, newer, larger trials, assessing the newer, longer-acting CCBs, now show that hypertensive treatment with Ca^{2+} channel blockade is actually superior to some other drugs (β-blockade) [4], including both primary and secondary prevention in patients with coronary

Anesthetic Pharmacology, 2nd edition, ed. Alex S. Evers, Mervyn Maze, Evan D. Kharasch. Published by Cambridge University Press. © Cambridge University Press 2011.

Table 46.1. Cardiovascular effects of different classes of calcium channel blockers

	Phenylalkylamines	Benzothiazepines	Dihydropyridines
Conduction	Decreased AV conduction	Mild decrease in conduction	None
Heart rate	Bradycardia	Bradycardia	Reflex tachycardia
Contractility	Decreased contractility	Mild decrease	No reflex effects
Afterload (SVR)	Major decrease	Major decrease	Major decrease

AV, atrioventricular; SVR, systemic vascular resistance.

artery disease [5]. Thus, concerns regarding the outcome efficacy and safety of CCBs should be laid to rest. It is reasonable to assume that long-acting CCBs will emerge as first-line treatment [6], since reports suggest that CCBs are associated with a decreased incidence of new-onset diabetes and fewer cerebral vascular accidents [4]. In the subpopulation of patients with both hypertension and diabetes, treatment should include an angiotensin-converting enzyme (ACE) inhibitor. In a meta-analysis comparing CCBs to ACE inhibitors, CCBs were associated with a twofold increase in morbidity [5]. In a prespecified substudy of INVEST, a randomized controlled assessment of antihypertensive therapy comparing verapamil to atenolol, patients were assessed for depressive symptoms. At 1 year patients randomized to verapamil had less depression than patients assigned to atenolol [7], suggesting that Ca^{2+} channel blockade may be a better alternative in patients with depressive symptoms.

Regression of left ventricular hypertrophy

The regression of left ventricular (LV) hypertrophy is thought to be a favorable prognostic sign. Studies assessing LV mass show that CCBs achieve a modest reduction in LV mass. However, blockade of the renin–angiotensin system is probably a superior method of achieving this goal [8].

Arrhythmias

Calcium channel blockers are considered to be class IV antiarrhythmic. This is related to their ability to decrease the firing rate of aberrant pacemaker sites within the heart, but more importantly their ability to decrease conduction velocity and prolong repolarization, especially at the AV node. Prolonging repolarization of the AV node helps to block reentry mechanisms, which can cause supraventricular tachycardia. CCBs bind directly to Ca^{2+} channels, lower diastolic membrane potential, and depress the slope of spontaneous depolarization in cells with slow-response action potentials (SA and AV nodes). SA rate is decreased, and AV conduction times and refractoriness are prolonged. Thus, these drugs have a role in the management of patients with inappropriate sinus tachycardia, reentrant arrhythmias involving the AV node, and ventricular rate control for atrial fibrillation and atrial flutter. Diltiazem has a more potent effect on the SA node than verapamil, whereas verapamil has a preferential effect on the AV node.

Angina

A variety of CCBs are currently available for use in angina; including amlodipine, diltiazem, nicardipine, nifedipine, and verapamil. Patients with stable angina benefit from dihydropyridine CCBs in combination with β-blockers. A necessary prerequisite for these combinations would be preserved LV function and preferably normal SA and AV nodal function. Alternatively, verapamil or diltiazem in combination with a nitrate may be indicated when β-blockers are contraindicated. Bradycardia, asystole, and complete heart block can occur when verapamil is either given alone or combined with a β-blocker, a result of combined inhibition of nodal function. Verapamil also can decrease β-blocker metabolism (leading to increased plasma concentrations), which potentially increases the interaction between these drugs. CCB antianginal effects are derived from their vasodilator and cardiodepressant actions. Systemic vasodilation reduces arterial pressure, with a concomitant reduction in afterload, and thereby oxygen demand. Calcium channel blockade with the cardioselective CCBs (verapamil and diltiazem) tends to decrease heart rate and contractility, also attenuating myocardial oxygen demand. CCBs also dilate coronary arteries and prevent or reverse the vasospasm associated with variant angina.

The early antihypertensive studies showing increased cardiac events in patients with coronary disease made the antianginal use of CCBs controversial. Studies had suggested that several mechanisms could be involved in the increased morbidity, including reflex tachycardia, a "coronary steal" phenomenon, and proarrhythmic and/or prohemorrhagic effects. We now realize that the mechanisms can be reconciled as follows [5,6,9]. The hemodynamic response to nifedipine is influenced by the rate of increase in plasma concentration of the drug. Heart rate is increased when nifedipine is administered rapidly [10], whereas newer slow-release formulations produce a sustained 24-hour therapeutic effect. These studies show that stable plasma levels of CCBs attenuate the increased sympathetic tone associated with fluctuating plasma concentrations [11]. This hypothesis is supported by the fact that the association between CCBs and cardiovascular events can only be demonstrated with older short-acting drugs. There are no direct comparisons between short-acting and long-acting dihydropyridines. There are no data to support the use of dihydropryidines in unstable angina [12]. In postinfarct care, β-blockers remain the drugs of choice. However, verapamil is indicated if β-blockers are contraindicated or not tolerated [13].

End-stage renal failure

Hypertension is an almost universal feature of end-stage renal disease (ESRD) patients. CCBs are useful drugs for the control of hypertension in ESRD, and have been extensively studied in controlled clinical trials in patients with ESRD [14]. These studies generally show that the pharmacokinetics of CCBs are not significantly altered, and they also suggest that the plasma concentration of CCBs is not decreased with dialysis. This pharmacologic profile simplifies the use of CCBs in ESRD and supports the clinical enthusiasm for using them in this situation, since dialysis-related hypotension occurs less frequently [15], and is also associated a 23% reduction in all-cause mortality [16]. However, neither the optimal blood pressure response nor the specific CCB of choice have been identified.

Perioperative cardioprotection

The American College of Cardiology/American Heart Association 2007 update of the guidelines for cardiac patients having noncardiac surgery made no recommendation concerning CCBs [17]. Eleven randomized controlled studies have been combined in a meta-analysis which shows that the use of CCBs in noncardiac surgery is associated with reduced ischemia and supraventricular arrhythmias, at the cost of increased hypotension and bradycardia [18]. The incidence of hypotension and bradycardia was similar to that found with β-blockers [19]. There was a trend towards reduced incidence of myocardial infarction, but the analysis was underpowered to provide useful information on infarction or death. A much larger meta-analysis of CCBs in cardiac surgery yielded essentially the same information [20]. In a separate propensity-matched cohort study in cardiac surgery, CCBs were associated with decreased incidence of supraventricular tachycardia and death [21]. In both the cardiac meta-analysis and the retrospective cohort study, all positive outcomes were achieved at the cost of an increase in the need for pacemaker support. In cardiac surgery the use of CCBs did not increase either the need for inotropic support or the incidence of a low cardiac output state. The comparative cardiovascular effects of CCBs during surgery are shown in Table 46.2.

Mechanisms of drug action

Calcium regulation and the calcium channel

Calcium channel structure and function, along with the concomitant cellular signaling mechanisms, are complex physiologic subjects. The area is the subject of intense and evolving knowledge, and readers with an interest in calcium

Table 46.2. Clinical effects of calcium channel blockers during surgery: relative risks based on meta-analysis of randomized controlled trials [18,20]

	Cardiac surgery RR (95% CI)	Noncardiac surgery RR (95% CI)
All-cause mortality	1.01 (0.46–2.22)	0.40 (0.14–1.16)
Myocardial infarction	0.58 (0.37–0.91)	0.25 (0.05–1.18)
Supraventricular arrhythmia (all drugs) (nondihydropyridines)	0.73 (0.48–1.12)	0.52 (0.37–0.78)
	0.62 (0.41–0.93)	
Congestive heart failure (low output state)	1.01 (0.25–4.11)	0.60 (0.08–4.81)
Hypotension (need for inotropes)	0.98 (0.63–1.53)	1.72 (0.28–10.8)
Bradycardia (need for pacing)	6.6 (3.5–12.2)	3.32 (0.70–15.6)

homeostasis and receptor signaling are referred to an excellent review for a more intensive treatment of the subject [22]. The following paragraphs are a short overview of the subject. See also Chapter 3 for a review of ion channels in general, and Fig. 46.1 for an illustration of the main interactions involved in Ca^{2+} homeostasis. The upstroke of the action potential causes the opening of the voltage-gated Ca^+ channel (VGCC), releasing calcium and eventually leading to the linking of excitation and contraction (EC coupling). Calcium channels comprise complex polypeptides, usually in four subunits (α_1, α_2/δ, β, and, in some tissues, γ subunits). Calcium enters the cell upon depolarization. The four subunits in excitable tissues make up the functional core of the Ca^{2+} channel. The physical properties of the α subunit are modulated by the accessory subunits (β, α_2/δ) which are bound to the α subunit. Four repeating subunits form the primary structure of the pore-forming structure, and each of these subunits is itself made up of six transmembrane segments. These six transmembrane segments are joined by cytoplasmic loops, named according to the subunits they link. The $\alpha_2\delta$ and γ subunits contain transmembrane domains, while the β subunit is entirely intracellular.

Each subunit possesses an ion-selective pore, voltage sensor, gating machinery, and binding sites for channel-modulating drugs. The pore is asymmetric. Each of the four repeating subunits contains a positively charged fourth transmembrane segment; this segment is highly conserved, likely forming a helix. It is thought that the α-helices traverse the membrane

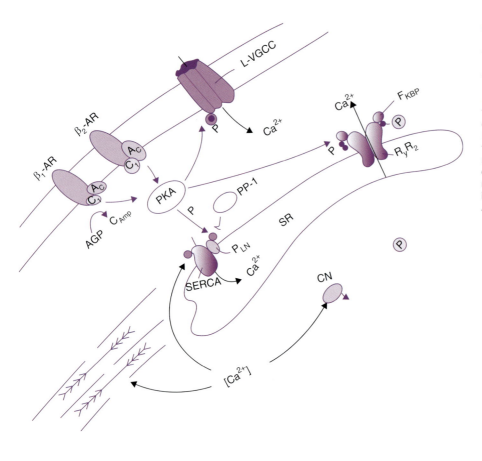

Figure 46.1. The main interactions in calcium homeostasis. Depolarization induces an inward Ca^{2+} current through the voltage-gated Ca^{2+} channel (VGCC). This induces a relatively small increase in Ca^{2+}, which interacts with the ryanodine receptor (RyR2) on the sarcoplasmic reticulum (SR). This in turn induces a Ca^{2+}-mediated Ca^{2+} release or an amplification in Ca^{2+} concentration ($[Ca^{2+}]$). This system can be modulated by the adrenergic system. Stimulation of the β-adrenoceptors (β-AR) activates protein kinases (PKA), which are important for the regulation of Ca^{2+} at the level of both the Ca^{2+} channel and the RyR2. Contraction is followed by release of Ca^{2+} from troponin. Reuptake into the SR is mediated through activation of the SR Ca^{2+} ATPase (SERCA2a) pump.

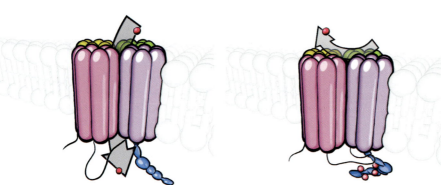

Figure 46.2. Upon depolarization, calcium enters the Ca^{2+} channel and binds to calmodulin. An interaction between the subunits prevents the channel from closing. As the Ca^{2+} concentration rises, the Ca^{2+}/calmodulin complex undergoes a Ca^{2+}-dependent conformational change. This conformational change is in turn associated with inactivation and closure of the Ca^{2+} channel.

electric field. Most structure–function studies support a conformational change of these α-helices in response to a depolarizing stimulus, initiating a change from nonconducting to conducting states, which in turn controls intracellular Ca^{2+} levels (Fig. 46.2).

The Ca^{2+} channels in cardiac tissue remain open for a relatively long duration and also possess a minor voltage-dependent inactivation component. In the heart, Ca^{2+}-dependent inactivation is compatible with the length of the Ca^{2+}-mediated plateau phase in the action potential. Ca^{2+}-induced inhibition of the cardiac Ca^{2+} channel plays a critical role in controlling Ca^{2+} entry and downstream control of contraction and relaxation. Calmodulin is thought to be the critical sensor during the inactivation process and in EC coupling.

The three classes of CCB interact with specific receptor portions of the membrane-spanning protein. These portions constitute most of the L-type Ca^{2+} channel, and these receptor sites are all located on the α subunit. The DHP receptor is located on the surface of the channel, making it easily accessible and therefore the most widely studied. The fact that it is easier to investigate may also explain the plethora of DHP derivatives designed to bind and inhibit (or, in selected cases, stimulate) these receptors.

The three CCB receptor sites maintain an important conformational relationship, and each site is also linked to the gating mechanism of the Ca^{2+} channel. Thus, drugs binding at the dihydropyridine site appear to increase the affinity of other drugs for the benzothiazepine site, and vice versa. However, verapamil seems to reduce the affinities of both diltiazem and the dihydropyridine CCBs for binding at their respective sites.

The activity of CCBs in particular tissues is likely dictated by the frequency of activity and hence the location of the receptor. Since the verapamil and diltiazem binding sites are located internally, deep within the channel, physical binding to the receptor is likely to be enhanced when the channel is open. Rapidly firing tissues of the myocardium and the AV node provide ample opportunity for the binding of these drugs, which are pharmacologically active in myocardial and cardiac conductive tissues. Thus, verapamil slows conduction through the AV node, producing a moderate bradycardia. Diltiazem binding is less specific than verapamil for nodal tissue and produces a mild bradycardia. The DHP class of CCBs is more dependent on the voltage-regulated state of the channel for high-affinity binding. Moreover the DHPs interact preferentially with vascular smooth muscle, which exists frequently in a depolarized state. These features explain how DHP CCBs can be associated with reflex tachycardia. This, as elaborated above, makes the DHP class relatively contraindicated where induction of a tachycardia (ischemia and tachyarrhythmias) would be considered deleterious.

Pharmacokinetics

The first-generation CCBs (diltiazem, nifedipine, and verapamil) are short-duration drugs with half-lives of 1.5–7 hours, and are therefore administered every 6–8 hours. They are associated with wide swings in plasma levels and consequently in blood pressure and heart rate. Extended-release formulations of these drugs (e.g., Calan SR, Cardizem CD, Procardia XL) have been developed to achieve stable plasma levels and once-daily administration. Isradipine, felodipine, and amlodipine have substantially longer elimination half-lives, but only amlodipine has a half-life consistent with once-daily administration.

CCBs are all well absorbed after oral administration, but there are differences in first-pass metabolism which affect bioavailability. The pharmacokinetic properties of selected CCBs are outlined in Table 46.3. Dihydropyridines are highly protein-bound [23–27], and binding with nifedipine and possibly other members of the DHP class is concentration-dependent, theoretically allowing for protein-binding interactions, although none of clinical significance have been reported. Conversely, protein binding of diltiazem [24] and verapamil [25] is not as high, but protein binding is independent of drug concentrations, making displacement interactions unlikely.

Drug metabolism

The dihydropyridines undergo metabolism by cytochrome P450 (CYP), most notably CYP3A4, which is found predominantly in the small bowel and liver [28]. There is significant potential for drug–drug interactions with the dihydropyridines. CYP3A4 inhibitors include itraconazole, ketoconazole, clarithromycin, erythromycin, nefazodone, ritonavir, and grapefruit juice. When CYP3A4 inhibitors are administered with a CCB, symptomatic hypotension has been reported. CCBs can also inhibit CYP3A4 activity, altering the disposition of other CYP3A4 substrates.

Some interactions with CYP3A4 inhibitors may also involve inhibition of the efflux transporter P-glycoprotein. P-glycoprotein, an intestinal efflux pump, counteracts passive CCB absorption and limits bioavailability. A strong overlap between P-glycoprotein and CYP3A in their substrate specificity and tissue distribution has been recognized. Mibefradil is a CCB that is a potent inhibitor of both cytochrome P450 and P-glycoprotein. Mibefradil was withdrawn from the market after drug interactions resulted in adverse events due to excessive plasma concentrations of coadministered drugs.

CCBs demonstrate age-dependent pharmacokinetic changes in association with age-related reductions in hepatic blood flow, leading to increases in bioavailability and decreases in systemic clearance [27]. This effect of age should be taken into consideration before presuming that alterations in CCB pharmacokinetics are solely renal-function-related, as most renal failure patients are older than the general population.

Adverse events

Adverse effects of CCBs have been reported to occur in 17% of patients using nifedipine, in 9% of patients using verapamil, and in 4% of those using diltiazem. The most common side effects are flushing, headache, hypotension, and pedal edema. Constipation is common with verapamil. Because of their negative inotropic effects, most CCBs, especially the non-DHPs, are contraindicated in patients with heart failure. Moreover, SA and AV nodal conduction is slowed with the use of non-DHPs, which may lead to bradycardia or heart block.

Proarrhythmia

CCBs and β-blockers account for approximately 40% of cardiovascular drug exposures reported to the American Association of Poison Control Centers. However, these drugs represent over 65% of deaths from cardiovascular medications. Diltiazem and especially verapamil tend to produce the most hypotension, bradycardia, conduction disturbances, and deaths due to CCBs. Nifedipine and other DHPs are generally less lethal and tend to produce sinus tachycardia instead of bradycardia, with fewer conduction disturbances. The proarrhythmic effects include ventricular or supraventricular arrhythmias and AV conduction disturbances. Proarrhythmia is increased in patients with structural heart disease. The

Table 46.3. Properties of selected calcium channel blockers

Drug	Volume of distribution (L kg⁻¹)	Protein binding (%)	Half-life (hours)	CYP interaction (severity/onset)	Changes in renal failure	Dosing changes with aging
Phenylalkylamines						
Verapamil	3–5	87		Minor/delayed	Minor increase	Yes
Benzothiazepines						
Diltiazem	4–7	80	25–65	Minor/delayed	No change	
Dihydropyridines (DHP)						
Amlodipine	21	98	40–50	Minor/delayed	No change	Yes
Felodipine	8–14	99	10–15	Moderate/rapid	Minor increase	Yes
Isradipine	4	96	8	Unavailable	No change	
Nicardipine	7	95	11–12	Moderate/rapid	NA	
Nifedipine	1–2	95	2	Minor/delayed	Increase	
Nimodipine	2	98	2–3	Moderate/rapid	Increase	Yes
Nisoldipine	6	99	15	Moderate/rapid		
Nitrendipine	5–6	98	3–4	Moderate/rapid		

dominant ventricular arrhythmias include torsades de pointes and ventricular tachycardia, with the commonest precipitating factors being bradyarrhythmia and hypokalemia. However, verapamil decreases torsades in animal and cellular experiments. In patients with Wolff–Parkinson–White syndrome, use of class IV drugs can be associated with decreased conduction through the AV node, which can potentially facilitate conduction over the bypass tract and result in rapid ventricular rates, which could transform into ventricular fibrillation. Diltiazem and verapamil have significant dromotropic effects and can precipitate advanced AV block in vulnerable patients. Most of the arrhythmic events are seen soon after initiation or a change in dose of these therapies, which suggests that extra vigilance is warranted at such times. Clinicians also need to be vigilant to prevent bradycardia and correct any electrolyte imbalances.

Bleeding
The non-DHPs have been linked to gastrointestinal hemorrhage in the elderly. This association is regarded as weak by the World Health Organization/International Society of Hypertension but supported by an observational study. In the case of verapamil, this possible risk did not alter the overall survival rate. Overall, the relative risk for gastrointestinal hemorrhage in observational studies with CCBs is close to unity. Nonetheless, prudence would suggest that administration of CCB be carefully considered in elderly patients with bleeding disorders.

Platelet function
All classes of CCBs inhibit ADP- and collagen-induced platelet aggregation in human blood. Diltiazem displayed the most

platelet inhibition, which was greater than that of verapamil and nifedipine [29]. The metabolites of diltiazem are powerful antiaggregatory agents, and the metabolites show greater activity than diltiazem itself. Verapamil (but not diltiazem or amlodipine) inhibited serotonin-induced platelet aggregation. One clinical study, which assessed the clinical effects of nimodopine in patients having elective valve surgery, was halted due to excess bleeding [30]. However, neither a meta-analysis of cardiac surgical patients utilizing all classes of CCBs [20] nor a propensity matched cohort study of cardiac surgery [21] exhibited excess bleeding or the need for excess transfusion. Finally, patients receiving clopidogrel and CCBs, after percutaneous coronary interventions, were found to have attenuated platelet aggregation tests compared to those who received clopidogrel alone [31].

Cancer
CCBs have been linked to cancer in the elderly, as one study with small numbers associated CCB usage with breast cancer. Five much larger studies have failed to confirm this association, and thus the risk of cancer does not appear to be increased [32].

Potentiation of anesthetic drugs
Analgesics
Numerous animal studies and several clinical studies have shown that CCBs augment opioid analgesia. However, studies in normal volunteers receiving an intravenous dose of morphine showed that pain ratings, subjective psychomotor, and physiological effects were unaffected by prior use of

CCBs. Morphine alone and in combination with the CCBs reduced pain ratings, with no statistically significant differences in the pain measures between morphine alone and CCB/morphine [33].

Muscle relaxants

The effects of verapamil and nicardipine on nondepolarizing muscle relaxants (vecuronium, atracurium, pancuronium) has been investigated using isolated rat phrenic nerve/hemidiaphragm preparations. Both CCBs caused significant depression of twitch amplitude. Verapamil significantly increased vecuronium- and atracurium-induced neuromuscular block. Nicardipine potentiated atracurium-induced neuromuscular block but had no effect on pancuronium- and vecuronium-induced twitch depression. Neostigmine did not produce any significant changes in the maximal recovery of twitch depression induced with CCBs and muscle relaxant combinations, nor did it affect maximal recovery time of twitch depression. Similarly, diltiazem has been implicated in causing increased plasma concentrations of methylprednisolone and enhanced suppression of morning plasma cortisol concentrations, suggesting caution should be used when methylprednisolone is coadministered with diltiazem [34].

Benzodiazepines

Diltiazem inhibits the metabolism of benzodiazepines, which likely occurs by inhibition of CYP3A. Patients anesthetized with midazolam and alfentanil, and concomitantly receiving diltiazem, experienced a significant delay in tracheal extubation [35].

Other drug interactions

Calcium channel antagonists are extensively metabolized by CYP3A. An important interaction occurs between grapefruit juice and DHP CCBs. For example, grapefruit juice selectively inhibits CYP3A4 in the small intestine wall and reduces first-pass metabolism, thereby increasing peak serum concentration and bioavailability. This interaction occurs more intensely with felodipine, nitrendipine, and nisoldipine than with nifedipine, nimodipine, and verapamil. Felodipine and grapefruit juice administered together resulted in lower blood pressures than felodipine alone. However this response was not sustained after 6 days of treatment with the same dose of felodipine [36]. Coadministration of CCBs and 3-hydroxy-3-methylglutaryl coenzyme A reductase inhibitors (statins) is associated with increased risk of developing myopathy or rhabdomyolysis [37].

Pharmacogenetics

Recognition of genetic differences may help explain the variability in response to CCBs and may potentially lead to individualized treatment. Several lines of evidence suggest that the variability in response to CCBs is linked to specific genes. Variability may occur in pharmacodynamics, pharmacokinetics, and consequently the magnitude of the antihypertensive response, or importantly in cardiovascular outcomes.

Calcium channels

As outlined above, calcium channels possess a regulatory β subunit. The gene that encodes the β subunit is *KCNMB1*, located on chromosome 5q34. Mice that do not express this gene have elevated blood pressure and cardiac hypertrophy. *KCNMB1* has two common single nucleotide polymorphisms (SNPs), Glu65Lys and Val110Leu. The Lys65 variant of the Glu65Lys polymorphism is associated with decreased hypertension. The protective effect of the Glu65Lys polymorphism appears to interact with age and sex, with the most significant effect being in women over 54 years old. INVEST-GENES, a randomized trial comparing verapamil to trandolapril, found that these two polymorphisms in hypertensive patients with coronary artery disease may account for the variability in response to verapamil SR [38]. The INVEST trial suggested that Val110Leu polymorphism may be associated with adverse outcomes. First, in the group randomized to verapamil, Lys65 variant carriers achieved blood pressure goals more rapidly, and required fewer drugs to achieve control. Second, the Leu110 variant allele was associated with a decreased risk of a composite cardiac outcome, which included myocardial infarction, stroke, and death.

Renal effects

There is mounting evidence that a widened pulse pressure, indicative of an increase in large-artery stiffness, is associated with cardiovascular morbidity, seen predominantly in the elderly. Pulse pressure is also a sexually dimorphic trait. Women have lower mean pulse pressure than men until their mid-50s, but it then increases with age at a rate greater than in men. Studies on pulse pressure have found associations with genes of the renin–angiotensin system. The candidate genes considered included an angiotensinogen single nucleotide polymorphism (AGT-6) on chromosome 1. The A/A genotype of the AGT-6 variant has been associated with hypertension in some studies. In the GenHAT study, a substudy of ALLHAT, the AGT-6 polymorphism showed a statistically significant genotype-by-sex interaction, where women with the G/G genotype had a lower adjusted mean pulse pressure after 6 months of treatment than women carrying an A allele. This effect was most pronounced in women randomized to amlodipine [39].

Atrial natriuretic peptide (ANP) controls fluid volume and electrolyte homeostasis. Genetically altered animals show that reduced ANP leads to hypertension, while increased ANP leads to hypotension. The plasma level of ANP has also been associated with cardiovascular events including hypertension, stroke, congestive heart failure, and hypertrophy, as well as with risk factors including insulin sensitivity. The atrial natriuretic precursor A (NPPA) gene encodes the precursor from which ANP is formed. In the GenHAT study, patients with the minor C allele had better outcomes when randomized to a diuretic, whereas patients with the TT allele (seen in approximately 50% of patients) had more favorable outcomes when receiving amlodipine [40].

Dantrolene

Malignant hyperthermia is a life-threatening sensitivity of skeletal muscles to volatile anesthetics and depolarizing neuromuscular blockers. The introduction of dantrolene decreased mortality from 80% to less than 10%. Dantrolene is the only available drug therapy for the effective treatment of malignant hyperthermia in humans.

Ryanodine receptors are channels that release Ca^{2+} from the sarcoplasmic reticulum. Activation of the L-type VGCC increases cytoplasmic Ca^{2+} concentration. Ryanodine detects this increase in Ca^{2+} concentration and amplifies this signal, releasing more Ca^{2+} from the sarcoplasmic reticulum. Mutations in ryanodine receptors have been linked to diseases including central core disease and malignant hyperthermia. The Ca^{2+} channel receptors are also peripherally involved in the mechanism of action of dantrolene. The α_1 subunit of the VGCC and RyR1 are intimate physiological partners. The opening of RyR1 induces the efflux of Ca^{2+} ions into the myoplasm.

Dantrolene attenuates the intrinsic mechanisms of excitation–contraction coupling in skeletal muscle by a mechanism thought to involve the ryanodine receptor. Inhibition of the ryanodine receptor, the major skeletal muscle Ca^{2+} release channel in the sarcoplasmic reticulum, is probably the basis of molecular action of dantrolene, sequestering intracellular Ca^{2+}. Dantrolene is also used for the treatment of spasticity and neuroleptic malignant syndrome, and it has been reported to be effective in the treatment of methylenedioxymethamphetamine ("ecstasy") intoxication.

In healthy volunteers, intravenous dantrolene 2.4 mg kg^{-1} results in plasma concentrations of 4.2 μg mL^{-1}, which were found to decrease skeletal muscle contraction by 75% [41]. Dantrolene cannot cause total paralysis regardless of the dose, which is attributed to the poor water solubility. Plasma concentrations remain within the therapeutic range for approximately 5 hours after a bolus dose. The elimination half-life time is estimated to be 12 hours [42] and approximately the same in children [43]. Dantrolene is metabolized by the liver to 5-hydroxydantrolene, which possesses muscle-relaxant properties. Dantrolene and its metabolites are excreted mainly via urine and bile. Dosing of dantrolene leads to the subjective feeling of weakness, confirmed by about a 50% reduction in grip strength.

The side effects that are most frequently observed include weakness, phlebitis, respiratory failure, and gastrointestinal upset [44]. Less frequently symptoms include confusion, dizziness, and drowsiness. Dantrolene in combination with verapamil is associated with a significant decrease in cardiac function in swine and dogs; this effect however, has not been described in humans. A marked prolongation of the neuromuscular junction recovery has been reported after vecuronium and dantrolene have been given in combination.

Dantrolene is thought to be universally effective in terminating a hyperthermic response. There have been occasional reports of death following malignant hyperthermia crisis even when treated with intravenous dantrolene. These deaths were thought to be the result of late recognition, delayed treatment, or inadequate dosage. Furthermore, deaths have been linked to inadequate supportive therapy, the development of renal failure, or the development of disseminated intravascular coagulopathy. There are no reliable data to rule out therapeutic failure. In addition, there are reports of fatality in malignant hyperthermia crisis, despite initial satisfactory response to intravenous dantrolene; these cases involve patients who could not be weaned from dantrolene therapy. A review published in 2004 provides an in-depth overview of malignant hyperthermia and dantrolene [45].

Summary

Calcium channel blockers (CCBs) are a heterogeneous group of drugs, differing in structure, Ca^{2+} channel binding sites, and tissue selectivity. They comprise three structural classes, the phenylalkylamines (i.e., verapamil), the benzothiazepines (i.e., diltiazem), and the dihydropyridines (i.e., nifedipine). The three classes interact with specific portions of the membrane-spanning region of the Ca^{2+} channel receptor protein, and each site is also linked to the gating mechanism of the Ca^{2+} channel. The dihydropyridine receptor is located on the surface of the channel, making it the most accessible and therefore widely studied. The pharmacologic profiles of phenylalkylamines and benzothiazepines are similar, but different from the dihydropyridines. In general, CCBs cause vasodilation, resulting in decreased vascular resistance with concomitantly increased blood flow, and have negative inotropic properties. Nifedipine is an effective coronary and peripheral vasodilator. Diltiazem produces coronary vasodilation but less peripheral vasodilation than nifedipine or verapamil. Verapamil is a weaker coronary vasodilator than diltiazem or nifedipine, with peripheral effects that are intermediate between the two, but is the most powerful negative inotrope. CCBs can be administered intravenously, and are all well absorbed after oral administration, but there are differences in first-pass metabolism which affect bioavailability. They undergo metabolism by cytochrome P450 3A4 (CYP3A4), and there are clinically significant drug–drug interactions with other CYP3A substrates.

Major clinical uses for CCBs include treatment of hypertension, arrhythmias (sinus tachycardia, AV nodal reentrant arrhythmias, and ventricular rate control for atrial fibrillation and atrial flutter, where diltiazem has a greater effect than verapamil on the sinus node, whereas verapamil has a preferential effect on the AV node), angina (where therapeutic effects derive from reduced oxygen demand due to decreased heart rate, contractility, and reduced arterial pressure, with a concomitant reduction in afterload, as well as coronary vasodilation), and perioperative cardioprotection.

Dantrolene, used primarily for the treatment of malignant hyperthermia, binds to the ryanodine receptor, an intracellular Ca^{2+} channel mediating excitation–contraction coupling in the sarcoplasmic reticulum, to reduce the skeletal muscle hypercontractility which occurs in an episode of malignant hyperthermia. Dantrolene is the only known treatment for malignant hyperthermia, and is highly effective, but early administration is important.

References

1. Schwartz A. Calcium antagonists: review and perspective on mechanism of action. *Am J Cardiol* 1989; **64**: 3I–9I.

2. Robertson DR, Waller DG, Renwick AG, George CF. Age-related changes in the pharmacokinetics and pharmacodynamics of nifedipine. *Br J Clin Pharm* 1988; **25**: 297–305.

3. Psaty BM, Smith NL, Siscovick DS, *et al.* Health outcomes associated with antihypertensive therapies used as first line agents: a systematic review and meta-analysis. *JAMA* 1997; **277**: 739–45.

4. Bangalore S, Sawhney S, Messerili FH. Relation of beta-blocker-induced heart rate lowering and cardioprotection in hypertension. *J Am Coll Cardiol* 2008; **52**: 1482–9.

5. Opie L, Schall R. Evidence based evaluation of calcium channel blockers for hypertension: equality of mortality and cardiovascular risk compared to conventional therapy. *J Am Coll Cardiol* 2002; **39**: 315–22.

6. Bradley H, Wiysonge CS, Volmink JA, Mayosi BM, Opie LH. How strong is the evidence for the use of beta blockers as first line therapy for hypertension? Systematic review and meta-analysis. *J Hypertens* 2006; **24**: 2131–41.

7. Reid LD, Tueth MJ, Handberg E, *et al.* A study of antihypertensive drugs and depressive symptoms (SADD-Sx) in patients treated with a calcium antagonist versus an atenolol hypertension treatment strategy in the International Vrapamil SR-Trandolapril Study (INVEST). *Psychosom Med* 2005; **67**: 398–406.

8. Yasunari K, Maeda K, Watanabe T, Nakamura M Yoshikawa J. Comparative effects of Valsartan versus Amlodipine on left ventricula mass and reactive oxygen species formation by monocytes in hypertensive patients with left ventricular hypertrophy. *J Am Coll Cardiol* 2004; **43**: 2116–23.

9. Messerli F, Bangalore S, Julius S. Should beta blockers and diuretics remain first line therapy for hypertension. *Circulation* 2008; **110**: 2707–15.

10. Kleinbloesem CH, van Brummelen P, Danhof M. Rate of increase in the plasma concentration of nifedipine as a major determinant of its hemodynamic effects in humans. *Clin Pharmacol Ther* 1987; **41**: 26–30.

11. Frohlich ED, McLoughlin MJ, Losem CJ. Hemodynamic comparison of two nifedipine formulations in patients with essential hypertension. *Am J Cardiol* 1991; **68**: 1346–50.

12. Eisenberg MJ, Brox A, Bestaros AJ. Calcium channel blockers: an update. *Am J Med* 2004; **116**: 35–43.

13. Jespersen CM, Hansen JF, Mortensen LS. The prognostic significance of post infarction angina pectoris and the effect of verapamil on the incidence of angina and prognosis. The Danish Study Group on Verapamil in Myocardial Infarction. *Eur Heart J* 1994; **15**: 270–6.

14. Sica DA, Geher TW. Calcium-channel blockers and end-stage renal disease: pharmacokinetic and pharmacodynamic considerations. *Curr Opin Nephrol Hypertens* 2003; **12**: 123–31.

15. Tisler A, Akocsi K, Harshegyi I. Comparison of dialysis and clinical characteristics of patients with frequent and occasional hemodialysis associated hypotension. *Kidney Blood Press Res* 2002; **25**: 97–102.

16. Kestenbaum B, Gillen DL, Sherrard DJ, *et al.* Calcium channel blocker use and mortality among patients with endstage renal disease. *Kidney Int* 2002; **61**: 2157–64.

17. Fleisher LA, Beckman JA, Brown KA, *et al.* ACC/AHA 2007 guidelines on perioperative cardiovascular evaluation and care for noncardiac surgery: executive summary: a report of the American College of Cardiology/ American Heart Association Task Force on Practice Guidelines. *Anesth Analg* 2008; **106**: 685–712.

18. Wijeysundera DN, Beattie WS. Calcium channel blockers for reducing cardiac morbidity after noncardiac surgery: a meta-analysis. *Anesth Analg* 2003; **97**: 634–41.

19. Devereaux PJ, Beattie WS, Choi PT, *et al.* How strong is the evidence for the use of perioperative beta blockers in non-cardiac surgery? Systematic review and meta-analysis of randomised controlled trials. *BMJ* 2005; **331**: 313–21.

20. Wijeysundera DN, Beattie WS, Rao V, Karski J. Calcium antagonists reduce cardiovascular complications after cardiac surgery: a meta-analysis. *J Am Coll Cardiol* 2003; **41**: 1496–505.

21. Wijeysundera DN, Beattie WS, Rao V, Ivanov J, Karkouti K. Calcium antagonists are associated with reduced mortality after cardiac surgery: a propensity analysis. *J Thorac Cardiovasc Surg* 2004; **127**: 755–62.

22. Bodi I, Mikala G, Koch SE, Akhter SA, Schwartz A. The L-type calcium channel in the heart: the beat goes on. *Journal Clin Invest* 2005; **115**: 3306–17.

23. Soons PA, Ankermann T, Breimer DD, Kirch W. Stereoselective pharmacokinetics of oral nitrendipine in elderly hypertensive patients with normal and impaired renal function. *Eur J Clin Pharm* 1992; **42**: 423–7.

24. Tawashi M, Marc-Aurele J, Bichet D, *et al.* Pharmacokinetics of intravenous diltiazem and five of its metabolites in patients with chronic renal failure and in healthy volunteers. *Biopharm Drug Dispo* 1991; **12**: 105–12.

25. Keefe DL, Yee YG, Kates RE. Verapamil protein binding in patients and in normal subjects. *Clinical Phamacol Ther* 1981; **29**: 21–6.

26. Wandel C, Kim RB, Guengrich FP, Wood AJ. Mibefradil is a P-glycoprotein

substrate and a potent inhibitor of both P-glycoprotein and CYP3A in vitro. *Drug Metab Dispos* 2000; **28**: 895–8.

27. Elliott HL, Meredith PA, Reid JL, Faulkner JK. A comparison of the disposition of single oral doses of amlodipine in young and elderly subjects. *Pharmacology* 1988; **12**: S64–6.

28. Zhang Y, Benet LZ. The gut as a barrier to drug absorption: combined role of cytochrome P450 3A and P-Glycoprotein. *Clin Pharmacokinet* 2001; **12**: 326–32.

29. Thaulow E. Pharmacologic effects of calcium channel blockers on restenosis. *J Cardiovasc Pharmacol* 1999; **33** (Suppl 2): S12–16.

30. Legault C, Furberg CD, Wagenknect LE. Nimodipine neuroprotectionin cardiac valve replacement: report of an early terminated trial. *Stroke* 1996; **27**: 593–8.

31. Siller-Mantula LM, Lang I, Christ G, Jilma B. Calcium channel blockers reduce the anti-platelet effect of clopidogrel. *J Am Coll Cardiol* 2008; **52**: 1557–63.

32. Assimes TL, Elstein E, Langleben A, Suissa S. Long-term use of antihypertensive drugs and the risk of cancer. *Pharmacoepidemiol Drug Saf* 2008; **11**: 1039–49.

33. Zarauza R, Sáez-Fernández AN, Iribarren M, *et al.* A comparative study with oral nifedipine, intravenous nimodipine, and magnesium sulfate in postoperative analgesia. *Anesth Analg* 2000; **91**: 938–43.

34. Booker BM, Magee MH, Blum RA, Lates CD, Jusko WJ. Pharmacokinetic and pharmacodynamic interactions between diltiazem and methylprednisolone in healthy volunteers. *Clin Pharmacol Ther* 2002; **72**: 370–82.

35. Ahonen J, Olkkola KT, Salmenpera M, Hynynen M, Neuvonen PJ. Effect of diltiazem on midazolam and alfentanil disposition in patients undergoing coronary artery bypass grafting. *Anesthesiology* 1996; **85**: 1246–52.

36. Sica D. Interaction of grapefruit juice and calcium channel blockers. *Am J Hypertens* 2006; **19**: 768–73.

37. Lewin JJ, Nappi JM, Taylor MH. Rhabdomyolysis with concurrent atorvastatin and diltiazem. *Ann Pharmacother* 2002; **36**: 1546–9.

38. Beitelshees A, Gong Y, Wang D, *et al.* KCNMB1 genotype influences response to verapamil SR and adverse outcomes in the International Verapamil SR/ Trandolapril Study (INVEST). *Pharmacogenet Genomics* 2007; **17**: 719–29.

39. Lynch AI, Arnett DK, Davis BR, *et al.* Sex-specific effects of AGT-6 and ACE I/D on pulse pressure after 6 months of antihypertensive therapy. *Ann Hum Genet* 2007; **71**: 735–45.

40. Lynch AI, Boerwinkle E, Davis BR, *et al.* Pharmacogenetic association of the NPPA T2238C genetic variant with cardiovascular disease outcomes in patients with hypertension. *JAMA* 2008; **299**: 296–307.

41. Flewellen EH, Nelson PE, Jones WP, Arens JF, Wagner DL. Dantrolene dose-response in awake man: implications for management of malignant hyperthermia. *Anesthesiology* 1983; **59**: 275–80.

42. Ellis KO, Carpenter JF. Mechanism of control of skeletal-muscle contraction by dantrolene sodium. *Arch Phys Med Rehabil* 1974; **55**: 362–9.

43. Lerman J, McLeod ME, Strong HA. Pharmacokinetics of intravenous dantrolene in children. *Anesthesiology* 1989; **70**: 625–9.

44. Brandom BW, Larach MG. The North American Malignant Hyperthermia Registry. Reassessment of the safety and efficacy of dantrolene. *Anesthesiology* 2002; **96**: A1199.

45. Krause T, Gerbershagen MU, Feige M, Weibhorn R, Wappler F. Dantrolene: a review of its pharmacology, therapeutic use and new developments. *Anesthesia* 2004; **59**: 364–73.

Introduction

In this chapter the various therapies for the chronic maintenance and acute exacerbations of asthmatic symptoms are explored by discussing (1) their mechanisms of drug action, (2) their preclinical pharmacology, and (3) their clinical pharmacology. The practical aspects of drug administration are also covered for β-adrenoceptor agonists, methylxanthines (theophylline), anticholinergics, corticosteroids, and anti-inflammatory drugs (nedocromil sodium, sodium cromoglycate, leukotriene antagonists, 5-lipoxygenase inhibitors, and omalizumab). Volatile anesthetics are also recognized as potent bronchodilators that are used when traditional therapies fail to relieve status asthmaticus, and promising emerging therapies are highlighted.

β-Adrenoceptor agonists

History and background

β-Adrenoceptor agonists, delivered via inhalation, are a mainstay in the treatment of asthma. Epinephrine was initially used systemically to achieve bronchodilation, but with the recognition of adrenoceptor classes (α and β) [1] the β-selective agonist isoproterenol evolved as the drug of choice [2]. However, its catecholamine structure rendered it unstable and it was replaced by the more chemically stable compound metaproterenol [3]. The discovery of subtypes of β-adrenoceptors led to the development of selective β_2-agonists devoid of the side effects of tachycardia that accompanied the nonselective β-agonists. Metaproterenol was the first β_2-selective agonist introduced for asthma therapy, followed by albuterol with increased β_2-selectivity, and despite the introduction of many other β_2-selective agonists (e.g., terbutaline, feneterol, procaterol), albuterol has remained the most widely used β_2-selective agonist in the acute treatment of asthma. Attempts to further enhance the selectivity of β_2-agonists (and presumably decrease side effects such as vasodilation and skeletal muscle tremor) led to the introduction of levalbuterol, a pure R-isomer of albuterol. Despite their high efficacy in achieving bronchodilation, albuterol and terbutaline have a relatively short duration of action (up to 4–6 hours),

which makes their clinical utility in asthma maintenance therapy limited. Therefore, long-duration β_2-selective agonists were introduced (salmeterol [4] and formoterol [5]) in an attempt to maintain β-agonist-mediated bronchodilation for up to 12 hours. Formoterol was developed due to its increased affinity for the β_2-adrenoceptor, while salmeterol contains a large lipophilic modification to facilitate binding to hydrophobic regions of the cell membrane. Although these long-acting formulations do provide extended relief, particularly useful in nocturnal asthma, they are not intended for acute rescue therapy during acute exacerbations of symptoms, because of their slower onset of action in comparison to albuterol or terbutaline.

Mechanisms of drug action

β_2-Adrenoeptors belong to a large family of proteins structurally characterized by seven transmembrane-spanning regions with a carboxy-terminal intracellular tail that couple to heterotrimeric G proteins to convey their signal to intracellular enzymes that effect second messengers. Indeed, it was studies of the β-adrenoceptor that elucidated classic receptor–G-protein interactions (discussed in Chapter 2) and mechanisms of receptor desensitization and downregulation.

Attempts to define the genetic determinants of asthma have evaluated the association of asthma with single nucleotide polymorphisms (SNPs) of the β_2-adrenoceptor. SNPs have been identified in both the promoter region and protein coding region of the human β_2-adrenoceptor gene. Nine different SNPs have been described within the protein coding region [6], the most frequent (30–45%) of which is substitution of a glycine residue for an arginine residue at amino acid position 16 in the receptor protein, resulting in an enhanced rate of receptor desensitization [6,7]. A second SNP results in the substitution of a glutamine residue for a glutamic acid residue at amino acid position 27, resulting in a decreased rate of receptor desensitization [6,7]. The most comprehensive studies to date have evaluated the incidence and severity of asthma and the response to therapy in subjects with the Gly16 and Glu27 polymorphisms. Multiple studies have shown that the presence of polymorphisms at these sites cannot alone account for the presence of

Anesthetic Pharmacology, 2nd edition, ed. Alex S. Evers, Mervyn Maze, Evan D. Kharasch. Published by Cambridge University Press. © Cambridge University Press 2011.

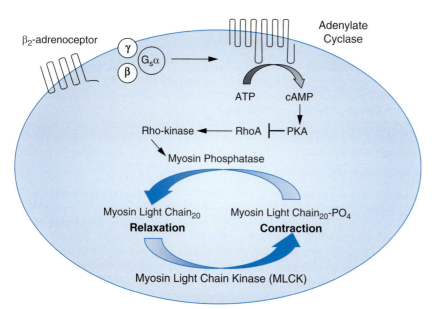

Figure 47.1. β-Adrenoceptor-mediated airway smooth-muscle relaxation. Rho-kinase normally phosphorylates and thus inhibits myosin phosphatase, favoring contraction. In the presence of β-adrenoceptor agonists, increased cyclic adenosine monophosphate (cAMP) and protein kinase A (PKA) inhibit RhoA, which inhibits Rho-kinase, increasing the activity of myosin phosphatase. The net result is dephosphorylation of myosin light chain$_{20}$ and relaxation. → indicates activation; ⊥ indicates inhibition.

asthma [8–11], but that these polymorphisms are associated with the severity of airway hyperresponsiveness [9,12] and predict airway responses to histamine constriction and β-agonist-mediated airway relaxation [13].

Preclinical pharmacology

β$_2$-adrenoceptors are widely expressed in many cell types, and activation universally results in increases in cellular levels of cyclic adenosine monophosphate (cAMP) (Fig. 47.1). However, the downstream signaling events that result from increased cellular levels of cAMP are cell-type-specific. For example, smooth-muscle cells of the airway and uterus relax in response to cAMP [14], while cardiac myocytes exhibit increased contractility [15].

Clinical pharmacology

The dose of a β-agonist aerosol deposited at the active site in the lungs (i.e., smooth muscle of large and intermediate-sized airways) is a fraction of the inhaled dose, which in turn is a fraction of the dose delivered with each actuation. The determinants of the amount of drug that reach target tissues include the particle size of the aerosol, the velocity at which it is released from the delivery device, the patient's inhalation technique, and the degree of airway narrowing. In some cases, the addition of a device-specific spacer increases the amount of aerosol reaching its airway target by keeping more of the drug aerosolized within the spacer, thus not allowing the drug to deposit in the oral cavity and oropharynx. The largest single factor that determines the amount and reproducibility of drug deposition at the smooth-muscle target is the patient's technique of inhaler use. Approximately 90 μg of albuterol is delivered per actuation of a metered dose inhaler, and it is estimated that with proper technique approximately 18 μg is deposited in the lung. Following its slow adsorption from

the lung, aerosolized albuterol achieves peak serum concentrations in 2–4 hours. Urinary excretion studies reveal a half-life of 3.8 hours. Within 24 hours of an inhaled dose, 72% is excreted in the urine, 28% as unchanged drug and 44% as metabolite. The time to onset of improved respiratory function following aerosolized albuterol is 15 minutes as determined by improvements in both forced expiratory volume in 1 second (FEV$_1$) and maximal midexpiratory flow rate (MMEF). Maximal improvement occurs within 60–90 minutes, with a duration of effect for 3–6 hours.

Adverse effects of β-agonists are attributable to elevation of cAMP levels in nontarget tissues and are typical of effects of sympathomimetic drugs. While tremor and nervousness are the most frequently reported adverse effects, tachycardia, hypertension, palpitations, nausea, and vomiting have also been reported.

Until recently, all marketed β-agonists were racemic preparations, even though they were historically designed to mimic the bronchodilatory effect of endogenous epinephrine, which is an isomerically pure R-isomer (R-epinephrine). Indeed, the bronchodilatory effects of albuterol are mediated by the R-isomer while the S-isomer has no therapeutic benefit. In fact, the S-isomer of albuterol has been shown to have effects on airway smooth muscle that would be expected to be detrimental to airway relaxation. The S-isomer of albuterol was shown to increase intracellular calcium concentrations accompanied by increased cell shortening [16]. Eosinophils exposed to S-albuterol exhibit enhanced superoxide production, a potential proinflammatory effect; this may partially account for the discrepancy between β-agonists' anti-inflammatory action in vitro and their lack of clinical anti-inflammatory effects [17]. The enhanced bronchodilatory effect of the R-isomer of albuterol on human airway smooth muscle has led to the clinical introduction of levalbuterol and

(R,R)-formoterol, which during phase II clinical studies demonstrated an increase in FEV$_1$ for 24 hours [18].

Practical aspects of drug administration

β-adrenergic agonists are the primary prescribed therapy for the chronic maintenance and acute exacerbations of asthmatic symptoms. Acute exacerbations are treated with rapidly acting drugs (e.g., albuterol, onset 5–7 minutes); however, their duration is limited (4–6 hours). Improved duration can be achieved with salmeterol or formoterol (10–12 hours), but because of their slow onset (35 minutes) they are not useful during acute exacerbations. Rapidly acting drugs (e.g., albuterol, levalbuterol, metaproterenol, pirbuterol) are available as sole drugs, while long-acting β$_2$-adrenoceptor agonists are combined with inhaled corticosteroids (salmeterol + fluticasone or formoterol + budesonide). Concerns over increased asthma deaths associated with the use of long-acting β$_2$ agonists [19] have led to restrictions in their use and formulations in the USA, with recommendations that long-acting β$_2$-agonists should only be used if combined with inhaled corticosteroids.

β-Agonists are available as oral, intravenous, subcutaneous, and inhalational formulations. Inhalational administration is generally preferred because it delivers larger doses directly to the airways, minimizing systemic toxicity, particularly on the cardiovascular system. Despite the relative β$_2$-selectivity of these drugs, higher systemic doses can stimulate both β$_1$ and β$_2$ cardiac adrenoceptors. Inhalation of albuterol (proventil or ventolin) by metered dose inhaler results in the delivery of 90–108 μg of albuterol per actuation. The speed of onset ranges from 6 to 15 minutes, with a duration of effect for 3–6 hours. Prophylactic administration of β-agonists before exercise is beneficial in exercise-induced asthma, and prophylactic administration of β-agonists or anticholinergic drugs 1 hour before induction of general anesthesia with intubation resulted in reduced airway resistance following endotracheal intubation [20].

Inhalational administration of β-agonists can be achieved using a pressurized metered dose inhaler (MDI) with or without a spacing device, a nebulizer, or a dry-powder inhaler. Albuterol, metaproterenol, pirbuterol, and salmeterol, are available in MDIs, while albuterol, pirbuterol, salmeterol, and formoterol are available in dry powder inhalers. Albuterol, metaproterenol, and levalbuterol are available for nebulization. MDIs have traditionally been powered by chlorofluorcarbons (CFCs), but international agreements targeted at eliminating CFCs because of their detrimental effects on the earth's ozone layer have resulted in reformulations of several β-agonists powered by hydrofluoroalkane (HFA) propellants. Additionally, dry-powder inhalers actuated by the patient's inspiratory flow rate are increasing in popularity for β-agonist and inhaled steroid delivery because they do not require a propellant and do not require close patient coordination between drug dispensing and the initiation of inspiration.

β-Agonists are available for oral administration in both tablet and syrup formulations. Albuterol (4–8 mg), metaproterenol (10 mg), and terbutaline (5 mg) are available in standard and delayed-release tablet form, while albuterol and metaproterenol are available in syrup formulation. β-Agonists are rapidly and well absorbed following oral administration, but the time of onset for bronchodilating properties is 30 minutes (as compared to 6–15 minutes via the aerosol route). Peak plasma levels following 2 mg and 4 mg albuterol doses are 6.7 and 14.8 ng mL^{-1}, respectively. Maximal serum levels occur 2–3 hours after dosing, with an elimination half-life of 5–6 hours. Albuterol has been formulated to provide a duration of action of up to 12 hours (Proventil Repetabs).

Terbutaline is the only selective β$_2$-adrenoceptor agonist available for parenteral (subcutaneous) use. It may be advantageous in acute exacerbations of asthma where inhaled β-agonists have not adequately reversed bronchospasm and oral therapy is not appropriate (e.g., anesthetized patients). Subcutaneous terbutaline is most widely used as a tocolytic drug, because of the relaxing effects of β-agonists on the smooth muscle of the uterus. The usual initial dose is 0.25 mg, which can be repeated in 15–30 minutes if no clinical improvement is seen. The total subcutaneous dose within 4 hours should not exceed 0.5 mg.

Methylxanthines

Theophylline is a methylxanthine derivative that inhibits adenosine receptors, facilitating release of catecholamines [21], and at very high concentrations inhibits phosphodiesterases, enzymes responsible for the degradation of cAMP. Aminophylline is a water-soluble salt of theophylline that can be administered orally or intravenously. Theophylline remains the mostly widely prescribed medication for asthma in the world because it is inexpensive. However, in industrialized countries theophylline is typically third-line therapy for bronchodilation because of systemic toxicity, and it is reserved for severe asthmatics not controlled with β-agonists and steroids. Although it is not typically the first choice for bronchodilating effects, the emerging understanding of theophylline's anti-inflammatory effects is contributing to a re-evaluation of its role in chronic asthma management.

Acute asthmatic exacerbations in anesthetized patients are typically treated with β-agonists and increased concentrations of volatile anesthetics. However, during emergence, in patients who are not candidates for deep extubation, the addition of theophylline may be of theoretical benefit during awakening with an endotracheal tube in place. However, the combination of theophylline and halothane can be quite proarrhythmogenic because of halothane's ability to sensitize the myocardium to the catecholamines released by theophylline [22]. The use of theophylline during the maintenance phase of inhalational anesthesia appears to have no added bronchodilator effect over that of the volatile drugs [23].

Preclinical pharmacology

Theophylline is a nonselective inhibitor of phosphodiesterases leading to increased cellular concentrations of cAMP and cyclic guanosine monophosphate (cGMP). Theophylline inhibits phosphodiesterases at high concentrations, but also increases the secretion of epinephrine from the adrenal medulla, inhibits adenosine receptors, and decreases airway inflammation. Despite 60 years of clinical use, the predominant mechanism of theophylline-induced bronchodilation remains in debate. The release of epinephrine from the adrenal medulla results in a small increase in plasma concentrations of epinephrine that may be too small to account for any bronchodilator effect. Theophylline, at therapeutic concentrations, inhibits only 5–10% of total phosphodiesterase activity in human lung extracts [24]. However, in vitro, the concentration of theophylline that inhibits phosphodiesterases is similar to the concentration that relaxes airway smooth muscle [25]. A theophylline derivative, 8-phenyltheophylline, inhibits adenosine receptors but does not inhibit phosphodiesterases and does not cause airway smooth-muscle relaxation, suggesting that adenosine receptor antagonism is not a mechanism by which xanthines promote bronchodilation [25]. Thus, it may be a combination of effects of theophylline including catecholamine release, phosphodiesterase inhibition, and inflammatory inhibition that contribute to smooth-muscle relaxation and bronchodilation.

Clinical pharmacology

Theophylline is rapidly and completely absorbed after oral administration whether in solution or tablet form. The drug distributes freely into fat-free tissues and is extensively metabolized in the liver. Its pharmacokinetics vary widely among similar patients and cannot be predicted based on gender, age, body weight, or other demographic characteristics. Moreover, its metabolism and clearance is greatly affected by concurrent disease states and altered physiology including liver disease, cystic fibrosis, pulmonary edema, chronic obstructive pulmonary disease (COPD), thyroid disease, pregnancy, and sepsis with multi-organ failure. Multiple concurrent medications are known to enhance (carbamazepine, rifampin) or inhibit (cimetidine, erythromycin, tacrine) the liver metabolism of theophylline. Specific drug interactions with numerous anesthetic-related medications have been described. An increased risk of ventricular arrhythmias occurs when theophylline is used in the presence of halothane because of the sensitizing effects of halothane on the myocardium to increased catecholamines released by theophylline. Larger doses of benzodiazepines may be needed to achieve the desired effect in the presence of theophylline, as benzodiazepines increase the central nervous system (CNS) concentrations of adenosine, a potent CNS depressant, while theophylline blocks adenosine receptors. Ketamine may lower the theophylline seizure threshold, and theophylline can antagonize the effect of nonpolarizing muscle relaxants, possibly due to phosphodiesterase inhibition.

Theophylline has effects on many physiological processes including CNS stimulation, tachycardia, decreased peripheral vascular resistance, increased cerebral vascular resistance, smooth-muscle relaxation, diuresis, and increased

secretion by endocrine and exocrine tissues (e.g., gastrin, parathyroid hormone). Theophylline serum concentrations only slightly above recommended therapeutic ranges (10–20 $\mu g\,mL^{-1}$) can produce nervousness, restlessness, insomnia, tremors, hyperesthesia. At higher serum concentrations, focal and generalized seizure activity can occur; seizures have been reported at serum concentrations only 50% above the upper limit of the accepted therapeutic range. Methylxanthines stimulate the medullary respiratory centers by increasing the sensitivity of these centers to CO_2. Theophylline-induced emesis is common when serum concentrations exceed 15 $\mu g\,mL^{-1}$, and this effect is likely centrally mediated. At therapeutic concentrations, theophylline produces a modest increase in heart rate [26]. At higher concentrations, tachycardia is experienced and some individuals may experience arrhythmias such as premature ventricular contractions. Therapeutic levels of theophylline reduce the left ventricular time index and isovolumetric contraction time, indicative of increased contractility and decreased preload [26]. Although some of these cardiac effects are likely due to direct effects on the heart, they are likely augmented by the release of catecholamines from the adrenal glands by theophylline. Methylxanthines decrease peripheral vascular resistance [26] but increase cerebrovascular resistance, with accompanying decreases in cerebral blood flow and brain oxygen tension [27]. This vasoconstriction is thought to account for the relief of hypertensive headaches by methlyxanthines and the relief of postdural puncture headaches caused by intracranial arterial and venous dilation [28]. Theophylline increases the production of urine by inhibiting solute reabsorption without changing total renal blood flow or glomerular filtration [29].

Practical aspects of drug administration

Theophylline preparations are indicated for the treatment of bronchospasm, but in developed countries its use has been largely supplanted by inhaled β-agonists and inhaled steroids. Its newly recognized effect as an anti-inflammatory drug has led some to suggest that it may reappear in the management of asthma. However, its narrow therapeutic index and vast range of serious systemic side effects may limit a renewed interest in this medication. Moreover, newer anti-inflammatory drugs directed against selective components of inflammation may dampen the enthusiasm for reintroducing theophylline as an anti-inflammatory drug. Methylxanthines have also been used in various respiratory failure syndromes, making use of its effect on the medullary respiratory centers of the CNS, its improvement in respiratory muscle mechanics, and its improvement in blood flow to muscles of respiration [30].

Anticholinergics

Mechanisms of drug action

Anticholinergic drugs promote airway relaxation by inhibiting M_2 and M_3 muscarinic receptors on airway smooth muscle

[31]. Normally the release of acetylcholine from parasympathetic nerves activates muscle M_3 muscarinic receptors which couple through the G_q protein to activate phospholipase C, which in turn liberates inositol trisphosphates, increasing intracellular calcium and initiating muscle contraction. Acetylcholine also activates muscle M_2 muscarinic receptors which act through G_i proteins to inhibit G_s-mediated relaxation and also activate the small G protein RhoA that ultimately inactivates a myosin phosphatase and maintains smooth-muscle contraction. Interestingly, M_2 muscarinic receptors also exist on the postganglionic prejunctional parasympathetic nerve itself to function as an autofeedback receptor inhibiting further acetylcholine release. The release of acetylcholine from parasympathetic nerves increases during exacerbations of asthma [32] and during the introduction of foreign substances into the well-innervated upper trachea (e.g., during endotracheal intubation) [33]. The systemic administration of anticholinergics is limited by systemic side effects, and therefore ipratropium bromide and tiotropium bromide are commonly administered via inhalation using either an MDI for ipratropium bromide or a dry-powder delivery device for tiotropium bromide.

Preclinical pharmacology

At least one animal study has shown that lower doses of ipratropium may cause bronchoconstriction (presumably due to blockade of prejunctional M_2 muscarinic autoreceptors on the parasympathetic nerve) while higher doses of ipratropium produce bronchodilation (presumably due to blockade of M_3 muscarinic receptors on airway smooth muscle) [34].

Clinical pharmacology

Most studies have suggested that inhaled anticholinergic drugs supplement rather than replace other bronchodilators (such as β-agonists). During acute exacerbations of asthma the combination of nebulized ipratropium with β-agonists has been shown in some studies to more quickly and completely relieve bronchoconstriction [35,36], while other studies have failed to show a benefit [37]. A meta-analysis of 10 studies showed a small benefit of ipratropium when added to β-agonists, but severe asthmatics benefited the most and the rate of hospital admissions from the emergency department was decreased [38].

Practical aspects of drug administration

Oral anticholinergics have only marginal anti-asthma activity and intolerable side effects such as urinary retention and visual accommodation impairments. Therefore, only the inhaled formulations of anticholinergics (ipratropium, oxitropium, tiotropium) are practical anti-asthma therapy. Inhaled anticholinergics have a slower time of onset and a slower time to peak effect than β-agonists, such that β-agonists are considered to be superior choices for acute rescue therapy. Anticholinergics (ipratropium bromide by aerosol or nebulizer or tiotropium bromide by dry powder inhalation) may be used as rescue therapy in patients who experience side effects from traditional β-agonist therapies or in patients who fail to completely respond to β-agonists, but they have found their highest efficacy in patients with COPD. Bronchospasm induced by the introduction of an endotracheal tube into the trachea, inducing an irritant reflex arc, may be particularly responsive to anticholinergic therapy since this reflex is thought to be mediated by acetylcholine from parasympathetic nerves acting on muscarinic receptors of airway smooth muscle. Indeed, nine asthmatics who developed bronchospasm following intubation improved with endotracheal ipratropium therapy [39] and prophylactic ipratropium before intubation was shown to reduce lung resistance following intubation in smokers [40]. Ipratropium bromide is available both in a metered dose inhaler and for nebulization. Tiotropium bromide has a longer duration of action (24 hours) than ipratropium, such that it is preferred as a component of long-term maintenance therapy in COPD with once-daily dosing using a proprietary inhaler [41].

Viral infections have been shown to cause dysfunction of the M_2 muscarinic autoreceptor of parasympathetic nerves resulting in increased release of acetylcholine [42]. Patients with recent upper respiratory tract infections may therefore have a greater benefit from anticholinergics than β-agonist therapy.

Volatile anesthetics as bronchodilators

Volatile anesthetics are such potent bronchodilators that they have been used when traditional therapies have failed to relieve status asthmaticus [43,44]. Animal studies have shown dose-dependent decreases in airway resistance with halothane and isoflurane [45]. The bronchodilatory effect of halothane was shown to be additive to that of β-agonists [46]. High-resolution computer tomography of small canine airways (<3 mm) during inhalational anesthesia revealed that halothane dilated histamine-constricted airways to a greater extent than isoflurane at 0.6 and 1.1 MAC concentrations. At 1.7 MAC the two drugs dilated histamine-constricted airways to a similar extent [45]. One MAC of sevoflurane was shown to be as effective as 1 MAC of isoflurane in attenuating bronchoconstriction caused by induced anaphylaxis in dogs [47]. Dilation of isolated human airways has been demonstrated with volatile anesthetics with an order of potency of halothane > isoflurane > desflurane [48]. In nonasthmatic humans, 1.1 MAC concentrations of halothane, isoflurane, and sevoflurane decreased respiratory system resistance following tracheal intubation, with sevoflurane exhibiting the greatest effect [49]. In another study of nonasthmatics, 1 MAC of sevoflurane but not desflurane was shown to decrease respiratory system resistance following intubation. In contrast, in a subset of patients who smoked, respiratory system resistance actually *increased* in the presence of desflurane [50].

The mechanism by which volatile anesthetics facilitate bronchodilation is incompletely understood. Relaxation is facilitated by both neural and direct muscle effects.

Sevoflurane, desflurane, and halothane have been shown to attenuate guinea pig tracheal contractions in response to both electrical field stimulation and direct addition of acetylcholine, suggesting an effect on neural release of acetylcholine from parasympathetic nerves and a direct effect on muscarinic receptor modulation of contraction in the airway smooth muscle itself [51]. Halothane decreases calcium sensitivity of the contractile apparatus in airway smooth muscle [52], at least in part due to decreases in regulatory myosin light chain phosphorylation resulting from increased smooth-muscle protein phosphatase activity [53]. Halothane appears to have a greater effect on calcium sensitivity than either sevoflurane or isoflurane [54]. An additional mechanism by which volatile anesthetics directly facilitate airway smooth-muscle relaxation is by impeding the entry of extracellular calcium via voltage-gated calcium channels (VGCCs). Halothane, isoflurane, and sevoflurane dose-dependently inhibit the entry of extracellular calcium in airway smooth muscle via VGCCs [55]. T-type VGCCs in bronchi were more sensitive to isoflurane and sevoflurane than L-type channels in trachea [56].

Corticosteroids

Inhaled corticosteroids are widely recommended as first-line therapy for persistent asthma. The benefits of steroids in asthma have been recognized for over 40 years. It is widely accepted that asthma is an inflammatory disease of the lung, and it is now apparent that the inclusion of inhaled steroids in an asthma management regimen reduces both hospitalization rates and mortality from asthma [57]. The realization of the combined benefit of inhaled corticosteroids and inhaled β-agonists has led to the development of inhalers that deliver both drugs simultaneously (e.g., budesonide/formoterol, fluticasone/salmeterol) [58,59].

Mechanisms of drug action
The mechanism of action of corticosteroids is reviewed in Chapter 51.

Preclinical pharmacology
Lymphocytes, eosinophils, neutrophils, macrophages, monocytes, mast cells, and basophils all have potential roles in the inflammatory response in the lung in asthma, and the contributions to inflammation of all of these cells are effected by steroids. Much attention has been focused on the role of cytokines liberated from specific subsets of T helper (Th) lymphocytes. Studies in mice [60] and humans have revealed that a component of airway inflammation in asthma is orchestrated by CD+ Th2 cells that secrete the cytokines IL-4, IL-5, and IL-13, while interferon γ (IFNγ), secreted by Th1 cells, suppresses the development and effector functions of Th2 cells. An attractive approach to modulating airway inflammation has been to selectively modulate the activity of Th1/Th2 lymphocytes [61]. The amount of eosinophils in peripheral blood and in bronchoalveolar lavage specimens has been correlated with the severity of asthma, and corticosteroids reduce their numbers [62]. Glucocorticoids also inhibit IL-4- and IL-5-mediated survival and enhance eosinophil apoptosis [63]. The roles of neutrophils in asthma is less clear, but infiltration of skin, airways, and mucosa has been demonstrated after inhaled antigen challenge. Neutrophil influx following nasal challenge was inhibited by topical corticosteroids [64]. Mast cells are known to be increased in both number and releasability of their inflammatory mediators in asthmatic airways [65]. Asthmatic airways are also more sensitive to the bronchospastic mediators released by mast cells [66]. The number of mast cells in the epithelium and mucosa of asthmatic patients is reduced by inhaled glucocorticoids, and mast cell apoptosis is increased by glucocorticoid-mediated withdrawal of IL-3 [67].

Numerous in-vivo animal studies have evaluated the benefit of corticosteroids on airway responses. Chronic systemic steroids (4–7 weeks) were shown to decrease methacholine-induced bronchoconstriction and to decrease propranolol-induced airway hyperresponsiveness in the Basenji-greyhound dog model of airway hyperresponsiveness [68]. These dogs also showed increased sensitivity to β-adrenoceptor bronchodilation following 48 hours of systemic corticosteroid therapy [69]. At least part of this in-vivo benefit of steroids on methacholine-induced bronchoconstriction may be accounted for by a reduced number of M_2 and M_3 muscarinic receptors in airway smooth muscle following 3 days of systemic glucocorticoid but not mineralocorticoid therapy [70]. An additional mechanism that may contribute to improved β-adrenoceptor response following glucocorticoid therapy is increased expression of β-adrenoceptors [71] and G_s protein [72]. The inhaled corticosteroid budesonide was shown to reduce both ozone- and allergen-induced increases in airway hyperresponsiveness in dogs [73,74]. In a model of antigen-challenged guinea pigs, whose airway dysfunction is mediated by eosinophil recruitment and neural M_2 muscarinic receptor dysfunction, systemic dexamethasone reduced eosinophil recruitment to the nerves and eliminated the neural M_2 receptor dysfunction [75]. Inhaled fluticasone decreased airway remodeling induced by ovalbumin sensitization in rats [76].

Clinical pharmacology
The clinical pharmacology is detailed in Chapter 51. Numerous studies have evaluated the effectiveness of inhaled steroids and the reduced risk of systemic complications with inhaled versus systemic steroid administration. Efficacy of inhaled corticosteroids has been shown in many studies [77,78], usually comparable to benefits demonstrated with systemic steroids but with fewer long-term side effects. Studies have shown patients discharged from the emergency room on either 40 mg of oral prednisone once a day or 600 μg of budesonide via inhalation four times a day had similar relapse rates of asthma, and similar improvements in FEV$_1$, asthma symptoms, and peak expiratory flow [77]. Inhaled steroids have also been

shown to reduce or eliminate the need for systemic steroids in severe asthmatics [79].

It is generally accepted that inhaled corticosteroid use has reduced the systemic complications of chronic systemic steroids, making routine steroids commonplace in the management of many asthmatic adults. However, it should not be assumed that inhaled steroids are without possible detrimental systemic effects when chronically used. Although some studies report no or minimal effects on the hypothalamic–pituitary–adrenal axis, bone density, cataracts, or glaucoma [80,81], other studies conclude that dose-related adrenal suppression, reduction in bone density, and posterior subcapsular cataracts occur with chronic use of all inhaled steroids [82]. The chronic effects of inhaled steroids in asthmatic children is of particular concern because of possible effects on skeletal development. Children treated for 20 months with beclomethasone, but not fluticasone, showed reduced skeletal growth rates during the final months of the study [83]. Serum cortisol significantly decreased with beclomethasone but not with fluticasone [84]. A comparison of fluticasone and budesonide in asthmatic adults, where doses effective for improvement of asthma symptoms were accounted for along with changes in serum cortisol and calcitonin, concluded that fluticasone had a more favorable therapeutic ratio [85].

Practical aspects of drug administration

Inhaled corticosteroids may be the sole drug therapy in asthma maintenance, or more commonly they are combined with inhaled β-agonists. The July 2007 National Heart, Lung, and Blood Institute's Expert Panel for the diagnosis and therapy for asthma recommends inhaled corticosteroids for asthma severity graded as mild persistent asthma or worse. Ciclesonide, fluticasone, budesonide, beclomethasone, triamcinolone, and flunisolide are corticosteroids available for inhalation. Drug delivery systems include both metered dose inhalers and dry-powder inhalers. Several formulations are available that combine glucocorticoid and β-agonist in the same inhalation delivery device. Improvement in asthma symptoms can occur as quickly as 1 day following initiation of inhaled corticosteroids (more quickly with systemic steroids) but maximum benefit may not be realized for 1–3 weeks. The chronic use of systemic glucocorticoids in asthmatic patients is reserved for those who fail combined therapy with inhaled steroids, inhaled β-agonists, perhaps inhaled anticholinergics, oral methylxanthines, oral leukotriene antagonists, 5-lipoxygenase inhibitors, or omalizumab. Systemic corticosteroids are a drug of last resort because of their devastating systemic effects with long-term use. Nonetheless, short courses (1–2 weeks) of oral corticosteroids are extremely effective in treating acute asthma exacerbations.

The need for preoperative systemic corticosteroids in all asthmatics is an important and unresolved clinical issue, especially for patients who are likely to have their airway instrumented with an endotracheal tube. Several studies have stressed the lack of serious side effects of prophylaxing all asthmatics with systemic steroids prior to surgery. It is also unknown if patients already on inhaled steroids would benefit from systemic steroids in the perioperative period. Despite the absence of a randomized clinical trial to prove their effectiveness, it is recommended that mild and moderate asthmatics receive 1 mg kg^{-1} of prednisone orally (up to 60 mg) for 3–7 days preoperatively and that severe asthmatics (defined as those that have ever needed systemic steroids for asthma control) receive increased doses of systemic steroids [86,87].

Anti-inflammatory drugs

Nedocromil sodium and sodium cromoglycate

One of the earliest clinical trials evaluating the effectiveness of sodium cromoglycate (cromolyn) was carried out in 10 severe, steroid-dependent asthmatics [88]. A larger study in 100 patients with a wider range of asthma severity and chronicity showed that cromolyn was of no benefit in nonallergic patients. However, 89% of allergic asthmatics had clinical improvement, younger patients tended to benefit more, and 88% of patients on steroids improved, with approximately one-third of these patients able to reduce their average steroid use by 40% [89]. In over 40 years since these original trials the clinical profile and utility of cromolyn has changed very little; cromolyn is most useful in younger patients who have an allergic basis for their asthma.

Sodium cromoglycate was synthesized in 1965 in an attempt to improve upon the bronchodilating properties of khellin, a naturally occurring chromone derived from the plant Ammi visnaga which has been known for centuries to function as a spasmolytic agent. Efforts ensued to improve upon the therapeutic profile of sodium cromoglycate, resulting in the synthesis of nedocromil sodium, which was released in the USA in 1992 [90].

Mechanisms of drug action

Electrophysiological studies have shown that antigen activation of mast cells results in intracellular influx of chloride via chloride channels, which in turn maintains activation of calcium channels, allowing intracellular entry of calcium leading to degranulation [91]. Cromolyn [92] and nedocromil [91] inhibit chloride channel activity in cultured mucosal-like mast cells and mouse 3T3 fibroblasts, respectively. It is unlikely that this fully explains the mechanism of action of these drugs, since both can inhibit mediator release in the absence of extracellular calcium. Another signaling pathway likely important in controlling mediator release involves a 78 kDa protein resembling moesin which is phosphorylated by protein kinase C in rat peritoneal mast cells following nedocromil or sodium cromoglycate exposure. It is proposed that this phosphorylated protein, which contains actin binding domains, attaches to the cytoskeleton, preventing degranulation [93]. In addition to mast cells, sodium cromoglycate and nedocromil are known to inhibit mediator release from airway epithelial cells and basophils, and to inhibit eosinophil chemotaxis and adherence to endothelial cells [94].

Preclinical pharmacology

Mast cells are located in the respiratory epithelium of the nasal and airway mucosa. Increased mast cells are present in the nasal mucosa of patients with seasonal and perennial rhinitis [95]. Sodium cromoglycate and nedocromil inhibit histamine release from human bronchoalveolar mast cells.

Clinical pharmacology

Both sodium cromoglycate and nedocromil sodium are administered by inhalation. Cromolyn inhibits both the immediate and late-phase bronchoconstrictive effects of inhaled antigen. It attenuates bronchospasm induced by exercise, aspirin, cold air, toluene diisocyanate, sulfur dioxide, and environmental pollutants. Approximately 8% of cromolyn inhaled is absorbed and rapidly excreted unchanged in both urine and bile. The remainder is exhaled or deposited in the oropharynx, swallowed, and excreted via the alimentary tract. Systemic bioavailability of nedocromil sodium is low. Peak mean serum concentrations of $1.6 \, ng \, mL^{-1}$ occurred 28 minutes after a 3.5 mg inhaled dose and had a half-life of 3.3 hours. Nedocromil is 89% protein-bound and is not metabolized. Adverse events with sodium cromoglycate or nedocromil sodium are uncommon and usually mild. Nausea, vomiting, dyspepsia, and unpleasant taste occurred more commonly with nedocromil than with placebo. Throat irritation or dryness, bad taste, cough, wheezing, and nausea are more common with sodium cromoglycate then with placebo. Uncommonly and paradoxically, severe asthma has been reported with sodium cromoglycate (presumably an airway irritant effect). Rarely laryngeal edema, nasal congestion, or pharyngeal irritation has been reported as an adverse effect of sodium cromoglycate.

Practical aspects of drug administration

Cromolyn and nedocromil have found their greatest clinical utility in the management of childhood asthma and exercise-induced asthma. Studies have shown an improvement in asthma symptom score and decreased use of albuterol in patients older than 12 years using cromolyn [96]. In children, cromolyn has been proposed as a first-line therapy to be used even before inhaled steroids [97] (because of concerns regarding effects of chronic inhaled steroids on skeletal development). Cromolyn is also known to reduce symptoms of exercise-induced bronchoconstriction in both children and adults [98]. Despite these beneficial findings, the efficacy of cromolyn in childhood asthma has been questioned by some investigators [99].

Three clinical studies have compared sodium cromoglycate to nedocromil sodium in the management of asthma. One hundred thirty-two adult asthmatics with moderately severe asthma had their inhaled glucocorticoid dose reduced by half and were then treated with either 16 mg per day nedocromil sodium, 8 mg per day sodium cromoglycate, or placebo.

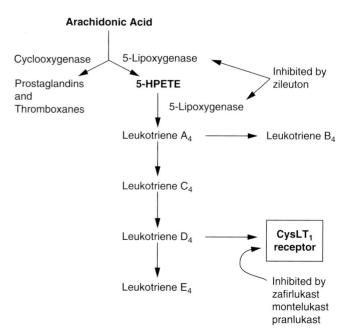

Figure 47.2. Biosynthetic pathway of leukotriene synthesis. Site of action of 5-lipoxygenase inhibitor (zileuton) and antagonists (zafirlukast, montelukast, pranlukast) of the cysteinyl/leukotriene 1 (CysLT$_1$) receptor are shown.

Both drugs were superior to placebo, and nedocromil produced greater improvements in asthma symptoms [100]. A comparison of 16 mg per day nedocromil sodium and 40 mg per day sodium cromoglycate in 77 patients already taking steroids and bronchodilators showed no difference between the two treatments [101]. Nedocromil sodium ($16 \, mg \, day^{-1}$), cromolyn sodium ($8 \, mg \, day^{-1}$) or placebo were compared in 306 patients over an 8-week period. Patients were selected who had a deterioration in their asthma symptoms after being switched from slow-release theophyllines to short-acting bronchodilators. Both drugs were better than placebo, and cromolyn was more effective than nedocromil in nighttime symptom control, FEV$_1$, and forced expiratory flow rate at 25–75% of forced vital capacity (FVC) [102].

Leukotriene antagonists, 5-lipoxygenase inhibitors

Leukotrienes belong to a family of compounds known as eicosanoids, a large group of products synthesized from arachadonic acid (Fig. 47.2). Other family members include prostaglandins, thromboxanes, lipoxins, and isoprostanes. Leukotrienes are synthesized from arachadonic acid, which is generated from membrane phospholipids by phospholipase A$_2$ when inflammatory cells are activated [103]. The first leukotriene identified was leukotriene B$_4$ (LTB$_4$) [104], followed by the discovery that LTC$_4$ was the slow-reacting substance of anaphylaxis (SRS-A) [105], long presumed to be a mediator of asthma and inflammation. It was subsequently determined that SRS-A was also composed of LTD$_4$ and LTE$_4$, products of LTC$_4$ [106] (Fig. 47.2).

Mechanisms of drug action

Two classes of leukotriene pathway inhibitors have been introduced for the clinical management of asthma. A 5-lipoxygenase inhibitor (zileuton) inhibits the conversion of arachadonic acid to leukotriene A_4, thus inhibiting the generation of LTB_4, LTC_4, LTD_4, and LTE_4. The second class of drugs are cysteinyl-leukotriene 1 ($CysLT_1$) antagonists and competitively block the ability of LTD_4 to bind to the $CysLT_1$ receptor. Bronchospasm, plasma exudation, vasoconstriction, and eosinophil recruitment are at least in part mediated by LTD_4 binding to the $CysLT_1$ receptor, and therefore either blockade of the synthesis of LTD_4 (zileuton) or blockade of the $CysLT_1$ target receptor (zafirlukast, montelukast, pranlukast) are therapeutic targets.

The CysLT1 receptor is a glycosylated G-protein-coupled receptor (GPCR) that initially had been identified as an orphan GPCR that could be activated by LTC_4 and LTD_4 [107]. Molecular cloning and characterization of this receptor identified it as a 337-amino-acid protein of approximately 38.5 kDa with seven putative transmembrane-spanning domains, potential N-glycosylation sites and potential phosphorylation sites by protein kinase A and protein kinase C. When this receptor was expressed in oocytes, it exhibited dose-dependent increases in calcium-activated chloride conductance in response to LTD_4 [108]. More recently this receptor has been shown to respond to the pyrimidinergic agonist uridine diphosphate (UDP) in addition to its classical activation by LTD_4 [109]. Activation of $CysLT_1$ receptors by pyrimidines is consistent with its protein homology to the purinergic family of receptors [109].

Preclinical pharmacology

Research interests in leukotrienes and asthma extends from the original observations that SRS-A (now known to be a mixture of LTC_4, LTD_4, and LTE_4) is a potent bronchoconstrictor [110]. Subsequently it was confirmed that the cysteinyl leukotrienes were potent constrictors of guinea pig airways in vivo and in vitro and that they constricted human bronchi in vitro [110]. LTC_4, LTD_4, and LTE_4 were each shown to increase extravasation of Evans blue dye in guinea pig airways, supporting a role for leukotriene-mediated increases in vascular permeability [111]. In humans, inhalation of LTE_4 increased the infiltration of eosinophils into the airway mucosa, while inhalation of LTD_4 increased eosinophil content of sputum from asthmatics [112]. Leukotrienes may also be involved in airway smooth-muscle hypertrophy and remodeling, hallmarks of chronic asthma [113]. Direct provocation of bronchoconstriction by leukotrienes in asthmatic subjects has been confirmed in many clinical studies [114,115].

Clinical pharmacology

Montelukast and zafirlukast are the $CysLT_1$ receptor antagonists currently available in the USA. Montelukast and zafirlukast are rapidly absorbed after oral administration with mean peak plasma concentrations achieved in 3–4 hours. Montelukast is 99% bound to plasma proteins, with a volume of distribution of 9–11 L. Montelukast and zafirlukast are extensively metabolized, and in-vitro studies with human liver microsomal membranes indicate that cytochromes P450 (CYP) 3A4 and 2C9 are primarily responsible for metabolism [116]. Metabolites of both drugs are excreted almost entirely in bile. Mean plasma half-life is 2.7–5.5 hours for both drugs, and their pharmacokinetics remain linear for doses up to 50 mg per day. While gender and age have not been shown to affect the pharmacokinetics of montelukast, clearance of zafirlukast decreases with age. Hepatic insufficiency and cirrhosis decrease the metabolism of both montelukast and zafirlukast, yet no dosage adjustment is recommended in patients with mild to moderate hepatic insufficiency. Since montelukast and zafirlukast and their metabolites are not excreted in urine, no changes in dosing are necessary in patients with renal failure.

Montelukast given at recommended amounts ($10\,mg\,day^{-1}$) did not influence the metabolism of a single intravenous dose of theophylline, or a single oral dose (30 mg) of warfarin, digoxin, or terfenadine, despite the fact that all of these drugs depend on CYP metabolism and warfarin and terfenadine are metabolized by the specific CYP subclasses implicated in the metabolism of montelukast (2C9 and 3A4, respectively). In contrast, the co-administration of zafirlukast and warfarin decreased the clearance of warfarin and increased the prothrombin time.

Adverse effects of montelukast and zafirlukast are uncommon and typically not severe, although severe liver injury has been reported with zafirlukast [117]. The commonest side effects with montelukast in over 2600 adults included headache (18.4% vs. 18.1% with placebo), cough/influenza symptoms (4.2% vs. 3.9% with placebo), abdominal pain/dyspepsia (2.9% vs. 2.5% with placebo), and elevation of alanine transaminase (ALT) (2.1% vs. 2.0% with placebo). Adverse effects of zafirlukast were of similar quality and frequency.

Zileuton is the only currently available inhibitor of 5-lipoxygenase, an enzyme responsible for the conversion of arachidonic acid to 5-HPETE and 5-HPETE to leukotriene A_4, a precursor to leukotriene D_4 (Fig. 47.2). It is rapidly absorbed after oral administration, with a peak serum concentration occurring at 1.7 hours. It is 93% bound to serum proteins and has a serum half-life of 2.5 hours. Zileuton is metabolized by CYP isoenzymes 1A2, 2C9, and 3A4, and metabolites are found in both urine and bile. Gender, age, and renal failure do not require changes in dosing, but zileuton is contraindicated in patients with hepatic insufficiency. The most common adverse effect of zileuton was dyspepsia, but arthralgias, chest pain, conjunctivitis, constipation, dizziness, fever, hypertonia, insomnia, lymphadenopathy, malaise, neck rigidity, nervousness, pruritus, somnolence, urinary tract infections, vaginitis and vomiting were all reported at an incidence of > 1% and at a greater frequency compared to placebo.

Practical aspects of drug administration

Corticosteroids do not suppress all inflammatory mediators involved in the asthmatic response. Asthmatic patients

deliver both drugs simultaneously. Systemic corticosteroids are a drug of last resort for treatment of asthma, because of their devastating adverse systemic effects with long-term use. Nonetheless, short courses (1–2 weeks) of oral corticosteroids are extremely effective in treating acute asthma exacerbations. Notably, it is recommended that patients who have received systemic steroids within the past 6 months should receive 100 mg hydrocortisone intravenously every 8 hours during the surgical period with a rapidly reduced dose within 24 hours of surgery.

Inhaled anticholinergic drugs (ipratropium bromide by aerosol or nebulizer, or tiotropium bromide by dry-powder inhalation) may be used as rescue therapy in patients who experience side effects from traditional β-agonist therapies or in patients who fail to completely respond to β-agonists, but they have found their highest efficacy in patients with chronic obstructive pulmonary disease (COPD). Inhaled anticolinergics have a slower onset and a longer time to peak effect than inhaled β-agonists and are thus considered second-line therapy. Bronchospasm induced by the introduction of an endotracheal tube into the trachea may be particularly responsive to anticholinergic therapy.

Theophylline is the mostly widely prescribed medication for asthma in the world, because it is inexpensive. However, in industrialized countries theophylline is typically third-line therapy for bronchodilation because of systemic toxicity, and it is reserved for severe asthmatics not controlled with β-agonists and corticosteroids. Volatile anesthetics are also potent bronchodilators that are occasionally used when traditional therapies have failed to relieve status asthmaticus.

Several targeted anti-inflammatory drugs are used in the treatment of asthma, including cromolyn, nedocromil, leukotriene antagonists, 5-lipoxygenase inhibitors, and omalizumab. Cromolyn and nedocromil are indicated in the prophylactic management of asthma, and cromolyn nasal spray is indicated in the treatment of allergic rhinitis. Leukotriene antagonists are typically used as an adjunct to asthma/allergy prevention or treatment, while 5-lipoxygenase inhibitors appear most efficacious in asthma patients with exercise-induced or aspirin-sensitive asthma. Omalizumab is a monoclonal antibody directed against IgE molecules administered in 1–3 injections every 2–4 weeks; this therapy is reserved for a subset of asthmatics not controlled with other combinations of therapies

Emerging therapies in asthma are focused on improved ultra-long-acting β$_2$-agonists, steroids with reduced systemic toxicity, and monoclonal antibodies, vaccines, and kinase inhibitors that inhibit specific subsets of inflammatory cells, chemokines, cytokines, and intracellular kinases.

References

1. Ahlquist RP. A study of the adrenotropic receptors. *Am J Physiol* 1948; **153**: 586–600.

2. Gay LN, Long JW. Clinical evaluation of isopropylepinephrine in management of bronchial asthma. *J Am Med Assoc* 1949; **139**: 452–7.

3. Engelhardt A, Hoefke W, Wick H. Zur pharmakologie des sympathomimeticums 1-(3,5-dihydroxylphenyl)-1-hydroxy-2-isopropyl aminoathan. *Arzneimittel-Forschung* 1961; **11**: 521–5.

4. Ullman A, Svedmyr N. Salmeterol, a new long acting inhaled beta 2 adrenoceptor agonist: comparison with salbutamol in adult asthmatic patients. *Thorax* 1988; **43**: 674–8.

5. Hekking PR, Maesen F, Greefhorst A, *et al*. Long-term efficacy of formoterol compared to salbutamol. *Lung* 1990; **168**: 76–82.

6. Reihsaus E, Innis M, MacIntyre N, Liggett SB. Mutations in the gene encoding for the β$_2$-adrenergic receptor in normal and asthmatic subjects. *Am J Respir Cell Mol Biol* 1993; **8**: 334–9.

7. Green SA, Turki J, Innis M, Liggett SB. Amino-terminal polymorphisms of the human β$_2$-adrenergic receptor impart distinct agonist-promoted regulatory properties. *Biochemistry* 1994; **33**: 9414–19.

8. Emala CW, McQuitty CK, Elleff SM, *et al*. Asthma, allergy and airway hyperresponsiveness are not linked to the β$_2$-adrenoceptor gene. *Chest* 2002; **121**: 722–31.

9. Weir TD, Mallek N, Sandiford AJ, *et al*. β$_2$ adrenergic receptor haplotypes in mild, moderate and fatal/near fatal asthma. *Am J Respir Crit Care Med* 1998; **158**: 787–91.

10. Dewar JC, Wheatley AP, Venn A, *et al*. Beta 2-adrenoceptor polymorphisms are in linkage disequilibrium, but are not associated with asthma in an adult population. *Clinical and Experimental Allergy* 1998; **28**: 442–8.

11. Turki J, Pak J, Green SA, Martin RJ, Liggett SB. Genetic polymorphisms of the beta 2-adrenergic receptor in nocturnal and nonnocturnal asthma. Evidence that Gly16 correlates with the nocturnal phenotype. *J Clin Invest* 1995; **95**: 1635–41.

12. Holloway JW, Dunbar PR, Riley GA, *et al*. Association of beta 2-adrenergic receptor polymorphisms with severe asthma. *Clin Exp Allergy* 2000; **30**: 1097–103.

13. Moore PE, Laporte JD, Abraham JH, *et al*. Polymorphism of the beta (2)-adrenergic receptor gene and desensitization in human airway smooth muscle. *Am J Respir Crit Care Med* 2000; **162**: 2117–24.

14. Bai TR, Mak JC, Barnes PJ. A comparison of β-adrenergic receptors and in vitro relaxant responses to isoproterenol in asthmatic airway smooth muscle. *Am J Respir Cell Mol Biol* 1992; **6**: 647–51.

15. Dorn GW, Tepe NM, Lorenz JN, Koch WJ, Liggett SB. Low- and high-level transgenic expression of beta 2-adrenergic receptors differentially affect cardiac hypertrophy and function in Galphaq- overexpressing mice. *Proc Natl Acad Sci U S A* 1999; **96**: 6400–5.

16. Mitra S, Ugur M, Ugur O, *et al*. (S)-Albuterol increases intracellular free calcium by muscarinic receptor activation and a phospholipase C-dependent mechanism in airway smooth muscle. *Mol Pharmacol* 1998; **53**: 347–54.

17. Handley DA, Anderson AJ, Koester J, Snider ME. New millennium bronchodilators for asthma: single-isomer beta agonists. *Curr Opin Pulm Med* 2000; **6**: 43–9.

18. Henriksen JM, Agertoft L, Pedersen S. Protective effect and duration of action of inhaled formoterol and salbutamol on exercise-induced asthma in children. *J Allergy Clin Immunol* 1992; **89**: 1176–82.

19. Cates CJ, Cates MJ. Regular treatment with salmeterol for chronic asthma: serious adverse events. *Cochrane Database Syst Rev* 2008; (3): CD006363.

20. Kil HK, Rooke GA, Ryan-Dykes MA, Bishop MJ. Effect of prophylactic bronchodilator treatment on lung resistance after tracheal intubation. *Anesthesiology* 1994; **81**: 43–8.

21. Higbee MD, Kumar M, Galant SP. Stimulation of endogenous catecholamine release by theophylline: a proposed additional mechanism of action for theophylline effects. *J Allergy Clin Immunol.* 1982; **70**: 377–82.

22. Zimmerman BL. Arrhythmogenicity of theophylline and halothane used in combination. *Anesthesia and Analgesia* 1979; **58**: 259–60.

23. Tobias JD, Kubos KL, Hirshman CA. Aminophylline does not attenuate histamine-induced airway constriction during halothane anesthesia. *Anesthesiology* 1989; **71**: 723–9.

24. Polson JB, Krzanowski JJ, Goldman AL, Szentivanyi A. Inhibition of human pulmonary phosphodiesterase activity by therapeutic levels of theophylline. *Clin Exp Pharmacol Physiol* 1978; **5**: 535–9.

25. Rabe KF, Magnussen H, Dent G. Theophylline and selective PDE inhibitors as bronchodilators and smooth muscle relaxants. *Eur Respir J* 1995; **8**: 637–42.

26. Ogilvie RI, Fernandez PG, Winsberg F. Cardiovascular response to increasing theophylline concentrations. *Eur J Clin Pharmacol* 1977; **12**: 409–14.

27. Robel-Tillig E, Vogtmann C. Aminophylline influences cerebral hyperperfusion after severe birth hypoxia. *Acta Paediatrica* 2000; **89**: 971–4.

28. Fernandez E. Headaches associated with low spinal fluid pressure. *Headache* 1990; **30**: 122–8.

29. Brater DC, Kaojarern S, Chennavasin P. Pharmacodynamics of the diuretic effects of aminophylline and acetazolamide alone and combined with furosemide in normal subjects. *J Pharmacol Exp Ther* 1983; **227**: 92–7.

30. Rochester DF, Arora NS. Respiratory muscle failure. *Med Clin North Am* 1983; **67**: 573–97.

31. Jacoby DB, Fryer AD. Anticholinergic therapy for airway diseases. *Life Sci* 2001; **68**: 2565–72.

32. Costello RW, Jacoby DB, Fryer AD. Pulmonary neuronal M2 muscarinic receptor function in asthma and animal models of hyperreactivity. *Thorax* 1998; **53**: 613–16.

33. Dohi S, Gold MI. Pulmonary mechanics during general anaesthesia. The influence of mechanical irritation on the airway. *Br J Anaesth* 1979; **51**: 205–14.

34. Groeben H, Brown RH. Ipratropium decreases airway size in dogs by preferential M2 muscarinic receptor blockade in vivo. *Anesthesiology* 1996; **85**: 867–73.

35. Lin RY, Pesola GR, Bakalchuk L, *et al.* Superiority of ipratropium plus albuterol over albuterol alone in the emergency department management of adult asthma: a randomized clinical trial. *Ann Emerg Med* 1998; **31**: 208–13.

36. Lanes SF, Garrett JE, Wentworth CE, Fitzgerald JM, Karpel JP. The effect of adding ipratropium bromide to salbutamol in the treatment of acute asthma: a pooled analysis of three trials. *Chest* 1998; **114**: 365–72.

37. Weber EJ, Levitt MA, Covington JK, Gambrioli E. Effect of continuously nebulized ipratropium bromide plus albuterol on emergency department length of stay and hospital admission rates in patients with acute bronchospasm. A randomized, controlled trial. *Chest* 1999; **115**: 937–44.

38. Rodrigo G, Rodrigo C, Burschtin O. A meta-analysis of the effects of ipratropium bromide in adults with acute asthma. *Am J Med* 1999; **107**: 363–70.

39. Ho WM, Wong KC. Ipratropium bromide and intraoperative bronchospasm. *Chung Hua I Hsueh Tsa Chih (Taipei)* 1995; **55**: 319–24.

40. Kil HK, Rooke GA, Ryan-Dykes MA, Bishop MJ. Effect of prophylactic bronchodilator treatment on lung resistance after tracheal intubation. *Anesthesiology* 1994; **81**: 43–8.

41. Tashkin DP, Celli B, Senn S, *et al.* A 4-year trial of tiotropium in chronic obstructive pulmonary disease. *N Engl J Med* 2008; **359**: 1543–54.

42. Fryer AD, Adamko DJ, Yost BL, Jacoby DB. Effects of inflammatory cells on neuronal M2 muscarinic receptor function in the lung. *Life Sciences* 1999; **64**: 449–55.

43. Parnass SM, Feld JM, Chamberlin WH, Segil LJ. Status asthmaticus treated with isoflurane and enflurane. *Anesth Analg* 1987; **66**: 193–5.

44. Restrepo RD, Pettignano R, DeMeuse P. Halothane, an effective infrequently used drug, in the treatment of pediatric status asthmaticus: a case report. *Journal of Asthma* 2005; **42**: 649–51.

45. Brown RH, Zerhouni EA, Hirshman CA. Comparison of low concentrations of halothane and isoflurane as bronchodilators. *Anesthesiology* 1993; **78**: 1097–101.

46. Tobias JD, Hirshman CA. Attenuation of histamine-induced airway constriction by albuterol during halothane anesthesia. *Anesthesiology* 1990; **72**: 105–10.

47. Mitsuhata H, Saitoh J, Shimizu R, *et al.* Sevoflurane and isoflurane protect against bronchospasm in dogs. *Anesthesiology* 1994; **81**: 1230–4.

48. Mercier FJ, Naline E, Bardou M, *et al.* Relaxation of proximal and distal isolated human bronchi by halothane, isoflurane and desflurane. *Eur Respir J* 2002; **20**: 286–92.

49. Rooke GA, Choi JH, Bishop MJ. The effect of isoflurane, halothane, sevoflurane, and thiopental/nitrous oxide on respiratory system resistance after tracheal intubation. *Anesthesiology* 1997; **86**: 1294–9.

50. Goff MJ, Arain SR, Ficke DJ, Uhrich TD, Ebert TJ. Absence of bronchodilation during desflurane anesthesia: a comparison to sevoflurane and thiopental. *Anesthesiology* 2000; **93**: 404–8.

51. Wiklund CU, Lim S, Lindsten U, Lindahl SG. Relaxation by sevoflurane, desflurane and halothane in the isolated guinea-pig trachea via inhibition of cholinergic neurotransmission. *Br J Anaesth* 1999; **83**: 422–9.

52. Kai T, Jones KA, Warner DO. Halothane attenuates calcium

sensitization in airway smooth muscle by inhibiting G-proteins. *Anesthesiology* 1998; **89**: 1543–52.

53. Hanazaki M, Jones KA, Perkins WJ, Warner DO. Halothane increases smooth muscle protein phosphatase in airway smooth muscle. *Anesthesiology* 2001; **94**: 129–36.

54. Kai T, Bremerich DH, Jones KA, Warner DO. Drug-specific effects of volatile anesthetics on Ca2+ sensitization in airway smooth muscle. *Anesth Analg* 1998; **87**: 425–9.

55. Yamakage M, Hirshman CA, Croxton TL. Volatile anesthetics inhibit voltage-dependent Ca2+ channels in porcine tracheal smooth muscle cells. *Am J Physiol* 1995; **268**: L187–L191.

56. Yamakage M, Chen X, Tsujiguchi N, Kamada Y, Namiki A. Different inhibitory effects of volatile anesthetics on T- and L-type voltage-dependent Ca^{2+} channels in porcine tracheal and bronchial smooth muscles. *Anesthesiology* 2001; **94**: 683–93.

57. Suissa S, Ernst P. Inhaled corticosteroids: impact on asthma morbidity and mortality. *J Allergy Clin Immunol* 2001; **107**: 937–44.

58. Markham A, Adkins JC. Inhaled salmeterol/fluticasone propionate combination. A pharmacoeconomic review of its use in the management of asthma. *Pharmacoeconomics* 2000; **18**: 591–608.

59. McGavin JK, Goa KL, Jarvis B. Inhaled budesonide/formoterol combination. *Drugs* 2001; **61**: 71–8.

60. Wills-Karp M, Luyimbazi J, Xu X, *et al.* Interleukin-13: central mediator of allergic asthma. *Science* 1998; **282**: 2258–61.

61. Ray A, Cohn L. Altering the Th1/Th2 balance as a therapeutic strategy in asthmatic diseases. *Curr Opin Investig Drugs* 2000; **1**: 442–8.

62. Robinson DS, Assoufi B, Durham SR, Kay AB. Eosinophil cationic protein (ECP) and eosinophil protein X (EPX) concentrations in serum and bronchial lavage fluid in asthma. Effect of prednisolone treatment. *Clin Exp Allergy* 1995; **25**: 1118–27.

63. Zhang X, Moilanen E, Kankaanranta H. Enhancement of human eosinophil apoptosis by fluticasone propionate, budesonide, and beclomethasone. *Eur J Pharmacol* 2000; **406**: 325–32.

64. Bascom R, Pipkorn U, Lichtenstein LM, Naclerio RM. The influx of inflammatory cells into nasal washings during the late response to antigen challenge. Effect of systemic steroid pretreatment. *Am Rev Respir Dis* 1988; **138**: 406–12.

65. Wardlaw AJ, Dunnette S, Gleich GJ, Collins JV, Kay AB. Eosinophils and mast cells in bronchoalveolar lavage in subjects with mild asthma. Relationship to bronchial hyperreactivity. *Am Rev Respir Dis* 1988; **137**: 62–9.

66. Boushey HA, Holtzman MJ. Experimental airway inflammation and hyperreactivity. Searching for cells and mediators. *Am Rev Respir Dis* 1985; **131**: 312–13.

67. Yoshikawa H, Tasaka K. Suppression of mast cell activation by glucocorticoid. *Arch Immunol Ther Exp (Warsz)* 2000; **48**: 487–95.

68. Tobias JD, Sauder RA, Hirshman CA. Methylprednisolone prevents propranolol-induced airway hyperreactivity in the Basenji-greyhound dog. *Anesthesiology* 1991; **74**: 1115–20.

69. Sauder RA, Lenox WC, Tobias JD, Hirshman CA. Methylprednisolone increases sensitivity to beta-adrenergic agonists within 48 hours in Basenji greyhounds. *Anesthesiology* 1993; **79**: 1278–83.

70. Emala CW, Clancy J, Hirshman CA. Glucocorticoid treatment decreases muscarinic receptor expression in canine airway smooth muscle. *Am J Physiol* 1997; **272**: L745–L751.

71. Hadcock JR, Wang HY, Malbon CC. Agonist-induced destabilization of beta-adrenergic receptor mRNA. Attenuation of glucocorticoid-induced up-regulation of beta-adrenergic receptors. *J Biol Chem* 1989; **264**: 19928–33.

72. Jiang P, Arinze IJ. Developmental and glucocorticoid modulation of the expression of mRNAs for Gs alpha and G beta subunits in neonatal liver. *Mol Cell Endocrinol* 1994; **99**: 95–102.

73. Stevens WH, Adelroth E, Wattie J, *et al.* Effect of inhaled budesonide on ozone-induced airway hyperresponsiveness and bronchoalveolar lavage cells in dogs. *J Appl Physiol* 1994; **77**: 2578–83.

74. Woolley MJ, Denburg JA, Ellis R, Dahlback M, O'Byrne PM. Allergen-induced changes in bone marrow progenitors and airway responsiveness in dogs and the effect of inhaled budesonide on these parameters. *Am J Respir Cell Mol Biol* 1994; **11**: 600–6.

75. Evans CM, Jacoby DB, Fryer AD. Effects of dexamethasone on antigen-induced airway eosinophilia and M(2) receptor dysfunction. *Am J Respir Crit Care Med* 2001; **163**: 1484–92.

76. Vanacker NJ, Palmans E, Kips JC, Pauwels RA. Fluticasone inhibits but does not reverse allergen-induced structural airway changes. *Am J Respir Crit Care Med* 2001; **163**: 674–9.

77. Fitzgerald JM, Shragge D, Haddon J, Jennings, *et al.* A randomized, controlled trial of high dose, inhaled budesonide versus oral prednisone in patients discharged from the emergency department following an acute asthma exacerbation. *Can Respir J* 2000; **7**: 61–7.

78. Pearlman DS, Noonan MJ, Tashkin DP, *et al.* Comparative efficacy and safety of twice daily fluticasone propionate powder versus placebo in the treatment of moderate asthma. *Ann Allergy Asthma Immunol* 1997; **78**: 356–62.

79. Fish JE, Karpel JP, Craig TJ, *et al.* Inhaled mometasone furoate reduces oral prednisone requirements while improving respiratory function and health-related quality of life in patients with severe persistent asthma. *J Allergy Clin Immunol* 2000; **106**: 852–60.

80. Wong CA, Walsh LJ, Smith CJ, *et al.* Inhaled corticosteroid use and bone-mineral density in patients with asthma. *Lancet* 2000; **355**: 1399–403.

81. Li JT, Ford LB, Chervinsky P, *et al.* Fluticasone propionate powder and lack of clinically significant effects on hypothalamic-pituitary-adrenal axis and bone mineral density over 2 years in adults with mild asthma. *J Allergy Clin Immunol* 1999; **103**: 1062–8.

82. Lipworth BJ. Systemic adverse effects of inhaled corticosteroid therapy: a systematic review and meta-analysis. *Arch Intern Med* 1999; **159**: 941–55.

83. Rao R, Gregson RK, Jones AC, *et al.* Systemic effects of inhaled corticosteroids on growth and bone turnover in childhood asthma: a comparison of fluticasone with beclomethasone. *Eur Respir J* 1999; **13**: 87–94.

84. Nielsen LP, Dahl R. Therapeutic ratio of inhaled corticosteroids in adult asthma. A dose- range comparison between fluticasone propionate and budesonide, measuring their effect on bronchial hyperresponsiveness and adrenal cortex function. *Am J Respir Crit Care Med* 2000; **162**: 2053–7.

85. Ellul-Micallef R. Pharmacokinetics and pharmacodynamics of glucocorticoids. In: Jenne JW, Murphy S, eds., *Drug Therapy for Asthma: Research and Clinical Practice.* New York, NY: Marcel Dekker, 1987: 463–516.

86. Pien LC, Grammer LC, Patterson R. Minimal complications in a surgical population with severe asthma receiving prophylactic corticosteroids. *J Allergy Clin Immunol* 1988; **82**: 696–700.

87. Kabalin CS, Yarnold PR, Grammer LC. Low complication rate of corticosteroid-treated asthmatics undergoing surgical procedures. *Arch Intern Med* 1995; **155**: 1379–84.

88. Howell JB, Altounyan RE. A double-blind trial of disodium cromoglycate in the treatment of allergic bronchial asthma. *Lancet* 1967; **2**: 539–42.

89. Altounyan RE, Howell JB. Treatment of asthma with disodium cromoglycate (FPL 670, "Intal"). *Respiration* 1969; **26**: 131–40.

90. Eady RP. The pharmacology of nedocromil sodium. *Eur J Respir Dis Suppl* 1986; **147**: 112–19.

91. Paulmichl M, Norris AA, Rainey DK. Role of chloride channel modulation in the mechanism of action of nedocromil sodium. *Int Arch Allergy Immunol* 1995; **107**: 416.

92. Romanin C, Reinsprecht M, Pecht I, Schindler H. Immunologically activated chloride channels involved in degranulation of rat mucosal mast cells. *EMBO J* 1991; **10**: 3603–8.

93. Pestonjamasp K, Amieva MR, Strassel CP, *et al.* Moesin, ezrin, and p205 are actin-binding proteins associated with neutrophil plasma membranes. *Mol Biol Cell* 1995; **6**: 247–59.

94. Vittori E, Sciacca F, Colotta F, Mantovani A, Mattoli S. Protective effect of nedocromil sodium on the interleukin-1-induced production of interleukin-8 in human bronchial epithelial cells. *J Allergy Clin Immunol* 1992; **90**: 76–84.

95. Abdelaziz MM, Devalia JL, Khair OA, *et al.* The effect of nedocromil sodium on human airway epithelial cell-induced eosinophil chemotaxis and adherence to human endothelial cell in vitro. *Eur Respir J* 1997; **10**: 851–7.

96. Furukawa C, Atkinson D, Forster TJ, *et al.* Controlled trial of two formulations of cromolyn sodium in the treatment of asthmatic patients > or = 12 years of age. Intal Study Group. *Chest* 1999; **116**: 65–72.

97. Korhonen K, Korppi M, Remes ST, Reijonen TM, Remes K. Lung function in school-aged asthmatic children with inhaled cromoglycate, nedocromil and corticosteroid therapy. *Eur Respir J* 1999; **13**: 82–6.

98. Kelly KD, Spooner CH, Rowe BH. Nedocromil sodium versus sodium cromoglycate in treatment of exercise-induced bronchoconstriction: a systematic review. *Eur Respir J* 2001; **17**: 39–45.

99. Tasche MJ, Uijen JH, Bernsen RM, de Jongste JC, van der Wouden JC. Inhaled disodium cromoglycate (DSCG) as maintenance therapy in children with asthma: a systematic review. *Thorax* 2000; **55**: 913–20.

100. Lal S, Dorow PD, Venho KK, Chatterjee SS. Nedocromil sodium is more effective than cromolyn sodium for the treatment of chronic reversible obstructive airway disease. *Chest* 1993; **104**: 438–47.

101. Boldy DA, Ayres JG. Nedocromil sodium and sodium cromoglycate in patients aged over 50 years with asthma. *Respir Med* 1993; **87**: 517–23.

102. Schwartz HJ, Blumenthal M, Brady R, *et al.* A comparative study of the clinical efficacy of nedocromil sodium and placebo. How does cromolyn sodium compare as an active control treatment? *Chest* 1996; **109**: 945–52.

103. Dennis EA. The growing phospholipase A2 superfamily of signal transduction enzymes. *Trends Biochem Sci* 1997; **22**: 1–2.

104. Borgeat P, Samuelsson B. Transformation of arachidonic acid by rabbit polymorphonuclear leukocytes. Formation of a novel dihydroxyeicosatetraenoic acid. *J Biol Chem* 1979; **254**: 2643–6.

105. Murphy RC, Hammarstrom S, Samuelsson B. Leukotriene C: a slow-reacting substance from murine mastocytoma cells. *Proc Natl Acad Sci U S A* 1979; **76**: 4275–9.

106. Morris HR, Taylor GW, Jones CM, *et al.* Slow reacting substances (leukotrienes): enzymes involved in their biosynthesis. *Proc Natl Acad Sci U S A* 1982; **79**: 4838–42.

107. Ellis C. EP874047A2: cDNA clone HMTMF81 that encodes a novel human 7-transmembrane receptor. *Eur Patent Applic* 1998; Ep0874047A2.

108. Heise CE, O'Dowd BF, Figueroa DJ, *et al.* Characterization of the human cysteinyl leukotriene 2 receptor. *J Biol Chem* 2000; **275**: 30531–6.

109. Mellor EA, Maekawa A, Austen KF, Boyce JA. Cysteinyl leukotriene receptor 1 is also a pyrimidinergic receptor and is expressed by human mast cells. *Proc Natl Acad Sci U S A* 2001; **98**: 7964–9.

110. Dahlen SE, Hedqvist P, Hammarstrom S, Samuelsson B. Leukotrienes are potent constrictors of human bronchi. *Nature* 1980; **288**: 484–6.

111. Hua XY, Dahlen SE, Lundberg JM, Hammarstrom S, Hedqvist P. Leukotrienes C4, D4 and E4 cause widespread and extensive plasma extravasation in the guinea pig. *Naunyn Schmiedebergs Arch Pharmacol* 1985; **330**: 136–41.

112. Diamant Z, Hiltermann JT, van Rensen EL, *et al.* The effect of inhaled leukotriene D4 and methacholine on sputum cell differentials in asthma. *Am J Respir Crit Care Med* 1997; **155**: 1247–53.

113. Wang CG, Du T, Xu LJ, Martin JG. Role of leukotriene D4 in allergen-induced increases in airway smooth muscle in the rat. *Am Rev Respir Dis* 1993; **148**: 413–17.

114. Holroyde MC, Altounyan RE, Cole M, Dixon M, Elliott EV. Bronchoconstriction produced in man by leukotrienes C and D. *Lancet* 1981; **2**: 17–18.

115. Weiss JW, Drazen JM, Coles N, *et al.* Bronchoconstrictor effects of leukotriene C in humans. *Science* 1982; **216**: 196–8.

116. Shader RI, Granda BW, von Moltke LL, Giancarlo GM, Greenblatt DJ: Inhibition of human cytochrome P450 isoforms in vitro by zafirlukast. *Biopharm Drug Dispos* 1999; **20**: 385–8.

117. Reinus JF, Persky S, Burkiewicz JS, *et al.* Severe liver injury after treatment with the leukotriene receptor antagonist zafirlukast. *Ann Intern Med* 2000; **133**: 964–8.

118. Salvi SS, Krishna MT, Sampson AP, Holgate ST. The anti-inflammatory effects of leukotriene-modifying drugs and their use in asthma. *Chest* 2001; **119**: 1533–46.

119. Coreno A, Skowronski M, Kotaru C, McFadden ER. Comparative effects of long-acting beta2-agonists, leukotriene receptor antagonists, and a 5-lipoxygenase inhibitor on exercise-induced asthma. *J Allergy Clin Immunol* 2000; **106**: 500–6.

120. Yamauchi K, Tanifuji Y, Pan LH, *et al.* Effects of pranlukast, a leukotriene receptor antagonist, on airway inflammation in mild asthmatics. *J Asthma* 2001; **38**: 51–7.

121. Yoo SH, Park SH, Song JS, *et al.* Clinical effects of pranlukast, an oral leukotriene receptor antagonist, in mild-to-moderate asthma: a 4 week randomized multicentre controlled trial. *Respirology* 2001; **6**: 15–21.

122. Busse W, Raphael GD, Galant S, *et al.* Low-dose fluticasone propionate compared with montelukast for first-line treatment of persistent asthma: a randomized clinical trial. *J Allergy Clin Immunol* 2001; **107**: 461–8.

123. Williams B, Noonan G, Reiss TF, *et al.* Long-term asthma control with oral montelukast and inhaled beclomethasone for adults and children 6 years and older. *Clin Exp Allergy* 2001; **31**: 845–54.

124. Christian VJ, Prasse A, Naya I, Summerton L, Harris A. Zafirlukast improves asthma control in patients receiving high-dose inhaled corticosteroids. *Am J Respir Crit Care Med* 2000; **162**: 578–85.

125. Centanni S, Santus P, Casanova F, *et al.* Evaluation of the effects of zafirlukast 40 mg b.i.d. in addition to preexisting therapy of high-dose inhaled steroids on symptomatic patients with reversible respiratory obstruction: preliminary data. *Drugs Exp Clin Res* 2000; **26**: 133–8.

126. Robinson DS, Campbell D, Barnes PJ. Addition of leukotriene antagonists to therapy in chronic persistent asthma: a randomised double-blind placebo-controlled trial. *Lancet* 2001; **357**: 2007–11.

127. Pauls JD, Simon RA, Daffern PJ, Stevenson DD. Lack of effect of the 5-lipoxygenase inhibitor zileuton in blocking oral aspirin challenges in aspirin-sensitive asthmatics. *Ann Allergy Asthma Immunol* 2000; **85**: 40–5.

128. Dahlen B, Nizankowska E, Szczeklik A, *et al.* Benefits from adding the 5-lipoxygenase inhibitor zileuton to conventional therapy in aspirin-intolerant asthmatics. *Am J Respir Crit Care Med* 1998; **157**: 1187–94.

129. Gomez FP, Iglesia R, Roca J, *et al.* The effects of 5-lipoxygenase inhibition by zileuton on platelet- activating-factor-induced pulmonary abnormalities in mild asthma. *Am J Respir Crit Care Med* 1998; **157**: 1559–64.

130. Hasday JD, Meltzer SS, Moore WC, *et al.* Anti-inflammatory effects of zileuton in a subpopulation of allergic asthmatics. *Am J Respir Crit Care Med* 2000; **161**: 1229–36.

131. Shields RL, Whether WR, Zioncheck K, *et al.* Inhibition of allergic reactions with antibodies to IgE. *Int Arch Allergy Immunol* 1995; **107**: 308–12.

132. Corren J, Shapiro G, Reimann J, *et al.* Allergen skin tests and free IgE levels during reduction and cessation of omalizumab therapy. *J Allergy Clin Immunol* 2008; **121**: 506–11.

133. Holgate ST, Chuchalin AG, Hebert J, *et al.* Efficacy and safety of a recombinant anti-immunoglobulin E antibody (omalizumab) in severe allergic asthma. *Clin Exp Allergy* 2004; **34**: 632–8.

134. Soler M, Matz J, Townley R, *et al.* The anti-IgE antibody omalizumab reduces exacerbations and steroid requirement in allergic asthmatics. *Eur Respir J* 2001; **18**: 254–61.

135. Busse W, Corren J, Lanier BQ, *et al.* Omalizumab, anti-IgE recombinant humanized monoclonal antibody, for the treatment of severe allergic asthma. *J Allergy Clin Immunol* 2001; **108**: 184–90.

136. Milgrom H, Fick RB, Su JQ, *et al.* Treatment of allergic asthma with monoclonal anti-IgE antibody. rhuMAb-E25 Study Group. *N Engl J Med* 1999; **341**: 1966–73.

137. Genentech. *Xolair.* Novartis Pharmaceutical Corporation, 2007: 1.

138. Winchester DE, Jacob A, Murphy T. Omalizumab for asthma. *N Engl J Med* 2006; **355**: 1281–2.

139. International consensus report on diagnosis and treatment of asthma. National Heart, Lung, and Blood Institute, National Institutes of Health. Bethesda, Maryland 20892. Publication no. 92–3091, March 1992. *Eur Respir J* 1992; **5**: 601–41.

140. Prenner BM. Asthma 2008: targeting immunoglobulin E to achieve disease control. *J Asthma* 2008; **45**: 429–36.

141. Holgate ST. Novel targets of therapy in asthma. *Curr Opin Pulm Med* 2009; **15**: 63–71.

142. Adcock IM, Caramori G, Chung KF. New targets for drug development in asthma. *Lancet* 2008; **372**: 1073–87.

143. Matera MG, Cazzola M. Ultra-long-acting beta 2-adrenoceptor agonists: an emerging therapeutic option for asthma and COPD? *Drugs* 2007; **67**: 503–15.

144. Flood-Page P, Swenson C, Faiferman I, *et al.* A study to evaluate safety and efficacy of mepolizumab in patients with moderate persistent asthma. *Am J Respir Crit Care Med* 2007; **176**: 1062–71.

145. Wark PA, Johnston SL, Bucchieri F, *et al.* Asthmatic bronchial epithelial cells have a deficient innate immune response to infection with rhinovirus. *J Exp Med* 2005; **201**: 937–47.

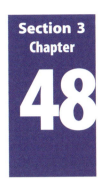

Section 3
Chapter
48

Essential drugs in anesthetic practice
Pulmonary vasodilators

Sunita Sastry and Ronald G. Pearl

Introduction

The pulmonary circulation is normally a low-pressure, low-resistance circulation. Pulmonary hypertension is defined as a mean pulmonary artery pressure (PAP) greater than 25 mmHg at rest or 30 mmHg with exercise. In patients with pulmonary hypertension, altered vascular endothelial and smooth-muscle function lead to a combination of vasoconstriction, localized thrombosis, and vascular growth and remodeling [1]. These processes increase pulmonary vascular resistance (PVR), resulting in right ventricular (RV) failure, inadequate oxygenation, and ultimately death [2]. Pulmonary vasodilator therapy is based on an understanding of the mechanisms of pulmonary hypertension [1–5].

Etiologic factors of pulmonary hypertension

The etiologic factors of pulmonary hypertension can be considered from the equation for PVR:

$$PVR = (PAP - LAP) \times 80/CO \qquad (48.1)$$

where PVR represents pulmonary vascular resistance (in dynes s cm^{-5}), PAP represents mean pulmonary artery pressure (in mmHg), LAP represents left atrial pressure (in mmHg), and CO represents cardiac output (in L min^{-1}).

Rearranging this equation for PAP demonstrates that:

$$PAP = LAP + (CO \times PVR)/80 \qquad (48.2)$$

Thus the three factors that cause pulmonary hypertension are increased LAP, increased CO, and increased PVR. For patients with chronic pulmonary hypertension, the common diagnoses can be considered in these three categories. Increased LAP includes left ventricular (LV) failure and valvular heart disease (particularly mitral stenosis or regurgitation). Increased CO primarily refers to patients with congenital heart disease with cardiac shunts producing increased pulmonary blood flow such as ventricular septal defects. The major categories

of chronically increased PVR are pulmonary disease (parenchymal or airway), hypoxia without pulmonary disease (hypoventilation syndromes, high altitude), pulmonary arterial obstruction (thromboembolism, schistosomiasis), and idiopathic pulmonary arterial hypertension (IPAH, formerly called primary pulmonary hypertension). The 2003 Third World Symposium on Pulmonary Hypertension divided pulmonary hypertension into five diagnostic categories: pulmonary arterial hypertension, pulmonary venous hypertension, pulmonary hypertension associated with hypoxemia, pulmonary hypertension due to chronic thrombotic or embolic disease, and miscellaneous (pulmonary hypertension caused by disorders directly affecting the pulmonary vasculature) (Table 48.1) [6].

In addition to the etiologies of chronic pulmonary hypertension, acute increases in PVR may result from hypoxia, hypercarbia, acidosis, increased sympathetic tone, and endogenous or exogenous pulmonary vasoconstrictors (catecholamines, serotonin, thromboxane, endothelin). Most patients with decompensated pulmonary hypertension will have a combination of chronic pulmonary hypertension plus an acute increase in PVR. In general, therapy will be directed at reversing this acute increase in PVR [7].

The pulmonary vascular endothelium is involved in the synthesis and removal of vasoactive substances that affect pulmonary vascular tone. A variety of abnormalities in endothelial cell function have been demonstrated in vessels from patients with pulmonary hypertension, including decreased production of vasodilator and antiproliferative substances such as prostacyclin and nitric oxide (NO) and increased production of vasoconstrictors such as thromboxane A_2, endothelin, serotonin, and norepinephrine [2,3,8–17]. Changes in the synthesis and release of these substances may alter pulmonary vascular tone. The lung is responsible for synthesizing and inactivating eicosanoids, including prostaglandins (PGs), thromboxanes, and leukotrienes. Metabolism of the eicosanoids through the cyclooxygenase pathway produces $PGF_2\alpha$, PGE_2, and thromboxane A_2, which are pulmonary vasoconstrictors; other prostaglandins such as PGE_1 and prostacyclin (PGI_2) are vasodilators. Leukotrienes are products of the lipoxygenase

Anesthetic Pharmacology, 2nd edition, ed. Alex S. Evers, Mervyn Maze, Evan D. Kharasch. Published by Cambridge University Press. © Cambridge University Press 2011.

Table 48.1. Classification of pulmonary hypertension according to the Third World Symposium on Pulmonary Hypertension, 2003 [6]

1. Pulmonary arterial hypertension (PAH)

   1.1. Idiopathic (IPAH)

   1.2. Familial (FPAH)

   1.3. Associated with

      1.3.1. Collagen vascular disease

      1.3.2. Congenital systemic to pulmonary shunts

      1.3.3. Portal hypertension

      1.3.4. HIV infection

      1.3.5. Drugs & toxins

      1.3.6. Other (thyroid disorders, glycogen storage disease, Gaucher's disease, hereditary hemorrhagic telangiectasia, hemoglobinopathies, myeloproliferative disorders, splenectomy)

   1.4. Associated with significant venous or capillary involvement

      1.4.1. Pulmonary veno-occlusive disease (PVO)

      1.4.2. Pulmonary capillary hemangiomatosis (PCH)

   1.5. Persistent pulmonary hypertension of the newborn

2. Pulmonary venous hypertension

   2.1. Left-sided atrial or ventricular heart disease

   2.2. Left-sided valvular heart disease

3. Pulmonary hypertension associated with hypoxemia

   3.1. Chronic obstructive pulmonary disease

   3.2. Interstitial lung disease

   3.3. Sleep-disordered breathing

   3.4. Alveolar hypoventilation disorders

   3.5. Chronic exposure to high altitude

   3.6. Developmental abnormalities

4. Pulmonary hypertension due to chronic thrombotic and/or embolic disease

   4.1. Thromboembolic obstruction of proximal pulmonary arteries

   4.2. Thromboembolic obstruction of distal pulmonary arteries

   4.3. Nonthrombotic pulmonary embolism (tumor, parasites, foreign material)

5. Miscellaneous: sarcoidosis, histiocytosis X, lymphangiomatosis, compression of pulmonary vessels (adenopathy, tumor, fibrosing mediastinitis)

pathway and produce pulmonary vasoconstriction. Thus a balance between the lipoxygenase and cyclooxygenase pathways may be an important determinant of the normally low resistance of the pulmonary circulation. Bradykinin is inactivated in the lungs by angiotensin-converting enzyme; bradykinin can produce direct pulmonary vasoconstriction through BK_2 receptors or indirect pulmonary vasodilation through endothelial NO production [18]. Histamine is produced by mast cells near the pulmonary arteries. Histamine is a strong pulmonary vasoconstrictor and systemic vasodilator. Histamine results in preferential pulmonary venoconstriction, thereby increasing capillary hydrostatic pressure and producing pulmonary edema [19]. Pulmonary vessels receive both sympathetic and parasympathetic innervation. α-adrenergic agonists such as norepinephrine produce pulmonary vasoconstriction, whereas β-adrenergic agonists such as isoproterenol produce vasodilation [20]. Sympathetic nervous system stimulation from stress and pain may exacerbate pulmonary hypertension [21].

Hypoxic pulmonary vasoconstriction

Acute hypoxia produces acute pulmonary hypertension due to hypoxic pulmonary vasoconstriction (HPV). Chronic hypoxia produces chronic pulmonary hypertension caused by the combination of HPV, pulmonary vascular remodeling from release of hypoxia inducible factor 1, and altered pulmonary vasoreactivity [22,23]. HPV was initially described in 1946 by von Euler and Liljestrand, who demonstrated an increase in PAP during hypoxic ventilation of the cat [24]. HPV was demonstrated in humans the next year. Studies since then have attempted to define the sensor, transducer, and effector mechanisms of HPV [25–31]. Although HPV was initially described in vivo, subsequent studies demonstrated that vasoconstriction in response to hypoxia occurs in isolated perfused lungs, in pulmonary artery strips, and in cultured pulmonary artery smooth-muscle cells (PASMCs). The small pulmonary arteries and arterioles (60–500 μm in diameter) have the strongest vasoconstrictor response and are primarily responsible for the increase in PVR. Large pulmonary arteries may not sense alveolar hypoxia in vivo because they receive perfusion with systemic blood through the vasa vasorum. Studies that divide PVR into arteriolar, capillary, and venous components have demonstrated that resistance increases in all segments in response to hypoxia, but the arteriolar segment constitutes the majority of the total increase [19]. As a result, pulmonary capillary pressure remains relatively constant during HPV [32].

The site of oxygen sensing for HPV is the small pulmonary arteries. These are surrounded by alveolar gas and are perfused with mixed venous blood. Both the alveolar oxygen tension (P_AO_2) and the mixed venous oxygen tension (P_vO_2) contribute to the stimulus for vasoconstriction. The P_AO_2 has a greater impact than the P_vO_2 so that the integrated response occurs to a sensed oxygen tension $(P_sO_2) = P_AO_2^{0.6} + P_vO_2^{0.4}$ [33]. The arterial oxygen tension (P_aO_2) has no direct effect on HPV. Vasoconstriction in response to the P_sO_2 has a sigmoidal relationship similar to the oxyhemoglobin dissociation curve so that there is little effect until P_sO_2 decreases to less than 70 mmHg, a half-maximal effect at a P_sO_2 of 30 mmHg, and essentially maximum effect at a P_sO_2 of 10 mmHg [33].

Studies examining the mechanisms of HPV have often produced conflicting results. There appear to be multiple redundant mechanisms and modulators of HPV, so the results may depend on the species, the experimental preparation (intact subject, perfused lung, pulmonary vessel, cultured PASMC), the vessel size (proximal pulmonary artery, distal pulmonary artery), and the specific experimental conditions (duration of hypoxia, precontraction stimulus, presence or inhibition of modulators). In many studies, HPV has a triphasic response (early transient contraction, relaxation, late sustained contraction), and the mechanisms responsible for each phase may differ. The hypoxic relaxation is primarily endothelium-independent and the late hypoxic contraction is primarily endothelium-dependent with a major component from endothelin 1 and a requirement for superoxide anion. In preparations with intact endothelium, hypoxia decreases NO release from endothelium because of the role of oxygen as a substrate in NO synthesis from L-citrulline.

PASMCs rapidly contract in response to hypoxia, a phenomenon that does not occur in smooth-muscle cells from systemic arteries. The basic explanation of HPV is that hypoxia inhibits voltage-gated potassium (K_v) channels, thereby producing membrane depolarization that activates voltage-dependent L-type calcium channels, resulting in increased calcium influx from the extracellular space. The increase in intracellular calcium results in calmodulin-mediated activation of myosin light-chain kinase and contraction. Contraction is caused by increased intracellular calcium concentration with no significant change in sensitivity. Some studies suggest that calcium release may occur from ryanodine-sensitive stores in the sarcoplasmic reticulum. The mechanisms by which hypoxia inhibits K_v remains controversial. The K_v channels in PASMCs are oxygen-sensitive, but whether the response is caused by decreased oxygen tension, by altered redox status, or by altered cellular energetic state is unresolved. K_v activity can be altered by oxidation of a cysteine residue in the N-terminal region. Hypoxia can alter the production of reactive oxygen species such as superoxide anion and hydrogen peroxide as a result of nicotinamide adenine dinucleotide or nicotinamide adenine dinucleotide phosphate oxidase activity. Studies suggest that the bioenergetic state of the cell is not a primary regulatory mechanism for HPV, because the contraction significantly precedes any decline in adenosine triphosphate.

Hypoxia causing pulmonary hypertension is most commonly seen in patients with chronic lung disease [34]. Continuous prolonged administration of oxygen decreases or prevents the progression of pulmonary hypertension [34,35]. Treatment of patients in whom pulmonary hypertension either develops acutely or becomes intensified as a result of bronchitis or pneumonia is aimed at maintaining arterial oxygenation. Such patients may not need and indeed may not respond to pulmonary vasodilator therapy unless oxygen is appropriately administered and the underlying infection is adequately treated. In general, maintenance of P_aO_2 at values greater than 50–60 mmHg minimizes hypoxic pulmonary vasoconstriction. In patients with chronic lung disease, these levels can generally be achieved by administering oxygen at low flow rates through nasal cannula. Hypercarbia may develop with excessive oxygen administration in patients with chronic obstructive pulmonary disease (COPD). This adverse effect is not primarily a result of decreased hypoxic respiratory drive, but instead results from worsened ventilation/perfusion mismatching during oxygen therapy [36].

Evaluation of pulmonary hypertension

Evaluation of the patient with pulmonary hypertension should determine the underlying diagnosis and the severity of the disease [1–6]. History and physical examination should focus on issues such as underlying lung disease, congenital heart disease, myocardial or valvular heart disease, thromboembolic disease, connective tissue disease, liver disease, human immunodeficiency virus infection, prior intravenous drug use, prior use of appetite-suppressant drugs, obstructive sleep apnea, and family history of pulmonary hypertension. Ventilation/perfusion lung scan or spiral computed tomography of the lung can be used to demonstrate chronic thromboembolic pulmonary hypertension; patients with this disorder who have proximal involvement should be considered for surgical thromboendarterectomy [37]. Echocardiography with Doppler measurements can determine RV function and RV systolic pressure. Pulmonary artery catheterization will demonstrate pulmonary hemodynamics, and whether the pulmonary circulation is reactive to vasodilators (normally tested with inhaled nitric oxide). Measurement of PAP, cardiac index, and right atrial pressure can be used to predict survival in the absence of disease-modifying therapy [38]. For evaluation of functional impairment and prognosis and in the evaluation of long-term treatment the 6-minute walk test is currently used [39].

Therapy of pulmonary hypertension

In the face of increased impedance to RV ejection, compensatory reserves of the RV are limited. Reduction in RV stroke volume and CO and ventricular interdependence with decreased LV filling and output occur [40]. RV dysfunction seen after cardiopulmonary bypass (CPB) either from pre-existing disease or inadequate myocardial RV protection, can be exacerbated by an increase in PVR caused by pulmonary vasoconstrictors or by decreased endogenous NO production from pulmonary endothelial injury during CPB. Traditional management of perioperative pulmonary hypertension involves optimization of acid–base status, oxygenation, ventilation, temperature, level of anesthesia and analgesia, and use of pulmonary vasodilators. Treatment of secondary pulmonary hypertension involves treatment of the underlying etiologic factors. In patients with IPAH, chronic anticoagulation therapy with a goal to achieve an international normalized ratio (INR) of 2–2.5 may improve survival [41].

Pulmonary vasodilator therapy

Because pulmonary vasoconstriction is a major factor in the development of pulmonary hypertension, vasodilators to reverse vasoconstriction were the first therapies used in the management of chronic pulmonary hypertension. As a general rule, all systemic vasodilator drugs are pulmonary vasodilators. Pulmonary vasodilators include direct-acting nitrovasodilators such as hydralazine, nitroglycerin, and nitroprusside; α-adrenergic blockers such as tolazoline and phentolamine; β-adrenergic agonists such as isoproterenol; calcium channel blockers (CCBs) such as nifedipine and diltiazem; prostaglandins such as prostacyclin and iloprost; adenosine; endothelin receptor antagonists; and indirect-acting vasodilators such as acetylcholine, which cause release of NO.

Pulmonary vasodilator therapy frequently results in major adverse effects. These adverse effects can be considered in four categories [42]:

(1) **Systemic hypotension** – In pulmonary hypertension, CO varies with right heart function. Both the pulmonary and systemic vasodilator effects of drugs are dose-dependent. For the majority of drugs, systemic vasodilator effects occur at doses that do not produce pulmonary vasodilation. Thus with a decrease in systemic vascular resistance (SVR) and no change in PVR, CO cannot increase and systemic blood pressure must decrease (BP = CO × SVR).

(2) **Pulmonary hypertension** – A drug-induced decrease in systemic blood pressure may increase PAP by increasing CO and sympathetic tone.

(3) **Decreased contractility** – This may occur from reduced RV coronary perfusion as a result of drug-induced hypotension, from loss of the contribution of the interventricular septum to RV ejection (paradoxical septal motion from decreased LV systolic pressure), or from direct negative inotropic effects as seen with verapamil.

(4) **Hypoxemia** – Pulmonary vasodilators may inhibit hypoxic pulmonary vasoconstriction and thereby adversely alter ventilation/perfusion matching. The degree of hypoxemia will depend on the degree of underlying ventilation/perfusion abnormalities.

All available intravenous vasodilators have one or more of these limitations. In general, the major limitation is the failure to produce selective pulmonary vasodilation. Approaches to develop selective pulmonary vasodilators have attempted to exploit either pharmacokinetic or pharmacodynamic aspects. Adenosine has extensive red blood cell and pulmonary endothelial metabolism, so pulmonary blood levels may exceed systemic blood levels and thereby produce selective pulmonary vasodilation [43,44]. Acetylcholine (because of pseudocholinesterase) and PGE_1 (because of pulmonary metabolism) may have selective effects [45–47]. However, this selectivity is frequently lost at doses that are required to produce adequate pulmonary vasodilation. Nitroglycerin and prostacyclin appear to have the best ratio of pulmonary to systemic vasodilator effects and are frequently used in patients with perioperative pulmonary hypertension [24,48–51].

For patients who respond to vasodilators, CCBs are the most effective option for chronic therapy. Due to the adverse effects of vasodilators and the limited vasodilator response of many patients with chronic pulmonary hypertension, measurement of vasodilator responsiveness should be performed before initiating such therapy. Measurement of vasodilator responsiveness should be performed with a short-acting vasodilator such as inhaled NO, intravenous prostacyclin, acetylcholine, or intravenous adenosine [1,4–6,44,45,52–55]. The purpose of vasodilator testing is primarily to determine whether the patient will be responsive to CCBs; in general, patients responsive to one vasodilator are responsive to all vasodilators. Vasodilator testing is currently performed during pulmonary artery catheterization, allowing measurement of PAP, pulmonary artery occlusion (wedge) pressure, CO, and PVR. A positive response requires a decrease in PAP as well as in PVR. Advances in echocardiography and noninvasive CO measurement may decrease the need for invasive hemodynamic monitoring.

Calcium channel blockers

The CCBs, including nifedipine, diltiazem, and verapamil, have both systemic and pulmonary vasodilating effects [56]. Reports of the acute and chronic use of CCBs in pulmonary hypertension began in the early 1980s [57]. Subsequent work demonstrated that high doses of CCBs are required to produce acute pulmonary vasodilation during studies of pulmonary vascular responsiveness [53,58–60]. In patients who respond to an acute vasodilator trial, chronic therapy with CCBs may result in sustained reduction of PAP, regression of RV hypertrophy, and increased survival [58,61]. Beneficial effects of calcium channel blockade occur in secondary PAH, as well as in IPAH [62–64]. Although initial reports indicated that approximately one-third of patients with IPAH were responsive to CCBs [59], subsequent studies suggest that the actual number is markedly lower [65]. Therefore an acute trial of a pulmonary vasodilator is indicated before initiating chronic therapy.

Although nifedipine is the most commonly used CCB for pulmonary hypertension [53,57–62], beneficial effects have been reported with diltiazem [59,66,67], verapamil [63], and amlodipine [68]. Adverse effects of CCBs include excessive systemic vasodilation, tachycardia, bradycardia, and negative inotropic effects [64,69–71]. These adverse effects, as well as the ratio of systemic to pulmonary vasodilation, may vary with the specific CCB used [59,64,69,71]. CCBs may worsen ventilation/perfusion matching in patients with underlying lung disease [66,67,72].

Nitrovasodilators

The nitrovasodilators include nitroprusside, nitroglycerin, and hydralazine. Nitrovasodilators produce both systemic and pulmonary vasodilation through activation of guanylate cyclase, resulting in increased intracellular cyclic guanosine monophosphate (cGMP). The combination of pulmonary and systemic vasodilation unloads both the right and the left ventricle and is particularly useful for patients with pulmonary hypertension caused by cardiac failure. Nitrovasodilators have been extensively studied in patients being considered for heart transplantation who have increased PVR because of remodeling. Nitroprusside is frequently used to determine pulmonary vasodilator responsiveness in this population [73]. Nitroprusside has a rapid onset of action and a short duration of effect because of the rapid breakdown of the unstable nitroprusside radical to produce cyanide [74]. Free cyanide ions can be converted to thiocyanate in the liver and kidney. Free cyanide that is not converted to thiocyanate can inhibit cytochrome oxidase and prevent cellular aerobic respiration. Prolonged administration of nitroprusside at moderate doses may result in cyanide and thiocyanate toxicity. Nitroprusside is therefore not a suitable drug for long-term infusion in patients with chronic pulmonary hypertension. In patients with acute or chronic lung disease, nitroprusside may produce hypoxemia by reversal of hypoxic pulmonary vasoconstriction [75]. The major limitation to the use of nitroprusside in patients with pulmonary hypertension is the potent systemic vasodilation that results in systemic hypotension, decreased RV coronary artery perfusion, and loss of the RV ejection contribution from the interventricular septum [70,76].

Nitroglycerin is a nitrovasodilator with preferential effects on the venous capacitance vessels and the large coronary arteries. Nitroglycerin can produce pulmonary vasodilation equivalent to the degree of systemic arterial dilation [48]. Nitroglycerin may therefore be preferable to nitroprusside in patients with pulmonary hypertension [48,77]. The reduction in PVR that occurs with nitroglycerin is proportional to the baseline PVR. When PVR decreases, RV output increases, allowing maintenance of blood pressure despite systemic vasodilation. However,

if PVR is only slightly increased at baseline, the venodilating effect of nitroglycerin predominates, reducing left ventricular preload and CO. Nitroglycerin is effective in patients with pulmonary hypertension secondary to chronic left heart failure [49]. A major limitation in the use of nitroglycerin and the related nitrates for therapy of chronic pulmonary hypertension is the rapid development of tolerance [78]. Similar to other vasodilators, nitroglycerin will inhibit hypoxic pulmonary vasoconstriction and worsen gas exchange in patients with acute respiratory distress syndrome [79]. The excess systemic vasodilation and the adverse effects on ventilation/erfusion matching do not occur when nitroglycerin or related nitrates are administered by inhalation [80–82]. The degree of systemic and pulmonary vasodilation that occurs in response to nitroglycerin and the related nitrovasodilators are dependent on endogenous NO production; therefore, inhibition (endogenous or exogenous) of NO synthase potentiates the effects of the nitrovasodilators [83].

Hydralazine is a direct systemic arterial vasodilator that works primarily by activating guanylate cyclase. The arterial vasodilation may produce reflex sympathetic activation with positive inotropic and chronotropic effects. The increased CO may increase PAP if pulmonary vasodilation does not occur. Hydralazine was one of the first vasodilators to be used in pulmonary hypertension [84–86]. However, hydralazine produces potent systemic vasodilation, which may result in severe hypotension and tachycardia [76,87]. As a result, hydralazine has not proven to be useful in patients with pulmonary hypertension.

Inhaled nitric oxide

NO is an endogenous vasodilator and inhibitor of platelet aggregation. NO is produced by the vascular endothelium, primarily in response to increased shear stress [10]. NO diffuses into the adjacent pulmonary vascular smooth-muscle cells, activating guanylate cyclase, resulting in increased cGMP. NO also causes inhibition of phosphoinositide 3-kinase and cyclooxygenase and impairs calcium flux across cell membranes. Intravenous nitrovasodilators such as nitroprusside produce pulmonary and systemic vasodilation caused by release of NO in both the pulmonary and systemic circulations. In contrast, inhaled NO produces selective pulmonary vasodilation [10,88,89]. Inhaled NO is lipid-soluble and diffuses across cell membranes from the alveoli into pulmonary vascular smooth muscle, where it produces pulmonary vasodilation. Inhaled NO does not produce systemic vasodilation because any NO that is absorbed into the pulmonary circulation is inactivated by binding to hemoglobin. Patients with pulmonary hypertension have decreased endogenous NO production [90–92]. In addition to its beneficial effects on pulmonary hypertension, NO may improve ventilation/perfusion matching in patients with lung disease [10,93–95]. Unlike intravenous vasodilators, which tend to increase blood flow to poorly ventilated alveoli, inhaled vasodilators are preferentially distributed to ventilated alveoli. By increasing blood flow to ventilated alveoli, there will be an improvement in ventilation/perfusion matching and a resulting improvement in gas exchange [93]. Although inhaled NO improves oxygenation and decreases pulmonary hypertension in the acute respiratory distress syndrome in adults, randomized studies have not demonstrated sustained improvement or improved outcome [96–98].

In general, the inhaled NO dose–response curve in patients with pulmonary hypertension demonstrates maximal responses at doses of 10 parts per million (ppm) or less and clinically significant responses at doses of 10–100 parts per billion (ppb). These doses of NO may be physiologic, because similar concentrations can occur as a result of production of NO by the pulmonary vascular endothelium and by bacteria in the nasal mucosa and sinuses. In clinical practice, tracheal intubation bypasses the nasopharynx and sinuses and thereby prevents autoinhalation of NO.

Inhaled NO is approved for therapy of pulmonary hypertension and hypoxemic respiratory failure in pulmonary hypertension of the newborn (persistent fetal circulation). In this disorder, pulmonary vasoconstriction and abnormal muscularization of peripheral pulmonary vessels lead to decreased pulmonary blood flow and increased anatomic shunting of desaturated venous blood across the ductus arteriosus or foramen ovale. The efficacy of inhaled NO in avoiding extracorporeal membrane oxygenation or death has been proven in many multicenter randomized controlled trials [88,99,100]. NO doses used varied from 5–20 ppm to as high as 80 ppm. A response rate in these trials was usually more than 50%. In the Neonatal Inhaled Nitric Oxide Study (NINOS) trial, the effects of 20 ppm inhaled NO were investigated in more than 200 full-term and nearly full-term neonates with hypoxic respiratory failure; significant improvement in oxygenation and reduced need for extracorporeal membrane oxygenation (39% NO group vs. 54% control) were demonstrated [101]. There was no effect on mortality alone.

Inhaled NO effectively decreases perioperative pulmonary hypertension in multiple settings, particularly after CPB, when PVR may be increased because of pulmonary endothelial dysfunction [46,50,102]. Selective pulmonary vasodilation with maintenance of systemic blood pressure and therefore coronary perfusion pressure makes inhaled NO an ideal agent in the setting of RV failure with increased PVR. In theory, NO may be useful in patients with allograft dysfunction after lung transplantation, because NO may decrease pulmonary hypertension, improve ventilation/perfusion mismatch, and decrease ischemia–reperfusion lung injury. However, randomized studies have not demonstrated clinical benefit in this setting [103,104]. In pediatric cardiac surgery, inhaled NO has been used for preoperative assessment of PVR reactivity, diagnosis of anatomic obstructions leading to pulmonary hypertension, treatment of pulmonary hypertension when weaning from CPB, and after surgery [105].

Inhaled NO is an ideal agent for screening for pulmonary vascular reactivity in patients with pulmonary hypertension because it produces rapid, maximal pulmonary vasodilation without systemic vasodilation [54,55,89]. Acute administration of inhaled NO can improve exercise tolerance in patients with pulmonary hypertension [106]. Pulsed delivery of NO through nasal prongs has been used for chronic outpatient use [107]. Chronic inhaled NO administration has been used in selected patient populations for chronic pulmonary hypertension. Potential beneficial effects of inhaled NO include selective pulmonary vasodilation, inhibition of platelet aggregation, and inhibition of cell proliferation.

Up to one-third of patients with perioperative pulmonary hypertension or acute respiratory failure have little or no response to inhaled NO. Possible explanations for a lack of response include an unreactive pulmonary circulation, rapid inactivation of NO, abnormalities in the guanylate cyclase system, or rapid metabolism of cGMP. Inhibition of cGMP phosphodiesterase with zaprinast or dipyridamole can increase the frequency, the magnitude, and the duration of response to inhaled NO. Combination of inhaled NO with an intravenous vasodilator that is not dependent on cGMP may produce additive pulmonary vasodilator effects [108,109]. Although inhaled NO normally produces acute pulmonary vasodilation in only a small minority of patients with IPAH, chronic NO may produce pulmonary vascular remodeling in some of these patients [14,107].

Adverse effects of inhaled NO include platelet inhibition during administration, and rebound hypoxemia and pulmonary hypertension with discontinuation. In patients with COPD, NO can produce a paradoxical worsening of oxygenation by reversal of hypoxic pulmonary vasoconstriction in lung areas with low ventilation/perfusion ratios. In patients with LV dysfunction, inhaled NO has been associated with episodes of LV failure and pulmonary edema. This occurs because the decrease of RV afterload augments pulmonary venous return to the left heart, thereby increasing LV filling pressures and precipitating LV failure. Multiple authors have reported severe rebound hypoxemia and pulmonary hypertension on inhaled NO withdrawal. The reasons for this phenomenon are not clear but may be related to suppression of endogenous NO synthase activity, downregulation of guanylate cyclase, and activation of endogenous vasoconstrictor systems. Several approaches are used to avoid clinical deterioration from this rebound effect. The easiest method is to discontinue inhaled NO after the patient has significantly improved and to increase the fraction of inspired oxygen (FIO_2) before discontinuation. Sildenafil, which inhibits phosphodiesterase 5, can attenuate rebound in patients with pulmonary hypertension but may itself produce systemic hypotension. Lepore et al. reported that the combination of inhaled NO and sildenafil produced greater pulmonary than systemic vasodilation, and that rebound pulmonary hypertension did not occur when oral sildenafil was administered before NO discontinuation [110].

Toxicity from inhaled NO administration includes methemoglobin formation, NO_2 production, peroxynitrite ($ONOO^-$)-related lung injury, and surfactant damage. Safe delivery of NO relies on a robust delivery system that includes monitoring of NO and NO_2 concentrations, analysis of methemoglobin levels, and minimizing the delivered NO concentration.

Prostacyclin

Prostacyclin (epoprostenol, PGI_2, Flolan) is a short-acting (half-life of 2–3 minutes) vasodilator produced by the vascular endothelium in response to increased shear stress. The main cellular target for prostacyclin is the prostaglandin I (IP) receptor which activates adenylate cyclase, leading to increased cyclic adenosine monophosphate (cAMP) levels [111]. Prostacyclin infusion decreases PAP and PVR in patients with pulmonary hypertension [45,52,85,111,112]. Prostacyclin synthase lung expression and circulating concentrations of endogenous prostacyclin are decreased in patients with IPAH [11]. Based on evidence that acute administration of intravenous prostacyclin produces pulmonary vasodilation, Higenbottam and colleagues initially demonstrated that continuous intravenous prostacyclin produced sustained beneficial effects in one patient with pulmonary hypertension [113]. Subsequent studies have demonstrated that continuous intravenous prostacyclin improves exercise tolerance, pulmonary hemodynamics, RV function, neurohumoral status, and survival in both primary and secondary pulmonary hypertension [114–120]. In the first of these reports, Rubin and colleagues reported that improvement in PVR and CO persisted with up to 18 months of continuous infusion, although dose requirements did increase in most cases [114]. Although initial studies focused on chronic therapy in patients with an acute response to prostacyclin, subsequent studies have demonstrated that patients who do not acutely respond to intravenous prostacyclin may have improvement after several weeks of chronic therapy. The beneficial effects of chronic prostacyclin may be related to a remodeling effect on the pulmonary vasculature. Prostacyclin is a potent inhibitor of platelet aggregation, which may explain the therapeutic benefit in patients with pulmonary hypertension secondary to thromboembolic diseases. Continuous intravenous prostacyclin has become standard therapy in patients with both primary and secondary pulmonary hypertension, particularly in patients who do not have an acute vasodilator response and are therefore not candidates for chronic oral CCB therapy. Prostacyclin has been used as a long-term therapy in patients with pulmonary hypertension or as a bridge to transplantation [121]. Continuous intravenous infusion of prostacyclin is indicated in patients with pulmonary hypertension with New York Heart Association (NYHA) class III and IV severity.

Failure to respond to prostacyclin is currently considered an indication for lung transplantation [122].

Adverse effects of chronic prostacyclin therapy include systemic hypotension, flushing, jaw pain, gastrointestinal distress, diarrhea, rash, arthralgias, ascites, and life-threatening catheter infections; in addition, infusion pump malfunction may result in immediate hemodynamic deterioration. Prostacyclin may cause pulmonary edema in patients with veno-occlusive disease, because an increased pulmonary blood flow will increase pulmonary capillary pressures when there is venous obstruction. Prostacyclin therapy is not suitable for patients with pulmonary hypertension resulting from pulmonary parenchymal disease, because it may increase intrapulmonary shunting as a result of increased blood to poorly ventilated areas.

Chronic administration of intravenous prostacyclin is an expensive therapy which requires a permanent central venous catheter, a portable infusion pump, and ice packs to keep the medication cold during administration. Patients need training in sterile techniques for mixing and setting up the infusion. Because of these issues, there has been interest in alternative prostanoids and mechanisms of delivery, including inhaled epoprostenol (prostacyclin), inhaled and intravenous iloprost, oral beraprost, and subcutaneous treprostinil. Mikhail and colleagues demonstrated that inhaled prostacyclin did not decrease systemic arterial pressure and did produce a greater reduction in PVR than either intravenous prostacyclin or inhaled NO [123]. Other studies have demonstrated beneficial effects of inhaled prostacyclin [124,125]. Iloprost is a longer-acting analog of prostacyclin and has been used in Europe, New Zealand, and Australia. It has similar hemodynamic effects as epoprostenol and is effective in improving pulmonary hemodynamics and symptoms in patients with pulmonary hypertension [126,127]. Iloprost can also be administered by inhalation. Hoeper and colleagues used inhaled aerosolized iloprost to treat 24 patients with IPAH and demonstrated significant improvements in pulmonary hemodynamics and exercise tolerance [128]. Benefits of inhaled iloprost in primary and secondary pulmonary hypertension have been confirmed in multiple studies [129–131]. Inhaled iloprost may have additive effects to intravenous prostacyclin [132] but may not necessarily be as effective during chronic administration [133]. Administration of iloprost requires a special inhalation device to produce particles of appropriate diameter and to prevent wastage of the drug. Inhaled iloprost has a short duration of effect and necessitates up to 12 inhalations per day to achieve adequate and consistent effect in some patients [128,129]. A long-term observational study in Germany involved patients who were started on inhaled iloprost between 1996 and 2002, with survival rates at 1, 2, and 3 years reported as 79%, 70%, and 59%, respectively [134].

Treprostinil (Uniprost, UT-15, Remodulin) is a long-acting subcutaneously administered analog of prostacyclin [135]. Treprostinil is infused subcutaneously by portable pumps, similar to those used for administering insulin. The pump must be refilled every 3 days but requires no other management. The most frequent side effect is pain and redness at the infusion site, which may limit dosage. McLaughlin and colleagues initially demonstrated the efficacy of chronic treprostinil infusion [136]. Recent retrospective and long-term studies of subcutaneous treprostinil suggest long-term clinical improvement and survival [137]. Barst et al. evaluated 860 patients of NYHA functional class II, III, and IV, and reported survival rates at 1–4 years of 88–70% [138]. This study did exclude patients who required additional agents or premature discontinuation due to adverse effects, most common of which was pain at the injection site. Treprostinil has been also been approved for intravenous use. The advantage over epoprostenol is that the drug delivery cassette can be changed every other day and the system does not require ice packs. The longer half-life of treprostinil may also decrease risk of cardiovascular collapse in case of disruption of the infusion [139,140].

Beraprost, an orally active and chemically stable analog of prostacyclin, was shown in an unblinded, noncontrolled dosing study to improve pulmonary hemodynamics and functional status in a group of 34 patients [141]. Beraprost may also improve survival rates for patients with IPAH [142]. One study demonstrated short- but not long-term benefit with beraprost [143]. A randomized double-blind placebo-controlled trial of oral beraprost also showed improvement in patients with IPAH, but not in patients with PAH from other causes [144]. Oral beraprost is not approved in the USA or in Europe but is approved in Japan.

Endothelin antagonists

Endothelin 1 is a powerful vasoconstrictor and proliferative agent [145]. Patients with pulmonary hypertension may have enhanced pulmonary production and increased circulating concentrations of endothelin 1 [12,14,90]. Intravenous infusion of oral bosentan, an endothelin receptor antagonist, improves pulmonary hemodynamics and exercise tolerance in patients with pulmonary arterial hypertension [146,147,148]. In the BREATHE-1 (Bosentan Randomized Trial of Endothelin Antagonist Therapy) trial, which included 213 patients, bosentan at a dose of either 125 or 250 mg orally twice daily increased 6-minute walk times and delayed the time to clinical worsening [149]. Because the greater dose resulted in more significant liver-function-test abnormalities, the study recommended 125 mg twice daily as the optimal dose.

Endothelin 1 activates two different endothelin receptors [150]. ET_A receptors are located primarily on vascular smooth-muscle cells, while ET_B receptors are located on both endothelial and vascular smooth-muscle cells. The vascular ET_A receptors mediate vasoconstriction and smooth-muscle proliferation, but the endothelial ET_B receptors produce release of vasodilator and antiproliferative modulators such as NO and

prostacyclin. Thus selective ET_A antagonists have been developed for pulmonary hypertension. The selective ET_A antagonists ambrisentan and sitaxsentan have been demonstrated to be effective in chronic therapy of patients with pulmonary hypertension, but studies have not convincingly demonstrated any clinical benefit compared to the nonselective blocker bosentan [151–153]. A recent study does suggest that ambrisentan may have a lower incidence of liver-function-test abnormalities than the other agents and may be used in patients who developed liver function test abnormalities on bosentan or sitaxsentan [154].

Phosphodiesterase inhibitors

Nitrovasodilators such as nitroglycerin produce pulmonary vasodilation by activating guanylate cyclase and thereby increasing cGMP. Prostacyclin, adenosine, and isoproterenol produce vasodilation by activating adenylate cyclase and increasing cAMP. Phosphodiesterases (PDEs) are enzymes that degrade cyclic nucleotides. The type 5 phosphodiesterase enzyme is selective for cGMP and is found in high concentrations in the lung [155]. PDE5 inhibitors therefore have the potential to produce pulmonary vasodilation when used as single-agent therapy, and to potentiate the magnitude and prolong the effect of nitrovasodilators when used as combination therapy. The effects of PDE5 inhibitors as selective pulmonary vasodilators were initially demonstrated in experimental pulmonary hypertension [156,157]. Sildenafil is a PDE5 inhibitor which was initially approved for the treatment of male erectile dysfunction and has now been demonstrated to be effective in idiopathic and secondary pulmonary hypertension [158–162]. Sildenafil has additive effects with intravenous prostacyclin [163], oral bosentan [164], and inhaled iloprost [165]; it increases the response to inhaled NO [166] and facilitates weaning of inhaled NO [167,168]. Other PDE5 inhibitors such as vardenafil and tadalafil may also be effective in patients with pulmonary hypertension [169,170].

Combination therapies

Combination therapies are being investigated as a means of inhibiting the multiple pathways that combine to produce pulmonary hypertension, thereby increasing efficacy while limiting side effects [171]. Some examples of combination therapy have been discussed under individual drugs. A combination of prostacyclin and endothelin antagonists has been investigated in the BREATHE-2 trial, in which patients with PAH received epoprostenol for 16 weeks and were then randomized to addition of either bosentan or placebo [172]. Although there were suggestive trends towards improvement, these were not statistically significant. However, two studies have reported improved maximal oxygen consumption [173] and pulmonary hemodynamics [174] with the addition of bosentan to prostacyclin in IPAH. Other combinations such

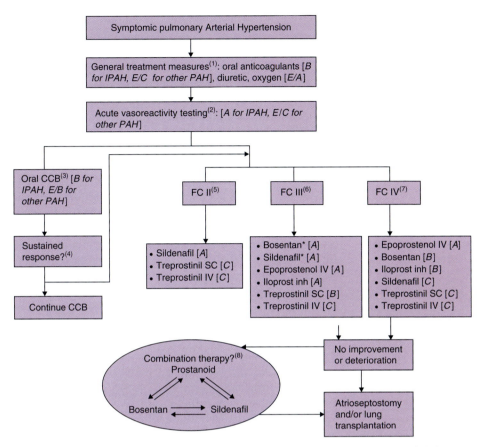

Figure 48.1. Treatment algorithm for pulmonary arterial hypertension (PAH). The recommended therapies presented here have been evaluated mainly in those with idiopathic PAH (IPAH), or PAH associated with connective tissue disease or anorexigen use. Extrapolation to other forms of PAH should be made with caution. Country-specific regulatory agency approval status and functional class indications for PAH medications vary. (1) Anticoagulation should be considered for patients with IPAH, and patients with an indwelling catheter for the administration of an intravenous (IV) prostanoid, in the absence of contraindications. Diuretics and oxygen should be added as necessary. (2) A positive acute vasodilator response is defined as a fall in mean pulmonary artery pressure $\geq$ 10 mmHg to $\leq$ 40 mmHg, with an unchanged or increased cardiac output when challenged with inhaled nitric oxide, IV epoprostenol, or IV adenosine. (3) Consideration should be given to using a PAH-specific medication such as a phosphodiesterase 5 inhibitor, endothelin receptor antagonist, or prostanoid as first-line treatment instead of a calcium channel blocker (CCB) in patients with PAH that is not IPAH or PAH associated with anorexigen use, or in those in an advanced functional class (FC), given the exceedingly low long-term response rate to CCB monotherapy in the former and poor prognosis in the latter. (4) Sustained response to CCB therapy is defined as being in functional class I or II with normal or near-normal hemodynamics after several months of treatment. (5) The risks and benefits of treatment in early PAH should be considered. (6) First-line therapy for functional class III includes bosentan, sildenafil, epoprostenol, inhaled (inh) iloprost, and treprostinil (see text for details). (7) Most experts recommend IV epoprostenol as first-line treatment for unstable patients in functional class IV. (8) RCTs studying add-on combination treatment regimens are under way. [A] strong recommendation; [B] moderate recommendation; [C] weak recommendation; [E/A] strong recommendation based on expert opinion only; [E/B] moderate recommendation based on expert opinion only; [E/C] weak recommendation based on expert opinion only; *, Not in order of preference; SC, subcutaneous. Reproduced with permission from Badesch et al. [4].

as subcutaneous treprostinil with oral bosentan may be another option [175], and there are reports of three-drug combinations being effective [176,177].

Approach to the patient with pulmonary hypertension

In contrast to the situation three decades ago, when there were no effective pharmacological therapies for pulmonary hypertension, there are now multiple drug classes and several drugs within each class to choose from. Severely symptomatic patients with a poor prognosis without effective therapy are therefore frequently started on continuous intravenous prostacyclin. In contrast,

based on the cost, complex administration, and adverse effects of continuous intravenous prostacyclin, less symptomatic patients are often started on oral, subcutaneous, or inhaled therapy. One approach to matching therapy to patient symptoms is presented in the ACCP guidelines (Fig. 48.1) [4].

Future therapies

Future therapy of the patient with pulmonary hypertension may involve novel pulmonary vasodilators such as potassium channel openers [178], antiproliferative agents such as triptolide, rapamycin, and the statins [179,180], Rho kinase inhibitors [181], adrenomedullin [182], and inhaled inovasodilators such as milrinone [183]. IPAH is often the result of a mutation in the bone morphogenetic type 2 receptor (BMPR-2) [184], and gene therapy may be used to restore BMPR-2 function [185], to increase the production of pulmonary vasodilator substances (NO synthase or prostacyclin synthase gene therapy) [186,187], or to alter vascular proliferation [188]. Finally, studies indicate that a fundamental problem in pulmonary hypertension is the loss of endothelial function, and transfusion of endothelial progenitor cells is already in clinical trials [189,190].

Summary

The pulmonary circulation is normally a low-pressure, low-resistance circulation. Pulmonary hypertension is potentially fatal and, unmitigated, can result in right ventricular (RV) failure and inadequate oxygenation. The three factors that cause pulmonary hypertension are increased left atrial pressure (LAP), as occurs in left ventricular (LV) failure or valvular heart disease; increased cardiac output (CO), such as occurs in patients with ventricular septal defects; and increased pulmonary vascular resistance (PVR), as seen in pulmonary disease, hypoxia, and pulmonary arterial obstruction. Most patients with decompensated pulmonary hypertension have a combination of chronic pulmonary hypertension plus an acute increase in PVR. Therapeutic interventions are generally directed at the acute increase in PVR.

Vascular endothelial cells, mast cells, the lungs, and the autonomic nervous system function to maintain the balance of synthesis, release, and removal of vasoactive substances. Abnormalities in endothelial cell function have been revealed in patients with pulmonary hypertension.

Both acute and chronic hypoxia cause hypoxic pulmonary vasoconstriction (HPV), while chronic hypoxia also leads to pulmonary vascular remodeling. In pulmonary artery smooth-muscle cells, hypoxia inhibits voltage-gated potassium channels, in turn activating voltage-dependent calcium channels. A calcium/calmodulin signaling pathway activates myosin light-chain kinase, culminating in contraction. Administration of oxygen can minimize HPV.

The patient should be evaluated to determine the underlying cause of pulmonary hypertension. Traditional management of perioperative pulmonary hypertension involves optimization of acid–base status, oxygenation, ventilation, temperature, level of anesthesia and analgesia, and use of pulmonary vasodilators. Each of the available intravenous pulmonary vasodilators is associated with at least one of the following adverse effects: systemic hypotension, pulmonary hypotension, decreased contractility, and hypoxemia due to poorer ventilation/perfusion matching. Improved selectivity for pulmonary vasodilation is desirable to minimize side effects.

For patients demonstrating responsiveness to vasodilators, there are a number of options. Calcium channel blockers such as nifedipine and diltiazem are the most effective option for

chronic therapy. Adverse effects and the ratio of systemic to pulmonary vasodilation may vary depending on the specific agent. Direct-acting nitrovasodilators are particulary useful for patients with pulmonary hypertension resulting from cardiac failure. Nitroprusside is not suitable for long-term therapy because of risks of cyanide and thiocyanate toxicity, and potent systemic vasodilation is a further limitation of this drug. Nitroglycerin may be preferable in this respect, although, as with the related nitrates, tolerance to nitroglycerin develops rapidly. Administration of nitroglycerin and related nitrates by inhalation prevents excess systemic vasodilation and adverse effects on ventilation/perfusion matching. Inhaled nitric oxide produces selective pulmonary vasodilation, and is approved for use in hypoxemic respiratory failure in pulmonary hypertension of the newborn. It is also effective in decreasing perioperative pulmonary hypertension in multiple settings; however, a proportion of patients have little or no response. Adverse effects include platelet inhibition, and rebound hypoxemia and pulmonary hypertension with discontinuation. Additional adverse effects can occur in patients with chronic obstructive pulmonary disease or LV dysfunction.

Prostacyclin targets prostaglandin I receptors, and continuous intravenous administration is standard therapy for patients with both primary and secondary pulmonary hypertension, particularly those who do not have an acute vasodilator response. However, prostacyclin may cause pulmonary edema in patients with veno-occlusive disease, and is also not suitable for use in pulmonary parenchymal disease. Furthermore, there are a number of adverse effects that can occur in chronic prostacyclin therapy, and continuous infusion is expensive and complicated, raising interest in alternative prostanoids and delivery mechanisms. Endothelin receptor antagonists such as ambrisentan and sitaxsentan selectively block endothelin A (ET$_A$) receptors on vascular smooth muscle. These receptors normally mediate vasoconstriction and smooth-muscle proliferation, and the selective antagonists have been shown to be effective in chronic therapy for pulmonary hypertension; however, convincing evidence is lacking of a clinical benefit compared to bosentan, a nonselective endothelin receptor blocker. While nitrovasodilators, prostacyclin, adenosine, and isoproterenol act to increase cyclic nucleotides, phosphodiesterases (PDEs) degrade these second messengers. The PDE5 inhibitor sildenafil has been shown to be effective in idiopathic and secondary pulmonary hypertension. It has additive effects when used in combination therapy with certain other agents.

Combination therapy aims to maximize efficacy by targeting multiple pathways involved in pulmonary hypertension, while simultaneously reducing side effects. Possible future therapies include potassium channel openers, antiproliferative agents, gene therapy, and progenitor cell therapy.

References

1. Chin KM, Rubin LJ. Pulmonary arterial hypertension. *J Am Coll Cardiol* 2008; **51**: 1527–38.

2. Michelakis ED, Wilkins MR, Rabinovitch M. Emerging concepts and translational priorities in pulmonary arterial hypertension. *Circulation* 2008; **118**: 1486–95.

3. Chan SY, Loscalzo J. Pathogenic mechanisms of pulmonary arterial hypertension. *J Mol Cell Cardiol* 2008; **44**: 14–30.

4. Badesch DB, Abman SH, Simonneau G, Rubin LJ, McLaughlin VV. Medical therapy for pulmonary arterial hypertension: updated ACCP evidence-based clinical practice guidelines. *Chest* 2007; **131**: 1917–28.

5. Benedict N, Seybert A, Mathier MA. Evidence-based pharmacologic management of pulmonary arterial hypertension. *Clin Ther* 2007; **29**: 2134–53.

6. Simonneau G, Galiè N, Rubin LJ, *et al.* Clinical classification of pulmonary hypertension. *J Am Coll Cardiol* 2004; **43**: 5S–12S.

7. Rodriguez RM, Pearl RG. Pulmonary hypertension and major surgery. *Anesth Analg* 1998; 87: 812–15.

8. Humbert M, Montani D, Perros F, *et al.* Endothelial cell dysfunction and cross talk between endothelium and smooth muscle cells in pulmonary arterial hypertension. *Vascul Pharmacol* 2008; **49**: 113–18.

9. Perros F, Dorfmüller P, Humbert M. Current insights on the pathogenesis of pulmonary arterial hypertension. *Semin Respir Crit Care Med* 2005; **26**: 355–64.

10. Steudel W, Hurford WE, Zapol WM. Inhaled nitric oxide: basic biology and clinical applications. *Anesthesiology* 1999; **91**: 1090–121.

11. Klinger JR. The nitric oxide/cGMP signaling pathway in pulmonary hypertension. *Clin Chest Med* 2007; **28**: 143–67.

12. Christman BW, McPherson CD, Newman JH, *et al.* An imbalance between the excretion of thromboxane and prostacyclin metabolites in pulmonary hypertension. *N Engl J Med* 1992; **327**: 70–5.

13. Price LC, Howard LS. Endothelin receptor antagonists for pulmonary arterial hypertension: rationale and place in therapy. *Am J Cardiovasc Drugs* 2008; **8**: 171–85.

14. Haynes WG, Webb DJ. Endothelin as a regulator of cardiovascular function in health and disease. *J Hypertens* 1998; **16**: 1081–98.

15. Giaid A, Yanagisawa M, Langleben D, *et al.* Expression of endothelin-1 in the lungs of patients with pulmonary hypertension. *N Engl J Med* 1993; **328**: 1732–9.

16. MacLean MR, Herve P, Eddahibi S, *et al.* 5-hydroxytryptamine and the pulmonary circulation: Receptors, transporters and relevance to pulmonary arterial hypertension. *Br J Pharmacol* 2000; **131**: 161–8.

17. Egermayer P, Town GI, Peacock AJ. Role of serotonin in the pathogenesis of acute and chronic pulmonary hypertension. *Thorax* 1999; **54**: 161–8.

18. Fischer LG, Hollmann MW, Horstman DJ, *et al.* Cyclooxygenase inhibitors attenuate bradykinin-induced vasoconstriction in septic isolated rat lungs. *Anesth Analg* 2000; **90**: 625–31.

19. Dawson CA, Linehan JH, Rickaby DA, *et al.* Effect of vasoconstriction on longitudinal distribution of pulmonary vascular pressure and volume. *J Appl Physiol* 1991; **70**: 1607–16.

20. Leblais V, Delannoy E, Fresquet F, *et al.* beta-adrenergic relaxation in pulmonary arteries: preservation of the endothelial nitric oxide-dependent beta2 component in pulmonary hypertension. *Cardiovasc Res* 2008; **77**: 202–10.

21. Mathew R, Altura BM. Physiology and pathophysiology of pulmonary circulation. *Microcirc Endothelium Lymphatics* 1990; **6**: 211–52.

22. Tuder RM, Yun JH, Bhunia A, Fijalkowska I. Hypoxia and chronic lung disease. *J Mol Med* 2007; **85**: 1317–24.

23. Pak O, Aldashev A, Welsh D, Peacock A. The effects of hypoxia on the cells of the pulmonary vasculature. *Eur Respir J* 2007; **30**: 364–72.

24. von Euler US, Liljestrand G. Observations on the pulmonary arterial blood pressure in the cat. *Acta Physiol Scand* 1946; **12**: 301.

25. Waypa GB, Schumacker PT. Oxygen sensing in hypoxic pulmonary vasoconstriction: using new tools to answer an age-old question. *Exp Physiol* 2008; **93**: 133–8.

26. Evans AM. Hypoxic pulmonary vasoconstriction. *Essays Biochem* 2007; **43**: 61–76.

27. Nozik-Grayck E, Stenmark KR. Role of reactive oxygen species in chronic hypoxia-induced pulmonary hypertension and vascular remodeling. *Adv Exp Med Biol* 2007; **618**: 101–12.

28. Mauban JR, Remillard CV, Yuan JX. Hypoxic pulmonary vasoconstriction: role of ion channels. *J Appl Physiol* 2005; **98**: 415–20.

29. Michelakis ED, Thébaud B, Weir EK, Archer SL. Hypoxic pulmonary vasoconstriction: redox regulation of O2-sensitive K+ channels by a mitochondrial O2-sensor in resistance artery smooth muscle cells. *J Mol Cell Cardiol* 2004; **37**: 1119–36.

30. Moudgil R, Michelakis ED, Archer SL. Hypoxic pulmonary vasoconstriction. *J Appl Physiol* 2005; **98**: 390–403.

31. Weissmann N, Sommer N, Schermuly RT, *et al.* Oxygen sensors in hypoxic pulmonary vasoconstriction. *Cardiovasc Res* 2006; **71**: 620–9.

32. Siegel LC, Pearl RG. Measurement of the longitudinal distribution of pulmonary vascular resistance from pulmonary artery occlusion pressure profiles. *Anesthesiology* 1988; **68**: 305–7.

33. Marshall BE, Clarke WR, Costarino AT, *et al.* The dose-response relationship for hypoxic pulmonary vasoconstriction. *Respir Physiol* 1994; **96**: 231–47.

34. Preston IR. Clinical perspective of hypoxia-mediated pulmonary hypertension. *Antioxid Redox Signal* 2007; **9**: 711–21.

35. Tarpy SP, Celli BR. Long-term oxygen therapy. *N Engl J Med* 1995; **14**: 710–14.

36. Hanson CW, Marshall BE, Frasch HF, Marshall C. Causes of hypercarbia with oxygen therapy in patients with chronic obstructive pulmonary disease. *Crit Care Med* 1996; **24**: 23–8.

37. Lang IM, Klepetko W. Chronic thromboembolic pulmonary

hypertension: an updated review. *Curr Opin Cardiol* 2008; **23**: 555–9.

38. D'Alonzo GE, Barst RJ, Ayres SM, *et al.* Survival in patients with primary pulmonary hypertension. Results from a national prospective registry. *Ann Intern Med* 1991; **115**: 343–9.

39. Miyamoto S, Nagaya N, Satoh T, *et al.* Clinical correlates and prognostic significance of six-minute walk test in patients with primary pulmonary hypertension. Comparison with cardiopulmonary exercise testing. *Am J Respir Crit Care Med* 2000; **161**: 487–92.

40. Haddad F, Doyle R, Murphy DJ, *et al.* Right ventricular function in cardiovascular disease, part II: pathophysiology, clinical importance, and management of right ventricular failure. *Circulation.* 2008; **117**: 1717–31.

41. Fuster V, Steele PM, Edwards WD, *et al.* Primary pulmonary hypertension: natural history and the importance of thrombosis. *Circulation* 1984; **70**: 580–7.

42. Granton J, Moric J. Pulmonary vasodilators: treating the right ventricle. *Anesthesiol Clin* 2008; **26**: 337–53.

43. Pearl RG. Adenosine produces pulmonary vasodilation in the perfused rabbit lung via an adenosine A2 receptor. *Anesth Analg* 1994; **79**: 46–51.

44. Nootens M, Schrader B, Kaufmann E, *et al.* Comparative acute effects of adenosine and prostacyclin in primary pulmonary hypertension. *Chest* 1995; **107**: 54–7.

45. Palevsky HI, Long W, Crow J, Fishman AP. Prostacyclin and acetylcholine as screening agents for acute pulmonary vasodilator responsiveness in primary pulmonary hypertension. *Circulation* 1990; **82**: 2018–26.

46. Schmid ER, Burki C, Engel MH, *et al.* Inhaled nitric oxide versus intravenous vasodilators in severe pulmonary hypertension after cardiac surgery. *Anesth Analg* 1999; **89**: 1108–15.

47. Tritapepe L, Voci P, Cogliati AA, *et al.* Successful weaning from cardiopulmonary bypass with central venous prostaglandin E1 and left atrial norepinephrine infusion in patients with acute pulmonary hypertension. *Crit Care Med* 1999; **27**: 2180–3.

48. Pearl RG, Rosenthal MH, Schroeder JS, Ashton JP. Acute hemodynamic effects of nitroglycerin in pulmonary hypertension. *Ann Intern Med* 1983; **99**: 9–13.

49. Bundgaard H, Boesgaard S, Mortensen SA, Arendrup H, Aldershvile J. Effect of nitroglycerin in patients with increased pulmonary vascular resistance undergoing cardiac transplantation. *Scand Cardiovasc J* 1997; **31**: 339–42.

50. Kieler-Jensen N, Lundin S, Ricksten SE. Vasodilator therapy after heart transplantation: effects of inhaled nitric oxide and intravenous prostacyclin, prostaglandin E1, and sodium nitroprusside. *J Heart Lung Transplant* 1995; **14**: 436–43.

51. Subramaniam K, Yared JP. Management of pulmonary hypertension in the operating room. *Semin Cardiothorac Vasc Anesth* 2007; **11**: 119–36.

52. Raffy O, Azarian R, Brenot F, *et al.* Clinical significance of the pulmonary vasodilator response during short-term infusion of prostacyclin in primary pulmonary hypertension. *Circulation* 1996; **93**: 484–8.

53. Schrader BJ, Inbar S, Kaufmann L, Vestal RE, Rich S. Comparison of the effects of adenosine and nifedipine in pulmonary hypertension. *J Am Coll Cardiol* 1992; **19**: 1060–4.

54. Sitbon O, Brenot F, Denjean A, *et al.* Inhaled nitric oxide as a screening vasodilator agent in primary pulmonary hypertension. A dose-response study and comparison with prostacyclin. *Am J Respir Crit Care Med* 1995; **151**: 384–9.

55. Morales-Blanhir J, Santos S, de Jover L, *et al.* Clinical value of vasodilator test with inhaled nitric oxide for predicting long-term response to oral vasodilators in pulmonary hypertension. *Respir Med* 2004; **98**: 225–34.

56. Eisenberg MJ, Brox A, Bestawros AN. Calcium channel blockers: an update. *Am J Med* 2004; **116**: 35–43.

57. Rich S, Ganz R, Levy PS. Comparative actions of hydralazine, nifedipine and amrinone in primary pulmonary hypertension. *Am J Cardiol* 1983; **52**: 1104–7.

58. Rich S, Kaufmann E, Levy PS. The effect of high doses of calcium-channel blockers on survival in primary pulmonary hypertension. *N Engl J Med* 1992; **327**: 76–81.

59. Rich S, Kaufmann E. High dose titration of calcium channel blocking agents for primary pulmonary hypertension: Guidelines for shortterm drug testing. *J Am Coll Cardiol* 1991; **18**: 1323–7.

60. Rich S, Brundage BH. High-dose calcium channel-blocking therapy for primary pulmonary hypertension: Evidence for long-term reduction in pulmonary arterial pressure and regression of right ventricular hypertrophy. *Circulation* 1987; **76**: 135–41.

61. Malik AS, Warshafsky S, Lehrman S. Meta-analysis of the long-term effect of nifedipine for pulmonary hypertension. *Arch Intern Med* 1997; **157**: 621–5.

62. Alpert MA, Pressly TA, Mukerji V, *et al.* Acute and long-term effects of nifedipine on pulmonary and systemic hemodynamics in patients with pulmonary hypertension associated with diffuse systemic sclerosis, the CREST syndrome and mixed connective tissue disease. *Am J Cardiol* 1991; **68**: 1687–91.

63. O'Brien JT, Hill JA, Pepine CJ. Sustained benefit of verapamil in pulmonary hypertension with progressive systemic sclerosis. *Am Heart J* 1985; **109**: 380–2.

64. Gassner A, Sommer G, Fridrich L. Differential therapy with calcium antagonists in pulmonary hypertension secondary to COPD. *Chest* 1990; **98**: 829–34.

65. Sitbon O, Humbert M, Jaïs X, *et al.* Long-term response to calcium channel blockers in idiopathic pulmonary arterial hypertension. *Circulation* 2005; **111**: 3105–11.

66. Clozel JP, Delorme N, Battistella P, Breda JL, Polu JM. Hemodynamic effects of intravenous diltiazem in hypoxic pulmonary vasoconstriction. *Chest* 1987; **91**: 171–5.

67. Crevey BJ, Dantzker DR, Bower JS, Popat KD, Walker SD. Hemodynamic and gas exchange effects of intravenous diltiazem in patients with pulmonary hypertension. *Am J Cardiol* 1982; **49**: 578–83.

68. Woodmansey PA, O'Toole L, Channer KS, Morice AH. Acute pulmonary vasodilatory properties of amlodipine in humans with pulmonary hypertension. *Heart* 1996; **75**: 171–3.

69. Packer M, Medina N, Yushak M. Adverse hemodynamic and clinical effects of calcium channel blockade in pulmonary hypertension secondary to obliterative pulmonary vascular disease. *J Am Coll Cardiol* 1984; **4**: 890–901.

70. Cockrill BA, Kacmarek RM, Fifer MA, *et al.* Comparison of the effects of nitric oxide, nitroprusside, and nifedipine on hemodynamics and right ventricular contractility in patients with chronic pulmonary hypertension. *Chest* 2001; **119**: 128–36.

71. Packer M, Medina N, Yushak M, Wiener I. Detrimental effects of verapamil in patients with primary pulmonary hypertension. *Br Heart J* 1984; **52**: 106–11.

72. Kennedy TP, Michael JR, Huang CK, *et al.* Nifedipine inhibits hypoxic pulmonary vasoconstriction during rest and exercise in patients with chronic obstructive pulmonary disease. A controlled double-blind study. *Am Rev Respir Dis* 1984; **129**: 544–51.

73. Costard-Jackle A, Fowler MB. Influence of preoperative pulmonary artery pressure on mortality after heart transplantation: Testing of potential reversibility of pulmonary hypertension with nitroprusside is useful in defining a high risk group. *J Am Coll Cardiol* 1992; **19**: 48–54.

74. Moffett BS, Price JF. Evaluation of sodium nitroprusside toxicity in pediatric cardiac surgical patients. *Ann Pharmacother* 2008; **42**: 1600–4.

75. Adnot S, Radermacher P, Andrivet P, *et al.* Effects of sodium-nitroprusside and urapidil on gas exchange and ventilation-perfusion relationships in patients with congestive heart failure. *Eur Respir J* 1991; **4**: 69–74.

76. McLean RF, Prielipp RC, Rosenthal MH, Pearl RG. Vasodilator therapy in microembolic porcine pulmonary hypertension. *Anesth Analg* 1990; **71**: 35–41.

77. Packer M, Halperin JL, Brooks KM, Rothlauf EB, Lee WH. Nitroglycerin therapy in the management of pulmonary hypertensive disorders. *Am J Med* 1984; **76**: 67–75.

78. Münzel T, Daiber A, Mülsch A. Explaining the phenomenon of nitrate tolerance. *Circ Res* 2005; **97**: 618–28.

79. Radermacher P, Santak B, Becker H, Falke KJ. Prostaglandin E1 and nitroglycerin reduce pulmonary capillary pressure but worsen ventilation-perfusion distributions in patients with adult respiratory distress syndrome. *Anesthesiology* 1989; **70**: 601–6.

80. Goyal P, Kiran U, Chauhan S, Juneja R, Choudhary M. Efficacy of nitroglycerin inhalation in reducing pulmonary arterial hypertension in children with congenital heart disease. *Br J Anaesth* 2006; **97**: 208–14.

81. Yurtseven N, Karaca P, Kaplan M, *et al.* Effect of nitroglycerin inhalation on patients with pulmonary hypertension undergoing mitral valve replacement surgery. *Anesthesiology* 2003; **99**: 855–8.

82. Yurtseven N, Karaca P, Uysal G, *et al.* A comparison of the acute hemodynamic effects of inhaled nitroglycerin and iloprost in patients with pulmonary hypertension undergoing mitral valve surgery. *Ann Thorac Cardiovasc Surg* 2006; **12**: 319–23.

83. Kavanagh BP, Thompson JS, Pearl RG. Inhibition of endogenous nitric oxide synthase potentiates nitrovasodilators in experimental pulmonary hypertension. *Anesthesiology* 1996; **85**: 860–6.

84. Rubin LJ, Peter RH. Oral hydralazine therapy for primary pulmonary hypertension. *N Engl J Med* 1980; **302**: 69–73.

85. Groves BM, Rubin LJ, Frosolono MF, Cato AE, Reeves JT. A comparison of the acute hemodynamic effects of prostacyclin and hydralazine in primary pulmonary hypertension. *Am Heart J* 1985; **110**: 1200–4.

86. Brent BN, Berger HJ, Matthay RA, *et al.* Contrasting acute effects of vasodilators (nitroglycerin, nitroprusside, and hydralazine) on right ventricular performance in patients with chronic obstructive pulmonary disease and pulmonary hypertension: A combined radionuclide-hemodynamic study. *Am J Cardiol* 1983; **51**: 1682–9.

87. Packer M, Greenberg B, Massie B, Dash H. Deleterious effects of hydralazine in patients with pulmonary hypertension. *N Engl J Med* 1982; **306**: 1326–31.

88. Ichinose F, Roberts JD, Zapol WM. Inhaled nitric oxide: a selective pulmonary vasodilator: current uses and therapeutic potential. *Circulation* 2004; **109**: 3106–11.

89. Griffiths MJ, Evans TW. Inhaled nitric oxide therapy in adults. *N Engl J Med* 2005; **353**: 2683–95.

90. Endo A, Ayusawa M, Minato M, *et al.* Endogenous nitric oxide and endothelin-1 in persistent pulmonary hypertension of the newborn. *Eur J Pediatr* 2001; **160**: 217–22.

91. Cella G, Bellotto F, Tona F, *et al.* Plasma markers of endothelial dysfunction in pulmonary hypertension. *Chest* 2001; **120**: 1226–30.

92. Giaid A, Saleh D. Reduced expression of endothelial nitric oxide synthase in the lungs of patients with pulmonary hypertension. *N Engl J Med* 1995; **333**: 214–21.

93. Rossaint R, Falke KJ, Lopez F, *et al.* Inhaled nitric oxide for the adult respiratory distress syndrome. *N Engl J Med* 1993; **328**: 399–405.

94. Payen DM. Inhaled nitric oxide and acute lung injury. *Clin Chest Med* 2000; **21**: 519–29.

95. Klinger JR. Inhaled nitric oxide in ARDS. *Crit Care Clin* 2002; **18**: 45–68.

96. Adhikari NK, Burns KE, Friedrich JO, *et al.* Effect of nitric oxide on oxygenation and mortality in acute lung injury: systematic review and meta-analysis. *BMJ* 2007; **334**: 779.

97. Sokol J, Jacobs SE, Bohn D. Inhaled nitric oxide for acute hypoxic respiratory failure in children and adults: a meta-analysis. *Anesth Analg* 2003; **97**: 989–98.

98. Taylor RW, Zimmerman JL, Dellinger RP, *et al.* Low-dose inhaled nitric oxide in patients with acute lung injury: a randomized controlled trial. *JAMA* 2004; **291**: 1603–9.

99. Barrington KJ, Finer NN. Inhaled nitric oxide for respiratory failure in preterm infants. *Cochrane Database Syst Rev* 2007; **3**: CD000509.

100. Clark RH, Kueser TJ, Walker MW, *et al.* Low-dose nitric oxide therapy for persistent pulmonary hypertension of the newborn. Clinical Inhaled Nitric Oxide Research Group. *N Engl J Med* 2000; **342**: 469–74.

101. Inhaled nitric oxide in full-term and nearly full-term infants with hypoxic respiratory failure. The Neonatal Inhaled Nitric Oxide Study Group. *N Engl J Med* 1997; **336**: 597–604.

102. Oz MC, Ardehali A. Collective review: perioperative uses of inhaled nitric oxide in adults. *Heart Surg Forum* 2004; **7**: E584–9.

103. Meade MO, Granton JT, Matte-Martyn A, *et al.* A randomized trial of inhaled nitric oxide to prevent ischemia-reperfusion injury after lung transplantation. *Am J Respir Crit Care Med* 2003; **167**: 1483–9.

104. Botha P, Jeyakanthan M, Rao JN, *et al.* Inhaled nitric oxide for modulation of ischemia-reperfusion injury in lung transplantation. *J Heart Lung Transplant* 2007; **26**: 1199–205.

105. Kawakami H, Ichinose F. Inhaled nitric oxide in pediatric cardiac surgery. *Int Anesthesiol Clin* 2004; **42**: 93–100.

106. Hasuda T, Satoh T, Shimouchi A, *et al.* Improvement in exercise capacity with nitric oxide inhalation in patients with precapillary pulmonary hypertension. *Circulation* 2000; **101**: 2066–70.

107. Pérez-Peñate G, Cabrera Navarro P, Ponce González M, *et al.* Long-term inhaled nitric oxide plus dipyridamole for pulmonary arterial hypertension. *Respiration* 2005; **72**: 419–22.

108. Aranda M, Bradford KK, Pearl RG. Continuous therapy with inhaled nitric oxide and intravenous vasodilators during experimental pulmonary hypertension. *Anesth Analg* 1999; **89**: 152–8.

109. Saji K, Sakuma M, Suzuki J, *et al.* Efficacy of acute inhalation of nitric oxide in patients with primary pulmonary hypertension using chronic use of continuous epoprostenol infusion. *Circ J.* 2005; **69**: 335–8.

110. Lepore JJ, Maroo A, Pereira NL, *et al.* Effect of sildenafil on the acute pulmonary vasodilator response to inhaled nitric oxide in adults with primary pulmonary hypertension. *Am J Cardiol.* 2002; **90**: 677–80.

111. Gomberg-Maitland M, Olschewski H. Prostacyclin therapies for the treatment of pulmonary arterial hypertension. *Eur Respir J* 2008; **31**: 891–901.

112. Rubin LJ, Groves BM, Reeves JT, *et al.* Prostacyclin-induced acute pulmonary vasodilation in primary pulmonary hypertension. *Circulation* 1982; **66**: 334–8.

113. Higenbottam TW, Wheeldon D, Wells FC, Wallwork J. Treatment of primary pulmonary hypertension with continuous intravenous epoprostenol (prostacyclin). *Lancet* 1984; **1**: 1046–7.

114. Rubin LJ, Mendoza J, Hood M, *et al.* Treatment of primary pulmonary hypertension with continuous intravenous prostacyclin (epoprostenol). *Ann Intern Med* 1990; **112**: 485–91.

115. Barst RJ, Rubin LJ, Long WA, *et al.* A comparison of continuous intravenous epoprostenol (prostacyclin) with conventional therapy for primary pulmonary hypertension: The primary pulmonary hypertension study group. *N Engl J Med* 1996; **334**: 296–302.

116. Rich S, McLaughlin VV. The effects of chronic prostacyclin therapy on cardiac output and symptoms in primary pulmonary hypertension. *J Am Coll Cardiol* 1999; **34**: 1184–7.

117. Barst RJ, Rubin LJ, McGoon MD, *et al.* Survival in primary pulmonary hypertension with long-term continuous intravenous prostacyclin. *Ann Intern Med* 1994; **121**: 409–15.

118. Aguilar RV, Farber HW. Epoprostenol (prostacyclin) therapy in HIV-associated pulmonary hypertension. *Am J Respir Crit Care Med* 2000; **162**: 1846–50.

119. Paramothayan NS, Lasserson TJ, Wells AU, Walters EH. Prostacyclin for pulmonary hypertension in adults. *Cochrane Database Syst Rev* 2005; **2**: CD002994.

120. Langleben D, Barst RJ, Badesch D, *et al.* Continuous infusion of epoprostenol improves the net balance between pulmonary endothelin-1 clearance and release in primary pulmonary hypertension. *Circulation* 1999; **99**: 3266–71.

121. Dandel M, Lehmkuhl HB, Mulahasanovic S, *et al.* Survival of patients with idiopathic pulmonary arterial hypertension after listing for transplantation: impact of iloprost and bosentan treatment. *J Heart Lung Transplant* 2007; **26**: 898–906.

122. Klepetko W, Mayer E, Sandoval J, *et al.* Interventional and surgical modalities of treatment for pulmonary arterial hypertension. *J Am Coll Cardiol* 2004; **43**: 73S–80S.

123. Mikhail G, Gibbs J, Richardson M, *et al.* An evaluation of nebulized prostacyclin in patients with primary and secondary pulmonary hypertension. *Eur Heart J* 1997; **18**: 1499–504.

124. Lowson SM. Inhaled alternatives to nitric oxide. *Crit Care Med* 2005; **33**: S188–95.

125. Siobal M. Aerosolized prostacyclins. *Respir Care* 2004; **49**: 640–52.

126. Higenbottam TW, Butt AY, McMahon A, Westerbeck R, Sharples L. Long term intravenous prostaglandin (epoprostenol or iloprost) for treatment of severe pulmonary hypertension. *Heart* 1998; **80**: 151–5.

127. Strauss WL, Edelman JD. Prostanoid therapy for pulmonary arterial hypertension. *Clin Chest Med* 2007; **28**: 127–42.

128. Hoeper MM, Schwarze M, Ehlerding S, *et al.* Long-term treatment of primary pulmonary hypertension with aerosolized iloprost, a prostacyclin analogue. *N Engl J Med* 2000; **342**: 1866–70.

129. Olschewski H, Ghofrani HA, Schmehl T, *et al.* Inhaled iloprost to treat severe pulmonary hypertension: An uncontrolled trial. German PPH Study Group. *Ann Intern Med* 2000; **132**: 435–43.

130. Baker SE, Hockman RH. Inhaled iloprost in pulmonary arterial hypertension. *Ann Pharmacother* 2005; **39**: 1265–74.

131. Hsu HH, Rubin LJ. Iloprost inhalation solution for the treatment of pulmonary arterial hypertension. *Expert Opin Pharmacother* 2005; **6**: 1921–30.

132. Petkov V, Ziesche R, Mosgoeller W, *et al.* Aerosolized iloprost improves pulmonary haemodynamics in patients with primary pulmonary

hypertension receiving continuous epoprostenol treatment. *Thorax* 2001; **56**: 734–6.

133. Schenk P, Petkov V, Madl C, *et al.* Aerosolized iloprost therapy could not replace long-term IV epoprostenol (prostacyclin) administration in severe pulmonary hypertension. *Chest* 2001; **119**: 296–300.

134. Opitz CF, Wensel R, Winkler J, *et al.* Clinical efficacy and survival with first-line inhaled iloprost therapy in patients with idiopathic pulmonary arterial hypertension. *Eur Heart J* 2005; **26**: 1895–902.

135. Skoro-Sajer N, Lang I. The role of treprostinil in the management of pulmonary hypertension. *Am J Cardiovasc Drugs* 2008; **8**: 213–17.

136. McLaughlin VV, Hess DM, Sigman J, *et al.* Long term effects of UT-15 on hemodynamics and exercise tolerance in primary pulmonary hypertension. *Eur Respir J* 2000; **16**: 394S.

137. Lang I, Gomez-Sanchez M, Kneussl M, *et al.* Efficacy of long-term subcutaneous treprostinil sodium therapy in pulmonary hypertension. *Chest* 2006; **129**: 1636–43.

138. Barst RJ, Galie N, Naeije R, *et al.* Long-term outcome in pulmonary arterial hypertension patients treated with treprostinil. *Eur Respir J* 2006; **28**: 1195–203.

139. Tapson VF, Gomberg-Maitland M, McLaughlin VV, *et al.* Safety and efficacy of IV treprostinil for pulmonary arterial hypertension: a prospective, multicenter, open-label, 12-week trial. *Chest* 2006; **129**: 683–8.

140. Gomberg-Maitland M, Tapson VF, Benza RL, *et al.* Transition from intravenous epoprostenol to intravenous treprostinil in pulmonary hypertension. *Am J Respir CritCare Med* 2005; **172**: 1586–9.

141. Vizza CD, Sciomer S, Morelli S, *et al.* Long term treatment of pulmonary arterial hypertension with beraprost, an oral prostacyclin analogue. *Heart* 2001; **86**: 661–5.

142. Nagaya N, Uematsu M, Okano Y, *et al.* Effect of orally active prostacyclin analogue on survival of outpatients with primary pulmonary hypertension. *J Am Coll Cardiol* 1999; **342**: 1188–92.

143. Barst RJ, McGoon M, McLaughlin V, *et al.* Beraprost therapy for pulmonary arterial hypertension. *J Am Coll Cardiol* 2003; **41**: 2119–25.

144. Galiè N, Humbert M, Vachiéry JL, *et al.* Effects of beraprost sodium, an oral prostacyclin analogue, in patients with pulmonary arterial hypertension: a randomized, double-blind, placebo-controlled trial. *J Am Coll Cardiol.* 2002; **39**: 1496–502.

145. Böhm F, Pernow J. The importance of endothelin-1 for vascular dysfunction in cardiovascular disease. *Cardiovasc Res* 2007; **76**: 8–18.

146. Liu C, Chen J. Endothelin receptor antagonists for pulmonary arterial hypertension. *Cochrane Database Syst Rev* 2006; **3**: CD004434.

147. Price LC, Howard LS. Endothelin receptor antagonists for pulmonary arterial hypertension: rationale and place in therapy. *Am J Cardiovasc Drugs* 2008; **8**: 171–85.

148. Dupuis J, Hoeper MM. Endothelin receptor antagonists in pulmonary arterial hypertension. *Eur Respir J* 2008; **31**: 407–15.

149. Rubin LJ, Badesch DB, Barst RJ, *et al.* Bosentan therapy for pulmonary arterial hypertension. *N Engl J Med* 2002; **346**: 896–903.

150. Abman SH. Role of endothelin receptor antagonists in the treatment of pulmonary arterial hypertension. *Annu Rev Med* 2009; **60**: 13–23.

151. Barst RJ, Langleben D, Badesch D, *et al.* Treatment of pulmonary arterial hypertension with the selective endothelin-A receptor antagonist sitaxsentan. *J Am Coll Cardiol* 2006; **47**: 2049–56.

152. Hrometz SL, Shields KM. Role of ambrisentan in the management of pulmonary hypertension. *Ann Pharmacother* 2008; **42**: 1653–9.

153. Opitz CF, Ewert R, Kirch W, Pittrow D. Inhibition of endothelin receptors in the treatment of pulmonary arterial hypertension: does selectivity matter? *Eur Heart J* 2008; **29**: 1936–48.

154. McGoon MD, Frost AE, Oudiz RJ, *et al.* Ambrisentan therapy in patients with pulmonary arterial hypertension who discontinued bosentan or

sitaxsentan due to liver function test abnormalities. *Chest* 2009; **135**: 122–9.

155. Kass DA, Champion HC, Beavo JA. Phosphodiesterase type 5: expanding roles in cardiovascular regulation. *Circ Res* 2007; **101**: 1084–95.

156. Weimann J, Ullrich R, Hromi J, *et al.* Sildenafil is a pulmonary vasodilator in awake lambs with acute pulmonary hypertension. *Anesthesiology* 2000; **92**: 1702–12.

157. Nagamine J, Hill LL, Pearl RG. Combined therapy with zaprinast and inhaled nitric oxide abolishes hypoxic pulmonary hypertension. *Crit Care Med* 2000; **28**: 2420–4.

158. Galiè N, Ghofrani HA, Torbicki A, *et al.* Sildenafil citrate therapy for pulmonary arterial hypertension. *N Engl J Med* 2005; **353**: 2148–57.

159. Sastry BK, Narasimhan C, Reddy NK, Raju BS. Clinical efficacy of sildenafil in primary pulmonary hypertension: a randomized, placebo-controlled, double-blind, crossover study. *J Am Coll Cardiol* 2004; **43**: 1149–53.

160. Singh TP, Rohit M, Grover A, *et al.* A randomized, placebo-controlled, double-blind, crossover study to evaluate the efficacy of oral sildenafil therapy in severe pulmonary artery hypertension. *Am Heart J* 2006; **151**: 851.e1–5.

161. Pepke-Zaba J, Gilbert C, Collings L, Brown MC. Sildenafil improves health-related quality of life in patients with pulmonary arterial hypertension. *Chest* 2008; **133**: 183–9.

162. Lewis GD, Shah R, Shahzad K, *et al.* Sildenafil improves exercise capacity and quality of life in patients with systolic heart failure and secondary pulmonary hypertension. *Circulation* 2007; **116**: 1555–62.

163. Simonneau G, Rubin LJ, Galiè N, *et al.* Addition of sildenafil to long-term intravenous epoprostenol therapy in patients with pulmonary arterial hypertension: a randomized trial. *Ann Intern Med* 2008; **149**: 521–30.

164. Mathai SC, Girgis RE, Fisher MR, *et al.* Addition of sildenafil to bosentan monotherapy in pulmonary arterial hypertension. *Eur Respir J* 2007; **29**: 469–75.

165. Ghofrani HA, Rose F, Schermuly RT, *et al.* Oral sildenafil as long-term adjunct therapy to inhaled iloprost in severe pulmonary arterial hypertension. *J Am Coll Cardiol* 2003; **42**: 158–64.

166. Bigatello LM, Hess D, Dennehy KC, *et al.* Sildenafil can increase the response to inhaled nitric oxide. *Anesthesiology* 2000; **92**: 1827–9.

167. Lee JE, Hillier SC, Knoderer CA. Use of sildenafil to facilitate weaning from inhaled nitric oxide in children with pulmonary hypertension following surgery for congenital heart disease. *J Intensive Care Med* 2008; **23**: 329–34.

168. Namachivayam P, Theilen U, Butt WW, *et al.* Sildenafil prevents rebound pulmonary hypertension after withdrawal of nitric oxide in children. *Am J Respir Crit Care Med* 2006; **174**: 1042–7.

169. Aizawa K, Hanaoka T, Kasai H, *et al.* Long-term vardenafil therapy improves hemodynamics in patients with pulmonary hypertension. *Hypertens Res* 2006; **29**: 123–8.

170. Tay EL, Geok-Mui MK, Poh-Hoon MC, *et al.* Sustained benefit of tadalafil in patients with pulmonary arterial hypertension with prior response to sildenafil: a case series of 12 patients. *Int J Cardiol* 2008; **125**: 416–17.

171. Taichman DB. Therapy for pulmonary arterial hypertension: the more, the merrier? *Ann Intern Med* 2008; **149**: 583–5.

172. Humbert M, Barst RJ, Robbins IM, *et al.* Combination of bosentan with epoprostenol in pulmonary arterial hypertension: BREATHE-2. *Eur Respir J* 2004; **24**: 353–9.

173. Hoeper MM, Taha N, Bekjarova A, Gatzke R, Spiekerkoetter E, Bosentan treatment in patients with primary pulmonary hypertension receiving nonparenteral prostanoids. *Eur Respir J* 2003; **22**: 330–4.

174. Akagi S, Matsubara H, Miyaji K, *et al.* Additional effects of bosentan in patients with idiopathic pulmonary arterial hypertension already treated with high-dose epoprostenol. *Circ J* 2008; **72**: 1142–6.

175. Benza RL, Rayburn BK, Tallaj JA, *et al.* Treprostinil-based therapy in the treatment of moderate-to-severe pulmonary arterial hypertension: long-term efficacy and combination with bosentan. *Chest* 2008; **134**: 139–45.

176. Austin MJ, McDougall NI, Wendon JA, *et al.* Safety and efficacy of combined use of sildenafil, bosentan, and iloprost before and after liver transplantation in severe portopulmonary hypertension. *Liver Transpl* 2008; **14**: 287–91.

177. Catapano-Minotti G, Corsonello A, Guadalupi G, Spani R, Antonelli-Incalzi R. Treatment of severe pulmonary hypertension secondary to scleroderma: a three-drug approach. *Intern Med* 2008; **47**: 511–13.

178. Moudgil R, Michelakis ED, Archer S. The role of K^+ channels in determining pulmonary vascular tone, oxygen sensing, cell proliferation, and apoptosis: implications in hypoxic pulmonary vasoconstriction and pulmonary arterial hypertension. *Microcirculation* 2006; **13**: 615–32.

179. Faul JL, Nishimura T, Berry GJ, *et al.* Triptolide attenuates pulmonary arterial hypertension and neointimal formation in rats. *Am J Respir Crit Care Med* 2000; **162**: 2252–8.

180. Kao PN. Simvastatin treatment of pulmonary hypertension: an observational case series. *Chest* 2005; **127**: 1446–52.

181. Oka M, Fagan KA, Jones PL, *et al.* Therapeutic potential of RhoA/Rho kinase inhibitors in pulmonary hypertension. *Br J Pharmacol* 2008; **155**: 444–54.

182. Murakami S, Kimura H, Kangawa K, Nagaya N. Physiological significance and therapeutic potential of adrenomedullin in pulmonary hypertension. *Cardiovasc Hematol Disord Drug Targets* 2006; **6**: 125–32.

183. Haraldsson A, Kieler-Jensen N, Ricksten S. The additive pulmonary vasodilatory effects of inhaled prostacyclin and inhaled milrinone in postcardiac surgical patients with pulmonary hypertension. *Anesth Analg* 2001; **93**: 1439–45.

184. Austin ED, Loyd JE. Genetics and mediators in pulmonary arterial hypertension. *Clin Chest Med* 2007; **28**: 43–57.

185. Reynolds AM, Xia W, Holmes MD, *et al.* Bone morphogenetic protein type 2 receptor gene therapy attenuates hypoxic pulmonary hypertension. *Am J Physiol Lung Cell Mol Physiol* 2007; **292**: L1182–92.

186. Champion HC, Bivalacqua TJ, D'souza FM, *et al.* Gene transfer of endothelial nitric oxide synthase to the lung of the mouse in vivo. Effect on agonist-induced and flow-mediated vascular responses. *Circ Res* 1999; **84**: 1422–32.

187. Nagaya N, Yokoyama C, Kyotani S, *et al.* Gene transfer of human prostacyclin synthase ameliorates monocrotaline-induced pulmonary hypertension in rats. *Circulation* 2000; **102**: 2005–10.

188. Zhao Q, Liu Z, Wang Z, *et al.* Effect of prepro-calcitonin gene-related peptide-expressing endothelial progenitor cells on pulmonary hypertension. *Ann Thorac Surg* 2007; **84**: 544–52.

189. Ward MR, Stewart DJ, Kutryk MJ. Endothelial progenitor cell therapy for the treatment of coronary disease, acute MI, and pulmonary arterial hypertension: current perspectives. *Catheter Cardiovasc Interv* 2007; **70**: 983–98.

190. Wang XX, Zhang FR, Shang YP, *et al.* Transplantation of autologous endothelial progenitor cells may be beneficial in patients with idiopathic pulmonary arterial hypertension: a pilot randomized controlled trial. *J Am Coll Cardiol* 2007; **49**: 1566–71.

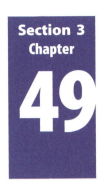

Essential drugs in anesthetic practice
Renal protection and pharmacology

Dean R. Jones and H. T. Lee

Introduction

The kidney is a remarkable organ, responsible for regulating the internal milieu, and playing an extraordinarily important role in regulating blood pressure, salt, and water homeostasis, as well as serving a number of endocrine functions [1]. These physiologic functions, and their attendant manipulation with diuretics, the drug class most traditionally associated with the kidney, are mostly issues of long-term homeostasis, with the exception of critical care medicine. Surgery and critical illness are major causes of acute kidney injury, which is associated with a high incidence of perioperative morbidity and mortality.

The concept of renal protection is not new. In many circumstances, however, clinically meaningful pharmacotherapy for renal protection remains an elusive goal. In its simplest form, renal protection means keeping the kidneys safe from harm, which can come in the form of a number of acute and chronic conditions. Accordingly, renal protection must be put into the context of a patient's underlying medical condition and the potential for further risk of renal injury in the perioperative period. From the perioperative and critical care perspective, renal pharmacology has evolved to focus more on preventing renal dysfunction.

This chapter addresses renal injury, reviewing chronic kidney disease and acute kidney injury as well as techniques for monitoring renal function and injury. We include a brief review of renal physiology and diuretic pharmacology, and focus on protection against renal injury, including nonpharmacologic techniques of renal protection and the current understanding of pharmacotherapy for renal protection.

Renal injury

The kidneys are responsible for a number of important functions including blood pressure modification, acid–base maintenance, and hormone production. Clinicians tend to focus on the kidneys' role in the regulation of fluid and solute composition and the excretion of metabolic wastes as measured with the surrogates of urine output (UO) and serum creatinine (SCr). Renal injury is generally defined in terms of a decrease in UO or an increase in SCr.

Chronic kidney disease

Chronic kidney disease (CKD) as defined in 2002 by the Kidney Disease Outcomes Quality Initiative (K/DOQI) of the National Kidney Foundation is either kidney damage or decreased kidney function for 3 or more months [2]. Proteinuria or abnormalities in imaging tests are markers for kidney damage, and a reduction in glomerular filtration rate (GFR) is a marker for decreased kidney function [3]. End-stage renal disease (ESRD) is a government-derived administrative term that only indicates chronic treatment by dialysis or transplantation. It does not refer to a specific degree of kidney function [3].

The National Kidney Foundation classifies CKD based on pathology:

- diabetic glomerulosclerosis
- glomerular diseases (primary or secondary)
- vascular diseases (e.g., hypertension and microangiopathy)
- tubulointerstitial diseases (e.g., obstructive or reflux nephropathy)
- cystic diseases
- diseases in renal transplant recipients (e.g., rejection, drug toxicity, recurrence of disease)

A GFR of less than $60 \, \text{mL} \, \text{min}^{-1} \, 1.73 \, \text{m}^{-2}$ is considered the threshold for CKD [4]. GFR varies on sex, age, and body size and is typically estimated with calculations based on serum creatinine (SCr). Two common formulas for this purpose are the Cockcroft–Gault formula and the Modification of Diet in Renal Disease (MDRD) equation. Proximal tubular cells in the kidney secrete creatinine, and therefore creatinine clearance surpasses GFR. However, in the steady state SCr is related to the reciprocal of GFR. There are five different stages of CKD (Table 49.1) [2]. Kidney failure is defined as either GFR $< 15 \, \text{mL} \, \text{min}^{-1} \, 1.73 \, \text{m}^{-2}$ or a need for dialysis or renal transplantation.

Acute kidney injury

Several different definitions for acute deterioration in renal function have been proposed. Previously the generic term used

Table 49.1. Stages of chronic kidney disease

Stage	Description	GFR (mL min⁻¹ 1.73 m⁻²)
1	Kidney damage with normal or ↑GFR	≥ 90
2	Kidney damage with mild ↓ GFR	60–69
3	Moderated ↓ GFR	30–59
4	Severe ↓ GFR	15–29
5	Kidney failure	< 15 (or dialysis)

Chronic kidney disease is defined as either kidney damage or glomerular filtration rate (GFR) $< 60 \, mL \, min^{-1} \, 1.73 \, m^{-2}$ for more than 3 months. Kidney damage is defined as pathologic abnormalities or markers of damage, including abnormalities in blood or urine tests or imaging studies.

to describe this situation was *acute renal failure* (ARF), even if the insult to the kidneys did not result in kidney failure.

In an attempt to standardize the classification of ARF, the Acute Dialysis Quality Initiative Group proposed the RIFLE criteria in 2004 [5]. RIFLE stands for *risk* of renal dysfunction, *injury* to the kidney, *failure* of kidney function, *loss* of kidney function, and *end-stage* kidney disease (Fig. 49.1). This classification relies on the measurement of GFR or SCr and UO to classify the severity of ARF. The RIFLE criteria have been validated in numerous studies of intensive care unit (ICU), postsurgical, and hospital patients as independent predictors of mortality [6]. In an effort to further standardize terminology, the term ARF has been replaced by **acute kidney injury** (AKI) [7]. AKI is meant to cover the entire range of ARF, from small changes in SCr to loss of function requiring dialysis.

The Acute Kidney Injury Network (AKIN) proposed a modification to the RIFLE criteria in 2007 [7]. The AKIN definition considers three different stages of AKI, adds a 48-hour time frame for the diagnosis of AKI, and changes the criteria for *risk*, or stage 1 AKI, to include patients with SCr increases of at least 0.3 mg dL⁻¹ (26.4 μmol L⁻¹) (Table 49.2). In a 5-year analysis of over 120 000 ICU admissions in Australia, investigators found no significant differences in the predictive ability of the RIFLE criteria as compared to the AKIN definition [8].

AKI can be classified according to prerenal, renal, and postrenal causes. Prerenal AKI is due to an absolute or relative decrease in renal perfusion. If the hypoperfusion is not corrected, ischemic acute tubular necrosis (ATN) will occur. Intrinsic renal causes of AKI can be divided into glomerular, tubular, vascular, or interstitial causes. Causes of postrenal AKI include bladder or ureter obstruction. Perioperatively the most common cause of AKI is secondary to ATN [9]. The resulting ischemia and inflammation from ATN lead to a cascade of effects: increased production of inflammatory mediators, impaired autoregulation, endothelial injury, decreased GFR, loss of tubular cell polarity, and ultimately cell death from necrosis and apoptosis [10].

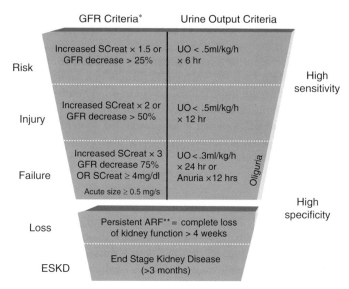

Figure 49.1. Proposed classification scheme for acute renal failure (ARF). The classification system includes separate criteria for serum creatinine (glomerular filtration rate: GFR) and urine ouput (UO). A patient can fulfill the criteria through changes in serum creatinine (SCreat) or changes in UO, or both. Reproduced with permission from Bellomo *et al*. [5].

Risk factors for AKI

Patients with kidney disease may present for a wide variety of surgical procedures. Access for dialysis is the most common procedure, followed by procedures for peripheral vascular disease, coronary artery disease, and kidney transplantation [11].

Overall, the risk of AKI in surgical patients has been estimated to be approximately 1%. However, certain patient populations are at much higher risk. Factors identified as increasing the risk of AKI include age, past history of kidney disease, left ventricular ejection fraction < 35%, cardiac index < 1.7 L min⁻¹ m⁻², hypertension, peripheral vascular disease, diabetes mellitus, emergency surgery, and type of surgery [12]. The highest-risk surgeries include coronary artery surgery, cardiac valve surgery, aortic aneurysm surgery, and liver transplant surgery. The literature is difficult to evaluate, given the many different definitions of AKI, but rates of AKI or need for postoperative dialysis range from 3–5% for cardiac surgery with cardiopulmonary bypass to well over 50% for emergency abdominal aortic aneurysm repair [12].

Perioperative morbidity of kidney disease

The United States Renal Data System (USRDS) collects data on the ESRD population in the United States. The 2007 USRDS report estimated that approximately 15% of the general population had CKD [13]. It is also estimated that all-cause hospitalization rates are three times higher for patients with CKD, and that rates of hospitalization due to AKI are approximately six times higher for patients with CKD.

The presence of CKD increases the rates of morbidity and mortality for a number of different surgical procedures.

Table 49.2. Classification staging system for acute kidney injury (AKI)

Stage	Serum creatinine criteria	Urine output criteria
1	Increase in serum creatinine of $\geq 0.3\,mg\,dL^{-1}$ ($\geq 26.4\,\mu mol\,L^{-1}$), or increase to $\geq 150–200\%$ (l.5- to 2-fold) from baseline	Less than $0.5\,mL\,kg^{-1}\,h^{-1}$ for more than 6 h
2	Increase in serum creatinine to $> 200–300\%$ (> 2- to 3-fold) from baseline	Less than $0.5\,mL\,kg^{-1}\,h^{-1}$ for more than 12 h
3[a]	Increase in serum creatinine to more than 300% (> 3-fold) from baseline, or serum creatinine $\geq 4.0\,mg\,dL^{-1}$ ($\geq 354\,\mu mol\,L^{-1}$) with an acute increase of at least $0.5\,mg\,dL^{-1}$ ($44\,\mu mol\,L^{-1}$)	Less than $0.3\,mL\,kg^{-1}\,h^{-1}$ for 24 h or anuria for 12 h

Modified from RIFLE (Risk, Injury, Failure, Loss, and End-stage kidney disease) criteria. The staging system proposed is a highly sensitive interim staging system and is based on recent data indicating that a small change in serum creatinine influences outcome. Only one criterion (creatinine or urine output) has to be fulfilled to qualify for a stage.
[a]Given wide variation in indications and timing of initiation of renal replacement therapy (RRT), individuals who receive RRT are considered to have met criteria for stage 3 irrespective of the stage they are in at the time of RRT.
Adapted with permission from Mehta *et al.* [7]

Investigators found estimated GFR (eGFR) calculated by the MDRD equation to be an independent predictor of mortality after coronary artery bypass graft surgery (CABG) [14]. The mean eGFR was $64.7\,mL\,min^{-1}\,1.73\,m^{-2}$ for survivors compared to $57.9\,mL\,min^{-1}\,1.73\,m^{-2}$ in the patients who died. Similar findings correlating eGFR with increased morbidity and mortality have also been published for elective major vascular surgery, hip fracture and repair, and endovascular aortic aneurysm surgery.

AKI (not limited to ARF) is an independent risk factor for increased length of hospital stay, in-hospital mortality, and long-term mortality. The overall mortality rate from AKI remained relatively unchanged between 1956 and 2003, at approximately 50%. AKI during the perioperative period had an even poorer prognosis, with mortality rates of 64–83% depending on the surgical population [15,16]. Even small changes in SCr correlate with a significant increase in the risk of death. In one study, patients with SCr increases of 0.3–$0.4\,mg\,dL^{-1}$ had a 70% increase in the risk for death compared to patients with little or no change in SCr [16].

The surgical period presents significant risks to patients with CKD or to those with, or at risk of, AKI. These risks need to be effectively communicated to patients. Moreover, when evaluating healthcare systems for patients with CKD, systems need to be in place to manage a potential deterioration in renal function in the perioperative period.

Monitoring renal injury

In the steady state, SCr is related to the reciprocal of GFR. However, in the acute setting of AKI, SCr is not a sensitive marker of renal function. For example, an abrupt decrease in GFR will cause only a slow rise in SCr over 48–72 hours (Fig. 49.2) [17].

Despite their use in the current definitions of AKI, SCr and UO are not the ideal markers for AKI, and significant research efforts are under way to identify biomarkers of AKI. Earlier recognition and treatment of AKI could potentially have a

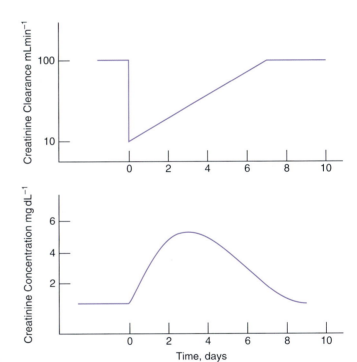

Figure 49.2. Relationship between glomerular filtration rate (GFR), creatinine clearance, and plasma creatinine levels. As depicted in the upper panel, a sudden decrease in GFR corresponds to a dramatic reduction in creatinine clearance. This in turn causes a slow increases in plasma creatinine levels, as depicted in the lower panel. Adapted with permission from Moran and Myers [17].

positive impact on outcome. Potential biomarkers of AKI include neutrophil gelatinase-associated lipocalin (NGAL), interleukin 18 (IL-18), cystatin C, and kidney injury molecule 1 (KIM-1) [18,19].

NGAL is an iron chelator/transporter expressed in the early phase of acute tubular injury. The exact role is unclear but it is thought to be involved in the repair processes after ischemia–reperfusion injury, perhaps with tubule re-epithelialization. Recent data suggest that NGAL is a sensitive marker of renal injury. In a study of renal transplant recipients, increases in both urinary NGAL and IL-18 predicted delayed graft function approximately 24 hours faster than the rise in serum creatinine. A prospective study of cardiac surgery patients found that urinary NGAL levels were significantly elevated within 1 hour after surgery [19].

Caspases are a family of intracellular cysteine proteases that are thought to play a role in a wide variety of cellular functions including apoptosis and inflammation. IL-18 is a proinflammatory cytokine produced by caspase 1 that has been implicated in the pathogenesis of AKI. Recent studies suggest that urine IL-18 is an early biomarker of acute kidney injury both in patients undergoing cardiopulmonary bypass and in ICU patients.

Cystatin C is a basic protein produced by nucleated cells that is freely filtered at the glomerulus then reabsorbed and catabolized by tubular epithelial cells. Studies evaluating whether serum cystatin C levels are an improvement over serum creatinine based measurements of GFR have provided conflicting results. With respect to cystatin C levels during AKI, an ICU-based study found it took 3 days for serum cystatin C to become significantly elevated, no different than for plasma creatinine.

KIM-1 is a transmembrane protein expressed in dedifferentiated proximal tubule epithelial cells after tubular injury and also in renal cell carcinoma patients. In AKI, KIM-1 could be detected within 12 hours of ischemic injury but larger prospective studies are needed to validate these initial findings [19].

Renal physiology

Salt and water homeostasis

The kidney receives about 20% of the total cardiac output (about $1\,L\,min^{-1}$), although it extracts relatively little oxygen, and therefore the renal arteriovenous oxygen difference $[(a - v)O_2]$ is only $1.5\,mL\,dL^{-1}$. There is nonuniform distribution of intrarenal blood flow and oxygen extraction. The cortex receives more than 90% of renal blood flow. In contrast, renal cortical oxygen extraction is low (< 20%) while that of the medulla is high (about 80%). Hence the outer medulla is susceptible to hypoxemia and reduced blood flow. The primary control mechanism for regulating systemic salt and water homeostasis involves complex interactions between opposing neurohumoral reflex systems [20].

Vasoconstrictor, salt-retaining systems, including the sympathoadrenal axis, the renin–angiotensin–aldosterone system, and arginine vasopressin (AVP), protect against hypovolemia, hypotension, and hyponatremia. Sympathoadrenal effects are mediated by circulating epinephrine and the release of norepinephrine from sympathetic nerve endings derived from the T12–L4 segments of the spinal cord. Low levels of sympathetic discharge preferentially constrict efferent arterioles, whereas high levels constrict the afferent arterioles as well. Angiotensinogen, synthesized in the liver, is cleaved by renin in the afferent arteriole to angiotensin I, which is further cleaved by angiotensin-converting enzyme (ACE) to angiotensin II [21]. Angiotensin II causes preferential efferent renal arteriolar constriction in low concentrations, while high concentrations constrict the afferent arteriole and the glomerular mesangial cells. Angiotensin II also contributes considerably to systemic arteriolar tone, as evidenced by the pronounced antihypertensive effect of ACE inhibitors and angiotensin II receptor antagonists (angiotensin receptor blockers, ARBs). In addition, angiotensin II promotes salt and water retention by stimulating the release of aldosterone secretion from the adrenal cortex, stimulating the release of AVP by the posterior pituitary, and enhancing proximal tubular sodium reabsorption [1]. Aldosterone is a steroid hormone produced in the adrenal cortex, released under the influence of adrenocorticotropic hormone (ACTH) and angiotensin II, which acts at the distal tubule to cause sodium reabsorption and potassium loss. Arginine vasopressin (AVP), previously known as antidiuretic hormone (ADH), is synthesized in the anterior hypothalamus, stored in the posterior pituitary gland, and released into the systemic circulation in response to increased serum osmolality, thereby regulating total body water. AVP acts at V_2 receptors in the collecting ducts to increase water reabsorption and concentrate urine. In higher concentrations AVP acts at systemic V_1 receptors to cause vasoconstriction.

Opposing the above systems are vasodilator salt-excreting systems, including prostaglandins, atrial natriuretic peptide (ANP), and endogenous dopamine, which protect against hypervolemia, hypertension, and hypernatremia. In addition, intrarenal synthesis of vasodilator prostaglandins (PGD_2 and PGE_2) and prostacyclin (PGI_2) promotes vasodilation and salt excretion, and also provides endogenous renal protection in response to oligemic stress by maintaining renal medullary perfusion [22,23]. ANP is synthesized in atrial myocytes, released in response to atrial stretch, and has both vasodilator and natriuretic activity, by causing afferent arteriolar vasodilation and inhibition of sodium absorption in the collecting duct [24]. Dopamine is produced in renal tubular cells and acts as an autocrine (i.e., intracellular) and paracrine (i.e., transcellular) factor that inhibits the activity of Na^+/K^+ ATPase and other sodium influx pathways [25]. Dopamine and ANP oppose the salt-retaining actions of norepinephrine and angiotensin II. Natriuretic effects of endogenous dopamine are most prominent with a high-salt diet to maintain sodium homeostasis and normal blood pressure.

Urine formation

The nephron is the basic functional unit of the kidney, consisting of a glomerulus and a tubule emptying into a collecting duct (Fig. 49.3). The kidneys contain approximately 2×10^6 nephrons. Urine is formed by the combination of glomerular ultrafiltration and tubular reabsorption and secretion.

The glomerulus is a highly convoluted tuft of capillary loops, supplied by an afferent arteriole and drained by an

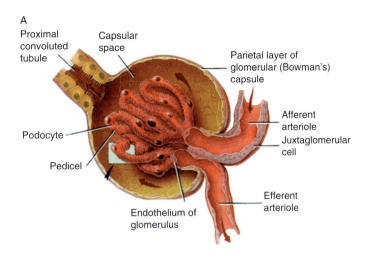

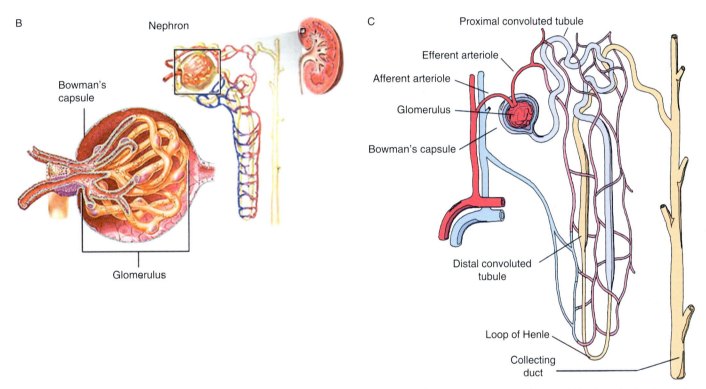

Figure 49.3. Anatomy of the functional units of the kidney: (A) renal corpuscle; (B) nephron; (C) functional arrangement of the renal blood supply, the glomerulus, and the collecting tubules.

efferent arteriole. In juxtamedullary nephrons, the efferent arteriole in turn drains into vasa recta, which line the loops of Henle that dive down into the medulla and create the countercurrent system which drives water reabsorption. Glomerular filtrate formation requires passage through three distinct layers, which are size- and charge-selective [26]. The fenestrated glomerular capillary endothelium restricts the passage of cells, the basement membrane filters plasma proteins, and the epithelial podocytes regulate pore size. Small molecules (< 36 Å diameter, e.g., water, sodium, urea, glucose, inulin)

are freely filtered, those > 72 Å (e.g., hemoglobin, albumin) are not, and filtration of those 36–72 Å depends on their electrical charge. Negatively charged glycoproteins retard the passage of other negatively charged proteins, so cations are filtered but anions are not. In glomerulonephritis, negatively charged glycoproteins are destroyed, polyanionic proteins are filtered, and proteinuria ensues.

Glomerular filtration rate (GFR) depends on the permeability of the filtration barrier and on the net difference between the hydrostatic forces pushing fluid into Bowman's space and the osmotic forces keeping fluid in the plasma. An important system for regulating GFR is the juxtaglomerular apparatus, which consists of the afferent and efferent arterioles and the macula densa, a modified portion of the loop of Henle interposed between the two arterioles. GFR is largely determined by the glomerular filtration pressure, which depends on the balance between afferent and efferent arteriolar tone. The afferent arterioles are innervated by sympathetic fibers, contain baroreceptors, and also release renin in response to arterial hypotension, sympathetic stimulation, or both, which triggers salt and water retention. A low level of sympathetic discharge and angiotensin II activation (e.g., mild hypovolemia, anesthetic induction, positive-pressure ventilation) causes preferential efferent arteriolar constriction, which increases filtration fraction and preserves GFR. Preferential efferent arteriolar constriction may be abolished by ACE inhibitors (e.g., captopril, enalapril, lisinopril) or ARBs (e.g., losartan) and may result in deteriorating GFR. Intense sympathoadrenal and angiotensin II activation (e.g., severe hypovolemia, sepsis, shock) also constricts the afferent arteriole, decreases filtration fraction, and worsens GFR already attenuated by renal hypoperfusion [27]. In addition, the glomerular mesangial cells contain actin fibers that constrict in response to norepinephrine, angiotensin II, and endothelin, which decreases glomerular surface area and further decreases GFR [28]. Of note, even at higher concentrations, AVP causes more selective efferent arteriolar vasoconstriction and is more likely to preserve GFR than norepinephrine or angiotensin II [29].

Renal function is autoregulated, and thus renal blood flow, GFR, and solute and water regulation are intrinsically maintained independently of mean arterial pressure (MAP) [30]. Autoregulation is not abolished by most anesthetic agents, but does appear impaired in severe sepsis [31], acute renal failure [32], and perhaps during cardiopulmonary bypass [33]. Absent autoregulation, renal blood flow is dependent on renal perfusion pressure, which is acutely decreased during hypotension and restored by vasoconstrictor therapy.

The renal tubule comprises four distinct segments: the proximal tubule, the loop of Henle (which includes the pars recta, descending and ascending thin limb segments, and the medullary thick ascending limb), the distal tubule, and the collecting duct (Figs. 49.3, 49.4). The last courses through the cortex and medulla before entering the renal pelvis at the papilla. The more numerous outer cortical nephrons have short loops of Henle and receive about 85% of the renal blood flow. The juxtamedullary nephrons, which receive less than 10% of the renal blood flow, have long loops of Henle. These dive deeply into the inner medulla together with the vasa recta and are responsible for the countercurrent mechanism that generates medullary hypertonicity and creates the concentrating ability of the kidney. The renal tubules absorb more than 99% of the salt and water in the 180 L day^{-1} of glomerular filtrate. Many other filtrates are completely reabsorbed, while some have a maximum rate of tubular reabsorption, such as

glucose, which spills into urine at concentrations greater than 375 mg dL^{-1}.

The proximal tubule reabsorbs about two-thirds of the filtered sodium, which draws with it water, chloride, and potassium, and reabsorbs almost 100% of the filtered glucose, lactate, and amino acids. The proximal tubule secretes many endogenous anions (bile salts, urate), cations (creatinine, dopamine), and drugs (diuretics, penicillin, probenecid, cimetidine).

The medullary thick ascending limb reabsorbs about 20% of filtered sodium, chloride, potassium, and bicarbonate. The medulla receives only 6% of the renal blood flow, but is highly metabolically active, extracts a large proportion of oxygen, has a tissue PO_2 of just 8 mmHg, and is thus particularly vulnerable to nephrotoxin-mediated ischemic injury [34]. For example, prostaglandin inhibitors such as nonsteroidal anti-inflammatory drugs (NSAIDs) can thus cause medullary ischemia. Urinary concentrating ability is dependent on the development of a hypertonic medullary interstitium, which is created by the countercurrent multiplier effect of the loop of Henle, in which solute is separated from water. The medullary thick ascending limb actively reabsorbs sodium from the lumen but is impermeable to water, which becomes trapped so that as the tubular fluid ascends in the thick ascending limb it becomes progressively more dilute. By the end of this "diluting segment," tubular fluid osmolality has decreased to less than 150 mOsm kg^{-1}. This in turn results in increased sodium chloride concentration and osmolality in the medullary interstitium. The descending loop of Henle is permeable to water, which diffuses out along the osmotic gradient so that the tubular fluid becomes maximally concentrated at the inferior pole of the loop. The vasa recta, which are a continuation of the efferent arteriole and surround the loops of Henle, maintain this condition by removing water and adding solute as they pass through the medullary interstitium. An osmotic gradient is established between the cortex (300 mOsm kg^{-1}), juxtamedullary zone (600 mOsm kg^{-1}), and deep medulla (1200 mOsm kg^{-1}), enhanced by the passive recycling of urea. In addition, AVP from the posterior pituitary acts on V_2 receptors in the distal tubule and collecting ducts and enhances their permeability to water, which is reabsorbed, resulting in an antidiuresis. Urinary concentrating ability can be abolished by diuretics, especially osmotic diuretics (e.g., mannitol), which "wash out" the hypertonic medulla, potentially resulting in intravascular hypovolemia. Concentrating ability is highly dependent on normal tubular function, and loss of concentrating ability is an early and singular sign of acute tubular injury.

The distal tubule initial segment is structurally and functionally similar to the thick ascending limb. About 5–8% of filtered sodium and chloride are actively reabsorbed. In the last part of the distal tubule, sodium is absorbed (and water follows) in exchange for potassium secretion. Aldosterone acts in the distal tubule to enhance cell permeability and stimulate sodium absorption and potassium excretion.

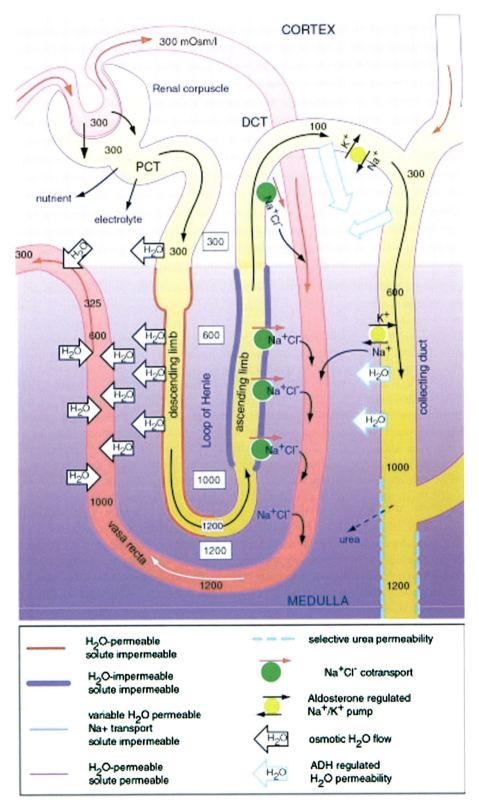

Figure 49.4. Water and electrolyte exchange across the renal tubules. Reproduced with permission from Metropolitan State College of Denver.

The collecting ducts (and distal tubules) contain specific V_2 vasopressin receptors, which respond to AVP, the endogenous hormone that controls the renal antidiuretic response to dehydration (hence the name *antidiuretic hormone*). AVP is synthesized in the anterior hypothalamus, stored in the posterior pituitary gland, and released in response to osmoreceptors in the hypothalamus that detect minute increases in serum osmolality. AVP increases collecting-duct permeability, resulting in water reabsorption and a decreased flow of concentrated urine. Antidiuresis is also triggered by hypovolemia and arterial hypotension, mediated by stretch receptors in the atria and great veins, or baroreceptors in the aortic arch and carotid sinuses.

Diuretics

Osmotic diuretics

Osmotic diuretics are small molecules that are freely filtered at the glomerulus, minimally reabsorbed, and increase tubular flow by drawing water into the renal tubule [35]. Mannitol is the prototypic osmotic diuretic, but others clinically used include urea, glycerin, and isosorbide. Additionally, any poorly reabsorbed solute that exceeds its transport maximum can also act as an osmotic diuretic. Thus in hyperglycemia, once the transport maximum for glucose has been surpassed, an osmotic diuresis will ensue, demarking one of the hallmark symptoms of diabetes mellitus. Mannitol prevents water (but not sodium) reabsorption in the segments of the tubule that are freely permeable to water – the proximal tubule, the descending loop of Henle, and the collecting duct. Water and solute reabsorption are coupled in these segments so that isotonicity is maintained. By osmotically obligating water to remain in the tubule, renal tubular flow increases and a marked diuresis occurs without natriuresis [36]. The osmotic diuresis "washes out" the countercurrent system that creates medullary hypertonicity, resulting in a loss of urinary concentrating ability and the production of dilute urine.

Mannitol also has numerous other effects, some of which contribute to diuresis [37–40]. It expands intravascular volume, vasodilates afferent arterioles, and increases renal blood flow and GFR, with a preferential shift of renal blood flow to the medulla. Mannitol has also been suggested to reduce cellular injury (swelling) during ischemia and protect against ischemia–reperfusion injury by scavenging free radicals (although this has been disputed [40,41]). Mannitol has also been suggested to prevent tubular obstruction from cellular debris than can occur in ischemic tubules and tubular injury by myoglobin, secondary to increased flow and flushing out of cellular debris [42].

Mannitol has been widely used in cardiac surgery as part of the cardiopulmonary bypass prime, in vascular surgery, in transplantation surgery, and in nephrotoxic situations, with the intent of renal protection. Mannitol causes a brisk and prolonged diuresis, to such an extent that volume replacement is often necessary. It may also be accompanied by hypokalemia. Patients who are given more than $1\,g\,kg^{-1}$ mannitol in the cardiopulmonary bypass prime are invariably volume- and potassium-depleted in the postoperative period. Because mannitol is rapidly redistributed, it may paradoxically cause

pulmonary or cerebral edema by translocation of fluid into the intracellular space. It should therefore be administered with caution in patients with poor left ventricular function or prior history of congestive heart failure, head injury, or intracranial mass.

Carbonic anhydrase inhibitors

Bicarbonate reabsorption occurs prominently in the proximal tubule, via the action of carbonic anhydrase. Carbonic anhydrase catalyzes the reversible combination of water and carbon dioxide to form carbonic acid, which serves as a source of hydrogen ions and is exchanged for filtered bicarbonate. Carbonic anhydrase inhibitors such as acetazolamide block bicarbonate reabsorption, resulting in obligatory bicarbonate loss, along with sodium loss, and resulting diuresis. Acetazolamide is a relatively weak diuretic, because most of the sodium that escapes the proximal tubule is reabsorbed more distally. Acetazolamide is usually indicated in the management of persistent metabolic alkalosis uncorrected by potassium chloride replacement, especially if it inhibits respiratory drive.

Loop diuretics

Loop diuretics such as furosemide, bumetanide, torasemide, and ethacrynic acid are the most efficacious diuretics available and generate the highest fractional excretion of sodium. They act at the loop of Henle, where up to 25% of all sodium reabsorption occurs, and there is very limited capability for compensatory reabsorption distally [35]. More specifically, they act at the medullary thick ascending limb, to inhibit the sodium/potassium chloride symporter situated at the luminal membrane and, to a lesser extent, the Na^+/K^+ ATPase pump at the basolateral cell membrane. Inhibition of solute reabsorption in the water-impermeable thick ascending limb dilutes the concentration gradient of the countercurrent mechanism, thus reducing the concentrating capacity and the amount of water that can be absorbed in the collecting duct. Loop diuretics also have some effects on vasodilation, the proximal tubule, and the distal tubule, which blunts the expected increase in sodium reabsorption due to increased downstream sodium load. Loop diuretics act at the luminal membrane of tubular epithelial cells, and not the basolateral aspect; therefore secretion is required for activity, and excretion of water and electrolytes is related to urinary concentrations of furosemide rather than the serum concentration [43].

Loop diuretics cause brisk diuresis, especially after an intravenous dosing, and should be administered only in patients with normal or increased intravascular volume. Acute hypovolemia may be a consequence of inappropriate administration of loop diuretics to "make urine" in hypovolemic states. Diuretic-induced dehydration and hypotension can cause pre-renal failure and further exacerbate ischemic injury. Excessive ongoing diuresis can induce hypokalemic metabolic alkalosis.

Chronic tolerance to loop diuretics can occur with prolonged use, requiring greater doses, and this is attributed to compensatory hypertrophy and increased reabsorptive activity of the distal tubule and collecting duct [44]. Tolerance can be overcome by concomitant administration of a thiazide diuretic, which may also actually prevent distal tubule hypertrophy [45]. This strategy, known as dual segment blockade, is also extremely effective in overcoming diuretic resistance in oliguria associated with renal insufficiency and low GFR.

Thiazide diuretics

Thiazides act in the early distal convoluted tubule to block sodium reabsorption at the luminal membrane of tubular cells. Because only 15% of the GFR is due to this segment and only 5–8% of tubular sodium reabsorption occurs here, thiazides have less diuretic and natriuretic efficacy than the loop diuretics [35]. Thiazides are mainly used for oral treatment of hypertension, in which the dual actions of diuresis/natriuresis and vasodilation are synergistic. Other uses include hypercalciuria and nephrolithiasis.

Potassium-sparing diuretics

Potassium-sparing diuretics are active in the distal tubule and collecting ducts [35]. They have weak diuretic activity because less than 5% of filtered sodium is reabsorbed in these segments. These drugs are used in combination with thiazides or loop diuretics to augment diuresis and restrict potassium loss which occurs in the distal tubule. They are not available for parenteral injection and are seldom used in the perioperative period.

There are two classes of potassium-sparing diuretics. Spironolactone is a competitive antagonist of aldosterone at the distal tubule. It binds to cytoplasmic mineralocorticoid receptors and prevents the aldosterone/receptor complex from translocating to the cell nucleus, and increasing gene expression. This explains why the onset of action requires 2–4 days for full effect and effects on aldosterone transport last for 2–3 days after the drug is discontinued. Spironolactone is used in primary and secondary hyperaldosteronism and is useful in reversing sodium retention and potassium excretion in edematous prerenal states characterized by excessive aldosterone secretion such as liver failure and congestive heart failure. Amiloride and triamterene inhibit the sodium channel in the luminal membrane of the distal tubule by a nonaldosterone-dependent mechanism, with a reduction in sodium reabsorption and potassium excretion [46]. These drugs are not available as intravenous formulations and are therefore not frequently used in the perioperative period or in critically ill patients.

Adult dosing guidelines for commonly used diuretics are provided in Table 49.3.

Renal dopamine

Renal effects of the dopaminergic system have been a focus in anesthesiology for decades. Endogenous dopamine plays an important role in salt and water homeostasis and renal function, by influencing sodium transport, vascular smooth muscle tone, renal blood flow, and the renin–angiotensin and sympathetic nervous systems. Dopamine receptors are classified into D_1-like (D_1 and D_5) and D_2-like (D_2, D_3, and D_4) subtypes based on their structure and pharmacology [47]. D_1-like receptors stimulate adenylate cyclase activity to increase intracellular cAMP concentrations. D_2-like receptors couple to inhibitory G-proteins and modulate ion channel activity and/or inhibit adenylate cyclase activity. Dopamine is synthesized in proximal tubular cells, and can act on local receptors and those in more distal segments of the nephron. Endogenous renal dopamine (via D_1 receptors) is a major regulator of renal sodium excretion.

Activation of D_1-like (D_1 and D_5) receptors causes renal vasodilation and increased renal blood flow, GFR, natriuresis, and diuresis. Dopamine-dependent natriuresis can also occur independently of renal blood flow changes. Relative contributions of D_1 and D_5 receptors to D_1-like receptor-mediated dopamine effects are not known. Whereas dopamine is a nonselective agonist, the drug fenoldopam is a selective D_1 agonist. Less is known about the physiologic effects of the D_2, D_3, and D_4 receptors, because of the lack of selective agonists and inhibitors; however, these appears to antagonize angiotensin II, affect renal blood flow and sodium excretion, and affect salt and water transport in the collecting duct, respectively.

Renal protection

Given the high mortality of AKI, an anesthesiologist's main objective for perioperative renal protection is prevention. Keys to this goal are maintenance of euvolemia and preservation of adequate renal perfusion.

Volume status

The face validity to "maintain adequate intravascular volume" seems irrefutable, yet debate continues as to the best strategy to manage patients at risk of AKI. Uncorrected hypovolemia and a reduction in oxygen delivery leave the renal medulla susceptible to ischemic ATN [12]. Clinical features of hypovolemia such as reduced skin turgor, collapsed peripheral veins, tachycardia, postural hypotension, reduced jugular venous pressure, and cool extremities can all be obscured by general or regional anesthesia and by surgery. Assessment of intravascular volume and left ventricular preload may be improved with invasive techniques such as central venous pressure monitoring, pulmonary artery wedge pressure monitoring, or transesophageal echocardiography [12]. Even with invasive monitoring, the clinician must remember that disease states, such as sepsis, can lead to regional maldistribution of intravascular volume and oxygen delivery due to vasodilation or altered capillary permeability. The implication is that the clinician must remain vigilant in assessment, and individualize therapy even in the setting of "normal" physiologic values.

The ideal fluid for maintenance and resuscitation of patients at risk of AKI is controversial. Crystalloids, colloids, and blood

Table 49.3. Adult dosing guidelines for commonly administered diuretics

Diuretic	Class	Indication	Dosage	Remarks
Mannitol	Osmotic	To promote diuresis in the prevention or treatment of the oliguric phase of acute renal failure	Test dose: 0.2 mg kg^{-1} IV over 3–5 min; may repeat one time Treatment of oliguria: 50–100 g of a 15–25% solution IV slowly	Include a filter when infusing concentrated mannitol
Furosemide	Loop	Treatment of edema associated with CHF, hepatic cirrhosis, or renal disease Treatment of hypertension	20–80 mg IM or IV slowly; dose may be increased by 20 mg and repeated in 2 h; may dose 1–2 times daily, 40 mg PO	Give intravenous injections slowly over 2 minutes For intravenous injections, do not exceed 1 g per day
Bumetanide	Loop	Same as furosemide	0.5–2 mg PO; may be repeated at 5 h intervals up to a maximum dose of I0 mg per day 0.5–1 mg IV or IM; may be repeated at 3 h intervals up to a maximum dose of I0 mg per day	Reserve IV or IM use for patients with impaired GI absorption Can be used in patients allergic to furosemide at 1:40 ratio of bumetanide to furosemide
Ethacrynic acid	Loop	Same as furosemide	50–200 mg per day PO 50 mg IV or 0.5–I mg kg^{-1} (usually only one IV dose necessary)	Do not give IM because of local pain and irritation. If second IV dose is necessary, use a new injection site to avoid thrombophlebitis
Chlorothiazide	Thiazide	Hypertension and edema associated with CHF, hepatic cirrhosis, or renal disease	0.5–1 0 g once or twice a day either PO or IV	Do not give IM IV is reserved for patients unable to take oral medications of emergency situations
Hydrochlorothiazide	Thiazide	Hypertension Edema associated with CHF, hepatic cirrhosis, or renal disease	12.5–50 mg per day PO 25–100 mg per day PO until dry weight is obtained	
Acetazol amide	Carbonic anhydrase inhibitor	Glaucoma Diuresis in CHF	250–1000 mg (5 mg kg^{-1}) per day PO or IV	IM administration is painful
Spironolactone	Potassium-sparing	Edema associated with CHF, hepatic cirrhosis, or renal disease	25–200 mg per day PO	If diuretic response has not occurred after 5 days, add a second diuretic that acts more proximally in the renal tubule
Amiloride	Potassium-sparing	Adjunctive therapy with thiazide or loop diuretics in CHF or hypertension	5–I0 mg per day	Useful for restoring normal serum potassium in patients with hypokalemia while taking diuretics
Triamterene	Potassium-sparing	Edema associated with CHF, hepatic cirrhosis, or renal disease	100–300 mg per day	May be used alone or with other diuretics for additive diuretic effect or antikaliuretic (potassium-sparing) effect

CHF, congestive heart failure; GI, gastrointestinal; IM, intramuscularly: IV, intravenously: PO, per os (by mouth).

products each have their own specific advantages and disadvantages. A recent Cochrane review on fluid resuscitation in critically ill patients concluded: "There is no evidence from randomized controlled trials that resuscitation with colloids reduces the risk of death, compared to resuscitation with crystalloids, in patients with trauma, burns or following surgery. As colloids are not associated with an improvement in survival, and as they are more expensive than crystalloids, it is hard to see how their continued use in these patients can be justified outside the context of randomized controlled trials" [48].

Nonetheless, crystalloids are far from perfect resuscitation fluids. The most commonly used intraoperative crystalloids include 0.9% normal saline (NS) and lactated Ringer's (LR). NS is both hypertonic and hyperchloremic compared to plasma, and in volumes greater than $30 \, \text{mL} \, \text{kg}^{-1}$ can lead to hyperchloremic metabolic acidosis and hyperkalemia. NS is commonly recommended over LR for renal transplant patients or for patients with renal failure, because of the hypothesized risk of hyperkalemia from the potassium-containing LR. This apprehension appears unfounded, as a prospective, randomized, double-blind clinical trial of NS compared to LR for intraoperative fluid therapy in kidney transplant patients found that NS was associated with more hyperkalemia and acidosis than LR [49]. Generally, hemodynamic parameters, UO, and invasive monitors direct the amount of crystalloid administered. It is commonly recommended to titrate crystalloid to maintain MAP $> 65–70 \, \text{mmHg}$, UO $> 0.5 \, \text{mL} \, \text{kg}^{-1} \, \text{h}^{-1}$, central venous pressure $10–15 \, \text{mmHg}$, and pulmonary artery wedge pressure $10–15$ mmHg [12]. Excessive fluid resuscitation may be harmful. For example, in a study of critically ill trauma patients goal-directed therapy to supranormal values resulted in administration of higher volumes of fluid with increased risk of abdominal compartment syndrome, organ failure, and death [50].

Hydroxyethyl starch (HES) solutions are also commonly used for intravascular volume expansion. Deleterious effects of HES solutions include coagulation derangements and allergic reactions. Other studies have also suggested an increased risk of AKI in association with the use of HES solutions, particularly in sepsis [51]. Overall this issue remains unresolved, as other studies conclude that HES does not influence renal outcome [52].

Renal perfusion

Blood flow to the kidney is autoregulated to maintain a stable GFR when MAP is within the range of $\sim 80–160 \, \text{mmHg}$. Autoregulation maintains fluid and salt balance or preserves glomerular structure via a myogenic response and tubuloglomerular feedback. Decreased renal perfusion can be due to decreased cardiac output, decreased MAP, or increased renal vasoconstriction [53]. An ideal MAP to optimize renal perfusion is not known. In patients with septic shock, a MAP of 85 mmHg compared to 65 mmHg produced no significant benefit in renal outcome [54]. Other researchers have used Doppler ultrasonography and calculated renal resistive index to monitor renal blood flow and individualize MAP goals [55]. This study

evaluated patients in septic shock who required fluids and norepinephrine to maintain a MAP greater than 65 mmHg. Increasing MAP from 65 to 75 mmHg resulted in significantly increased UO and decreased resistive index. No further improvement was found when MAP was increased from 75 to 85 mmHg.

Given the concern of maintaining renal perfusion within the limits of autoregulation, hypotensive anesthesia is generally avoided in patients with chronic renal insufficiency. A study of hypotensive anesthesia induced with volatile anesthetics in patients with normal renal function found a short-term reversible alteration in tubular function as measured by urinary N-acetyl-β-D-glucosaminidase [56]. Other studies contend that hypotensive epidural anesthesia augmented with intravenous epinephrine infusion does not predispose patients with chronic renal insufficiency to AKI [57]. In general, more research is required before these findings can be applied to broader surgical populations.

Abdominal laparoscopic surgical techniques may also influence renal perfusion. There is evidence to suggest that both renal blood flow and renal function are decreased during pneumoperitoneum, although the clinical significance of this is uncertain. Even though urine output decreases as intra-abdominal pressure increases, abdominal insufflation pressures of less than 15 mmHg are considered safe [58]. To alleviate the effects of elevated intra-abdominal pressure, euvolemia or fluid loading is advocated. An animal model of hemorrhagic shock demonstrated that abdominal insufflation of pressures of 15 mmHg significantly decreased renal perfusion, and therefore careful monitoring of trauma laparoscopy patients is advised [59]. There is one case report of kidney graft loss after laparoscopic donor nephrectomy that suggests prolonged insufflation pressures of 15 mmHg as contributory [60]. Other studies of laparoscopic live-donor nephrectomies found that laparoscopic procurement may be an independent risk factor for rejection in pediatric recipients [61]. This finding was not replicated in an adult study that showed equivalent early and late outcomes between laparoscopic and open procurement [62]. Gasless laparoscopy may be an alternative for patients at high risk of renal ischemia. Further research to delineate whether there are other populations at risk of renal injury during laparoscopy is needed.

Pharmacotherapy for renal protection

Before reviewing pharmacotherapy for renal protection, an area that should not be overlooked is the avoidance of nephrotoxins. An enormous number of over-the-counter medications, prescription medications, and herbal medications can potentially cause AKI. In patients with CKD, and in those at risk of AKI, appropriate dosing of antibiotics, avoidance of contrast dyes as permitted, and avoidance of NSAIDs are all recommended. Pharmacotherapy for renal protection can be considered in two categories: halting the progression of CKD, and prevention and/or treatment of AKI.

Chronic kidney disease

Given the epidemiology of CKD, treatment of the underlying cause often revolves around management of hypertension and type 2 diabetes. Whether lipid-lowering therapy can protect against the progression of CKD remains unanswered [63]. Tight glycemic control may lead to a reduction in diabetic nephropathy but without an overall benefit in mortality [64,65].

The seventh report of the Joint National Committee on prevention, detection, evaluation, and treatment of high blood pressure (JNC VII) recommends patients with CKD or diabetes have a blood pressure < 130/80 mmHg [66]. ACE inhibitors and ARBs slow the progression of nephropathy in type 1 and 2 diabetics [67]. This renal protection means they are commonly used to treat hypertension in patients with CKD. Recently a new drug class, direct renin inhibitors (DRI), has been approved for treatment of hypertension. Aliskiren is a direct renin inhibitor that may prove to have additional renal protective effect alone or in combination with ACE inhibitors and ARBs [68].

Patients with preoperative hypertension and diabetes undergoing noncardiac surgery with MAP > 110 mmHg are at increased risk of intraoperative hypotension. Furthermore, intraoperative hypotension and hypertension are associated with higher rates of cardiovascular and renal complications [69]. Intraoperative hypotension and decreased renal perfusion are often considered risk factors for the development of perioperative AKI.

This dual goal of adequate preoperative treatment of hypertension and simultaneous avoidance of hypotension in the perioperative period can be difficult to achieve with patients treated with ACE inhibitors and ARBs. The preoperative use of these drugs is commonly associated with intraoperative hypotension, particularly with induction of general anesthesia. Discontinuation of ACE inhibitor and ARB therapy for at least 10 hours before general anesthesia is recommended to reduce the risk of postinduction hypotension [70].

Acute kidney injury

There is a great deal of research aimed at finding pharmacotherapeutic options for prevention and/or treatment of AKI. Many promising treatments for AKI in animal models have failed to translate into successful clinical therapies. Suggested therapies include diuretics, dopaminergic agents, antioxidants, atrial natriuretic peptide, and a range of more experimental therapies.

Diuretics

Loop diuretics, as monotherapy or in conjunction with mannitol and dopaminergic agents, are commonly used in the treatment of AKI. A cohort study of 552 patients with AKI, after adjusting for covariates and propensity scores, found that diuretic use was associated with increased risk of death and nonrecovery of renal function [71]. In contrast, a more recent prospective multicenter study found that diuretic use was not associated with increased mortality in AKI patients [72]. In a rat ischemia–reperfusion model of AKI, furosemide was found to increase renal blood flow and to attenuate ischemia-induced gene expression [73]. In patients with established AKI requiring dialysis, furosemide did not alter survival or renal recovery [74]. A meta-analysis of loop diuretics in the management of AKI found that loop diuretics were associated with a decreased duration of renal replacement therapy (dialysis) and increased UO but no improvement in mortality or independence from renal replacement therapy [75]. Overall, there remains no compelling evidence to recommend the routine use of loop diuretics in patients with AKI. Despite promising animal studies with diuretics, this research has not led to similar results in human studies of AKI.

Dopaminergic agents

"Renal dose" dopamine does not protect patients from AKI and has numerous side effects [76]. Previous meta-analyses of low-dose dopamine have failed to find any clinical benefit and its routine use is not recommended [77]. Fenoldopam mesylate, a D_1-receptor agonist initially approved for treatment of hypertensive emergencies, has been studied in a variety of surgical and intensive care populations at risk of AKI. A meta-analysis of 16 randomized studies found that fenoldopam reduced the risk of AKI, renal replacement therapy, and in-hospital death [78]. Many of the positive trials used a dose of fenoldopam of approximately 0.1 $\mu g\ kg^{-1}\ min^{-1}$ and initiated treatment with the induction of surgery [79]. This finding, if replicated in a larger multicenter randomized trial, would be a breakthrough in the treatment of AKI.

Antioxidants

Contrast-induced nephropathy (CIN) is a form of ATN caused by free radical injury. It is associated with the use of radiocontrast dyes [80]. Radiocontrast leads to hyperosmolar stress and hypoxia in the renal medulla and subsequent free radical production. Risk factors for the development of CIN include chronic renal insufficiency, diabetes mellitus, dehydration, poor cardiac performance, contrast volume, and high osmolar contrast. Multiple studies and meta-analyses have attempted to determine if prophylactic strategies of intravenous hydration, N-acetylcysteine (NAC), or other agents can reduce the incidence of CIN. Since hypovolemia or a reduction in effective circulating volume are known risks for CIN, hydration with normal saline is thought to work by maintenance of renal perfusion by expansion of intravascular volume. However, the optimal type of hydration fluid, route (intravenous or oral), volume, and timing of hydration remain to be determined.

NAC is an antioxidant that has been evaluated for the prevention of CIN in both oral and intravenous protocols. Its mechanism of action is thought to be scavenging of oxygen-derived free radicals in the renal tubule. Another strategy for CIN is the use of sodium bicarbonate. Suggested mechanisms of action for sodium bicarbonate include an alkalinizing effect to decrease free radical production and a direct scavenging action to reduce reactive oxygen species. Studies suggest that hydration with sodium bicarbonate may be more efficacious than with sodium chloride alone in high-risk populations [81].

Overall the best evidence seems to indicate that pre- and postprocedure hydration with normal saline or sodium bicarbonate solutions is efficacious [82]. There are positive and negative studies of prophylaxis with adequate hydration and NAC to reduce the incidence of CIN [80]. There are few side effects reported with the use of NAC or sodium bicarbonate. NAC may increase the frequency of nausea, and sodium bicarbonate treatment carries the risks of alkalosis or volume overload. Ultimately, more research is required for a definitive answer to this question.

In animal studies, NAC had a positive effect on renal blood flow and GFR in an ischemic model of AKI [83]. An ischemia-reperfusion model of ARF found that NAC failed to improve renal hemodynamics after reperfusion but decreased interstitial inflammation and oxidative stress [84]. When extended to surgical patients undergoing open repair of abdominal aortic aneurysm or coronary artery bypass graft, NAC treatment failed to show benefit [85,86].

Atrial natriuretic peptide

A recent study of recombinant human atrial natriuretic peptide, anaritide, found that an infusion of 50 ng kg^{-1} min^{-1} decreased the probability of dialysis in a study of postcardiac surgical heart-failure patients with AKI [87]. Two previous trials of anaritide failed to show a benefit in outcome for patients with AKI [88,89]. The studies differ in that the positive study used a lower dose of anaritide in a highly selected group of patients on inotropic support after cardiac surgery. More recent studies with B-type natriuretic peptide, nesiritide, also suggest a renal protective effect for patients with congestive heart failure undergoing cardiac surgery [90].

Experimental pharmacotherapy for acute kidney injury

The efficacy of therapies in animal models of AKI must be tempered with the realization that many successful treatment strategies in animals have not translated to successful clinical studies in humans.

Volatile anesthetics protect against renal ischemia-reperfusion injury in rats. Sevoflurane has direct anti-inflammatory and antinecrotic effects in vitro in human kidney proximal tubule cells [91]. In clinically relevant doses, 4 hours of sevoflurane anesthesia activated prosurvival kinases ERK and Akt and upregulation of heat shock protein 70 (HSP70) [91].

Erythropoietin receptors are expressed in multiple tissues, including the human kidney. In animal models of ischemia-reperfusion injury, erythropoietin can reduce damage at the endothelial and tubular level. An in-vivo model of ischemia-reperfusion injury found that the delayed administration of either darbepoietin or erythropoietin significantly inhibited apoptotic cell death and augmented functional recovery [92]. A retrospective cohort study did not find that erythropoietin administration was associated with renal recovery in critically ill patients with AKI requiring dialysis [93]. A prospective randomized controlled trial is needed to address the potential benefits of erythropoietin in AKI.

The role of adenosine in kidney function has been extensively reviewed [94]. Adenosine can mediate a variety of effects in the kidney depending on the receptor subtype involved, including vasoconstriction, vasodilation, tubuloglomerular feedback, and inhibition of renin secretion. Adenosine's role in ischemia-reperfusion injury is complex as beneficial effects have been reported with A_1-receptor agonists, A_{2A}-receptor agonists, and the unselective adenosine-receptor antagonist theophylline. The role of adenosine receptors in treatment of ischemia-reperfusion injury in AKI holds potential but remains to be determined.

Another strategy in the treatment of AKI is to supply stem cells to aid in regeneration of damaged tubular cells. Studies have provided evidence in animal models of ischemia-reperfusion injury and cisplatin nephrotoxicity that mesenchymal stem cells improve renal function and recovery [95,96]. Recent studies also suggest that mesenchymal stem cells may act via a paracrine mechanism in the kidney rather than by transdifferentiating into renal tubule cells [96].

Summary

The kidneys are responsible for a number of important functions in addition to fluid and electrolyte homeostasis, including blood pressure modulation, acid-base maintenance, and hormone production. Renal injury is generally defined in terms of a decrease in urine output or increase in serum creatinine. Either kidney damage or decreased renal function for 3 or more months is considered to be chronic kidney disease (CKD), defined as a glomerular filtration rate of < 60 mL min^{-1} 1.73 m^{-2}, while renal failure is either a glomerular filtration rate < 15 mL min^{-1} 1.73 m^{-2} or a need for dialysis or renal transplantation. End-stage renal disease (ESRD) is a term that indicates chronic treatment by dialysis or transplantation, but does not infer any specific degree of renal dysfunction. Acute kidney injury (AKI) encompasses the entire functional range from increases in serum creatinine (> 0.3 mg dL^{-1}) to the requirement for dialysis, and is classified according to prerenal, renal, and postrenal causes. Prerenal AKI is due to an absolute or relative decrease in renal perfusion. Intrinsic renal causes of AKI can be divided into glomerular, tubular, vascular, or interstitial causes, while causes of postrenal AKI include bladder or ureter obstruction. Standardization of disease definitions and terminology is an important step forward for future clinical and basic science research studies.

CKD and AKI are significant causes of patient morbidity and mortality. The overall risk of AKI in surgical patients is approximately 1%, although certain populations are at higher risk, such as cardiopulmonary bypass surgery (3–5%) and emergency abdominal aortic aneurysm repair (>50%). CKD also increases morbidity and mortality for a number of different surgical procedures.

Despite their use in the current definitions of AKI, serum creatinine (SCr) and urine output (UO) are suboptimal markers. At steady state, serum creatinine reflects glomerular filtration rate (GFR), but with acute changes in renal function an abrupt decrease in GFR will cause only a slow rise in SCr over 2–3 days. Significant research efforts are under way to identify improved biomarkers, with the hope that earlier recognition and treatment of AKI could potentially have a positive impact on outcome. Potential biomarkers of AKI include neutrophil gelatinase-associated lipocalin (NGAL), interleukin 18 (IL-18), cystatin C, and kidney injury molecule 1 (KIM-1).

An anesthesiologist's main objective for perioperative renal protection is prevention, keys to which are maintenance of euvolemia, preservation of adequate renal perfusion, and avoidance of nephrotoxins. Nevertheless, optimal strategies to manage patients and the ideal fluid remain controversial, and the ideal blood pressure to optimize renal perfusion is similarly unknown. In patients with chronic renal insufficiency, hypotension is generally best avoided.

Pharmacotherapy for renal protection generally includes halting the progression of CKD, and treatment of hypertension and diabetes, and prevention and/or treatment of AKI. Many attempted treatments for AKI in animal models, such as diuretics, dopaminergic agents, antioxidants, atrial natriuretic peptide, and a range of more experimental therapies, have failed to translate into successful clinical therapies. For example, "renal dose" dopamine does not protect patients from AKI and has numerous side effects. Loop diuretics, although commonly used, have evidence to support their use in AKI. Conversely, fenoldopam may reduce the risk of acute renal injury. N-acetylcysteine and intravenous hydration with normal saline or sodium bicarbonate solutions may reduce the risk of contrast-induced nephropathy. Human natriuretic peptides have been evaluated with varying outcomes. Basic science research is evaluating several strategies that may provide a breakthrough in the treatment of AKI.

Acknowledgments
The authors are grateful to Drs. Robert Sladen, Susan Garwood, and Terri G. Monk, whose chapters on renal physiology and diuretics in the first edition provided some of the material for this update.

References
1. Levens NR, Peach MJ, Carey RM. Role of the intrarenal reninangiotensin system in the control of renal function. *Circ Res* 1981; **48**: 157–67.
2. K/DOQI clinical practice guidelines for chronic kidney disease: evaluation, classification, and stratification. *Am J Kidney Dis* 2002; **39** (2 Suppl 1): S1–266.
3. Levey AS, Coresh J, Balk E, *et al.* National Kidney Foundation practice guidelines for chronic kidney disease: evaluation, classification, and stratification. *Ann Intern Med* 2003; **139**: 137–47.
4. Stevens LA, Coresh J, Greene T, Levey AS. Assessing kidney function – measured and estimated glomerular filtration rate. *N Engl J Med* 2006; **354**: 2473–83.
5. Bellomo R, Ronco C, Kellum JA, Mehta RL, Palevsky P. Acute renal failure – definition, outcome measures, animal models, fluid therapy and information technology needs: the Second International Consensus Conference of the Acute Dialysis Quality Initiative (ADQI) Group. *Crit Care*; **8**: R204–12.
6. Uchino S, Bellomo R, Goldsmith D, Bates S, Ronco C. An assessment of the RIFLE criteria for acute renal failure in hospitalized patients. *Crit Care Med* 2006; **34**: 1913–17.
7. Mehta RL, Kellum JA, Shah SV, *et al.* Acute Kidney Injury Network: report of an initiative to improve outcomes in acute kidney injury. *Crit Care* 2007; **11**: R31.
8. Bagshaw SM, George C, Bellomo R. A comparison of the RIFLE and AKIN criteria for acute kidney injury in critically ill patients. *Nephrol Dial Transplant* 2008; **23**: 1569–74.
9. Lameire N, Van Biesen W, Vanholder R. Acute renal failure. *Lancet* 2005; **365**: 417–30.
10. Schrier RW, Wang W, Poole B, Mitra A. Acute renal failure: definitions, diagnosis, pathogenesis, and therapy. *J Clin Invest* 2004; **114**: 5–14.
11. Krishnan M. Preoperative care of patients with kidney disease. *Am Fam Physician* 2002; **66**: 1471–6, 1379.
12. Carmichael P, Carmichael AR. Acute renal failure in the surgical setting. *ANZ J Surg* 2003; **73**: 144–53.
13. US Renal Data System. *USRDS 2007 Annual Data Report: Atlas of Chronic Kidney Disease and End-Stage Renal Disease in the United States.* Bethesda, MD: NIH, National Institute of Diabetes and Digestive and Kidney Diseases, 2007.
14. Hillis GS, Croal BL, Buchan KG, *et al.* Renal function and outcome from coronary artery bypass grafting: impact on mortality after a 2.3-year follow-up. *Circulation* 2006; **113**: 1056–62.
15. Ympa YP, Sakr Y, Reinhart K, Vincent JL. Has mortality from acute renal failure decreased? A systematic review of the literature. *Am J Med* 2005; **118**: 827–32.
16. Chertow GM, Burdick E, Honour M, Bonventre JV, Bates DW. Acute kidney injury, mortality, length of stay, and costs in hospitalized patients. *J Am Soc Nephrol* 2005; **16**: 3365–70.
17. Moran SM, Myers BD. Course of acute renal failure studied by a model of

creatinine kinetics. *Kidney Int* 1985; **27**: 928–37.

18. Hewitt SM, Dear J, Star RA. Discovery of protein biomarkers for renal diseases. *J Am Soc Nephrol* 2004; **15**: 1677–89.

19. Jones DR, Lee HT. Protecting the kidney during critical illness. *Curr Opin Anaesthesiol* 2007; **20**: 106–12.

20. Sladen RN, Landry D. Renal blood flow regulation, autoregulation, and vasomotor nephropathy. *Anesthesiol Clin North America* 2000; **18**: 791–807.

21. Ballerman BJ, Zeidel ML, Gunning ME, Brenner BM. Vasoactive peptides and the kidney. In: Brenner BM, Rector FCJ, eds., *The Kidney*, 4th edn. Philadelphia, PA: WB Saunders, 1991: 510–83.

22. Gerber JG, Olsen RD, Nies AS. Interrelationship between prostaglandins and renin release. *Kidney Int* 1981; **19**: 816–21.

23. Garella S, Matarese RA. Renal effects of prostaglandins and clinical adverse effects of nonsteroidal anti-inflammatory agents. *Medicine* 1984; **63**: 165–81.

24. Rubattu S, Sciarretta S, Valenti V, Stanzione R, Volpe M. Natriuretic peptides: an update on bioactivity, potential therapeutic use, and implication in cardiovascular diseases. *Am J Hypertens* 2008; **21**: 733–41.

25. Holtbäck U, Kruse MS, Brismar H, Aperia A. Intrarenal dopamine coordinates the effect of antinatriuretic and natriuretic factors. *Acta Physiol Scand* 2000; **168**: 215–18.

26. Stanton BA, Koeppen BM. Elements of renal function. In: Berne RM, Levy MN, eds., *Physiology*, 3rd edn. St Louis, MO: Mosby Year-Book, 1993: 719–53.

27. Schrier RW. Effects of the adrenergic nervous system and catecholamines on systemic and renal hemodynamics, sodium and water excretion and renin secretion. *Kidney Int* 1974; **6**: 291–306.

28. Maddox DA, Brenner BM. Glomerular ultrafiltration. In: Brenner BM, Rector FCJ, eds., *The Kidney*, 4th edn. Philadelphia, PA: WB Saunders, 1992: 215–31.

29. Edwards RM, Rizna W, Kinter LB. Renal microvascular effects of vasopressin and vasopressin antagonist. *Am J Physiol* 1989; **256**: F526–34.

30. Shipley RE, Study RS. Changes in renal blood flow, extraction of inulin, glomerular filtration rate, tissue pressure and urine flow with acute alterations of renal artery pressure. *Am J Physiol* 1951; **167**: 676–88.

31. Desjars PH, Pinaud M, Bugnon D, *et al.* Norepinephrine has no deleterious renal effects in human septic shock. *Crit Care Med* 1989; **17**: 426–9.

32. Kelleher SP, Robinette JB, Miller F, Conger JD. Effect of hemorrhagic reduction in blood pressure on recovery from acute renal failure. *Kidney Int* 1987; **31**: 725–30.

33. Mackay JH, Feerick AE, Woodson LC, *et al.* Increasing organ blood flow during cardiopulmonary bypass in pigs: comparison of dopamine and perfusion pressure. *Crit Care Med* 1995; **23**: 1090–8.

34. Brezis M, Rosen S. Hypoxia of the renal medulla: its implications for disease. *N Engl J Med* 1995; **332**: 647–55.

35. Puschett JB. Pharmacological classification and renal actions of diuretics. *Cardiology* 1994; **84**: 4–13.

36. Behnia R, Koushanpoor E, Brunner EA. Effects of hyperosmotic mannitol infusion on hemodynamics of dog kidney. *Anesth Analg* 1996; **82**: 902–8.

37. Johnson PA, Barnard DB, Perrin NS, Levinsky NG. Prostaglandins mediate the vasodilatory effect of mannitol in the hypoperfused rat kidney. *J Clin Invest* 1981; **68**: 127–33.

38. Blantz CA. Effect of mannitol on glomerular ultrafiltration in the hydropenic rat. *J Clin Invest* 1974; **54**: 1135–43.

39. Lang F. Osmotic diuresis. *Renal Physiol* 1987; **10**: 160–73.

40. Schrier RW, Arnold PE, Gordon JA, Burke TJ. Protection of mitochondrial function by mannitol in ischemic acute renal failure. *Am J Physiol* 1984; **247**: F365–9.

41. Zager RA, Foerder C, Bredl C. The influence of mannitol on myoglobinuric acute renal failure: functional, biochemical, and morphological assessments. *J Am Soc Nephrol* 1991; **2**: 848–55.

42. Mason J. The pathophysiology of ischemic acute renal failure: a new hypothesis about the initiation phase. *Ren Physiol* 1986; **9**: 129–47.

43. Burg M, Stoner L. Renal tubular chloride transport and the mode of action of some diuretics. *Annu Rev Physiol* 1976; **38**: 37–45.

44. Kaissling B, Stanton BA. Adaptation of distal tubule and collecting duct to increased sodium delivery. I. Ultrastructure. *Am J Physiol* 1985; **248**: F374–81.

45. Sica DA, Gehr TW. Diuretic combinations in refractory oedema states: pharmacokinetic–pharmacodynamic relationships. *Clin Pharmacokinet* 1996; **30**: 229–49.

46. Chambrey R, Achard JM, St John PL, *et al.* Evidence for an amiloride-insensitive Na/H exchanger in rat renal cortical tubules. *Am J Physiol* 1997; **273**: C1064–74.

47. Zeng C, Zhang M, Asico LD, Eisner GM, Jose PA. The dopaminergic system in hypertension. *Clin Sci (Lond)* 2007; **112**: 583–97.

48. Roberts I, Alderson P, Bunn F, *et al.* Colloids versus crystalloids for fluid resuscitation in critically ill patients. *Cochrane Database Syst Rev* 2004 (4): CD000567.

49. O'Malley CM, Frumento RJ, Hardy MA, *et al.* A randomized, double-blind comparison of lactated Ringer's solution and 0.9% NaCl during renal transplantation. *Anesth Analg* 2005; **100**: 1518–24.

50. Balogh Z, McKinley BA, Cocanour CS, *et al.* Supranormal trauma resuscitation causes more cases of abdominal compartment syndrome. *Arch Surg* 2003; **138**: 637–42; discussion 42–3.

51. Schortgen F, Lacherade JC, Bruneel F, *et al.* Effects of hydroxyethylstarch and gelatin on renal function in severe sepsis: a multicentre randomised study. *Lancet* 2001; **357**: 911–16.

52. Sakr Y, Payen D, Reinhart K, *et al.* Effects of hydroxyethyl starch administration on renal function in critically ill patients. *Br J Anaesth* 2007; **98**: 216–24.

53. Mockel M, Scheinert D, Potapov EV, *et al.* Continuous measurements of renal perfusion in pigs by means of intravascular Doppler. *Kidney Int* 2001; **59**: 1439–47.

54. Bourgoin A, Leone M, Delmas A, et al. Increasing mean arterial pressure in patients with septic shock: effects on oxygen variables and renal function. Crit Care Med 2005; 33: 780–6.

55. Deruddre S, Cheisson G, Mazoit JX, et al. Renal arterial resistance in septic shock: effects of increasing mean arterial pressure with norepinephrine on the renal resistive index assessed with Doppler ultrasonography. Intensive Care Med 2007; 33: 1557–62.

56. Hara T, Fukusaki M, Nakamura T, Sumikawa K. Renal function in patients during and after hypotensive anesthesia with sevoflurane. J Clin Anesth 1998; 10: 539–45.

57. Sharrock NE, Beksac B, Flynn E, Go G, Della Valle AG. Hypotensive epidural anaesthesia in patients with preoperative renal dysfunction undergoing total hip replacement. Br J Anaesth 2006; 96: 207–12.

58. Nguyen NT, Wolfe BM. The physiologic effects of pneumoperitoneum in the morbidly obese. Ann Surg 2005; 241: 219–26.

59. Pastor CM, Morel DR, Clergue F, Mentha G, Morel P. Effects of abdominal Co2 insufflation on renal and hepatic blood flows during acute hemorrhage in anesthetized pigs. Crit Care Med 2001; 29: 1017–22.

60. Nakache R, Szold A, Merhav H, Klausner JM. Kidney graft loss after laparoscopic live donor nephrectomy. Transplant Proc 2000; 32: 683.

61. Troppmann C, McBride MA, Baker TJ, Perez RV. Laparoscopic live donor nephrectomy: a risk factor for delayed function and rejection in pediatric kidney recipients? A UNOS analysis. Am J Transplant 2005; 5: 175–82.

62. Derweesh IH, Goldfarb DA, Abreu SC, et al. Laparoscopic live donor nephrectomy has equivalent early and late renal function outcomes compared with open donor nephrectomy. Urology 2005; 65: 862–6.

63. Wheeler DC. Does lipid-lowering therapy slow progression of chronic kidney disease? Am J Kidney Dis 2004; 44: 917–20.

64. Gerstein HC, Miller ME, Byington RP, et al. Effects of intensive glucose lowering in type 2 diabetes. N Engl J Med 2008; 358: 2545–59.

65. Patel A, MacMahon S, Chalmers J, et al. Intensive blood glucose control and vascular outcomes in patients with type 2 diabetes. N Engl J Med 2008; 358: 2560–72.

66. Chobanian AV, Bakris GL, Black HR, et al. Seventh report of the Joint National Committee on Prevention, Detection, Evaluation, and Treatment of High Blood Pressure. Hypertension 2003; 42: 1206–52.

67. Mann JF, Schmieder RE, McQueen M, et al. Renal outcomes with telmisartan, ramipril, or both, in people at high vascular risk (the ONTARGET study): a multicentre, randomised, double-blind, controlled trial. Lancet 2008; 372: 547–53.

68. Pool JL. Direct renin inhibition: focus on aliskiren. J Manag Care Pharm 2007; 13: 21–33.

69. Charlson ME, MacKenzie CR, Gold JP, et al. Preoperative characteristics predicting intraoperative hypotension and hypertension among hypertensives and diabetics undergoing noncardiac surgery. Ann Surg 1990; 212: 66–81.

70. Comfere T, Sprung J, Kumar MM, et al. Angiotensin system inhibitors in a general surgical population. Anesth Analg 2005; 100: 636–44.

71. Mehta RL, Pascual MT, Soroko S, Chertow GM. Diuretics, mortality, and nonrecovery of renal function in acute renal failure. JAMA 2002; 288: 2547–53.

72. Uchino S, Doig GS, Bellomo R, et al. Diuretics and mortality in acute renal failure. Crit Care Med 2004; 32: 1669–77.

73. Aravindan N, Shaw A. Effect of furosemide infusion on renal hemodynamics and angiogenesis gene expression in acute renal ischemia/reperfusion. Ren Fail 2006; 28: 25–35.

74. Cantarovich F, Rangoonwala B, Lorenz H, Verho M, Esnault VL. High-dose furosemide for established ARF: a prospective, randomized, double-blind, placebo-controlled, multicenter trial. Am J Kidney Dis 2004; 44: 402–9.

75. Bagshaw SM, Delaney A, Haase M, Ghali WA, Bellomo R. Loop diuretics in the management of acute renal failure: a systematic review and meta-analysis. Crit Care Resusc 2007; 9: 60–8.

76. Jones D, Bellomo R. Renal-dose dopamine: from hypothesis to paradigm to dogma to myth and, finally, superstition? J Intensive Care Med 2005; 20: 199–211.

77. Friedrich JO, Adhikari N, Herridge MS, Beyene J. Meta-analysis: low-dose dopamine increases urine output but does not prevent renal dysfunction or death. Ann Intern Med 2005; 142: 510–24.

78. Landoni G, Biondi-Zoccai GG, Tumlin JA, et al. Beneficial impact of fenoldopam in critically ill patients with or at risk for acute renal failure: a meta-analysis of randomized clinical trials. Am J Kidney Dis 2007; 49: 56–68.

79. Morelli A, Ricci Z, Bellomo R, et al. Prophylactic fenoldopam for renal protection in sepsis: a randomized, double-blind, placebo-controlled pilot trial. Crit Care Med 2005; 33: 2451–6.

80. Pannu N, Wiebe N, Tonelli M. Prophylaxis strategies for contrast-induced nephropathy. JAMA 2006; 295: 2765–79.

81. Masuda M, Yamada T, Mine T, et al. Comparison of usefulness of sodium bicarbonate versus sodium chloride to prevent contrast-induced nephropathy in patients undergoing an emergent coronary procedure. Am J Cardiol 2007; 100: 781–6.

82. Pannu N, Tonelli M. Strategies to reduce the risk of contrast nephropathy: an evidence-based approach. Curr Opin Nephrol Hypertens 2006; 15: 285–90.

83. Conesa EL, Valero F, Nadal JC, et al. N-acetyl-L-cysteine improves renal medullary hypoperfusion in acute renal failure. Am J Physiol Regul Integr Comp Physiol 2001; 281: R730–7.

84. Nitescu N, Ricksten SE, Marcussen N, et al. N-acetylcysteine attenuates kidney injury in rats subjected to renal ischaemia-reperfusion. Nephrol Dial Transplant 2006; 21: 1240–7.

85. Macedo E, Abdulkader R, Castro I, et al. Lack of protection of N-acetylcysteine (NAC) in acute renal failure related to elective aortic aneurysm repair: a randomized controlled trial. Nephrol Dial Transplant 2006; 21: 1863–9.

86. Burns KE, Chu MW, Novick RJ, *et al.* Perioperative N-acetylcysteine to prevent renal dysfunction in high-risk patients undergoing CABG surgery: a randomized controlled trial. *JAMA* 2005; **294**: 342–50.

87. Sward K, Valsson F, Odencrants P, Samuelsson O, Ricksten SE. Recombinant human atrial natriuretic peptide in ischemic acute renal failure: a randomized placebo-controlled trial. *Crit Care Med* 2004; **32**: 1310–15.

88. Allgren RL, Marbury TC, Rahman SN, *et al.* Anaritide in acute tubular necrosis. Auriculin Anaritide Acute Renal Failure Study Group. *N Engl J Med* 1997; **336**: 828–34.

89. Lewis J, Salem MM, Chertow GM, *et al.* Atrial natriuretic factor in oliguric acute renal failure. Anaritide Acute Renal Failure Study Group. *Am J Kidney Dis* 2000; **36**: 767–74.

90. Mentzer RM, Oz MC, Sladen RN, *et al.* Effects of perioperative nesiritide in patients with left ventricular dysfunction undergoing cardiac surgery: the NAPA Trial. *J Am Coll Cardiol* 2007; **49**: 716–26.

91. Lee HT, Kim M, Jan M, Emala CW. Anti-inflammatory and antinecrotic effects of the volatile anesthetic sevoflurane in kidney proximal tubule cells. *Am J Physiol Renal Physiol* 2006; **291**: F67–78.

92. Johnson DW, Pat B, Vesey DA, *et al.* Delayed administration of darbepoetin or erythropoietin protects against ischemic acute renal injury and failure. *Kidney Int* 2006; **69**: 1806–13.

93. Park J, Gage BF, Vijayan A. Use of EPO in critically ill patients with acute renal failure requiring renal replacement therapy. *Am J Kidney Dis* 2005; **46**: 791–8.

94. Vallon V, Muhlbauer B, Osswald H. Adenosine and kidney function. *Physiol Rev* 2006; **86**: 901–40.

95. Morigi M, Imberti B, Zoja C, *et al.* Mesenchymal stem cells are renotropic, helping to repair the kidney and improve function in acute renal failure. *J Am Soc Nephrol* 2004; **15**: 1794–804.

96. Togel F, Hu Z, Weiss K, *et al.* Administered mesenchymal stem cells protect against ischemic acute renal failure through differentiation-independent mechanisms. *Am J Physiol Renal Physiol* 2005; **289**: F31–42.

Section 3
Chapter

50

Essential drugs in anesthetic practice
Fluids and electrolytes

Robert G. Hahn

Introduction

Many pharmacologists do not consider infusion fluids to be drugs. However, it soon becomes evident for the clinical anesthesiologist that fluids operate as drugs, as they have life-saving properties in many situations. They are also needed for maintenance of fluid balance in patients undergoing lengthy surgery and in the critically ill.

The main component of infusion fluids is sterile water. Molecules of various sizes are added to prevent hemolysis, raising the osmolality to (usually) the same level as the body fluids (295 mOsm kg^{-1}). The added molecules also govern the distribution and elimination of the infusion fluid, which are important characteristics. In addition, they may directly or indirectly affect physiological systems, such as the coagulation cascade, which is usually regarded as an adverse effect.

Physiological principles of fluid distribution

There are three body fluid volumes between which infusion fluids become distributed. The first two are the intravascular volume (**plasma volume**, PV) and the **interstitial fluid volume** (IFV), which together are called the **extracellular fluid volume** (ECV). These two can be estimated to be roughly 4% and 13% of the body weight, respectively. The third body fluid space of relevance to infusion fluids is the **intracellular fluid volume** (ICV), which makes up approximately 40% of the body weight. The sum of these body fluid spaces constitutes the **total body water**, which corresponds to 50% of the body weight in adult females and 60% in adult males. Some reduction of these percentages occurs with age.

The permeability of the membranes that separate these body fluid volumes is crucial to the distribution of infusion fluids. The one that separates the PV from the IFV is simply the lining of the vascular system, the **capillary membrane**. This endothelium is fenestrated with pores that allow water and small molecules, like sodium and glucose, to pass with great ease. Therefore, an infusion fluid that only contains water and small molecules, a **crystalloid fluid**, distributes freely between the PV and the IFV.

A fluid that contains macromolecules, such as albumin and hetastarch (HES), becomes more consistently distributed inside the PV, since these molecules pass the capillary membrane only with difficulty, or not at all. A fluid that contains macromolecules is called a **colloid fluid**. A problem is that they only raise the osmolality of a fluid to a very small extent. Therefore, a colloid fluid also contains small molecules in order to be nonhemolytic.

The forces that distribute fluid across the capillary membrane are expressed mathematically in the Starling equation, which holds that a balance is created by the sum of the hydrostatic pressure and the osmotic pressure created by macromolecules (oncotic pressure) on either side. The hydrostatic fluid pressure in this part of the cardiovascular system (the capillaries) is *not* equivalent to the arterial pressure, since the pressure is greatly affected by precapillary sphincters sensitive to adrenergic stimulation.

The ECV is separated from the ICV by the **cell membrane**. A system of channels that operate with quite sophisticated energy-consuming pumping mechanisms regulates the distribution of ions, amino acids, and other substrates across this membrane. These pumps modify the osmolality on either side of the membrane, changing the distribution of water between the cells and non-cells in a finely graded manner. Changes in osmolality redistribute water across the cell membrane within seconds, while the pumping mechanisms may require hours to restore the original situation (Fig. 50.1) [1].

Calculation of plasma volume expansion

The expansion of the PV is an important issue in fluid therapy. In hemorrhage, the therapeutic goal is to rapidly restore the circulating blood volume. However, when a fluid is used merely to hydrate a debilitated patient the clinician may only want to maintain steady state. In the patient with cardiac

Anesthetic Pharmacology, 2nd edition, ed. Alex S. Evers, Mervyn Maze, Evan D. Kharasch. Published by Cambridge University Press. © Cambridge University Press 2011.

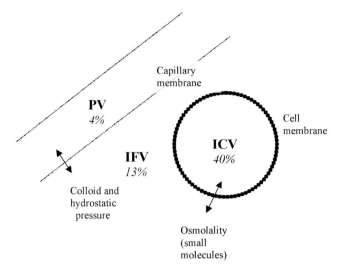

Figure 50.1. Basic principles of fluid distribution between body fluid spaces. ICV, intracellular fluid volume; IFV, interstitial fluid volume; PV, plasma volume.

insufficiency, a fluid with strong PV expansion properties might even induce life-threatening pulmonary edema. Therefore, the choice of fluid and the infusion rate should always be guided by having the PV expansion in mind. Several methods may be used to calculate plasma or blood volume expansion.

In the 1950s and 1960s, PV expansion was often assessed by serial measurements of blood volume using a **radioactive tracer**, such as radioiodine-labeled human serum albumin [2]. Many measurements have to be made to account for the slow loss of tracer from the bloodstream, and clinical situations rarely offer the physiological stability required for safe backward extrapolation to the time of injection [3]. Using the dye **indocyanine green** as a tracer reduces the time required for a single blood volume measurement from 20–30 minutes to 2–5 minutes, which better captures dynamic events [4]. Measurement of indocyanine green concentrations in blood requires blood sampling and later analysis in the laboratory. Pulse dye densitometry has, more recently, made it possible to analyze the blood indocyanine green concentration noninvasively [5].

Comparisons between different fluids can also be made by infusing them until a predetermined **physiological target** is reached [6]. This is based on the fact that the PV expanding property of an infusion fluid is essential to its capacity to restore the compromised circulation.

The most widely used method today for estimating PV changes is to make calculations based on measurements of the **blood hemoglobin** (Hgb) concentration. This approach is simplistic but has the benefit of making it possible to perform quite elaborate calculations to obtain various forms of information. The text below describes methods for estimation of the PV expansion resulting from infusion of a fluid, as well as the PV expanding efficacy of that fluid. The baseline blood volume (BV) is preset at baseline (time 0) by using a multiple regression equation based on the weight and height of the subject. Many equations of this kind have been derived from

analyses of the BV by isotopes in a large number of individuals [3,7]. Further calculations are not very sensitive to which equation is used. By obtaining a Hgb value at time 0 and at any time (t), the BV change during this period of time can be calculated as:

$$\Delta BV(t) = BV_0(\mathrm{Hgb}_0/\mathrm{Hgb}(t)) - BV_0 \qquad (50.1)$$

The amount of fluid retained in the bloodstream (efficacy of the fluid) is given by [7,8]:

$$\text{Fluid retained}(\%) = 100 \times \Delta BV(t)/\text{infused volume} \qquad (50.2)$$

Time (t) might be at the very end of the infusion. The sampling technique and the Hgb assay must be highly accurate in order to provide meaningful results, since the hemodilution resulting from a fluid load is in the range of only 10–20%. Duplicate samples for Hgb analysis may be drawn to reduce variability.

An extension of these calculations can be made if urine output is known and an isotonic fluid that distributes outside the cells is used, such as Ringer's solution. The expansion of the IFV can then be calculated by subtracting the urine volume and the increase in BV from the total amount of infused fluid [9,10]. This provides a "spotlight" view of the distribution and elimination of an infusion fluid at a specific point in time during or after infusion. Moreover, it can easily be repeated many times.

In the examples given above, the change in PV is the same as the change in BV, since no simultaneous hemorrhage occurs. If Hgb is lost between time 0 and time (t), however, modified equations should be applied [3,11].

Even in case of blood loss, the Hgb calculations can be further extended to estimate the average BV expanding property of an infusion fluid during dynamic conditions, such as during surgery. The tendency for a fluid to increase the blood volume can then be regarded as a vector, and blood loss as another vector that acts to reduce it. This can be expressed as:

$$\Delta BV(t) = A \times (\text{infused fluid volume}) - B \times (\text{blood loss}) \qquad (50.3)$$

The PV expanding efficacy of acetated Ringer's solution during 30 transurethral resections of the prostate performed during general anesthesia was calculated using this method. By applying data on $\Delta BV(t)$, infused fluid volume, and blood loss for each 10-minute period of all operations, multiple regression analysis was used to yield the average values of A and B. The number obtained for A showed that approximately 60% of the infused fluid volume remained in the bloodstream at any time, while the value obtained for B showed that the blood volume decreased by as much as the amount of blood lost [12]. Hence, the PV expansion efficacy of Ringer's is much greater during general anesthesia with an ongoing blood loss than under experimental conditions. This type of calculation can be applied with insignificant ethical problems and overcomes many methodological difficulties associated with using radioactive tracers to capture the dynamic situation during surgery.

Many animals, such as sheep and dogs, have considerable reserves of erythrocytes in the spleen that become released during hemorrhage and other stressful events. These animals must be splenectomized before they can participate in fluid balance studies based on Hgb changes. In humans, the role of the spleen in temporarily raising the Hgb level is very small, or even absent [13].

Fluid pharmacokinetics

Drug regimens are commonly based on pharmacokinetic analysis. Conventional kinetic methods may be applied to the molecules added to the water component of an infusion fluid, such as glucose or HES. However, these calculations do not adequately reflect the kinetics of the main therapeutic component of the infusion fluid, which is the infused volume. Certain theoretical problems must be solved before such calculations can be made. In drug kinetics the main input in most calculations is the plasma **concentration** of the drug. Volume kinetics uses **dilution** instead of concentration as input data, because the infused water volume is dissolved in the blood, which already contains 80% water. Hgb is a useful index of dilution, since this molecule is exclusively confined to the vascular space. However, it is the plasma that equilibrates with the other fluid spaces in the body. Therefore, the hemodilution developing between time 0 and time (t) needs to be converted to the corresponding plasma dilution before being used in further calculations:

$$\text{Plasma dilution}(t) = [(\text{Hgb}_0 - \text{Hgb}_{(t)})/\text{Hgb}_{(t)}]/$$

$$(1 - \text{baseline hematocrit}) \quad (50.4)$$

During the past decade, volume kinetics has evolved as a means of estimating the distribution and elimination of the volume component of infusion fluids [10,11–18]. This uses repeated Hgb concentrations over several hours and (at best) simultaneous collection of urine as the input data. The key equation (see below) indicates that the fluid is distributed over two body fluid spaces which become expanded from a baseline size V to an expanded size v. Elimination in this **two-volume kinetic model** is governed by a zero-order rate parameter (mainly evaporation) termed k_b and also by dilution-dependent rate, k_r. Exchange between v_1 and v_2 is proportional to the difference in dilution between them with a rate parameter k_t. Hence, the volume changes in the central body fluid space (v_1) and the peripheral body fluid space (v_2) are given by the following equations:

$$\frac{dv_1}{dt} = k_i - k_b - k_r \frac{(v_1 - V_1)}{V_1} - k_t \left[\frac{(v_1 - V_1)}{V_1} - \frac{(v_2 - V_2)}{V_2} \right] \quad (50.5)$$

$$\frac{dv_2}{dt} = k_t \left[\frac{(v_1 - V_1)}{V_1} - \frac{(v_2 - V_2)}{V_2} \right] \quad (50.6)$$

Since the plasma is a part of v_1, the measured plasma dilution equals the dilution of v_1, which is $(v_1 - V_1)/V_1$ in the kinetic model. The optimal values of the unknown parameters V_1, V_2,

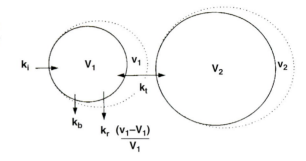

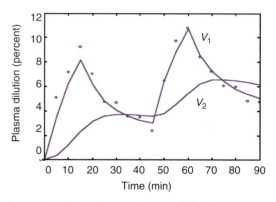

Figure 50.2. (*Top*) Schematic drawing of the volume kinetic model used to analyze the distribution and elimination of crystalloid solutions with electrolytes. (*Bottom*) Experimental data on plasma dilution during two short infusions of acetated Ringer's (points) and the best fit of the kinetic model to data, the solid lines showing the dilution of V_1 and V_2, respectively (principally the plasma volume and interstitial fluid space). Rapid changes in the dilution of the IFV can only be captured by calculations of this type.

k_t, and k_r are then calculated by using a least-squares regression program on a personal computer (Fig. 50.2).

The rate parameter k_r can also be obtained as the **renal clearance** of the infused volume. It is given by the urine volume divided by the area under the curve for the dilution–time profile. The difference between the k_r calculated by using the data on plasma dilution and that obtained by the urinary excretion may be used to quantify "third-spacing" of fluid [10,11]. This term denotes accumulation of fluid outside the kinetic system, which might occur, for example, in the gut, the pleura, and the intraperitoneal space.

The two-fluid space model is usually applicable for crystalloid solutions in stressful conditions such as during surgery [11] and hemorrhage [15]. Colloid solutions are often better described by a **one-volume kinetic model** where the single expandable fluid space v_1 corresponds to the PV [16]. The one-volume model is also applicable when crystalloid solutions are eliminated fast, which is often the case in well-hydrated volunteers studied in the laboratory and under preoperative conditions [17]. The size of v_1 is then approximately twice the expected size of the PV.

Volume kinetics allows qualitative and quantitative comparisons between different infusion fluids. Simulations of expected hydration of all body fluid compartments resulting from the infusion can be conducted. Experiments to compare physiological effects of infusion fluids can be simulated so that the actual volumes achieved will be comparable. Without such comparability it is difficult to know which effects are attributed to the volume effect of the fluid and which are due to the fluid composition itself. These aspects of how to best compare two fluids are poorly understood in many fields of science. One example is the study of artificial oxygen carriers, which are typically colloids, but where a crystalloid fluid is used as control infusion. If infused in similar amounts, it is no wonder that the effect of using the artificial oxygen carrier in hemorrhaged animals is always better than the control infusion. Moreover, the duration of the PV expansion is very different between the fluids, which can be controlled for by volume kinetics but not by guessing.

Intracellular fluid flux

Osmotic forces act to translocate fluid into ICF when small molecules are taken up by the cells. An example is **glucose**, which is a component of many fluids used for maintenance of fluid balance. When isotonic 5% glucose is administered, the infused volume initially expands the ECV and, as insulin gradually reduces the plasma glucose level, the same volume will be translocated to the ICV. Finally, as the glucose is metabolized, the water volume redistributes evenly throughout the entire ICV. However, the initial PV expansion also stimulates excretion of fluid by the kidneys, with the k_r for 2.5% and 5% glucose solutions being similar to those for other crystalloid solutions [18].

Another example is **glycine**, which is used in a 1.5% solution that might be accidentally infused into the vascular system from the operating site during transurethral operations. The time frame for distribution and intracellular uptake is similar to that for glucose, but metabolism is slower and occurs mainly in the liver and the kidneys. Hence, the cellular edema is more long-lasting for glycine solutions than for glucose [19].

Certain small molecules that enter cells very easily will create no gradient in osmolality across the cell membrane. These compounds do not produce fluid shifts between the ECV and ICV, although the serum osmolality might be considerably raised. **Ethanol** is an example of such a compound.

The **sodium ion** can be used as an endogenous tracer of fluid transfer between the ICV and ECV. Calculations require knowledge of the amount of sodium and fluid that has been infused and excreted between time 0 and time (t) and also the serum sodium (S-Na) concentration at time 0 and time (t). An assumption is that the ECV is 20% of the body weight at baseline. The change in ICV is calculated by rearrangement of the following basic equation [11]:

$$S - Na(t) = \frac{(S - Na_o \times ECV_o + Na\ infused - Na\ excreted)}{(ECV_o + infused\ fluid - urine\ volume - \Delta ICV)} \quad (50.7)$$

The calculation is not robust enough for safely quantifying small fluid shifts (100–200 mL) in single patients due to the variability inherent in measuring the S-Na concentration.

The fluids

Crystalloid solutions with electrolytes

Ringer's solution is available without buffer, but more commonly as lactated Ringer's and acetated Ringer's. These are composed to be as similar as possible to the extracellular fluid. The buffered solutions contain 130 mmol of sodium, 110 mmol of chloride, and 30 mmol of lactate or acetate, as well as small amounts of potassium, calcium, and (sometimes) magnesium (Table 50.1). Both lactate and acetate are metabolized to bicarbonate to prevent the dilution of extracellular buffer capacity when the fluid is infused. Lactated Ringer's is most widely used. Enthusiasts for acetated Ringer's refer to animal experiments suggesting that acetate may have benefits when the circulation is compromised [20]. The diagnosis of hypoxia by measuring lactate in the blood becomes confused by an ongoing rapid infusion of lactated Ringer's.

Table 50.1. Composition of the most common crystalloid solutions

	Osmolality (mOsm kg^{-1})	pH	Na$^+$ (mmol L^{-1})	K$^+$ (mmol L^{-1})	HCO$_3^-$ (mmol L^{-1})	Cl$^-$ (mmol L^{-1})	Glucose (mmol L^{-1})
Lactated Ringer's	273	6.5	130	4	30	110	0
Acetated Ringer's	270	6	130	4	30	110	0
0.9% saline	308	5	154	0	0	154	0
7.5% saline	2400	3.5–7	1250	0	0	1250	0
5% glucose	278	5	0	0	0	0	278
2.5% glucose + electrolytes	280	6	70	0	25	45	139

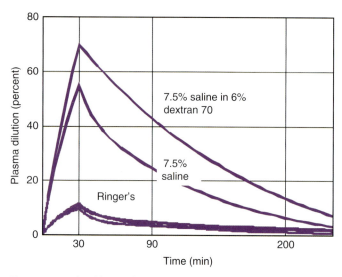

Figure 50.4. The dilution of venous plasma induced by infusing 1 L of 7.5% saline with and without 6% dextran 70 as compared to Ringer's lactate and Ringer's acetate over 30 minutes in volunteers. Computer simulation based on kinetic data from Drobin and Hahn [23]. To obtain the PV expansion one must multiply the plasma dilution by the PV, which should average 3.6 L, as the volunteers weighed 80 kg.

The PV expanding efficacy of 7.5% saline is 3.2 times stronger than 0.9% saline in humans, whereas 7.5% saline with 6% dextran is 6 times stronger (Fig. 50.4) [25]. The duration of PV expansion is approximately 4 hours in male volunteers [25]. Osmotic forces act quickly to fill both V_2 and V_1 with water from the ICV. This means that hypertonic electrolyte solutions do not share the distribution phase of 25–30 minutes for equilibration between the PV and IFV that is typical for the isotonic or nearly isotonic crystalloid fluids. The decline of the PV expansion after infusion is strongly dependent on the body's capacity to excrete sodium [53]. Hypertonic saline solutions have been claimed to exert beneficial effects on the immune system, but results are not consistent and a clinical effect questionable.

Clinical use

A commonly used dose of hypertonic saline is 250 mL, which can be repeated if necessary. The recommended infusion time is 2–5 minutes. A standard 250 mL infusion raises the serum sodium concentration by approximately 10 mmol L^{-1}. Hypertonic saline has found limited use in vascular and cardiac surgery. For example, it has been used as a rapidly acting PV expander when the clamp is removed in aortic surgery. Several studies have been performed to demonstrate better survival by using hypertonic fluids in prehospital resuscitation, but none has shown a statistically significant reduction in mortality. A major multicenter study is currently being performed in the USA and Canada by the Resuscitation Outcome Consortium to revalidate this hypothesis [54]. Sub-analyses of earlier trauma trials suggest that hypertonic saline dextran promotes patient survival in patients with head trauma [55,56].

Adverse effects

The most common adverse effect is pain on infusion, which can be prevented by slowly injecting 0.5–1 mL of local anesthetic at the site of infusion. Warm sensations and headache may be complaints in awake patients. Dextran, which is marketed as a mixture with 7.5% NaCl, occasionally gives rise of anaphylaxis – which has, however, not been described in trauma patients. Nevertheless, as a precaution if time permits, a hapten (dextran 1) should be used to block irregular antibodies against dextran.

Glucose solutions

Glucose solutions are indicated for hydration when the intake of calories is nil or very low. It is often infused in an isotonic 5% solution without electrolytes. To allow more rapid administration, the bag sometimes contains only 2.5% glucose together with electrolytes (Table 50.1). For postoperative use, the infused fluid might contain as much as 10% glucose, which is a hypertonic concentration. Patients who have very low glycogen stores in the liver after fasting overnight might, in theory, be at risk of developing hypoglycemia. When surgery starts, however, the hormonal changes associated with surgery raise the blood glucose level by stimulating glycogenolysis and gluconeogenesis.

The basic glucose need corresponds to 1 L of 5% glucose every 6 hours. However, the amount provided to hospital patients is 2–3 L per 24 hours. This amount provides 400–600 kcal of energy, which is much less energy than the body utilizes, but the glucose supplementation still reduces the muscle-wasting characteristic of starvation [57]. Thus, administration of glucose inhibits gluconeogenesis and makes nitrogen available for incorporation in proteins. While this nitrogen-sparing effect is apparent in starvation per se, it has been more difficult to demonstrate in association with surgery, because of the effects of accompanying physiological stress.

Pharmacokinetics

Glucose rapidly distributes over a volume approximately two-thirds of the expected ECV [18,58,59]. Elimination results from cellular uptake, and it occurred with a half-life of 12–16 minutes in healthy volunteers [18,58] but required 30 minutes during laparoscopic cholecystectomy [59]. The clearance constant for the volume component of glucose 2.5% with electrolytes is similar to that for Ringer's, while glucose 5% is eliminated at a slightly lower rate [18].

The metabolism of the administered glucose should not be confused with the distribution of the water volume. Glucose in isotonic 5% or 2.5% solutions initially expands the PV as effectively as Ringer's, but the duration is shorter [18]. In addition to renal excretion, glucose metabolism also results in uptake of some of the fluid by the cells. Infused volume first becomes distributed in the ECV, and some of it gradually enters cells along with the glucose, because of the osmotic strength of the molecule.

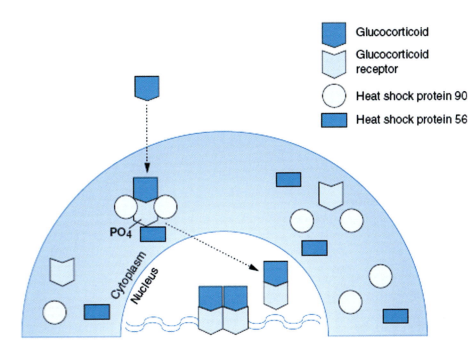

Glucocorticoid

Glucocorticoid receptor

Heat shock protein 90

Heat shock protein 56

Figure 51.1. Mechanism of glucocorticoid action. After entry of the glucocorticoid molecule into the cell, its receptor must be phosphorylated and bind two large (90 kDa) and one small (56 kDa) molecules of heat shock proteins (HSP). This complex binds the corticosteroid molecule with high affinity and functions as a cytoplasmic chaperone. Disassembly of this glucocorticoid/receptor/HSP complex is required before nuclear entry, where the glucocorticoid/receptor complex binds to specific DNA sequences to act as activators or repressors of transcription of specific genes.

Binding of intracellular glucocorticoid molecules to GRs is initiated by phosphorylation of the soluble receptor (GCR) located in the cytoplasm [7–10]. After phosphorylation the receptor binds to two heat shock protein 90 (HSP90) molecules followed by binding of one HSP56 molecule. This complex is able to bind to GCs with high affinity (Fig. 51.1) [11]. Before transport to the nucleus of the cell the GC/GCR complex must undergo what is probably a conformational change resulting from an alteration in receptor charge. The precise mechanism of this transformation is incompletely understood but may involve dephosphorylation after which the hormone/receptor complex disassociates from its chaperone HSPs [12]. The transformed GC/GCR complex translocates to the nucleus where it binds to glucocorticoid response elements (GREs) – specific DNA consensus sequences located within the promoter regions of target genes [13] (Fig. 51.1). GREs exist within a myriad of genes, and binding of GC/GCR can result in expression or repression of specific gene products [14]. Interaction of the GC/GCR complex with GREs modulates transcription of mRNAs encoding multiple cytokines known to be important in inflammation [15–17]. Further, GCs inhibit several signaling pathways important in the activation of such diverse inflammatory mediators as leukotrienes, prostaglandins, platelet activating factor, inducible nitric oxide, NFκB, and adhesion molecules [17–20]. Glucocorticoids also can alter transcription by interacting directly with transcription factors such as activating protein 1 or NFκB [16]. Importantly, GCs seem to possess activity that does not result from altered transcription [21–26]. In particular, the GC/GCR complex can directly stimulate and repress signal transduction in a number of important inflammatory pathways. This also may occur via post-translational modification of proteins [6].

Production, circulation, and inactivation

Glucocorticoids are produced in the zona fasciculata of the adrenal cortex under the control of adrenocorticotropic hormone (ACTH). This pituitary hormone (see below) is the rate-limiting step in biosynthesis. It governs the conversion of cholesterol to prenenolone [27,28]. The newly synthesized hormone is not stored in appreciable quantities but diffuses into the blood. Cortisol production and release from the adrenal gland is episodic. Although the frequency over a 24-hour period is usually constant, these pulses change in amplitude. As a result, serum cortisol levels are circadian. Increases in cortisol levels in response to stressful stimuli largely result from alterations in the amplitude of the pulses, although in some instances the frequency of the pulses may also change [29]. This circadian rhythm is linked to the sleep/wake cycle, with maximal levels (140–180 ng mL^{-1}) occurring just before waking and the lowest levels (20–40 ng mL^{-1}) occurring 8–10 hours later. Significant changes in this profile occur in subjects whose sleep patterns have been disrupted, for example, by shift work or travel. Stress-induced changes in serum levels of cortisol are superimposed on the circadian tone and vary in onset, magnitude, and duration depending on the nature, intensity, and duration of the stress [29].

At low to moderate concentrations nearly all released cortisol is transported bound to corticosteroid-binding globulin (CBG) (95%) and albumin. These carriers are synthesized by hepatocytes. Thus, they are decreased under inflammatory and hypermetabolic conditions or during starvation. At greater doses, however, CBG becomes saturated and the concentration of free steroid increases in the blood [30]. Importantly, many important synthetic GCs (methylprednisolone, dexamethasone) bind only weakly to albumin and do not bind to CBG at all [30].

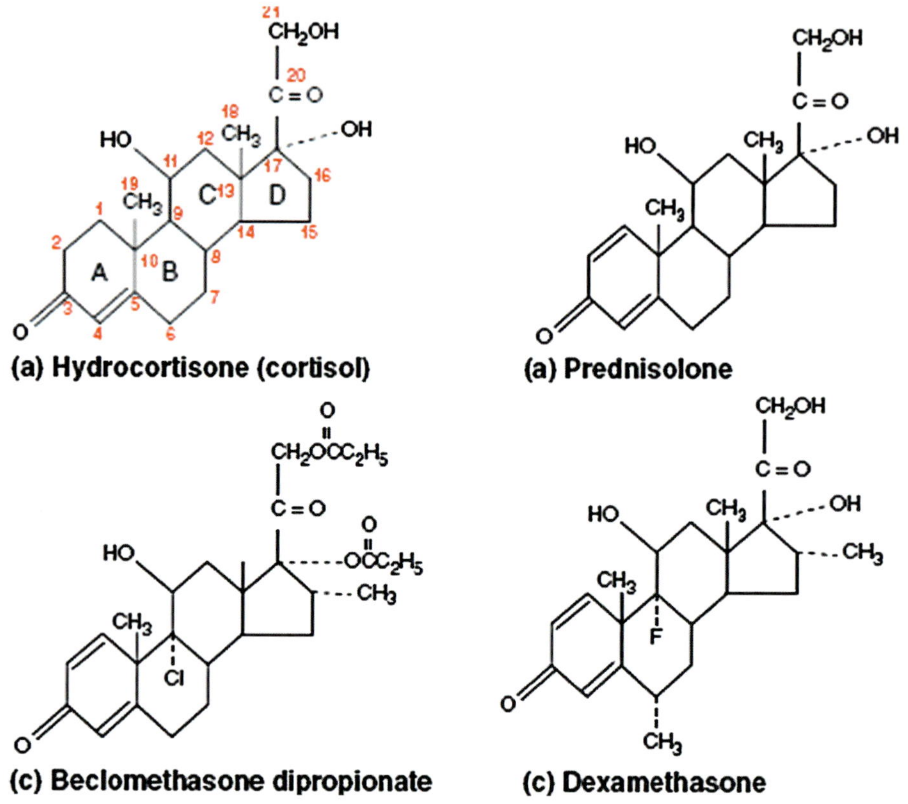

Figure 51.2. Structures of selected glucocorticoids.

(a) Hydrocortisone (cortisol)

(a) Prednisolone

(c) Beclomethasone dipropionate

(c) Dexamethasone

Cortisol (Fig. 51.2) is inactivated in the liver. The principal step is reduction of the A ring and, after other modifications, conjugation. The resulting tetrahydro-metabolites are excreted in the urine and through the bile. Although the serum half-life of cortisol is approximately 90 minutes, its biologic actions persist for several hours [27,28].

Organ-specific and physiologic responses

GCs affect a large number of physiologic functions (Table 51.1) [6,27]. Steroids are powerful catabolic agents that promote the breakdown of carbohydrates, proteins, and fats. Thus they partially antagonize the physiologic effects of insulin. GCs also are important regulators of immune and inflammatory processes involved in host defense. In addition, GCs have complex effects on bone, exert both positive and negative effects on cell growth, and modulate blood pressure. Within the central nervous system, GCs target both neuronal and glial cells. During prenatal and postnatal development, GCs effect brain organization and contribute to adult neuronal plasticity and the processes of neural degeneration. Other central effects include complex changes on mood and behavior, temperature, and neuroendocrine function.

GCs affect homeostasis during stress in at least two ways [4,27,31,32]. At lower physiologic concentrations they are "permissive" in that they potentiate the activities of other important metabolic regulators. For example, they enhance the effects of endogenous catecholamines on lipid and carbohydrate

metabolism. In addition, they prepare the body for a response to altered homeostasis by upregulating the expression of receptors for inflammatory mediators, and act centrally to aid the processes underlying integration of sensory information as well as response selection. In addition, GCs may be "protective." This response occurs when GC activity is elevated. Included in these responses are the potent anti-inflammatory and immunosuppressive actions of GCs that may serve as a form of inhibitory feedback response [31,32]. At the same time, GCs redirect metabolism to meet energy demands during stress, enhance memory processes, and impair nonessential activities such as growth and reproduction.

The permissive and protective actions of the glucocorticoids are complementary and enable the organism to mount an appropriate stress response and to maintain homeostasis. Dysregulation of these actions by genetic or environmental factors, or by prolonged administration of exogenous GCs, may be harmful and may predispose the individual to a variety of untoward outcomes. Deleterious effects that result from long-term increases in serum GCs are detailed in Table 51.2.

Equally important is adrenal insufficiency. This may result from Addison's disease, congenital adrenal hyperplasia, postpartum pituitary or adrenal dysfunction, or abrupt discontinuation of exogenous steroid therapy. The result may include an increased white blood cell count, lymphoid tissue hypertrophy, hypotension, depression, weakness, lethargy, hypoglycemia, and other pathologies. Most importantly, patients with severe

Table 51.1. Responses to acute and long-term increases in glucocorticoid secretion/activity

System	Acute	Long-term
Host defense	Protection from potentially harmful inflammatory mediators	Immunosuppression and vulnerability to infection Poor tissue repair/wound healing
Metabolism	Mobilization of energy stores: ↑ glycogen stores, ↑ gluconeogenesis, ↑ blood glucose, ↑ lipolysis,↑ protein catabolism, ↑ peripheral glucose uptake/ utilization	Insulin-resistant "steroid" diabetes mellitus Centripetal obesity, moonface Protein depletion in muscle, connective, and other tissues
Musculoskeletal	Protein catabolism Altered Ca^{2+} nomeostatis	Increased serum lipids and cholesterol Impaired growth Muscle wasting Loss of connective tissue Osteoporosis and disturbed Ca^{2+} homeostasis
Central nervous system	Improved cognitive function	Mood changes (depression and psychotic episodes) Neurodegeneration
Cardiovascular	Salt and water retention Inhibition of the production of vasoactive inflammatory mediators	Hypertension and other cardiovascular disease
Reproductive	Inhibition of hypothalamic– pituitary–gonadal function	Menstrual irregularities Infertility (male and female)
Gastrointestinal tract	Reduced bicarbonate and mucus production	Increased susceptibility to ulcers

Table 51.2. Unwanted effects of prolonged systemic treatment with supraphysiologic doses of glucocorticoids

Dose-dependent effects

Na^+ and H_2O retention, K^+ loss (mineralocorticoid action)

Hyperglycemia, glucose intolerance, "steroid diabetes"

Redistribution of fat, moon face, buffalo hump, centripetal obesity

Muscle wasting, particularly in limbs

Suppression of the HPA axis

Collagen loss → thin skin, easy bruising

Impaired wound healing

Immunosuppression and increased susceptibility to infection

Osteoporosis

Menstrual irregularities

Growth retardation

Dose-independent effects

Mood swings, psychoses

Increased risk for peptic ulcers

Increased risk for cataracts and glaucoma

Benign intracranial hypertension

Hypertension

Acute pancreatitis

Steroid withdrawal

Withdrawal "syndrome" characterized by rheumatoid symptoms

Sustained HPA suppression[a]

[a]The hypothalamic–pituitary–adrenal (HPA) axis may take weeks or even months to recover from long-term steroid treatment. During this phase, patients are unable to respond appropriately to stress and require exogenous steroids for "protection," for example, perioperatively. If possible, steroids should be withdrawn slowly by reducing the dose over a period of months.

adrenal insufficiency may experience a potentially fatal "adrenal crisis" characterized by a sudden decrease in blood pressure [33–37].

Exogenous GCs most often are given for their anti-inflammatory and immunosuppressive properties. Glucocorticoids attenuate both the early and the late stages of inflammation. They suppress the initial vasodilation, infiltration of leukocytes,

and pain. In addition, GCs limit the proliferative events associated with wound healing and tissue repair. GCs also oppose inflammation-mediated changes in vascular permeability and thus reduce edema.

GCs are potent inhibitors of immune responses mediated by T cells and may also modulate B-cell-mediated humoral responses [38]. These actions extend to the growth, differentiation, distribution, and function of monocytes, macrophages, and neutrophils. GCs enhance movement of monocytes and lymphocytes into lymphoid tissues, particularly the bone marrow, and increase apoptosis of these cell populations. In contrast, the concentration of neutrophils in the blood increases as steroids inhibit migration of cells into inflamed tissues. This effect appears to result from reduced expression of cell-surface adhesion molecules, thus impairing attachment. GCs inhibit neutrophil apoptosis, which normally is initiated on release from the bone marrow, thus prolonging circulating half-life.

GCs suppress cell-mediated immunity in three ways: (1) they direct the development of undifferentiated T helper (Th0) cells away from the Th1 (γ-interferon-dependent) phenotype and towards the Th2 (IL-4) phenotype, (2) they inhibit the synthesis of interleukins 1 and 2 (IL-1 and IL-2), thus impairing antigen presentation and T-cell proliferation, and (3) they induce T-cell apoptosis [38,39]. The resulting inhibition of alloreactive and cytotoxic T-cell proliferation provides the basis for GC use in the treatment of allograft rejection, autoimmune disorders, and leukemia. High doses of GCs also may depress synthesis of cytokines and therefore of immunoglobulins. This in time may decrease serum immunoglobulin levels. Yet lower doses of GCs may stimulate antibody production, probably because of the positive effect of such doses on Th2 cells.

Other immune-cell functions influenced by GCs include phagocytosis and processing of antigens. GCs decrease expression of Fc receptors on macrophages and thus prevent the recognition of particulate antigens that are bound to antibodies or opsonized for subsequent clearance. GCs also affect mast-cell and basophil function by inhibiting IgE-dependent degranulation and hence the release of histamine and leukotrienes. In addition, steroids impair fibroblast function and reduce the production of collagen, glycosaminoglycans, and other components of the extracellular matrix [38,39].

GCs also inhibit synthesis, release, and activity of many other inflammatiory mediators. In particular GCs inhibit the generation of eicosaniods (prostanoids, leukotrienes and epoxides) and platelet activating factor (PAF) by inhibiting the enzyme phospholipase A_2. Further, GCs suppress production of prostanoids by repressing the expression of the inducible form of cyclooxygenase, normally expressed in abundance by activated macrophages, fibroblasts, and endothelial cells. GCs limit synthesis of NO by suppressing inducible NO synthase (iNOS) expression and promote the degradation of nonlipid inflammatory mediators via upregulation of degradative enzymes [28,29]. GCs reduce serum complement components, acute phase proteins, and heat shock proteins, limit release of serotonin, and impair the production or/or activity of proteolytic enzymes such as elastase and collagenase in late inflammation [28,29,39].

Physiology of the hypothalamic–pituitary–adrenal (HPA) axis

Control of secretion

Synthesis and release of cortisol is governed mainly by ACTH. This polypeptide hormone is produced in specialized cells (corticotrophs) and secreted by the anterior pituitary gland. ACTH production is regulated by post-translational cleavage of a precursor molecule, pro-opiomelanocortin (POMC). POMC also

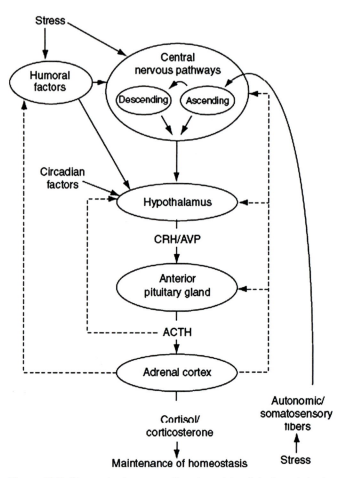

Figure 51.3. The mechanisms controlling the activity of the hypothalamic–pituitary–adrenal (HPA) axis. The *intact line* shows the stimulatory pathway, and the *dotted line* the inhibitory pathway. ACTH, adrenocorticotropic hormone; AVP, arginine vasopressin; CRH, corticotrophin-releasing hormone.

gives rise to a number of other peptides. These are released along with ACTH. Some of these peptides (e.g., g-melanocyte-stimulating hormone) also exert regulatory effects on adrenal function that augment the production of steroids [29].

The secretion of ACTH by corticotrophs in the anterior pituitary gland is governed largely by two hypothalamic neurohormones (Fig. 51.3). These proteins, corticotropin-releasing hormone (CRH) [40] and arginine vasopressin (AVP) [41], act synergistically. They are synthesized in parvocellular neurons that project from the median paraventricular nucleus (PVN) to the external lamina of the median eminence. The peptides are then secreted into the hypothalamic–hypophyseal portal vessels for transport to the anterior pituitary gland. This arrangement assures that the concentrations of CRH and AVP directed to the pituitary are high. CRH and AVP may be cosecreted, but the absence of AVP from some CRH-positive neurons accounts for some variation in the AVP/CRH ratio [28,29].

The actions of CRH and AVP on the corticotrophs are mediated by specific G-protein/adenylate cyclase/phospholipase C-coupled receptors, the type 1 CRH receptor and the V1b AVP receptor. Although release of ACTH is triggered by either receptor, stimulation of both receptors provides a synergistic response. The biochemical basis for this phenomenon is unknown. Importantly, the synergy between CRH and AVP affects only ACTH release and does not alter POMC gene expression or proliferation of corticotrophs. These latter responses are CRH-dependent and are not altered by AVP [28,29].

CRH also is expressed within the hypothalamus, where it is found in magnocellular neurons that project from the posterior PVN and in the supraoptic nucleus with projections to the posterior pituitary. Some CRH-containing neurons within the PVN also are concerned with the regulation of autonomic outflow. CRH production in the limbic system, particularly the amygdala and the cortex, may be involved in the behavioral and autonomic responses to stress and in the concomitant suppression of the growth hormone and pituitary gonadal axes. Indeed, CRH is sometimes termed the executive organizer of the stress response.

In states of acute inflammation, responses in the HPA are altered. This reflects the fact that inflammatory cytokines, notably tumor necrosis factor α (TNFα), IL-1β, and IL-6, directly stimulate release of CRH, ACTH, and cortisol [42–44]. This has important consequences for management during surgery or following injury.

Feedback inhibition

The adrenocortical responses to incoming stimuli are tightly controlled by the ability of GCs and the other hormones of the HPA axis to inhibit axis activation [42,45]. The POMC-derived peptides ACTH and β-endorphin inhibit hypothalamic secretion of CRH. In addition, CRH and AVP may modulate their own secretion. However, the most important feedback effects are those exerted by the GCs themselves. Increases in circulating GCs, as occurs in the presence of adrenal tumors or following administration of exogenous steroids, effectively suppress the circadian increase in pituitary–adrenocortical activity and the HPA responses to many kinds of stress. In contrast, adrenocortical insufficiency, as occurs in Addison's disease, results in a sustained hypersecretion of ACTH and an exaggerated ACTH response to pituitary stimulation. This is corrected by GC replacement therapy. The feedback actions of steroids are complex. GCs affect multiple sites within the axis and involve multiple molecular mechanisms that operate over at least three time domains, (1) rapid or fast, (2) early delayed, and (3) late delayed.

Rapid feedback inhibition reflects a response to the rate of change of GCs in the systemic venous system and in blood entering the hypothalamic–hypophyseal portal circulation. This is independent of actual GC concentration in the blood. A rapid change in this concentration decreases secretion of CRH, ACTH, and cortisol. However, the major effect is on ACTH release. In contrast, early delayed inhibition results from a change in the absolute circulating level of cortisol and also decreases secretion of CRH, ACTH, and cortisol itself.

These actions depend in part on the translation of a protein, annexin 1 (also called lipocortin 1), that appears to interfere with the processes of exocytosis [45]. In addition, glucocorticoids induce regulatory actions within the hippocampus and other parts of the central nervous system (e.g., amygdala, cerebral cortex, brainstem nuclei) that repress functional activity of the HPA axis. Late delayed inhibition alters the CRH/AVP-mediated expression of genes encoding POMC and cortisol as well as production of the neurohormones themselves. Thus, while early and late delayed mechanisms both decrease cortisol release, late mechanisms also affect the production of both ACTH and cortisol. Thus, a late delayed response, as may occur when exogenous steroids are chronically administered, depletes ACTH and cortisol content. The induced suppression of HPA activity by serum glucocorticoids, including those resulting from hypoglycemia or exogenous steroids, is mediated principally by GRs expressed in abundance in the anterior pituitary gland, the hypothalamus, and elsewhere [4].

As mentioned, in states of acute inflammation the HPA directly responds to inflammatory mediators such as TNFα, IL-1β, and IL-6 [42–44]. This response may override normal feedback mechanisms. Indeed, it may make the practice of administering "stress dose" steroids unnecessary (see below). Fortunately, the anti-inflammatory effects of GCs in the periphery function as a second level of feedback inhibition. That is, glucocorticoids may act within the periphery to quench the transmission of information to the brain by suppressing the generation of inflammatory mediators or limiting the passage of substances across the blood–brain barrier [29].

Effects of anesthetics on normal physiology

Anesthetic effects on HPA function are unclear. This in part reflects the inability, in clinical studies, to separate anesthetic effects from the inflammatory response induced by surgery. Practitioners have long been aware that even a single dose of the induction drug etomidate suppresses cortisol secretion [46]. Similar effects on adrenal activity have been reported in experimental studies examining benzodiazepines [47]. The effects of inhaled or other intravenous anesthetics are less clear. Animal studies examining anesthetics alone indicate that inhaled anesthetics decrease serum corticosteroid levels and perhaps other components of the HPA axis. However, these studies are complicated by differences in both the type of GC secreted (for example, rodents do not make cortisol) and differences in control mechanisms. Most investigations exploring the combined effects of anesthesia and surgery in humans reveal increased cortisol levels. For example, both propofol and desflurane were associated with increased cortisol levels following colorectal surgery of relatively short duration [48]. An investigation into the effects of different doses of desflurane revealed that this drug is associated with increases in serum cortisol levels in women undergoing abdominal hysterectomy [49]. A similar study investigating patients undergoing long (> 10 h) resections of head and neck tumors indicated that both

Table 51.3. (cont.)

Drug	Dose	Duration	Administration	Indication	Side effects
		5-day course		Wean babies off a ventilator	Endocrine effects include adrenal suppression, hirsutism, hypokalemla, diabetes, menstrual irregularities; increased susceptibility to and severity of infection
	200 µg kg^{-1} day^{-1}	3 days	IV		
	100 µg kg^{-1} day^{-1}	1 day	IV		
	50 µg kg^{-1} day^{-1}	1 day	IV		Ophthalmic effects include corneal and scleral thinning and glaucoma
Betamethasone sodium phosphate (4 mg mL^{-1}) Soluble in 1 in 2 of water, 1 in 470 of alcohol; insoluble in acetone or chloroform	12 mg	Twice a day to the mother	IM	Threatened premature delivery	General side effects include suppression of the mother's HPA axis
Betamethasone sodium phosphate (0.1%)		2–3 drops every 2–3 hours; frequency reduced when relief is seen	In the ear, eyes, and nose	Eczematous inflammation in otitis externa and other allergic or inflammatory conditions of the eyes and nose	
		0.5–5 mg daily	Mouth		
		4–20 mg repeated up to 4 times a day in 24 hours	IV, IM, or infusion	Suppression of inflammatory and allergic disorders	
		4–8 mg repeated 3 or 4 times in 24 hours depending on severity of condition	Local injection into soft tissues	Relieve the pain and stiffness of rheumatoid arthiritis and other forms of joint inflammation	
Betamethasone benzoate, dipropionate, and valerate esters	Topical application of 0.025% betamethasone benzoate, 0.05% diproplonate, and 0.025% or 0.1% valerate	As indicated by the physician	Cream or gel	Skin complaints such as eczema and psoriasis	Other side effects include skin atrophy, acne, impaired healing.

Table 51.3. (cont.)

Drug	Dose	Duration	Administration	Indication	Side effects
Beclometasone diproplonate	Starting dose is dependent on severity of the disease; usual starting dose for adults is 200 μg; hi a severe case, dose can be increased to 600–800 μg	Up to 2 times a day	Oral inhalation (aerosol)	Preventive treatment for asthma, anti-inflammatory	Bronchospasm can occur with an immediate increase in wheezing after dosing
					In some patients. candidiasis of the mouth and throat can occur
					In overdose, temporary adrenal suppression may occur
	400 μg	2 sprays into each nostril twice	Intranasal route (aqueous nasal spray)	Prophylaxis and treatment of perennial and seasonal allergic rhinitis including hayfever, and vasomotor rhinitis	As with other nasal sprays, there can be dryness and irritation of the nose and throat
					Overdose can rarely result in the suppression of the HPA axis
Hydrocortisone cream		A thin layer of cream applied to the affected area 2–3 times a day; treatment should be limited to 10–14 days and up to 7 days if applied to the face	Skin	Eczema and dermatitis of all types including atopic eczema, photodermatitis, primary irritant and allergic dermatitis, prurigo and insect bite reactions.	Burning sensation and itching can occur at the site of application
					Long-term use can lead to permanent thinning of the skin and rarely to adrenal suppression.
Hydrocortisone 10 mg tablets	20–30 mg	Daily	Mouth	Adrenal replacement therapy in deficiency states	As for dexamethasone
Hydrocortisone sodium phosphate (l00 mg mL^{-1})	100–500 mg	3–4 times a day in 24 hours	IM, IV, or infusion	Injections may also be given to relieve severe attacks of asthma	As for dexamethasone

Table 51.4. Relative anti-inflammatory and salt-retaining properties of corticosteroids

Drug	Anti-inflammatory	Salt-retaining	Equivalent oral dose (mg)	Forms available
Short-acting glucocorticoids				
Hydrocortisone	1	1	20	O, I, T
Cortisone	0.8	0.8	25	O, I, T
Prednisone	4	0.8	5	O
Prednisolone	4	0.8	5	O, I, T
Methylprednisolone	5	0.5	4	O, T
Intermediate-acting glucocorticoids				
Triamcinolone	5	0	4	O, I, T
Paramethasone	10	0	2	O
Long-acting glucocorticoids				
Betamethasone	25	0	0.75	O, I, T
Dexamethasone	25	0	0.75	O, I, T
Mineralocorticoids				
Fludrocortisone	10	250	2	O, I, T
Desoxycorticosterone	0	100	0	O, I
Aldosterone	?	3000	—	—

I, injectable; O, oral; T, topical.

the primary drugs themselves (Table 51.4). Serum half-lives of commonly used synthetic corticosteroids range from 90 to 240 minutes [65]. Importantly, prednisone is unique among the synthetic glucocorticoids in that it is a prodrug that must be converted to an active form, prednisolone, in tissues.

Glucocorticoid metabolism and elimination

Metabolism of exogenous GCs is principally in the liver. Compounds are reduced and conjugated to form water-soluble derivatives that are excreted in the urine. Therefore the rate of elimination can be affected by liver disease. Concurrent medications that rely on liver metabolism can also alter the clearance of glucocorticoids. Phenytoin, phenobarbital, carbamazepine, and rifampin can increase the elimination rate for dexamethasone, prednisolone, and methylprednisolone [66,67]. Ketoconazole [68,69], erythromycin, troleandomycin [70], and oral contraceptives [71] can reduce clearance of glucocorticoids, resulting in increased serum concentrations.

Side effects of corticosteroid administration

The side effects of commonly used steroid preparations also are noted in Table 51.3. Importantly, most of these are not toxic responses but rather exaggerations of normal hormonal activity. These include redistribution of fat from extremities to face and trunk, increased fine hair growth, acne, insomnia, increased appetite, protein breakdown, and increased gluconeogenesis leading to diabetes and osteoporosis. Other complications include peptic ulcers, infections, psychosis, cataracts, glaucoma, growth retardation in children, and a hypokalemic/hypochloremic alkalosis. Long-term use of high doses of exogenous steroids may lead to iatrogenic Cushing's syndrome. Systemic corticosteroids used for short periods (less than a week), even at high doses, are unlikely to cause serious side effects.

Perioperative management of the patient receiving corticosteroids

Perioperative patients may be taking GCs for a number of reasons. For example, these drugs are frequently used for a short period of time to treat swelling or allergic reactions. The management of patients who have been receiving GCs for a limited time is similar to that of patients taking most other medications. That is, the GC should be taken at the normal time or prior to surgery and continued as directed. The likelihood that a short course of exogenous GCs will alter HPA reactivity or affect outcome is small [72].

The need to administer preoperative steroids to patients with reactive airway disease is an important and unresolved clinical issue. Many practitioners prescribe a 3-week course of GCs for asthmatics scheduled for a procedure that will require endotracheal intubation. The data supporting this practice, however, are less than robust. Steroids clearly reduce airway responses in animals. Chronic systemic steroids (4–7 weeks) have been shown to decrease methacholine-induced broncho-constriction and to decrease propranolol-induced airway hyperresponsiveness in the Basenji-greyhound dog model of airway hyperresponsiveness [73,74]. Human data are less clear. Several studies have stressed the lack of serious side effects associated with pre-emptively treating all patients with asthma with systemic steroids before surgery. In one study of 68 patients with asthma, 100 mg hydrocortisone was administered intravenously beginning the night before surgery, and rates of wound infection and delayed wound healing were not different compared with historical control patient populations [75]. This study did not, however, assess the effects of treatment on respiratory complications (e.g., bronchospasm). A second study evaluated the incidence of bronchospasm, infection, and adrenocortical insufficiency in patients with asthma treated with corticosteroids before surgery and found no differences between patients prophylactically treated with steroids and control patients not treated with steroids [72]. Again, this study did not examine the effects of treatment on perioperative respiratory complications. It also is unknown if patients already on inhaled steroids benefit from systemic steroids in the perioperative period. Despite the absence of a randomized clinical trial to prove their effectiveness, most studies recommended that mild and moderate asthmatics receive 1 mg kg^{-1} prednisone orally (up to 60 mg) for 3–7 days before surgery, and that patients with severe asthma (defined as those needing systemic steroids for asthma control) receive increased doses of systemic corticosteroids [72,75]. Indeed, the International Consensus Report on Diagnosis and Treatment of Asthma generated by the National Heart, Lung, and Blood Institute (NHLBI) of the National Institutes of Health recommends that (1) all patients with asthma be seen before the day of surgery and that a measure of pulmonary function be performed and (2) if possible attempts should be made to improve lung function to their predicted values or their personal best level, including a short course of systemic steroids to optimize function [76,77]. These recommendations are not, however, supported by high-level evidence.

Perioperative management of the patient taking glucocorticoids for a prolonged period of time is also controversial. The most common approach has been for patients taking CGs preoperatively to receive "stress doses" of steroids, that is 100 mg of hydrocortisone every 8 hours for some period of time. For example, The NHLBI International Consensus Report on Diagnosis and Treatment of Asthma recommends that patients who have received systemic steroids within the past 6 months should receive 100 mg hydrocortisone intravenously every 8 hours during the surgical period with a rapidly reduced dose within 24 hours of surgery [76,77]. The data supporting this practice are sparse. The dosage appears to be based on a very old study examining GC secretion in the terminally ill [78]. Serum cortisol levels were measures in these patients just before they expired. The measurement was used to derive a 24-hour dose with the assumption that this represented the adrenal response to maximal stress. These finding then were extrapolated to surgical and critically ill patients. In fact, any GC supplementation may be unnecessary.

It has long been known that the absence of an adrenocortical response in the perioperative period may be fatal [33,34,79]. It also is clear that some patients taking corticosteroids for prolonged periods of time may become hypotensive during or after surgery, and that this hypotension will respond to GC administration [34,35]. What is unclear, however, is the existence of a cause-and-effect relationship. Indeed, given what is known about the permissive effects of GCs on catecholamine-induced vasoconstriction (see above) the improvement in blood pressure would be expected with GC administration in the face of hypotension from any cause. Several older studies examined potential causes of hypotension in perioperative patients who had been taking steroids at the time of surgery [35,36]. Winstone and Brooke found that, of 17 patients chronically taking GCs who did not receive any perioperative steroids, two "collapsed in a state of pituitary–adrenal failure and died" [35]. However, the diagnosis of "pituitary-adrenal failure" is presumed – no testing to confirm this was performed. In contrast, Knudsen et al. carefully examined the perioperative records of 250 operations on 95 patients who were on chronic steroid therapy for inflammatory bowel disease [36]. Of these, 50 received perioperative steroids. Hypotension was noted in 29 operations. When data were corrected for severity of disease, lack of GC cover was not associated with hypotension. Indeed, this investigation demonstrated that hypotension during and after surgery most often results from something (hemorrhage, septicemia, hypovolemia, cardiogenic shock, anesthetic overdose) other than adrenal insufficiency. Importantly, data on activation of the HPA by cytokines make it clear that there are profound immune effects on endogenous GC secretion [80]. Thus, surgical "stress," especially if it involves the gastrointestinal tract, may be sufficient to overcome suppression of the HPA induced by exogenous corticosteroids. Clearly the practice of routinely administering large doses of cortisone equivalents to patients in the perioperative period is questionable.

What, then, is the prudent practitioner to do? The answer was first provided by a landmark study conducted in monkeys. Udelsman et al. subjected cynomolgus monkeys to bilateral adrenalectomy [37]. These animals were allowed to recover for 4 months while receiving physiologic doses of glucocorticoids. Animals were then randomized to three groups. One group received one-tenth of the physiologic dose of GCs, another the normal physiologic dose, and the final group 10 times the normal dose. After 4 days of treatment, a cholecystectomy was performed on each animal. The selected dose was continued throughout the recovery phase of 3 weeks. Mortality in the subphysiologic dose was 37.5% as opposed to 12.5% in monkeys receiving both the physiologic and supraphysiologic doses. The undertreated animals developed vasodilatory shock.

Table 51.5. Recommendations for perioperative glucocorticoid coverage [82]

Level of surgical stress	Daily hydrocortisone equivalent dose	Duration
Minor (e.g., inguinal herniorrhaphy)	25 mg	Day of surgery
Moderate (cholecystectomy, lower extremity revascularization, total joint replacement, abdominal hysterectomy, segmental colon resection)	50–75 mg	1–2 days
Major (e.g., Whipple procedure, total colectomy, esophageal resection, cardiac surgery involving bypass)	100–150 mg	2–3 days

This accounted for the deaths. No difference in hemodynamics was noted in animals treated with either physiologic or supra-physiologic GCs. This study suggests that, while a subphysiologic adrenal response may result in shock, replacement above the physiologic range adds no additional benefit.

The study by Udelsman *et al.* led to a reassessment of the use of stress-dose steroids in the perioperative period. Bromberg and colleagues prospectively evaluated a different approach in 40 renal transplant patients presenting for a variety of operations [81]. These patients received only their baseline dose of prednisone on the day of surgery. No evidence of adrenal insufficiency was detected. Five episodes of hypotension and five episodes of hyponatremia responded to treatment that did not include additional GCs. All patients demonstrated elevations (above baseline) of serum and urinary free cortisol levels following surgery. Interestingly, ACTH levels did not rise, suggesting that the response to surgery involved direct adrenal stimulation, bypassing the HPA. Additional, the ACTH stimulation test predicted adrenal insufficiency in 63% of patients. These data suggest that additional supplementation beyond the usual daily dose in patients on chronic GC therapy is unnecessary. Further, they cast doubt on the value of the ACTH stimulation test, suggesting that it is of little clinical value. This interpretation, however, carries important caveats. The majority of operations were not extensive or prolonged. Further, the transplant patient population

may be unique. This led Salem *et al.* to propose a scheme that incorporates the basal dose of GCs taken, the preoperative duration of GC treatment, and the nature and anticipated duration of the operation [82]. These recommendations are summarized in Table 51.5.

It is important to remember that these recommendations are not based on high-quality data. A randomized prospective trial would be useful. In general, a reasonable approach is to have patients take their usual dose of steroids just prior to surgery and supplement in the presence of otherwise unexplained hypotension. Again, this recommendation is purely anecdotal and without evidence-based support.

Summary

Glucocorticoids (GCs) are frequently administered in the operating room and ICU. Therefore, anesthesiologists and perioperative physicians need to have a firm understanding of their physiology and pharmacology. GCs influence intracellular activity by binding to specific cytoplasmic receptors, exerting their effects via transcriptional and nontranscriptional pathways. GCs affect a large number of physiologic functions. These include the breakdown of carbohydrates, proteins, and fats; regulation of immune and inflammatory processes; and complex effects on bone, cell growth, and blood pressure. GCs contribute to adult neuronal plasticity and neural degeneration and induce complex changes on mood and behavior, temperature and neuroendocrine function.

Synthesis and release of cortisol are governed mainly by adrenocorticotropic hormone (ACTH). However, cortisol secretion is also influenced by inflammatory mediators. GC release is tightly controlled via feedback inhibition at the level of the cortex, hypothalamus, pituitary, and adrenal cortex. It is unclear how or to what extent anesthetics affect GC release and activity. Critical illness is associated with an endocrinopathy that may decrease release and activity of GCs.

A number of different GC preparations are available. Patients taking these medications may present for perioperative care. Several forms of GCs are available for intravenous use during the perioperative period. These have different potencies and also different degrees of mineralocorticoid activity. Absent or severely impaired GC responses are associated with poor perioperative outcome. Levels approaching the "normal" physiologic range are necessary and likely sufficient; the use of "stress dose" steroids in the perioperative period is likely unnecessary.

References

1. Furu K, Kilvik K, Gautvik K, Haug E. The mechanism of [3H]dexamethasone uptake into prolactin producing rat pituitary cells (GH3 cells) in culture. *J Steroid Biochem* 1987; **28**: 587–91.

2. Mendel D, Orti E. Isoform composition and stoichiometry of the approximately 90-kDa heat shock protein associated with glucocorticoid receptors. *J Biol Chem* 1988; **263**: 6695–702.

3. Johnson D, Newby R, Bourgeois S. Membrane permeability as a determinant of dexamethasone resistance in murine thymoma cells. *Cancer Res* 1984; **44**: 2435–40.

4. De Kloet E, Vreugdenhil E, Citzl M, Joëls M. Brain corticosteroid receptor balance in health and disease. *Endocr Rev* 1998; **19**: 269–301.

5. Seckl J. 11β-hydroxysteroid dehydrogenase in the brain: a novel regulator of glucocorticoid action? *Front Neuroendocrinol.* 1997; **18**: 49–99.

6. Oakley R, Cidlowski A. The glucocorticoid receptor: expression, function, and regulation of glucocorticoid responsiveness. In: Goulding NJ, Flower RJ, eds., *Glucocorticoids.* Switzerland: Birkhauser Verlig, 2001.

7. Haske T, Nakao M, Moudgil V. Phosphorylation of immunopurified rat liver glucocorticoid receptor by the catalytic subunit of cAMP-dependent protein kinase. *Mol Cell Biochem* 1994; **132**: 163–71.

8. Nielsen C, Sando J, Pratt W. Evidence that dephosphorylation inactivates glucocorticoid receptors. *Proc Natl Acad Sci U S A* 1977; **74**: 1398–402.

9. Sando J, Hammond N, Stratford C, Pratt WB. Activation of thymocyte glucocorticoid receptors to the steroid binding form: the roles of reduction agents, ATP, and heat-stable factors. *J Biol Chem* 1979; **254**: 4779–89.

10. Sando J, La Forest A, Pratt W. ATP-dependent activation of L cell glucocorticoid receptors to the steroid binding form. *J Biol Chem* 1979; **254**: 4772–8.

11. Nemoto T, Ohara-Nemoto Y, Denis M, Gustafsson JA. The transformed glucocorticoid receptor has a lower steroid-binding affinity than the nontransformed receptor. *Biochemistry* 1990; **29**: 1880–6.

12. Muller M, Renkawitz R. The glucocorticoid receptor. *Biochim Biophys Acta* 1991; **1088**: 171–82.

13. Bloom J, Meisfeld R. Molecular mechanisms of glucocorticoid action. In: Szefler SJ, Leung DY, eds., *Severe Asthma Pathogenisis and Clinical Management.* New York, NY: Marcel Dekker, 1996: 255–84.

14. Yamamoto K. Steroid receptor regulated transcription of specific genes and gene networks. *Annu Rev Genet* 1985; **19**: 209–52.

15. Mozo L, Gayo A, Suarez A, *et al.* Glucocorticoids inhibit IL-4 and mitogen-induced IL-4R alpha chain expression by different posttranscriptional mechanisms.

J Allergy Clin Immunol 1998; **102**: 968–76.

16. Guyre P, Girard M, Morganelli P, Manganiello PD. Glucocorticoid effects on the production and actions of immune cytokines. *J Steroid Biochem* 1988; **30**: 89–93.

17. Barnes P. Molecular mechanisms of steroid action in asthma. *J Allergy Clin Immunol* 1996; **97**: 159–68.

18. Cronstein B, Kimmel S, Levin R, Martiniuk F, Weissmann G. A mechanism for the anti-inflammatory effects of corticosteroids: the glucocorticoid receptor regulates leukocyte adhesion to endothelial cells and expression of endothelial-leukocyte adhesion molecule 1 and intercellular adhesion molecule 1. *Proc Natl Acad Sci U S A* 1992; **89**: 9991–5.

19. Scheinman R, Gualberto A, Jewell C, Cidlowski JA, Baldwin AS. Characterization of mechanisms involved in transrepression of NF-kappa B by activated glucocorticoid receptors. *Mol Cell Biochem* 1995; **15**: 943–53.

20. Zhang H, Kumar S, Barnett A, Eggo MC. Dexamethasone inhibits tumor necrosis factor-alpha-induced apoptosis and interleukin-1 beta release in human subcutaneous adipocytes and preadipocytes. *J Clin Endocrinol Metab* 2001; **86**: 2817–25.

21. Molnar G, Lindschau C, Dubrovska G, *et al.* Glucocorticoid-related signaling effects in vascular smooth muscle cells. *Hypertension* 2008; **51**: 1372–8.

22. Levin E. Rapid signaling by steroid receptors. *Am J Physiol Regul Integr Comp Physiol* 2008; **295**: R1425–30.

23. Matthews L, Berry A, Ohanian V, *et al.* Caveolin mediates rapid glucocorticoid effects and couples glucocorticoid action to the antiproliferative program. *Mol Endocrinol* 2008; **22**: 1320–30.

24. Malcher-Lopes R, Franco A, Tasker J. Glucocorticoids shift arachidonic acid metabolism toward endocannabinoid synthesis: a non-genomic anti-inflammatory switch. *Eur J Pharmacol* 2008; **583**: 322–39.

25. Hu G, Lian Q, Lin H, *et al.* Rapid mechanisms of glucocorticoid signaling

in the Leydig cell. *Steroids* 2007; **73**: 1018–24.

26. Lowenberg M, Verhaar A, van den Brink G, Hommes DW. Glucocorticoid signaling: a nongenomic mechanism for T-cell immunosuppression. *Trends Mol Med* 2007; **13**: 158–63.

27. Buckingham J. Glucocorticoids: role in stress of. In: Fink G, ed., *The Encyclopaedia of Stress.* New York, NY: Academic Press, 1999.

28. Buckingham J, Christian H, Gillies G, *et al.* The hypothalamo-pituitary-adrenocortical immune axis. In: Marsh JA, Kendall MD, eds., *The Physiology of Immunity.* Boca Raton FL:, CRC Press, 1996.

29. Buckingham J. Glucocorticoids: effects of stress on. In: Fink G, ed., *The Encyclopaedia of Stress.* New York NY: Academic Press, 1999.

30. Parente L. The development of synthetic glucocorticoids. In: Goulding NJ, Flower RJ, eds., *Glucocorticoids.* Switzerland: Birkhauser, 2001.

31. Munck A, Guyre P, Holbrook N. Physiological functions of glucocorticoids and their relation to pharmacological actions. *Endocr Rev* 1984; **51**: 25–44.

32. Munck A, Naraj-Fejes-Toth A. The ups and downs of glucocorticoid physiology: permissive and suppressive effects revisited. *Mol Cell Endocrinol* 1992; **90**: C1–4.

33. Sampson P, Brooke B, Winstone N. Biochemical conformation of collapse due to adrenal failure. *Lancet* 1961; **1**: 1377–9.

34. Sampson P, Winstone N, Brooke B. Adrenal function in surgical patients after steroid therapy. *Lancet* 1962; **2**: 322–5.

35. Winstone N, Brooke B. Effects of steroid treatment on patients undergoing operation. *Lancet* 1961; **1**: 973–5.

36. Knudsen L, Christiansen L, Lorentzen J. Hypotension during and after operation in glucocorticoid-treated patients. *Br J Anaesth* 1981; **53**: 295–301.

37. Udelsman R, Ramp J, Gallucci W, *et al.* Adaptation during surgical stress: a reevaluation of the role of

glucocorticoids. *J Clin Invest* 1986; **77**: 1377–81.

38. Rook G. Glucocorticoids and immune function. *Balliere's Clin Endocrinol* 1999; **13**: 567–81.

39. Paliogianni F, Boumpas D. Molecular and cellular aspects of cytokine regulation by glucocorticoids. In: Goulding NJ, Flower RJ, eds., *Glucocorticoids*. Switzerland: Birkhauser Verlig, 2001.

40. Vale W, Spiess J, Rivier L, Rivier J. Characterization of a 41-residue ovine hypothalmic peptide that stimulates secretion of corticotropin and β -endorphin. *Science* 1981; **213**: 1394–7.

41. Gillies G, Linton E, Lowry P. Corticotropin releasing activity of the new CRF is potentiated several times by vasopressin. *Nature* 1982; **299**: 355–7.

42. Keller-Wood M, Dallman M. Corticosteroid inhibition of ACTH secretion. *Endocr Rev* 1984; **5**: 1–24.

43. Mastorakos G, Chrousos G, Webere J. Recombinant interleukin-6 activates the hypothalamic-pituitary-adrenal in humans. *J Clin Endocrinol Metab* 1993; **77**: 1690–4.

44. Bateman A, Singh A, Kral T, Solomon S. The immune-hypothalamic-pituitary-adrenal axis. *Endocr Rev* 1989; **10**: 92–112.

45. Buckingham J. Stress and the neuroendocrine immune axis: the pivotal role of glucocorticoids and lipocortin 1. *Br J Pharmacol* 1996; **118**: 1–19.

46. Hildreth A, Mejia V, Maxwell R, *et al.* Adrenal suppression following a single dose of etomidate for rapid sequence induction: a prospective randomized study. *J Trauma* 2008; **65**: 573–9.

47. Irwin M, Hauger R, Britton K. Benzodiazepines antagonize central corticotropin releasing hormone-induced suppression of natural killer cell activity. *Brain Res* 1993; **631**: 114–18.

48. Schricker T, Latterman R, Fiset P, Wykes L, Carli F. Integrated analysis of protein and glucose metabolism during surgery: effects of anesthesia. *J Appl Physiol* 2001; **91**: 2523–30.

49. Baldini G, Bagry H, Carli F. Depth of anesthesia with desflurane does not influence the endocrine-metabolic response to pelvic surgery. *Acta Anaesthesiol Scand* 2008; **52**: 99–105.

50. Nishiyama T, Yamashita K, Yokoyama T. Stress hormone changes in general anesthesia of long duration: isoflurane-nitrous oxide vs sevoflurane-nitrous oxide anesthesia. *J Clin Anesth* 2005; **17**: 586–91.

51. Goldmann A, Hoehne C, Fritz G, *et al.* Combined vs. isoflurane/fentanyl anesthesia for major abdominal surgery: effects on hormones and hemodynamics. *Med Sci Monit* 2008; **14**: CR445–52.

52. Breslow MJ, Miller CF, Parker SD, Walman AT, Traystman RJ. Effect of vasopressors on organ blood flow during endotoxin shock in pigs. *Am J Physiol* 1987; **252**: H291–300.

53. Landry DW, Levin HR, Gallant EM, *et al.* Vasopressin deficiency contributes to the vasodilation of septic shock. *Circulation* 1997; **95**: 1122–5.

54. Malay MB, Ashton JL, Dahl K, *et al.* Heterogeneity of the vasoconstrictor effect of vasopressin in septic shock. *Crit Care Med* 2004; **32**: 1327–31.

55. Russell JA, Walley KR, Singer J, *et al.* VASST Investigators. Vasopressin versus norepinephrine infusion in patients with septic shock. *N Engl J Med* 2008; **358**: 877–87.

56. Mebis L, Debaveye Y, Visser TJ, Van den Berghe G. Changes within the thyroid axis during the course of critical illness. *Endocrinol Metab Clin North Am* 2006; **35**: 807–21.

57. Mesotten D, Van Den Berghe G. Changes within the growth hormone/insulin-like growth factor I/IGF binding protein axis during critical illness. *Endocrinol Metab Clin North Am* 2006; **35**: 793–805.

58. Van den Berghe G, Weekers F, Baxter RC, *et al.* Five-day pulsatile gonadotropin-releasing hormone administration unveils combined hypothalamic-pituitary-gonadal defects underlying profound hypoandrogenism in men with prolonged critical illness. *J Clin Endocrinol Metab* 2001; **86**: 3217–26.

59. Knöferl MW, Angele MK, Diodato MD, *et al.* Female sex hormones regulate macrophage function after trauma-hemorrhage and prevent increased death rate from subsequent sepsis. *Ann Surg* 2002; **235**: 105–12.

60. Van den Berghe G, de Zegher F, Lauwers P, Veldhuis JD. Luteinizing hormone secretion and hypoandrogenaemia in critically ill men: effect of dopamine. *Clin Endocrinol* 1994; **41**: 563–9.

61. Van den Berghe G, Wouters P, Weekers F, *et al.* Intensive insulin therapy in the critically ill patients. *N Engl J Med* 2001; **345**: 1359–67.

62. Van den Berghe G, Wilmer A, Hermans G, *et al.* Intensive insulin therapy in the medical ICU. *N Engl J Med* 2006; **354**: 449–61.

63. Annane D, Sébille V, Charpentier C, *et al.* Effect of treatment with low doses of hydrocortisone and fludrocortisone on mortality in patients with septic shock. *JAMA* 2002; **288**: 862–71. .

64. Sprung CL, Annane D, Keh D, *et al.* CORTICUS Study Group. Hydrocortisone therapy for patients with septic shock. *N Engl J Med* 2008; **358**: 111–24.

65. Ellul-Micallef R. Pharmacokinetics and pharmacodynamics of glucocorticoids. In: Jenne JW, Murphy S, eds., *Drug Therapy for Asthma: Research and Clinical Practice*. New York, NY: Marcel Dekker, 1987: 463–516.

66. Brooks S, Werk E, Ackerman S, Sullivan I, Thrasher K. Adverse effects of phenobarbital on corticosteroid metabolism in patients with bronchial asthma. *N Engl J Med* 1972; **286**: 1125–8.

67. Bartoszek M, Brenner A, Szefler S. Prednisolone and methylprednisolone kinetics in children receiving anticonvulsant therapy. *Clin Pharmacol Ther* 1987; **42**: 424–32.

68. Glynn A, Slaughter R, Brass C, D'Ambrosio R, Jusko WJ. Effects of ketoconazole on methylprednisolone pharmacokinetics and cortisol secretion. *Clin Pharmacol Ther* 1986; **39**: 654–9.

69. Zurcher R, Frey B, Frey F. Impact of ketoconazole on the metabolism of prednisolone. *Clin Pharmacol Ther* 1989; **45**: 366–72.

70. Szefler S, Ellis E, Brenner M, *et al.* Steroid-specific and anticonvulsant interaction aspects of troleandomycin-

steroid therapy. *J Allergy Clin Immunol* 1982; **69**: 455–60.

71. Boekenoogen S, Szefler S, Jusko W. Prednisolone disposition and protein binding in oral contraceptive users. *J Clin Endocrinol Metab* 1983; **56**: 702–9.

72. Kabalin C, Yarnold P, Grammer L. Low complication rate of corticosteroid-treated asthmatics undergoing surgical procedures. *Arch Intern Med* 1995; **155**: 1379–84.

73. Tobias J, Sauder R, Hirshman C. Methylprednisolone prevents propranolol-induced airway hyper-reactivity in the Basenji-greyhound dog. *Anesthesiology* 1991; **74**: 1115–20.

74. Darowski M, Hannon V, Hirshman C. Corticosteroids decrease airway hyperresponsiveness in the Basenji-greyhound dog model of asthma. *J Appl Physiol* 1989; **66**: 1120–6.

75. Pien L, Grammer L, Patterson R. Minimal complications in a surgical population with severe asthma receiving prophylactic corticosteroids. *J Allergy Clin Immunol* 1988; **82**: 696–700.

76. International consensus report on diagnosis and treatment of asthma. *Clin Exp Allergy* 1992; **22** (Suppl 1): 1–72.

77. International consensus report on diagnosis and treatment of asthma. National Heart, Lung, and Blood Institute, National Institutes of Health. *Eur Respir J* 1992; **5**: 601–41.

78. Sandberg A, Eik-Nes K, Migeon C, Samuels LT. Metabolism of adrenal steroids in dying patients. *J Clin Endocrinol Metab* 1956; **16**: 1001–16.

79. Fraser C, Preus F, Bigford W. Adrenal atrophy and irreversible shock associated with cortisone therapy. *JAMA* 1952; **149**: 1542–3.

80. Spath-Schwalbe E, Born J, Schrezenmeier H, *et al.* Interleukin-6 stimulates the hypothalamic-pituitary-adrenocortical axis in man. *J Clin Endocrinol Metab* 1994; **79**: 1212–14.

81. Bromberg J, Alfrey E, Barker C, *et al.* Adrenal suppression and steroid supplementation in renal transplant recipients. *Transplantation* 1991; **51**: 385–90.

82. Salem M, Tainsh R, Bromberg J, Loriaux DL, Chernow B. Perioperative glucocorticoid coverage: a reassessment 42 years after emergence of a problem. *Ann Surg* 1994; **219**: 416–25.

Nándor Marczin and Kristof Racz

Introduction

Despite major advances in general and specialized medicine in the last century, there is no definite cure for many degenerative diseases. For a significant number of patients presenting with end-stage organ failure, only organ transplantation provides hope for increased survival. The transplant of a tissue from one individual to another with a fully functional immune system, however, is followed almost invariably by rejection of the graft because of the relentless aggression of immunocompetent cells and their mediators against the foreign tissue, resulting in acute damage, loss of function, and death in most instances.

Depending on the timing and principal mechanisms of the immune response, three forms of rejections are distinguished [1,2] (Figs. 52.1, 52.2). **Hyperacute rejection** occurs within the first 48 hours and is related to preformed antibodies against well-characterized donor antigens causing complement activation and graft thrombosis. The most common form of rejection, termed **acute rejection**, occurs mainly within the first year and is characterized by vascular and parenchymal inflammatory reactions orchestrated primarily by T lymphocytes (Fig. 52.1). Finally, a more chronic loss of graft function termed **chronic rejection** is characterized by microvascular proliferation leading to vascular occlusion through a complex interaction of cellular and humoral immune and nonspecific injurious mechanisms [2] (Fig. 52.1D). A similar proliferative mechanism affecting the small airways exists in the lung, manifesting chronic rejection in the form of obliterative bronchiolitis (Fig. 52.1H).

The pivotal event in the initiation of the complex immunologic process that ultimately leads to destruction of invading foreign pathogen or recognized self-antigen is antigen-induced activation, proliferation, and differentiation of T lymphocytes [3,4]. The engagement between the antigen and T-cell receptor at the specialized area between the antigen-presenting cell (APC) and T cell (immunological synapse) is followed by activation of the T cells, which involves intricate signal transduction mechanisms leading to upregulation of T-cell-derived cytokines, among them the potent T-cell growth factor

interleukin 2 (IL-2) [5–8]. These in turn initiate a series of events underlying proliferation and differentiation of T cells to helper and effector cells, which, in concert with B-cell-mediated humoral response, results in elimination of the initiating antigen. The cascade of T-cell-centered events presents a number of targets for immunosuppression. Current strategies inhibit T-cell effects by depleting T cells, inhibiting T-cell activation pathways, or interrupting the trafficking of T cells into allografts [2,9,10].

Mechanisms of drug action

Antigen presentation and cell-surface events in T lymphocytes

The principal immune reaction after allograft engraftment is the recognition and response to donor antigens that are part of the major histocompatibility complex (MHC). Generally, T cells recognize the donor MHC antigens through APCs. In the process of direct allorecognition, T cells recognize determinant peptides on the intact donor MHC molecules on the surface of the transplanted donor cells. There is, however, an alternative mechanism in which the *donor's* MHC molecules are processed and presented as peptides by the *host's* MHC molecules at the surface of the *host's* APCs, thereby eliciting a T-cell response that is restricted to the host rather than the donor ("indirect pathway") [11]. Evidence suggest that direct antigen recognition is responsible for the initial in-vivo sensitization of recipient T cells to allograft MHC antigens, whereas the indirect pathway might play a key role in the actual rejection process.

During the recognition step, the MHC antigen becomes engaged with the T-cell antigen receptor (TCR) complex [3,5,6]. Allorecognition stimulates a redistribution of cell-surface proteins and coclustering of the TCR complex with crucial signal transduction proteins, resulting in highly organized molecular assemblies termed supramolecular activation clusters [5].

Engagement of the donor MHC antigenic peptides and the TCR, however, only results in weak stimulation of T-cell

---

Anesthetic Pharmacology, 2nd edition, ed. Alex S. Evers, Mervyn Maze, Evan D. Kharasch. Published by Cambridge University Press. © Cambridge University Press 2011.

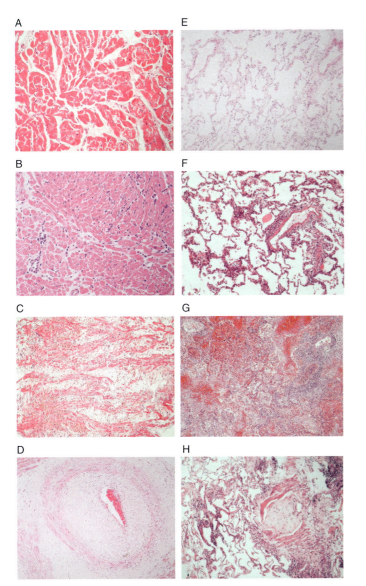

Figure 52.1. The spectrum of acute and chronic rejection in heart and lung transplantation.
(A–D) Heart transplantation: (A) normal endomyocardial biopsy (grade 0); (B) mild acute cellular rejection (grade 1R), with a sparse infiltrate of lymphocytes around a vessel and elsewhere in interstitium; (C) severe acute rejection (grade 3R) with extensive haemorrhage into the interstitium between myocytes: there is often necrosis of myocytes and an acute inflammatory infiltrate around them; (D) chronic rejection, also known as graft vascular disease: the epicardial coronary arteries are diffusely thickened by proliferation of myofibroblasts in the intima of the artery; often there is a T-lymphocytic infiltrate immediately beneath the endothelium (not shown).
(E–H) Lung transplantation: (E) normal alveolated transbronchial lung biopsy (grade 0); (F) mild acute cellular rejection (grade A1), with a sparse infiltrate of lymphocytes around septal venules; often there is lymphocytic endothelialitis (not shown); (G) severe acute rejection (grade A4), in which there is extensive destruction of lung by diffuse alveolar damage; the only clue that this is due to acute rejection is the presence of large lymphocytes around a venule in one corner of the frame; hyaline membranes are plentiful; (H) chronic rejection, also known as obliterative bronchiolitis (grade C2), with almost total obliteration of the lumen of a bronchiole by dense fibrous tissue; there is acute rejection in nearby lung. Courtesy of Dr. Margaret Burke, consultant histopathologist, Harefield Hospital.

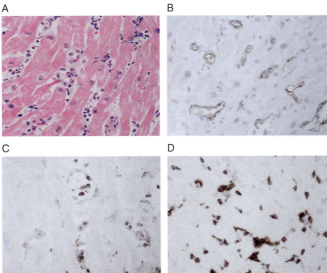

Figure 52.2. Antibody-mediated rejection in the heart: (A) there is a sparse mononuclear cell infiltrate in the interstitium adjacent to capillaries with prominent endothelial cells; (B) antibodies to the split component of complement C4 (C4d) show deposition in the myocardial capillaries; (C) antibodies to macrophages (CD68) show macrophages in both capillaries and interstitium; (D) there is also acute cellular rejection, as shown by the diffuse interstitial infiltrate of T cells using antibodies to CD3.

responses and anergy or paralysis in most instances [4]. Sufficient T-cell activation requires the presence of supplementary costimulatory signals in addition to the antigenic signals [12]. This is usually brought about by cell-to-cell interactions among the antigen-specific T cells and APCs because of interactions of a number of cognate cell-surface proteins on both. In addition to direct cell–cell interactions, APC-derived soluble cytokines such as IL-1β and IL-6 provide costimulatory signals that result in T-cell activation, resulting in effective signal transduction in the T cells and upregulation of pivotal T-cell activation genes such as *IL-2*.

T-cell receptor signaling

Following T-cell stimulation, the cell-surface signal generated from the TCR and its coreceptors on the T-cell surface is transmitted through the cytoplasm into the nucleus, resulting in global reprogramming of gene expression, including both up- and downregulation of gene transcription. Although the signal transduction process leads to the production of various cytokines, which, in turn, help to drive the proliferation of T cells, the central event in T-cell activation is that of *IL-2* gene expression [3,7].

Activation of at least three major different families of transcription factors and their nuclear translocation and cooperative binding to the *IL-2* enhancer region is required to cause transcriptional activation of the *IL-2* gene [5,8,13,14] (Fig. 52.3). They are the nuclear factor of the activated T cells (NFAT) family, the activating protein 1 (AP-1) family, and the nuclear factor κB (NFκB) family. In resting T cells, both NFAT and NFκB are kept in the cytosol in an inactive form by

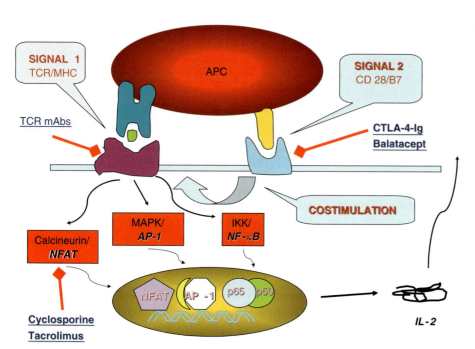

Figure 52.3. Mechanisms of T-cell activation, part 1. A signal transduction cascade leading from the T-cell receptor (TCR) to interleukin (IL)-2 secretion. Shown are the immunological synapse, stimulation of TCR by MHC peptides on an antigen-presenting cell (APC), the role of costimulation, transcription-factor regulation of IL-2 secretion, and targets of immunosuppressants. NFAT, nuclear factor of activated T cells; MAPK, mitogen-activated protein kinase; IKK, inhibitor κB kinase; NF-κB, nuclear factor κB; AP-1, activator protein 1.

their negative regulators, which mitigate their nuclear localization signals. AP-1 is absent in resting T lymphocytes and is transcriptionally induced only by appropriate TCR signaling.

Various intracellular mechanisms, frequently involving complex protein kinase and phosphatase cascades, are responsible for transcription-factor activation following allorecognition and engagement of TCR and costimulation receptors. A Ca^{2+}/calmodulin and calcineurin pathway is the major determinant of NFAT activation, whereas mitogen-activated protein kinase (MAP kinase) pathways have been implicated in AP-1 and NFκB activation, nuclear translocation, and binding to a promoter element of the *IL-2* gene.

Calcium/calmodulin/calcineurin-induced nuclear factor of activated T cells

Within 1–100 seconds of T-cell receptor engagement, tyrosine kinases become activated, leading to the generation of inositol 1,4,5-trisphosphate (IP_3) and subsequent intracellular release of Ca^{2+} and the increase in cytoplasmic Ca^{2+} concentration $[Ca^{2+}]_i$. The increase in intracellular calcium activates calmodulin, a Ca^{2+}-binding protein, and this in turn interacts with calcineurin, which belongs to a superfamily of protein serine/threonine phosphatases [15]. Binding of activated calmodulin to the catalytic subunit of calcineurin (calcineurin A, CnA) releases the autoinhibitory domain from its active site, bringing about an increase in its phosphatase activity. One of the substrates of calcineurin's phosphatase activity is the NFAT family of transcription factors [16]. Dephosphorylation of NFAT allows translocation of the *cis*-acting NFAT into the nucleus, with activation of gene expression (Fig. 52.3).

Interleukin 2 receptor signaling and cell-cycle regulation in T cells

Secreted IL-2 from activated T cells acts as a major growth factor producing mitogenesis and proliferation of T cells. This involves entry from a resting G_0 cell-cycle phase into a cell-cycle progression through G_1 phase and DNA synthesis followed by cell division.

Mechanism of this mitogenic effect of IL-2 involves activation of IL-2 receptor (IL-2R) and signaling events activating a distinct set of transcription factors leading to upregulation of genes responsible for G_0/G_1 transition and progression through G_1 phase [7]. Among the transcription factors, phosphorylation and nuclear translocation of STAT-3 and STAT-5 – two members of the transcription-factor family known as signal transducers and activators of transcription (STATs) – appear to be the most important [17–19] (Fig. 52.4). The functional consequence of IL-2 signaling is upregulation of genes involved in cell-cycle progression. This includes upregulation of genes that promote cell-cycle progression, control cell survival, and increase synthetic and metabolic processes during proliferation, and also suppression of genes that block cell-cycle progression and promote cell death.

Cellular proliferation depends not only on the appropriate genetic environment of the cells but also on increased metabolism, including appropriate rate of synthesis of nucleic acid building blocks such as purine and pyrimidine nucleotides [20]. Particularly, dividing lymphocytes increase both their pyrimidine and purine pools dramatically after stimulation. All cells in the body are able to synthesize nucleotides by two pathways, de-novo synthesis and the salvage pathway [21].

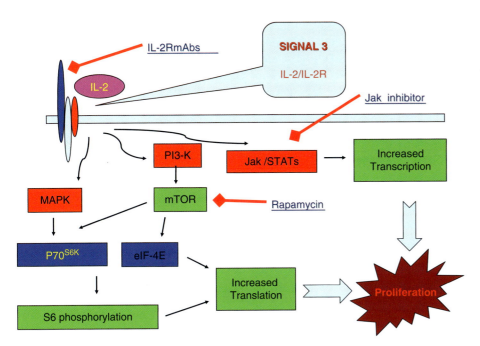

Figure 52.4. Mechanisms of T-cell activation, part 2. Orchestration of T-cell proliferation by the IL-2/IL-2 receptor system. Shown are major events underlying transcriptional and translational regulation of T-cell proliferation. MAPK, mitogen-activated protein kinase; mTOR, mammalian target of rapamycin.

There are indications that lymphocytes might become more dependent on the de-novo purine and pyrimidine pathway during proliferation. This might offer important opportunities for immunosuppression based on inhibitors of crucial enzymes in the de-novo nucleotide synthetic pathways.

Preclinical pharmacology

Two main classes of drugs have been the focus of immunosuppressive drug development: **biologics** and **xenobiotics**. Biologics are naturally occurring mammalian proteins or peptides, or modified forms of these, whereas xenobiotics are drugs produced from microorganisms or chemically synthesized molecules that are structurally dissimilar from naturally occurring mammalian molecules. These drugs target one or more molecular events in lymphocyte activation. Table 52.1 summarizes potential events to interfere with untoward T-cell activation, drugs affecting these events that are already in clinical use, and molecules in development that target these steps.

Drugs affecting the T-cell receptor complex

The monoclonal antibody (mAb) OKT3 targets one of the four conserved proteins of the T-cell antigen receptor complex. When given in vivo, OKT3 causes profound immunosuppression by three basic mechanisms: reduction in T-cell numbers, modulation of the TCR, and blocking the T-cell response by anergy [22,23].

CD4 and CD8 proteins are important functional members of the receptor complex, and they are involved in effective signal transduction initiation after antigenic recognition. Prevention of CD4 and MHC class II interaction by mAbs has been shown to prolong graft survival and to cause tolerance induction in different animal models. Clinical

Table 52.1. Immunosuppressants and their molecular and physiologic targets

Targets	Immunosuppressants
Antigen presentation and allorecognition	MHC protein, peptides, anti-T-lymphocyte globulin, mAb OKT3, mAb CD4
Costimulation	Anti-CD40, CTLA4-Ig, antimonokine antibodies, glucocorticoids
TCR signaling	Cyclosporine, tacrolimus, MAPK inhibitors, NFκB inhibitors
IL-2 binding	mAb-IL2R, daclizumab
IL-2R signaling	Rapamycin, JAK 3 inhibitors
Clonal expansion	Azathioprine, mycophenolate mofetil, leflunomide

IL-2R, interleukin-2 receptor; mAb, monoclonal antibody; MAPK, mitogen-activated protein kinase; MHC, major histocompatibility complex; NFκB, nuclear factor κB; TCR, T-cell receptor.

studies have addressed the potential roles of these mAbs as adjuvant therapy [24].

Drugs affecting costimulation

The dimeric fusion protein abatacept (CTLA4-Ig) targets the interaction of the T-cell-based CD28 molecule and its counter receptors CD80 or CD86 on APCs. Although rodent transplant models were promising, this drug failed further development in the transplantation arena. However, it slowed disease progression in autoimmune disease models and it is now approved for the treatment of rheumatoid arthritis [12,14].

Based on better preclinical profile, belatacept, a more potent drug with increased binding avidity to CD86, has progressed into clinical trials, where it performed with equivalent efficacy to cyclosporine but was associated with better renal function and histology in renal transplants. Various phase II and III trials are now ongoing in renal and liver transplantation [14].

Drugs affecting signaling underlying interleukin-2 gene transcription

Cyclosporine (cyclosporine A, CsA), a neutral lipophilic cyclic undecapeptide isolated from the fungus *Tolypocladium inflatum*, has revolutionized treatment of allograft rejection since the late 1970s, when studies revealed that CsA inhibits T-cell activation by blocking the transcription of cytokine genes, including *IL-2* and *IL-4* [15,25–27]. The major mechanism of action of CsA involves binding to the cytosolic 17 kDa cyclophilin A and the inhibition of the phosphatase activity of calcineurin by the CsA/cyclophilin A complex [27]. By preventing their calcineurin-mediated dephosphorylation of NFAT transcription factor, CsA inhibits the nuclear translocation of NFAT family members and subsequent gene expression in activated T cells [26].

Although structurally different from CsA, tacrolimus (FK506) also binds to immunophilins, termed FK506 binding proteins, and shares with CsA the inhibition of calcineurin as a molecular mechanism underlying its immunosuppressant activity (28,29).

Drugs affecting the interleukin-2 receptor complex

IL-2 and IL-2R are not expressed by resting T cells, but are expressed by T cells activated by interaction with alloantigens [30]. Murine mAbs directed against this inducible IL-2R inhibit the proliferation of alloantigen-activated T cells and have been proven effective in animal models of transplantation. To overcome the host immune response against the murine protein, humanized antibodies (daclizumab) were introduced with better pharmacokinetics and longer half-life [30,31]. In phase III trials daclizumab significantly reduced the frequency of renal allograft rejection when compared with a placebo, leading to approval by the US Food and Drug Administration (FDA). Daclizumab is now being evaluated for other organ transplants and in autoimmune disorders. There is evidence for the efficacy of daclizumab in reducing acute rejection episodes; however, an increased incidence of serious infections has been uncovered in both heart and lung transplantation [32,33].

Drugs affecting T-cell clonal proliferation

Rapamycin (sirolimus) and its structural relative everolimus block signal transduction mediated by IL-2 through the IL-2R complex, and hence they are termed proliferation signal inhibitors [34,35]. The cellular receptor(s) for the rapamycin/FKBP complex appears to be a 289 kDa phosphatidylinositol-3-kinase (PI3K)-related kinase, termed mammalian target of rapamycin, mTOR. The antiproliferative activity of rapamycin appears to be a consequence of the rapamycin/FKBP complex blocking the activation of the 70 kDa S6 protein kinases, selective inhibition of the synthesis of several ribosomal proteins ultimately affecting protein synthesis [20,34–36].

Interestingly, treatment of vascular smooth-muscle cells with rapamycin resulted in reduced growth-factor-stimulated proliferation in vitro [35,37]. This represents an additional therapeutic potential of rapamycin to control the intimal thickening of graft vascular disease and potentially prevent chronic rejection in other forms of organ transplantation.

Another class of drugs, which interferes with proliferation of T cells, targets the nucleotide metabolism necessary to provide building blocks for the DNA synthetic phase of the cell cycle. The antimetabolite azathioprine is a thioguanine derivative of 6-mercaptopurine. This purine analog acts as a purine antagonist and is the oldest – but still effective – antiproliferative drug [2,10,13].

Newer members of the antimetabolite group are mycophenolate mofetil (MMF) and leflunomide (LFM) [20,20,38–40]. In addition to their effectiveness in several animal models of arthritis, autoimmune disease, and allograft and xenograft rejection, they may inhibit chronic rejection manifested by vascular and airway narrowing [41–43]. This may be explained by direct inhibition of the proliferation of smooth-muscle cells.

Clinical pharmacology

Cyclosporine
Pharmacokinetics
Cyclosporine has a complex pharmacokinetic profile with poor absorption, formulation-dependent bioavailability, extensive metabolism to more than 30 metabolites, and considerable interpatient and intrapatient variability [44]. It has a narrow therapeutic range with adverse clinical consequences after either underdosing or overdosing.

Because of limitations in bioavailability and pharmacokinetics that were associated with the original formulation of cyclosporine, a microemulsion formulation was developed to improve bioavailability [45]. Neoral, the microemulsion formulation, exhibits significantly faster and more extensive absorption than the original oil-based formulation. Because of the more rapid and complete absorption of cyclosporine from Neoral, patients are exposed to greater peak blood concentrations and to greater areas under the curve of the drug, with a consequent reduction in acute rejection episodes [46].

Metabolism and drug interactions
Cyclosporine is primarily eliminated through biotransformation by cytochrome P450 (CYP) 3A in the gut wall and liver

[46]. In addition, P-glycoprotein (MDR1) located in the gastrointestinal epithelium can affect blood concentrations of cyclosporine after oral administration of the drug, presumably by countertransporting the drug from the systemic circulation back into the gastrointestinal lumen. CYP3A4 oxidizes a broad spectrum of drugs by a number of metabolic processes. The location of CYP3A4 in the small bowel and liver permits both to exert an effect on orally administered drugs. Thus drugs inhibiting or inducing CYP activity are expected to interact and modulate CsA levels. The implications of these interactions are twofold: they might increase CsA levels to toxic concentrations, and they might be used to allow a reduction in the dosage of cyclosporine while maintaining therapeutic blood cyclosporine (cyclosporine-sparing drugs) [47,48]. Included in this list are the azole *antifungal drugs* (ketoconazole, fluconazole, itraconazole), *the calcium channel blockers* (diltiazem, verapamil, nicardipine), and the *macrolide antibacterials* (erythromycin and related compounds). Studies of various regimens involving the combined use of ketoconazole and cyclosporine have shown that cyclosporine dosages can be reduced by approximately 70–85% while maintaining therapeutic blood concentrations in patients who received kidney, heart, or liver transplant [49]. The calcium channel blocker diltiazem allows a decrease in cyclosporine dosage by approximately 30–50% in patients who have received an organ transplant.

Contrastingly, CYP inducers, including rifampicin and the majority of anticonvulsants, can decrease cyclosporine blood concentrations to undetectable levels [50]. Other drugs that have been reported to decrease cyclosporine concentration include sulfadimidine, trimethoprim, nafcillin, and octreotide. Because of the numerous interactions with cyclosporine, clinicians should monitor the concentration of this drug more frequently when another drug is added or discontinued, and cyclosporine dosage should be adjusted when appropriate, because sustained departure from optimal concentrations can result in either graft rejection or increased renal toxicity.

Adverse effects

Benefits of cyclosporine-based immunosuppression are hampered by a broad adverse-effect profile that includes nephrotoxicity, neurotoxicity, and adverse cardiovascular risk profile such as diabetes, hypercholesterolemia, and hypertension [51–54].

Tacrolimus

Tacrolimus is a very potent immunosuppressant, with a 10- to 100-fold greater in-vitro immunosuppressive activity than cyclosporine. Consistent with its greater potency, therapeutic whole-blood through concentrations for tacrolimus are ~ 20-fold less than the corresponding cyclosporine concentrations.

In general, the clinical efficiency of tacrolimus is similar to that of cyclosporine. Both drugs provide comparable 1-year graft and patient survival rate. However, in patients who received renal transplant tacrolimus is more powerful in preventing severe and refractory rejections, even when compared with the new cyclosporine microemulsion formulation. Both drugs are equally nephrotoxic, but tacrolimus induces less hypertension, and less pronounced hyperlipidemia, gingival hyperplasia, and hirsutism [53].

Azathioprine

Azathioprine is a prodrug that is converted in vivo to 6-mercaptopurine, which is subsequently metabolized to the pharmacologically active 6-thioguanine nucleotides. The latter is also responsible for the cytotoxic side effects associated with this drug, which include bone-marrow depression [55]. Measuring blood counts has, therefore, been a part of routine monitoring during azathioprine therapy. Immunosuppressive efficacy of azathioprine can be obtained through pharmacodynamic measurements such as thiopurine S-methyltransferase activity and the quantification of intracellular 6-thioguanine nucleotide concentrations in red blood cells.

Azathioprine is largely inactivated by xanthine oxidase, and the product, 6-thiouric acid, is excreted by the kidneys. Toxicity is increased twofold in renal failure and fourfold by inhibiting xanthine oxidase. Thus one of the most important drug interactions of azathioprine is with allopurinol in patients treated for hyperuricemia.

Rapamycin

Rapamycin has been shown to produce a significant reduction in acute rejection (7% vs. 36%) in clinical trials, when used in combination with other immunosuppressants such as CsA and prednisone. It also allowed early withdrawal of steroid therapy in a large number of patients (78%), demonstrating a great clinical impact [35,56].

Gastrointestinal absorption of rapamycin is rapid, and it reaches peak concentrations within 1 hour in 70% of patients. Its systemic availability is low (14%). The majority of drug is sequestered in red blood cells, causing plasma concentrations to be lower than in whole blood. It is primarily metabolized by the same CYP3A4 enzyme involved in the metabolism of calcineurin inhibitors, thus exhibiting large intersubject and intrasubject variability because of genetic differences in the activity of this system. The drug has a relatively long half-life (62 hours). The side-effect profile of rapamycin indicates no increased incidence of hypertension, nephrotoxicity, or hepatotoxicity. However, rapamycin causes leukopenia, thrombocytopenia, and a marked hyperlipidemia [34,35]. The main mechanism of this latter effect is interference with lipid clearance by inhibiting lipoprotein lipase and blocking insulin-like growth-factor-induced signaling underlying the uptake of fatty acids.

Mycophenolate mofetil

Initial multicenter clinical studies in renal transplantation showed significant reduction of acute rejection episodes (by 40%) in patients treated with mycophenolate, and histology showed less extensive disease. Recent randomized clinical trials also have demonstrated that mycophenolate, when used with cyclosporine and steroids, reduces the frequency and severity of acute rejection episodes in kidney, heart, and lung transplants [57]. It also improved patient and graft survival rates in heart allograft recipients and increased renal allograft survival [9]. In addition, mycophenolate has been effective in reversing acute and resistant rejection episodes in patients who received heart, kidney, or liver transplants. The ability of MMF to facilitate sparing of other immunosuppressive drugs, particularly in CsA-related nephrotoxicity, is also promising [51]. By permitting reduction in CsA doses, MMF may stabilize or improve renal graft function in patients with CsA-related nephrotoxicity or chronic allograft nephropathy. The main adverse effects of mycophenolate include gastrointestinal and hematologic complications [58].

Immunosuppression protocols

Current protocols rely on combinations of immunosuppressive drugs to produce an additive or synergistic effect while minimizing toxicity. Drugs with different mechanisms of action and preferably nonoverlapping toxicity are combined so that the doses of the individual drugs can be reduced to levels below toxicity.

The role of a strict early immunosuppression regimen, termed **induction immunosuppression**, is being increasingly recognized in the immediate and critical postoperative period to minimize the initial strong immune response to the plethora of newly transplanted antigens and donor APCs. Over the past decade, the use of this strategy has increased for nearly all organs, with over 70% of kidney and pancreas transplant patients, 50% of heart, lung, and intestine recipients, and about 20% of liver recipients now receiving induction therapy. In addition to steroids and calcineurin inhibitors, polyclonal antibody induction with antithymocyte globulin is the most frequent choice for kidney and pancreas transplantation, while anti-IL-2 receptor antibody induction with basiliximab or daclizumab is more common for liver, heart, and lung recipients (Fig. 52.5).

Maintenance immunosuppression refers to lifelong prophylactic therapy against rejection. Calcineurin inhibitors are prescribed for 90% or more of all categories of solid-organ recipients at discharge from the initial transplant hospitalization. There is an important trend away from cyclosporine towards tacrolimus. Antimetabolite usage varies from a low of 9% for intestine recipients to a high of 95% for heart recipients (Fig. 52.6). Again the trend away from azathiprine to MMF is evident in nearly all but lung transplantation. Sirolimus use has gained acceptance as part of many combination regimens, but it only accounts for around 10–20% of maintenance protocols.

Anesthetic implications of immunosuppressive drugs

Apart from specialized transplant anesthesiologists, the large majority of anesthesiologists face the issues of maintenance immunosuppression and its sequelae only when a transplant recipient or a patient with autoimmune disease is presented for nontransplant surgery. Detailed and systematic analysis of individual organ dysfunction after transplantation is beyond the scope of this chapter, but there are excellent anesthetic reviews available on the topic [60–62]. Here we emphasize the side effects of immunosuppressants on different organ systems, and potential drug interactions that may be important to the anesthesiologist.

Cyclosporine causes at least 20% decrease in **renal function** in almost all patients, an effect shared with tacrolimus [53]. Renal insufficiency partly attributable to immunosuppression, mainly nephrotoxicity induced by calcineurin inhibitors, is an unfortunate feature that plagues both kidney and nonrenal solid-organ recipients. In the renal scenario, the combined effects of immunosuppression and chronic rejection lead to late renal allograft dysfunction, termed chronic renal allograft nephropathy. This is the primary cause of late graft loss, accounting up to 50% of cases. In those patients who require dialysis for failed graft, the risk of death is more than three times higher than before graft loss. In the case of nonrenal solid-organ transplants, the 5-year incidence of renal failure is organ-dependent, developing in 11% of heart, 16% of lung, and 18% of liver transplant recipients. Approximately one-third of these patients require dialysis or renal transplantation. Development of renal failure is associated with more than a fourfold increase in mortality.

As in the general population, traditional risk factors for **cardiovascular disease** are relevant for the development of atherosclerosis, ischemic heart disease, and cardiovascular mortality in transplant recipients. However, transplanted patients are at two- to fourfold higher relative risk for major cardiovascular events.

Hypertension might be caused by renal mechanisms but could be related to generalized vasoconstriction caused by interference with endogenous nitric oxide mechanisms or overproduction of vasoconstrictor endothelins or angiotensins [63].

Type 2 **diabetes mellitus** occurs in up to 30% of recipients 2 years after transplantation. Risk factors for development include older age, African-American race, increased body mass index, the use of tacrolimus, and hepatitis C infection. The development of post-transplant diabetes mellitus is associated with a 63% increase in kidney graft failure and a nearly doubled mortality rate in transplant recipients [64].

Immunosuppressant-induced **hyperlipidemia** is a commonly reported adverse event following steroid, cyclosporine, and proliferation signal inhibitor treatment [65]. However,

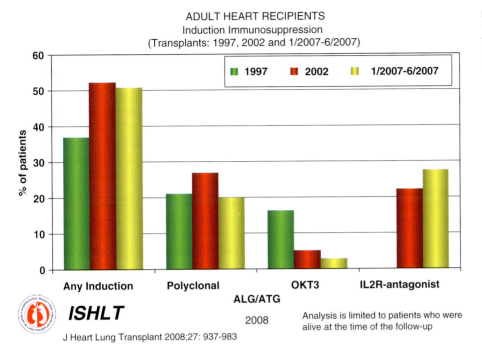

ADULT HEART RECIPIENTS
Induction Immunosuppression
(Transplants: 1997, 2002 and 1/2007-6/2007)

ISHLT   2008   Analysis is limited to patients who were alive at the time of the follow-up

J Heart Lung Transplant 2008;27: 937-983

Figure 52.5. The changing face of induction immunosuppression in heart transplantation. Reproduced with permission from Registry of the International Society for Heart and Lung Transplantation [59].

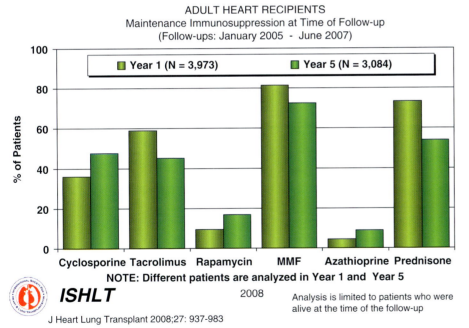

ADULT HEART RECIPIENTS
Maintenance Immunosuppression at Time of Follow-up
(Follow-ups: January 2005 - June 2007)

NOTE: Different patients are analyzed in Year 1 and Year 5

ISHLT   2008   Analysis is limited to patients who were alive at the time of the follow-up

J Heart Lung Transplant 2008;27: 937-983

Figure 52.6. Components of maintenance immunosuppression in heart transplantation. Reproduced with permission from Registry of the International Society for Heart and Lung Transplantation [59].

everolimus or sirolimus inhibit local and systemic inflammation and smooth-muscle proliferation and may ultimately exert beneficial effects on the risk profile. Nevertheless, the use of long-term statin therapy seems essential, as shown by a 50% reduction in transplant vasculopathy and a 30% increase in late patient survival rates in heart transplantation [65].

Immunosuppressant-induced **liver disease** can be a major problem in many transplant patients, and preoperative checks should include an assessment of cellular integrity, as well as of synthetic, detoxification, and excretion capacity. This can be done by measuring aminotransferases, bilirubins, and clotting profile. This is especially important in anesthesia for surveillance or diagnostic biopsy procedures. As discussed earlier, several of the immunosuppressants influence **bone-marrow function**, and a full blood count is required to assess acceptable reserve. A leukocyte count of less than 2000 μL^{-1} in patients receiving azathioprine is usually a contraindication to surgery, which should be postponed until recovery is achieved after dose adjustment.

Most recipients of solid-organ transplants experience an increased frequency of **fractures** post-transplant. A unique feature of these fractures is the predominance of fractures in the appendicular skeleton, especially the feet. The phenomenon appears multifactorial. Loss of bone mineral density, diabetic neuropathy, advanced age, decreased muscle mass, poor mobility, and poor balance have been demonstrated to play a major role in fracture risk.

Conduct of anesthesia

It is advisable to maintain the patient's regular medications until surgery, because sudden changes might greatly influence serum levels of immunosuppressants. Usual premedication is appropriate in most cases. Most intravenous anesthetic drugs can be used, and isoflurane is commonly and safely delivered as the primary inhalation drug. Although there are reports of some degree of interaction between volatiles and cyclosporine, these are likely of academic rather than clinical importance. There is also some theoretical reason to avoid enflurane and sevoflurane because of potential liberation of nephrotoxic inorganic fluoride.

Among muscle relaxants, succinylcholine is appropriate for short procedures if serum potassium levels are in the normal range, while atracurium is useful for longer procedures. Renal dysfunction and cyclosporine might increase the duration of pancuronium- and vecuronium-induced neuromuscular blockade, and liver dysfunction should be taken into consideration in dosing vecuronium. In general, smaller doses of nondepolarizing muscle relaxants are required, and monitoring neuromuscular blockade is essential. Regarding postoperative pain control, nonsteroidal anti-inflammatory drugs should be avoided because in conjunction with cyclosporine they might precipitate renal failure. Perhaps the best solution is opiate-based patient-controlled analgesia for intermediate and painful operations.

One of the most important aspects of the conduct of anesthesia is infection control and prophylaxis. Invasive monitoring should be used judiciously when hemodynamic instability is anticipated, but it should be kept to a minimum. Most centers have relaxed extra measures for sterility, but anesthetic personnel should adopt strict aseptic procedures. Most of these patients are already receiving antibacterial, viral, and fungal prophylaxis, but if bacteremia is anticipated during the surgery, extra antibiotic prophylaxis is recommended, with the initial dose given before surgery and cover for the postoperative period. In this regard, potential drug interactions with cyclosporine should be taken into account.

In summary, anesthetizing an immunosuppressed patient presents multiple challenges. Understanding the impact of immunosuppression and transplantation-related system dysfunction should prompt a perioperative plan in which careful assessment of metabolic and electrolyte status, optimal fluid balance and aggressive hemodynamic monitoring and management, infection control and general attention to details appear more important than the actual choice of anesthetic drug. However, vigilance is paramount, as on rare occasions anesthetic drugs may even trigger fatal myopathy in the setting of polypharmacy comprising high-dose steroids, cyclosporine, and statins.

Anesthetic drugs as immunosuppressants

The evidence to support a clinically significant direct immunosuppressant effect of inhalation or intravenous anesthetics after surgery is inconclusive [66–68]. There is evidence that a variety of anesthetics produce a considerable suppression of both nonspecific and antigen-specific cellular immune mechanisms in vitro. In the concentrations used in a clinical setting, however, these negative effects are rapidly and completely reversible. No clinically relevant adverse effects on the immune system have been identified that are conclusively attributable to short-term anesthesia. However, the situation might be different with high doses of anesthetic used for long-term sedation, during which thiobarbiturates or diazepam can reach tissue concentrations sufficient to cause suppression of cellular immune mechanisms. This has been shown in patients with craniocerebral trauma, in whom high doses of thiopental were associated with an increased incidence of bacterial pneumonias [69].

Acute and chronic opioid administration is known to have inhibitory effects on humoral and cellular immune responses, including antibody production, natural killer cell activity, cytokine expression, and phagocytic activity [70–72]. Opiate-related immunosuppression may be relevant to increased infections in addicts and patients receiving long-term opioid therapy for malignant and nonmalignant pain.

The relative contribution of anesthesia itself and the surgical trauma and stress in causing immunosuppression remains controversial. Many findings seem to point to an essential role played by surgical factors, as well as by the preoperative immune status of the patient, in the occurrence of subsequent infectious complications [68].

Summary

Organ transplantation can increase survival in patients with end-stage organ failure. First, however, the problem of immunological rejection must be overcome. Hyperacute rejection involves preformed antibodies. Chronic rejection results from microvascular proliferation. Acute rejection is the most commonly observed, involving inflammatory processes orchestrated by T cells. Activation of a T-cell response is a pivotal event in complex immunologic processes, and strategies for immunosuppression include depleting T cells, inhibiting T-cell activation pathways, and interrupting T-cell trafficking.

Host T cells recognize donor major histocompatibility complex (MHC) antigen by direct allorecognition or as processed peptide fragments presented by host antigen-presenting cells (APC). T-cell receptor (TCR) engagement, together with costimulatory signals, activates protein kinase signaling cascades and a Ca^{2+}/calmodulin and calcineurin pathway. These pathways culminate in the activation of several families of transcription factors, including nuclear factor of activated T cells (NFAT), activating protein 1 (AP-1), and nuclear factor κB (NFκB) families. The resulting alterations in gene expression include upregulation of interleukin 2 (IL-2). IL-2 signaling acts via activation of transcription factors such as STAT-3 and STAT-5, to have a mitogenic effect on T cells.

Molecules targeting T-cell signaling include monoclonal antibodies which bind to conserved regions of the TCR (OKT-3), and those which interfere with the CD4 coreceptor binding to MHC class II. Drugs which bind CD80 and CD86 on APCs interfere with signaling through the T-cell costimulatory receptor CD28 – an example is belatacept, currently in phase II and III trials.

Cyclosporine and tacrolimus (FK506) are approved immunosuppressants which act to inhibit the phosphatase activity of calcineurin, blocking NFAT-mediated gene expression. The microemulsion formulation of cyclosporine (Neoral) exhibits better absorption than the original formulation, but cyclosporine-based immunosuppression has a broad adverse-effect profile. Tacrolimus generally has similar clinical efficiency, and while it is equally nephrotoxic, other adverse effects are less pronounced. More frequent monitoring of cyclosporine blood concentration is recommended after any drug regimen change, becauase of the many drug interactions reported.

Humanized monoclonal antibodies to the IL-2 receptor (daclizumab) and drugs which block signal transduction through the IL-2 receptor (rapamycin and everolimus) also inhibit T-cell proliferation. There is evidence that rapamycin may also have the potential to control the intimal thickening of graft vascular disease. Leukopenia, thrombocytopenia, and hyperlipidemia are side effects of rapamycin.

T-cell proliferation requires an increased abundance of nucleotides, suggesting potential immunosuppression strategies based on inhibition of enzymes in nucleotide synthetic pathways. The antimetabolite azathioprine acts as a purine antagonist with antiproliferative effects. Cytotoxic side effects of azathioprine include bone-marrow depression, hence monitoring of blood counts is routine. Mycophenolate mofetil (MMF) and leflunomide (LFM) are more recent additions to the antimetabolite group. MMF used in combination with other drugs may permit reductions in their doses; this holds promise for patients with cyclosporine-related nephrotoxicity or chronic allograft nephropathy. Adverse effects include gastrointestinal and hematologic complications.

Immunosuppressive protocols use combinations of drugs that act synergistically while reducing individual doses to below threshold levels for toxicity. Induction immunosuppression is a strict regimen followed in the immediate postoperative period. Maintenance immunosuppression involves lifelong prophylactic therapy, and can have implications for anesthesiologists presented with a transplant recipient or autoimmune-disease patient for nontransplant surgery. The perioperative plan should include close monitoring of the patient. Potential complications include renal dysfunction, cardiovascular dysfunction, hypertension, diabetes mellitus, hyperlipidemia, and bone disease. Preoperative checks for liver and hematological dysfunction should be carried out, and it is advisable to continue the patient's regular medications until surgery. Usual premedication is generally appropriate, although for anesthesia there is an argument for avoiding enflurane and sevoflurane. Choice and dosing of muscle relaxant is dependent upon the length of the procedure and whether renal or liver dysfunction is present. Nonsteroidal anti-inflammatory drugs should be avoided for postoperative pain control. Invasive monitoring should be limited to the minimum necessary and strict asepsis adhered to by anesthetic personnel. In some circumstances, additional antibiotic prophylaxis is recommended. It is important to be aware that anesthetic drugs can trigger fatal myopathy when used in combination with high-dose steroids, cyclosporine, and statins.

Although there is evidence that anesthetics may have immunosuppressive effects, particularly with long-term use of certain drugs, the relative contribution of anesthesia to postoperative immunosuppression is unclear.

References

1. Moller E, Soderberg-Naucler C, Sumitran-Karuppan S. Role of alloimmunity in clinical transplantation. *Rev Immunogenet* 1999; **1**: 309–22.

2. Snell GI, Westall GP. Immunosuppression for lung transplantation: evidence to date. *Drugs* 2007; **67**: 1531–9.

3. Suthanthiran M. Signaling features of T cells: implications for the regulation of the anti-allograft response. *Kidney Int Suppl* 1993; **43**: S3–11.

4. Choi S, Schwartz RH. Molecular mechanisms for adaptive tolerance and other T cell anergy models. *Semin Immunol* 2007; **19**: 140–52.

5. Dustin ML. T-cell activation through immunological synapses and kinapses. *Immunol Rev* 2008; **221**: 77–89.

6. Grakoui A, Bromley SK, Sumen C, et al. The immunological synapse: a molecular machine controlling T cell activation. *Science* 1999; **285**: 221–27.

7. Taniguchi T, Minami Y. The IL-2/IL-2 receptor system: a current overview. *Cell* 1993; **73**: 5–8.

8. Viola JP, Rao A. Molecular regulation of cytokine gene expression during the immune response. *J Clin Immunol* 1999; **19**: 98–108.

9. Knoll G. Trends in kidney transplantation over the past decade. *Drugs* 2008; **68**: 3–10.

10. Ciancio G, Burke GW, Miller J. Current treatment practice in immunosuppression. *Expert Opin Pharmacother* 2000; **1**: 1307–30.

11. Benichou G. Direct and indirect antigen recognition: the pathways to allograft immune rejection. *Front Biosci* 1999; **4**: D476–80.

12. Vincenti F, Luggen M. T cell costimulation: a rational target in the therapeutic armamentarium for autoimmune diseases and transplantation. *Annu Rev Med* 2007; **58**: 347–58.

13. Marder W, McCune WJ. Advances in immunosuppressive therapy. *Semin Respir Crit Care Med* 2007; **28**: 398–417.

14. Vincenti F. Costimulation blockade in autoimmunity and transplantation. *J Allergy Clin Immunol* 2008; **121**: 299–306.

15. Clipstone NA, Crabtree GR. Identification of calcineurin as a key signalling enzyme in T-lymphocyte activation. *Nature* 1992; **357**: 695–7.

16. Flanagan WM, Corthesy B, Bram RJ, Crabtree GR. Nuclear association of a T-cell transcription factor blocked by FK-506 and cyclosporin A. *Nature* 1991; **352**: 803–7.

17. Nelson BH, Willerford DM. Biology of the interleukin-2 receptor. *Adv Immunol* 1998; **70**: 1–81.

18. Johnston JA, Bacon CM, Finbloom DS, *et al.* Tyrosine phosphorylation and activation of STAT5, STAT3, and Janus kinases by interleukins 2 and 15. *Proc Natl Acad Sci U S A* 1995; **92**: 8705–9.

19. Kim HP, Imbert J, Leonard WJ. Both integrated and differential regulation of components of the IL-2/IL-2 receptor system. *Cytokine Growth Factor Rev* 2006; **17**: 349–66.

20. Brazelton TR, Morris RE. Molecular mechanisms of action of new xenobiotic immunosuppressive drugs: tacrolimus (FK506), sirolimus (rapamycin), mycophenolate mofetil and leflunomide. *Curr Opin Immunol* 1996; **8**: 710–20.

21. Sharma VK, Li B, Khanna A, Sehajpal PK, Suthanthiran M. Which way for drug-mediated immunosuppression? *Curr Opin Immunol* 1994; **6**: 784–90.

22. Norman DJ. Mechanisms of action and overview of OKT3. *Ther Drug Monit* 1995; **17**: 615–20.

23. Bonnefoy-Berard N, Revillard JP. Mechanisms of immunosuppression induced by antithymocyte globulins and OKT3. *J Heart Lung Transplant* 1996; **15**: 435–42.

24. Webster A, Pankhurst T, Rinaldi F, Chapman JR, Craig JC. Polyclonal and monoclonal antibodies for treating acute rejection episodes in kidney transplant recipients. *Cochrane Database Syst Rev* 2006; **19**: CD004756.

25. Borel JF, Feurer C, Gubler HU, Stahelin H. Biological effects of cyclosporin A: a new antilymphocytic agent. 1976. *Agents Actions* 1994; **43**: 179–86.

26. Matsuda S, Koyasu S. Mechanisms of action of cyclosporine. *Immunopharmacology* 2000; **47**: 119–25.

27. Liu J, Farmer JD, Lane WS, *et al.* Calcineurin is a common target of cyclophilin-cyclosporin A and FKBP-FK506 complexes. *Cell* 1991; **66**: 807–15.

28. Goto T, Kino T, Hatanaka H, *et al.* Discovery of FK-506, a novel immunosuppressant isolated from Streptomyces tsukubaensis. *Transplant Proc* 1987; **19**: 4–8.

29. Ochiai T, Nakajima K, Nagata M, *et al.* Effect of a new immunosuppressive agent, FK 506, on heterotopic cardiac allotransplantation in the rat. *Transplant Proc* 1987; **19**: 1284–6.

30. Waldmann TA, O'shea J. The use of antibodies against the IL-2 receptor in transplantation. *Curr Opin Immunol* 1998; **10**: 507–12.

31. Vincenti F, Kirkman R, Light S, *et al.* Interleukin-2-receptor blockade with daclizumab to prevent acute rejection in renal transplantation. Daclizumab Triple Therapy Study Group. *N Engl J Med* 1998; **338**: 161–5.

32. Hershberger RE, Starling RC, Eisen HJ, *et al.* Daclizumab to prevent rejection after cardiac transplantation. *N Engl J Med* 2005; **352**: 2705–13.

33. Mullen JC, Oreopoulos A, Lien DC, *et al.* A randomized, controlled trial of daclizumab vs anti-thymocyte globulin induction for lung transplantation. *J Heart Lung Transplant* 2007; **26**: 504–10.

34. Chan M, Pearson GJ. New advances in antirejection therapy. *Curr Opin Cardiol* 2007; **22**: 117–22.

35. Zuckermann A, Manito N, Epailly E, *et al.* Multidisciplinary insights on clinical guidance for the use of proliferation signal inhibitors in heart transplantation. *J Heart Lung Transplant* 2008; **27**: 141–9.

36. Terada N, Takase K, Papst P, Nairn AC, Gelfand EW. Rapamycin inhibits ribosomal protein synthesis and induces G1 prolongation in mitogen-activated T lymphocytes. *J Immunol* 1995; **155**: 3418–26.

37. Morris RE, Cao W, Huang X, *et al.* Rapamycin (sirolimus) inhibits vascular smooth muscle DNA synthesis in vitro and suppresses narrowing in arterial allografts and in balloon-injured carotid arteries: evidence that rapamycin antagonizes growth factor action on immune and nonimmune cells. *Transplant Proc* 1995; **27**: 430–1.

38. Ransom JT. Mechanism of action of mycophenolate mofetil. *Ther Drug Monit* 1995; **17**: 681–4.

39. Zwerner J, Fiorentino D. Mycophenolate mofetil. *Dermatol Ther* 2007; **20**: 229–38.

40. Cherwinski HM, McCarley D, Schatzman R, Devens B, Ransom JT. The immunosuppressant leflunomide inhibits lymphocyte progression through cell cycle by a novel mechanism. *J Pharmacol Exp Ther* 1995; **272**: 460–8.

41. Nair RV, Cao W, Morris RE. The antiproliferative effect of leflunomide on vascular smooth muscle cells in vitro is mediated by selective inhibition of pyrimidine biosynthesis. *Transplant Proc* 1996; **28**: 3081.

42. Fraser-Smith EB, Rosete JD, Schatzman RC. Suppression by mycophenolate mofetil of the neointimal thickening caused by vascular injury in a rat

arterial stenosis model. *J Pharmacol Exp Ther* 1995; **275**: 1204–8.

43. Allison AC, Eugui EM. Mechanisms of action of mycophenolate mofetil in preventing acute and chronic allograft rejection. *Transplantation* 2005; **80**: S181–90.

44. Kahan BD, Welsh M, Schoenberg L, *et al.* Variable oral absorption of cyclosporine. A biopharmaceutical risk factor for chronic renal allograft rejection. *Transplantation* 1996; **62**: 599–606.

45. Ritschel WA. Microemulsion technology in the reformulation of cyclosporine: the reason behind the pharmacokinetic properties of Neoral. *Clin Transplant* 1996; **10**: 364–73.

46. Fahr A. Cyclosporin clinical pharmacokinetics. *Clin Pharmacokinet* 1993; **24**: 472–95.

47. Trotter JF. Drugs that interact with immunosuppressive agents. *Semin Gastrointest Dis* 1998; **9**: 147–53.

48. Martin JE, Daoud AJ, Schroeder TJ, First MR. The clinical and economic potential of cyclosporin drug interactions. *Pharmacoeconomics* 1999; **15**: 317–37.

49. Keogh A, Spratt P, McCosker C, *et al.* Ketoconazole to reduce the need for cyclosporine after cardiac transplantation. *N Engl J Med* 1995; **333**: 628–33.

50. Campana C, Regazzi MB, Buggia I, Molinaro M. Clinically significant drug interactions with cyclosporin: an update. *Clin Pharmacokinet* 1996; **30**: 141–79.

51. Flechner SM, Kobashigawa J, Klintmalm G. Calcineurin inhibitor-sparing regimens in solid organ transplantation: focus on improving renal function and nephrotoxicity. *Clin Transplant* 2008; **22**: 1–15.

52. Bechstein WO. Neurotoxicity of calcineurin inhibitors: impact and clinical management. *Transpl Int* 2000; **13**: 313–26.

53. Olyaei AJ, de Mattos AM, Bennett WM. Immunosuppressant-induced nephropathy: pathophysiology, incidence and management. *Drug Saf* 1999; **21**: 471–88.

54. Meraw SJ, Sheridan PJ. Medically induced gingival hyperplasia. *Mayo Clin Proc* 1998; **73**: 1196–9.

55. Schutz E, Gummert J, Armstrong VW, Mohr FW, Oellerich M. Azathioprine pharmacogenetics: the relationship between 6-thioguanine nucleotides and thiopurine methyltransferase in patients after heart and kidney transplantation. *Eur J Clin Chem Clin Biochem* 1996; **34**: 199–205.

56. Calne RY, Collier DS, Lim S, *et al.* Rapamycin for immunosuppression in organ allografting. *Lancet* 1989; **2**: 227.

57. Knight SR, Morris PJ. Does the evidence support the use of mycophenolate mofetil therapeutic drug monitoring in clinical practice? A systematic review. *Transplantation* 2008; **85**: 1675–85.

58. Staatz CE, Tett SE. Clinical pharmacokinetics and pharmacodynamics of mycophenolate in solid organ transplant recipients. *Clin Pharmacokinet* 2007; **46**: 13–58.

59. Registry of the International Society for Heart and Lung Transplantation. *J Heart Lung Transplant* 2008; **27**: 937–83.

60. Sharpe MD. Anaesthesia and the transplanted patient. *Can J Anaesth* 1996; **43**: R89–98.

61. Kostopanagiotou G, Smyrniotis V, Arkadopoulos N, *et al.* Anesthetic and perioperative management of adult transplant recipients in nontransplant surgery. *Anesth Analg* 1999; **89**: 613–22.

62. Toivonen HJ. Anaesthesia for patients with a transplanted organ. *Acta Anaesthesiol Scand* 2000; **44**: 812–33.

63. MacDonald AS. Impact of immunosuppressive therapy on hypertension. *Transplantation* 2000; **70**: SS70–6.

64. Aliabadi AZ, Zuckermann AO, Grimm M. Immunosuppressive therapy in older cardiac transplant patients. *Drugs Aging* 2007; **24**: 913–32.

65. Ballantyne CM, el Masri B, Morrisett JD, Torre-Amione G. Pathophysiology and treatment of lipid perturbation after cardiac transplantation. *Curr Opin Cardiol* 1997; **12**: 153–60.

66. Thomson DA. Anesthesia and the immune system. *J Burn Care Rehabil* 1987; **8**: 483–7.

67. Hunter JD. Effects of anaesthesia on the human immune system. *Hosp Med* 1999; **60**: 658–63.

68. Procopio MA, Rassias AJ, DeLeo JA, *et al.* The in vivo effects of general and epidural anesthesia on human immune function. *Anesth Analg* 2001; **93**: 460–5.

69. Stover JF, Stocker R. Barbiturate coma may promote reversible bone marrow suppression in patients with severe isolated traumatic brain injury. *Eur J Clin Pharmacol* 1998; **54**: 529–34.

70. Peterson PK, Molitor TW, Chao CC. The opioid-cytokine connection. *J Neuroimmunol* 1998; **83**: 63–9.

71. Gaveriaux-Ruff C, Matthes HW, Peluso J, Kieffer BL. Abolition of morphine-immunosuppression in mice lacking the mu-opioid receptor gene. *Proc Natl Acad Sci U S A* 1998; **95**: 6326–30.

72. Reece AS. Clinical implications of addiction related immunosuppression. *J Infect* 2008; **56**: 437–45.

Antimotility and antisecretory drugs

Robert P. Walt and Eugene B. Campbell

Introduction

Anesthetists may be presented with surgical and critical care patients suffering high enterostomy efflux or diarrhea, and investigations should be undertaken to determine and treat the underlying cause of such disturbances. Disorders such as irritable bowel syndrome (IBS), short bowel syndrome, and diarrhea can benefit from pharmacologic intervention to slow gut motility and reduce some gastrointestinal secretions. Therapy to reduce gastric acid secretion, in particular, can be beneficial in short bowel syndrome, gastroesophageal reflux disease, and gastroduodenal ulcers. Treatment to reduce volume and acidity of the gastric contents may also have applications prior to elective surgery to reduce severity of aspiration pneumonitis. It is important to understand the gastrointestinal system and the various mechanisms of action of antimotility and antisecretory drugs, as well as their pharmacokinetics, interactions, side effects, and clinical applications.

For decades the main therapies available to alter gut motility and secretion were opiates and antimuscarinic drugs. In the 1970s, histamine (H_2)-receptor antagonists provided effective suppression of gastric acid secretion for the first time. A decade later, proton pump inhibitors (PPIs) went a step further in efficacy. With further recognition of the transmitters and receptors involved in secretion and motility, further advances seem likely.

The normal gut

The major function of the gut is ingestion, digestion, absorption, and defecation. The stomach provides a highly acidic environment, primarily to provide an antimicrobial barrier.

The small bowel consists of duodenum, jejunum, and ileum. The duodenum is about 25 cm in length, absorbs iron, and allows mixing of pancreatic enzymes, bile salts, and food. The jejunum is 250 cm in length and is responsible for the majority of nutrient absorption. The ileum is longer, at 350 cm, and, with slower intrinsic motility and the ileocecal valve acting as an *ileal brake*, it slows transit in the upper gut when carbohydrate and fats enter the ileum, thereby allowing

more time for nutrient absorption. The ileum is also specialized to absorb vitamin B_{12} and bile salts. The colon, 150 cm in length, absorbs water and stores feces until defecation.

Motility

Transit of luminal contents depends on contractions and relaxations of the smooth muscles. These are integrated to both mix and propel the bowel contents. This is under central control via the vagus nerve, and locally by the enteric nerves. The enteric nervous system contains about 10^8 neurons, approximately the same number as in the spinal cord. These form neural circuits that control motor functions, blood flow, secretions, and absorption, and interact with other organs such as the pancreas and gall bladder. There are many transmitters and receptors identified in the gut wall, but their physiological roles are not all understood [1]. Metoclopramide (see Chapter 54) may have an effect on gastric motility. Gut transit time is not typically measured in clinical practice, but research studies utilize radiolabeled meals, passage of inert particles, or breath hydrogen peaks after lactulose ingestion as approximate measures of transit time.

Secretions and fluid turnover

The normal small intestine is presented with about 9 L of fluid a day, 2 L from the diet and the rest in the form of secretions from saliva, stomach, bile, and pancreas (Table 53.1). Currently, gastric acid secretion can be effectively controlled by proton pump inhibitors (PPIs). Octreotide, a synthetic somatostatin analog, may reduce pancreatic secretions.

The small intestine is the site of active and passive absorption of fluids, electrolytes, and nutrients. Transport proteins, ion channels, and tight junctions participate in regulating these fluxes. Net absorption is such that out of 9 L influx only 1.5 L reaches the colon. Any disturbances in small-bowel absorption can result in significant symptomatic diarrhea and fluid and electrolyte losses. Opiates can alter small-bowel motility, and drugs to alter secretory capacity are under development.

The colon has a large capacity to absorb fluids: up to 6 L per 24 hours provided it is presented evenly and not in large fluxes. Normal human colonic microflora contains over

Anesthetic Pharmacology, 2nd edition, ed. Alex S. Evers, Mervyn Maze, Evan D. Kharasch. Published by Cambridge University Press. © Cambridge University Press 2011.

Table 53.1. Daily fluid turnover in the gut (mL)

Ingested		2000
Endogenous secretions	Saliva	1500
	Stomach	2500
	Bile	500
	Pancreas	1500
	Intestine	1000
Total input		9000
Absorbed	Jejunum	5500
	Ileum	2000
	Colon	1300
Total absorbed		8800
Balance in stool		200

500 species of bacteria, yet peaceful coexistence rather than inflammation is the norm. However, disturbances of colonic microflora may result in altered colonic function.

Gastric acid secretion

The human stomach contains 1 billion parietal cells, each capable of secreting 3.3 billion hydrogen ions per second. Hydrochloric acid is produced at a pH of 0.8, or 150 mmol L^{-1}. Gastric acid serves several purposes, aiding digestion and preventing bacterial colonization of the small bowel.

Acid secretion is controlled by three pathways: neurocrine, paracrine, and endocrine. The major neurocrine transmitter is acetylcholine, secreted from postganglionic vagal neurones. Histamine is the primary paracrine transmitter; it binds to histamine receptors, raising cellular cyclic adenosine monophosphate (cAMP) levels and stimulating acid secretion. Endocrine control is mediated via gastrin, secreted from the gastric antral cells. Gastrin causes acid secretion by stimulating histamine secretion from enterochromaffin-like (ECL) cells and by binding to gastrin receptors on parietal cells.

The final step in acid production is H^+/K^+ ATPase, an enzyme/proton pump that secretes hydrogen ions on the tubulovesicular and canalicular structures. When acid secretion is stimulated, the H^+/K^+ ATPase undergoes at least two conformational changes, and H^+ is released in exchange for K^+. A further conformational change translocates the K^+ intracellularly where it is released. Concurrently, Cl^- and K^+ channels are activated, leading to efflux of these ions along their concentration gradient to the outside of the cell [2].

Practical approach to patients

Anesthetists will come across disorders of gut motility and secretion mainly in the context of surgical or critical care patients with high ileostomy efflux or diarrhea.

One of the commonest causes of diarrhea is *Clostridium difficile*-associated diarrhea (CDAD). A number of studies have shown high false-negative rates for toxin-A and toxin-B ELISAs. A single negative stool test is inadequate to exclude CDAD, and several samples should be examined. Flexible sigmoidoscopy has been proposed in those patients with negative stool tests as the next investigation [3]. This can demonstrate the classic pseudomembranous colitis and allow biopsies to exclude other conditions such as inflammatory bowel disease or even microscopic colitis. This latter can be caused by many drugs, including statins, nonsteroidal anti-inflammatory drugs (NSAIDs), and even some PPIs.

Histamine receptor antagonists

Histamine has long been known to play a role in acid secretion, but it was not until 1966 that H_1 and H_2 receptors were described [4]. Histamine released from ECL cells activates H_2 receptors on the parietal cell to elevate cAMP and switch on acid production. Cimetidine, ranitidine, famotidine, and nizatidine are all competitive H_2 receptor antagonists.

Cimetidine

Cimetidine contains the imidazole ring of histamine with a bulky substituted side chain producing its competitive antagonism for histamine at the H_2 receptor.

Clinical pharmacology

- After oral absorption bioavailability is 60%. Time to peak serum concentration is 1–2 hours. Volume of distribution is 0.8–2.1 L kg^{-1}. Serum half-life is 1.5–2.5 hours.
- Elimination occurs by a combination of hepatic metabolism (60%) and renal clearance (40%) after oral doses. For intravenous doses the figures are 25–40% and 50–80%, respectively. No dose adjustment is normally needed in hepatic dysfunction.
- In renal impairment the dose should be halved if creatinine clearance is less than 15 mL min^{-1} [4].
- Cimetidine crosses the placenta and the blood–brain barrier, and is excreted in breast milk.

Adverse effects

- Central nervous system (CNS) – Cimetidine interacts with cerebral H_2 receptors. Headaches, somnolence, confusion and delirium may occur [5]. The distribution of cimetidine in cerebrospinal fluid is increased in severe hepatic dysfunction, and dose reduction may be needed if confusion occurs [6].
- Cardiovascular – Bradycardia and hypotension may occur due to interactions with cardiac H_2 receptors. These events have generally been associated with rapid intravenous infusion; thus, when used intravenously, cimetidine should be given by slow infusion over 15–30 minutes [7].

- Endocrine – Cimetidine may cause impotence, loss of libido, gynecomastia and a fall in sperm count in males. In females and males hyperprolactinemia may occur. These effects may be due to decreased testosterone synthesis or inhibition of estradiol metabolism [8].
- Other reported adverse effects of cimetidine include acute pancreatitis, reversible rises in transaminases, leukopenia, thrombocytopenia, pancytopenia and agranulocytosis, diarrhea, rash, dizziness, alopecia, and interstitial nephritis.
- Alcohol dehydrogenase may be inhibited by cimetidine, and this theoretically leads higher plasma levels at lower doses of alcohol [9].

Interactions

- Cimetidine is metabolized in the liver, where it binds to the heme group of cytochrome P450 (CYP) and thereby interferes with the metabolism of many CYP drugs [4]; however, only a few interactions are clinically relevant. The metabolism of warfarin, theophylline, phenytoin, carbamazepine, lidocaine, quinidine, tricyclic antidepressants, and propanolol are reduced. Consequently, serum levels of these drugs may rise and produce adverse effects.
- Concurrent sucralfate or antacid use decreases absorption of cimetidine by 10–30%. Because many people take H_2-blockers in conjunction with antacids at night (see below), cimetidine's effectiveness may be reduced [10].

Practical aspects

- The longest period of basal acid secretion is at night. Nocturnal doses of H_2-antagonists suppress nocturnal acid secretion, leaving daytime secretion virtually unchanged. Despite this, diurnal functional ulcer healing is faster. Bedtime is the optimal time for giving H_2-blockers [11].

Dosage and administration

- Benign gastroduodenal ulceration – 400 mg twice daily or 800 mg at night for 4–8 weeks.
- Reflux disease – 400 mg four times daily for 4–8 weeks.

Ranitidine

The imidazole ring of histamine is replaced by a furan ring to produce ranitidine. Like cimetidine, ranitidine is an H_2-antagonist, but it is 5–10 times more potent.

Clinical pharmacology

- After oral administration, bioavailability is 50%. Time to peak serum concentration is 1–3 hours. Volume of distribution is 1.0–1.9 L kg^{-1}. Serum half-life is 1.6–3.1 hours. Elimination occurs by a combination of hepatic metabolism (73%), and renal clearance (23%) after oral doses. For intravenous doses the figures are 30% and 50% respectively. No dose adjustment is needed in hepatic dysfunction.

- In renal impairment the dose should be halved if creatinine clearance is less than 30 mL min^{-1} [4].

Adverse effects

- Ranitidine binds less avidly (5- to 10-fold) to CYP than cimetidine, and has no clinically significant interactions.

Practical aspects

- Similar to cimetidine.

Dosage and administration

- Benign gastric and duodenal ulceration – 150 mg twice daily or 300 mg at night for 4–8 weeks.
- Reflux esophagitis – 150 mg twice daily or 300 mg at night for up to 8 weeks. The dose can be doubled and the course extended to 12 weeks in severe disease. For maintenance of reflux disease, 150 mg twice daily. In resistant cases, 150 mg three times daily, but doses up to 6 g daily have been used.
- An intravenous formulation is available in 50 mg ampoules. This should be diluted in 20 mL normal saline 0.9% or glucose 5% and given over 2 minutes by slow injection.

Nizatidine

The imidazole ring of histamine is replaced by a thiazole ring to produce nizatidine, which is 5–10 times more potent than cimetidine.

Clinical pharmacology

- After oral administration, bioavailability is 95%. The greater bioavailability compared to the other H_2-blockers is due to lesser first-pass hepatic metabolism. Time to peak serum concentration is 1–3 hours. Volume of distribution is 1.2–1.6 L kg^{-1}. Serum half-life is 1.1–2 hours.
- Elimination occurs by a combination of hepatic metabolism (22%) and renal clearance (65%) after oral doses. The figures are similar after intravenous use. No dose reduction is needed for hepatic dysfunction.
- In renal impairment the dose should be halved if creatinine clearance is less than 50 mL min^{-1} [4].

Adverse effects

- Similar to cimetidine. There is no interference with CYP.

Practical aspects

- Similar to cimetidine.

Dosage and administration

- Benign gastric and duodenal ulceration – 300 mg at night or 150 mg twice daily for 4–8 weeks.

- Gastroesophageal reflux disease – 150–300 mg twice daily for up to 12 weeks.

Famotidine

The imidazole ring of histamine is replaced by a thiazole ring to produce famotidine, which is about 30 times more potent than cimetidine.

Clinical pharmacology

- After oral administration, bioavailability is 45%. Time to peak serum concentration is 1–3.5 hours. Volume of distribution is 1.1–1.3 L kg^{-1}. Serum half-life is 2.5–4 hours.
- Elimination occurs by a combination of hepatic metabolism (75%) and renal clearance (25%) after oral doses. After intravenous doses the figures are 30% and 70%, respectively. No dose reduction is needed for hepatic dysfunction.
- In renal impairment the dose should be halved if creatinine clearance is less than 50 mL min^{-1} [4].

Adverse effects

- Similar to cimetidine. There is no interference with CYP.

Practical aspects

- The indications are similar to cimetidine.

Dosage and administration

- Benign gastric and duodenal ulceration – 40 mg at night for 6–8 weeks.
- Reflux esophagitis – 20–40 mg twice daily for 6–8 weeks.

Proton pump inhibitors

Proton pump inhibitors (PPIs) bind irreversibly and inhibit acid secretion until new pumps become available. Omeprazole is the prototype PPI, and is described here in more detail.

Omeprazole

Omeprazole is a pyridyl methylsulfinyl benzamidazole. It is a lipophilic weak base, $pK_a \sim 4.0$, that is membrane-permeable in the nonprotonated form but impermeable when protonated. Omeprazole preparations are produced with an enteric coat that releases the drug when the pH is above 6, in the small intestine. Otherwise the acid environment of the stomach converts it to the nonabsorbable protonated form. Thus there is greater bioavailability after the first few doses than initially. Esomeprazole (see below) is the S-isomer of omeprazole, which is a mixture of the S- and R-isomers. The S- and R-isomers are metabolized differently by the liver, resulting in higher plasma levels of the S- than of the R-isomer [12].

Omeprazole is absorbed in the small bowel and reaches the parietal cells from the circulation. It diffuses into the parietal cell and accumulates in the secretory canaliculus, where in the acid environment it is converted to a sulfenamide, the active component. This binds covalently to exposed cysteine residues on the luminal α domain of the H^+/K^+ ATPase and stops the pump functioning [13]. Three cysteine residues are accessible, but cys 813 is critical to all PPIs. It is unclear whether binding to other cysteine residues is pharmacologically or clinically relevant.

Preclinical pharmacology

- Animal studies demonstrated that omeprazole was a potent inhibitor of gastric acid secretion. Furthermore, in spite of a short half-life ($t_{1/2} = 60$ minutes in dogs), omeprazole has a long duration of action and the acid-inhibitory effect increases with repeated dosing [14].

Clinical pharmacology

- After oral administration, bioavailability is 60%. Time to peak serum concentration is 2–4 hours. More than 90% bound to plasma proteins. Serum half-life 0.5–1.0 hours.
- Omeprazole is eliminated by CYPs in the liver. Metabolites are excreted in urine, feces, and breast milk.
- No dose reduction is needed in renal failure, and omeprazole is not detected in dialysis fluid. Although hepatic dysfunction can prolong the elimination half-life slightly, no dose reduction is necessary.

Contraindications

- Hypersensitivity to omeprazole. Caution in lactation and pregnancy.

Adverse effects

- CNS – Omeprazole crosses the blood–brain barrier, and headache, dizziness, agitation, and confusion may occur.
- Gastrointestinal (GI) – 3% of patients taking omeprazole may experience GI effects including nausea, vomiting, diarrhea, constipation, flatulence, or abdominal pain. Small-bowel bacterial overgrowth may occur.
- Endocrine – Serum gastrin rises as a consequence of acid suppression because the inhibitory effect of gastric acid is lost. Rat studies with high-dose omeprazole produced hyperplasia of ECL cells and carcinoid tumors. However, humans have lower gastrin secretion in response to acid inhibition than rats [15], and despite omeprazole doubling gastrin levels, no clinically significant ECL changes have been seen after long-term use and gastrin levels are usually maintained within the normal range.

Interactions

- Omeprazole is metabolized by CYPs in the liver. Despite a theoretical risk of drug interactions, in clinical practice these are rare. Metabolism of the R-isomer of warfarin may be inhibited, but clinical studies suggest the effect is not great. Similarly, omeprazole may reduce the metabolism of phenytoin and diazepam but in-vivo studies show this to be minor. Profound acid suppression may interfere with the absorption of certain drugs for which a low gastric pH is needed, e.g., ketoconazole, itraconazole, ampicillin esters, and iron.

Practical aspects

- Omeprazole is indicated to heal benign gastroduodenal ulceration and maintenance to prevent recurrence, in combination with antibiotics in *Helicobacter pylori* eradication regimes, gastroesophageal reflux disease, Zollinger–Ellison syndrome, and prophylaxis for NSAID-induced ulceration.
- The potency of omeprazole is theoretically reduced in patients who are fasting or concomitantly taking H_2-blockers, as the initial dose of omeprazole will not inhibit all proton pumps, only those present and working on the luminal surface. As pumps are generated and inserted into the membrane, further doses are required to inhibit these new pumps. Omeprazole thus takes several days to exert its maximal inhibitory effect on gastric acid secretion [16]. Once-daily dosing gives 66% inhibition after 5 days. Likewise, once omeprazole has been stopped, acid secretion will not return to normal for several days until new pumps are generated [17].

Dosage and administration

- Benign gastroduodenal ulceration and NSAID-induced erosions and ulcers – 20 mg daily for 4–8 weeks. In severe cases up to 40 mg daily may be required.
- Zollinger–Ellison syndrome – initially 60 mg daily, up to 120 mg (in 2 divided doses) if needed.
- Gastroesophageal reflux – 20 mg daily for 4 weeks, up to 40 mg in resistant cases. 10 mg daily for long-term maintenance.
- Capsules can be opened and the granules passed down a nasogastric tube with a neutral liquid such as water if capsules cannot be swallowed.
- An intravenous formulation is available in 40 mg vials. This requires reconstitution in normal saline 0.9% or glucose 5% solution and infused in 100 mL over 30 minutes.
- For high-risk upper GI bleeds – an 80 mg bolus of omeprazole, followed by a continous infusion over 72 hours of omeprazole 8 mg h^{-1} (e.g., 40 mg omeprazole in 100 mL normal saline infused over 5 hours).

Esomeprazole

Esomeprazole is the S-enantiomer of omeprazole. A similar dose of esomeprazole can be expected to produce greater inhibition of acidity than omeprazole. Clinical pharmacology is similar to omperazole

Contraindications

- Similar to omeprazole.

Adverse effects

- Similar to omeprazole.

Interactions

- Similar to omeprazole.

Dosage and administration

- Gastroesophageal reflux disease – 20–40 mg daily for 4–8 weeks.
- *Helicobacter* eradication regimes – 40 mg twice daily.

Lansoprazole

Lansoprazole is a substituted benzimidazole which inhibits the H^+/K^+ ATPase. It is a weak base with a $pK_a \sim 4.0$.

Clinical pharmacology

- After oral administration, bioavailability is 85%. Time to peak serum concentration is 1.5–3 hours. 97% bound to plasma protein. Serum half-life 1.5 hours.
- Eliminated by CYPs in the liver. Lansoprazole induces some forms of CYP but rarely causes significant interactions. 14–25% is excreted in urine as metabolites. Some is eliminated in bile, feces, and breast milk. No dose reduction needed in renal failure or hepatic dysfunction [18].

Contraindications

- Hypersensitivity to lansoprazole, pregnancy, and lactation.

Adverse effects

- Similar to omeprazole.

Interactions

- May decrease theophylline levels and interfere with absorption of ketoconazole, digoxin, and ampicillin. Food reduces peak lansoprazole level by 50%. Sucralfate decreases bioavailability. No significant CYP interactions.

Practical aspects

- Indicated for benign gastroduodenal ulceration, *Helicobacter* eradication regimes, NSAID-induced ulcer healing, Zollinger–Ellison syndrome, and gastroesophageal reflux disease.

Dosage and administration

- Benign gastroduodenal ulceration – 30 mg daily for 4–8 weeks.
- Gastroesophageal reflux disease – 30 mg daily for 4–8 weeks; 15 mg daily for long-term maintenance.
- *Helicobacter* eradication regimes – 30 mg twice daily.

Pantoprazole

Pantoprazole is a substituted benzimidazole which inhibits the H^+/K^+ ATPase. It is a weak base with a $pK_a \sim 4.0$.

Clinical pharmacology

- After oral administration, bioavailability is 77%. Time to peak serum concentration is 2.5 hours. 98% protein-bound. Serum half-life 1.9 hours.
- Eliminated by CYP in the liver. No clinically significant interactions have been reported. Metabolites are excreted in

urine, feces, and breast milk. No dose reduction is needed in renal failure and hepatic dysfunction [18].

Contraindications
- Hypersensitivity to pantoprazole. Caution in lactation and pregnancy.

Adverse effects
- Similar to omeprazole.

Interactions
- Similar to omeprazole. No significant CYP interactions.

Practical aspects
- Indicated for benign gastroduodenal ulcer healing, *Helicobacter* eradication regimes, and gastroesophageal reflux disease.

Dosage and administration
- Supplied as tablets containing 40 mg or 20 mg. An intravenous formulation is available in 40 mg vials. This requires reconstitution in normal saline 0.9% or glucose 5% and should be infused in 100 mL over 2–15 minutes.
- Benign gastroduodenal ulceration – 40 mg daily for 4–6 weeks.
- Gastroesophageal reflux disease – 40 mg daily for 4–8 weeks; 20 mg daily for long-term maintenance.
- *Helicobacter* eradication regimes – 40 mg twice daily.

Rabeprazole
Rabeprazole is a substituted benzimidazole which inhibits the H^+/K^+ ATPase. It is a weak base with a $pK_a \sim 5.0$.

Clinical pharmacology
- After oral administration, bioavailability is 85%. Time to peak serum concentration is 2.9–3.8 hours. 96% bound to plasma protein. Serum half-life is 1 hour.
- Eliminated by CYPs in the liver. No clinically significant interactions have been reported. Some is eliminated in bile, feces, and breast milk. No dose reduction needed in renal failure and hepatic dysfunction [18].

Contraindications
- Hypersensitivity to rabeprazole. Caution in lactation and pregnancy.

Adverse effects
- Similar to omeprazole.

Interactions
- May interfere with absorption of ketoconazole and digoxin.

Practical aspects
- Indicated for benign gastroduodenal ulcer healing, *Helicobacter* eradication regimes, and gastroesophageal reflux disease.

Dosage and administration
- Benign gastroduodenal ulceration – 20 mg daily for 4–6 weeks.
- Gastroesophageal reflux disease – 20 mg daily for 4–8 weeks.
- Helicobacter eradication regimes – 20 mg daily.

Histamine receptor antagonists versus proton pump inhibitors

PPIs have virtually replaced H_2-receptor antagonists, as they are vastly more effective. However, some patients are intolerant of PPIs, making H_2-receptor antagonists their drug of choice for acid suppression.

Gastroesophageal reflux disease
PPIs are more effective than H_2-antagonists at healing esophagitis and preventing relapse. There are no significant differences between PPIs [19–21]. Consequently, PPIs are the treatment of choice.

Gastroduodenal ulcers
PPIs are more effective than H_2-antagonists at healing gastroduodenal ulcers. No one PPI is better than another. The use of H_2-antagonists and PPIs for maintenance therapy has largely become obsolete since the role of *Helicobacter pylori* in gastroduodenal ulceration was discovered [22]. Eradication of *H. pylori* results in significantly fewer relapses and is more cost-effective than maintenance treatment.

Helicobacter eradication regimes
Seven days treatment with:
- amoxicillin 1 g twice daily (or metronidazole 400 mg twice daily if penicillin allergic), *plus*
- clarithromycin 500mg twice daily, *plus*
- a PPI twice daily

Zollinger–Ellison syndrome
High doses of H_2-antagonists were used with some benefit, but PPIs are the treatment of choice in Zollinger–Ellison syndrome because of their potent acid suppression.

Acute upper gastrointestinal hemorrhage
Studies have not conclusively demonstrated an important benefit from H_2-antagonists in upper GI bleeding, and their routine use cannot be recommended [23]. There are theoretical reasons why stronger acid suppression could be beneficial, with improved platelet function and reduced clot lysis. Guidelines based on meta-analyses recommend infusion of PPI after endoscopic treatment of bleeding ulcers [24].

NSAID-associated ulceration
NSAIDS may cause 30% of gastroduodenal ulcers. Risk factors are previous ulcer disease, age, particular "high-risk" NSAIDs such as azapropazone and piroxicam, and concurrent use of

warfarin or corticosteroids. Omeprazole can heal both gastric and duodenal ulcers despite continued NSAID use and is superior to ranitidine. Omeprazole is also significantly better at preventing ulcer recurrence [25,26]. However, the optimal strategy to prevent NSAID-ulceration is to avoid NSAIDs if possible.

Stress ulcers

Stress ulcers are superficial erosions precipitated by reduced mucosal blood flow in critically ill patients. Those most at risk have a coagulopathy and require mechanical ventilation. Several studies have examined H_2-antagonist use and have shown a benefit. A meta-analysis has suggested that they do reduce the incidence of bleeding but at increased risk of pneumonia [27]. Their use does not reduce mortality.

Although omeprazole reduced stress ulceration in animal experiments, there is still a lack of evidence of clinical benefit. PPIs are more effective at acid suppression and raising mean gastric pH, but again their use does not translate into lower mortality or reduce ICU stay.

Short bowel syndrome

Acid suppression may reduce enterostomy output by reducing the volume and osmolality of fluid entering the upper GI tract. These effects may be enough to reduce jejunostomy output by up to 300 mL per day. PPIs are more effective and recommended over H_2-blockers. High-dose loperamide should also be given.

Aspiration pneumonitis

Volume of aspirated contents and acidity of contents influences the severity of aspiration pneumonitis. Cimetidine, as well as other H_2-blockers, can reduce the volume and acidity of gastric contents when given electively.

There are theoretical reasons why omeprazole may not be effective, in that it takes up to 5 days to achieve full acid suppression. However, omeprazole can reduce acidity and volume if given at high dose, 40 mg on the preceding evening and 40 mg 2–6 hours before surgery [28]. However, in emergency use, neither H_2-antagonists nor PPIs alter what is already present in the stomach, and this still presents a risk of aspiration.

Somatostatin and analogs

Somatostatin is a naturally occurring tetradecapeptide with many effects on the bowel. It stimulates water and salt absorption, and inhibits small-bowel motility and secretion of several gut hormones [29–31]. The short half-life of 2–3 minutes makes somatostatin unsuitable for many applications, as it requires continuous intravenous infusion. Consequently, longer-acting analogs have been developed.

Octreotide

Studies of somatostatin analogs established that a four-amino-acid sequence was essential for biologic activity. This sequence, Phe-Trp-Lys-Thr, formed the basis for synthetic analogs. Furthermore, substituting the native L-amino acids for D-amino acids makes peptides more resistant to peptidases whilst retaining

biological activity. Substitution by D-Thr-ol at the carboxy terminal led to an extra increase in in-vitro and in-vivo activity. This is the basis for octreotide acetate.

Octreotide activates the inhibitory G protein, G_i, thereby inhibiting adenylate cyclase. Somatostatin and octreotide have slightly different affinities for somatostatin receptors, which may account for differences in effects. There are five different receptors for somatostatin (sst_1 to sst_5). Octreotide is selective for sst_2, less potent on sst_3, and inactive on sst_1 and sst_4 [32].

Clinical pharmacology

- Octreotide exerts a long-lasting inhibitory action on gastric acid secretion. It inhibits biliary secretion and gall-bladder contraction. It inhibits the release of neuropeptides and hormones such as insulin, glucagon, pancreatic polypeptide, gastrin, and gastric inhibitory polypeptide. Octreotide reduces splanchnic blood flow and inhibits pancreatic exocrine function, diminishing secretions of amylase, trypsin and lipase. It can prolong transit time and decrease fluid secretion in the jejunum and ileum, thus increasing the absorption of water and electrolytes [33,34].
- After subcutaneous injection, peak plasma concentrations are seen within 30 minutes, with a half-life of about 100 minutes. After intravenous bolus injection the elimination is biphasic, with half-lives of 10 minutes and 80 minutes, respectively. About 65% octreotide is plasma protein-bound. The volume of distribution is 0.27 L kg^{-1}. No dose adjustment is needed in renal and hepatic dysfunction.

Contraindications

- Pregnancy and lactation.

Adverse effects

- When given subcutaneously, up to a third of patients experience side effects. Nausea, vomiting, pain, tingling at injection site, diarrhea, and abdominal discomfort occur in 10% of patients. Headaches, hyperglycemia, hypoglycemia, hair loss, elevated transaminases, and hyperbilirubinemia have been described, as has steatorrhea and increased risk of gallstone formation [35]. Side effects tend to improve with time or dose reduction.

Interactions

- May reduce intestinal absorption of cyclosporine.

Practical aspects

- Indicated for relief of symptoms associated with gastroenteropancreatic endocrine tumors, including VIPomas, glucagonomas, and carcinoid tumors with features of carcinoid syndrome.
- Octreotide has been used in short bowel syndrome [36]. It successfully reduces enterostomy output but at the risk of

retarding the physiological process of adaptation [37,38]. Even so, it may still offer patients benefit in reducing stomal efflux and improving quality of life.

- Newer long-acting preparations are available. Octreotide is available as Sandostatin LAR. Lanreotide, another synthetic octapeptide derivative of somatostatin, is available as Somatuline LA and Autogel. They are used to treat acromegaly secondary to growth-hormone-secreting tumors, but data in support of their use in gut disorders are lacking.

Dosage and administration

- Initially 50 μg once or twice daily by subcutaneous injection. Dosage increased gradually up to 200 μg three times daily, depending on response.
- To reduce local discomfort let the solution reach room temperature before injection. For intravenous use, octreotide should be diluted with normal saline solution. Glucose solution is not recommended.

Antimuscarinic drugs

Antimuscarinic drugs (anticholinergics) block the effects of acetylcholine and reduce secretory and motility responses. Their use is limited by side effects and there are doubts about their efficacy. Even so, they may prove beneficial in some patients.

Hyoscine butylbromide

Hyoscine butylbromide is a quaternary ammonium compound. It is an antimuscarinic drug. It does not cross the blood–brain barrier (unlike hyoscine hydrobromide).

Pharmacology

- After oral administration, less than 10% is absorbed, with 90% lost in feces and 2% in urine. Following intravenous bolus, 42% is recovered in urine and 37% in feces. The serum half-life is 8 hours. There is no relationship between plasma concentration and clinical activity. Liver metabolism produces unknown inactive compounds. No dose reduction is needed in renal and hepatic dysfunction.

Contraindications

- Glaucoma, prostatism, paralytic ileus. Caution in lactation, pregnancy.

Adverse effects

- Dry mouth, pupillary dilation, urinary urgency and retention.

Practical aspects

- Hyoscine butylbromide may be used as an adjunct in irritable bowel syndrome (IBS), and as an aid to gastrointestinal endoscopy. It may help cannulation of

the ampulla during ERCP, by producing a hypotonic duodenum [39].

Dosage and administration

- IBS – 20 mg up to four times daily.
- Endoscopy – 20 mg by intravenous injection. May be repeated as necessary.

Dicyclomine hydrochloride

Dicyclomine is a synthetic tertiary amine. It is an antimuscarinic with an additional antispasmodic effect on smooth muscle [40].

Pharmacology

- Dicyclomine is absorbed in the gut. Time to peak serum concentration is 1.5 hours. Volume of distribution is 3.65 L kg^{-1}. Serum half-life is 4–6 hours.
- The metabolism is uncertain, but 80% of a dose appears in urine and 10% in feces. No dose adjustment is needed for renal and hepatic dysfunction. It has not been studied in pregnancy and lactation – caution is advised.

Contraindications

- Similar to hyoscine.

Adverse effects

- Similar to hyoscine.

Practical aspects

- May be useful adjunct to treating IBS.

Dosage and administration

- 10–20 mg three times daily in adults.

Propantheline bromide

Propantheline bromide is a synthetic quaternary ammonium compound. It is an antimuscarinic drug.

Pharmacology

- Propantheline bromide is incompletely absorbed from the GI tract. Time to peak serum concentration 2 hours. Serum half-life is 1.6 hours.
- The distribution and metabolism are not fully determined. 50% is metabolized in the GIT and is excreted primarily in urine. No dose adjustment is needed in hepatic and renal dysfunction.

Contraindications

- Similar to hyoscine.

Adverse effects

- Similar to hyoscine.

Practical aspects

- May be useful in IBS.

Dosage and administration

- Up to 15 mg three times daily and 30 mg at night, taken an hour before meals. Maximum 120 mg daily.

5-HT₃ antagonists

Type 3 serotonin receptors (5-HT₃) are nonselective cation channels that are extensively distributed on enteric neurons within the GI tract and within the brain. The 5-HT₃ receptor antagonists have shown great efficacy in the treatment of chemotherapy-induced emesis and have been found to have effects on GI motility and visceral sensation. Ondansetron is covered in more detail in Chapter 54. It has been shown to have benefit in reducing stool frequency and improving consistency [41]. This spurred the development of more potent drugs. Alosetron and cilansetron have been trialed in humans but only alosetron has been licensed (but under restricted circumstances: see below).

Alosetron

5-HT₃-antagonists cause constipation, and increase thresholds for sensation and discomfort of the rectum [42,43]. These findings promoted the trial of 5-HT₃-receptor antagonists for IBS, particularly in diarrhea-predominant IBS. Alosetron was the first 5-HT₃ receptor antagonist licensed for use in IBS.

Preclinical pharmacology

- Alosetron has effects on visceral nociception in rats and dogs, attenuating the effects of rectal distension. These effects also occur in humans, were alosetron increases rectal compliance, delays colonic transit and reduces visceral sensitivity to rectal distension [44–46]. Clinical trials have shown that alosetron is well tolerated and effective in alleviating pain and reducing bowel frequency in IBS, particularly in diarrhea-predominant IBS. These effects are mainly seen in women. It is not known if men derive equal benefit [47,48].

Clinical pharmacology

- Alosetron has good oral bioavailability, approximately 50–60%. Peak plasma levels are reached within 1 hour and steady-state plasma levels are achieved within 1 day.
- The elimination half-life is 93 hours. Alosetron is eliminated largely by the kidneys (73%), with the remainder lost through fecal excretion. The long half-life allows for twice-daily dosing. No dose adjustment is needed for elderly patients, nor for renal or hepatic impairment.
- Animal studies show that alosetron is present in breast milk. No human studies have been done in lactation and pregnancy.

Contraindications

- Caution in pregnancy and lactation. Contraindicated with a history of intestinal obstruction, stricture, toxic megacolon, GI perforation, GI adhesions, ischemic colitis, active diverticulitis, and inflammatory bowel disease.

Interactions

- No clinically important interactions have been reported.

Adverse reactions

- Headache, anorexia, nausea, dizziness, loose stools, abdominal cramping, and flatulence. Severe constipation, fecal impaction, and ischemic colitis have been reported, and consequently alosetron should not be commenced when patients are constipated.

Practical aspects

- Alosetron is indicated for use in diarrhea-predominant IBS, where its effects on slowing bowel transit and reducing visceral pain sensation are helpful. Due to reports of ischemic colitis [49], alosetron was voluntarily withdrawn by Glaxo Wellcome, but has since been reapproved by the US Food and Drug Administration (FDA) under restricted prescribing. It has been included here as an indication of future drug avenues.

Dosage and administration

- Commence at a dose of 0.5 mg twice daily. If response is inadequate after 4 weeks, the dose can be increased to 1 mg twice daily. It should be discontinued after 4 weeks if no response on 1 mg twice daily or if constipation or signs of ischemic colitis develop.

Opiates

Morphine and opiates produce constipation in all mammalian species, although there are variations in its actions between species. However, concern over addictive potential means synthetic alternatives have been sought.

Loperamide

Loperamide hydrochloride is a synthetic piperidine opioid used primarily for treatment of acute or chronic diarrhea.

Animal experiments have shown that opiates decrease luminal fluid content by actions on mucosal ion transport processes [50]. Loperamide may also have some nonopioid antidiarrheal effects, inhibiting calmodulin and preventing activation of Ca^{2+}/calmodulin-dependent protein kinases [51].

Preclinical pharmacology

- Loperamide mediates most of its action through binding to the μ opioid receptor in the GI tract, but also interacts with δ receptors. Loperamide affects mucosal transport of water and solutes by slowing transit time, allowing lumen contents more time to be absorbed, and stimulates μ and δ receptors, resulting in decreased secretion of Na^+, K^+, and Cl^-, but not $HCO3^-$ [52]. This effect is maximal in the jejunum and colon. Loperamide also affects the rectum, increasing anal tone and decreasing urgency in patients with urge incontinence [53].

Clinical pharmacology

- Loperamide is absorbed in the gut and is extensively metabolized by the liver. Due to first-pass effects, peak plasma levels are low, corresponding to less than 0.5% of the administered dose. Consequently, CNS side effects are rare.
- The half-life of loperamide in humans is 10.8 hours (range 9–14 hours). Loperamide is metabolized in the liver, where it is conjugated and excreted via bile. Loperamide is secreted in small amounts in breast milk.

Contraindications

- Children younger than 4 years. Caution in lactation and pregnancy.

Adverse effects

- Abdominal cramps, nausea, vomiting, fatigue, drowsiness, dizziness, dry mouth, and skin reactions including urticaria have been reported. Paralytic ileus and bloating may occur.
- Overdosage produces somnolence, myosis, and bradypnea which responds to naloxone. The duration of loperamide is longer than naloxone, so repeated doses or naloxone infusion may be required. In hepatic insufficiency overdosage may occur due to decreased metabolism.
- Reports of opiate-toxicity symptoms mean loperamide should not be prescribed to children younger than 4 years.

Interactions

- No interactions have been reported.

Practical aspects

- Loperamide can be used for acute and chronic diarrhea. If used for diarrhea it is important to search for the underlying cause.
- It can help in diarrhea-predominant IBS and short bowel syndrome.
- For short bowel syndrome, higher doses of loperamide have been used in some centers, up to 64 mg daily in combination with codeine phosphate to reduce stomal output and fluid losses [54].
- Loperamide is not routinely advised in inflammatory bowel disease, as it may precipitate toxic megacolon [55].
- Diphenoxylate is described below, but two trials comparing loperamide and diphenoxylate have shown loperamide to be more effective at reducing diarrhea and better tolerated by patients, with fewer side effects [56,57].

Dosage and administration

- Child under 4 – not recommended. Children 4–8 years – 1 mg 3–4 times daily for up to 3 days only. Children 9–12 years – 2 mg 4 times daily for up to 5 days.

- Acute diarrhea in adults – 4 mg initially followed by 2 mg after each loose stool. Usual dose 6–8 mg daily. Max 16 mg daily.
- Chronic diarrhea in adults – up to 16 mg daily in divided doses. Adjust according to response.
- Loperamide is available as capsules and syrup, which can be given down nasogastric or percutaneous endoscopic gastrostomy (PEG) feeding tubes.

Diphenoxylate hydrochloride and atropine sulfate

Diphenoxylate hydrochloride is a synthetic piperidine opioid used to treat diarrhea. The anticholinergic effects of atropine may help reduce GI motility and secretions, but the main reason for its addition is to discourage opiate abuse by causing unpleasant side effects such as dry mouth and blurred vision.

The mechanism of action is similar to that of loperamide, by binding to opioid receptors in the bowel.

Pharmacology

- Peak plasma concentrations occur within 2 hours, and plasma half-life is 2 hours. Diphenoxylate is metabolized to an active metabolite, diphenoxylic acid, which has a half-life of 3–14 hours. The clinical onset of action occurs within 45 minutes to 1 hour, and duration of action is approximately 3–4 hours.
- Diphenoxylate metabolites and their conjugates are excreted in bile. Smaller amounts appear in urine.
- No studies have looked at safety in pregnancy, and the manufacturers advise caution. Both diphenoxylate and atropine are excreted in breast milk, and infants may exhibit effects of the drugs.

Adverse effects

- Both diphenoxylate and atropine produce effects in overdoses. Diphenoxylate causes ileus and narcosis, and will respond to naloxone. Onset may be delayed 12–30 hours after ingestion. Duration of action of naloxone is shorter than duration of diphenoxylate, and repeated doses or naloxone infusion may be necessary.
- Atropine side effects include flushing, dry skin and mucous membranes, tachycardia, urinary retention, and hyperthermia. Hyperthermia occurs especially in children.

Interactions

- Because the chemical structure is similar to meperidine, concurrent use with monoamine oxidase inhibitors (MAOIs) could precipitate a hypertensive crisis. Diphenoxylate may potentiate the action of CNS depressants such as barbiturates and alcohol.

Practical aspects

- For treatment of acute or chronic diarrhea.

Dosage and administration

- Diphenoxylate is supplied as tablets containing diphenoxylate hydrochloride 2.5 mg and atropine sulfate 25 µg.
- Children under 4 years – not recommended. Children 4–8 years – 1 tablet 3 times daily. Children 9–12 years – 1 tablet 4 times daily. Children 13–16 years – 2 tablets 3 times daily.
- Adults – initially 4 tablets, followed by 2 tablets every 6 hours until diarrhea is controlled.

Prebiotics and probiotics

Prebiotics are nondigestible oligosaccharides which selectively stimulate the growth and/or activity of probiotic-like bacteria already present in the human gut. Probiotics may be defined as living organisms which, upon ingestion, exert health benefits beyond inherent basic nutrition.

Interest in the use of probiotics has risen recently. Both bacteria and yeasts have been used, although the majority tried are lactic-acid-producing bacteria and bifidobacteria. Probiotic trials have been studied in inflammatory bowel disease, CDAD, and IBS [58–60]. There is some evidence that probiotics may have beneficial effects on symptoms and on inflammatory status. However, many of the studies of probiotics on gut function are underpowered, have a short follow-up period, or use different preparations. It is not known if efficacy relates to a particular strain, composition, or concentration of probiotic preparation. Currently, no single probiotic preparation can be recommended on the basis of available evidence. One fatal fungemia has been reported during treatment, so probiotics cannot be considered absolutely safe [61].

New and emerging concepts

Only a small number of drugs are available to alter motility and secretion in the gut. Opiates and atropine have been established for decades, H$_2$-receptor antagonists since the 1960s, and proton pump inhibitors since the 1980s. As greater understanding of the enteric nervous system and interactions with gut flora develops, we expect new drugs in the future.

The most promising avenue is likely to be drugs affecting the enteric nervous system. Antagonists of neurokinin receptors, vasoactive intestinal polypeptide (VIP), and enkephalinase are under development and have shown promise in early studies, but it is too early to speculate on their full clinical role [62].

Summary

The gastrointestinal tract facilitates ingestion, digestion, absorption, and defecation, as well as providing an antimicrobial barrier. The enteric nervous system and the vagus nerve control smooth-muscle function, mediating both mixing and peristaltic actions. Endogenous secretions represent a substantial proportion of the fluid passing through the small intestine. Here, fluids, electrolytes, and nutrients are absorbed, leaving just 1.5 L of fluid to pass daily into the colon, where further fluid is absorbed. Gastric acid is secreted by parietal cells of the stomach, under neurocrine, paracrine, and endocrine control by acetylcholine, histamine, and gastrin, respectively. Acid is produced by an ATP-dependent proton pump which exchanges hydrogen for potassium ions.

Pharmacologic interventions for suppression of acid secretion include histamine H$_2$-receptor antagonists (e.g., cimetidine, ranitidine, famotidine, and nizatidine) and proton pump inhibitors (PPIs) (e.g., omeprazole, esomeprazole, lansoprazole, pantoprazole, and rabeprazole). In general, the PPIs are superior, and are the treatment of choice for gastroesophageal reflux disease, healing gastroduodenal ulcers (along with an *H. pylori* eradication regime), Zollinger–Ellison syndrome, acute upper gastrointestinal bleeding (along with endoscopic treatment), and short bowel syndrome (along with loperamide). However, for patients intolerant of PPIs, H$_2$-antagonists offer an alternative. Furthermore, the H$_2$-antagonist omeprazole has been shown to heal nonsteroidal anti-inflammatory drug (NSAID)-associated ulcers, and other H$_2$-blockers, such as cimetidine, can reduce the volume and acidity of gastric contents, thereby reducing the severity of aspiration pneumonitis.

Of the H$_2$-antagonists described, cimetidine is notable for its potential to alter serum levels of drugs metabolized by hepatic cytochrome P450 (CYP) enzymes. Clinically relevant interactions of cimetidine include warfarin, theophylline, phenytoin, carbamazepine, lidocaine, quinidine, tricyclic antidepressants, and propranolol. Ranitidine binds less avidly to CYPs, while famotidine and nizatidine show no interference with CYP-mediated metabolism.

PPIs function by covalently binding the ATPase and inhibiting secretion. The prototype PPI, omeprazole, takes several days to achieve maximal acid suppression, as its inhibitory properties are restricted to those proton pumps present on the luminal surface; newly expressed pumps require additional doses in order to be rendered inactive. Omeprazole is metabolized by CYPs in the liver, but in clinical practice drug interactions are rare or minor, although acid suppression can interfere with absorption of drugs which require a low gastric pH (e.g., ketoconazole, itraconazole, ampicillin esters, and iron).

Several drugs are available to inhibit both gut motility and secretions. Octreotide acetate is an analog of the naturally occurring peptide hormone somatostatin. It acts via inhibitory G protein, Gi, to inhibit secretion of gastric acid and multiple other gastrointestinal and endocrine secretions, as well as inhibiting pancreatic exocrine function and prolonging transit time. Antimuscarinic drugs, such as hyoscine butylbromide, dicyclomine hydrochloride, and propantheline bromide, also reduce secretion and motility.

Serotonin (5-HT$_3$) antagonists, in addition to their antiemetic properties, have been shown to slow bowel transit.

Alosetron is licensed for use in irritable bowel syndrome under restricted prescribing conditions, following reports of ischemic colitis. Opiates such as loperamide and diphenoxylate hydrochloride act on opioid receptors in the gut, slowing transit time and reducing urgency, and are therefore used in the treatment of acute and chronic diarrhea. Atropine sulfate is added to diphenoxylate hydrochloride, and its anticholinergic effects may help to reduce gastrointestinal motility and secretions.

There is interest in the use of probiotics to benefit gut function. However, more extensive studies are required to determine the safety and efficacy of the various probiotic preparations. Future developments may also include drugs that affect the enteric nervous system.

References

1. Tack J. Receptors of the enteric nervous system: potential targets for drug therapy. *Gut* 2000; **47**: 20–2.

2. Wallmark B, Lorentzon P, Sachs G. The gastric H^+, K^+-ATPase. *J Intern Med* 1990; **228**: 3–8.

3. Monaghan T, Boswell T, Mahida YR. Recent advances in *Clostridium difficile*-associated disease. *Gut* 2008; **57**: 850–60.

4. Feldman M, Burton ME. Histamine$_2$-receptor antagonists. Standard therapy for acid-peptic diseases. *N Eng J Med* 1990; **323**: 1672–80.

5. Cantu TG, Korek JS. Central nervous system reactions to histamine-2 receptor blockers. *Ann Intern Med* 1991; **114**: 1027–34.

6. Somogyi A, Gugler R. Clinical pharmacokinetics of cimetidine. *Clin Pharmacokinet* 1983; **8**: 463–95.

7. Hughes DG, Dowling EA, DeMeersman RE, Garnett WR, Karnes HT. Cardiovascular effects of H2-receptor antagonists. *J Clin Pharmacol* 1989; **29**: 472–7.

8. McGuigan JE. A consideration of the adverse effects of cimetidine. *Gastroenterology* 1981; **80**: 181–92.

9. Hernandez-Monoz R, Cabacleria J, Baraona E, *et al*. Human gastric alcohol dehydrogenase: its inhibition by H$_2$-receptor antagonists, and its effect on the bioavailability of ethanol. *Alcoholism* 1990; **14**: 946–50.

10. Steinberg WM, Lewis JH, Katz DM. Antacids inhibit absorption of cimetidine. *N Eng J Med* 1982; **307**: 400–4.

11. Damman HG, Muller P, Simon B. 24 hour intragastric acidity and single night-time dose of three H2 blockers. *Lancet* 1983; **2**: 1078.

12. Spencer CM, Foulds D. Esomeprazole. *Drugs* 2000; **60**; 321–9.

13. Lorentzon P, Jackson R, Wallmark B, Sachs G. Inhibition of H K-ATPase by omeprazole in isolated gastric vesicles requires proton transport. *Biochem Biophys Acta* 1987; **897**: 41–51.

14. Larsson H, Carlsson E, Junggren U, *et al*. Animal studies with omeprazole, a potent inhibitor of gastric acid secretion. *Scand J Gastroenterol* 1982; **17** (Suppl): 76.

15. Carlsson E, Larsson H, Mattsson H, Ryberg B, Sundell G. Pharmocology and toxicology of omeprazole-with special reference to the effects on the gastric mucosa. *Scand J Gastroenterol* 1986; **118**: 31–8.

16. Howden CW, Forrest JA, Reid JL. Effects of single and repeated doses of omeprazole on gastric and pepsin secretion in man. *Gut* 1984; **25**: 707–10.

17. Sachs G. Proton pump inhibitors and acid related diseases. *Pharmacotherapy* 1997; **17**: 22–37.

18. Richardson P, Hawkey CJ, Stack WA. Proton pump inhibitors: pharmacology and rationale for use in gastrointestinal disorders. *Drugs* 1998; **56**; 307–35.

19. Petite JP, Salducci J, Grimaud JC, *et al*. Lansoprazole versus omeprazole in the treatment of reflux oesophagitis. *Med Chir Dig* 1995; **24**: 291–4.

20. Corinaldesi R, Valentini M, Belaiche J, *et al*. Pantoprazole and omeprazole in the treatment of reflux oesophagitis: a European multicentre study. *Aliment Pharmacol Ther* 1995; **9**: 667–71.

21. Thjodleifsson B, Beker JA, Dekkers C, *et al*. Rabeprazole versus omeprazole in preventing relapse of erosive or ulcerative gastroesophageal reflux disease. *Dig Dis Sci* 2000; **45**: 845–53.

22. Marshall BJ, Warren JR. Unidentified curved bacilli in the stomach of patients with gastritis and peptic ulceration. *Lancet* 1984; **1**: 1311–15.

23. Collins R, Langman M. Treatment with histamine H2 antagonists in acute upper gastrointestinal hemorrhage: implications of randomised trials. *N Eng J Med* 1985; **313**: 660–6.

24. Leontiadis GI, Sreedharan A, Dorward S, *et al*. Systematic reviews of the clinical effectiveness and cost-effectiveness of proton pump inhibitors in acute upper gastrointestinal bleeding. *Health Technol Assess* 2007; **11**: 1–164.

25. Hawkey CJ, Karrasch JA, Szczepanski L, *et al*. Omeprazole compared to misoprostol for ulcers associated with nonsteroidal antiinflammatoro drugs. *N Eng J Med* 1998; **338**: 727–34.

26. Yeomans ND, Tulassay Z, Juhasz L, *et al*. A comparison of omeprazole with ranitidine for ulcers associated with nonsteroidal anti-inflammatory drugs. *N Eng J Med* 1998; **338**: 719–26.

27. Cook DJ, Reeve BK, Guyatt GH, *et al*. Stress ulcer prophylaxis in critically ill patients: resolving discordant meta-analysis. *JAMA* 1996: **275**: 308–14.

28. Ewart MC, Yau G, Gin T, Kotur CF, Oh TE. A comparison of the effects of omeprazole and ranitidine on gastric secretion in women undergoing elective caesarian section. *Anesthesiology* 1990; **45**: 527–30.

29. Ruskone A, Rene E, Chayvialle JA, *et al*. Effect of somatostatin on diarrhoea and on small intestinal water and electrolyte transport in a patient with pancreatic cholera. *Dig Dis Sci* 1982: **27**: 459–66.

30. Efendic S, Mattson O. Effect of somatostatin on intestinal motility. *Acta Radiol Diag* 1978: **19**: 348–52.

31. Bloom SR. Somatostatin and the gut. *Gastroenterology* 1978: **75**: 145–7.

32. Viollet C, Prevost G, Maubert E, *et al*. Molecular pharmacology of somatostatin receptors. *Fundam Clin Pharmacol* 1995; **92**: 107–113.

33. Gyr KE, Meier R. Pharmacodynamic effects of sandostatin in the

gastrointestinal tract. *Digestion* 1993; **54**: 14–19.

34. Harris AG. Somatostatin and somatostatin analogues: pharmacokinetics and pharmacodynamic effects. *Gut* 1994; **35**: S1–4.

35. Bornschein J, Drozdov I, Malfertheiner P. Octreotide LAR: safety and tolerability issues. *Expert Opin Drug Saf* 2009; **8**: 755–68.

36. O'Keefe SJ, Peterson ME, Fleming CR. Octreotide as an adjunct to home parenteral nutrition in the management of permanent end-jejunostomy syndrome. *J Parenter Enteral Nutr* 1994; **18**: 26–34.

37. Seydel AS, Miller JH, Sarac TP, *et al.* Octreotide diminishes luminal nutrient transport activity, which is reversed by epidermal growth factor. *Am J Surg* 1996; **172**: 267–71.

38. O'Keefe SJD, Haymond MW, Bennet WM, *et al.* Long-acting somatostatin analogue therapy and protein metabolism in patients with jejunostomies. *Gastroenterology* 1994; **107**: 379–88.

39. Cotton PB. Progress report. ERCP. *Gut* 1977; **18**: 316–41.

40. McGrath WR, Lewis RE, Kuhn WL. The dual mode of the antispasmodic efffct of dicyclomine hydrochloride. *J Pharmacol Exp Ther* 1964; **146**: 354–8.

41. Maxton DG, Morris J, Whorwell PJ. Selective 5-hydroxytryptamine antagonism: a role in irritable bowel syndrome and functional dyspepsia? *Aliment Pharmacol Ther* 1996; **10**: 595–9.

42. Prior A, Read NW. Reduction of rectal sensitivity and post-prandial motility by granisetron, a 5-HT3 receptor antagonist, in patients with irritable bowel syndrome. *Aliment Pharmacol Ther* 1993: **7**: 175–80.

43. Goldberg PA, Kamm MA, Setti-Carraro P, van der Sijp JR, Roth C. Modification of visceral sensitivity and pain and irritable bowel syndrome by 5-HT3 antagonism (ondansetron). *Digestion* 1996: **57**: 478–83.

44. Kozlowski CM, Green A, Grundy D, Boissonade FM, Bountra C. The 5-HT₃ receptor antagonist alosetron inhibits the colorectal induced depressor response and spinal c-fos expression in the anaesthetised rat. *Gut* 2000; **46**: 474–80.

45. Balfour JA, Goa KL, Perry CM. Alosetron (review). *Drugs* 2000; **59**; 511–18.

46. Miura M, Lawson DC, Clary DM, Mangel AW, Pappas TN. Central modulation of rectal distension-induced blood pressure changes by alosetron, a 5HT₃ receptor antagonist. *Dig Dis Sci* 1999; **44**: 20–4.

47. Camilleri M, Mayer E, Drossman D, *et al.* Improvement in pain with alosetron, a 5-HT3-receptor antagonist. *Aliment Pharmacol Ther* 1999; **14**: 1149–51.

48. Camilleri M, Northcutt AR, Kong GE, McSorley D, Mangel AW. Efficacy and safety of alosetron in women with irritable bowel syndrome: a randomised, placebo-controlled trial. *Lancet* 2000; **355**: 1035–40.

49. Friedel D, Thomas R, Fisher RS. Ischaemic colitis during treatment with Alosetron. *Gastroenterology* 2001; **120**: 557–60.

50. Coupar IM. Opioid action on the intestine: the importance of the intestinal mucosa. *Life Sci* 1987; **41**: 917–25.

51. Jaffe JH, Martin WR. Opioid analgesics and antagonists. In: Gilman AG, Goodman LS, Rall TW, Murad F, eds., *The Pharmacological Basis of Therapeutics*, 7th edn. New York, NY: Macmillan, 1985: 491–531.

52. Burleigh DE. Loperamide but not morphine has anti-secretory effects in human colon in vitro. *Eur J Pharmacol* 1991: **202**: 277–280.

53. Read M, Read NW, Barber DC, Duthie HL. Effects of loperamide on anal sphincter function in patients complaining of chronic diarrhoea with faecal incontinence and urgency. *Dig Dis Sci* 1982: **27**: 807–14.

54. Forbes A. *Clinicians' Guide to Inflammatory Bowel Disease.* London: Chapman & Hall, 1997.

55. Brown JW. Toxic megacolon associated with loperamide therapy. *J Am Med Assoc* 1979: **241**: 501–2.

56. Palmer KR, Corbett CL, Holdsworth CD. Double-blind crossover study comparing loperamide, codeine and diphenoxylate in the treatment of chronic diarrhoea. *Gastroenterology* 1980; **79**: 1272–5.

57. Pelemans W, Vantrappen G. A double blind crossover comparison of loperamide with diphehoxylate in the symptomatic treatment of chronic diarrhoea. *Gastroenterology* 1976; **70**: 1030–4.

58. Schulz H. Clinical use of E. coli Nissle 1917 in inflammatory bowel disease. *Inflamm Bowel Dis* 2008; **14**: 1012–18.

59. O'Mahony L, McCarthy J, Kelly P, *et al.* Lactobacillus and bifidobacterium in irritable bowel syndrome: symptom responses and relationship to cytokine profiles. *Gastroenterology* 2005; **128**: 541–51.

60. McFarland LV, Surawicz CM, Greenberg RN, *et al.* A randomised placebo-controlled trial of Saccharomyces boulardii in combination with standard antibiotics for Clostridium difficile disease. *JAMA* 1994; **271**: 1913–18.

61. Cherifi S, Robberecht J, Miendje Y. *Saccharomyces cerevisiae* fungemia in an elderly patient with Clostridium difficile colitis. *Acta Clin Bel* 2004; **59**: 223–4.

62. Sanger GJ, Alpers DH. Development of drugs for gastrointestinal motor disorders: translating science to clinical need. *Neurogastroenterol Motil* 2008; **20**: 177–84.

Essential drugs in anesthetic practice
Antiemetics

Jens Scholz, Markus Steinfath, and Patrick Meybohm

Introduction

The decrease in the incidence of life-threatening anesthetic-related complications has led anesthesiologists to focus on the less dangerous but more common distressing symptoms, including pain and nausea and vomiting after surgery. With respect to postoperative pain management, several convincing concepts have already been introduced into clinical practice, and postoperative pain should no longer be the most common sequel following surgery. This chapter deals with antiemetics in the prevention and therapy of postoperative nausea and vomiting (PONV).

Nausea and vomiting have long been associated with anesthesia and surgery. In 1848, Snow recognized severe nausea and vomiting after ether inhalation and proposed wine and other pharmacologic solutions for postoperative treatment. Surgical patients with previous experience of PONV invariably rate nausea and vomiting as the most unpleasant consequence of their surgery. This complication is not only unpleasant and aesthetically displeasing to patients and their caregivers, but can also be associated with stress on suture lines, wound dehiscence, bleeding, electrolyte disturbances, dehydration, and pulmonary aspiration of gastric contents [1]. Further, high-risk cardiovascular patients may be exposed to additional perioperative stress leading to myocardial ischemia [2]. Frequently, PONV delays discharge from the postanesthesia care unit (PACU) and ambulatory surgery center, and results in an increased use of resources of both supplies and personnel, each of which has financial implications. Furthermore, after ambulatory anesthesia, PONV may occur at home, resulting in an unplanned hospital admission [1,3]. Consequently, prevention and appropriate management of PONV are highly relevant.

Definitions

The terms *nausea, vomiting*, and *retching* are not synonymous. **Nausea** is a subjectively unpleasant sensation in the epigastrium and throat associated with the urge to vomit, whereas **vomiting** or emesis is the forceful expulsion of upper gastrointestinal contents through the mouth, caused by the powerful sustained contraction of the abdominal muscles. **Retching** refers to the labored rhythmic activity of the respiratory muscles, including the diaphragm and abdominal muscles, without expulsion of gastric contents. This sensation usually precedes vomiting [4].

Incidence

During the early days of anesthesia with ether, the incidence rate of PONV was estimated at 75–80% [4]. Despite major advances in surgical techniques and the introduction of new anesthetic drugs with reduced emetogenicity, the global incidence of PONV in an adult surgical population receiving general anesthesia has been estimated at 20–30%, differing considerably among institutions and even among anesthesiologists within the same hospital [1,3–6]. If less precise definitions are used, the incidence rates of PONV vary from 14% to 82% [3,7], and this wide range may also be due to the variety of anesthetic drugs and different types of surgery or populations undergoing surgical procedures. In contrast, PONV was observed in only 12–22% of patients undergoing short surgical procedures such as dental extraction, minor gynecologic surgery, or joint arthroscopy [3].

Physiology

Vomiting is a complex process coordinated by the vomiting center in the lateral reticular formation of the medulla (Fig. 54.1) [8]. The theory of such a center is based on studies using electrical stimulation and brainstem lesion. This center receives input from (1) the chemoreceptor trigger zone of the area postrema on the floor of the fourth ventricle, (2) the vestibular apparatus through the nucleus vestibularis and cerebellum, (3) higher brainstem and cortical structures, and (4) afferents from the gastrointestinal tract (mainly serotoninergic), pharynx, and mediastinum. The area postrema is highly enriched in vascular structures, and the vessels terminate in fenestrated capillaries surrounded by large perivascular spaces. Further, the blood–brain barrier is poorly developed in

Anesthetic Pharmacology, 2nd edition, ed. Alex S. Evers, Mervyn Maze, Evan D. Kharasch. Published by Cambridge University Press. © Cambridge University Press 2011.

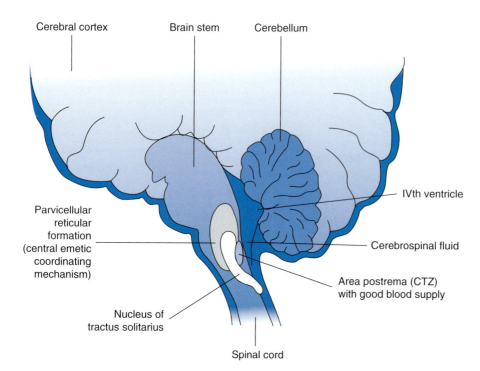

Figure 54.1. The structures within the brain involved in the control of emesis. Reproduced with permission from Simpson and Lynch [8].

the area postrema; therefore, the chemoreceptor trigger zone is readily accessible to emetic substances (e.g., opioids) of the systemic circulation or cerebrospinal fluid. Destruction of this area would block opioid-induced vomiting. In addition, some peripheral signals bypass the trigger zone, reaching the vomiting center through the nucleus tractus solitarius from the pharynx, stomach, and small intestine.

Knowledge of the neuropharmacology of pathways leading to and from the vomiting center is incomplete, but a complex concept has evolved that provides a rational basis for current antiemetic therapy. Serotonin (5-hydroxytryptamine [5-HT], acting at 5-HT receptor subtype 3, 5-HT$_3$) is an important emetic transmitter in the afferent pathway from the gastro-intestinal tract terminating in the chemoreceptor trigger zone and in the nucleus tractus solitarius. Dopamine (acting at D$_2$ receptors), acetylcholine (acting at muscarinic [M] receptors), histamine (acting at H$_1$ receptors), and substance P (acting at neurokinin 1 [NK$_1$] receptors) are also implicated in emetic signaling at the chemoreceptor trigger zone and in the nucleus tractus solitarius (Fig. 54.2) [1,9]. Antagonism of these path-ways contributes to the antiemetic effects of 5-HT$_3$ and D$_2$ receptor antagonists [10]. Cholinergic and histaminergic syn-apses seem to be involved in transmission from the vestibular apparatus to the vomiting center, suggesting a basis for the particular use of H$_1$ receptor-directed antihistaminic and mus-carinic anticholinergic drugs in motion sickness. NK$_1$ receptor antagonists have been suggested to be effective in the preven-tion of postoperative emesis because of their ability to block input from emetic stimuli in the central nervous system [11]. Other useful antiemetic drugs, including corticosteroids, do not fit into the scheme shown in Fig. 54.2, but it is likely that

such drugs derive their antiemetic efficacy from other sites and mechanisms of action that have yet to be elucidated. Moreover, the role of specific opioid receptor subtypes within various brainstem structures in the genesis of the emetic response is not yet resolved.

After stimulation of the vomiting center, either directly or indirectly through neural pathways, various efferent pathways, including the vagus, the phrenic nerves, and innervation to the abdominal musculature, mediate vomiting. The initial manifestation often involves nausea, in which gastric tone is reduced, gastric peristalsis is reduced or absent, and the tone of the duodenum and upper jejunum is increased, so that, finally, gastric reflux occurs. Ultimately, the upper portion of the stomach relaxes while the pylorus constricts, and the coordin-ated contraction of the diaphragm and abdominal muscles leads to expulsion of gastric contents.

Patient- and surgery-related risk factors

Several risk factors for PONV have been claimed in a large series of investigations [1,3,4,8].

Age

A greater risk for PONV has been reported in children than in adults. Within the pediatric population, postoperative emesis increases with age to reach a peak incidence in the preadoles-cent age group [12]. The incidence rates have been estimated at 5% in infants younger than 12 months old, 20% in children 1–5 years old, 34% in children 6–10 years old, and 32% in

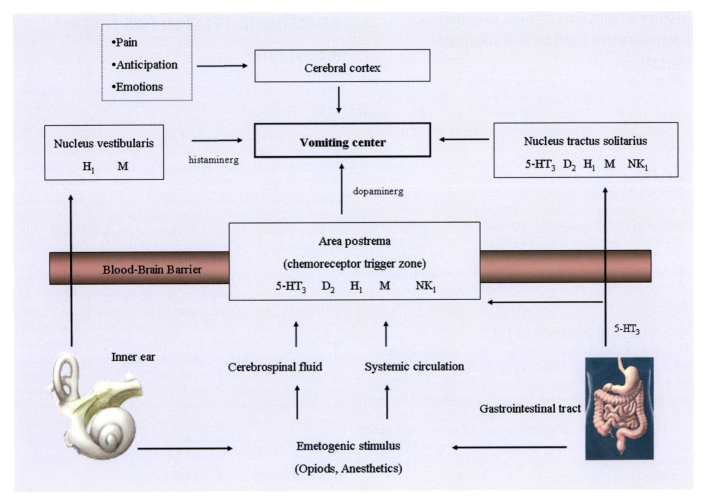

Figure 54.2. Schematic representation of the complex pathophysiology of postoperative nausea and vomiting. 5-HT$_3$, serotonin subtype 3 receptor; D$_2$, dopamine subtype 2 receptor; H$_1$, histamine subtype 1 receptor; M, muscarinic cholinergic receptor; NK$_1$, neurokinin subtype 1 receptor. Adapted from Scholz *et al.* [1]; Kreis [9].

children older than 11 years. However, the lack of relevant pediatric PONV data remains a major drawback and is highly unsatisfactory [13].

Sex

PONV is approximately 2–3 times more prevalent in adult women than in men, and the severity of vomiting is greater [14]. There is no significant sex difference in children, but the incidence of PONV increases in girls as menarche approaches. Because PONV varies according to the phase of the menstrual cycle, with a fourfold increased incidence during menses [15], it has been suggested that the increasing levels of estrogen, combined with decreasing levels of follicle-stimulating hormone, may sensitize chemoreceptors, or the vomiting center, or both.

Body weight

Obesity, defined by body mass index greater than 30 kg m^{-2} (weight divided by height squared), has been assumed to be associated with increased PONV in previous reports [4].

This correlation is explained by the fact that adipose tissue acts as a reservoir for anesthetic drugs, from which they continue to enter the circulation even after their administration has been discontinued. Other explanations for an increased incidence of PONV in obese patients include a larger residual gastric volume, increased incidence of esophageal reflux, and other gastrointestinal diseases. In addition, compared with nonobese subjects, these patients have a higher incidence of difficult airway management, and thereby more gastric insufflation may occur during facemask ventilation. However, a systematic review failed to demonstrate a significant influence of body weight on frequency of PONV. Furthermore, several evaluations also failed to demonstrate obesity as a predictor for PONV [16].

Smoking status

A few investigations have shown that PONV is more frequently observed in patients who do not smoke [17,18]. The reason why nonsmoking status is a risk factor for PONV is currently not understood.

History of motion sickness or previous postoperative nausea and vomiting sensations

Patients with a history suggesting that they have a low threshold for vomiting are at increased risk for development of emetic symptoms. These include patients with a prior history of PONV after anesthesia or patients who usually experience motion sickness [4].

Anxiety

Patients with undue anxiety about the forthcoming surgical procedure are at greater risk for emesis [19]. It has been suggested that PONV in anxious patients may be related to an increase in gastric fluid volume caused by increased circulating stress hormones. Anxiety may also provoke air swallowing, resulting in gut distension and activation of mechanoreceptors. Decreased PONV risk was noted when hypnosis or sedation techniques were used to reduce perioperative anxiety [19].

Presence and absence of food

Patients who have had recent food or fluid intake, e.g., emergency patients, are often found to be at risk for PONV. Apart from the high risk for aspiration into the bronchial tree, this is another reason to advocate fasting before elective surgery. However, prolonged fasting also tends to increase the incidence of nausea, particularly in women. Therefore, both children and adults who are considered to be at normal risk of aspiration/regurgitation during anesthesia benefit from unlimited fluid uptake up to 2 hours preoperatively [20,21].

Gastroparesis

Patients with delayed gastric emptying secondary to an underlying disease (e.g., ileus) may be at increased risk for PONV after surgery [3]. These disease processes include gastrointestinal obstruction, chronic cholecystitis, neuromuscular disorder, and intrinsic neuropathies. Gastric hypomotility can complicate conditions such as scleroderma, myotonic dystrophy, progressive muscular dystrophies, amyloidosis, and familial visceral myopathies. Gastroparesis also can be associated with pylorospasm and isolated antral hypomotility in patients with diabetes mellitus [3].

Type and duration of surgery

PONV is more often observed in patients undergoing abdominal versus nonabdominal surgery, with a markedly increased incidence in women undergoing laparoscopic procedures [22]. Pediatric patients undergoing strabismus repair, adenotonsillectomy, orchidopexy, middle-ear surgery, and laparotomy are also at increased risk [23,24]. The duration of surgery also has an effect on the incidence of PONV, with more frequent emesis being reported after longer operations, possibly because patients may receive a larger number and volume of potentially emetic anesthetic drugs [25].

Anesthesia-related risk factors

Nitrous oxide

The results of studies investigating the influence of nitrous oxide (N_2O) on PONV are inconsistent. Several fairly outdated studies suggest an independent contribution of N_2O for PONV [25]. For example, the high incidence of PONV during laparoscopic procedures was thought to be further exacerbated by the introduction of N_2O in this particular high-risk population. Contrarily, other investigators failed to demonstrate a significant increase in PONV after addition of N_2O to other anesthetic drugs [3]. In addition, in an investigation dealing with the detection of relevant risk factors for PONV using multiple logistic regression analysis, N_2O was not identified as a significant risk factor in this regard [26]. Nevertheless, meta-analyses of existing studies support the view that addition of N_2O may lead to increased nausea and vomiting [27,28]. Thus, N_2O has to be considered as a risk factor for PONV, and omitting N_2O may decrease the incidence of PONV [29]. Omitting N_2O was also shown to be more effective in protecting against vomiting rather than from nausea; its prophylactic effect was most effective in patients at high risk for PONV.

Nitrous oxide may cause PONV through both central and peripheral mechanisms. This may involve stimulation of the sympathetic nervous system with catecholamine release, changes in middle ear pressure with stimulation of the vestibular system, and increased distension of the gastrointestinal tract due to diffusion into air-filled spaces [3].

Inhalational anesthetic drugs

For a long time volatile anesthetics were not considered to have a significant impact on PONV. In fact, the well-known lower incidence of PONV after total intravenous anesthesia (TIVA) compared to volatile anesthetic drugs was attributed to antiemetic effects of propofol rather than proemetic effects of volatile anesthetics [30]. There is now strong evidence that volatile anesthetics are emetogenic [31]. Thus, volatile anesthetics per se are strongly responsible for induction of PONV, such that avoidance of volatile anesthetics alone reduced the incidence of PONV by 19% [6]. Kaplan–Meier curves demonstrated for the first time that the main difference between propofol and inhalational anesthesia occurred within the first 2 hours, when pharmacokinetic effects are most likely to account for differences (Fig. 54.3) [32]. Thereafter, there is a parallel trend, suggesting that the chosen anesthetics do not cause this difference; this finding was supported by multivariate analyses of the data from the delayed period. In order to distinguish between pro- and antiemetic effects of volatile and intravenous anesthetics, five percentile groups were constructed for each anesthetic according to the degree of exposure with the outcome of early vomiting (Fig. 54.4) [31]. With respect to emetogenic potency of individual inhalational anesthetic drugs, results of several studies may be controversial; however, it is safe to conclude that the emetic effect of all

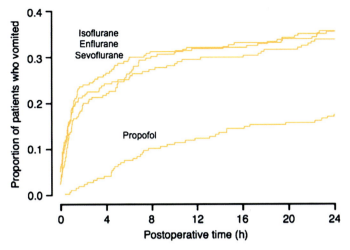

Figure 54.3. Kaplan–Meier curves representing the proportion of patients who vomited over time broken down by the type of maintenance anesthetics. Note that the difference between propofol and volatile anesthetics is related only to the early postoperative period. Reproduced with permission from Apfel *et al.* [32].

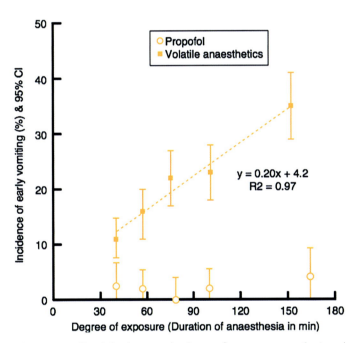

Figure 54.4. Correlation between the degree of exposure to anesthesia and early postoperative vomiting in the first 2 hours. In order to compare inhalational and propofol anesthesia, five percentile groups were formed for each, as a function of the anesthesia duration. Note that the incidence of early vomiting correlates positively with the degree of exposure to inhalational anesthesia but not to propofol anesthesia. Reproduced with permission from Apfel *et al.* [32].

volatile anesthetics appears to be roughly the same [31,33]. In terms of noble gases, xenon has been proved to be safe and efficacious for general anesthesia in numerous trials [34,35]. Though experimental studies indicate that xenon inhibits the 5-HT$_3$ receptor [36], its use was associated with a higher incidence of nausea and emetic episodes compared with propofol-based TIVA [37].

Opioid analgesics

Opioids are well documented as powerful emetogenic drugs [3,4,38]. Fentanyl has been associated with an incidence of approximately 25% for nausea and 18% for vomiting. The more lipid-soluble drugs, alfentanil and sufentanil, have also been associated with similar incidences of PONV [39]. Alfentanil infusions have been used instead of halothane for short surgical procedures in children and were associated with a greater incidence rate of PONV (45% vs. 15%). Remifentanil, a new ultra-short-acting opioid, resulted in less PONV after propofol/remifentanil versus propofol/fentanyl anesthesia during plastic surgery [40]. In contrast, more recent studies revealed a comparable incidence of PONV after remifentanil compared to sufentanil [41]. Thus, it seems unimportant which opioid is used, because they are all associated with similar incidence rates of PONV [42].

Other anesthetic drugs

Administration of traditional intravenous anesthetic drugs, including barbiturates and etomidate, can also be associated with PONV [3,4]. In contrast, propofol has been shown to exhibit antiemetic properties [43]. Neostigmine in doses of more than 2.5 mg is thought to induce PONV [44]; however, coadministration of atropine rather than glycopyrrolate may nullify the results, because atropine has antiemetogenic effects, whereas glycopyrrolate does not [45]. Thus, although the emetogenic effect of neostigmine and pyridostigmine is documented, it may not be important clinically [46]. Sugammadex (designation Org 25969) is a novel drug for reversal of neuromuscular blockade by the drug rocuronium in general anesthesia. With respect to PONV, a recent study failed to demonstrate a reduction in the incidence of PONV with sugammadex compared to standard cholinesterase inhibitors, though this study was clearly underpowered to demonstrate a difference [47]. A larger multicenter, randomized study comparing sugammadex and neostigmine is currently evaluating PONV as a secondary outcome parameter (NCT 00675792).

Pharmacology of antiemetics and therapeutic approach

Several strategies in PONV prophylaxis and therapy have been adapted from techniques used in the prevention or treatment of chemotherapy-induced nausea and vomiting (CINV). A panel of clinical, health-economic, and basic scientists with expertise in various oncology disciplines reviewed published literature to develop evidence-based consensus guidelines for the prevention and treatment of CINV [48]. Currently, 5-HT receptor antagonists and corticosteroids are the two categories of antiemetics that are most effective; they have the fewest side effects and are the most convenient to use.

Similar evidence-based consensus guidelines for the prevention and treatment of PONV are now available [49–51].

Table 54.1. Various antiemetics and their interaction with different specific receptor sites

Antiemetic	Receptor site of action				
	H_1	M	D_2	5-HT_3	NK_1
Antihistamines					
Promethazine	++++	++	++	–	–
Dimenhydrinate	++++	++	+	–	–
Anticholinergics					
Scopolamine	+	++++	+	–	–
Benzamides					
Metoclopramide	+	–	+++	++	–
Neuroleptics					
Droperidol	+	–	++++	+	–
Triflupromazine	+	–	++++	–	–
5-HT_3 antagonists					
Ondansetron	–	–	–	++++	–
Tropisetron	–	–	–	++++	–
Granisetron	–	–	–	++++	–
Dolasetron	–	–	–	++++	–
Palonosetron	–	–	–	++++	–
NK_1 antagonists					
Aprepitant	–	–	–	–	++++
Glucocorticoids					
Dexamethasone	–	–	–	–	–

+, positive interaction; –, no interaction; 5-HT_3, serotonin subtype 3 receptor; D_2, dopamine subtype 2 receptor; H_1, histamine subtype 1 receptor; M, muscarinic cholinergic receptor; NK_1, neurokinin subtype 1 receptor.

Three major groups of drugs –benzamides, neuroleptics, and 5-HT_3 receptor antagonists – are most frequently used in the management of PONV in daily clinical practice. Dimenhydrinate and corticosteroids are also used, but predominantly as adjuvants. As mentioned earlier, transdermal muscarinic receptor antagonists and antihistaminics are effective in both the prevention of motion sickness and the treatment of postoperative vomiting related to vestibular stimulation [52–56]. A new class of antiemetics, NK_1 receptor antagonists, has recently evolved for the prevention of vomiting in the first 48 hours postoperatively [57,58]. The various antiemetic drugs are summarized in Table 54.1 in relation to their interaction with different receptor sites.

Benzamides

The substituted benzamides, particularly metoclopramide (Fig. 54.5), are widely used in CINV and in some countries for the prevention and therapy of PONV. Although structurally related to procainamide, metoclopramide lacks significant local anesthetic or antiarrhythmic actions. Metoclopramide is

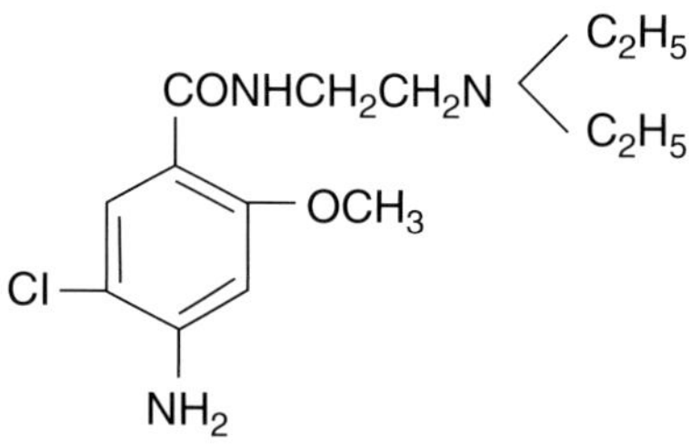

Figure 54.5. Chemical structure of metoclopramide.

rapidly and completely absorbed after oral administration, but hepatic first-pass metabolism reduces its bioavailability to about 75%. Metoclopramide is rapidly distributed into most tissues and readily crosses the blood–brain barrier and the placenta; the concentration of the drug in breast milk may exceed that in plasma. Up to 30% of metoclopramide is excreted unchanged in the urine, and the remainder is eliminated in the urine and the bile after conjugation with sulfate or glucuronic acid. The half-life of the drug in the circulation is about 4–6 hours, but it may be as much as 24 hours in patients with impaired renal function.

The efficacy of metoclopramide in preventing PONV is equivocal [23]. Nevertheless, some investigators found metoclopramide at doses of 0.25 mg kg^{-1} or 10 mg intravenously to be more effective in preventing PONV than 0.1 mg kg^{-1} tropisetron or 8 mg ondansetron, which are potent 5-HT$_3$ receptor antagonists. Further, the addition of 50 mg metoclopramide to 8 mg dexamethasone (given intraoperatively) has been shown to be an effective, safe, and cheap way to prevent PONV [59]. Another study demonstrated metoclopramide to be of no or limited value when compared with other antiemetics, including 5-HT$_3$ receptor antagonists and droperidol [60]. At high concentrations, metoclopramide has been shown to have a weak 5-HT$_3$ receptor antagonistic effect, which may account for some of its antiemetic properties when used at high doses in CINV. However, in a systematic review of randomized, placebo-controlled studies, metoclopramide was shown to have no clinically relevant antiemetic effect [61].

As metoclopramide antagonizes the action of dopamine, typical side effects of the dopamine antagonists, such as extrapyramidal reactions and sedation, may also occur in patients receiving metoclopramide. Intravenous application may be associated with significant cardiovascular side effects, which include hypotension and bradycardia or tachycardia. Metoclopramide should not be used after gastrointestinal surgery, such as pyloroplasty or intestinal anastomosis, because it stimulates gastric motility and may delay healing.

Other benzamide derivates have been synthesized (e.g., trimethobenzamide and cisapride) with the two aims of increasing the antiemetic efficacy and reducing side effects; however, these hopes have not been realized.

Neuroleptics

The butyrophenones are potent neuroleptics that were developed primarily for use in patients with schizophrenia and other psychoses, but they also have antiemetic properties mediated by their powerful D$_2$ receptor antagonism. Most studies involving dopamine antagonists have used droperidol (Fig. 54.6). The total-body clearance of droperidol is limited to hepatic blood flow, emphasizing the importance of hepatic metabolism in elimination of this drug (perfusion- rather than capacity-dependent); thus accumulation of droperidol is more likely to occur when the hepatic blood flow is decreased rather than with an alteration in hepatic enzyme activity. The elimination half-life of droperidol is about 100 minutes, the clearance is 14 mL kg^{-1} min^{-1}, and the volume of distribution is 2 L kg^{-1}. The short elimination half-life is not consistent with the prolonged central nervous system (CNS) effects of droperidol,

which may reflect slow dissociation of the drug from receptors or retention of droperidol in the brain.

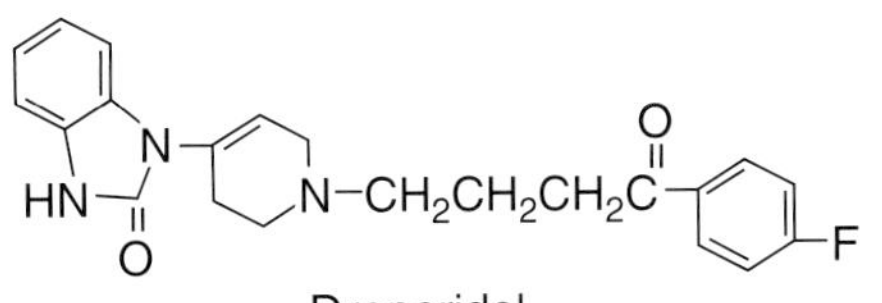

Droperidol has been widely used in adults and children for the prevention and treatment of PONV over several decades, and previously for the prevention of opioid-induced PONV during postoperative patient-controlled analgesia (PCA) in adults [62]. In unpremedicated children undergoing elective strabismus surgery, 0.075 mg kg^{-1} droperidol intravenously decreased the incidence of PONV and did not delay awaking from anesthesia. In outpatient gynecologic surgery, 0.625 mg droperidol intravenously provided antiemetic prophylaxis comparable to that of 4 mg ondansetron without increasing side effects or delaying discharge, and it was more cost-effective [62]. These results were previously confirmed by Chan and colleagues, indicating an additive interaction between ondansetron and droperidol for preventing PONV in laparoscopic gynecologic surgery [55]. Droperidol also effectively reduced the risk of opioid-induced nausea and vomiting, with a number needed to treat (NNT) of approximately 3, when given concomitantly with PCA [63].

In contrast, other studies failed to demonstrate an efficacy of droperidol administration in preventing PONV [3,4]. However, in these studies, droperidol was given during induction of anesthesia, and it was suggested that efficacy might be improved if droperidol was to be administered toward the end of prolonged surgical intervention. Nevertheless, most single studies found a beneficial effect of droperidol when compared with placebo in the prevention of PONV, and efficacy has also been demonstrated when droperidol was administered before and at the end of surgery. In an earlier systematic review, Henzi and coworkers concluded that droperidol is antiemetic in the surgical setting, and the effect on nausea is short-lived but more pronounced than the effect on vomiting [64]. Labyrinthine-induced vomiting (motion sickness) is not influenced by droperidol.

In December 2001, the US Food and Drug Administration (FDA) imposed a black-box warning for droperidol. According to the FDA, droperidol should only be used with continuous ECG monitoring. The drug may extend the QT interval, which can lead to torsades de pointes and, in rare cases, death. The provocation of torsades de pointes is very rare and depends on the dose of droperidol. So far, this arrhythmic disorder was largely described in patients who took very high antipsychotic doses of droperidol over days or weeks. In contrast, the droperidol dose used for the management of PONV is extremely low, and at this dosing level droperidol is unlikely to be associated with significant cardiovascular events [65–67].

Neuroleptics can also induce extrapyramidal side effects that are extremely unpleasant [64]. A few case reports have further focused upon their ability to cause an uncommon disorder, the neuroleptic malignant syndrome, which includes fluctuating level of consciousness, hyperthermia, muscular rigidity, and autonomic instability postoperatively [68,69]. In addition, high doses of droperidol can cause hypotension (as a result of peripheral α-adrenergic blockade), prolonged

Figure 54.6. Chemical structure of droperidol.

Droperidol

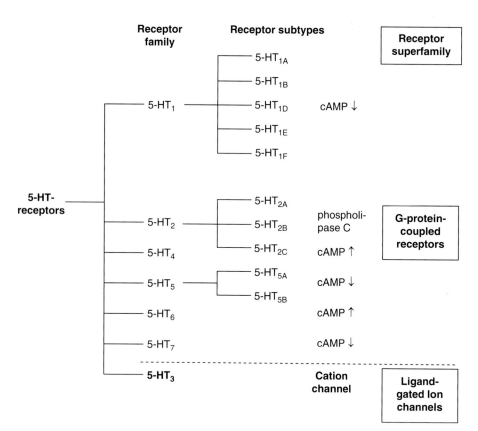

Figure 54.7. Serotonin (5-HT) receptor subtypes.

tiredness, or dysphoria. However, droperidol is generally well tolerated in low doses, and the incidence of adverse effects is similar to that observed with placebo and the serotonin 5-HT₃ receptor antagonists [62,70]. A preliminary meta-analysis has further indicated that dexamethasone, droperidol, and 5-HT₃ receptor antagonists have comparable safety profiles [71]. Moreover, Nuttall *et al.*, in the first epidemiologic study over 300 000 patients, addressed the issue of sudden death and torsades associated with the use of droperidol [72], and indicated that the FDA black-box warning for low-dose droperidol might be excessive and unnecessary. However, this study does not in itself justify removal of the warning on droperidol use. Although the precise format of the warning certainly remains a matter for debate, the warning itself may be still justified, because one has to be more stringent on safety issues than on efficacy issues [73].

Other neuroleptic drugs exhibiting antiemetic properties are the phenothiazines – triflupromazine, chlorpromazine, perphenazine, and levomepromazine. Their antiemetic effects are primarily caused by an interaction with dopaminergic receptors of the CNS. They seem to be most effective in preventing opioid-related nausea and vomiting. Although their antiemetic effects are achieved at low doses, all phenothiazines are capable of producing significant adverse effects, including extrapyramidal effects and sedation. Thus the phenothiazines may complicate postoperative care and result in prolonged hospitalization [4].

Serotonin type 3 receptor antagonists

The role of 5-HT in drug-induced emesis has received increased attention. As 5-HT is rapidly removed from plasma by platelets, endothelium, and the liver, peripheral 5-HT release is reflected by analyzing its major metabolite 5-hydroxyindole acetic acid (5-HIAA). Levels of 5-HIAA are significantly increased in patients with PONV sensations compared with patients without PONV [74].

Twenty-three 5-HT receptor subtypes have been described, among which the 5-HT₃ receptor occupies a special place (Fig. 54.7) [75–77]. The 5-HT₃ receptor is phylogenetically much older than the other 5-HT receptors, all of which have developed from a single primordial 5-HT receptor. The 5-HT₃ receptor is a ligand-gated ion channel and thereby differs from other serotonin receptors (5-HT₁ to 5-HT₇), whose actions are mediated via G-proteins. The structure of 5-HT₃ receptors shows that they are members of the Cys-loop family of ligand-gated ion channel, which includes glycine, γ-aminobutyric acid (GABA), and nicotinic acetylcholine receptors. Members of this family share a structure that is composed of five pseudosymmetrically arranged subunits surrounding a central ion-conducting pore. Each subunit is composed of extracellular, a transmembrane, and intracellular domains. The extracellular domain contains the binding site for agonists and competitive antagonists; it is the major therapeutic target for 5-HT₃ receptor antagonists (Fig. 54.8) [77].

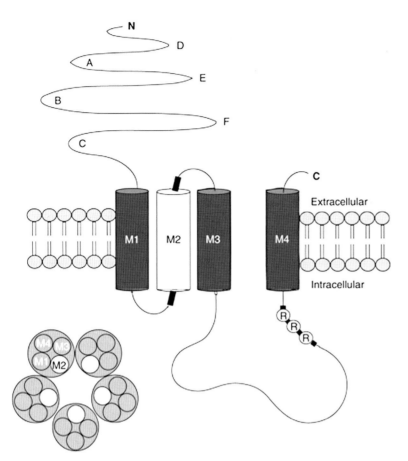

Figure 54.8. Schematic representation of the serotonin subtype 3 (5-HT$_3$) receptor with a typical Cys-loop receptor subunit. The diagram at the lower left is a cross-section of the transmembrane region indicating how five subunits form a central ion-conducting pore that is lined by M2 α-helices. Six loops (A–F) form the ligand binding site for agonists and competitive antagonists. Reproduced with permission from Thompson and Lummis [77].

With respect to 5-HT$_3$ receptor heterogeneity, five different human 5-HT$_3$ receptor subunit genes have been characterized (A–E) [78–81]. Concerning the distribution of 5-HT$_3$ receptor subunit genes, 5-HT$_{3A}$ receptor subunit mRNA has been found to be widely distributed in the adult human brain and internal organs. The distribution of 5-HT$_{3B}$ receptor subunit mRNA is not as widespread but it is still detectable across a range of adult brain regions and kidney [78]. 5-HT$_{3C}$ receptor subunit mRNA has a relatively wide distribution within adult brain, colon, intestine, lung, muscle, and stomach, while 5-HT$_{3D}$ mRNA has been indentified in kidney, colon, and liver, and 5-HT$_{3E}$ mRNA in the colon, intestine, and stomach [82]. Thus, high densities of 5-HT$_{3A-C}$ receptor subunits have been located in brain areas including the hippocampus, cortex, and amygdala, with highest levels in the brainstem, especially areas involved in the vomiting reflex such as the area postrema and the nucleus tractus solitarius [77]. The 5-HT$_{3B}$, 5-HT$_{3C}$, 5-HT$_{3D}$, and 5-HT$_{3E}$ subunits alone cannot form homomeric functional receptors, but coexpression with 5-HT$_{3A}$ has been demonstrated to result in the formation of functional heteromeric complexes with different serotonin efficacies [78,80].

Four 5-HT$_3$ antagonists are available for PONV in the USA at present: ondansetron, dolasetron, granisetron, and palonosetron (Fig. 54.9). In Europe, tropisetron is also approved for PONV, but palonosetron is only approved for CINV.

Other drugs in this class include azasetron and ramosetron, which are available in the Far East, and alosetron, which has been approved for the treatment of irritable bowel syndrome in the USA [77]. 5-HT$_3$ receptor antagonists are very specific drugs with almost no significant interaction with other 5-HT receptor subtypes or other specific receptor binding sites [76]. The 5-HT$_3$ receptor antagonists may be advantageous in the management of emesis because of their high effectiveness and low side-effect profile, especially when compared with benzamides and neuroleptics. The 5-HT$_3$ receptor antagonists are readily absorbed after oral administration. The blood–brain barrier is easily crossed, and the maximum CNS concentration is reached within a few minutes after intravenous injection. The compounds exhibit moderately strong protein binding of about 60–75%. Different subtypes of the cytochrome P450 (CYP) enzyme system metabolize the drugs, and the biodegradation products are predominantly eliminated by the renal route [76].

Ondansetron was the first drug of this class, and its efficacy has been established in large studies of various populations [76,83–85], not only in CINV but also in the prevention and therapy of PONV. Ondansetron is a carbazalone derivative that is structurally related to 5-HT and possesses specific 5-HT$_3$ subtype receptor antagonist properties, without affecting dopamine, histamine, adrenergic, or cholinergic receptor

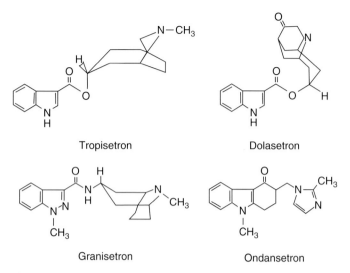

Figure 54.9. Chemical structures of serotonin subtype 3 (5-HT$_3$) receptor antagonists.

activity (Table 54.1). It can be administered orally or intravenously and has an oral bioavailability of about 60%, with effective blood levels appearing 30–60 minutes after administration. This drug is metabolized extensively by the liver, with a plasma half-life of 3–4 hours [86].

Superior effects in the prevention of PONV have been observed after administration of ondansetron in comparison with droperidol and metoclopramide [84]. In a dose-finding study examining both antiemetic efficacy and side effects, it has been shown that ondansetron at a dose of 4 mg is associated with the lowest emesis rate along with comparable side-effect profiles at various doses ranging from 1 to 8 mg. Ondansetron 4–8 mg administered intravenously over 2–5 minutes immediately before the induction of anesthesia is highly effective in decreasing the incidence of PONV in patients undergoing ambulatory gynecologic surgery or middle-ear surgery. Oral (0.15 mg kg^{-1}) or intravenous (0.05–0.15 mg kg^{-1}) administration of ondansetron was effective in decreasing the incidence of PONV in preadolescent children undergoing ambulatory surgery including tonsillectomy and strabismus surgery. In addition to prophylaxis, 1–8 mg ondansetron is highly effective in the treatment of PONV [84]. In a systematic review it has been demonstrated that ondansetron could prevent further PONV in one of four patients who would otherwise continue to have these symptoms. Whereas Tramer and colleagues claim that ondansetron did not differ from metoclopramide or droperidol in controlling further emetic symptoms when administered to patients with established PONV [27], another study has shown ondansetron to provide better and longer-lasting control of PONV than metoclopramide [60]. Although the antiemetic effects of ondansetron appear to be superior to those of other prophylactic antiemetics in many studies, previous data suggest that small doses of droperidol (0.625–1.25mg) may be equally effective. Another study has also demonstrated that droperidol

seems to be as effective as ondansetron in preventing PONV and that significant cost savings can be realized if droperidol is used rather than ondansetron [87]. On the other hand, in pediatric surgical patients prophylactic ondansetron (0.1 mg kg^{-1} intravenously) significantly decreased PONV compared with placebo and droperidol (0.75 mg kg^{-1}) and reduced hospital length of stay compared with droperidol.

Ondansetron is generally well tolerated, causing only transient, mild adverse effects, including headache, constipation, and dizziness. Because this drug is not an antagonist of dopamine receptors, it does not cause the extrapyramidal side effects associated with metoclopramide or droperidol. In other words, the most significant feature of ondansetron prophylaxis and treatment is the relative freedom from side effects compared with other classes of antiemetic drugs. Increased liver enzymes have been reported only in patients receiving antineoplastic drugs at the same time, and it is unclear whether this effect is a result of the chemotherapy or ondansetron. Ondansetron and other 5-HT$_3$ receptor antagonists such as tropisetron and granisetron can cause slight QT prolongation and reduced heart rate [66]. In some cases, cardiac conduction disorders (atrioventricular block) and arrhythmias have been documented during treatment with 5-HT$_3$ receptor antagonists [76,88].

Other 5-HT$_3$ receptor antagonists can be summarized as follows:

- Tropisetron is an indoleacetic acid ester of tropine with a longer half-life (8–30 hours) than ondansetron. Beneficial effects of tropisetron have been reported for CINV and after gynecologic procedures [89].
- Granisetron is more selective, and also has a longer half-life (9 hours) than ondansetron, and thus may also require less frequent dosing. Concomitant administration of dexamethasone significantly improved the acute antiemetic efficacy of granisetron [90,91].
- Dolasetron is rapidly metabolized to hydrodolasetron, which is responsible for the antiemetic effect and is approximately 100 times more potent as a 5-HT$_3$ receptor antagonist than the parent compound. Its elimination half-time is approximately 8 hours. Dolasetron 12.5 mg should be administered intravenously for the prevention and therapy of PONV, according to current recommendations [51,84,92].
- Palonosetron was introduced to the US market in 2003, and was found to be effective in preventing acute and delayed CINV [93]. It is now also approved in the USA for PONV.

Neurokinin type 1 receptor antagonists

CP-122,721, a nonpeptide antagonist of the NK$_1$ receptor, was the first NK$_1$ antagonist to be approved for clinical testing in North America. Oral administration of 200 mg of CP-122,721 decreased emetic episodes compared with ondansetron (4 mg intravenously) during the first 24 hours after gynecologic surgery; however, there was no difference in patient satisfaction [11]. In the case of the NK$_1$ receptor antagonist aprepitant (Fig. 54.10), Diemunsch *et al.* demonstrated that a single oral

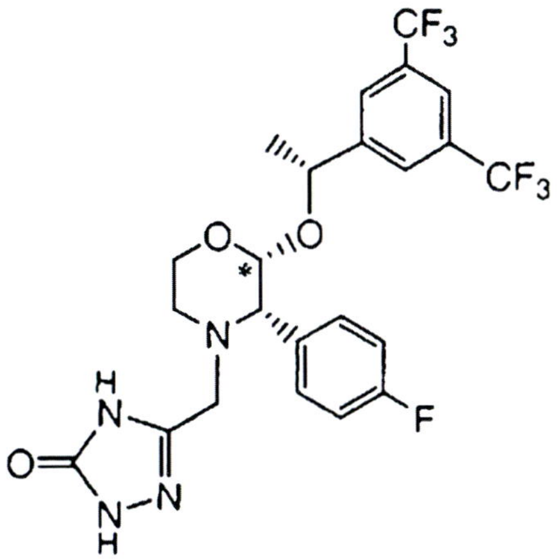

Figure 54.10. Chemical structure of the neurokinin subtype 1 (NK_1) receptor antagonist, aprepitant.

Anesthetic and pharmacologic strategies in the management of postoperative nausea and vomiting

The high incidence of PONV is due to a variety of factors, and a range of effective antiemetics is available for its prevention and therapy. Pharmacologic strategies in PONV management should be considered before a patient is transferred to the PACU or surgical ward. If PONV prophylaxis fails, PONV treatment should be started postoperatively with the first episode of vomiting or when a moderate degree of nausea occurs, because without therapy further episodes of PONV will occur in over 50% of all cases.

Premedication

Anesthesiologists usually order a premedication, to be given before induction of anesthesia. Before the advent of benzodiazepines, it was traditional to use opioids for preanesthetic sedation, but this practice is associated with increased PONV. The benzodiazepines have become popular because they are associated with reduced anxiety, amnesia, and PONV sensations [107,108]. Similarly, preoperative use of the α_2-receptor agonist clonidine for sedation seems to be associated with decreased PONV, partly because it results in reduced consumption of anesthetic drugs and opioids [109].

Anesthesia

Regional anesthesia is usually associated with a lower incidence of PONV than general anesthesia [32]. A variety of techniques, including inhalational anesthesia (potent volatile anesthetic with or without N_2O), balanced anesthesia (a combination of inhaled drugs and opioid analgesics), and total intravenous anesthesia (TIVA), produce general anesthesia. If general anesthesia is essential, the anesthesiologist should use techniques known to reduce the risk for PONV. When antiemetic drugs have not been administered prophylactically, the incidence of PONV has been reported as greatest with balanced anesthesia, intermediate with inhalational anesthesia, and least with propofol-based TIVA [4]. This observation is supported by several additional investigations. Watcha and colleagues demonstrated that there was a lower incidence of PONV in children undergoing day-case strabismus surgery if propofol was used for both induction and maintenance of anesthesia than for induction alone followed by inhalational drugs for anesthesia maintenance [110]. In a study comparing TIVA with propofol and isoflurane anesthesia, TIVA reduced the absolute risk of PONV up to 72 hours by 15% among inpatients (from 61% to 46%) and by 18% among outpatients (from 46% to 28%) [111]. In a systematic review propofol has been shown to provide a clinically relevant effect on PONV. This was, however, limited to studies with a continuous

preoperative dose of 40–125 mg was significantly more effective than 4 mg intravenous ondansetron for preventing vomiting at 24 and 48 hours after major abdominal surgery, and in reducing nausea severity in the first 48 hours after surgery [57,58]. Aprepitant was generally well tolerated.

Recent analysis of the 5-HT_3 antagonists suggests that, like other antiemetics [94], they reduce the relative risk for both nausea and vomiting similarly [95]. NK_1 receptor antagonists are different in this respect [96]. For example, aprepitant and ondansetron are similarly efficacious against nausea, but aprepitant is considerably more efficacious than ondansetron against vomiting [97]. The considerably higher efficacy against vomiting seems to be a class effect, as it is also supported by a recently completed phase II trial of casopitant [98].

Corticosteroids

Dexamethasone and other glucocorticoids (5–20 mg dexamethasone, 125–375 mg methylprednisolone) have significant antiemetic effects both when administered before chemotherapy and in the postoperative period [4,99]. Further, efficacy in preventing PONV is still present for up to 24 hours [100]. In patients undergoing thyroidectomy, the minimum effective dose in preventing PONV was found to be 5 mg dexamethasone [101]. The mechanisms by which corticosteroids exert their antiemetic effects currently are not completely understood. However, dexamethasone is known to have multiple CNS effects, including effects on mood and sense of well-being [4]. Further, dexamethasone has been claimed to prevent PONV mainly when given near the beginning of surgery, probably by reducing surgery-induced inflammation [102]. Although corticosteroids are effective alone, they are more commonly used in combination with other antiemetics [4,103,104]. Dexamethasone was shown to increase the antiemetic efficacy of both 5-HT_3 receptor antagonists and droperidol when given for prophylaxis of PONV [100,105]. In addition, combinations of dexamethasone with dolasetron or dexamethasone with haloperidol have been demonstrated to be superior to dolasetron or haloperidol alone for the treatment of established PONV, when PONV prophylaxis failed [106].

infusion, and only in settings where the rate for emesis was greater than 20%. Propofol may have a greater effect on the control of nausea than of emesis in low-risk patients. Conversely, it has been shown that the use of propofol for induction and maintenance of anesthesia may be as effective as ondansetron in preventing PONV [4]. Moreover, even subhypnotic doses of propofol administered after surgery have been shown to result in an antiemetic effect. Overall, there is considerable evidence that propofol-based TIVA should be the principal anesthetic technique for general anesthesia in patients at high risk for PONV [32].

Propofol seems to provide an antiemetic effect that may be mediated by GABA influences on the 5-HT system [112]. Propofol binds to a specific site on the $GABA_A$ receptor to potentiate GABA-activated chloride flux. In addition, 5-HT release is reduced by GABA-mediated inhibition. Cechetto and coworkers postulated that propofol inhibits the release of 5-HT from the dorsal raphe nucleus through an enhancement of the $GABA_A$ synaptic activity [112]. This results in a reduction of the 5-HT released into the cerebrospinal fluid from the serotonergic supraependymal fibers that, in turn, causes a reduction of the 5-HT sequestered by the area postrema.

Scoring systems for a holistic approach

Routine antiemetic prophylaxis is not warranted for all surgical patients, as the global incidence of PONV is about one-third of the overall population scheduled for surgical and diagnostic procedures under general anesthesia. However, it is still a matter of debate which patients should receive an antiemetic prophylaxis, which antiemetic drugs are most suitable, and when the drug should be administered [113]. In addition, the clinical relevance of individual risk factors should be viewed with caution, since even well-proven risk factors, such as a history of PONV, do not allow the

identification of patients at risk for PONV with a satisfactory sensitivity or specificity. Therefore, it might be helpful to have a scoring system which considers several risk factors simultaneously, thereby the probability of PONV, and which leads the anesthesiologist to administer an adequate antiemetic prophylaxis. Several risk models have been developed [1,114–116]. While some scores are based on complex calculations, simplified risk scores allow a valid and objective assessment of the patient's risk for PONV at the bedside [18,114,117].

Koivuranta and coworkers published a simplified score based on the five strongest predictors of PONV, each having the same weight [114]. These factors were female sex, non-smoking status, previous PONV, history of motion sickness, and duration of operation longer than 60 minutes (Fig. 54.11). The presence of one of these factors increased the risk of nausea from 17% (no factor present) to 18%, 42%, 54%, 74%, and finally to 87% when all five risk factors were present. Correspondingly, the risk for vomiting was 7%, 7%, 17%, 25%, 38%, and 61% for none up to five risk factors. The risk scores were based on surgical patients undergoing general anesthesia using an inhalational technique. This included a benzodiazepine for premedication, induction with 3–5 mg kg^{-1} thiopental and either up to 2 μg kg^{-1} fentanyl or up to 20 μg kg^{-1} alfentanil, and the use of a volatile anesthetic (isoflurane, enflurane, or sevoflurane). No prophylactic antiemetics were given. Postoperative pain was treated with non-steroidal analgesic drugs or opioid analgesics if needed. The risk score evaluation published by Koivuranta and coworkers has been proven to be attractive for clinical practice [114].

Apfel and collegues have published the results of two centers that independently developed a risk score for predicting PONV [6,26]. The final score consisted of four predictors: female sex, nonsmoking status, history of motion sickness or

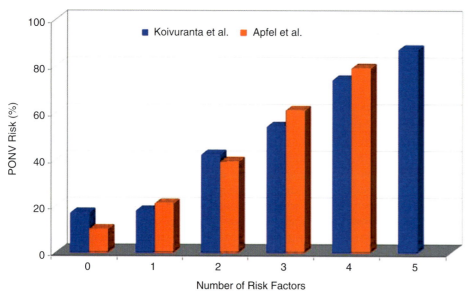

Figure 54.11. Simplified risk score for PONV in adults from Koivuranta *et al.* [114] and Apfel *et al.* [26] to predict a patient's risk for PONV. When 0, 1, 2, 3, 4, or 5 of the depicted independent predictors are present, the corresponding risk for PONV is approximately 10%, 20%, 40%, 55%, 80%, or 87%.

PONV, and the use of postoperative opioids. If none, one, two, three, or four of these risk factors was present, the incidence of PONV was 10%, 21%, 39%, 61%, and 79%, respectively. Anesthesia was comparable to the strategy mentioned earlier. This study demonstrated that risk scores derived from one center were able to predict PONV from the other center (Fig. 54.11). Nevertheless, van den Bosch and coworkers have shown that neither of two established scoring systems provided a risk threshold for administering antiemetic prophylaxis yielding satisfying results in terms of predictive values, sensitivity, and specificity [118]. The area under the receiver operator curve was 0.63 for the scoring system of Apfel et al. [26] and 0.66 for that of Koivuranta et al. [114].

In a prospective evaluation including 17 638 consecutive outpatients undergoing surgical procedures, Sinclair and coworkers found that a 10-year increase in age decreased the likelihood of PONV by 13% [116]. A 30-minute increase in the duration of balanced general anesthesia increased the likelihood of PONV by 59%. Balanced general anesthesia increased the probability of PONV 11 times compared with other types of anesthesia.

Although there are numerous risk scores available for adults, only a few studies have exclusively focused on a pediatric

patient population (postoperative vomiting in children [POVOC] score) [119,120]. This is important, because it has been shown that transferring risk scores for adults to children yields no meaningful predictive conclusion [120]. The POVOC score is a simplified risk score considering the following clinical risk factors: (1) duration of surgery > 30 min, (2) age > 3 year, (3) strabismus surgery, and (4) a positive history of motion sickness or history of PONV in parents or siblings. Depending on the presence of none, one, two, three, or four risk factors the estimated incidence for PONV in the pediatric patient is 9%, 10%, 30%, 55%, and 70%, respectively. Further, the POVOC score has previously been validated [12].

In summary, scoring systems can give some information on the probability of PONV, and can clearly point out patients at high risk. But all score evaluations were based on general anesthesia using inhalational techniques. Therefore, additional evaluations are needed to reveal the risk for PONV in patients with multiple risk factors undergoing propofol-based TIVA.

Risk-adapted antiemetic prophylaxis
Prophylaxis and therapy of PONV in individual patients should take into account evidence-based guidelines, including a standardized algorithm (Fig. 54.12) [49–51]. Administration

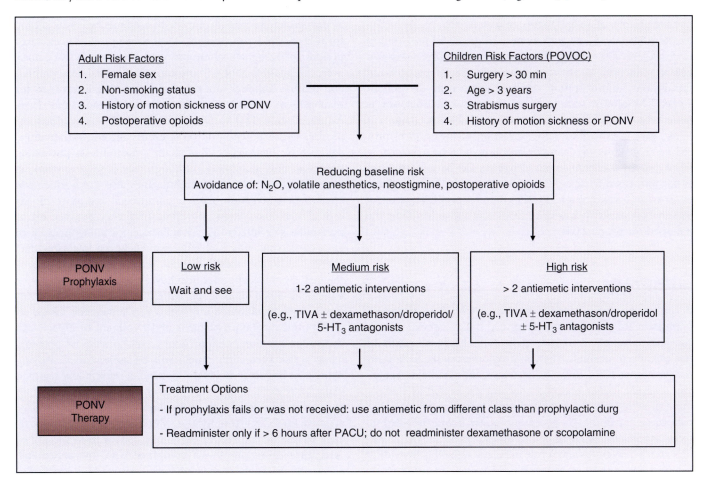

Figure 54.12. Algorithm for prophylaxis and therapy of postoperative nausea and vomiting (PONV). Adapted from Gan et al. [49].

of antiemetic prophylaxis to patients with a low baseline risk for PONV is not justified, whereas high-risk patients should be treated with an antiemetic combination (multimodal approach). As mentioned previously, patients can be classified according to their risk factors. The simplified risk score of Apfel and colleagues showed simplicity and practicability in practice and in several multicenter studies [6,26]. Medium-risk patients (existence of one or two risk factors, with a risk between 20% and 40%) may benefit from 1–2 antiemetic interventions. Based on the results from the IMPACT study [121], each tested antiemetic drug (dexamethason, droperidol, ondansetron) and the use of TIVA reduced the relative risk of nausea and vomiting to a similar extent, i.e., by 26% [6]. The logical sequence is to use the least expensive or safest intervention first. For children with medium risk, 5-HT$_3$ receptor antagonists (e.g., 50–100 μg kg^{-1} ondansetron intravenously) have been shown to be useful. Multiple interventions should generally be reserved for patients at high risk for PONV. However, the absolute risk reduction provided by a second or third intervention is less than that provided by the initial intervention (irrespective of which combination is chosen). A 70% reduction in the relative risk of PONV is thus the best that can be expected, even when TIVA is used in combination with three antiemetics [18,32,122].

The timing of prophylactic antiemetic therapy is still a matter of debate. Some authors prefer the oral administration of 5-HT$_3$ receptor antagonists together with premedication before induction of anesthesia, whereas others recommend intravenous administration of these drugs near the end of surgery. Moreover, some authors administer neuroleptics as antiemetic drugs during induction of anesthesia, whereas others give neuroleptics before cessation of the surgical procedure. Currently, a definitive recommendation concerning when prophylactic antiemetic drugs should be administered is not warranted by scientific studies. Nevertheless, if patients experience breakthrough PONV despite prophylaxis, they should be treated with a drug from a group other than the one used for prophylaxis.

Summary

Postoperative nausea and vomiting (PONV) is not only unpleasant for patients and caregivers, but is associated with complications that can delay patient discharge or result in readmission to hospital. The vomiting center in the brainstem receives input from the area postrema, the vestibular apparatus, and the higher brainstem and cortex, as well as afferent input directly from the gastrointestinal tract. Serotonin 5-HT$_3$ receptors, dopamine D$_2$ receptors, acetylcholine muscarinic receptors, histamine H$_1$ receptors, and substance P NK$_1$ receptors are all thought to play a role in emetic signaling, providing a rationale for the use of certain antagonists in prophylaxis and treatment.

Studies of risk factors for PONV have, in some cases, produced mixed findings or suffered from a lack of relevant data. Proposed risk factors include age, sex, body weight, smoking status, history of a low threshold for vomiting, anxiety, food or fluid intake, gastroparesis, type of surgery, and duration of surgery. Anesthetic drugs may also have emetic effects. Though studies have produced conflicting findings regarding nitrous oxide (N$_2$O), meta-analyses indicate that it may be considered a risk factor for PONV. There is also strong evidence that volatile anesthetic drugs are emetogenic. The powerful emetic effects of opioid analgesics are mediated by their actions on the area postrema. Some intravenous anesthetic drugs may be emetogenic (e.g., barbiturates and etomidate), while others have antiemetic properties (e.g., propofol).

Benzamides, neuroleptics, and 5-HT$_3$ receptor antagonists are the most commonly used drug groups in the management of PONV. Metoclopramide is a benzamide used widely in the treatment of chemotherapy-induced nausea and vomiting (CINV); however, the efficacy of the drug in preventing PONV is uncertain. Furthermore, it is associated with a number of potential side effects, including extrapyramidal symptoms, sedation, and cardiovascular effects. Metoclopramide is contraindicated after gastrointestinal surgery since its actions stimulating gastric motility can delay healing. Butyrophenones such as droperidol are neuroleptics, with antiemetic actions arising from D$_2$ receptor antagonism. Most single studies found droperidol to be beneficial in the prevention of PONV; however, the possibility of QT prolongation, torsades de pointes, and death – although unlikely to occur at the levels used for management of PONV – have led the Food and Drug Administration (FDA) to impose a black-box warning on its use. Other potential adverse events include extrapyramidal effects, neuroleptic malignant syndrome, hypotension, tiredness, and dysphoria, although low-dose droperidol is generally well tolerated. Phenothiazines also exert antiemetic effects via interaction with dopaminergic receptors of the central nervous system, and thus may also produce extrapyramidal side effects. The 5-HT$_3$ receptor antagonists, such as ondansetron, have high effectiveness and a low side-effect profile, although some cardiac effects have been documented. Some corticosteroids have also been shown to be antiemetic when used alone, although they are more commonly used in combination with other antiemetic drugs.

Optimizing the prophylaxis and treatment of PONV will depend on a number of approaches. First, emetic risk profiling using a risk prediction model will be useful for identifying patients at high risk of PONV. Second, a multimodal regimen using antiemetic drugs with different mechanisms of action and the avoidance of emetogenic anesthetic techniques will be effective for PONV prophylaxis. Moderate-risk patients (existence of one or two risk factors) may benefit from the use of total intravenous anesthesia combined with one antiemetic, e.g., corticosteroids (dexamethasone), droperidol, or 5-HT$_3$ receptor antagonists. Patients at high risk for PONV should receive a multimodal approach composed of intravenous anesthesia and two or three antiemetic drugs (e.g., dexamethasone plus ondansetron). A new class of antiemetics, NK_1 receptor antagonists (e.g., aprepitant), has been shown to be more effective than ondansetron for preventing vomiting after major abdominal surgery, but further studies are required.

References

1. Scholz J, Steinfath M, Tonner PH. Postoperative nausea and vomiting. *Curr Opin Anaesthesiol* 1999; **12**: 657–61.

2. Priebe HJ. Perioperative myocardial infarction: aetiology and prevention. *Br J Anaesth* 2005; **95**: 3–19.

3. Scholz J, Steinfath M. Prophylaxis and therapy of postoperative nausea and vomiting. In: Herbert M, Holzer P, Roewer N, eds., *Problems of the Gastrointestinal Tract in Anesthesia, the Perioperative Period, and Intensive Care*. Berlin: Springer, 1999: 313–26.

4. Rose J, Watcha M. Postoperative nausea and vomiting. In: Benumof J, Saidman L, eds., *Anesthesia and Perioperative Complications*, 2nd edn. St Louis, MO: Mosby, 1999: 425–40.

5. Golembiewski J, Chernin E, Chopra T. Prevention and treatment of postoperative nausea and vomiting. *Am J Health Syst Pharm* 2005; **62**: 1247–60.

6. Apfel CC, Korttila K, Abdalla M, *et al.* A factorial trial of six interventions for the prevention of postoperative nausea and vomiting. *N Engl J Med* 2004; **350**: 2441–51.

7. Silva AC, O'Ryan F, Poor DB. Postoperative nausea and vomiting (PONV) after orthognathic surgery: a retrospective study and literature review. *J Oral Maxillofac Surg* 2006; **64**: 1385–97.

8. Simpson K, Lynch L. Physiology and pharmacology of nausea and vomiting. In: Hemmings HJ, Hopkins P, eds., *Foundations of Anesthesia: Basic and Clinical Sciences*, 2nd edn. St Louis, MO: Mosby, 2005: 623–30.

9. Kreis ME. Postoperative nausea and vomiting. *Auton Neurosci* 2006; **129**: 86–91.

10. Gan TJ. Mechanisms underlying postoperative nausea and vomiting and neurotransmitter receptor antagonist-based pharmacotherapy. *CNS Drugs* 2007; **21**: 813–33.

11. Gesztesi Z, Scuderi PE, White PF, *et al.* Substance P (neurokinin-1) antagonist prevents postoperative vomiting after abdominal hysterectomy procedures. *Anesthesiology* 2000; **93**: 931–7.

12. Kranke P, Eberhart LH, Toker H, *et al.* A prospective evaluation of the POVOC score for the prediction of postoperative vomiting in children. *Anesth Analg* 2007; **105**: 1592–7.

13. Tramer MR. [Prevention and treatment of postoperative nausea and vomiting in children: an evidence-based approach]. *Ann Fr Anesth Reanim* 2007; **26**: 529–34.

14. Fujii Y. Prophylaxis of postoperative nausea and vomiting in patients scheduled for breast surgery. *Clin Drug Investig* 2006; **26**: 427–37.

15. Fujii Y, Toyooka H, Tanaka H. Prevention of postoperative nausea and vomiting in female patients during menstruation: comparison of droperidol, metoclopramide and granisetron. *Br J Anaesth* 1998; **80**: 248–9.

16. Kranke P, Apefel CC, Papenfuss T, *et al.* An increased body mass index is no risk factor for postoperative nausea and vomiting: a systematic review and results of original data. *Acta Anaesthesiol Scand* 2001; **45**: 160–6.

17. Choi DH, Ko JS, Ahn HJ, Kim JA. A korean predictive model for postoperative nausea and vomiting. *J Korean Med Sci* 2005; **20**: 811–15.

18. Pierre S, Corno G, Benais H, Apfel CC. A risk score-dependent antiemetic approach effectively reduces postoperative nausea and vomiting – a continuous quality improvement initiative. *Can J Anaesth* 2004; **51**: 320–5.

19. Chen CC, Lin CS, Ko YP, *et al.* Premedication with mirtazapine reduces preoperative anxiety and postoperative nausea and vomiting. *Anesth Analg* 2008; **106**: 109–13.

20. Brady M, Kinn S, O'Rourke K, Randhawa N, Stuart P. Preoperative fasting for preventing perioperative complications in children. *Cochrane Database Syst Rev* 2005; **4**: CD005285.

21. Brady M, Kinn S, Stuart P. Preoperative fasting for adults to prevent perioperative complications. *Cochrane Database Syst Rev* 2003; **4**: CD004423.

22. Scholz J, Hennes HJ, Steinfath M, *et al.* Tropisetron or ondansetron compared with placebo for prevention of postoperative nausea and vomiting. *Eur J Anaesthesiol* 1998; **15**: 676–85.

23. Bolton CM, Myles PS, Carlin JB, Nolan T. Randomized, double-blind study comparing the efficacy of moderate-dose metoclopramide and ondansetron for the prophylactic control of postoperative vomiting in children after tonsillectomy. *Br J Anaesth* 2007; **99**: 699–703.

24. Kovac AL. Management of postoperative nausea and vomiting in children. *Paediatr Drugs* 2007; **9**: 47–69.

25. Gan TJ. Risk factors for postoperative nausea and vomiting. *Anesth Analg* 2006; **102**: 1884–98.

26. Apfel CC, Laara E, Koivuranta M, Greim CA, Roewer N. A simplified risk score for predicting postoperative nausea and vomiting: conclusions from cross-validations between two centers. *Anesthesiology* 1999; **91**: 693–700.

27. Tramer M, Moore A, McQuay H. Meta-analytic comparison of prophylactic antiemetic efficacy for postoperative nausea and vomiting: propofol anaesthesia vs omitting nitrous oxide vs total i.v. anaesthesia with propofol. *Br J Anaesth* 1997; **78**: 256–9.

28. Myles PS, Leslie K, Chan MT, *et al.* Avoidance of nitrous oxide for patients undergoing major surgery: a randomized controlled trial. *Anesthesiology* 2007; **107**: 221–31.

29. Myles PS, Leslie K, Silbert B, Paech MJ, Peyton P. A review of the risks and benefits of nitrous oxide in current anaesthetic practice. *Anaesth Intensive Care* 2004; **32**: 165–72.

30. Sneyd JR, Carr A, Byrom WD, Bilski AJ. A meta-analysis of nausea and vomiting following maintenance of anaesthesia

with propofol or inhalational agents. *Eur J Anaesthesiol* 1998; **15**: 433–45.

31. Apfel CC, Kranke P, Katz MH, *et al.* Volatile anaesthetics may be the main cause of early but not delayed postoperative vomiting: a randomized controlled trial of factorial design. *Br J Anaesth* 2002; **88**: 659–68.

32. Apfel CC, Stoecklein K, Lipfert P. PONV: a problem of inhalational anaesthesia? *Best Pract Res Clin Anaesthesiol* 2005; **19**: 485–500.

33. Wallenborn J, Rudolph C, Gelbrich G, *et al.* The impact of isoflurane, desflurane, or sevoflurane on the frequency and severity of postoperative nausea and vomiting after lumbar disc surgery. *J Clin Anesth* 2007; **19**: 180–5.

34. Rossaint R, Reyle-Hahn M, Schulte Am Esch J, *et al.* Multicenter randomized comparison of the efficacy and safety of xenon and isoflurane in patients undergoing elective surgery. *Anesthesiology* 2003; **98**: 6–13.

35. Wappler F, Rossaint R, Baumert J, *et al.* Multicenter randomized comparison of xenon and isoflurane on left ventricular function in patients undergoing elective surgery. *Anesthesiology* 2007; **106**: 463–71.

36. Suzuki T, Koyama H, Sugimoto M, Uchida I, Mashimo T. The diverse actions of volatile and gaseous anesthetics on human-cloned 5-hydroxytryptamine3 receptors expressed in Xenopus oocytes. *Anesthesiology* 2002; **96**: 699–704.

37. Coburn M, Kunitz O, Apfel CC, *et al.* Incidence of postoperative nausea and emetic episodes after xenon anaesthesia compared with propofol-based anaesthesia. *Br J Anaesth* 2008; **100**: 787–91.

38. Roberts GW, Bekker TB, Carlsen HH, *et al.* Postoperative nausea and vomiting are strongly influenced by postoperative opioid use in a dose-related manner. *Anesth Analg* 2005; **101**: 1343–8.

39. Langevin S, Lessard MR, Trepanier CA, Baribault JP. Alfentanil causes less postoperative nausea and vomiting than equipotent doses of fentanyl or sufentanil in outpatients. *Anesthesiology* 1999; **91**: 1666–73.

40. Rama-Maceiras P, Ferreira TA, Molins N, *et al.* Less postoperative nausea and vomiting after propofol + remifentanil versus propofol + fentanyl anaesthesia during plastic surgery. *Acta Anaesthesiol Scand* 2005; **49**: 305–11.

41. Martorano PP, Aloj F, Baietta S, *et al.* Sufentanil-propofol vs remifentanil-propofol during total intravenous anesthesia for neurosurgery. A multicentre study. *Minerva Anestesiol* 2008; **74**: 233–43.

42. Unkel W, Peters J. [Postoperative nausea and emesis: mechanisms and treatment]. *Anasthesiol Intensivmed Notfallmed Schmerzther* 1998; **33**: 533–44.

43. Tramer M, Moore A, McQuay H. Propofol anaesthesia and postoperative nausea and vomiting: quantitative systematic review of randomized controlled studies. *Br J Anaesth* 1997; **78**: 247–55.

44. Tramer MR, Fuchs-Buder T. Omitting antagonism of neuromuscular block: effect on postoperative nausea and vomiting and risk of residual paralysis. A systematic review. *Br J Anaesth* 1999; **82**: 379–86.

45. Chhibber AK, Lustik SJ, Thakur R, Francisco DR, Fickling KB. Effects of anticholinergics on postoperative vomiting, recovery, and hospital stay in children undergoing tonsillectomy with or without adenoidectomy. *Anesthesiology* 1999; **90**: 697–700.

46. Cheng CR, Sessler DI, Apfel CC. Does neostigmine administration produce a clinically important increase in postoperative nausea and vomiting? *Anesth Analg* 2005; **101**: 1349–55.

47. Sacan O, White PF, Tufanogullari B, Klein K. Sugammadex reversal of rocuronium-induced neuromuscular blockade: a comparison with neostigmine-glycopyrrolate and edrophonium-atropine. *Anesth Analg* 2007; **104**: 569–74.

48. Herrstedt J, Dombernowsky P. Anti-emetic therapy in cancer chemotherapy: current status. *Basic Clin Pharmacol Toxicol* 2007; **101**: 143–50.

49. Gan TJ, Meyer TA, Apfel CC, *et al.* Society for Ambulatory Anesthesia guidelines for the management of postoperative nausea and vomiting. *Anesth Analg* 2007; **105**: 1615–28.

50. Habib AS, Gan TJ. Evidence-based management of postoperative nausea and vomiting: a review. *Can J Anaesth* 2004; **51**: 326–41.

51. Gan TJ, Meyer T, Apfel CC, *et al.* Consensus guidelines for managing postoperative nausea and vomiting. *Anesth Analg* 2003; **97**: 62–71.

52. Kranke P, Morin AM, Roewer N, Eberhart LH. Dimenhydrinate for prophylaxis of postoperative nausea and vomiting: a meta-analysis of randomized controlled trials. *Acta Anaesthesiol Scand* 2002; **46**: 238–44.

53. Kranke P, Morin AM, Roewer N, Wulf H, Eberhart LH. The efficacy and safety of transdermal scopolamine for the prevention of postoperative nausea and vomiting: a quantitative systematic review. *Anesth Analg* 2002; **95**: 133–43.

54. Turner KE, Parlow JL, Avery ND, Tod DA, Day AG. Prophylaxis of postoperative nausea and vomiting with oral, long-acting dimenhydrinate in gynecologic outpatient laparoscopy. *Anesth Analg* 2004; **98**: 1660–4.

55. Chan MT, Choi KC, Gin T, *et al.* The additive interactions between ondansetron and droperidol for preventing postoperative nausea and vomiting. *Anesth Analg* 2006; **103**: 1155–62.

56. Jones S, Strobl R, Crosby D, *et al.* The effect of transdermal scopolamine on the incidence and severity of postoperative nausea and vomiting in a group of high-risk patients given prophylactic intravenous ondansetron. *AANA J* 2006; **74**: 127–32.

57. Diemunsch P, Apfel C, Gan TJ, *et al.* Preventing postoperative nausea and vomiting: post hoc analysis of pooled data from two randomized active-controlled trials of aprepitant. *Curr Med Res Opin* 2007; **23**: 2559–65.

58. Diemunsch P, Gan TJ, Philip BK, *et al.* Single-dose aprepitant vs ondansetron for the prevention of postoperative nausea and vomiting: a randomized, double-blind phase III trial in patients undergoing open abdominal surgery. *Br J Anaesth* 2007; **99**: 202–11.

59. Wallenborn J, Gelbrich G, Bulst D, *et al.* Prevention of postoperative nausea and vomiting by metoclopramide combined with dexamethasone: randomised

double blind multicentre trial. *BMJ* 2006; **333**: 324.

60. Leksowski K, Peryga P, Szyca R. Ondansetron, metoclopramid, dexamethason, and their combinations compared for the prevention of postoperative nausea and vomiting in patients undergoing laparoscopic cholecystectomy: a prospective randomized study. *Surg Endosc* 2006; **20**: 878–82.

61. Henzi I, Walder B, Tramer MR. Metoclopramide in the prevention of postoperative nausea and vomiting: a quantitative systematic review of randomized, placebo-controlled studies. *Br J Anaesth* 1999; **83**: 761–71.

62. McKeage K, Simpson D, Wagstaff AJ. Intravenous droperidol: a review of its use in the management of postoperative nausea and vomiting. *Drugs* 2006; **66**: 2123–47.

63. Culebras X, Corpataux JB, Gaggero G, Tramer MR. The antiemetic efficacy of droperidol added to morphine patient-controlled analgesia: a randomized, controlled, multicenter dose-finding study. *Anesth Analg* 2003; **97**: 816–21.

64. Henzi I, Sonderegger J, Tramer MR. Efficacy, dose-response, and adverse effects of droperidol for prevention of postoperative nausea and vomiting. *Can J Anaesth* 2000; **47**: 537–51.

65. White PF, Song D, Abrao J, Klein KW, Navarette B. Effect of low-dose droperidol on the QT interval during and after general anesthesia: a placebo-controlled study. *Anesthesiology* 2005; **102**: 1101–5.

66. Charbit B, Albaladejo P, Funck-Brentano C, *et al.* Prolongation of QTc interval after postoperative nausea and vomiting treatment by droperidol or ondansetron. *Anesthesiology* 2005; **102**: 1094–100.

67. Gan TJ. Postoperative nausea and vomiting – can it be eliminated? *JAMA* 2002; **287**: 1233–6.

68. So PC. Neuroleptic malignant syndrome induced by droperidol. *Hong Kong Med J* 2001; **7**: 101–3.

69. Edgar J. Droperidol-induced neuroleptic malignant syndrome. *Hosp Med* 1999; **60**: 448–9.

70. Habib AS, Gan TJ. Food and drug administration black box warning on the perioperative use of droperidol: a review of the cases. *Anesth Analg* 2003; **96**: 1377–9.

71. Leslie JB, Gan TJ. Meta-analysis of the safety of 5-HT3 antagonists with dexamethasone or droperidol for prevention of PONV. *Ann Pharmacother* 2006; **40**: 856–72.

72. Nuttall GA, Eckerman KM, Jacob KA, *et al.* Does low-dose droperidol administration increase the risk of drug-induced QT prolongation and torsade de pointes in the general surgical population? *Anesthesiology* 2007; **107**: 531–6.

73. Charbit B, Funck-Brentano C. Droperidol-induced proarrhythmia: the beginning of an answer? *Anesthesiology* 2007; **107**: 524–6.

74. Laer S, Scholz J, Ritterbach C, *et al.* Association between increased 5-HIAA plasma concentrations and postoperative nausea and vomiting in patients undergoing general anaesthesia for surgery. *Eur J Anaesthesiol* 2001; **18**: 833–5.

75. Meneses A. Physiological, pathophysiological and therapeutic roles of 5-HT systems in learning and memory. *Rev Neurosci* 1998; **9**: 275–89.

76. Wolf H. Preclinical and clinical pharmacology of the 5-HT3 receptor antagonists. *Scand J Rheumatol Suppl* 2000; **113**: 37–45.

77. Thompson AJ, Lummis SC. The 5-HT3 receptor as a therapeutic target. *Expert Opin Ther Targets* 2007; **11**: 527–40.

78. Davies PA, Pistis M, Hanna MC, *et al.* The 5-HT3B subunit is a major determinant of serotonin-receptor function. *Nature* 1999; **397**: 359–63.

79. Brady CA, Dover TJ, Massoura AN, *et al.* Identification of 5-HT3A and 5-HT3B receptor subunits in human hippocampus. *Neuropharmacology* 2007; **52**: 1284–90.

80. Niesler B, Walstab J, Combrink S, *et al.* Characterization of the novel human serotonin receptor subunits 5-HT3C,5-HT3D, and 5-HT3E. *Mol Pharmacol* 2007; **72**: 8–17.

81. Stewart A, Davies PA, Kirkness EF, Safa P, Hales TG. Introduction of the 5-HT3B subunit alters the functional properties of 5-HT3 receptors native to neuroblastoma cells. *Neuropharmacology* 2003; **44**: 214–23.

82. Niesler B, Frank B, Kapeller J, Rappold GA. Cloning, physical mapping and expression analysis of the human 5-HT3 serotonin receptor-like genes HTR3C, HTR3D and HTR3E. *Gene* 2003; **310**: 101–11.

83. Neufeld SM, Newburn-Cook CV. The efficacy of 5-HT3 receptor antagonists for the prevention of postoperative nausea and vomiting after craniotomy: a meta-analysis. *J Neurosurg Anesthesiol* 2007; **19**: 10–17.

84. Ho KY, Gan TJ. Pharmacology, pharmacogenetics, and clinical efficacy of 5-hydroxytryptamine type 3 receptor antagonists for postoperative nausea and vomiting. *Curr Opin Anaesthesiol* 2006; **19**: 606–11.

85. Carlisle JB, Stevenson CA. Drugs for preventing postoperative nausea and vomiting. *Cochrane Database Syst Rev* 2006; **3**: CD004125.

86. Somers GI, Harris AJ, Bayliss MK, Houston JB. The metabolism of the 5HT3 antagonists ondansetron, dolasetron and GR87442 I: a comparison of in vitro and in vivo metabolism and in vitro enzyme kinetics in rat, dog and human hepatocytes, microsomes and recombinant human enzymes. *Xenobiotica* 2007; **37**: 832–54.

87. Tang J, Wang B, White PF, *et al.* The effect of timing of ondansetron administration on its efficacy, cost-effectiveness, and cost-benefit as a prophylactic antiemetic in the ambulatory setting. *Anesth Analg* 1998; **86**: 274–82.

88. Kuryshev YA, Brown AM, Wang L, Benedict CR, Rampe D. Interactions of the 5-hydroxytryptamine 3 antagonist class of antiemetic drugs with human cardiac ion channels. *J Pharmacol Exp Ther* 2000; **295**: 614–20.

89. Gan TJ. Selective serotonin 5-HT3 receptor antagonists for postoperative nausea and vomiting: are they all the same? *CNS Drugs* 2005; **19**: 225–38.

90. Moussa AA, Oregan PJ. Prevention of postoperative nausea and vomiting in patients undergoing laparoscopic bariatric surgery–granisetron alone vs granisetron combined with

dexamethasone/droperidol. *Middle East J Anesthesiol* 2007; **19**: 357–67.

91. Fujii Y, Saitoh Y, Tanaka H, Toyooka H. Granisetron/dexamethasone combination for the prevention of postoperative nausea and vomiting after laparoscopic cholecystectomy. *Eur J Anaesthesiol* 2000; **17**: 64–8.

92. Apfel CC, Kranke P, Piper S, *et al.* [Nausea and vomiting in the postoperative phase. Expert- and evidence-based recommendations for prophylaxis and therapy]. *Anaesthesist* 2007; **56**: 1170–80.

93. Rubenstein EB, Slusher BS, Rojas C, Navari RM. New approaches to chemotherapy-induced nausea and vomiting: from neuropharmacology to clinical investigations. *Cancer J* 2006; **12**: 341–7.

94. Apfel CC, Cakmakkaya OS, Frings G, *et al.* Droperidol has comparable clinical efficacy against both nausea and vomiting. *Br J Anaesth* 2009; **103**: 359–63.

95. Jokela R, Kranke P, Danzeisen O, *et al.* Ondansetron has similar clinical efficacy against both nausea and vomiting. *Anaesthesia* 2009; **64**: 147–51.

96. Apfel CC, Malhotra A, Leslie JB. The role of neurokinin-1 receptor antagonists for the management of postoperative nausea and vomiting. *Curr Opin Anaesthesiol* 2008; **21**: 427–32.

97. Gan TJ, Apfel CC, Kovac A, *et al.* A randomized, double-blind comparison of the NK1 antagonist, aprepitant, versus ondansetron for the prevention of postoperative nausea and vomiting. *Anesth Analg* 2007; **104**: 1082–9.

98. Singla NK, Singla SK, Chung F, *et al.* Phase II study to evaluate the safety and efficacy of the oral neurokinin-1 receptor antagonist casopitant (GW679769) administered with ondansetron for the prevention of postoperative and postdischarge nausea and vomiting in high-risk patients. *Anesthesiology* 2010; **113**: 74–82.

99. Warren A, King L. A review of the efficacy of dexamethasone in the prevention of postoperative nausea and vomiting. *J Clin Nurs* 2008; **17**: 58–68.

100. Henzi I, Walder B, Tramer MR. Dexamethasone for the prevention of postoperative nausea and vomiting: a quantitative systematic review. *Anesth Analg* 2000; **90**: 186–94.

101. Wang JJ, Ho ST, Lee SC, Liu YC, Ho CM. The use of dexamethasone for preventing postoperative nausea and vomiting in females undergoing thyroidectomy: a dose-ranging study. *Anesth Analg* 2000; **91**: 1404–7.

102. Wang JJ, Ho ST, Tzeng JI, Tang CS. The effect of timing of dexamethasone administration on its efficacy as a prophylactic antiemetic for postoperative nausea and vomiting. *Anesth Analg* 2000; **91**: 136–9.

103. Gan TJ, Coop A, Philip BK. A randomized, double-blind study of granisetron plus dexamethasone versus ondansetron plus dexamethasone to prevent postoperative nausea and vomiting in patients undergoing abdominal hysterectomy. *Anesth Analg* 2005; **101**: 1323–9.

104. Fujii Y, Nakayama M. Dexamethasone for reduction of nausea, vomiting and analgesic use after gynecological laparoscopic surgery. *Int J Gynaecol Obstet* 2008; **100**: 27–30.

105. Paech MJ, Rucklidge MW, Lain J, *et al.* Ondansetron and dexamethasone dose combinations for prophylaxis against postoperative nausea and vomiting. *Anesth Analg* 2007; **104**: 808–14.

106. Rusch D, Arndt C, Martin H, Kranke P. The addition of dexamethasone to dolasetron or haloperidol for treatment of established postoperative nausea and vomiting. *Anaesthesia* 2007; **62**: 810–17.

107. Bauer KP, Dom PM, Ramirez AM, O'Flaherty JE. Preoperative intravenous midazolam: benefits beyond anxiolysis. *J Clin Anesth* 2004; **16**: 177–83.

108. Lee Y, Wang JJ, Yang YL, Chen A, Lai HY. Midazolam vs ondansetron for preventing postoperative nausea and vomiting: a randomised controlled trial. *Anaesthesia* 2007; **62**: 18–22.

109. Oddby-Muhrbeck E, Eksborg S, Bergendahl HT, Muhrbeck O, Lonnqvist PA. Effects of clonidine on postoperative nausea and vomiting in breast cancer surgery. *Anesthesiology* 2002; **96**: 1109–14.

110. Watcha MF, Simeon RM, White PF, Stevens JL. Effect of propofol on the incidence of postoperative vomiting after strabismus surgery in pediatric outpatients. *Anesthesiology* 1991; **75**: 204–9.

111. Visser K, Hassink EA, Bonsel GJ, Moen J, Kalkman CJ. Randomized controlled trial of total intravenous anesthesia with propofol versus inhalation anesthesia with isoflurane-nitrous oxide: postoperative nausea with vomiting and economic analysis. *Anesthesiology* 2001; **95**: 616–26.

112. Cechetto DF, Diab T, Gibson CJ, Gelb AW. The effects of propofol in the area postrema of rats. *Anesth Analg* 2001; **92**: 934–42.

113. Tramer MR. A rational approach to the control of postoperative nausea and vomiting: evidence from systematic reviews. Part I. Efficacy and harm of antiemetic interventions, and methodological issues. *Acta Anaesthesiol Scand* 2001; **45**: 4–13.

114. Koivuranta M, Laara E, Snare L, Alahuhta S. A survey of postoperative nausea and vomiting. *Anaesthesia* 1997; **52**: 443–9.

115. Junger A, Michel A, Benson M, *et al.* Evaluation of the suitability of a patient data management system for ICUs on a general ward. *Int J Med Inform* 2001; **64**: 57–66.

116. Sinclair DR, Chung F, Mezei G. Can postoperative nausea and vomiting be predicted? *Anesthesiology* 1999; **91**: 109–18.

117. Apfel CC, Kranke P, Eberhart LH, Roos A, Roewer N. Comparison of predictive models for postoperative nausea and vomiting. *Br J Anaesth* 2002; **88**: 234–40.

118. van den Bosch JE, Kalkman CJ, Vergouwe Y, *et al.* Assessing the applicability of scoring systems for predicting postoperative nausea and vomiting. *Anaesthesia* 2005; **60**: 323–31.

119. Eberhart LH, Geldner G, Kranke P, *et al.* The development and validation of a risk score to predict the probability of postoperative vomiting in pediatric patients. *Anesth Analg* 2004; **99**: 1630–7.

120. Eberhart LH, Morin AM, Guber D, *et al.* Applicability of risk scores for postoperative nausea and vomiting in

adults to paediatric patients. *Br J Anaesth* 2004; **93**: 386–92.

121. Apfel CC, Korttila K, Abdalla M, *et al.* An international multicenter protocol to assess the single and combined benefits of antiemetic interventions in a controlled clinical trial of a 2×2×2×2×2×2 factorial design (IMPACT). *Control Clin Trials* 2003; **24**: 736–51.

122. Habib AS, White WD, Eubanks S, Pappas TN, Gan TJ. A randomized comparison of a multimodal management strategy versus combination antiemetics for the prevention of postoperative nausea and vomiting. *Anesth Analg* 2004; **99**: 77–81.

Section 3
Chapter

55

Essential drugs in anesthetic practice
Insulin and antihyperglycemic drugs

Nick Oliver, Martin Smith, and Stephen Robinson

Introduction

To use insulin appropriately it is necessary to understand how glucose uptake and utilization is regulated. Insulin is administered for the treatment of insulin deficiency and insulin resistance in diabetes mellitus. Type 1 and type 2 diabetes represent chronic disorders with symptoms associated with acute metabolic complications, chronic complications, and increased mortality rates. The chronic complications can be classified into microvascular (retinopathy, nephropathy, and neuropathy) and macrovascular (atherosclerosis causing coronary artery, cerebrovascular, and peripheral vascular disease). The metabolic actions of insulin are summarized in Table 55.1. The diabetic patient undergoing surgery is in a vulnerable state brought about by derangements in glucose uptake and utilization that complicate the perioperative period. These need to be fully understood if the diabetic surgical patient is to avoid adverse consequences.

Glucose homeostasis

Pancreatic islets of Langerhans have three cell populations involved in the synthesis, storage, and secretion of hormones responsible for glucose homeostasis. Alpha cells synthesize glucagon, β cells synthesize insulin, and δ cells synthesize somatostatin. The islets are innervated by parasympathetic and sympathetic neurons. Insulin and glucagon operate in a reciprocal manner to maintain blood glucose concentration within the physiological range, and they directly modify the secretion of one another by paracrine and endocrine action. Somatostatin inhibits the secretions of insulin and glucagon.

Intact homeostatic mechanisms maintain plasma glucose within the range of 4–8 mmol L^{-1} despite wide variation in dietary intake and metabolic expenditure to ensure continuous delivery of glucose to the central nervous system (CNS). Glucose is taken up from the plasma in an insulin-independent manner by the glucose 1 transporter (GLUT1) within the blood–brain barrier and enters the CNS along a concentration gradient. When plasma glucose decreases to less than

Table 55.1. The physiological effects of insulin

Stimulation	Inhibition
Glucose uptake into skeletal muscle and adipose tissue (GLUT-4-mediated)	Gluconeogenesis
Amino acid uptake and protein synthesis in muscle	Proteolysis
Lipogenesis	Lipolysis and ketogenesis
Glycogen synthesis	Glycogenolysis
Activity of Na^+/K^+ ATPase pump	Glucagon secretion
Nitric oxide synthesis	
Renal sodium reabsorption	

3.7 mmol L^{-1}, GLUT1 activity becomes rate-limiting for cerebral function [1].

Postprandial state

The most potent stimulus for insulin secretion is an increase in plasma glucose. This is achieved through two mechanisms:

- Increased peripheral glucose uptake, predominantly into muscle, mediated through the GLUT4 transporter.
- Suppression of hepatic glucose output by inhibition of gluconeogenesis and glycogenolysis.

The postprandial actions of insulin are summarized in Fig. 55.1.

The insulin response to glucose is larger for an oral load than for an intravenous infusion. This is referred to as the *incretin effect*, and is because oral intake causes the release of glycogen-like peptide 1 (GLP-1) and glucose-dependent insulinotropic polypeptide (GIP) from the gastrointestinal mucosa, which augment the β-cell response.

Fasted state

During the fasted state, reduced insulin concentration and the counterregulatory hormones glucagon, epinephrine, growth hormone, and cortisol are required for the maintenance

Anesthetic Pharmacology, 2nd edition, ed. Alex S. Evers, Mervyn Maze, Evan D. Kharasch. Published by Cambridge University Press. © Cambridge University Press 2011.

A

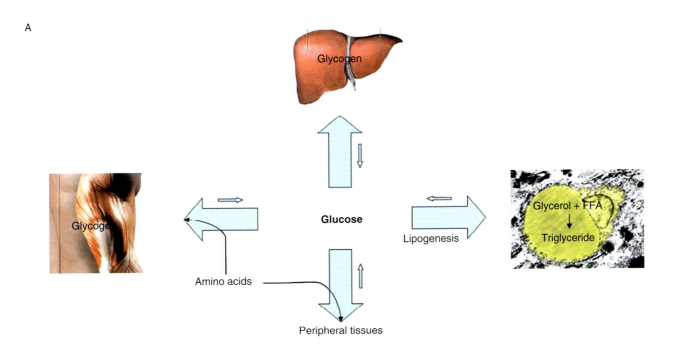

B

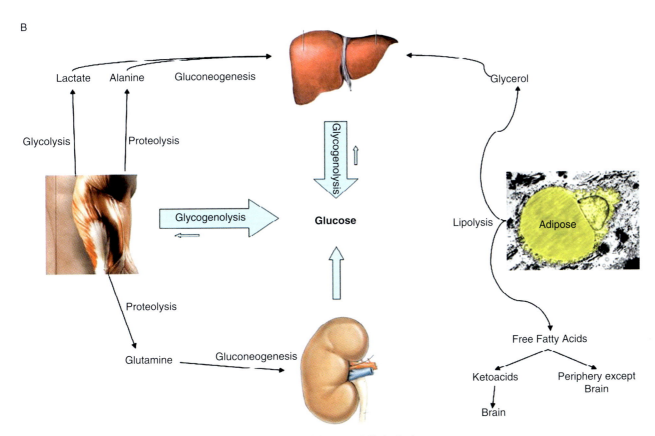

Figure 55.1. Summary of glucose metabolism in (A) the postprandial state and (B) the fasting state.

of normoglycemia. Fasting glucose homeostasis is summarized in Fig. 55.1.

Glycogen provides the most immediately accessible source of energy consumed during fasting. A decrease in plasma glucose concentration inhibits insulin secretion and stimulates release of glucagon. Glucagon acts through generation of cyclic adenosine monophosphate (cAMP), increasing hepatic glucose output by stimulation of hepatic glycogenolysis. Physical activity depletes muscle glycogen and increases the delivery of lactate to the liver, where it is used as substrate for gluconeogenesis.

During a prolonged fast, hepatic glycogen stores become exhausted. The combination of increased concentrations of glucagon, epinephrine, growth hormone, and cortisol with a low concentration of insulin promotes lipolysis and proteolysis. Hormone-sensitive lipase is activated, which metabolizes triglyceride in adipose tissue to glycerol and free fatty acids (FFAs). Glycerol is metabolized in the liver by gluconeogenic pathways, increasing hepatic glucose output. FFAs are used as an alternative energy substrate to glucose by most tissues except the brain.

Ketoacids are produced from fatty acids, as a result of chronic lipolysis, when the capacity of the Krebs cycle to metabolize acetyl coenzyme A is exceeded. In these circumstances, acetyl coenzyme A is metabolized to the ketoacids acetoacetate and 3-hydroxybutyrate. A small proportion of acetoacetate is spontaneously broken down to acetone, which is exhaled. Ketogenesis is important because the brain is able to use ketoacids as an alternative fuel source. Proteolysis of skeletal muscle provides substrate for gluconeogenesis by increasing hepatic delivery of alanine. Significant gluconeogenesis occurs also in the kidney, where glutamine is the preferred substrate.

Glucose intolerance and insulin resistance

Glucose intolerance may be a consequence of two processes: insulin resistance or insulin deficiency. Insulin resistance is common in conditions such as sepsis, hypertension, ischemic heart disease, and pregnancy, or during such procedures as cardiac surgery.

Insulin resistance occurs when a cell, tissue, system, or whole body requires increased insulin concentration for a given effect. It is strongly associated with an increased cardiovascular risk [2] and is associated with polycystic ovary syndrome and reduced postprandial energy expenditure [3]. The main defect is an impaired insulin-mediated phosphatidylinositol-3-kinase (PI3K) signal that leads to a decrease in the recruitment of GLUT4 transport proteins to the plasma membrane and consequently reduced glucose uptake [1]. Compensatory hyperinsulinemia is required to overcome the peripheral resistance to insulin action and maintain normoglycemia.

Insulin resistance reduces feedback inhibition of glucagon production. Increased glucagon concentrations stimulate hepatic glycogenolysis and gluconeogenesis, and insulin resistance leads to reduced insulin-induced suppression of hepatic glucose output. Chronic hyperglycemia downregulates the

glucose transport system and exacerbates the tendency to hyperglycemia also [4]. This is glucose toxicity, which is alleviated by restoration to euglycemia [5].

Insulin resistance is associated with a prothrombotic disposition and increased inflammation. An increased fibrinogen concentration is seen along with a decreased capacity for fibrinolysis secondary to a rise in plasminogen activator inhibitor 1 (PAI-1). In addition to this, platelet aggregation is increased.

The metabolic syndrome

The metabolic syndrome is a cluster of related cardiovascular risk factors with several diagnostic criteria. In 2006, the International Diabetes Federation defined the metabolic syndrome as central obesity plus any two of raised triglyceride concentration, reduced high-density lipoprotein (HDL) cholesterol concentration, raised blood pressure, or raised fasting plasma glucose [6].

The metabolic syndrome is also a proinflammatory state. Inflammatory cytokines including adipocyte tumor necrosis factor α (TNFα), interleukin 6 (IL-6), and C-reactive protein are all increased and adiponectin concentration is reduced. These circulating inflammatory changes alter insulin cell signaling and increase FFA flux.

Insulin resistance, where a greater amount of insulin is required for the same physiological effect, is a prominent feature of the metabolic syndrome and is related to the central adiposity seen. Patients with the metabolic syndrome are at a greater risk of developing coronary artery disease than controls and have a threefold increase in the risk of myocardial infarction or stroke, with double the mortality of patients without the syndrome following such an event [7].

Metabolic response to surgery and trauma

Trauma and surgery, changes in circulating volume with hemorrhage, and infection (local or systemic) all lead to a stress response. The increased concentrations of catecholamines and glucocorticoids seen in stress contribute to or exacerbate insulin resistance. Sympathetic activity, through stimulation of α_2-adrenoceptors in the pancreas, reduces insulin secretion, contributing to relative insulin deficiency.

Relative and absolute insulin deficiencies lead to catabolism with lipolysis in adipocytes and ketogenesis. Proteolysis occurs, and increased hepatic glucose output from gluconeogenesis and glycogenolysis is seen. These changes are more pronounced in individuals with pre-existing diabetes, leading to increased insulin requirements at times of surgery, trauma, and acute physiological stress.

During surgery, blood loss has an independent correlation with postoperative insulin resistance [8], and the stress response seen is proportional to the duration of surgery, with reduced glucose utilization after longer surgical procedures [9]. Plasma insulin and IL-6 concentration changes are matched during the perioperative period. IL-6, an inflammatory cytokine, reduces insulin sensitivity by an effect on GLUT4 activity and lipid metabolism, while adipokines secreted during surgery such as TNFα have a similar action [10].

In the perioperative insulin-resistant state, FFA concentrations rise. FFAs and their metabolites reduce PI3K activity, further reducing GLUT4 expression and exacerbating ongoing insulin resistance [11].

Clinical data from studies of outcomes following surgery in patients with diabetes suggest that suboptimal perioperative glycemic control is an independent risk factor for unfavorable outcomes including cardiovascular events, infection, prolonged hospital stay, and death [12,13]. Hyperglycemia perioperatively impairs monocyte activation and oxidative burst and leads to glycosylation of immunoproteins [14]. Amplification of injury-induced inflammation has also been observed in hyperglycemia.

Patients with pre-existing diabetic states frequently require insulin during surgery, regardless of preoperative treatment. At present, there is not an evidence base to support the use of insulin for surgery in the insulin-resistant patient without hyperglycemia.

Insulin biosynthesis and release

Insulin is cosecreted with C-peptide in equimolar concentrations. Only insulin that has intrinsic biologic activity and products of insulin protein biosynthesis (proinsulin, split fragments, and C-peptide) have no effect on glucose homeostasis.

Depolarization of the β-cell membrane is coupled to exocytosis of secretory granules containing mature insulin when blood glucose rises to > 7 mmol L^{-1}. These secretory granules contain a rapidly available store of insulin, allowing large changes in the magnitude of insulin secretion.

Regulation of insulin action

Insulin delivery to target tissues

Optimal delivery of insulin to target tissues is dependent on an adequate circulation to capillary beds, migration across the endothelium, and passage through interstitial fluid to the target insulin receptor. The major rate-limiting sites for insulin action are at the postreceptor level in the target cell [15].

The insulin signal

Insulin's major actions on carbohydrate, lipid, and protein metabolism are initiated through binding to cell-membrane insulin receptors in muscle, liver, and adipose tissue. This triggers a cascade of intracellular events mediated by tyrosine kinase activation and involving multiple pathway activation, including protein synthesis, glycogen synthesis, lipid synthesis, and translocation of the glucose transport protein, GLUT4, to the plasma membrane [16].

Insulin degradation

The plasma half-life of insulin, after endogenous β-cell secretion, is estimated at 4–6 minutes, with a plasma clearance of 8–18 mL min^{-1} kg^{-1} [17]. Metabolism of insulin by intracellular proteolysis is the predominant method of elimination. Excretion of intact insulin by the kidney is minimal. Subsequent to the binding of insulin to its receptor, proteolysis occurs in liver (80%) and kidney (15%), with the liver removing 50% of the portal secreted load of insulin through a first-pass effect. The kidney, however, removes 50% of insulin that enters the systemic circulation, leading to decreased exogenous insulin requirements in renal disease [18]. Skeletal muscle, adipose tissue, and skin also make minor contributions to insulin degradation.

Within the physiological range, elimination of insulin is linear, but in the presence of persistently high concentrations of insulin (supraphysiological or pharmacological), the relation between clearance and concentration becomes nonlinear, demonstrating saturation kinetics.

There is evidence that insulin resistance is associated with slower metabolic clearance of insulin, and this may contribute to the peripheral hyperinsulinemia. This has been demonstrated in type 2 diabetes, obesity, and hypertension [19,20]. In obesity, reduction of body mass index is associated with reduced insulin concentration, predominantly through increased clearance [21].

Development and administration of insulin as a drug

Insulin is manufactured in solution or suspension standardized to a concentration of 100 U mL^{-1} (U100), although more concentrated solutions (U500) are available for those whose insulin requirements are exceptionally high. Insulin should be stored in a refrigerator. The "insulin unit" is an expression of bioequivalence among different insulin preparations.

The manufacture of human insulin by recombinant DNA technology enables mass production of a variety of insulins on a scale not possible with the previous methods of extraction and purification of animal insulin. Human insulin causes fewer hypersensitivity reactions than animal insulin, and lipoatrophy of injection sites is not seen. Lipohypertrophy is a consequence of subcutaneous insulin.

Routes of administration

The major routes of administration of insulin are subcutaneous, intravenous, and intramuscular. Insulin is inactivated rapidly by proteases in the upper gastrointestinal tract and therefore cannot be given orally. The delivery of insulin into either the upper or lower respiratory tract can produce systemic insulin concentrations similar to subcutaneous administration.

Subcutaneous is the most widely used route of administration. Administration into the subcutaneous tissues differs from endogenous insulin secretion in two significant aspects: the kinetics do not mimic the normal rapid increase and decrease of native insulin secretion in response to ingestion of food, and the insulin diffuses into the systemic rather than the portal circulation. Therefore, the first-pass effects of insulin action on the liver that obtains during a meal do not occur.

The recommended sites for subcutaneous administration are the anterior abdominal wall, anterior or lateral aspect of the thigh, or the upper lateral aspect of the arm. Some variability of absorption occurs between sites. With repeated insulin administration at one site, lipohypertrophy may develop. Therefore, it is recommended that injection sites are rotated. Lipohypertrophy may cause variability in insulin absorption.

Continuous subcutaneous insulin infusion (CSII) is achieved using a syringe pump, which delivers soluble regular insulin or a rapid acting insulin analog at a basal rate that attempts to mimic background endogenous insulin secretion. This is typically within the range of 0.1–1.0 U per hour. In addition, the pump is able to administer intermittent bolus doses given before meal times or to correct hyperglycemia [22]. Because the insulin administered has a short duration of action and there is only a minimal subcutaneous insulin depot, there is a faster onset of ketoacidosis should there be a failure of insulin delivery.

The intravenous route of administration is used in the management of diabetic hyperglycemic emergencies and in the perioperative period, when the patient is unable, or not permitted, to take food by mouth. Soluble or rapid-acting analog insulin is given intravenously because the short half-life allows rapid adjustment of insulin delivery according to blood glucose concentration and the clinical condition.

The intramuscular route of administration of soluble insulin may be used in diabetic hyperglycemic emergency states, when there is delay in the administration of intravenous insulin. The absorption of insulin from muscle can be compromised significantly in circulatory failure, and therefore intravenous administration is the preferred route.

Pharmacokinetics of the available insulin

The kinetics of synthetic insulin can be altered either through changes to the amino acid sequence of insulin or by the addition of a zinc salt or protamine to form a suspension. Moreover, the degree of crystallization of zinc insulin suspension is also important. These modifications have a major impact on the speed of onset, time to peak effect, and duration of action of subcutaneous insulin (Table 55.2).

Soluble regular insulin

Human, porcine, and bovine insulin are available as soluble insulin to be injected 30 minutes before meals. The time for hexameric insulin aggregates to dissociate into insulin monomers and their consequent absorption is responsible for the delay in onset of action [23].

Table 55.2. Pharmacokinetic characteristics of the commonly used insulins

	Onset (h)	Peak (h)	Duration (h)
Soluble regular	0.5–1	2–3	4–6
Rapid-acting analog	<0.25–0.5	0.5–1.5	2–3
Long-acting analog	1–2	Peakless	20–24
Isophane	2–4	4–8	10–15
Insulin zinc suspension	2–4	7–15	15–24

Long-acting analog insulins glargine and detemir are closer to a square wave response.

Soluble regular insulin is used in subcutaneous multiple insulin injection regimens, when it is administered before meals and long-acting insulin is injected at night.

Isophane protamine insulin (NPH insulin)

NPH (neutral protamine Hagedorn) insulin is a suspension of human, porcine, or bovine isophane insulin with protamine. The addition of protamine slows the speed of onset of action and lengthens the duration of effect of this insulin.

Isophane insulin is most commonly administered in a manufactured mixture with soluble regular insulin (biphasic isophane insulin) or with an analog (biphasic isophane insulin analog). When used in combination with an insulin analog, there is a faster onset of action and time to peak effect.

Insulin zinc suspension and protamine zinc insulin suspension

Human, porcine, and bovine insulin are available as salts in combination with zinc and protamine. This prolongs the action of insulin over 24 hours but increases the risk of hypoglycemia.

Insulin analogs

Insulin analogs are molecular-engineered human insulin. The amino acid sequence of analogs may be changed, or they may be bound to moieties that alter the pharmacology of the insulin. Insulin analogs may be rapid-acting or long-acting and are available in premixed form.

Rapid-acting analogs

Rapid-acting insulin analogs exist as monomeric insulin only. This ensures a faster onset of action and time to peak effect, with a shorter duration of action than soluble regular insulin. Their kinetic profile is therefore similar to that of endogenous insulin and helps to reduce postprandial glucose excursions. They are also associated with a lower incidence of hypoglycemia and improved patient compliance, as they may be administered during or even after a meal. Insulin lispro and insulin aspart are the most widely prescribed rapid analogs.

Rapid-acting analogs are used in multiple injection regimens, CSII, and twice-daily insulin regimens.

Long-acting analogs

Insulin glargine and insulin detemir are the most commonly used long-acting insulins. Insulin glargine has an amino acid substitution, with two amino acids added to the carboxy terminal of the B chain. This allows the formation of hexamers subcutaneously which are slow to dissociate. Peakless absorption occurs over a period of up to 24 hours. Insulin detemir is created by attaching a C_{14} fatty acid moiety. Insulin detemir is albumin-bound in plasma, slowing its action. These long-acting analogs provide peakless basal insulin profiles, improving glycemic control and reducing the likelihood of fasting hypoglycemia.

Maintenance treatment of diabetes mellitus

Type 1 diabetes mellitus

Type 1 diabetes mellitus is a state of absolute insulin deficiency caused by failure of the islet β cells. The incidence is less than 0.5% of the population, although the rate is increasing. All patients require lifelong insulin therapy.

The destruction of the β-cell unit is a cell-mediated autoimmune response associated with circulating antibodies to its structural components and secretions. The precipitant of this autoimmune process is unknown, but there is a genetic susceptibility operating through the HLA-DR4 genotype.

The Diabetes Control and Complications Trial (DCCT) showed conclusively that intensive glycemic control of type 1 diabetes mellitus, with either bolus subcutaneous insulin or CSII, reduces the incidence rates of microvascular complications by 60–70% [24].

There are three subcutaneous insulin regimens that attempt to achieve this goal:

(1) **Basal bolus** – Soluble or rapid-acting analog insulin is given before meals and long-acting insulin at night.
(2) **Twice daily** – Biphasic mixed insulin is given before breakfast and evening meal.
(3) **CSII** – Continuous infusion (see above).

Type 2 diabetes mellitus

Type 2 diabetes mellitus is a progressive metabolic disorder of insulin resistance, in association with hyperglycemia, which is accompanied commonly by progressive β-cell failure and relative insulin deficiency [25]. It is a multifactorial disorder, with genetic and environmental factors playing a significant role [26]. The prevalence varies with ethnic group from 2% in Europeans to 35% in Pima Indians.

Treatment consists of diet and weight reduction, in combination with oral hypoglycemic drugs (Table 55.3).

Metformin is the only available biguanide. It activates protein kinase A (PKA), decreasing hepatic glucose production, increasing peripheral insulin sensitivity, and reducing fatty acid oxidation. It is first-line management in type 2 diabetes, particularly in overweight patients as it limits weight gain, in contrast with other therapies for type 2 diabetes which increase weight. In addition to its use in diabetes, metformin is also used in polycystic ovarian syndrome. It is contraindicated in moderate renal impairment and should be stopped for the duration of any radiological investigation requiring radio-opaque contrast media. Metformin is associated with an increased risk of lactic acidosis and should be avoided in patients with a history of lactic acidosis or with comorbidities increasing their risk.

The commonest side effects of metformin include nausea, abdominal cramp, and diarrhea that may limit the dose tolerated. Modified-release metformin is available with an improved gastrointestinal side-effect profile.

Sulfonylureas are insulin secretagogues acting on the pancreatic β cell through ATP-dependent potassium channels to cause tonic depolarization. Sulfonylureas reduce glucose and may cause hypoglycemia, particularly in the elderly and particularly in long-acting formulations. They are associated with weight gain, and do not have evidence supporting their use in improving diabetes-related outcomes. They are, however, a very useful treatment of hyperglycemia and are, in many patients, second-line management, added to metformin. Sulfonylureas should be avoided in liver failure because of the significantly increased risk of hypoglycemia.

Thiazolidinediones (TZD) are insulin sensitizers which bind to peroxisome proliferator-activated receptor γ (PPARγ), modulating gene transcription. In common with sulfonylureas, TZDs treat hyperglycemia but cause weight gain. TZDs are also associated with edema and increased hospital admissions for congestive heart failure. Two TZDs are available: rosiglitazone and pioglitazone. Pioglitazone has been shown to reduce fatal and nonfatal myocardial infarction in type 2 diabetes patients in one study, but this was a secondary endpoint [27]. Rosiglitazone has shown no cardiovascular benefit in clinical trials.

Postprandial glucose regulators include the meglitinides and α-glucosidase inhibitors. Meglitinides are short-acting insulin secretagogues with a similar mode of action to sulfonylureas. They reduce postprandial glucose excursions but are associated with weight gain and hypoglycemia. α-glucosidase inhibitors act in the gastrointestinal tract to inhibit disaccharide hydrolysis, slowing carbohydrate absorption postprandially. They cause a small fall in HbA1c but are associated with significant dose-related flatulence.

Glycogen-like peptide 1 (GLP-1) analogs have been licensed for use in the treatment of type 2 diabetes. GLP-1 increases insulin secretion in a glucose-dependent manner (thereby minimizing the risk of hypoglycemia), reduces glucagon secretion, and delays gastric emptying, increasing satiety.

Table 55.3. Oral hypoglycemic drugs

Class	Example	Mechanism of action	Duration of action	Additional benefits	Principal side effects	Contraindications
Biguanide	Metformin	Intracellular cAMP messaging	3–4 h	Reduced macrovascular risk	Nausea, gastrointestinal disturbance	Renal impairment
Insulin sensitizer						
Sulfonylurea	Gliclazide	Bind to K$_{ATP}$ on β cell membrane	12–24 h	Nil	Hypoglycemia	Liver disease
Insulin secretagogue	Glibenclamide				Weight gain	
Thiazolidinediones	Pioglitazone	PPARγ agonist	12–24 h	Pioglitazone – reduction in fatal/ nonfatal MI (secondary endpoint)	Edema	Cardiac failure
Insulin sensitizer	Rosiglitazone				Weight gain	Insulin treatment
DPP4 inhibitor	Sitagliptin	DPP4 inhibition	6–12 h	Weight-neutral	Nausea	—
Potentiates endogenous GLP-1	Vildagliptin					
Meglitinides	Repaglinide	Bind to K$_{ATP}$ on β cell membrane	2–3 h	Nil	Hypoglycemia	—
Insulin secretagogue	Nateglinide				Weight gain	
α-Glucosidase inhibitor	Acarbose	α-Glucosidase inhibition	3–4 h	Nil	Flatulence	—
Postprandial glucose regulator					Diarrhea	

GLP-1 is rapidly metabolized by dipeptidyl peptidase 4 (DPP4), with a half-life of approximately 2 minutes. Modified analogs are injected subcutaneously. Glycemic control is improved with GLP-1 analogs to a level comparable with that provided by insulin, but they are associated with weight loss, providing a major advantage.

DPP4 inhibitors are also licensed for use in type 2 diabetes. These are oral drugs which prolong the activity of endogenous GLP-1. They have similar effects to the GLP-1 analogs, with improved glycemic control and weight loss. DPP4 is a ubiquitous enzyme involved in multiple pathways, but no effects of inhibition on other systems have been demonstrated.

The UK Prospective Diabetes Study established that intensive glycemic control reduces the incidence of microvascular complications in type 2 diabetes, and intensive control achieved with metformin reduces macrovascular events [28]. In addition, intensive blood pressure treatment reduces the incidence of microvascular and macrovascular events [29].

The principal indication for insulin therapy in type 2 diabetes is unsatisfactory glycemic control, despite attention to diet and compliance with maximal oral medication. Insulin therapy is associated with weight gain, which is undesirable in the patient who is already overweight and insulin-resistant. Insulin can be used in combination with metformin or a sulfonylurea, which may reduce insulin requirements [30]. In the patient who is overweight, the combination of metformin or an insulin sensitizer with one or two injections of insulin daily is an effective treatment for patients requiring insulin [31].

Perioperative management of diabetes mellitus

In contrast to the patient with normal glucose tolerance, the patient with diabetes mellitus is at greater risk for an adverse event during the perioperative period. Some of this risk is predictable and is caused by preoperative factors that can be modified or assessed before surgery.

Preoperative factors

Patients with diabetes carry a significant cardiovascular risk and are therefore more likely to suffer an acute coronary event, cardiac failure, or a stroke. Attempts should be made to assess and minimize this risk before elective surgery, with attention to blood pressure control, weight reduction, left ventricular function, coronary ischemia, renal function, proteinuria, and hyperlipidemia. Unless the medical and metabolic states are optimal, it is generally safer to delay surgery.

Obesity may lead to problems with intubation, ventilation, and postoperative atelectasis and pulmonary infection. There is the additional risk for thromboembolic disease and skin necrosis over pressure points, which should be prevented with appropriate prophylaxis. The obese patient also may be slower to rehabilitate after major surgery.

Delayed wound healing and sepsis are more common in diabetes, and this relates in part to poor glycemic control and ischemia, but there is an increased susceptibility to wound complications from the diabetic state. Glycemic control should be optimized before surgery to minimize this risk, and optimal metabolic control should be the aim over the entire perioperative period.

Subjects with insulin-treated diabetes mellitus should be admitted 24 hours before elective major surgery. If metabolic control is poor, then admission may need to be earlier. Subjects taking long-acting sulfonylureas should be changed to short-duration drugs to reduce the risk of fasting hypoglycemia in the preoperative period.

Perioperative and postoperative metabolic control

The management of perioperative glycemic control is best considered according to the treatment used to manage diabetes before surgery, the nature of the surgical procedure, and its anticipated duration. The risk for hypoglycemia as a result of fasting on the day of surgery can be minimized. Not all patients require treatment with intravenous insulin. Some surgical procedures, particularly cardiac surgery, cause particular insulin resistance. The glucose-rich solutions, inotropes, and metabolic consequences of hypothermia all contribute to this process. Surgery is a catabolic process, being performed during fasting and stimulating catecholamines, cortisol, and inflammatory changes with rises in anorectic cytokines such as TNF. These catabolic factors occur in all surgery, but in absolute insulin deficiency must be counteracted with insulin. In states of relative insulin deficiency, an insulin infusion should be considered.

If an intravenous insulin infusion is required, capillary glucose monitoring at least every 2 hours is essential. Intravenous insulin should not be discontinued in insulin-treated patients; if hypoglycemia occurs despite low intravenous insulin infusion rates, the dextrose infusion should be increased.

- **Glucose–insulin–potassium infusion regimen** – This is the simpler of the intravenous regimens because the infusates are all contained within one infusion bag. It is infused at a constant rate of 100mL h^{-1}. Because only one intravenous line is required, this eliminates the risk for an unidentified line or pump failure (increasing the risk for hypoglycemia or hyperglycemia) with the use of multiple lines. If adjustments are required to achieve target glucose concentrations, a different glucose–insulin–potassium mixture is made up. Potassium is required to prevent insulin-induced hypokalemia.
- **Intravenous insulin sliding scale** – Intravenous soluble insulin (1 U mL^{-1}) is given as an infusion using a pump adjusted to a rate appropriate to ambient capillary glucose measurements. A 5% glucose solution is co-infused to prevent hypoglycemia. This regimen provides more flexibility for insulin adjustment and is the ideal regimen if large fluctuations in blood glucose are anticipated (e.g., cardiopulmonary bypass surgery or parenteral nutrition therapy). Intravenous insulin requirements for sliding scales can be estimated in patients treated with insulin from the total daily maintenance subcutaneous dose. The intravenous insulin infusion rate per hour required for an ambient capillary glucose of 4–8 mmol L^{-1} approximates to the maintenance hourly subcutaneous insulin requirement.

No specific medical therapy (diet-controlled)

If minor surgery is planned, and prior glycemic control is satisfactory, patients may require no specific intervention, other than capillary glucose monitoring, for a short procedure. With major surgery, blood glucose concentrations should be checked up to four times per hour; if persistent hyperglycemia develops (glucose > 10 mmol L^{-1}), intravenous insulin should be considered.

There is no evidence to suggest that insulin should be used in all patients with diabetes undergoing surgery, and hypoglycemia is associated with poor outcomes and should be avoided.

In all patients with diabetes undergoing surgery it is important to consider cardiovascular risk, and for this reason adequate hypertensive and lipid control must be considered perioperatively. It has been suggested that statins improve postoperative outcomes and should be restarted as soon as possible postoperatively [32].

Oral drugs

Oral drugs should be discontinued on the day of surgery. Long-acting sulfonylureas should have been changed previously to short-duration drugs. Metformin should be discontinued before a procedure involving contrast media if the creatinine is elevated.

If minor surgery is planned, and prior glycemic control is satisfactory, patients may require no specific intervention for a short procedure. Blood glucose concentrations should be checked up to four times per hour; if persistent hyperglycemia develops (glucose > 10 mmol L^{-1}), intravenous insulin should be considered. If major surgery is planned, intravenous insulin should be commenced before surgery. When the patient is eating and drinking normally after surgery, oral therapy can be restarted. Patients are more insulin-resistant in the postoperative period due to an increase in stress hormone (cortisol, epinephrine, growth hormone) secretion and inflammation which downregulates GLUT4 expression and increases FFA concentrations. Therefore, patients may require subcutaneous insulin for a short time if oral therapy does not ensure euglycemia.

Insulin therapy

Ideally, patients treated with insulin should be first on a morning operating schedule. This reduces the inconvenience of an insulin infusion in preparation for later surgery. In addition, the risk for overnight and early morning hypoglycemia should be reduced by a small meal at night if blood glucose levels are less than 8 mmol L^{-1}. If patients are scheduled for afternoon surgery, an early light breakfast should be offered with administration of subcutaneous soluble insulin. An insulin infusion should be started from mid-morning.

The normal dose of subcutaneous insulin should be restarted when the patient is eating and drinking adequately. There should be an overlap of 30 minutes between the administration of subcutaneous insulin and the discontinuation of the intravenous infusion, to prevent insulin deficiency. Subcutaneous insulin requirements in the postoperative period can be estimated from the amount of intravenous insulin required

during the previous 24 hours. Maintenance insulin can then be adjusted in accordance with the amount of additional soluble insulin required during the previous day.

Emergency management of diabetes mellitus

The common metabolic emergencies of diabetes are:
- diabetic ketoacidosis
- hyperglycemic hyperosmolar state
- hypoglycemia

The management of hyperglycemic emergencies is summarized in Table 55.4.

Diabetic ketoacidosis

Diabetic ketoacidosis (DKA) occurs following prolonged insulin deficiency. It is characterized by the presence of ketoacids and acidosis, and usually occurs with hyperglycemia, which may be marked. Mortality rates have been quoted at 1–4% in unselected cases, but prognosis is significantly worse in advanced ketoacidosis (5–10%) [33]. Adverse outcomes are related to infection, multiple organ failure, adult respiratory distress syndrome, acute pancreatitis, cerebral edema, coronary heart and cerebrovascular disease, coma, or electrolyte disturbance. In children, there is a greater frequency of cerebral edema as a cause of death [34].

Table 55.4. Management of hyperglycemic emergencies

Intervention	Diabetic ketoacidosis	Hyperglycemic hyperosmolar state
Fluid resuscitation	Normal saline	Normal saline
	Can be infused rapidly	Infuse slowly with close monitoring
	Apparent hyperkalemia may mask total-body potassium deficit	Correct osmolality by maximum 5 mOsm per hour
	Aggressive potassium replacement with regular monitoring	Normal potassium requirement 5% dextrose when capillary glucose < 10–15 mmol L^{-1}
	5% dextrose when capillary glucose < 10–15 mmol L^{-1}	Hypotonic saline used with caution
Insulin	Intravenous insulin	Low-dose intravenous insulin
	Intramuscular insulin if delay	Correct osmolality by maximum 5 mOsm per hour
	Acidosis is insulin-resistant state, may need to titrate insulin dose	
	Intravenous insulin can be stopped when normoglycemic, nonketotic, and eating	
Other measures	Low threshold for antibiotics	Broad-spectrum antibiotics recommended in all cases
	Anticoagulant prophylaxis	Full anticoagulation
		Assess for complications including pancreatitis, rhabdomyolysis, arterial thrombus, acute coronary syndrome

Seventeen percent of patients with diabetic ketoacidosis have new-onset type 1 diabetes. The common causes of decompensation of known diabetes are infection, noncompliance with treatment, inappropriate insulin dose alteration, and new diagnosis. In older patients, acute coronary events and stroke also are likely causes.

Hyperglycemia in DKA may only be modest; it is the metabolic acidosis and ketonemia that lead to the early presentation of DKA compared with the relatively late presentation of the hyperglycemic hyperosmolar state in type 2 diabetes. Euglycemic ketoacidosis occurs in malnutrition, liver disease and in patients who have ingested excess alcohol, preventing gluconeogenesis. Ketoacidosis must, therefore, be excluded in any unwell diabetic, regardless of glucose concentration. Euglycemic ketoacidosis has a worse prognosis than hyperglycemic ketoacidosis.

Four clinical factors contribute to the development of ketoacidosis:
(1) Insulin deficiency occurs with β-cell loss.
(2) Increased stress hormones (e.g., catecholamines, cortisol, glucagon, and growth hormone) exacerbate hyperglycemia, causing an osmotic diuresis with water and electrolyte loss.
(3) The insulin deficiency and stress hormones accelerate lipolysis and ketogenesis, which in turn will be exacerbated by fasting.
(4) Dehydation is a late additional insult. The kidney is able to buffer ketoacids until dehydration leads to poor renal perfusion with failed distal convoluted tubule function.
Hyperkalemia results from the systemic acidosis and Na^+/K^+ ATPase pump failure. There will be a total-body deficit of potassium that must be addressed.

Ketoacidosis can occur also in type 2 diabetes and is therefore not entirely indicative of the true insulin dependency of type 1 diabetes. In Afro-Caribbean and Chinese patients, ketoacidosis as the presentation of type 2 diabetes is being increasingly recognized [35]. This syndrome is more common in obese patients and in the presence of acanthosis nigricans.

The management of the patient with DKA involves general aspects of the resuscitation of the unwell or patients in coma, in addition to the specific management of hyperglycemia, electrolyte disturbances, and metabolic acidosis.

The assessment of airway protection, oxygenation, gas exchange, and adequacy of the circulation should proceed as for any acutely ill patient. History, clinical examination, initial laboratory investigations, and radiology should be directed toward the identification of a precipitant of the decompensation (e.g., infection, myocardial infarction, stroke, or pancreatitis) and complications of the adverse clinical state (e.g., arrhythmia, organ failure, aspiration, electrolyte disturbance, and metabolic acidosis).

Increased concentrations of amylase and lipase are seen in up to 30% of presentations with ketoacidosis; however, only one-third of these patients have acute pancreatitis confirmed.

The osmotic diuresis and vomiting of advanced DKA lead to profound deficiencies principally of sodium, potassium, and water, with significant losses of phosphate, calcium, and magnesium also. These total-body deficits on average amount to 7 L water, 700 mEq sodium, 350 mEq potassium, 500 mEq phosphate, 100 mEq magnesium, and 100 mEq calcium in a 70 kg individual [36].

Fluid resuscitation is one of the mainstays of management of DKA, insulin being the other. The choice of fluid and rate of administration should be judged clinically. Not all patients with DKA require a urinary catheter. Central venous pressure measurements are justified in elderly patients or those in whom there is concern regarding cardiac, renal, or fluid status. The use of intravenous colloid in preference to crystalloid infusions in initial fluid resuscitation is not advocated.

DKA is treated optimally with a continuous intravenous infusion of soluble insulin through a delivery system that allows easy and frequent adjustments of the infusion rate. The most convenient method is the use of a syringe-driver pump administering a 1 U mL^{-1} solution of soluble insulin. Insulin will cause a rapid decrease in serum potassium concentration, which may precipitate cardiac arrhythmia if there is significant pre-existing hypokalemia. Insulin requirements can be large during the initial stage of treatment because of insulin resistance caused by metabolic acidosis, high concentrations of counterregulatory hormones, infection, tissue hypoxia, and glucose toxicity. If glucose concentrations do not decrease after the start of the infusion, the rate of infusion should be increased. Once blood glucose concentrations are reduced to less than 12–15 mmol L^{-1}, the intravenous crystalloid should be changed from 0.9% saline to 5% dextrose to maintain normoglycemia in the presence of continuous intravenous insulin. If intravenous insulin therapy is delayed during the initial treatment phase, 10 U soluble insulin can be administered intramuscularly.

The initiation of intravenous insulin therapy for DKA immediately terminates ketogenesis; however, ketones can persist in the urine for a further 72 hours. Insulin will immediately inhibit glycogenolysis and gluconeogenesis and stimulate glucose uptake to correct hyperglycemia. Correction of dehydration and restoration of renal perfusion pressure with fluid replacement will encourage excretion of ketones and hydrogen ions, the generation of bicarbonate, and therefore restoration of normal blood and cellular pH.

When acidosis has been corrected, ketonuria has resolved, and the patient is eating and drinking normally, subcutaneous insulin can be started.

One of the principal causes of early morbidity and mortality in DKA is cardiac arrhythmias caused by hypokalemia. At presentation with ketoacidosis, all patients have a whole-body deficit of potassium. Insulin deficiency and metabolic acidosis cause redistribution of potassium across plasma membranes, which may result in hyperkalemia. Insulin replacement drives potassium into cells and causes an immediate decrease in the serum potassium concentration. Intravenous potassium replacement is usually required after the first 500 mL of 0.9% saline. Oliguria and hyperkalemia may dictate a different strategy in the context of acute renal failure.

Potassium requirements are considerable in the initial stages of management of ketoacidosis to restore and maintain normokalemia. To ensure adequate rates of replacement, serum electrolytes must be checked frequently (2–4 hourly) in the first 24–48 hours and infusion rates adjusted accordingly.

Administration of intravenous sodium bicarbonate to rapidly increase the arterial pH in cases of advanced ketoacidosis has been advocated by some authors. Concerns regarding bicarbonate therapy are exacerbation of hypokalemia and hyperosmolality, and an increase in intracellular acidosis (especially within the CNS) despite an increase in arterial pH (paradoxic cerebrospinal fluid acidosis). The administration of bicarbonate may also delay recovery from ketosis by the stimulation of hepatic ketogenesis [37].

Studies of administration of bicarbonate to patients with advanced diabetic ketoacidosis (pH 6.9–7.1), have shown no improvement in morbidity or mortality rates, nor an increase in the frequency of adverse outcomes [38]. Therefore, its use is only advocated if the pH is less than 6.9 with no improvement in the metabolic parameters during insulin and fluid therapy. Failure to improve acidosis despite adequate management is usually related to an unidentified source of sepsis or tissue necrosis (e.g., intra-abdominal abscess, foot sepsis, bowel infarction, pancreatitis).

The identification of sepsis may be difficult during the initial clinical and biochemical assessment of patients with DKA. Ketoacidosis can cause pyrexia, increased C-reactive protein, and leukocytosis, which may be difficult to differentiate from infection. It may be associated also with peripheral vasodilation, which can cause hypothermia and mask the presence of infection. Because sepsis is an important precipitant of increasing insulin requirements and consequent metabolic decompensation, most patients with ketoacidosis receive broad-spectrum antibiotics.

Ketoacidosis is a prothrombotic state, and management of all episodes of DKA should include thromboprophylaxis with low-molecular-weight heparin.

Gastric stasis and reduced gastric emptying consequent to ketoacidosis make the risk of vomiting, with consequent inhalation, considerable in the absence of stomach aspiration.

Phosphate deficiency is commonly seen at presentation with ketoacidosis, but there is no evidence that replacement improves outcome. Severe deficiency of phosphate is associated with respiratory and skeletal muscle weakness and reduced cardiac function [39]. Some advocate phosphate replacement in diabetic ketoacidosis if there is associated cardiorespiratory failure.

An important aspect to be addressed with the patient before discharge from the hospital is the reason for the development of ketoacidosis and how it could be avoided in the future. This may involve improvements in the day-to-day management and monitoring of diabetes, the management of "sick days" and reiteration of the signs of imminent metabolic decompensation, and when to seek medical assistance.

Hyperglycemic hyperosmolar state

The hyperglycemic hyperosmolar state describes the metabolic decompensation of type 2 diabetes. It is characterized by severe hyperglycemia (> 40 mmol L^{-1}), hyperosmolality of the plasma (> 320 mOsm kg^{-1}), and dehydration sufficient to cause renal failure. It is differentiated clinically from DKA by an arterial pH greater than 7.30 and the presence of no more than mild dipstick ketonuria. It is not exclusive to type 2 diabetes, because some patients with type 1 diabetes can present with a similar syndrome. DKA and hyperglycemic hyperosmolar syndrome represent a spectrum of hyperglycemic crises in diabetes, and there is potential for overlap between types 1 and 2 diabetes in their clinical and metabolic presentation.

Precipitants induce hyperglycemic crises by increasing insulin resistance. Common precipitants include sepsis, acute coronary syndromes, stroke, trauma, corticosteroids, and alcohol abuse [40].

The prognosis for hyperglycemic hyperosmolar state is worse than ketoacidosis because patients are typically older and more hyperglycemic, dehydrated, and hyperosmolar. They are likely to have significant coexisting disease that contributes to an adverse clinical course [41]. Mortality rates from 15% to 50% have been quoted.

The development of the hyperglycemic hyperosmolar state results from the combination of inadequate insulin action and increased concentrations of the counterregulatory hormones, glucagon, epinephrine, cortisol, and growth hormone. The presence of insulin is able to prevent the transition from ketogenesis to ketoacidosis.

Patients present with the symptoms of hyperglycemia. The degree of hyperglycemia can be extreme, and the chronic osmotic diuresis leads to dehydration, significant loss of electrolytes, and renal failure. The combination of hyperglycemia, uremia, and hypernatremia (from water depletion) results in plasma hyperosmolality, and this is a major contributing factor toward the high mortality rate of this condition. Severe hyperosmolality leads to altered consciousness and coma [41]. Elderly patients may have dehydration exacerbated by hypodipsia. Coexisting disease contributes to the adverse prognosis.

The general aspects of management and supportive care are as for ketoacidosis. Precipitants for the decompensation should be identified and treated; pneumonia and urinary tract sepsis remain the most common. Abdominal pain is less common than in ketoacidosis and its presence is more indicative of underlying pathology. Drowsiness or coma occur more frequently and focal neurologic signs may be apparent, although these can be transient (e.g., hemiparesis).

The dehydration and electrolyte losses of the hyperglycemic hyperosmolar state are greater than for DKA. This relates to the longer passage of time before disease presentation. Average fluid depletion is 9 L, and average electrolyte losses are 5–13 mEq kg^{-1} sodium, 4–6 mEq kg^{-1} potassium, 3–7 mEq kg^{-1} phosphate, 1–2 mEq kg^{-1} magnesium, and 1–2 mEq kg^{-1} calcium.

Fluid replacement should commence with isotonic 0.9% saline. Central venous pressure monitoring should be considered in all patients to ensure optimal rates of fluid replacement, as should a urinary catheter. Isotonic saline restores circulating volume, which independently improves insulin sensitivity and reduces the concentration of the counterregulatory hormones. Rapid correction of plasma hyperosmolality with hypotonic saline may cause a significant cerebrospinal fluid/plasma osmotic gradient that may precipitate cerebral edema. Hypotonic saline may be used in hypernatremic patients but must be used cautiously. The hyperosmolality should be corrected at a rate no greater than 5 mOsm per hour.

When plasma glucose concentration decreases to less than 12–15 mmol L^{-1}, 5% dextrose should be substituted for saline to reduce the risk of hypoglycemia and to enable the continuation of intravenous insulin.

Fluid replacement and gradual correction of plasma hyperosmolality is of greater importance than rapid achievement of euglycemia. Fluid replacement and treatment of precipitants of the hyperglycemic state will cause improvement in insulin sensitivity.

The role of intravenous insulin in the hyperglycemic hyperosmolar state has been a subject of controversy, with some suggesting that insulin is not required as part of the management of patients already hyperinsulinemic. However, the physiological hyperinsulinemia is insufficient to overcome the insulin resistance of the acute illness, leading to hyperglycemia which subsequently contributes to the hyperosmolar state. The glucose concentration should not be reduced rapidly, but low rates of insulin infusion are safe and appropriate.

Patients are likely to require subcutaneous insulin during the acute illness because of significant insulin resistance. However, most can be managed with oral hypoglycemic drugs or diet alone at the time of discharge from hospital.

The risk for venous or arterial thromboembolic events (myocardial infarction, cerebral thrombosis, pulmonary embolism, and systemic arterial thromboembolism) in the hyperglycemic hyperosmolar state is significant and is a cause of the heightened mortality of the condition [40]. Systemic, formal anticoagulation with low-molecular-weight or intravenous heparin should be used in all patients with plasma osmolality greater than 330 mOsm kg^{-1}.

Hypoglycemia

Hypoglycemia is the most common metabolic emergency in diabetes. Fear of hypoglycemia or recurrent, unpredictable hypoglycemia is one of the major limiting factors for the achievement of desirable glycemic control [42].

For ease of description, hypoglycemia can be classified as:

- **Asymptomatic** – This requires the confirmation of a low plasma glucose in the absence of symptoms.
- **Mild to moderate** – Recognition of symptoms of hypoglycemia that allows self-treatment.
- **Severe** – The help of another individual is required in the treatment of hypoglycemia.

There is not a clear relation between plasma glucose concentration and the clinical features in any individual.

The intensive treatment group in the DCCT trial had 62 episodes of severe hypoglycemia per 100 patient-years [24]. The conventional-treatment group had 19 episodes. The true prevalence may be greater, because those with recurrent episodes were excluded from the main study [43].

The prevalence of hypoglycemia in type 2 diabetes is less than in type 1 [44]. The rate of severe hypoglycemia with sulfonylurea treatment is approximately 2 episodes per 100 patient years.

Hypoglycemia results from administration of insulin or its secretagogues without normal feedback control. It is defined as plasma glucose less than 3.9 mmol L^{-1}; symptoms relating to hypoglycemia may not be experienced. The common causes are:

(1) Food intake is insufficient or ill-timed for the hypoglycemic drug administered.
(2) Hypoglycemic drug dose is excessive or ill-timed for a given meal.
(3) Glucose utilization is excessive for given doses of insulin (e.g., exercise).
(4) Hepatic glucose production is reduced (e.g., alcohol).
(5) Insulin resistance is reduced (e.g., GLP-1 analog, weight loss, thiazolidinediones, hypopituitarism, hypoadrenalism).
(6) Insulin elimination rate is reduced (e.g., chronic renal failure).

In type 1 diabetes, the best predictive factors for severe hypoglycemia were a previous episode and longer duration of diabetes [45].

Mechanisms for recurrent severe hypoglycemia may involve dysfunctional counterregulatory hormones. In type 1 diabetes, the glucagon and epinephrine response to acute hypoglycemia is defective after a 5- to 10-year duration of disease. This is a selective glucose-sensing defect, because other stimuli remain able to provoke a normal physiologic response from the α cells and adrenal medulla.

When plasma glucose concentration decreases to less than 4.6 mmol L^{-1}, the brain initiates counterregulatory responses that aim to maintain normoglycemia and glucose delivery to the CNS. In individuals with diabetes these involve inhibition of insulin secretion initially. When plasma glucose decreases to less than 3.9 mmol L^{-1}, secretion of glucagon, epinephrine, growth hormone, and cortisol begins [46]. Recruitment of these hormones causes the neurogenic symptoms of hypoglycemia: anxiety, sweating, tremor, palpitations, pallor, piloerection, mydriasis, and hunger. When plasma glucose decreases to less than 2.8 mmol L^{-1}, cognition and the sensorium become impaired. These neuroglycopenic symptoms include confusion, disorientation, agitation, poor concentration, incoordination, speech disturbance, automatism, and personality and behavioral changes. Seizures may occur, while irreversible severe hypoglycemia leads to coma and death.

Hypoglycemia unawareness in type 1 diabetes is common and may affect up to 25% of all patients [47]. Patients do not experience the neurogenic symptoms, and hypoglycemia becomes apparent only with the appearance of neuroglycopenic symptoms. It seems related to metabolic factors and autonomic neuropathy. There are no good data to suggest that it is related to insulin species [48].

The treatment route of hypoglycemia is dependent on the patient's ability to protect his or her airway. In the alert, cooperative individual, hypoglycemia can be treated by the consumption of a rapid-acting source of glucose (e.g., sugary drink). This should be followed by a meal of complex carbohydrate to replete hepatic glycogen stores.

Third-party assistance will be required if neuroglycopenic symptoms render the patient unable to self-treat. With an uncooperative patient, or if the airway is compromised, intravenous glucose should be given as a 10–20% solution. Extravasation of 50% glucose can cause loss of tissue or even a limb.

When it proves difficult or impossible to secure venous access, 1 mg glucagon can be given by intramuscular injection. This stimulates hepatic glucose production through glycogenolysis. Improvement in the clinical condition should occur within 5–10 minutes. If hepatic glycogen stores are depleted (e.g., catabolic state, prolonged fasting, alcohol excess, or eating disorders), glucagon will be ineffective. The most common adverse effect of glucagon is nausea and vomiting.

All patients should eat a substantial carbohydrate meal to prevent recurrence of hypoglycemia. The possible precipitants should be examined. Hospital admission should be arranged if the patient is taking sulfonylureas as there is significant risk for recurrence of hypoglycemia. Patients treated with insulin do not require admission unless there are confounding factors such as advanced age, complex psychosocial factors, or lack of supervision. With repeated hypoglycemic episodes, the diabetologist will review diet, lifestyle, and treatment.

Additional indications for insulin therapy

Hyperkalemia
Plasma potassium is a poor guide to total-body potassium, especially in the sick or insulin-deficient patient. The Na^+/K^+ ATPase cotransporter of plasma membranes is important in the maintenance of the transmembrane electrochemical gradient. Insulin stimulates activity of this pump in the liver and in muscle, driving potassium into cells. This action is used in the treatment of acute

hyperkalemia. A total of 15 U of soluble insulin is added to 50 mL of 50% dextrose and infused over 30 minutes. This will reduce the serum potassium concentration by 1–1.5 mmol L^{-1} over 60–120 minutes, but the effect is temporary.

Acute myocardial infarction in diabetes
Initial studies suggested that the prognosis of acute myocardial infarction in diabetes can be improved with insulin therapy initiated during the immediate postinfarction period. The use of a continuous intravenous glucose–potassium–insulin infusion during the acute treatment phase and treatment with subcutaneous insulin for a further 12 months caused a 30% reduction in mortality [49]. There may be longer-term benefits to insulin beyond improvement in glycemia, although this has not been confirmed [50]. This was attributed to a reduced incidence of cardiac failure after infarction. The mechanism proposed was that early insulin therapy reduced the extent of myocardial damage. Similar benefit was seen also in patients without diabetes with admission blood glucose concentrations greater than 11.1 mmol L^{-1}. Further studies assessing insulin treatment in the acute phase of acute coronary syndromes have suggested that tight glycemic control and aggressive risk-factor modulation are more important than the use of insulin [51].

Insulin in acute severe illness
The use of insulin to overcome insulin resistance in acute severe illness has been studied. In the surgical intensive care unit (ICU), the use of insulin to achieve intensive control in patients with glucose concentrations greater than 12 mmol L^{-1} reduced in-hospital mortality, acute renal failre, critical illness, polyneuropathy, and episodes of septicemia [52]. However, the study required intensive input with a staff-to-patient ratio of 2 : 1, and 63% of the population had cardiac surgery. A follow-up study, using the same protocol, in the medical ICU showed no difference in overall mortality and morbidity between groups, although patients in the intensive insulin-treatment arm took fewer days to wean from artificial ventilation and had less acute renal failure. However, intensive insulin treatment was also associated with increased mortality in patients requiring ICU care for less than 3 days [53]. The data suggest that intensive glucose control on the ICU using insulin has benefit in surgical patients, particularly those undergoing cardiac surgery, but the benefits are less clear in medical patients.

Summary
Glucagon and insulin, produced by pancreatic islet α and β cells, respectively, mediate reciprocal actions to maintain glucose homeostasis. Increased plasma glucose stimulates release of insulin and consequent reduction of hepatic glucose output and increased glucose uptake into muscle; conversely, decreased plasma glucose inhibits insulin secretion, and causes the release of glucagon, which in turn stimulates hepatic

glycogenolysis. Insulin and glucagon each directly modify secretion of the other. Insulin resistance, which occurs under a number of conditions, including during cardiac surgery, results in compensatory hyperinsulinemia, while the reduced feedback inhibition of glucagon production results in hyperglycemia. Insulin resistance is a feature of the metabolic syndrome, a cluster of related cardiovascular abnormalities. The stress response to surgery and trauma can exacerbate insulin resistance, and sympathetic activity also reduces insulin secretion; optimal perioperative glycemic control is important in minimizing the risk for adverse events.

Exogenous insulin is most commonly administered via the subcutaneous route. However, for diabetic hyperglycemic emergencies and the management of blood glucose during the perioperative fasting period, intravenous administration of soluble or rapid-acting analog insulin is used, to facilitate adjustment of delivery according to clinical needs. A range of insulin and insulin analog preparations with distinct pharmacokinetic properties are available.

The underlying cause of type 1 diabetes mellitus is autoimmune destruction of pancreatic islet β cells and their consequent failure to produce insulin, necessitating lifelong insulin therapy. Type 2 diabetes mellitus is the result of progressive insulin resistance with hyperglycemia, commonly accompanied by progressive β-cell failure. This condition is managed with dietary adjustment, weight reduction, and treatment with oral hypoglycemic drugs such as biguanides (e.g., metformin), sulfonylureas, thiazolidinediones (e.g., rosiglitazone and pioglitazone), meglitinides, α-glucosidase inhibitors, GLP-1 analogs, and DPP4 inhibitors. Unsatisfactory glycemic control, despite adherence to diet and drug regimen, is an indication for insulin therapy.

The increased risk for adverse events amongst diabetic patients undergoing surgery can be reduced by preoperative blood pressure control, weight reduction, and attention to left ventricular function, renal function, coronary ischemia, proteinuria, and hyperlipidemia. Surgery should generally be delayed until optimal medical states and satisfactory glycemic control are achieved. Surgery is a catabolic process, requiring insulin infusion and capillary glucose monitoring at least every 2 hours in patients with absolute insulin deficiency. This approach should also be considered for those patients with relative insulin deficiency. For surgery on patients with diet-controlled diabetes or those taking oral hypoglycemic drugs, assessment of glycemic control and the duration and nature of the planned surgery is required to determine the perioperative strategy; depending on these factors, capillary glucose monitoring alone may be sufficient, or insulin may be required. Long-acting oral sulfonylureas should be changed in advance for short-duration drugs in preparation for surgery, and all oral drugs should be discontinued on the day of surgery.

Common metabolic emergencies of diabetes are diabetic ketoacidosis (DKA), hyperglycemic hyperosmolar state, and hypoglycemia. DKA follows prolonged insulin deficiency, and treatment involves general aspects of resuscitation and management of hyperglycemia, electrolyte disturbances, and metabolic acidosis, as well as addressing the underlying cause of the decompensation. The hyperglycemic hyperosmolar state is a metabolic decompensation occurring predominantly but not exclusively in type 2 diabetes patients, and management of this condition involves aspects similar to those described for ketoacidosis. Hypoglycemia results from the administration of insulin or its secretagogues (e.g., sulfonylureas, meglitinides) in the absence of normal feedback control. Self-treatment involves replenishment of glucose, for example with a sugary drink, followed by complex carbohydrate intake; however, in severe cases self-treatment will not be possible, and intravenous glucose should be given. Intramuscular administration of glucagon is an alternative option if venous access is precluded.

Insulin is also indicated in the treatment of acute hyperkalemia. Furthermore, insulin may have benefits for acute myocardial infarction and glucose control in insulin-resistant patients in an intensive care setting, although studies into these effects have produced mixed results.

References

1. Cheatham B, Kahn CR. Insulin action and the insulin signalling network. *Endocrin Rev* 1995; **16**: 117–42.

2. Reaven GM. Pathophysiology of insulin resistance in human disease. *Physiol Rev* 1995; **75**: 473–86.

3. Robinson S, Niththyananthan R, Anyaoku V, *et al*. Reduced postprandial energy expenditure in women predisposed to type 2 diabetes. *Diabet Med* 1994; **11**: 545–50.

4. Yki-Jarvinen H. Acute and chronic effects of hyperglycemia on glucose metabolism. *Diabetologia* 1990; **33**: 579–85.

5. Yki-Jarvinen H. Glucose toxicity. *Endocrin Rev* 1992; **13**: 415–31.

6. International Diabetes Federation. *The IDF Consensus Worldwide Definition of the Metabolic Syndrome*. Brussels: IDF, 2006.

7. Isomaa B, Almgren P, Tuomi T, *et al*. Cardiovascular morbidity and mortality associated with the metabolic syndrome. *Diabetes Care* 2001; **24**: 683–9.

8. Thorell A, Nygren J, Ljungqvist O. Insulin resistance: a marker of surgical stress. *Curr Opin Nutr Metab Care* 1999; **2**: 69–78.

9. Tsubo T, Kudo T, Matsuki A, Oyama T. Decreased glucose utilization during prolonged anesthesia and surgery. *Can J Anaesth* 1990; **37**: 645–9.

10. Thorell A, Loftenius A, Andersson B, Ljungqvist O. Postoperative insulin resistance and circulating concentrations of stress hormones and cytokines. *Clin Nutr* 1996; **15**: 75–9.

11. Avramoglu RK, Basciano H, Adeli K. Lipid and lipoprotein dysregulation in insulin resistant states. *Clinica Chimica Acta* 2006; **368**: 1–19.

12. McGirt MJ, Woodworth GF, Brooke BS, *et al.* Hyperglycemia independently increases the risk of perioperative stroke, myocardial infarction, and death after carotid endarterectomy. *Neurosurgery* 2006; **58**: 1066–73.

13. Malmstedt J, Wahlberg E, Jorneskog G, Swedenborg J. Influence of perioperative blood glucose levels on outcome after infrainguinal bypass surgery in patients with diabetes. *Br J Surg* 2006; **93**: 1360–7.

14. McGirt MJ, Woodworth GF, Brooke BS, *et al.* Hyperglycemia independently increases the risk of perioperative stroke, myocardial infarction, and death after carotid endarterectomy. *Neurosurgery* 2006; **58**: 1066–73.

15. Ziereth JR, He L, Guma A, *et al.* Insulin action on glucose transport and plasma membrane GLUT 4 content in skeletal muscle from patients with NIDDM. *Diabetologia* 1996; **39**: 1180–9.

16. Shepherd PR, Kahn BB. Glucose transporters and insulin action. Implications for insulin resistance and diabetes mellitus. *N Eng J Med* 1999; **341**: 248–57.

17. Castillo MJ, Scheen AJ, Letiexhe MR, *et al.* How to measure insulin clearance. *Diabetes Metab Rev* 1994; **10**: 119–50.

18. Duckworth WC, Bennett RG, Hamel FG. Insulin degradation: progress and potential. *Endocrin Rev* 1998; **19**: 608–24.

19. Lender D, Arauz-Pacheco C, Adams-Huet B, *et al.* Essential hypertension is associated with decreased insulin clearance and insulin resistance. *Hypertension* 1997; **29**: 111–14.

20. Jiang X, Srinivasan SR, Berenson GS. Relation of obesity to insulin secretion and clearance in adolescents: The Bogalusa Heart Study. *Int J Obes Relat Metab Disord* 1996; **20**: 951–6.

21. Letiexhe MR, Scheen AJ, Gerard PL, *et al.* Insulin secretion, clearance and action before and after gastroplasty in severely obese subjects. *Int J Obes Relat Metab Disord* 1994; **18**: 295–300.

22. Boland EA, Grey M, Oesterle A, *et al.* Continuous subcutaneous insulin infusion. A new way to lower risk of severe hypoglycemia, improve metabolic control and enhance coping in adolescents with type 1 diabetes. *Diabetes Care* 1999; **22**: 1779–84.

23. Brange J, Owens DR, Kang S, *et al.* Monomeric insulins and their experimental and clinical implications. *Diabetes Care* 1990; **13**: 923–54.

24. The Diabetes Control and Complications Trial Research Group. The effect of intensive treatment of diabetes on the development and progression of long-term complications in insulin-dependent diabetes mellitus. *N Eng J Med* 1993; **329**: 977–86.

25. Ferrannini E. Insulin resistance versus insulin deficiency in non-insulin dependent diabetes mellitus: problems and prospects. *Endocr Rev* 1998; **19**: 477–90.

26. McCarthy MI, Froguel P, Hitman GA. The genetics of non-insulin-dependent diabetes mellitus: tools and aims. *Diabetologia* 1994; **37**: 959–68.

27. Wilcox R, Kupfer S, Erdmann E; PROactive Study investigators. Effects of pioglitazone on major adverse cardiovascular events in high-risk patients with type 2 diabetes: results from PROspective pioglitAzone Clinical Trial In macro Vascular Events (PROactive 10). *Am Heart J* 2008; **155**: 712–17.

28. UK Prospective Diabetes Study (UKPDS) Group. Effect of intensive blood glucose control with metformin on complications in overweight patients with type 2 diabetes (UKPDS 34). *Lancet* 1998; **352**: 854–65.

29. UK Prospective Diabetes Study Group. Tight blood pressure control and risk of macrovascular and microvascular complications in type 2 diabetes: UKPDS 38. *BMJ* 1998; **317**: 703–13.

30. Bell DSH. Prudent utilization of the presently available treatment modalities for type 2 diabetes. *Endocrinologist* 1998; **8**: 332–41.

31. Robinson A, Burke J, Robinson S, *et al.* The effects of metformin on glycaemic control and serum lipids in insulin treated NIDDM patients with suboptimal metabolic control. *Diabetes Care* 1998; **21**: 701–5.

32. Hindler K, Shaw AD, Samuels J, *et al.* Improved postoperative outcomes associated with preoperative statin therapy. *Anesthesiology* 2006; **105**: 1260–72.

33. Wagner A, Risse A, Brill HL, *et al.* Therapy of severe diabetic ketoacidosis. Zero-mortality under very-low-dose insulin application. *Diabetes Care* 1999; **22**: 674–7.

34. Edge JA. Cerebral oedema during treatment of diabetic ketoacidosis: are we any nearer finding a cause? *Diabetes Metab Res Rev* 2000; **16**: 316–24.

35. Davis SN, Umpierrez GE. Diabetic Ketoacidosis in type 2 diabetes mellitus – pathophysiology and clinical presentation. *Nat Clin Endocrinol Metab* 2007; **3**: 730–1.

36. Kitabchi AE, Umpierrez GE, Murphy MB, *et al.* Management of hyperglycaemic crises in patients with diabetes. *Diabetes Care* 2001; **24**: 131–53.

37. Okuda Y, Adrogue HJ, Field JB, *et al.* Counterproductive effects of sodium bicarbonate in diabetic ketoacidosis. *J Clin Endocrinol Metab* 1996; **81**: 314–20.

38. Viallon A, Zeni F, Lafond P, *et al.* Does bicarbonate therapy improve the management of severe diabetic ketoacidosis? *Crit Care Med* 1999; **27**: 2690–3.

39. Miller DW, Slovis CM. Hypophosphatemia in the emergency department therapeutics. *Am J Emerg Med* 2000; **18**: 457–61.

40. Lorber D. Nonketotic hypertonicity in diabetes mellitus. *Med Clin North Am* 1995; **79**: 39–52.

41. Pinies JA, Cairo G, Gaztambide S, *et al.* Course and prognosis of 132 patients with diabetic nonketotic hyperosmolar state. *Diabetes Metab* 1994; **20**: 43–8.

42. Cox DJ, Gonder-Frederick L, Antoun B, *et al.* Psychobehavioral metabolic parameters of severe hypoglycaemic episodes. *Diabetes Care* 1990; **13**: 458–9.

43. The Diabetes Control and Complications Trial research Group. Diabetes Control and Complications Trial (DCCT): results of feasibility study. *Diabetes Care* 1987; **10**: 1–19.

44. Bell DSH, Yumuk V. Frequency of severe hypoglycemia in patients with non-insulin dependent diabetes mellitus

treated with sulphonylureas or insulin. *Endocr Pract* 1997; **3**: 281–3.

45. The Diabetes Control and Complications Trial Research Group. Epidemiology of severe hypoglycemia in the Diabetes Control and Complications Trial. *Am J Med* 1991; **90**: 450–9.

46. Thompson CJ, Baylis PH. Endocrine changes during insulin-induced hypoglycemia. In: Frier BM, Fisher BM, eds., *Hypoglycemia and Diabetes.* London: Edward Arnold, 1993: Cant find page numbers.

47. Gerich JE, Mokan M, Veneman T, *et al.* Hypoglycemia unawareness. *Endocrin Rev* 1991; **12**: 356–71.

48. Colagiuri S, Miller JJ, Petocz P, *et al.* Double blind crossover comparison of human and porcine insulins in patients reporting hypoglycemia unawareness. *Lancet* 1992; **339**: 1432–5.

49. Malmberg K, Ryden L, Efendic S, *et al.* Randomized trial of insulin-glucose infusion followed by subcutaneous insulin treatment in diabetic patients with acute myocardial infarction (DIGAMI study): effects on mortality at 1 year. *J Am Coll Cardiol* 1995; **26**: 57–65.

50. Malmberg K, Norhammar A, Wedel H, *et al.* Glycometabolic state at admission: important risk factor of mortality in conventionally treated patients with diabetes mellitus and acute myocardial infarction: long term results from the Diabetes and Insulin-Glucose Infusion in Acute Myocardial Infarction (DIGAMI) study. *Circulation* 1999; **99**: 2626–32.

51. Malmberg K, Ryden L, Wedel H, *et al.* DIGAMI 2 Investigators. Intense metabolic control by means of insulin in patients with diabetes mellitus and acute myocardial infarction (DIGAMI 2): effects on mortality and morbidity. *Eur Heart J* 2005; **26**: 650–61.

52. Van den Berghe G, Wouters P, Weekers F, *et al.* Intensive insulin therapy in critically ill patients. *N Engl J Med* 2001; **345**: 1359–67.

53. Van den Berghe G, Wilmer A, Hermans G, *et al.* Intensive insulin therapy in the medical ICU. *N Engl J Med* 2006; **354**: 449–61.

Essential drugs in anesthetic practice
Nutritional pharmacology

Paul Wischmeyer

Introduction

The last 100 years of medicine have brought great pharmacologic advances in the treatment of disease. Largely ignored has been the vital role of basic nutrients and nutrition in the maintenance of health and treatment of illness. Traditionally, this has been due to the observation that in nature, illness reduces food intake by inducing anorexia and loss of appetite, or simply not permitting the organism to forage for food. At its discovery, tumor necrosis factor α (TNFα) was known as cachexin. This vital cytokine, released at the initiation of stress and injury, induces anorexia and catabolism, and this inflammatory pathway has been preserved through many years of evolution. Thus the body utilizes anorexia and catabolism in the face of stress and injury as key survival mechanisms. However, it must be realized that until 100–150 years ago, if an individual was attacked by the proverbial "saber-tooth tiger" he or she had perhaps 48 hours to recover before dying (or being left behind by the tribe as a liability). This involved achieving hemostasis and preventing rapid, overwhelming infection. Eating and anabolism were not part of this desperate fight for survival.

Our understanding and management of this survival mechanism has changed dramatically since the evolution of emergency medicine, surgery, and critical care. Now, severely ill and injured individuals are supported through these massive insults. Thus, while we have learned to accept that lean body-mass catabolism is mandatory, long-term survival mandates that lean body-mass loss is minimized by early enteral/oral feeding in the acute phase and aggressive feeding and proanabolic therapy in the recovery or convalescent phase. Also, adequate acute-care nutrition hinges, not only on how many calories are provided, but also on our ability to provide key pharmacologic-acting nutrients that the body rapidly becomes deficient in following an insult. This chapter delineates these phenomena by describing (1) the pharmacology of nutrients and nutrition, (2) the practical aspects of nutrient administration, and (3) the challenges in nutritional therapy. For example, mobilization of amino acids stored in muscle is a vital mechanism for survival, as these amino acids are utilized

as obligate nutrient sources for the immune system and gut. The recent data indicating that amino acids also serve as stress signals that initiate activation of fundamental cell protective pathways following an insult have spawned a new field of "nutritional pharmacology."

Significant mortality occurs after critically ill patients are discharged from the hospital. More than 50% of the 6-month mortality following severe sepsis occurs after the patient has been discharged from the intensive care unit (ICU) [1]. Recent data also reveal that one-third of patients discharged following community-acquired pneumonia are dead at 1 year [2]. These deaths are thought to occur indirectly as a result of catabolism, loss of lean body mass, lack of therapeutic physical activity, and ultimately weakness and inability to walk [2,3]. These patients often go to rehabilitation centers or go home only to die of pulmonary embolus or pneumonia because they are unable to stand, get out of bed, or perform activities of daily life. It is important not only to provide care for the acute phase of illness with vasopressors, resuscitation, ventilation, and antibiotics to enhance survival, but also to minimize the mandatory catabolism that occurs during the acute phase and to learn to manage the convalescent phase of severe illness when the key intervention becomes nutrition, anabolism, and rehabilitation. The key to providing this care is initiation of enteral or oral feeding within hours of surgery or admission to the ICU. Data will also likely reveal that administration of certain key nutrients such as omega-3 fatty acids, glutamine, and antioxidants may be vitally important. The practices of maintaining prolonged nil-by-mouth periods after surgery and awaiting "bowel sounds" to initiate feeding are not supported by clinical or scientific data. This does not mean the patient must achieve full nutritional needs in the first few days after injury or illness, but nutrition, perhaps as trophic feeds, must be initiated. This is to prevent the intractable ileus that delayed feeding induces, to help support the body's obligate need for key nutrients, and to attenuate loss of the lean body mass that will be required for recovery.

Presently, we are in a "revival" period of interest in clinical nutrition, particularly in the area of "pharmaconutrition" [4]

Anesthetic Pharmacology, 2nd edition, ed. Alex S. Evers, Mervyn Maze, Evan D. Kharasch. Published by Cambridge University Press. © Cambridge University Press 2011.

(or "nutritional pharmacology"). Further, years of poorly designed or nongeneralizable trials in fundamental feeding and nutrition support are being re-explored using modern clinical trial methods and employing newly discovered mechanistic science.

Pharmacology of nutrients and nutrition

This section will cover the pharmacology of specific nutrients. However, the effect of illness on nutrient metabolism and energy expenditure deserves a brief review (Table 56.1).

Energy expenditure

The response to stress is characterized by hypermetabolism [5]. After elective surgery resting energy expenditure (REE) increases 10–20% above preoperative values [5]. Septic patients can have increases of 20–40% [6], while patients with burns have increases up to 120%, with the increase proportional to the extent of the burns [7]. The early phase of sepsis is characterized by small increases in REE [6,8]. As sepsis progresses to septic shock, the increase in REE remains negligible [9]. This is consistent with early appearance of cachexin (TNFα) in this phase of illness. However, in the recovery phase of septic shock REE increases to 161% of basline [9]. This is consistent with the transition from an acute, survival phase to a convalescent

Table 56.1. Energy expenditure and caloric intake

Caloric requirements

Estimating resting energy expenditure (Harris–Benedict equation)

Males: EBEE (kcal day^{-1}) = 66 + (13.7 × W) + (5 × H) – (6.8 × A)

Females: EBEE (kcal day^{-1}) = 655 + (9.6 × W) + (1.7 × H) – (4.7 × A)

Estimated resting energy expenditure (EREE) = EBEE × stress factor

Estimated total energy expenditure (ETEE) = EREE × activity factor

A, age (years); EBEE, estimated basal energy expenditure; H, height (cm); W, weight (kg).

Stress factors

Spontaneously breathing, nonsedated patients (for sedated mechanically ventilated patients subtract 10–15%)

Major surgery: 15–25%

Burns: up to 120% depending on extent

Infection: 20%

Sepsis (post septic-shock and acute phase): 30–55%

Long bone fracture: 20–35%

Major trauma: 20–35%

Malnutrition: subtract 10–15%

COPD: 10–15%

Activity factors

Sedated mechanically ventilated patients: 0–5%

Bed-ridden, spontaneously breathing nonsedated patients: 10–15%

Sitting in chair: 15–20%

Ambulating patients: 20–25%

Measuring energy expenditure (EE)

Indirect calorimetry involves measuring oxygen consumption (VO_2) and carbon dioxide production (VCO_2)

Weir equation: EE (kcal day^{-1}) = 1.44 (3.9 × VO_2) + (1.1 × VCO_2)

Measurements made at rest provide the REE. To determine the total energy expenditure: REE × activity factor

Continuous measurement made over 24 hours provides the total energy expenditure

Measuring nitrogen balance

N balance = [N intake] – [N output]

where [N intake] = all protein/amino acid intake over 24 hours whether enteral or parenteral

[N output] = [UUN + 4 + EL]

UUN = urine urea nitrogen over 24 hours; 4 g average fecal and cutaneous losses

Table 56.1. *(cont.)*

Caloric requirements	
EL = excessive losses, such as protein rich drainages (e.g., pus)	
6.25 g protein/amino acids = 1 g nitrogen	

Daily caloric requirements

Sedated mechanically ventilated patients	1.0–1.2 × REE
Nonsedated mechanically ventilated patients	1.2 × REE
Spontaneously breathing critically ill patients	1.2–1.3 × REE
Spontaneously breathing ward patients (maintenance)	1.3 × REE
Spontaneously breathing ward patients (repletion)	1.5–1.7 × REE

To gain 1 lb of body weight would need a cumulative excess greater than TEE of approximately 3500 kcal

Caloric properties of food

	Energy (kcal g^{-1})
Carbohydrate	4.0
Dextrose (glucose monohydrate)	3.4
Fat	9.0
Protein	4.0
Alcohol	7.0

phase that must be approached from a different nutritional perspective. In surgical illness, peak REE occurs about the third postoperative day and hypermetabolism may last up to 21 days in critically ill trauma and burn patients [10,11]. Burn and trauma patients have, on average, a much larger increase in REE than patients with sepsis alone [6]. Head injury and other neurological problems increase REE secondary to marked outpouring of catecholamines. For at least 5 days after subarachnoid hemorrhage REE was 18% greater than predicted values [12]. Mechanically ventilated patients have lower increases in REE than spontaneously breathing patients because of sedation and decreased work of breathing [13].

Clinical pharmacology of carbohydrates
Metabolism and pathophysiology
Carbohydrate metabolism is significantly altered during stress by the increased secretion of cortisol, catecholamines, and glucagon [14]. These hormones increase endogenous glucose production (hepatic gluconeogenesis) in proportion to the degree of stress. Insulin concentrations are normal or mildly increased but not sufficiently elevated to prevent hyperglycemia. This is in part due to the insulin resistance that accompanies significant injury or illness.

Glucose and carbohydrate nutrition
Administering exogenous glucose and carbohydrates to injured or septic patients minimally diminishes the rates of gluconeogenesis and lipolysis [15]. This contrasts with starvation, during which carbohydrate administration reduces gluconeogenesis and lipolysis. Despite reduced glucose utilization, it is still important to administer carbohydrates because some body tissues (such as the brain) are unable to readily use other substrates. Hyperglycemia often limits the amount of glucose and carbohydrate that can be administered. It is important to understand that nondiabetic patients who have new-onset hyperglycemia (> 200 mg dL^{-1}) in the ICU have significantly increased mortality compared with nondiabetic patients who do not develop hyperglycemia [16]. This increased mortality is not observed in known diabetics who are hyperglycemic while in the ICU [16]. Thus, excessive glucose infusions that lead to hyperglycemia in nondiabetics are best avoided. Further, any nondiabetic patient with a glucose value over 200 mg dL^{-1} should likely be treated aggressively with insulin to a glucose value of 140–180 mg dL^{-1} as neither tight glucose control (< 110 mg dL^{-1}) nor moderate glucose control (< 150 mg dL^{-1}) has shown benefit on ICU mortality in a recent meta-analysis [17].

Critically ill patients often receive carbohydrates from sources other than the glucose in parenteral nutrition (PN) or carbohydrates in enteral nutrition. Five-percent dextrose infusions contain 170 kcal L^{-1}. Overfeeding glucose (> 4 mg kg^{-1} min^{-1}) to acutely stressed patients, receiving a total caloric intake greater than resting energy expenditure, results in further increase of blood glucose concentrations and production of additional CO_2 [18]. This CO_2 must be excreted through the lungs and, if inadequately excreted, can contribute to ventilatory failure. Such carbohydrate overfeeding is not uncommon. A survey of US teaching hospitals demonstrated that many patients are fed with more than 4.5 mg kg^{-1} min^{-1} glucose [19].

Clinical pharmacology of lipids
Metabolism and pathophysiology
Lipid metabolism is substantially affected during stress [20], particularly by accelerated lipolysis secondary to β_2-adrenergic stimulation [21]. Glucagon, cortisol, TNFα, interleukin 1 (IL-1), and interferon γ (IFNγ) may also stimulate lipolysis [22,23].

During stress, the relative caloric contribution of fat oxidation to resting energy expenditure is increased, while the contribution of glucose oxidation decreases [24]. Fatty acids released by lipolysis undergo β-oxidation, which in the stressed patient is the predominant ATP-producing pathway. This situation is seen after esophagectomy, in which there is a gradual decrease in the contribution of fat oxidation and increase in glucose oxidation during convalescence [25].

Lipid nutrition
In North America, intravenous lipid is currently only administered as an emulsion of omega-6-based long-chain triglycerides (LCTs). These emulsions contain soybean oil and an emulsifier (egg phospholipid). In most other countries in the world omega-3 lipids and omega-6/omega-3 combinations of lipids are available. Intravenous lipid emulsions are calorie-dense (e.g., 10% and 20% solutions contain 1.0 and 2.0 kcal mL^{-1}, respectively). Lipid emulsions are also the vehicle for lipid-soluble drugs, such as propofol [26]. In patients receiving infusions of propofol for sedation, the amount of lipid calories may be significant and should be included when calculating caloric intake [27].

In patients with minimal or no oral intake, exogenous lipid is needed to prevent essential free fatty acid deficiency. Therefore, patients receiving PN should be administered a lipid emulsion infusion of at least 1.2–2.4 g of lipid per kg body weight biweekly to prevent essential fatty acid deficiency [28]. Lipid emulsion is also an energy substrate, given that lipid oxidation is a predominant energy-producing pathway during stress. There has been debate whether exogenous lipids (LCT) are useful energy substrates, driven by observation that exogenous LCT failed to suppress glucose oxidation in the critically ill so that 45% of the administered fat was stored [29,30]. Others observed that fat emulsions were well oxidized when administered to septic and trauma patients even when glucose was administered [31,32].

Past practice has prescribed lipid administration that contributes 30–40% of total PN calories. Newer studies have revealed that reducing or withholding lipids in states of critical illness may reduce infection and improve outcome [33]. These data are a result of concern over possible immunosuppressive effects of solely omega-6-based lipid emulsions. Ex-vivo studies demonstrated decreased neutrophil bacterial killing, depressed monokine expression, and other immune-depressant effects [34]. A study of trauma patients attributed increased infections to lipid emulsions [33]. This has led to recommendations in clinical guidelines to reduce lipid administration to once a week in critically ill patients (data and guidelines available at www.criticalcare-enutrition.com; Table 56.2). The availability of omega-3-based lipid infusions in Europe and on other continents may alleviate this concern around omega-6-based lipids. There is a growing body of literature showing beneficial effects of these omega-3 lipids in surgical and critically ill populations [35–37].

As described previously, the soybean-derived fat emulsions used exclusively in North America for parenteral nutrition contain high proportions of omega-6 polyunsaturated fatty acids, specifically linoleic acid (53%). Linoleic acid is the precursor of thromboxane A$_2$ and prostaglandin E$_1$, which cause platelet aggregation and inflammation. Alternatively, fish and olive oils containing omega-3 fatty acids are precursors of another class of prostaglandins, including thromboxane A$_3$, which have less platelet-aggregating and inflammatory activity. There has been interest in using omega-3 fatty acids, particularly eicosapentaenoic acid (EPA) and γ-linolenic acid (GLA), in acute respiratory distress syndrome (ARDS) to reduce pulmonary microvascular permeability and alveolar macrophage prostaglandin and leukotriene synthesis [38,39]. Data from three randomized controlled clinical trials of EPA/GLA-enriched enteral formulas revealed statistically significant reductions in time of mechanical ventilation, length of ICU stay, organ failure, and in some cases mortality [40–42]. The meta-analysis of these data reveals that EPA/GLA-supplemented enteral formulas lead to a risk reduction of 43% in 28-day in-hospital all-cause mortality (RR 0.57, 95% CI 0.41–0.79, $p = 0.001$). Similar statistically significant reductions were seen in length of ICU stay, ventilator time, and organ failure in this analysis [43]. Existing clinical guidelines (available at www.criticalcarenutrition.com) recommend the use of a specialized EPA/GLA in patients with acute lung injury or ARDS. There are currently available enteral formulas that are EPA/GLA fatty-acid-enriched (Table 56.3).

Clinical pharmacology of protein and amino acids
Metabolism and pathophysiology
One of the hallmarks of the response to injury is catabolism caused by accelerated proteolysis of skeletal muscle. This is thought to be modulated by cortisol and cytokines (TNFα, IL-1, IL-6, and IFNγ [44]). It is the balance between these catabolic substances and anabolic hormones, such as insulin and insulin-like growth factor 1 (IGF-1) that determines the degree of catabolism. The degree of nitrogen loss is proportional to the degree of stress and abates as patients convalesce [45].

Protein and amino acid nutrition
Amino acids and protein are basic ingredients of all nutritional support regimens. Parenteral formulas contain amino acid mixtures, whereas enteral formulas contain free amino acids,

Table 56.2. Summary of recommendations from the Canadian Critical Care Nutrition Guidelines, the only fully evidence-based guidelines in critical care nutrition therapy: 2009 guidelines (www.criticalcarenutrition.com)

Topic	Question	Recommendation
1. Enteral nutrition vs. parenteral nutrition	Does enteral nutrition compared to parenteral nutrition result in better outcomes in the critically ill adult patient?	Based on 1 level 1 study and 12 level 2 studies, when considering nutrition support for critically ill patients, we strongly recommend the use of enteral nutrition over parenteral nutrition.
2. Early vs. delayed nutrient intake	Does early enteral nutrition compared to late enteral nutrition result in better outcomes in the critically ill adult patient?	Based on 14 level 2 studies, we recommend early enteral nutrition (within 24–48 hours following admission to ICU) in critically ill patients.
3.1 Dose of EN: use of indirect calorimetry vs. predictive equation for EN	Does the use of indirect calorimetry vs. a predictive equation for determining energy needs result in better outcomes in the critically ill adult patient?	There are insufficient data to make a recommendation on the use of indirect calorimetry vs. predictive equations for determining energy needs for enteral nutrition in critically ill patients.
3.2 Dose of EN: achieving target dose of EN *	Does achieving target dose of enteral nutrition result in better outcomes in the critically ill adult patient?	Based on 2 level 2 studies and 2 cluster randomized controlled trials, when starting enteral nutrition in critically ill patients, strategies to optimize delivery of nutrients (starting at target rate, higher threshold of gastric residual volumes, use of prokinetics and small bowel feedings) should be considered.
4.1(a) Composition of EN: immune enhancing diets: diets supplemented with arginine and other select nutrients	Compared to standard enteral feeds, do diets supplemented with arginine and other select nutrients result in improved clinical outcomes in the critically ill adult patient?	Based on 4 level 1 studies and 18 level 2 studies, we recommend that diets supplemented with arginine and other select nutrients* not be used for critically ill patients.
4.1(b) Composition of EN: immune enhancing diets: fish oils	Does the use of an enteral formula with fish oils, borage oils, and antioxidants result in improved clinical outcomes in the critically ill adult patient?	Based on 1 level 1 study and 4 level 2 studies, we recommend the use of an enteral formula with fish oils, borage oils and antioxidants in patients with Acute Lung Injury (ALI) and acute respiratory distress syndrome (ARDS).
4.1(c) Composition of EN: immune enhancing diets: glutamine	Compared to standard care, does glutamine-supplemented EN result in improved clinical outcomes in the critically ill adult patient?	Based on 2 level 1 and 7 level 2 studies, enteral glutamine should be considered in burn and trauma patients. There are insufficient data to support the routine use of enteral glutamine in other critically ill patients.
4.1(d) Composition of EN: ornithine ketoglutarate (OKG)	Does supplementation of enteral nutrition with ornithine ketoglutarate (OKG) influence outcomes in the critically ill adult patient?	There are insufficient data to make a recommendation regarding the use of ornithine ketoglutarate in burn patients and other critically ill patients.
4.2(a) Composition of EN: CHO/FAT: high fat, low CHO	Does a high fat/low carbohydrate enteral formula influence outcomes in the critically ill adult patient?	There are insufficient data to recommend high fat/low CHO diets for critically ill patients.
4.2(b) Composition of EN: CHO/FAT: low fat, high CHO	Does a low fat/high carbohydrate enteral formula influence outcomes in the critically ill adult patient?	There are insufficient data to make a recommendation regarding the use of a low fat formula in critically ill patients.
4.2(c) Composition of EN: high protein vs. low protein	Does the use of a higher protein enteral formula, compared to a lower protein enteral formula, result in better outcomes in the critically ill adult patient?	There are insufficient data to make a recommendation regarding the use of high protein diets for head-injured and other critically ill patients.

Table 56.2. (cont.)

Topic	Question	Recommendation
4.3 Composition of EN: protein/peptides	Does the use of peptide based enteral formula, compared to a whole protein formula, result in better outcomes in the critically ill adult patient?	Based on 4 level 2 studies, when initiating enteral feeds, we recommend the use of whole protein formulas (polymeric) in critically ill patients.
4.4 Composition of EN: pH	Do acidified feeds (low pH) compared to standard feeds result in better outcomes in the critically ill adult patient?	There are insufficient data to make a recommendation regarding the use of low pH feeds in critically ill patients.
4.5 Composition of EN: fibre	Do enteral feeds with fibre, compared to standard feeds result in better outcomes in the critically ill adult patient?	There are insufficient data to support the routine use of fibre (pectin or soy polysaccharides) in enteral feeding formulas in critically ill patients.
5.1 Strategies to optimize delivery and minimize risks of EN: feeding protocols	Does the use of a feeding protocol result in better outcomes in the critically ill adult patient?	Based on 1 level 2 study and 2 cluster randomized controlled trials, an evidence-based feeding protocol that incorporates prokinetics at initiation and a higher gastric residual volume (250 mls) and the use of post pyloric feeding tubes, should be considered as a strategy to optimize delivery of enteral nutrition in critically ill adult patients.
5.2 Strategies to optimize delivery and minimize risks of EN: motility agents	Compared to standard practice (placebo), does the routine use of motility agents result in better clinical outcomes in the critically ill adult patient?	Based on 1 level 1 study and 5 level 2 studies, in critically ill patients who experience feed intolerance (high gastric residuals, emesis), we recommend the use of a promotility agent. Given the safety concerns associated with erythromycin, the recommendation is made for metoclopramide. There are insufficient data to make a recommendation about the use of combined use of metoclopramide and erythromycin.
5.3 Strategies to optimize delivery and minimize risks of EN: small bowel feeding	Does enteral feeding via the small bowel compared to gastric feeding result in better outcomes in the critically ill adult patient?	Based on 11 level 2 studies, small bowel feeding compared to gastric feeding may be associated with a reduction in pneumonia in critically ill patients. In units where obtaining small bowel access is feasible, we recommend the routine use of small bowel feedings. In units where obtaining access involves more logistical difficulties, small bowel feedings should be considered for patients at high risk for intolerance to EN (on inotropes, continuous infusion of sedatives, or paralytic agents, or patients with high nasogastric drainage) or at high risk for regurgitation and aspiration (nursed in supine position). Finally, in units where obtaining small bowel access is not feasible (no access to fluoroscopy or endoscopy and blind techniques not reliable), small bowel feedings should be considered for those select patients who repeatedly demonstrate high gastric residual volumes and are not tolerating adequate amounts of EN delivered into the stomach.
5.4 Strategies to optimize delivery and minimize risks of EN: body position	Do alterations in body position result in better outcomes in the critically ill adult patient?	Based on 1 level 1 and 1 level 2 study, we recommend that critically ill patients receiving enteral nutrition have the head of the bed elevated to 45 degrees. Where this is not possible, attempts to raise the head of the bed as much as possible should be considered.
6.1 EN other: closed vs. open system	Does the use of a closed system for enteral feeding result in better outcomes when compared to an open system in the critically ill adult patient?	There are insufficient data to make a recommendation on the administration of EN via a closed vs. open system in critically ill patients.
6.2 EN other: prebiotics/probiotics/synbiotics	Does the addition of prebiotics/probiotics/synbiotics to enteral nutrition result in better outcomes in the critically ill adult patient?	There are insufficient data to make a recommendation on the use of prebiotics/probiotics/synbiotics in critically ill patients.

Table 56.2. *(cont.)*

Topic	Question	Recommendation
6.3 EN other: continuous vs. other methods of administration	Does continuous administration of enteral nutrition compared to other methods of administration result in better outcomes in the critically ill adult patient?	There are insufficient data to make a recommendation on enteral feeds given continuously vs. other methods of administration in critically ill patients.
6.4 EN other: gastrostomy vs. nasogastric feeding	Does enteral feeding via a gastrostomy compared to nasogastric feeding result in better outcomes in the critically ill adult patient?	There are insufficient data to make a recommendation on gastrostomy feeding vs. nasogastric feeding in the critically ill.
7. EN in combination with PN	Does the use of parenteral nutrition in combination with enteral nutrition result in better outcomes in the critically ill adult patient?	Based on 5 level 2 studies, for critically ill patients starting on enteral nutrition, we recommend that parenteral nutrition not be started at the same time as enteral nutrition. In the patient who is not tolerating adequate enteral nutrition, there are insufficient data to put forward a recommendation about when parenteral nutrition should be initiated. Practitioners will have to weigh the safety and benefits of initiating PN in patients not tolerating EN on an individual case-by-case basis. We recommend that PN not be started in critically ill patients until all strategies to maximize EN delivery (such as small bowel feeding tubes, motility agents) have been attempted.
8. PN: PN vs. standard care	Compared to standard care (IV fluids, oral diet, etc.), does parenteral nutrition result in better outcomes in critically ill patients who have an intact GI tract?	Based on 5 level 2 studies, in critically ill patients with an intact gastrointestinal tract, we recommend that parenteral nutrition not be used routinely.
9.1 Composition of PN: branched chain amino acids (BCAA)	Does the addition of BCAA to parenteral nutrition influence outcomes in the critically ill adult patient?	In critically ill patients who are receiving parenteral nutrition, there are insufficient data to make a recommendation regarding the use of branched chain amino acids.
9.2 Composition of PN: type of lipids	Does the type of lipids in parenteral nutrition influence outcomes in the critically ill adult patient?	There are insufficient data to make a recommendation on the type of lipids to be used in critically ill patients who are receiving parenteral nutrition.
9.3 Composition of PN: zinc	Does zinc supplementation (via IV/PN) given either alone or in combination with other nutrients result in better outcomes in the critically ill patient?	There are insufficient data to make a recommendation regarding IV/PN zinc supplementation in critically ill patients.
9.4 Composition of PN: glutamine	Does glutamine supplementation of parenteral nutrition influence outcomes in the critically ill adult patient?	Based on 4 level 1 studies and 13 level 2 studies, when parenteral nutrition is prescribed to critically ill patients, parenteral supplementation with glutamine, where available, is strongly recommended. There are insufficient data to generate recommendations for intravenous glutamine in critically ill patients receiving enteral nutrition.
10.1 Strategies to optimize benefits and minimize risks of PN: dose of PN	Does the dose parenteral nutrition influence outcomes in the critically ill adult patient?	Based on 4 level 2 studies, in critically ill patients who are not malnourished, are tolerating some EN, or when parenteral nutrition is indicated for short-term use (< 10 days), low dose parenteral nutrition should be considered. There are insufficient data to make recommendations about the use of low-dose parenteral nutrition in the following patients: those requiring PN for long term (> 10 days), obese critically ill patients, and malnourished critically ill patients. Practitioners will have to weigh the safety and benefits of low dose PN on an individual case-by-case basis in these latter patient populations.

Table 56.2. *(cont.)*

Topic	Question	Recommendation
10.2 Use of lipids	Does the presence of lipids in parenteral nutrition affect outcomes in the critically ill adult patient?	Based on 2 level 2 studies, in critically ill patients who are not malnourished, are tolerating some EN, or when parenteral nutrition is indicated for short term use (< 10 days), withholding lipids high in soybean oil should be considered. There are insufficient data to make a recommendation about withholding lipids high in soybean oil in critically ill patients who are malnourished or those requiring PN for long term (> 10 days). Practitioners will have to weigh the safety and benefits of withholding lipids high in soybean oil on an individual case-by-case basis in these latter patient populations.
10.3 Strategies to optimize benefits and minimize risks of PN: mode of lipid delivery	Does the mode of delivery of lipids influence outcomes in the critically ill adult patient?	There are insufficient data to make a recommendation on mode of lipid delivery in critically ill patients who are receiving parenteral nutrition.
10.4 Strategies to optimize benefits and minimize risks of PN: intensive insulin therapy	Does tight blood sugar control result in better outcomes in the critically ill adult patient?	We recommend that hyperglycemia (blood sugars > 10 mmol L^{-1}) be avoided in all critically ill patients. Based on the NICE-SUGAR study and a recent meta-analysis, we recommend a blood glucose target of around 8.0 mmol L^{-1} (or 7–9 mmol L^{-1}), rather than a more stringent target range (4.4–6.1 mmol L^{-1}) or a more liberal target range (10–11.1 mmol L^{-1}).
11.1 Supplemental antioxidant nutrients: combined vitamins and trace elements	Does the addition of supplemental antioxidant combined vitamins and trace elements result in better outcomes in the critically ill patient?	Based on 3 level 1 and 13 level 2 studies, the use of supplemental combined vitamins and trace elements should be considered in critically ill patients.
11.2 Supplemental antioxidant nutrients: parenteral selenium	Does parenteral selenium supplementation (alone or in combination with other antioxidants) result in better outcomes in the critically ill patient?	There are insufficient data to make a recommendation regarding IV/PN selenium supplementation alone, or in combination with other antioxidants, in critically ill patients.

peptides, or whole proteins (Table 56.3). The aim of administering protein or amino acids to stressed patients is to attenuate (but not block) the breakdown of endogenous proteins by providing an alternative source of amino acids for gluconeogenesis and protein synthesis. Further, there are particular amino acids, such as glutamine and arginine, which have clear pharmacologic effects following illness and injury [46,47]. It appears that supplementation of these amino acids can be used to cause specific pharmacologic effects independent of their effect on protein anabolism/catabolism and energy substrate. In the stressed state, exogenous amino acids and protein will not inhibit proteolysis. However, amino acid supplementation can be used to attenuate the body's inherent protein catabolism and reduce lean body-mass loss. Severe loss of lean body mass has long been correlated with poor outcomes following insult [48]. Catabolism persists well into the convalescent period and may last for as long as 9–12 months after severe (> 40%) burns in children [49]. In the persistent catabolic state, intake of 1.5–2.0 g kg^{-1} day^{-1} protein/amino acid is recommended. Large external losses of protein, such as from extensive burns and draining abscesses, make it necessary to increase protein/amino acid intake.

In the early acute phase of the stress response nitrogen loss is inevitable, and patients should be supported with early protein supplementation. However, attempting to make a patient anabolic in this phase of illness is neither possible nor safe. This is exemplified by the increased mortality observed in critically ill patients administered growth hormone (GH). In the chronic or convalescent phase of illness nutritional goals change, and methods to decrease proteolysis, increase protein synthesis, and promote anabolism become paramount. Anabolic substances such as GH have been investigated in a number of trials. During catabolism, GH concentrations are reduced and there is resistance to its actions [50]. The aim of its administration is to increase nitrogen retention and promote wound healing. However, a large randomized study showed that in critically ill patients GH was associated with increased mortality because of infection and multiple organ failure [51]. There remains interest in using hypothalamic-releasing hormones to induce GH and thyroid hormone release during the anabolic, convalescent phase of illness. These releasing hormones lead to the physiologic, pulsatile release of hormones, which may prove more beneficial than bolus doses of these hormones [51]. More recent trials have looked at anabolic agents administered later in

Table 56.3. Typical enteral nutrition formulary (University of Colorado Hospital Formulary)

Formula	Characteristics	Cost	kcal mL⁻¹	Recommended tube size (Pump)	Recommended tube size (Gravity)	Protein (g L⁻¹)	N₂ (g L⁻¹)	CHO %	Fat %	Osmolality (mOsm kg⁻¹)	Na (mEq L⁻¹)	K⁺ (mEq L⁻¹)	PO₄ (mg L⁻¹)	Volume to meet RDI (mL day⁻¹)	Free water (mL L⁻¹)
Primary tube feed															
		$	1.06	≥5 Fr	≥8 Fr	37.1	5.93	57	29	300	27.8	26.1	535	1887	841
Osmolite 1.2	High protein, low residue. Contains MCT oil.	$	1.2	≥5 Fr	≥8 Fr	55.5	8.8	53	29	360	58.3	46.4	1200	1000	820
Standard high-nitrogen tube feed															
Fibersource HN	Semi-conc., moderate N₂, fiber (10 g fiber L⁻¹)	$	1.2	≥5 Fr	≥8 Fr	53	8.5	53	29	490	52	51	1000	1165	814
High-fiber tube feed															
Nutren 2.0	Concentrated, 2 kcal mL⁻¹ formula (can be used as oral supplement, vanilla flavor); 75% of fat is MCT oil	$	2.0	≥5 Fr	≥8 Fr	80	12.8	39	45	745	56.5	49.2	1340	750	700
For fluid-restricted patients/calorically dense															
Diabetisource AC	Moderate carbohydrate, diabetic formula. Contains FOS, fiber (15 g L⁻¹), arginine (9 g L⁻¹), fish oil (1 g L⁻¹)	$$	1.2	≥5 Fr	≥8 Fr	60	9.6	36	44	450	46	44	800	1250	818
For diabetic patients/low carbohydrate															
Secondary tube feed															
Nutren Renal (or NutriRenal: same product)	Moderate protein for chronic/acute renal failure with hemodialysis. Vanilla flavor, can be used as an oral supplement	$$	2.0	≥5 Fr	≥8 Fr	70	11.2	40	46	650	32.1	32.2	700	750	704
For renal failure patients															
Vivonex RTF	Elemental, low fat, arginine (5.8 g L⁻¹); no additional glutamine, 100% free amino acids.	$$$$	1.0	≥5 Fr	≥8 Fr	50	8	70	10	630	29	31	670	1500	848
Free AA tube feed/pancreatitis/poor GI tolerance															
Oxepa	Modulates inflammation in sepsis, SIRS, acute lung injury, ARDS. 4.6g L⁻¹ EPA, 4 g L⁻¹ GLA.	$$$$	1.5	≥8 Fr	≥10 Fr	62.7	10	28	55.2	493	57	50.1	1060	947	785

For ARDS/ALI/SIRS/sepsis patients

Modular protein supplements

Product	Description	Cost									
Protein Powder (Beneprotein)	Recommended to use as flush. *Mix with at least 60 ml water. Do not mix directly with TF formula.*	$		6 g/sc	0.96 g/sc				1.5	0.18	3.5
Pro-Stat 64	Suitable with fluid restriction or intolerance of protein powder. Sugar free. Contains arginine, glutamine. Each tube is 30 mL. *Do not mix directly with TF formula, no mixing required.*	$$$		15 g/tube				1.7/ tube		0.1/tube	5.9/tube

Oral supplements

Product	Description	Cost									
Ensure Plus	350 kcal, 13 g protein per serving. Chocolate, strawberry, vanilla. Lactose-free, gluten-free, low residue	$	1.5	54	8.64	56	29	43	47	833	750
Resource Breeze	250 kcal, 9 g protein per serving, clear liquid, fat free. Orange, peach, berry. Lactose-free, low residue	$$	1.06	38	6.08	86	0	<15	<2.2	680	750
Boost Diabetic	237 kcal with 13.8 g of protein, 20 g total carb/8 oz. 3.5 g fiber/8 oz, 4 g arginine/L. Choc and vanilla. Contains FOS. Lactose-free	$$	1.06	58.2	9.3	36	42	47.8 (van) 54 (choc)	28.1	928	400 / 1180 / 847
Scandishake-Regular	High calorie powder mixed with 8oz whole milk. Provides 600 calories with 14 g protein	$$$	600/svg	13/svg		39	45	9/svg	17/ svg	1094	478 / NA

High-calorie oral supplement

Product	Description	Cost									
High Kcal Shake	High-calorie shakes: (a) peaches & cream, (b) peanut butter cup, or (c) Christmas in a cup. (Derived from 2cal HN, not lactose free). *Nutr info is per serving*	$		(a) 22 (b) 27 (c) 22						(a) 681 (b) 707 (c) 584	(a) 34 (b) 439 (c) 319

AA, amino acid; ALI, acute lung injury; ARDS, adult respiratory distress syndrome; CHO, carbohydrate; EPA, eicosapentaenoic acid; GLA, γ-linolenic acid; MCT, medium-chain triglyceride; SIRS, systemic inflammatory response syndrome.

the progression of illness/injury. A multicenter trial of oxandrolone (a testosterone derivative) in burn injury demonstrated a reduction in hospital length of stay and the number of operative procedures in patients receiving oxandrolone [52]. As opposed to purely anabolic agents, a new area of research has looked at anti-catabolic agents to reduce hypermetabolism and improve outcome. A trial demonstrated that propranolol can reduce resting energy expenditure in severely burned children [53]. Further, propranolol increased protein synthesis to a point where these burned children were anabolic at 2 weeks post-injury, as opposed to the continued catabolism at 2 weeks that persisted in the control group. Finally, the deposition of lean body mass versus fat deposition (primarily in the liver) was significantly improved by propranalol therapy.

Specific pharmacologically active amino acids
Glutamine

To help maintain gut integrity, it has been recommended for many years that glutamine (GLN) be added to both enteral and parenteral nutrition regimens. GLN, the most abundant free amino acid in the blood and skeletal muscle, is a primary fuel for rapidly dividing cells such as enterocytes and immunocytes and is a precursor of purines, pyrimidines, and nucleotides [54]. Plasma GLN levels decrease significantly following critical illness and remain decreased for more than 21 days because of marked increases in utilization and decreased GLN synthesis [55]. This deficiency is associated with increased mortality in critically ill patients [56]. A meta-analysis demonstrated a strong trend toward benefit of GLN supplementation in clinical trials of critically ill subjects [57]. When more recent trials of GLN in the critical care setting are added to this analysis, GLN therapy leads to a statistically significant effect in reducing mortality in critically ill patients (RR 0.75, 95% CI 0.59–0.76) (available at www.criticalcarenutrition.com). This 25% reduction in mortality is associated with no sign of harm or adverse events in any of the trials performed to date. This meta-analysis indicated that GLN was most beneficial when given in larger parenteral doses.

Multiple mechanistic explanations for this beneficial effect of GLN have been proposed, including improved tissue protection, immune modulation, preservation of glutathione and antioxidant capacity, and preservation of metabolism [58]. One possible central theme in these proposed mechanisms may involve the requirement of GLN for induction of heat shock proteins (HSPs), specifically HSP70 [47,59,60]. HSPs are a family of highly conserved proteins involved in the most basic mechanisms of cellular protection. Data in experimental injury models indicate that induction of HSP70 protects proteins from damage, allows for restoration of function to damaged proteins, reduces stress-related increases in gut permeability, prevents post-injury metabolic dysfunction, attenuates proinflammatory response, and prevents cellular injury and death [61–66]. Enhanced HSP expression has been hypothesized to be beneficial in numerous clinical settings including sepsis, shock, tissue ischemia–reperfusion injury, and autoimmune/inflammatory diseases. It appears that critically ill patients who are GLN-deficient (which virtually all are) will be unable to generate an adequate HSP response, placing them at greater risk for organ failure. It has been shown that GLN can induce HSP expression in unstressed animals as well as in clinically relevant models of critical illness [67–73]. This induction is correlated with decreased organ injury and improved survival. GLN administration to critically ill patients has also been shown to enhance HSP70 expression, and this correlates with improved ICU outcome [74]. There are numerous large, randomized, multi-institutional studies currently ongoing, which will further refine our understanding of how to utilize this emerging "phamaconutrient."

Arginine

Arginine is another key nutrient in the body's response to injury. Arginine is metabolized by a number of pathways following injury. One leads to formation of nitric oxide (NO), which is vital to appropriate vascular and immune function following stress, but can lead to adverse consequences when NO is overexpressed [75]. The second pathway is the ornithine pathway, which is vital to wound healing and recovery [75]. Finally, arginine is vital for T-cell division and maintenance of lymphocyte counts, particularly following trauma and surgery [46]. A great deal of controversy has surrounded arginine supplementation in recent years. A meta-analysis of arginine supplementation indicated that enteral formulas containing high amounts of arginine administered in patients with sepsis or septic shock led to increased mortality and worsened outcomes [76]. However, data from this same group reveal that arginine supplementation prior to and/or following major abdominal surgery leads to large statistically significant reductions in postoperative infection and length of stay [76].

How do we explain this apparent dichotomy? More recent laboratory data have begun to provide an answer [46]. Following trauma and surgery, large decreases in plasma arginine occur. This is driven by the appearance of a new class of T cells known as myeloid suppressor cells, which express arginase, an enzyme that breaks down arginine rapidly. These cells are not present in sepsis, and concomitantly arginine deficiency does not occur in isolated sepsis or septic shock. This newly defined "arginine deficiency syndrome" following trauma or surgery, as well as in cancer, leads to loss of T cells in the spleen and lymph nodes and apparent immunosuppression. This contributes to the common occurrence of infection in the post-trauma and postoperative setting. This provides a very likely explanation for why arginine supplementation is beneficial following surgical illness, because these patients are arginine-deficient [77]. However, septic patients do not exhibit arginine deficiency and thus supplementation is likely unnecessary and may drive pathologic increases in NO [77]. Current data strongly support that all patients having major abdominal surgery should receive arginine-enriched nutritional supplements preoperatively.

Trace elements (micronutrients) and vitamins

There has been a recent revival of interest in the use of antioxidants as therapeutic agents in critical illness [78]. Studies of specific antioxidants are lacking, but meta-analysis data have implied that there may be a survival benefit to regimens containing selenium, and numerous trials are currently ongoing (see www.criticalcarenutrition.com). It appears that doses of selenium in the 500 µg per day range may be of benefit in critical illness [78]. Larger doses can become pro-oxidant and create risk for the patients [78]. See Table 56.4 for trace elements and vitamins when designing nutritional support regimens.

Practical aspects of nutrient administration

Indications for nutrition

A many as 50–70% of hospitalized patients may be malnourished [79,80]. A recent study emphasizes the importance of providing adequate enteral/oral nutrition to all hospitalized patients [81]. This trial examined hospitalized patients for the occurrence of "gut failure" or inadequate gut function. "Gut failure" was defined in this study as patients who failed to achieve 80% of goal enteral feeds for at least 48 hours at any time during their hospital stay. Patients diagnosed with gut failure had a mortality of greater than 80%, whereas those able to be fed near goal for at least 48 hours had less than a 20% mortality. The occurrence of gut failure led to significant increases in mortality and sepsis. By univariate analysis, gut failure was associated with a 16-fold increased risk of death [81].

Surgical patients

Preoperative malnutrition is associated with poor surgical outcome [82]. Even in apparently well-nourished patients, preoperative nutritional intervention has been shown to be improve outcome [83]. Preoperative nutrition with an oral arginine-enriched formula for 5–7 days prior to surgery leads to significant reductions in postoperative infection and hospital length of stay [83–85]. To date over 25 trials of arginine-enriched enteral nutrition have been published, all showing a benefit in incidence of infection and length of stay. This benefit is primarily in patients having major abdominal surgery. However, it is not limited to malnourished patients. Patients with less than a 10% weight loss prior to surgery appear to benefit equally from arginine-enriched oral supplements as compared with patients with more significant preoperative malnutrition [83].

The benefit of preoperative parenteral nutrition in malnourished patients has been difficult to demonstrate, except in severely malnourished patients, who have been shown to have fewer noninfectious complications after 7–10 days of nutritional repletion. It is also beneficial to continue total parenteral nutrition (TPN) during and after surgery in these patients [86]. In normally nourished patients, typically defined as patients with a body mass index (BMI) > 25, postoperative parenteral nutritional support is typically not indicated unless it is anticipated that patients will be unable to resume adequate oral or enteral feeding within 7–10 days of surgery. However, it is routine to administer at least 2 L per day of a 5% dextrose solution, which has some protein-sparing effects. Patients not expected to resume adequate oral feedings within 7–10 days of surgery, or with significant preoperative malnutrition (> 10% of body weight loss or BMI < 20), should have enteral nutritional support attempted immediately (0–2 days) after surgery. There are extensive data indicating that the practice of keeping patients nil-by-mouth until the return of bowel sounds or passage of gas should be abandoned [87,88]. This is particularly true in high-risk surgical patients with malnutrition at time of surgery. The fear of anastomotic dehiscence if patients were fed too early has not been confirmed in clinical trials. In fact, data reveal that enteral feedings started immediately postoperatively improve anastomotic healing and reduce anastomotic dehiscence [87,88]. A Cochrane review group examined the effect of very early enteral feeding versus delayed enteral feeding following gastrointestinal surgery, and their meta-analysis revealed that early enteral nutrition led to a 59% relative risk reduction (RR 0.41, 95% CI 0.18–0.93, $p < 0.03$) of complications following gastrointestinal surgery [87]. Modern thinking preaches that "ileus begets ileus," and the longer one waits to feed following surgery or other injury the greater the chance of persistent gastroparesis and ileus. Burn care provides the most useful example of this phenomenon. Patients in major burn centers with the most massive injury known to be survivable by a human (up to and beyond 90% burns) are fed within hours of admission and tolerate this well. If feeding is delayed even for short periods of time, significant ileus and gastroparesis set in, making feeding more difficult. Thus, if one wishes to be consistently successful in enterally feeding sick patients, early feeding (even if it is only trophic in nature) gives the greatest chance of success. Sufficient early nutritional support of surgical patients not expected to eat soon after surgery has also reduced hospital length of stay and decreased costs [89].

Critical care patients

Malnutrition has been observed in 38–100% of mechanically ventilated patients in the ICU [90]. Therefore it is mandatory to begin enteral nutrition within 24 hours of ICU admission in patients without significant contraindications (see recommendations at www.criticalcarenutrition.com). This is to attempt to prevent further loss of lean body mass and provide key pharmacologically active nutrients that can be depleted rapidly

Table 56.4. Considerations when designing nutritional support regimens

Considerations	Issues	Recommendations
Route of administration	Enteral vs. parenteral vs. both	Enteral is always preferred to parenteral with functioning gut
Caloric requirements	Measure energy expenditure using indirect calorimetry or estimate energy expenditure using established equations (see Table 56.1).	
Protein/amino acids	Evaluate degree of stress, measure nitrogen balance	Unstressed patients: 1.0–1.5 g kg^{-1} day^{-1} protein
	Parenteral nutrition: amino acid solutions	Stressed patients: 1.5–2.0 g kg^{-1} day^{-1} protein
	Enteral nutrition: standard vs. high-protein formulas; amino acids (elemental diet) peptides vs. protein hydrolysates. If protein losses are excessive then need increased protein	
Calorie/protein ratio	Expressed as calorie/nitrogen ratio:	
	Standard enteral formulas: 150:1	
	Enteral stress formulas: 125–100:1	
Carbohydrates	Parenteral nutrition: glucose is only available nutrient	Glucose intake not to exceed 4 mg kg^{-1} min^{-1} during stress
	Enteral nutrition: oligosaccharides and starches	
Lipid	Parenteral nutrition: LCT emulsions	Consider reducing parenteral lipids in critical care to once a week administration
	Enteral formulas: contain LCT or LCT/MCT; some enriched with omega-3 fatty acids	Use omega-3 enriched formulas in ALI/ARDS and sepsis?
Lipid/carbohydrate ratio	Parenteral nutrition: 30:70 to 60:40	
	Enteral nutrition: depends on formula. Calorie-dense formulas have higher fat ratios	
Electrolytes	Parenteral nutrition: sodium (NaCl, Na acetate), potassium (KCl, K acetate), PO$_4$ (NaPO$_4$, KPO$_4$), MgSO$_4$, calcium (Ca-gluconate)	K: 1–1.2 mEq kg^{-1}
	Enteral nutrition: as per formulation. May add electrolytes, if needed	Mg: 8–20 mEq
		Ca: 10–15 mEq
		PO$_4$: 20–30 mmol day^{-1}
Trace elements	Trace elements are minerals with requirements < 100 mg day^{-1}	
	Parenteral nutrition: additives contain copper, selenium, zinc, manganese, chromium. Cobalt is given as vitamin B$_{12}$.	
	Check zinc, copper, selenium with prolonged admnistration	
	Enteral nutrition: also contain iron, molybdenum, iodine	
	Critical Care: selenium/zinc may be vital	
Vitamins	Parenteral nutrition: commercial preparations usually contain all vitamins (except vitamin K). Monitor PT weekly and give vitamin K, if indicated.	
	Enteral nutrition: contain all vitamins including vitamin K; the volume of formula that provides the recommended daily requirements depends on the formula (see Table 56.3).	
	Vitamin C: needs are increased during wound repair	
	Vitamin B (esp. thiamine): important in alcoholics	
Water	Parenteral nutrition: dilute vs. concentrated formulas. Dilute for peripheral vein administration. Concentrated for fluid restriction and high caloric intakes.	
	Standard enteral nutrition (1.06 kcal mL^{-1}) vs. calorie-dense (2.0 kcal mL^{-1}).	

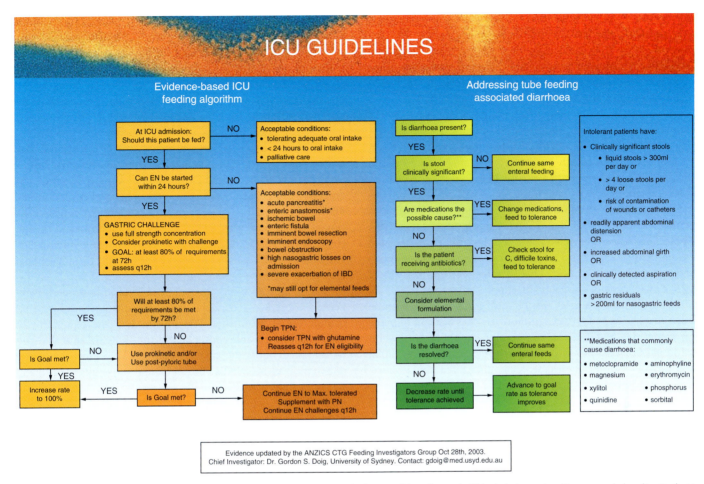

Figure 56.1. Critical care feeding protocol and feeding intolerance protocol. Ideal protocol form for use in ICU admission orders. Recommended prokinetic drugs are erythromycin for first-line prokinetic therapy. Metoclopramide may be used as second-line drug. Reproduced from www.evidencebased.net, courtesy of Dr. Gordon S. Doig and Dr. Andrew Davies.

or those that appear to improve outcome (e.g., glutamine and omega-3 fatty acids). This is not a new concept. Data from the early 1980s showed that patients who accumulated a caloric deficit of greater the 10 000 kcal during their ICU stay had a mortality of 76% [91]. All major nutrition and critical care society clinical guidelines recommend the early initiation of enteral feeding. A useful flow-sheet guideline for the initiation of critical care nutrition therapy is shown in Fig. 56.1 (available for download from www.evidencebased.net).

Route of administration

A major decision in the nutritional support of seriously ill patients is the route of administration. If patients are eating on their own, it is necessary to monitor their actual intake to assess its adequacy. Many of these patients have little appetite and thus may need nutritional supplements to increase their caloric intake. There are commercially available nutritional supplements that provide a balanced intake (Table 56.3). Patients who do not sustain adequate caloric intake by eating may require either enteral or parenteral nutrition.

Enteral nutrition

The enteral route is preferred over the parenteral because it is the natural portal for exogenous nutrients. The enteral route obviates the need for intravascular access and its attendant propensity for infections. Also, the variety of nutrients that can be administered via the gastrointestinal tract is greater than those available for parenteral use, allowing for better tailoring of nutrient intake. Other advantages of the enteral route include lower cost [92], ease of administration, and maintenance of gut function.

There has been a great deal of interest in enteral nutrition being utilized to maintain gut integrity and therefore lessen the translocation of bacteria from the gut [93]. Animal experiments show that translocation of bacteria from the intestines leads to local activation of the gut's immune inflammatory system (Peyer's patches and hepatic Kupffer cells [93]). The released cytokines then exacerbate the already existing systemic inflammatory response, leading to multiple organ failure [93]. However, there is no significant evidence of translocation in humans [94]. One important trial that examined this question studied patients following major torso trauma [95]. The patients in the trial had a catheter placed in their portal vein following trauma laparotomy. Blood was sampled on multiple occasions looking for the presence of bacteria or increased levels of endotoxin/cytokines versus systemic blood samples. No meaningful bacteremia was found in any of the 212 samples, with one exception (one positive culture for *Staphylococcus aureus* in a patient with *S. aureus* pneumonia). Further, no increases in endotoxin or cytokine presence were found in the portal circulation versus systemic blood samples. However, extensive laboratory data implicate the translocation of inflammatory and toxic mediators from the gut into the lymph as a primary cause of organ failure, particularly lung injury [96]. These mediators are likely secreted by the gut-associated lymph tissue (GALT) and carried by the lymph to the pulmonary and central circulation. This hypothesized mechanism of injury may provide impetus to supply enteral nutrition in order to protect the gut barrier and regulate gut immune function. The fear of reduced gut integrity has been an impetus for recommending that enteral nutrition should begin as soon as possible, even when it is possible to administer only small amounts [97]. In the latter case, concomitant parenteral nutrition may be needed to provide adequate caloric intake.

Timing and initiation of enteral feeding

Another key consideration when initiating nutrition support is timing and how to advance nutritional delivery. A growing body of literature indicates that early or immediate initiation of nutrition support postoperatively or at admission to the ICU improves patient outcome. Recent meta-analysis data reveal that early feeding shows a nonsignificant trend towards reduction in mortality in ICU patients (RR 0.69, 95% CI 0.45–1.05, $p = 0.08$) (available at www.criticalcarenutrition.com). These data suggest that enteral feeding should be initiated within 24 hours of ICU admission. What is not well understood is how aggressively enteral feeding should be advanced once begun. The chart shown in Fig. 56.1 provides the best available guide to the initiation of enteral feeding. Standard of practice should be to attempt to advance all patients to goal feeds over 72 hours, particularly if a small-bowel feeding tube is in place. Monitoring of gastric residual volumes, abdominal distension, nausea/vomiting, and diarrhea are useful guides to patient tolerance. As will be discussed subsequently, the most current data indicate that feeding should only be suspended or decreased when gastric residuals are greater than 500 mL for one measurement [98].

Parenteral nutrition

The key to successful PN administration is a nutrition therapy team with a certified nutrition support dietician (CNSD) and/or a pharmacist expert in PN prescription. Very few practicing physicians are expert in writing in PN. PN is indicated when the enteral route cannot provide or sustain sufficient caloric intake. Although the current approach is to attempt to use the gut, there are situations in which PN is mandatory. Patients with short bowel syndrome require PN after surgery and may require it for life if the remaining bowel does not undergo sufficient adaptation to sustain adequate oral intake. Other absolute indications for PN are prolonged small-bowel obstruction, active gastrointestinal bleeding, pseudo-obstruction with complete intolerance to food, and high-output enterocutaneous fistulae (unless a feeding tube can be passed distal to the fistula). In partial large-bowel obstruction it may or may not be possible to feed with a low-residue diet. Relative indications for PN include nonhealing, moderate-output, enterocutaneous fistulae; acute radiation enteritis; marked abdominal distension and ileus caused by intra-abdominal sepsis; continued distention after relief of intestinal obstruction; and chylothorax unresponsive to a medium-chain triglyceride diet. PN is also indicated when adequate nutrition cannot be sustained through the enteral route.

PN is administered through either central or peripheral venous catheters. Peripheral veins are unable to tolerate an osmolarity of more than 750 mOsm L^{-1} (the equivalent of 12.5% dextrose), and consequently the fluid volume that can be tolerated limits the calories that can be administered. No data have ever revealed a clinical benefit to peripheral PN, and its use is therefore strongly discouraged except for very short-term use (i.e., while awaiting central venous access). Central venous catheters are the main route of PN administration. The catheter should have the least number of lumens possible and have a lumen dedicated for PN administration only. This lumen should have no other medications or "piggy-back" drugs given other than the PN. The catheter should have antibacterial coatings (silver or antibiotics) to lessen the risk of infection. Multi-lumen catheters and multipurpose single-lumen catheters have high infection rates. For long-term use, silastic Hickman or Broviac catheters should be inserted using a subcutaneous tunnel. These catheters have a Dacron cuff at the proximal end of the tunnel to reduce infections.

Monitoring of nutrition support

In the acutely ill patient, the effects of enteral and parenteral nutrition must be monitored. The most basic monitoring is quantifying the actual caloric intake. This is especially important during enteral nutrition because it is difficult to achieve and maintain adequate intake using only the enteral route [99]. With large losses of enteric content, serum zinc and selenium levels should be measured after a few weeks of nutritional support. In long-term PN support, copper deficiency has been described as far more common than previously recognized [100]. A trace element panel should be checked regularly in patients on long-term PN. As glutamine is not contained in typical PN solutions in North America it may also become deficient. This is often true in oncology patients and ICU patients. Two meta-analyses of the data in this population support the routine use of glutamine in these populations when they require PN [57,101]. Stable and viable L-glutamine solutions are available in North America from PN compounding agencies. However, these come as 2.5% solutions and thus are quite dilute. This can make delivering the 0.3–0.5 g kg^{-1} day^{-1} of GLN required for optimal clinical effect challenging in fluid-restricted patients.

During the initial phase of PN, plasma triglyceride should be monitored weekly in patients with potential fat clearance problems, such as those with hyperlipidemia, diabetes, sepsis, and impaired renal or hepatic function. Liver function tests should be monitored weekly during the initial month of nutritional support. Increases of aminotransferases and alkaline phosphatase may occur secondary to hepatic steatosis, especially if large glucose loads are administered. Liver function tests should continue to be monitored monthly in patients on long-term PN, because intrahepatic cholestasis may develop.

Assessing the direct effects of nutritional support in the short term (days to weeks) is difficult. In severely ill catabolic patients, the aim of feeding is not to restore lost body mass but to attenuate further losses. Therefore, initial evidence of lean body-mass restoration should not be expected. In one study, it took 2 weeks to show even a slight improvement in nutritional status [102]. Short-term changes in body weight in acutely ill patients reflect mainly fluid balance, and anthropometric measurements (e.g., triceps skin thickness) often reflect the degree of edema. Measurements of nitrogen balance assess catabolic/anabolic state and guide adjustments in protein/ amino acid intake. Serum albumin (normal $t_{1/2}$ 21 days) concentrations are decreased in acute illness because of decreased synthetic rate, shortened half-life, and redistribution into the extracellular fluid. Therefore, acute changes in plasma albumin concentrations after surgery or trauma are caused by the redistribution of albumin into the expanded extracellular fluid. Proteins with short half-lives, e.g., prealbumin ($t_{1/2}$ 2–3 days) and transferrin ($t_{1/2}$ 8 days), are better indicators of protein synthesis. It is currently the standard of practice in most academic centers to obtain a weekly prealbumin and C-reactive protein (CRP) to measure nutritional delivery [103]. The prealbumin reflects nutritional status accurately in non-inflamed/noninfected patients. However, in patients with systemic inflammatory response or SIRS an elevation of the CRP will be noted and the prealbumin will always be low and not reflect nutritional delivery. This is due to the fact that when the body is focused on making "inflammatory" proteins it will not produce "anabolic" proteins such as prealbumin. Thus, when the CRP is greater than ~ 5 mg dL^{-1} the prealbumin will not be an accurate reflection of nutritional delivery. In these cases, the cause of the inflammation must be found (e.g., alleviating pancreatitis or a wound infection) and nutritional delivery should be based on a dietician's or physician's assessment of needs. Increases in caloric intake should not be based on a low prealbumin in the face of an elevated CRP if the predictive equations or metabolic cart data judge the caloric intake to be adequate.

As patients convalesce, the type, amount, and composition of the nutritional support may need to be changed. The proportion of carbohydrate calories might be increased as glucose intolerance abates. One might also consider increasing intravenous lipid intake in patients on PN. Overfeeding must be avoided.

Complications of nutritional therapy

Parenteral nutrition: gastrointestinal system complications

Parenteral nutrition is associated with hepatobiliary complications whose causes may be multifactorial. The most important factors in the development of hepatobiliary dysfunction are the underlying disease and its severity, omega-6-based lipid infusion, intercurrent sepsis, and drugs [104]. Large glucose loads (> 4 mg kg^{-1} min^{-1}) can result in hepatic steatosis and steatohepatitis. The latter is accompanied by increases in ALT, AST, and alkaline phosphatase [105]. Intrahepatic cholestasis with increased alkaline phosphatase and bilirubin may occur 3–6 weeks after TPN is started. Large lipid loads (> 2 g day^{-1}) administered for prolonged periods can also cause cholestasis. In PN-dependent pediatric short-bowel patients, cholestasis and subsequent liver failure often results in the need for liver transplantation or ultimately the death of the child [106]. However, an exciting new therapeutic option is now available to treat and prevent this PN-related life-threatening liver failure. An intravenous fish oil preparation that has been used for many years in Europe is now available for compassionate use in North America. In a large series of PN-dependent children at the Boston Children's Hospital, intravenous fish oil has been shown to completely reverse PN-related liver disease in an average of 12 weeks of therapy [106]. This therapy is not effective once these children have progressed to cirrhosis with portal flow abnormalities. However, for children treated prior to the terminal stages of liver failure, it appears that this is a safe and truly life-saving intervention.

Enteral nutrition: gastrointestinal system complications

Gastric residuals and increased risk of aspiration have long been a reason cited for poor delivery of enteral nutrition. Recent data from multiple studies reveal that gastric residuals of under 500 mL do not increase the risk of aspiration [98]. Thus, tube feedings should not be routinely held or stopped for gastric residuals less than 500 mL. If gastric residuals and gastroparesis do become issues, the most effective treatment appears to be erythromycin, which acts to increase motility in the stomach and proximal small bowel [107]. Metoclopramide is a second choice that can be added to the erythromycin to improve feeding tolerance [107].

A frequent and particularly unpleasant (for patient and staff) complication of enteral nutrition is diarrhea. Its reported incidence, depending on the definition of diarrhea, ranges from 2% to as high as 53% and 38% of feeding days [108,109]. The definition of diarrhea is important, because many enteral products are "low-residual," i.e., they do not contain fiber and may not cause formed stools. Diarrhea is caused both by the feeds and by other factors [110]. Formula-related causes include hyperosmolar feeds and contamination of feedings with enterotoxigenic or pathogenic organisms. To prevent the latter, feeds should be sterile and not allowed to hang more than 8 hours. Other causes include *Clostridium difficile* enterocolitis, broad-spectrum antibiotics, and hypoalbuminemia. *C. difficile* enterocolitis, once a minor annoyance in sick patients, has become a more serious and even fatal complication and should be checked for any time new-onset diarrhea is noted in the ICU setting [111]. A protocol for evaluation of enteral feeding intolerance and diarrhea is included in Fig. 56.1.

Metabolic complications of nutrition therapy: feeding in the operating room and glycemic control

Metabolic complications of nutritional support occur with some frequency. Thus in acutely ill patients it is important to monitor electrolytes and glucose daily, especially when initiating support. Hyperglycemia is a frequent problem, especially with severe stress, steroid use, and diabetes mellitus. These patients often require insulin treatment. Importantly, as the stress response abates, the degree of glucose intolerance lessens and insulin requirements decrease. Therefore it is imperative to monitor blood glucose closely to reduce insulin treatment and prevent hypoglycemia.

Hypoglycemia may occur on the abrupt discontinuation of continuous feedings containing significant amounts of carbohydrate. Continuous feedings result in high blood insulin concentrations so that hypoglycemia intervenes when the carbohydrate intake stops. Therefore, when stopping continuous parenteral and enteral nutrition, any concomitant insulin infusion should be stopped, intravenous glucose should be infused, and blood glucose monitored frequently. In the operative setting it is probably safer to keep PN infusions running in the operating room. This is particularly true in patients on insulin infusions. The risk of hypoglycemia causing a poor outcome or mortality in sick patients is discussed below. Enteral nutrition should be discontinued 6 hours before surgery and a glucose infusion should be started to prevent hypoglycemia in patients who are not intubated. In intubated patients who have a cuffed endotracheal tube there is no clear indication to stop enteral feeds unless the patient is having a gastrointestinal operation and needs a bowel preparation or the patient will be going prone and is at greater risk for unexpected extubation.

In the last 10 years significant interest and controversy have surrounded the use of "tight glucose control" in the critical care setting. The seminal publication of van den Berghe and colleagues in 2001 demonstrated that in a surgical ICU population of predominantly cardiac surgery patients insulin infusion to reduce glucose to 80–110 mg dL^{-1} led to major reductions in mortality, organ failure, and infectious complications [112]. Tight glucose control became widespread in virtually all ICUs worldwide almost immediately following this publication. Van den Berghe subsequently published a medical ICU trial which showed no effect of tight glucose control in the intention-to-treat data, but a significant reduction of mortality in patients in the ICU for 3 or more days [113]. Despite their widespread acceptance, neither of these trials was generalizable to the majority of other ICUs in the world. This was due to the fact that both trials initiated PN with high dextrose loads on day 1 of every ICU admission. This is a significant limitation, as fewer than 10% of North American patients receive TPN during their ICU stay (see survey results at www.criticalcarenutrition.com). Further, almost no critical care units in North America initiate TPN in all patients on day 1 of admission to ICU. Thus, it is possible that the tight glucose control trials were improving outcome because the control group was experiencing increased morbidity due to large early infusions of PN (which has been associated with increased ICU complications). Conversely, the experimental group experienced less caloric debt due to more aggressive PN feeding. It is possible that the improved outcomes observed are due to decreased caloric debt and treatment of associated hyperglycemia with insulin. This question remains unanswered. It should also be noted that although both studies enrolled over 1000 patients, they were both single-center trials (the same center in both trials). This question has recently been addressed in a more generalizable fashion by two large multicenter trials of tight glucose control in critically ill patients, the VISEP and Glucontrol trials [114]. Both trials were stopped due to lack of efficacy and unanticipated risk of hypoglycemia in the tight control or intensive insulin therapy groups. In both of these the trials the majority of patients received early enteral nutrition and very limited PN calories. Neither trial showed a mortality benefit from intensive insulin therapy. Further, the Glucontrol trial showed a twofold increase in the risk of death for any patient experiencing hypoglycemia of < 60 mg dL^{-1}. Forty-one percent of patients in the intensive insulin group experienced a hypoglycemic episode of this magnitude during the study. Meta-analysis of all trials of tight glucose control showed no beneficial effect of tight glucose control on mortality [17]. The recently published multinational NICE-SUGAR trial studied over 6000 patients and revealed that tight glucose control (TGC: 81–108 mg dL^{-1}) led to a significant increase in 90-day post-ICU mortality compared with moderate glucose control (MGC: < 180 mg dL^{-1}) [115]. Mortality was 27.5% with TGC versus 24.9% with MGC (OR 1.14, 95% CI 1.02–1.28, $p = 0.02$). Thus it appears that until the issue of the risks of hypoglycemia and tight glucose control can be resolved, the latest recommendations suggest maintaining glucose levels below 180 mg dL^{-1} in ICU patients.

108. Edes TE, Walk BE, Austin JL. Diarrhea in tube-fed patients: feeding formula not necessarily the cause. *Am J Med* 1990; **88**: 91–3.

109. Medley F, Stechmiller J, Field A. Complications of enteral nutrition in hospitalized patients with artificial airways. *Clin Nurs Res* 1993; **2**: 212–23.

110. Heimburger DC, Sockwell DG, Geels WJ. Diarrhea with enteral feeding: prospective reappraisal of putative causes. *Nutrition* 1994; **10**: 392–6.

111. Taubes G. Collateral damage. The rise of resistant C. difficile. *Science* 2008; **321**: 360.

112. van den Berghe G, Wouters P, Weekers F, *et al.* Intensive insulin therapy in the critically ill patients. *N Eng J Med* 2001; **345**: 1359–67.

113. van den Berghe G, Wilmer A, Hermans G, *et al.* Intensive insulin therapy in the medical ICU. *N Eng J Med* 2006; **354**: 449–61.

114. Brunkhorst FM, Engel C, Bloos F, *et al.* Intensive insulin therapy and pentastarch resuscitation in severe sepsis. *N Eng J Med* 2008; **358**: 125–39.

115. Finfer S, Chittock DR, Su SY, *et al.* Intensive versus conventional glucose control in critically ill patients. *N Engl J Med* 2009; **360**: 1283–97.

116. Frankenfield DC, Reynolds HN. Nutritional effect of continuous hemodiafiltration. *Nutrition* 1995; **11**: 388–93.

117. Druml W. Protein metabolism in acute renal failure. *Miner Electrolyte Metab* 1998; **24**: 47–54.

118. Fortin MC, Amyot SL, Geadah D, Leblanc M. Serum concentrations and clearances of folic acid and pyridoxal-5-phosphate during venovenous continuous renal replacement therapy. *Intensive Care Med* 1999; **25**: 594–8.

Troy Wildes, Michael Avidan, and George Despotis

Physiology of hemostasis

The vascular endothelium serves as a protective layer and prevents activation of the coagulation system. When vascular integrity is compromised, the coordinated actions of platelets, the blood vessel wall, von Willebrand factor (vWF), and other coagulation factors trigger thrombus formation (Fig. 57.1), thus limiting hemorrhage. The endothelium contains important antiplatelet regulators, including nitric oxide (NO) [1], prostacyclin (PGI_2) [2], adenosine, and the ectonucleotidase CD39 [3]. PGI_2 and NO, which are released in response to shearing forces, are labile vasorelaxant and antiaggregatory substances [4]. The endothelium is also a source of anticoagulant factors such as antithrombin, heparin cofactor II, tissue plasminogen activator (tPA), tissue factor pathway inhibitor (TFPI), and thrombomodulin as well as procoagulant factors such as factor VIII and vWF and subendothelial tissue factor (Fig. 57.2).

Platelets are integrally involved in the initial response to vessel injury and play a pivotal role in hemostasis. Inactivated, they float inert as smooth discs in the blood. In response to numerous stimuli, they change shape, form pseudopods, extrude their granular contents, and bind avidly both to subendothelial surfaces and to one another. When endothelium is denuded, activated platelets adhere to exposed subendothelium, a reaction largely mediated by collagen and vWF, and then aggregate to provide initial hemostasis (Fig. 57.1). Platelets also provide an active phospholipid surface for interaction with coagulation factors, such as factor Va/Xa prothrombinase complex, that are activated by tissue factor. Platelet receptors are membrane glycoproteins (GPs) that bind to vWF, to collagen, and to fibrinogen (Fig. 57.2). Activated platelets express adhesins and integrins, members of the superfamily of adhesion molecules. Collagen binding to the platelet GPIa receptor and vWF binding to the GPIb receptor, both located on the surface of the activated platelet, facilitate both adhesion and further activation of platelets. The platelet, once activated, initiates an amplification process of further platelet aggregation and binding. There is release of platelet agonists from

alpha and dense storage granules in the platelet, including adenosine diphosphate (ADP) and serotonin. Thrombin, a key regulator of the coagulation cascade, is one of the most powerful platelet activators. The platelet GPIIb/IIIa receptor acts as a binding site for fibrinogen and fibrin, facilitating the linkage of platelets to one another and stabilizing the platelet plug.

Exposed collagen triggers the accumulation and activation of platelets, whereas exposed tissue factor initiates the generation of thrombin [5]. The interactions of platelet glycoprotein VI with the collagen of the exposed vessel wall and of platelet glycoprotein Ib-V-IX with collagen-bound vWF result in adhesion of platelets to the site of injury. Tissue factor forms a complex with factor VIIa, the enzymatically active form of factor VII, and this tissue factor–factor VIIa complex activates factor IX, thereby initiating a proteolytic cascade that generates thrombin [5]. Thrombin cleaves protease-activated receptor 1 on the platelet surface, thereby activating platelets [6] and causing them to release ADP, serotonin, and thromboxane A_2 (TxA_2). Thrombin promotes the activation of factors V and VIII, which leads to a massive amplification of further thrombin production. The rate of thrombin generation is less than 1% of the rate in the presence of thrombin-activated factor Va [7,8].

The coagulation system consists of a number of clotting active zymogens and cofactors and has classically been subdivided into the intrinsic, extrinsic, and common pathways that lead to formation of a fibrin clot (Fig. 57.1). Tissue factor binds to and activates factor VII, and drives the extrinsic pathway to form fibrin, which activates platelets and stabilizes the hemostatic platelet plug. Tissue factor can exist in a latent (or "encrypted") form that lacks coagulant activity or in an active form that initiates blood coagulation [5]. Tissue factor is the sole initiator of thrombin generation and fibrin formation. The contact or collagen or intrinsic pathway of blood coagulation [9,10], a powerful tool for in-vitro studies of the coagulation cascade, is not required for initiation of hemostasis in vivo [11]. A complete deficiency of factor XII, high-molecular-weight kininogen, or prekallikrein is associated with major defects in the initiation of the contact pathway of

Anesthetic Pharmacology, 2nd edition, ed. Alex S. Evers, Mervyn Maze, Evan D. Kharasch. Published by Cambridge University Press. © Cambridge University Press 2011.

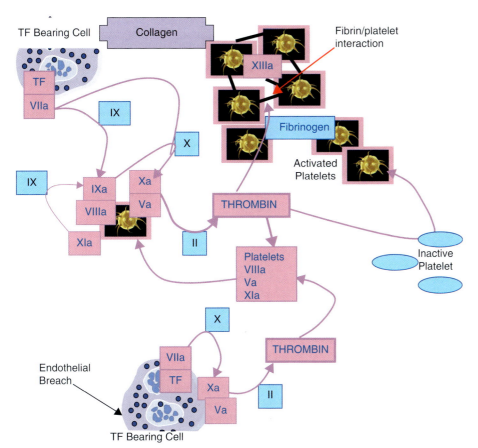

Figure 57.1. Normal clotting mechanisms. Inactivated clotting factors are blue and activated clotting factors are pink. The figure shows predominantly the cellular injury or extrinsic or tissue factor pathway. When the endothelium is denuded, cells bearing tissue factor (TF) and collagen are exposed. TF binds to and activates factor VII, and collagen provides a surface for platelets. This TF-VIIa complex in turn activates factors X and IX. Factor Xa activates factor V, and they then activate thrombin. The small amount of thrombin produced sends out an array of activating signals, most notably to platelets, FVIII and FV, fibrinogen/fibrin, FXIII and FXI. Activated platelets aggregate, exude sticky pseudopods, extrude granules (e.g., ADP, TXA$_2$, PAF), and attract more platelets to plug the breech by combining with fibrin. FXIIIa stabilizes the fibrin–platelet clot. FVa and FVIIIa complex with Xa and IXa respectively, and bind to activated platelets. On the activated platelet surface, a massive thrombin burst occurs, which sends out its signals and accelerates clotting.

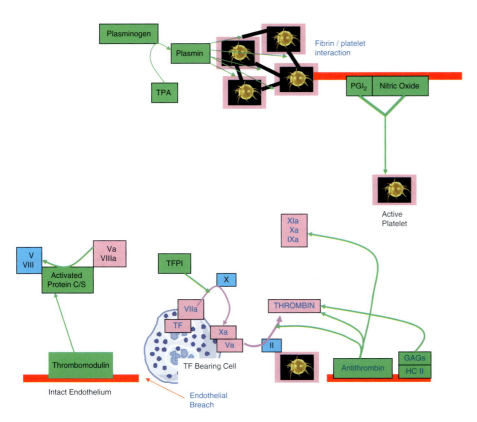

Figure 57.2. Normal anticlotting mechanisms. Inactivated clotting factors are blue, anticlotting factors are green, and activated clotting factors are pink. The intact endothelium usually prevents clotting. Nitric oxide and prostacyclin (PGI$_2$) are constitutively produced, and prevent platelet aggregation and adhesion. Tissue factor pathway inhibitor (TFPI) opposes the TF/VIIa/Xa complex. In areas where the endothelium has not been breeched, thrombomodulin receives signals from thrombin, and protein C and protein S inactivate the "amplification factors," VIIIa and Va. Antithrombin (AT), heparin cofactor II (HC II), and glycosaminoglycans (GAGs), such as heparan sulfate and dermatan sulfate, are also released by intact endothelium to oppose clotting agents. HC II potentiates the antithrombin action of the GAGs. Plasmin, a proteolytic enzyme, is activated by tissue plasminogen activator (TPA). Plasmin prevents rampant clot extension and promotes clot lysis or cleavage.

coagulation, as manifested by a markedly prolonged partial-thromboplastin time. Nevertheless, patients with any one of these deficiencies do not have a hemorrhagic disorder. Activated factor XII might be an example of a target for new inhibitors of thrombin generation: occlusive thrombi do not form in mice lacking factor XII [12,13], and neither mice nor humans who are deficient in factor XII have a hemostatic defect. The ideal drug for prophylaxis and treatment of thrombotic disease remains one that will inhibit thrombosis but not hemostasis.

PGI$_2$ and NO inhibit platelets, whereas proteins C and S in concert with thrombomodulin, antithrombin, heparin cofactor II, and TFPI, inhibit or degrade coagulation proteins (Fig. 57.2). The fibrinolytic system consists of several plasmatic factors, including tPA and plasminogen, that interact to produce plasmin, which lyses clots and potentially prevents vaso-occlusion at the site of vessel injury. The fibrinolytic system is regulated by factors such as plasminogen activator inhibitor and either α_1-antiplasmin or thrombin activatable fibrinolytic inhibitor (TAFI), which bind and inhibit tPA and plasmin, respectively.

There are many congenital and acquired causes of hemostatic abnormalities, including deficiencies or abnormal function of platelets, vWF, coagulation proteins, anticoagulants, or fibrinolytic peptides. With disseminated intravascular coagulopathy (DIC), excessive bleeding occurs after consumption of clotting factors and platelets. Thrombotic complications can also result from DIC-related excessive activation of the hemostatic system. Congenital abnormalities of platelets or coagulation factors are rare, with the most common involving defects in factor VIII (1 in 10 000 individuals) and vWF (which has been estimated to be present in as much as 1.5% of the general population). Acquired abnormalities of the hemostatic system occur with liver, renal, bone-marrow, or B-cell dysfunction, deficiencies of key nutrients such as proteins, folate, vitamin K, consumption of clotting factors or platelets with DIC, and with therapeutic use of anticoagulant or antiplatelet drugs. Significant hepatic dysfunction can result in reduced synthesis of all of the coagulation proteins with the exception of factor VIII, accelerated clearance of platelets with splenomegaly, or abnormal platelet function related to reduced hepatic clearance of fibrinogen/fibrin split products. Uremia secondary to renal failure can affect platelet function and interaction of platelets with vWF. Impairment of hepatic or renal function may affect the clearance of drugs that affect clotting and bleeding. Deficiency of a protein substrate or key cofactors, such as vitamin K, impairs coagulation factor synthesis, whereas vitamin B$_{12}$ and folate are required for platelet production. In certain clinical situations, there is a loss of platelets and coagulation factors that is not related to DIC. Such circumstances include volume resuscitation for bleeding, and pre-eclampsia. Other clinical conditions such as abruptio placentae, hypoperfusion, organ ischemia, ABO-incompatible transfusion, trauma, and use of cardiopulmonary bypass (CPB) with cardiac surgery can result in development of a consumptive process similar to DIC that depletes coagulation factors and platelets.

Numerous drugs have been developed to modify hemostasis (Fig. 57.3). Warfarin prevents coagulation-factor synthesis; heparin and thrombin inhibitors oppose coagulation-factor activity; and aspirin, ADP receptor blockers, and glycoprotein IIb/IIIa (GPIIb/IIa) antagonists inhibit platelet function, whereas tPA and streptokinase (SK) accelerate clot lysis. New drugs, the most advanced of which are directed against factor Xa or thrombin [14], have the potential to replace warfarin, heparin, and low-molecular-weight heparin for the treatment of and prophylaxis against thromboembolic disease.

Drugs that inhibit coagulation factors (Table 57.1) or platelet function are administered to prevent thromboses or complications relating to existing clots. Patients with established thromboses in the deep veins, arteries, and the heart require anticoagulant medication. In addition, patients who are at high risk for thromboses may require anticoagulation. Examples include patients with a history of recurrent thromboses, those with known thrombophilia, patients undergoing orthopedic surgery or other operative procedures that involve an extended period of immobilization, patients with prosthetic cardiac valves, abnormal cardiac function, or atrial fibrillation, patients with acute ischemic stroke, patients with arterial vaso-occlusive disease, patients with acute coronary syndromes, patients undergoing either percutaneous angioplasty or stenting procedures, and patients undergoing operative revascularization procedures or other cardiac surgical procedures.

As the physiology of platelets has been elucidated, targets for therapeutic intervention have been realized (Fig. 57.3). There has been an explosion of drugs that work in concert with aspirin to prevent or attenuate platelet activation by acting on different pathways. Examples include ticlopidine and clopidogrel, which block the platelet ADP receptor. The recently developed GPIIb/IIIa receptor blockers result in virtually complete inhibition of platelet-to-fibrinogen and platelet-to-platelet binding. This has been invaluable for interventional cardiology, in which early restenosis was a common event after coronary angioplasty. With GPIIb/IIIa receptor blockers, coronary angioplasty and stenting has become as successful in treating coronary artery disease, in many instances, as bypass surgery at a fraction of the cost and with considerably less morbidity.

There are also medications that oppose the actions of anticoagulants or prevent excessive bleeding. Protamine reverses the anticoagulant properties of heparin, ε-aminocaproic acid (EACA) and tranexamic acid (TA) inhibit physiologic or excessive fibrinolysis, and desmopressin (DDAVP) augments endothelial release of vWF, vWF/platelet interactions, or platelet function (enhanced platelet microtubule function, platelet expression of Ib receptors). Aprotinin is a broad-spectrum drug that affects hemostasis in multiple ways. Aprotinin has fallen into disfavor over concerns of renal dysfunction, thrombotic complications, and increased mortality.

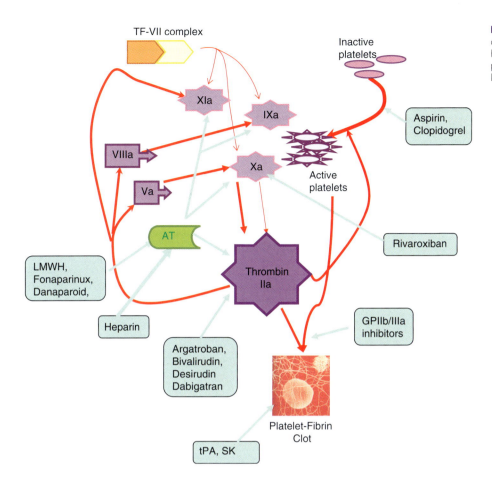

Figure 57.3. Sites of action of anticoagulant medications. AT, antithrombin; LMWH, low-molecular-weight heparin; SK, streptokinase; TF, tissue factor; tPA, tissue plasminogen activator; thick red arrows, amplification; light green arrows, inhibition.

Recombinant factor VIIa is increasingly being used off-label to treat life-threatening hemorrhage.

Heparin and related compounds

Unfractionated heparin (UFH) was first isolated by Howell in 1922. UFH and the low-molecular-weight heparin (LMWH) preparations are two of the most commonly prescribed medications in hospital, and indications for their use are increasing [15].

Mechanisms of action

Heparin, a glycosaminoglycan, is contained within mast-cell secretory granules and requires a cofactor, antithrombin (AT), to inhibit activated coagulation factors and result in an anticoagulant effect (Fig. 57.3) [16]. UFH is a mixture of low- and high-molecular-weight fractions that range from 3000 to 30 000 Da, whereas LMWH consists of fractions ranging from 2000 to 10 000 Da. Greater-molecular-weight fractions (with a minimum chain length of 18 oligosaccharide units) preferentially inhibit thrombin (factor IIa) [17]. Chain length is important because thrombin inhibition requires simultaneous binding of thrombin and AT by heparin. Conversely, inhibition of factor Xa does not require simultaneous heparin binding to Xa and AT. Therefore, lower-molecular-weight heparin fractions selectively inhibit factor Xa (Fig. 57.3).

The antithrombotic properties of heparin are predominantly mediated by the binding of a specific pentasaccharide sequence on heparin to AT. This complex inhibits both factor Xa and thrombin [18,19], in addition to several other sites in the intrinsic coagulation pathway such as factors IXa, XIa, and XIIa. Heparin indirectly suppresses thrombin-induced activation of factors V and VIII by binding thrombin.

A minimum chain length of six oligosaccharide units is essential for heparin to catalyze the inhibition of thrombin by heparin cofactor II, another in-vivo inhibitor of hemostasis [20]. Inhibition of thrombin through heparin cofactor II is optimal with a chain length of 20–24 oligosaccharide units. The ability of heparin cofactor II to inhibit clot-bound thrombin at greater heparin concentrations may be important in some clinical settings, such as during extracorporeal circulation with cardiac surgery. The extrinsic coagulation pathway can also be inhibited by heparin-mediated release of TFPI [21]. UFH may inhibit or activate platelets, affect endothelial function or vessel wall permeability, initiate fibrinolysis, and augment inhibition of fibrinolysis by plasminogen activator inhibitor 1 [22,23].

Preclinical pharmacology

The dose of UFH used to treat patients with venous thromboembolism or unstable angina is based on maintenance of

915

Table 57.1. Anticoagulant medications

Drug	Mechanism	Metabolism	Dose for DVT prophylaxis	Dose for therapeutic anticoagulation	Therapeutic target	Reversal agent
Heparin	Potentiates antithrombin: IIa, Xa, IXa, XIa, XIIa inhibition	Hepatic, reticuloendothelial system, and 50% renal excretion	5000 U SC twice to thrice daily	Bolus = 80 U kg^{-1} Infusion = 18 U kg^{-1} h^{-1}; adjust to target PTT	aPTT = 60–80 seconds	Protamine: start with 25–50 mg
LMWH (e.g., enoxaparin)	Potentiates antithrombin: Xa inhibition	Mainly renal excretion	40 mg SC once daily	1 mg kg^{-1} SC twice daily	Chromogenic anti-Xa assay: 0.6–1.0 anti-Xa U mL^{-1}	None
Danaparoid	Potentiates antithrombin: Xa inhibition, and IIa to a lesser extent	Renal	750 units twice daily	750–1250 units three times daily	Chromogenic anti-Xa assay: 0.5–0.8 anti-Xa U mL^{-1}	None
Fondaparinux	Potentiates antithrombin: Xa inhibition	Renal	2.5 mg SC once daily	5, 7.5, or 10 mg SC once daily	Chromogenic anti-Xa assay	None
Rivaroxiban	Direct Xa inhibition	Likely liver	10 mg PO once daily		Chromogenic anti-Xa assay	None
Warfarin	Prevents carboxylation of X, IX, VII, II, protein C & S	Hepatic, marked genetic variability		2–10 mg PO daily; adjust to target INR	INR = 2 to 4	Vitamin K: 1–10 mg PO or plasma; start with 2–4 units
Bivalirudin	Direct thrombin Inhibition	Proteolytic cleavage & renal (20%)		Bolus = 1 mg kg^{-1} Infusion = 0.2 mg kg^{-1} h^{-1}; adjust to target PTT	aPTT = 60–80 seconds	None
Desirudin	Direct thrombin inhibition	Renal	10–15 mg SC twice daily		Prolongs the aPTT	None
Argatroban	Direct thrombin inhibition	Hepatic		Infusion = 2 µg kg^{-1} min^{-1}; adjust to target PTT	aPTT = 60–80 seconds; may prolong INR	None
Dabigatran (etexilate)	Direct thrombin inhibition	Renal (unchanged) & some conjugation with glucuronic acid	150 mg PO once daily	150 mg PO twice daily	Fixed dosing; no laboratory monitoring required	None

^{a}PTT, activated partial thromboplastin time; DVT, deep vein thrombosis; INR, international normalized ratio; LMWH, low-molecular-weight heparin; PO, per os (by mouth); PTT, partial thromboplastin time; SC, subcutaneous.

activated partial thromboplastin time (aPTT) values in the range of 1.5–2.5 × control (consistent with anti-Xa heparin levels in the range of 0.2–0.7 U mL^{-1}). This therapeutic range is based on early animal studies [24,25]. Activated coagulation time (ACT) values of approximately 350 seconds are considered therapeutic for coronary interventions such as angioplasty or stenting procedures [26]. Anticoagulation is used during cardiac surgery to prevent overt thrombosis of the extracorporeal circuit and to minimize excessive CPB-related activation of the hemostatic system. In this setting, higher heparin concentrations (3–8 U mL^{-1}) are maintained to offset the extraordinary activation of coagulation that occurs. Early human studies demonstrated that fibrin formation during extracorporeal circulation could be avoided when ACT values exceeded 280–300 seconds [27]; in an attempt to provide a margin of safety, this led to the recommendation that ACT values exceed 480 seconds in this setting [27,28]. Subsequent studies have demonstrated that ACT values can be extremely misleading during CPB with respect to heparin-mediated anticoagulation because of the effects of hypothermia and hemodilution to prolong ACT values independent of heparin [29].

Clinical pharmacology

Unfractionated heparin is normally present within mast cells and is synthesized from UDP-sugar precursors as a polymer of alternating N-acetyl-D-glucosamine and D-glucuronic acid residues. The commercial heparin preparations are derived from either bovine lung or porcine intestinal mucosa and have biologic activities similar to those of endogenous heparin. Although UFH is metabolized in the reticuloendothelial system and liver, at least 50% is eliminated unchanged through the kidneys. Generally, the plasma elimination half-life of UFH is 1–2 hours; however, the half-life increases with significant hepatic or renal dysfunction or with heparin doses greater than 100 U kg^{-1} [30]. In contrast to UFH, LMWH compounds such as enoxaparin or dalteparin, which are derived from UFH, have a longer half-life of 4–5 hours. These drugs also have a more consistent pharmacokinetic profile because of the lower protein binding, lower affinity for platelets, vWF and endothelial cells, and predictable clearance, which is primarily renal [31,32].

Heparin is administered by deep subcutaneous injection, or IV bolus or infusion, because it is not absorbed through the gastrointestinal tract. When administered parenterally, heparin has an immediate onset, whereas subcutaneous administration results in variable bioavailability with an onset delay of 1–2 hours. Intravenous heparin is used when therapeutic anticoagulation is needed, as in deep venous thrombosis (DVT), pulmonary embolism, interventional cardiology, cardiac surgery, and vascular surgery. Heparin loading doses vary between 80 and 400 U kg^{-1} depending on the clinical setting. In settings such as DVT or acute coronary syndromes, heparin infusions are used to maintain a steady state, because of heparin's short half-life and the importance of maintaining anticoagulation. Monitoring systems are generally not used for subcutaneous heparin or LMWH administration, unless there is renal dysfunction, in which case chromogenic factor Xa assays or protamine titration assays are useful to quantify heparin concentration.

The anticoagulant properties of UFH are monitored with tests that assess the intrinsic coagulation pathway. The test used depends on the heparin concentration required for particular clinical situations. The aPTT is generally maintained at 1.5–2.5 × control values, which is consistent with heparin levels of 0.2–0.7 U mL^{-1} (anti-Xa activity), in patients receiving heparin for the management of DVT/pulmonary embolism, as well as with noninterventional acute coronary syndromes (e.g., unstable angina) [33]. The ACT or heparin concentration methods (e.g., Hepcon automated protamine titration) are used when greater heparin concentrations are required during interventional cardiology procedures (ACT values of 200–400 seconds, heparin concentrations of 1–3 U mL^{-1}) or cardiac surgical procedures (ACT values > 400–500 seconds, heparin concentrations of 3–8 U mL^{-1}) [34].

There is substantial variability of heparin anticoagulant responsiveness among patients, with some patients exhibiting heparin resistance, which is attributed either to AT deficiency or to increases in one or more heparin binding proteins [35]. AT activity levels as low as 40–50% of normal, similar to those in patients with heterozygotic hereditary deficiency, are commonly seen during cardiac surgery [36]. Acquired reductions in plasma AT concentrations have been related to preoperative heparin use, hemodilution, or consumption during extracorporeal circulation. The heparin tissue source (intestinal vs. lung, porcine vs. bovine), method of preparation, molecular-weight distribution of heparin used, and possibly the use of nitroglycerin infusions may also contribute to impaired responsiveness to heparin [37]. In addition to congenital deficiency, AT levels may be low in patients with nephrotic syndrome, hepatic cirrhosis, DIC, or prolonged heparin infusion.

Adverse effects

Heparin and related compounds can be associated with bleeding complications. The risk increases with the intensity of anticoagulation, pre-existing defects in hemostasis, concurrent antithrombotic or antiplatelet use, and instrumentation, such as biopsies, surgery, or neuraxial anesthetic techniques. Advantages of UFH are that its anticoagulant properties can be assessed with routine tests (e.g., aPTT, thrombin time, ACT), its short half-life, and the availability of protamine as an immediate reversal drug. LMWHs, fondaparinux, and danaparoid do not have these advantages; this has proven to be important in patients receiving LMWH, in whom there have been multiple reports of epidural/spinal hematomas leading to paraplegia in the setting of neuraxial anesthetic blocks [38], or in patients who have demonstrated excessive bleeding after cardiac surgery if this drug was administered within 24 hours prior to surgery.

Hypersensitivity reactions to heparin consist of heparin-induced thrombocytopenia (HIT), allergic vasculitis, hypereosinophilia, immediate hypersensitivity, as well as delayed-type skin reactions. Hypersensitivity to unfractionated and low-molecular-weight heparins and semisynthetic heparinoids is increasingly common. However, the pathogenesis is still not fully understood. Clinically, this phenomenon is of relevance because of its increasing incidence and the resulting therapeutic difficulties that arise because cross-reactions between unfractionated and low-molecular-weight heparins as well as between various heparins and heparinoids have been observed [39]. In addition to hemorrhagic complications, heparin has limitations based on its pharmacokinetic properties; its ability to induce immune-mediated platelet activation, which can lead to thrombosis with HIT; and its effect on bone metabolism, which can lead to osteoporosis [40]. Osteoporosis is caused by binding of heparin to osteoblasts, which then release factors that activate osteoclasts [41].

Heparin-induced thrombocytopenia

A serious and potentially life-threatening complication of treatment with UFH or LMWH is immune-mediated heparin-induced thrombocytopenia (HIT). It is associated with significant morbidity and mortality if unrecognized [42]. Patient groups at the highest risk for developing HIT (estimated incidence of 1–5%) include postoperative orthopedic, cardiac, and vascular surgery patients who are receiving heparin for as little as 2 days up to 1–2 weeks [43,44]. Approximately one-fifth of patients undergoing CPB surgery have detectable heparin-induced platelet antibodies before the procedure as a result of prior heparin exposure, and many more develop antibodies after surgery (ranging from 35% to 65% by days 7–10) even when heparin thrombosis prophylaxis is not used [45,46].

HIT usually develops within 3–15 days after first exposure in patients receiving UFH, or as early as 12–24 hours with repeated exposure [47,48]. In addition to thrombocytopenia, HIT can lead to severe arterial or venous thrombosis in a significant proportion of patients [47]. Serious sequelae associated with HIT can potentially be avoided with early recognition and appropriate treatment [49].

HITT, or HIT with thrombosis, involves an IgG immune response in which antibodies bind to a conformationally modified epitope on platelet factor 4 (PF4) bound to heparin and simultaneously to Fc receptors on the platelet surface, causing platelet activation, platelet aggregation, the generation of procoagulant platelet microparticles, generation of thrombin, and activation of leukocytes and endothelial cells. Activated platelets are removed from the circulation, which causes thrombocytopenia [40]. Early diagnosis is imperative, but limitations of the laboratory assays and atypical clinical presentations can make the diagnosis difficult. Improving the pretest probability for laboratory tests based on "4 Ts" (thrombocytopenia, thrombosis, time course, and no other cause) has been proposed. Clinical management of patients with HIT is with a nonheparin anticoagulant such as a direct thrombin inhibitor (DTI) or danaparoid followed by warfarin for long-term treatment [50].

Rarely, patients develop acute inflammatory (e.g., fever, chills) or cardiorespiratory (e.g., hypertension, tachycardia, dyspnea, chest pain, cardiorespiratory arrest) symptoms and signs within 30 minutes following an intravenous heparin bolus [51]. Termed acute systemic reactions, these can also mimic acute pulmonary embolism (pseudopulmonary embolism) and strongly suggest acute in-vivo platelet activation secondary to HIT [44]. The platelet count may be informative in this setting [44].

Thrombocytopenia is not necessary for the diagnosis of HIT. A 50% and perhaps even 30% reduction in platelet count from pre-heparin levels is more specific. Warfarin should not be used until the platelet count has recovered to more than $150 \times 10^9 \text{ L}^{-1}$, since it reduces protein C and S levels within several hours [44,52]. Accordingly, patients taking warfarin at the time of HIT diagnosis should receive vitamin K (10 mg PO or 5–10 mg IV) to restore these critical anticoagulants, especially if patients display evidence of thrombosis [44].

HIT antibodies are transient and typically disappear within 3–6 months. However, in patients with lingering antibodies, heparin re-exposure can be catastrophic, and moreover thrombosis unrelated to heparin re-exposure is possible if antibody titers are high as evidenced by ELISA optical density (OD) values > 1.0 or serotonin release assay (SRA) values > 70%. With strong clinical suspicion of HIT (high pretest probability), heparin should be discontinued and a parenteral alternative anticoagulant initiated, even before laboratory confirmation. Subsequent laboratory test results may help with the decision to continue with HIT treatment or to restart heparin. Heparin avoidance in patients with current HIT is preferable in most clinical situations. If surgery requiring anticoagulation cannot be delayed until HIT antibodies have disappeared, alternative anticoagulants, such as bivalirudin, are recommended; however, bleeding related to the nonreversible nature of these drugs is problematic [53].

Because the diagnosis is based on both clinical and serologic findings, clinicians should consider HIT a clinicopathologic syndrome [54]. The most important possible clinical features of HIT include anaphylactoid reactions, thromboses, and skin lesions at heparin injection sites [47]. A false diagnosis of HIT is possible in about one-third to two-thirds of patients who are antibody-positive by ELISA [55]. Interestingly, there is a correlation between the degree of reactivity in the ELISA, expressed in OD units, as well as the degree of serotonin release with the SRA method, and the presence of platelet-activating anti-PF4/heparin antibodies [44,55]. Negative HIT ELISA results generally exclude HIT, especially in a setting of a low pretest probability. In addition, because the magnitude of a positive test result correlates with greater likelihood of HIT, a Bayesian diagnostic approach that combines pretest probability and the magnitude of a positive test result is recommended. Recent studies suggest that presence of ELISA-detected antibodies in certain clinical settings confers an adverse prognosis, even without clinically evident HIT [56]. Diagnostic specificity can be increased by use of either new ELISA methods that only detect pathologic IgG HIT antibodies or a sensitive washed platelet activation assay; a positive platelet activation assay is much more specific for clinical HIT than a positive HIT ELISA [56,57]. Only a subset of anti-PF4/heparin antibodies activate platelets (especially IgG and not other immunoglobulin subclasses), which explains the greater diagnostic specificity of certain platelet activation assays, such as platelet serotonin release assay and heparin-induced platelet activation (HIPA) assay, for HIT compared with the HIT ELISA [43].

Dosage and administration

Lower heparin doses (e.g., 5000–7500 U every 12 hours) are administered subcutaneously to prevent DVT, whereas higher subcutaneous doses (e.g., 17 000 U every 12 hours) can be used for long-term anticoagulation when warfarin is contraindicated. Generally, monitoring is not used in these two scenarios.

An initial intravenous bolus dose (5000 U or 80 U kg^{-1}) followed by a continuous intravenous infusion (1200–1600 U h^{-1}) is used when immediate anticoagulation is required. Greater initial intravenous doses are administered for interventional cardiology procedures (100–200 U kg^{-1}) and during cardiac surgery (300–400 U kg^{-1}); subsequent doses of 5000–10 000 units are administered to maintain sufficient anticoagulation. This is usually guided by near-patient anticoagulation assessment using monitoring systems such as ACT or heparin concentration through an automated protamine titration method.

LMWHs can be used for thrombosis prophylaxis or systemic anticoagulation. For example, 40 mg once a day or 30 mg twice a day of enoxaparin can be administered as a subcutaneous injection for thrombosis prophylaxis. For therapeutic anticoagulation, enoxaparin 1.5 mg kg^{-1} daily or 1 mg kg^{-1} twice a day is effective, and monitoring is typically not required unless the patient has reduced clearance owing to renal dysfunction.

New and emerging concepts

The effects of various heparinoids (heparin, tinzaparin, enoxaparin, danaparoid, and fondaparinux) on the aPTT, anti-Xa assays, and the calibrated automated thrombogram have been evaluated. The calibrated automated thrombogram was the only test to detect both the coagulopathy and potentially the successful reversal of these anticoagulants [58]. With the exception of standard UFH, protamine sulfate had limited efficacy in reversing anticoagulation with the other drugs. Recombinant factor VIIa may have a role in treating coagulopathy and bleeding with nonheparin heparinoids [58]. Correction of thrombin-generating capacity following fondaparinux has been found with low doses of FEIBA (factor eight inhibitor bypassing activity) [59].

There is an urgent need to confirm that oversulfated chondroitin sulfate (OSCS), a compound contaminating heparin supplies worldwide, is the cause of the severe and fatal anaphylactoid reactions that have occurred after intravenous heparin administration in the United States and Germany. OSCS found in contaminated lots of UFH, as well as a synthetically generated OSCS reference standard, directly activated the kinin–kallikrein pathway in human plasma, which can lead to the generation of bradykinin, a potent vasoactive mediator. In addition, OSCS induced generation of C3a and C5a, potent anaphylatoxins derived from complement proteins [60]. This impurity has also contaminated LMWH obtained by chemical and enzymatic depolymerization of heparin [61].

Protamine

Protamine sulfate is a low-molecular-weight cationic protein that is derived from salmon sperm.

Mechanisms of action

Protamine is used to reverse heparin and does so by ionic binding to acidic polyanionic heparin to form a stable salt without any anticoagulant activity. Protamine has two active binding sites. One binds to heparin and the other exerts mild anticoagulant and antiplatelet effects. Every milligram of protamine neutralizes approximately 80–100 USP units of heparin. Of importance, protamine inadequately and inconsistently reverses the anticoagulant (anti-factor Xa) activity of LMWH. If protamine is administered alone or in excess of what is needed to reverse heparin, it has antiplatelet activity which may aggravate a bleeding diathesis [62]. This is evident with circulating levels as low as 30 μg mL^{-1}, which can be attained with as little as 50–60 mg protamine. At doses in excess of 600–800 mg, protamine also displays anticoagulant activity.

Clinical pharmacology

Protamine has a rapid onset of action, with neutralization of heparin occurring within 5 minutes. The fate of the heparin–protamine complex has not been clearly elucidated. Isolated protamine or the heparin–protamine complex are cleared through the reticuloendothelial system within 10–20 minutes, which is more rapid than heparin clearance [63]. This may in part explain the phenomenon of "heparin rebound." Heparin rebound has been described predominantly after cardiac surgery and refers to heparin-related anticoagulation and bleeding that occurs 30 minutes to 9 hours after protamine administration. The etiology of heparin rebound is likely related to release of heparin from intravascular or extravascular protein binding sites or from heparin–protamine complexes that occurs after clearance of unbound protamine.

The full protamine dose should be administered slowly through an intravenous catheter over 20–30 minutes (about 5 mg min^{-1}) after confirming that there is no reaction when a small (10 mg) test dose is administered. The patient should be carefully observed for development of any hypersensitivity or nonimmunologic reactions. Several reports have summarized relatively uncommon (< 1%) immunologic reactions involving classic anaphylaxis mediated through antiprotamine IgE. Other reports have described catastrophic but rare hemodynamic reactions, possibly mediated through antiprotamine IgG or complement activation, consisting of thromboxane-mediated development of noncardiogenic pulmonary edema, severe pulmonary vasoconstriction, right heart decompensation, hypotension, and cardiovascular collapse. This immunologic reaction may be more common in patients who have received insulin that contains protamine (NPH, isophane), those with a previous exposure to protamine, those with fish allergies, or in male vasectomized patients, of whom 22–33% have antiprotamine antibodies. Protamine has also been shown to result in direct activation of the complement cascade, which can lead to noncardiogenic pulmonary edema. More commonly, protamine-induced hypotension and bronchospasm may be related to nonimmunologic mechanisms (direct physicochemical displacement of histamine from mast cells) that are generally related to total dose and rate of administration.

Dosage and administration

When heparin has been administered by deep subcutaneous injection, 1–1.2 mg protamine should be administered for every 100 U heparin measured within the circulation. Similarly, when heparin has been given intravenously, 1–1.2 mg protamine should be administered for every 100 U heparin within the systemic circulation, or 0.5 mg protamine for every 100 U heparin administered over the last 4 hours. During cardiac surgery, several different approaches have been used. Empiric dosing schedules such as administration of 0.5–1.0 mg protamine for every 100 U heparin administered throughout the procedure or 1 mg protamine for every 100 U heparin administered initially (before initiation) and during CPB have been described. Ideally, test systems, such as the Hepcon automated protamine titration method, that quantify the circulating concentration of heparin should be used to identify the accurate dose of protamine required to neutralize heparin. Although not consistently observed within the literature, optimizing protamine dose seems to be supported by several studies that have demonstrated either reduced bleeding or transfusion when lower doses of protamine are administered [64]. The decreases in perioperative blood loss associated with reduced doses of protamine may be related to less complement activation, less protamine-induced platelet dysfunction, or decreased thrombin inhibition. Heparin rebound can be successfully countered with administration of additional doses based on sensitive methods for detection of heparin rebound (e.g., heparinase ACT) or with 25 mg h^{-1} of protamine for 6 hours postoperatively [65].

Tests that are sensitive to low concentrations (0.1 U mL^{-1}) of heparin, such as the aPTT, the thrombin time, the automated protamine titration, the heparinase ACT, and the heparin-neutralized thrombin time, should be used to confirm adequacy of heparin reversal in the operating room or to assess heparin rebound in the postoperative setting. When patients (those receiving NPH insulin) are at increased risk for an adverse hemodynamic reaction to protamine, antihistamine blockers and steroids should be considered in addition to a protamine test dose.

New and emerging concepts

Hemodynamic perturbations after protamine administration are independently related to in-hospital mortality after primary coronary artery bypass surgery [66]. Protamine inhibits the carboxypeptidase N-mediated degradation of bradykinin, a peptide that causes vasodilation and tPA release. Early research suggests that blocking the bradykinin B [2] receptor attenuates protamine-related hypotension [67]. Inducible nitric oxide synthase (iNOS) has also been implicated in protamine-associated hemodynamic instability [68].

Danaparoid

With the recognition of HIT, as well as for other reasons, investigators and clinicians have pursued alternative anticoagulant drugs. Danaparoid, derived from porcine intestinal mucosa, is a glycosaminoglycuronan that consists of a mixture of heparan sulfate (84%), dermatan sulfate (12%), and chondroitin sulfate (4%). This low-molecular-weight heparinoid compound has a molecular weight of approximately 5500–6000 Da, and does not contain any heparin or heparin fragments. Danaparoid is not presently licensed for use in the United States.

Mechanisms of action

Similar to heparin, the antithrombotic properties of danaparoid relate to attenuation of fibrin formation through inhibition of Xa and thrombin. The main anti-Xa activity of danaparoid is related to binding of AT by heparan sulfate, whereas its anti-IIa activity is related to dermatan sulfate, which binds to AT and heparin cofactor II [69]. Danaparoid has substantially greater inhibitory effects on Xa activity than either standard UFH or LMWH.

Clinical pharmacology

Subcutaneously administered danaparoid has a bioavailability of 100%. The volume of distribution is 9 L, and peak plasma levels are achieved within 4–5 hours (maximum anti-Xa activity in 2–5 hours) with linear kinetics. Elimination of danaparoid is predominantly through the kidneys, and the terminal half-lives for anti-Xa and anti-IIa activity are 24 and 7 hours, respectively.

Compared with placebo, danaparoid has been shown to reduce the incidence of DVT from 57% to 15% in the setting of total hip arthroplasty [70]. In a randomized trial in the setting of hip replacement, there was a 17% incidence of DVT with danaparoid compared with a 32% incidence with UFH [71]. Similarly, in the setting of hip fracture surgery, danaparoid reduced the incidence of DVT from 35% to 13% compared with dextran and from 21% to 7% compared with warfarin, without an increase in bleeding complications [72,73]. Less impressive reductions in the incidence of perioperative DVT were observed when danaparoid was compared with heparin in the setting of abdominothoracic surgery [74]. After ischemic stroke, danaparoid has been shown to reduce DVT occurrence from 31% to 9% compared with heparin [69].

The antithrombotic effects of danaparoid should be monitored using an anti-Xa method, because routine tests that assess AT activity such as aPTT and the thrombin time are minimally affected by danaparoid.

Dosage and administration

The recommended dosage of danaparoid for prevention of DVT is 750 anti-Xa units by subcutaneous injection before surgery, 2 hours after surgery, and then daily for 7–14 days. Dosage should be adjusted for patients with significant renal insufficiency. As with LMWH, no drugs are currently available to reverse danaparoid, which is problematic since there are several reports of life-threatening bleeding that have occurred with its use during cardiac surgery.

New and emerging concepts
Danaparoid, unlike other anticoagulants approved for the treatment of HIT, uniquely interferes with the pathogenesis of HIT through several mechanisms at therapeutic concentrations. It disrupts PF4-containing immune complexes, decreases PF4 binding to platelets, displaces PF4–heparin complexes from platelets, inhibits HIT antibody binding to PF4–heparin complexes, and prevents platelet activation by HIT antibodies. It is possible that these effects contribute to its therapeutic efficacy [75].

Fondaparinux

Fondaparinux is a synthetic pentasaccharide, antithrombin-dependent, selective factor Xa inhibitor, approved by the US Food and Drug Administration (FDA) for treatment of venous thrombosis and for thrombosis prophylaxis after orthopedic surgery [76]. Recent trials have demonstrated the ability of fondaparinux to prevent venous thromboembolism (VTE) in other surgical and medical settings and to treat established VTE.

Mechanism of action
Heparin fragments with a high affinity for AT have been identified, and the minimum heparin fragment necessary for high-affinity binding to AT consists of a pentasaccharide [77]. Fondaparinux binds to AT and produces a conformational change at the reactive site of AT that enhances its reactivity with factor Xa [78]. AT then forms a covalent complex with factor Xa. Fondaparinux is released from AT and is available to activate additional AT molecules. Because it is too short to bridge AT to thrombin, fondaparinux does not increase the rate of thrombin inhibition by AT [40].

Clincal pharmacology
Fondaparinux may improve and simplify the prevention and treatment of thrombosis in a large range of medical and surgical settings [79], and specifically may be a suitable alternative anticoagulant to UFH, LMWH, or bivalirudin in the setting of unstable angina and non-ST-elevation myocardial infarction (NSTEMI). Fondaparinux may be associated with less risk of bleeding than other anticoagulants [80], but concerns about hemorrhage, even at low dosages, remain, especially since it has a long half-life and has no effective reversal drug [76]. Fondaparinux has not been shown to be associated with immune-mediated thrombocytopenia, and can potentially be used for the treatment of patients with HIT [50,81].

A steady state is reached after the third or fourth daily dose, and fondaparinux is excreted unchanged in the urine. The terminal half-life is 17 hours in young subjects and 21 hours in elderly volunteers [40]. As there is minimal nonspecific binding to plasma proteins other than AT, fondaparinux produces a predictable anticoagulant response and exhibits linear pharmacokinetics when given in subcutaneous doses of 2–8 mg or in intravenous doses of 2–20 mg [82,83]. If severe bleeding occurs with fondaparinux, protamine is ineffective, but recombinant factor VIIa may be somewhat effective [84].

Dosage and administration
Fondaparinux is given at a fixed dose of 2.5 mg for thromboprophylaxis. For treatment of DVT or pulmonary embolism, the drug is given at a dose of 7.5 mg for patients with a body weight of 50–100 kg; the dose is decreased to 5 mg for patients weighing less than 50 kg and increased to 10 mg for those weighing more than 100 kg [40]. Although routine coagulation monitoring is not recommended, there may be circumstances when it is useful to determine the anticoagulant activity of fondaparinux, which can be measured using anti-Xa assays [40].

Rivaroxaban

Rivaroxaban is a small-molecule orally administered inhibitor of activated factor Xa that is in advanced clinical development for the prevention and treatment of arterial and venous thromboembolic disorders [85]. Rivaroxaban does not cause platelet activation or aggregation in the presence of anti-PF4/heparin antibodies, unlike heparin and enoxaparin, suggesting lack of cross-reactivity. Furthermore, rivaroxaban does not cause the release of PF4 from platelets and does not interact with PF4. Rivaroxaban may be a suitable oral anticoagulant for the management of patients with HIT [86].

Clinical pharmacology
In a recent study of 4500 patients, a 10 mg oral daily dose of rivaroxaban was more effective for extended thromboprophylaxis than a 40 mg daily subcutaneous dose of enoxaparin in patients undergoing elective total hip arthroplasty. The two drugs had similar safety profiles [87]. Rivaroxaban is being evaluated for the treatment of pulmonary embolism, secondary prevention after acute coronary syndromes, and the prevention of stroke and non-CNS embolism in patients with nonvalvular atrial fibrillation. The drug may have its greatest impact in providing a much-needed and attractive alternative to warfarin [85].

Argatroban

Argatroban is an arginine derivative that is a highly specific direct thrombin inhibitor [88]. Direct thrombin inhibitors do not stimulate formation of the antibody that causes HIT [89]. Unlike the hirudin derivatives, neutralizing antibodies to argatroban have not been detected following administration [90].

Mechanisms of action
Argatroban is a synthetic, small molecule that binds to the catalytic but not the exo 1 or exo 2 sites of thrombin and inhibits its activity. Argatroban is a competitive inhibitor of

thrombin and binds reversibly to the active site of thrombin [91]. Argatroban's binding site on thrombin and pharmacologic characteristics are different from those of hirudin. In addition to its antithrombin activity, argatroban has also been shown to promote NO release, which may partially explain the improved perfusion seen when it is administered to patients with peripheral vascular disease [92].

Preclinical pharmacology

In rabbit models of arterial but not venous thrombosis, argatroban is a more potent antithrombotic drug than heparin, with antithrombotic effects at a much lower degree of systemic anticoagulation [93]. Argatroban was compared with heparin for anticoagulation in a dog model of CPB. There was less activation of coagulation and fibrinolysis and better preservation of platelet number and function in the argatroban group, without any clotting in the extracorporeal circuit [94].

Clinical pharmacology

The pharmacokinetics of argatroban are well described by a two-compartment model with first-order elimination [91]. Plasma drug concentrations increase linearly with dose, and weight-adjusted plasma clearance is dose-independent [95]. The elimination half-life is 40–50 minutes. Argatroban is distributed mainly in the extracellular space and is readily metabolized in the liver via cytochrome P450 (CYP) 3A4/5 to an active M1-metabolite that has pharmacologically distinct characteristics [91,96]. In patients with liver dysfunction, the half-life is increased two- to threefold and clearance is 25% that of healthy volunteers [91]. Renal function, age, and sex do not significantly affect the pharmacokinetics of argatroban; it is particularly useful in patients with HIT who have severe renal impairment [40,91]. Argatroban anticoagulation, compared with historical control subjects, was found to improve clinical outcomes in patients diagnosed with HIT, without increasing bleeding risk [97,98].

Argatroban has been proposed as an alternative to heparin for anticoagulation during CPB. One of the main disadvantages with argatroban, as with the other direct thrombin inhibitors, is that there is no available drug that reverses its anticoagulant action. Nonetheless, its reversible binding to thrombin, coupled with its rapid clearance from circulation, suggest that it may be a viable anticoagulant in this setting [99]. There is more clinical experience currently with bivalirudin than argatroban in this setting.

Adverse effects

The major adverse effect related to argatroban is bleeding [100]. All of the direct thrombin inhibitors increase the international normalized ratio (INR), albeit to a variable extent. When given in therapeutic doses, argatroban has the greatest effect on the INR [40]. This makes it difficult to make a safe transition between argatroban and warfarin therapy, which has led to the recommendation to overlap the use of the two drugs for 3–5 days.

Dosage and administration

For anticoagulation in patients with HIT, an initial infusion of $2\ \mu g\ kg^{-1}\ min^{-1}$ is recommended, and the dose is adjusted to maintain the aPTT ratio in the 1.5–3.0 range [40]. For patients with hepatic dysfunction, the initial infusion rate should be decreased to $0.5\ \mu g\ kg^{-1}\ min^{-1}$. The maximum advisable dose is $10\ \mu g\ kg^{-1}\ min^{-1}$. When argatroban is used to treat patients who have heart failure, multiple organ system failure, or severe anasarca, or after cardiac surgery, the suggested initial infusion rate is between 0.5 and $1.2\ \mu g\ kg^{-1}\ min^{-1}$, with subsequent adjustments according to the target aPTT [44].

New and emerging concepts

When assessing the independent effect of warfarin when patients are anticoagulated with argatroban, the argatroban infusion can be paused and the INR assessed. However, this introduces a risk of thrombosis. Another option is to continue argatroban therapy and to monitor the therapeutic effect of warfarin with a chromogenic factor X assay [40]. In this setting, factor X levels less than 45% have been associated with INR values greater than 2 when the effect of argatroban has been eliminated [101]. Monitoring factor X levels may be safer than aiming for an INR of 4 or higher when warfarin is given in conjunction with argatroban [102].

Dabigatran

Dabigatran etexilate is an orally administered prodrug, which is rapidly absorbed and converted by esterase-mediated hydrolysis to the active form, dabigatran, which specifically and reversibly inhibits thrombin [103,104].

Clinical pharmacology

Dabigatran and its prodrug, dabigatran etexilate, demonstrate concentration-dependent anticoagulant effects in various species, with a dose-dependent prolongation of the aPTT [105]. In humans, time curves for aPTT, INR, thrombin time, and ecarin clotting time parallel plasma concentration–time curves [106]. Dabigatran has predictable pharmacokinetic and pharmacodynamic profiles, allowing for a fixed-dose regimen [107]. Peak plasma concentrations are reached approximately 0.5–2 hours after oral administration, with no accumulation after multiple dosing [108]. Administration with food has no effect on the extent of dabigatran absorption, but there is a moderate decrease when dabigatran is coadministered with drugs that modulate gastric pH such as pantoprazole [109]. Steady-state conditions are reached within 3 days with multiple dosing [106]. Dabigatran etexilate pharmacokinetics are linear across a wide dosage range [110]. Excretion as unchanged drug is predominantly renal, and differences in dabigatran pharmacokinetics are attributable to variations in renal function [103]. Dabigatran is not metabolized by CYP isoenzymes, and moderate hepatic impairment produces no effect [107]. Dabigatran undergoes some conjugation with glucuronic acid to form pharmacologically active conjugates that account for approximately 20% of total dabigatran in plasma [106]. Dabigatran etexilate has estimated half-lives of 8–10 hours and 14–17 hours with single and multiple dose administrations, respectively [106]. The pharmacodynamic profile of dabigatran demonstrates effective anticoagulation combined with a low risk of bleeding [103,110,111]. The mean terminal half-life of dabigatran is 8 hours [104]. Dabigatran etexilate has demonstrated superiority or noninferiority to enoxaparin as prophylaxis for venous thromboembolism in patients undergoing orthopedic surgery, with the most frequent adverse effects being gastrointestinal complaints [108,110,112,113]. The overall rates of bleeding have been low. Results of short-term efficacy and safety trials are promising [108], and dabigatran is undergoing extensive evaluation for prophylaxis and treatment in various clinical settings [114,115].

Hirudin-related compounds

Direct thrombin inhibitors offer benefits over drugs like heparin and warfarin. They inhibit both circulating and clot-bound thrombin, have a more predictable anticoagulant response (because they do not bind to plasma proteins and are not neutralized by PF4), lack a requirement for cofactors (such as antithrombin or heparin cofactor II), inhibit thrombin-induced platelet aggregation, and do not cause immune-mediated thrombocytopenia [116]. Hirudin is a direct-acting thrombin inhibitor derived from the leech, *Hirudo medicinalis*. Using polymerase chain reaction technology, recombinant hirudin (desirudin, lepirudin) has been synthesized in yeast. Lepirudin is identical to natural hirudin, except for the substitution of leucine for isoleucine at the N-terminus and the elimination of a sulfate group on the tyrosine at position 63. Desirudin is identical to hirudin, except for a valine–valine at the N-terminus and the absence of the sulfate group on tyrosine at position 63. Bivalirudin is a synthetic peptide based on hirudin [117]. In a seminal trial, intravenous lepirudin was shown to be effective in treating patients with HIT, resulting in decreased mortality and a rapid and sustained increase in platelet count [118]. Bivalirudin in combination with aspirin has been approved in the United States for use in patients with unstable angina who are undergoing percutaneous transluminal coronary angioplasty [100]. Like UFH, LMWH, and fondaparinux, desirudin can be dosed intermittently by subcutaneous injection, and is efficacious for thrombosis prophylaxis following orthopedic surgery [119].

Mechanisms of action

Hirudin-related compounds are direct thrombin inhibitors that bind thrombin itself and do not depend on AT for their anticoagulant activity. Although hirudin and bivalirudin both inhibit thrombin by attaching to the exo I (fibrinogen binding site) and catalytic sites, bivalirudin has a shorter biologic half-life, which is in part related to its reversible inhibition of thrombin. Conversely, hirudin irreversibly inhibits thrombin by forming a 1 : 1 complex. Hirudin has also been found to stimulate PGI_2 production, which may contribute to its antithrombotic activity because PGI_2 promotes vasodilation and prevents platelet aggregation [120].

Clinical pharmacology

Hirudin and bivalirudin are administered by intravenous infusion, while desirudin is given via the subcutaneous route. Onset of action after intravenous administration is rapid, and the peak effect occurs after about 4 hours. Distribution is mainly to the extracellular space. Hirudin undergoes some metabolism by hydrolysis, but is mainly excreted unchanged in the urine. When renal function is normal, plasma clearance is rapid and the hirudin-related compounds obey a first-order or concentration-dependent pharmacokinetic model. The plasma half-lives of hirudin and bivalirudin are about 1.5 hours and 30 minutes, respectively. As with other small polypeptides, bivalirudin is filtered at the glomerulus, secreted in the proximal convoluted tubule, reabsorbed in the distal convoluted tubule, and degraded within intracellular lysosomes to constituent amino acids [121,122]. When there is severe renal impairment (creatinine clearance < 15 mL min^{-1}), hirudin's elimination half-life may be extended to days. While bivalirudin undergoes renal excretion, it also undergoes significant proteolysis, which may explain its successful use in patients with renal dysfunction [123,124]. Hirudin-related compounds can be cleared from plasma by hemodialysis.

The clinical niche for hirudin-related compounds has yet to be fully determined. Hirudin may be an alternative to heparin when there is heparin resistance or HIT. Lepirudin has been used successfully for the management of HIT in cardiac surgery, but at the cost of increased bleeding [125]. Hirudin-related compounds should be used with caution during surgery in patients who are at increased risk for life-threatening bleeding or in patients with renal dysfunction, as there is no pharmacological antagonist. Bivalirudin, with its shorter half-life, has been shown to be a viable alternative to heparin for both on- and off-pump cardiac surgery in patients with and without HIT [126–129]; however, average blood loss is doubled and 6/98 patients had excessive (i.e., > 2500 mL) 24-hour chest tube drainage with use of this drug with CPB [127].

The Thrombin Inhibition in Myocardial Ischemia (TIMI-7) trial demonstrated that bivalirudin was a valuable adjunct to aspirin in the treatment of unstable angina [117]. In the Global Use of Strategies to Open Occluded Coronary Arteries (GUSTO 2b) trial, patients treated with streptokinase and adjunctive hirudin after myocardial infarction had reduced myocardial damage compared with adjunctive heparin [130,131]. The Hirulog/Early Reperfusion Occlusion (HERO-1) study similarly showed improved arterial patency and decreased bleeding when bivalirudin was used as opposed to heparin in combination with aspirin and SK for acute myocardial infarction [132].

For both hirudin and bivalirudin, there is a correlation between plasma concentrations, the aPTT, and the ACT [121]. The aPTT is sensitive for monitoring low doses of desirudin [133]. In the noncardiac surgical setting, prothrombin time or aPTT values are maintained at 2–3 × control, and these values are generally associated with hirudin levels of approximately 1–1.5 μg mL^{-1} [118]. With cardiac surgery, maintenance of hirudin levels of 4–5 μg mL^{-1} has been suggested [118]. A plasma-modified ACT may be useful in monitoring hirudin and bivalurudin anticoagulation during CPB [134]. Patients who receive either lepirudin or desirudin and have a creatinine clearance less than 60 mL min^{-1} should receive a reduced dose and monitoring with aPTT [40]. These drugs should be avoided when the creatinine clearance is less than 30 mL min^{-1} [40].

Adverse effects

Use of these drugs may increase the risk of bleeding. Liver dysfunction and skin rashes have been reported. Severe hypersensitivity reactions can also occur. Bleeding is significantly increased when hirudin or bivalirudin are administered to patients with impaired renal function [121], and these drugs should not be used in patients with renal failure. Antihirudin neutralizing antibodies that reduce effectiveness develop in 40% of patients, but this has not been associated with adverse events. Ten percent of patients who received desirudin subcutaneously following orthopedic hip surgery developed antihirudin antibodies, the significance of which is unknown [135]. In contrast to hirudin, bivalirudin is not immunogenic [40]. Hirudin has been shown in vitro to cause endothelium-independent coronary artery contraction, the significance of which is uncertain [136].

Dosage and administration

In view of the extracellular distribution, dosage should be calculated according to lean body mass. The suggested hirudin dose is 0.4 mg kg^{-1} followed by an infusion at a rate of 0.15 mg kg^{-1} h^{-1} [118]. The dosage for anticoagulation for CPB is not well established. In one study with eight patients, an initial dose of 0.25 mg kg^{-1} was administered followed by 5 mg increments as needed [118]. With bivalirudin, an initial 1 mg kg^{-1} dose followed by 2.5 mg kg^{-1} h^{-1} is advocated. Dosages of both drugs should be adjusted according to point-of-care coagulation tests, and should be decreased for patients with renal impairment. For patients undergoing percutaneous coronary interventions and off-pump cardiac surgery, the recommended bivalirudin dose is a bolus of 0.7 mg kg^{-1} followed by an infusion of 1.75 mg kg^{-1} h^{-1} for the duration of the procedure [40,129]. When given for thromboprophylaxis after elective hip replacement surgery, desirudin is given subcutaneously at a dose of 15 mg twice daily; routine aPTT monitoring is unnecessary with this dose [40].

New and emerging concepts

The antiplatelet, anticoagulant, and pharmacokinetic properties of bivalirudin support its use for both low- and high-risk patients, including those undergoing percutaneous coronary intervention (PCI) [137]. If antibodies are formed to lepirudin or desirudin, dosing may need to be adjusted, and subsequent administration should be with caution in view of the hypothetical risk of anaphylaxis [40].

Warfarin

Schofield first reported hemorrhage in cattle secondary to ingestion of spoiled sweet clover silage; Roderick traced the cause of bleeding to reduced levels of prothrombin; and Link determined that bishydroxycoumarin (dicoumarol) formed in the spoilage process of sweet clover was responsible for development of hypoprothrombinemia, and that this effect could be reversed by vitamin K [138]. The coumarin drugs were introduced into clinical practice in the early 1940s for the management of myocardial infarction and cerebral embolism, and a derivative of dicoumarol (warfarin) was introduced in 1948 as a rodenticide. Warfarin is presently the only commonly used oral anticoagulant with reasonably predictable onset of action, good bioavailability, and fairly predictable duration of action [139]. Like heparin, warfarin is inexpensive and widely prescribed, but there is a greater than 10-fold interindividual variability in the dose required to attain a therapeutic response [140].

Mechanisms of action

The 4-hydroxycoumarin compounds (warfarin, acenocoumarol, ethyl biscoumacetate, and phenprocoumon), as well as dicoumarol, inhibit the hepatic conversion of four vitamin-K-dependent coagulation proteins (factors II, VII, IX, and X) and two anticoagulant proteins (protein C and S) to active forms. Specifically, these drugs inhibit the cyclic interconversion of vitamin K and vitamin K epoxide. Vitamin K plays an essential role in the synthesis of the vitamin-K-dependent coagulant proteins by acting as a cofactor for the post-translational carboxylation of glutamate residues to γ-carboxyglutamate on the N-terminal regions of these proteins. γ-carboxylation is essential in that it enables these coagulation proteins to undergo a conformational change in the presence of calcium, which is critical for their biologic activity and binding of these proteins to their cofactors on phospholipid surfaces [141,142].

The therapeutic anticoagulant effect of warfarin is achieved after several days when the vitamin K-dependent procoagulant proteins (factors II, VII, IX, and X) are reduced by 50–70%, which is consistent with INR values in the range of 2–3. The antithrombotic effects of warfarin are predominantly mediated by reducing plasma concentrations of factor II and, to a lesser extent, factor X. The time required for each vitamin-K-dependent protein to be substantially reduced and reach a steady state depends on the half-lives of the respective protein. The half-lives of the vitamin-K-dependent procoagulant and anticoagulant proteins vary substantially as follows: factor VII,

6 hours; factor IX, 24 hours; factor X, 36 hours; factor II, 40 hours; protein C, 8 hours; protein S, 30 hours.

Clinical pharmacology

Warfarin consists of a racemic mixture of two optically active isomers – designated R and S forms – which have different pharmacologic properties. These two forms are cleared by different pathways; S-warfarin is five times more potent with respect to vitamin K antagonism and is metabolized primarily by CYP2C9 [143,144]. The target for warfarin's inhibitory effect on the vitamin K cycle is the vitamin K oxide reductase (VKOR) enzyme first described in 1974 [145]. The gene coding for the VKOR protein was recently identified and found to be located on the short arm of chromosome 16 [146]. The gene encodes for several isoforms of the protein that collectively are termed the VKOR complex 1 (VKORC1).

After rapid absorption in the gastrointestinal tract, which may be slowed by food, blood concentrations usually peak 2–8 hours after ingestion, and the plasma half-life is approximately 40 hours [143,147]. Warfarin is an organic acid (pK_a 5.1), which accumulates rapidly in the liver, is highly protein-bound (99%) to plasma albumin, and has a volume of distribution similar to albumin (12–13% of body weight or 0.14 L kg^{-1}). Plasma concentrations of warfarin within a fetus approximate maternal levels. Warfarin, unlike other coumarins, is not present in breast milk.

Warfarin is metabolized into byproducts that have little anticoagulant activity. The average rate of clearance from plasma is 0.045 mL min^{-1} kg^{-1}, the biologic half-life ranges from 25 to 60 hours (mean 40 hours), and the duration of action is 2–5 days. The metabolic byproducts are excreted in the urine or stool after some degree of conjugation with glucuronic acid.

High variability in between-subject and within-subject dose–response relations is frequently observed with warfarin, which necessitates ongoing monitoring of anticoagulant response. Several factors affect the pharmacokinetic and pharmacodynamic profiles of warfarin, including the metabolic clearance of warfarin, the pharmacologic profile of vitamin K (intake, absorption, concurrent use of antibiotics), factors that influence the vitamin-K-dependent clotting factors (synthesis, clearance, liver disease), and numerous causes of hemostatic system malfunction (drugs, acquired and inherited disorders). The relationship between the dose of warfarin and the response is modified by genetic and environmental factors that can influence the absorption of warfarin, its pharmacokinetics, and its pharmacodynamics [144]. The significance of these factors cannot be overemphasized, given the potential for both bleeding (supratherapeutic anticoagulation) and thrombotic complications (subtherapeutic anticoagulation). This emphasizes the importance of monitoring the anticoagulant properties of warfarin and related compounds, especially when the status of the patient changes. People receiving long-term warfarin therapy are sensitive to fluctuating levels of dietary

vitamin K [148], which is derived predominantly from phylloquinones in plant material [148].

The anticoagulant effects of warfarin are routinely assessed using the prothrombin time (PT). Prolongation of the PT depends on the stage of therapy (initiation vs. maintenance) based on the different half-lives of the respective vitamin-K-dependent coagulation factors. To standardize the PT, the World Health Organization has used a reference preparation of thromboplastin to develop an international normalized ratio (INR), which can be reliably used to measure warfarin anticoagulation [149]. The optimal INR depends on the clinical indication for warfarin therapy, and accordingly guidelines by several organizations have been generated. The American College of Chest Physicians has suggested INR values ranging from 1.5–2.5 to as high as 3.0–4.5, based on the intensity of anticoagulation required for different clinical situations. For example, the target INR varies widely for treatment of venous thromboembolism, patients with mechanical heart valves, atrial fibrillation, and after acute myocardial infarction [150]. The evidence for maintaining the INR within specific therapeutic ranges in patients who are treated with warfarin is strong because it is based on consistent results of randomized trials and case–control studies [40].

Although prolongation of the PT or INR is frequently observed within 1–2 days after initiation of therapy, reflecting the reduction in factor VII, it generally takes an additional 2–3 days to achieve therapeutic anticoagulation based on the slower reductions in factors X and II. Because protein C and S have shorter half-lives than factors X and II, initiation of warfarin therapy may result in a period of hypercoagulability in the first 24–48 hours. This has led to the recommendation that heparin therapy should be initiated before administration of warfarin or related compounds and then discontinued when the INR is in the therapeutic range, typically requiring about 4 days.

Adverse effects

Bleeding is the most common complication related to warfarin therapy. Several studies have demonstrated that greater-intensity anticoagulation with warfarin may result in increases in bleeding rates when INR values range from 3 to 4.5 [151,152]. Although periprocedure bleeding secondary to warfarin therapy can occur, empiric reversal of warfarin anticoagulation with plasma is not indicated, based on several studies that have not demonstrated a relation between low coagulation-factor levels and bleeding [153,154]. Reversal of warfarin-induced anticoagulation depends on the relative urgency, which is predominantly driven by the presence or absence of clinical bleeding or the requirement for a surgical procedure. In nonurgent situations, discontinuation of warfarin will result in normalization of the INR in 3 days unless the patient has substantial liver disease or vitamin K deficiency. When warfarin reversal is required more rapidly, administration of vitamin K (preferably orally) can result in normalization of INR values within 6–24 hours. Low doses of vitamin K (0.5–1.0 mg) should be used if moderate normalization of the INR is required or if warfarin therapy is to be reinitiated. Otherwise, 5–10 mg vitamin K can be administered. Urgent reversal of warfarin anticoagulation in cases of warfarin overdosage, active or life-threatening bleeding, or high-risk surgical procedures such as craniotomy procedures can be achieved by administering 2–4 units of fresh frozen plasma (or 15 mL kg^{-1}), which should increase coagulation-factor levels by 20–30% or 0.2–0.3 U mL^{-1}.

An uncommon, nonhemorrhagic side effect of warfarin (which may be more likely in patients with protein C or protein S deficiency, or factor V Leiden) involves skin necrosis caused by extensive thrombosis of the venules and capillaries within subcutaneous fat in the third to eighth day after initiating therapy [155–157]. This complication can be managed with heparin or alternative therapy (direct thrombin inhibitors), while restoration of protein C or S levels can be achieved with fresh frozen plasma.

Dosage and administration

The initial dosage of warfarin is 5–10 mg day^{-1} for the first 2–4 days, followed by 2–10 mg day^{-1} as directed by prolongation of the INR. Although the average dose of warfarin required to maintain an INR of 2–3 is between 4 and 5 mg day^{-1}, a small percentage of patients may require substantially less (1–3 mg day^{-1}) because of slower hepatic metabolism.

New and emerging concepts

The recently updated warfarin package insert highlights the potential role of pharmacogenetics in improving the safety and effectiveness of warfarin [158]. Two key genes have been identified that influence the individual's response to warfarin: the cytochrome P450 2C9 gene, *CYP2C9*, and the vitamin K epoxide reductase complex 1 gene, *VKORC1*. Single nucleotide polymorphisms (SNPs) in these genes affect warfarin metabolism or sensitivity [159]. There are a number of common mutations in the gene coding for the CYP2C9 hepatic microsomal enzyme, which is responsible for the oxidative metabolism of the more potent warfarin S-enantiomer, and these mutations alter the pharmacokinetics of warfarin [160–162]. *CYP2C9* variant genotypes have been associated with a significantly increased risk of serious bleeding events. SNPs in *VKORC1* correlate with warfarin sensitivity [159]. Evidence has not yet demonstrated an added benefit of incorporating genotype-guided therapy in improving anticoagulation control or in preventing or reducing the risk of hemorrhagic or thromboembolic complications, but research is ongoing [158]. In 2007, the FDA updated the label of warfarin to include information on pharmacogenetic testing and to encourage, but not require, the use of this information in dosing individual patients initiating warfarin therapy [159]. A free website, WarfarinDosing.org, has been created to help clinicians initiate warfarin therapy. Warfarin dosing estimates are based on clinical factors and, when available, genotypes of

the two important genes, *CYP2C9* and *VKORC1*. Since vitamin K levels can vary substantially with intake of various food products, another novel concept involves stabilization of the anticoagulant effects of warfarin by maintaining a steady dietary intake of vitamin K. There is less variability in INR values when patients receive a consistent daily intake of 150 µg of vitamin K, which may translate into less bleeding and thrombotic complications.

Aspirin

Aspirin is the most widely used antiplatelet drug. Aspirin is useful in the treatment of myocardial ischemia and in other patients at risk for vascular morbidity. Specific indications include acute myocardial infarction, unstable angina, PCI, prevention of cerebrovascular events, and polycythemia vera.

Mechanisms of action

Aspirin irreversibly inactivates cyclooxygenase 1 and 2 (COX-1 and COX-2) via acetylation of serine residues (Ser530 and Ser516, respectively), thus blocking the synthesis of downstream eicosanoids that modulate platelet and vascular function [163,164]. Thromboxane A$_2$ (TxA$_2$), the major eicosanoid produced by platelets, is largely dependent on COX-1 for synthesis and induces platelet aggregation and vasoconstriction. Conversely, prostacyclin (PGI$_2$) is the chief eicosanoid produced by endothelial cells and is derived from both the COX-1 and COX-2 pathways. PGI$_2$ leads to vasodilation and inhibition of platelet aggregation. Low-dose aspirin therapy predominantly effects acetylation of the more susceptible COX-1 enzyme, resulting in relatively greater suppression of TxA$_2$ production. Additionally, while platelets are unable to resynthesize COX during their lifespan (about 10 days), endothelial cells rapidly replace COX, enabling PGI$_2$ production. (See Chapter 34 for further discussion of aspirin's mechanism of action and its use as an anti-inflammatory drug.)

Clinical pharmacology

Aspirin is available in oral and rectal formulations. Enteric-coated and buffered preparations are also produced, to minimize gastrointestinal complications. Ingested aspirin has a systemic bioavailability of 40–50% [165]. In many patients, enteric-coated aspirin preparations result in inferior suppression of thromboxane production when compared to standard dispersible aspirin, likely because of lower bioavailability of these preparations [166]. Aspirin is rapidly and widely distributed into most body tissues and fluids. The volume of distribution of aspirin is 0.15–0.2 L kg^{-1}. A high proportion of aspirin in the blood is bound to albumin.

Aspirin undergoes extensive first-pass metabolism and is rapidly hydrolyzed to salicylic acid in the liver, plasma, and red blood cells. Aspirin and its metabolites are excreted in the urine, with about 1% being excreted as aspirin. While salicylic acid has similar anti-inflammatory potency to aspirin, aspirin is a considerably more potent inhibitor of thromboxane production [167]. The plasma half-life of aspirin is 15 minutes and that of salicylate is dose-dependent, ranging between 2 and 12 hours. Though aspirin has a brief half-life, the duration of action is prolonged because platelet inhibition far outlasts the physical presence of the drug in the body [168].

The antithrombotic indications for aspirin are diverse. The ISIS-2 study showed that aspirin improves short- and long-term mortality when given to patients presenting with acute myocardial infarction [169]. Additionally, a meta-analysis including nearly 50 000 high-risk patients randomized to aspirin or placebo demonstrated a 23% odds reduction (SE 2%) in nonfatal MI, nonfatal stroke, or vascular death [170]. Aspirin is part of the antiplatelet regimen used for PCI. The role of aspirin in primary prevention is less clear. The Physician's Health Study demonstrated a 44% reduction in myocardial infarction when used for primary prevention [171]. However, when the risk of hemorrhage is considered, aspirin may not be beneficial in primary prevention for patients at low risk of thrombosis.

Aspirin may be added to warfarin anticoagulation in patients with mechanical heart valves and other high-risk features for thrombosis [172]. A large randomized prospective study suggested that aspirin decreases the incidence of venous thrombosis after surgery for hip fracture, irrespective of the use of other antithrombotic drugs [173]. However, aspirin is not recommended as a sole drug for the prevention of venous thromboembolism. The role of aspirin in atrial fibrillation is controversial, where it is not as protective as warfarin.

Monitoring

The effects of aspirin on platelet function are not detected by routine laboratory tests of coagulation. Use of the template bleeding time has been advocated, but results have been inconsistent [174,175]. Platelet aggregometry induced by epinephrine and low concentrations of collagen, but not induced by thrombin or high concentrations of collagen, detect an aspirin effect [176]. The PFA-100 platelet function analyzer detects the antiplatelet effect of aspirin [177,178]. The ACT and thromboelastography are generally unaffected by aspirin [179].

Surgery

There are several potential issues regarding antiplatelet drugs in the perioperative period. These include which drugs (if any) should be stopped, how early drugs should be stopped, when drugs should be restarted, whether the use of "bridging" antithrombotic therapies should be used, and whether regional anesthetic techniques are contraindicated. The cessation of aspirin therapy has been associated with a high risk of cardiovascular events, especially in patients with intracoronary stents [180–182]. Though definitive evidence is not yet available, aspirin therapy should be continued perioperatively except in patients at low coronary risk or for procedures with catastrophic bleeding risk (i.e., intracranial surgery, intramedullary spinal surgery, posterior-chamber eye surgery) [183]. Perioperative aspirin use is associated with a small increased risk of surgical bleeding and transfusion but a low risk of

perioperative cardiac events [183]. Early postoperative use of aspirin following coronary artery bypass grafting (CABG) seems to be gaining widespread acceptance, as receiving aspirin within 48 hours of CABG has been associated with a decreased incidence of myocardial infarction and mortality [184]. Aspirin has not been implicated in an increased incidence of epidural hematoma after neuraxial blockade, and most practitioners would not consider aspirin therapy alone to be a contraindication to spinal or epidural anesthesia [185,186].

Adverse effects

Adverse effects of aspirin, including erosion of the gastrointestinal mucosa and bleeding, are discussed in more detail in Chapter 34. The adverse effects relate predominantly to COX inhibition. Histamine-2 antagonists and proton pump inhibitors are helpful in decreasing gastrointestinal tract mucosal damage and upper gastrointestinal bleeding in the high-risk patient taking aspirin [187]. Enteric-coated or buffered aspirin is sometimes used to lower the risk of gastrointestinal hemorrhage, though evidence is lacking to support this practice [188].

Low-dose aspirin does not adversely affect antihypertensive therapy or renal function, unlike other nonsteroidal anti-inflammatory drugs [189]. Increased leukotriene synthesis secondary to COX inhibition can precipitate bronchospasm in patients with aspirin sensitivity or asthma [190]. Aspirin is not licensed for use in children because it has been associated with a syndrome of life-threatening acute liver failure known as Reye's syndrome [191].

Patients with an aspirin overdose may present with renal failure, complex acid–base abnormalities, dehydration, deranged blood glucose, seizures, or coma. Activated charcoal may prevent the systemic absorption of ingested aspirin [192]. Treatment should include intensive care unit admission and forced alkaline diuresis, and hemodialysis may be necessary [193].

There is a small subset of patients who display dramatic increases in bleeding time after administration of routine doses of aspirin and who may be susceptible to an increased incidence of bleeding complications. This hyperresponse may be related to either the presence of concurrent intrinsic platelet defects (e.g., storage pool disease, Glanzman's or Bernard–Soulier disease) or other defects within the hemostatic system (e.g., von Willebrand disease).

Dosage and administration

For almost all of its antiplatelet indications, a daily dose of aspirin of 80–325 mg is recommended. The antithrombotic effect of aspirin does not appear to be dose-related over a wide range of daily doses, an observation consistent with saturability of platelet COX-1 inhibition by aspirin at very low doses. In contrast, gastrointestinal toxicity of the drug does appear to be dose-related.

New and emerging concepts

The occurrence of cardiovascular events in some patients despite aspirin therapy has generated numerous recent publications regarding a potential role of aspirin resistance. The FDA has issued a warning regarding the potential detrimental effect of concomitant ibuprofen on aspirin antiplatelet therapy [7]. Currently, the clinical significance of aspirin resistance remains unclear.

Dipyridamole

Dipyridamole has antithrombotic and vasodilator actions and is usually used in combination with aspirin in clinical practice, most commonly for the secondary prevention of transient ischemic attack (TIA) and ischemic stroke.

Mechanisms of action

The mechanism by which dipyridamole reduces cardiovascular events is controversial [194]. Potential mechanisms include increasing cyclic adenosine monophosphate (cAMP) by phosphodiesterase (PDE) inhibition and also increasing plasma adenosine levels by inhibiting the uptake of adenosine by platelets. The increase in platelet cAMP inhibits calcium release and decreases secretion of serotonin and ADP. Therefore the broad actions of dipyridamole include vasodilation, inhibition of platelet adhesion, PGI_2 potentiation, and enhanced action of cAMP [195]. These actions result in a greater inhibition of platelet adhesion than aspirin, but less effect on aggregation. There is also recent evidence that dipyridamole inhibits inflammatory gene expression by platelet–monocyte aggregates, providing a new potential mechanism of cardiovascular disease modulation [196].

Clinical pharmacology

Oral absorption is slow, and dipyridamole is extensively protein-bound, mainly to α_1-acid glycoprotein (AAG) [195]. Dipyridamole is metabolized in the liver through glucuronic acid conjugation and is excreted in bile [195]. There is minimal urinary excretion. The time to peak effect is about 1.5 hours after ingestion and rapid (< 5 minutes) after intravenous administration. Elimination half-life is 10 hours.

A reformulation of dipyridamole that offers higher bioavailability than the orginal formulation (modified-release) has been used in more recent clinical trials, renewing interest in its use. In the ESPS-2 trial, including 6602 patients receiving placebo, aspirin, modified-release dipyridamole, or combination therapy, the use of aspirin–dipyridamole was associated with a relative risk of 0.76 for stroke (95% CI 0.63–0.93) without a significant increase in bleeding events when compared to aspirin monotherapy [197]. A Cochrane systematic review did not find evidence for a benefit over aspirin monotherapy outside of cerebral ischemic events, though this could relate to the use of the lower-bioavailability preparation in a majority of trials [198].

Adverse effects

The most common limiting side effect is headache. Other adverse effects include hypotension, bronchospasm, nausea, vomiting, and diarrhea. Cardiac ischemia, arrhythmias, and angina pectoris may be precipitated by dipyridamole, possibly as a result of coronary steal [199]. When adenosine is administered to patients taking dipyridamole, it should be given in reduced doses, because dipyridamole can potentiate the action of adenosine.

Dosage and administration

When used for the secondary prevention of cerebral ischemic events, 200 mg of modified-release dipyridamole (combined with aspirin 25 mg) is administered twice daily. Dipyridamole has also been used in combination with warfarin or aspirin for thromboprophylaxis of prosthetic cardiac valves, usually at a dose of 75–100 mg four times daily.

Prostacyclin

Prostacyclin (PGI_2, also known as epoprostenol) is an important physiologic inhibitor of platelet activation and aggregation. The triad of PGI_2, nitric oxide (NO), and tissue plasminogen activator (tPA) constitute key endothelial mediators that inhibit platelet activation and intravascular thrombosis [200]. The recent development of stable PGI_2 analogs has facilitated the exogenous administration of this crucial prostaglandin.

Mechanisms of action

PGI_2 binds to receptors on platelets that activate adenylate cyclase and increase intracellular cAMP. This in turns leads to a decrease in intracellular free calcium and inhibition of platelet activity.

Clinical pharmacology

PGI_2 has a half-life of only 3 minutes in plasma and is thus given by continuous intravenous infusion. PGI_2 is a potent vasodilator, and its side effects include flushing, headache, nausea, vomiting, and hypotension. PGI_2 can be given to inhibit platelet aggregation during renal dialysis either alone or with heparin. The use of exogenous PGI_2 as an antithrombotic drug is limited by its chemical instability and its vasodilatory actions [201].

Dosage and administration

PGI_2 may be initiated at a rate of 2 ng kg^{-1} min^{-1} and increased in increments of 2 ng kg^{-1} min^{-1} every 15 minutes. Infusion rate may be limited by hemodynamic instability or other side effects.

Thienoypyridines

The thienopyridine adenosine diphosphate (ADP) receptor antagonists inhibit a pathway of platelet activation parallel to the TxA_2 pathway. Drugs in this class include clopidogrel (Plavix) and ticlopidine and they are often used in combination with aspirin to produce additive antiplatelet effects. The use of ticlopidine has largely been supplanted by clopidogrel because of the higher potential for serious adverse effects such as thrombotic thrombocytopenic purpura (TTP). Indications for clopidogrel include primary prevention in patients intolerant to aspirin, acute myocardial infarction, and prior to PCI.

Mechanisms of action

Clopidogrel and ticlopidine are prodrugs. Their active metabolites irreversibly inhibit the P2Y$_{12}$ ADP receptor expressed on the platelet surface membrane. As such, they block the actions of ADP on platelets, namely promotion of platelet activation, aggregation, and degranulation [202–204]. ADP-induced binding of fibrinogen to the platelet GPIIb/IIIa receptor is inhibited [202]. Other pathways of platelet activation are also affected because of inhibition of ADP-mediated amplification.

Clinical pharmacology

A minority of absorbed clopidogrel is metabolized in the liver to the pharmacologically active compound, predominantly by CYP3A4 [205]. Clopidogrel has an onset of about 2 hours following ingestion. Peak platelet inhibition occurs approximately 4 days after initiation of therapy, though the onset can be dramatically shortened (i.e., hours) with the use of large loading doses. The peak effect of ticlopidine occurs at least several days after initiation, and loading doses are not used because of concern for adverse reactions [194]. Though the active metabolite of clopidogrel has a short half-life, the antiplatelet effect lasts for the life of the platelet, with a clinical duration of action of approximately 5 days, dependent on the formation of new platelets. Both clopidogrel and ticlopidine are more than 98% protein-bound and are metabolized in the liver followed by excretion in the urine and feces. The half-life of clopidogrel is approximately 8 hours. Ticlopidine has an elimination half-life between 8 and 13 hours after a single dose and 4–5 days with repeated dosing.

The CAPRIE study demonstrated a small benefit for clopidogrel over aspirin for patients with ischemic heart disease, cerebrovascular disease, and peripheral vascular disease for the primary outcomes (ARR 0.5%, 95% CI 0.02–0.98%) [206]. However, most indications for clopidogrel are in combination with aspirin. In acute myocardial infarction, the COMMIT trial demonstrated an early reduction in myocardial infarction, stroke, or death without an excess in bleeding events when clopidogrel was added to aspirin therapy [207]. However, in clinical practice, clopidogrel is frequently withheld in acute coronary syndromes because of the potential for urgent coronary bypass grafting. The CREDO trial demonstrated the benefit of adding clopidogrel to aspirin in patients undergoing PCI, and a subgroup analysis demonstrated the benefit of receiving a clopidogrel loading dose at least 6 hours prior to PCI [208]. Dual antiplatelet therapy with clopidogrel and aspirin is recommended for at least 12 months following coronary stent placement in the absence of an elevated risk for bleeding [209].

Surgery and anesthesia

Thienopyridines are usually stopped 5–10 days prior to surgery, because of an increased risk of bleeding. Although not well studied, the risk of transfusion is probably increased by around 50% in patients who continue clopidogrel perioperatively [183]. However, some patients have significant risks associated with clopidogrel discontinuation, especially patients with recently placed coronary stents. Premature cessation of antiplatelet therapy is the strongest predictor of stent thrombosis following coronary stent placement and carries a significant mortality risk [210]. If surgery cannot be postponed beyond 1 year after stent placement (minimums of 6 weeks following bare metal stent and 12 months following drug-eluting stent), dual antiplatelet therapy (including clopidogrel) should ideally be continued perioperatively. Riddell et al. discuss a rational approach to antiplatelet therapy management in these high-risk patients [211]. Oral antiplatelet therapy should probably never be interrupted for surgeries associated with a low bleeding risk, unless the antiplatelet therapy is being used strictly for primary prevention. When excess bleeding is encountered in patients who have recently received thienopyridines, platelet transfusion may be effective in improving hemostasis [212]. Regional anesthesia is best avoided until the effects of these drugs have dissipated (at least 7 days for clopidogrel and 14 days for ticlopidine).

Adverse effects

Ticlopidine has been largely replaced by clopidogrel, because of the frequency of neutropenia and TTP with ticlopidine. TTP can also occur with clopidogrel, usually in the first 2 weeks of therapy. Intracranial, gastrointestinal, and surgical bleeding are also potential serious complications. Bleeding may be especially problematic, given the long duration of action of the thienopyridines. Patients who present with an acute coronary syndrome and subsequently undergo bypass grafting within 5 days of receiving clopidogrel have a higher risk of reoperation (OR 4.60, 95% CI 1.45–14.55) [213]. These drugs should be avoided in patients with severe hepatic insufficiency.

Dosage and administration

The dose for clopidogrel is 75 mg orally once daily. The use of a large loading dose achieves a more rapid clinical effect, and a 600 mg loading dose is currently advocated prior to PCI [214]. Ticlopidine is administered as 250 mg orally twice daily with food.

New and emerging concepts

As with aspirin, the variable inhibition of platelet action associated with clopidogrel therapy is under examination. Potentially important pharmacologic mechanisms of antiplatelet attenuation include variable bioavailability, P2Y$_{12}$ receptor polymorphisms [215], CYP polymorphisms [216], and drug interactions involving CYP metabolism [217].

The new thienopyridine prasugrel is more potent than clopidogrel and ticlopidine, has a faster onset of action, and achieves a more uniform antiplatelet effect. The TRITON-TIMI 38 trial demonstrated a reduction in cardiovascular events with prasugrel compared to clopidogrel in patients undergoing PCI, but this was accompanied by an increased risk of major bleeding events [218].

Glycoprotein IIb/IIIa receptor inhibitors

The GPIIb/IIIa receptor inhibitors in current use are intravenous drugs and are predominantly used in patients undergoing PCI, especially in patients who present with acute coronary syndromes. These drugs block GPIIb/IIIa-mediated platelet binding and therefore target the final common pathway of platelet aggregation. Though early trials demonstrating a marked benefit of GPIIb/IIIa inhibitors led to burgeoning use, their use has declined in recent years with increased use of clopidogrel. When used in concert with dual-antiplatelet therapy (including preprocedural clopidogrel), trials have shown that benefits are confined to specific patient groups. Oral short-acting GPIIb/IIIa inhibitors have been developed but clinical results have been inconsistent.

Mechanisms of action

Abciximab is a chimeric human-murine monoclonal antibody that binds avidly to the platelet GPIIb/IIIa receptor. Eptifibatide (Integrilin) is a reversible peptide antagonist of the GPIIb/IIIa receptor. Tirofiban (Aggrastat) is a reversible nonpeptide antagonist of the GPIIb/IIIa receptor. The GPIIb/IIa receptor is the major surface receptor responsible for platelet aggregation [219]. All three drugs prevent binding of fibrinogen, vWF, and other adhesive molecules to activated platelets. Pharmacologically, these drugs do not all have equal efficacy, with abciximab displaying the greatest antiplatelet effect [220].

Clinical pharmacology

All three drugs are administered by intravenous infusion. Abciximab has the highest affinity for the GPIIb/IIIa receptor, whereas eptifibatide has the lowest affinity of the three drugs. The onset of action of abciximab is almost immediate, and although the duration of action after cessation of the infusion is up to 48 hours, most of the platelet inhibition dissipates after about 12 hours [221]. Abciximab is cleared by the kidneys. The onset of action of eptifibatide is within 15 minutes, the time to reach peak effect may be as long as 6 hours, and clinical effect continues for 4–6 hours after discontinuation. Up to 50% of the drug is excreted unchanged in the urine. Tirofiban achieves peak platelet inhibition rapidly and its effect lasts 4–8 hours after discontinuation. The elimination half-life of tirofiban is 2 hours, and it is mainly excreted unchanged in urine and feces. Eptifibatide and tirofiban may be cleared from plasma by dialysis.

Clinical benefits of the GPIIb/IIIa inhibitors have been demonstrated in several large clinical studies. A long-term follow-up study of three of the large early randomized trials (EPIC, EPILOG, and EPISTENT) examining abciximab use in patients underoing PCI demonstrated a survival benefit with abciximab (hazard ratio 0.82, 95% CI 0.70–0.96) [222]. However, the efficacy of these drugs has been re-examined in varying risk populations following the advent of clopidogrel loading doses prior to interventional procedures. The ISAR-REACT and ISAR-SWEET trials studied stable patients and stable diabetic patients, respectively, and found no benefit with GPIIb/IIIa inhibitors [223,224]. However, high-risk patients with acute coronary syndromes did have a reduction in ischemic events in the ISAR-REACT-2 trial. Though the role of GPIIb/IIIa inhibitors in elective PCI is not clear, they are generally indicated in patients with acute coronary syndromes for whom interventional management is planned. Specific recommendations are available for the selection of drugs in ST-elevation myocardial infarction (STEMI) and acute coronary syndromes [225,226].

Adverse effects

Bleeding represents the most likely complication encountered with any of the GPIIb/IIIa receptor inhibitors and occurs most frequently with abciximab [227]. Acute severe thrombocytopenia is a class effect of these drugs and occurs in 0.5% of cases. This risk may be compounded when they are given together with other drugs that carry this risk, such as ticlopidine or clopidogrel [228]. Thrombocytopenia can reportedly be treated successfully with a combination of platelet transfusion and steroid therapy [229].

Monitoring

The ACT has been used for near-patient monitoring of patients receiving GPIIb/IIIa receptor inhibitors along with other anticoagulants during PCI. Newer point-of-care assays may be more specific as a monitor of platelet function. Insufficient platelet inhibition during GPIIb/IIIa therapy, when measured with the Ultegra rapid platelet function analyzer, has been associated with adverse cardiac events after PCI [230]. The platelet count should be monitored during therapy.

Surgery and anesthesia

Some patients who receive GPIIb/IIIa receptor inhibitors will require subsequent surgery. When a sufficient time interval prior to surgery is not possible, the antiplatelet effects can be reversed with platelet transfusions or potentially cryoprecipitate (tirofiban, eptifibatide). An early report indicated that the use of abciximab may increase perioperative bleeding, especially if administered within 12 hours of surgery [231]. There are other data suggesting that there is no increased bleeding during cardiac surgery after administration of GPIIb/IIIa receptor inhibitors [232]. However, the lack of increased bleeding in this trial might be a result of pre-emptive platelet transfusions. Although abciximab may be associated with increased hemorrhage [231], the GPIIb/IIIa receptor inhibitors may protect platelets, preventing sequestration during CPB

[232,233]. There is a suggestion that heparin dosage for CPB should be reduced in patients who have received GPIIb/IIIa receptor inhibitors [231]. The combination of UFH with GPIIb/IIIa receptor inhibitors during CPB may be an alternative to other anticoagulation strategies in patients with HIT [234]. Regional anesthesia is best avoided when patients have recently received GPIIb/IIIa antagonists.

Dosage and administration

The GPIIb/IIIa antagonists are not intended as monotherapy and should be given in conjunction with other drugs, such as aspirin and heparin. The usual doses are:

Abciximab – Loading dose of 0.4 µg kg^{-1} min^{-1} for 30 minutes, administered 10–60 minutes before the start of the procedure, followed by an infusion of 0.125 µg kg^{-1} min^{-1} (maximum 10 µg min^{-1}) for 12 hours.

Eptifibatide – Loading dose of 180 µg kg^{-1} followed by an infusion of 2 µg min^{-1} for 12–24 hours. The dosage should be adjusted in renal failure.

Tirofiban – Intravenous infusion of 25 µg kg^{-1} followed by 0.15 µg kg^{-1} min^{-1} for 24 hours. Decrease the infusion rate by 50% in patients with creatinine clearance less than 30 mL min^{-1}.

Thrombolytic drugs

Thrombolytic drugs such as streptokinase (SK), urokinase, anisoylated plasminogen streptokinase activator complex (APSAC), and tissue plasminogen activator (tPA) are used for thrombolysis of arterial or venous clots in several clinical settings. The thrombolytic drugs have revolutionized the treatment of STEMI, as it has been decisively established that these drugs can significantly improve survival, especially when timely PCI is not an option [235]. Although also used as a therapy for acute ischemic stroke and pulmonary embolism, efficacy for these indications is less clear. Thrombolysis using these drugs carries a significant risk of bleeding and allergic reactions.

Mechanisms of action

Fibrinolysis occurs when circulating and fibrin-bound plasminogen activators enzymatically convert plasminogen into plasmin. Plasmin, a serine protease, hydrolyzes fibrin to dissolve clot. All thrombolytic drugs promote thrombolysis through this plasmin-mediated degradation of fibrinogen, circulating fibrin monomers/polymers, and clot-bound fibrin. They are much more capable of dissolving newly formed "white" clot – that is, platelet-rich clot (formed by weaker fibrinogen bonds) – than the older, more stable "red" clot that is tightly bound with fibrin [236]. Therefore, to be most effective, thrombolytic drugs must be given soon after thrombus formation.

Plasminogen activators act either directly (tPA, reteplase, urokinase, tenecteplase, and lanoteplase) or indirectly (SK and staphylokinase). Indirect activators (SK) are proteins that form a complex with plasminogen to catalyze the conversion of

additional, uncomplexed plasminogen to plasmin. This indirect action makes SK much less fibrin-specific by enabling action upon free and clotbound plasminogen. In contrast, the direct activators (tPA) cleave plasminogen into plasmin directly. Their activity is preferential to plasminogen already bound to fibrin, and this makes tPA more clot-specific than SK. When interacting within a clot, the presence of these drugs effectively shields plasmin from circulating plasmin inhibitors [236]. These drugs can be administered intravenously or delivered more specifically (e.g., intracoronary injections).

APSAC (anistreplase) is the preformed complex that SK forms in vivo and does not necessitate the presence of free circulating plasminogen to be effective.

Preclinical pharmacology
Development of genetically engineered mutants

In an effort to provide more quick-acting, more specific, and longer-acting thrombolytic drugs, researchers have created a number of plasminogen activators by genetically engineering human tPA with sequence deletions and substitutions. The first commercially available drug was reteplase (rPA), a deletion mutant with a longer half-life than human tPA [237]. Another genetic variation is tenecteplase (TNK-tPA), offering a 14-fold increase in fibrin specificity in vitro, which should theoretically reduce systemic plasminogen activation [238]. Both have equivalent infarct artery patency rates and patient survival data to human tPA (alteplase), but they can be administered as a bolus injection and thus may provide faster onset in clinical settings.

Laboratory evaluation of therapy

The thrombolytic state created by the thrombolytic drugs affects the coagulation system and laboratory tests of hemostatic function. Thrombolysis results in a depletion of plasma fibrinogen levels, factor V, and factor VIII. Low levels of fibrinogen (as low as 50mg dL^{-1} or less) can persist for more than 24 hours. Laboratory evaluation has demonstrated increased levels of fibrinogen degradation products and prolonged thrombin time, PT, and aPTT. Such laboratory tests are nonspecific and generally not useful in guiding therapy.

Clinical pharmacology

Each drug has relative advantages and disadvantages based on its fibrin specificity, biologic half-life, cost, ease of administration, and risk for allergic and other adverse reactions. FDA-approved indications for usage include the treatment of acute myocardial infarction and acute pulmonary embolism. SK, tPA, anistreplase, reteplase, and tenecteplase are used in the United States in acute myocardial infarction. Alteplase (tPA) is the only approved drug for the treatment of acute ischemic stroke. The novel genetically engineered versions of tPA are also undergoing study in the setting of acute ischemic stroke. SK is approved for the treatment of DVT and arterial thrombosis.

Pharmacokinetics

For the treatment of thrombosis, thrombolytic drugs can be delivered intravenously or directly via therapeutic catethers (e.g., coronary artery, pulmonary artery, cerebral artery). Although directed administration minimizes bleeding risks, the intravenous route is more suitable for providing early therapy and may avoid added procedural risks.

SK has a half-life of approximately 23 minutes, and its infusion may decrease vascular resistance and cause hypotension. SK is eliminated by the liver without detectable metabolites. Antistreptococcal antibodies contribute significantly to its inactivation. APSAC, which is SK precomplexed with plasminogen, demonstrates a longer half-life than SK.

Alteplase (recombinant human tPA) is cleared from the plasma primarily by the liver, with a half-life of 5 minutes and a volume of distribution approximating plasma volume. Tenecteplase is a bioengineered version of tPA that is more fibrin-specific and has a longer half-life than tPA [238]. Reteplase is a deletion mutant of tPA for which the deletion results in decreased hepatic elimination and thus a longer half-life, permitting bolus dosing [237]. Urokinase occurs in a low- and a high-molecular-weight form and has an approximate half-life of 15 minutes [239].

Adverse effects

All thrombolytic drugs may cause major bleeding complications, including intracranial hemorrhage. Severe bleeding can be treated with transfusions of fresh frozen plasma, cryoprecipitate, or platelets and drugs that have antifibrinolytic properties (e.g., ε-aminocaproic acid, EACA). Other adverse reactions include reperfusion arrhythmias, hypotension, cholesterol embolism, and allergic reaction. Allergic reactions are most commonly seen with SK (1–4% develop fever and shivering, while < 0.5% develop true anaphylaxis), because many patients have varying levels of antistreptococcal antibodies from previous bacterial infections. Repeat administration of SK carries greater risk for allergic reaction, including serum sickness and hypersensitivity vasculitis [169]. SK and APSAC are contraindicated when patients have had exposure greater than 5 days prior. The risk for allergic reaction to tPA is less than 0.2%.

Dosage and administration
Streptokinase

In the setting of acute STEMI, dosage for intravenous administration is 1 500 000 U over 60 minutes; intracoronary delivery is 20 000 U bolus followed by a 2000 U min^{-1} infusion for 60 minutes. For pulmonary embolism, DVT, or arterial thrombosis, the loading dose is 250 000 U intravenous infusion over 30 minutes followed by a 100 000 U infusion for 24–72 hours. To treat occlusion of vascular cannulae, 250 000 U in 2 mL of solution should be instilled and left in the clamped-off cannula for 2 hours. Then the contents of the cannula should be aspirated – not flushed – and then, if clear, flushed with saline and reconnected.

Alteplase

For the treatment of acute STEMI, a total of no more than 100 mg is administered over 90 minutes: a 15 mg bolus is followed by 0.75 mg kg^{-1} over 30 minutes (maximum 50 mg), followed by 0.5 mg kg^{-1} (maximum 35 mg) over 60 minutes [235]. The dose should not exceed 100 mg because of the increased risk of intracranial hemorrhage. For pulmonary embolism, infusion of 100 mg over 2 hours is recommended. For the treatment of acute ischemic stroke, 0.9 mg kg^{-1} of alteplase should be given (maximum 90 mg), with 10% of the dose given as a bolus followed by infusion of the remaining 90% over 60 minutes [240].

Reteplase

For the treatment of acute STEMI, two bolus doses of 10 000 000 U (each given over 2 minutes) should be administered 30 minutes apart [235].

Tenecteplase

For the treatment of acute STEMI, tenecteplase is administered as a bolus dose, with the dose varying from 30 to 50 mg depending on body weight [235].

Desmopressin

Desmopressin (DDAVP) is a synthetic polypeptide structurally related to arginine vasopressin (antidiuretic hormone). As a hemostatic drug, it is indicated for the treatment of bleeding associated with mild hemophilia, type 1 von Willebrand disease (vWD), uremia-induced platelet dysfunction, antiplatelet drugs, and platelet dysfunction after surgery [241,242].

Mechanisms of action

Desmopressin causes a dose-dependent increase in clotting factor VIII, plasminogen activator, factor VIII-related antigen, and vWF activity. Desmopressin increases plasma vWF concentrations through receptor-mediated release from endothelial cells [243].

Although increases in vWF can improve platelet–subendothelium and platelet–platelet interactions, other mechanisms may contribute, such as desmopressin-mediated generation of platelet microparticles or enhanced procoagulant activity, improvement of platelet retention, increased release of vWF from platelets, and increased expression of GPIb receptors [244–247].

Clinical pharmacology

After intranasal administration of desmopressin, 10–20% is absorbed through the nasal mucosa. Bioavailability is 3.3–4.1% and peak plasma concentrations are attained after 40–45 minutes. After both intranasal and intravenous administration, increases in plasma concentrations of factor VIII and vWF are evident within 30 minutes and peak between 90 minutes and 3 hours. Plasma concentrations of desmopressin decline in a biphasic manner, with a mean initial plasma half-life of 8 minutes and a mean plasma elimination half-life of 75 minutes. The metabolic fate of desmopressin is unknown. Large intravenous doses of desmopressin increase factor VIII activity in healthy individuals, in patients with mild hemophilia A and B, in patients with certain types of vWD, and in patients with uremia. The effect of desmopressin on platelet function lasts for about 3 hours, but may be prolonged by a repeat dose [248].

The increase in factor VIII activity is dose-dependent, with a 300–400% maximum increase occurring after intravenous administration of a 0.4 μg kg^{-1} dose. Desmopressin is only beneficial for treatment of hemophilia A when baseline plasma factor VIII activity is greater than 5%. Although desmopressin is useful with type I vWD (75% of patients with vWD have this type), it should be used judiciously in patients with type 2B vWD, because there may be an increased risk for thrombocytopenia or thrombosis. In patients with type 2B and pseudo-vWD, desmopressin may induce platelet aggregation and thrombocytopenia secondary to release of abnormal forms of very high-molecular-weight multimers. Desmopressin is ineffective for type 3 vWD. Tachyphylaxis occurs if desmopressin is administered more than once within a 48-hour period.

With large doses administered rapidly (< 30 minutes), tachycardia, hypotension, facial flushing, headache, water retention, and hyponatremia have been reported [249]. Hypotension may be related to the rate of administration and release of vasodilating prostaglandins from endothelial cells [250]. Desmopressin can also result in release of tPA via the endothelium, which may result in fibrinolysis. The risk for water intoxication and hyponatremia increases with doses greater than 0.5 μg kg^{-1}. Hemodynamic side effects can be attenuated by slow intravenous administration [242].

Dosage and administration

The intranasal dosage of desmopressin for the management of hemophilia A or type 1 vWD is 0.3 mg (0.1 mL or one spray from the spray pump into each nostril of a solution containing 1.5 mg mL^{-1}). A dosage of 0.15 mg may be sufficient in patients who weigh less than 50 kg. The usual parenteral dose for those older than 3 months with hemophilia A or type 1 vWD is 0.3–0.4 μg kg^{-1} given by slow intravenous infusion over 30 minutes [242].

In patients with hemophilia A, factor VIII and vWF activities, factor VIII antigen levels, and aPTT should be monitored during desmopressin therapy. In patients with vWD, factor VIII and vWF antigen and activities should be monitored. Tests of platelet function such as the bleeding time, platelet aggregometry, the HemoSTATUS, and the PFA-100 platelet function analyzer may be useful [242].

If desmopressin is used before surgery for bleeding prophylaxis, the nasal drug should be administered 2 hours before surgery and the intravenous infusion 30 minutes before surgery. Desmopressin is well established in the prevention of bleeding for patients with inherited bleeding abnormalities, especially vWD [251]. In the perioperative period, patients are particularly vulnerable to electrolyte and fluid imbalances, and desmopressin increases these risks.

There is much controversy surrounding the ability of desmopressin to decrease perioperative bleeding when patients are not known to have a specific bleeding diathesis. Most of the studies, including spinal, aortic, and liver surgery, have not shown a reduction in blood loss after routine desmopressin administration [252–254]. The composite evidence does not support the routine use of desmopressin, unless there is a specific indication such as vWD, patients at high risk for bleeding (e.g., uremia, long CPB intervals), or in-vitro evidence of platelet dysfunction [242,255–257].

New and emerging concepts

For high-risk surgery, desmopressin is associated with a modest reduction in blood loss and transfusion requirements [258]. Desmopression may be specifically useful in conditions where the shear rate of flowing blood is increased and there is mechanical destruction of large vWF multimers or an acquired vWD state, an example of which is aortic stenosis [259].

ε-Aminocaproic acid and tranexamic acid

The fibrinolytic pathway leads to clot lysis and is important in preventing occlusion at sites of vessel injury. However, excessive fibrinolysis can lead to a bleeding diathesis by depleting fibrinogen, factors V, and VIII. Further, circulating fibrinogen/fibrin degradation products can inhibit platelet function. Surgery, organic diseases, and drugs can initiate and promote fibrinolysis, with CPB representing the most extensively studied clinical situation. Antifibrinolytic drugs can inhibit this activity and aid in reducing the associated bleeding. These drugs include the synthetic lysine analogs – ε-aminocaproic acid (EACA) and tranexamic acid (trans-4-aminomethylcyclohexane-1-carboxylic acid; TA) – and the nonspecific serine protease inhibitor, aprotinin. Although their mechanisms of action, efficacy, adverse effects, and cost have been most extensively studied in the cardiac surgical setting, they have also been examined in other procedures associated with significant bleeding.

Mechanisms of action

All antifibrinolytic drugs competitively inhibit the degradation of fibrin and fibrinogen by plasmin. The method of inhibition differs between the lysine analogs and aprotinin, and their effects may be additive or even synergistic.

EACA is a synthetic chemical analog of the amino acid lysine. It acts by binding to the kringles, or lysine-binding sites, of plasminogen and plasmin. Once bound, EACA displaces plasminogen from fibrin, thus inhibiting its ability to split fibrinogen [260]. Another proposed mechanism of action involves the ability of EACA to bind to fibrin and protect it from plasmin degradation. The mechanism of action of TA is identical to that of EACA, but TA is approximately 10 times more potent on a molar basis. Both TA and EACA preferentially inhibit the cleavage of plasminogen to plasmin by clot-bound tissue plasminogen activator (tPA) rather than circulating tPA; accordingly, they may not be as effective as aprotinin in inhibiting systemic fibrinolysis when high levels of tPA result in systemic plasmin generation and prolongation of bleeding times secondary to increased fibrinogen degradation products [261].

Clinical pharmacology

EACA is a water-soluble drug with a volume of distribution of approximately 30 L. It is primarily eliminated unchanged (65%) in urine and has a terminal half-life of approximately 2 hours.

TA has a volume of distribution of about 9–12 L. About 3% of circulating TA is bound to plasminogen. It is almost entirely excreted unchanged through the kidney (90–95%). Its terminal elimination half-life is about 2 hours [262]. A study of the pharmacokinetics of tranexamic acid in relation to cardiopulmonary bypass suggested that a low-dose strategy (334 μM target) of 12.5 mg kg^{-1} loading dose, 6.5 mg kg^{-1} h^{-1} maintenance infusion, and 1 mg kg^{-1} in pump prime would yield more stable TA concentrations than traditional regimens [263]. For a high-dose strategy (800 μM target), a regimen of 30 mg kg^{-1} loading dose, 16 mg kg^{-1} h^{-1} maintenance infusion, and 2 mg kg^{-1} in pump prime is suggested [263]. Given the high degree of renal excretion, the doses of both EACA and TA should be reduced or limited to a loading dose in patients with renal insufficiency.

EACA and TA have been used in treatment and prophylaxis of bleeding in numerous clinical situations. They have been helpful as adjunctive therapy in disease states such as hemophilia, vWD, and uremia [264]. They have been administered to reduce risk for rebleeding in upper gastrointestinal bleeding, severe epistaxis, menorrhagia, hemorrhagic laryngitis/tonsillitis, traumatic hyphema, and subarachnoid hemorrhage from cerebral aneurysm [265]. In the surgical setting, these drugs have been given to reduce perioperative bleeding in major orthopedic joint replacement, liver transplantation, and most extensively with cardiac surgery and the use of extracorporeal membrane oxygenation. The potential role of lysine analogs has been studied in patients with 4G and 5G plasminogen activator inhibitor 1 (PAI-1) polymorphisms who underwent cardiac surgery. Patients homozygous for the 5G allele and receiving placebo had the highest blood loss, but elevated blood loss was not observed in 5G homozygotes who received TA [266].

Concerns have been raised regarding using the lysine analogs in settings involving secondary fibrinolysis such as DIC. The administration of antifibrinolytic drugs in this setting can potentially lead to be catastrophic thrombotic complications, especially if given without concomitant heparin. However, these drugs have been extensively used in cardiac surgery (which routinely leads to secondary fibrinolysis) without an apparent increased risk for thrombotic complications. This may be because of the routine use of high-dose heparin for systemic anticoagulation and the hypocoagulable state (i.e., up to 80% reduction in coagulation factors and quantitative and qualitative platelet abnormalities) commonly observed after CPB. However, judicious use of these drugs should be considered, since the lack of association with target organ injury or thrombotic complications has not been formally evaluated with randomized controlled trials.

EACA and TA have little effect on the laboratory evaluation of coagulation. Tests of platelet function, including aggregation and thromboelastograph curves, are unchanged in vivo when standard dosing is used [267,268]. Intraoperative point-of-care testing with ACTs is also unaffected by EACA [262,269]. EACA activity can be demonstrated ex vivo by a decrease in circulating fibrin degradation products when compared with placebo [262,268].

Surgery

Numerous studies have been performed to evaluate the efficacy of EACA and TA in reducing blood loss during and after cardiac surgery. The evidence for a transfusion-sparing effect in cardiac surgery is stronger for TA than for EACA, with a Cochrane systematic review of randomized trials yielding relative risks of transfusion of 0.61 for TA (95% CI 0.54–0.69) and 0.75 for EACA (95% CI 0.58–0.96) [270]. This difference may be related to potency or dosing issues.

The antifibrinolytic drugs have been used to limit hemorrhage in spine and large joint surgery. Proponents theorize that use of tourniquet and traumatic exposure of marrow can promote fibrinolysis. A recent meta-analysis of EACA, TA, and aprotinin in spine surgery demonstrated a beneficial effect upon blood transfusion and blood loss with each drug [271]. The synthetic lysine analogs have not been noted to increase the risk of venous thromboembolic complications with orthopedic surgery.

Antifibrinolytic drugs have been administered to neurosurgical patients to decrease the risk for rebleeding from cerebral aneurysm while awaiting surgery. In patients with subarachnoid hemorrhage, antifibrinolytic therapy reduced the risk for rebleeding by 45% when compared with placebo. The beneficial effect on rebleeding is, however, offset by an increased risk for cerebral ischemia, and there is no overall improvement in mortality rate [265]. In addition, Kang and colleagues demonstrated that an EACA-modified thromboelastograph can be used to identify patients with hyperfibrinolysis during the anhepatic stage of liver transplantation [272]. These authors also demonstrated that use of this technique reduced bleeding when EACA was administered on the basis of thromboelastogram results [273].

Adverse effects

Antifibrinolytic drugs have occasionally been implicated in thrombotic complications. One pooled analysis of EACA in cardiac surgery demonstrated an increased incidence of perioperative myocardial infarction [274]. Other randomized clinical trials and meta-analyses have not revealed any increased incidence of thrombotic complications when routine dosing has been used [275]. In unique clinical situations such as ongoing DIC or concomitant treatment with coagulation factor concentrates, such as factor IX concentrate in patients with hemophilia, caution should be exercised, as an increased incidence of thrombotic complications has been observed.

Other rare but serious adverse effects have been reported. Hyperkalemic arrest after CPB has been attributed to the structural similarity of EACA with the cationic amino acid lysine. Lysine has been shown in isolated rat muscle and intact animals to increase serum potassium by an electroneutral exchange of intracellular potassium for extracellular lysine. The resultant increase in potassium can be rapid and can be worse in patients with significant reduction in renal function [276]. Intravenous EACA has been linked with postoperative proteinuria and with skeletal muscle injury, ranging from myalgias to myonecrosis and rhabdomyolysis [277,278].

Dosage and administration

EACA is available as a 250 mg mL^{-1} injectable solution, with benzyl alcohol as a preservative (thus not recommended for use in newborns). For oral administration, EACA is available as a 25% syrup and as 500 mg tablets. TA is available in injectable form, in a 100 mg mL^{-1} concentration, and in 50 mg tablets.

For the control of local fibrinolysis, the recommended dosing regimen for EACA is a 4–5 g loading dose infused intravenously over 1 hour followed by a 1 g h^{-1} infusion for 8 hours or until the bleeding is controlled. TA dosing has been recommended as 0.5–1 g slow intravenous infusion twice daily or as 1–1.5 g orally two or three times daily. TA, as indicated for tooth extraction prophylaxis, is a 10 mg kg^{-1} intravenous bolus given just before surgery, followed by 25 mg kg^{-1} orally or 10 mg kg^{-1} intravenously three or four times daily for 2–8 days.

For the inhibition of general fibrinolysis associated with CPB, EACA can be given as a 75–150 mg kg^{-1} intravenous loading dose over 15–30 minutes, followed by a 10–15 mg kg^{-1} h^{-1} infusion [279]. More recent evidence indicates that to maintain a reasonable level of this drug, the bolus dose should be reduced to 50 mg kg^{-1} and the infusion rate should be increased to 25 mg kg^{-1} h^{-1} [280]. The most common TA dosing for cardiac surgery is a 10–15 mg kg^{-1} intravenous loading dose with a 1 mg kg^{-1} h^{-1} infusion [262], though alternative dosing regimens have been advocated [263].

New and emerging concepts

The lysine analogs reduce bleeding in cardiac surgery. However, the use of these drugs may still have a negative mortality effect in cardiac surgery, as the safety of these drugs versus placebo has not been adequately studied in large trials. This is especially an area of concern in coronary bypass grafting, where impairment of fibrinolysis could contribute to ischemic morbidity. Results from the ongoing ATACAS trial will help to answer these questions [281].

Aprotinin

Although aprotinin has antifibrinolytic properties, it is clearly a broad-spectrum drug on the basis of its anticoagulant and anti-inflammatory properties. Aprotinin has been withdrawn by the manufacturer because of safety concerns.

Mechanisms of action

Aprotinin is a strongly basic polypeptide isolated from bovine lung [282]. In addition to its antifibrinolytic properties (plasmin inhibition), aprotinin also inhibits trypsin, chymotrypsin, thrombin, kallikrein, bradykinin, elastase, activated protein C, and urokinase. Overall, aprotinin is categorized as an antifibrinolytic, anticoagulant, platelet-protective, and anti-inflammatory drug.

Plasmin is aprotinin's major site of action. Aprotinin binds plasmin bound to fibrin and to cell receptors, where plasmin is usually protected from the body's naturally occurring inhibitors (such as α_2-antiplasmin and α_2-macroglobulin). Aprotinin can also prevent fibrinolysis by a nonplasmin pathway by inhibiting kallikrein (and therefore the contact activation coagulation system) [279,282].

Aprotinin may also reduce tissue-factor-mediated activation of the hemostatic system by directly inhibiting the tissue factor–factor VIIa complex and factor VIII [283]. This action on the coagulation cascade is also intertwined with aprotinin's other mechanisms: decreasing thrombin-induced platelet activation and inhibiting kallikrein activation of fibrinolysis. By acting on plasmin, aprotinin can protect platelets because plasmin and thrombin can induce platelet activation, release, and aggregation. Potential explanations for the ability of aprotinin to preserve platelets include attenuation of TxA$_2$ release, inhibition of thrombin formation, preservation of GPIIb/IIIa receptors, and protection against heparin-induced platelet dysfunction. In addition, one of the most important mechanisms related to aprotinin may involve its ability to inhibit thrombin-mediated platelet activation/destruction through a dose-dependent inhibition of the platelet PAR1 receptor [284], which is important since thrombin is systemically active with cardiac surgery involving CPB.

Clinical pharmacology

After intravenous injection, aprotinin is rapidly distributed throughout the extracellular compartment. This distribution phase has a half-life of approximately 20–30 minutes. Aprotinin has a plasma half-life of approximately 150 minutes and a terminal elimination half-life of 7–10 hours unless there is substantial renal insufficiency. Aprotinin requires repeated boluses or maintenance infusion to maintain therapeutic plasma concentrations.

Aprotinin is reabsorbed by the renal proximal tubular system, with 80–90% stored in phagosomes found in the tubules' ciliated border cells. These border cells accumulate aprotinin for the first 12–24 hours to be later metabolized and eliminated during the next 4–5 days [282]. The remainder is excreted unchanged in the urine, with the excreted fraction increasing as the dose increases.

Monitoring

Aprotinin prolongs celite activated clotting time (ACT) in a dose-dependent manner. It is recommended that in patients receiving aprotinin and heparin anticoagulation for CPB, celite ACT values should exceed 750 seconds and kaolin ACT should be more than 450 seconds [285].

Adverse effects

Two observational studies reported on cardiac surgery patients receiving EACA, TA, aprotinin, or no antifibrinolytic. The use of aprotinin was associated with an increased risk of renal failure, myocardial infarction or heart failure, and stroke or encephalopathy while significantly reducing blood loss [286]. Aprotinin was also associated with an increased risk of mortality after propensity adjustment (adjusted odds ratio 1.48, 95% CI 1.13–1.93) [287]. Finally, a blinded trial of EACA, TA, or aprotinin in cardiac surgery patients at high risk for bleeding was terminated early, following randomization of 2331 patients, because of an elevated 30-day mortality in patients receiving aprotinin (relative risk vs. EACA or TA 1.53, 95% CI 1.06–2.22) [288]. Aprotinin has subsequently been withdrawn by the manufacturer.

Aprotinin is a foreign protein and can cause allergic reactions. The overall risk of allergic reaction has been estimated to be about 2.8% [289,290]. There is strong evidence that repeated exposure within 3–6 months carries the greatest risk for reaction.

Summary

There is a delicate balance between procoagulant and anticoagulant pathways. The intact endothelium releases powerful antiplatelet compounds and peptides that promote the inactivation of clotting factors. When the endothelium is denuded or platelets are activated, clotting is initiated. Cells presenting tissue factor bind to and activate factor VII, which initiates a cascade resulting in thrombin and fibrin production. Fibrin binds to activated platelets to form clot, and thrombin sends an array of signals, which lead to amplification of clotting where tissue is damaged, and inhibition of clotting where endothelium is intact.

Heparin and low-molecular-weight heparin (LMWH) potentiate the anticoagulant properties of antithrombin, and are administered commonly for thrombosis prophylaxis and therapeutic anticoagulation. The anticoagulant effect of heparin can be reversed with protamine. Low-molecular-weight heparins are easy to dose and have developed a track record for safety. Heparin-induced thrombocytopenia (HIT) is a potentially life-threatening complication of heparin-like medications.

Protamine is an intravenous cationic protein that binds to heparin and facilitates the complete antagonism of heparin-induced coagulation. Protamine is itself a weak anticoagulant and is occasionally associated with severe hemodynamic instability.

Danaparoid is a low-molecular-weight heparinoid that exerts its anticoagulant action primarily through indirect factor Xa inhibition and partly through indirect thrombin inhibition. Danaparoid has proven efficacy as an anticoagulant for patients with HIT. Fondaparinux is a synthetic pentasaccharide, antithrombin-dependent, selective factor Xa inhibitor that is effective for thrombosis prophylaxis as a once-daily subcutaneous injection. Rivaroxaban is an orally administered direct inhibitor of activated factor Xa that may be a suitable alternative to warfarin and may be safe in the setting of HIT.

Argatroban is a synthetic intravenous direct thrombin inhibitor that is used anticoagulation of patients with HIT. Argatroban is metabolized by the liver, and is useful in the setting of renal dysfunction. Dabigatran etexilate, the prodrug of dabigatran, is a new orally administered direct thrombin inhibitor that has predictable pharmacokinetics and pharmacodynamics and has promising efficacy for thrombosis prophylaxis.

Hirudin-related compounds are direct thrombin inhibitors that may be useful in several settings, especially for patients with HIT. Bivalirudin has a relatively short half-life and has even been used in cardiac surgery with favorable outcomes. Desirudin is an alternative to heparin in that effective thrombosis prophylaxis can be achieved with twice-daily subcutaneous injection.

Warfarin is a cheap and widely tested oral anticoagulant drug that prevents the carboxylation (activation) of vitamin-K-dependent clotting factors. Owing to genetic and environmental factors, there is a wide interindividual variability in the dose required to attain a therapeutic response to warfarin. There is a strong impetus to consider relevant genotypic information when dosing warfarin.

Aspirin is the most commonly used antiplatelet drug and acts by irreversibly acetylating cyclooxygenase (COX), thus modulating the production of downstream eicosanoids which affect platelet and vascular function. Platelet COX-1 is predominantly affected by low-dose aspirin, which leads to decreased thromboxane A_2 (TxA_2), while prostacyclin (PGI_2) is relatively preserved. Aspirin has a short half-life but achieves a lengthy clinical effect because of irreversible modification of platelet COX-1, persisting for the life of the platelet. The antiplatelet effects of aspirin are dose-independent across a broad low-dose range, while adverse gastrointestinal effects are dose-dependent. Because of the risk of cardiovascular events, aspirin should generally be continued perioperatively, unless the bleeding risk is prohibitive or aspirin is prescribed for primary prevention only.

Dipyridamole increases cAMP and leads to vasodilation and inhibition of platelet adhesion. A modified-release formulation is used for secondary prevention of cerebral ischemic events in combination with aspirin. Prostacyclin is an antiplatelet drug which can be administered by intravenous infusion and effects short-lived inhibition of platelet aggregation.

The thienopyridines irreversibly inhibit the $P2Y_{12}$ ADP receptor, which blocks ADP-mediated platelet activation and also inhibits the amplification of platelet activation by other ligands. Clopidogrel is a prodrug (metabolized to its active compound by cytochrome P450). It has a short half-life but a long effective clinical duration (5–7 days) because of irreversible platelet inhibition. Clopidogrel is often initiated with a loading dose (150–600 mg) to shorten the time to effective antiplatelet inhibition. Premature cessation of dual antiplatelet therapy (aspirin and thienopyridine) following percutaneous cardiac intervention (PCI) is associated with a significant risk of adverse cardiovascular events.

The glycoprotein IIb/IIIa inhibitors inhibit the final common pathway of platelet aggregation: GPIIb/IIIa-mediated linkage of platelets, fibrinogen, and von Willebrand factor (vWF). The currently used drugs are administered via intravenous infusion in patients undergoing PCI or in acute coronary syndromes when invasive management is planned. The duration of platelet inhibition following drug discontinuation is longest with abciximab (about 12 hours) and shorter with tirofiban and eptifibatide (4–8 hours). Acute severe thrombocytopenia can occur with GPIIb/IIIa inhibitor therapy.

The thrombolytic drugs are intravenous drugs that are chiefly used for acute myocardial infarction, especially when PCI is not immediately available. They act either directly (tissue plasminogen activator, tPA) upon plasminogen to conver it to plasmin or indirectly (streptokinase, SK), by first forming a complex with plasminogen before acting on additional plasminogen. They are contraindicated in postoperative patients or in other patients at risk of bleeding. The structures of newer thrombolytics can allow differing fibrin-selectivity, differing metabolism, and reduced susceptibility to plasminogen activator inhibitor-1 (PAI-1). SK and anisoylated plasminogen streptokinase activator complex (APSAC) should not be re-dosed after 5 days because of a risk of anyphylaxis.

Desmopressin is a hemostatic drug that is useful for treating bleeding associated with mild hemophilia, type 1 von Willebrand disease, renal insufficiency, and CPB-associated platelet dysfunction. Overall, desmopressin is associated with a minor reduction in blood loss and transfusion with major surgery. The antifibrinolytic drugs ε-aminocaproic acid (EACA) and tranexamic acid (TA) bind to the lysine-binding sites of plasminogen and plasmin, displacing fibrin. They decrease the generation of fibrinogen degradation products, which inhibit platelet function, and attenuate the depletion of clotting factors (e.g., factors V, VIII, fibrinogen). Tranexamic acid has been shown to be more effective in reducing blood loss and transfusion after cardiac surgery. Use of the antifibrinolytic drugs carries a risk of thrombosis.

The serine protease inhibitor aprotinin decreases perioperative blood loss, but has been withdrawn by the manufacturer following an increase in mortality (versus EACA and TA) in a randomized trial involving high-risk cardiac surgical patients.

References

1. Ignarro LJ, Buga GM, Wood KS, Byrns RE, Chaudhuri G. Endothelium-derived relaxing factor produced and released from artery and vein is nitric oxide. *Proc Natl Acad Sci U S A* 1987; **84**: 9265–9.

2. Marcus AJ, Broekman MJ, Pinsky DJ. COX inhibitors and thromboregulation. *N Engl J Med* 2002; **347**: 1025–6.

3. Marcus AJ, Broekman MJ, Drosopoulos JH, *et al.* The endothelial cell ecto-ADPase responsible for inhibition of platelet function is CD39. *J Clin Invest* 1997; **99**: 1351–60.

4. Vane JR, Botting RM. Formation by the endothelium of prostacyclin, nitric oxide and endothelin. *J Lipid Mediat* 1993; **6**: 395–404.

5. Furie B, Furie BC. Mechanisms of thrombus formation. *N Engl J Med* 2008; **359**: 938–49.

6. Vu TK, Hung DT, Wheaton VI, Coughlin SR. Molecular cloning of a functional thrombin receptor reveals a novel proteolytic mechanism of receptor activation. *Cell* 1991; **64**: 1057–68.

7. Nesheim ME, Taswell JB, Mann KG. The contribution of bovine Factor V and Factor Va to the activity of prothrombinase. *J Biol Chem* 1979; **254**: 10952–62.

8. Orfeo T, Brufatto N, Nesheim ME, *et al.* The factor V activation paradox. *J Biol Chem* 2004; **279**: 19580–91.

9. Davie EW, Ratnoff OD. Waterfall sequence for intrinsic blood clotting. *Science* 1964; **145**: 1310–12.

10. Macfarlane RG. An enzyme cascade in the blood clotting mechanism, and its function as a biochemical amplifier. *Nature* 1964; **202**: 498–9.

11. Furie B, Furie BC. Molecular and cellular biology of blood coagulation. *N Engl J Med* 1992; **326**: 800–6.

12. Renne T, Pozgajova M, Gruner S, *et al.* Defective thrombus formation in mice lacking coagulation factor XII. *J Exp Med* 2005; **202**: 271–81.

13. Kleinschnitz C, Stoll G, Bendszus M, *et al.* Targeting coagulation factor XII provides protection from pathological thrombosis in cerebral ischemia without interfering with hemostasis. *J Exp Med* 2006; **203**: 513–18.

14. Hirsh J, O'Donnell M, Eikelboom JW. Beyond unfractionated heparin and

warfarin: current and future advances. *Circulation* 2007; **116**: 552–60.

15. Bartholomew JR. Heparin-induced thrombocytopenia: 2008 update. *Curr Treat Options Cardiovasc Med* 2008; **10**: 117–27.

16. Brinkhous KM, Smith HP, Warner ED, Seegers WH. Heparin and Blood Clotting. *Science* 1939; **90**: 539.

17. Bray B, Lane DA, Freyssinet JM, Pejler G, Lindahl U. Anti-thrombin activities of heparin. Effect of saccharide chain length on thrombin inhibition by heparin cofactor II and by antithrombin. *Biochem J* 1989; **262**: 225–32.

18. Choay J, Petitou M, Lormeau JC, *et al.* Structure–activity relationship in heparin: a synthetic pentasaccharide with high affinity for antithrombin III and eliciting high anti-factor Xa activity. *Biochem Biophys Res Commun* 1983; **116**: 492–9.

19. Hirsh J, Raschke R, Warkentin TE, *et al.* Heparin: mechanism of action, pharmacokinetics, dosing considerations, monitoring, efficacy, and safety. *Chest* 1995; **108**: 258S–275S.

20. Tollefsen DM. Insight into the mechanism of action of heparin cofactor II. *Thromb Haemost* 1995; **74**: 1209–14.

21. Abildgaard U. Heparin/low molecular weight heparin and tissue factor pathway inhibitor. *Haemostasis* 1993; **23**: 103–6.

22. John LC, Rees GM, Kovacs IB. Inhibition of platelet function by heparin. An etiologic factor in postbypass hemorrhage. *J Thorac Cardiovasc Surg* 1993; **105**: 816–22.

23. Khuri SF, Valeri CR, Loscalzo J, *et al.* Heparin causes platelet dysfunction and induces fibrinolysis before cardiopulmonary bypass. *Ann Thorac Surg* 1995; **60**: 1008–14.

24. Basu D, Gallus A, Hirsh J, Cade J. A prospective study of the value of monitoring heparin treatment with the activated partial thromboplastin time. *N Engl J Med* 1972; **287**: 324–7.

25. Hull RD, Raskob GE, Hirsh J, *et al.* Continuous intravenous heparin compared with intermittent subcutaneous heparin in the initial treatment of proximal-vein thrombosis. *N Engl J Med* 1986; **315**: 1109–14.

26. Chew DP, Bhatt DL, Lincoff AM, *et al.* Defining the optimal activated clotting time during percutaneous coronary intervention: aggregate results from 6 randomized, controlled trials. *Circulation* 2001; **103**: 961–6.

27. Bull BS, Korpman RA, Huse WM, Briggs BD. Heparin therapy during extracorporeal circulation. I. Problems inherent in existing heparin protocols. *J Thorac Cardiovasc Surg* 1975; **69**: 674–84.

28. Bull BS, Huse WM, Brauer FS, Korpman RA. Heparin therapy during extracorporeal circulation. II. The use of a dose-response curve to individualize heparin and protamine dosage. *J Thorac Cardiovasc Surg* 1975; **69**: 685–9.

29. Despotis GJ, Summerfield AL, Joist JH, *et al.* Comparison of activated coagulation time and whole blood heparin measurements with laboratory plasma anti-Xa heparin concentration in patients having cardiac operations. *J Thorac Cardiovasc Surg* 1994; **108**: 1076–82.

30. de Swart CA, Nijmeyer B, Roelofs JM, Sixma JJ. Kinetics of intravenously administered heparin in normal humans. *Blood* 1982; **60**: 1251–8.

31. Boneu B, Caranobe C, Cadroy Y, *et al.* Pharmacokinetic studies of standard unfractionated heparin, and low molecular weight heparins in the rabbit. *Semin Thromb Hemost* 1988; **14**: 18–27.

32. Sobel M, McNeill PM, Carlson PL, *et al.* Heparin inhibition of von Willebrand factor-dependent platelet function in vitro and in vivo. *J Clin Invest* 1991; **87**: 1787–93.

33. Cruickshank MK, Levine MN, Hirsh J, Roberts R, Siguenza M. A standard heparin nomogram for the management of heparin therapy. *Arch Intern Med* 1991; **151**: 333–7.

34. Despotis GJ, Gravlee G, Filos K, Levy J. Anticoagulation monitoring during cardiac surgery: a review of current and emerging techniques. *Anesthesiology* 1999; **91**: 1122–51.

35. Despotis GJ, Levine V, Joist JH, Joiner-Maier D, Spitznagel E. Antithrombin III during cardiac surgery: effect on response of activated clotting time to heparin and relationship to markers of hemostatic activation. *Anesth Analg* 1997; **85**: 498–506.

36. Hashimoto K, Yamagishi M, Sasaki T, Nakano M, Kurosawa H. Heparin and antithrombin III levels during cardiopulmonary bypass: correlation with subclinical plasma coagulation. *Ann Thorac Surg* 1994; **58**: 799–804; discussion 804–5.

37. Anderson EF. Heparin resistance prior to cardiopulmonary bypass. *Anesthesiology* 1986; **64**: 504–7.

38. Wysowski DK, Talarico L, Bacsanyi J, Botstein P. Spinal and epidural hematoma and low-molecular-weight heparin. *N Engl J Med* 1998; **338**: 1774–5.

39. Jappe U. Allergy to heparins and anticoagulants with a similar pharmacological profile: an update. *Blood Coagul Fibrinolysis* 2006; **17**: 605–13.

40. Hirsh J, Bauer KA, Donati MB, Gould M, Samama MM, Weitz JI. Parenteral anticoagulants: American College of Chest Physicians Evidence-Based Clinical Practice Guidelines, 8th edn. *Chest* 2008; **133**: 141S–159S.

41. Bhandari M, Hirsh J, Weitz JI, *et al.* The effects of standard and low molecular weight heparin on bone nodule formation in vitro. *Thromb Haemost* 1998; **80**: 413–17.

42. Franchini M. Heparin-induced thrombocytopenia: an update. *Thromb J* 2005; **3**: 14.

43. Warkentin TE, Sheppard JA, Horsewood P, *et al.* Impact of the patient population on the risk for heparin-induced thrombocytopenia. *Blood* 2000; **96**: 1703–8.

44. Warkentin TE, Greinacher A, Koster A, Lincoff AM. Treatment and prevention of heparin-induced thrombocytopenia: American College of Chest Physicians Evidence-Based Clinical Practice Guidelines (8th Edition). *Chest* 2008; **133**: 340S–380S.

45. Bauer TL, Arepally G, Konkle BA, *et al.* Prevalence of heparin-associated antibodies without thrombosis in patients undergoing cardiopulmonary bypass surgery. *Circulation* 1997; **95**: 1242–6.

46. Pouplard C, May MA, Iochmann S, et al. Antibodies to platelet factor 4-heparin after cardiopulmonary bypass in patients anticoagulated with unfractionated heparin or a low-molecular-weight heparin: clinical implications for heparin-induced thrombocytopenia. *Circulation* 1999; **99**: 2530–6.

47. Singer RL, Mannion JD, Bauer TL, Armenti FR, Edie RN. Complications from heparin-induced thrombocytopenia in patients undergoing cardiopulmonary bypass. *Chest* 1993; **104**: 1436–40.

48. Lubenow N, Kempf R, Eichner A, et al. Heparin-induced thrombocytopenia: temporal pattern of thrombocytopenia in relation to initial use or reexposure to heparin. *Chest* 2002; **122**: 37–42.

49. Greinacher A, Warkentin TE. Recognition, treatment, and prevention of heparin-induced thrombocytopenia: review and update. *Thromb Res* 2006; **118**: 165–76.

50. Prechel M, Walenga JM. The laboratory diagnosis and clinical management of patients with heparin-induced thrombocytopenia: an update. *Semin Thromb Hemost* 2008; **34**: 86–96.

51. Ansell JE, Clark WP, Compton CC. Fatal reactions associated with intravenous heparin. *Drug Intell Clin Pharm* 1986; **20**: 74–5.

52. Ahmed I, Majeed A, Powell R. Heparin induced thrombocytopenia: diagnosis and management update. *Postgrad Med J* 2007; **83**: 575–82.

53. Levy JH, Tanaka KA, Hursting MJ. Reducing thrombotic complications in the perioperative setting: an update on heparin-induced thrombocytopenia. *Anesth Analg* 2007; **105**: 570–82.

54. Warkentin TE, Chong BH, Greinacher A. Heparin-induced thrombocytopenia: towards consensus. *Thromb Haemost* 1998; **79**: 1–7.

55. Warkentin TE, Sheppard JI, Moore JC, Sigouin CS, Kelton JG. Quantitative interpretation of optical density measurements using PF4-dependent enzyme-immunoassays. *J Thromb Haemost* 2008; **6**: 1304–12.

56. Warkentin TE, Sheppard JA. Testing for heparin-induced thrombocytopenia antibodies. *Transfus Med Rev* 2006; **20**: 259–72.

57. Warkentin TE, Sheppard JA, Moore JC, et al. Laboratory testing for the antibodies that cause heparin-induced thrombocytopenia: how much class do we need? *J Lab Clin Med* 2005; **146**: 341–6.

58. Gatt A, van Veen JJ, Woolley AM, et al. Thrombin generation assays are superior to traditional tests in assessing anticoagulation reversal in vitro. *Thromb Haemost* 2008; **100**: 350–5.

59. Desmurs-Clavel H, Huchon C, Chatard B, Negrier C, Dargaud Y. Reversal of the inhibitory effect of fondaparinux on thrombin generation by rFVIIa, aCCP and PCC. *Thromb Res* 2009; **5**: 796–8.

60. Kishimoto TK, Viswanathan K, Ganguly T, et al. Contaminated heparin associated with adverse clinical events and activation of the contact system. *N Engl J Med* 2008; **358**: 2457–67.

61. Zhang Z, Weiwer M, Li B, et al. Oversulfated chondroitin sulfate: impact of a heparin impurity, associated with adverse clinical events, on low-molecular-weight heparin preparation. *J Med Chem* 2008; **51**: 5498–501.

62. Ammar T, Fisher CF. The effects of heparinase 1 and protamine on platelet reactivity. *Anesthesiology* 1997; **86**: 1382–6.

63. DeLucia A, Wakefield TW, Kadell AM, et al. Tissue distribution, circulating half-life, and excretion of intravenously administered protamine sulfate. *Asaio J* 1993; **39**: M715–18.

64. Guffin AV, Dunbar RW, Kaplan JA, Bland JW. Successful use of a reduced dose of protamine after cardiopulmonary bypass. *Anesth Analg* 1976; **55**: 110–13.

65. Teoh KH, Young E, Blackall MH, Roberts RS, Hirsh J. Can extra protamine eliminate heparin rebound following cardiopulmonary bypass surgery? *J Thorac Cardiovasc Surg* 2004; **128**: 211–19.

66. Welsby IJ, Newman MF, Phillips-Bute B, et al. Hemodynamic changes after protamine administration: association with mortality after coronary artery bypass surgery. *Anesthesiology* 2005; **102**: 308–14.

67. Pretorius M, Scholl FG, McFarlane JA, Murphey LJ, Brown NJ. A pilot study indicating that bradykinin B2 receptor antagonism attenuates protamine-related hypotension after cardiopulmonary bypass. *Clin Pharmacol Ther* 2005; **78**: 477–85.

68. Takakura K, Mizogami M, Fukuda S. Protamine sulfate causes endothelium-independent vasorelaxation via inducible nitric oxide synthase pathway. *Can J Anaesth* 2006; **53**: 162–7.

69. Turpie AG, Gent M, Cote R, et al. A low-molecular-weight heparinoid compared with unfractionated heparin in the prevention of deep vein thrombosis in patients with acute ischemic stroke. A randomized, double-blind study. *Ann Intern Med* 1992; **117**: 353–7.

70. Hoek JA, Nurmohamed MT, Hamelynck KJ, et al. Prevention of deep vein thrombosis following total hip replacement by low molecular weight heparinoid. *Thromb Haemost* 1992; **67**: 28–32.

71. Leyvraz P, Bachmann F, Bohnet J, et al. Thromboembolic prophylaxis in total hip replacement: a comparison between the low molecular weight heparinoid Lomoparan and heparin-dihydroergotamine. *Br J Surg* 1992; **79**: 911–14.

72. Bergqvist D, Kettunen K, Fredin H, et al. Thromboprophylaxis in patients with hip fractures: a prospective, randomized, comparative study between Org 10172 and dextran 70. *Surgery* 1991; **109**: 617–22.

73. Gerhart TN, Yett HS, Robertson LK, et al. Low-molecular-weight heparinoid compared with warfarin for prophylaxis of deep-vein thrombosis in patients who are operated on for fracture of the hip: a prospective, randomized trial. *J Bone Joint Surg Am* 1991; **73**: 494–502.

74. Gallus A, Cade J, Ockelford P, et al. Orgaran (Org 10172) or heparin for preventing venous thrombosis after elective surgery for malignant disease? A double-blind, randomised, multicentre comparison. ANZ-Organon Investigators. *Group Thromb Haemost* 1993; **70**: 562–7.

75. Krauel K, Furll B, Warkentin TE, et al. Heparin-induced thrombocytopenia – therapeutic concentrations of

danaparoid, unlike fondaparinux and direct thrombin inhibitors, inhibit formation of PF4/heparin complexes. *J Thromb Haemost* 2008; **6**: 2160–7.

76. Fareed J, Hoppensteadt DA, Fareed D, *et al.* Survival of heparins, oral anticoagulants, and aspirin after the year 2010. *Semin Thromb Hemost* 2008; **34**: 58–73.

77. Choay J, Lormeau JC, Petitou M, Sinay P, Fareed J. Structural studies on a biologically active hexasaccharide obtained from heparin. *Ann N Y Acad Sci* 1981; **370**: 644–9.

78. Boneu B, Necciari J, Cariou R, *et al.* Pharmacokinetics and tolerance of the natural pentasaccharide (SR90107/ Org31540) with high affinity to antithrombin III in man. *Thromb Haemost* 1995; **74**: 1468–73.

79. Bauersachs RM. Fondaparinux: an update on new study results. *Eur J Clin Invest* 2005; **35**: 27–32.

80. Coons JC, Battistone S. 2007 Guideline update for unstable angina/non-ST-segment elevation myocardial infarction: focus on antiplatelet and anticoagulant therapies. *Ann Pharmacother* 2008; **42**: 989–1001.

81. Kuo KH, Kovacs MJ. Fondaparinux: a potential new therapy for HIT. *Hematology* 2005; **10**: 271–5.

82. Lieu C, Shi J, Donat F, *et al.* Fondaparinux sodium is not metabolised in mammalian liver fractions and does not inhibit cytochrome P450-mediated metabolism of concomitant drugs. *Clin Pharmacokinet* 2002; **41**: 19–26.

83. Paolucci F, Clavies MC, Donat F, Necciari J. Fondaparinux sodium mechanism of action: identification of specific binding to purified and human plasma-derived proteins. *Clin Pharmacokinet* 2002; **41**: 11–18.

84. Bijsterveld NR, Moons AH, Boekholdt SM, *et al.* Ability of recombinant factor VIIa to reverse the anticoagulant effect of the pentasaccharide fondaparinux in healthy volunteers. *Circulation* 2002; **106**: 2550–4.

85. Piccini JP, Patel MR, Mahaffey KW, Fox KA, Califf RM. Rivaroxaban, an oral direct factor Xa inhibitor. *Expert Opin Investig Drugs* 2008; **17**: 925–37.

86. Walenga JM, Prechel M, Jeske WP, *et al.* Rivaroxaban--an oral, direct Factor Xa inhibitor--has potential for the management of patients with heparin-induced thrombocytopenia. *Br J Haematol* 2008; **143**: 92–9.

87. Eriksson BI, Borris LC, Friedman RJ, *et al.* Rivaroxaban versus enoxaparin for thromboprophylaxis after hip arthroplasty. *N Engl J Med* 2008; **358**: 2765–75.

88. Fitzgerald D, Murphy N. Argatroban: a synthetic thrombin inhibitor of low relative molecular mass. *Coron Artery Dis* 1996; **7**: 455–8.

89. Matthai WH. Use of argatroban during percutaneous coronary interventions in patients with heparin-induced thrombocytopenia. *Semin Thromb Hemost* 1999; **25**: 57–60.

90. Walenga JM, Ahmad S, Hoppensteadt D, *et al.* Argatroban therapy does not generate antibodies that alter its anticoagulant activity in patients with heparin-induced thrombocytopenia. *Thromb Res* 2002; **105**: 401–5.

91. Swan SK, Hursting MJ. The pharmacokinetics and pharmacodynamics of argatroban: effects of age, gender, and hepatic or renal dysfunction. *Pharmacotherapy* 2000; **20**: 318–29.

92. Ueki Y, Matsumoto K, Kizaki Y, *et al.* Argatroban increases nitric oxide levels in patients with peripheral arterial obstructive disease: placebo-controlled study. *J Thromb Thrombolysis* 1999; **8**: 131–7.

93. Berry CN, Girard D, Girardot C, *et al.* Antithrombotic activity of argatroban in experimental thrombosis in the rabbit. *Semin Thromb Hemost* 1996; **22**: 233–41.

94. Sakai M, Ohteki H, Narita Y, *et al.* Argatroban as a potential anticoagulant in cardiopulmonary bypass-studies in a dog model. *Cardiovasc Surg* 1999; **7**: 187–94.

95. Swan SK, St Peter JV, Lambrecht LJ, Hursting MJ. Comparison of anticoagulant effects and safety of argatroban and heparin in healthy subjects. *Pharmacotherapy* 2000; **20**: 756–70.

96. Ahmad S, Ahsan A, George M, *et al.* Simultaneous monitoring of argatroban and its major metabolite using an HPLC method: potential clinical applications. *Clin Appl Thromb Hemost* 1999; **5**: 252–8.

97. Lewis BE, Wallis DE, Berkowitz SD, *et al.* Argatroban anticoagulant therapy in patients with heparin-induced thrombocytopenia. *Circulation* 2001; **103**: 1838–43.

98. Lewis BE, Wallis DE, Leya F, Hursting MJ, Kelton JG. Argatroban anticoagulation in patients with heparin-induced thrombocytopenia. *Arch Intern Med* 2003; **163**: 1849–56.

99. Kawada T, Kitagawa H, Hoson M, Okada Y, Shiomura J. Clinical application of argatroban as an alternative anticoagulant for extracorporeal circulation. *Hematol Oncol Clin North Am* 2000; **14**: 445–57.

100. Shen GX. Inhibition of thrombin: relevance to anti-thrombosis strategy. *Front Biosci* 2006; **11**: 113–20.

101. Arpino PA, Demirjian Z, Van Cott EM. Use of the chromogenic factor X assay to predict the international normalized ratio in patients transitioning from argatroban to warfarin. *Pharmacotherapy* 2005; **25**: 157–64.

102. Hursting MJ, Lewis BE, Macfarlane DE. Transitioning from argatroban to warfarin therapy in patients with heparin-induced thrombocytopenia. *Clin Appl Thromb Hemost* 2005; **11**: 279–87.

103. Stangier J. Clinical pharmacokinetics and pharmacodynamics of the oral direct thrombin inhibitor dabigatran etexilate. *Clin Pharmacokinet* 2008; **47**: 285–95.

104. Blech S, Ebner T, Ludwig-Schwellinger E, Stangier J, Roth W. The metabolism and disposition of the oral direct thrombin inhibitor, dabigatran, in humans. *Drug Metab Dispos* 2008; **36**: 386–99.

105. Wienen W, Stassen JM, Priepke H, Ries UJ, Hauel N. In-vitro profile and ex-vivo anticoagulant activity of the direct thrombin inhibitor dabigatran and its orally active prodrug, dabigatran etexilate. *Thromb Haemost* 2007; **98**: 155–62.

106. Stangier J, Rathgen K, Stahle H, Gansser D, Roth W. The pharmacokinetics, pharmacodynamics and tolerability of

dabigatran etexilate, a new oral direct thrombin inhibitor, in healthy male subjects. *Br J Clin Pharmacol* 2007; **64**: 292–303.

107. Stangier J, Stahle H, Rathgen K, Roth W, Shakeri-Nejad K. Pharmacokinetics and pharmacodynamics of dabigatran etexilate, an oral direct thrombin inhibitor, are not affected by moderate hepatic impairment. *J Clin Pharmacol* 2008; **48**: 1411–19.

108. Baetz BE, Spinler SA. Dabigatran etexilate: an oral direct thrombin inhibitor for prophylaxis and treatment of thromboembolic diseases. *Pharmacotherapy* 2008; **28**: 1354–73.

109. Stangier J, Eriksson BI, Dahl OE, *et al.* Pharmacokinetic profile of the oral direct thrombin inhibitor dabigatran etexilate in healthy volunteers and patients undergoing total hip replacement. *J Clin Pharmacol* 2005; **45**: 555–63.

110. Sanford M, Plosker GL. Dabigatran etexilate. *Drugs* 2008; **68**: 1699–709.

111. Stangier J, Stahle H, Rathgen K, Fuhr R. Pharmacokinetics and pharmacodynamics of the direct oral thrombin inhibitor dabigatran in healthy elderly subjects. *Clin Pharmacokinet* 2008; **47**: 47–59.

112. Eriksson BI, Dahl OE, Rosencher N, *et al.* Oral dabigatran etexilate vs. subcutaneous enoxaparin for the prevention of venous thromboembolism after total knee replacement: the RE-MODEL randomized trial. *J Thromb Haemost* 2007; **5**: 2178–85.

113. Eriksson BI, Dahl OE, Rosencher N, *et al.* Dabigatran etexilate versus enoxaparin for prevention of venous thromboembolism after total hip replacement: a randomised, double-blind, non-inferiority trial. *Lancet* 2007; **370**: 949–56.

114. Eriksson BI, Dahl OE, Buller HR, *et al.* A new oral direct thrombin inhibitor, dabigatran etexilate, compared with enoxaparin for prevention of thromboembolic events following total hip or knee replacement: the BISTRO II randomized trial. *J Thromb Haemost* 2005; **3**: 103–11.

115. Hoppensteadt DA, Jeske W, Walenga J, Fareed J. The future of anticoagulation.

Semin Respir Crit Care Med 2008; **29**: 90–9.

116. Nutescu EA, Shapiro NL, Chevalier A. New anticoagulant agents: direct thrombin inhibitors. *Cardiol Clin* 2008; **26**: 169–87.

117. Fuchs J, Cannon CP. Hirulog in the treatment of unstable angina. Results of the Thrombin Inhibition in Myocardial Ischemia (TIMI) 7 trial. *Circulation* 1995; **92**: 727–33.

118. Greinacher A, Volpel H, Janssens U, *et al.* Recombinant hirudin (lepirudin) provides safe and effective anticoagulation in patients with heparin-induced thrombocytopenia: a prospective study. *Circulation* 1999; **99**: 73–80.

119. Deitcher SR. Clinical utility of subcutaneous hirudins. *Am J Health Syst Pharm* 2003; **60**: S27–31.

120. Turunen P, Mikkola T, Ylikorkala O, Viinikka L. Hirudin stimulates prostacyclin but not endothelin-1 production in cultured human vascular endothelial cells. *Thromb Res* 1996; **81**: 635–40.

121. Robson R. The use of bivalirudin in patients with renal impairment. *J Invasive Cardiol* 2000; **12**: 33F–36F.

122. Robson R, White H, Aylward P, Frampton C. Bivalirudin pharmacokinetics and pharmacodynamics: effect of renal function, dose, and gender. *Clin Pharmacol Ther* 2002; **71**: 433–9.

123. Shammas NW. Bivalirudin: pharmacology and clinical applications. *Cardiovasc Drug Rev* 2005; **23**: 345–60.

124. Chew DP, Lincoff AM, Gurm H, *et al.* Bivalirudin versus heparin and glycoprotein IIb/IIIa inhibition among patients with renal impairment undergoing percutaneous coronary intervention (a subanalysis of the REPLACE-2 trial). *Am J Cardiol* 2005; **95**: 581–5.

125. Riess FC, Poetzsch B, Madlener K, *et al.* Recombinant hirudin for cardiopulmonary bypass anticoagulation: a randomized, prospective, and heparin-controlled pilot study. *Thorac Cardiovasc Surg* 2007; **55**: 233–8.

126. Dyke CM, Smedira NG, Koster A, *et al.* A comparison of bivalirudin to heparin

with protamine reversal in patients undergoing cardiac surgery with cardiopulmonary bypass: the EVOLUTION-ON study. *J Thorac Cardiovasc Surg* 2006; **131**: 533–9.

127. Smedira NG, Dyke CM, Koster A, *et al.* Anticoagulation with bivalirudin for off-pump coronary artery bypass grafting: the results of the EVOLUTION-OFF study. *J Thorac Cardiovasc Surg* 2006; **131**: 686–92.

128. Koster A, Dyke CM, Aldea G, *et al.* Bivalirudin during cardiopulmonary bypass in patients with previous or acute heparin-induced thrombocytopenia and heparin antibodies: results of the CHOOSE-ON trial. *Ann Thorac Surg* 2007; **83**: 572–7.

129. Palmer GJ, Sankaran IS, Sparkman GM, *et al.* Routine use of the direct thrombin inhibitor bivalirudin for off-pump coronary artery bypass grafting is safe and effective. *Heart Surg Forum* 2008; **11**: E24–9.

130. A comparison of recombinant hirudin with heparin for the treatment of acute coronary syndromes. The Global Use of Strategies to Open Occluded Coronary Arteries (GUSTO) IIb investigators. *N Engl J Med* 1996; **335**: 775–82.

131. Metz BK, White HD, Granger CB, *et al.* Randomized comparison of direct thrombin inhibition versus heparin in conjunction with fibrinolytic therapy for acute myocardial infarction: results from the GUSTO-IIb Trial. Global Use of Strategies to Open Occluded Coronary Arteries in Acute Coronary Syndromes (GUSTO-IIb) Investigators. *J Am Coll Cardiol* 1998; **31**: 1493–8.

132. White HD, Aylward PE, Frey MJ, *et al.* Randomized, double-blind comparison of hirulog versus heparin in patients receiving streptokinase and aspirin for acute myocardial infarction (HERO). Hirulog Early Reperfusion/Occlusion (HERO) Trial Investigators. *Circulation* 1997; **96**: 2155–61.

133. Mazoyer E, Drouet L, Delahousse B, Gruel Y, Rouyrre N. Activated partial thromboplastin time is more sensitive than ecarin clotting time for monitoring low doses of desirudin. *Thromb Res* 2002; **106**: 271–2.

134. Despotis GJ, Hogue CW, Saleem R, *et al.* The relationship between hirudin and activated clotting time: implications

for patients with heparin-induced thrombocytopenia undergoing cardiac surgery. *Anesth Analg* 2001; **93**: 28–32.

135. Greinacher A, Eichler P, Albrecht D, *et al.* Antihirudin antibodies following low-dose subcutaneous treatment with desirudin for thrombosis prophylaxis after hip-replacement surgery: incidence and clinical relevance. *Blood* 2003; **101**: 2617–19.

136. Sorajja P, Cable DG, Hamner CE, Schaff HV. Hirudin (desulfated, 54–65) contracts canine coronary arteries: extracellular calcium influx mediates hirudin-induced contractions. *J Surg Res* 2004; **121**: 38–41.

137. Lepor NE. Anticoagulation for acute coronary syndromes: from heparin to direct thrombin inhibitors. *Rev Cardiovasc Med* 2007; **8**: S9–S17.

138. Link KP. The discovery of dicumarol and its sequels. *Circulation* 1959; **19**: 97–107.

139. O'Reilly RA. Vitamin K and the oral anticoagulant drugs. *Annu Rev Med* 1976; **27**: 245–61.

140. Yin T, Miyata T. Warfarin dose and the pharmacogenomics of CYP2C9 and VKORC1 – rationale and perspectives. *Thromb Res* 2007; **120**: 1–10.

141. Nelsestuen GL. Role of gamma-carboxyglutamic acid. An unusual protein transition required for the calcium-dependent binding of prothrombin to phospholipid. *J Biol Chem* 1976; **251**: 5648–56.

142. Borowski M, Furie BC, Bauminger S, Furie B. Prothrombin requires two sequential metal-dependent conformational transitions to bind phospholipid. Conformation-specific antibodies directed against the phospholipid-binding site on prothrombin. *J Biol Chem* 1986; **261**: 14969–75.

143. Breckenridge A, Orme M, Wesseling H, Lewis RJ, Gibbons R. Pharmacokinetics and pharmacodynamics of the enantiomers of warfarin in man. *Clin Pharmacol Ther* 1974; **15**: 424–30.

144. Ansell J, Hirsh J, Hylek E, *et al.* Pharmacology and management of the vitamin K antagonists: American College of Chest Physicians Evidence-Based Clinical Practice Guidelines, 8th edn. *Chest* 2008; **133**:160S–198S.

145. Zimmermann A, Matschiner JT. Biochemical basis of hereditary resistance to warfarin in the rat. *Biochem Pharmacol* 1974; **23**: 1033–40.

146. Li T, Chang CY, Jin DY, *et al.* Identification of the gene for vitamin K epoxide reductase. *Nature* 2004; **427**: 541–4.

147. Kelly JG, O'Malley K. Clinical pharmacokinetics of oral anticoagulants. *Clin Pharmacokinet* 1979; **4**: 1–15.

148. Suttie JW, Mummah-Schendel LL, Shah DV, Lyle BJ, Greger JL. Vitamin K deficiency from dietary vitamin K restriction in humans. *Am J Clin Nutr* 1988; **47**: 475–80.

149. Taberner DA, Poller L, Thomson JM, Darby KV. Effect of international sensitivity index (ISI) of thromboplastins on precision of international normalised ratios (INR). *J Clin Pathol* 1989; **42**: 92–6.

150. ACCP-NHLBI National Conference on Antithrombotic Therapy. American College of Chest Physicians and the National Heart, Lung and Blood Institute. *Chest* 1986; **89**: 1S–106S.

151. Hull R, Hirsh J, Jay R, *et al.* Different intensities of oral anticoagulant therapy in the treatment of proximal-vein thrombosis. *N Engl J Med* 1982; **307**: 1676–81.

152. Saour JN, Sieck JO, Mamo LA, Gallus AS. Trial of different intensities of anticoagulation in patients with prosthetic heart valves. *N Engl J Med* 1990; **322**: 428–32.

153. Friedman EW, Sussman, II. Safety of invasive procedures in patients with the coagulopathy of liver disease. *Clin Lab Haematol* 1989; **11**: 199–204.

154. Foster PF, Moore LR, Sankary HN, *et al.* Central venous catheterization in patients with coagulopathy. *Arch Surg* 1992; **127**: 273–5.

155. Tollefson DF, Friedman KD, Marlar RA, Bandyk DF, Towne JB. Protein C deficiency. A cause of unusual or unexplained thrombosis. *Arch Surg.*1988; **123**: 881–4.

156. Grimaudo V, Gueissaz F, Hauert J, *et al.* Necrosis of skin induced by coumarin in a patient deficient in protein S. *BMJ*1989; **298**: 233–4.

157. Ng T, Tillyer ML. Warfarin-induced skin necrosis associated with Factor V Leiden and protein S deficiency. *Clin Lab Haematol* 2001; **23**: 261–4.

158. Limdi NA, Veenstra DL. Warfarin pharmacogenetics. *Pharmacotherapy* 2008; **28**: 1084–97.

159. Gage BF, Lesko LJ. Pharmacogenetics of warfarin: regulatory, scientific, and clinical issues. *J Thromb Thrombolysis* 2008; **25**: 45–51.

160. Takahashi H, Echizen H. Pharmacogenetics of warfarin elimination and its clinical implications. *Clin Pharmacokinet* 2001; **40**: 587–603.

161. Herman D, Peternel P, Stegnar M, Breskvar K, Dolzan V. The influence of sequence variations in factor VII, gamma-glutamyl carboxylase and vitamin K epoxide reductase complex genes on warfarin dose requirement. *Thromb Haemost* 2006; **95**: 782–7.

162. Mannucci PM. Genetic control of anticoagulation. *Lancet* 1999; **353**: 688–9.

163. Loll PJ, Picot D, Garavito RM. The structural basis of aspirin activity inferred from the crystal structure of inactivated prostaglandin H2 synthase. *Nat Struct Biol* 1995; **2**: 637–43.

164. Roth GJ, Majerus PW. The mechanism of the effect of aspirin on human platelets. I. Acetylation of a particulate fraction protein. *J Clin Invest* 1975; **56**: 624–32.

165. Pedersen AK, FitzGerald GA. Dose-related kinetics of aspirin. Presystemic acetylation of platelet cyclooxygenase. *N Engl J Med* 1984; **311**: 1206–11.

166. Cox D, Maree AO, Dooley M, *et al.* Effect of enteric coating on antiplatelet activity of low-dose aspirin in healthy volunteers. *Stroke* 2006; **37**: 2153–8.

167. Higgs GA, Salmon JA, Henderson B, Vane JR. Pharmacokinetics of aspirin and salicylate in relation to inhibition of arachidonate cyclooxygenase and antiinflammatory activity. *Proc Natl Acad Sci U S A* 1987; **84**: 1417–20.

168. Pedersen AK, FitzGerald GA. The human pharmacology of platelet inhibition: pharmacokinetics relevant to drug action. *Circulation* 1985; **72**: 1164–76.

169. Randomised trial of intravenous streptokinase, oral aspirin, both, or neither among 17,187 cases of suspected acute myocardial infarction: ISIS-2. ISIS-2 (Second International Study of Infarct Survival) Collaborative Group. *Lancet* 1988; **2**: 349–60.

170. Collaborative meta-analysis of randomised trials of antiplatelet therapy for prevention of death, myocardial infarction, and stroke in high risk patients. Antithrombotic Trialists' Collaboration. *BMJ* 2002; **324**: 71–86.

171. Final report on the aspirin component of the ongoing Physicians' Health Study. Steering Committee of the Physicians' Health Study Research Group. *N Engl J Med* 1989; **321**: 129–35.

172. Salem DN, O'Gara PT, Madias C, Pauker SG. Valvular and structural heart disease: American College of Chest Physicians Evidence-Based Clinical Practice Guidelines, 8th edn. *Chest* 2008; **133**: 593S–629S.

173. Prevention of pulmonary embolism and deep vein thrombosis with low dose aspirin: Pulmonary Embolism Prevention (PEP) trial. *Lancet* 2000; **355**: 1295–302.

174. Michelson AD, Barnard MR, Khuri SF, *et al.* The effects of aspirin and hypothermia on platelet function in vivo. *Br J Haematol* 1999; **104**: 64–8.

175. Pogliani EM, Fowst C, Bregani R, Corneo G. Bleeding time and antiplatelet agents in normal volunteers. *Int J Clin Lab Res* 1992; **22**: 58–61.

176. Sathiropas P, Marbet GA, Sahaphong S, Duckert F. Detection of small inhibitory effects of acetylsalicylic acid (ASA) by platelet impedance aggregometry in whole blood. *Thromb Res* 1988; **51**: 55–62.

177. Gum PA, Kottke-Marchant K, Poggio ED, *et al.* Profile and prevalence of aspirin resistance in patients with cardiovascular disease. *Am J Cardiol* 2001; **88**: 230–5.

178. Homoncik M, Jilma B, Hergovich N, *et al.* Monitoring of aspirin (ASA) pharmacodynamics with the platelet function analyzer PFA-100. *Thromb Haemost* 2000; **83**: 316–21.

179. Orlikowski CE, Payne AJ, Moodley J, Rocke DA. Thrombelastography after aspirin ingestion in pregnant and non-

pregnant subjects. *Br J Anaesth* 1992; **69**: 159–61.

180. Biondi-Zoccai GG, Lotrionte M, Agostoni P, *et al.* A systematic review and meta-analysis on the hazards of discontinuing or not adhering to aspirin among 50,279 patients at risk for coronary artery disease. *Eur Heart J* 2006; **27**: 2667–74.

181. Collet JP, Montalescot G, Blanchet B, *et al.* Impact of prior use or recent withdrawal of oral antiplatelet agents on acute coronary syndromes. *Circulation* 2004; **110**: 2361–7.

182. Ferrari E, Benhamou M, Cerboni P, Marcel B. Coronary syndromes following aspirin withdrawal: a special risk for late stent thrombosis. *J Am Coll Cardiol* 2005; **45**: 456–9.

183. Chassot PG, Delabays A, Spahn DR. Perioperative antiplatelet therapy: the case for continuing therapy in patients at risk of myocardial infarction. *Br J Anaesth* 2007; **99**: 316–28.

184. Mangano DT. Aspirin and mortality from coronary bypass surgery. *N Engl J Med* 2002; **347**: 1309–17.

185. Horlocker TT, Wedel DJ, Schroeder DR, *et al.* Preoperative antiplatelet therapy does not increase the risk of spinal hematoma associated with regional anesthesia. *Anesth Analg* 1995; **80**: 303–9.

186. Wulf H. Epidural anaesthesia and spinal haematoma. *Can J Anaesth* 1996; **43**: 1260–71.

187. Lanas AI. Current approaches to reducing gastrointestinal toxicity of low-dose aspirin. *Am J Med* 2001; **110**: 70S–73S.

188. Kelly JP, Kaufman DW, Jurgelon JM, *et al.* Risk of aspirin-associated major upper-gastrointestinal bleeding with enteric-coated or buffered product. *Lancet* 1996; **348**:1413–16.

189. Mene P, Pugliese F, Patrono C. The effects of nonsteroidal anti-inflammatory drugs on human hypertensive vascular disease. *Semin Nephrol* 1995; **15**: 244–52.

190. Babu KS, Salvi SS. Aspirin and asthma. *Chest* 2000; **118**: 1470–6.

191. Heubi JE, Partin JC, Partin JS, Schubert WK. Reye's syndrome: current concepts. *Hepatology* 1987; **7**: 155–64.

192. Barone JA, Raia JJ, Huang YC. Evaluation of the effects of multiple-dose activated charcoal on the absorption of orally administered salicylate in a simulated toxic ingestion model. *Ann Emerg Med* 1988; **17**: 34–7.

193. Higgins RM, Connolly JO, Hendry BM. Alkalinization and hemodialysis in severe salicylate poisoning: comparison of elimination techniques in the same patient. *Clin Nephrol* 1998; **50**: 178–83.

194. Patrono C, Baigent C, Hirsh J, Roth G. Antiplatelet drugs: American College of Chest Physicians Evidence-Based Clinical Practice Guidelines 8th edn. *Chest* 2008; **133**: 199S–233S.

195. FitzGerald GA. Dipyridamole. *N Engl J Med* 1987; **316**: 1247–57.

196. Weyrich AS, Denis MM, Kuhlmann-Eyre JR, *et al.* Dipyridamole selectively inhibits inflammatory gene expression in platelet-monocyte aggregates. *Circulation* 2005; **111**: 633–42.

197. Diener HC, Cunha L, Forbes C, *et al.* European Stroke Prevention Study. 2. Dipyridamole and acetylsalicylic acid in the secondary prevention of stroke. *J Neurol Sci* 1996; **143**: 1–13.

198. De Schryver EL, Algra A, van Gijn J. Dipyridamole for preventing stroke and other vascular events in patients with vascular disease. *Cochrane Database Syst Rev* 2006; (2): CD001820.

199. Younis LT, Chaitman BR. Update on intravenous dipyridamole cardiac imaging in the assessment of ischemic heart disease. *Clin Cardiol* 1990; **13**: 3–10.

200. Gryglewski RJ. Interactions between endothelial secretogues. *Ann Med* 1995; **27**: 421–7.

201. Saniabadi AR, Belch JJ, Lowe GD, Barbenel JC, Forbes CD. Comparison of inhibitory actions of prostacyclin and a new prostacyclin analogue on the aggregation of human platelet in whole blood. *Haemostasis* 1987; **17**: 147–53.

202. Defreyn G, Bernat A, Delebassee D, Maffrand JP. Pharmacology of ticlopidine: a review. *Semin Thromb Hemost* 1989; **15**: 159–66.

203. Defreyn G, Gachet C, Savi P, *et al.* Ticlopidine and clopidogrel (SR 25990C) selectively neutralize ADP inhibition of PGE1-activated platelet

adenylate cyclase in rats and rabbits. *Thromb Haemost* 1991; **65**: 186–90.

204. Gachet C, Cazenave JP, Ohlmann P, *et al.* The thienopyridine ticlopidine selectively prevents the inhibitory effects of ADP but not of adrenaline on cAMP levels raised by stimulation of the adenylate cyclase of human platelets by PGE1. *Biochem Pharmacol* 1990; **40**: 2683–7.

205. Lau WC, Gurbel PA, Watkins PB, *et al.* Contribution of hepatic cytochrome P450 3A4 metabolic activity to the phenomenon of clopidogrel resistance. *Circulation* 2004; **109**: 166–71.

206. **A randomised**, blinded, trial of clopidogrel versus aspirin in patients at risk of ischaemic events (CAPRIE). CAPRIE Steering Committee. *Lancet* 1996; **348**: 1329–39.

207. Chen ZM, Jiang LX, Chen YP, *et al.* Addition of clopidogrel to aspirin in 45,852 patients with acute myocardial infarction: randomised placebo-controlled trial. *Lancet* 2005; **366**: 1607–21.

208. Steinhubl SR, Berger PB, Mann JT, *et al.* Early and sustained dual oral antiplatelet therapy following percutaneous coronary intervention: a randomized controlled trial. *JAMA* 2002; **288**: 2411–20.

209. Grines CL, Bonow RO, Casey DE, *et al.* Prevention of premature discontinuation of dual antiplatelet therapy in patients with coronary artery stents: a science advisory from the American Heart Association, American College of Cardiology, Society for Cardiovascular Angiography and Interventions, American College of Surgeons, and American Dental Association, with representation from the American College of Physicians. *Circulation* 2007; **115**: 813–18.

210. Iakovou I, Schmidt T, Bonizzoni E, *et al.* Incidence, predictors, and outcome of thrombosis after successful implantation of drug-eluting stents. *JAMA* 2005; **293**: 2126–30.

211. Riddell JW, Chiche L, Plaud B, Hamon M. Coronary stents and noncardiac surgery. *Circulation* 2007; **116**: e378–82.

212. Vilahur G, Choi BG, Zafar MU, *et al.* Normalization of platelet reactivity in clopidogrel-treated subjects. *J Thromb Haemost* 2007; **5**: 82–90.

213. Berger JS, Frye CB, Harshaw Q, *et al.* Impact of clopidogrel in patients with acute coronary syndromes requiring coronary artery bypass surgery: a multicenter analysis. *J Am Coll Cardiol* 2008; **52**: 1693–701.

214. King SB, Smith SC, Hirshfeld JW, *et al.* 2007 Focused Update of the ACC/AHA/SCAI 2005 Guideline Update for Percutaneous Coronary Intervention: a report of the American College of Cardiology/American Heart Association Task Force on Practice Guidelines. *Circulation* 2008; **117**: 261–95.

215. Staritz P, Kurz K, Stoll M, *et al.* Platelet reactivity and clopidogrel resistance are associated with the H2 haplotype of the P2Y(12)-ADP receptor gene. *Int J Cardiol* 2008; **133**: 341–5.

216. Giusti B, Gori AM, Marcucci R, *et al.* Cytochrome P450 2C19 loss-of-function polymorphism, but not CYP3A4 IVS10 + 12G/A and P2Y12 T744C polymorphisms, is associated with response variability to dual antiplatelet treatment in high-risk vascular patients. *Pharmacogenet Genomics* 2007; **17**: 1057–64.

217. Lau WC, Waskell LA, Watkins PB, *et al.* Atorvastatin reduces the ability of clopidogrel to inhibit platelet aggregation: a new drug-drug interaction. *Circulation* 2003; **107**: 32–7.

218. Wiviott SD, Trenk D, Frelinger AL, *et al.* Prasugrel compared with high loading- and maintenance-dose clopidogrel in patients with planned percutaneous coronary intervention: the Prasugrel in Comparison to Clopidogrel for Inhibition of Platelet Activation and Aggregation-Thrombolysis in Myocardial Infarction 44 trial. *Circulation* 2007; **116**: 2923–32.

219. Topol EJ, Califf RM, Weisman HF, *et al.* Randomised trial of coronary intervention with antibody against platelet IIb/IIIa integrin for reduction of clinical restenosis: results at six months. The EPIC Investigators. *Lancet* 1994; **343**: 881–6.

220. Lages B, Weiss HJ. Greater inhibition of platelet procoagulant activity by antibody-derived glycoprotein IIb--IIIa inhibitors than by peptide and peptidomimetic inhibitors. *Br J Haematol* 2001; **113**: 65–71.

221. Ellis SG, Bates ER, Schaible T, *et al.* Prospects for the use of antagonists to the platelet glycoprotein IIb/IIIa receptor to prevent post-angioplasty restenosis and thrombosis. *J Am Coll Cardiol* 1991; **17**: 89B–95B.

222. Topol EJ, Lincoff AM, Kereiakes DJ, *et al.* Multi-year follow-up of abciximab therapy in three randomized, placebo-controlled trials of percutaneous coronary revascularization. *Am J Med* 2002; **113**: 1–6.

223. Kastrati A, Mehilli J, Schuhlen H, *et al.* A clinical trial of abciximab in elective percutaneous coronary intervention after pretreatment with clopidogrel. *N Engl J Med* 2004; **350**: 232–8.

224. Mehilli J, Kastrati A, Schuhlen H, *et al.* Randomized clinical trial of abciximab in diabetic patients undergoing elective percutaneous coronary interventions after treatment with a high loading dose of clopidogrel. *Circulation* 2004; **110**: 3627–35.

225. Anderson JL, Adams CD, Antman EM, *et al.* ACC/AHA 2007 guidelines for the management of patients with unstable angina/non-ST-Elevation myocardial infarction: a report of the American College of Cardiology/American Heart Association Task Force on Practice Guidelines (Writing Committee to Revise the 2002 Guidelines for the Management of Patients With Unstable Angina/Non-ST-Elevation Myocardial Infarction) developed in collaboration with the American College of Emergency Physicians, the Society for Cardiovascular Angiography and Interventions, and the Society of Thoracic Surgeons endorsed by the American Association of Cardiovascular and Pulmonary Rehabilitation and the Society for Academic Emergency Medicine. *J Am Coll Cardiol* 2007; **50**: e1–157.

226. Smith SC, Feldman TE, Hirshfeld JW, *et al.* ACC/AHA/SCAI 2005 guideline update for percutaneous coronary intervention: a report of the American College of Cardiology/American Heart Association Task Force on Practice Guidelines (ACC/AHA/SCAI Writing Committee to Update 2001 Guidelines for Percutaneous Coronary Intervention). *Circulation* 2006; **113**: e166–286.

227. Jong P, Cohen EA, Batchelor W, *et al.* Bleeding risks with abciximab after full-dose thrombolysis in rescue or urgent angioplasty for acute myocardial infarction. *Am Heart J* 2001; **141**: 218–25.

228. Dillon WC, Eckert GJ, Dillon JC, Ritchie ME. Incidence of thrombocytopenia following coronary stent placement using abciximab plus clopidogrel or ticlopidine. *Catheter Cardiovasc Interv* 2000; **50**: 426–30.

229. Nguyen N, Salib H, Mascarenhas DA. Acute profound thrombocytopenia without bleeding complications after re-administration of abciximab. *J Invasive Cardiol* 2001; **13**: 56–8.

230. Steinhubl SR, Talley JD, Braden GA, *et al.* Point-of-care measured platelet inhibition correlates with a reduced risk of an adverse cardiac event after percutaneous coronary intervention: results of the GOLD (AU-Assessing Ultegra) multicenter study. *Circulation* 2001; **103**: 2572–8.

231. Gammie JS, Zenati M, Kormos RL, *et al.* Abciximab and excessive bleeding in patients undergoing emergency cardiac operations. *Ann Thorac Surg* 1998; **65**: 465–9.

232. Lincoff AM, LeNarz LA, Despotis GJ, *et al.* Abciximab and bleeding during coronary surgery: results from the EPILOG and EPISTENT trials. Improve long-term outcome with abciximab GP IIb/IIIa blockade. Evaluation of platelet IIb/IIIa inhibition in STENTing. *Ann Thorac Surg* 2000; **70**: 516–26.

233. Silvestry SC, Smith PK. Current status of cardiac surgery in the abciximab-treated patient. *Ann Thorac Surg* 2000; **70**: S12–19.

234. Koster A, Kukucka M, Bach F, *et al.* Anticoagulation during cardiopulmonary bypass in patients with heparin-induced thrombocytopenia type II and renal impairment using heparin and the platelet glycoprotein IIb-IIIa antagonist tirofiban. *Anesthesiology* 2001; **94**: 245–51.

235. Goodman SG, Menon V, Cannon CP, *et al.* Acute ST-segment elevation myocardial infarction: American College of Chest Physicians Evidence-Based Clinical Practice Guidelines, 8th edn. *Chest* 2008; **133**: 708S–775S.

236. Tsikouris JP, Tsikouris AP. A review of available fibrin-specific thrombolytic agents used in acute myocardial infarction. *Pharmacotherapy* 2001; **21**: 207–17.

237. Nordt TK, Bode C. Thrombolysis: newer thrombolytic agents and their role in clinical medicine. *Heart* 2003; **89**: 1358–62.

238. Tanswell P, Modi N, Combs D, Danays T. Pharmacokinetics and pharmacodynamics of tenecteplase in fibrinolytic therapy of acute myocardial infarction. *Clin Pharmacokinet* 2002; **41**: 1229–45.

239. Baruah DB, Dash RN, Chaudhari MR, Kadam SS. Plasminogen activators: a comparison. *Vascul Pharmacol* 2006; **44**: 1–9.

240. Albers GW, Amarenco P, Easton JD, Sacco RL, Teal P. Antithrombotic and thrombolytic therapy for ischemic stroke: American College of Chest Physicians Evidence-Based Clinical Practice Guidelines, 8th edn. *Chest* 2008; **133**: 630S–669S.

241. Mannuccio PM, Altieri D, Faioni E. Vasopressin analogues. Their role in disorders of hemostasis. *Ann N Y Acad Sci* 1987; **509**: 71–81.

242. Despotis GJ, Levine V, Saleem R, Spitznagel E, Joist JH. Use of point-of-care test in identification of patients who can benefit from desmopressin during cardiac surgery: a randomised controlled trial. *Lancet* 1999; **354**: 106–10.

243. Czer LS, Bateman TM, Gray RJ, *et al.* Treatment of severe platelet dysfunction and hemorrhage after cardiopulmonary bypass: reduction in blood product usage with desmopressin. *J Am Coll Cardiol* 1987; **9**: 1139–47.

244. Cattaneo M, Mannucci PM. Desmopressin and blood loss after cardiac surgery. *Lancet* 1993; **342**: 812.

245. Horstman LL, Valle-Riestra BJ, Jy W, *et al.* Desmopressin (DDAVP) acts on platelets to generate platelet microparticles and enhanced procoagulant activity. *Thromb Res* 1995; **79**: 163–74.

246. Lethagen S, Nilsson IM. DDAVP-induced enhancement of platelet retention: its dependence on platelet-von Willebrand factor and the platelet

receptor GP IIb/IIIa. *Eur J Haematol* 1992; **49**: 7–13.

247. Sloand EM, Alyono D, Klein HG, *et al.* 1-Deamino-8-D-arginine vasopressin (DDAVP) increases platelet membrane expression of glycoprotein Ib in patients with disorders of platelet function and after cardiopulmonary bypass. *Am J Hematol* 1994; **46**: 199–207.

248. Lethagen S, Olofsson L, Frick K, Berntorp E, Bjorkman S. Effect kinetics of desmopressin-induced platelet retention in healthy volunteers treated with aspirin or placebo. *Haemophilia* 2000; **6**: 15–20.

249. Humphries JE, Siragy H. Significant hyponatremia following DDAVP administration in a healthy adult. *Am J Hematol* 1993; **44**: 12–15.

250. Johns RA. Desmopressin is a potent vasorelaxant of aorta and pulmonary artery isolated from rabbit and rat. *Anesthesiology* 1990; **72**: 858–64.

251. Nitu-Whalley IC, Griffioen A, Harrington C, Lee CA. Retrospective review of the management of elective surgery with desmopressin and clotting factor concentrates in patients with von Willebrand disease. *Am J Hematol* 2001; **66**: 280–4.

252. Alanay A, Acaroglu E, Ozdemir O, *et al.* Effects of deamino-8-D-arginin vasopressin on blood loss and coagulation factors in scoliosis surgery. A double-blind randomized clinical trial. *Spine* 1999; **24**: 877–82.

253. Theroux MC, Corddry DH, Tietz AE, *et al.* A study of desmopressin and blood loss during spinal fusion for neuromuscular scoliosis: a randomized, controlled, double-blinded study. *Anesthesiology* 1997; **87**: 260–7.

254. Clagett GP, Valentine RJ, Myers SI, Chervu A, Heller J. Does desmopressin improve hemostasis and reduce blood loss from aortic surgery? A randomized, double-blind study. *J Vasc Surg* 1995; **22**: 223–9.

255. Letts M, Pang E, D'Astous J, *et al.* The influence of desmopressin on blood loss during spinal fusion surgery in neuromuscular patients. *Spine* 1998; **23**: 475–8.

256. Laupacis A, Fergusson D. Drugs to minimize perioperative blood loss in

cardiac surgery: meta-analyses using perioperative blood transfusion as the outcome. The International Study of Peri-operative Transfusion (ISPOT) Investigators. *Anesth Analg* 1997; **85**: 1258–67.

257. Carless PA, Henry DA, Moxey AJ, *et al.* Desmopressin for minimising perioperative allogeneic blood transfusion. *Cochrane Database Syst Rev* 2004; **1**: CD001884.

258. Crescenzi G, Landoni G, Biondi-Zoccai G, *et al.* Desmopressin reduces transfusion needs after surgery: a meta-analysis of randomized clinical trials. *Anesthesiology* 2008; **109**: 1063–76.

259. Michiels JJ, Budde U, van der Planken M, *et al.* Acquired von Willebrand syndromes: clinical features, aetiology, pathophysiology, classification and management. *Best Pract Res Clin Haematol* 2001; **14**: 401–36.

260. Attar S, Hammon JW. Pharmacologic agents in perioperative bleeding. In: Attar S, ed., *Hemostasis in Cardiac Surgery.* Armonk, NY: Futura Publishing, 1999: 203–14.

261. de Bono DP, Pringle S. Local inhibition of thrombosis using urokinase linked to a monoclonal antibody which recognises damaged endothelium. *Thromb Res* 1991; **61**: 537–45.

262. Dunn CJ, Goa KL. Tranexamic acid: a review of its use in surgery and other indications. *Drugs* 1999; **57**: 1005–32.

263. Dowd NP, Karski JM, Cheng DC, *et al.* Pharmacokinetics of tranexamic acid during cardiopulmonary bypass. *Anesthesiology* 2002; **97**: 390–9.

264. Mezzano D, Panes O, Munoz B, *et al.* Tranexamic acid inhibits fibrinolysis, shortens the bleeding time and improves platelet function in patients with chronic renal failure. *Thromb Haemost* 1999; **82**: 1250–4.

265. Roos Y. Antifibrinolytic treatment in subarachnoid hemorrhage: a randomized placebo-controlled trial. STAR Study Group. *Neurology* 2000; **54**: 77–82.

266. Iribarren JL, Jimenez JJ, Hernandez D, *et al.* Postoperative bleeding in cardiac surgery: the role of tranexamic acid in

patients homozygous for the 5G polymorphism of the plasminogen activator inhibitor-1 gene. *Anesthesiology* 2008; **108**: 596–602.

267. Troianos CA, Sypula RW, Lucas DM, *et al.* The effect of prophylactic epsilon-aminocaproic acid on bleeding, transfusions, platelet function, and fibrinolysis during coronary artery bypass grafting. *Anesthesiology* 1999; **91**: 430–5.

268. Vander Salm TJ, Kaur S, Lancey RA, *et al.* Reduction of bleeding after heart operations through the prophylactic use of epsilon-aminocaproic acid. *J Thorac Cardiovasc Surg* 1996; **112**: 1098–107.

269. Saleem R, Bigham M, Spitznagel E, Despotis GJ. The effect of epsilon-aminocaproic acid on HemoSTATUS and kaolin-activated clotting time measurements. *Anesth Analg* 2000; **90**: 1281–5.

270. Henry DA, Carless PA, Moxey AJ, *et al.* Anti-fibrinolytic use for minimising perioperative allogeneic blood transfusion. *Cochrane Database Syst Rev* 2007; (**4**): CD001886.

271. Gill JB, Chin Y, Levin A, Feng D. The use of antifibrinolytic agents in spine surgery. A meta-analysis. *J Bone Joint Surg Am* 2008; **90**: 2399–407.

272. Kang Y, Lewis JH, Navalgund A, *et al.* Epsilon-aminocaproic acid for treatment of fibrinolysis during liver transplantation. *Anesthesiology* 1987; **66**: 766–73.

273. Kang YG, Martin DJ, Marquez J, *et al.* Intraoperative changes in blood coagulation and thrombelastographic monitoring in liver transplantation. *Anesth Analg* 1985; **64**: 888–96.

274. Wells PS. Safety and efficacy of methods for reducing perioperative allogeneic transfusion: a critical review of the literature. *Am J Ther* 2002; **9**: 377–88.

275. Munoz JJ, Birkmeyer NJ, Birkmeyer JD, O'Connor GT, Dacey LJ. Is epsilon-aminocaproic acid as effective as aprotinin in reducing bleeding with cardiac surgery? A meta-analysis. *Circulation* 1999; **99**: 81–9.

276. Perazella MA, Biswas P. Acute hyperkalemia associated with

intravenous epsilon-aminocaproic acid therapy. *Am J Kidney Dis* 1999; **33**: 782–5.

277. Britt CW, Light RR, Peters BH, Schochet SS. Rhabdomyolysis during treatment with epsilon-aminocaproic acid. *Arch Neurol* 1980; **37**: 187–8.

278. Stafford-Smith M, Phillips-Bute B, Reddan DN, Black J, Newman MF. The association of epsilon-aminocaproic acid with postoperative decrease in creatinine clearance in 1502 coronary bypass patients. *Anesth Analg* 2000; **91**: 1085–90.

279. Levy JH, Morales A, Lemmer JH. Pharmacologic approaches to prevent or decrease bleeding in surgical patients. In: BD Speiss RC, SA Gould, eds., *Perioperative Transfusion Medicine.* Baltimore, MD: Williams & Wilkins, 1998: 383–97.

280. Butterworth J, James RL, Lin Y, Prielipp RC, Hudspeth AS. Pharmacokinetics of epsilon-aminocaproic acid in patients undergoing aortocoronary bypass surgery. *Anesthesiology* 1999; **90**: 1624–35.

281. Myles PS, Smith J, Knight J, *et al.* Aspirin and Tranexamic Acid for Coronary Artery Surgery (ATACAS) Trial: rationale and design. *Am Heart J* 2008; **155**: 224–30.

282. Levy JH. Hemostatic agents and their safety. *J Cardiothorac Vasc Anesth* 1999; **13**: 6–11; discussion 36–7.

283. Menichetti A, Tritapepe L, Ruvolo G, *et al.* Changes in coagulation patterns, blood loss and blood use after cardiopulmonary bypass: aprotinin vs tranexamic acid vs epsilon aminocaproic acid. *J Cardiovasc Surg (Torino)* 1996; **37**: 401–7.

284. Poullis M, Manning R, Laffan M, *et al.* The antithrombotic effect of aprotinin: actions mediated via the proteaseactivated receptor 1. *J Thorac Cardiovasc Surg* 2000; **120**: 370–8.

285. Hunt BJ, Segal H, Yacoub M. Aprotinin and heparin monitoring during cardiopulmonary bypass. *Circulation* 1992; **86**: II410–12.

286. Mangano DT, Miao Y, Vuylsteke A, *et al.* Mortality associated with

aprotinin during 5 years following coronary artery bypass graft surgery. *JAMA* 2007; **297**: 471–9.

287. Mangano DT, Tudor IC, Dietzel C. The risk associated with aprotinin in cardiac surgery. *N Engl J Med* 2006; **354**: 353–65.

288. Fergusson DA, Hebert PC, Mazer CD, *et al*. A comparison of aprotinin and lysine analogues in high-risk cardiac surgery. *N Engl J Med* 2008; **358**: 2319–31.

289. Dietrich W, Spath P, Ebell A, Richter JA. Prevalence of anaphylactic reactions to aprotinin: analysis of two hundred forty-eight reexposures to aprotinin in heart operations. *J Thorac Cardiovasc Surg* 1997; **113**: 194–201.

290. Dietrich W, Spath P, Zuhlsdorf M, *et al*. Anaphylactic reactions to aprotinin reexposure in cardiac surgery: relation to antiaprotinin immunoglobulin G and E antibodies. *Anesthesiology* 2001; **95**: 64–71.

Introduction

Pharmacology in the obstetric patient is complex and challenging. Many physiological changes occur during pregnancy which may alter the pharmacokinetics and pharmacodynamics of many drugs. Medications given to the mother may affect the fetus directly after placental transfer, or indirectly by altering uterine and placental function. Some obstetric drugs will complicate anesthetic management, while others may cause serious adverse events requiring anesthetic intervention. Even after delivery, drug effects may be modified by the rapid changes that occur in maternal physiology, and drug transfer to breast milk must be remembered.

Despite these major changes in pharmacology, there has been little high-quality anesthetic research during pregnancy, because of obvious practical and ethical concerns regarding obtaining such data. Animal studies may not be that relevant because of species differences in physiology. The relative lack of information means that many drugs are labeled as not approved for use in pregnancy because of unknown effects on the fetus, even though they may have a long-established and uncomplicated history of successful use unlicensed or "off-label" [1]. For example, opioids are usually not licensed for epidural or intrathecal use. Pregnancy restrictions are a factor which influences the choice of drugs administered. Regulatory agencies such as the US Food and Drug Administration (FDA) also have classification systems for drugs regarding their use in pregnancy and possible fetal effects. There are five simple categories, A, B, C, D, and X (Table 58.1), but in 2008 the FDA proposed a more useful and detailed labeling that would include a summary of risks to the fetus and breastfeeding infant, and a discussion of the data supporting that summary [2].

The first section of this chapter describes how variation in drug response may occur in pregnancy because of pharmacogenetic, pharmacokinetic, and pharmacodynamic factors. The second section presents the pharmacology of obstetric drugs relevant to the anesthesiologist. The last section describes some current controversies about the choice of anesthetic drugs in pregnancy.

Variations in drug disposition and response during pregnancy

Pharmacogenetics

Some of the variation among individuals in drug response arises from genetic differences. One would expect these differences to manifest whether or not the patient is pregnant, but some are still very relevant to obstetric pharmacology and anesthesia [3]. The β_2-adrenoceptor may have an arginine-to-glycine substitution at codon 16 (Arg16Gly) and a glutamine-to-glutamate substitution at codon 27 (Gln27Glu). Arg16 homozygotes given β_2-agonists for tocolysis had prolonged gestation and significantly better neonatal outcome [4]. During spinal anesthesia for cesarean delivery, Gly16 homozygotes required less ephedrine for the management of hypotension compared with the Arg16 homozygotes and Arg16Gly heterozygotes [5]. Glu27 homozygotes similarly required less ephedrine [5]. Patients with the 894T allele in the endothelial nitric oxide synthase gene had increased response to phenylephrine (during cardiac surgery) [6]. The μ-opioid receptor gene at nucleotide position 118 may have an adenine-to-guanine substitution (A118G). In vitro, the G118 allele increases the binding and potency of β-endorphin, but clinical results have been conflicting. In laboring women, the AA homozygote had an increased intrathecal fentanyl requirement for effective analgesia [7]. In women who received intrathecal morphine for analgesia after cesarean delivery, the AA genotype had less pain, required less morphine by patient-controlled analgesia, and had a higher incidence of nausea and vomiting [8]. It is not known whether pregnancy may accentuate some of these variations in drug response.

Pharmacokinetic changes

The large physiological changes that occur throughout pregnancy should have a significant influence on the disposition of drugs [9,10]. However, it is difficult to easily summarize the effect of pregnancy on pharmacokinetics because the magnitude and time course of the different physiological changes

Anesthetic Pharmacology, 2nd edition, ed. Alex S. Evers, Mervyn Maze, Evan D. Kharasch. Published by Cambridge University Press. © Cambridge University Press 2011.

Table 58.1. FDA categories for drug use in pregnancy

Category	Description
A	Adequate, well-controlled studies in pregnant women have not shown an increased risk of fetal abnormalities.
B	Animal studies have revealed no evidence of harm to the fetus. However, there are no adequate and well-controlled studies in pregnant women. *or* Animal studies have shown an adverse effect, but adequate and well-controlled studies in pregnant women have failed to demonstrate a risk to the fetus.
C	Animal studies have shown an adverse effect and there are no adequate and well-controlled studies in pregnant women. *or* No animal studies have been conducted and there are no adequate and well-controlled studies in pregnant women.
D	Studies, adequate well-controlled or observational, in pregnant women have demonstrated a risk to the fetus. However, the benefits of therapy may outweigh the potential risk.
X	Studies, adequate well-controlled or observational, in animals or pregnant women have demonstrated positive evidence of fetal abnormalities. The use of the product is contraindicated in women who are or may become pregnant.

vary throughout pregnancy and among individuals. There are obvious ethical and practical problems with research in pregnancy, and older studies with small sample sizes and limited measurements often produced conflicting results. Our knowledge of maternal physiology and pharmacology is continually being updated as better measurements are made, but this unfortunately means that even recent reviews may contain outdated information. There are relatively few pharmacokinetic studies, and these are concentrated on drugs that need to be prescribed during pregnancy. Much of the data are also more limited and of lower quality than those expected from modern pharmacokinetic research. Thus, some of the general pharmacokinetic changes described below are more theoretical and based on limited data.

Maternal pharmacokinetics
Absorption/uptake
Intestinal motility and gastric acidity are decreased but oral absorption and bioavailability are not usually affected. However, gastric emptying is delayed during labor or after opioid drugs. Nausea and vomiting may also limit the oral intake of

drugs. Cardiac output is increased by 30–50% by the end of the first trimester, and the increased blood flow to skin and mucous membranes will enhance absorption from these sites. Minute ventilation is increased by 20–40%, and this will increase the pulmonary uptake of gases, especially as functional residual capacity is also decreased and cardiac output increased. However, the rate of induction with inhalational anesthetics will not necessarily be faster, because this depends on tissue distribution as well as pulmonary uptake.

Distribution
Intravascular plasma volume is increased by 40%, and extravascular volume by a variable amount depending on weight gain and edema. The average gain of 8 L in total body water will significantly increase the volume of distribution of hydrophilic drugs such as neuromuscular blockers. Body fat is increased by 4 kg on average, but this is relatively unimportant given the large volume of distribution of lipophilic drugs. The presence of fetal and placental tissues does provide another compartment where drugs are distributed (see below). The increased cardiac output may hasten the onset of action of intravenous drugs, but this depends to some extent on regional distribution of the increased flow. Increased cardiac output is generally associated with an increased dose requirement for intravenous induction drugs. Increased peripheral perfusion promotes the return of drug from tissue reservoirs during the elimination phase.

The concentration of albumin is reduced to about 70% of normal, while that of α_1-acid glycoprotein (AAG) is variable but nearly unchanged. Increased concentrations of free fatty acids and other endogenous displacing substances may decrease protein binding. However, with chronic drug administration, an increase in free drug concentration is compensated for by increased clearance, and clinically relevant changes in protein binding are restricted to a few drugs such as valproate and phenytoin. It is important to know whether concentrations used for therapeutic monitoring are for free or total drug.

Metabolism
The metabolism of drugs via some cytochrome P450 (CYP) isoenzymes (CYP3A4, CYP2D6, and CYP2C9) and uridine diphosphate glucuronosyltransferase (UGT) isoenzymes (UGT1A4 and UGT2B7) is increased during pregnancy [9,11]. Examples are phenytoin (CYP2C), midazolam (CYP3A4), and morphine (UGT2B7). In contrast, CYP1A2 and CYP2C19 activity is decreased during pregnancy, and this reduces the metabolism of drugs such as caffeine and theophylline (CYP1A2).

There is decreased pseudocholinesterase activity, but this does not lead to prolonged block after succinylcholine [12]. Diminished elimination may be offset by an increased volume of distribution. However, block is prolonged in postpartum patients who still have decreased pseudocholinesterase, but a volume of distribution that has not yet decreased to normal.

The metabolism of some drugs is dependent on hepatic blood flow. Although cardiac output is markedly increased, any change in liver blow flow is still uncertain. Two studies using clearance of markers concluded that hepatic blood flow was unchanged [13,14], while one using Doppler ultrasonography reported increased portal venous flow after 28 weeks gestation but unchanged hepatic arterial flow [15].

Elimination

Renal blood flow is increased by 60–80% and glomerular filtration rate by 50%, although this decreases near term. The renal excretion of unchanged drugs such as β-lactam cephalosporin antibiotics is increased. Clearance of digoxin is also increased in pregnancy, and this is consistent with increased renal P-glycoprotein activity [16]. Increased minute ventilation will enhance elimination of inhalational anesthetics.

The complex physiological changes will have different effects on drugs depending on their characteristics such as lipid solubility, degree of protein binding, and metabolic pathways. In general, the bioavailability of drugs is not changed during pregnancy. Increased plasma volume and protein binding changes can alter the apparent volume of distribution of drugs but the significance of this is limited. Drugs excreted unchanged by the kidneys will require an increased dose, but for other drugs dose depends on which isoenzymes are involved in the metabolism of the drug. Pharmacokinetic studies in pregnant women are still relatively simple, but there is increasing interest in modeling to make the most of the limited data [17,18].

Placental transfer and metabolism

Our understanding of placental transfer and metabolism is changing rapidly [19]. Early research was often limited to measuring drug concentrations in the umbilical vessels and maternal vein at delivery. Many pairs of samples were required to provide an estimate of umbilical-to-maternal concentration ratios. Results could be very variable and difficult to interpret, especially for drugs such as anesthetics that are administered shortly before delivery. Umbilical blood samples are obtained at variable times after drug exposure, well before steady-state conditions can be achieved. The finding that maternal and fetal concentrations were often different led to the theory of a placental barrier. However it is differences in concentrations of binding proteins that are responsible for the fetal/maternal distribution of drugs at steady state [20]. The fetal concentration of albumin is slightly greater than in the mother, but AAG concentrations are a third of maternal values at term. To complicate matters, fetal binding proteins may have drug affinities that are different from maternal proteins, and the placenta may also sequester drugs. Umbilical-to-maternal ratios of total drug may also be misleading because equilibrium across the placenta is established on free drug concentrations. Maternal-to-fetal ratios of drugs are still reported, but these data are generally not that helpful. The rate of drug transfer and the amount of drug that has already been transferred to the fetus is not known. This has led to the development of models to study drug transfer and metabolism such as the in-vitro perfused placental cotyledon. Many studies have been conducted in sheep, but there are major differences in placental structure and human data are more relevant. The human placenta is classified as hemochorial, where the fetal tissue is in direct contact with the maternal blood, whereas the sheep has an epitheliochorial structure with three additional maternal layers that drugs must traverse.

Until recently, drug transfer across the placenta was thought to occur mainly by diffusion. This would favor the movement of lipophilic drugs, and placental perfusion would be an important factor governing transfer. Fetal pH is lower than maternal pH and "ion trapping" is possible. Weak bases are more ionized in the fetus and this would limit their transfer back across the placenta. Normally the difference in pH is only 0.1 and ion trapping irrelevant, but fetal acidosis can lead to significant increases in the fetal concentration of drugs such as local anesthetics.

With the advent of transplacental pharmacotherapy, such as the treatment of sustained fetal tachyarrhythmia, there has been renewed interest in placental transfer and metabolism [21]. Membrane-associated drug-transporting proteins have been found in the syncytiotrophoblast, and their localization and mode of drug transport affect the direction of net drug transfer. For example, the syncytiotrophoblast expresses P-glycoprotein on the brush-border membrane. P-glycoprotein is an adenosine triphosphate (ATP)-dependent drug efflux pump, reducing net transfer of substrates such as digoxin and verapamil from maternal to fetal compartments.

The placenta also contains many enzymes, including UGT [19]. Clearance of a substrate for UGT in full-term placentas ranged from 7.5% to 43% of an adult female liver, so it is possible that the placenta may contribute to overall maternal metabolism.

Fetal and neonatal elimination

The fetus and neonate are capable of metabolizing drugs, but at a reduced rate compared with adults [22–24]. The fetal circulation causes some of the drug transferred across the placenta to undergo first-pass hepatic metabolism, while some may bypass the liver. Renal blood flow is minimal until near term, but nonetheless the excreted products just pass into the amniotic fluid to be swallowed. Elimination of drugs by the fetus is thus mainly reliant on placental transfer. It would seem prudent to minimize the amount of drug transferred to the neonate, and to choose anesthetic drugs that are eliminated rapidly. The neonate has a relatively large minute ventilation, which promotes elimination of inhalational anesthetics. Elimination may be further enhanced by assisted maternal ventilation.

Transfer to breast milk

Most drugs are transferred to milk by passive diffusion, but there are also transporter systems [25]. For most drugs the amount ingested by the infant rarely attains therapeutic concentrations. Anesthetic drugs are also only given for a short duration, so the amount of drug transferred is very low and no adverse neonatal effects are expected.

However, neonates of mothers receiving meperidine by intravenous patient-controlled analgesia after cesarean delivery had significant neurobehavioral depression by the third day [26]. The cumulative maternal meperidine dose at 48 hours postpartum was 14 mg kg^{-1}. No neonatal depression was seen in a morphine group where the cumulative maternal dose at 48 hours was 2.1 mg kg^{-1}. Both opioids and their major metabolites accumulated in colostrum. In a subsequent study, the cumulative opioid doses at 48 hours were lower (meperidine 4.7 mg kg^{-1} and morphine 0.54 mg kg^{-1}), but infants in the morphine group were still more alert and oriented [27]. With lower maternal morphine doses, concentrations in colostrum may even be undetectable [28].

Recently, it has been recognized that infants of breastfeeding mothers taking codeine may have central nervous system depression, and even death from opioid poisoning has been reported. Codeine is metabolized to morphine by CYP2D6, and 1–16% of mothers may be ultrarapid CYP2D6 metabolizers. In addition, genetic variability in UGT2B7 may increase the formation of active morphine-6-glucuronide. It is estimated that 1.4% of Western European women would have both the CYP2D6 and UGT2B7 variants promoting neonatal depression [29].

Pharmacodynamic changes
General anesthesia
Animal studies several decades ago showed that maternal anesthetic requirements were reduced during pregnancy. Minimum alveolar concentration (MAC) values for inhalational anesthetics were reduced in pregnant ewes by 25–40% [30], and in rats by 16–19% [31]. Ethical and practical difficulties with research in pregnant women delayed confirmation of this finding in humans. As a first step, it was shown that isoflurane MAC in women undergoing termination of pregnancy at 8–12 weeks gestation was decreased by 28% [32]. MAC was determined using transcutaneous electrical stimulation instead of the classical skin incision for the noxious stimulus. Similar reductions in MAC were found for enflurane (30%) and halothane (27%) [33]. MAC was also reduced by approximately 30% in the immediate postpartum period, with a return to nonpregnant values by 12–72 hours after delivery (Fig. 58.1) [34,35].

Studies in rabbits suggested that the reduced anesthetic requirements could be caused by progesterone, because chronic progesterone administration reduced MAC [36]. Similar experiments cannot be performed in humans, and studies have not found a good correlation between progesterone concentrations and the reduction in anesthetic requirement. However, the effect of progesterone need not be dose-dependent, and the increase in progesterone during pregnancy may simply exceed a threshold concentration above which anesthetic requirements are reduced. Even nonpregnant women have

differing sevoflurane requirements for maintaining anesthesia depending on the phase of the menstrual cycle [37]. Less sevoflurane was used in the luteal phase when the progesterone concentrations were greater.

Another possible explanation for reduced MAC is that it is related to endogenous endorphins that mediate the increase in nociceptive threshold during pregnancy. The stimuli used to determine MAC are noxious, and an increase in endogenous opioid activity would obviously decrease the amount of anesthetic required to prevent a reaction to the stimulus.

Apart from MAC, pregnancy also influences other measures of anesthetic effect. In early pregnancy, the isoflurane concentration required for hypnosis was reduced by 31%, and the Bispectral Index (BIS) was decreased at isoflurane concentrations over the range 0.1–2.0% [38]. During the second trimester, the amount of sevoflurane required to achieve a targeted BIS of 50 was reduced by 31% in pregnant women compared with nonpregnant controls [39]. Both early and term pregnancy increased the sedative effects of N_2O as measured by a reduction of 25–27% in the median concentration required for loss of consciousness (MAC-awake) and lower BIS [40].

Less information is available for intravenous anesthetics. At the induction of anesthesia, the bolus dose of thiopental for hypnosis (open eyes to command) was 17% less, and that for anesthesia (no purposeful movement to a transcutaneous electrical stimulus) was 18% less in early pregnancy compared with nonpregnant women [41] (Fig. 58.2). Using a slow infusion for induction of anesthesia, the propofol dose for loss of consciousness and the calculated effect site concentrations at loss of consciousness were 8% lower than in nonpregnant women [42].

Studies with intravenous anesthetics are more challenging to perform than with inhalational anesthetics because it is difficult to produce a stable effect-site concentration of the intravenous drug to allow accurate measurement of drug effect. Pregnant patients also have an increased cardiac output, which may increase the dose of intravenous anesthetic required to produce central effects, and hence bias the results. Pharmacokinetic models for propofol may also be inaccurate in pregnancy, especially when there is already some misspecification of the pharmacokinetic parameters during rapid changes in concentration such as occur at induction. These methodological problems may be the reason that one study did not find differences in the concentration of propofol required for loss of consciousness in early pregnancy [43]. The reduction in anesthetic requirements for intravenous drugs appears to be less (8–18%) than that for inhalational anesthetics (~30%). It is not known whether this reflects real differences between the drugs or the methodological problems outlined above.

Local anesthesia
It is well accepted clinically that pregnant women require less local anesthetic for epidural or intrathecal anesthesia. This may be related to greater spread of local anesthetic resulting from factors such as increased epidural venous blood volume.

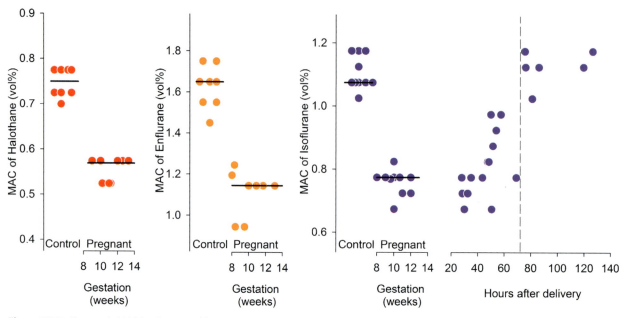

Figure 58.1. Changes in MAC (as determined by response to transcutaneous electrical stimulation) for halothane, enflurane, and isoflurane in early pregnancy, and for isoflurane in the early postpartum period [30–35].

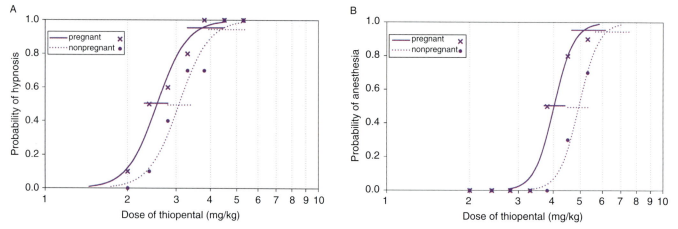

Figure 58.2. Calculated dose–response curves (log dose scale) for (A) hypnosis and (B) anesthesia in pregnant and nonpregnant women. The 95% confidence intervals for the ED50s and ED95s are also displayed, slightly offset for clarity [41].

Increased spread of block from intrathecal anesthetics can occur by the second trimester [44]. However, several studies have concluded that the nerves are also more sensitive to local anesthetics during pregnancy. The onset of conduction block to bupivacaine was faster in the vagus nerves of pregnant rabbits [45,46]. In women receiving median nerve block at the wrist with lidocaine, sensory nerve action potentials were inhibited to a greater extent in pregnant women [47]. The mechanism of increased susceptibility is not clear. Exogenously administered progesterone increased the susceptibility of rabbit vagus nerves to bupivacaine [48]. In pregnant rats, sciatic nerve block was of longer duration and the lidocaine content in the nerves was lower at the time of return of deep pain [49]. This was consistent with a pharmacodynamic rather than a pharmacokinetic mechanism for the increased block. However, other studies found no changes in conduction block [50]. Increased epidural block may simply be related to an increased spread of local anesthetic [51]. Other proposals are that pregnancy-induced changes may facilitate diffusion of local anesthetic and hasten the onset of block, or that increased block may be the result of an interaction with endogenous analgesic systems.

Analgesia

Pregnancy is associated with increases in nociceptive response thresholds that are mediated by endogenous opioid systems [52,53]. The threshold elevations result from changes in estrogen and progesterone with pregnancy, and these can be reproduced using exogenous hormones. The main pathways involved are spinal cord κ- and δ-opioid systems, but interaction with descending spinal α_2-noradrenergic pathways is also important [54]. Despite the good animal evidence for pregnancy-induced nociception, early human studies produced mixed results, probably because of methodological problems. A controlled study showed that heat pain tolerance was increased in term pregnant women, and this persisted during the first 24–48 hours after delivery [55]. There are no data to suggest how this change in pain threshold might influence analgesic requirements. It would also be difficult to account for factors that would influence pain behavior in pregnant women.

We can conclude that pregnancy reduces inhalational anesthetic requirements by 25–30%, and this is apparent from the end of the first trimester through to a few days after delivery. There is less of a reduction in intravenous anesthetic requirements, but further research is required to separate pharmacokinetic from pharmacodynamic factors. Pregnancy also decreases sensitivity to pain, especially near term. Progesterone is probably mainly responsible for these changes, because exogenously administered progesterone can produce most of these effects.

Obstetric drugs relevant to the anesthesiologist

Obstetric patients may be receiving a variety of drugs that have implications for anesthetic management [56]. The anesthesiologist should be familiar with the pharmacological management of common complications of pregnancy such as pre-eclampsia, hypertensive disorders, preterm labor, and obstetric hemorrhage.

Drugs in pre-eclampsia

Pre-eclampsia complicates 2–7% of pregnancies in developed countries and is a leading cause of maternal death. The treatment of pre-eclampsia is delivery of the placenta and fetus. Before delivery, management is aimed at prevention of seizures, control of blood pressure, and maintenance of placental perfusion. Anticonvulsants are used to prevent recurrent convulsions in eclampsia, or to prevent initial convulsions in pre-eclampsia. Magnesium sulfate is the drug of choice, although it may not be effective in all cases [57,58].

Magnesium sulfate

The main cellular actions of magnesium are the regulation of transmembrane movement of calcium, sodium, and potassium, regulation and blockage of calcium channels, and activation of hundreds of enzymatic reactions involving ATP [59,60]. Magnesium often opposes the actions of calcium and can thus regulate diverse events such as contractile activity and the release of neurotransmitters that are calcium-dependent. Normal serum magnesium concentrations are 0.75–1.0 mmol L^{-1} (1.5–2.5 mEq L^{-1} or 1.8–2.4 mg dL^{-1}), with 62% ionized,

33% bound to plasma proteins, and 5% in anion complexes. Magnesium deficiency is associated with poorer outcomes after diverse neurological injury. Magnesium has various therapeutic applications [59,60]. It has been extensively studied in cardiology, with a role in managing arrhythmias and in cardiac surgery, and magnesium replacement is an important part of intensive care management.

Magnesium has been used in obstetrics for anticonvulsant, antihypertensive, and tocolytic purposes [61,62]. The best evidence supports the use of magnesium in the treatment of convulsions in eclampsia. The antihypertensive effect of magnesium is relatively mild, and it should not be used for this primary purpose. However, magnesium decreases the release of catecholamines and has been used to attenuate the sympathetic response to laryngoscopy and tracheal intubation in parturients with hypertensive disease [63]. Although magnesium sulfate is now considered inappropriate as a tocolytic for preterm birth [64,65], earlier studies showed that it substantially reduced the risk of cerebral palsy in the child (RR 0.68, 95% CI 0.54–0.87, five trials, 6145 infants) [66]. There was also a significant reduction in the rate of substantial gross motor dysfunction (RR 0.61, 95% CI 0.44–0.85, four trials, 5980 infants). There was no effect on infant mortality.

Eclampsia and pre-eclampsia – There is universal agreement that patients with eclampsia should receive magnesium sulfate. However, only a small proportion of patients with pre-eclampsia progress to eclampsia, so the prophylactic administration of magnesium in pre-eclampsia is controversial. The mechanism of action in preventing eclamptic seizures is unclear [67]. Magnesium is much less effective as an anticonvulsant outside eclampsia. Abnormal electroencephalograms are frequent in pre-eclampsia and eclampsia, but they are not altered by magnesium sulfate. Magnesium may vasodilate smaller-diameter intracranial blood vessels and thus relieve cerebral ischemia. Magnesium increases prostacyclin release by vascular endothelium, which may inhibit platelet aggregation and vasoconstriction. Magnesium may limit the formation of cerebral edema by actions at the blood–brain barrier. Some of the mechanisms postulated here are inhibition of myosin light chain phosphorylation that will inhibit paracellular movement of solutes through the tight junctions of cerebral endothelial cells, decreased pinocytosis that will also restrict movement of water and solutes, and downregulation of aquaporin-4 expression in astrocytes [67]. Magnesium may also have a central anticonvulsant action through antagonism of N-methyl-D-aspartate (NMDA) receptors.

Magnesium is usually given as an intravenous loading dose followed by an infusion, although intramuscular administration is an alternative. A typical regimen is a loading dose of 4–6 g IV over 20 minutes followed by maintenance at 1–2 g h^{-1}. An intramuscular regimen is 4 g every 4 hours (1 g magnesium sulfate = 98 mg = 4.06 mmol = 8.12 mEq elemental magnesium). Magnesium is rapidly excreted by the kidney. The half-life in patients with normal renal function is 4 hours, and

90% of the dose is excreted by 24 hours after the infusion [68]. The dose should be reduced and serum concentrations monitored if there is renal impairment. A suggested target serum concentration for severe pre-eclampsia is 2–3.5 mmol L^{-1} (4–7 mEq L^{-1} or 4.8–8.4 mg dL^{-1}).

Magnesium toxicity is associated with muscle weakness, areflexia (4–5 mmol L^{-1}) and respiratory paralysis (> 7.5 mmol L^{-1}). Increased conduction time with increased PR and QT intervals and QRS duration can lead to sinoatrial and atrioventricular block (> 7.5 mmol L^{-1}) and cardiac arrest in diastole (> 12.5 mmol L^{-1}). Toxicity is unlikely when deep tendon reflexes are present. Magnesium toxicity can be treated with small intravenous doses of calcium. Other reported adverse effects of magnesium include death from overdose, increased bleeding, slowed cervical dilation, and pulmonary edema. Magnesium crosses the placenta and can cause neonatal flaccidity and respiratory depression. Although magnesium decreases systemic vascular resistance, cardiac output is often increased, and its effect as a hypotensive drug is relatively modest.

Magnesium therapy can complicate anesthesia. Magnesium decreases presynaptic acetylcholine release at the neuromuscular junction. However, the duration of action of succinylcholine is not affected, although fasciculations may be reduced. Neuromuscular block is prolonged with nondepolarizing neuromuscular blocking drugs but this can be monitored and managed with a peripheral nerve stimulator. The cardiovascular effects of magnesium could theoretically modify hemodynamic responses during regional anesthesia, but little effect is normally seen.

Other anticonvulsants

If seizures continue despite therapeutic levels of magnesium, phenytoin may be used. The initial intravenous loading dose is 10 mg kg^{-1}, followed 2 hours later by 5 mg kg^{-1}. The electrocardiogram and arterial pressure must be monitored. Maintenance doses of 200 mg orally or intravenously are started 12 hours after the second bolus and given every 8 hours. Phenytoin may also be useful when there is renal failure complicating magnesium therapy. Diazepam has also been used as an infusion 40 mg in 500 mL normal saline titrated to keep patients sedated.

Antihypertensive therapy

The general pharmacology of antihypertensives was presented in Chapters 42, 45, and 46. The most commonly used drugs in obstetrics are hydralazine, labetalol, and nifedipine [69]. Hydralazine is a direct arteriolar vasodilator with a long history of use in pre-eclampsia. The initial dose is 5 mg intravenous bolus followed by 5–10 mg every 20 minutes. Adverse effects include headache, tachycardia, tremor, nausea, and rare cases of neonatal thrombocytopenia. Labetalol is a nonselective β-adrenoceptor blocker with some α_1-blocking effect. The initial dose is 20–40 mg intravenously every 10–15 minutes followed by an infusion at 0.5–2 mg min^{-1}. Labetalol preserves uteroplacental blood flow and, although it crosses the placenta, neonatal bradycardia and hypoglycemia are

rarely seen. Nifedipine is a calcium channel blocker that relaxes arterial smooth muscle. Nifedipine 10 mg is usually given orally and repeated after 30 minutes as required. Nifedipine given sublingually or chewed may cause sudden hypotension and fetal compromise. Patients also receiving magnesium sulfate may have increased hypotension and potentiation of neuromuscular block. Nifedipine also relaxes uterine muscle and this may increase the risk of postpartum hemorrhage.

Tocolytics

Tocolytics are drugs that decrease uterine tone. Their major indication is the management of preterm labor. The anesthesiologist may also have to decrease uterine tone to facilitate cesarean delivery or surgical access during fetal surgery.

Preterm labor is the main cause of perinatal morbidity and mortality in the developed world. Unfortunately, the etiology of preterm labor is not well understood, and the management of preterm labor has concentrated on trying to reduce uterine contractions, even though this does not address the primary cause of preterm labor. The physiology of uterine contraction is complex, and many drugs with different mechanisms of action have been used with limited success [70]. Tocolytics have usually not been successful in delaying labor by more than 48 hours. This short delay may however provide sufficient time to administer corticosteroids to assist with fetal lung maturation, and to transport the mother to a more specialized maternity unit for obstetric care. The use of tocolytics in preterm labor remains controversial, because current tocolytic therapy may have side effects and preterm labor may resolve spontaneously in 30–50% of cases [71].

β-Adrenoceptor agonists

Although ritodrine is the only drug approved by the FDA for preterm labor, other drugs such as terbutaline and salbutamol have often been used. They increase intracellular cyclic adenosine monophosphate (cAMP), which activates protein kinase, thus inactivating myosin light-chain kinase and decreasing contractility. The main side effects are maternal and fetal tachycardia. Pulmonary edema is an uncommon (1 in 400 pregnancies) but serious complication of tocolytic therapy with β-adrenergic agonists [72]. The underlying mechanism for the pulmonary edema is unclear but it is probably related to fluid overload and increased hydrostatic pressure rather than increased pulmonary capillary permeability or left ventricular dysfunction. The initial management is stopping the β-adrenergic agonist and providing oxygen therapy, with further monitoring, diuretics, and respiratory support as necessary.

Calcium channel blockers

Nifedipine has been used in the majority of clinical trials. It reduces intracellular calcium influx and inhibits myosin light-chain kinase, causing uterine relaxation. Nifedipine can also be given orally and is relatively inexpensive. Nifedipine has obvious cardiovascular effects and may not be indicated in some women. Common adverse effects include dizziness, hypotension, headache, flushing, and edema.

Cyclooxygenase inhibitors
These drugs decrease the production of prostaglandins and thus the transmembrane influx and sarcolemmal release of calcium. Indomethacin is the most commonly used drug in this class.

Magnesium sulfate
Although magnesium has a long history of use for this purpose, the evidence is clear that it is ineffective for tocolysis.

Nitric oxide donors
These cause an increase in cyclic guanosine monophosphate (cGMP) that inactivates myosin light-chain kinase and decreases contractility. Nitroglycerin can be given transdermally, sublingually, or intravenously. In the acute situation of fetal distress during labor, or request for rapid uterine relaxation at delivery, nitroglycerin 100 µg can be given intravenously.

Oxytocin-receptor antagonists
Atosiban is a synthetic competitive oxytocin inhibitor, although it also inhibits vasopressin. It is given intravenously and rapidly eliminated with a short initial half-life. Adverse effects include headache, nausea, vomiting, and dizziness but it does not appear to have anesthetic implications. It does not reduce the incidence of preterm birth or improve neonatal outcome. There are newer oxytocin antagonists such as barusiban that have a higher selectivity for the oxytocin receptor.

Oxytocics
Oxytocics are drugs that stimulate uterine contraction. Apart from oxytocin and its analogs, some ergot alkaloids and prostaglandins also induce uterine contractions. Clinical indications for oxytocics include the induction of abortion, induction and augmentation of labor, and the management of postpartum bleeding.

Oxytocin
Oxytocin is a hormone and neurotransmitter best known for its role in uterine contraction and breastfeeding, but recent studies have shown it involved in diverse behaviors including social recognition, bonding, anxiety, trust, and maternal behaviors [73,74]. Oxytocin is a cyclic nonapeptide (molecular weight 1007 Da, 1 international unit equivalent to 2 µg) that is very similar to vasopressin. It is synthesized as a large precursor molecule in cell bodies of the paraventricular and supraoptic hypothalamic nuclei, and stored in Herring bodies at the axon terminals in the posterior pituitary. Oxytocin is packaged bound to the carrier protein neurophysin I, both being cleavage products from the same precursor, and secretion is regulated by the oxytocin cells in the hypothalamus that depolarize the nerve terminals and cause exocytosis of the vesicles. Oxytocin is released in large amounts after distension of the cervix

and vagina during labor, and after stimulation of the nipples, facilitating breastfeeding. Oxytocin is also made by neurons in the paraventricular nucleus that project to other parts of the brain and spinal cord, as well as by the corpus luteum, endometrium, and placenta.

The actions of oxytocin are mediated by the rhodopsin-type (class I) group of G-protein-coupled receptors and inositol trisphosphate (IP$_3$) and diacylglycerol (DAG) [75]. IP$_3$ triggers calcium release to initiate the contraction of smooth-muscle cells, while DAG activates protein kinase C for continued longer-term effects. Oxytocin receptors are expressed by the myoepithelial cells of the mammary gland, and the myometrium and endometrium at the end of pregnancy. Oxytocin receptors are also widely distributed throughout the central nervous system. Recently, oxytocin receptors found in the heart have been linked to the release of atrial natriuretic peptide.

Oxytocin causes uterine contraction and is important for cervical dilation before birth as well as contractions during the second and third stages of labor. Oxytocin mediates the letdown reflex in lactating mothers. Infant sucking at the nipple causes release of oxytocin that acts at the mammary glands, causing milk to be "let down." Oxytocin release during breastfeeding also causes mild uterine contractions during the first few weeks of lactation.

The important central effects of oxytocin are being recognized, and are the subject of intense research. Oxytocin secreted from the pituitary gland cannot re-enter the brain because of the blood–brain barrier, and thus the behavioral effects of oxytocin are thought to reflect release from centrally projecting oxytocin neurons. Some of the behaviors affected include appetite, sexual arousal, bonding, autism and other disorders, maternal bonding, increasing trust, and reducing fear [73,74].

Clinically, oxytocin is used for the induction and augmentation of labor. There is considerable debate among obstetricians about the dosage and administration of oxytocin because of the potential for various adverse maternal and fetal effects during labor [76]. Because of its structural similarity to vasopressin, oxytocin has antidiuretic effects and can cause hyponatremia if hypotonic fluids are used.

Oxytocin is also used to contract the uterus in the management of the third stage of labor. The recommended dose of oxytocin for uterine contraction after cesarean delivery is 5 units intravenously, given slowly. Previously, it was not uncommon in the United Kingdom for 10 units to be given rapidly, but the risks of hypotension and even death from this practice were highlighted in the 1997–99 report of the Confidential Enquiries into Maternal Deaths [77]. Various infusion regimens may also be used by obstetricians. Carbetocin is a longer-acting analog of oxytocin.

Ergot alkaloids
Ergot is the common name of a fungus that grows on some grains and grasses. The fungus synthesizes derivatives of the compound ergoline that have a wide range of effects due to

their structural similarities to norepinephrine, dopamine, and serotonin [78,79]. Ergot poisoning or ergotism can be associated with convulsive or gangrenous symptoms. Historically, controlled doses of ergot were used to induce abortions and to stop maternal bleeding after childbirth. The exact mechanism for uterine contraction is uncertain, but it is probably partially mediated by serotonin receptors. Ergoline derivatives are also used clinically to cause vasoconstriction, and in the treatment of migraine and Parkinson's disease. In addition to the naturally occurring ergotamine and ergonovine (also known as ergometrine), important synthetic derivatives are methylergonivine (methergine), bromocriptine, and psychedelic drugs such as lysergic acid diethylamide (LSD).

Ergotamine was first isolated from the ergot fungus in 1918. It is used to treat acute migraine attacks, and less commonly to prevent postpartum hemorrhage. The antimigraine effect is through vasoconstriction of cerebral vessels mediated by serotonin receptors. The main side effect is peripheral vasoconstriction.

Ergonovine and methylergonovine are primarily used as oxytocics. Side effects include hypertension, coronary artery spasm, bronchospasm, and nausea and vomiting. Syntometrine is a combination of synthetic oxytocin 5 IU mL^{-1} and ergometrine 0.5 mg mL^{-1} given intramuscularly for the prevention and treatment of postpartum hemorrhage.

Prostaglandins (PG) and analogs

Prostaglandins have an essential role in reproduction and parturition. Their effects are diverse because the different prostaglandins interact in different ways with a large family of G-protein-coupled receptors. Responsiveness to prostaglandins also varies during the menstrual cycle and pregnancy. In pregnant women, PGE_2 and $PGF_{2\alpha}$ produce dose-dependent increases in uterine tone and frequency and intensity of uterine contractions.

PGE_1 (alprostadil) is mainly used for erectile dysfunction, but analogs of PGE_1 have obstetric indications. Misoprostol is a synthetic PGE_1 analog. It was initially used as a cytoprotective drug, reducing the risk of gastric ulcers in patients taking nonsteroidal anti-inflammatory drugs. In the gastric parietal cell, misoprostol inhibits the secretion of gastric acid via G-protein-coupled receptor (GPCR)-mediated inhibition of adenylate cyclase. Misoprostol is also used for the induction of labor, where it promotes the ripening of the cervix and uterine contractions. Misoprostol may be used for medical abortions instead of surgical evacuation, and it may have a role in preventing postpartum hemorrhage in community births. Gemeprost (16,16-dimethyl-trans-delta2 PGE_1 methyl ester) is an analog of PGE_1 used for abortion and postpartum bleeding. PGE_2 (dinoprostone) is available as a vaginal suppository to prepare the cervix for labor and to induce labor. Sulprostone is an analog of PGE_2 used as an oxytocic. $PGF_{2\alpha}$ (dinoprost) effects are mainly uterine contraction, but it may also cause bronchoconstriction. It has largely been replaced by carboprost (15-methyl-$PGF_{2\alpha}$) for the management of postpartum bleeding.

Progesterone antagonists

There is now a large class of synthetic drugs that bind to the progesterone receptor, including pure antagonists and mixed agonist-antagonists (named selective progesterone receptor modulators) [80]. Mifepristone was the first antiprogestin synthesized, and controversy about this drug probably inhibited the early development of related drugs. Diverse applications for these drugs include medical termination of pregnancy, emergency contraception, estrogen-free contraception, and the management of myomas and endometriosis. Mifepristone is a 19-nor steroid with some partial agonist activity but it acts as a competitive progesterone antagonist with more than twice the relative binding affinity of progesterone. It also has some antiglucocorticoid and weak antiandrogen activity. Mifeprostone is used in the medical termination of pregnancy, causing endometrial decidual degeneration and cervical softening and dilation, and it often generated widespread social debate where it was to be introduced. After mifeprostone, a prostaglandin (e.g., misoprostol) is usually administered to cause uterine contraction and complete the abortion.

Gonadotropins

Gonadotropins are hormones secreted by the pituitary or placenta that influence gonadal activity, e.g., follicle-stimulating hormone (FSH), luteinizing hormone (LH), and human chorionic gonadotrophin (hCG). These glycoproteins have identical α subunits but distinct β subunits that are responsible for their unique properties [81].

The anesthesiologist may encounter women receiving hCG. This hormone is normally produced by the developing embryo and syncytiotrophoblast. It binds with the LH/choriogonadotrophin (LHCG) receptor to maintain the corpus luteum at the start of pregnancy, causing it to secrete progesterone. Early pregnancy testing is often based on the detection of hCG. Because of its similarity to LH, hCG is used clinically to induce ovulation in the ovaries during infertility treatment (and in males to stimulate the Leydig cells to produce testosterone for the treatment of hypogonadism and infertility). Performance-enhancing drug regimens may also use hCG. It was formerly prepared from the urine of pregnant women, but a recombinant product is now available.

Ovarian hyperstimulation syndrome (OHSS) is an unpredictable and incompletely understood complication of ovarian stimulation [82]. The syndrome is associated with increased capillary permeability, leading progressively to hypovolemia with hemoconcentration, edema and accumulation of fluid in the abdomen and pleural spaces. A possible mediator is vascular endothelial growth factor (VEGF), but many interacting cytokines and endocrine factors may be involved. Subclinical OHSS may be found in most patients, while a small number may require admission for fluid management to restore circulating volume, heparin for prevention of thrombosis, and paracentesis for treatment of ascites. Severe OHSS may cause renal failure, respiratory failure, or thromboembolism.

Choice of anesthetic drugs in pregnancy

Some anesthetic techniques used during pregnancy have not changed for several decades, but more of these are being challenged. This section briefly introduces some of the current controversies.

Vasopressor treatment of hypotension from spinal anesthesia

Spinal anesthesia for cesarean delivery is often associated with maternal hypotension. Arterial vasodilation will decrease systemic vascular resistance while venous vasodilation will decrease venous return. Among the treatment options, the vasopressor of choice has long been believed to be ephedrine. This was based on early studies that showed ephedrine did not reduce uterine blood flow as much as other direct α-adrenergic agonists such as metaraminol and phenylephrine [83]. However, ephedrine may not always be effective in treating hypotension [84,85]. This is partly because ephedrine has a slower indirect action and tachyphylaxis may occur, but also because ephedrine is a mixed α- and β-adrenergic agonist. The β$_2$-adrenergic effect is vasodilation, and there may be little net increase in the (low) systemic vascular resistance [86–88]. If this occurs, ephedrine will only maintain arterial pressure by increasing the heart rate and cardiac output, but this requires adequate fluid volume. More recent studies found that direct α-adrenergic agonists such as metaraminol and phenylephrine were effective for managing maternal hypotension without adverse neonatal effects [89–91]. On reviewing the early literature on ephedrine it was apparent that the experimental conditions in those studies (standing sheep that had their arterial pressure raised above normal) were different from the clinical problem of trying to return low maternal arterial pressure back to normal. Ephedrine is also associated with dose-dependent fetal acidosis [85], unlike phenylephrine [90,91]. Ephedrine is transferred across the placenta [92] and probably has a direct stimulating effect on fetal metabolism. Although phenylephrine may not have replaced ephedrine, the latter is no longer considered the vasopressor of choice in obstetrics [93]. Various dosing strategies have been reported, including a simple closed-loop computer-controlled infusion [94]. Combinations of phenylephrine and ephedrine are not superior to phenylephrine alone [95]. Some clinicians may still use ephedrine, especially when the maternal heart rate is relatively low, because the direct α-adrenergic agonists will cause a reactive bradycardia. There may be additional maternal or fetal considerations during nonelective surgery, and a recent report concluded that both vasopressors were still suitable for treating hypotension [96].

Propofol for the induction and maintenance of anesthesia

The main reservation about the use of propofol in obstetrics arises from the warning in the product prescribing information for propofol. The original text used nearly 20 years ago read: "Diprivan should not be used in pregnancy. Diprivan crosses the placenta and may be associated with neonatal depression. It should not be used for obstetric anaesthesia." This author was unable to persuade the manufacturer to change this warning despite having conducted much of the early research with propofol in obstetrics. There was no good evidence that propofol caused more neonatal depression than thiopental when given at equipotent doses, and one suspects that the choice of words in the original prescribing information was a defensive decision by the manufacturer. Unfortunately, these statements are still found in the current global prescribing information for Diprivan [97]. Exactly the same warning is even found in prescribing information for other preparations of propofol marketed in these countries.

Fortunately, the product sheet in the United States is more reasonable [98], and contains the common caveats found for many drugs in pregnancy: "Diprivan Injectable Emulsion is not recommended for obstetrics, including cesarean section deliveries. Diprivan Injectable Emulsion crosses the placenta, and as with other general anesthetics, the administration of Diprivan Injectable Emulsion may be associated with neonatal depression."

Compared with thiopental, some early data suggested that Apgar scores were lower with propofol, but high propofol doses (2.8 mg kg^{-1} pregnant body weight) were used [99]. The same authors have published other reports of transient neonatal depression after propofol [100], but all other investigators found no difference in Apgar scores or neonatal behavioral scores after propofol or thiopental [101–104]. In vitro, propofol 10 μg mL^{-1} reduced human pregnant uterine muscle tension but propofol 2 μg mL^{-1} did not [105]. There has been no suggestion that uterine blood loss may be increased after propofol. Maternal and neonatal elimination of propofol is rapid [106] and faster than thiopental. A feature of propofol is rapid recovery from anesthesia, but it has been argued that this might not be ideal during an operation where there has been a high incidence of awareness. However, this reservation should not be relevant given the modern general anesthetic technique for cesarean delivery using sufficient concentrations of volatile anesthetic before delivery. The only study reporting a high incidence of awareness after propofol actually discontinued the volatile anesthetic for 1–4 minutes between uterine incision and delivery [107]. Although previously more controversial [108], propofol is currently widely used in obstetric anesthesia off-label, despite the warning in the product prescribing information. This probably reflects a worldwide preference for propofol over thiopental rather than any specific advantage in obstetric anesthesia.

Propofol infusions can be used for the maintenance of anesthesia [109–110]. The main problem with this technique is that maintaining an elevated concentration of propofol in the maternal blood will lead to continued transfer of propofol across the placenta and increased fetal concentrations at delivery [111]. Clinical studies using propofol infusions have been able to detect some neonatal depression compared with maintenance of anesthesia using volatile anesthetics [109,112]. Neonatal recovery from propofol will depend on the neonatal redistribution and elimination of propofol. In contrast, inhalational anesthetics transferred to the fetus can be rapidly eliminated via the lungs after delivery, and alveolar ventilation can be controlled to further enhance elimination. The ability to rapidly eliminate inhalational anesthetics from the neonate makes them an inherently more attractive option than propofol for maintenance of anesthesia.

Remifentanil in obstetric general anesthesia

Opioids are an integral component of general anesthetic techniques for major surgery. They are usually given during induction of anesthesia, permitting a reduction in the dose of other anesthetics because of synergistic drug interactions [113], and attenuating the hemodynamic and catecholamine ("stress") response to tracheal intubation [114]. In obstetric general anesthesia, opioids have not been given until after delivery because of concerns about neonatal respiratory depression. However, plasma concentrations of catecholamines increase after tracheal intubation in pregnant women having cesarean section [115], and uterine blood flow is decreased by 20%–35% [116]. Preventing this increase in catecholamines may be beneficial for placental perfusion. There has been a long history of using opioids successfully in selected patients where maternal hemodynamic stress is best avoided. Is it possible to use opioids routinely at induction of anesthesia for cesarean delivery, as one would normally for other major operations?

This idea was tested initially using alfentanil 10 μg kg^{-1} at induction of anesthesia, but this was associated with transiently lower Apgar scores [117]. It was hoped that the shorter-acting remifentanil would be less likely to cause neonatal depression. However, two studies using remifentanil by bolus (1 μg kg^{-1}) [118] and by bolus and infusion (0.5 μg kg^{-1} then 0.15 μg kg^{-1} min^{-1}) [119] have also reported a few cases of transient neonatal depression. The maternal stress response was attenuated as expected. A study using both remifentanil and propofol infusions before delivery also found brief neonatal depression, and the authors did not recommend routine use of their anesthetic technique [120]. Appropriate dosing regimens are still being evaluated, but remifentanil is being used widely off-label for obstetric anesthesia and analgesia [121].

Summary

Obstetric pharmacology is complex and challenging. Physiological changes during pregnancy may affect the pharmacokinetics and pharmacodynamics of many drugs. The magnitude and time course of these physiological changes vary throughout pregnancy and among individuals. High-quality pharmacologic data are difficult to obtain due to the practical and ethical challenges of clinical research during pregnancy.

Pregnancy alters drug disposition. Most notably, the average 8 L gain in total body water, including a 40% increase in intravascular volume and a more variable increase in extravascular volume depending on weight gain and edema, will significantly increase the volume of distribution of hydrophilic drugs such as neuromuscular blockers. Drug metabolism is variably affected, depending on the specific enzymes responsible. Pseudocholinesterase activity is reduced, although this does not prolong block after succinylcholine. Renal excretion of drugs is increased, because of a 50% increase in glomerular filtration rate. Due to recent improvements in research methodology, understanding of placental drug transfer and fetal metabolism in humans is rapidly changing. Simple reporting of maternal/fetal drug concentration ratios is now considered uninformative. Until recently, placental drug transfer was thought to occur mainly by passive diffusion, but a role for membrane-associated drug-transporting proteins has been increasingly recognized. The fetus and neonate metabolize drugs at lower rates than adults. The fetal circulation causes some transplacentally transferred drugs to undergo first-pass hepatic metabolism, while some may bypass the liver. Fetal drug elimination relies mainly on placental transfer. Maternal drug transfer to breast milk is typically not a concern, except for certain opioids such as meperidine and codeine (due to its metabolism to morphine).

Pregnancy reduces inhalational anesthetic requirements by 25–30% from the end of the first trimester until a few days after delivery. Less information is available for intravenous anesthetics, although there appears to be a small reduction in anesthetic requirements. Pregnant women require less local anesthetic for epidural or intrathecal anesthesia, which may be related to greater spread of local anesthetic, and/or greater sensitivity of nerves to local anesthetics during pregnancy. Pregnancy also decreases sensitivity to pain, especially near term, likely due primarily to increased endogenous progesterone.

Practitioners should be familiar with the pharmacological management of common pregnancy complications such as pre-eclampsia, hypertensive disorders, preterm labor, and obstetric hemorrhage. The definitive treatment of pre-eclampsia, which affects about 1 in 20 pregnancies, is delivery of the placenta and fetus, although predelivery management targets the prevention of seizures, control of blood pressure, and maintenance of placental perfusion. Magnesium sulfate is the drug of choice for prophylaxis and treatment of seizures. While there is agreement that patients with eclampsia should receive magnesium, prophylactic administration of magnesium in pre-eclampsia is controversial because only a small proportion of pre-eclamptic patients progress to eclampsia. Magnesium is a poor antihypertensive and not indicated for this primary purpose, and is now considered inappropriate as a tocolytic for preterm birth. Magnesium therapy can complicate anesthesia, for example by prolonging the effects of nondepolarizing neuromuscular blocking drugs. The most commonly used antihypertensives in obstetrics are hydralazine, labetalol, and nifedipine.

Tocolytics, drugs that decrease uterine tone, are used primarily to delay preterm labor, but also to facilitate cesarean delivery or surgical access during fetal surgery. The use of tocolytics in preterm labor remains controversial. The only FDA-approved drug for preterm labor is the β-receptor agonist ritodrine, although others (terbutaline, salbutamol, nifedipine, cyclooxygenase inhibitors, nitroglycerin, and oxytocin-receptor antagonists) have been used. Oxytocin stimulates uterine contraction, and is used most commonly for induction and augmentation of labor and the management of postpartum bleeding, and also for the induction of abortion.

Whereas some anesthetic techniques used during pregnancy have remained constant for decades and remain so, others are being challenged. Treatment of hypotension from spinal anesthesia was long treated with ephedrine as the vasopressor of choice, based on early studies showing that it did not reduce uterine blood flow as much as other direct α-adrenergic agonists. More recently, direct α-adrenergic agonists such as metaraminol and phenylephrine were found to be effective for managing maternal hypotension, and without adverse neonatal effects, and they may be preferred. For induction of anesthesia in parturients, propofol is widely used, off-label, despite the warning in the product prescribing information. There appears no specific advantage over thiopental in obstetric anesthesia, so this may simply reflect a generalized preference for propofol. For maintenance of anesthesia, however, the ability to rapidly eliminate inhalational drugs from the neonate makes them an inherently more attractive option than propofol for maintenance of anesthesia. Opioids have traditionally not been given until after delivery because of concerns about neonatal respiratory depression. It is possible to use opioids routinely at induction of anesthesia for cesarean delivery, and remifentanil is widely used, off-label, although ideal dosing regimens are still under evaluation.

References

1. Howell PR, Madej TH. Administration of drugs outside of Product Licence: awareness and current practice. *Int J Obstet Anesth* 1999; **8**: 30–6.

2. Food and Drug Administration. Pregnancy and Lactation Labeling. www.fda.gov/Drugs/DevelopmentApprovalProcess/DevelopmentResources/Labeling/ucm093307.htm (accessed June 30, 2010).

3. Landau R. Pharmacogenetics and obstetric anesthesia. *Int Anesthesiol Clin* 2007; **45**: 1–15.

4. Landau R, Morales MA, Antonarakis SE, Blouin JL, Smiley RM. Arg16 homozygosity of the beta2-adrenergic receptor improves the outcome after beta2-agonist tocolysis for preterm labor. *Clin Pharmacol Ther* 2005; **78**: 656–63.

5. Smiley RM, Blouin JL, Negron M, Landau R. Beta2-adrenoceptor genotype affects vasopressor requirements during spinal anesthesia for cesarean delivery. *Anesthesiology* 2006; **104**: 644–50.

6. Philip I, Plantefeve G, Vuillaumier-Barrot S, *et al.* G894T polymorphism in the endothelial nitric oxide synthase gene is associated with an enhanced vascular responsiveness to phenylephrine. *Circulation* 1999; **99**: 3096–8.

7. Landau R, Kern C, Columb MO, Smiley RM, Blouin JL. Genetic variability of the mu-opioid receptor influences intrathecal fentanyl analgesia requirements in laboring women. *Pain* 2008; **139**: 5–14.

8. Sia AT, Lim Y, Lim EC, *et al.* A118G single nucleotide polymorphism of human mu-opioid receptor gene influences pain perception and patient-controlled intravenous morphine consumption after intrathecal morphine for postcesarean analgesia. *Anesthesiology* 2008; **109**: 520–6.

9. Anderson GD. Pregnancy-induced chages in pharmacokinetics. A mechanistic-based approach. *Clin Pharmacokinet* 2005; **44**: 989–1008.

10. Frederiksen MC. Physiological changes in pregnancy and their effect on drug disposition. *Semin Perinatology* 2001; **25**: 120–3.

11. Tracy TS, Venkataramanan R, Glover DD, Caritis SN, National Institute for Child Health and Human Development Network of Maternal-Fetal-Medicine Units. Temporal changes in drug metabolism (CYP1A2, CYP2D6 and CYP3A activity) during pregnancy. *Am J Obstet Gynecol* 2005; **192**: 633–9.

12. Leighton BL, Cheek TG, Gross JB, *et al.* Succinylcholine pharmacodynamics in peripartum patients. *Anesthesiology* 1986; **64**: 202–5.

13. Munnell EW, Taylor HC. Liver blood flow in pregnancy – hepatic vein catheterization. *J Clin Invest* 1947; **26**: 952–6.

14. Robson SC, Mutch E, Boys RJ, Woodhouse KW. Apparent liver blood flow during pregnancy: a serial study using indocyanine green clearance. *Br J Obstet Gynaecol* 1990; **97**: 720–4.

15. Nakai A, Sekiya I, Oya A, Koshino T, Araki T. Assessment of the hepatic arterial and portal venous blood flows during pregnancy with Doppler ultrasonography. *Arch Gynecol Obstet* 2002; **266**: 25–9.

16. Hebert MF, Easterling TR, Kirby B, *et al.* Effects of pregnancy on CYP3A and P-glycoprotein activities as measured by disposition of midazolam and digoxin: a University of Washington specialized center of research study. *Clin Pharm Ther* 2008; **84**: 248–53.

17. Wyska E, Jusko WJ. Approaches to pharmacokietic/pharmacodymanic modeling during pregnancy. *Semin Perinatology* 2001; **25**: 124–32.

18. Andrew MA, Herbert MF, Vicini P. Physiologically based pharmacokinetic model of midzolam disposition during pregnancy. *Conf Proc IEEE Eng Med Biol Soc 2008*; **2008**: 5454–7.

19. Syme MR, Paxton JW, Keelan JA. Drug transfer and metabolism by the human placenta. *Clin Pharmacokinet* 2004; **43**: 487–514.

20. Hill MD, Abramson FP. The significance of plasma protein binding on the fetal/maternal distribution of

drugs at steady state. *Clin Pharmacokinet* 1988; **14**: 156–70.

21. Ito S. Transplacental treatment of fetal tachycardia: implications of drug transporting proteins in placenta. *Semin Perinatology* 2001; **25**: 196–201.

22. Morgan DJ. Drug disposition in mother and foetus. *Clin Exp Pharmacol Physiol* 1997; **24**: 869–73.

23. Alcorn J, McNamara PJ. Pharmacokinetics in the newborn. *Adv Drug Del Rev* 2003; **55**: 667–86.

24. Besunder JB, Reed MD, Blumer JL. Principles of drug biodisposition in the neonate. A clinical evaluation of the pharmacokinetic-pharmacodynamic interface (Part I). *Clin Pharmacokinet* 1988; **14**: 189–216.

25. Ito S, Alcorn A. Xenobiotic transporter expression and function in the human mammary gland. *Adv Drug Del Rev* 2003; **55**: 653–5.

26. Wittels B, Scott DT, Sinatra RS. Exogenous opioids in human breast milk and acute neonatal neurobehavior: a preliminary study. *Anesthesiology* 1990; **73**: 864–9.

27. Wittels B, Glosten B, Faure EA, *et al.* Postcesarean analgesia with both epidural morphine and intravenous patient controlled analgesia: neurobehavioral outcomes among nursing mothers. *Anesth Analg* 1997; **85**: 600–6.

28. Baka NE, Bayoumeu F, Boutroy MJ, Laxenaire MC. Colostrum morphine concentrations during postcesarean intravenous patient-controlled analgesia. *Anesth Analg* 2002; **94**: 184–7.

29. Madadi P, Ross CJD, Hayden MR, *et al.* Pharmacogenetics of neonatal opioid toxicity following maternal use of codeine during breastfeeding: a case-control study. *Clin Pharmacol Ther* 2009; **85**: 31–5.

30. Palahniuk RJ, Shnider SM, Eger EI. Pregnancy decreases the requirement for inhaled anesthetic agents. *Anesthesiology* 1974; **41**: 82–3.

31. Strout CD, Nahrwold ML. Halothane requirement during pregnancy and lactation in rats. *Anesthesiology* 1981; **55**: 322–3.

32. Gin T, Chan MT. Decreased minimum alveolar concentration of isoflurane in pregnant humans. *Anesthesiology* 1994; **81**: 829–32.

33. Chan MT, Mainland P, Gin T. Minimum alveolar concentration of halothane and enflurane are decreased in early pregnancy. *Anesthesiology* 1996; **85**; 782–6.

34. Chan MT, Gin T. Postpartum changes in the minimum alveolar concentration of isoflurane. *Anesthesiology* 1995; **82**: 1360–3.

35. Zhou HH, Norman P, DeLima LG, Mehta M, Bass D. The minimum alveolar concentration of isoflurane in patients undergoing bilateral tubal ligation in the postpartum period. *Anesthesiology* 1995; **82**: 1364–8.

36. Datta S, Migliozzi RP, Flanagan HL, Krieger NR. Chronically administered progesterone decreases halothane requirements in rabbits. *Anesth Analg* 1989; **68**: 46–50.

37. Erden V, Yangin Z, Erkalp K, *et al.* Increased progesterone production during the luteal phase of menstruation may decrease anesthetic requirement. *Anesth Analg* 2005; **101**: 1007–11.

38. Gin T, Chan MTV. Pregnancy reduces the bispectral index during isoflurane anesthesia. *Anesthesiology* 1997; **87**: A305.

39. Chan MT, Gin T. Pregnancy potentiates the sedative effects of sevoflurane. *Anesthesiology* 2008; A616.

40. Gin T, Chan MTV, Lau TK, Lam KK. Pregnancy potentiates the sedative effects of nitrous oxide. *Anesthesiology* 1998; **89**: A1042.

41. Gin T, Mainland P, Chan MTV, Short TG. Decreased thiopental requirements in early pregnancy. *Anesthesiology* 1997; **86**: 73–8.

42. Mongardon N, Servin F, Perrin M, *et al.* Predicted propofol effect-site concentration for induction and emergence of anesthesia during early pregnancy. *Anesth Analg* 2009; **109**: 90–5.

43. Higuchi H, Adachi Y, Arimura S, Kanno M, Satoh T. Early pregnancy does not reduce the C50 of propofol for loss of consciousness. *Anesth Analg* 2001; **93**: 1565–9.

44. Hirabayashi Y, Shimizu R, Saitoh K, Fukuda H. Spread of subarachnoid

methocaine in pregnant women. *Br J Anaesth* 1995; **74**: 384–6.

45. Datta S, Lambert DH, Gregus J, Gissen AJ, Covino BG. Differential sensitivities of mammalian nerve fibres during pregnancy. *Anesth Analg* 1983; **62**: 1070–2.

46. Flanagan HL, Datta S, Lambert DH, Gissen AJ, Covino BG. Effect of pregnancy on bupivacaine-induced conduction blockade in the isolated rabbit vagus nerve. *Anesth Analg* 1987; **66**: 123–6.

47. Buterworth JF, Walker FO, Lysak SZ. Pregnancy increases median nerve susceptibility to lidocaine. *Anesthesiology* 1990; **72**: 962–5.

48. Flanagan HL, Datta S, Moller RA, Covino BG. Effect of exogenously administered progesterone on susceptibility of rabbit vagus nerves to bupivacaine. *Anesthesiology* 1988; **69**: A676.

49. Popitz-Bergez FA, Leeson S, Thalhammer JG, Strichartz GR. Intraneural lidocaine uptake compared with analgesic differences between pregnant and nonpregnant rats. *Reg Anesth* 1997; **22**: 363–71.

50. Arakawa M. Does pregnancy increase the efficacy of lumbar epidural anesthesia? *Int J Obstet Anesth* 2004; **13**: 86–90.

51. Dietz FB, Jaffe RA. Pregnancy does not increase susceptibility to bupivacaine in spinal root axons. *Anesthesiology* 1997; **87**: 610–16.

52. Gintzler AR. Endorphin–mediated increases in pain threshold during pregnancy. *Science* 1980; **210**: 193–5.

53. Jayaram A, Singh P, Carp H. SCH 32615, an enkephalinase inhibitor, enhances pregnancy-induced analgesia in mice. *Anesth Analg* 1995; **80**: 944–8.

54. Gintzler AR, Liu NJ. The maternal spinal cord: biochemical and physiological correlates of steroid-activated antinociceptive processes. *Prog Brain Res* 2001; **133**: 83–97.

55. Carvalho B, Angst MS, Fuller AJ, *et al.* Experimental heat pain for detecting pregnancy-induced analgesia in humans. *Anesth Analg* 2006; **103**: 1283–7.

56. Vercauteren M, Palit S, Soetens F, Jacquemyn Y, Alahuhta

S. Anaesthesiological considerations on tocolytic and uterotonic therapy in obstetrics. *Acta Anaesthesiol Scand* 2009; **53**: 701–9.

57. Collaborative Eclampsia Trial. Which anticonvulsant for women with eclampsia? Evidence from the Collaborative Eclampsia Trial. *Lancet* 1995; **345**: 1455–63.

58. Sibai BM. Magnesium sulfate prophylaxis in preeclampsia: evidence from randomized trials. *Clin Obstet Gynecol* 2005; **48**: 478–88.

59. Fawcett WJ, Haxby EJ, Male DA. Magnesium: physiology and pharmacology. *Br J Anaesth* 1999; **83**: 302–20.

60. Dubé L, Granry JC. The therapeutic use of magnesium in anesthesiology, intensive care and emergency medicine: a review. *Can J Anesth* 2003; **50**: 732–46.

61. James MFM. Magnesium in obstetric anesthesia. *Int J Obstet Anesth* 1998; **7**: 115–23.

62. Idama TO, Lindow SW. Magnesium sulphate: a review of clinical pharmacology applied to obstetrics. *Br J Obstet Gynaecol* 1998; **105**: 260–8.

63. Ashton WB, James MFM, Janicki PK, Uys PC. The control of the hypertensive response to intubation in hypertensive pregnant patients with magnesium sulphate with and without alfentanil. *Br J Anaesth* 1991; **67**: 741–7.

64. Crowther CA, Hiller JE, Doyle LW. Magnesium sulphate for preventing preterm birth in threatened preterm labour. *Cochranr Database Syst Rev* 2002; **4**: CD001060.

65. Grimes DA, Nanda K. Magnesium sulphate tocolysis: time to quit. *Obstet Gynecol* 2006; **108**: 986–9.

66. Doyle LW, Crowther CA, Middleton P, Marret S, Rouse D. Magnesium sulphate for women at risk of preterm birth for neuroprotection of the fetus. *Cochrane Database Syst Rev* 2009; **1**: CD004661.

67. Euser AG, Cipolla MJ. Magnesium sulfate for the treatment of eclampsia. A brief review. *Stroke* 2009; **40**: 1169–75.

68. Lu JF, Nightingale CH. Magnesium sulfate in eclampsia and pre-eclampsia: pharmacokinetic principles. *Clin Pharmacokinet* 2000; **38**: 305–14.

69. Duley L, Henderson-Smart DJ, Meher S. Drugs for treatment of very high blood pressure during pregnancy. *Cochrane Database Syst Rev* 2006; **3**: CD001449.

70. López Bernal A. The regulation of uterine relaxation. *Semin Cell Dev Biol* 2007; **18**: 340–7.

71. Simhan HN, Caritis SN. Prevention of preterm delivery. *N Engl J Med* 2007; **357**: 477–87.

72. Lamont RF. The pathophysiology of pulmonary oedema with the use of beta-agonists. *Br J Obstet Gynaecol* 2000; **107**: 439–44.

73. Lee HJ, Macbeth AH, Pagani JH, Young WS. Oxytocin: the great facilitator of life. *Prog Neurobiol* 2009; **88**: 127–51.

74. Leng G, Meddle SL, Douglas AJ. Oxytocin and the maternal brain. *Clin Opin Pharmacol* 2008; **8**: 731–4.

75. Maybauer MO, Maybauer DM, Enkhbaatar P, Traber DL. Physiology of the vasopressin receptors. *Best Pract Res Clin Anaesthesiol* 2008; **22**: 253–63.

76. Clark SL, Simpson KR, Knox GE, Garite TJ. Oxytocin: new perspectives on an old drug. *Am J Obstet Gynecol* 2009; **200**: 35.e1–6.

77. *Why Mothers Die 1997–1999: the Confidential Enquiries into Maternal Deaths in the United Kingdom.* RCOG Press, London 2001.

78. Schiff PL. Ergot and its alkaloids. *Am J Pharm Educ* 2006; **70**: 98.

79. Haarmann T, Rolke Y, Giesbert S, Tudzynski P. Ergot: from witchcraft to biotechnology. *Mol Plant Pathol* 2009; **10**: 563–77.

80. Chabbert-Buffet N, Meduri G, Bouchard P, Spitz IM. Selective progesterone receptor modulators and progesterone antagonists: mechanisms of action and clinical applications. *Hum Reprod Update* 2005; **11**: 293–307.

81. The Practice Committee of the American Society for Reproductive Medicine. Gonadotropin preparations: past, present, and future perspectives. *Fertil Steril* 2008; **90**: S13–20.

82. Avecillas JF, Falcone T, Arroliga AC. Ovarian hyperstimulation syndrome. *Crit Care Clin* 2004; **20**: 679–95.

83. Ralston DH, Shnider SM, deLorimier AA. Effects of equipotent ephedrine, metaraminol, mephentermine, and methoxamine on uterine blood flow in the pregnant ewe. *Anesthesiology* 1974; **40**: 354–70.

84. Lee A, Ngan Kee WD, Gin T. Prophylactic ephedrine prevents hypotension during spinal anesthesia for Cesarean delivery but does not improve neonatal outcome: a quantitative systematic review. *Can J Anaesth* 2002; **49**: 588–99.

85. Lee A, Ngan Kee WD, Gin T. Dose-response meta-analysis of prophylactic intravenous ephedrine for the prevention of hypotension during spinal anesthesia for elective cesarean delivery. *Anesth Analg* 2004; **98**: 483–90.

86. Critchley LA, Short TG, Gin T. Hypotension during subarachnoid anaesthesia: haemodynamic analysis of three treatments. *Br J Anaesth* 1994; **72**: 151–5.

87. Park GE, Haunch MA, Curlin F, Datta S, Bader AM. The effects of varying volumes of crystalloid administration before cesarean delivery on maternal hemodynamics and colloid osmotic pressure. *Anesth Analg* 1996; **83**: 299–303.

88. Tsen LC, Boosalis P, Segal S, Datta S, Bader AM. *J Clin Anesth* 2000; **12**: 378–82.

89. Ngan Kee WD, Lau TK, Khaw KS, Lee BB. Comparison of metaraminol and ephedrine infusions for maintaining arterial pressure during spinal anesthesia for elective cesarean section. *Anesthesiology* 2001; **95**: 307–13.

90. Cooper DW, Carpenter M, Mowbray P, *et al.* Fetal and maternal effects of phenylephrine and ephedrine during spinal anesthesia for cesarean delivery. *Anesthesiology* 2002; **97**: 1582–90.

91. Lee A, Ngan Kee WD, Gin T. A quantitative systematic review of randomized controlled trials of ephedrine versus phenylephrine for the management of hypotension during spinal anesthesia for cesarean delivery. *Anesth Analg* 2002; **94**: 920–6.

92. Ngan Kee WD, Khaw KS, Tan PE, Ng FF, Karmakar MK. Placental transfer and fetal metabolic effects of phenylephrine and ephedrine during spinal anesthesia for cesarean delivery. *Anesthesiology* 2009; **111**: 506–12.

961

93. Riley ET. Spinal anaesthesia for caesarean delivery: keep the pressure up and don't spare the vasoconstrictors. *Br J Anaesth* 2004; **92**: 459–61.

94. Ngan Kee WD, Tam YH, Khaw KS, *et al.* Closed-loop feedback computer controlled infusion of phenylephrine for maintaining blood pressure during spinal anesthesia for caesarean section: a preliminary descriptive study. *Anaesthesia* 2007; **62**: 1251–6.

95. Ngan Kee WD, Lee A, Khaw KS, *et al.* A randomized double-blinded comparison of phenylephrine and ephedrine infusion combinations to maintain blood pressure during spinal anesthesia for cesarean delivery: the effects on fetal acid-base status and hemodynmaic control. *Anesth Analg* 2008; **107**: 1295–302.

96. Ngan Kee WD, Khaw KS, Lau TK, *et al.* Randomised double-blinded comparison of phenylephrine and ephedrine for maintaining blood pressure during spinal anaesthesia for non-elective caesarean section. *Anaesthesia* 2008; **63**: 1319–26.

97. Anaesthesia-AZ: Diprivan. AstraZeneca. www.anaesthesia-az.com/510827/510897?itemId=676595 (accessed June 30, 2010).

98. Diprivan. www1.astrazeneca-us.com/PI/diprivan.pdf (accessed June 30, 2010).

99. Celleno D, Capogna G, Tomassetti M, *et al.* Neurobehavioural effects of propofol on the neonate following elective caesarean section. *Brit J Anaesth* 1989; **62**: 649–54.

100. Celleno D, Capogna G, Emanuelli M, *et al.* Which induction drug for Cesarean section? A comparison of thiopental sodium, propofol and midazolam. *J Clin Anesth* 1993; **5**: 284–8.

101. Moore J, Bill KM, Flynn RJ, McKeating KT, Howard PJ. A comparison between propofol and thiopentone as induction agents in obstetric anaesthesia. *Anaesthesia* 1989; **44**: 753–7.

102. Valtonen M, Kanto J, Rosenberg P. Comparison of propofol and thiopentone for induction of anaesthesia for elective caesarean section. *Anaesthesia* 1989; **44**: 758–62.

103. Gin T, O'Meara ME, Kan AF, *et al.* Plasma catecholamines and neonatal condition after induction of anaesthesia with propofol or thiopentone at caesarean section. *Br J Anaesth* 1993; **70**: 311–16.

104. Gin T. Propofol during pregnancy. *Acta Anaesthesiologica Sin* 1994; **32**: 127–32.

105. Shin YK, Kim YD, Collea JV. The effect of propofol on isolated human prenant uterine muscle. *Anesthesiology* 1998; **89**: 105–9.

106. Gin T, Yau G, Jong W, *et al.* Disposition of propofol at caesarean section and in the postpartum period. *Br J Anaesth* 1991; **67**: 49–53.

107. Dailland P, Cockshott ID, Lirzin JD, *et al.* Intravenous propofol during Cesarean section: placental transfer, concentrations in breast milk and neonatal effects. A preliminary study. *Anesthesiology* 1989; **71**: 827–34.

108. Duggal K. Propofol should be the induction agent of choice for caesarean section under general anaesthesia. *Int J Obstet Anesth* 2003; **12**: 275–6.

109. Yau G, Gin T, Ewart MC, *et al.* Propofol for induction and maintenance of anaesthesia at caesarean section. A comparison with thiopentone/enflurane. *Anaesthesia* 1991; **46**: 20–3.

110. Abboud TK, Zhu J, Richardson M, *et al.* Intravenous propofol vs thiamylal-isoflurane for caesarean section, comparative maternal and neonatal effects. *Acta Anaesthesiol Scand* 1995; **39**: 205–9.

111. Gin T, Yau G, Chan K, Gregory MA, Oh TE. Disposition of propofol infusions for caesarean section. *Can J Anaesth* 1991; **38**: 31–6.

112. Gregory MA, Gin T, Yau G, *et al.* Propofol infusion anaesthesia for caesarean section. *Can J Anaesth* 1990; **37**: 514–20.

113. Glass PSA. Anesthetic drug interactions: an insight into general anesthesia – its mechanism and dosing strategies. *Anesthesiology* 1998; **88**: 5–6.

114. Kovac AL. Controlling the hemodynamic response to laryngoscopy and endotracheal intubation. *J Clin Anesth* 1996; **8**: 63–79.

115. Loughran PG, Moore J, Dundee JW. Maternal stress response associated with caesarean delivery under general and epidural anaesthesia. *Br J Obstet Gynecol* 1986; **93**: 943–9.

116. Jouppila P, Kuikka J, Jouppila R, Hollmén A. Effect of induction of general anesthesia for cesarean section on intervillous blood flow. *Acta Obstet Gynecol Scand* 1979; **58**: 249–53.

117. Gin T, Ngan Kee WD, Siu YK, *et al.* Alfentanil given immediately before the induction of anesthesia for elective cesarean delivery. *Anesth Analg* 2000; **90**: 1167–72.

118. Ngan Kee WD, Khaw KS, Ma KC, *et al.* Maternal and neonatal effects of remifentanil at induction of general anesthesia for cesarean delivery. *Anesthesiology* 2006; **104**: 14–20.

119. Draisci G, Valente A, Suppa E, *et al.* Remifentanil for cesarean section under general anesthesia: effects on maternal stress hormone secretion and neonatal well-being: a randomized trial. *Int J Obstet Anesth* 2008; **17**: 130–6.

120. Van de Velde M, Teunkens A, Kuypers M, Dewinter T, Vandermeersch E. General anaesthesia with target controlled infusion of propofol for planned caesarean section: maternal and neonatal effects of a remifentanil-based technique. *Int J Obstet Anesth* 2004; **13**: 153–8.

121. Hill D. The use of remifentanil in obstetrics. *Anesthesiol Clin* 2008; **26**: 169–82.

Section 3
Chapter
59

Essential drugs in anesthetic practice
Antimicrobial therapy

Conan MacDougall, B. Joseph Guglielmo, and Jeanine Wiener-Kronish

Introduction

Approximately half of all hospitalized patients, including the vast majority of those undergoing surgical procedures, receive at least one antimicrobial drug during their hospital stay [1]. As a result, understanding the spectrum of activity, pharmacokinetics, toxicities, and drug interactions of antimicrobials is essential in the surgical suite or the critical care setting. Increasing antimicrobial resistance also complicates antimicrobial selection. While the development pipeline for antiretrovirals, antifungals, and antibacterials targeting Gram-positive pathogens is robust, there is a paucity of upcoming drugs targeting Gram-negative bacteria [2]. Considering the development of multidrug resistance among the latter pathogens, appropriate antimicrobial use is essential to preserve the activity of currently available drugs. This chapter aims to equip the reader with a fundamental understanding of antimicrobial clinical pharmacology, and to address some of the important scenarios in which anesthesiologists are asked to select antimicrobial therapy.

Overview of mechanisms of action and preclinical pharmacology

Major antimicrobial targets

Most antibacterial targets have been discovered not through rational drug design but through "reverse engineering" those natural products found to have antibacterial activity through exhaustive screening programs. The major targets of **antibacterials** are listed in Table 59.1. Targets of **antifungals** and **antivirals** are discussed in their respective sections.

Predictors of antimicrobial effect

The most common in-vitro predictor of antimicrobial effect is the minimum inhibitory concentration (MIC), i.e., the lowest antimicrobial concentration which prevents visible bacterial growth in liquid medium (Fig. 59.1). Each antimicrobial/ organism pair is associated with a specific MIC at which the

organism is considered susceptible, i.e., the **breakpoint** [3]. For example, the breakpoint for susceptibility for ceftriaxone for *E. coli* is 8 µg mL^{-1}, while for *Streptococcus pneumoniae*, it is 0.5 mg dL^{-1}. While different antibiotics achieve substantially different serum and tissue concentrations, the antibiotic with the lowest MIC is generally the best choice.

The inhibition quantified by the MIC may be associated with inhibition of bacterial growth without killing the organism (a **bacteriostatic** effect) or rendering the organisms nonviable (a **bactericidal** effect) [4]. Bactericidal activity is determined by taking a sample of the broth at the MIC and below and spreading the broth on agar plates (Fig. 59.1). The number of bacterial colonies on the plates is counted and the concentration corresponding to a 99.9% reduction in the original bacterial inoculums is the minimum bactericidal concentration (MBC). In general, if the MBC is four times the MIC or less, the drug is considered to be bactericidal; if the MBC/MIC ratio is greater than four, it is considered bacteriostatic. For certain infections, including endocarditis, meningitis, and infections in neutropenic patients, bactericidal therapy is preferred. Table 59.1 lists drugs as either bacteriostatic or bactericidal. However, static/cidal activity can vary by pathogen.

Antimicrobials also differ in how they manifest their effects with respect to time and concentration (pharmacokinetic/ pharmacodynamic relationships) (Fig. 59.2) [5]. For some antimicrobials, continually increasing drug concentration above the MIC predictably increases killing: these drugs are considered to have **concentration-dependent** activity. Antibacterial effect for these drugs is often best predicted by the peak-concentration to MIC ratio (**peak/MIC**). For other drugs, there is a ceiling effect at approximately 4 × MIC; increasing the concentration beyond this point does not lead to increased killing. For these drugs, considered to have **time-dependent** activity, the duration that the drug concentration remains above the MIC (**time > MIC**) is usually predictive of efficacy. For some drugs from these two groups, the ratio of the total drug exposure (area under the curve, AUC) to MIC (**AUC/ MIC**) is the best predictor of efficacy. The practical implications of these findings are in the design of antibiotic dosing

Anesthetic Pharmacology, 2nd edition, ed. Alex S. Evers, Mervyn Maze, Evan D. Kharasch. Published by Cambridge University Press. © Cambridge University Press 2011.

Table 59.1. Antibacterial targets and pharmacodynamics by drug class

Target and group	Drugs	Mechanism	Pharmacodynamics
Cell wall			
β-Lactams	Penicillins, cephalosporins, carbapenems, monobactams	Inhibition of transpeptidases responsible for peptidoglycan cross-linking → loss of structural integrity	Bactericidal Time-dependent Time > MIC
Glycopeptides	Vancomycin	Inhibition of peptidoglycan cross-linking by steric inhibition → loss of structural integrity	Bactericidal Time-dependent AUC/MIC
Cell membrane			
Lipopeptides	Daptomycin	Destabilization of inner cell membrane → leakage of ions and membrane depolarization	Bactericidal Concentration-dependent Peak/MIC
Polymyxins	Colistin, polymyxin B	Disruption of outer cell membrane of Gram-negative bacteria → altered cell membrane permeability	Bactericidal Concentration-dependent Peak/MIC
Ribosome			
Aminoglycosides	Gentamicin, tobramycin, amikacin, streptomycin	Binding to 30S ribosomal subunit → inhibition of protein synthesis, production of mistranslated proteins	Bactericidal Concentration-dependent Peak/MIC
Macrolides	Azithromycin, clarithromycin, erythromycin	Binding to 50S ribosomal subunit → inhibition of protein synthesis	Bacteriostatic Time-dependent AUC/MIC or Time > MIC
Tetracyclines & Glycylcyclines	Doxycycline, tigecycline	Binding to 30S ribosomal subunit → inhibition of protein synthesis	Bacteriostatic Time-dependent AUC/MIC
Oxazolidinones	Linezolid	Binding to 50S ribosomal subunit → inhibition of protein synthesis	Bacteriostatic Time-dependent AUC/MIC or Time > MIC
Streptogramins	Quinupristin/ dalfoprstin	Sequential binding to 50S ribosomal subunit → synergistic inhibition of protein synthesis	Bactericidal/static Time-dependent AUC/MIC
Lincosamides	Clindamycin	Binding to 50S ribosomal subunit → inhibition of protein synthesis	Bacteriostatic Time-dependent Time > MIC
DNA synthesis and structure			
Fluoroquinolones	Ciprofloxacin, levofloxacin, moxifloxacin	Inhibition of bacterial topoisomerases, preventing DNA uncoiling → DNA strand breakage	Bactericidal Concentration-dependent AUC/MIC
Antifolates	Trimethoprim/ sulfa-methoxazole	Sequential inhibition of nucleotide precursors → interruption of DNA synthesis	Bactericidal Concentration-dependent Peak/MIC
Nitroimidazoles	Metronidazole	Generation of free radicals → DNA destabilization and strand breakage	Bactericidal Concentration-dependent Peak/MIC

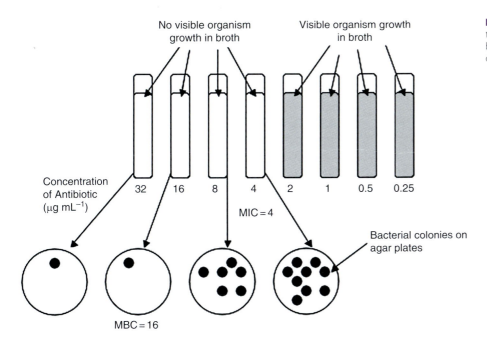

No visible organism growth in broth

Visible organism growth in broth

Concentration of Antibiotic (μg mL⁻¹)

32 16 8 4 2 1 0.5 0.25

MIC = 4

Bacterial colonies on agar plates

MBC = 16

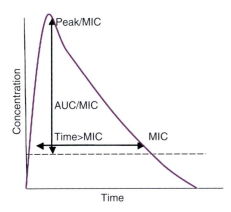

Figure 59.2. Pharmacokinetic/pharmacodynamic parameters. AUC, area under the concentration–time curve; MIC, minimum inhibitory concentration.

Peak/MIC

AUC/MIC

Time>MIC   MIC

Concentration

Time

schedules. Aminoglycosides generally should be administered as a single large dose daily to leverage the concentration-dependent activity [6]. In contrast, β-lactam drugs, such as ceftazidime, may be administered as continuous infusions because of their time-dependent activity [7,8], and vancomycin dosing should be tailored to maximize the AUC/MIC ratio [9,10]. Considering the increased recognition of the importance of pharmacokinetic/pharmacodynamic parameters to outcome, individualization of antimicrobial dosing will become an important consideration in designing dosage regimens, particularly in critically ill patients.

Principles of antimicrobial allergy

Allergic reactions, particularly to β-lactams, are among the most common and important toxicities of antimicrobial drugs. As an example, up to 10% of patients report a "penicillin allergy" [11–13]. However, the nature of allergic reactions is often poorly documented, is subject to inaccurate recall by patients, varies greatly in severity and clinical importance, and may change over time [11–13]. Documentation of the nature and timing of the initial reaction and whether the patient has been re-exposed to the drug are crucial in determining the clinical significance of an allergy. Patients inaccurately labeled with allergies face a restricted choice of antimicrobials for future infections, possibly leading to suboptimal therapy. While avoiding rechallenge with an individual drug allergen is relatively straightforward, many antimicrobials share a common pharmacophore, which makes the administration of structurally related drugs potentially perilous. This problem of cross-reactivity has been most thoroughly investigated for β-lactams [14]. Estimates of the probability of cross-reactivity are available only for patients with known penicillin allergies who receive cephalosporins or carbapenems, and vary widely. For patients with a penicillin allergy, the likelihood of allergic reaction to cephalosporins has been variably reported, ranging from 1% to almost 20%; for patients receiving carbapenems, from 10% to 50% [14–17]. However, the probability of cross-reactivity between cephalosporins and carbapenems, or the probability of those with a documented cephalosporin allergy reacting to a penicillin, has not been extensively investigated. Further, many of these studies have relied on patient self-report of allergy rather than using antigen skin testing. The monobactam class (aztreonam) has a unique pharmacophore and is generally considered to have a low risk of cross-reactivity with penicillins and cephalosporins (ceftazidime, which has an identical side chain to aztreonam, may be an exception [18]), although published clinical experience with this drug in β-lactam-allergic patients is limited [19–21]. Cross-allergenicity between drugs in other classes (e.g., fluoroquinolones) is far less well defined.

Antimicrobial drugs

The following sections review the clinical pharmacology of antimicrobial drugs. Clinicians should note particularly that spectrum of activity may be variable by geographic area, patient-care site (ambulatory versus inpatient), and patient-specific risk factors. Whenever possible, data on local antimicrobial susceptibility patterns should be incorporated into decision-making when selecting antimicrobial therapy. Because of space limitations, the general pharmacologic characteristics of the antimicrobials will not be extensively referenced; readers are referred to excellent texts in infectious diseases therapy for more in-depth information [22–25].

Antibacterials: cell-wall-active drugs

β-Lactams: penicillins
Spectrum of activity

The spectrum of activity of the penicillin class of β-lactams steadily increases proceeding from the oldest to the newest drugs (Table 59.2). The spectrum of the **natural penicillins** (various salts of penicillin G and V) has diminished over time due to antimicrobial resistance, but these drugs still possess potent activity against most streptococci, including *S. pyogenes* and *S. pneumoniae*, and the most common enterococcal species, *E. faecalis*. Most (~ 90%) strains of *Staphylococcus aureus* produce a β-lactamase that inactivates penicillin, although for isolates that have documented susceptibility, penicillin is an option. The **antistaphylococcal penicillins** (nafcillin, oxacillin, dicloxacillin, methicillin) are stable to the staphylococcal β-lactamase and reliably active against non-methicillin-resistant (MRSA) strains. The activity of the antistaphylococcal penicillins is otherwise similar to the natural penicillins, but they have no activity against enterococci.

The **aminopenicillins** (ampicillin, amoxicillin) have similar activity against streptococci and enterococci as the natural penicillins, as well as modest Gram-negative activity including non-β-lactamase producing *Haemophilus influenzae*, *Proteus mirabilis*, and some isolates of *E. coli*. Activity against most Gram-negative bacilli is limited by the production of β-lactamases, so the formulation of these aminopenicillins into combinations with β-lactamase inhibitors (ampicillin/sulbactam, amoxicillin/clavulanate) greatly expands their spectrum of activity, including *Klebsiella pneumoniae*, *Bacteroides fragilis*, and methicillin-susceptible *Staphylococcus aureus* (MSSA). The broadest-spectrum penicillins are the **antipseudomonal penicillins** combined with β-lactamase inhibitors (piperacillin/tazobactam, ticarcillin/clavulanate). These drugs expand the Gram-negative activity of the aminopenicillin/β-lactamase inhibitor combinations by adding activity against *Pseudomonas aeruginosa* and some *Enterobacter*, *Citrobacter*, and *Serratia marsescens*.

Pharmacokinetics, toxicity, and drug interactions

Oral absorption of the penicillins, while good, is associated with substantial interpatient variability. The procaine and benzathine forms of penicillin are designed to provide a slow, steady release of drug over days to weeks when given as an intramuscular administration. Penicillins are eliminated primarily through renal excretion and require dosage adjustment in renal dysfunction, with the exception of the antistaphylococcal penicillins (nafcillin, oxacillin) (Table 59.3).

Adverse effects are generally similar between the various penicillins. Administration of the oral forms of these drugs frequently causes mild to moderate gastrointestinal distress; this complication is more common for amoxicillin/clavulanate. Rashes are also frequent, usually manifesting as maculopapular eruptions. Peculiar to the aminopenicillins is the "ampicillin rash," a maculopapular reaction occurring frequently (25–100%) among patients receiving aminopenicillins, particularly with concomitant viral illness (especially mononucleosis) or leukemia, or who are taking allopurinol [26]. If rechallenged in the absence of the aforementioned predisposing conditions, in most instances the rash will not recur. Neutropenia (primarily nafcillin) and interstitial nephritis (primarily methicillin) also occur. High-dose penicillins are associated with seizures, hypokalemia, and inhibition of platelet aggregation, particularly in the face of renal failure. Immediate hypersensitivity reactions, including anaphylaxis, occur in approximately 0.05% of the population receiving natural penicillins. Patients who experience anaphylaxis due to a penicillin should receive other β-lactams only under special circumstances (see *Principles of antimicrobial allergy*, above).

Clinically significant drug interactions with the penicillins, and most β-lactams, are minimal (Table 59.3). Probenecid blocks tubular secretion of some β-lactams, prolonging their half-life. Aminoglycosides can provide synergistic killing of organisms when combined with cell-wall-active drugs; penicillin–aminoglycoside combinations are regularly used for treatment of certain severe infections (e.g., enterococcal endocarditis).

β-Lactams: cephalosporins
Spectrum of activity

The cephalosporins are divided into "generations," largely on the basis of their spectrum of activity (Table 59.4). However, there may be substantial differences between individual drugs within each generation. The most commonly used **first-generation cephalosporins** are cefazolin (parenteral) and cephalexin (oral). These drugs are active against streptococci and MSSA. Like all currently available cephalosporins, they are inactive against MRSA, all enterococci, and *Listeria* species. Their Gram-negative activity is limited to variable coverage of *Proteus*, *E. coli*, and *Klebsiella*. The **second-generation cephalosporins**, such as cefuroxime, expand upon the Gram-negative activity of the first-generation: their spectrum includes *Haemophilus influenzae* as well as *Neisseria* spp.

Table 59.2. Spectrum of activity of penicillins

Organism	Drug				
	Penicillin	*Nafcillin*	*Ampicillin Amoxicillin*	*Amp/sulbactam Amox/clavulante*	*Piperacillin/tazobactam*
Gram-positive					
Streptococus pyogenes	++	++	++	++	++
Streptococcus pneumoniae	++	++	++	++	++
Viridans streptococci	++	++	++	++	++
Staph aureus (MSSA)	–	++	–	++	++
Staph aureus (MRSA)	×	×	×	×	×
Enterococcus faecalis	++	–	++	++	++
Enterococcus faecium (VRE)	–	–	–	–	–
Gram-negative					
H. influenzae	–	–	+	++	++
Proteus mirabilis	×	×	+	++	++
E. coli	×	×	–	++	++
Klebsiella spp.	×	×	×	+	+++
Serratia	×	×	×	+	++
Pseudomonas	×	×	×	×	++
Entero/Citro/Acinetobacter	×	×	×	–	++
Bacteroides fragilis	–	–	–	++	++

++, drug of choice and/or reliable susceptibility; +, alternative drug and/or variable susceptibility; – , rare in-vitro activity, not reliable for empiric therapy; ×, intrinsic resistance.

Table 59.3. Pharmacokinetics, toxicity, and drug interactions of penicillins

Drug	Dose adjustment in organ dysfunction	Toxicity/drug interactions
Penicillin G IV (generic)	Renal	*Common*: nausea/vomiting/diarrhea
Penicillin VK PO (generic)		*Uncommon*: rash, neutropenia
Penicillin G benzathine IM		*Rare*: anaphylaxis, encephalopathy, seizures, interstitial nephritis
Penicillin G procaine IM		
Nafcillin IV	Combined renal + hepatic	
Dicloxacillin PO		Drug interactions
Amoxicillin PO	Renal	*Probenecid*: increased serum levels of penicillins
Ampicillin IV, PO		
Amoxicillin/clavulanate PO (Augmentin)	Renal	
Ampicillin/sulbactam IV (Unasyn)		
Piperacillin/tazobactam IV (Zosyn)	Renal	

Table 59.4. Spectrum of activity of cephalosporins

Organism	Drug				
	1st-Gen	**2nd-Gen**	**3rd-Gen**		**4th-Gen**
	Cefazolin	Cefuroxime	Ceftriaxone Ceftriaxone	Ceftazidime	Cefepime
Gram-positive					
Streptococus pyogenes	++	++	++	++	++
Streptococcus pneumoniae	++	+	++	+	++
Viridans streptococci	++	+	++	–	++
Staph aureus (MSSA)	++	+	+	–	++
Staph aureus (MRSA)	×	×	×	×	×
Enterococcus faecalis	×	×	×	×	×
Enterococcus faecium (VRE)	×	×	×	×	×
Gram-negative					
H. influenzae	–	+	++	++	++
Proteus mirabilis	+	++	++	++	++
E. coli	+	+	++	++	++
Klebsiella spp.	+	+	++	++	++
Serratia	–	–	++	++	++
Pseudomonas	×	×	×	++	++
Entero/Citro/Acinetobacter	×	–	+	+	++
Bacteroides fragilis	×	×	×	×	×

++, drug of choice and/or reliable susceptibility; +, alternative drug and/or variable susceptibility, – , rare in vitro activity, not reliable for empiric therapy; ×, intrinsic resistance.

The Gram-positive potency of most second-generation drugs is reduced relative to the first-generation drugs. However, cefuroxime is equal in Gram-positive activity when compared with first-generation drugs. Two cephamycins (drugs structurally very similar to cephalosporins), cefoxitin and cefotetan, are grouped with the second-generation cephalosporins. Their distinguishing characteristic is enhanced activity against *Bacteroides fragilis*. The **third-generation cephalosporins**, such as cefotaxime and ceftriaxone, combine broad coverage of many aerobic Gram-negative pathogens, with the most notable exception of *Pseudomonas*, with good activity against *Streptococcus pneumoniae*. In contrast, ceftazidime has good antipseudomonal activity but poor activity against streptococci and staphylococci. The **fourth-generation cephalosporin** cefepime combines many of the characteristics of ceftriaxone and ceftazidime, with broad Gram-positive and Gram-negative coverage, including third-generation resistant pathogens, such as *Pseudomonas* and *Enterobacter*. A potential **fifth-generation cephalosporin**, ceftobiprole, is in clinical trials.

This drug is similar to cefepime but uniquely active against MRSA and enterococci.

Pharmacokinetics, toxicity, and drug interactions

Only a few cephalosporins are available as both intravenous and oral dosage formulations. Considering that oral drugs in a given generation generally have lower MICs than the intravenous drugs, and variable oral bioavailability, caution should be taken when transitioning a patient from intravenous to oral cephalosporins. Most cephalosporins are eliminated primarily through renal excretion and require dosage adjustment in renal dysfunction; ceftriaxone is eliminated via biliary mechanisms (Table 59.5).

The toxicity profile of cephalosporins overlaps generally with those of penicillins (Table 59.5). Allergic reactions, including immediate hypersensitivity reactions, occur with cephalosporins, although the incidence of these reactions is lower than that observed with penicillins. Some toxicities unique to particular drugs are worth highlighting. Ceftriaxone

Table 59.5. Pharmacokinetics, toxicity, and drug interactions of cephalosporins

Drug	Dose adjustment in organ dysfunction	Toxicity/drug interactions
1st-generation cephalosporins	Renal	*Common*: nausea/vomiting/diarrhea
Cefazolin IV		*Uncommon*: rash, neutropenia
Cephalexin PO		*Rare*: anaphylaxis, encephalopathy, seizures, interstitial nephritis, bleeding (cefotetan), biliary sludging (ceftriaxone)
2nd-generation cephalosporins	Combined renal + hepatic	
Cefuroxime IV, PO		
Cefoxitin IV		Drug interactions
Cefotetan IV		Minimal
3rd-generation cephalosporins	Renal	
Ceftriaxone IV		
Cefotaxime IV		
Ceftazidime IV		
4th-generation cephalosporins	Renal	
Cefepime IV		

Table 59.6. Spectrum of activity of monobactams and carbapenems

Organism	Drug		
	Aztreonam	Ertapenem	Imipenem Meropenem
Gram-positive			
Streptococus pyogenes	×	++	++
Streptococcus pneumoniae	×	++	++
Viridans streptococci	×	++	++
Staph aureus (MSSA)	×	++	++
Staph aureus (MRSA)	×	×	×
Enterococcus faecalis	×	×	+
Enterococcus faecium (VRE)	×	×	×
Gram-negative			
H. influenzae	++	++	++
Proteus mirabilis	++	++	++
E. coli	++	++	++
Klebsiella spp.	++	++	++
Serratia	++	++	++
Pseudomonas	++	×	++
Entero/Citro/Acinetobacter	+	+	++
Bacteroides fragilis	–	++	++

++, drug of choice and/or reliable susceptibility; +, alternative drug and/or variable susceptibility, – , rare in vitro activity, not reliable for empiric therapy; ×, intrinsic resistance.

has been associated with metastatic precipitation in neonates, due to complexing with ionic calcium [27]. Ceftriaxone also displaces bilirubin from serum albumin, and has been associated with jaundice in neonates, particularly those with pre-existing hyperbilirubinemia [28]. Consequently, cefotaxime is preferred in this patient population. Cefotetan possesses a side chain that can interfere with prothrombin, prolonging the prothrombin time with potential bleeding risk. This effect is reversible with administration of vitamin K.

β-Lactams: monobactams
Spectrum of activity
The spectrum of activity of the one monobactam, aztreonam, closely parallels that of ceftazidime, possessing potent Gram-negative (including antispseudomonal) activity (Table 59.6). However, aztreonam is completely inactive against Gram-positive organisms.

Pharmacokinetics, toxicity, and drug interactions
Aztreonam is administered parenterally and is eliminated via the kidneys (Table 59.7). Its most distinguishing feature is its low incidence of cross-allergenicity with other β-lactams, such that patients with documented anaphylactic reactions to other β-lactams have safely received aztreonam [19–21]. This is due to the different structure of the β-lactam ring of monobactams. One caution is that aztreonam and ceftazidime share identical chemical side chains off the β-lactam ring, and allergic reactions to aztreonam have been observed in patients whose hypersensitivity is to the ceftazidime side chain [18]. Otherwise aztreonam toxicity follows the generic adverse effect profile of β-lactams (rash, rare neutropenia).

Table 59.7. Pharmacokinetics, toxicity, and drug interactions of monobactams and carbapenems

Drug	Dose adjustment in organ dysfunction	Toxicity/drug interactions
Aztreonam IV (Azactam)	Renal	*Common*: nausea/vomiting/diarrhea
Imipenem IV (Primaxin)	Renal	*Uncommon*: rash, neutropenia
Meropenem IV (Merrem)		*Rare*: anaphylaxis, encephalopathy, seizures (especially imipenem), interstitial nephritis
Ertapenem IV (Invanz)		
		Drug interactions Minimal

Table 59.8. Spectrum of activity of glycopeptides and lipopeptides

Organism	Drug	
	Vancomycin	*Daptomycin*
Gram-positive		
Streptococus pyogenes	++	++
Streptococcus pneumoniae	++	++
Viridans streptococci	++	++
Staph aureus (MSSA)	++	++
Staph aureus (MRSA)	++	++
Enterococcus faecalis	++	++
Enterococcus faecium (VRE)	++	+

++, drug of choice and/or reliable susceptibility; +, alternative drug and/or variable susceptibility.

β-Lactams: carbapenems
Spectrum of activity

Carbapenems are the broadest-spectrum β-lactam drugs available (Table 59.6). The drugs imipenem, meropenem, and doripenem have excellent activity against both aerobic and anaerobic Gram-positive and Gram-negative organisms. They are generally active against strains of *Acinetobacter*, *Enterobacter*, *Pseudomonas*, *E. coli*, and *Klebsiella* resistant to other β-lactam drugs. Among common pathogens, only MRSA and *Enterococcus faecium* are consistently resistant to these drugs. Differences in activity between imipenem, meropenem, and doripenem are minor; however, there are major differences between these drugs and ertapenem. Ertapenem is a "narrow-spectrum" carbapenem in that it lacks activity against *Acinetobacter*, *Pseudomonas*, and *Enterococcus faecalis*.

Pharmacokinetics, toxicity, and drug interactions

The carbapenems are all intravenously administered and eliminated via the kidneys (Table 59.7). It should be noted that imipenem is coformulated with cilastatin, which inhibits renal dihydropeptidase, thus prolonging imipenem's half-life; cilastatin does not have antibacterial activity. Ertapenem has the longest half-life of the carbapenems, allowing for convenient once-daily dosing. Hypersensitivity reactions to carbapenems occur, with a higher risk among patients with pre-existing β-lactam allergies (although the precise incidence of cross-allergenicity is not well characterized) [16]. Central nervous system adverse effects, including seizures, may be more common with the carbapenems at doses used clinically than other β-lactams [29]. The risk appears to be highest with imipenem, lower with meropenem, and unclear for ertapenem and doripenem, although estimates of risk are generally derived from studies that did not compare the drugs directly [30,31]. Risk factors for seizures include the presence of a pre-existing seizure disorder and excessive drug exposure, particularly large doses in renal failure. Meropenem has been safely used in patients with meningitis [32], while imipenem is contraindicated in these patients because of enhanced seizure risk.

Glycopeptides
Spectrum of activity

Vancomycin, the predominant glycopeptide in clinical use in the United States, has activity against the vast majority of aerobic Gram-positive organisms (Table 59.8) and historically has been the standard treatment of severe infections due to MRSA. High-level resistance to vancomycin is extremely rare in *Staphylococcus aureus*. However, a rise in isolates with intermediate resistance to vancomycin has been described by some investigators [33,34]. Some data suggest patients with intermediate or borderline susceptible isolates may be more likely to fail therapy [9,10]. Optimization of vancomycin dosing or choice of another drug should be considered for these isolates. About 50–75% of isolates of *Enterococcus faecium* are vancomycin-resistant (VRE), but the vast majority of isolates of *E. faecalis* are susceptible. Vancomycin has in-vitro activity but unknown utility for infections due to *Listeria*. Vancomycin has no activity against Gram-negative organisms.

A number of newer glycopeptides have been recently introduced into clinical practice (dalbavancin, telavancin) or are in late-stage clinical development (oritavancin). These drugs have a similar overall spectrum of activity to vancomycin, although they possess more potent activity against vancomycin-resistant *Staphylococcus* and *Enterococcus*.

Table 59.9. Pharmacokinetics, toxicity, and drug interactions of glycopeptides and lipopeptides

Drug	Dose adjustment in organ dysfunction	Toxicity/drug interactions
Vancomycin IV (generic)	Renal	*Uncommon*: rash, infusion-related reactions ("red man syndrome") *Rare*: neutropenia, nephrotoxicity, ototoxicity Drug interactions *Aminoglycosides*: increased nephro- and ototoxicity
Daptomycin IV (Cubicin)	Renal	*Uncommon*: myalgias *Rare*: rhabdomyolysis Drug interactions *Statins*: increased myopathy

Pharmacokinetics, toxicity, and drug interactions

Vancomycin is administered via the intravenous route when used to treat systemic infections, with elimination via the kidneys (Table 59.9). Despite the availability of an oral capsule formulation, vancomycin is not appreciably absorbed through this route of administration; rather, oral vancomycin is used for the intraluminal treatment of *Clostridium difficile* disease of the colon. Vancomycin has modest penetration into the cerebrospinal fluid in meningitis; aggressive, weight-based dosing should be used to ensure that adequate levels are achieved. The new glycopeptides have longer half-lives than vancomycin, allowing for once-daily, or in the case of dalbavancin once-weekly, dosing.

The most common adverse effect of vancomycin is the development of "red man syndrome," characterized by flushing and erythema of the upper torso (Table 59.9). More severe reactions may be accompanied by hypotension. The reaction typically occurs during or soon after the drug is infused and is thought to be caused by vancomycin-induced histamine release. The reaction is not considered a hypersensitivity reaction, and reduction of the rate of infusion (no faster than 1 g per hour) and premedication with diphenhydramine usually allow patients to receive subsequent doses. In past years, vancomycin developed a reputation for nephrotoxicity, partly due to the presence of toxic impurities in early preparations. Modern formulations lack such impurities, reducing the incidence of nephrotoxicity; however, a more recent increase in

vancomycin-associated nephrotoxicity has been suggested and attributed to the use of higher dosages [35]. Neutropenia and thrombocytopenia attributable to vancomycin are uncommon but well described. Vancomycin appears to have minimal ototoxicity or nephrotoxicity as monotherapy; however, vancomycin may increase the oto- and nephrotoxicity of aminoglycosides when used in combination.

Antibacterials: cell-membrane-active drugs

Lipopeptides
Spectrum of activity

Daptomycin, the only lipopeptide in current clinical use, is rapidly bactericidal against streptotocci, staphylococci (including MRSA), and enterococci (including VRE) (Table 59.8). Daptomycin lacks activity against Gram-negative organisms.

Pharmacokinetics, toxicity, and drug interactions

Daptomycin is administered intravenously, with elimination via the kidneys (Table 59.9). Although daptomycin penetrates modestly into the lungs, the drug is inactivated by pulmonary surfactant [36]. Animal models and human studies have confirmed the significance of this effect, and daptomycin should not be used for the treatment of pneumonia. Based on the clinical experience to date, daptomycin appears to be well tolerated. The most characteristic adverse effect is skeletal-muscle toxicity, generally after several days of therapy. In most instances, the toxicity is a reversible myalgia, and monitoring of CPK enzymes is recommended for long-term therapy.

Polymyxins
Spectrum of activity

The polymyxins (polymyxin B and polymyxin E, also known as colistin) were introduced in the 1960s but soon fell out of favor as systemic antibacterials because of their toxicity. Possibly because of the minimal systemic use of these drugs over this period of time, they have retained activity against a number of multidrug-resistant Gram-negative pathogens (Table 59.10). Thus there has been a revival of use of these drugs for treatment of *Pseudomonas* and *Acinetobacter*. They do not have useful activity against Gram-positive organisms.

Pharmacokinetics, toxicity, and drug interactions

Polymyxins are used parenterally for the treatment of invasive infections (they have been commonly used in topical antibacterial formulations). The intravenous form is sometimes adapted for use as an aerosol for inhalation for prophylaxis in high-risk populations (transplant, cystic fibrosis). These drugs are eliminated via the kidneys (Table 59.11). While the drugs are nephrotoxic, more recent experience suggests that,

Table 59.13. Pharmacokinetics, toxicity, and drug interactions of macrolides and tetracyclines/glycylcyclines

Drug	Dose adjustment in organ dysfunction	Toxicity/drug interactions
Azithromycin IV, PO (Zithromax)		*Common*: nausea/vomiting/diarrhea
Clarithromycin PO (Biaxin)	Renal (clarithromycin)	*Rare*: hepatotoxicity
		Drug interactions
		Serotoninergic drugs: risk of serotonin syndrome
Doxycycline IV, PO (generic)		*Common*: nausea/vomiting/diarrhea
Tigecycline IV (Tygacil)	Hepatic (tigecycline)	*Uncommon*: esophagitis (doxycycline)
		Rare: hepatotoxicity
		Drug interactions
		Oral cations (Ca, Mg, Fe, Al, Zn): reduced absorption of oral doxycycline

Table 59.14. Spectrum of activity of oxazolidinones, streptogramins, and lincosamides

Organism	Drug		
	Linezolid	Quinupristin/ dalfopristin	Clindamycin
Gram-positive			
Streptococus pyogenes	++	++	++
Streptococcus pneumoniae	++	++	+
Viridans streptococci	++	++	+
Staph aureus (MSSA)	++	++	+
Staph aureus (MRSA)	++	++	+
Enterococcus faecalis	++	×	×
Enterococcus faecium (VRE)	++	++	×

++, drug of choice and/or reliable susceptibility; +, alternative drug and/or variable susceptibility; ×, intrinsic resistance.

(Table 59.12). Coverage of *Streptococcus pneumoniae* is variable, and doxycycline is unreliable against other streptococci. Like the macrolides, doxycycline has good coverage of atypical respiratory pathogens. Doxycycline is a primary therapy option for a number of unusual pathogens, including the agents of Rocky Mountain spotted fever, bartonellosis, brucellosis, anthrax, and tularemia. Increasing levels of resistance have eroded the Gram-negative spectrum of doxycycline such that it is only occasionally useful for treatment of infections due to these organisms.

The glycylcycline subclass arose from modifications to the tetracycline core structure, allowing these drugs to overcome common tetracycline resistance mechanisms and enhancing the spectrum of activity. Tigecycline, the first available glycylcycline, displays excellent activity against a variety of aerobic and anaerobic Gram-positive and Gram-negative pathogens. Major holes in the spectrum of activity include *Pseudomonas* and *Proteus* species.

Pharmacokinetics, toxicity, and drug interactions

Doxycycline is available both as a well-absorbed oral formulation and as an intravenous preparation, while tigecycline is only available for intravenous administration. Both drugs distribute deeply into tissue. For tigecycline, tissue distribution is so complete that serum levels of the drug are low, potentially reducing utility in infections with an intravascular source. Both drugs are cleared via hepatic metabolism (Table 59.13). The most common toxicity for these drugs is gastrointestinal distress. Children under 8 years of age should not receive these drugs because of associated teeth mottling. The most important drug interaction with tetracyclines is the chelation of orally administered tetracyclines by orally administered divalent and trivalent cations (calcium, magnesium, aluminum, iron, zinc). Absorption of the tetracycline is significantly decreased, potentially leading to clinical failure. Oral administration of tetracyclines and cations should be separated by at least 2 hours.

Oxazolidinones
Spectrum of activity

Linezolid is the oxazolidinone in current clinical use. Linezolid has broad activity against Gram-positive organisms, including a number of organisms resistant to multiple drugs, such as VRE and MRSA (Table 59.14). Linezolid has poor activity against Gram-negative pathogens.

Pharmacokinetics, toxicity, and drug interactions

Linezolid is available as an intravenous formulation and a 100% bioavailable oral form. The drug undergoes wide distribution into many tissue compartments including the lungs and is inactivated by non-CYP hepatic enzymes in the liver (Table 59.15).

Table 59.15. Pharmacokinetics, toxicity, and drug interactions of oxazolidinones, streptogramins, and lincosamides

Drug	Dose adjustment in organ dysfunction	Toxicity/drug interactions
Linezolid IV, PO (Zyvox)	Not required	*Uncommon*: thrombocytopenia *Rare*: lactic acidosis, peripheral neuropathy, optic neuritis Drug interactions *Serotoninergic drugs*: risk of serotonin syndrome
Quinupristin/ dalfopristin IV (Synercid)	Not required	*Common*: myalgias, infusion site reactions *Rare*: hepatotoxicity Drug interactions *Antiarrhythmics*: potential increase in antiarrhythmic serum levels *Immunosuppressants*: potential increase in immunosuppressant levels
Clindamycin IV, PO (generic)	Not required	*Common*: nausea/ vomiting/diarrhea *Uncommon*: Clostridium difficile-associated diarrhea *Rare*: Clostridium difficile-associated colitis Drug interactions Minimal

Linezolid is generally well tolerated during short courses of therapy. Dose- and duration-dependent hematologic toxicity, primarily thrombocytopenia, may occur after 10–14 days of treatment, but this is reversible on drug discontinuation. Prolonged linezolid therapy (on the order of months) has been associated with a variety of toxicities thought to result from interference with mitochondrial processes. These include optic neuritis, peripheral neuropathy, and lactic acidosis; these effects have sometimes been irreversible or fatal [40].

Linezolid is a minor to moderate inhibitor of monoamine oxidase, an enzyme responsible for the metabolism of serotonin, and case reports of serotonin syndrome have been reported in patients receiving linezolid and selective serotonin reuptake inhibitors (SSRIs) [41]. Close monitoring for symptoms of serotonin syndrome during therapy with linezolid, or discontinuation of one or both drugs, is recommended.

Streptogramins
Spectrum of activity
Quinupristin/dalfopristin is a coformulation of two streptogramins that act in synergy to produce antibacterial effects. The combination has activity against streptococci, staphylococci (including MRSA), and *Enterococcus faecium* (including VRE), though not *Enterococcus faecalis* or Gram-negative bacteria (Table 59.14).

Pharmacokinetics, toxicity, and drug interactions
Quinupristin/dalfopristin is administered intravenously, with clearance via hepatic metabolism (Table 59.15). The adverse-effect profile of this drug includes a high incidence of myalgias and arthralgias (approximately half of patients), often treatment-limiting. Pain and irritation at the infusion site are also common; consequently the drug generally is administered through central venous catheters. Quinupristin/dalfopristin is an inhibitor of CYP and should be used cautiously with concomitant antiarrhythmics, antretrovirals, immunosuppressives, and other narrow-therapeutic-index drugs.

Lincosamides
Spectrum of activity
Clindamycin is the only lincosamide currently available, with a spectrum of activity encompassing a variety of aerobic and anaerobic Gram-positive organisms including streptococci and staphylococci, although not *Enterococcus* (Table 59.14). Clindamycin is active against some anaerobic Gram-negative organisms, such as *Bacteroides fragilis*, although it is not as active as metronidazole or β-lactam/β-lactamase inhibitor combinations. It is not active against aerobic Gram-negative organisms. Clindamycin has activity against some nonbacterial pathogens, including *Pneumocystis jirovecii* (used in combination with primaquine).

Pharmacokinetics, toxicity, and drug interactions
Clindamycin can be administered intravenously or orally, with clearance via hepatic metabolism and biliary excretion (Table 59.15). Nausea, vomiting, and diarrhea are frequent complaints, especially with administration of the oral formulation. In most cases the etiology of this toxicity is unknown and attributed to direct toxic effects of the drug on the gastrointestinal tract or drug-induced alterations of the gastrointestinal flora. However, a substantial fraction of cases of clindamycin-associated diarrhea is due to overgrowth of toxin-producing *Clostridium difficile*. Infection due to *C. difficile* can present over a range of severity from diarrhea to life-threatening colitis. Thus, patients experiencing diarrhea while receiving

Table 59.16. Spectrum of activity of fluoroquinolones and trimethoprim/sulfamethoxazole (TMP/SMX)

Organism	Drug			
	Ciprofloxacin	Levofloxacin	Moxifloxacin	TMP/SMX
Gram-positive				
Streptococus pyogenes	++	++	++	–
Streptococcus pneumoniae	–	++	++	+
Viridans streptococci	+	++	++	–
Staph aureus (MSSA)	–	+	+	+
Staph aureus (MRSA)	–	–	–	+
Enterococcus faecalis	–	–	–	×
Enterococcus faecium (VRE)	–	–	–	×
Gram-negative				
H. influenzae	++	++	++	+
Proteus mirabilis	++	++	+++	++
E. coli	++	++	++	+
Klebsiella spp.	++	++	++	+
Serratia	++	++	++	++
Pseudomonas	++	++	×	×
Entero/Citro/Acinetobacter	++	++	+	+
Bacteroides fragilis	–	–	+	–

++, drug of choice and/or reliable susceptibility; +, alternative drug and/or variable susceptibility; –, rare in-vitro activity, not reliable for empiric therapy; ×, intrinsic resistance.

clindamycin (and up to several weeks afterwards) should be carefully evaluated to exclude *C. difficile* disease. While clindamycin's association with *C. difficile* disease is often highlighted, it should be noted that essentially all antimicrobials, including β-lactam drugs and fluoroquinolones, have been associated with *C. difficile* disease [42].

Antibacterials: drugs targeting DNA synthesis and structure

Fluoroquinolones
Spectrum of activity
Ciprofloxacin has moderate to excellent Gram-negative activity, including activity against *Pseudomonas*, but its potency against streptococci and staphylococci is generally poor (Table 59.16). Levofloxacin and moxifloxacin (often referred to as **respiratory fluoroquinolones**) more potently inhibit streptococci, especially *S. pneumoniae*. These drugs have modest activity against staphylococci, but emergence of resistance is well described. Levofloxacin maintains activity against *Pseudomonas*, whereas moxifloxacin has minimal activity against this organism. Moxifloxacin has modest but variable activity against anaerobic organisms, including *B. fragilis*. The respiratory fluoroquinolones have excellent activity against the "atypical" respiratory pathogens. Note that there is increasing resistance to fluoroquinolones among Gram-negative organisms, especially *E. coli* and *Pseudomonas*. Depending on local susceptibility patterns, these drugs may not be reliable choices for empiric therapy of hospitalized patients.

Pharmacokinetics, toxicity, and drug interactions
All commonly used fluoroquinolones have excellent oral bioavailability – serum levels achieved from oral administration are very similar to those achieved via intravenous administration. Unlike moxifloxacin, ciprofloxacin and levofloxacin require dosage reduction in renal dysfunction (Table 59.17). Considering the minimal renal excretion and associated low urinary levels, moxifloxacin is not approved for treatment of urinary tract infections.

The most common toxicities of fluoroquinolones include gastrointestinal distress, photosensitivity, and central nervous system symptoms (headache, dizziness, confusion). Fluoroquinolones can also cause arthralgias and have been generally contraindicated in children because of concerns over their potential cartilage toxicity. However, considerable experience

Table 59.17. Pharmacokinetics, toxicity, and drug interactions of fluoroquinolones and trimethoprim/sulfamethoxazole

Drug	Dose adjustment in organ dysfunction	Toxicity/drug interactions
Ciprofloxacin IV, PO (generic, Cipro)	Renal (ciprofloxacin, levofloxacin)	*Uncommon*: nausea/vomiting/diarrhea, headache/dizziness/confusion, arthralgias
Levofloxacin IV, PO (Levaquin)	Not required (moxifloxacin)	*Rare*: Achilles tendon rupture, seizures, QT prolongation, dysglycemia
Moxifloxacin IV, PO (Avelox)		Drug interactions
		Oral cations (Ca, Mg, Fe, Al, Zn): reduced absorption of oral fluoroquinolones
		Warfarin: increased INR (ciprofloxacin)
Trimethoprim/ sulfamethoxazole IV, PO (generic, Bactrim, Septra)	Renal	*Common*: rash
		Uncommon: hyperkalemia, increased serum creatinine, neutropenia
		Rare: nephrotoxicity
		Drug interactions
		Warfarin: increased INR

in children with cystic fibrosis confirms that these drugs can safely be used in most children [43]. Tendonitis and acute tendon rupture is a well-described, though rare, adverse effect of fluoroquinolones. Fluoroquinolones can prolong the QT interval to varying degrees, although torsades de pointes is rare in the absence of predisposing conditions. Dysglycemias (hypo- and hyperglycemia) may occur on occasion with the currently available drugs.

Similar to the tetracyclines, the most important drug interaction with fluoroquinolones is the chelation of orally administered fluoroquinolones by orally administered divalent and trivalent cations (calcium, magnesium, aluminum, iron, zinc) (Table 59.17). Oral administration of fluoroquinolones and cations should be separated by at least 2 hours.

Trimethoprim/sulfamethoxazole (TMP/SMX)
Spectrum of activity
Over the years, the spectrum of antibacterial activity has narrowed due to the spread of antimicrobial resistance including S. pneumoniae, E.coli, and H. influenzae. However, TMP/SMX has retained good activity against S. aureus, including methicillin-susceptible and methicillin-resistant isolates (Table 59.16). Although TMP/SMX has been a mainstay for the treatment of urinary tract infections due to Gram-negative bacteria, such as E. coli, Proteus, and Klebsiella, there is increasing resistance among these pathogens. TMP/SMX has no antipseudomonal activity, and variable activity against Citrobacter and Enterobacter. TMP/SMX also

has activity against some nonbacterial pathogens, notably Pneumocystis and Toxoplasma.

Pharmacokinetics, toxicity, and drug interactions
TMP/SMX is well absorbed, with serum levels achieved with oral administration approximately 90% of those obtained with intravenous administration of equivalent doses. Both TMP and SMX are eliminated through renal clearance, either primarily as an unchanged drug (TMP) or as metabolites (SMX).

Although TMP/SMX is generally well-tolerated, there are a number of adverse effects that may require discontinuation or dosage modification (Table 59.17). Dermatologic reactions, ranging from uncomplicated maculopapular rashes to life-threatening toxic epidermal necrolysis, are likely attributable to the sulfamethoxazole component. Desensitization, consisting of administration of slowly escalating doses in a supervised setting, may be considered in those instances in which TMP/SMX absolutely must be used. TMP/SMX can cause bone-marrow suppression, usually in a dose-dependent fashion. TMP may cause hyperkalemia and "pseudorenal failure," where the serum creatinine becomes elevated even without a change in glomerular filtration rate, due to inhibition of creatinine secretion in the renal tubules [44]. Rarely, acute interstitial nephritis or crystalluria attributable to SMX may cause true renal insufficiency.

There are several clinically important drug interactions with TMP/SMX (Table 59.17). TMP/SMX potentiates the effects of the antifolate chemotherapy drug methotrexate and

Table 59.18. Spectrum of activity of antifungals

Organism	Drug				
	Fluconazole	Voriconazole	Posaconazole	Amphotericin	Echinocandins
Yeasts					
Candida albicans, tropicalis, parapsilosis	++	++	++	++	++
Candida glabrata	+	++	++	++	++
Candida kruseii	×	++	++	++	++
Cryptococcus	++	++	++	++	×
Molds					
Aspergillus	×	++	++	+	+
Fusarium	×	+	+	+	−
Zygomyces	×	−	+	++	−

++, drug of choice and/or reliable susceptibility; +, alternative drug and/or variable susceptibility; −, rare in-vitro activity, not reliable for empiric therapy; ×, intrinsic resistance.

should not be coadministered with this drug. The anticoagulant effects of warfarin may be increased by TMP/SMX, so careful monitoring of the prothrombin time is recommended during coadministration. TMP/SMX reduces the metabolism of phenytoin; dosage modification may be required.

Nitroimidazoles
Spectrum of activity
There are two nitroimidazoles in current clinical practice, metronidazole and tinidazole. Metronidazole is the drug with the most experience in hospitalized patients. Metronidazole's bacterial spectrum is solely limited to anaerobic organisms; it is active against essentially all Gram-negative anaerobes, including *Bacteroides fragilis*. Metronidazole has activity against a number of Gram-positive anaerobes, including *Clostridium difficile*; however, some Gram-positive anaerobes, such as *Propionibacterium* and *Lactobacillus*, are usually resistant. Metronidazole is also active against a number of protozoa, including *Giardia*, *Trichonomonas*, *Entamoeba*, and *Blastocystis*.

Pharmacokinetics, toxicity and drug interactions
Metronidazole has excellent oral absorption; serum levels achieved with oral administration approximate those achieved with intravenous administration. The drug has excellent penetration into the central nervous system, with concentrations in brain abscesses similar to those observed in serum. Metronidazole is extensively metabolized by the liver, and dosage reduction may be necessary in severe hepatic disease.

Adverse effects attributable to metronidazole are uncommon. Gastrointestinal disturbances, including a metallic taste, are the most frequently reported toxicity. During prolonged therapy, neurologic adverse effects, including paresthesias and peripheral neuropathy, have been reported. Metronidazole

inhibits enzymes responsible for the metabolism of warfarin, tacrolimus, cyclosporine, and phenytoin.

Antifungals: mechanisms of action
Most available antifungals target ergosterol, a component of the fungal cell membrane that plays a similar role to cholesterol in mammalian cells. The azoles and allylamines (such as terbinafine) inhibit steps in the biosynthesis of ergosterol, leading to depletion of the molecule in the fungal cell membrane and membrane instability. The polyene drugs, such as amphotericin B, bind to ergosterol in the fungal cell membrane resulting in leakage of cellular contents. Pyrimidine drugs such as flucytosine inhibit thymidylate synthetase, ultimately interfering with DNA and protein synthesis. The echinocandin drugs (anidulafungin, caspofungin, micafungin) target β-glucan in the fungal cell wall.

Antifungals: drugs targeting the fungal cell membrane
Azoles
Spectrum of activity
There are important differences in spectrum of activity between the various azole antifungals (Table 59.18). Fluconazole has activity against yeasts (such as *Candida*) and dimorphic fungi (such as *Blastomyces*, *Coccidioides*, and *Histoplasma*). This drug lacks activity against molds (such as *Aspergillus*) and has poor activity against certain species of *Candida*, including *C. glabrata* and *C. kruseii*. Voriconazole substantially improves on this activity, including potent activity against *Aspergillus* and *C. kruseii*. Voriconazole is inactive

Table 59.19. Pharmacokinetics, toxicity, and drug interactions of antifungals

Drug	Dose adjustment in organ dysfunction	Toxicity/drug interactions
Fluconazole IV, PO (Diflucan)	Renal (fluconazole)	*Common*: transient visual changes (voriconazole)
Voriconazole IV, PO (Vfend)	Hepatic (voriconazole)	*Uncommon*: GI disturbances, hepatotoxicity
Posaconazole PO (Noxafil)		*Rare*: visual hallucinations (voriconazole)
		Drug interactions
		Rifampin: decreased azole levels
		Immunosuppressants: increased immunosuppressant levels
		Statins: increased statin levels
		Phenytoin: decreased azole levels
Amphotericin B deoxycholate IV (generic)	Not required	*Common*: infusion-related reactions, nephrotoxicity
Amphotericin B colloidal dispersion IV (Amphotec)		Drug interactions
		Other nephrotoxins: increased nephrotoxicity
Amphotericin B lipid complex IV (Abelcet)		
Liposomal amphotericin B IV (AmBisome)		
Caspofungin IV (Cancidas)	Hepatic (caspofungin, micafungin)	*Rare*: hepatotoxicity
Micafungin IV (Mycamine)		
Anidulafungin IV (Eraxis)		

against zygomycetes. Posaconazole offers similar activity as voriconazole, but it is active against zygomycetes.

Pharmacokinetics, toxicity, and drug interactions

Fluconazole and voriconazole achieve similar concentrations when administered intravenously or orally. Posaconazole is only available as an oral suspension; the drug should be administered with a high-fat meal to enhance absorption. Azoles, particularly fluconazole and voriconazole, achieve good penetration into cerebrospinal fluid. Fluconazole is primarily eliminated via the kidneys, whereas voriconazole and posaconazole are eliminated by hepatic metabolism (Table 59.19). Of note, the intravenous formulation of voriconazole includes a cyclodextran carrier that accumulates in renal dysfunction and is toxic in laboratory animals [45]. The oral formulation is recommended for patients with renal failure whenever possible, although one study did not observe any adverse effects in a group of critically ill patients with renal dysfunction receiving the intravenous formulation [46].

All azoles have some potential for hepatotoxicity, including rare cases of fatal liver failure. Hepatic transaminases should be monitored for patients receiving extended courses of therapy. Voriconazole is unique among the azoles in causing visual disturbances. Approximately half of patients report transient

alterations in their vision, usually manifesting as altered light and color perception and blurry vision. These effects are most common around the time of dosing and at the initiation of treatment, and usually subside as patients continue on the drug. Rarely, visual hallucinations of a different nature than the transient visual disturbances may occur.

All the azoles have some potential for drug interactions, although they vary in degree (Table 59.19). These drugs inhibit drug-metabolizing enzymes in the CYP family, voriconazole and posaconazole being much more potent inhibitors than fluconazole. Drugs such as rifampin or phenytoin that induce hepatic drug-metabolizing enzymes can reduce the serum concentrations of azoles, with voriconazole most strongly affected and fluconazole least affected. Depending on the degree of enzyme inhibition, azoles may also substantially increase the serum concentrations of other drugs, including a number of narrow-therapeutic-index drugs such as cyclosporine and warfarin. Thus, patients started on azoles require careful screening of their drug profile to avoid potentially dangerous drug interactions.

Polyenes
Spectrum of activity
Amphotericin B has a broad spectrum of activity against both yeasts and molds (Table 59.18). Only a few

uncommon fungi, such as *Candida lusitanae, Aspergillus terreus*, and *Scedosporium prolificans*, are fully resistant to amphotericin.

Pharmacokinetics, toxicity, and drug interactions

Amphotericin B must be administered intravenously in the treatment of systemic fungal infections. The elimination of amphotericin B is not well characterized, although the drug does not accumulate in renal dysfunction (Table 59.19). However, amphotericin is associated with a high incidence of dose-related nephrotoxicity. Thus, dosage reduction may be required if renal dysfunction occurs. Administering infusions of normal saline before and/or after the amphotericin B infusion may reduce renal toxicity [47]. In addition, amphotericin is associated with infusion-related reactions, including fever, hypotension, chills, and rigors. Paracetamol (acetaminophen), hydrocortisone, diphenydramine, and meperidine (for chills) may be used as treatment for and/or prophylaxis against these reactions.

The highest incidence of renal and infusion-related reactions occurs with administration of conventional amphotericin B (amphotericin B deoxycholate). Lipid-associated formulations of amphotericin B reduce the incidence of nephrotoxicity relative to conventional amphotericin B, and liposomal amphotericin may reduce infusion-related reactions as well. These drugs are much more expensive by acquisition cost when compared with conventional amphotericin.

Antifungals: drugs targeting the fungal cell wall

Echinocandins
Spectrum of activity

Anidulafungin, caspofungin, and micafungin have equivalent spectra of activity (Table 59.18). They have potent fungicidal activity against many yeasts, including all species of *Candida*, but lack activity against *Cryptococcus*. Echinocandins have activity against *Aspergillus*, although not against many other molds.

Pharmacokinetics, toxicity, and drug interactions

The echinocandins are administered intravenously. Caspofungin and micafungin undergo substantial hepatic metabolism, although not through the CYP group of enzymes (Table 59.19). Micafungin is cleared through plasma esterases. An important characteristic of the echinocandins is their excellent tolerability relative to the other antifungal drugs. Occasional infusion-related reactions and rare hepatotoxicity have been reported. Drug interactions are generally minimal, although doses of caspofungin may need to be increased when coadministered with enzyme-inducing drugs.

Antivirals
Antiretrovirals

Over the last decade there has been an explosion in the development of antiretroviral drugs targeting the human immunodeficiency virus (HIV). Selection of an antiretroviral regimen (usually at least three drugs from at least two different classes) is an extremely complex task best left to HIV specialists. Patients on antiretroviral regimens pose a challenge for anesthesiologists because of the myriad toxicities and drug interactions these drugs possess. Characteristics of antiretrovirals relevant to anesthesiologists, including selected toxicities and major drug interactions, are summarized in Table 59.20. Abbreviations commonly used for antiretroviral drugs are provided, along with their brand names; however, the abbreviations should not be used when writing orders for these drugs. Note that many antiretroviral drugs are now provided as coformulations to improve patient adherence (e.g., the Atripla combination pill of efavirenz, tenofovir, and emtricitabine). Zidovudine is the only antiretroviral available in intravenous as well as oral formulations; enfurvitidine is only available as a subcutaneous injection. Thus, interruption in antiretroviral therapy may take place among patients undergoing surgery or the critically ill. Interruption of therapy, when it does occur, should involve stopping all components of a regimen, and should occur for the shortest duration to avoid development of antiretroviral resistance. Because of the rapidly changing nature of this field, clinicians are encouraged to consult experts or the latest government guidelines (available at aidsinfo.nih.gov).

Anti-herpesvirus drugs

Antivirals active against herpesviruses (herpes simplex virus, cytomegalovirus, varicella-zoster virus) are the most commonly used antivirals in hospitalized patients. Characteristics of these drugs are outlined in Table 59.21. Acyclovir is the least toxic of the available drugs, but lacks sufficient potency against cytomegalovirus for use in infections due to this pathogen. Of note, the oral valine-esterified prodrugs of acyclovir and ganciclovir (valacyclovir and valganciclovir) improve substantially on the absorption of their parent drugs. After absorption, the valine moiety is immediately hydrolyzed, resulting in the same spectrum of activity and toxicity profile as the parent drug. Because of the substantial renal toxicity of cidofovir and foscarnet, prehydration is recommended prior to infusion of these drugs. In the case of cidofovir, coadministration of probenecid is required to reduce nephrotoxicity (also prolonging the serum half-life such that the drug may be administered once weekly).

Anti-influenza drugs

Two classes of drugs with activity against the influenza virus are available, the **adamantanes** (amantadine and rimantadine) and the **neuraminidase inhibitors** (oseltamivir and zanamavir). The adamantanes lack intrinsic activity against influenza

Table 59.20. Pharmacology of antiretrovirals

Group and drugs	Mechanism	Toxicities	Drug interactions
Nucleoside and nucleotide reverse transcriptase inhibitors (NRTI)			
Zidovudine (AZT, Retrovir)	Competitive inhibition of HIV reverse transcriptase → interruption of viral DNA synthesis	*Common*: nausea/vomiting/diarrhea (all) *Uncommon*: Anemia (AZT), nephrotoxicity (TDF) *Rare*: lactic acidosis (all); peripheral neuropathy, pancreatitis (d4T, ddI); rash (FTC); hypersensitivity syndrome (ABC)	*Atazanavir*: reduced atazanavir levels (ddI, TDF) *Methadone*: increased AZT levels (AZT) *Ribavirin*: pharmacologic antagonism (ddI, AZT)
Didanosine (ddI, Videx EC)			
Stavudine (d4T, Zerit)			
Lamivudine (3TC, Epivir)			
Emtricitabine (FTC, Emtriva)			
Abacavir (ABC, Ziagen)			
Tenovovir (TDF, Viread)			
Non-nucleoside reverse transcriptase inhibitors (NNRTI)			
Efavirenz (EFV, Sustiva)	Non-competitive inhibition of HIV reverse transcriptase → interruption of viral DNA synthesis	*Common*: dizziness/insomnia/vivid dreams (EFV) *Uncommon*: Rash, elevations in hepatic transmaminases (all) *Rare*: hepatic failure (all)	Numerous, including: *Rifampin*: decreased NNRTI levels Statins: increased or decreasesd statin levels *Phenytoin/ carbamezapine*: decreased NNRTI levels
Nevirapine (NVP, Viramune)			
Etravirine (ETR, Intelence)			
Protease inhibitors (PI)			
Ritonavir (RTV)	Competitive inhibition of HIV protease → failure to process viral proteins into functional units	*Common*: nausea/vomiting/diarrhea, hyperglycemia, fat redistribution (all); hyperlipidemia (all except ATV); indirect hyperbilirubinemia (ATV); *Uncommon*: elevations in hepatic transmaminases (all); rash (DRV, FPV, TPV); PR prolongation (ATV) *Rare*: intracranial hemorrhage (TPV)	Numerous, including: *Rifampin*: decreased PI levels *Statins*: increased statin levels *Midazolam/ triazolam*: increased benzodiazepine levels Phenytoin/ carbamezapine: decreased PI levels *Azole antifungals*: increased or decreased azole levels
Atazanavir (ATV, Reyataz)			
Lopinavir (LPV, Kaletra)			
Fosamprenavir (FPV, Lexiva)			
Darunavir (DRV, Prezista)			
Tipranavir (TPV, Aptivus)			
Entry inhibitors			
Maraviroc (MVC, Selzentry)	Blockade of coreceptor required for viral entry → inhibition of cell infection	*Uncommon*: elevations in hepatic transaminases *Rare*: allergic-type hepatic failure	*Rifampin*: decreased MVC levels Phenytoin/ carbamezapine: decreased MVC levels *Azole antifungals*: increased MVC levels

Table 59.20. *(cont.)*

Group and drugs	Mechanism	Toxicities	Drug interactions
Fusion inhibitors			
Enfurvitide (T20, Fuzeon)	Blockade of coreceptor required for viral entry → inhibition of cell infection	*Common*: injection site reactions *Rare*: hypersensitivity syndrome	Minimal
Integrase inhibitors			
Raltegravir (RAL, Isentress)	Inhibition of viral integrase enzyme → prevents free HIV DNA from merging with host cell NDA	*Common*: hyperlipidemia *Uncommon*: hyperglycemia, nausea/vomiting/diarrhea, CPK elevations *Rare*: myopathy, rhabdomyolysis	*Rifampin*: decreased RAL levels

B, have an unfavorable toxicity profile, and have been limited by the emergence of resistance among influenza A strains. Thus, current recommendations do not include the adamantanes in the treatment of influenza, including that associated with avian flu [48]. The strongest efficacy data for the neuraminidase inhibitors is in the reduction of influenza symptoms (by 1–2 days) among ambulatory patients starting the drugs within 24 hours of symptom onset, and in prevention of spread of influenza among nonvaccinated institutional residents [49]. The evidence for a reduction in complications in hospitalized patients with severe influenza is less robust; nevertheless, some clinicians consider the risk/benefit ratio to favor treatment in severely ill patients. Characteristics of the neuraminidase inhibitors are summarized in Table 59.21.

Key scenarios for anesthesiologists involving antibiotics and quality metrics

Surgical antibiotic prophylaxis

Surgical site infections (SSIs) are now the second most common nosocomial infections [50]. The incidence of SSIs appears to vary, affected by factors including the site of the operation, the surgeon, and the hospital where the procedures are performed. The anesthesiologist has the ability to control factors that are involved in SSIs, including the timing of administration of the antibiotics, the temperature of the patient, the oxygen level of the patient, the glucose concentration in the patient, and the number of transfusions the patient receives [51–71].

The anesthesiologist must administer the prophylactic perioperative antibiotics so that the blood and tissue antibiotic concentrations exceed the minimum inhibitory concentration (MIC: see above) of the bacteria that are likely to cause an infection. There is a United States program to reduce SSIs, the National Surgical Infection Prevention Project, that includes the Centers for Disease Control and Prevention (CDC), Medicare, and both surgical and anesthesia societies. This program has a website and a number of publications [72–74] that clearly state the recommended antibiotics for different surgical procedures. The general concept is that antibiotic prophylaxis in clean procedures is usually done with cefazolin, because skin microbes are killed by this antibiotic and tend to be involved in SSIs. However, those hospitals with high rates of MRSA may preferentially use vancomycin prophylaxis in these clean procedures. In contrast, surgeries that involve the intestines will require Gram-negative and anaerobic coverage, utilizing drugs such as cefotetan or cefoxitin. Finally, as suggested above, patients chronically colonized with MRSA likely should be given vancomycin for their prophylaxis; there are contradictory studies in this area, with marginal evidence of improvement in SSIs with vancomycin administration and a study that did not document a benefit from universal surveillance for MRSA in perioperative patients [75,76].

Cefazolin should be given within 1 hour prior to the incision; much of the evidence for this comes from an investigation completed in 1969 [77]. If vancomycin is administered, it should be given over 120 minutes to avoid producing the "red man syndrome" (see above). Antibiotics need to be administered prior to the inflation of tourniquets. Finally, antibiotic administration should be discontinued after 24 hours in almost all procedures.

Issues in antibiotic prophylaxis

For patients with confirmed β-lactam allergies, clindamycin or vancomycin can be given as the prophylactic antibiotic in clean procedures [73]. It is not clear what the optimal dose of antibiotic is for morbidly obese patients; doses may have to be increased to achieve optimal drug levels [78,79]. Consultation with clinical pharmacists should be considered, as these patients have multiple factors that may lead to an increase incidence of SSIs, including diabetes, metabolic syndrome, and an inability to properly warm their tissues [80]. The morbidly obese patient may require continuous infusions to achieve optimal concentrations [78,79].

Table 59.21. Pharmacology of anti-herpesvirus and anti-influenza antivirals

Group and drugs	Mechanism	Toxicities	Drug interactions
Anti-herpesvirus antivirals			
Acyclovir IV, PO (generic) Valacyclovir PO (Valtrex)	Competitive inhibition of viral DNA polymerase → decrease in viral DNA replication	*Uncommon*: headache *Rare*: nephrotoxicity	Minimal
Ganciclovir IV, PO (generic, Cytovene) Valganciclovir PO (Valcyte)		*Uncommon*: bone marrow suppression, nausea/vomiting/diarrhea *Rare*: paresthesias	Minimal
Cidofovir IV (generic, Vistide)		*Common*: nephrotoxicity, electrolyte wasting *Uncommon*: neutropenia	*Other nephrotoxins*: increased nephrotoxicity
Foscarnet IV (generic, Foscavir)	Non-competitive inhibition of viral DNA polymerase → decrease in viral DNA replication	*Common*: nephrotoxicity, electrolyte wasting, fatigue, headache *Uncommon*: anemia, leukopenia	*Other nephrotoxins*: increased nephrotoxicity
Anti-influenza antivirals			
Oseltamivir PO (Tamiflu)	Inhibition of neuraminidase → impaired viral release from infected cells	*Uncommon*: nausea/vomiting/diarrhea (oseltamivir)	Minimal
Zanamavir INH (Relenza)		*Rare*: psychiatric effects (oseltamivir), bronchospasm (zanamivir)	

Summary

The vast majority of patients undergoing a surgical procedure receive at least one antimicrobial drug. Consequently, understanding the spectrum of antibiotic activity, pharmacokinetics, toxicities, and drug interactions is essential to medical practice in the operating room or the critical care unit. The basic principle of antimicrobial therapy is to administer an antibiotic such that its blood and tissue concentrations exceed the minimum inhibitory concentration (MIC) for the bacteria that are likely to cause an infection. The MIC is the lowest antimicrobial concentration that prevents visible bacterial growth in liquid medium. Different antibiotics achieve substantially different serum and tissue concentrations, and the antibiotic with the lowest MIC is generally the best choice. The inhibition quantified by the MIC may be associated with a bacteriostatic effect (inhibition of bacterial growth without killing the organism) or a bactericidal effect (rendering the organism nonviable). Whenever possible, data on local antimicrobial susceptibility patterns should be incorporated into decision-making when selecting antimicrobial therapy.

Allergic reactions, particularly to β-lactams, are among the most common and important antibiotic toxicities. Documentation of the nature and timing of an initial reaction to an antibiotic and whether the patient has been re-exposed to the drug are crucial in determining the clinical significance of an allergy. It is also important to carefully consider the likelihood of cross-reactivity between various β-lactam antibiotics, before selecting antibiotics for patients with a history of allergic reaction to a penicillin or cephalosporin.

Antimicrobial drugs can be classified according to their mechanisms of action. Broad classes of antibacterial drugs include cell-wall-active drugs (penicillins, cephalosporins, monobactams, carbapenems, glycopeptides), cell-membrane-active drugs (lipopeptides, polymixins), inhibitors of ribosomal protein synthesis (aminoglycosides, macrolides, tetracyclines and glycylcyclines, oxazolidiones, streptogramins, lincosamides), and drugs targeting DNA synthesis and structure (fluoroquinolones, trimethoprim/sulfamethoxazole, nitroimidazoles).

Most available antifungals target ergosterol, a component of the fungal cell membrane. The azoles and allylamines inhibit the biosynthesis of ergosterol, leading to fungal cell membrane instability, whereas the polyene drugs bind to ergosterol in the fungal cell membrane, resulting in leakage of cellular contents. Pyrimidine drugs such as flucytosine inhibit thymidylate synthetase, ultimately interfering with DNA and protein synthesis, and the echinocandin drugs target β-glucan in the fungal cell wall.

The explosion in the development of antiretroviral drugs targeting the human immunodeficiency virus (HIV) makes the selection of an antiretroviral regimen (usually at least three drugs from at least two different classes) an extremely complex task best left to HIV specialists. In general, antiretroviral regimens pose a challenge for anesthesiologists because of the myriad toxicities and drug interactions these drugs possess. Other antiviral drugs include anti-herpesvirus drugs and anti-influenza drugs.

Surgical antibiotic prophylaxis is a key clinical scenario encountered daily by anesthesiologists. Antibiotic prophylaxis for clean procedures is usually done with cefazolin. If a hospital has a particularly high rate of MRSA, vancomycin may be the preferred drug. Antibiotic prophylaxis for surgery involving the intestines requires Gram-negative and anaerobic coverage, usually with cefotetan or cefoxitin. Cefazolin should be administered within 1 hour prior to incision, and vancomycin should be given over 120 minutes. All prophylactic antibiotics should be discontinued within 24 hours.

References

1. MacDougall C, Polk RE. Variability in rates of use of antibacterials among 130 US hospitals and risk-adjustment models for interhospital comparison. *Infect Control Hosp Epidemiol* 2008; **29**: 203–11.

2. Spellberg B, Powers JH, Brass EP, Miller LG, Edwards JE. Trends in antimicrobial drug development: implications for the future. *Clin Infect Dis* 2004; **38**: 1279–86.

3. Turnidge J, Paterson DL. Setting and revising antibacterial susceptibility breakpoints. *Clin Microbiol Rev* 2007; **20**: 391–408.

4. Finberg RW, Moellering RC, Tally FP, *et al.* The importance of bactericidal drugs: future directions in infectious disease. *Clin Infect Dis* 2004; **39**: 1314–20.

5. Ambrose PG, Bhavnani SM, Rubino CM, *et al.* Pharmacokinetics-pharmacodynamics of antimicrobial therapy: it's not just for mice anymore. *Clin Infect Dis* 2007; **44**: 79–86.

6. Bailey TC, Little JR, Littenberg B, Reichley RM, Dunagan WC. A meta-analysis of extended-interval dosing versus multiple daily dosing of aminoglycosides. *Clin Infect Dis* 1997; **24**: 786–95.

7. Lipman J, Gomersall CD, Gin T, Joynt GM, Young RJ. Continuous infusion ceftazidime in intensive care: a randomized controlled trial. *J Antimicrob Chemother* 1999; **43**: 309–11.

8. Lorente L, Jimenez A, Palmero S, *et al.* Comparison of clinical cure rates in adults with ventilator-associated pneumonia treated with intravenous ceftazidime administered by continuous or intermittent infusion: a retrospective, nonrandomized, open-label, historical chart review. *Clin Ther* 2007; **29**: 2433–9.

9. Sakoulas G, Moise-Broder PA, Schentag J, *et al.* Relationship of MIC and bactericidal activity to efficacy of vancomycin for treatment of methicillin-resistant Staphylococcus aureus bacteremia. *J Clin Microbiol* 2004; **42**: 2398–402.

10. Moise-Broder PA, Forrest A, Birmingham MC, Schentag JJ. Pharmacodynamics of vancomycin and other antimicrobials in patients with Staphylococcus aureus lower respiratory tract infections. *Clin Pharmacokinet* 2004; **43**: 925–42.

11. Gadde J, Spence M, Wheeler B, Adkinson NF. Clinical experience with penicillin skin testing in a large inner-city STD clinic. *JAMA* 1993; **270**: 2456–63.

12. Kerr JR. Penicillin allergy: a study of incidence as reported by patients. *Br J Clin Pract* 1994; **48**: 5–7.

13. Salkind AR, Cuddy PG, Foxworth JW. The rational clinical examination. Is this patient allergic to penicillin? An evidence-based analysis of the likelihood of penicillin allergy. *JAMA* 2001; **285**: 2498–505.

14. Robinson JL, Hameed T, Carr S. Practical aspects of choosing an antibiotic for patients with a reported allergy to an antibiotic. *Clin Infect Dis* 2002; **35**: 26–31.

15. Apter AJ, Kinman JL, Bilker WB, *et al.* Is there cross-reactivity between penicillins and cephalosporins? *Am J Med* 2006; **119**: 354, e11–9.

16. Prescott WA, Kusmierski KA. Clinical importance of carbapenem hypersensitivity in patients with self-reported and documented penicillin allergy. *Pharmacotherapy* 2007; **27**: 137–42.

17. DePestel DD, Benninger MS, Danziger L, *et al.* Cephalosporin use in treatment of patients with penicillin allergies. *J Am Pharm Assoc (2003)* 2008; **48**: 530–40.

18. Perez Pimiento A, Gomez Martinez M, Minguez Mena A *et al.* Aztreonam and ceftazidime: evidence of in vivo cross allergenicity. *Allergy* 1998; **53**: 624–5.

19. Patriarca G, Schiavino D, Lombardo C, *et al.* Tolerability of aztreonam in patients with IgE-mediated hypersensitivity to beta-lactams. *Int J Immunopathol Pharmacol* 2008; **21**: 375–9.

20. Jensen T, Koch C, Pedersen SS, Hoiby N. Aztreonam for cystic fibrosis patients who are hypersensitive to other beta-lactams. *Lancet* 1987; **1**: 1319–20.

21. Moss RB. Sensitization to aztreonam and cross-reactivity with other beta-lactam antibiotics in high-risk patients with cystic fibrosis. *J Allergy Clin Immunol* 1991; **87**: 78–88.

22. Yu VL. *Antimicrobial Therapy and Vaccines: Volume 2: Antimicrobial Agents.*, 2nd edn. Pittsburgh, PA: ESun Technologies, 2004.

23. Kucers A. *The Use of Antibiotics: a Clinical Review of Antibacterial, Antifungal, and Antiviral Drugs*, 5th edn. Oxford; Boston: Butterworth-Heinemann, 1997.

24. Bryskier A. *Antimicrobial Agents: Antibacterials and Antifungals.* Washington, DC: ASM Press, 2005.

25. Mandell GL, Douglas RG, Bennett JE, Dolin R. *Mandell, Douglas, and Bennett's Principles and Practice of Infectious Diseases.*, 5th edn. Philadelphia, PA: Churchill Livingstone, 2000.

26. Romano A, Quaratino D, Papa G, Di Fonso M, Venuti A. Aminopenicillin allergy. *Arch Dis Child* 1997; **76**: 513–17.

27. Monte SV, Prescott WA, Johnson KK, Kuhman L, Paladino JA. Safety of ceftriaxone sodium at extremes of age. *Expert Opin Drug Saf* 2008; 7: 515–23.

28. Martin E, Fanconi S, Kalin P, et al. Ceftriaxone – bilirubin-albumin interactions in the neonate: an in vivo study. *Eur J Pediatr* 1993; **152**: 530–4.

29. Norrby SR. Neurotoxicity of carbapenem antibacterials. *Drug Saf* 1996; **15**: 87–90.

30. Calandra G, Lydick E, Carrigan J, Weiss L, Guess H. Factors predisposing to seizures in seriously ill infected patients receiving antibiotics: experience with imipenem/cilastatin. *Am J Med* 1988; **84**: 911–18.

31. Linden P. Safety profile of meropenem: an updated review of over 6,000 patients treated with meropenem. *Drug Saf* 2007; **30**: 657–68.

32. Odio CM, Puig JR, Feris JM, et al. Prospective, randomized, investigator-blinded study of the efficacy and safety of meropenem vs. cefotaxime therapy in bacterial meningitis in children. Meropenem Meningitis Study Group. *Pediatr Infect Dis J* 1999; **18**: 581–90.

33. Steinkraus G, White R, Friedrich L. Vancomycin MIC creep in non-vancomycin-intermediate Staphylococcus aureus (VISA), vancomycin-susceptible clinical methicillin-resistant S. aureus (MRSA) blood isolates from 2001–05. *J Antimicrob Chemother* 2007; **60**: 788–94.

34. Wang G, Hindler JF, Ward KW, Bruckner DA. Increased vancomycin MICs for Staphylococcus aureus clinical isolates from a university hospital during a 5-year period. *J Clin Microbiol* 2006; **44**: 3883–6.

35. Lodise TP, Lomaestro B, Graves J, Drusano GL. Larger vancomycin doses (at least four grams per day) are associated with an increased incidence of nephrotoxicity. *Antimicrob Agents Chemother* 2008; **52**: 1330–6.

36. Silverman JA, Mortin LI, Vanpraagh AD, Li T, Alder J. Inhibition of daptomycin by pulmonary surfactant: in vitro modeling and clinical impact. *J Infect Dis* 2005; **191**: 2149–52.

37. Falagas ME, Kasiakou SK. Toxicity of polymyxins: a systematic review of the evidence from old and recent studies. *Crit Care* 2006; **10**: R27.

38. Selimoglu E. Aminoglycoside-induced ototoxicity. *Curr Pharm Des* 2007; **13**: 119–26.

39. Brogard JM, Conraux C, Collard M, Lavillaureix J. Ototoxicity of tobramycin in humans: influence of renal impairment. *Int J Clin Pharmacol Ther Toxicol* 1982; **20**: 408–16.

40. Narita M, Tsuji BT, Yu VL. Linezolid-associated peripheral and optic neuropathy, lactic acidosis, and serotonin syndrome. *Pharmacotherapy* 2007; **27**: 1189–97.

41. Lawrence KR, Adra M, Gillman PK. Serotonin toxicity associated with the use of linezolid: a review of postmarketing data. *Clin Infect Dis* 2006; **42**: 1578–83.

42. Owens RC, Donskey CJ, Gaynes RP, Loo VG, Muto CA. Antimicrobial-associated risk factors for Clostridium difficile infection. *Clin Infect Dis* 2008; **46**: S19–S31.

43. Grady R. Safety profile of quinolone antibiotics in the pediatric population. *Pediatr Infect Dis J* 2003; **22**: 1128–32.

44. Andreev E, Koopman M, Arisz L. A rise in plasma creatinine that is not a sign of renal failure: which drugs can be responsible? *J Intern Med* 1999; **246**: 247–52.

45. von Mach MA, Burhenne J, Weilemann LS. Accumulation of the solvent vehicle sulphobutylether beta cyclodextrin sodium in critically ill patients treated with intravenous voriconazole under renal replacement therapy. *BMC Clin Pharmacol* 2006; **6**: 6.

46. Alvarez-Lerma F, Allepuz-Palau A, Garcia MP, et al. Impact of intravenous administration of voriconazole in critically ill patients with impaired renal function. *J Chemother* 2008; **20**: 93–100.

47. Branch RA. Prevention of amphotericin B-induced renal impairment. A review on the use of sodium supplementation. *Arch Intern Med* 1988; **148**: 2389–94.

48. Fiore AE, Shay DK, Broder K, et al. Prevention and control of influenza: recommendations of the Advisory Committee on Immunization Practices (ACIP), 2008. *MMWR Recomm Rep* 2008; **57**: 1–60.

49. Jefferson TO, Demicheli V, Di Pietrantonj C, Jones M, Rivetti D. Neuraminidase inhibitors for preventing and treating influenza in healthy adults. *Cochrane Database Syst Rev* 2006; **3**: CD001265.

50. Mauermann WJ, Nemergut EC. The anesthesiologist's role in the prevention of surgical site infections. *Anesthesiology* 2006; **105**: 413–21.

51. Belda FJ, Aguilera L, García de la Asunción J, et al. Supplemental perioperative oxygen and the risk of surgical wound infection: a randomized controlled trial. *JAMA* 2005; **294**: 2035–42.

52. Greif R, Akça O, Horn EP, Kurz A, Sessler DI. Supplemental perioperative oxygen to reduce the incidence of surgical-wound infection. Outcomes Research Group. *N Eng J Med* 2000; **342**: 161–7.

53. Kurz A, Sessler DI, Lenhardt R. Perioperative normothermia to reduce the incidence of surgical-wound infection and shorten hospitalization. Study of Wound Infection and Temperature Group. *N Engl J Med* 1996; **334**: 1209–15.

54. Leaper D. Effects of local and systemic warming on postoperative infections. *Surg Infect (Larchmt)* 2006; **7**: S101–3.

55. Sessler DI. Complications and treatment of mild hypothermia. *Anesthesiology* 2001; **95**: 531–43.

56. Sessler DI. Non-pharmacologic prevention of surgical wound infection. *Anesthesiol Clin* 2006; **24**: 279–97.

57. Xiao H, Remick DG. Correction of perioperative hypothermia decreases experimental sepsis mortality by modulating the inflammatory response. *Crit Care Med* 2005; **33**: 161–7.

58. Brandstrup B, Tønnesen H, Beier-Holgersen R. Effects of intravenous fluid restriction on postoperative complications:comparison of two perioperative fluid regimens-a randomized assessor-blinded multicenter trial. *Ann Surg* 2003; **238**: 641–8.

59. Furnary AP, Zerr KJ, Grunkemeier GL, Starr A. Continuous intravenous insulin infusion reduces the incidence of deep sternal wound infection in diabetic patients after cardiac surgical procedures. *Ann Thorac Surg* 1999; **67**: 352–60.

60. Holte K, Foss NB, Andersen J, *et al.* Liberal or restrictive fluid administration in fast track colonic surgery: a randomized double-blind study. *Brit J Anaesthesia* 2007; **99**: 500–8.

61. Agarwal N, Murphy JG, Cayten CG, Stahl WM. Blood transfusion increases the risk of infection after trauma. *Arch Surg* 1993; **128**: 171–6.

62. Ali ZA, Lim E, Motalleb-Zadeh R*et al.* Allogenic blood transfusion does not predispose to infection after cardiac surgery. *Ann Thorac Surg* 2004; **78**: 1542–6.

63. Fergusson D, Hébert PC, Lee SK, *et al.* Clinical outcomes following institution of universal leukoreduction of blood transfusions for premature infants. *JAMA* 2003; **289**: 1950–6.

64. Hébert PC, Fergusson D, Blajchman MA, *et al.* Clinical outcomes following institution of the Canadian universal leukoreduction program for red blood cell transfusions. *JAMA* 2003; **289**: 1941–9.

65. Houbiers JG, van de Velde CJ, van de Watering LM, *et al.* Transfusion of red cells is associated with increased incidence of bacterial infection after colorectal surgery: a prospective study. *Transfusion* 1997; **37**: 126–34.

66. Ouattara A, Lecomte P, Le Manach Y, *et al.* Poor intraoperative blood glucose control is associated with a worsened hospital outcome after cardiac surgery in diabetic patients. *Anesthesiology* 2005; **103**: 687–94.

67. Raghavan M, Marik PE. Anemia, allogenic blood transfusion, and immunomodulation in the critically ill. *Chest* 2005; **127**: 295–307.

68. van den Berghe G, Wouters P, Weekers F, *et al.* Intensive insulin therapy in the critically ill patients. *N Eng J Med* 2001; **345**: 1359–67.

69. Vriesendorp TM, Morélis QJ, Devries JH, Legemate DA, Hoekstra JB. Early post-operative glucose levels are an independent risk factor for infection after peripheral vascular surgery. *Eur J Vasc Endovasc Surg* 2004; **28**: 520–5.

70. Zerr KJ, Furnary AP, Grunkemeier GL, *et al.* Glucose control lowers the risk of wound infection in diabetics after open heart operations. *Ann Thorac Surg* 1997; **63**: 356–61.

71. Lang K, Boldt J, Suttner S, Haisch G. Colloids versus crystalloids and tissue oxygen tension in patients undergoing major abdominal surgery. *Anesth Analg* 2001; **93**: 405–9.

72. Bratzler DW, Houck PM, Surgical Infection Prevention Guidelines Writers Workgroup. Antimicrobial prophylaxis for surgery: an advisory statement from the National Surgical Infection Prevention Project. *Clin Infect Dis* 2004; **38**: 1706–15.

73. Bratzler DW, Houck PM, Surgical Infection Prevention Guidelines Writers Workgroup. Antimicrobial prophylaxis for surgery: an advisory statement from the National Surgical Infection Prevention Project. *Am J Surg* 2005; **189**: 395–404.

74. Dellinger EP, Hausmann SM, Bratzler DW, *et al.* Hospitals collaborate to decrease surgical site infections. *Am J Surg* 2005; **190**: 9–15.

75. Harbarth S, Fankhauser C, Schrenzel J, *et al.* Universal screening for methicillin-resistant Staphylococcus aureus at hospital admission and nosocomial infection in surgical patients. *JAMA* 2008; **299**: 1149–57.

76. Robicsek A, Beaumont JL, Paule SM, *et al.* Universal surveillance for methicillin-resistant Staphylococcus aureus in 3 affiliated hospitals. *Ann Intern Med* 2008; **148**: 1–46.

77. Polk HC, Lopez-Mayor JF. Postoperative wound infection: a prospective study of determinant factors and prevention. *Surgery* 1969; **66**: 97–103.

78. Bamgbade OA, Rutter TW, Nafiu OO, Dorje P. Postoperative complications in obese and nonobese patients. *World J Surg* 2007; **31**: 556–60.

79. Edmiston CE, Krepel C, Kelly H, *et al.* Perioperative antibiotic prophylaxis in the gastric bypass patient: do we achieve therapeutic levels? *Surgery* 2004; **136**: 738–47.

80. Szmuk P, Rabb MF, Baumgartner JE, *et al.* Body morphology and the speed of cutaneous rewarming. *Anesthesiology* 2001; **95**: 18–21.

Clinical applications: evidence-based anesthesia practice
Preoperative drug management

Laureen Hill

Introduction

It is critical that clinicians understand the complex issues surrounding the use of chronic medications in the perioperative period in order to make safe and effective decisions regarding therapeutic drug management. Over 26 million surgical procedures are performed in the USA annually, and it is estimated that over 46% of the population uses at least one prescription drug, with over 63% of persons age 65 years or older taking three or more prescribed drugs [1]. Surveys of selected prescription and nonprescription medications based on records collected during physician office and outpatient hospital department visits reveal that, on average, patients over 45 years of age report concurrent use of nine medications, while patients over 65 years of age report concurrent use of 20 different medications. The potential for complications arising from chronic medication use during the perioperative period is significant.

Important considerations regarding chronic drug management include any potential effects, positive or negative, on proposed surgical and anesthetic procedures or on the patient's response to illness or surgical stress. One must also consider the potential for withdrawal symptoms or undesired physiologic consequences if a drug is to be withheld. In addition, decisions regarding the timing of safe, practical reinstitution of any medications during the postoperative period must be factored into the preoperative assessment and plan, with a focus on interactions between medications and likely postoperative conditions such as drug-induced bleeding with neuraxial catheter use, postoperative ileus, and tolerance or efficacy of orally administered drugs.

The focus of this chapter is to review general principles in the evaluation and management of chronic medications in the perioperative period, with particular emphasis on preoperative management. While earlier chapters have reviewed in great detail the preclinical and clinical pharmacology of specific classes of drugs, this chapter will emphasize practical aspects of drug administration and management strategies in the preoperative setting. There are few published randomized controlled trials regarding drug management in the perioperative period, and even fewer studies of drug–drug interactions in this same context. Recommendations here are based on existing evidence, expert opinions, and clinical application of available information.

Cardiovascular drugs

Given that the prevalence of cardiovascular disease increases with age, and that the number of patients over age 65 presenting for noncardiac surgery in the United States could conceivably reach 12 million per year, clinicians will certainly encounter high-risk surgical patients in whom the incidence of major complications can exceed 11% [2]. Drugs used in the treatment of cardiovascular pathophysiology have important effects, and potential interactions, that will be reviewed here (Fig. 60.1).

β-Adrenergic antagonists

The use of perioperative β-blockade has been widely demonstrated to reduce the incidence of cardiovascular complications associated with noncardiac surgery [3–5].

As discussed in Chapter 42, β-adrenoceptor antagonists reduce myocardial oxygen consumption via numerous mechanisms including reductions in heart rate, contractility, and afterload. While tight heart-rate control with β-blockade has been associated with improved short- and long-term cardiac outcomes in noncardiac surgery patients [6–8], the widespread and nonselective use of perioperative β-blockade has also been called into question based on lack of benefit and potential harm in low-risk patients [9] and an increased incidence of clinically relevant bradycardia, hypotension, and stroke [10]. While the best approach to reduce perioperative cardiac risk remains unresolved, the weight of the evidence would suggest that β-blockers should be administered throughout the perioperative period and titrated to maintain heart rate 60–65 bpm in high-risk patients (i.e., history of ischemic heart disease, congestive heart failure, cerebrovascular disease, insulin-requiring diabetes, renal insufficiency with baseline creatinine > 2.0 mg dL^{-1}, or planned vascular surgery), patients identified to have ischemic heart disease on preoperative testing, and

Anesthetic Pharmacology, 2nd edition, ed. Alex S. Evers, Mervyn Maze, Evan D. Kharasch. Published by Cambridge University Press. © Cambridge University Press 2011.

strategy, with or without anticoagulation, or a rhythm-control strategy. β-Adrenergic antagonists are the most effective single drugs used for rate control [49], although nondihydropyridine CCBs may be commonly used as well. Digoxin, while less effective than either β-blockers or CCBs, is another atrioventricular-nodal blocking drug that may be encountered, particularly in patients with heart failure or intolerance to the β-blockers or CCBs. In general, these drugs may be safely continued in the perioperative period, with special attention to electrolyte and acid–base balance and careful titration of anesthetic drugs to avoid precipitous decreases in heart rate or blood pressure.

For patients in whom therapy is aimed at restoring and maintaining sinus rhythm, a number of antiarrhythmic drugs may be used, and their selection is usually guided by the presence or absence of underlying cardiac disease. The class IC drugs, (flecainide, propafenone) are recommended as first-line drugs in patients without evidence of underlying structural heart disease [50]. These drugs do have negative inotropic and proarrhythmic properties. Amiodarone is a class III antiarrhythmic drug and is the most effective drug for preventing recurrence of AF [51–53]. Despite its demonstrated efficacy when compared to other rhythm-control drugs, amiodarone is not recommended as a first-line drug because of extensive potential adverse effects including neuropathy, interstitial pneumonitis, hepatotoxicity, and thyroid dysfunction. Like other class III drugs (sotalol and dofetilide), amiodarone is associated with QT prolongation and torsades de pointes and may increase sensitivity to hypotensive and bradycardic effects of volatile anesthetics during general anesthesia.

Preoperative evaluation in patients taking antiarrhythmics should include careful assessment for possible end-organ effects as described above, including 12-lead electrocardiography. Caution must be used with the continued administration of all of these drugs in the perioperative setting, but risks of recurrent AF must be considered before withdrawing these drugs prior to surgery. Many of the antiarrhythmics, including amiodarone, sotalol, β-blockers, and nondihydropyridine CCBs, have been associated with a reduction in postoperative AF [19,54–58], which complicates up to 8% of all noncardiac surgeries and is associated with increased morbidity, mortality, and hospital length of stay [59]. Given its extremely long half-life, routine discontinuation of amiodarone in the immediate preoperative period has little benefit and cannot be recommended.

Antilipemic drugs

There is strong evidence to support continued use of statins (3-hydroxy-3-methylglutaryl coenzyme A reductase inhibitors) in the perioperative period [11,60,61]. In addition to their lipid-lowering effects, statins reduce the harmful consequences of inflammation, thrombosis, platelet reactivity and ischemia–reperfusion injury observed during the surgical stress response [62]. A number of investigators have shown in multiple observational cohort studies and two small randomized controlled trials that even short-term treatment with statins reduces adverse cardiovascular outcomes in high-risk patients undergoing either cardiac or noncardiac surgery [63–66]. Furthermore, acute statin withdrawal in patients with acute coronary syndrome is associated with a higher rate of cardiovascular complications compared to patients who continue statin therapy and even those never treated with statins [67–69]. Surgical patients, in whom oral medications may be difficult to resume in the early postoperative course, have been shown to have increased risk of myonecrosis when statin resumption was delayed for an average of 4 days [70]. Despite earlier concerns about the risk of myositis and rhabdomyolysis with ongoing statin therapy during hospitalization for surgery [71], the weight of evidence supports current recommendations to continue statin therapy during the perioperative period to reduce cardiovascular morbidity and mortality [11,72].

Studies evaluating the use of other antilipemic drugs including bile-acid sequestrants, fibric-acid derivatives, and miscellaneous drugs such as ezetimibe have failed to demonstrate a role for the perioperative use of these drugs. The primary side effects of these drugs are gastrointestinal, including abdominal pain, bloating, nausea/vomiting, and constipation. Fibrates are associated with a significantly higher risk of rhabdomyolysis compared to statin monotherapy in hospitalized patients, and the risk is increased when statins and fibrates are used concurrently [73]. It is recommended to withhold all of these drugs prior to surgery.

The nicotinic acid drugs such as niaspan often produce "flushing" due to cutaneous and peripheral vasodilation, effects which may lead to hypotension in patients undergoing general anesthesia. In addition, nicotinic acid may cause decreases in platelet count or increases in prothrombin time and should be avoided in the preoperative period.

Diuretics

Typically it is recommended to withhold diuretics in the immediate preoperative period, to avoid presumed hypovolemia and electrolyte disturbances in fasting patients about to undergo surgery and anesthesia. It is interesting to note that in experimental studies furosemide has been shown to have dose-related direct effects at the neuromuscular junction, with depressant effects at low doses and increased force of contraction at higher doses [74]. Considering the typical therapeutic dose range of chronic loop diuretic drugs and the use of intraoperative neuromuscular blockade (NMB) monitoring to guide NMB dosing, the clinical relevance of this effect remains unclear.

Antiplatelet drugs, anticoagulants, hematologic drugs

Antiplatelet drugs

Increasing numbers of patients are receiving antiplatelet drugs for both primary and secondary prevention of myocardial infarction and stroke, and a large number of patients will

Table 60.1. Oral antiplatelet drugs: mechanisms of action and preoperative considerations

Drug	Mechanism of action	Time prior to surgery to withhold drug for return of platelet function
Aspirin	Irreversibly inhibits cyclooxygenase production of thromboxane A_2 (TxA$_2$) and TxA$_2$-mediated platelet aggregation	7–10 days
Cilastazol	Reversibly inhibits platelet aggregation via inhibition of phosphodiesterase leading to increased cAMP levels	2–3 days
Clopidogrel	Inhibits ADP-induced activation of glycoprotein IIb/IIIa complex	5–7 days
Dipyridamole	Stimulates release of prostacyclin, presumably inhibits adenosine deaminase, leading to accumulation of adenosine, and inhibits phosphodiesterase, leading to increased cAMP	2–3 days
NSAIDs	Reversibly inhibits cyclooxygenase production of TxA$_2$	24 hours for most drugs Ketorolac requires 24–48 hours Naproxen requires 2–3 days

present for noncardiac surgery within 12 months after coronary stent placement [75], many of whom will be receiving one or more antiplatelet drugs for prevention of stent thrombosis. Decisions concerning the preoperative management of patients receiving antiplatelet medications must be guided by a number of important factors, including clinical indications for therapy, risk of surgical bleeding, potential for thrombotic complications with drug interruption, regional anesthesia considerations [76,77], and individual drug pharmacokinetics (Table 60.1). Surgical stimulation confers a prothrombotic state that may persist for days, placing patients who are already at risk for coronary artery thrombosis or stroke at even greater risk of perioperative cardiovascular complications. In this context, it is

important to consider that abrupt withdrawal of either aspirin or clopidogrel leads to a rebound phenomenon resulting in increased thrombin generation and platelet aggregation [78–80]. Patients receiving antiplatelet drugs for primary prevention of myocardial infarction or stroke are probably at low risk for adverse cardiovascular events during temporary medication cessation, but patients receiving these drugs following an ischemic event or coronary stent placement are at much greater risk and must be managed more cautiously [81].

The risks of discontinuing antiplatelet therapy for noncardiac surgery in patients with either bare metal stents (BMS) or drug-eluting stents (DES) have been well described, and the reader is referred to a recent review article on the subject [82]. The risk of stent thrombosis is greatest prior to stent endothelialization, estimated to be 6 weeks in the case of BMS and 12 months or more with DES, although there is no readily available diagnostic test to evaluate the degree to which stent endothelialization has occurred [75,83–85]. Other factors that increase the risk of perioperative DES thrombosis include off-label uses such as placement of multiple stents, overlapping stents, stents implanted in bifurcations or branch points, and stent penetration of the necrotic core, information which may be unknown or unavailable during routine preoperative assessment [86]. It is estimated that 60–70% of patients receiving DES are in off-label populations [87], so this is not a trivial problem.

It is recommended that elective surgery be postponed in patients following percutaneous coronary intervention (PCI) for 6 weeks in the case of BMS and 12 months for DES placement [11,88]. If surgical delay is not possible within those time frames, it is recommended that both aspirin and clopidogrel be continued throughout the perioperative period [11,88]. While this approach raises concerns about surgical bleeding, studies looking at the bleeding risk from antiplatelet therapy in the perioperative period are conflicting and suggest greater surgical bleeding risk with continued use of clopidogrel when compared to aspirin [89,90]. In their review and meta-analysis of perioperative cardiovascular and bleeding risks in patients on low-dose aspirin for secondary cardiovascular prevention, Burger and colleagues found that with the exception of intracranial and transurethral prostate surgery, low-dose aspirin confers no increase in severity of bleeding or perioperative morbidity/mortality due to bleeding complications [91]. In vascular and coronary bypass surgery, the efficacy of continued aspirin therapy to improve graft patency, reduce incidence of transient ischemic attacks and stroke, and lower risk of perioperative morbidity and mortality is well documented [89,91,92].

On the basis of these and other studies, the recommendation for patients in whom surgery cannot be safely postponed and surgical bleeding risk is estimated to be unacceptably high is to continue aspirin if at all possible throughout the perioperative period while withholding clopidogrel until it can be safely resumed when hemostasis is achieved postoperatively.

Alternative bridging approaches to reduce stent thrombosis risk with unfractionated heparin (UFH), low-molecular-weight heparin (LMWH) or short-acting glycoprotein IIb/IIIa antagonists (tirofiban, eptifibitide) have also been proposed but remain poorly studied with insufficient evidence for recommendation [11,93].

Anticoagulants

As discussed above, many factors must be considered when making perioperative anticoagulation management decisions, including clinical indications for anticoagulation, surgical procedure and potential for significant bleeding, risk of adverse thromboembolic events, regional anesthesia considerations [76,77,94], and drug pharmacokinetics. Certain procedures are considered a low risk for significant periprocedural bleeding, including dental, cataract, dermatologic, and diagnostic gastrointestinal procedures, and therefore continued oral anticoagulation is recommended [95–97]. For all other procedures where surgical bleeding is a significant concern, risk stratification and management based on thromboembolic risk is advised.

In general, patients considered to have higher risk for thromboembolic events include those with recent pulmonary embolism (PE) or deep venous thrombosis (DVT), mechanical aortic valve with prior stroke, mechanical mitral valve, ventricular assist devices, or atrial fibrillation with prior stroke. These patients should have alternative therapies when possible (e.g., vena cava filter) and/or bridging therapy with shorter-acting anticoagulants while longer-acting drugs are withheld [88,98]. Vitamin K antagonists such as warfarin should be discontinued 5 days prior to surgery to allow adequate time for the INR to normalize. Temporary bridging anticoagulation with LMWH should be discontinued 24 hours prior to surgery, while UFH should be discontinued approximately 4 hours prior to surgery. Direct thrombin inhibitors are shorter-acting anticoagulants that may be encountered in patients with documented or suspected heparin-induced thrombocytopenia. Bivalirudin has an elimination half-life of 25 minutes in patients with normal renal function, and argatroban has a terminal elimination half-life of approximately 45 minutes in patients with normal hepatic function, so discontinuation of these drugs for 4 hours (longer in patients with renal or hepatic impairment) should be adequate for reversal of anticoagulant effects. Patients at lower risk, including those with aortic valve prosthesis, isolated atrial fibrillation, and remote DVT/PE, may suspend anticoagulation preoperatively without need for bridging therapy [88,99]. Patients with other indications for anticoagulation (e.g., pulmonary hypertension, cardiomyopathy, transient ischemic attack, etc.) must be considered individually. Decisions regarding reinstitution of anticoagulation will depend on surgical hemostasis and likely bleeding risk and are likely to vary widely.

With respect to the use of antithrombotic drugs and neuraxial anesthesia, the American Society of Regional Anesthesia (ASRA) has published guidelines for preoperative management [76].

In general, there is no contraindication to performing neuraxial anesthesia in patients receiving aspirin or nonsteroidal anti-inflammatory drugs (NSAIDs) as monotherapy, but the concurrent use of other antithrombotic drugs does confer increased risk of spinal hematoma. ASRA recommends that prior to neuraxial procedures, ticlopidine should be withheld 14 days, clopidogrel 7 days, and GPIIa/IIIb inhibitors for anywhere between 8 and 48 hours depending on the particular drug. Vitamin K antagonists, LMWH, and UFH should be managed according to the recommendations discussed above, with prothrombin (PT) and activated partial thromboplastin (aPTT) times used to verify restoration of normal clotting.

Pentoxifylline

Pentoxifylline is a methylxanthine derivative that has rheologic effects which may be useful in the management of patients with peripheral vascular disease and claudication, cerebrovascular insufficiency, or even sickle cell disease. Pentoxifylline acts to increase erythrocyte flexibility, decrease blood viscosity, decrease fibrinogen concentration, and increase fibrinolytic activity. While it has no direct effects on platelet function, it may produce additive or synergistic effects when use concomitantly with antiplatelet, antithrombotic, or certain herbal products such as gingko, garlic, or ginger, so caution is advised. Patients presenting for surgery with bleeding risk, especially patients at risk for intracranial and retinal bleeding should not receive pentoxifylline. Given the elimination half-life of 2 hours for active metabolites, it is reasonable to withhold this drug for 1 day prior to surgery.

Antidiabetic drugs

Glucose management in the perioperative period is a major determinant of postoperative outcomes [100–102]. Surgical stress and critical illness have been shown to induce a catabolic state and development of insulin resistance, contributing to glucose derangements in diabetic and nondiabetic patients [103–105]. The positive effects of intraoperative and postoperative insulin administration on stress metabolism have been well described [103,106–108], and strategies aimed at blood glucose control are advocated. Preoperative strategies, in contrast, are often aimed at minimizing the risk of hypoglycemia during a fasting state, although a number of investigators are challenging traditional paradigms and have shown that minimizing fasting and administering preoperative carbohydrate will significantly reduce insulin resistance and improve a number of postoperative outcomes in orthopedic, colorectal, cardiac, and general surgical patients [109–112]. Decisions about preoperative management of antidiabetic drugs should integrate an assessment of the individual's level of glucose control, risk for hypoglycemia, surgical procedure, and the type and route of drug administration.

Sulfonylureas act on adenosine-triphosphate-sensitive potassium (K_{ATP}) channels in the pancreas to cause β-cell depolarization and insulin release. The magnitude of insulin resistance during surgical stress often renders these drugs ineffective at achieving desired metabolic control. Sulfonylureas also act on cardiomyocyte K_{ATP} channels and potentially reduce or prevent the protective effects of ischemic or anesthetic preconditioning. Sulfonylureas are not recommended in the perioperative or acute care setting and should be discontinued preoperatively.

Metformin works by increasing insulin sensitivity in target tissues and reducing hepatic gluconeogenesis. Metformin has been linked to an increased incidence of lactic acidosis and death, but this is extremely rare when the drug is used as labeled [113,114]. The accumulation of metformin due to renal impairment may contribute to lactic acidosis, and its use should be avoided in surgical patients in whom fluid shifts, blood loss, and other factors may increase the likelihood of renal injury.

The thiazolidinediones enhance insulin sensitivity in target tissues and have a slow onset due to extensive protein binding. Pioglitazone induces cytochrome P450 (CYP) activity and may decrease effects of certain anesthetic drugs metabolized by this enzyme such as midazolam and fentanyl. As with all oral drugs, these drugs should be suspended in the preoperative period when patients are fasting and risk of hypoglycemia is increased.

In general, insulin is the preferred drug for glucose management in the perioperative period because of the relative ease with which administration can be titrated to achieve glucose levels within the desired range. Short- and rapid-acting drugs like regular insulin, insulin aspart, insulin lispro, and insulin glulisine are appropriate therapeutic adjuncts when food and fluid intake are restricted and during periods of physiologic stress when glucose levels may fluctuate significantly. Patients using intermediate-acting insulin such as neutral protamine Hagedorn (NPH) or long-acting drugs such as insulin detemir or insulin glargine should be instructed to reduce dosing preoperatively to avoid dangerous decreases in blood glucose levels during periods of fasting. Patients using insulin pumps for continuous infusion should be advised to continue the basal infusion but to eliminate intermittent bolus dosing until a steady diet is resumed.

Central and peripheral nervous system drugs

Many patients presenting for surgery are likely to be taking psychotropic medications, with one study demonstrating 43% of adults surveyed in a preoperative assessment clinic reporting use of at least one psychotropic drug and 11% reporting use of multiple psychotropic drugs [115]. The potential for significant physiologic effects, hazardous drug interactions, or important withdrawal events must be considered in managing these drugs in the perioperative setting [116,117].

Antidepressants
Tricyclic antidepressants

Tricyclic antidepressants (TCAs) inhibit presynaptic uptake of norepinephrine and serotonin and block postsynaptic cholinergic, histaminergic, and α_1-adrenergic receptors. They lower the seizure threshold, may cause orthostatic hypotension, and slow cardiac conduction, prolonging the QT interval. TCAs may potentiate direct-acting sympathomimetics while blunting the response of indirect-acting drugs. Rapid discontinuation of TCAs may lead to withdrawal symptoms and increased relapse rates and is therefore not recommended [118].

Monoamine oxidase inhibitors

Monoamine oxidase inhibitors (MAOIs) are probably most recognized for their potential hazardous interactions with a number of drugs commonly used in anesthesia and the perioperative setting. Both reversible and irreversible MAOIs act by preventing the degradation of norepinephrine and serotonin. These drugs potentiate the effects of all sympathomimetics, and use of indirect-acting sympathomimetic drugs has led to hypertensive crises [119]. Concomitant use of drugs that block presynaptic serotonin reuptake, such as meperidine, dextromethorphan, TCAs, and selective serotonin reuptake inhibitors (SSRIs), may precipitate serotonin syndrome, a serious condition associated with stupor, muscle rigidity, severe agitation, and fever [120,121]. Severe withdrawal symptoms including suicidal ideation, hallucinations, paranoia, and major depression may accompany abrupt withdrawal from MAOIs, so discontinuation is not advised. Avoidance of "triggering" drugs is recommended in the perioperative period.

Selective serotonin reuptake inhibitors

The SSRIs exert their effects through presynaptic inhibition of serotonin reuptake. Although this class is generally better tolerated and safer in overdose than the TCAs or MAOIs, important side effects do occur, including platelet dysfunction and bleeding and syndrome of inappropriate antidiuretic hormone hypersecretion (SIADH). Important anesthetic interactions are only notable for possible serotonin syndrome with concomitant use of drugs like meperidine which also block serotonin reuptake. Withdrawal symptoms may be severe, especially with the shorter-acting drugs, so discontinuation is not recommended.

Miscellaneous antidepressants

Mirtazapine, venlafaxine, and bupropion are antidepressants that do not belong to any of the other classes of drugs described. In general, they have few serious side effects or drug interactions with anesthetic drugs and may be continued in the preoperative period. One important exception applies to bupropion, which has a greater potential to produce seizures and should be avoided or used with caution in patients at risk.

Antipsychotics

Antipsychotics exert their effects primarily through antagonism at the dopamine (D_2) receptor, although they also have important anticholinergic and anti-α-adrenergic effects. Newer atypical drugs possess less potency at the D_2 receptor and produce fewer extrapyramidal effects. All of the antipsychotics have the potential to prolong the QTc interval, and careful ECG monitoring is warranted. Some of these drugs lower the seizure threshold, and seizures have been reported in combination with desflurane [122]. Antipsychotics potentiate the effects of sedatives and analgesics and may lead to excessive anticholinergic effects when used with other dopamine antagonists such as phenothiazines or scopolamine in the treatment of nausea. Neuroleptic malignant syndrome (NMS) is a serious condition associated with use of antipsychotic drugs and is manifest by muscle rigidity, altered mental status, fever, elevated creatine phosphokinase (CPK), tachycardia, diaphoresis, tachypnea, and leukocytosis. NMS is not necessarily due to overdosage and in fact has been described with abrupt cessation of therapy [123]. Given the potential for withdrawal symptoms and early relapse, discontinuation is not advised, but caution must be exercised during the perioperative period in patients receiving chronic antipsychotic therapy.

Lithium

Lithium is used as a mood-stabilizing and antimanic drug. It competes with sodium, potassium, magnesium, and calcium at various cellular binding and transport sites, although its exact mechanism of action in bipolar disorder is unknown. It has a narrow therapeutic window, and plasma concentrations may change rapidly with changes in fluid balance and renal function. Important interactions exist with NSAIDs, ACE inhibitors, thiazide diuretics, drugs which may decrease glomerular filtration or alter fluid and sodium balance. Withdrawal symptoms are not significant, although risk of relapse is increased with abrupt discontinuation. In surgical patients at increased risk for hypovolemia or renal impairment, it is reasonable to decrease or discontinue lithium in the perioperative period and to follow lithium levels frequently when treatment resumes.

Benzodiazepines

Benzodiazepines are used primarily for their anxiolytic properties, although they also have anticonvulsant and muscle-relaxant effects. Benzodiazepines exert their anxiolytic effects through enhancement of the benzodiazepine/γ-aminobutyric acid (GABA)$_A$ receptor complex. Their CNS-depressant properties are additive with those of other CNS-depressant anesthetic drugs. Withdrawal symptoms may be severe and potentially life-threatening, particularly with shorter-acting drugs, and abrupt discontinuation in the perioperative period should be avoided.

Anticonvulsants

Anticonvulsant drugs have many therapeutic applications including treatment and prevention of seizures, mood stabilization, treatment of cardiac dysrhythmias associated with QT prolongation, and management of chronic neuropathic pain syndromes. This is a broad category comprising many drugs with differing chemical structures, mechanisms of action, and side-effect profiles. In general, these drugs should be continued in the preoperative period to avoid precipitating seizures or other unwanted withdrawal symptoms. Gabapentin is a second-generation anticonvulsant that, in addition to its chronic use in seizure disorders and neuropathic pain syndromes, may be useful as an acute therapeutic to reduce preoperative anxiety and postoperative pain, nausea, vomiting, and delirium [124]. Therapeutic levels of anticonvulsant drugs should be monitored where applicable. Chronic exposure to certain anticonvulsants (carbamazepine, phenytoin, and phenobarbital in particular) may result in resistance and increased requirements for nondepolarizing neuromuscular blocking drugs [125].

Antiparkinson drugs

The pathophysiology of Parkinson's disease is a deficiency of dopamine in the basal ganglia. The mainstay of therapy is with levodopa, a prodrug which is converted into dopamine in the CNS. Combination with carbidopa prevents peripheral conversion of levodopa, resulting in greater concentrations in the CNS where it has its therapeutic effect. Orthostatic hypotension is a common side effect, although hypertension and tachyarrhythmias are reported and may affect intraoperative management. Abrupt discontinuation of levodopa or carbidopa/levodopa may result in NMS and should be avoided [123].

Skeletal muscle relaxants

This class of drugs includes a wide variety of drugs with different chemical structures, mechanisms of action, and side-effect profiles. Cyclobenzaprine is similar in structure and function to TCAs and is used to treat painful musculoskeletal conditions. Baclofen is a structural analog of the inhibitory neurotransmitter GABA and is used as an oral or intrathecal drug to treat spasticity and improve mobility in patients with spinal cord pathology. Tizanidine is a central-acting α_2-adrenergic agonist used to treat spasticity associated with cerebral or spinal cord disorders. Dantrolene interferes with calcium release from the sarcoplasmic reticulum in skeletal muscle cells and is useful in treating muscle spasm associated with upper motor neuron disorders, although it is associated with significant hepatotoxicity, limiting its chronic therapeutic use. Anesthesiologists are most familiar with the use of intravenous dantrolene to treat malignant hyperthermia. Abrupt discontinuation of baclofen is associated with severe withdrawal reactions and has in rare cases progressed to rhabdomyolysis, multi-organ failure, and death. There is limited experience with withdrawal of tizanidine, but caution is advised because of adverse withdrawal reactions in animal studies. All of these drugs should be continued in the perioperative period.

Cholinesterase inhibitors

Myasthenia gravis is an autoimmune disease characterized by production of antibodies against acetylcholine receptors at the motor endplate. Treatment consists primarily of cholinesterase inhibitors used to potentiate the action of acetylcholine at the nicotinic receptors on the skeletal muscle. Muscarinic cholinergic effects occur as well. Use of cholinesterase inhibitors in myasthenic patients in the immediate preoperative period is generally advocated to minimize risk of muscle weakness and respiratory embarrassment immediately following surgery, but intraoperative use of neuromuscular blockers and reversal drugs must be done with extreme caution if at all. Excessive anticholinesterase effects (cholinergic crisis) are difficult to distinguish from residual neuromuscular blockade or inadequate anticholinesterase effects (myasthenic crisis), as all will produce extreme muscle weakness.

Alzheimer's disease drugs

Patients with Alzheimer's disease have limited drug therapy options. Two centrally acting cholinesterase inhibitors have been approved by the US Food and Drug Administration (FDA) for the treatment of Alzheimer's disease. Depression and insomnia are often present in early stages and may be treated with antidepressant drugs. The MAOI selegiline may be used to slow the rate of decline in people with more advanced disease. All of these drugs should be managed as described in earlier sections.

CNS stimulants

Amphetamines are noncatecholamine sympathomimetic drugs used in the treatment of attention-deficit hyperactivity disorder and narcolepsy, and as such they have significant cardiovascular affects. These drugs, including amphetamine, dextroamphetamine, and methamphetamine, generally cause increases in blood pressure and heart rate, and at higher doses cardiac dysrhythmias may occur. Despite the potential for hemodynamic instability during the perioperative period, they should not be discontinued abruptly because of the potential for significant and possibly severe withdrawal symptoms.

Anti-infective drugs

Antibiotics are recommended as prophylaxis in surgical patients, depending on multiple factors including wound classification, risk of endocarditis, procedures involving infected tissues or spaces, and patient immune competence. Indications, dosing, and timing of antibiotic prophylaxis are reviewed in Chapter 59.

Antiretroviral drugs and antituberculous drugs may be encountered in the surgical patient, and while disease status and coexisting processes are most relevant to appropriate preoperative management, a few important drug interactions are worth noting. The non-nucleoside reverse transcriptase inhibitor, nevirapine, and rifampin both cause CYP enzyme induction and can decrease serum levels of drugs metabolized by this enzyme, including midazolam, fentanyl, and barbiturates. The protease inhibitors and isoniazid have the opposite effect, competitively inhibiting CYP and increasing the effects of these drugs. Many of the retroviral drugs can produce hyperglycemia, and careful blood glucose monitoring is warranted. These medications should be continued in the perioperative period, as discontinuation may contribute to development of resistance.

Antineoplastics

The pharmacologic interactions between anesthetic and chemotherapeutic drugs are not well described and are understandably difficult to study or confirm because of the high incidence of adverse effects from both the underlying malignancy and the drugs used in cancer treatment [126]. A few drugs have known important effects that anesthesiologists should understand, and these will be described here, but in general discontinuation of antineoplastic drugs may lead to important disruptions in cancer treatment and cannot be recommended. Instead, preoperative evaluation should aim to identify any current or potential organ-system dysfunction due to chemotherapy and to address possible important interactions (Table 60.2) [127]. Most antineoplastic drugs are potent myelosuppressants and may affect any or all of the bone-marrow cell lines. Anthracycline antibiotics, cyclophosphamide, and 5-fluorouracil (5-FU) are cardiotoxic and can produce heart failure or enhance any cardiac-depressant effects of general anesthetic drugs. Bleomycin causes a dose-related interstitial pneumonitis which can be aggravated by high inspired oxygen concentrations [128]. Lidocaine has been shown to enhance bleomycin-induced cytotoxicity [129,130]. A number of drugs including cisplatin, carboplatin, paclitaxel, and methotrexate are nephrotoxic, and renal function should be assessed. Methotrexate may also lead to mild, reversible hepatic dysfunction, although cirrhosis can occur with prolonged use. The cytotoxic effects of methotrexate, particularly on proliferating cells such as bone-marrow and mucosal cells, are potentiated by previous or concomitant use of nitrous oxide [131]. Peripheral neurotoxicity may be pronounced with vincristine or paclitaxel, and a careful neurologic assessment should be performed, particularly if a regional anesthetic technique is considered. Cyclophosphamide is a pseudocholinesterase inhibitor and may prolong the effects of succinylcholine for up to 4 weeks following its use.

Immunosuppressants

As with anticancer drugs, maintenance immunosuppressive drugs have few known specific interactions with anesthetic drugs, but they do have several important organ-system effects that should be considered during the preoperative evaluation [132,133]. Cyclosporine and tacrolimus are calcineurin

Table 60.2. Antineoplastic drugs: major organ-system toxicities and preoperative considerations

Class	Drug	Cardiac toxicity	Pulmonary toxicity	Renal/genitourinary toxicity	Hepatotoxicity	Neurotoxicity	Myelosuppression
Alkylating drugs	Cyclophosphamide	●	●				●
	Busulfan		●		●	●	●
	Carboplatin			●	●		●
	Cisplatin			●		●	
Antibiotics	Bleomycin		●				
	Doxorubicin	●					●
Antimetabolites	Methotrexate		●	●	●		●
	5-Fluorouracil	●				●	●
Biologic response modifiers	Imitinab	●			●		●
	Rituximab	●	●		●	●	●
	Interferon-α		●		●	●	●
Epipodophylatoxins	Etoposide						●
Taxanes	Paclitaxel	●			●	●	●
	Docetaxel				●	●	●
Vinca alkaloids	Vinblastine					●	●
	Vincristine					●	

inhibitors that have significant neurotoxicity including generalized seizures. Nephrotoxicity is another potential complication of calcineurin inhibitors, and electrolytes and renal function should be monitored closely. These drugs are metabolized by the CYP system and may have significant interactions with other drugs that also undergo CYP biotransformation. Cyclosporine and its solvent, Cremophor, prolong the duration of nondepolarizing muscle relaxants. Azathioprine and mycophenolate interfere with purine synthesis and can cause significant bone-marrow suppression. Azathioprine can also lead to hepatobiliary dysfunction. Corticosteroids have many known side effects including hyperglycemia, hypertension, osteoporosis, and adrenal suppression. All of these drugs should be continued in the perioperative period, using intravenous substitution intraoperatively and postoperatively as necessary to avoid inadequate blood levels and possible rejection.

Antithymocyte globulin (ATG), OKT3, and the interleukin 2 (IL-2) receptor monoclonal antibodies, basiliximab and daclizumab, are typically used as induction therapy for a limited time following transplantation. Side effects are typically related to a cytokine release syndrome including fever, rigors, and hemodynamic lability. Marrow suppression may occur with ATG, and cell counts should be evaluated preoperatively.

Hormones and metabolics

Estrogens
Estrogens are partially metabolized by CYP enzymes and may have significant interactions with other drugs that undergo biotransformation by CYP enzymes including benzodiazepines, barbiturates, and potent synthetic opiates. Estrogens are associated with increased thromboembolic risk [134,135] and may place surgical patients at greater risk due to the prothrombotic state associated with surgical stress and decreased mobilization during and after surgery. It is not clear whether stopping estrogens shortly before surgical intervention reduces this risk, or what adverse effects may be associated with abrupt withdrawal. In addition, there is no evidence that suggests venous thromboembolism (VTE) prophylaxis is not effective in surgical patients taking estrogens in the perioperative period. It is reasonable to discuss alternatives with patients and to develop an individualized plan that incorporates VTE prophylaxis to minimize risk.

Thyroid preparations
Levothyroxine has a half-life of several days, so a brief interruption in daily dosing should have little impact. Intervals longer than 7 days may lead to hypothyroidism, so intravenous drugs should be substituted if oral dosing is not possible, and

dosing should be halved due to greater bioavailability with intravenous administration compared to the oral route [136]. Patients taking medications for hyperthyroidism should continue these drugs in the preoperative period [136].

Glucocorticoids

Patients taking steroids prior to surgery should continue these drugs perioperatively to prevent adrenal crisis. The duration of treatment with corticosteroids that results in hypothalamic–pituitary–adrenal axis suppression has not been precisely defined, but steroid use for greater than 5 days may place a patient at risk for adrenal suppression [137]. Stress-dose steroid coverage is no longer routinely recommended, but providers should have a high index of suspicion for adrenal insufficiency in surgical or critically ill patients with refractory hypotension, and supplement with intravenous steroid drugs.

Gout preparations

Colchicine is used chronically in the treatment of gout and works through an antimitotic mechanism to prevent neutrophil migration and thus inflammatory response in areas of urate crystal deposition. Colchicine exhibits diverse pharmacologic effects, and in addition to its antimitotic activity in proliferating tissues, including bone marrow, it may cause hypothermia, respiratory center suppression, and vasomotor stimulation, all of which may be detrimental in the surgical patient [138]. Adverse gastrointestinal effects are quite common, and colchicine is likely poorly tolerated in fasting patients. Colchicine may be safely discontinued in the preoperative period. When it is resumed, peak anti-inflammatory effect will require 24–48 hours. Allopurinol is used for the treatment of signs and symptoms of gout, including acute attacks, tophi, joint destruction, uric acid lithiasis, and/or uric acid nephropathy. It inhibits xanthine oxidase to reduce uric acid synthesis. Allopurinol therapy should be constant to avoid increases in serum urate concentrations, but since it should be administered after meals and with plenty of fluids, it is not appropriate in the fasting surgical patient. Intravenous allopurinol is available, although the FDA has designated it an orphan drug indicated for use to prevent acute hyperuricemia during chemotherapy in patients at risk for tumor lysis syndrome.

Respiratory drugs

Inhaled drugs

For the prevention of bronchospasm due to reactive airways disease, scheduled use of inhaled longer-acting β-agonists and/or inhaled corticosteroids is recommended [139]. These drugs should be continued throughout the perioperative period. For treatment of acute bronchospasm, short-acting β-agonists are the therapy of choice. Inhaled anticholinergic therapy may have added benefit in treating severe acute exacerbations in the perioperative period [139].

Leukotriene antagonists

Leukotriene antagonists are alternative treatment for the prophylaxis and chronic management of asthma and allergic rhinitis, and may be safely continued in the perioperative period for patients who can tolerate oral medications.

Theophylline

Theophylline is a xanthine derivative that is recommended as an alternative, adjunct therapy with low-dose inhaled corticosteroids for inadequately controlled moderate persistent asthma [139]. Theophylline relaxes airway smooth muscle and appears to possess anti-inflammatory and immunomodulatory activity [140], although its mechanism of action is complex and not completely understood. Theophylline exerts stimulant effects on the CNS, and on cardiac and skeletal muscle. Chronic toxicity may lead to seizures, cardiac dysrhythmias, and hemodynamic instability. Interactions with volatile anesthetics may precipitate tachyarrhythmias, and concurrent use with ketamine reduces seizure threshold. Theophylline is metabolized by CYP enzymes and may have significant interactions with several drugs, including anesthetic drugs that undergo biotransformation by the same enzyme system, such as potent synthetic opiates, benzodiazepines, and barbiturates. Theophylline may decrease enzymatic metabolism of ropivacaine via competitive inhibition. Given that several studies have failed to demonstrate a benefit of theophylline in the management of acute bronchospasm, and the potential for several adverse effects, it is prudent to withhold theophylline prior to surgery and to monitor levels closely when the drug is resumed postoperatively.

Acetylcysteine

Acetylcysteine is a mucolytic drug that may be used in patients with cystic fibrosis or COPD. It is thought to react with disulfide linkages of mucoproteins in bronchial secretions to decrease viscosity and facilitate removal. It is typically administered via inhalation, although oral and intravenous preparations are available and used for a variety of indications including prevention of hepatotoxicity in paracetamol (acetaminophen) overdose and prevention of nephrotoxicity in high-risk patients when used with hydration prior to radiocontrast administration. Important interactions in the perioperative period have not been reported and inhalational therapy may be continued. Oral preparations have an unpleasant odor and may induce vomiting, so their use prior to induction of general anesthesia is undesirable.

Analgesics and anti-inflammatory drugs

Opiates

Patients taking chronic opiate analgesics should have these medications continued in the perioperative period to prevent the adverse consequences of opiate withdrawal.

It is generally recommended that usual dosing be continued prior to surgery, with additional opiates as necessary to manage acute surgical pain intra- and postoperatively. It is important to recognize that prolonged activation of opioid receptors can lead to tolerance, or apparent loss of effectiveness of opioid agonists, and increased drug administration may be required in surgical patients with chronic opiate use for adequate pain relief.

Nonsteroidal anti-inflammatory drugs

These drugs act by inhibiting cyclooxygenase enzymes responsible for production of prostaglandins and thromboxanes involved the inflammatory response. In addition to their anti-inflammatory properties, NSAIDs are effective analgesics and antipyretics, may lead to decreased renal perfusion and glomerular filtration, and may produce gastrointestinal irritation and inhibit platelet aggregation. The antiplatelet properties may be relevant in the surgical patient and are reversible within 1–10 days depending on the drug in question. For patients in whom a high degree of hemostasis is desired, these drugs should be discontinued preoperatively, allowing adequate time for recovery of platelet function (Table 60.1).

Tumor necrosis factor α inhibitors

Tumor necrosis factor α (TNFα) inhibitors have become fairly commonplace in the treatment of rheumatoid arthritis (RA). They act through disruption of multiple important cell-signaling pathways in the inflammatory and immune cascades. In theory, patients receiving these drugs would be presumed to be at higher risk for poor wound healing and wound infections following surgery, but the literature is conflicting [141,142]. Other important factors that may contribute more significantly to surgical wound complications include documented history of wound infections or poor wound healing, low albumin, diabetes, tobacco use, or anticipated difficult dissection and/or prolonged tourniquet time [141]. In many patients, RA symptoms are disabling when medications are discontinued, so decisions to continue or withhold RA therapy should be made based on a careful assessment of all risk factors.

Ophthalmic drugs

Ophthalmic drugs used chronically in the treatment of glaucoma reduce intraocular pressure by either decreasing aqueous humor production (β-adrenergic antagonists, carbonic anhydrase inhibitors, α2-adrenergic agonists) or increasing aqueous humor outflow (prostaglandins, cholinergic agonists, anticholinesterases). Perioperative use of these drugs is advised to minimize increases in intraocular pressure, but most of these drugs are systemically absorbed, and systemic effects should be anticipated.

Tobacco- and alcohol-cessation drugs

Nicotine

Nicotine acts on nicotinic cholinergic receptors in the CNS, autonomic ganglia, adrenal medullary cells, and neuromuscular junction. Nicotine produces an increase in circulating cortisol and catecholamine levels, increasing vasomotor tone, chronotropy, and inotropy, and its neuroendocrine effects aggravate insulin resistance. Concerns about the use of nicotine transdermal systems in the perioperative period are related to the consequences of vasoconstriction on myocardial perfusion and tissue perfusion and potential adverse effects on cardiac function and wound healing. While it would appear that discontinuing nicotine in the surgical patient would be advised, some investigators have reported on the use of transdermal or transnasal nicotine as a useful analgesic to reduce postoperative opiate requirements [143]. Consideration of potential risks and benefits in any given case should inform decisions regarding perioperative nicotine use. Tobacco smoke contains hydrocarbons that induce hepatic CYP enzymes, so sudden cessation of smoking may reduce clearance of several important drugs used in anesthesia and increase their effects, and caution is advised. These microsomal enzyme effects are not related to the nicotine component of tobacco, so substitution of nicotine for tobacco would not decrease the expected risks of tobacco cessation on drug clearance.

Disulfiram

Disulfiram interferes with hepatic oxidation of acetaldehyde, a product of ethanol metabolism. Increasing levels of acetaldehyde due to alcohol ingestion produce unpleasant symptoms such as headache, nausea, vomiting, diaphoresis, and palpitations, and may progress to cardiopulmonary collapse. It is used as an adjunctive treatment in alcoholics to discourage alcohol ingestion. Disulfiram itself is rather nontoxic and has no known interactions with general anesthesia. It may compete for CYP binding sites with benzodiazepines that undergo biotransformation by CYP enzymes, increasing their plasma concentrations and effects. It has also been reported to exacerbate hepatic dysfunction. Disulfiram may have biologic activity for as long as 2 weeks from the last dose. It is reasonable to discontinue in the perioperative period to minimize interactions with sedative drugs and risks of hepatic insufficiency, particularly in hospitalized patients with limited access to alcohol and low risk of relapse.

Herbal preparations

The history of herbal medicine use in the United States dates back to the early colonial days when health care was largely provided in the home. Today, it is estimated that over 20–30% of adults in the USA take herbal supplements in a market that has grown into a multi-billion-dollar industry [144]. The FDA considers herbals as foods, so they do not undergo rigorous testing before going to market. Unfortunately, many patients also do not consider these products "medicines" and may not mention their use during preoperative evaluation. Many of the effects and interactions of these products may still be unrecognized, although a few commonly used herbal preparations do have known and significant consequences in surgical patients. Many of them interfere with normal platelet function, and several may alter CYP activity [144–146]. It is recommended that a careful history, including the use of herbal supplements, be sought at the time of preoperative assessment, and that these products be discontinued for 2–3 weeks prior to surgery when at all possible [147].

Echinacea is used primarily for its immunostimulant properties. It has potential hepatotoxicity, particularly if used along with anesthetic or nonanesthetic drugs that may affect hepatic function [148]. Garlic has been used for "heart health" by patients seeking antiplatelet, antioxidant, and fibrinolytic effects. Garlic-induced decreases in platelet aggregation have been described in vitro [149], and spontaneous epidural hematoma has been reported in an 87-year-old man with excessive garlic ingestion [150]. Ginger is used in the treatment of gastrointestinal upset, but has been shown to be a potent inhibitor of thromboxane synthetase and platelet aggregation [151].Gingko biloba is used for a number of ailments including claudication, vertigo, sexual dysfunction, and memory impairment. It is becoming increasingly popular because of its purported effectiveness on cognitive performance in patients with dementia [152]. Unfortunately it inhibits platelet-activating factor (153) and has been linked to intracranial hemorrhage [154,155]. St. John's wort has been used for a number of psychiatric disorders including depression, anxiety, and insomnia. Its mechanism of action remains unclear, but it can cause serotonin syndrome in patients taking SSRIs. Ginseng is used to increase energy levels and reduce stress. It may have untoward effects on blood pressure and glucose regulation. There may be clinically relevant interactions with warfarin [156] and antiplatelet drugs [157]. Kava kava is used for anxiety disorders and may have important interactions with other CNS depressants [158]. Ma-huang is used for a number of ailments including viral infections, fever, and arthritis and as a diet aid. It can produce adverse cardiovascular and CNS effects, including hypertension, tachyarrhythmias, seizures, stroke, myocardial infarction, and death [159]. Use of indirect-acting sympathomimetics during surgery may be completely ineffective due to depletion of norepinephrine stores at autonomic nerve terminals.

Summary

The potential for complications arising from chronic medication use during the perioperative period is significant. Therefore it is critical that clinicians understand the complex issues surrounding the use of chronic medications, in order to make safe and effective preoperative decisions regarding therapeutic drug management throughout the perioperative period. A particularly important consideration is the potential for withdrawal symptoms or undesired physiologic consequences if a drug is withheld.

Cardiovascular drugs

β-Adrenergic antagonists – Perioperative β-blockade has been demonstrated to reduce the incidence of cardiovascular complications associated with noncardiac surgery. While the best approach to reduce perioperative cardiac risk remains unresolved, the weight of evidence suggests that β-blockers should be administered throughout the perioperative period, as β-blocker withdrawal is associated with increased mortality risk.

Calcium channel blockers – In general, calcium channel blockers (CCB) are well tolerated perioperatively.

Renin angiotensin system (RAS) antagonists – Patients with low normal baseline blood pressure, those receiving neuraxial local anesthetics as part of the planned anesthetic technique, or those with anticipated significant blood and third-space losses are at risk for intraoperative hypovolemia and hypotension and should have renin–angiotensin system antagonist therapy temporarily suspended prior to surgery.

α-Adrenergic antagonists – Although there have been suggestions to withhold α₁-adrenoceptor antagonists and other dilating drugs prior to ocular surgery, there are no prospective trials to support this practice. Perioperative use of α₂-agonists has been shown to reduce cardiac morbidity and mortality. Prophylactic use may reasonably be considered in patients with or at risk for coronary artery disease.

Nitrates – Patients receiving chronic nitrate therapy should not be withdrawn from their nitrates prior to surgery. Patients receiving nitrates as single-drug therapy for angina are potentially at increased risk, and additional anti-ischemic therapies may be warranted.

Pulmonary vasodilators – These drugs should be continued to prevent rebound pulmonary hypertension, but potential undesirable effects of oral medications such as systemic vasodilation and inhibition of platelet aggregation must be considered.

Antiarrhythmics – These drugs may be safely continued, with special attention to electrolyte and acid–base balance.

Antilipemic drugs – Statins should be continued. Studies evaluating the use of other antilipemic drugs, including bile-acid sequestrants, fibric-acid derivatives, and miscellaneous drugs such as ezetimibe, have failed to demonstrate a role for perioperative use. Nicotinic acid may cause decreases in platelet count or increases in prothrombin time and should be avoided.

Diuretics – Diuretics should generally be held in the immediate preoperative period to avoid hypovolemia and electrolyte disturbances in fasting patients.

Antiplatelet drugs, anticoagulants, hematologic drugs

Anticoagulants – Many factors must be considered when making perioperative anticoagulation management decisions, including clinical indications for anticoagulation, surgical procedure and potential for significant bleeding, risk of adverse thromboembolic events, regional anesthesia considerations, and drug pharmacokinetics.

Central and peripheral nervous system drugs

Antidepressants – Rapid discontinuation of tricyclic antidepressants may lead to withdrawal symptoms and increased relapse rates and is therefore not recommended. Monoamine oxidase inhibitors are recognized for their potential hazardous interactions with a number of drugs commonly used in anesthesia and the perioperative setting, so discontinuation is not advised and avoidance of "triggering" drugs is recommended. In the case of selective serotonin reuptake inhibitors, withdrawal symptoms may be severe, especially with the shorter-acting drugs, so discontinuation is not recommended. Withdrawal symptoms are not significant with lithium, although risk of relapse is increased with abrupt discontinuation. In surgical patients at increased risk for hypovolemia or renal impairment, it is reasonable to decrease or discontinue lithium perioperatively, and to follow lithium levels frequently when treatment resumes.

Benzodiazepines – Benzodiazepine withdrawal symptoms may be severe and potentially life-threatening, particularly with shorter-acting drugs, and abrupt discontinuation should be avoided.

Anticonvulsants – In general, anticonvulsants should be continued to avoid precipitating seizures or other unwanted withdrawal symptoms.

Antiparkinson drugs – Abrupt discontinuation of levodopa or carbidopa/levodopa should be avoided.

Cholinesterase inhibitors and Alzheimer's disease drugs – Use of cholinesterase inhibitors in myasthenic patients in the immediate preoperative period is generally advocated, to minimize risk of muscle weakness and respiratory problems, but intraoperative administration of neuromuscular blockers and reversal drugs should be minimized, and avoided if possible.

CNS stimulants – Despite the potential for hemodynamic instability, CNS stimulants should not be discontinued abruptly, given the potential for significant and possibly severe withdrawal symptoms.

Hormones and metabolics

Antidiabetic drugs – Decisions about preoperative management of antidiabetic drugs should integrate an assessment of the individual's level of glucose control, risk for hypoglycemia, surgical procedure, and the type and route of drug administration. In general, insulin is the preferred drug for glucose management in the perioperative period, because of the relative ease with which administration can be titrated to achieve glucose levels within the desired range. Oral hypoglycemic drugs should be discontinued prior to surgery.

Thyroid preparations – A brief interruption in daily dosing of thyroid drugs should have little impact. Patients taking medications for hyperthyroidism should continue these drugs.

Glucorticoids – Patients taking steroids should continue to do so perioperatively to prevent adrenal crisis.

Respiratory drugs

Inhaled drugs – These drugs should be continued throughout the perioperative period.

Leukotriene antagonists – These drugs may be safely continued in patients who can tolerate oral medications.

Theophylline – It is prudent to withhold theophylline prior to surgery and to monitor levels closely when the drug is resumed postoperatively.

Other drugs

Anti-infective drugs – These drugs should be continued, as discontinuation may contribute to development of resistance.

Cancer chemotherapy drugs – Discontinuation of antineoplastic drugs may lead to important disruptions in cancer treatment and cannot be recommended.

Immunosuppressants – All of these drugs should be continued, using intravenous substitution intra- and postoperatively as necessary to avoid inadequate blood levels and possible rejection.

Analgesics and anti-inflammatory agents – Patients taking chronic opiate analgesics should have these medications continued to prevent the adverse consequences of opiate withdrawal. For patients in whom a high degree of hemostasis is desired, NSAIDs should be discontinued preoperatively, allowing adequate time for recovery of platelet function. Rheumatoid arthritis symptoms are often disabling when medications are discontinued, so decisions to continue or withhold anti-TNFα drugs should be made based on a careful assessment of all risk factors.

Ophthalmic drugs – Perioperative use of these drugs is advised, to minimize increases in intraocular pressure, but most of these drugs are systemically absorbed, and systemic effects should be anticipated.

Nicotine – While it would appear that discontinuing nicotine in the surgical patient is advisable, transdermal or transnasal nicotine may reduce postoperative opiate requirements. Sudden cessation of smoking may reduce clearance of several important drugs used in anesthesia and increase their effects, so caution is advised.

Disulfiram – It is reasonable to discontinue disulfiram in the perioperative period to minimize interactions with sedative drugs and risk of hepatic insufficiency, particularly in hospitalized patients with limited access to alcohol and low risk of relapse.

Herbal preparations – It is recommended that any use of herbal preparations should be identified at the time of preoperative assessment, and that these products be discontinued for 2–3 weeks prior to surgery.

References

1. National Center for Health Statistics. *Health, United States, 2009: With Special Feature on Medical Technology.* Hyattsville, MD: CDC, 2010. www.cdc.gov/nchs/data/hus/hus09.pdf (accesed May 31, 2010).

2. Lee TH, Marcantonio ER, Mangione CM, *et al.* Derivation and prospective validation of a simple index for prediction of cardiac risk of major noncardiac surgery. *Circulation* 1999; **100**: 1043–9.

3. Auerbach AD, Goldman L. beta-Blockers and reduction of cardiac events in noncardiac surgery: scientific review. *JAMA* 2002; **287**: 1435–44.

4. Poldermans D, Boersma E, Bax JJ, *et al.* The effect of bisoprolol on perioperative mortality and myocardial infarction in high-risk patients undergoing vascular surgery. Dutch Echocardiographic Cardiac Risk Evaluation Applying Stress Echocardiography Study Group. *N Engl J Med* 1999; **341**: 1789–94.

5. Mangano DT, Layug EL, Wallace A, Tateo I. Effect of atenolol on mortality and cardiovascular morbidity after noncardiac surgery. Multicenter Study of Perioperative Ischemia Research Group. *N Engl J Med* 1996; **335**: 1713–20.

6. Feringa HH, Bax JJ, Boersma E, *et al.* High-dose beta-blockers and tight heart rate control reduce myocardial ischemia and troponin T release in vascular surgery patients. *Circulation* 2006; **114**: I344–9.

7. Poldermans D, Bax JJ, Schouten O, *et al.* Should major vascular surgery be delayed because of preoperative cardiac testing in intermediate-risk patients receiving beta-blocker therapy with tight heart rate control? *J Am Coll Cardiol* 2006; **48**: 964–9.

8. Beattie WS, Wijeysundera DN, Karkouti K, McCluskey S, Tait G. Does tight heart rate control improve beta-blocker efficacy? An updated analysis of the noncardiac surgical randomized trials. *Anesth Analg* 2008; **106**: 1039–48.

9. Lindenauer PK, Pekow P, Wang K, *et al.* Perioperative beta-blocker therapy and mortality after major noncardiac surgery. *N Engl J Med* 2005; **353**: 349–61.

10. Devereaux PJ, Yang H, Yusuf S, *et al.* Effects of extended-release metoprolol succinate in patients undergoing non-cardiac surgery (POISE trial): a randomised controlled trial. *Lancet* 2008; **371**: 1839–47.

11. Fleisher LA, Beckman JA, Brown KA, *et al.* ACC/AHA 2007 guidelines on perioperative cardiovascular evaluation and care for noncardiac surgery: a report of the American College of Cardiology/American Heart Association Task Force on Practice Guidelines. *Circulation* 2007; **116**: e418–99.

12. Hoeks SE, Scholte Op Reimer WJ, van Urk H, *et al.* Increase of 1-year mortality after perioperative beta-blocker withdrawal in endovascular and vascular surgery patients. *Eur J Vasc Endovasc Surg* 2007; **33**: 13–19.

13. Shammash JB, Trost JC, Gold JM, *et al.* Perioperative beta-blocker withdrawal and mortality in vascular surgical patients. *Am Heart J* 2001; **141**: 148–53.

14. Salpeter S, Ormiston T, Salpeter E. Cardioselective beta-blockers for chronic obstructive pulmonary disease. *Cochrane Database Syst Rev* 2005; **4**: CD003566.

15. Albouaini K, Andron M, Alahmar A, Egred M. Beta-blockers use in patients with chronic obstructive pulmonary disease and concomitant cardiovascular conditions. *Int J Chron Obstruct Pulmon Dis* 2007; **2**: 535–40.

16. Andrus MR, Loyed JV. Use of beta-adrenoceptor antagonists in older patients with chronic obstructive pulmonary disease and cardiovascular co-morbidity: safety issues. *Drugs Aging* 2008; **25**: 131–44.

17. Wijeysundera DN, Beattie WS. Calcium channel blockers for reducing cardiac morbidity after noncardiac surgery: a meta-analysis. *Anesth Analg* 2003; **97**: 634–41.

18. Wijeysundera DN, Beattie WS, Rao V, Ivanov J, Karkouti K. Calcium antagonists are associated with reduced mortality after cardiac surgery: a propensity analysis. *J Thorac Cardiovasc Surg* 2004; **127**: 755–62.

19. Wijeysundera DN, Beattie WS, Rao V, Karski J. Calcium antagonists reduce cardiovascular complications after cardiac surgery: a meta-analysis. *J Am Coll Cardiol* 2003; **41**: 1496–505.

20. Saltzman LS, Kates RA, Corke BC, Norfleet EA, Heath KR. Hyperkalemia and cardiovascular collapse after verapamil and dantrolene administration in swine. *Anesth Analg* 1984; **63**: 473–8.

21. Rubin AS, Zablocki AD. Hyperkalemia, verapamil, and dantrolene. *Anesthesiology* 1987; **66**: 246–9.

22. Tuman KJ, McCarthy RJ, O'Connor CJ, Holm WE, Ivankovich AD. Angiotensin-converting enzyme inhibitors increase vasoconstrictor requirements after cardiopulmonary bypass. *Anesth Analg* 1995; **80**: 473–9.

23. Colson P, Ryckwaert F, Coriat P. Renin angiotensin system antagonists and anesthesia. *Anesth Analg* 1999; **89**: 1143–55.

24. Colson P, Saussine M, Seguin JR, Cuchet D, Chaptal PA, Roquefeuil B. Hemodynamic effects of anesthesia in patients chronically treated with

angiotensin-converting enzyme inhibitors. *Anesth Analg* 1992; **74**: 805–8.

25. Coriat P, Richer C, Douraki T, *et al.* Influence of chronic angiotensin-converting enzyme inhibition on anesthetic induction. *Anesthesiology* 1994; **81**: 299–307.

26. Licker M, Schweizer A, Hohn L, Farinelli C, Morel DR. Cardiovascular responses to anesthetic induction in patients chronically treated with angiotensin-converting enzyme inhibitors. *Can J Anaesth* 2000; **47**: 433–40.

27. Pigott DW, Nagle C, Allman K, Westaby S, Evans RD. Effect of omitting regular ACE inhibitor medication before cardiac surgery on haemodynamic variables and vasoactive drug requirements. *Br J Anaesth* 1999; **83**: 715–20.

28. Brabant SM, Bertrand M, Eyraud D, Darmon PL, Coriat P. The hemodynamic effects of anesthetic induction in vascular surgical patients chronically treated with angiotensin II receptor antagonists. *Anesth Analg* 1999; **89**: 1388–92.

29. Bertrand M, Godet G, Meersschaert K, *et al.* Should the angiotensin II antagonists be discontinued before surgery? *Anesth Analg* 2001; **92**: 26–30.

30. Colson P, Ribstein J, Mimran A, *et al.* Effect of angiotensin converting enzyme inhibition on blood pressure and renal function during open heart surgery. *Anesthesiology* 1990; **72**: 23–7.

31. Joob AW, Harman PK, Kaiser DL, Kron IL. The effect of renin-angiotensin system blockade on visceral blood flow during and after thoracic aortic cross-clamping. *J Thorac Cardiovasc Surg* 1986; **91**: 411–18.

32. Licker M, Bednarkiewicz M, Neidhart P, *et al.* Preoperative inhibition of angiotensin-converting enzyme improves systemic and renal haemodynamic changes during aortic abdominal surgery. *Br J Anaesth* 1996; **76**: 632–9.

33. Booker PD, Davis AJ, Franks R. Gut mucosal perfusion in infants undergoing cardiopulmonary bypass: effect of preoperative captopril. *Br J Anaesth* 1997; **79**: 14–18.

34. Chang DF, Campbell JR. Intraoperative floppy iris syndrome associated with tamsulosin. *J Cataract Refract Surg* 2005; **31**: 664–73.

35. Stuhmeier KD, Mainzer B, Cierpka J, Sandmann W, Tarnow J. Small, oral dose of clonidine reduces the incidence of intraoperative myocardial ischemia in patients having vascular surgery. *Anesthesiology* 1996; **85**: 706–12.

36. Wallace AW, Galindez D, Salahieh A, *et al.* Effect of clonidine on cardiovascular morbidity and mortality after noncardiac surgery. *Anesthesiology* 2004; **101**: 284–93.

37. Wijeysundera DN, Naik JS, Beattie WS. Alpha-2 adrenergic agonists to prevent perioperative cardiovascular complications: a meta-analysis. *Am J Med* 2003; **114**: 742–52.

38. Oliver MF, Goldman L, Julian DG, Holme I. Effect of mivazerol on perioperative cardiac complications during non-cardiac surgery in patients with coronary heart disease: the European Mivazerol Trial (EMIT). *Anesthesiology* 1999; **91**: 951–61.

39. Dodds TM, Stone JG, Coromilas J, Weinberger M, Levy DG. Prophylactic nitroglycerin infusion during noncardiac surgery does not reduce perioperative ischemia. *Anesth Analg* 1993; **76**: 705–13.

40. Thomson IR, Mutch WA, Culligan JD. Failure of intravenous nitroglycerin to prevent intraoperative myocardial ischemia during fentanyl-pancuronium anesthesia. *Anesthesiology* 1984; **61**: 385–93.

41. Gallagher JD, Moore RA, Jose AB, Botros SB, Clark DL. Prophylactic nitroglycerin infusions during coronary artery bypass surgery. *Anesthesiology* 1986; **64**: 785–9.

42. Fusciardi J, Godet G, Bernard JM, *et al.* Roles of fentanyl and nitroglycerin in prevention of myocardial ischemia associated with laryngoscopy and tracheal intubation in patients undergoing operations of short duration. *Anesth Analg* 1986; **65**: 617–24.

43. Sear JW, Howell SJ, Sear YM, *et al.* Intercurrent drug therapy and perioperative cardiovascular mortality in elective and urgent/emergency surgical patientst. *Br J Anaesth* 2001; **86**: 506–12.

44. DeMots H, Glasser SP. Intermittent transdermal nitroglycerin therapy in the treatment of chronic stable angina. *J Am Coll Cardiol* 1989; **13**: 786–95.

45. Thadani U, Lipicky RJ. Short and long-acting oral nitrates for stable angina pectoris. *Cardiovasc Drugs Ther* 1994; **8**: 611–23.

46. Thadani U, Rodgers T. Side effects of using nitrates to treat angina. *Expert Opin Drug Saf* 2006; **5**: 667–74.

47. Lange RL, Reid MS, Tresch DD, *et al.* Nonatheromatous ischemic heart disease following withdrawal from chronic industrial nitroglycerin exposure. *Circulation* 1972; **46**: 666–78.

48. Savelieva I, Camm J. Anti-arrhythmic drug therapy for atrial fibrillation: current anti-arrhythmic drugs, investigational agents, and innovative approaches. *Europace* 2008; **10**: 647–65.

49. Wyse DG, Waldo AL, DiMarco JP, *et al.* A comparison of rate control and rhythm control in patients with atrial fibrillation. *N Engl J Med* 2002; **347**: 1825–33.

50. Fuster V, Ryden LE, Cannom DS, *et al.* ACC/AHA/ESC 2006 guidelines for the management of patients with atrial fibrillation: full text: a report of the American College of Cardiology/American Heart Association Task Force on practice guidelines and the European Society of Cardiology Committee for Practice Guidelines (Writing Committee to Revise the 2001 guidelines for the management of patients with atrial fibrillation) developed in collaboration with the European Heart Rhythm Association and the Heart Rhythm Society. *Europace* 2006; **8**: 651–745.

51. Naccarelli GV, Wolbrette DL, Khan M, *et al.* Old and new antiarrhythmic drugs for converting and maintaining sinus rhythm in atrial fibrillation: comparative efficacy and results of trials. *Am J Cardiol* 2003; **91**: 15D–26D.

52. Roy D, Talajic M, Dorian P, *et al.* Amiodarone to prevent recurrence of atrial fibrillation. Canadian Trial of Atrial Fibrillation Investigators. *N Engl J Med* 2000; **342**: 913–20.

53. Singh BN, Singh SN, Reda DJ, *et al.* Amiodarone versus sotalol for atrial fibrillation. *N Engl J Med* 2005; **352**: 1861–72.

54. Auer J, Weber T, Berent R, *et al.* A comparison between oral antiarrhythmic drugs in the prevention of atrial fibrillation after cardiac surgery: the pilot study of prevention of postoperative atrial fibrillation (SPPAF), a randomized, placebo-controlled trial. *Am Heart J* 2004; **147**: 636–43.

55. Gomes JA, Ip J, Santoni-Rugiu F, *et al.* Oral d,l sotalol reduces the incidence of postoperative atrial fibrillation in coronary artery bypass surgery patients: a randomized, double-blind, placebo-controlled study. *J Am Coll Cardiol* 1999; **34**: 334–9.

56. Amar D, Roistacher N, Rusch VW, *et al.* Effects of diltiazem prophylaxis on the incidence and clinical outcome of atrial arrhythmias after thoracic surgery. *J Thorac Cardiovasc Surg* 2000; **120**: 790–8.

57. Amar D. Prevention and management of perioperative arrhythmias in the thoracic surgical population. *Anesthesiol Clin* 2008; **26**: 325–35.

58. Crystal E, Connolly SJ, Sleik K, Ginger TJ, Yusuf S. Interventions on prevention of postoperative atrial fibrillation in patients undergoing heart surgery: a meta-analysis. *Circulation* 2002; **106**: 75–80.

59. Mayson SE, Greenspon AJ, Adams S, *et al.* The changing face of postoperative atrial fibrillation prevention: a review of current medical therapy. *Cardiol Rev* 2007; **15**: 231–41.

60. Kapoor AS, Kanji H, Buckingham J, Devereaux PJ, McAlister FA. Strength of evidence for perioperative use of statins to reduce cardiovascular risk: systematic review of controlled studies. *Bmj* 2006; **333**: 1149.

61. Le Manach Y, Coriat P, Collard CD, Riedel B. Statin therapy within the perioperative period. *Anesthesiology* 2008; **108**: 1141–6.

62. Ray KK, Cannon CP. The potential relevance of the multiple lipid-independent (pleiotropic) effects of statins in the management of acute coronary syndromes. *J Am Coll Cardiol* 2005; **46**: 1425–33.

63. Hindler K, Shaw AD, Samuels J, *et al.* Improved postoperative outcomes associated with preoperative statin therapy. *Anesthesiology* 2006; **105**: 1260–72; quiz 1289–90.

64. Poldermans D, Bax JJ, Kertai MD, *et al.* Statins are associated with a reduced incidence of perioperative mortality in patients undergoing major noncardiac vascular surgery. *Circulation* 2003; **107**: 1848–51.

65. Durazzo AE, Machado FS, Ikeoka DT, *et al.* Reduction in cardiovascular events after vascular surgery with atorvastatin: a randomized trial. *J Vasc Surg* 2004; **39**: 967–75.

66. Lindenauer PK, Pekow P, Wang K, Gutierrez B, Benjamin EM. Lipid-lowering therapy and in-hospital mortality following major noncardiac surgery. *JAMA* 2004; **291**: 2092–9.

67. Heeschen C, Hamm CW, Laufs U, *et al.* Withdrawal of statins increases event rates in patients with acute coronary syndromes. *Circulation* 2002; **105**: 1446–52.

68. Spencer FA, Allegrone J, Goldberg RJ, *et al.* Association of statin therapy with outcomes of acute coronary syndromes: the GRACE study. *Ann Intern Med* 2004; **140**: 857–66.

69. Schouten O, Hoeks SE, Welten GM, *et al.* Effect of statin withdrawal on frequency of cardiac events after vascular surgery. *Am J Cardiol* 2007; **100**: 316–20.

70. Le Manach Y, Godet G, Coriat P, *et al.* The impact of postoperative discontinuation or continuation of chronic statin therapy on cardiac outcome after major vascular surgery. *Anesth Analg* 2007; **104**: 1326–33, table of contents.

71. Pasternak RC, Smith SC, Bairey-Merz CN, *et al.* ACC/AHA/NHLBI Clinical Advisory on the Use and Safety of Statins. *Circulation* 2002; **106**: 1024–8.

72. Schouten O, Kertai MD, Bax JJ, Durazzo AE, Biagini E, Boersma E, *et al.* Safety of perioperative statin use in high-risk patients undergoing major vascular surgery. *Am J Cardiol* 2005; **95**: 658–60.

73. Graham DJ, Staffa JA, Shatin D, *et al.* Incidence of hospitalized rhabdomyolysis in patients treated with lipid-lowering drugs. *JAMA* 2004; **292**: 2585–90.

74. Scappaticci KA, Ham JA, Sohn YJ, Miller RD, Dretchen KL. Effects of furosemide on the neuromuscular junction. *Anesthesiology* 1982; **57**: 381–8.

75. Vicenzi MN, Meislitzer T, Heitzinger B, *et al.* Coronary artery stenting and non-cardiac surgery: a prospective outcome study. *Br J Anaesth* 2006; **96**: 686–93.

76. Horlocker TT, Wedel DJ, Benzon H, *et al.* Regional anesthesia in the anticoagulated patient: defining the risks (the second ASRA Consensus Conference on Neuraxial Anesthesia and Anticoagulation). *Reg Anesth Pain Med* 2003; **28**: 172–97.

77. Llau JV, De Andres J, Gomar C, *et al.* Anticlotting drugs and regional anaesthetic and analgesic techniques: comparative update of the safety recommendations. *Eur J Anaesthesiol* 2007; **24**: 387–98.

78. Biondi-Zoccai GG, Lotrionte M, Agostoni P, *et al.* A systematic review and meta-analysis on the hazards of discontinuing or not adhering to aspirin among 50,279 patients at risk for coronary artery disease. *Eur Heart J* 2006; **27**: 2667–74.

79. Collet JP, Montalescot G, Blanchet B, *et al.* Impact of prior use or recent withdrawal of oral antiplatelet agents on acute coronary syndromes. *Circulation* 2004; **110**: 2361–7.

80. Angiolillo DJ, Fernandez-Ortiz A, Bernardo E, *et al.* Clopidogrel withdrawal is associated with proinflammatory and prothrombotic effects in patients with diabetes and coronary artery disease. *Diabetes* 2006; **55**: 780–4.

81. Berger JS, Roncaglioni MC, Avanzini F, *et al.* Aspirin for the primary prevention of cardiovascular events in women and men: a sex-specific meta-analysis of randomized controlled trials. *JAMA* 2006; **295**: 306–13.

82. Newsome LT, Weller RS, Gerancher JC, Kutcher MA, Royster RL. Coronary artery stents: II. Perioperative considerations and management. *Anesth Analg* 2008; **107**: 570–90.

83. Wilson SH, Fasseas P, Orford JL, *et al.* Clinical outcome of patients undergoing non-cardiac surgery in the two months following coronary stenting. *J Am Coll Cardiol* 2003; **42**: 234–40.

84. McFadden EP, Stabile E, Regar E, *et al.* Late thrombosis in drug-eluting

coronary stents after discontinuation of antiplatelet therapy. *Lancet* 2004; **364**: 1519–21.

85. Compton PA, Zankar AA, Adesanya AO, Banerjee S, Brilakis ES. Risk of noncardiac surgery after coronary drug-eluting stent implantation. *Am J Cardiol* 2006; **98**: 1212–13.

86. Win HK, Caldera AE, Maresh K, *et al.* Clinical outcomes and stent thrombosis following off-label use of drug-eluting stents. *JAMA* 2007; **297**: 2001–9.

87. Grines CL, Bonow RO, Casey DE, *et al.* Prevention of premature discontinuation of dual antiplatelet therapy in patients with coronary artery stents: a science advisory from the American Heart Association, American College of Cardiology, Society for Cardiovascular Angiography and Interventions, American College of Surgeons, and American Dental Association, with representation from the American College of Physicians. *Circulation* 2007; **115**: 813–18.

88. Douketis JD, Berger PB, Dunn AS, *et al.* The perioperative management of antithrombotic therapy: American College of Chest Physicians Evidence-Based Clinical Practice Guidelines, 8th edn. *Chest* 2008; **133**: 299S–339S.

89. Mangano DT. Aspirin and mortality from coronary bypass surgery. *N Engl J Med* 2002; **347**: 1309–17.

90. Mehta RH, Roe MT, Mulgund J, *et al.* Acute clopidogrel use and outcomes in patients with non-ST-segment elevation acute coronary syndromes undergoing coronary artery bypass surgery. *J Am Coll Cardiol* 2006; **48**: 281–6.

91. Burger W, Chemnitius JM, Kneissl GD, Rucker G. Low-dose aspirin for secondary cardiovascular prevention – cardiovascular risks after its perioperative withdrawal versus bleeding risks with its continuation – review and meta-analysis. *J Intern Med* 2005; **257**: 399–414.

92. Jackson MR, Clagett GP. Antithrombotic therapy in peripheral arterial occlusive disease. *Chest* 2001; **119**: 283S–299S.

93. Chun R, Orser BA, Madan M. Platelet glycoprotein IIb/IIIa inhibitors: overview and implications for the anesthesiologist. *Anesth Analg* 2002; **95**: 879–88.

94. Horlocker TT. Low molecular weight heparin and neuraxial anesthesia. *Thromb Res* 2001; **101**: V141–54.

95. Eisen GM, Baron TH, Dominitz JA, *et al.* Guideline on the management of anticoagulation and antiplatelet therapy for endoscopic procedures. *Gastrointest Endosc* 2002; **55**: 775–9.

96. Alam M, Goldberg LH. Serious adverse vascular events associated with perioperative interruption of antiplatelet and anticoagulant therapy. *Dermatol Surg* 2002; **28**: 992–8.

97. Gainey SP, Robertson DM, Fay W, Ilstrup D. Ocular surgery on patients receiving long-term warfarin therapy. *Am J Ophthalmol* 1989; **108**: 142–6.

98. Vitin AA, Dembo G, Vater Y, *et al.* Anesthetic implications of the new anticoagulant and antiplatelet drugs. *J Clin Anesth* 2008; **20**: 228–37.

99. Wysokinski WE, McBane RD, Daniels PR, *et al.* Periprocedural anticoagulation management of patients with nonvalvular atrial fibrillation. *Mayo Clin Proc* 2008; **83**: 639–45.

100. van den Berghe G, Wouters P, Weekers F, *et al.* Intensive insulin therapy in the critically ill patients. *N Engl J Med* 2001; **345**: 1359–67.

101. Gandhi GY, Nuttall GA, Abel MD, *et al.* Intraoperative hyperglycemia and perioperative outcomes in cardiac surgery patients. *Mayo Clin Proc* 2005; **80**: 862–6.

102. Lazar HL, Chipkin SR, Fitzgerald CA, *et al.* Tight glycemic control in diabetic coronary artery bypass graft patients improves perioperative outcomes and decreases recurrent ischemic events. *Circulation* 2004; **109**: 1497–502.

103. Hinton P, Allison SP, Littlejohn S, Lloyd J. Insulin and glucose to reduce catabolic response to injury in burned patients. *Lancet* 1971; **1**: 767–9.

104. Thorell A, Nygren J, Ljungqvist O. Insulin resistance: a marker of surgical stress. *Curr Opin Clin Nutr Metab Care* 1999; **2**: 69–78.

105. Nygren J. The metabolic effects of fasting and surgery. *Best Pract Res Clin Anaesthesiol* 2006; **20**: 429–38.

106. Brandi LS, Frediani M, Oleggini M, *et al.* Insulin resistance after surgery: normalization by insulin treatment. *Clin Sci (Lond)* 1990; **79**: 443–50.

107. Hansen TK, Thiel S, Wouters PJ, Christiansen JS, Van den Berghe G. Intensive insulin therapy exerts anti-inflammatory effects in critically ill patients and counteracts the adverse effect of low mannose-binding lectin levels. *J Clin Endocrinol Metab* 2003; **88**: 1082–8.

108. Woolfson AM, Heatley RV, Allison SP. Insulin to inhibit protein catabolism after injury. *N Engl J Med* 1979; **300**: 14–17.

109. Nygren J, Thorell A, Ljungqvist O. Are there any benefits from minimizing fasting and optimization of nutrition and fluid management for patients undergoing day surgery? *Curr Opin Anaesthesiol* 2007; **20**: 540–4.

110. Henriksen MG, Hessov I, Dela F, *et al.* Effects of preoperative oral carbohydrates and peptides on postoperative endocrine response, mobilization, nutrition and muscle function in abdominal surgery. *Acta Anaesthesiol Scand* 2003; **47**: 191–9.

111. Yuill KA, Richardson RA, Davidson HI, Garden OJ, Parks RW. The administration of an oral carbohydrate-containing fluid prior to major elective upper-gastrointestinal surgery preserves skeletal muscle mass postoperatively: a randomised clinical trial. *Clin Nutr* 2005; **24**: 32–7.

112. Breuer JP, von Dossow V, von Heymann C, *et al.* Preoperative oral carbohydrate administration to ASA III-IV patients undergoing elective cardiac surgery. *Anesth Analg* 2006; **103**: 1099–108.

113. Misbin RI, Green L, Stadel BV, *et al.* Lactic acidosis in patients with diabetes treated with metformin. *N Engl J Med* 1998; **338**: 265–6.

114. Misbin RI. The phantom of lactic acidosis due to metformin in patients with diabetes. *Diabetes Care* 2004; **27**: 1791–3.

115. Scher CS, Anwar M. The self-reporting of psychiatric medications in patients scheduled for elective surgery. *J Clin Anesth* 1999; **11**: 619–21.

116. Huyse FJ, Touw DJ, van Schijndel RS, de Lange JJ, Slaets JP. Psychotropic

drugs and the perioperative period: a proposal for a guideline in elective surgery. *Psychosomatics* 2006; **47**: 8–22.

117. Desan PH, Powsner S. Assessment and management of patients with psychiatric disorders. *Crit Care Med* 2004; **32**: S166–73.

118. Kudoh A, Katagai H, Takazawa T. Antidepressant treatment for chronic depressed patients should not be discontinued prior to anesthesia. *Can J Anaesth* 2002; **49**: 132–6.

119. Stack CG, Rogers P, Linter SP. Monoamine oxidase inhibitors and anaesthesia. A review. *Br J Anaesth* 1988; **60**: 222–7.

120. Bowdle TA. Adverse effects of opioid agonists and agonist-antagonists in anaesthesia. *Drug Saf* 1998; **19**: 173–89.

121. Gillman PK. Monoamine oxidase inhibitors, opioid analgesics and serotonin toxicity. *Br J Anaesth* 2005; **95**: 434–41.

122. Dawson J, Karalliedde L. Drug interactions and the clinical anaesthetist. *Eur J Anaesthesiol* 1998; **15**: 172–89.

123. Stonecipher A, Galang R, Black J. Psychotropic discontinuation symptoms: a case of withdrawal neuroleptic malignant syndrome. *Gen Hosp Psychiatry* 2006; **28**: 541–3.

124. Kong VK, Irwin MG. Gabapentin: a multimodal perioperative drug? *Br J Anaesth* 2007; **99**: 775–86.

125. Soriano SG, Martyn JA. Antiepileptic-induced resistance to neuromuscular blockers: mechanisms and clinical significance. *Clin Pharmacokinet* 2004; **43**: 71–81.

126. Zaniboni A, Prabhu S, Audisio RA. Chemotherapy and anaesthetic drugs: too little is known. *Lancet Oncol* 2005; **6**: 176–81.

127. Kvolik S, Glavas-Obrovac L, Sakic K, Margaretic D, Karner I. Anaesthetic implications of anticancer chemotherapy. *Eur J Anaesthesiol* 2003; **20**: 859–71.

128. Ingrassia TS, Ryu JH, Trastek VF, Rosenow EC. Oxygen-exacerbated bleomycin pulmonary toxicity. *Mayo Clin Proc* 1991; **66**: 173–8.

129. Kennedy KA, Hait WN, Lazo JS. Chemical modulation of bleomycin induced toxicity. *Int J Radiat Oncol Biol Phys* 1986; **12**: 1367–70.

130. Chlebowski RT, Block JB, Cundiff D, Dietrich MF. Doxorubicin cytotoxicity enhanced by local anesthetics in a human melanoma cell line. *Cancer Treat Rep* 1982; **66**: 121–5.

131. Goldhirsch A, Gelber RD, Tattersall MN, Rudenstam CM, Cavalli F. Methotrexate/nitrous-oxide toxic interaction in perioperative chemotherapy for early breast cancer. *Lancet* 1987; **2**: 151.

132. Kostopanagiotou G, Smyrniotis V, Arkadopoulos N, *et al.* Anesthetic and perioperative management of adult transplant recipients in nontransplant surgery. *Anesth Analg* 1999; **89**: 613–22.

133. Denton MD, Magee CC, Sayegh MH. Immunosuppressive strategies in transplantation. *Lancet* 1999; **353**: 1083–91.

134. Grady D, Wenger NK, Herrington D, *et al.* Postmenopausal hormone therapy increases risk for venous thromboembolic disease. The Heart and Estrogen/progestin Replacement Study. *Ann Intern Med* 2000; **132**: 689–96.

135. Anderson FA, Spencer FA. Risk factors for venous thromboembolism. *Circulation* 2003; **107**: I9–16.

136. Spell NO. Stopping and restarting medications in the perioperative period. *Med Clin North Am* 2001; **85**: 1117–28.

137. Axelrod L. Perioperative management of patients treated with glucocorticoids. *Endocrinol Metab Clin North Am* 2003; **32**: 367–83.

138. Putterman C, Ben-Chetrit E, Caraco Y, Levy M. Colchicine intoxication: clinical pharmacology, risk factors, features, and management. *Semin Arthritis Rheum* 1991; **21**: 143–55.

139. National Institutes of Health. *Expert Panel Report 3: Guidelines for the Diagnosis and Management of Asthma.* National Heart, Lung, and Blood Institute Publication 07–405. Bethesda, MD: NIH, 2007.

140. Weinberger M, Hendeles L. Theophylline in asthma. *N Engl J Med* 1996; **334**: 1380–8.

141. Bibbo C. Wound healing complications and infection following surgery for rheumatoid arthritis. *Foot Ankle Clin* 2007; **12**: 509–24.

142. Escalante A, Beardmore TD. Risk factors for early wound complications after orthopedic surgery for rheumatoid arthritis. *J Rheumatol* 1995; **22**: 1844–51.

143. Benowitz NL. Nicotine and postoperative management of pain. *Anesth Analg* 2008; **107**: 739–41.

144. Kaye AD, Baluch A, Kaye AJ, Frass M, Hofbauer R. Pharmacology of herbals and their impact in anesthesia. *Curr Opin Anaesthesiol* 2007; **20**: 294–9.

145. Skinner CM, Rangasami J. Preoperative use of herbal medicines: a patient survey. *Br J Anaesth* 2002; **89**: 792–5.

146. Kaye AD, Kucera I, Sabar R. Perioperative anesthesia clinical considerations of alternative medicines. *Anesthesiol Clin N Am* 2004; **22**: 125–39.

147. American Society of Anesthesiologists. Anesthesiologists warn: if you're taking herbal products, tell your doctor before surgery. www.asahq.org/PublicEducation/herbal.html. (accessed May 31, 2008).

148. Miller LG. Herbal medicinals: selected clinical considerations focusing on known or potential drug-herb interactions. *Arch Intern Med* 1998; **158**: 2200–11.

149. Bordia A. Effect of garlic on human platelet aggregation in vitro. *Atherosclerosis* 1978; **30**: 355–60.

150. Rose KD, Croissant PD, Parliament CF, Levin MB. Spontaneous spinal epidural hematoma with associated platelet dysfunction from excessive garlic ingestion: a case report. *Neurosurgery* 1990; **26**: 880–2.

151. Backon J. Ginger: inhibition of thromboxane synthetase and stimulation of prostacyclin: relevance for medicine and psychiatry. *Med Hypotheses* 1986; **20**: 271–8.

152. Le Bars PL, Katz MM, Berman N, *et al.* A placebo-controlled, double-blind, randomized trial of an extract of Ginkgo biloba for dementia. North American EGb Study Group. *JAMA* 1997; **278**: 1327–32.

153. Lachachi H, Plantavid M, Simon MF, *et al.* Inhibition of transmembrane movement and metabolism of platelet

activating factor (PAF-acether) by a specific antagonist, BN 52021. *Biochem Biophys Res Commun* 1985; **132**: 460–6.

154. Vale S. Subarachnoid haemorrhage associated with *Ginkgo biloba*. *Lancet* 1998; **352**: 36.

155. Rowin J, Lewis SL. Spontaneous bilateral subdural hematomas associated with chronic *Ginkgo biloba* ingestion. *Neurology* 1996; **46**: 1775–6.

156. Janetzky K, Morreale AP. Probable interaction between warfarin and ginseng. *Am J Health Syst Pharm* 1997; **54**: 692–3.

157. Kimura Y, Okuda H, Arichi S. Effects of various ginseng saponins on 5-hydroxytryptamine release and aggregation in human platelets. *J Pharm Pharmacol* 1988; **40**: 838–43.

158. Almeida JC, Grimsley EW. Coma from the health food store: interaction between kava and alprazolam. *Ann Intern Med* 1996; **125**: 940–1.

159. Nightingale SL. From the Food and Drug Administration. *JAMA* 1997; **278**: 15.

61

Clinical applications: evidence-based anesthesia practice
Induction of anesthesia

T. Andrew Bowdle

Introduction

Induction of anesthesia refers to the transition from consciousness to unconsciousness at the outset of a general anesthetic. Induction drugs can be administered by virtually every route, but intravenous administration is currently the most popular. Drugs that were specifically developed as intravenous induction drugs, such as thiopental, ketamine, etomidate, and propofol, are often referred to as "induction drugs," although this classification has limited utility since some induction drugs are also used for maintenance of anesthesia (e.g., propofol infusion), and drugs that are more typically used for maintenance of anesthesia (e.g., inhaled anesthetics) are also used for induction of anesthesia. Drugs that are often used adjunctively, and not usually regarded as primary anesthetic drugs, such as opioids and benzodiazepines, can also be used to induce anesthesia. This chapter will emphasize the practical clinical application of anesthetic pharmacology during induction of anesthesia. For a more detailed discussion of the pharmacology of individual drugs the reader is referred to the chapters of Section 3.

History

Many anesthesiologists would consider the introduction of thiopental by Lundy at the Mayo Clinic in 1934 [1] as beginning the era of intravenous drugs for induction of anesthesia. However, the first attempt at intravenous anesthesia occurred in 1665, when Sigismund Elsholtz injected an opioid [2]. Oré published a monograph in 1875 advocating the use of intravenous chloral hydrate. In 1939 less than 10% of anesthetics administered in Great Britain included a barbiturate (hexobarbital or thiopental), and 73 patients were anesthetized with thiopental at the Mayo Clinic in 1934, but this had grown to 7310 by 1941. Enthusiasm for thiopental was tempered by experience during World War II, when the cardiovascular-depressant properties of thiopental became evident in combat casualties. Payne wrote that "i.v. anaesthesia was the cause of more fatal casualties among the servicemen at Pearl Harbor than were the enemy bombs" [3]. A re-examination of first-

hand accounts and official records concluded, however, that the death rate from thiopental at Pearl Harbor was "greatly exaggerated" [4,5]. Nevertheless, the potential cardiovascular-depressant effects of thiopental became well recognized. The shortcomings of intravenous induction (specifically thiopental) were addressed decisively by the synthesis of etomidate [6,7], which was introduced into clinical use in 1977 and remains the intravenous induction drug with the fewest cardiovascular side effects.

Choice of induction drugs

There are remarkably few good studies that examine clinical outcomes as they relate to the choice of anesthetic induction drug, and historically it has generally been difficult to show substantial differences in clinical outcomes even for such seemingly disparate choices as regional versus general anesthesia. Some anesthesiologists use the same induction drug for every patient, and would claim that by judicious choice of dose they are able to get satisfactory results under virtually all circumstances. However, there are good reasons to prefer certain drugs or to avoid certain drugs in particular clinical circumstances [8]. Reasons for choosing particular induction drugs are given in Table 61.1, and further details are provided throughout this chapter.

Speed of onset

In general, fast speed of onset is an asset when inducing anesthesia. The factors determining speed of onset are quite complex, and not entirely understood. The major factors to consider would include the dose, the rate of administration of the chosen dose, the time course of plasma concentrations, and the time course of equilibration between plasma and the effect site. Traditional pharmacokinetic models, based on blood samples obtained after drug effects have peaked, tend to overestimate the central volume of distribution, thereby underestimating the peak plasma and effect-site concentrations [9,10]. However, some general pharmacokinetics concepts are useful. If there is a very rapid decline in plasma concentration following a bolus dose, the effect-site concentration will reach

Anesthetic Pharmacology, 2nd edition, ed. Alex S. Evers, Mervyn Maze, Evan D. Kharasch. Published by Cambridge University Press. © Cambridge University Press 2011.

Table 61.1. Properties of drugs for induction of anesthesia

Drug	Speed of onset	Duration of effect[a]	Pain on injection	Myoclonus	Cardiovascular side effects	Cerebral blood flow	Drug-specific side effects	Recommended for	Avoid for
Thiopental	Fast	Short	No	Unlikely	Hypotension, vasodilation, myocardial depression, tachycardia	Decreased	Inadvertent subcutaneous or intraarterial administration may injure tissue	Increased intracranial pressure	Hemodynamic compromise
Ketamine [racemic or S(+)]	Fast	Short	No	Yes	Tachycardia, hypertension[b], myocardial depression[c], pulmonary hypertension[b]	Increased	Psychedelic (LSD-like) in subanesthetic doses; Bronchodilator; May have neuroprotective properties	Asthma; Trauma; Cardiac tamponade	Pulmonary hypertension[b]; Psychotomimetic side effects may be undesirable; Tachycardia and/or hypertension[b] may be undesirable; May be hazardous if intracranial compliance is decreased
Etomidate	Fast	Short	Yes	Yes	Minimal	Decreased	Inhibits cortisol biosynthesis	Hemodynamic compromise of all kinds	May interfere with cosyntropin stimulation testing
Propofol	Fast	Short	Yes	Yes	Hypotension, vasodilation	Decreased	May reduce incidence of postoperative nausea	Ambulatory surgery; LMA insertion	Hemodynamic compromise
Fentanyl analogs	Fast	Variable[d]	No	Yes	Bradycardia[e]; Vasodilation[f]	Conflicting data	Rigidity	Preventing responses to laryngoscopy	Hypovolemia
Benzodiazepines	Fast	Long	No[g]	No	Vasodilation[f]	Decreased			Hypovolemia

[a]Duration of effect of a typical induction dose.
[b]Increased sympathetic tone.
[c]Direct myocardial depression.
[d]Duration of effect of fentanyl analogs is significantly dependent upon dose, except for remifentanil, which is an ultrashort acting drug.
[e]Increased vagal tone.
[f]Decreased sympathetic tone may produce hypotension, especially in hypovolemic patients.
[g]Diazepam produces pain on injection, but midazolam, which has largely replaced diazepam in clinical practice, does not.

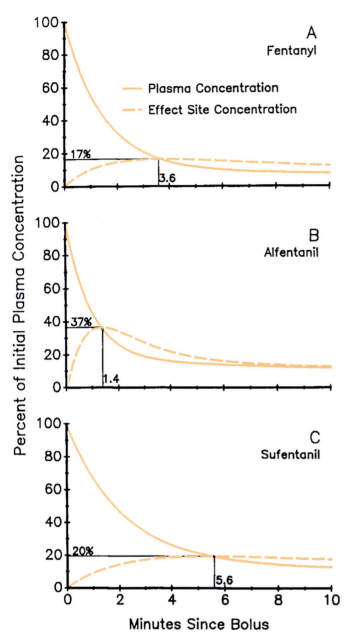

Figure 61.1. Plasma and effect-site opioid concentrations as a percentage of the initial plasma concentration following a bolus dose, for (A) fentanyl, (B) alfentanil, and (C) sufentanil. The time at which the peak effect concentration occurs depends upon the k_{e0} (equilibration between plasma and effect site) and the plasma pharmacokinetics. Alfentanil, which has the most rapid decline in plasma concentrations and the most rapid transfer from plasma to effect site, has the earliest peak effect. Reproduced with permission from Shafer and Varvel [11].

a peak very quickly, regardless of the rate of equilibration between plasma and effect site, since the driving force for transfer of drug from plasma to the effect site wanes very quickly. If decline in plasma concentration is slow, the time of peak effect will be determined primarily by the rate of equilibration between plasma and effect site. For drugs with a relatively fast equilibration between plasma and effect site and a relatively rapid decline in plasma concentration

following a bolus, the time to peak effect will be determined by a combination of the equilibration rate and the plasma pharmacokinetics (Fig. 61.1) [11]. Equilibration between plasma and effect site is rapid ($t_{1/2ke0} < 3$ minutes) for remifentanil, alfentanil, propofol, thiopental, and ketamine, intermediate ($t_{1/2ke0} < 6$ minutes) for fentanyl, sufentanil, methadone, and midazolam. Morphine equilibrates very slowly with the effect site (median $t_{1/2ke0} = 2.8$ hours) [12,13], which is one of the main reasons that it is seldom used as an induction drug.

Rate of administration of induction drugs is a critical consideration that is seldom fully taken into account. Rate of administration can vary widely, from "push" boluses in which the drug is administered from a syringe as rapidly as possible, to syringe-delivered boluses which are given quite slowly, to brief infusions delivered by pumps. The rate of administration from hand-delivered boluses is generally not quantified or standardized. Several studies have served to define more precisely the effect of administration rate. When 2.5% thiopental, 0.5% methohexital, or 0.2% etomidate were infused at 1200, 600, and 300 mL h^{-1} until loss of consciousness, the fastest administration rate resulted in the fastest onset of unconsciousness, but also the largest accumulated dose [14]. Interestingly, there was no significant difference in heart rate or mean arterial pressure for the three different rates of administration. Studies of propofol found similar results [15,16]. When propofol was administered at 25, 50, or 100 mg min^{-1}, induction times were shortest and the total dose was largest with the fastest infusion rate [15]. When the dose was fixed (1.46 mg kg^{-1} for patients 18–50 years or 0.82 mg kg^{-1} for patients older than 60 years) and given as a bolus over 5 seconds or as an infusion at 25 mg min^{-1}, the induction times were shorter for the bolus (approximately 30 seconds for the bolus versus 2 minutes for the infusion) [15]. There were no differences or only minor differences in heart rate or blood pressure related to speed of administration of propofol [15,16]. Another study of propofol examined a fixed dose (2 mg kg^{-1}) administered over 5, 20, or 60 seconds. Induction time increased from 21 to 35 to 50 seconds as the rate of administration slowed. There was no significant difference in blood pressure or heart rate related to speed of administration [17]. In a study of induction of anesthesia with remifentanil, using target-controlled infusion (TCI) to achieve an effect-site concentration of 15 ng mL^{-1}, the effect of limiting the plasma concentration to 15 ng mL^{-1} was compared with faster remifentanil administration without a limit on the plasma concentration [18]. Final effect-site concentration was reached in 7.3 minutes in the slower group and 2.2 minutes in the faster group. There were no significant differences in heart rate or blood pressure. Together, these studies suggest that more rapid administration of an induction drug results in faster induction of anesthesia.

Hypothetically there could also be pharmacologic significance to the rate of change of effect-site concentration, such that the pharmacologic effects would depend upon not only the peak effect-site concentration but also the speed with which the peak effect-site concentration is reached. However, the author is not aware of specific examples of this applying to anesthetic drugs. A study of propofol pharmacodynamics found that effect-site concentrations of propofol associated with particular pharmacologic effects were not affected by the rate of increase of propofol effect-site concentration [19].

If reproducibility were the goal, this would seem least likely with slower, hand-delivered boluses, in which the rate of administration could easily vary significantly from one administration to the next. Logically, the most reproducible approaches would appear to be either rapid push boluses (in which the drug is given as rapidly as possible, and the intensity of drug effect is manipulated by altering the dose) or the use of a brief infusion delivered by a pump (see *Target-controlled infusion*, below).

Opioids as sole induction drugs

Although opioids are thought of more for analgesia than for hypnosis, larger doses of opioids can produce unconsciousness, and opioids can be used as the sole drug for induction of anesthesia. Since an initial suggestion that "there is no evidence to suggest that narcotic anesthesia should produce unconsciousness and amnesia" [20], several studies have demonstrated the hypnotic properties of opioids. For induction of anesthesia by alfentanil alone in unpremedicated young adults, the ED50 and ED90 were 92 and 111 μg kg^{-1} respectively for loss of response to verbal stimulus, and 111 and 169 μg kg^{-1} respectively for loss of response to oral airway placement [21]. The response to an oral airway might be a more appropriate surrogate endpoint, prior to laryngoscopy and intubation. Another investigation found a similar ED50 for induction of anesthesia with alfentanil (130 μg kg^{-1}) [22]. The ED50 for loss of consciousness with remifentanil was reported to be 12 μg kg^{-1}, compared to 176 μg kg^{-1} for alfentanil in the same study [23]. These authors also found a striking reduction in the dose of thiopental required to produce unconsciousness in those patients who were not unconscious following administration of remifentanil or alfentanil (Fig. 61.2). Equipotent doses of other fentanyl analogs produced similar results. For example, sufentanil (1.3 μg kg^{-1}) produced unconsciousness in 9/10 patients, and fentanyl (13 μg kg^{-1}) produced unconsciousness in 8/10 patients [24].

In the author's experience, induction of anesthesia with an opioid alone does not suppress the eyelash reflex that is often used to indicate unconsciousness following administration of intravenous induction drugs such as thiopental and proprofol. Placement of an oral airway or some other substantial stimulus should probably be used instead.

While an opioid can be used as the sole induction drug, it is an uncommon practice, because the relatively weak hypnotic effect of opioids (compared to intravenous induction drugs) is disadvantageous. The risk of awareness during intubation with an opioid induction alone is probably greater than when a

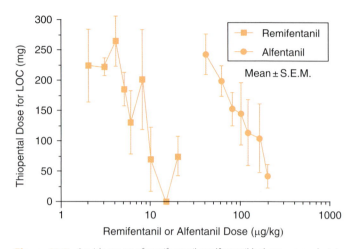

Figure 61.2. A wide range of remifentanil or alfentanil boluses were administered over 2 minutes to unpremedicated healthy patients. The patients were observed for 30 seconds following the end of the bolus. If not unconscious 30 seconds after the end of the bolus, thiopental 2 mg kg^{-1} min^{-1} was administered until loss of consciousness (LOC) occurred. For those patients receiving thiopental, there was a striking reduction in the mean dose of thiopental required to produce unconsciousness that was inversely related to the dose of opioid. Reproduced with permission from Jhaveri *et al.* [23].

hypnotic drug is added, or used alone, although there are no data. Most anesthesiologists combine a sedative-hypnotic, such as propofol or etomidate, with an opioid for induction of anesthesia. The interaction between opioids and sedative-hypnotics is usually synergistic (see *Anesthetic drug interactions*, below).

Induction by inhaled anesthetic

Induction of anesthesia by inhaling a gaseous anesthetic is usually reserved for situations where intravenous access cannot be obtained prior to induction of anesthesia, a situation that typically applies in younger children. The anesthetic drugs used for inhalational induction of anesthesia must be reasonably pleasant to breathe and cannot be irritating to the airway, otherwise coughing, laryngospasm and breath-holding can interfere with smooth induction. Currently, the inhaled anesthetics useful for induction of anesthesia are isoflurane, sevoflurane, and nitrous oxide (N_2O). Nitrous oxide would virtually never be used alone, since it is not potent enough to induce anesthesia by itself, but it may be used in combination with one of the more potent anesthetic gases. Sevoflurane is preferred because it has a somewhat faster onset than isoflurane. Techniques for inhalation induction include progressively increasing the inspired concentration (incremental induction) or use of high inspired concentrations administered with a vital-capacity breath (vital-capacity or "single-breath" induction). There are several studies which describe so-called "single-breath" inhalation induction with sevoflurane or sevoflurane combined with N_2O [25–29]. After the anesthesia circuit is primed with 7–8% sevoflurane (with or without N_2O), the patient exhales to residual volume, and then inhales from the circuit to vital capacity, followed by a breath hold.

Onset of anesthesia is somewhat faster than with tidal breathing of sevoflurane, although generally not as fast as an intravenous induction with propofol. Despite the moniker, loss of consciousness does not necessarily occur with a single breath. A meta-analysis compared sevoflurane and propofol induction [30]. Induction with 7–8% sevoflurane and N_2O administered with the vital-capacity technique was similar to propofol in effectiveness, but patient satisfaction was lower. Addition of an opioid to an inhalational drug reduces the dose of inhalational drug needed for induction of anesthesia, much as the addition of an opioid to an intravenous hypnotic drug reduces the required dose of the hypnotic drug (see *Anesthetic drug interactions*, below). For example, the addition of remifentanil (1 µg kg^{-1} bolus and 0.25 µg kg^{-1} min^{-1} infusion) reduced the end-tidal sevoflurane concentration required for intubation (without a muscle relaxant) from 4.5% to 2.5% [31].

Induction of anesthesia by other than intravenous administration

Intravenous induction drugs can also be given by other routes, such as rectal, nasal, or intramuscular, or even by inhalation, although these routes are seldom as practical as the intravenous route.

In 2002 the Russian military attempted to free more than 800 people held hostage by Chechen rebels in a Moscow theater by introducing an unidentified anesthetic gas through the ventilation system [32,33]. This tactic was partially successful, although more than 120 hostages died and hundreds were taken to local hospitals. Although the details are still unclear, the Russians announced that a "fentanyl derivative" was used. Some news reports suggested that a combination of anesthetics was used, possibly a fentanyl analog with halothane. Some experts believed that the most likely fentanyl analog was carfentanil (Wildnil; Wildlife Pharmaceuticals), which is approved in the United States only for immobilizing certain wild animals. Carfentanil is 80–100 times more potent than fentanyl, and had been shown previously to be effective in anesthetizing primates when nebulized and administered by inhalation [33].

Intubation without neuromuscular blocking drugs

Discussions of pharmacology related to producing good conditions for intubation tend to focus on neuromuscular blocking drugs, their speed of onset, duration of action, and effect on muscle twitch. Frequently ignored in these discussions is the important role of anesthetic drugs in facilitating intubation. Most experienced anesthesia practitioners have had the experience of intubating patients entirely without neuromuscular blocking drugs, and consequently have had the opportunity to make the observation that perfectly good intubating conditions can be had without any neuromuscular blocking drugs at all. An observational study of 612 consecutive patients, 68% intubated without muscle relaxation, found no significant difference in adequate intubating conditions or postoperative laryngeal symptoms between patients intubated with and without muscle relaxants [34]. A number of investigations have suggested that propofol may be superior to thiopental or etomidate for achieving adequate intubating conditions without muscle relaxants [35,36], but these studies typically compare a fixed dose of each drug, based on assumptions about equipotency that may not be justified. It should be noted that in these studies the hypnotic drugs were combined with substantial doses of opioid (e.g., remifentanil 2–3 µg kg^{-1} [35,36], sufentanil 0.2–0.4 µg kg^{-1} [34]), which undoubtedly contributed significantly to the quality of intubating conditions.

Anesthetic drug interactions

Although it is possible to achieve anesthesia with a single intravenous or inhaled anesthetic drug, modern anesthetic practice usually involves the coadministration of several or even numerous anesthetic drugs. When more than one anesthetic drug is given to induce anesthesia, the term "co-induction" is sometimes applied, although the use of multiple drugs during induction is so common that this terminology is seldom used in ordinary conversation. Sometimes the effects of more than one anesthetic drug are additive, as typically occurs when combining two drugs from the same class (e.g., two opioids or two inhalational anesthetics). When drugs from different classes are combined the effects are often (but not always) synergistic, which means that the combined effect of two (or more) drugs exceeds what would be expected from simply adding the individual effects of each drug.

Anesthetic interactions for the endpoints of hypnosis and immobility have been extensively reviewed [37]. Synergy is common when drugs acting on GABA$_A$ receptors are combined with drugs acting on non-GABA$_A$ receptors, but there are exceptions to this rule, especially where ketamine is used. Ketamine interacts additively or infra-additively. Intravenous anesthetics usually interact synergistically with inhaled anesthetics, while inhaled anesthetics interact additively with each other. In some cases, different results may be seen depending upon whether the endpoint is hypnosis or immobility.

There is a marked synergistic interaction between opioids and commonly used hypnotics such as thiopental, propofol or midazolam. For example, the ED50 of alfentanil for induction of anesthesia, using response to verbal command as an endpoint, was reduced from 130 to 28 µg kg^{-1} by administering one-third the ED50 of midazolam (0.07 mg kg^{-1}) 1 minute before alfentanil [38]. Similarly, the ED50 of midazolam for induction of anesthesia was reduced from.0.22 to 0.14 mg kg^{-1} by a subanalgesic dose of alfentanil, 3 µg kg^{-1} [38]. Propofol reduced remifentanil [39,40] or alfentanil [41] requirements for suppression of responses to laryngoscopy, intubation, and intra-abdominal surgical stimulation in a synergistic manner.

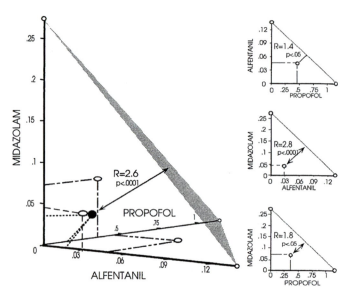

Figure 61.3. This somewhat complicated figure describes the hypnotic effects of propofol, alfentanil, and midazolam, each drug given by itself, in binary combinations (alfentanil/propofol, midazolam/alfentanil, midazolam/propofol) and all three drugs given together. On the right side of the figure are three isobolograms for the binary combinations. The circles on the x- and y-axes represent the ED50 (the dose that produces hypnosis in 50% of subjects) of each individual drug. The line drawn between the circles would represent all of the combinations of doses that would result in ED50, assuming that the effects of the drugs are additive. If the effects are supra-additive (synergistic) then any combination of doses producing an ED50 will fall to the left of the line. For the binary combinations tested, an ED50 pair of doses (open circle) did fall to the left of the line of additivity, showing that there is a synergistic interaction between the binary combinations. On the left side of the figure, the three-dimensional plot is an assemblage of the binary combinations shown on the right side of the figure. The three-dimensional plot has a triangular plane or surface connecting the ED50 of each individual drug, representing all of the combinations of doses that would result in ED50 if the effects of the drugs are additive. Synergy is indicated by points below the surface. For example, an ED50 combination of doses of the three drugs indicated by a dark circle demonstrates synergy. Reproduced with permission from Vinik et al. [45].

Etomidate interacted synergistically with morphine or fentanyl in rats [42], but there do not appear to be any studies of etomidate interactions in humans [37].

There is a synergistic interaction between benzodiazepines and the intravenous induction drugs, such as thiopental and propofol. A subhypnotic dose of midazolam (0.02 mg kg^{-1}) reduced the ED90 of thiopental for induction of anesthesia from 3.9 to 2.0 mg kg^{-1} [43]. There is also a similar synergistic interaction between midazolam and propofol. The ED50 that was expected if the effects were simply additive was reduced by 37% for combinations of midazolam and propofol [44].

Studies of combinations of three intravenous drugs, such as propofol, midazolam, and alfentanil, suggest that there is a synergistic interaction, but not beyond what would be expected from the synergistic interaction between two drugs, such as midazolam and alfentanil (Fig. 61.3) [44,45]. The addition of propofol to midazolam and alfentanil produced an additive, rather than a synergistic, effect.

Interestingly, ketamine combined with either thiopental [46] or midazolam [47] produced only an additive, not a

synergistic interaction for both hypnosis and antinociception. Combinations of thiopental and propofol also were additive rather than synergistic [48].

Several studies of induction and intubation with sevoflurane have shown that opioids improve intubating conditions (in the absence of muscle relaxants) and reduce the required dose of sevoflurane. Remifentanil administered by TCI at 3 and 5 ng mL^{-1} (effect site) with sevoflurane 1 MAC (age-adjusted) provided excellent intubating conditions in 50% and 95% of adult patients respectively [49]. An effect-site concentration of 5 ng mL^{-1} could be achieved without TCI by infusing remifentanil 1 µg kg^{-1} over 60 seconds followed by 0.23 µg kg^{-1} min^{-1} [49]. Fentanyl [50] and alfentanil [51] have also been shown to blunt hemodynamic responses or improve intubating conditions in combination with sevoflurane.

Interactions between anesthetic drugs also affect cardiovascular and respiratory side effects. Fentanyl 25 µg kg^{-1} combined with diazepam 0.125–0.5 mg kg^{-1} produced a synergistic reduction in blood pressure (mean arterial pressure was reduced from about 100 mmHg to about 60 mmHg) related to reduced peripheral vascular resistance, with no change in cardiac index, while fentanyl alone or diazepam alone produced no significant change in blood pressure (Fig. 61.4) [52]. Propofol alone (3 or 3.5 mg kg^{-1}) reduced systolic blood pressure prior to intubation, while lower doses (2 or 2.5 mg kg^{-1}) did not [53]. When fentanyl 2 or 4 µg kg^{-1} was given 5 minutes prior to these propofol doses, systolic blood pressure decreased by about 50 mmHg prior to intubation, irrespective of the dose of fentanyl or propofol [53]. The increase in blood pressure and heart rate (above baseline) that occurred with intubation was not attenuated by any dose of propofol alone, but was significantly attenuated, in a dose-dependent fashion, by the addition of fentanyl 2 or 4 µg kg^{-1} [53].

Administration of midzolam 0.05 mg kg^{-1} or fentanyl 2.0 µg kg^{-1} to volunteers produced either no significant respiratory effects (midazolam alone) or hypoxemia ($S_pO_2 < 90$) without apnea in half of the subjects (fentanyl alone). Combining midazolam and fentayl produced hypoxemia in 11/12 subjects and apnea in 6/12 subjects. The authors concluded that "combining midazolam with fentanyl or other opioids produces a potent drug interaction that places patients at high risk for hypoxemia and apnea" [54].

Cardiovascular side effects of induction of anesthesia

Cardiovascular side effects may be an important consideration in selecting an induction regimen, particularly in elderly, debilitated, or hemodynamically compromised patients. As noted earlier, anesthesiologists became acutely aware of the cardiovascular-depressant effects of thiopental, and other similar barbiturates, soon after their introduction into clinical

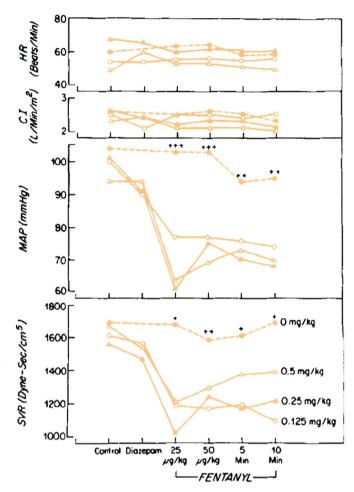

Figure 61.4. Patients undergoing induction of anesthesia for cardiac surgery were randomly assigned to 0 1.5, 2.5, or 5 mg of diazepam, followed by fentanyl 50 µg kg^{-1} given at a rate of 400 µg min^{-1}. Hemodynamic parameters were determined at baseline, following administration of diazepam, after 25 µg kg^{-1} of fentanyl, after 50 µg kg^{-1} of fentanyl, and 5 and 10 minutes following completion of the fentanyl dose. Diazepam alone or fentanyl alone did not produce any significant changes in hemodynamics. Fentanyl combined with diazepam (in any of the doses tested) produced statistically and clinically significant reductions in systemic vascular resistance and blood pressure. Significant intergroup differences are designated by + ($p < 0.05$), ++ ($p < 0.01$), or +++ ($p < 0.001$). Reproduced with permission from Tomicheck *et al.* [52].

practice. The two intravenous induction drugs that followed thiopental into widespread clinical use, ketamine and etomidate, were distinguished in large measure by having less of a cardiovascular-depressant side effect. Judging from animal studies, and from largely anecdotal information about clinical application, ketamine and etomidate are much less likely than thiopental to produce or exacerbate hypotension or shock in a wide variety of abnormal hemodynamic states, including hypovolemia, congestive heart failure, cardiac tamponade, and sepsis. Ketamine appears to accomplish this by increasing sympathetic tone, thus compensating for its underlying direct cardiovascular-depressant effects. However, the compensatory effects of increased sympathetic tone are limited. Ketamine has a direct myocardial-depressant effect. In isolated perfused

guinea pig heart, the S(+) isomer of ketamine produces less myocardial depression than the R(–) isomer, but this applies only because of an increase in available catecholamines; if catecholamines are depleted, the enantiomers of ketamine produce comparable myocardial depression [55]. Therefore ketamine is not a perfect drug in the hemodynamically compromised patient, and may produce hemodynamic decompensation [56]. Etomidate probably has the least effect on the cardiovascular system of any of the intravenous induction drugs. Etomidate has little or no direct cardiovascular-depressant effect [57]. Etomidate may lower blood pressure slightly by producing peripheral vasodilation, but this effect may be opposed by an apparent α_{2B}-adrenoceptor agonist action [58]. Thus etomidate has emerged as hypothetically the safest intravenous induction drug for patients with cardiovascular compromise [58] (however, see further comments about etomidate under *Critical illness, adrenal insufficiency, and etomidate*, below).

Propofol, like thiopental, has significant cardiovascular side effects, although the mechanisms are different. Thiopental causes significant myocardial depression, while propofol causes little if any myocardial depression [57]. However, propofol reduces blood pressure significantly by reducing sympathetic tone [59].

While opioids, particularly the fentanyl analogs, are reputed to cause minimal hemodynamic side effects during induction of anesthesia, there are notable exceptions to this general rule. Fentanyl analogs reduce sympathetic tone [60,61], and increase vagal tone. The increase in vagal tone frequently results in a reduction in heart rate, which is often regarded as a beneficial effect, particularly in patients with coronary disease. Rarely, however, the reduction in heart rate can be extreme, even to the point of sinus arrest and asystole [62–64]. Hypnotic and neuromuscular blocking drugs given at the same time may mitigate these effects. Fentanyl analogs combined with pancuronium tend to produce less heart-rate depression during induction of anesthesia compared to vecuronium [65,66], presumably because of the sympathetic ganglionic stimulating effects of pancuronium. Therefore some have advocated using pancuronium as an "antagonist" to the heart-rate-lowering effects of fentanyl analogs during induction of anesthesia. However, this tactic is not without risk, because elevation of heart rate attributed to pancuronium during induction of anesthesia with fentanyl analogs and pancuronium has been implicated in causing coronary ischemia in some patients undergoing coronary artery bypass surgery [67]. Laryngoscopy can sometimes provoke a vagal response, so the administration of a fentanyl analog followed by larnygoscopy may result in bradycardia or asystole at the time of laryngoscopy [68,69]. Since the anesthesia provider may be preoccupied with laryngoscopy at the time of intubation, and unable to observe the physiologic monitor screen, it is important to always have an audible indication of heart rate during induction, laryngoscopy, and intubation, so that if bradycardia or asystole occurs it is detected immediately. The reduction in sympathetic tone caused by fentanyl analogs generally does not produce hypotension in patients with normal cardiac preload. However, if hypovolemia is present or if cardiac filling is compromised, such as by pericardial effusion (cardiac tamponade), the reduction in sympathetic tone produced by even relatively small doses of opioids may produce dramatic reductions in blood pressure. Under such circumstances, inducing anesthesia with etomidate alone, without any fentanyl, and then adding fentanyl to the anesthetic once hemodynamic stability has been achieved, may be a useful approach.

Other important side effects during induction of anesthesia

In addition to hemodynamic side effects, there are some other common side effects that are clinically important.

Pain on injection

Propofol and etomidate produce a significant burning sensation, especially when injected into a small vein or a slow-flowing intravenous line. This does not occur nearly as frequently with thiopental, ketamine, opioids, or midazolam. A survey ranked pain on injection of propofol as the seventh most important problem in clinical anesthesiology [70], and more than 400 clinical and preclinical studies on propofol pain have been published [71]. Mixing propofol or etomidate with lidocaine, or injecting lidocaine into the intravenous line prior to injecting the anesthetic drug, variably attenuates the discomfort [72].

Diazepam, the predecessor to midazolam, also produced both significant pain on injection and vein damage resulting in painful phlebitis. This was due primarily to the propylene glycol solvent that was necessary to formulate diazepam for intravenous injection, due to its very low aqueous solubility. An alternative formulation of diazepam in a fat emulsion (Diazemuls) [73], analogous to the emulsion used to solubilize propofol, is apparently less irritating [74]. Midazolam is more water-soluble than diazepam because the pK_a of the imidazole ring of midazolam is approximately 6 (compared to approximately 3 for diazepam) and because at pH < 4 the diazepine ring of midazolam opens spontaneously, resulting in a more water-soluble molecule. At a pH of 2.5, approximately 50% of midazolam is in the open-ring form (benzophenone) [75,76]. Hence midazolam can be formulated in an aqueous solution that does not produce much pain on injection or venous irritation. Following injection of midazolam, under conditions of physiologic pH, diazepine ring closure occurs, and the equilibrium shifts towards the nonionized imidazole group, resulting in a more highly lipid-soluble molecule that easily crosses the blood–brain barrier.

Another strategy for overcoming the problem of formulating a highly lipid-soluble drug is to create a prodrug which is water-soluble. This was done successfully with fosphenytoin, the phosphono-O-methyl prodrug of phenytoin. The same tactic has been applied to propofol. Fospropofol is hydrolyzed by alkaline phosphatase to propofol, formaldehyde, and phosphate. The formaldehyde is rapidly converted to formate. Fospropofol (Aquavan) appears to produce much less discomfort on injection than propofol emulsion. The pharmacokinetic properties of fospropofol are somewhat different from propofol emulsion, in part due to the time required to metabolize fospropofol to propofol, resulting in a slightly delayed peak propofol level following bolus administration of fospropofol [77–79]. However, recently revealed problems with the fospropofol assay may result in reinterpretation of fospropofol pharmacokinetics [80].

Thiopental may be damaging to tissues if inadvertently administered into an artery or if extravasated into tissues from an infiltrated intravenous line. Since thiopental does not ordinarily produce discomfort on injection into a free-flowing intravenous line, should a patient complain of pain during injection of thiopental, the injection should be stopped and intra-arterial injection or tissue extravasation should be ruled out.

Myoclonus and rigidity

Tonic–clonic movement (also known as myoclonus) is not uncommon during induction of anesthesia, and can occur with any of the intravenous induction drugs. Movement, predominantly myoclonus, was observed in 87% of unpremedicated patients who received 0.3 mg kg^{-1} etomidate, 17% after thiopental, 12% after methohexital, and 6% after propofol [81]. Myoclonus could be prolonged, up to 4.2 minutes. While movement was common, electroencephalogram (EEG) recordings during induction found no evidence of cortical seizure activity [81]. While etomidate is an attractive drug for cardioversion in patients with serious cardiac disease, because of its lack of cardiovascular side effects, myoclonus may be a nuisance because of movement artifact on the electrocardiogram, sometimes causing difficulty in interpretation of the postcardioversion cardiac rhythm. Opioids may also produce myoclonus. Opioids in very large doses have produced seizure activity in laboratory animals. However, there appears not to be any EEG evidence that opioids produce generalized cortical seizure activity in humans, despite many studies of opioids in which EEG recordings have been made [82] (an exception is that the meperidine metabolite normeperidine does produce neuroexcitatory effects, by a nonopioid-receptor-mediated mechanism [83]). Opioid-induced myoclonus has been observed during simultaneous EEG recording, in the absence of EEG evidence of seizure activity [84]. Fentanyl (mean dose 25 μg kg^{-1}) [85], alfentanil (50 μg kg^{-1}) [86], and remifentanil [87] have been reported to produce localized temporal lobe epileptiform activity in patients with complex partial epilepsy, but this was not accompanied by motor activity. Occasionally opioid-induced myoclonus may be profound enough to be a significant nuisance, but it can be eliminated quickly by administration of an

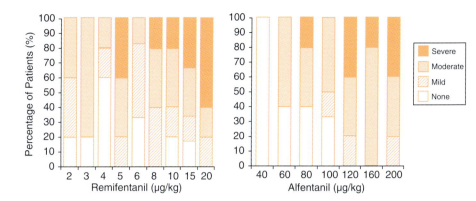

Figure 61.5. Remifentanil or alfentanil boluses were administered over 2 minutes to unpremedicated healthy patients. The patients were observed for 30 seconds following the end of the bolus. If not unconscious 30 seconds after the end of the bolus, thiopental 2 mg kg^{-1} min^{-1} was administered until loss of consciousness occurred. Rigidity during the 30-second observation period was graded as none, mild, moderate, or severe (the criteria for grading the ridity were not specified). The figure shows the percentage of patients in each dosing group with the various grades of rigidity. The relationship between the drug dose and the severity of rigidity was statistically significant ($p < 0.001$). Reproduced with permission from Jhaveri et al. [23].

intubating dose of muscle relaxant. The main importance of appreciating that induction drugs can produce myoclonus is to avoid confusing drug-induced myoclonus with tonic–clonic seizure activity, which may result in a needless neurological evaluation.

Opioids can produce tonic rigidity as well as myoclonus. Muscle rigidity is seen commonly during induction of anesthesia with larger doses of opioids. Administration of fentanyl 15 µg kg^{-1} at a rate of 150 µg min^{-1} resulted in rigidity (and unconsciousness) in 6/12 unpremedicated volunteers [88]. Smaller doses of fentanyl averaging 7.3 [89] or 8 µg kg^{-1} [90] administered more slowly, at 30 or 50 µg min^{-1}, produced chest-wall rigidity but not unconsciousness. Ascending doses of remifentanil (2–20 µg kg^{-1}) or alfentanil (40–200 µg kg^{-1}) were administered over 2 minutes to unpremedicated healthy patients [23]. The incidence and severity of rigidity were found to be dose-related (Fig. 61.5). A simple experiment convincingly demonstrated that opioid rigidity is central in origin. After a tourniquet was applied to prevent circulation to the arm, alfentanil produced rigidity in the entire body, including the isolated extremity [91]. Studies in rodents suggest that opioid rigidity is mediated by µ receptors in brainstem midline nuclei; since a naloxone analog applied by microinjection to these brain areas antagonized alfentanil-induced rigidity [92]. The basal ganglia have also been implicated in opioid rigidity. Because opioid rigidity may prevent ventilation of the lungs with a bag and mask, it has often been associated primarily with the chest-wall muscles. However, opioid rigidity affects not only the chest muscles but virtually all of the major muscle groups in the body [91]. Rigidity during induction of anesthesia with alfentanil (175 µg kg^{-1}) was quantified by electromyogram (EMG) recording from sternocleidomastoid, deltoid, biceps, forearm flexors, intercostal, rectus abdominus, vastus medialis/lateralis, and gastrocnemius muscles. Rigidity occurred in all muscles, beginning first in the upper body (sternocleidomastoid, deltoid, biceps, forearm). Ridigity was often sudden in onset and could be provoked by stimulation such as passive movement of an extremity, manipulation of the anesthesia mask, or a loud sound. Stereotyped postures were noted: flexion of the upper extremity, extension of the lower extremity, rigid immobility of the head, flexion of the neck

with chin on chest, and severe rigidity of the abdomen and chest wall.

The only reliable treatment for opioid-induced rigidity currently available is the administration of neuromuscular blocking drugs, in doses large enough to facilitate intubation. A very small dose of pancuronium, 1.5 mg per 70 kg body weight, (e.g., for defasciculation) was reported to attenuate rigidity [93], but it is difficult to explain how a dose of neuromuscular blocker that is generally too small to prevent voluntary movement could significantly affect the considerable motor activity necessary to produce rigidity. Another study using electromyography to quantify rigidity found that small doses of neuromuscular blockers did not significantly attenuate rigidity [94]. Considering the neuroanatomical basis of opioid rigidity, drugs that act on GABAergic, serotonergic, or adrenergic pathways might be expected to affect rigidity. The serotonin receptor antagonist ketanserin and the α_2-adrenergic agonist dexmedetomidine prevented opioid-induced rigidity in rats [95,96]. Benzodiazepines and thiopental (GABAergic mechanisms of action) have also been reported to attenuate rigidity in rats and humans, although this finding has not been consistent [97].

Psychotomimetic effects

Ketamine can produce psychotomimetic effects, like its analog and predecessor, phencyclidine. These effects may be evident when ketamine is administered in subanesthetic doses [98], or following emergence from anesthesia. Whether these effects are objectionable depends upon the dose of ketamine that is used, individual patient characteristics, and the concomitant effects of other drugs.

Induction in special circumstances

Trauma and the hemodynamically unstable patient

The goal of anesthesic induction in trauma patients or other hemodynamically unstable patients is to avoid further deterioration in cardiovascular physiology. Considerations for induction of anesthesia in trauma patients or other hemodynamically unstable patients are based on an understanding of the cardiovascular side effects of induction drugs, as presented in the section on *Cardiovascular side effects of induction of anesthesia*, above. There are no outcome studies that compare the various drugs directly in relevant clinical settings, so the approach has to be guided by knowledge of the underlying pharmacology of the drugs and clinical experience. Etomidate has the fewest cardiovascular side effects, and is frequently chosen for that reason.

A swine model of hemorrhagic shock has been used to study the pharmacokinetics and pharmacodynamics of propofol [99], etomidate [100], fentanyl [101], and remifentanil [102]. In the presence of acute blood loss (30 mL kg^{-1}), propofol pharmacokinetics and pharmacodynamics were altered. Plasma propofol concentrations were higher due to decreased propofol clearance, and there was increased sensitivity to propofol manifested by a 2.7-fold decrease in the effect-site concentration required to produce 50% of the maximum effect on the Bispectral Index (BIS) [99]. A combined pharmacokinetic/pharmacodynamic model predicted that the dose of propofol would have to be reduced by 5.4 times to produce the same effect on BIS. In an important side note to this study, the authors reported that in pilot studies, when swine were bled to a mean arterial pressure of 40 mmHg, animals survived infusions of fentanyl 10 µg kg^{-1} min^{-1} for 5 minutes or remifentanil 10 µg kg^{-1} min^{-1} for 10 minutes but did not survive propofol administration because of cardiovascular collapse. When swine were subjected to blood loss of 42 mL kg^{-1} and then resuscitated with lactated Ringer's solution to maintain a mean blood pressure of 70 mmHg, propofol pharmacokinetics were not significantly altered compared to controls, but there was a 1.5-fold decrease in the effect-site concentration required to produce 50% of the maximum effect on the BIS [103].

Similar results were obtained in patients undergoing elective surgery, where blood loss (30 mL kg^{-1}) was replaced with lactated Ringer's solution to maintain cardiac output and blood pressure [104]. A balanced anesthetic was given consisting of N$_2$O, fentanyl 10–20 µg kg^{-1}, and propofol 8 µg kg^{-1} min^{-1}. Total plasma propofol concentrations remained constant, but mean unbound propofol significantly increased from 0.10 to 0.17 µg mL^{-1} and mean BIS index decreased from 47 to 39. The authors interpreted these results to suggest that the potency of propofol was increased, resulting in decreased BIS index values, perhaps because of increased concentration of the unbound drug in plasma (plasma protein binding of propofol was not determined in the previous study of hemorrhaged swine) [104].

When swine were subject to blood loss sufficient to lower mean blood pressure to 40 mmHg, fentanyl concentrations following a 5-minute infusion were twofold higher than in controls [101]. Similar results were found for remifentanil [102]. The sensitivity to remifentanil at the effect site, assessed by EEG, was not altered by hemorrhagic shock.

When swine were subject to blood loss of 30 mL kg^{-1}, only minor differences in etomidate pharmacokinetics were found compared to controls [100]. There was no change in etomidate pharmacodynamics. Interestingly, administration of etomidate actually increased mean blood pressure 20% because of an increase in systemic vascular resistance.

Rapid sequence induction

The goal of rapid sequence induction is to achieve intubation of the trachea as rapidly as possible in order to prevent or reduce the likelihood of aspirating gastric contents. Patients are usually selected for rapid sequence induction based on risk factors for aspiration, such as a recent meal, diabetic gastroparesis, morbid obesity, pregnancy, or gastrointestinal pathology. Following preoxygenation, induction drugs and a neuromuscular blocker are given by push bolus in rapid succession (not waiting for unconsciousness to occur prior to administering the neuromuscular blocker) and the trachea is intubated as soon as possible, usually in 60–120 seconds. Rapid sequence induction of anesthesia is often combined with other measures that are intended to reduce the likelihood of aspiration, such as cricoid pressure or drugs that reduce gastric volume or acidity. The efficacy of rapid sequence induction or any of the adjunctive practices has not been established by adequate clinical trials [105,106]. The use of cricoid pressure [107–110] or drugs that reduce gastric volume or acidity [111] is particularly controversial.

Thiopental, propofol, etomidate, ketamine, midazolam, and the fentanyl analogs all have sufficiently fast onset to be used for rapid sequence induction of anesthesia. As noted under *Speed of onset*, above, remifentanil and alfentanil have faster equilibration with the effect site than fentanyl or sufentanil, but the difference is not critically important and fentanyl or sufentanil can be used for rapid sequence induction. Succinylcholine has the fastest onset of the neuromuscular blockers and is the traditional choice for rapid sequence induction, although nondepolarizing neuromuscular blocking drugs can be used as an alternative. Rocuronium is the most likely choice due to its relatively rapid onset [112]. As noted under *Intubation without neuromuscular blocking drugs*, above, intubating conditions depend critically upon anesthesia as well as neuromuscular blockade. For example, a prospective, randomized and double-blinded comparison of three anesthetic regimens for induction (etomidate 0.3 mg kg^{-1}, etomidate plus fentanyl 1.5 µg kg^{-1}, or etomidate plus S-ketamine 0.5 mg kg^{-1}, each given with rocuronium 0.6 mg kg^{-1}) showed that intubating conditions after 1 minute were significantly improved by addition of fentanyl or S-ketamine to etomidate [113].

Open eye injury

The goal of induction of anesthesia in the patient with an open eye injury is to avoid large increases in intraocular pressure by achieving a smooth induction which avoids dramatic increases in blood pressure, coughing, or bucking (which increases venous pressure), any of which may increase intraocular

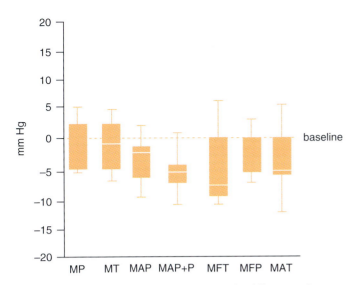

Figure 61.6. Intraocular pressure was measured after different combinations of induction drugs and succinylcholine, prior to intubation. A, alfentanil; F, fentanyl; M, midazolam; P, propofol; T, thiopental; +P, additional propofol. Reproduced with permission from Vinik *et al.* [115].

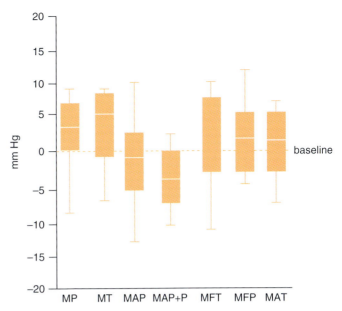

Figure 61.7. Intraocular pressure was measured after intubation with various combinations of induction drugs and succinylcholine. A, alfentanil; F, fentanyl; M, midazolam; P, propofol; T, thiopental; +P, additional propofol Reproduced with permission from Vinik *et al.* [115].

pressure. No intravenous anesthetic drug is particularly indicated. Thiopental, propofol, and etomidate may lower intraocular pressure. Ketamine may raise intraocular pressure by raising blood pressure. There has been an ongoing discussion over many years about the advisability of using succinylcholine in the patient with an open eye. Succinylcholine does cause a relatively small increase in intraocular pressure, although some authors have argued persuasively that extrusion of intraocular contents is extremely unlikely, based on the small increase in intraocular pressure caused by succinylcholine alone [114]. Avoidance of coughing and bucking during induction may be relatively more important. Intraocular pressure was measured after succinylcholine and after intubation with different combinations of induction drugs (Figs. 61.6, 61.7). A combination of midazolam, alfentanil, and propofol maintained intraocular pressure below baseline during induction, but additional propofol was needed to control intraocular pressure during intubation [115].

Asthma

The goal of induction of anesthesia in the patient with asthma is to avoid increasing airway resistance, particularly during manipulation of the airway. Ketamine relaxes bronchiolar muscle and prevents bronchoconstriction induced by histamine, apparently by a direct action, and indirectly by increasing sympathetic tone [116]. Ketamine may increase bronchial secretions (which would be undesirable), an effect which can be antagonized by atropine or glycopyrrolate. Propofol also has a direct airway smooth-muscle relaxing effect [117]. Compared to etomidate or thiopental, induction of anesthesia with propofol results in lower airway resistance following intubation [118]. Based on these considerations, ketamine or propofol may be preferable to etomidate or thiopental for induction of anesthesia in patients with asthma. Inhalational

anesthetics such as halothane, isoflurane, and sevoflurane have bronchodilating effects, decrease airway responsiveness, and attenuate histamine-induced bronchospasm [119]. Conversely, desflurane can increase airway resistance and narrowing and cause coughing, laryngospasm, and bronchospasm [120]. Opioids and lidocaine may be very useful adjuncts in asthmatic patients by virtue of reducing airway reflexes. Opioids that do not release histamine (fentanyl analogs) would be preferable to those that have the potential to release histamine (morphine, meperidine [121], methadone [122]). Muscle relaxants that release histamine, such as atracurium and mivacurium, should be avoided. Attaining adequate depth of anesthesia to attenuate airway reflexes prior to airway instrumentation is probably much more important in avoiding bronchospasm than the choice of any particular anesthetic drug. Many practitioners would invoke the effects of multiple drugs during induction. An example of such an approach might include propofol, fentanyl, and lidocaine given intravenously, followed by administration of an inhalational drug by bag and mask prior to airway instrumentation. Intubation of the trachea is more likely to produce bronchospasm than placement of a laryngeal mask airway [123].

Critical illness, adrenal insufficiency, and etomidate

Patients with bacterial sepsis, trauma, and other critical illnesses are often given anesthetics to facilitate intubation, either for ventilatory support or for surgery. Etomidate is an ideal drug to induce anesthesia for this purpose from the standpoint of maintaining hemodynamic stability, since such patients are often hemodynamically compromised, and etomidate produces minimal hemodynamic side effects. However, etomidate does suppress cortisol biosynthesis by inhibiting 11β-hydroxylase, the enzyme involved in the final step in cortisol synthesis, leading to concern about whether etomidate could produce harmful adrenal insufficiency. The question of whether the interference of etomidate in cortisol biosynthesis is harmful is an old issue. One editorial stated, "I shall not use etomidate in my practice until there are convincing data that refute the current concerns about its influences on the adrenal cortex and their possible implications for postoperative morbidity and/or mortality" [124]. Despite this editorial, etomidate gradually gained widespread acceptance, because there did not appear to be a clinically significant problem related to inhibition of cortisol biosynthesis. Cortisol concentrations do not fall below normal following a single bolus of etomidate, while the rise in cortisol that usually occurs in response to surgery is suppressed [125], and there are no convincing data to indicate that short-term suppression of cortisol biosynthesis is harmful to surgical patients. Nonetheless, there is renewed concern about etomidate adrenal suppression in septic patients, trauma patients, and perhaps others with critical illness. Because some patients with critical illness may be adrenally insufficient, the question has been raised whether additional adrenal suppression related to etomidate administration might be harmful in these patients [126–131]. Not surprisingly, response to adrenal stimulation testing by cosyntropin (synthetic adrenocorticotrophic hormone) may be attenuated following etomidate. However, there is no evidence from adequately designed prospective trials demonstrating that a single bolus of etomidate is harmful in trauma, sepsis, or other critical illness [132]. Concerns about possible adverse effects of 11β-hydroxylase inhibition by etomidate should be weighed against the possible adverse hemodynamic side effects of the alternative induction drugs, such as thiopental, etomidate, and ketamine. Ironically, while clinicians have been debating whether etomidate inhibition of 11β-hydroxylase is clinically significant, medicinal chemists have been creating more potent selective analogs of etomidate for the treatment of conditions that induce hypercortisolemia [133,134].

Induction of anesthesia for LMA insertion

There are numerous studies comparing anesthetic drugs for insertion of a laryngeal mask airway (LMA) [135]. Propofol alone appears to produce superior conditions to thiopental alone for induction of anesthesia for LMA placement, based on several comparative studies. However, the conclusions of these studies are somewhat limited because most often only a single dose of each drug was compared. In the absence of more extensive dose–response data it is difficult to know whether the doses that were compared are equipotent. In several studies, addition of an opioid or lidocaine to thiopental resulted in LMA insertion conditions similar to propofol alone. A comparison of manual versus target-controlled infusion of

propofol reported that a larger mean propofol dose was given by TCI (201 vs. 160 mg), and that insertion of an LMA therefore occurred earlier (114 vs. 132 seconds) [136]. Blood pressure and heart rate were not significantly different in the two groups. The participating anesthesiologists expressed a clear preference for TCI (see additional comments under *Target-controlled infusion*, below).

Maintaining spontaneous ventilation during induction of anesthesia

Some clinicians have advocated maintaining spontaneous ventilation during induction of anesthesia in the presence of certain pathological conditions, such as large mediastinal masses, bronchopleural fistula, upper-airway masses such as tumors, or infections. Generally, this involves an inhalational induction, since it is fairly difficult (although not impossible) to administer just the right bolus dose of an intravenous induction drug to produce unconsciousness while maintaining spontaneous breathing.

The putative advantage of maintaining spontaneous breathing depends upon the situation. The idea with mediastinal masses is that maintaining negative intrathoracic pressure may help to stent bronchi open and oppose airway collapse caused by the mass. In the case of bronchopleural fistula, the idea is that maintaining negative intrathoracic pressure may reduce the size of the leak through the bronchopleural fistula, compared with positive-pressure ventilation. In the case of upper-airway masses, the idea is that maintaining spontaneous ventilation and some laryngeal muscle tone may tend to stent the airway open and prevent obstruction. While these ideas may have appeal, and are frequently cited in textbooks and review articles, there does not appear to be any evidence from clinical studies showing that an inhalational induction is any safer than an intravenous one in these circumstances. Case reports suggest that airway obstruction can occur during inhalation or intravenous induction. A review cited 22 case reports of anesthetic complications from medistinal masses published between 1969 and 1983 [137]. There were three cases, including the case reported by the authors, in which airway obstruction occurred during an inhalational induction. In eight cases, the airway obstruction occurred postoperatively, requiring reintubation.

There are counterarguments to the use of inhalational induction. An inhalational induction does not guarantee that spontaneous ventilation can be maintained. As anesthetic depth increases, airway obstruction may take place in the case of mediastinal or upper-airway masses, and spontaneous ventilation may cease to be effective. Inhalational induction may be quite slow in a patient with a partially obstructed airway, and light planes of inhalational anesthesia may be associated with coughing, bucking, or laryngospasm, which may be difficult to manage. There are alternative strategies to inhalational induction. These would include standard intravenous induction of patients with mediastinal masses, with a surgeon standing by with a rigid bronchoscope, should complete airway obstruction occur at the carinal level (rapid institution of cardiopulmonary bypass is a more extreme form of treatment in this circumstance; the necessity of this would be vanishingly rare in adult patients [138]). Standard intravenous induction of anesthesia in patients with bronchopleural fistula can be followed by placement of a double-lumen endotracheal tube, which allows selective ventilation of the lung with and without the bronchopleural fistula. Upper-airway masses may be managed by awake intubation with topical anesthesia and sedation, usually with the aid of a fiberoptic bronchoscope.

Induction of anesthesia in patients with increased intracranial pressure or decreased intracranial compliance

Determining the effect of anesthetic drugs on intracranial pressure can be difficult because of the complex interrelationship between blood pressure, cerebral vascular tone, intracranial compliance, and intracranial pressure. Direct cerebral vasodilators generally increase intracranial pressure in the presence of decreased intracranial compliance by increasing intracranial blood volume. The effects of blood pressure are complicated. Reduction of blood pressure may cause cerebral vasodilation due to autoregulation, which can increase intracranial pressure in the presence of decreased intracranial compliance. Hypertension may increase intracranial blood volume if autoregulation is impaired or if the blood pressure exceeds the autoregulatory threshold.

Many, but not all, anesthetic drugs cause cerebral vasoconstriction by decreasing neuronal acitivity and thereby reducing cerebral metabolic oxygen demand, which is linked to cerebral vascular tone. Thiopental, etomidate, and propofol all reduce cerebral metabolic oxygen demand and can produce cerebral vasoconstriction. Ketamine is exceptional because it may increase cerebral metabolic activity, and therefore may produce cerebral vasodilation and increased intracranial pressure. Therefore ketamine has traditionally been regarded as a drug to avoid in patients with intracranial pathology. This notion has been re-evaluated, and some have suggested that ketamine might be a reasonable choice, at least under certain circumstances [139, 140]. A review concluded that ketamine did not actually increase intracranial pressure when used with controlled ventilation and coadministration of a GABA-receptor agonist (e.g., propofol, thiopental) and without N$_2$O, and that ketamine may increase cerebral perfusion by increasing blood pressure [139]. Another review drew similar conclusions, that ketamine generally improves cerebral perfusion, and maintained that ketamine has been shown to raise intracranial pressure significantly only in patients with obstruction to cerebrospinal fluid flow and redistribution [140]. Ketamine may have neuroprotective effects at the cellular level, unrelated to its effects on cerebral hemodynamics. Whether or not ketamine has clinically useful neuroprotective effects in

humans remains to be proven. While some recent studies have suggested that ketamine may be safer than previously thought, ketamine may not be an ideal drug for induction of anesthesia in patients with decreased intracranial compliance. Readers contemplating the use of ketamine in patients with intracranial pathology are urged to carefully and critically review the relevant literature.

Opioids decrease cerebral metabolic oxygen demand, and do not appear to have direct effects on cerebral vascular tone, but indirect effects caused by changes in blood pressure may alter intracranial pressure. Most studies have suggested that opioids can be safely used for induction of anesthesia in patients with decreased intracranial compliance, although data regarding the effects of opioids on cerebral hemodynamics are conflicting. For example, sufentanil caused substantial increases in cerebral blood flow in normocapnic dogs anesthetized with small doses of halothane [141]. The increase in cerebral blood flow was not explained by concomitant changes in cerebral oxygen consumption, implying that sufentanil directly dilated cerebral vessels [141]. In patients with severe head trauma, paralyzed with vecuronium, intracranial pressure controlled using standard clinical procedures (including hyperventilation, osmotic drugs, elevation of the head, sedation with midazolam), and intracranial pressure monitored by a subarachnoid bolt device, administration of fentanyl (3 µg kg^{-1}) or sufentanil (0.6 µg kg^{-1}) resulted in a mean intracranial pressure increase of about 10 mmHg [142], while mean blood pressure declined by about 10 mmHg. The maximum increase in intracranial pressure occurred about 5 minutes after opioid administration and persisted for about 20 minutes. The explanation for the apparent increase in cerebral blood flow or intracranial pressure in these studies is unknown. Alterations in blood pressure caused by opioids may indirectly change cerebrovascular tone, due to cerebral autoregulation of blood flow. There is also some evidence for neuroexcitatory effects of opioids, including localized electrical (but not motor) seizure activity in neurosurgical patients that could be associated with increases in regional cerebral blood flow [85,86]. However, it is important to note that there is no evidence for cortical or motor seizure activity caused by fentanyl analogs in nonepileptic patients, although opioid-induced myoclonus has often been confused with seizure activity [143]. It is generally concluded that fentanyl analogs do not have harmful effects on cerebral hemodynamics as long as blood pressure (and therefore cerebral perfusion pressure) are controlled [144,145].

Target-controlled infusion (TCI) for induction of anesthesia

Target-controlled infusion (TCI) has been used extensively for administration of propofol [146–158]. There is some evidence that TCI is superior to boluses administered by hand for induction of anesthesia, but a recent Cochrane meta-analysis was

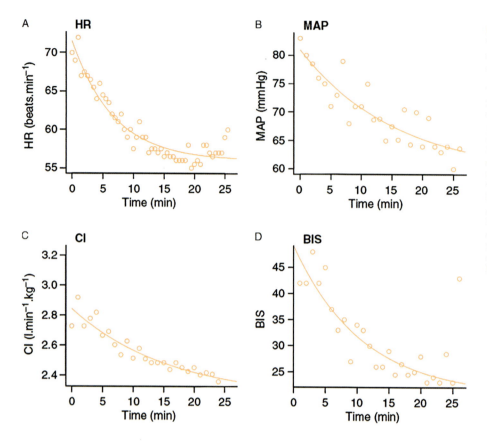

Figure 61.8. Anesthesia was induced and maintained with propofol (effect-site target 5 μg mL^{-1}) and remifentanil (effect-site target 2 ng mL^{-1}) administered by target-controlled infusion (TCI) in 10 healthy patients. Vecuronium was used to facilitate intubation and ventilation. 6.5 minutes after starting induction of anesthesia, at which time effect-site concentrations of propofol and remifentanil were predicted to be constant, the patients were left unstimulated for 25 minutes, during which time heart rate (HR), mean arterial pressure (MAP), cardiac index (CI), and Bispectral Index (BIS) were recorded. All of these variables declined during the study period. Whether the continued change in hemodynamic variables and BIS was due to the anesthetic effect-site concentrations not actually being constant is unknown, since no plasma drug concentrations were measured. Regardless of the mechanism, the result is interesting and may reflect some fundamental problems with the TCI concept. Reproduced with permission from Jack *et al.* [160].

unable to draw definite conclusions [159]. Interestingly, a recent study suggested that TCI administration of propofol and remifentanil, intended to produce a steady level of drugs at the effect site, did not result in stability of BIS or cardiovascular parameters following intubation of surgical patients who were otherwise unstimulated during the period of data collection [160]. Heart rate continued to decline for 20 minutes, BIS declined for 32 minutes, and cardiac index and mean arterial pressured declined for 47 minutes after effect-site drug concentrations were hypothetically stable (Fig. 61.8). This result was not expected, and calls into question whether the understanding of TCI is adequate. TCI is not commercially available in the United States at this time due to regulatory issues [161,162].

Remifentanil infusion without TCI

The key concept underlying TCI is to combine a loading dose with a variable-rate infusion in order to quickly and smoothly attain a new higher plasma or effect-site concentration, while minimizing overshooting or undershooting of the target concentration. If a drug has a very short elimination half-life, a relatively small volume of distribution, and a rapid transfer from plasma to effect site, then new higher steady-state plasma or effect-site concentrations can be obtained very quickly simply by turning on an infusion, or increasing an ongoing infusion, without the need to give loading doses by bolus or rapid infusion. In this case, TCI adds little or no value. Remifentanil is such a drug. As shown in the simulation illustrated in

Fig. 61.9, simply starting or increasing a remifentanil infusion, without giving any loading dose, will result in a very rapid rise in plasma and effect-site concentrations towards a new steady-state level. While the original trials of total intravenous anesthesia with remifentanil and propofol involved a bolus loading dose of remifentanil during induction of anesthesia [163], very satisfactory results can be attained without the need for boluses. For example, a remifentanil infusion may be started at approximately 0.5 μg kg^{-1} min^{-1} during preoxygenation. After several minutes of preoxygenation, a hypnotic drug may be given to induce anesthesia, followed by a muscle relaxant. By the time the laryngoscope is inserted and the trachea intubated, remifentanil concentrations will have attained roughly 60% or more of the steady-state level (Fig. 61.9). Following intubation, the remifentanil infusion can usually be reduced during the period of reduced stimulation associated with prepping and draping the surgical field.

Summary

This chapter synthesizes information on several classes of drugs, presenting practical clinical application of anesthetic pharmacology during induction of general anesthesia – the transition from consciousness to unconsciousness. Individual practitioners have myriad reasons to prefer or avoid certain induction drugs in particular clinical circumstances. However, there are remarkably

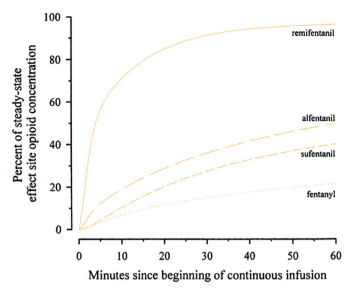

Figure 61.9. A computer simulation compares constant-rate infusions of remifentanil, alfentanil, fentanyl, and sufentanil. The percentage of steady-state effect-site concentration is plotted against time. Because of its relatively small volume of distribution and very short elimination half-life, remifentanil approaches steady state very rapidly, despite the lack of a loading dose. Reproduced with permission from Weiss and Gerber [106].

few methodical studies that examine clinical outcomes as they relate to the choice of anesthetic induction drugs.

Rapid speed of onset is generally desirable when inducing anesthesia. Anesthetic induction is typically performed with intravenous drugs, specifically a sedative-hypnotic, often also with an opioid, and also neuromuscular blocking drug if intubation is planned. Induction can also be performed by spontaneous ventilation and inhalation of a volatile anesthetic. More rapid intravenous drug administration typically results in faster loss of consciousness but also higher drug doses, although the hemodynamic consequence of such higher doses appears negligible. Large opioid doses can produce unconsciousness, and can be used as the sole drug for induction of anesthesia. Nevertheless, because the interaction between opioids and sedative-hypnotics is synergistic, and addition of

an opioid to an intravenous sedative-hypnotic reduces the required dose of the hypnotic drug and associated hemodynamic effects, drug combinations for induction are more common. Similarly, addition of an opioid during an inhalation induction reduces the dose of volatile drug needed for induction of anesthesia. Induction of anesthesia can cause cardiovascular side effects, pain on injection, myoclonus and rigidity, and psychotomimetic effects, depending on the drugs used, and these side effects are important considerations when selecting an induction regimen. Excellent intubating conditions can be achieved without a neuromuscular blocking drug, using a combination of a sedative-hypnotic and a substantial dose of opioid. Intravenous induction drugs can also be given by routes other than intravenous injection, such as rectal, nasal, or intramuscular, or even by inhalation, although these routes are less practical and have longer induction times.

Induction of anesthesia may occur during special circumstances. The goal in trauma or other hemodynamically unstable patients is to avoid further deterioration in cardiovascular physiology. The goal of rapid sequence induction is to achieve intubation of the trachea as rapidly as possible in order to prevent or reduce the likelihood of aspirating gastric contents. The goal of induction of anesthesia in the patient with an open eye injury is to avoid large increases in intraocular pressure by achieving a smooth induction, which avoids dramatic increases in blood or venous pressure. The goal of induction of anesthesia in the patient with asthma is to avoid increasing airway resistance, particularly during manipulation of the airway. Understanding the underlying pharmacology of the drugs and relying on clinical experience can meet each of these goals.

Since the introduction of thiopental by Lundy at the Mayo Clinic in 1934, the pharmacology of induction of anesthesia has gradually evolved with the development of several intravenous and inhaled anesthetic drugs, followed by progressively improved understanding of the pharmacology of these drugs. The future will undoubtedly bring new drugs, and a better understanding of the drugs currently available.

References

1. Lundy JS. Intravenous anesthesia: preliminary report of the use of two new thiobarbiturates. *Proc Staff Meet Mayo Clin* 1935; **10**: 536–43.

2. Price HL. General anesthetics, cont.: Intravenous anesthetics. In: Goodman LS, Gilman A, Gilman AG, Koelle GB, eds., *The Pharmacological Basis of Therapeutics*, 5th edn. New York, NY: MacMillan, 1975: 97–101.

3. Payne JP. Awareness and its medicolegal implications. *Br J Anaesth* 1994; **73**: 38–45.

4. Bennetts FE. Thiopentone anaesthesia at Pearl Harbor. *Br J Anaesth* 1995; **75**: 366–8.

5. Kidd AG, Restall J. Thiopentone anaesthesia at Pearl Harbor. *Br J Anaesth* 1995; **75**: 823.

6. Janssen PA, Niemegeers CJ, Schellekens KH, Lenaerts FM. Etomidate, R-(+)-ethyl-1-(-methyl-benzyl)imidazole-5-carboxylate (R 16659), a potent, short-acting and relatively atoxic intravenous hypnotic agent in rats. *Arzneimittelforschung* 1971; **21**: 1234–43.

7. Stanley TH, Egan TD, Van Aken H. A tribute to Dr. Paul A. J. Janssen:

entrepreneur extraordinaire, innovative scientist, and significant contributor to anesthesiology. *Anesth Analg* 2008; **106**: 451–62.

8. Nathan N, Odin I. Induction of anaesthesia: a guide to drug choice. *Drugs* 2007; **67**: 701–23.

9. Struys MM, Coppens MJ, De Neve N, *et al.* Influence of administration rate on propofol plasma-effect site equilibration. *Anesthesiology* 2007; **107**: 386–96.

10. Henthorn TK, Krejcie TC, Avram MJ. Early drug distribution: a generally

neglected aspect of pharmacokinetics of particular relevance to intravenously administered anesthetic agents. *Clin Pharmacol Ther* 2008; **84**: 18–22.

11. Shafer SL, Varvel JR. Pharmacokinetics, pharmacodynamics, and rational opioid selection. *Anesthesiology* 1991; **74**: 53–63.

12. Groenendaal D, Freijer J, Rosier A, *et al.* Pharmacokinetic/pharmacodynamic modelling of the EEG effects of opioids: the role of complex biophase distribution kinetics. *Eur J Pharm Sci* 2008; **34**: 149–63.

13. Lotsch J, Skarke C, Schmidt H, Grosch S, Geisslinger G. The transfer half-life of morphine-6-glucuronide from plasma to effect site assessed by pupil size measurement in healthy volunteers. *Anesthesiology* 2001; **95**: 1329–38.

14. Berthoud MC, McLaughlan GA, Broome IJ, *et al.* Comparison of infusion rates of three i.v. anaesthetic agents for induction in elderly patients. *Br J Anaesth* 1993; **70**: 423–7.

15. Peacock JE, Spiers SP, McLauchlan GA, *et al.* Infusion of propofol to identify smallest effective doses for induction of anaesthesia in young and elderly patients. *Br J Anaesth* 1992; **69**: 363–7.

16. Stokes DN, Hutton P. Rate-dependent induction phenomena with propofol: implications for the relative potency of intravenous anesthetics. *Anesth Analg* 1991; **72**: 578–83.

17. Rolly G, Versichelen L, Huyghe L, Mungroop H. Effect of speed of injection on induction of anaesthesia using propofol. *Br J Anaesth* 1985; **57**: 743–6.

18. Schmartz D, Ferring M, Ducart A, Barvais L. Haemodynamics during remifentanil induction by high plasma or effect-site target controlled infusion. *Acta Anaesthesiol Belg* 2007; **58**: 15–18.

19. Doufas AG, Bakhshandeh M, Bjorksten AR, Shafer SL, Sessler DI. Induction speed is not a determinant of propofol pharmacodynamics. *Anesthesiology* 2004; **101**: 1112–21.

20. Wong KC. Narcotics are not expected to produce unconsciousness and amnesia. *Anesth Analg* 1983; **62**: 625–6.

21. McDonnell TE, Bartkowski RR, Williams JJ. ED50 of alfentanil for induction of anesthesia in unpremedicated young adults. *Anesthesiology* 1984; **60**: 136–40.

22. Vinik HR, Bradley EL, Kissin I. Midazolam-alfentanil synergism for anesthetic induction in patients. *Anesth Analg* 1989; **69**: 213–17.

23. Jhaveri R, Joshi P, Batenhorst R, Baughman V, Glass PS. Dose comparison of remifentanil and alfentanil for loss of consciousness. *Anesthesiology* 1997; **87**: 253–9.

24. Bowdle TA, Ward RJ. Induction of anesthesia with small doses of sufentanil or fentanyl: dose versus EEG response, speed of onset and thiopental requirement. *Anesthesiology* 1989; **70**: 26–30.

25. Baum VC, Yemen TA, Baum LD. Immediate 8% sevoflurane induction in children: a comparison with incremental sevoflurane and incremental halothane. *Anesth Analg* 1997; **85**: 313–16.

26. Hall JE, Stewart JI, Harmer M. Single-breath inhalation induction of sevoflurane anaesthesia with and without nitrous oxide: a feasibility study in adults and comparison with an intravenous bolus of propofol. *Anaesthesia* 1997; **52**: 410–15.

27. Lejus C, Bazin V, Fernandez M, *et al.* Inhalation induction using sevoflurane in children: the single-breath vital capacity technique compared to the tidal volume technique. *Anaesthesia* 2006; **61**: 535–40.

28. Philip BK, Lombard LL, Roaf ER, *et al.* Comparison of vital capacity induction with sevoflurane to intravenous induction with propofol for adult ambulatory anesthesia. *Anesth Analg* 1999; **89**: 623–7.

29. Thwaites A, Edmends S, Smith I. Inhalation induction with sevoflurane: a double-blind comparison with propofol. *Br J Anaesth* 1997; **78**: 356–61.

30. Joo HS, Perks WJ. Sevoflurane versus propofol for anesthetic induction: a meta-analysis. *Anesth Analg* 2000; **91**: 213–19.

31. Cros AM, Lopez C, Kandel T, Sztark F. Determination of sevoflurane alveolar concentration for tracheal intubation with remifentanil, and no muscle relaxant. *Anaesthesia* 2000; **55**: 965–9.

32. Wax PM, Becker CE, Curry SC. Unexpected "gas" casualties in Moscow: a medical toxicology perspective. *Ann Emerg Med* 2003; **41**: 700–5.

33. Stanley T. Human immobilization: is the experience in Moscow just the beginning? *Eur J Anaesthesiol* 2003; **20**: 427–8.

34. Baillard C, Adnet F, Borron SW, *et al.* Tracheal intubation in routine practice with and without muscular relaxation: an observational study. *Eur J Anaesthesiol* 2005; **22**: 672–7.

35. Erhan E, Ugur G, Gunusen I, Alper I, Ozyar B. Propofol – not thiopental or etomidate – with remifentanil provides adequate intubating conditions in the absence of neuromuscular blockade. *Can J Anaesth* 2003; **50**: 108–15.

36. Taha S, Siddik-Sayyid S, Alameddine M, *et al.* Propofol is superior to thiopental for intubation without muscle relaxants. *Can J Anaesth* 2005; **52**: 249–53.

37. Hendrickx JF, Eger EI, Sonner JM, Shafer SL. Is synergy the rule? A review of anesthetic interactions producing hypnosis and immobility. *Anesth Analg* 2008; **107**: 494–506.

38. Vinik HR, Bradley EL, Kissin I. Midazolam–alfentanil synergism for anesthetic induction in patients. *Anesth Analg* 1989; **69**: 213–17.

39. Mertens MJ, Olofsen E, Engbers FH, *et al.* Propofol reduces perioperative remifentanil requirements in a synergistic manner: response surface modeling of perioperative remifentanil-propofol interactions. *Anesthesiology* 2003; **99**: 347–59.

40. Johnson KB, Syroid ND, Gupta DK, *et al.* An evaluation of remifentanil propofol response surfaces for loss of responsiveness, loss of response to surrogates of painful stimuli and laryngoscopy in patients undergoing elective surgery. *Anesth Analg* 2008; **106**: 471–9.

41. Vuyk J, Lim T, Engbers FH, *et al.* The pharmacodynamic interaction of propofol and alfentanil during lower abdominal surgery in women. *Anesthesiology* 1995; **83**: 8–22.

42. Kissin I, Brown PT, Bradley EL. Morphine and fentanyl anesthetic interactions with etomidate. *Anesthesiology* 1987; **67**: A383.

43. Tverskoy M, Fleyshman G, Bradley EL, Kissin I. Midazolam-thiopental

anesthetic interaction in patients. *Anesth Analg* 1988; **67**: 342–5.

44. Short TG, Plummer JL, Chui PT. Hypnotic and anaesthetic interactions between midazolam, propofol and alfentanil. *Br J Anaesth* 1992; **69**: 162–7.

45. Vinik HR, Bradley EL, Kissin I. Triple anesthetic combination: propofol–midazolam–alfentanil. *Anesth Analg* 1994; **78**: 354–8.

46. Roytblat L, Katz J, Rozentsveig V, *et al.* Anaesthetic interaction between thiopentone and ketamine. *Eur J Anaesthesiol* 1992; **9**: 307–12.

47. Hong W, Short TG, Hui TW. Hypnotic and anesthetic interactions between ketamine and midazolam in female patients. *Anesthesiology* 1993; **79**: 1227–32.

48. Vinik HR, Bradley EL, Kissin I. Isobolographic analysis of propofol–thiopental hypnotic interaction in surgical patients. *Anesth Analg* 1999; **88**: 667–70.

49. Sztark F, Chopin F, Bonnet A, Cros AM. Concentration of remifentanil needed for tracheal intubation with sevoflurane at 1 MAC in adult patients. *Eur J Anaesthesiol* 2005; **22**: 919–24.

50. Katoh T, Nakajima Y, Moriwaki G, *et al.* Sevoflurane requirements for tracheal intubation with and without fentanyl. *Br J Anaesth* 1999; **82**: 561–5.

51. Sivalingam P, Kandasamy R, Dhakshinamoorthi P, Madhavan G. Tracheal intubation without muscle relaxant: a technique using sevoflurane vital capacity induction and alfentanil. *Anaesth Intensive Care* 2001; **29**: 383–7.

52. Tomicheck RC, Rosow CE, Philbin DM, *et al.* Diazepam–fentanyl interaction: hemodynamic and hormonal effects in coronary artery surgery. *Anesth Analg* 1983; **62**: 881–4.

53. Billard V, Moulla F, Bourgain JL, Megnigbeto A, Stanski DR. Hemodynamic response to induction and intubation. Propofol/fentanyl interaction. *Anesthesiology* 1994; **81**: 1384–93.

54. Bailey PL, Pace NL, Ashburn MA, *et al.* Frequent hypoxemia and apnea after sedation with midazolam and fentanyl. *Anesthesiology* 1990; **73**: 826–30.

55. Graf BM, Vicenzi MN, Martin E, Bosnjak ZJ, Stowe DF. Ketamine has stereospecific effects in the isolated perfused guinea pig heart. *Anesthesiology* 1995; **82**: 1426–37; discussion 25A.

56. Weiskopf RB, Bogetz MS, Roizen MF, Reid IA. Cardiovascular and metabolic sequelae of inducing anesthesia with ketamine or thiopental in hypovolemic swine. *Anesthesiology* 1984; **60**: 214–19.

57. Gelissen HP, Epema AH, Henning RH, *et al.* Inotropic effects of propofol, thiopental, midazolam, etomidate, and ketamine on isolated human atrial muscle. *Anesthesiology* 1996; **84**: 397–403.

58. Vanlersberghe C, Camu F. Etomidate and other non-barbiturates. *Handb Exp Pharmacol* 2008; **182**: 267–82.

59. Ebert TJ. Sympathetic and hemodynamic effects of moderate and deep sedation with propofol in humans. *Anesthesiology* 2005; **103**: 20–4.

60. Flacke JW, Davis LJ, Flacke WE, Bloor BC, Van Etten AP. Effects of fentanyl and diazepam in dogs deprived of autonomic tone. *Anesth Analg* 1985; **64**: 1053–9.

61. Flacke JW, Flacke WE, Bloor BC, Olewine S. Effects of fentanyl, naloxone, and clonidine on hemodynamics and plasma catecholamine levels in dogs. *Anesth Analg* 1983; **62**: 305–13.

62. Cardinal V, Martin R, Tetrault JP, *et al.* [Severe bradycardia and asystole with low dose sufentanil during induction with sevoflurane: a report of three cases]. *Can J Anaesth* 2004; **51**: 806–9.

63. Egan TD, Brock-Utne JG. Asystole after anesthesia induction with a fentanyl, propofol, and succinylcholine sequence. *Anesth Analg* 1991; **73**: 818–20.

64. Starr NJ, Sethna DH, Estafanous FG. Bradycardia and asystole following the rapid administration of sufentanil with vecuronium. *Anesthesiology* 1986; **64**: 521–3.

65. O'Connor JP, Ramsay JG, Wynands JE, *et al.* The incidence of myocardial ischemia during anesthesia for coronary artery bypass surgery in patients receiving pancuronium or vecuronium. *Anesthesiology* 1989; **70**: 230–6.

66. Gravlee GP, Ramsey FM, Roy RC, *et al.* Rapid administration of a narcotic and neuromuscular blocker: a hemodynamic comparison of fentanyl, sufentanil, pancuronium, and vecuronium. *Anesth Analg* 1988; **67**: 39–47.

67. Thomson IR, Putnins CL. Adverse effects of pancuronium during high-dose fentanyl anesthesia for coronary artery bypass grafting. *Anesthesiology* 1985; **62**: 708–13.

68. Podolakin W, Wells DG. Precipitous bradycardia induced by laryngoscopy in cardiac surgical patients. *Can J Anaesth* 1987; **34**: 618–21.

69. Mizuno J, Mizuno S, Ono N, *et al.* [Sinus arrest during laryngoscopy for induction of general anesthesia with intravenous fentanyl and propofol]. *Masui* 2005; **54**: 1030–3.

70. Macario A, Weinger M, Truong P, Lee M. Which clinical anesthesia outcomes are both common and important to avoid? The perspective of a panel of expert anesthesiologists. *Anesth Analg* 1999; **88**: 1085–91.

71. Akeson J. Pain on injection of propofol – why bother? *Acta Anaesthesiol Scand* 2008; **52**: 591–3.

72. Lee P, Russell WJ. Preventing pain on injection of propofol: a comparison between lignocaine pre-treatment and lignocaine added to propofol. *Anaesth Intensive Care* 2004; **32**: 482–4.

73. Thorn-Alquist AM. Parenteral use of diazepam in an emulsion formulation. A clinical study. *Acta Anaesthesiol Scand* 1977; **21**: 400–4.

74. Schou Olesen A, Huttel MS. Local reactions to i.v. diazepam in three different formulations. *Br J Anaesth* 1980; **52**: 609–11.

75. Andersin R. Solubility and acid-base behaviour of midazolam in media of different pH, studied by ultraviolet spectrophotometry with multicomponent software. *J Pharm Biomed Anal* 1991; **9**: 451–5.

76. Gerecke M. Chemical structure and properties of midazolam compared with other benzodiazepines. *Br J Clin Pharmacol* 1983; **16**: 11S–16S.

77. Gibiansky E, Struys MM, Gibiansky L, *et al.* AQUAVAN injection, a water-soluble prodrug of propofol, as a bolus injection: a phase I dose-escalation comparison with DIPRIVAN (part 1): pharmacokinetics. *Anesthesiology* 2005; **103**: 718–29.

78. Struys MM, Vanluchene AL, Gibiansky E, *et al.* AQUAVAN injection, a water-soluble prodrug of propofol, as a bolus injection: a phase I dose-escalation comparison with DIPRIVAN (part 2): pharmacodynamics and safety. *Anesthesiology* 2005; **103**: 730–43.

79. Gan TJ. Pharmacokinetic and pharmacodynamic characteristics of medications used for moderate sedation. *Clin Pharmacokinet* 2006; **45**: 855–69.

80. Shah A, Mistry B, Gibiansky E, Gibiansky L. Fospropofol assay issues and impact on pharmacokinetic and pharmacodynamic evaluation. *Anesthesiology* 2008; **109**: 937.

81. Reddy RV, Moorthy SS, Dierdorf SF, Deitch RD, Link L. Excitatory effects and electroencephalographic correlation of etomidate, thiopental, methohexital, and propofol. *Anesth Analg* 1993; **77**: 1008–11.

82. Smith NT, Benthuysen JL, Bickford RG, *et al.* Seizures during opioid anesthetic induction: are they opioid-induced rigidity? *Anesthesiology* 1989; **71**: 852–62.

83. Armstrong PJ, Bersten A. Normeperidine toxicity. *Anesth Analg* 1986; **65**: 536–8.

84. Bowdle TA. Myoclonus following sufentanil without EEG seizure activity. *Anesthesiology* 1987; **67**: 593–5.

85. Tempelhoff R, Modica PA, Bernardo KL, Edwards I. Fentanyl-induced electrocorticographic seizures in patients with complex partial epilepsy. *J Neurosurg* 1992; **77**: 201–8.

86. Cascino GD, So EL, Sharbrough FW, *et al.* Alfentanil-induced epileptiform activity in patients with partial epilepsy. *J Clin Neurophysiol* 1993; **10**: 520–5.

87. Wass CT, Grady RE, Fessler AJ, *et al.* The effects of remifentanil on epileptiform discharges during intraoperative electrocorticography in patients undergoing epilepsy surgery. *Epilepsia* 2001; **42**: 1340–4.

88. Streisand JB, Bailey PL, LeMaire L, *et al.* Fentanyl-induced rigidity and unconsciousness in human volunteers. Incidence, duration, and plasma concentrations. *Anesthesiology* 1993; **78**: 629–34.

89. Grell FL, Koons RA, Denson JS. Fentanyl in anesthesia: a report of 500 cases. *Anesth Analg* 1970; **49**: 523–32.

90. Waller JL, Hug CC, Nagle DM, Craver JM. Hemodynamic changes during fentanyl–oxygen anesthesia for aortocoronary bypass operation. *Anesthesiology* 1981; **55**: 212–17.

91. Benthuysen JL, Smith NT, Sanford TJ, Head N, Dec-Silver H. Physiology of alfentanil-induced rigidity. *Anesthesiology* 1986; **64**: 440–6.

92. Weinger MB, Smith NT, Blasco TA, Koob GF. Brain sites mediating opiate-induced muscle rigidity in the rat: methylnaloxonium mapping study. *Brain Res* 1991; **544**: 181–90.

93. Bailey PL, Wilbrink J, Zwanikken P, Pace NL, Stanley TH. Anesthetic induction with fentanyl. *Anesth Analg* 1985; **64**: 48–53.

94. Blasco TA, Smith NT, Sanford TJ, *et al.* A clinical study of the effects of various pretreatment agents on alfentanil-induced rigidity: EMG data *Anesthesiology* 1985; **63**: A380.

95. Weinger MB, Segal IS, Maze M. Dexmedetomidine, acting through central alpha-2 adrenoceptors, prevents opiate-induced muscle rigidity in the rat. *Anesthesiology* 1989; **71**: 242–9.

96. Weinger MG, Cline EJ, Smith NT, Koob GF. Ketanserin pretreatment reverses alfentanil-induced muscle rigidity. *Anesthesiology* 1987; **67**: 348–54.

97. Vacanti CA, Silbert BS, Vacanti FX. The effects of thiopental sodium on fentanyl-induced muscle rigidity in a human model. *J Clin Anesth* 1991; **3**: 395–8.

98. Bowdle TA, Radant AD, Cowley DS, *et al.* Psychedelic effects of ketamine in healthy volunteers: relationship to steady-state plasma concentrations. *Anesthesiology* 1998; **88**: 82–8.

99. Johnson KB, Egan TD, Kern SE, *et al.* The influence of hemorrhagic shock on propofol: a pharmacokinetic and pharmacodynamic analysis. *Anesthesiology* 2003; **99**: 409–20.

100. Johnson KB, Egan TD, Layman J, *et al.* The influence of hemorrhagic shock on etomidate: a pharmacokinetic and pharmacodynamic analysis. *Anesth Analg* 2003; **96**: 1360–8.

101. Egan TD, Kuramkote S, Gong G, *et al.* Fentanyl pharmacokinetics in hemorrhagic shock: a porcine model. *Anesthesiology* 1999; **91**: 156–66.

102. Johnson KB, Kern SE, Hamber EA, *et al.* Influence of hemorrhagic shock on remifentanil: a pharmacokinetic and pharmacodynamic analysis. *Anesthesiology* 2001; **94**: 322–32.

103. Johnson KB, Egan TD, Kern SE, *et al.* Influence of hemorrhagic shock followed by crystalloid resuscitation on propofol: a pharmacokinetic and pharmacodynamic analysis. *Anesthesiology* 2004; **101**: 647–59.

104. Takizawa E, Takizawa D, Hiraoka H, Saito S, Goto F. Disposition and pharmacodynamics of propofol during isovolaemic haemorrhage followed by crystalloid resuscitation in humans. *Br J Clin Pharmacol* 2006; **61**: 256–61.

105. Neilipovitz DT, Crosby ET. No evidence for decreased incidence of aspiration after rapid sequence induction. *Can J Anaesth* 2007; **54**: 748–64.

106. Weiss M, Gerber AC. Rapid sequence induction in children: it's not a matter of time! *Paediatr Anaesth* 2008; **18**: 97–9.

107. Smith KJ, Ladak S, Choi PT, Dobranowski J. The cricoid cartilage and the esophagus are not aligned in close to half of adult patients. *Can J Anaesth* 2002; **49**: 503–7.

108. Garrard A, Campbell AE, Turley A, Hall JE. The effect of mechanically-induced cricoid force on lower oesophageal sphincter pressure in anaesthetised patients. *Anaesthesia* 2004; **59**: 435–9.

109. Ellis DY, Harris T, Zideman D. Cricoid pressure in emergency department rapid sequence tracheal intubations: a risk-benefit analysis. *Ann Emerg Med* 2007; **50**: 653–65.

110. Butler J, Sen A. Best evidence topic report. Cricoid pressure in emergency rapid sequence induction. *Emerg Med J* 2005; **22**: 815–16.

111. Engelhardt T, Webster NR. Pulmonary aspiration of gastric contents in anaesthesia. *Br J Anaesth* 1999; **83**: 453–60.

112. Perry JJ, Lee JS, Sillberg VA, Wells GA. Rocuronium versus succinylcholine for rapid sequence induction intubation. *Cochrane Database Syst Rev* 2008; **2**: CD002788.

113. Ledowski T, Wulf H. The influence of fentanyl vs. s-ketamine on intubating conditions during induction of anaesthesia with etomidate and

rocuronium. *Eur J Anaesthesiol* 2001; **18**: 519–23.

114. Chidiac EJ, Raiskin AO. Succinylcholine and the open eye. *Ophthalmol Clin North Am* 2006; **19**: 279–85.

115. Vinik HR. Intravenous Drug Interactions. In: White PF, ed., *Textbook of Intravenous Anesthesia*. Baltimore, MD: Williams and Wilkins, 1997: 447–58.

116. Brown RH, Wagner EM. Mechanisms of bronchoprotection by anesthetic induction agents: propofol versus ketamine. *Anesthesiology* 1999; **90**: 822–8.

117. Ouedraogo N, Roux E, Forestier F, *et al.* Effects of intravenous anesthetics on normal and passively sensitized human isolated airway smooth muscle. *Anesthesiology* 1998; **88**: 317–26.

118. Eames WO, Rooke GA, Wu RS, Bishop MJ. Comparison of the effects of etomidate, propofol, and thiopental on respiratory resistance after tracheal intubation. *Anesthesiology* 1996; **84**: 1307–11.

119. Burburan SM, Xisto DG, Rocco PR. Anaesthetic management in asthma. *Minerva Anestesiol* 2007; **73**: 357–65.

120. Goff MJ, Arain SR, Ficke DJ, Uhrich TD, Ebert TJ. Absence of bronchodilation during desflurane anesthesia: a comparison to sevoflurane and thiopental. *Anesthesiology* 2000; **93**: 404–8.

121. Flacke JW, Flacke WE, Bloor BC, Van Etten AP, Kripke BJ. Histamine release by four narcotics: a double-blind study in humans. *Anesth Analg* 1987; **66**: 723–30.

122. Bowdle TA, Even A, Shen DD, Swardstrom M. Methadone for the induction of anesthesia: plasma histamine concentration, arterial blood pressure, and heart rate. *Anesth Analg* 2004; **98**: 1692–7.

123. Kim ES, Bishop MJ. Endotracheal intubation, but not laryngeal mask airway insertion, produces reversible bronchoconstriction. *Anesthesiology* 1999; **90**: 391–4.

124. Longnecker DE. Stress free: to be or not to be? *Anesthesiology* 1984; **61**: 643–4.

125. Absalom A, Pledger D, Kong A. Adrenocortical function in critically ill patients 24 h after a single dose of etomidate. *Anaesthesia* 1999; **54**: 861–7.

126. Sacchetti A. Etomidate: not worth the risk in septic patients. *Ann Emerg Med* 2008; **52**: 14–16.

127. Hildreth AN, Mejia VA, Maxwell RA, *et al.* Adrenal suppression following a single dose of etomidate for rapid sequence induction: a prospective randomized study. *J Trauma* 2008; **65**: 573–9.

128. Mohammad Z, Afessa B, Finkielman JD. The incidence of relative adrenal insufficiency in patients with septic shock after the administration of etomidate. *Crit Care* 2006; **10**: R105.

129. den Brinker M, Joosten KF, Liem O, *et al.* Adrenal insufficiency in meningococcal sepsis: bioavailable cortisol levels and impact of interleukin-6 levels and intubation with etomidate on adrenal function and mortality. *J Clin Endocrinol Metab* 2005; **90**: 5110–17.

130. Cotton BA, Guillamondegui OD, Fleming SB, *et al.* Increased risk of adrenal insufficiency following etomidate exposure in critically injured patients. *Arch Surg* 2008; **143**: 62–7.

131. Schenarts CL, March JA. Corticosteroids for patients with septic shock. *JAMA* 2003; **289**: 41; author reply 43–4.

132. Walls RM, Murphy MF. Clinical controversies: etomidate as an induction agent for endotracheal intubation in patients with sepsis: continue to use etomidate for intubation of patients with septic shock. *Ann Emerg Med* 2008; **52**: 13–14.

133. Igaz P, Tombol Z, Szabo PM, Liko I, Racz K. Steroid biosynthesis inhibitors in the therapy of hypercortisolism: theory and practice. *Curr Med Chem* 2008; **15**: 2734–47.

134. Zolle IM, Berger ML, Hammerschmidt F, *et al.* New selective inhibitors of steroid 11beta-hydroxylation in the adrenal cortex. Synthesis and structure–activity relationship of potent etomidate analogues. *J Med Chem* 2008; **51**: 2244–53.

135. Brimacombe JR. Placement Phase. In: *Laryngeal Mask Anesthesia: Principles and Practice*, 2nd edn., Philadelphia, PA: Saunders, 2005: 191–240.

136. Russell D, Wilkes MP, Hunter SC, *et al.* Manual compared with target-controlled infusion of propofol. *Br J Anaesth* 1995; **75**: 562–6.

137. Mackie AM, Watson CB. Anaesthesia and mediastinal masses: a case report and review of the literature. *Anaesthesia* 1984; **39**: 899–903.

138. Slinger P, Karsli C. Management of the patient with a large anterior mediastinal mass: recurring myths. *Curr Opin Anaesthesiol* 2007; **20**: 1–3.

139. Himmelseher S, Durieux ME. Revising a dogma: ketamine for patients with neurological injury? *Anesth Analg* 2005; **101**: 524–34.

140. Sehdev RS, Symmons DA, Kindl K. Ketamine for rapid sequence induction in patients with head injury in the emergency department. *Emerg Med Australas* 2006; **18**: 37–44.

141. Milde LN, Milde JH, Gallagher WJ. Effects of sufentanil on cerebral circulation and metabolism in dogs. *Anesth Analg* 1990; **70**: 138–46.

142. Sperry RJ, Bailey PL, Reichman MV, *et al.* Fentanyl and sufentanil increase intracranial pressure in head trauma patients. *Anesthesiology* 1992; **77**: 416–20.

143. Bowdle TA. Adverse effects of opioid agonists and agonist-antagonists in anaesthesia. *Drug Safety* 1998; **19**: 173–89.

144. Artru AA. Effects of fentanyl, sufentanil, and alfentanil on epileptiform EEG activity, cerebral blood flow, and intracranial pressure. In: Hines R, Bowdle TA. , eds., *Anesthesiology Clinics of North America Annual of Anesthetic Pharmacology*. Philadelphia, PA: WB Saunders, 1997: 117–54.

145. Fodale V, Schifilliti D, Pratico C, Santamaria LB. Remifentanil and the brain. *Acta Anaesthesiol Scand* 2008; **52**: 319–26.

146. Coates D. "Diprifusor" for general and day-case surgery. *Anaesthesia* 1998; **53**: 46–8.

147. Engbers F. Practical use of "Diprifusor" systems. *Anaesthesia* 1998; **53**: 28–34.

148. Glen JB. The development of "Diprifusor": a TCI system for propofol. *Anaesthesia* 1998; **53**: 13–21.

149. Gray JM, Kenny GN. Development of the technology for "Diprifusor" TCI systems. *Anaesthesia* 1998; **53**: 22–7.

150. Huggins NJ. "Diprifusor" for neurosurgical procedures. *Anaesthesia* 1998; **53**: 53–5.

151. Milne SE, Kenny GN. Future applications for TCI systems. *Anaesthesia* 1998; **53** : 56–60.

152. Richards AL, Orton JK, Gregory MJ. Influence of ventilatory mode on target concentrations required for anaesthesia using a "Diprifusor" TCI system. *Anaesthesia* 1998; **53**: 77–81.

153. Russell D. Intravenous anaesthesia: manual infusion schemes versus TCI systems. *Anaesthesia* 1998; **53**: 42–5.

154. Servin FS. TCI compared with manually controlled infusion of propofol: a multicentre study. *Anaesthesia* 1998; **53**: 82–6.

155. Servin FS, Marchand-Maillet F, Desmonts JM. Influence of analgesic supplementation on the target propofol concentrations for anaesthesia with "Diprifusor" TCI. *Anaesthesia* 1998; **53**: 72–6.

156. Struys M, Versichelen L, Rolly G. Influence of pre-anaesthetic medication on target propofol concentration using a "Diprifusor" TCI system during ambulatory surgery. *Anaesthesia* 1998; **53**: 68–71.

157. Sutcliffe NP, Hyde R, Martay K. Use of "Diprifusor" in anaesthesia for ophthalmic surgery. *Anaesthesia* 1998; **53**: 49–52.

158. Swinhoe CF, Peacock JE, Glen JB, Reilly CS. Evaluation of the predictive performance of a "Diprifusor" TCI system. *Anaesthesia* 1998; **53**: 61–7.

159. Leslie K, Clavisi O, Hargrove J. Target-controlled infusion versus manually-controlled infusion of propofol for general anaesthesia or sedation in adults. *Cochrane Database Syst Rev* 2008; (**3**): CD006059.

160. Jack ES, Shaw M, Harten JM, Anderson K, Kinsella J. Cardiovascular changes after achieving constant effect site concentration of propofol. *Anaesthesia* 2008; **63**: 116–20.

161. Manberg PJ, Vozella CM, Kelley SD. Regulatory challenges facing closed-loop anesthetic drug infusion devices. *Clin Pharmacol Ther* 2008; **84**: 166–9.

162. Bazaral MG, Ciarkowski A. Food and drug administration regulations and computer-controlled infusion pumps. *Int Anesthesiol Clin* 1995; **33**: 45–63.

163. Hogue CW, Bowdle TA, O'Leary C, *et al.* A multicenter evaluation of total intravenous anesthesia with remifentanil and propofol for elective inpatient surgery. *Anesth Analg* 1996; **83**: 279–85.

Clinical applications: evidence-based anesthesia practice
Maintenance of and emergence from anesthesia

J. Lance Lichtor

Introduction

Maintenance of and emergence from general anesthesia is a large topic, and the intent of this chapter is to provide a basic understanding of how to manage a general anesthetic. For the purpose of presentation, assume that induction of anesthesia has occurred and the airway has been secured. Now, how does the anesthesiologist move forward? What needs to be done so that the patient is awake and ready to go to the postanesthesia care unit (PACU) when the procedure is complete? Both intravenous and inhalation approaches will be considered, as well as the fluid intake and ventilation method. Wake-up tests, the use of vasoactive substances as additions to maintenance drugs, and monitoring will also be considered. Drug costs are briefly considered, although these are a small component of perioperative costs [1].

The primary anesthetic choice: inhalation drugs or propofol

Stability of the patient during surgery

Intraoperative blood pressure is one of the concerns of the anesthesiologist. Cardiovascular effects of the different anesthetics have been considered in other chapters. Both inhalation drugs and propofol cause vasodilation, and this vasodilation is dose-dependent. Reflex tachycardia is variable: isoflurane causes reflex tachycardia, sevoflurane and propofol do not, and propofol may actually result in bradycardia.

Patients can cough with any anesthetic, though coughing is less with propofol. In one study, for example, during emergence from anesthesia, a propofol-based anesthetic was associated with less coughing than that consisting primarily of sevoflurane [2]. Patients cough during anesthesia most likely because there is some fluid in the oropharynx. This was illustrated in one study in which coughing frequency during dental treatments was correlated with the amount of water in the oropharynx [3]. Patients with an upper respiratory tract infection or a history of smoking also have a greater incidence of coughing. It is unclear, however, which volatile anesthetic is

better for smokers. In one study of active smokers where a laryngeal mask airway was used, evidence of airway irritation during anesthesia was modest and it made no difference whether desflurane or sevoflurane was used [4]. Yet, in another study of smokers, patients who received sevoflurane intraoperatively had less coughing than those who received isoflurane [5].

Speed and quality of emergence and awakening

Time to recovery may be measured by various criteria. For an ambulatory center, a patient may be considered awake when able to leave the center. For an inpatient, this may be time for discharge from the PACU or, if a patient is to go to the intensive care unit (ICU), the only concern may be whether a patient requires mechanical ventilation. Actual discharge from an ambulatory center or PACU, though, may depend on administrative issues, such as a written order from a surgeon or anesthesiologist. The time necessary before a patient can be taken from the operating room after completion of surgery, or, for the ambulatory patient, a patient's ability to skip the PACU and go directly to a step-down unit, may be directly related to the anesthetic, and it may result in cost savings for an institution.

Does choice of maintenance drug affect recovery after anesthesia? Propofol, desflurane, and sevoflurane have characteristics that make them ideal for maintenance of anesthesia for ambulatory surgery because of their short-lived effects. Propofol has a short context-sensitive half-time and, when used as a maintenance drug, results in rapid recovery and few side effects. Desflurane and sevoflurane, halogenated ether anesthetics with low blood/gas partition coefficients, also result in rapid emergence. Wake-up times, however, may have different definitions. Patients may emerge from anesthesia with desflurane and nitrous oxide (N_2O) significantly faster than after propofol or after sevoflurane and N_2O, though the ability to sit up, stand, and tolerate fluids and the time to fitness for discharge may be no different. In one study, for patients undergoing surgery for at least 2.5 hours, initial recovery

Anesthetic Pharmacology, 2nd edition, ed. Alex S. Evers, Mervyn Maze, Evan D. Kharasch. Published by Cambridge University Press. © Cambridge University Press 2011.

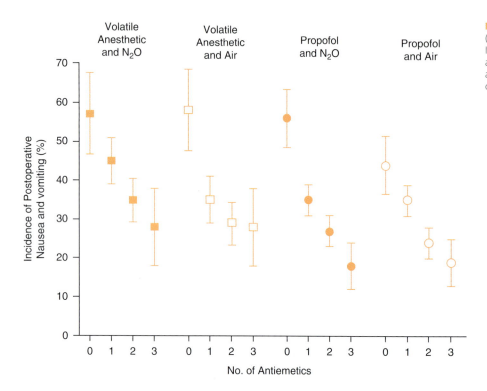

Figure 62.1. Postoperative nausea and vomiting (PONV) is least after a propofol anesthetic with air. Illustrated is the incidence of PONV when different anesthetics and different numbers of prophylactic antiemetic treatments are administered. Reproduced with permission from Apfel *et al.* [8].

variables such as time to extubate the trachea and time to state name were faster after desflurane than after propofol [6]. But in a study comparing sevoflurane (set initially at 2% end-tidal), to target-controlled propofol infusion in patients undergoing craniotomy, times to open eyes, extubation, and obey commands were no different between the two groups [7].

Postoperative nausea and vomiting

Postoperative nausea and vomiting (PONV) is less after a propofol than after an inhalation anesthetic. In one study of patients undergoing surgery for at least 2.5 hours, the incidence of PONV after desflurane was 33%, compared with 0% after propofol [6]. In another study of 5161 patients, propofol, compared with a volatile anesthetic, reduced nausea and vomiting by 19% (Fig. 62.1) [8].

Postoperative pain

Choice of anesthetic may have an influence on postoperative opioid requirement or postoperative pain. Women undergoing open uterine surgery who received propofol for anesthesia maintenance reported less pain and used less morphine during the first day after surgery than those who received isoflurane [9]. In contrast, among patients who received either sevoflurane, desflurane, or propofol for maintenance of anesthesia, postoperative morphine use and patient assessment of pain did not differ between anesthetics [10].

Risk of malignant hyperthermia

Propofol is not a trigger for malignant hyperthermia. All of the inhalation drugs are triggers for malignant hyperthermia.

Salivation

Whether salivation is increased after propofol is questionable. In patients undergoing laryngeal surgery, salivation was greater after a propofol anesthetic than after a sevoflurane anesthetic [11]. In another study, where salivation after isoflurane and propofol anesthesia were compared, stimulated salivation postoperatively was decreased after either anesthetic and did not return to baseline until the fourth postoperative day [12].

Rare adverse effects

Overall, anesthetic drugs that are currently used are generally considered safe. Rare adverse events include anesthesia-induced hepatitis and propofol infusion syndrome. Anesthesia-induced hepatitis is most commonly seen after halothane, though the drug is no longer available in the United States. Anesthesia-induced hepatitis has also been reported after exposure to isoflurane, desflurane, and sevoflurane. In the propofol infusion syndrome, patients develop metabolic acidosis, bradyarrhythmias, and progressive myocardial failure frequently followed by death [13]. Usually, patients have received larger doses of propofol for more than 48 hours, though this syndrome has also been described in patients who have received propofol for shorter periods. In one case, after 3 hours of a propofol anesthetic, a patient developed lactic acidosis; several hours later, after the propofol was stopped, the acid–base status returned to normal [14].

Ultimately, the decision whether to use a particular inhalation drug or propofol is up to the individual directing anesthesia care. Clearly, with propofol, both PONV and the risk of triggering malignant hyperthermia is less compared to any inhalation drug.

Cost

Cost is sometimes used as an argument for or against certain anesthetics, though the cost of a drug cannot be considered in isolation, as certain anesthetic techniques or drugs can have effects long after the surgery. Propofol is now generic, with attendant cost reductions. Moreover, drug costs are a small component of perioperative costs, and the major cost of an anesthetic is the anesthesiologist's professional fee [1].

Medicinal supplements to the primary anesthetic

Blood pressure control

There are many different definitions of intraoperative hypotension, including a blood pressure below a certain value or a decrease relative to the patient's baseline blood pressure. One group of authors who studied the problem of defining intraoperative hypotension found that if hypotension was defined as a greater than 10% decrease from baseline, 99% of the patients would be categorized as having hypotension. If a mean arterial pressure of 70 mmHg was used as the definition, only 5% of the patients were considered hypotensive [15]. An accompanying editorial stated that a better definition of intraoperative hypotension is needed [16]. In some instances, e.g., tympanoplasty, blood pressure might be kept below a certain value to decrease blood loss. Or a patient whose blood pressure is poorly controlled preoperatively may also be hypertensive while undergoing general anesthesia.

Generally, tight blood pressure control is probably not necessary. A patient can develop side effects after any drug that is used to lower blood pressure. For example, when β-blockers are used, some patients might develop congestive heart failure [17]. Cardiovascular drugs are not the only drugs that can be used to lower blood pressure. Analgesics in general can be used for this purpose, and also to help control blood loss [18]. When blood pressure is lowered with a cardiovascular drug instead of an anesthetic, however, assuming that the elevated blood pressure is not due to inadequate anesthesia, recovery is faster and there are fewer side effects [19].

Vasopressors can be used to help raise blood pressure. Phenylephrine and ephedrine are the most commonly used drugs for that purpose. Only one study has compared the two drugs, though the primary purpose of the study was to compare Bispectral Index (BIS) values [20]. Blood pressure increased after both drugs, though BIS increased only after ephedrine. Vasopressor use may be associated with worse outcome. In retrospective analysis of 65 000 noncardiac surgery patients between 2003 and 2006, total vasopressor dose and use of a vasopressor infusion was associated with a greater

incidence of postoperative acute renal failure as well as increased mortality [21]. In low-risk patients undergoing elective cardiac surgery with cardiopulmonary bypass, perioperative dobutamine use that was simply based on the clinical judgement of the attending anesthesiologist was associated with adverse postoperative cardiac outcome [22]. Fluids can also be administered to help raise blood pressure, and fluid administration is discussed below. The most important concept to remember is that drugs should not be given "because we do it this way" but based on medical indication.

Higher blood pressure may have some advantages. Blood pressure, or more accurately cardiac output, can affect the onset time of drugs given during an anesthetic. For example, rocuronium onset time is faster after ephedrine administration [23]. Yet with higher blood pressure there is risk of myocardial ischemia, stroke, neurocognitive dysfunction, bleeding, and even prolonged hospital stay. Opioids, sedatives, ketamine, β-blockers, nitroglycerin, sodium nitroprusside, and calcium channel blockers can help reduce blood pressure.

Hypertension can sometimes be an issue towards the end of a procedure and in the PACU. In one study, intraoperative dexmedetomidine when combined with a sevoflurane and reminfentanil anesthetic was associated with better control of hypertension both intra- and postoperatively in the PACU [24].

Postoperative nausea and vomiting

Patients hate vomiting. When patients are asked how much they would pay to avoid PONV or postoperative pain, they are willing to pay the most to prevent either of these outcomes, though the actual amount is a function, in part, of patient income [25]. Women, especially those who are pregnant, have a higher incidence of PONV. Other risk factors include a previous history of motion sickness or postanesthetic emesis, surgery within 1–7 days of the menstrual cycle, not smoking, and procedures such as laparoscopy, lithotripsy, major breast surgery, and ear, nose, or throat surgery. The greater the number of risk factors, the greater the risk of nausea or vomiting after surgery. Inhalation drugs are associated with an increased risk of PONV, particularly in the early stages of recovery, and postoperative opioid use is associated with PONV more than 2 hours after surgery [26].

PONV is multifactorial, and several drug classes have been used for prophylaxis and treatment of PONV (see Chapter 54). The selective serotonin antagonists ondansetron, dolasetron, and granisetron have been shown to have equivalent efficacy. Dopamine antagonists, antihistamines, and anticholinergic drugs are useful and are generally less expensive, but are associated with extensive side effects. Neurokinin type 1 receptor antagonists may also be useful to control PONV. Other therapies useful in controlling PONV include acupuncture [28], supplemental fluid therapy [29], clonidine (perhaps in part because it decreases anesthetic requirement) [30], and dexamethasone [8,31]. Some studies have found that steroids

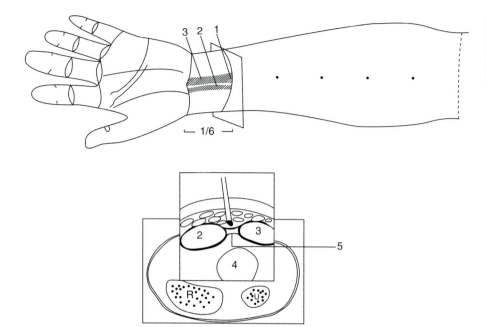

Figure 62.2. The P6 acupuncture point in relation to other hand structures is illustrated: (1) P6 acupuncture point, (2) palmaris longus tendon, (3) flexor carpi radialis tendon, (4) median nerve, (5) palmar aponeurosis. Reproduced with permission from Wang and Kain [27].

may impair wound healing and increase the risk of postoperative infection. Yet recent meta-analyses of perioperative high-dose methylprednisolone or dexamethasone did not find increases in infection or other complications [31,32].

Stimulation of the P6 acupoint on the wrist has received the most study, although other acupoints might also help reduce PONV. The P6 acupoint is located 4 cm proximal to the wrist crease between the tendons of palmaris longus and flexor carpi radialis muscles (Fig. 62.2). In a Cochrane review, P6 accupoint stimulation was compared to both sham therapy and other antiemetics [33]. P6 stimulation was more effective than sham treatment. The type of P6 acupoint stimulation, e.g., invasive or noninvasive, made no difference; and the need for rescue antimetic with P6 stimulation was reduced. Therefore, antiemetic drug cost may be reduced with P6 stimulation. When P6 stimulation was compared to other prophylactic antiemetics, there was no difference in outcome, although the number of trials and the number of participants were both small. In studies comparing antiemetic drugs to P6 stimulation, nausea but not vomiting risk was lower in patients who received P6 stimulation than in patients who received prophylactic antiemetics. In one study, acupuncture therapy was effective in controlling both PONV and postoperative pain [34]. Acupressure is most effective when it is administered after surgery [35], although if neuromuscular transmission (NMT) leads are placed intraoperatively at the P6 acupuncture point, PONV is reduced [36]. That study, in which NMT leads were placed at the P6 acupuncture point, gives another reason to monitor neuromuscular function (see below), though it should be noted that in that study the frequency of single twitch stimulation was 1 Hz, a frequency for NMT monitoring that is not commonly used.

Droperidol is an effective treatment for the prevention of PONV. In December 2001 the US Food and Drug Administration (FDA) issued a "black-box" warning for the drug due to the potential for drug-induced QT prolongation and torsades de pointes. This warning was controversial because of the droperidol 30-year safety record and because the serotonin (5-hydroxytryptamine) type 3 (5-HT$_3$) antagonists which became first-line drugs for prevention and treatment have also been shown to prolong the QT interval. It is important to note that the black-box warning only referred to droperidol doses ≥ 2.5 mg, because doses < 2.5 mg are off-label, and black-box warnings only apply to label indications [37]. When patients were compared before and after the black-box warning, when droperidol use decreased from 12% to 0%, the incidence of torsades de pointes did not change [38].

Combination therapy is the most effective way to control PONV. PONV is reduced with avoidance of N$_2$O, and with inhalation anesthetics, anticholinesterases for muscle relaxant reversal, and opioids. PONV is also reduced by fluid hydration and administration of a 5-HT$_3$ antagonist, an antiemetic from a different drug class, and dexamethasone [39]. When combination therapy was used, nausea incidence was less than 10%, and even lower for certain procedures and types of patients [40].

Paralysis

Should the longer-acting neuromuscular blockers no longer be used? There is in fact little evidence to show that longer-acting drugs such as pancuronium should be abandoned in favor of intermediate acting drugs such as vecuronium or rocurnoium. In one study, after a fast-track protocol for cardiac surgery patients that used rocuronium instead of pancuronium was implemented, duration of mechanical ventilation after surgery was shortened [41]. Duration of action and recovery time of muscle relaxants is significantly increased when a patient is hypothermic, even as little as 2 °C less than normal [42]. Although the nondepolarizing drugs may provide surgical paralysis for only 25–40 minutes, residual paralysis may last much longer. Neuromuscular-blocker reversal drugs should always be used unless there is unequivocal evidence of full neuromuscular function.

Pain control

Intraoperative opioids are useful to supplement both intra-operative and postoperative analgesia. Fentanyl is probably the most popular drug, although all other intravenous opioids can be used. All opioids can cause nausea, sedation, and dizziness, which can delay discharge. Nonsteroidal analgesics are not effective as supplements during general anesthesia, although they are useful in controlling postoperative pain, particularly when given before skin incision. To control post-operative pain, combination therapy is most useful.

The time to return of consciousness after propofol/opioid anesthesia is influenced more by the opioid and less by the duration of propofol infusion [43]. Remifentanil is the opioid associated with the most rapid return to consciousness (Fig. 62.3). This is particularly evident for longer cases. For example, in a study of fast-track management of patients undergoing cardiac surgery, when remifentanil replaced sufentanil, extubation time and PACU time were both reduced [41].

Perioperative administration of intravenous lidocaine has recently been shown to decrease postoperative pain and also improve bowel function in patients undergoing laparoscopic colectomy. When patients scheduled to undergo laparoscopic colectomy received intravenous lidocaine (bolus injection of 1.5 mg kg^{-1} lidocaine at induction of anesthesia, then a continuous infusion of 2 mg kg^{-1} h^{-1} intraoperatively and 1.33 mg kg^{-1} h^{-1} for 24 hours postoperatively), postoperative bowel function and analgesia were improved, fatigue was less, and length of hospital stay was reduced [45]. More study is needed to show whether this therapy is effective for other types of surgery, and how this therapy compares with epidural nerve blocks or epidural analgesia. Nonsteroidal anti-inflammatory drugs are useful for postoperative pain control, although they should be started before or during surgery and then continued postoperatively.

Nitrous oxide

N_2O has been used as supplement for general anesthesia for 150 years. Though it does allow the dose of the primary inhalation or intravenous anesthetic to be reduced, it is not without hematologic, neurologic, immunologic, and/or myocardial risks. Air-filled spaces can expand. Long-lasting cognitive deficits have been reported in older patients. Postoperative infections and pulmonary complications were greater after 70% nitrous oxide/30% oxygen compared to 20% nitrogen/80% oxygen [46]. Admittedly, a more appropriate comparison

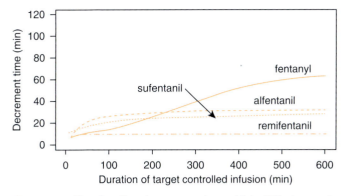

Figure 62.3. Time for effect-site concentration to fall by 50% after steady-state effect-site concentration for 300 minutes with propofol and one of the following: fentanyl, alfentanil, sufentanil, remifentanil [44]. Of the opioids, remifentanil is associated with the most rapid return to consciousness.

would have been with 80% nitrogen instead of 80% oxygen, since oxygen itself may have affected outcome. Postoperative nausea and vomiting is greater when N_2O is used for maintenance. In patients undergoing laparoscopic gynecologic surgery, N_2O increased PONV in a dose-dependent fashion [47].

There is an occupational exposure risk with N_2O, although it is probably minimal because scavenging is used in operating rooms. Some have recently suggested that N_2O should no longer be used, while others feel that exclusion from clinical practice is not warranted and future research is needed [48].

The importance of normal temperature

Anesthesia impairs thermoregulation. For that reason, if patients are not warmed, they become hypothermic. Even a body temperature less than 2 °C from normal in patients with cardiac risk factors undergoing noncardiac surgery is associated with an increased incidence of morbid cardiac events and ventricular tachycardia [49]. Mild hypothermia increases the risk of surgical wound infection [50]. Mild hypothermia (< 1 °C) increases blood loss and increases the risk for transfusion [51]. When patients are both acidotic and hypothermic, the two act synergistically to impair coagulation [52]. Hypothermia begins during the first 30 minutes after anesthesia induction when there is an internal core-to-peripheral redistribution of body heat. Temperature should be monitored for all cases that last 30 minutes or more (see below for details of temperature monitoring).

Thermal management of patients has been reviewed [53]. Forced air warmers are the most effective and most common way to warm patients and prevent hypothermia. They work by convection, since warm air is blown over the skin, and by radiation, since a warm cover is over the body. Recently, elective-resistive heating blankets have been introduced: carbon-fiber patient covers are powered by battery-powered electrical heaters. Warming fluids is not really effective in warming patients unless the administered solution is cold, e.g., blood, or large amounts of fluid are administered.

Monitors

Since the anesthesiologist does not usually choose what type of ECG, inspired gas, ventilation, or blood pressure monitor will be used, these will not be discussed. Though the American Society of Anesthesiologists (ASA) has not stated that depth of anesthesia or twitch monitors are standard, since many use them and there are reasons why some might even think they should be considered standard, they will be discussed.

Depth of anesthesia

Should the vaporizer be turned to give a patient 1–2 MAC of anesthesia? In the case of total intravenous anesthesia (TIVA), is propofol 150 μg kg^{-1} min^{-1} sufficient? Every patient is different and some need more anesthesia than others. Patient age, height, weight, administration of other drugs besides the primary anesthetic, and type of surgery are just some of the factors that govern the decision about anesthetic dosing. The proper depth of anesthesia suppresses relevant clinical responses to noxious stimuli which include patient movement, an increase in blood pressure, pulse, or minute ventilation. If a patient is paralyzed some of these responses (e.g., movement or change in minute ventilation) might not be apparent. Though vital signs have been used for over 150 years as surrogates for depth of anesthesia, these clinical signs may not really be reliable to measure the hypnotic component of anesthesia.

Electroencephalography-derived variables such as the Bispectral Index (BIS; Aspect Medical Systems), patient state index (PSI), the Narcotrend, cerebral state index, and entropy monitors are examples of brain-based monitors of depth of anesthesia. Auditory evoked potentials might also be used.

Depth of anesthesia monitors can decrease anesthesia requirement without sacrificing amnesia during general anesthesia. Because less anesthesia is used, titration of anesthesia with these monitors results in earlier emergence from anesthesia. For example, when anesthesia care is managed with the BIS, patients wake up faster and do not stay in the recovery room as long as when anesthesia depth is monitored clinically [54]. In a meta-analysis of BIS monitoring for ambulatory anesthesia, BIS monitoring was shown to reduce anesthetic use by 19%, with more modest decreases in PACU duration (4 minutes) and PONV (6%) (Fig. 62.4) [55]. In another meta-analysis, amount of anesthesia, time for eye-opening, time to respond to verbal command, and time to extubate were all reduced when a BIS monitor was used [56]. Results are even more modest, albeit mixed, for later recovery endpoints.

Anesthesia awareness may be less when a depth of anesthesia monitor is used. In a study of almost 5000 patients who underwent general anesthesia and who were paralyzed and/or intubated, awareness was significantly reduced in the group of patients who were monitored with a BIS compared with the group who were not so monitored [57]. But in a study of 1941 patients at high risk for awareness in which a BIS-guided protocol was compared to measuring end-tidal anesthetic gases, anesthesia awareness was no different [58]. Because these monitors result in less use of anesthesia, there is the possibility that intraoperative awareness and myocardial ischemia might be increased. In addition, these monitors do not always correlate with anesthesia depth, because of insensitivity to different anesthesia combinations, improper monitor application, or artifact. An ASA practice advisory on intraoperative awareness and brain function monitoring concluded that brain function monitors should not be routinely used to monitor anesthesia depth and to prevent intraoperative awareness, but individual physicians should be able to decide whether they should be used [59].

At present, no depth of anesthesia monitor seems any better than another, though few studies have actually compared the different monitors. When BIS and PSI monitors were compared in patients receiving sevoflurane, both predicted depth of anesthesia well [60]. In a study in which BIS and entropy monitors were compared in patients who received propofol and then desflurane for maintenance of anesthesia, detection of changes in anesthesia depth were the same, but electrical interference during electrocautery use was less with the entropy monitor [61].

Temperature

Temperature should be measured to make sure a patient is not developing malignant hyperthermia, and to quantify both hypo- and hyperthermia. Core temperature can be measured in the pulmonary artery, distal esophagus, nasopharynx, or tympanic membrane. If the patient's trachea is intubated, distal esophageal temperature measurements are easy. If the probe is incorporated into an esophageal stethoscope, the probe should be placed where heart sounds are maximal. Nasopharyngeal probes should be placed a few centimeters beyond the nares. Use of the tympanic membrane for temperature monitoring can be problematic if the probe is not actually placed on the tympanic membrane. Axillary temperature measurement is reasonably accurate, though the temperature probe must be placed near the axillary artery and the patient's arm should be placed to the side. Infrared temperature monitors are not precise [62]. Forehead skin temperature monitors are easy to place. Forehead temperatures measured are about 2 °C less than core temperature. Since the skin-to-core temperature gradient is linear over the temperature range usually encountered in the operating room, it is reasonable to simply add 2 °C to the skin temperature to obtain core temperature.

Neuromuscular function monitoring

Neuromuscular function must be monitored when patients are paralyzed. While some practitioners still do not routinely

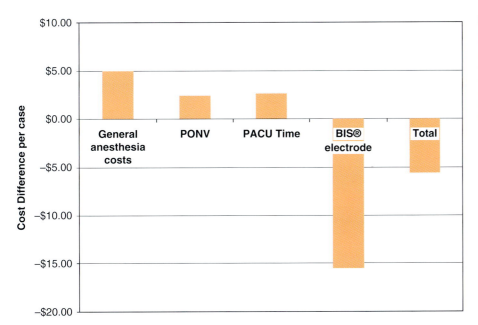

Figure 62.4. Bispectral Index (BIS) monitoring reduces anesthetic consumption, cost to treat nausea and vomiting, and postanesthesia care unit (PACU) time; the cost of the electrode reverses cost savings. The ordinate represents cost difference per case pooled from three studies (i.e., costs for the control group minus cost for the group that used BIS). The capital cost for the BIS monitor was not included. Data from Liu [55].

monitor neuromuscular function, evidence shows that this practice is not safe, even when short- and intermediate-acting muscle relaxants are used [63].

Acceleromyography, the most widely available objective measure of neuromuscular function, measures acceleration of the thumb (Fig. 62.5). When using this technique, the thumb must be allowed to move freely. The unit requires calibration before paralysis. In addition, once calibration has started, to accurately measure how twitch and train-of-four (TOF) has changed from baseline, the position of the hand cannot change. Compared to usual clinical tests such as head lift and grip strength or visual or tactile evaluation of the response to nerve stimulation, there is good evidence that acceleromyography is more sensitive in diagnosing and detecting postoperative residual neuromuscular block [64]. In one study after neostigmine reversal, residual block was more common when neuromuscular function was monitored using a conventional nerve stimulator; in addition, the group monitored using acceleromyography had a lower incidence of adverse respiratory events [65]. In that study, patients who were monitored using acceleromyography were not extubated until they had a TOF ratio > 0.8.

Fluids

For most patients, before the start of an anesthetic, an intravenous catheter is or already has been inserted and an intravenous solution that usually contains lactated Ringer's solution is attached. Lactated Ringer's electrolyte composition includes sodium 130 mEq L^{-1}, potassium 4 mEq L^{-1}, calcium 3 mEq L^{-1}, and chloride 110 mEq L^{-1}, and is therefore closer to the electrolyte composition of blood than normal saline (0.9%), which includes sodium 154 mEq L^{-1} and cholride

154 mEq L^{-1}. Normal saline use is associated with hyperchloremic metabolic acidosis, so it is usually not used for intraoperative fluid therapy, except to reconstitute packed red blood cells, for patients with hyponatremia, hypochloremic metabolic alkalosis, or brain injury. Lactated Ringer's solution should not be used to reconstitute blood because it contains calcium, which might cause clotting,

The primary intent of fluid therapy is to optimize preload. Before a case starts, preload may be low because the patient has fasted before the procedure and/or due to bowel preparation. Intraoperatively, preload may be low because of the anesthetic (e.g., vasodilation) or the procedure (e.g., evaporation or blood loss), or it may be too low because of anesthetic effects on the heart (e.g., anesthetic-induced changes in myocardial contractility necessitating a higher preload). The first line of fluid therapy to optimize preload is lactated Ringer's solution, and then, as needed, either colloid or blood.

In everyday management, assuming that lactated Ringer's solution is the first line of therapy, the question is how much fluid is appropriate, particularly for cases where there is minimal fluid loss due to the surgical procedure. Patients who fast do not necessarily have low intravascular volume. For example, in a study of otherwise healthy patients with cervical cancer who were undergoing hysterectomy, where blood volume was measured using indocyanine green dilution and erythrocytes labeled with fluorescein, even after fasting for 10 hours before surgery, patients were not intravascularly hypovolemic [66]. Yet studies of fluid administration to account for flood loss due to fasting have found that fluid boluses at the start of surgery have effects beyond changes in preload. In one study, administration of 1 L of fluid for patients who fasted preoperatively improved early symptoms of dehydration such as drowsiness and dizziness [67]. In another study, patients who were

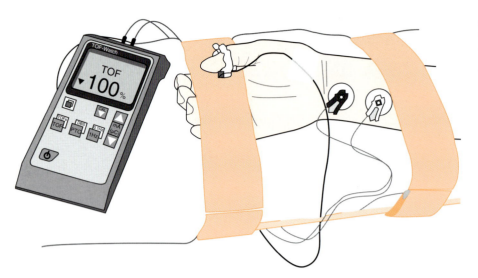

Figure 62.5. To set up the acceleromyograph, two electrodes are placed along the ulnar nerve and the piezoelectrode acceleration trandsducer is positioned on the volar side of the thumb. The thumb must be allowed to move freely and the hand position must be fixed. Reproduced with permission from Claudius and Viby-Mogensen [64].

to undergo gynecologic laparoscopy who received 2 mL kg^{-1} sodium lactate 20 minutes preoperatively had less PONV and postoperative pain [68]. Adequate blood flow to vital organs is the ultimate determinant of how much fluid is appropriate. Hypervolemia is usually not problematic, since the kidney can regulate fluid overload [69]. To prevent postoperative renal dysfunction, urine output should be maintained at 0.5 mL kg^{-1} h^{-1}, though there is no randomized clinical trial to prove this assertion. There is also little evidence to back such strategies as mannitol, "renal doses" of dopamine, and loop diuretics, which have been recommended to decrease postoperative renal function. Certainly, however, maintenance of normovolemia will minimize postoperative renal dysfunction, and this topic is discussed in more detail in an excellent review [70].

There are some special instances, e.g., patients who undergo pulmonary surgery, where lesser amounts of fluid are desirable. Patients with acute lung injury who received conservative fluid therapy for 1 week had a shortened duration of mechanical ventilation and a decreased length of stay in the ICU [71]. Relative fluid restriction during major intraabdominal surgery is also associated with reduced complications, time to recovery of gastrointestinal function, and time to hospital discharge [72].

In some types of surgery, more liberal fluid administration of fluids is associated with improved outcome. For example, patients undergoing laparoscopic cholecystectomy who intraoperatively received 40 mL kg^{-1} instead of 15 mL kg^{-1} lactated Ringer's, postoperatively had better pulmonary function and exercise capacity, less nausea, thirst, dizziness, drowsiness, and fatigue, better balance function and general well-being, and greater likelihood of being discharged on the day of surgery [73]. In a study of patients undergoing knee arthroplasty, patients who received liberal compared to restrictive fluid therapy had better coagulability and a reduction in vomiting, though other recovery variables and length of hospital stay were no different between groups [74].

The discussion about colloid versus crystalloid continues. There appears to be little difference in terms of long-term outcome [75]. For patients with traumatic brain injury, however, saline seems preferable to albumin during acute resuscitation [76].

How is one to know if enough fluids have been administered or more fluids are needed? Hematocrit can be followed to determine fluid volume, but this only works if there is no blood loss, and hematocrit only represents intravascular volume. Delta pulse pressure, defined as the difference between the maximal and minimal pulse pressure during one breathing cycle divided by the mean of the two numbers, is useful as a nonivasive indicator of vascular volume. It can be used to predict the hemodynamic response to volume expansion if a patient is mechanically ventilated [77]. A change in pulse oximetry plethysmographic waveform amplitude of at least 13% can also predict response to volume expansion and can quantify the effects of volume expansion on hemodynamic parameters (Fig. 62.6) [78]. Esophageal Doppler monitoring used for patients undergoing major elective surgery led to decreased postoperative morbidity, earlier return to normal bowel function, less PONV, and shorter hospital stay [79]. An excellent review on indices that can be used to assesses preload has been published [80].

In the ASA's updated guidelines for blood transfusion, blood administration is recommended if the hemoglobin is less than 6 g dL^{-1} and is not recommended if it is greater than 10 g dL^{-1} [81]. For surgical or obstetric patients, platelet transfusion is usually indicated if the platelet count is less than 50×10^9 in the presence of excessive bleeding or if there is known or suspected platelet dysfunction, and is rarely indicated if the platelet count is greater than 100×10^9. Fresh frozen plasma (FFP) administration is indicated if there is coagulopathy with a prothrombin time (PT) greater than 1.5 times normal; an INR greater than 2 or aPTT $> 2 \times$ normal; if there is coagulopathy after blood transfusion greater

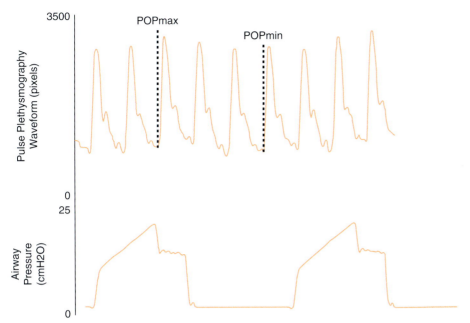

Figure 62.6. Respiratory variations in pulse oximetry plethysmographic waveform amplitude can be calculated. POPmax and POPmin are defined as the maximum and minimum pulse oximetry plethysmographic waveform amplitude over a single respiratory cycle. $\Delta POP = (POPmax - POPmin)/[(POPmax + POPmin)/2]$. Reproduced with permission from Cannesson et al. [78].

than 70 mL kg^{-1}; to urgently reverse warfarin; if there are coagulation factor deficiencies and specific concentrates are not available; and for heparin resistance.

Ventilation

When considering ventilator parameters for mechanical ventilation, it is important to remember that lung volume is proportional to patient height, rather than weight. If using weight, consider a tidal volume based on ideal body weight. With some anesthesia machines, delivered tidal volume may be different from the tidal volume set on the ventilator.

In patients with lung injury, lower tidal volumes and positive end-expiratory pressure (PEEP) may limit pulmonary inflammation. Even in patients without pre-existing lung injury, mechanical ventilation was associated with significant inflammatory changes in the lung, and mechanical ventilation with lower tidal volumes and PEEP helped to limit inflammatory changes [82]. There is no difference in oxygenation between pressure-controlled and volume-controlled ventilation in patients with lung disease or during one-lung ventilation [83].

Patient position may affect pulmonary function. In morbidly obese patients undergoing laparoscopic gastric banding who were paralyzed for the procedure, the beach-chair position and PEEP both improved respiratory function, and both maneuvers were needed together during pneumoperitoneum to improve oxygenation [84].

There are no accepted standards for the desired carbon dioxide partial pressure (PCO_2) in the blood, and permissive hypercapnia may have some advantages. Hypercapnia may improve resistance to surgical wound infections because tissue oxygen partial pressure, skin blood-flow velocity, cardiac index, and muscle oximeter saturation all increase linearly as a function of PCO_2 [85,86]. In one ovine model of septic shock, hypercapnia had similar effects to dobutamine for hemodynamic variables and lactic acidosis, and improved tissue oxygenation and reduced lung edema formation more than dobutamine administration [87].

Emergence issue: reversal of paralysis

Some practitioners believe that if only one dose of an intermediate-acting neuromuscular blocking drug is used and the patient's endotracheal tube is to be removed more than 1.5 hours after the drug was administered, then the drug does not have to be reversed. Yet there are examples of residual paralysis lasting more than 3 hours after a single intubating dose [88]. In one study of patients with critical respiratory events in the PACU, hypoxemia and respiratory obstruction were more commonly observed in patients whose paralysis was not reversed. Incomplete neuromuscular blockade is an important contributing factor for development of adverse respiratory events in the PACU [89].

Acetylcholinesterase inhibitors, edrophonium, and most commonly neostigmine, are used to reverse muscle paralysis. Muscle paralysis should be reversed to improve patient comfort and safety. Even if the patient's TOF ratio is 0.9 without pharmacologic reversal, pharmacologic reversal is necessary, since impaired pharyngeal function and airway protection has been found even at a TOF ratio of 0.9 [90]. Conversely, if neuromuscular blockade is profound, anticholinesterase inhibitors are ineffective. Acetylcholinesterase inhibitors also stimulate muscarinic receptors, which can cause cardiovascular, gastrointestinal, and respiratory complications. For that reason, when acetylcholinesterase inhibitors are administered, muscarnic anatagonists such as glycopyrrolate or atropine should also be given. Muscarinic antagonists can also cause tachycardia, blurred vision, and sedation. When patients are cold, even in the range commonly encountered in the operating room, reversal or neuromuscular blockade can be delayed. Complete reversal of neuromuscular blockade will not occur until a patient's temperature is greater than 36 °C [42].

When neuromuscular blockade is profound and it is not advisable to use an anticholinesterase inhibitor, sugammadex may be an option. Sugammadex is a selective relaxant-binding drug. It acts by forming a tight complex with unbound neuromuscular blocking drug (NMBD) molecules, which then cannot act at the neuromuscular junction. Sugammadex, compared to neostigmine, can rapidly reverse profound rocuronium neuromuscular blockade [91,92]. Some evidence suggests that suggamadex can also reverse moderate vecuronium-induced neuromuscular block [93]. Sugammadex dose is dependent on the intensity of blockade, and re-paralysis may be apparent if the dose is inadequate. Sugammadex is not yet available in the United States, in part because of hypersensitivity/allergic reactions. In one study, hypertension for up to 15 minutes was noted in two patients after sugammadex injection [92].

Special concern: posterior scoliosis correction and the wake-up test

After posterior scoliosis correction, there is a risk of paraplegia. Spinal cord assessment during the procedure can help determine whether intraoperative damage to the spinal cord has occurred. Somatosensory evoked potential (SSEP) and transcranial electric motor evoked potential monitoring both are sensitive predictions of postoperative neurologic dysfunction. If damage is found, then early revision of the repair can hopefully minimize postoperative neurologic deficits. Anesthetics have a dose-dependent effect on ability to record evoked potential responses. Generally, 0.5–1.0 MAC isoflurane, desflurane, or sevoflurane allows satisfactory monitoring of evoked potentials. N_2O compounds the effect of the inhalation drugs. Intravenous anesthetics affect evoked potentials less than inhalation drugs. For example, when BIS was used to guide isoflurane or propofol administration during SSEP monitoring, at equivalent BIS levels, isoflurane caused a greater decrease in amplitude and increase in the latency of the SSEP than propofol [94]. Opioids have trivial effects on evoked potentials. Dexmedetomidine in doses up to 0.6 ng mL^{-1} also has minimal effects on somatosensory or motor evoked potentials [95]. An excellent review of pharmacologic and physiologic influences that affect evoked potentials has been published [96].

For a wake-up test, the anesthetic is stopped until the patient can voluntarily move all extremities. After movement is verified, propofol 1–2 mg kg^{-1} can be used to deepen the anesthetic. If remifentanil was used before patient wake-up, a remifentanil bolus is also administered. If sufentanil was used, then an additional bolus of 0.3 μg kg^{-1} is appropriate. Some also administer midazolam 1–2 mg along with propofol, but this is probably not indicated, since midazolam is not associated with retrograde amnesia. When wake-up tests are used, impaired sleep quality is apparent postoperatively. In one study, postoperative sleep quality was less impaired if sufentanil was used instead of remifentanil [97].

Summary

General anesthesia was developed almost 150 years ago, though the specialty and the management of patients continues to evolve. Contemporary anesthetic management, even when compared to 20 years ago, has changed. As new drugs and techniques are introduced, evidence-based clinical practice will be the key to success for optimal patient management during general anesthesia.

Many factors affect the choice of primary drugs for maintenance of anesthesia. The principal concerns are hemodynamic stability during surgery, speed and quality of emergence and awakening, and how the primary anesthetic drugs may affect postoperative recovery. With the inhaled anesthetics, blood pressures are generally stable and emergence and awakening are relatively rapid. Though malignant hyperthermia is always a possibility, the likelihood that it will develop is low. Other complications, such as anesthesia-induced hepatitis, are unusual. When propofol is used for maintenance, a pump is usually required. With propofol, nausea and vomiting are less frequent, and malignant hyperthermia is not a risk. Propofol is now generic, with attendant cost reductions.

Any of the inhalation or sedative-hypnotic anesthetics can be used as the sole drug for maintenance of anesthesia, but other drugs are also usually included. During anesthesia, medications are frequently administered to increase or lower blood pressure, though the first question to ask is what blood pressure is considered appropriate, excluding patients who have organ damage, e.g., brain, where organ flow is dependent on blood pressure. Nausea, with or without vomiting, is probably the most important factor contributing to a delay in discharge of patients and an increase in unanticipated admissions of both children and adults after ambulatory surgery. Neuromuscular blockers are frequently used to facilitate intubation of the trachea, though they are also used to maintain paralysis throughout a procedure. Neuromuscular blocking drugs should be reversed, and adequate reversal should be demonstrated using neuromuscular monitoring and documented on the anesthetic record.

References

1. Demeere JL, Merckx C, Demeere N. Cost minimisation and cost effectiveness in anaesthesia for total hip replacement surgery, in Belgium? A study comparing three general anaesthesia techniques. *Acta Anaesthesiol Belg* 2006; **57**: 145–51.

2. Hohlrieder M, Tiefenthaler W, Klaus H, *et al.* Effect of total intravenous anaesthesia and balanced anaesthesia on the frequency of coughing during emergence from the anaesthesia. *Br J Anaesth* 2007; **99**: 587–91.

3. Kohjitani A, Egusa M, Shimada M, Miyawaki T. Accumulated oropharyngeal water increases coughing during dental treatment with intravenous sedation. *J Oral Rehabil* 2008; **35**: 203–8.

4. McKay RE, Bostrom A, Balea MC, McKay WR. Airway responses during desflurane versus sevoflurane administration via a laryngeal mask airway in smokers. *Anesth Analg* 2006; **103**: 1147–54.

5. Wild MR, Gornall CB, Griffiths DE, Curran J. Maintenance of anaesthesia with sevoflurane or isoflurane effects on adverse airway events in smokers. *Anaesthesia* 2004; **59**: 891–3.

6. Rohm KD, Piper SN, Suttner S, Schuler S, Boldt J. Early recovery, cognitive function and costs of a desflurane inhalational vs. a total intravenous anaesthesia regimen in long-term surgery. *Acta Anaesthesiol Scand* 2006; **50**: 14–18.

7. Sneyd JR, Andrews CJ, Tsubokawa T. Comparison of propofol/remifentanil and sevoflurane/remifentanil for maintenance of anaesthesia for elective intracranial surgery. *Br J Anaesth* 2005; **94**: 778–83.

8. Apfel CC, Korttila K, Abdalla M, *et al.* A factorial trial of six interventions for the prevention of postoperative nausea and vomiting. *N Engl J Med* 2004; **350**: 2441–51.

9. Cheng SS, Yeh J, Flood P. Anesthesia matters: patients anesthetized with propofol have less postoperative pain than those anesthetized with isoflurane. *Anesth Analg* 2008; **106**: 264–9.

10. Fassoulaki A, Melemeni A, Paraskeva A, Siafaka I, Sarantopoulos C. Postoperative pain and analgesic requirements after anesthesia with sevoflurane, desflurane or propofol. *Anesth Analg* 2008; **107**: 1715–19.

11. Kang JG, Kim JK, Jeong HS, *et al.* A prospective, randomized comparison of the effects of inhaled sevoflurane anesthesia and propofol/remifentanil intravenous anesthesia on salivary excretion during laryngeal microsurgery. *Anesth Analg* 2008; **106**: 1723–7.

12. Lahteenmaki M, Salo M, Tenovuo J. Mucosal host defence response to hysterectomy assessed by saliva analyses: a comparison of propofol and isoflurane anaesthesia. *Anaesthesia* 1998; **53**: 1067–73.

13. Fong JJ, Sylvia L, Ruthazer R, *et al.* Predictors of mortality in patients with suspected propofol infusion syndrome. *Crit Care Med* 2008; **36**: 2281–7.

14. Salengros JC, Velghe-Lenelle CE, Bollens R, Engelman E, Barvais L. Lactic acidosis during propofol–remifentanil anesthesia in an adult. *Anesthesiology* 2004; **101**: 241–3.

15. Bijker JB, van Klei WA, Kappen TH, *et al.* Incidence of intraoperative hypotension as a function of the chosen definition: literature definitions applied to a retrospective cohort using automated data collection. *Anesthesiology* 2007; **107**: 213–20.

16. Warner MA, Monk TG. The impact of lack of standardized definitions on the specialty. *Anesthesiology* 2007; **107**: 198–9.

17. Beattie WS, Wijeysundera DN, Karkouti K, McCluskey S, Tait G. Does tight heart rate control improve beta-blocker efficacy? An updated analysis of the noncardiac surgical randomized trials. *Anesth Analg* 2008; **106**: 1039–48.

18. Richa F, Yazigi A, Sleilaty G, Yazbeck P. Comparison between dexmedetomidine and remifentanil for controlled hypotension during tympanoplasty. *Eur J Anaesthesiol* 2008; **25**: 369–74.

19. White PF, Wang B, Tang J, *et al.* The effect of intraoperative use of esmolol and nicardipine on recovery after ambulatory surgery. *Anesth Analg* 2003; **97**: 1633–8.

20. Ishiyama T, Oguchi T, Iijima T, *et al.* Ephedrine, but not phenylephrine, increases bispectral index values during combined general and epidural anesthesia. *Anesth Analg* 2003; **97**: 780–4.

21. Kheterpal S, Tremper KK, Englesbe MJ, *et al.* Predictors of postoperative acute renal failure after noncardiac surgery in patients with previously normal renal function. *Anesthesiology* 2007; **107**: 892–902.

22. Fellahi JL, Parienti JJ, Hanouz JL, *et al.* Perioperative use of dobutamine in cardiac surgery and adverse cardiac outcome: propensity-adjusted analyses. *Anesthesiology* 2008; **108**: 979–87.

23. Han DW, Chun DH, Kweon TD, Shin YS. Significance of the injection timing of ephedrine to reduce the onset time of rocuronium. *Anaesthesia* 2008; **63**: 856–60.

24. Bekker A, Sturaitis M, Bloom M, *et al.* The effect of dexmedetomidine on perioperative hemodynamics in patients undergoing craniotomy. *Anesth Analg* 2008; **107**: 1340–7.

25. Macario A, Fleisher LA. Is there value in obtaining a patient's willingness to pay for a particular anesthetic intervention? *Anesthesiology* 2006; **104**: 906–9.

26. Apfel CC, Kranke P, Katz MH, *et al.* Volatile anaesthetics may be the main cause of early but not delayed postoperative vomiting: a randomized controlled trial of factorial design. *Br J Anaesth* 2002; **88**: 659–68.

27. Wang SM, Kain ZN. P6 acupoint injections are as effective as droperidol in controlling early postoperative nausea and vomiting in children. *Anesthesiology* 2002; **97**: 359–66.

28. Turgut S, Ozalp G, Dikmen S, *et al.* Acupressure for postoperative nausea and vomiting in gynaecological patients receiving patient-controlled analgesia. *Eur J Anaesthesiol* 2007; **24**: 87–91.

29. Magner JJ, McCaul C, Carton E, Gardiner J, Buggy D. Effect of intraoperative intravenous crystalloid infusion on postoperative nausea and vomiting after gynaecological laparoscopy: comparison of 30 and 10 mL kg-1. *Br J Anaesth* 2004; **93**: 381–5.

30. Oddby-Muhrbeck E, Eksborg S, Bergendahl HT, Muhrbeck O, Lonnqvist PA. Effects of clonidine on postoperative nausea and vomiting in

breast cancer surgery. *Anesthesiology* 2002; **96**: 1109–14.

31. Henzi I, Walder B, Tramer MR. Dexamethasone for the prevention of postoperative nausea and vomiting: a quantitative systematic review. *Anesth Analg* 2000; **90**: 186–94.

32. Sauerland S, Nagelschmidt M, Mallmann P, Neugebauer EA. Risks and benefits of preoperative high dose methylprednisolone in surgical patients: a systematic review. *Drug Saf* 2000; **23**: 449–61.

33. Lee A, Done ML. Stimulation of the wrist acupuncture point P6 for preventing postoperative nausea and vomiting. *Cochrane Database Syst Rev* 2004; (2): CD003281.

34. Gan TJ, Jiao KR, Zenn M, Georgiade G. A randomized controlled comparison of electro-acupoint stimulation or ondansetron versus placebo for the prevention of postoperative nausea and vomiting. *Anesth Analg* 2004; **99**: 1070–5.

35. White PF, Hamza MA, Recart A, *et al.* Optimal timing of acustimulation for antiemetic prophylaxis as an adjunct to ondansetron in patients undergoing plastic surgery. *Anesth Analg* 2005; **100**: 367–72.

36. Arnberger M, Stadelmann, K, Alischer, P, *et al.* Monitoring of neuromuscular blockade at the P6 acupuncture point reduces the incidence of postoperative nausea and vomiting. *Anesthesiology* 2007; **107**: 903–8.

37. Ludwin DB, Shafer SL. Con: The black box warning on droperidol should not be removed (but should be clarified!). *Anesth Analg* 2008; **106**: 1418–20.

38. Nuttall GA, Eckerman KM, Jacob KA, *et al.* Does low-dose droperidol administration increase the risk of drug-induced QT prolongation and torsade de pointes in the general surgical population? *Anesthesiology* 2007; **107**: 531–6.

39. Gan TJ, Meyer TA, Apfel CC, *et al.* Society for Ambulatory Anesthesia guidelines for the management of postoperative nausea and vomiting. *Anesth Analg* 2007; **105**: 1615–28.

40. Skledar SJ, Williams BA, Vallejo MC, *et al.* Eliminating postoperative nausea and vomiting in outpatient surgery with multimodal strategies including low doses of nonsedating, off-patent antiemetics: is "zero tolerance" achievable? *ScientificWorldJournal* 2007; **7**: 959–77.

41. Ender J, Borger MA, Scholz M, *et al.* Cardiac surgery fast-track treatment in a postanesthetic care unit: six-month results of the Leipzig fast-track concept. *Anesthesiology* 2008; **109**: 61–6.

42. Heier T, Caldwell JE. Impact of hypothermia on the response to neuromuscular blocking drugs. *Anesthesiology* 2006; **104**: 1070–80.

43. Vuyk J, Mertens MJ, Olofsen E, Burm AG, Bovill JG. Propofol anesthesia and rational opioid selection: determination of optimal EC50-EC95 propofol-opioid concentrations that assure adequate anesthesia and a rapid return of consciousness. *Anesthesiology* 1997; **87**: 1549–62.

44. Minto CF, Schnider TW. Contributions of PK/PD modeling to intravenous anesthesia. *Clin Pharmacol Ther* 2008; **84**: 27–38.

45. Kaba A, Laurent SR, Detroz BJ, *et al.* Intravenous lidocaine infusion facilitates acute rehabilitation after laparoscopic colectomy. *Anesthesiology* 2007; **106**: 11–18.

46. Myles PS, Leslie K, Chan MT, *et al.* Avoidance of nitrous oxide for patients undergoing major surgery: a randomized controlled trial. *Anesthesiology* 2007; **107**: 221–31.

47. Mraovic B, Simurina T, Sonicki Z, Skitarelic N, Gan TJ. The dose-response of nitrous oxide in postoperative nausea in patients undergoing gynecologic laparoscopic surgery: a preliminary study. *Anesth Analg* 2008; **107**: 818–23.

48. Sanders RD, Weimann J, Maze M. Biologic effects of nitrous oxide: a mechanistic and toxicologic review. *Anesthesiology* 2008; **109**: 707–22.

49. Frank SM, Fleisher LA, Breslow MJ, *et al.* Perioperative maintenance of normothermia reduces the incidence of morbid cardiac events. A randomized clinical trial. *JAMA* 1997; **277**: 1127–34.

50. Kurz A, Sessler DI, Lenhardt R. Perioperative normothermia to reduce the incidence of surgical-wound infection and shorten hospitalization. Study of Wound Infection and Temperature Group. *N Engl J Med* 1996; **334**: 1209–15.

51. Rajagopalan S, Mascha E, Na J, Sessler DI. The effects of mild perioperative hypothermia on blood loss and transfusion requirement. *Anesthesiology* 2008; **108**: 71–7.

52. Dirkmann D, Hanke AA, Gorlinger K, Peters J. Hypothermia and acidosis synergistically impair coagulation in human whole blood. *Anesth Analg* 2008; **106**: 1627–32.

53. Lenhardt R. Monitoring and thermal management. *Best Pract Res Clin Anaesthesiol* 2003; **17**: 569–81.

54. Mayer J, Boldt J, Schellhaass A, Hiller B, Suttner SW. Bispectral index-guided general anesthesia in combination with thoracic epidural analgesia reduces recovery time in fast-track colon surgery. *Anesth Analg* 2007; **104**: 1145–9.

55. Liu SS. Effects of Bispectral Index monitoring on ambulatory anesthesia: a meta-analysis of randomized controlled trials and a cost analysis. *Anesthesiology* 2004; **101**: 311–15.

56. Punjasawadwong Y, Boonjeungmonkol N, Phongchiewboon A. Bispectral index for improving anaesthetic delivery and postoperative recovery. *Cochrane Database Syst Rev* 2007; **4**: CD003843.

57. Ekman A, Lindholm ML, Lennmarken C, Sandin R. Reduction in the incidence of awareness using BIS monitoring. *Acta Anaesthesiol Scand* 2004; **48**: 20–6.

58. Avidan MS, Zhang L, Burnside BA, *et al.* Anesthesia awareness and the bispectral index. *N Engl J Med* 2008; **358**: 1097–108.

59. Practice advisory for intraoperative awareness and brain function monitoring: a report by the American Society of Anesthesiologists Task Force on IntraOperative Awareness. *Anesthesiology* 2006; **104**: 847–64.

60. Soehle M, Ellerkmann RK, Grube M, *et al.* Comparison between bispectral index and patient state index as measures of the electroencephalographic effects of sevoflurane. *Anesthesiology* 2008; **109**: 799–805.

61. White PF, Tang J, Romero GF, *et al.* A comparison of state and response entropy versus bispectral index values

during the perioperative period. *Anesth Analg* 2006; **102**: 160–7.

62. Cattaneo CG, Frank SM, Hesel TW, *et al.* The accuracy and precision of body temperature monitoring methods during regional and general anesthesia. *Anesth Analg* 2000; **90**: 938–45.

63. Eriksson LI. Evidence-based practice and neuromuscular monitoring: it's time for routine quantitative assessment. *Anesthesiology* 2003; **98**: 1037–9.

64. Claudius C, Viby-Mogensen J. Acceleromyography for use in scientific and clinical practice: a systematic review of the evidence. *Anesthesiology* 2008; **108**: 1117–40.

65. Murphy GS, Szokol JW, Marymont JH, *et al.* Intraoperative acceleromyographic monitoring reduces the risk of residual neuromuscular blockade and adverse respiratory events in the postanesthesia care unit. *Anesthesiology* 2008; **109**: 389–98.

66. Jacob M, Chappell D, Conzen P, Finsterer U, Rehm M. Blood volume is normal after pre-operative overnight fasting. *Acta Anaesthesiol Scand* 2008; **52**: 522–9.

67. Holte K, Kehlet H. Compensatory fluid administration for preoperative dehydration: does it improve outcome? *Acta Anaesthesiol Scand* 2002; **46**: 1089–93.

68. Maharaj CH, Kallam SR, Malik A, *et al.* Preoperative intravenous fluid therapy decreases postoperative nausea and pain in high risk patients. *Anesth Analg* 2005; **100**: 675–82.

69. Chappell D, Jacob M, Hofmann-Kiefer K, Conzen P, Rehm M. A rational approach to perioperative fluid management. *Anesthesiology* 2008; **109**: 723–40.

70. Sear JW. Kidney dysfunction in the postoperative period. *Br J Anaesth* 2005; **95**: 20–32.

71. Wiedemann HP, Wheeler AP, Bernard GR, *et al.* Comparison of two fluid-management strategies in acute lung injury. *N Engl J Med* 2006; **354**: 2564–75.

72. Nisanevich V, Felsenstein I, Almogy G, *et al.* Effect of intraoperative fluid management on outcome after

intraabdominal surgery. *Anesthesiology* 2005; **103**: 25–32.

73. Holte K, Klarskov B, Christensen DS, *et al.* Liberal versus restrictive fluid administration to improve recovery after laparoscopic cholecystectomy: a randomized, double-blind study. *Ann Surg* 2004; **240**: 892–9.

74. Holte K, Kristensen BB, Valentiner L, *et al.* Liberal versus restrictive fluid management in knee arthroplasty: a randomized, double-blind study. *Anesth Analg* 2007; **105**: 465–74.

75. Finfer S, Bellomo R, Boyce N, *et al.* A comparison of albumin and saline for fluid resuscitation in the intensive care unit. *N Engl J Med* 2004; **350**: 2247–56.

76. Myburgh J, Cooper DJ, Finfer S, *et al.* Saline or albumin for fluid resuscitation in patients with traumatic brain injury. *N Engl J Med* 2007; **357**: 874–84.

77. Deflandre E, Bonhomme V, Hans P. Delta down compared with delta pulse pressure as an indicator of volaemia during intracranial surgery. *Br J Anaesth* 2008; **100**: 245–50.

78. Cannesson M, Attof Y, Rosamel P, *et al.* Respiratory variations in pulse oximetry plethysmographic waveform amplitude to predict fluid responsiveness in the operating room. *Anesthesiology* 2007; **106**: 1105–11.

79. Noblett SE, Snowden CP, Shenton BK, Horgan AF. Randomized clinical trial assessing the effect of Doppler-optimized fluid management on outcome after elective colorectal resection. *Br J Surg* 2006; **93**: 1069–76.

80. Bendjelid K, Romand JA. Fluid responsiveness in mechanically ventilated patients: a review of indices used in intensive care. *Intensive Care Med* 2003; **29**: 352–60.

81. Practice guidelines for perioperative blood transfusion and adjuvant therapies: an updated report by the American Society of Anesthesiologists Task Force on Perioperative Blood Transfusion and Adjuvant Therapies. *Anesthesiology* 2006; **105**: 198–208.

82. Wolthuis EK, Choi G, Dessing MC, *et al.* Mechanical ventilation with lower tidal volumes and positive end-expiratory pressure prevents pulmonary inflammation in patients without

preexisting lung injury. *Anesthesiology* 2008; **108**: 46–54.

83. Unzueta MC, Casas JI, Moral MV. Pressure-controlled versus volume-controlled ventilation during one-lung ventilation for thoracic surgery. *Anesth Analg* 2007; **104**: 1029–33.

84. Valenza F, Vagginelli F, Tiby A, *et al.* Effects of the beach chair position, positive end-expiratory pressure, and pneumoperitoneum on respiratory function in morbidly obese patients during anesthesia and paralysis. *Anesthesiology* 2007; **107**: 725–32.

85. Akca O, Doufas AG, Morioka N, *et al.* Hypercapnia improves tissue oxygenation. *Anesthesiology* 2002; **97**: 801–6.

86. Fleischmann E, Herbst F, Kugener A, *et al.* Mild hypercapnia increases subcutaneous and colonic oxygen tension in patients given 80% inspired oxygen during abdominal surgery. *Anesthesiology* 2006; **104**: 944–9.

87. Wang Z, Su F, Bruhn A, Yang X, Vincent JL. Acute hypercapnia improves indices of tissue oxygenation more than dobutamine in septic shock. *Am J Respir Crit Care Med* 2008; **177**: 178–83.

88. Claudius C, Karacan H, Viby-Mogensen J. Prolonged residual paralysis after a single intubating dose of rocuronium. *Br J Anaesth* 2007; **99**: 514–17.

89. Murphy GS, Szokol JW, Marymont JH, *et al.* Residual neuromuscular blockade and critical respiratory events in the postanesthesia care unit. *Anesth Analg* 2008; **107**: 130–7.

90. Sundman E, Witt H, Olsson R, *et al.* The incidence and mechanisms of pharyngeal and upper esophageal dysfunction in partially paralyzed humans: pharyngeal videoradiography and simultaneous manometry after atracurium. *Anesthesiology* 2000; **92**: 977–84.

91. Jones RK, Caldwell JE, Brull SJ, Soto RG. Reversal of profound rocuronium-induced blockade with sugammadex: a randomized comparison with neostigmine. *Anesthesiology* 2008; **109**: 816–24.

92. Puhringer FK, Rex C, Sielenkamper AW, *et al.* Reversal of profound, high-dose rocuronium-induced neuromuscular

blockade by sugammadex at two different time points: an international, multicenter, randomized, dose-finding, safety assessor-blinded, phase II trial. *Anesthesiology* 2008; **109**: 188–97.

93. Suy K, Morias K, Cammu G, *et al*. Effective reversal of moderate rocuronium- or vecuronium-induced neuromuscular block with sugammadex, a selective relaxant binding agent. *Anesthesiology* 2007; **106**: 283–8.

94. Liu EH, Wong HK, Chia CP, *et al*. Effects of isoflurane and propofol on cortical somatosensory evoked potentials during comparable depth of anaesthesia as guided by bispectral index. *Br J Anaesth* 2005; **94**: 193–7.

95. Bala E, Sessler DI, Nair DR, *et al*. Motor and somatosensory evoked potentials are well maintained in patients given dexmedetomidine during spine surgery. *Anesthesiology* 2008; **109**: 417–25.

96. Banoub M, Tetzlaff JE, Schubert A. Pharmacologic and physiologic influences affecting sensory evoked potentials: implications for perioperative monitoring. *Anesthesiology* 2003; **99**: 716–37.

97. Rehberg S, Weber TP, Van Aken H, *et al*. Sleep disturbances after posterior scoliosis surgery with an intraoperative wake-up test using remifentanil. *Anesthesiology* 2008; **109**: 629–41.

Clinical applications: evidence-based anesthesia practice

Management of sedation, analgesia, and delirium

Christopher G. Hughes, Stuart McGrane, E. Wesley Ely, and Pratik P. Pandaharipande

Introduction

Sedation and analgesia are administered to patients to provide comfort and ensure safety of the patients, especially when mechanically ventilated [1]. Optimal sedation and analgesia regimens need to be individualized in the critically ill, taking into consideration the presenting condition, the severity of illness, and the intensity of treatment. As a first step it is important that the healthcare provider determine the specific problem requiring sedation in order to determine the appropriate treatment strategy [1]. However, history, institutional bias, and individual patient variability contribute to wide variation in the approach to sedation of the critically ill. Furthermore, differences in resources, technology, and culture create major differences in the practice of sedation and analgesia in the United States and among different countries [1–5].

The Society of Critical Care Medicine (SCCM) guidelines recommend routine monitoring and management of sedation, analgesia, and delirium in all patients admitted to the intensive care unit (ICU) [1]. Existing disease, surgical procedures, trauma, invasive monitors, endotracheal intubation, and nursing interventions are only a few sources of discomfort commonly experienced by patients in the ICU. In addition to patient discomfort, inadequately treated pain leads to an increased stress response, with resultant tachycardia, increased oxygen consumption, hypercoagulability, immunosuppression, hypermetabolism, and increased endogenous catecholamine activity [1,6,7]. Insufficient pain relief can also contribute to deficient sleep, disorientation, and anxiety [1,6]. Recent studies have shown that sedatives and analgesics can decrease oxygen consumption by about 15% from baseline, highlighting the importance of adequate analgesia in patients in a stressed state [6].

Sedation is often used to treat anxiety and agitation in the ICU. The sources of anxiety are multifactorial and may be related to the patient's physical condition (metabolic derangements, hypoxemia, head injury), emotional status (confusion, inability to communicate, lack of control), environment (excessive noise, alarms, continuous lighting, temperature), or therapy (repositioning, frequent vital signs, medications) [1].

Additionally, coughing and sense of dyspnea can lead to ventilator dysynchrony, increasing work of breathing and oxygen consumption [1,7]. Adequate sedation and analgesia is further needed to facilitate nursing care including dressing changes and baths, to prevent adverse events such as removal of endotracheal tubes and central venous catheters, and to reduce patient discomfort during such procedures [1,7].

Sedatives can also be utilized to achieve amnesia, which is mandatory only when neuromuscular blocking drugs are administered [1,7]. Unpleasant memories of the ICU stay may contribute to post-traumatic stress disorder (PTSD) symptoms in survivors [8,9], though data have shown that PTSD is more often related to having delusional memories of the ICU stay, and that factual memories, even if painful, are less likely to cause PTSD [10,11].

Delirium is a frequent complication of critical illness, occurring in 50–80% of mechanically ventilated patients [12,13], and it is often treated with the administration of sedative medications [14]. Recent data suggest that benzodiazepines may be associated with an increased risk of development of delirium [12,15], and these should be therefore be avoided or minimized in the management of delirium unless specifically used for benzodiazepine or alcohol withdrawal [16]. Inadequate analgesia has also been shown to be a risk factor for delirium [17]. Morrison et al. conducted a prospective cohort study that enrolled 541 patients with hip fracture and without delirium [17]. Patients who received less than 10 mg of parenteral morphine sulfate equivalents per day were more likely to develop delirium than patients who received more analgesia (RR 5.4, 95% CI 2.4–12.3). However, providing adequate analgesia needs to be balanced with the potential risk for predisposing patients to delirium due to excess opiate administration [12,17,18].

Complications of sedative administration in critically ill patients

The unpredictability of pharmacokinetics and pharmacodynamics in critically ill patients, secondary to drug interactions,

Anesthetic Pharmacology, 2nd edition, ed. Alex S. Evers, Mervyn Maze, Evan D. Kharasch. Published by Cambridge University Press. © Cambridge University Press 2011.

organ dysfunction, absorption, protein binding, and hemodynamic instability, leads to the development of complications when administering sedative and analgesic medications in the ICU [7]. Because most sedatives and analgesics are administered as continuous infusions, drug accumulation, redistribution, and tachyphylaxis also confound their utilization.

Deep sedation, especially with the use of continuous infusions, has been shown to be associated with prolongation of mechanical ventilation and ICU length of stay, and an inability to perform adequate daily patient assessments, thus resulting in increased need for neuroradiological procedures such as computed axial tomography (CAT) scans and magnetic resonance imaging (MRI) [19,20]. Patients receiving prolonged sedative infusions may also experience withdrawal symptoms upon removal of the medication [1,7]. Symptoms of depression and PTSD have been positively associated to the number of days of sedation in the ICU [21]. Similarly, another study has shown that patients who had recall of their ICU stay had less cognitive dysfunction than patients who had no recall of their ICU experience, further emphasizing that excessive sedation may have prolonged neuropsychological and cognitive effects [22].

As alluded to above, associations between psychoactive medications and worsening cognitive outcomes have been published in postsurgical patients. Marcantonio *et al.* studied postoperative patients who developed delirium, and found an association between benzodiazepines and meperidine use and the occurrence of delirium [18]. Dubois *et al.* have shown that opiates (morphine and meperidine) administered either intravenously or via an epidural route may be associated with the development of delirium in medical/surgical patients [23]. Studies such as these have generated concern regarding whether these drugs were actually responsible for the development of delirium or were given as a result of delirium. To study the temporal association between administration of sedatives and the transition to delirium, one needs to have repeated cognitive assessments and be able to assess the risk factors which a patient is exposed to, in between these assessments. In one of the first such studies, Pandharipande *et al.* found that lorazepam was an independent risk factor for daily transition to delirium after adjusting for important covariates such as age, severity of illness, and presence of sepsis (Fig. 63.1) [15]. Fentanyl, morphine, and propofol were associated with higher but not statistically significant odds ratios [15]. Similar associations between midazolam and worse delirium outcomes have been found in a more recently completed study in trauma and surgical ICU patients [12]. It is important to note that the data on opioids and delirium are not as consistent as those for the benzodiazepines. While meperidine has been associated with delirium in most of the published studies, findings with fentanyl and morphine have been less convincing, and there are some studies suggesting a beneficial effect of morphine [12,17,18,23].

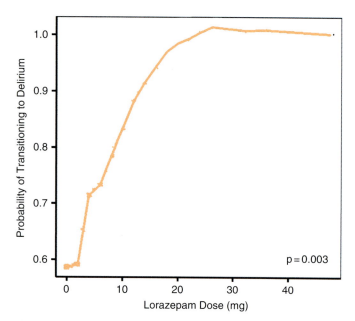

Figure 63.1. Lorazepam and the probability of transitioning to delirium. The probability of transitioning to delirium increased with the dose of lorazepam administered in the previous 24 hours. This *incremental* risk was large at low doses and plateaued at around 20 mg per day. Reproduced from Pandharipande *et al.* [15], with the permission of Lippincott Williams & Wilkins.

Pharmacology of drugs for sedation and analgesia in the critically ill

A detailed discussion of the pharmacology of medications used for sedation and analgesia in the ICU has been covered elsewhere (see especially Chapters 27–33). Here, we confine ourselves to a brief overview.

Opioids

Opioids have been utilized in the ICU for many years, taking advantage of their analgesic, anxiolytic, antitussive, and sedative properties. The most commonly used opiates in the ICU are morphine, hydromorphone, and fentanyl, though remifentanil is gaining popularity as an ultra-short-acting analgesic/sedative drug. All these drugs provide less sedation than the commonly used hypnotics or anesthetic drugs, and patients receiving analgesic-based regimens with opioids are more likely to have accurate memory and less likely to suffer from PTSD [24].

Morphine is a naturally occurring opioid from the opium poppy. It is 40% protein-bound and has a large volume of distribution [25]. Morphine is metabolized by glucuronidation to form morphine-3 and morphine-6 glucuronides, with the morphine-6-glucuronide metabolite having greater pharmacological activity than morphine itself [25]. This metabolite can accumulate in those with renal dysfunction, as this is the main method of excretion of the glucuronides. Morphine can also cause histamine release with subsequent hypotension [25].

Hydromorphone is a congener of morphine. It is more potent than morphine but otherwise has a very similar pharmacokinetic and pharmacodynamic profile [25]. It is metabolized to the inactive hydromorphone-3-glucuronide, which is eliminated by the kidneys [25]. This metabolite is associated with dose-dependent neuroexcitation when accumulation occurs secondary to renal failure [26].

Fentanyl is a lipophilic, semisynthetic opioid with a rapid onset of action. It is highly protein-bound and has a very high volume of distribution because of its lipophilicity [25]. Fentanyl is metabolized by cytochrome P450 (CYP) 3A4, which has decreased function in critically ill patients, and this can contribute to the prolonged effect of this drug in ICU patients [24]. Fentanyl pharmacokinetics, however, are not changed in those with renal insufficiency [25]. Fentanyl administration can lead to hypotension, and compensatory intracranial vasodilation may result, potentially increasing intracranial pressures (ICP) [27].

Remifentanil is a 4-anilidopiperidine derivative of fentanyl with an ester linkage to propanoic acid [27]. It displays three-compartment kinetics in those with normal renal function, but two-compartment kinetics in those with severe renal dysfunction [28]. Because it is metabolized by nonspecific blood and tissue esterases, the elimination half-life of remifentanil is under 10 minutes regardless of the infusion duration [29]. Remifentanil acid is the one active metabolite, but it has negligible effects even in those with chronic renal failure [30,31]. Hypotension and bradycardia are the most common side effects of remifentanil administration, and supplemental analgesic medication is usually required at the conclusion of a remifentanil infusion [27].

Common side effects of all opioids include nausea and vomiting, constipation, pruritus, dose-related respiratory depression, sedation, miosis, and urinary retention. Hypotension can result, especially in those with hypovolemia, and the vasodilation can lead to increased ICP, as previously mentioned [25].

Benzodiazepines

Benzodiazepines bind to the benzodiazepine (BZD) subunit on the γ-aminobutyric acid (GABA) receptor, producing a conformational change that results in an increased affinity for GABA [32]. This increases chloride conductance, producing hyperpolarization of the neuron, which results clinically in anxiolysis and sedation [32]. Lorazepam and midazolam are the two main benzodiazepines utilized for sedation in the ICU.

Lorazepam is one of the most potent benzodiazepines, and it is metabolized to inactive products by glucuronidation. This is unique among the benzodiazepines, and hence it has few drug interactions [32]. The conjugative metabolic pathways are preserved even in severe liver failure, making lorazepam the benzodiazepine of choice in liver failure patients. These conjugated inactive metabolites are renally cleared, and lorazepam's pharmacokinetics do not change significantly in critically ill

populations [1,32,33]. Because of its poor lipid solubility relative to the other benzodiazepines, it provides a much longer duration of amnesia [33]. However, this delayed uptake and clearance make it a poor choice if rapid onset and offset are desired [33]. Patients who receive large doses of lorazepam for long periods can develop a lactic acidosis, especially if they have renal failure [34]. This is due to the metabolism of propylene glycol, which is used as a solvent for lorazepam, and patients can also develop hyperosmolarity from the propylene glycol [34].

Midazolam has anxiolytic, muscle-relaxant, and sedative properties. In its packaged form (pH 3.5), midazolam is water-soluble, but when it is injected into blood (pH 7.4) it undergoes a conformational change which increases its lipid solubility [33]. It is metabolized by hepatic microsomal oxidation by the isoenzyme CYP3A4 [33]. Midazolam has an active metabolite, α-hydroxymidazolam, which has a shorter half-life and is only 20% as potent [35]. Metabolism of midazolam is delayed by many drugs, including propofol, cimetidine, and erythromycin [33]. Clearance is dependent on hepatic blood flow and is prolonged in those with cirrhosis [35,36]. Changes in albumin concentration can greatly affect the free fraction of midazolam and therefore alter its dose-response attributes [37]. There is also an increased free fraction in those with renal failure [38,39]. Given these two characteristics, a large pharmacokinetic variation exists amongst ICU patients and the half-time of midazolam is often significantly prolonged [38,39]. Volumes of distribution are greatly increased in the obese, and women have been shown to have increased volumes of distribution, clearance, and elimination half-lives when compared to men [40]. In critically ill patients, the volume of distribution can be greater than three times that of healthy volunteers, causing extensively prolonged elimination [41].

Propofol

Propofol is a diisopropylphenol prepared in a lipid emulsion formula containing soybean, egg phosphatide, and glycerol. Propofol can behave as an immunosuppressant and hence increase the risk of infection [32,42–44]. It mainly exerts its action through $GABA_A$ receptors, but propofol also has actions at other central nervous system (CNS) receptor sites such as glycine, nicotinic, and muscarinic receptors [45]. Infusions of propofol follow a three-compartment model that includes a central intravascular compartment and two peripheral redistribution compartments. It has a large volume of distribution, is 97% protein-bound, and has a terminal elimination half-life that can be very long. Clearance of propofol is rapid from the plasma, and it is metabolized mainly in the liver by conjugation to inactive metabolites [42,46].

A propofol bolus can rapidly lead to sedation after a single arm–brain circulation and lasts up to 8 minutes [42,46]. Sedation onset is within 10 minutes after commencement of an infusion, and the peak sedative effects occur within 30 minutes. It decreases both cerebral blood flow and cerebral

The **bispectral analysis** of the EEG with a Bispectral Index monitor (BIS) is an example of the tools available to process EEG data. This monitor detects a signal through a frontal temporal sensor and provides a digital score from 100 (completely awake) to 0 (isoelectric EEG, deep sedation) [62], derived by incorporating several EEG components including the degree of suppression, the relative power in several frequency ranges, and additional bispectral components. The BIS monitor also records the presence of burst suppression, a severely decreased brain activity on the EEG. The burst suppression is characterized by periods of suppressed EEG activity alternated with periods of higher-amplitude EEG activity. The presence of this EEG pattern is considered to be a good indicator of deep drug-induced coma [63,64]. A burst suppression ratio > 0 can be considered as a threshold positive for burst suppression.

Benefits of goal-directed and protocolized sedation

Studies evaluating the efficacy of sedation protocols and target-based sedation have all shown tremendous benefits with regard to shorter time on mechanical ventilation and less time in the ICU and in hospital [65,66]. However, subjective sedation scales that depend on patient behavior and clinical examination may be insensitive during deep sedation [67]. This is evident from a recent study that showed that almost 40% of patients admitted to a medical ICU had episodes of burst suppression on their EEG, despite being managed by the use of targeted sedation with sedation scales. More alarmingly, burst suppression was associated with an increased in-hospital and 6-month mortality [68].

Simmons *et al.* evaluated mechanically ventilated patients using the BIS and the Riker Sedation–Agitation Scale (SAS) and found a significant correlation between the two [69]. Similarly, Riker *et al.* studied 39 patients with short-term ICU sedation after cardiac surgery and showed significant changes in the BIS values as patients awoke and were weaned, with a significant agreement between BIS and SAS [70]. While the BIS and sedation level are correlated, however, there is little evidence about the efficacy of the BIS in assisting in the titration of sedation in ICU. In one of the first studies, Weatherburn *et al.* evaluated the use of the BIS monitor in supporting clinical sedation management decisions in mechanically ventilated ICU patients, and concluded that the use of BIS monitoring did not reduce the amount of sedation used, the length of mechanical ventilation time, or the length of ICU stay [71]. Further studies on the applicability of neurological monitoring beyond sedation scales are under way, given that despite the use of targeted sedation, occurrence of deep sedation still occurs. However, in the interim, sedation protocols and scales need to be implemented to prevent unnecessary administration of sedatives and analgesics to critically ill patients.

Changing sedation paradigms to improve patient outcomes

Modifying the delivery pattern of sedatives and analgesics

A landmark study evaluated the role of daily interruptions of continuous sedative infusions in critically ill patients [20,72]. The study protocol mandated the stopping of sedation and analgesia on a daily basis, with restart of the medications at half of the original dose once patients were able to follow simple commands. Patients managed with sedation cessation had a significant reduction in the duration of mechanical ventilation, ICU and hospital length of stay, neuroradiological procedures, and the need for tracheostomy, without any long-term sequelae due to the daily "wake-ups" [20,72].

The multicenter Awakening Breathing Controlled (ABC) trial built on the benefits of daily spontaneous breathing trials and of the daily wake-up trials (Fig. 63.2) [73]. This study tested the results of linking sedation and ventilator weaning protocols using a "wake up and breathe" approach. In both groups, patients were managed by a "targeted-sedation" strategy, and all patients in the control group received a daily spontaneous breathing trial (SBT). Patients managed with the ABC intervention had a mandatory spontaneous awakening trial (SAT) as step A, consisting of total cessation of sedation long enough to wake to verbal stimulus or tolerate for 4 hours, followed by the SBT as step B. The ABC "wake up and breathe" intervention resulted in a 3-day reduction of mechanical ventilation, 1 day less in coma, 4 days less in the ICU and hospital, and a 14% absolute reduction in the risk of death within 1 year (58% in control reduced to 44% in treatment group) (Fig. 63.3) [73].

Altering the choice of sedative regimens to improve patient outcomes

Strategies that focus on provision of adequate analgesia likely result in less sedative requirement. Few comparative trials of opioid infusions have been performed. Traditionally, the selection of an opioid depended on the likely duration of analgesic infusion and the pharmacology of the specific opioid. Morphine and hydromorphone are typically utilized for cases of prolonged infusions, because of their longer duration of action [1]. The advantages of hydromorphone over morphine include hydromorphone's lack of histamine release and its lack of a clinically active metabolite. This may result in less vasodilation and hypotension and less prolonged sedation in patients with renal insufficiency. Fentanyl's rapid onset and short duration of action make it more suitable for shorter periods of infusion. Its ease of titration and lack of histamine release also make it preferred in the hemodynamically unstable patient [1].

Remifentanil is one of the newest μ-agonists, with a rapid onset and offset of action, and its lack of accumulation makes

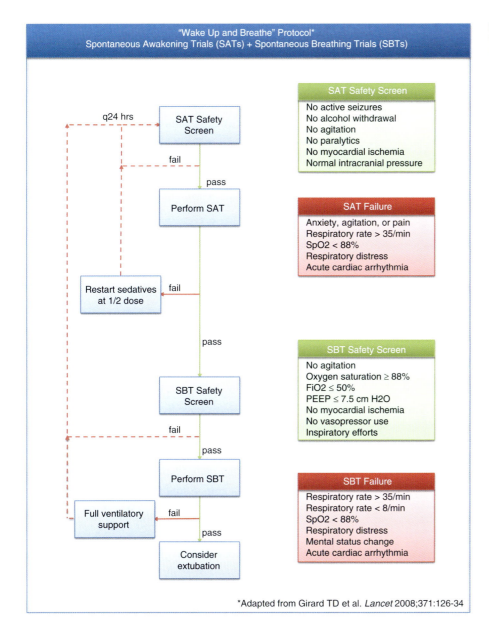

Figure 63.2. The ABC study protocol. Reproduced from www.icudelirium.org, with permission from Drs. Ely and Girard.

it a promising drug for continuous infusion in the ICU. In a randomized double-blind study, the mean percentage hours of optimal sedation was significantly longer for patients receiving remifentanil versus morphine, and the duration of mechanical ventilation and extubation time were shorter for patients receiving remifentanil [74]. More patients in the morphine group also required the addition midazalom for supplemental sedation. When compared with fentanyl, efficacy of achieving sedation goals was similar with remifentanil, though more breakthrough propofol was required in the fentanyl group [75]. There were no differences in time to extubation in both groups, but the percentage of patients experiencing pain after extubation was significantly higher among those receiving remifentanil, indicating the need for proactive pain management when weaning remifentanil [75].

The safety and efficacy of analgesia-based sedation with remifentanil has been compared to conventional sedation with hypnotic-based regimens for patients with brain injury requiring prolonged sedation for mechanical ventilation [27]. Neurological assessment times and time to extubation were significantly shorter for patients receiving remifentanil than for those receiving propofol or midazolam supplemented with morphine or fentanyl [27]. In another study comparing remifentanil-based sedation with a midazolam-based regime, the duration of mechanical ventilation and duration of weaning were significantly shorter in patients receiving remifentanil, and a trend towards shortened ICU stay was also observed [76].

Several comparative trials between hypnotic sedative regimens have been performed. A study of short-duration sedation

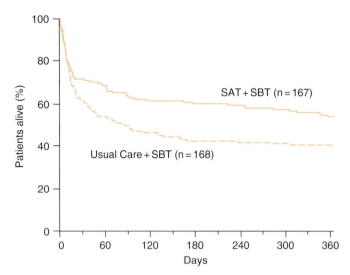

Figure 63.3. Mortality benefit in the Awakening and Breathing Controlled (ABC) trial. The ABC "wake up and breathe" intervention resulted in a 14% absolute reduction in the risk of death within 1 year (58% in control reduced to 44% in treatment group). Reproduced from Girard *et al.* [73], with the permission of Elsevier.

(8 hours) revealed no significant differences between intermittent lorazepam and continuous-infusion midazolam in terms of quality of sedation, anxiolysis, hemodynamic and oxygen transport variables, and patient and nurse satisfaction [77]. However, lorazepam was deemed more cost-effective because of the larger doses of midazolam required to produce the desired level of sedation. Utilizing a pharmacologic model to compare lorazepam and midazolam infusions, lorazepam was found to have twice the sedative potency and four times the amnestic potency of midazolam [78]. The emergence times for light and deep sedation were significantly longer for lorazepam than for midazolam. In a prospective randomized controlled study in trauma patients comparing infusions of lorazepam, midazolam, and propofol, oversedation occurred most frequently with lorazepam, and the greatest number of dosage adjustments was required by the lorazepam group [79]. Undersedation occurred most often with propofol, and the cost of sedation was also greatest with propofol. This study indicated midazolam as the most titratable drug with the least amount of oversedation or undersedation, and suggested that lorazepam was the most cost-effective drug for sedation [79].

Propofol has been compared to individual benzodiazepines in several studies. Carson *et al.* conducted a randomized trial comparing intermittent lorazepam boluses to propofol infusion, with daily interruption of sedatives in both groups [80]. Patients in the propofol group had fewer mechanical ventilation days, with a trend towards a greater number of ventilator-free survival days. In an economic evaluation of propofol versus lorazepam, propofol was determined to be over US $6000 less costly per patient than lorazepam despite the considerably lower pharmacy unit cost of lorazepam [81]. The lower costs were likely attributable to the greater number of ventilator-free days in patients treated with propofol [81].

When compared to midazolam infusion, patients sedated by propofol infusion were found to have faster and more reliable wake-up times [82]. Average time to sedation and change in oxygen consumption were similar between the groups. In a second study, propofol was demonstrated to have equal efficacy in achieving sedation goals as midazolam, but required more frequent dose adjustments and had a lower nurse-rated quality of sedation [83]. Propofol was also observed to cause more cardiovascular depression and less amnesia than midazolam, with higher costs. The Canadian multicenter randomized controlled trial comparing propofol to midazolam further demonstrated that patients sedated with propofol spent a larger percentage of time at their target sedation goal than patients sedated with midazolam [84]. The use of propofol sedation also led to a more rapid extubation, but this did not correlate with earlier ICU discharge. In a systematic review of the trials comparing sedation with propofol and midazolam, the duration of adequate sedation was found to be greater with propofol independent of the length of sedation [85]. The weaning times were found to be shorter with propofol, but this was only statistically significant in patients sedated for less than 36 hours. The review surmised that effective sedation was possible with both propofol and midazolam, and it also determined that 1 of 12 patients sedated with propofol was likely to have hypotension that would not have been experienced with midazolam.

The introduction of dexmedetomidine into clinical practice has provided clinicians with an alternative to GABA-agonist sedative medications. In one of the first comparative studies against propofol, Venn *et al.* found that patients sedated with dexmedetomidine were adequately sedated and required three times less opiates than patients sedated with propofol [86]. While patients on dexmedetomidine had lower heart rates, there were no difference in arterial blood pressure among the group. Additionally, sedation with dexmedetomidine, unlike other sedative medications, did not depress respiration [87]. Interestingly, dexmedetomidine, when compared to propofol, decreases interleukin 6, with no differences in adrenocortical function, suggesting possible immunomodulatory properties [53]. Dexmedetomidine has also been studied in patients after coronary artery bypass surgery, with similar times to weaning and extubation in patients treated with dexmedetomidine or propofol, though there was a significant reduction in the utilization of opioids, β-blockers, antiemetics, nonsteroidal anti-inflammatory drugs, epinephrine, and diuretics in patients receiving dexmedetomidine [88]. Corbett *et al.* evaluated patient ratings of sedation during mechanical ventilation and found that patients on dexmedetomidine perceived a shorter length of intubation despite no actual difference in length of intubation or length of ICU stay [89]. Awareness as an indicator of amnesia did not differ between groups, despite deeper level of sedation in patients sedated with propofol. Patients treated with dexmedetomidine, however, expressed more discomfort and sleeping difficulty, and patients treated

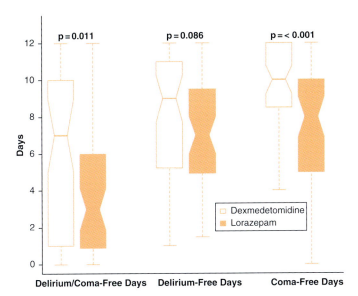

Figure 63.4. Duration of the cognitive outcomes in the MENDS trial. The notches on the sides of the boxes allow visual assessment of the significance in difference between the two medians. If the notches do not overlap, then the two medians are significantly different at least for the $p = 0.05$ level. "Delirium/coma-free days" is a composite score to assess duration of being alive and without delirium or coma over a 12-day evaluation period (i.e., 1 week beyond the maximum 120-hour study drug protocol). The primary outcome measured in this study showed that dexmedetomidine-treated patients had significantly more days alive without delirium or coma than lorazepam-treated patients. Reproduced from Pandharipande et al. [52], with the permission of the American Medical Association.

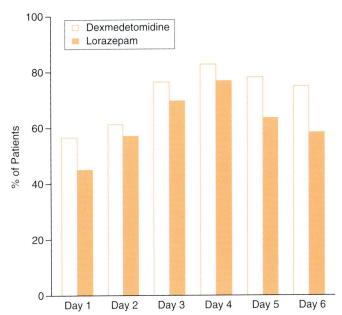

Figure 63.5. Percentage of patients within one point of the ICU team's clinically determined target (goal) RASS sedation score. On any given day, dexmedetomidine-treated patients had a 4–17% higher likelihood of being at the target sedation score than lorazepam-treated patients. Patients in the study were permitted to be on the study drug for 120 hours. Some patients received the study drug till day 6, reflecting enrollment and start of study drug late on day 1, and hence requiring drug infusion till day 6 for completion of 120 hours. Reproduced from Pandharipande et al. [52], with the permission of the American Medical Association.

with propofol tended to have greater ability to rest. Pandharipande et al. recently performed one of the first double-blind randomized controlled trials comparing long-term (up to 5 days) sedation with dexmedetomidine to lorazepam in mechanically ventilated surgical and medical ICU patients [52], and showed that sedation with dexmedetomidine resulted in more days alive without delirium or coma (Fig. 63.4), a lower prevalence of coma, greater achievement of target sedation (Fig. 63.5), and an important trend towards reduction in mortality in the dexmedetomidine group (27% in lorazepam and 17% in dexmedetomidine group). A further subgroup analysis of septic patients revealed improvements in acute brain dysfunction (delirium and coma), shorter time on mechanical ventilation, and improved survival in the dexmedetomidine group without any differences in hemodynamic profiles or cardiovascular and hepatic adverse events, attesting to the fact that choice of sedative regimens is even more important in our sickest critically ill patients [90].

Diagnosis and management of delirium

Diagnosis
The development of tools such as the Intensive Care Delirium Screening Checklist [91] and the Confusion Assessment

Method for the ICU (CAM-ICU) [13] have allowed for the rapid diagnosis of delirium by nonpsychiatric physicians and other healthcare personnel, even while the patient is mechanically ventilated.

Diagnosis of delirium is a two-step process. Level of arousal is first measured by using a standardized sedation scale such as the Richmond Agitation–Sedation Scale (RASS: Table 63.1) [60,61]. If the patient is a RASS –4 or –5, no further evaluation for delirium is performed, since the patient is comatose and is unable to be assessed for delirium. For patients with a RASS score of –3 and lighter (or responsive to verbal stimulus with other sedation scales), delirium can be assessed by the CAM-ICU (Fig. 63.4 Fig. 63.6) [13] or the ICDSC (Table 63.2) [91]. A complete description of the CAM-ICU, the ICDSC, and training materials (including translations of the CAM-ICU and clinical vignettes) can be found at our website, www.icudelirium.org.

Prevention and management
Primary prevention and nonpharmacologic approaches
Protocols targeting risk factors for delirium have shown varied degrees of success in non-ICU cohorts, though few data exist concerning the efficacy of these in ICU patients [93–98]. Clearly such investigations need to be designed and conducted in the ICU setting (rather than simply extrapolated from non-ICU studies).

Step One: Sedation Assessment

The Richmond Agitation and Sedation Scale: The RASS*

Score	Term	Description
+4	Combative	Overtly combative, violent, immediate danger to staff
+3	Very agitated	Pulls or removes tube(s) or catheter(s); aggressive
+2	Agitated	Frequent non-purposeful movement, fights ventilator
+1	Restless	Anxious but movements not aggressive vigorous
0	Alert and calm	
−1	Drowsy	Not fully alert, but has sustained awakening (eye-opening/eye contact) to *voice* (≥ 10 seconds)
−2	Light sedation	Briefly awakens with eye contact to *voice* (< 10 seconds)
−3	Moderate sedation	Movement or eye opening to *voice* (but no eye contact)
−4	Deep sedation	No response to voice, but movement or eye opening to *physical* stimulation
−5	Unarousable	No response to *voice or physical* stimulation

Verbal Stimulation (−1, −2, −3)

Physical Stimulation (−4)

If RASS is −4 or −5, then **Stop** and **Reassess** patient at later time
If RASS is above −4 (−3 through +4) then **Proceed to Step 2**

*Sessler, et al. AJRCCM 2002; 166:1338 –1344.
*Ely, et al. JAMA 2003; 289:2983–2991.

Step Two: Delirium Assessment

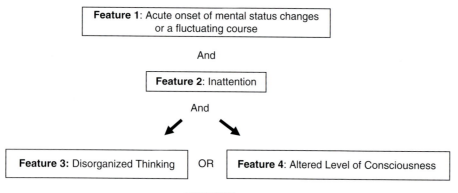

Feature 1: Acute onset of mental status changes or a fluctuating course

And

Feature 2: Inattention

And

Feature 3: Disorganized Thinking   OR   **Feature 4:** Altered Level of Consciousness

= DELIRIUM

Figure 63.6. Richmond Agitation–Sedation Scale (RASS) and the Confusion Assessment Method for the ICU (CAM-ICU). This sedation scale and delirium instrument can be used together as a two-step approach to assess consciousness and diagnose delirium. Patients are considered to have delirium if they have RASS scores of −3 and above and are CAM-ICU positive by having features 1 and 2, and either 3 or 4 positive. Reproduced from www.icudelirium.org, with permission from Dr. E Wesley Ely.

Additionally it should be emphasized that though sedatives and analgesics have a very important role in patient comfort, healthcare professionals must also strive to achieve the right balance of administrating these drugs through greater focus on reducing unnecessary or overzealous use. Instituting daily interruption of sedatives and analgesics, protocolizing their delivery, and instituting target-based sedation have all been shown to improve patient outcomes, though these have not specifically looked at delirium rates or duration [19,20,66]. Studies have also shown a benefit of pain control using morphine in the prevention of delirium, since pain itself can be a risk factor for the development of delirium [17].

Pharmacologic therapy

Medications should be used only after giving adequate attention to correction of modifiable contributing factors (e.g., sleep disturbance, restraints, etc.) as discussed above. It is important to recognize that delirium could be a manifestation of an acute, life-threatening problem that requires immediate attention (such as hypoxia, hypercarbia, hypoglycemia, metabolic derangements, or shock). After addressing such concerns,

Table 63.2. The Intensive Care Delirium Screening Checklist (ICDSC)

Patient evaluation

Altered level of consciousness (A–E)	A: No response, score: none
	B: Response to intense and repeated stimulation (loud voice and pain), score: none
	C: Response to mild or moderate stimulation, score 1
	D: Normal wakefulness, score: 0
	E: Exaggerated response to normal stimulation, score: 1
Inattention	Difficulty in following a conversation or instructions. Easily distracted by external stimuli. Difficulty in shifting focuses. Any of these scores 1 point.
Disorientation	Any obvious mistake in time, place or person scores 1 point.
Hallucinations-delusion-psychosis	The unequivocal clinical manifestation of hallucination or of behavior probably due to hallucination or delusion. Gross impairment in reality testing. Any of these scores 1 point.
Psychomotor agitation or retardation	Hyperactivity requiring the use of additional sedative drugs or restraints in order to control potential danger to oneself or others. Hypoactivity or clinically noticeable psychomotor slowing.
Inappropriate speech or mood	Inappropriate, disorganized or incoherent speech. Inappropriate display of emotion related to events or situation. Any of these scores 1 point.
Sleep/wake cycle disturbance	Sleeping less than 4 h or waking frequently at night (do not consider wakefulness initiated by medical staff or loud environment). Sleeping during most of the day. Any of these scores 1 point.
Symptom fluctuation	Fluctuation of the manifestation of any item or symptom over 24 h scores 1 point.
Total score (0–8)	**A score of 4 or greater is consistent with a diagnosis of delirium**
	A score of 1–3 is considered to be subsyndromal delirium [92]

Adapted from Bergeron *et al.* [91].

delirious patients should be considered for pharmacologic management. It should be recognized that while drugs used to treat delirium are intended to improve cognition, they all have psychoactive effects which may further cloud the sensorium and promote a longer overall duration of cognitive impairment. Therefore, until we have outcomes data that confirm beneficial effects of treatment, these drugs should be used judiciously in the smallest possible dose and for the shortest time necessary, a practice *infrequently* adhered to in most ICUs. Indeed, some patients will prove refractory to all "cocktail" approaches to sedation and delirium therapy, and these patients should be considered for a trial of complete cessation of all psychoactive drugs. There are reports that have described the utility of dexmedetomidine (an α_2-agonist) as an adjunct to assist with weaning patients of all psychoactive medications [99]. The MENDS study has further shown us that dexmedetomidine can decrease the duration of brain dysfunction, as described above (Fig. 63.4) [52]. A comparator study of dexmedetomidine and midazolam is ongoing, and preliminary results show similar improvement in resolution of delirium, making this an attractive drug in the management of patients with delirium.

Benzodiazepines, which are used most commonly in the ICU for sedation, are not recommended for the management of delirium because of the likelihood of oversedation,

exacerbation of confusion, and respiratory suppression. However, they remain the drugs of choice for the treatment of delirium tremens (and other withdrawal syndromes) and seizures. The amnestic qualities of benzodiazepines make these drugs especially useful when noxious or unpleasant procedures are required. It is likely, however, that residual accumulation of these drugs may lead to prolonged delirium long after the drugs have been discontinued. In certain populations, particularly elderly patients with underlying dementia, benzodiazepines may lead to increased confusion and agitation. In such cases, one may try to take advantage of the sedative effects of haloperidol in lieu of continued benzodiazepines.

There are currently no US Food and Drug Administration (FDA)-approved drugs for the treatment of delirium. The SCCM guidelines recommend haloperidol as the drug of choice [1], though it is acknowledged that this is based on sparse outcomes data from nonrandomized case series and anecdotal reports (i.e., level C data). Nevertheless, haloperidol is a butyrophenone "typical" antipsychotic, which is the most widely used neuroleptic drug for delirium [100]. It does not suppress the respiratory drive and works as a dopamine receptor antagonist by blocking the D_2 receptor, which results in treatment of positive symptomatology (hallucinations, unstructured thought patterns, etc.) and produces a variable sedative effect.

In the non-ICU setting, the recommended starting dose of haloperidol is 0.5–1.0 mg orally or parenterally, with repeated doses every 20–30 minutes until the desired effect is achieved. In the ICU setting, a recommended starting dose would be 2–5 mg every 6–12 hours (intravenous or oral), with maximal effective doses usually in the neighborhood of 20 mg per day. This dose range will usually be adequate to achieve the "theoretically optimal" 60% D_2 receptor blockage [101], while avoiding complete D_2 receptor saturation associated with the adverse effects cited below. Given the urgency of the situation in many ICU patients – because of the potential for inadvertent removal of central lines, endotracheal tubes, or even aortic balloon pumps – much higher doses of haloperidol or a sedative are often used. Unfortunately, there are few data in the way of formal pharmacologic investigations to guide dosage recommendations in the ICU. Once calm, the patient can usually be managed with much lower maintenance doses of haloperidol.

Neither haloperidol nor similar drugs (e.g., droperidol and chlorpromazine) have been extensively studied in the ICU [1]. Newer "atypical" antipsychotic drugs (e.g., risperidone, ziprasidone, quetiapine, and olanzapine) may also prove helpful for delirium [102]. The rationale behind use of the atypical antipsychotics over haloperidol (especially in hypoactive/mixed subtypes of delirium) is theoretical and centers on the fact that they affect not only dopamine but also other potentially key neurotransmitters such as serotonin, acetylcholine, and norepinephrine [102–106]. Use of haloperidol has been shown to have a mortality benefit in a retrospective analysis of critically ill patients [107]. Kalisvaart et al. showed that low-dose haloperidol prophylaxis reduced the duration and severity of delirium in elderly hip surgery patients, even though the actual prevalence of delirium was not reduced [108]. Skrobik and colleagues reported that olanzapine and haloperidol were equally efficacious in treating ICU delirium in both medical and surgical patients, but that olanzapine was associated with fewer side effects [102]. The results of this initial study in ICU patients should be tested in larger more robust trials with a placebo group. Kato et al. reported a case study that suggests that genotyping may affect the choice of antipsychotic drugs [109]. The researchers showed that a patient with the CYP2D6 genotype had persistent delirium and developed severe extrapyramidal symptoms when treated with risperidone. The patient was switched to quetiapine (metabolized by CYP3A4) and the delirium cleared within 2 days without side effects. This case report is not proof of a positive effect of antipsychotics, yet it is interesting and hypothesis-generating in that pharmacogenetics may play an important role in medication choices in the near future. Adequately powered prospective randomized controlled trials of these drugs are not available to date and need to be performed to provide clinicians with evidence-based guidelines for preventing and treating delirium.

Adverse effects of typical and atypical antipsychotics include hypotension, acute dystonias, extrapyramidal effects, laryngeal spasm, malignant hyperthermia, glucose and lipid dysregulation, and anticholinergic effects such as dry mouth, constipation, and urinary retention. Perhaps the most immediately life-threatening adverse effect of antipsychotics is torsades de pointes, and these drugs should not be given to patients with prolonged QT intervals unless thought to be absolutely necessary. Patients who receive substantial quantities of typical or atypical antipsychotics or coadministered arrhythmogenic drugs should be monitored closely with electrocardiography. In early 2005 the FDA issued an alert that atypical antipsychotic medications are associated with a mortality risk among elderly patients. This warning was supported by a meta-analysis of a large volume of data from outpatient treatment of dementia patients who were experiencing psychotic symptoms that resulted in their receiving antipsychotic medications [110]. Similar associations with increased stroke risk and mortality have been reported by other investigators [111,112]. Subsequently, investigators have reported that such an increased risk of death in non-ICU elderly patients treated with antipsychotics may not be limited to the atypical class, as they found that the conventional antipsychotic haloperidol had an even higher mortality risk than atypical antipsychotics [111].

Protocols and evidence-based strategies for prevention and treatment of delirium will no doubt emerge as more evidence becomes available from ongoing randomized clinical trials of both nonpharmacologic and pharmacologic strategies. To assist readers in developing a delirium management algorithm in their respective clinical arena, we have included an empiric protocol (Fig. 63.7), largely based on the current SCCM clinical practice guidelines. At this time, we have few data regarding the use of antipsychotic medications that are most suitable for delirium. While the nonpharmacologic interventions recommended in this protocol have shown beneficial results in non-ICU patients, the extrapolation to ICU populations is speculative. Nevertheless, such data emphasize the need for more research in this area and underscore the importance of exercising caution when treating delirium. We emphasize that protocols such as this need to be updated regularly with new data and also personalized at each medical center according to thought leaders at that center to form your own integrated approach to delirium monitoring, sedation targeting, and delirium management in critically ill ICU patients.

Procedural sedation

Sedation for awake fiberoptic intubation

Awake fiberoptic intubation is often the technique of choice for securing the airway in patients with known or suspected difficult airway or in patients with cervical spine disease/

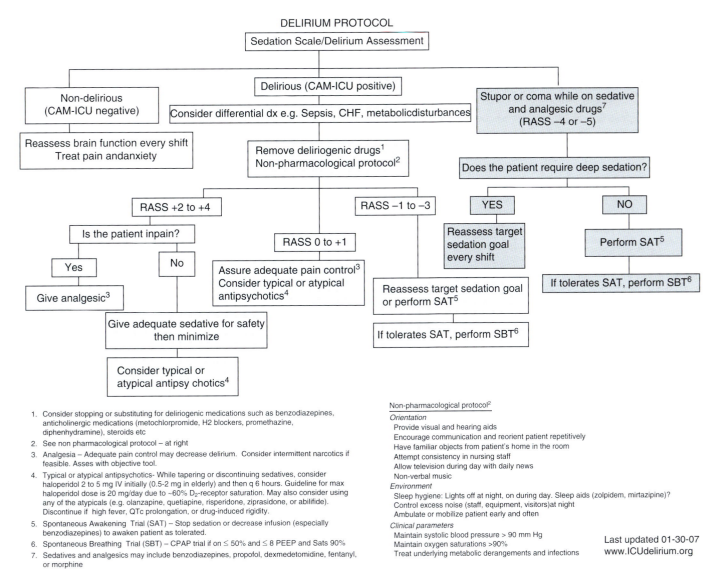

DELIRIUM PROTOCOL

Sedation Scale/Delirium Assessment

Non-delirious (CAM-ICU negative)

Delirious (CAM-ICU positive)

Consider differential dx e.g. Sepsis, CHF, metabolicdisturbances

Stupor or coma while on sedative and analgesic drugs[7] (RASS −4 or −5)

Reassess brain function every shift Treat pain andanxiety

Remove deliriogenic drugs[1] Non-pharmacological protocol[2]

Does the patient require deep sedation?

RASS +2 to +4

RASS −1 to −3

YES

NO

Is the patient inpain?

RASS 0 to +1

Reassess target sedation goal every shift

Perform SAT[5]

Yes

No

Assure adequate pain control[3] Consider typical or atypical antipsychotics[4]

Reassess target sedation goal or perform SAT[5]

If tolerates SAT, perform SBT[6]

Give analgesic[3]

Give adequate sedative for safety then minimize

If tolerates SAT, perform SBT[6]

Consider typical or atypical antipsy chotics[4]

1. Consider stopping or substituting for deliriogenic medications such as benzodiazepines, anticholinergic medications (metochlorpromide, H2 blockers, promethazine, diphenhydramine), steroids etc
2. See non pharmacological protocol – at right
3. Analgesia – Adequate pain control may decrease delirium. Consider intermittent narcotics if feasible. Asses with objective tool.
4. Typical or atypical antipsychotics- While tapering or discontinuing sedatives, consider haloperidol 2 to 5 mg IV initially (0.5-2 mg in elderly) and then q 6 hours. Guideline for max haloperidol dose is 20 mg/day due to ~60% D_2-receptor saturation. May also consider using any of the atypicals (e.g. olanzapine, quetiapine, risperidone, ziprasidone, or abilifide). Discontinue if high fever, QTc prolongation, or drug-induced rigidity.
5. Spontaneous Awakening Trial (SAT) – Stop sedation or decrease infusion (especially benzodiazepines) to awaken patient as tolerated.
6. Spontaneous Breathing Trial (SBT) – CPAP trial if on ≤ 50% and ≤ 8 PEEP and Sats 90%
7. Sedatives and analgesics may include benzodiazepines, propofol, dexmedetomidine, fentanyl, or morphine

Non-pharmacological protocol[2]

Orientation
 Provide visual and hearing aids
 Encourage communication and reorient patient repetitively
 Have familiar objects from patient's home in the room
 Attempt consistency in nursing staff
 Allow television during day with daily news
 Non-verbal music
Environment
 Sleep hygiene: Lights off at night, on during day. Sleep aids (zolpidem, mirtazipine)?
 Control excess noise (staff, equipment, visitors)at night
 Ambulate or mobilize patient early and often
Clinical parameters
 Maintain systolic blood pressure > 90 mm Hg
 Maintain oxygen saturations >90%
 Treat underlying metabolic derangements and infections

Last updated 01-30-07
www.ICUdelirium.org

Figure 63.7. Delirium protocol. This empiric protocol, which is largely based on the current SCCM clinical practice guidelines, is the algorithm the authors use to treat delirium in their ICUs. Such protocols need to be updated regularly with new data and also personalized to each medical center. Specific recommendations about the choice of antipsychotics to treat delirium have not been described, since there are limited data available regarding the appropriate drug to use in ICU patients. The nonpharmacologic interventions recommended in this protocol have shown beneficial results in non-ICU patients, but the extrapolation to ICU populations is speculative. Reproduced from www.icudelirium.org, with permission from Drs. Ely and Pandharipande.

trauma necessitating postintubation neurological exam [113]. Utilization of local anesthetics for nerve blocks, nebulization, and topicalization is advantageous for both the patient and the proceduralist. Many excellent review articles and book chapters are dedicated to proper airway preparation for awake fiberoptic intubation [113,114]. However, techniques for sedation during awake fiberoptic intubation receive relatively little attention, and few comparative trials have been reported.

Providing adequate sedation for both the airway preparation and the procedure itself will greatly improve patients' comfort levels and cooperation [113]. Thorough explanation of the procedure is the initial step in providing a comfortable atmosphere for the patient [114,115]. Traditionally, combinations of

benzodiazepines and opioids have been used to provide sedation and analgesia for awake intubation, but the development of newer drugs has led to alternative regimens that can also be utilized [114,115].

Benzodiazepines can produce significant sedation and amnesia but can also produce unconsciousness and an uncooperative patient if titrated incorrectly. Midazolam is the recommended benzodiazepine, because of its quick onset, lack of pain on injection, and short duration of action. An intravenous dose of 1–3 mg for adult patients is usually sufficient to produce a relaxed patient, but an opioid is often required, as benzodiazepines do not produce analgesia and will not blunt airway reflexes [114,115].

Opioids are useful in the sedation of patients by providing analgesia and cough suppression during awake fiberoptic intubation. They produce dose-dependent respiratory depression which can lead to apnea. However, they do not produce unconsciousness, and apneic patients will frequently breathe if encouraged. Although any opioid can be used in this setting, fentanyl in a dose of 0.5–2 $\mu g\ kg^{-1}$ is frequently used because of its familiarity, hemodynamic stability, and low cost [114,115].

More recently, remifentanil has been utilized as both an individual drug [116] and in combination with other drugs [117] to provide conscious sedation for awake intubation, because of its short-acting profile and ease of titration. Hemodynamic stability and adequate intubating conditions have been shown to result from regimens as low as 0.75 $\mu g\ kg^{-1}$ initial bolus followed by a continuous infusion of 0.075 $\mu g\ kg^{-1}$ min^{-1} when combined with midazolam [117]. When used as a single drug, higher doses of remifentanil (0.25–0.5 $\mu g\ kg^{-1}$ min^{-1}) were found to better suppress the hemodynamic response to nasal intubation than a combination of midazolam and fentanyl [116]. Remifentanil did produce a much higher incidence of recall, which was to be expected [116]. Finally, remifentanil target-controlled infusion provided better conditions, shorter endoscopy time, and shorter intubation times than propofol target-controlled infusion [118]. Patient tolerance of the awake intubation was greater with remifentanil, and despite the higher level of recall, no difference in patient satisfaction scores existed [118].

Propofol is another common sedative frequently used for awake fiberoptic intubation. It can be used to achieve rapid sedation, as a bolus can lead to sedation in one circulation time and an infusion within 10 minutes [119]. Propofol can cause a decrease in blood pressure, decrease in cardiac output, and increase in heart rate, though in one study these hemodynamic perturbations were less than those seen in patients intubated using midazolam [120]. Propofol (2 $mg\ kg^{-1}\ h^{-1}$) and remifentanil (0.05 $\mu g\ kg^{-1}\ min^{-1}$) have also been used together effectively for fiberoptic intubation. Careful monitoring should be performed since propofol does produce dose-dependent respiratory depression and unconsciousness. These characteristics create a fairly narrow therapeutic window for the use of propofol for awake intubation.

The most recent addition to the sedatives utilized for awake fiberoptic intubation is the selective α_2-receptor agonist dexmedetomidine. An infusion of dexmedetomidine provides sedation characterized by an easily arousable, communicative, and cooperative patient [121–123]. It has anxiolytic and analgesic effects without causing respiratory depression. These characteristics lend themselves well to utilization for awake intubation, and several case reports have been published highlighting its potential use. A bolus dose of dexmedetomidine of 0.5–1 $\mu g\ kg^{-1}$ administered over 10 minutes followed by an infusion ranging from 0.2 to 0.7 $\mu g\ kg^{-1}\ h^{-1}$ has been shown to be effective in providing adequate sedation for awake fiberoptic intubations [121–123].

Sedation outside the operating room

Advances in medical technology have allowed medically complex patients to undergo diagnostic and therapeutic procedures outside the operating room. With the considerable increase in the number and scope of these procedures, anesthesiologists frequently are required to provide anesthesia and/or analgesia outside the operating room [124]. The choice of anesthetic technique will vary greatly, depending on the requirements of the procedure and the health of the patient, but several underlying themes are present for the clinician providing sedation for these cases.

The preparation and setup for sedation outside the operating room should be no different than sedation in the operating room, as sedation has the potential to become general anesthesia at any point [124]. According to the Joint Commission on Accreditation of Hospital Organizations, clinicians administering deep sedation (sedation which could inadvertently progress to general anesthesia) are required to possess the skills necessary to rescue unstable patients [125]. Upon review of the American Society of Anesthesiology (ASA) closed claims database, the severity of complications for patients undergoing general anesthesia and monitored anesthetic care were comparable [125]. The greatest number of claims (33%) for non-operating-room anesthesia (NORA) was from inadequate oxygenation or ventilation secondary to the effects administered drugs, and the proportion of death was significantly increased in NORA claims when compared to operating-room claims (54% vs. 24%) [124]. This illustrates the need for trained anesthesia staff experienced in airway management and cardiopulmonary resuscitation to perform safe sedation for NORA. Negative events were associated with increased age (> 70 years), ASA physical status III or higher, and obesity [124,125]. Other specific conditions that warrant special care when performing NORA include uncooperative patients, severe gastroesophageal reflux, orthopnea, decreased mental status, known or suspected difficult airway, obstructive sleep apnea, prone position, and acute trauma. Few data exist comparing monitored anesthesia care to general anesthesia for NORA, but resuscitation medication and equipment must be immediately available whenever and wherever either technique is performed [124,125].

Sedation for radiology procedures

Anesthesia or sedation is often required for patients undergoing MRI or CAT scanning to prevent movement during examination and to relieve anxiety and symptoms of claustrophobia [124,126,127]. The efficiency of the procedure depends on the interval from drug administration to the patient being ready to scan and the time required for emergence after the procedure [126]. Chloral hydrate, benzodiazepines, and barbiturates have been found to have a high percentage of prolonged sedation, unsteadiness, and hyperactivity, thus decreasing their efficacy for radiological testing [126]. Propofol has the advantage of a short recovery profile, but relatively high doses (approximately 100 µg kg^{-1} min^{-1}) are required to prevent involuntary movement, increasing the incidence of respiratory depression [126]. The inaccessibility of patients in the scanner, especially for MRIs, can create problems with patient visualization and airway management [128]. This has led many centers to conclude that with the proper equipment in the radiology suite, general anesthesia offers a safe efficient technique to provide optimal scan conditions and quick recovery [126].

For interventional radiology and neuroradiology, the severity of the underlying medical condition and the urgency of the procedure often determine the optimal anesthetic plan [124,129]. The primary goals of the anesthetic choice are to alleviate patient anxiety and discomfort, and to provide immobility. Neuroradiology procedures additionally require rapid awakening to obtain neurological exams [127,130]. General anesthesia is preferred for cerebral angiograms and aneurysm coiling, given the requirement for an immobile patient and control of respiratory and hemodynamic profiles [124,127,130]. Maintenance of anesthesia for neuroradiology with sevoflurane has been shown to lead to a more rapid recovery than propofol infusion in one study [131]. Sedation can allow neurological testing during the procedure, but an unprotected airway also increases the risk of aspiration and the potential for hypoxemia and hypercapnia [127,130]. Dexmedetomidine may be advantageous in patients receiving sedation, because patients retain their respiratory drive and are often arousable and cooperative when stimulated [130].

Endoscopy in the gastrointestinal suite

Cardiopulmonary problems account for a large percentage of complications and death in gastrointestinal endoscopy cases, with precipitating events including arterial desaturations, tachycardia, and hypertension [126]. Sedation is recommended to counteract the stress response associated with the procedure, and patient tolerance was found to be significantly higher when sedation was provided initially as opposed to upon request by the patient [126]. The anesthetic plan should be determined after discussion of the patient's position and the required depth of sedation [124]. If deep sedation in the prone position is required, general anesthesia may be necessary. Traditionally, benzodiazepines and opioids are used for the majority of endoscopies, but propofol utilization has rapidly increased in recent years [125,126]. While the combination of meperidine and midazolam was found to produce deep sedation in 68% or patients planned to receive moderate sedation [132], the quality of sedation was higher and recovery time shorter in a study of patients sedated with propofol versus midazolam plus meperidine [133]. Two large studies have reported the safety of nurse-administered propofol infusions, but not all these studies employed capnography or elucidated the total number of patients with hypoxemia, thus likely grossly underestimating the number of respiratory events [125,134,135]. A quality assurance review of NORA with

benzodiazepines and opioids found a comparable respiratory event incidence to that reported with propofol, and because of propofol's narrow therapeutic index, debate continues as to whether it should be administered only be trained anesthesia personnel [125,136].

In examining remifentanil infusion versus propofol infusion for colonoscopy, the respiratory rate, oxygen saturation, and pain scores of the remifentanil group were found to be lower than those of the propofol group. Patients receiving propofol had increased amnesia and lower nausea and vomiting, and overall the discharge times were similar in the two groups [137]. Conscious sedation with remifentanil and propofol versus total intravenous anesthesia (TIVA) with midazolam, fentanyl, and propofol has been compared for colonoscopy, with the conscious-sedation group reporting higher pain intensity scores; however, this group was discharged from the recovery room approximately 15 minutes faster than the TIVA group [138]. The combination of remifentanil and propofol had less change in mean arterial pressure, heart rate, and respiratory depression than the TIVA technique [138]. In addition to the traditional administration of benzodiazepines, opioids, and propofol, patient-controlled sedation and analgesia with propofol and fentanyl has been shown to be effective and safe for upper gastrointestinal endoscopy [139–141]. Studies are conflicting as to whether topical pharyngeal local anesthetic improves tolerance of upper gastrointestinal endoscopy in unsedated patients [142–144], but topical anesthesia has been shown to increase obstructive and central apnea in patients receiving sedation [126].

Although inhaled anesthetics can be utilized effectively for NORA, the requirement and cost for additional specialized equipment and the likely lack of a scavenging system lead most providers to prefer intravenous anesthetics for the majority of non-operating-room procedures [145].

Sedation in the cardiology suite

Anesthesiologists are frequently consulted to provide sedation for transesophageal echocardiography in the cardiology suite. Given the comorbid conditions associated with these patients, care must be taken to ensure proper resuscitative equipment is available at all times. While many centers utilize topicalization and intermittent doses of benzodiazepines and fentanyl, propofol is an attractive drug in these patients, with initial bolus doses of 0.5–0.75 mg kg^{-1} followed by intermittent doses of 0.25 mg kg^{-1} [125,126]. These doses of propofol can also be utilized to provide sedation for cardioversion in patients with atrial fibrillation or flutter [125,126]. For insertion of implantable defibrillators, most cases can be performed under moderate sedation, with deepening of sedation during the defibrillator check. Because of its rapid onset and offset, propofol infusions with boluses during defibrillation check work well for this procedure.

Summary

Sedation and analgesia are routinely administered to mechanically ventilated critically ill patients to prevent pain and anxiety, permit invasive procedures, reduce stress and oxygen consumption, and prevent ventilator/patient dyssynchrony. Oversedation is associated with worse clinical outcomes, including longer time on mechanical ventilation and in the ICU, greater need for neuroradiological evaluations of mental status, and higher probability of developing delirium and potentially long-term neurocognitive impairment, affecting longevity and quality of life.

Modifying sedation delivery by incorporating sedation and analgesia protocols, targeted sedation, daily wake-up trials, and linking spontaneous awakening trials with spontaneous breathing trials have all been associated with improvements in patient outcomes and should be incorporated into clinical management of critically ill patients. Altering conventional sedation paradigms by reducing benzodiazepine exposure and utilizing regimens incorporating propofol, remifentanil or dexmedetomidine have all shown reduction in times on mechanical ventilation. Studies with dexmedetomidine have additionally shown an improvement in brain dysfunction outcomes.

Acute brain dysfunction (delirium and coma) is a frequent complication of critical illness, with rates of delirium as high as 80% in mechanically ventilated patients. Delirium is an independent predictor of longer time in the ICU, greater costs, and higher risk of dying. Benzodiazepines appear to be potentially modifiable risk factors for delirium. Preventive protocols including reorientation, improving sleep architecture, geriatric consultation, and reducing medications with anticholinergic side effects have shown some benefit in non-ICU patients, though not studied in ICU patients. There are no differences in outcomes between typical and atypical antipsychotics for treating delirium in ICU patients.

Various pharmacologic techniques can be utilized for sedation outside the ICU. Proper equipment and monitoring is important to prevent complications.

References

1. Jacobi J, Fraser GL, Coursin DB, *et al.* Clinical practice guidelines for the sustained use of sedatives and analgesics in the critically ill adult. *Crit Care Med* 2002; **30**: 119–41.

2. Weinert CR, Chlan L, Gross C. Sedating critically ill patients: factors affecting nurses' delivery of sedative therapy. *Am J Crit Care* 2001; **10**: 156–65.

3. Weinert CR, Calvin AD. Epidemiology of sedation and sedation adequacy for mechanically ventilated patients in a medical and surgical intensive care unit. *Crit Care Med* 2007; **35**: 393–401.

4. Payen JF, Chanques G, Mantz J, *et al.* Current practices in sedation and analgesia for mechanically ventilated critically ill patients: a prospective multicenter patient-based study. *Anesthesiology* 2007; **106**: 687–95.

5. Mehta S, Burry L, Fischer S, *et al.* Canadian survey of the use of sedatives, analgesics, and neuromuscular blocking agents in critically ill patients. *Crit Care Med* 2006; **34**: 374–80.

6. Kress JP, Pohlman AS, Hall JB. Sedation and analgesia in the intensive care unit. *Am J Respir Crit Care Med* 2002; **166**: 1024–8.

7. Gehlbach BK, Kress JP. Sedation in the intensive care unit. *Curr Opin Crit Care* 2002; **8**: 290–8.

8. Weinert CR, Sprenkle M. Post-ICU consequences of patient wakefulness and sedative exposure during mechanical ventilation. *Intensive Care Med* 2008; **34**: 82–90

9. Rotondi AJ, Chelluri L, Sirio C, *et al.* Patients' recollections of stressful experiences while receiving prolonged mechanical ventilation in an intensive care unit. *Crit Care Med* 2002; **30**: 746–52.

10. Jones C, Griffiths RD, Humphris G. Disturbed memory and amnesia related to intensive care. *Memory* 2000; **8**: 79–94.

11. Jones C, Griffiths RD, Humphris G, Skirrow PM. Memory, delusions, and the development of acute posttraumatic stress disorder-related symptoms after intensive care. *Crit Care Med* 2001; **29**: 573–80.

12. Pandharipande P, Cotton B, Shintani A, *et al.* Prevalence and risk factors for development of delirium in surgical and trauma intensive care unit patients. *J Trauma* 2008; **65**: 34–41.

13. Ely EW, Inouye SK, Bernard GR, *et al.* Delirium in mechanically ventilated patients: validity and reliability of the confusion assessment method for the intensive care unit (CAM-ICU). *JAMA* 2001; **286**: 2703–10.

14. Wijdicks EFM. *Neurologic Complications of Critical Illness*, 2nd edn. New York, NY: Oxford University Press, 2002.

15. Pandharipande P, Shintani A, Peterson J, *et al.* Lorazepam is an independent risk factor for transitioning to delirium in intensive care unit patients. *Anesthesiology* 2006; **104**: 21–6.

16. Moss M, Burnham EL. Alcohol abuse in the critically ill patient. *Lancet* 2006; **368**: 2231–42.

17. Morrison RS, Magaziner J, Gilbert M, *et al.* Relationship between pain and opioid analgesics on the development of delirium following hip fracture. *J Gerontol A Biol Sci Med Sci* 2003; **58**: 76–81.

18. Marcantonio ER, Juarez G, Goldman L, *et al.* The relationship of postoperative delirium with psychoactive medications. *JAMA* 1994; **272**: 1518–22.

19. Kollef MH, Levy NT, Ahrens TS, *et al.* The use of continuous i.v. sedation is associated with prolongation of mechanical ventilation. *Chest* 1998; **114**: 541–8.

20. Kress JP, Pohlman AS, O'Connor MF, Hall JB. Daily interruption of sedative infusions in critically ill patients undergoing mechanical ventilation. *N Engl J Med* 2000; **342**: 1471–7.

21. Nelson BJ, Weinert CR, Bury CL, Marinelli WA, Gross CR. Intensive care unit drug use and subsequent quality of

life in acute lung injury patients. *Crit Care Med* 2000; **28**: 3626–30.

22. Larson MJ, Weaver LK, Hopkins RO. Cognitive sequelae in acute respiratory distress syndrome patients with and without recall of the intensive care unit. *J Int Neuropsychol Soc* 2007; **13**: 595–605.

23. Dubois MJ, Bergeron N, Dumont M, Dial S, Skrobik Y. Delirium in an intensive care unit: a study of risk factors. *Intensive Care Med* 2001; **27**: 1297–304.

24. Park G, Lane M, Rogers S, Bassett P. A comparison of hypnotic and analgesic based sedation in a general intensive care unit. *Br J Anaesth* 2007; **98**: 76–82.

25. Horn E, Nesbit SA. Pharmacology and pharmacokinetics of sedatives and analgesics. *Gastrointest Endosc Clin N Am* 2004; **14**: 247–68.

26. Patel S, Roshan VR, Lee KC, Cheung RJ. A myoclonic reaction with low-dose hydromorphone. *Ann Pharmacother* 2006; **40**: 2068–70.

27. Karabinis A, Mandragos K, Stergiopoulos S, *et al.* Safety and efficacy of analgesia-based sedation with remifentanil versus standard hypnotic-based regimens in intensive care unit patients with brain injuries: a randomised, controlled trial [ISRCTN50308308]. *Crit Care* 2004; **8**: R268–80.

28. Battershill AJ, Keating GM. Remifentanil: a review of its analgesic and sedative use in the intensive care unit. *Drugs* 2006; **66**: 365–85.

29. Kapila A, Glass PS, Jacobs JR, *et al.* Measured context-sensitive half-times of remifentanil and alfentanil. *Anesthesiology* 1995; **83**: 968–75.

30. Breen D, Wilmer A, Bodenham A, *et al.* Offset of pharmacodynamic effects and safety of remifentanil in intensive care unit patients with various degrees of renal impairment. *Crit Care* 2004; **8**: R21–30.

31. Pitsiu M, Wilmer A, Bodenham A, *et al.* Pharmacokinetics of remifentanil and its major metabolite, remifentanil acid, in ICU patients with renal impairment. *Br J Anaesth* 2004; **92**: 493–503.

32. Young C, Knudsen N, Hilton A, Reves JG. Sedation in the intensive care unit. *Crit Care Med* 2000; **28**: 854–66.

33. Young CC, Prielipp RC. Benzodiazepines in the intensive care unit. *Crit Care Clin* 2001; **17**: 843–62.

34. Angelini G, Ketzler JT, Coursin DB. Use of propofol and other nonbenzodiazepine sedatives in the intensive care unit. *Crit Care Clinics* 2001; **17**: 863–80.

35. Fragen RJ. Pharmacokinetics and pharmacodynamics of midazolam given via continuous intravenous infusion in intensive care units. *Clin Ther* 1997; **19**: 405–19.

36. MacGilchrist AJ, Birnie GG, Cook A, *et al.* Pharmacokinetics and pharmacodynamics of intravenous midazolam in patients with severe alcoholic cirrhosis. *Gut* 1986; **27**: 190–5.

37. Khanderia U, Pandit SK. Use of midazolam hydrochloride in anesthesia. *Clin Pharm* 1987; **6**: 533–47.

38. Vinik HR, Reves JG, Greenblatt DJ, Abernethy DR, Smith LR. The pharmacokinetics of midazolam in chronic renal failure patients. *Anesthesiology* 1983; **59**: 390–4.

39. Driessen JJ, Vree TB, Guelen PJ. The effects of acute changes in renal function on the pharmacokinetics of midazolam during long-term infusion in ICU patients. *Acta Anaesthesiol Belg* 1991; **42**: 149–55.

40. Greenblatt DJ, Abernethy DR, Locniskar A, *et al.* Effect of age, gender, and obesity on midazolam kinetics. *Anesthesiology* 1984; **61**: 27–35.

41. Malacrida R, Fritz ME, Suter PM, Crevoisier C. Pharmacokinetics of midazolam administered by continuous intravenous infusion to intensive care patients. *Crit Care Med* 1992; **20**: 1123–6.

42. Barr J. Propofol: a new drug for sedation in the intensive care unit. *Int Anesthesiol Clin* 1995; **33**: 131–54.

43. Mikawa K, Akamatsu H, Nishina K, *et al.* Propofol inhibits human neutrophil functions. *Anesth Analg* 1998; **87**: 695–700.

44. Pirttikangas CO, Perttila J, Salo M. Propofol emulsion reduces proliferative responses of lymphocytes from intensive care patients. *Intensive Care Med* 1993; **19**: 299–302.

45. Trapani G, Altomare C, Liso G, Sanna E, Biggio G. Propofol in anesthesia.

Mechanism of action, structure–activity relationships, and drug delivery. *Curr Med Chem* 2000; **7**: 249–71.

46. Barr J, Egan TD, Sandoval NF, *et al.* Propofol dosing regimens for ICU sedation based upon an integrated pharmacokinetic-pharmacodynamic model. *Anesthesiology* 2001; **95**: 324–33.

47. Bentley GN, Gent JP, Goodchild CS. Vascular effects of propofol: smooth muscle relaxation in isolated veins and arteries. *J Pharm Pharmacol* 1989; **41**: 797–8.

48. Vasile B, Rasulo F, Candiani A, Latronico N. The pathophysiology of propofol infusion syndrome: a simple name for a complex syndrome. *Intensive Care Med* 2003; **29**: 1417–25.

49. Maze M, Scarfini C, Cavaliere F. New agents for sedation in the intensive care unit. *Crit Care Clin* 2001; **17**: 881–97.

50. Bekker AY, Kaufman B, Samir H, Doyle W. The use of dexmedetomidine infusion for awake craniotomy. *Anesth Analg* 2001; **92**: 1251–3.

51. Bekker AY, Basile J, Gold M, *et al.* Dexmedetomidine for awake carotid endarterectomy: efficacy, hemodynamic profile, and side effects. *J Neurosurg Anesthesiol* 2004; **16**: 126–35.

52. Pandharipande PP, Pun BT, Herr DL, *et al.* Effect of sedation with dexmedetomidine vs lorazepam on acute brain dysfunction in mechanically ventilated patients: the MENDS randomized controlled trial. *JAMA* 2007; **298**: 2644–53.

53. Venn RM, Bryant A, Hall GM, Grounds RM. Effects of dexmedetomidine on adrenocortical function, and the cardiovascular, endocrine and inflammatory responses in post-operative patients needing sedation in the intensive care unit. *Br J Anaesth* 2001; **86**: 650–6.

54. Taniguchi T, Kidani Y, Kanakura H, Takemoto Y, Yamamoto K. Effects of dexmedetomidine on mortality rate and inflammatory responses to endotoxin-induced shock in rats. *Crit Care Med* 2004; **32**: 1322–6.

55. Nelson LE, Lu J, Guo T, *et al.* The α_2-adrenoceptor agonist dexmedetomidine converges on an endogenous sleep-promoting pathway to exert its sedative effects. *Anesthesiology* 2003; **98**: 428–36.

56. Sanders RD, Ma D, Hossain M, Maze M. Dexmedetomodine is neuroprotective against wortmannin and staurosporine-induced apoptosis in vitro. *ASA Abstract* 2004; A778.

57. Engelhard K, Werner C, Kaspar S, *et al.* Effect of the alpha2-agonist dexmedetomidine on cerebral neurotransmitter concentrations during cerebral ischemia in rats. *Anesthesiology* 2002; **96**: 450–7.

58. Ramsay MA, Savege TM, Simpson BR, Goodwin R. Controlled sedation with alphaxalone-alphadolone. *Br Med J* 1974; **2**: 656–9.

59. Riker RR, Picard JT, Fraser GL. Prospective evaluation of the Sedation-Agitation Scale for adult critically ill patients. *Crit Care Med* 1999; **27**: 1325–9.

60. Ely EW, Truman B, Shintani A, *et al.* Monitoring sedation status over time in ICU patients: reliability and validity of the Richmond Agitation-Sedation Scale (RASS). *JAMA* 2003; **289**: 2983–91.

61. Sessler CN, Gosnell MS, Grap MJ, *et al.* The Richmond Agitation-Sedation Scale: validity and reliability in adult intensive care unit patients. *Am J Respir Crit Care Med* 2002; **166**: 1338–44.

62. Sigl JC, Chamoun NG. An introduction to bispectral analysis for the electroencehpalogram. *J Clin Monit* 1994; **10**: 392–404.

63. Wolter S, Friedel C, Bohler K, *et al.* Presence of 14Hz spindle oscillations in the human EEG during deep anesthesia. *Clin Neurophysiol* 2006; **117**: 157–68.

64. Leistritz L, Jager H, Schelenz C, *et al.* New approaches for the detection and analysis of electroencephalographic burst-suppression patterns in patients under sedation. *J Clin Monit Comput* 1999; **15**: 357–67.

65. Brattebo G, Hofoss D, Flaatten H, *et al.* Effect of a scoring system and protocol for sedation on duration of patients' need for ventilator support in a surgical intensive care unit. *BMJ* 2002; **324**: 1386–9.

66. Brook AD, Ahrens TS, Schaiff R, *et al.* Effect of a nursing-implemented sedation protocol on the duration of mechanical ventilation. *Crit Care Med* 1999; **27**: 2609–15.

67. De Deyne C, Struys M, Decruyenaere J, *et al.* Use of continuous bispectral EEG monitoring to assess depth of sedation in ICU patients. *Intensive Care Med* 1998; **24**: 1294–8.

68. Watson PL, Shintani A, Tyson R, *et al.* Presence of EEG burst suppression in critically ill patients is associated with increased mortality. *Crit Care Med* 2008; **36**: 3171–7.

69. Simmons LE, Riker R, Prato M, Fraser G. Assessing sedation during intensive care unit mechanical ventilation with the bispectral index and the sedation-agitation scale. *Crit Care Med* 1999; **27**: 1499–504.

70. Riker RR, Fraser GL, Simmons LE, Wilkins ML. Validating the sedation-agitation scale with the bispectral index and visual analog scale in adult ICU patients after cardiac surgery. *Intensive Care Med* 2001; **27**: 853–8.

71. Weatherburn C, Endacott R, Tynan P, Bailey M. The impact of bispectral index monitoring on sedation administration in mechanically ventilated patients. *Anaesth Intensive Care* 2007; **35**: 204–8.

72. Kress JP, Gehlbach B, Lacy M, *et al.* The long-term psychological effects of daily sedative interruption on critically ill patients. *Am J Respir Crit Care Med* 2003; **168**: 1457–61.

73. Girard TD, Kress JP, Fuchs BD, *et al.* Efficacy and safety of a paired sedation and ventilator weaning protocol for mechanically ventilated patients in intensive care (Awakening and Breathing Controlled trial): a randomised controlled trial. *Lancet* 2008; **371**: 126–34.

74. Dahaba AA, Grabner T, Rehak PH, List WF, Metzler H. Remifentanil versus morphine analgesia and sedation for mechanically ventilated critically ill patients: a randomized double blind study. *Anesthesiology* 2004; **101**: 640–6.

75. Muellejans B, Lopez A, Cross MH, *et al.* Remifentanil versus fentanyl for analgesia based sedation to provide patient comfort in the intensive care unit: a randomized, double-blind controlled trial [ISRCTN43755713]. *Crit Care* 2004; **8**: R1–11.

76. Breen D, Karabinis A, Malbrain M, *et al.* Decreased duration of mechanical ventilation when comparing analgesia-based sedation using remifentanil with standard hypnotic-based sedation for up to 10 days in intensive care unit patients: a randomised trial [ISRCTN47583497]. *Crit Care* 2005; **9**: R200–10.

77. Cernaianu AC, DelRossi AJ, Flum DR, *et al.* Lorazepam and midazolam in the intensive care unit: a randomized, prospective, multicenter study of hemodynamics, oxygen transport, efficacy, and cost. *Crit Care Med.* 1996; **24**: 222–8.

78. Barr J, Zomorodi K, Bertaccini EJ, Shafer SL, Geller E. A double-blind, randomized comparison of i.v. lorazepam versus midazolam for sedation of ICU patients via a pharmacologic model. *Anesthesiology* 2001; **95**: 286–98.

79. McCollam JS, O'Neil MG, Norcross ED, Byrne TK, Reeves ST. Continuous infusions of lorazepam, midazolam, and propofol for sedation of the critically ill surgery trauma patient: a prospective, randomized comparison. *Crit Care Med* 1999; **27**: 2454–8.

80. Carson SS, Kress JP, Rodgers JE, *et al.* A randomized trial of intermittent lorazepam versus propofol with daily interruption in mechanically ventilated patients. *Crit Care Med* 2006; **34**: 1326–32.

81. Barrientos-Vega R, Mar Sanchez-Soria M, Morales-Garcia C, *et al.* Prolonged sedation of critically ill patients with midazolam or propofol: impact on weaning and costs. *Crit Care Med* 1997; **25**: 33–40.

82. Kress JP, O'Connor MF, Pohlman AS, *et al.* Sedation of critically ill patients during mechanical ventilation. A comparison of propofol and midazolam. *Am J Respir Crit Care Med* 1996; **153**: 1012–18.

83. Weinbroum AA, Halpern P, Rudick V, *et al.* Midazolam versus propofol for long-term sedation in the ICU: a randomized prospective comparison. *Intensive Care Med* 1997; **23**: 1258–63.

84. Hall RI, Sandham D, Cardinal P, *et al.* Propofol vs midazolam for ICU sedation: a Canadian multicenter randomized trial. *Chest* 2001; **119**: 1151–9.

85. Walder B, Elia N, Henzi I, Romand JR, Tramer MR. A lack of evidence of superiority of propofol versus

midazolam for sedation in mechanically ventilated critically ill patients: a qualitative and quantitative systematic review. *Anesth Analg* 2001; **92**: 975–83.

86. Venn RM, Grounds RM. Comparison between dexmedetomidine and propofol for sedation in the intensive care unit: patient and clinician perceptions. *Br J Anaesth* 2001; **87**: 684–90.

87. Venn RM, Hell J, Grounds RM. Respiratory effects of dexmedetomidine in the surgical patient requiring intensive care. *Crit Care* 2000; **4**: 302–8.

88. Herr DL, Sum-Ping ST, England M. ICU sedation after coronary artery bypass graft surgery: dexmedetomidine-based versus propofol-based sedation regimens. *J Cardiothorac Vasc Anesth* 2003; **17**: 576–84.

89. Corbett SM, Rebuck JA, Greene CM, *et al.* Dexmedetomidine does not improve patient satisfaction when compared with propofol during mechanical ventilation. *Crit Care Med* 2005; **33**: 940–5.

90. Pandharipande PP, Girard T, Sanders RD, *et al.* Comparison of sedation with dexmedetomidine versus lorazepam in septic ICU patients. *Crit Care* 2008; **12**: P275

91. Bergeron N, Dubois MJ, Dumont M, Dial S, Skrobik Y. Intensive Care Delirium Screening Checklist: evaluation of a new screening tool. *Intensive Care Med* 2001; **27**: 859–64.

92. Ouimet S, Riker R, Bergeron N, *et al.* Subsyndromal delirium in the ICU: evidence for a disease spectrum. *Intensive Care Med* 2007; **33**: 1007–13.

93. Inouye SK, Bogardus ST, Charpentier PA, *et al.* A multicomponent intervention to prevent delirium in hospitalized older patients. *N Engl J Med* 1999; **340**: 669–76.

94. Bogardus ST, Desai MM, Williams CS, *et al.* The effects of a targeted multicomponent delirium intervention on postdischarge outcomes for hospitalized older adults. *Am J Med* 2003; **114**: 383–90.

95. Marcantonio ER, Flacker JM, Wright RJ, Resnick NM. Reducing delirium after hip fracture: a randomized trial. *J Am Geriatr Soc* 2001; **49**: 516–22.

96. Cole MG, McCusker J, Bellavance F, *et al.* Systematic detection and

multidisciplinary care of delirium in older medical inpatients: a randomized trial. *CMAJ* 2002; **167**: 753–9.

97. Milisen K, Foreman MD, Abraham IL, *et al.* A nurse-led interdisciplinary intervention program for delirium in elderly hip-fracture patients. *J Am Geriatr Soc* 2001; **49**: 523–32.

98. Lundstrom M, Edlund A, Karlsson S, *et al.* A multifactorial intervention program reduces the duration of delirium, length of hospitalization, and mortality in delirious patients. *J Am Geriatr Soc* 2005; **53**: 622–8.

99. Siobal MS, Kallet RH, Kivett VA, Tang JF. Use of dexmedetomidine to facilitate extubation in surgical intensive-care-unit patients who failed previous weaning attempts following prolonged mechanical ventilation: a pilot study. *Respir Care* 2006; **51**: 492–6.

100. Ely EW, Stephens RK, Jackson JC, *et al.* Current opinions regarding the importance, diagnosis, and management of delirium in the intensive care unit: a survey of 912 healthcare professionals. *Crit Care Med* 2004; **32**: 106–12.

101. Kapur S, Remington G, Jones C, *et al.* High levels of dopamine d2 receptor occupancy with low-dose haloperidol treatment: a pet study. *Am J Psychiatry* 1996; **153**: 948–50.

102. Skrobik YK, Bergeron N, Dumont M, Gottfried SB. Olanzapine vs haloperidol: treating delirium in a critical care setting. *Intensive Care Med* 2004; **30**: 444–9.

103. Alao AO, Soderberg M, Pohl EL, Koss M. Aripiprazole in the treatment of delirium. *Int J Psychiatry Med* 2005; **35**: 429–33.

104. Foreman M, Milisen K, Marcantonia EM. Prevention and treatment strategies for delirium. *Primary Psychiatry* 2004; **11**: 52–8.

105. Tune L. The role of antipsychotics in treating delirium. *Curr Psychiatry Rep* 2002; **4**: 209–12.

106. Tune LE, Damlouji NF, Holland A, *et al.* Association of postoperative delirium with raised serum levels of anticholinergic drugs. *Lancet* 1981; **2**: 651–3.

107. Milbrandt EB, Kersten A, Kong L, *et al.* Haloperidol use is associated with lower

hospital mortality in mechanically ventilated patients. *Crit Care Med* 2005; **33**: 226–9.

108. Kalisvaart KJ, de Jonghe JF, Bogaards MJ, *et al.* Haloperidol prophylaxis for elderly hip-surgery patients at risk for delirium: a randomized placebo-controlled study. *J Am Geriatr Soc* 2005; **53**: 1658–66.

109. Kato D, Kawanishi C, Kishida I, *et al.* Delirium resolving upon switching from risperidone to quetiapine: implication of the CYP2D6 genotype. *Psychosomatics* 2005; **46**: 374–5.

110. Wang PS, Schneeweiss S, Avorn J, *et al.* Risk of death in elderly users of conventional vs. atypical antipsychotic medications. *N Engl J Med* 2005; **353**: 2335–41.

111. Schneider LS, Dagerman KS, Insel P. Risk of death with atypical antipsychotic drug treatment for dementia: meta-analysis of randomized placebo-controlled trials. *JAMA* 2005; **294**: 1934–43.

112. Sink KM, Holden KF, Yaffe K. Pharmacological treatment of neuropsychiatric symptoms of dementia: a review of the evidence. *JAMA* 2005; **293**: 596–608.

113. Benumof JL. Management of the difficult adult airway. With special emphasis on awake tracheal intubation. *Anesthesiology* 1991; **75**: 1087–110.

114. Simmons ST, Schleich AR. Airway regional anesthesia for awake fiberoptic intubation. *Reg Anesth Pain Med* 2002; **27**: 180–92.

115. Morris IR. Fibreoptic intubation. *Can J Anaesth* 1994; **41**: 996–1007.

116. Puchner W, Egger P, Puhringer F, *et al.* Evaluation of remifentanil as single drug for awake fiberoptic intubation. *Acta Anaesthesiol Scand* 2002; **46**: 350–4.

117. Machata AM, Gonano C, Holzer A, *et al.* Awake nasotracheal fiberoptic intubation: patient comfort, intubating conditions, and hemodynamic stability during conscious sedation with remifentanil. *Anesth Analg* 2003; **97**: 904–8.

118. Rai MR, Parry TM, Dombrovskis A, Warner OJ. Remifentanil target-controlled infusion vs propofol target-controlled infusion for conscious

sedation for awake fibreoptic intubation: a double-blinded randomized controlled trial. *Br J Anaesth* 2008; **100**: 125–30.

119. Andel H, Klune G, Andel D, *et al.* Propofol without muscle relaxants for conventional or fiberoptic nasotracheal intubation: a dose-finding study. *Anesth Analg* 2000; **91**: 458–61.

120. Ozturk T, Cakan A, Gulerce G, *et al.* Sedation for fiberoptic bronchoscopy: fewer adverse cardiovascular effects with propofol than with midazolam. *Anasthesiol Intensivmed Notfallmed Schmerzther* 2004; **39**: 597–602.

121. Abdelmalak B, Makary L, Hoban J, Doyle DJ. Dexmedetomidine as sole sedative for awake intubation in management of the critical airway. *J Clin Anesth* 2007; **19**: 370–3.

122. Avitsian R, Lin J, Lotto M, Ebrahim Z. Dexmedetomidine and awake fiberoptic intubation for possible cervical spine myelopathy: a clinical series. *J Neurosurg Anesthesiol* 2005; **17**: 97–9.

123. Bergese SD, Khabiri B, Roberts WD, *et al.* Dexmedetomidine for conscious sedation in difficult awake fiberoptic intubation cases. *J Clin Anesth* 2007; **19**: 141–4.

124. Robbertze R, Posner KL, Domino KB. Closed claims review of anesthesia for procedures outside the operating room. *Curr Opin Anaesthesiol* 2006; **19**: 436–42.

125. Pino RM. The nature of anesthesia and procedural sedation outside of the operating room. *Curr Opin Anaesthesiol* 2007; **20**: 347–51.

126. Melloni C. Anesthesia and sedation outside the operating room: how to prevent risk and maintain good quality. *Curr Opin Anaesthesiol* 2007; **20**: 513–19.

127. Hashimoto T, Gupta DK, Young WL. Interventional neuroradiology: anesthetic considerations. *Anesthesiol Clin North America* 2002; **20**: 347–59, vi.

128. Gooden CK. Anesthesia for magnetic resonance imaging. *Curr Opin Anaesthesiol* 2004; **17**: 339–42.

129. Kotob F, Twersky RS. Anesthesia outside the operating room: general overview and monitoring standards. *Int Anesthesiol Clin* 2003; **41**: 1–15.

130. Varma MK, Price K, Jayakrishnan V, Manickam B, Kessell G. Anaesthetic considerations for interventional neuroradiology. *Br J Anaesth* 2007; **99**: 75–85.

131. Castagnini HE, van EF, Salevsky FC, Nathanson MH. Sevoflurane for interventional neuroradiology procedures is associated with more rapid early recovery than propofol. *Can J Anaesth* 2004; **51**: 486–91.

132. Patel S, Vargo JJ, Khandwala F, *et al.* Deep sedation occurs frequently during elective endoscopy with meperidine and midazolam. *Am J Gastroenterol* 2005; **100**: 2689–95.

133. Sipe BW, Rex DK, Latinovich D, *et al.* Propofol versus midazolam/meperidine for outpatient colonoscopy: administration by nurses supervised by endoscopists. *Gastrointest Endosc* 2002; **55**: 815–25.

134. Rex DK, Heuss LT, Walker JA, Qi R. Trained registered nurses/endoscopy teams can administer propofol safely for endoscopy. *Gastroenterology* 2005; **129**: 1384–91.

135. Walker JA, McIntyre RD, Schleinitz PF, *et al.* Nurse-administered propofol sedation without anesthesia specialists in 9152 endoscopic cases in an ambulatory surgery center. *Am J Gastroenterol* 2003; **98**: 1744–50.

136. Lazzaroni M, Bianchi PG. Preparation, premedication and surveillance in gastrointestinal endoscopy. *Endoscopy* 1994; **26**: 3–8.

137. Akcaboy ZN, Akcaboy EY, Albayrak D, *et al.* Can remifentanil be a better choice than propofol for colonoscopy during monitored anesthesia care? *Acta Anaesthesiol Scand* 2006; **50**: 736–41.

138. Rudner R, Jalowiecki P, Kawecki P, *et al.* Conscious analgesia/sedation with remifentanil and propofol versus total intravenous anesthesia with fentanyl, midazolam, and propofol for outpatient colonoscopy. *Gastrointest Endosc* 2003; **57**: 657–63.

139. Agostoni M, Fanti L, Arcidiacono PG, *et al.* Midazolam and pethidine versus propofol and fentanyl patient controlled sedation/analgesia for upper gastrointestinal tract ultrasound endoscopy: a prospective randomized controlled trial. *Dig Liver Dis* 2007; **39**: 1024–9.

140. Fanti L, Agostoni M, Arcidiacono PG, *et al.* Target-controlled infusion during monitored anesthesia care in patients undergoing EUS: propofol alone versus midazolam plus propofol. A prospective double-blind randomised controlled trial. *Dig Liver Dis* 2007; **39**: 81–6.

141. Fanti L, Agostoni M, Casati A, *et al.* Target-controlled propofol infusion during monitored anesthesia in patients undergoing ERCP. *Gastrointest Endosc* 2004; **60**: 361–6.

142. Hedenbro JL, Ekelund M, Jansson O, Lindblom A. A randomized, double-blind, placebo-controlled study to evaluate topical anaesthesia of the pharynx in upper gastrointestinal endoscopy. *Endoscopy* 1992; **24**: 585–7.

143. Campo R, Brullet E, Montserrat A, *et al.* Topical pharyngeal anesthesia improves tolerance of upper gastrointestinal endoscopy: a randomized double-blind study. *Endoscopy* 1995; **27**: 659–64.

144. Dhir V, Swaroop VS, Vazifdar KF, Wagle SD. Topical pharyngeal anesthesia without intravenous sedation during upper gastrointestinal endoscopy. *Indian J Gastroenterol* 1997; **16**: 10–11.

145. Melloni C. Morbidity and mortality related to anesthesia outside the operating room. *Minerva Anestesiol* 2005; **71**: 325–34.

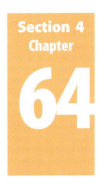

Clinical applications: evidence-based anesthesia practice
Postoperative analgesia

Richard W. Rosenquist and Ellen W. King

Introduction

Pain is the inevitable result of all surgical procedures – or is it? Historically, this has been the expected result of all surgical interventions. Although a good understanding of the conceptual basis for pain is lacking, there has been an ongoing effort to gain a better understanding of the physiologic, sensory, affective, cognitive, behavioral, and sociocultural events leading to the pain response [1]. While our knowledge has advanced significantly in the past decade, we are still largely relegated to the use of existing techniques to control symptoms rather than applying new techniques or combinations to modify the physiologic events that occur in response to acute trauma with the goal of reducing pain and preventing long-term complications or chronic pain. This is slowly changing, and there is at least preliminary evidence that appropriate use of regional blocks or medications may impact the duration of pain as a major component of the recovery process and the risk of developing chronic pain. The importance of a good understanding of acute perioperative pain management cannot be overstated. In the United States, this has been recognized by the Accreditation Council for Graduate Medical Education (ACGME), and residents training in accredited anesthesiology residencies are required to have significant experience in acute postoperative pain management. This chapter addresses the broad range of techniques used to control acute postoperative pain and prevent the development of chronic pain, and describes the application of these techniques in special patient populations.

Systemic analgesics

Opioids and patient-controlled analgesia

Opioid analgesics are the gold standard for the treatment of cancer-related and non-cancer nociceptive pain. Morphine was first isolated from the opium poppy in the early 1800s, and since that time many derivatives of morphine and synthetic opioid analogs have been developed and used to treat nociceptive pain. This includes drugs such as morphine, codeine,

hydrocodone, oxycodone, hydromorphone, oxymorphone, nicomorphine, fentanyl, sufentanil, meperidine, diacetylmorphine, methadone, tramadol, and propoxyphene.

Opioids are a popular choice for analgesia because they are familiar to most physicians and can be delivered in a variety of fashions depending on the clinical situation. Routes of administration include transdermal, oral, rectal, intranasal, intramuscular, intravenous, sublingual, epidural, and intrathecal. The route of administration has a significant impact on the apparent relative potency of the drug (based on dose). Potency ratios for morphine are 3:1 parenteral to oral, 10:1 epidural to parenteral, and 10:1 intrathecal to epidural administration. Thus a 1 mg intrathecal morphine dose is approximately equivalent to 300 mg of oral morphine.

In the postoperative setting, opioids are commonly administered using intravenous patient-controlled analgesia (PCA). Once postoperative oral intake has resumed, or when postoperative pain is mild, patients are converted to oral analgesics. In some situations, moderate to severe pain is expected to persist for extended periods of time, and oral analgesic regimens must be developed to address these long-term needs. In order to provide continuous adequate postoperative pain control, it is important to be able to rapidly and accurately convert the dose of one opioid to another and from one route of administration to another. A common practice is to convert all administered opioid analgesics to morphine equivalents (Table 64.1) before converting to the new drug dose and route needed for the desired opioid analgesic. Incomplete tolerance between opioids should be assumed in most cases, and new opioid analgesics should be started at two-thirds of the calculated equianalgesic dose (Box 64.1).

Although opioids are effective analgesics, they are not without side effects. The most common side effects include pruritus, nausea and/or vomiting, constipation, urinary retention, and respiratory depression. Side effects occur regardless of route of administration, and in most situations the frequency, severity, and duration of the side effects is dose-related. Many side effects can be prevented or minimized by concurrently administering adverse-effect-specific prophylaxis.

Anesthetic Pharmacology, 2nd edition, ed. Alex S. Evers, Mervyn Maze, Evan D. Kharasch. Published by Cambridge University Press. © Cambridge University Press 2011.

Table 64.1. Equianalgesic chart

Analgesic	Dosage Parenteral	Oral
Fentanyl (Sublimaze)	0.1–0.2 mg	—
Hydrocodone (Vicodin)	—	30 mg
Hydromorphone (Dilaudid)	1.5 mg	7.5 mg
Meperidine (Demerol)	75–100 mg	300 mg[a]
Morphine	10 mg	30 mg[b]
Oxycodone	—	20 mg

Doses listed are equivalent to 10 mg of parenteral morphine. Doses should be titrated according to individual response.
[a]Dosage in this range may lead to neuroexcitability.
[b]For a single dose, 10 mg intravenous morphine = 60 mg oral morphine. For chronic dosing, 10 mg intravenous morphine = 30 mg oral morphine.

Intravenous PCA devices have been in use for more than 25 years and have become widely accepted as the preferred means for delivering opioid analgesics for postoperative analgesia, as well as other acute-pain conditions. These devices allow the patient to self-administer an opioid analgesic on an as-needed basis within the parameters set by the ordering physician and avoid the inconsistent delivery and absorption associated with intermittent subcutaneous and intramuscular administration. In most settings, the readily available drug afforded by the PCA device has the potential to allow safe individualization of opioid analgesic dosing, improve pain control, and increase patient satisfaction. An inherent safety feature of a PCA is that if the patient is too sedated as a side effect of the medication, he or she will not push the button to deliver more medication. This safety feature is absent when patients receive basal infusion rates, or when the PCA device is activated by other authorized or unauthorized care providers.

PCA leads to improved patient outcomes when compared with nurse-controlled analgesia (NCA) in both randomized trials and meta-analyses. In addition to improved pain control, this outcome may reflect satisfaction regarding the ability to maintain a degree of control during hospitalization, especially over something as individual as pain control. The value of self-determination is reflected in the wide variability of total opioid use by individuals undergoing the same surgical procedure. This variable cannot be predicted in advance in most cases and may cause some patients to be undertreated if a one-size-fits-all approach is used to order postoperative analgesics. In most studies, patients using PCA obtained better pain relief without an increase in undesirable side effects [2,3].

The use of PCA does not appear to lead to clear improvement in other outcomes. However, the potential benefits outlined in some small studies include improved pulmonary function, provision for a wide variability in opioid dose, and reduced hospital stay. The absence of clearly defined and widely accepted measures of patient outcomes limits comparisons

Box 64.1. Example of opioid conversion

(1) Patient is receiving a total of 5 mg of parenteral hydromorphone in a 24-hour period via a PCA pump. The goal is to convert this to oral morphine for discharge. When converting from PCA administration, add the total amount of opioid that the patient received in the last 24 hours, including:
  (a) basal infusion
  (b) demand boluses administered by the patient
  (c) bolus doses administered by the medical/nursing staff
(2) The equianalgesic chart (Table 64.1) indicates that 1.5 mg of parenteral hydromorphone equals 7.5 mg of oral hydromorphone (a fivefold increase).
(3) The patient's current dose of 5 mg per day of parenteral hydromorphone is equal to 25 mg per day of oral hydromorphone.
(4) The next step is to convert 25 mg of oral hydromorphone to the daily oral morphine equivalent dose (DOMED).
(5) The equianalgesic chart indicates that 7.5 mg of oral hydromorphone is equal to 30 mg of oral morphine.
(6) The patient's calculated dose of 25 mg of oral hydromorphone is equal to 100 mg of oral morphine.
(7) The oral dose of morphine should be reduced by 33% to reduce the risk of overdose after the conversion, since opioids do not have complete cross-tolerance. A 33% dose reduction from the calculated dose of 100 mg is equal to 67 mg of oral morphine per day.
(8) The recommended dosing frequency of long-acting morphine (MS Contin) is every 12 hours (two doses per day).
(9) MS Contin is available in 15 mg, 30 mg, 100 mg, and 200 mg controlled-release tablets. The tablet strength closest to the calculated dose is 30 mg. The proper starting dose should therefore be 30 mg of sustained-release morphine every 12 hours. This may be supplemented with immediate-release oral morphine in a dose of 15 mg every 3 hours as needed for breakthrough pain and to determine if the total daily dose given as sustained-release morphine should be increased.

between studies and makes accumulation of sufficient patient numbers to draw clear conclusions a challenge.

Morphine and hydromorphone are the two most common opioids used in intravenous PCA, with fentanyl running a distant third. Most often, PCA devices are programmed to deliver on-demand dosing only with a given lockout interval to prevent overdosing. Continuous basal rates are sometimes combined with on-demand dosing to achieve better analgesia in patients with large opioid requirements. Ketamine has been used as an adjuvant medication in combination with morphine for PCA delivery. However, the benefit of including ketamine with morphine for PCA administration is unclear [4,5].

Caregiver-controlled analgesia (CCA) or "PCA by proxy" is a unique form of self-administered analgesia. Medical personnel or caregivers assist patients with "self"-delivery of pain medication when they can no longer do so for themselves. It has been used to help manage postoperative pain in patients without the ability to do so, or in end-of-life situations. Ideally, the PCA device is activated only by direct request of the patient or in response to clearly identified indications of pain. CCA is controversial for a variety of reasons, including marginally educated PCA activators, handing off responsibility to other family members or caregivers who have not received appropriate training, and excessive dosing in response to the wrong cues leading to patient injury or death. PCA by proxy was the topic of a sentinel alert issued by the Joint Commission on Accreditation of Healthcare Organizations (JCAHO) in 2004 [6] and a safety alert from the Institute for Safe Medication Practices (ISMP) in 2005 [7].

Other issues regarding the inherent safety of PCA devices need to be resolved for the future but are not widely reported in the medical literature. These complications include overdose, drug switches, inaccurate drug delivery, and others. Improved devices capable of recognizing the drug, its concentration, and common dosing, in addition to improved delivery accuracy, may reduce device-related and human-related errors but may not make significant changes in most routine outcomes [8].

Tramadol is a "minor" synthetic opioid and is often used for moderate postoperative pain. Tramadol does not cause respiratory depression like its opioid cousins and may therefore confer an advantage over other opioids in the treatment of postoperative pain. Tramadol is manufactured in oral, rectal, and injectable forms. The oral form can be immediate release or extended release. The immediate-release formulation is administered every 6 hours and the extended-release formulation is given once a day. For moderate to moderately severe postoperative pain, 50–100 mg every 4–6 hours can be administered, not to exceed 400 mg per day. Outside the United States, tramadol has been administered rectally, intravenously, and epidurally as well. Studies have shown that tramadol added to morphine PCA reduces the total dose of morphine required [9]. Tramadol has also been used effectively for PCA following major surgical procedures and may be associated with improved cognitive function [10,11]. Tramadol has a better side-effect profile than traditional opioids. However, they still occur. Common side effects include nausea, vomiting, dry mouth, dizziness, drowsiness, and sedation, as well as orthostatic hypotension. More serious side effects include angioedema and serotonin toxicity. Tramadol should not be given in combination with monoamine oxidase inhibitors and should be used with caution in patients receiving tricyclic antidepressants. It should also be used in caution in people with liver or kidney dysfunction.

NSAIDs

Nonsteroidal anti-inflammatory drugs (NSAIDs) are a diverse group of drugs commonly used as adjuncts for postoperative analgesia. They include aspirin, the cyclooxygenase (COX-1 and COX-2) mixed drugs, and the COX-2 selective inhibitors. For mild to moderate postoperative pain, they can be used as a sole analgesic. However, because there is a limit to their analgesic efficacy but not their toxicity, NSAIDs are often used in combination with other analgesics. NSAIDs have been shown to have a synergistic effect on analgesia when combined with opioids, resulting in an opioid-sparing effect. The effects of nonselective NSAIDs on platelet function have been the source of some controversy regarding their use in the perioperative period to provide analgesia and reduce opioid requirements. In studies examining the use of ketorolac in a variety of surgical procedures, no adverse effects on bleeding have been demonstrated [12,13].

Aspirin irreversibly binds to cyclooxygenase and has prolonged adverse effects on platelet function. Other NSAIDs reversibly bind to cyclooxygenase and may be safer in the pre- and postoperative setting with respect to their effects on platelet function. Ketorolac is a potent analgesic that has the unique advantage of availability in both an oral and parenteral form. However, it has a limited duration of use, with sustained administration associated with significant risk for ulcer and/or gastrointestinal bleeding.

The newer, selective COX-2 inhibitors provide effective analgesia while minimizing the adverse gastrointestinal effects common with nonselective NSAIDs. In addition, they do not affect platelet function as do the nonselective NSAIDs.

There has been a theoretical concern that mixed COX-1/2 and COX-2 inhibitors inhibit bone healing via their prostaglandin effects. As a result, there has been controversy over whether COX-2 inhibitors should be used in surgical procedures such as spinal fusion surgery. Studies regarding the effects of nonselective NSAIDs on bone healing after spinal fusion surgery have conflicting conclusions [14,15]. COX-2 inhibitors have been used preoperatively as well as postoperatively as part of a multimodal analgesic regimen for a wide variety of orthopedic surgical procedures without significant evidence of bony ingrowth inhibition.

Paracetamol (acetaminophen) is an NSAID often used in conjunction with other analgesics. It provides analgesia similar to other NSAIDs, with no effects on platelet function and little risk of gastrointestinal bleeding. It also has antipyretic properties, which makes it an alluring choice of analgesic in clinical situations where fever and pain coexist. There are many combination over-the-counter products containing paracetamol, and one must use caution when administering paracetamol or paracetamol/opioid combination analgesics to postoperative patients. Accidental overdose is a common adverse event associated with paracetamol-containing preparations.

Other drugs

Ketamine is phencyclidine derivative with NMDA-receptor antagonist properties, commonly used intraoperatively as part of a balanced anesthetic. Used in conjunction with opioids and local anesthetics, ketamine may reduce postoperative opioid requirements. Ketamine has been used in conjunction with patient-controlled opioids. Its efficacy in improving postoperative analgesia is controversial. Ketamine is frequently associated with bad dreams and hallucinations when administered as a sole drug at anesthetic doses. Subanesthetic doses used for postoperative analgesia do not tend to cause these side effects. Some studies suggest an improvement in postoperative analgesia, reduced opioid requirements, and a better side-effect profile, while others show no significant benefit [16,17].

Clonidine and dexmedetomidine are α_2-agonists that may be used as adjuncts for postoperative analgesia. Clonidine stimulates α_2-receptors in the dorsal horn and has some local anesthetic effects. It is manufactured in numerous forms and has been utilized for neuraxial analgesia and prolongation of peripheral nerve-block analgesia, as well as for intravenous and transdermal administration [18,19]. The transdermal patch is easy to use and is the preferred route for clonidine administration. It has been shown to be efficacious when used for pre-emptive analgesia. Clonidine can cause hypotension and bradycardia. Caution must be taken with use in the postoperative patient who has been volume-restricted or who had a large intraoperative blood loss and is already hemodynamically unstable. Other common side effects include dry mouth, fatigue, headache, and dizziness.

Dexmedetomidine is approved by the US Food and Drug Administration (FDA) for sedation in the intensive care setting and in nonintubated patients before and/or during surgical and other procedures. It is commonly used for conscious sedation and as an off-label adjunct to postoperative analgesia. It has been administered intravenously, added to epidural solutions, and given pre-emptively to reduce the total amount of morphine required postoperatively. Side effects of this drug, including sedation and hypertension, may limit its use [20].

Regional anesthesia

Techniques

Regional anesthesia is seeing tremendous growth in its use as an integral part of the postoperative analgesic plan. Brachial plexus blocks (e.g., cervical paravertebral, interscalene, infraclavicular, supraclavicular) and axillary plexus blocks are routinely used, either as single-shot injections with long-acting local anesthetics or as continuous catheter approaches for prolonged analgesia. Brachial plexus block selection is dependent on individual patient anatomy and the planned surgical procedure. For procedures involving the shoulder, cervical paravertebral or interscalene blocks are the most appropriate. For procedures involving the arm, the forearm, and the hand, supraclavicular or infraclavicular blocks are more useful.

A wide variety of lower extremity blocks are available. For surgical procedures involving the hip, thigh, and knee, blocks of the lumbar plexus such as a psoas compartment or lumbar paravertebral block and femoral nerve block are appropriate.

In the case of pain involving the posterior thigh or the leg below the knee, blocks of the sciatic nerve such as parasacral, Labat, subgluteal, or popliteal are all appropriate.

Regional analgesia has also seen growing use for procedures involving the chest, including breast surgery and thoracotomy. In this setting thoracic paravertebral blocks may be very helpful, either as single injections at the desired level or in combination with the insertion of a catheter for continuous infusion. These blocks may reduce the risk of sympathetic block and hemodynamic compromise commonly associated with epidural analgesia for similar procedures.

Local anesthetic infusions in peripheral nerve catheters are the norm, and in some cases they may include the addition of clonidine, though evidence for its use is weak [21]. Most peripheral nerve catheters can be maintained with infusion rates of 3–5 mL h^{-1}. In some cases it is beneficial to use patient-controlled regional analgesics in which a small infusion rate such as 3 mL h^{-1} is supplemented by intermittent boluses of 5–10 mL on patient demand. Although there is a role for increased infusion rates for blocks such as psoas compartment or thoracic paravertebral blocks, in general low-volume infusions are satisfactory for well-placed catheters. Increasing infusion rates for poorly placed catheters does little to maintain or salvage the block, and a better strategy may be either to implement patient-controlled regional analgesia or to manually bolus the catheter as needed and maintain the same infusion. Total dose of local anesthetic should be taken into consideration when determining infusion rates, especially in patients with more than one peripheral nerve catheter. Patients receiving peripheral nerve blocks should have special attention paid to padding of the extremities, especially those that have significant motor block and loss of sensation. In some cases, anesthetized limbs fall off pillows or lean up against the bed rails. In the absence of tactile sensation and position sense, the patient may not move the limb, and may develop pressure-related injury of the soft tissues or nerves.

There is growing use of peripheral nerve block analgesia on an outpatient basis, and in some cases its use has the theoretical ability to convert an inpatient procedure to an outpatient procedure [22–24].

Epidural analgesia has been used to provide high-quality postoperative analgesia following many types of surgical procedures. Epidural catheters can be successfully inserted in multiple regions of the spine, either percutaneously or under direct vision during spine surgery. One of the most important steps in obtaining successful postoperative analgesia with an epidural catheter is to choose the correct insertion site. For example, in patients undergoing thoracic surgical procedures, catheter insertion sites at T5–6 or T6–7 are utilized to provide metameric analgesia over the thorax. In patients undergoing abdominal surgical procedures, insertion sites from T7–8 to T10–11 are commonly used to provide metameric analgesia over the abdomen. This focused approach to catheter insertion site provides effective analgesia as well as motor and sensory sparing of the lower extremities, allowing the patient to ambulate without difficulty. In the case of lower extremity surgery, catheter insertion sites in the lumbar region produce effective analgesia, but often limit ambulation because of motor and sensory effects. Regardless of insertion site, the use of epidural analgesia often produces urinary retention requiring Foley catheterization.

Once the epidural catheter has been inserted, the choice of epidural infusion solution often varies widely from institution to institution and from patient to patient, depending on the patient's particular needs. Common epidural infusion solution components include local anesthetics, opioids, epinephrine, and clonidine. In general, combinations of local anesthetics and opioids are the most frequently used epidural infusion solutions and their relative amounts are often modified to reduce unwanted side effects or improve analgesia. Opioids commonly used in these solutions include hydrophilic drugs such as morphine and hydromorphone or the more lipophilic drugs such as fentanyl or occasionally sufentanil. The most common local anesthetics include bupivacaine, levobupivacaine, or ropivacaine, with infusion rates varying from 5 to $12\,mL\,h^{-1}$ in most adult patients. There is a wide variety of solutions used in various institutions, with no perfect solution available. One approach is to use a solution containing a mixture of bupivacaine and hydromorphone. If there are no contraindications, a relatively healthy patient may be given an epidural bolus of hydromorphone $10\,\mu g\,kg^{-1}$ followed by an infusion of hydromorphone $10\,\mu g\,mL^{-1}$ with bupivacaine 0.05% starting at $7\,mL\,h^{-1}$. If pain control is inadequate, the infusion rate may be increased in increments until it reaches $14\,mL\,h^{-1}$. If analgesia is inadequate despite changes in infusion rate and a patient's blood pressure will tolerate it, the infusion solution may be changed to hydromorphone $10\,\mu g\,mL^{-1}$ with bupivacaine 0.1%. The increased concentration of local anesthetic may produce improved analgesia, and in many cases it provides improved analgesia during activity as compared to solutions with more dilute local anesthetic. If a patient reports significant opioid-related side effects, it may be helpful to reduce the concentration of the opioid or remove it from the infusion altogether. There are many other opioid/local anesthetic combinations in common use that are also effective in providing analgesia.

If patient-controlled epidural analgesia (PCEA) is to be used, initial infusion rates of $3–5\,mL\,h^{-1}$ with patient-demand boluses of 2–4 mL every 20 minutes may be ordered. In children, infusion rates may be much lower and are often dependent on avoiding toxic local anesthetic concentrations based on body weight. Epidurals can either be run as continuous infusions or as PCEA [25]. More recently, there has been an effort to produce prolonged analgesia via a slow-release epidural opioid product. Extended-release epidural morphine has been utilized to provide successful analgesia for 48–72 hours following a single epidural administration of the compound [26]. There have been issues related to correct dose selection

and respiratory depression, in addition to the inability to safely use the compound in the epidural space in the presence of local anesthetic, that have limited its use. However, additional extended-release products are highly likely to be seen in the future. Routine monitoring for these patients needs to be part of the postoperative pain orders. This includes traditional vital signs with special attention to respiratory rate and level of alertness. This should be done hourly during the first 24 hours in patients receiving intraspinal opioids to facilitate detection of respiratory depression. Current practice guidelines for the prevention, detection, and management of respiratory depression associated with neuraxial opioid administration were approved by the American Society of Anesthesiologists (ASA) in October 2008 and published in 2009 [27].

Intrathecal analgesia has seen widespread use for postoperative analgesia since its first description in 1979 [28]. In early trials with intrathecal morphine, doses were quite large and profound sedation and respiratory depression was common. Subsequent study has clearly demonstrated that relatively small doses of intrathecal opioids are capable of producing prolonged, high-quality analgesia. In most patients, 200–250 μg of preservative-free intrathecal morphine provides adequate analgesia, and the efficacy of doses larger than this in opioid-naive patients is often limited by side effects. More recently, clinical trials have attempted to establish optimal dosing regimens for specific surgical procedures. Intrathecal morphine analgesia has been studied for pain control after cesarean section, a variety of orthopedic procedures, thoracotomy, and cardiac surgery. Optimal doses vary to a significant degree. Doses <100 μg are often sufficient for pain control following cesarean section [29].

Infusions of local anesthetics via catheters placed within surgical wounds or joints, and along various nerves and nerve plexuses, have become commonplace for a wide variety of surgical procedures [30–35]. The development of elastometric pumps with continuous infusion rates, variable infusion rates, and the ability to deliver intermittent boluses has fostered increased use. In addition, a wide variety of disposable electronic infusion devices or electronic infusion pumps with disposable cassettes are now available. In most cases, a long-lasting local anesthetic such as bupivacaine or ropivacaine is used for the infusions. Inpatient catheters are usually followed by the surgical service or an acute postoperative pain service. Infusion catheters are left in for 2–3 days and in the outpatient setting are removed by the patient or a family member at home following written and verbal instructions given at the time of discharge, with telephone support available if necessary. However, home infusions of local anesthetics or opioids into the epidural space for postoperative analgesia are extremely uncommon.

Clinical outcomes

There is a strong belief that epidural and peripheral regional analgesia produces improved outcomes for postoperative recovery. In many cases beliefs exceed the available data, although there are areas in which clear efficacy has been established. Epidural analgesia has been associated with a reduction in systemic opioid requirements for postoperative analgesia. A meta-analysis examined the effects of postoperative analgesic therapies on pulmonary outcome. Compared with systemic opioids, epidural opioids decreased the incidence of atelectasis and had a weak tendency to reduce the incidence of pulmonary infections [36]. Epidural local anesthetics increased P_aO_2, and decreased the incidence of pulmonary infections and pulmonary complications overall compared with systemic opioids. A meta-analysis examining the efficacy of postoperative epidural analgesia found that regardless of analgesic drug, catheter location, and type and time of pain assessment, epidural analgesia provided better postoperative analgesia than parenteral opioids [37]. Another meta-analysis evaluating analgesia after abdominal surgery found that continuous epidural analgesia was superior to intravenous opioid PCA for up to 72 hours, but was associated with a higher incidence of pruritus [38]. The ability of epidural analgesia to reduce postoperative ileus is controversial, and it is most likely to be successful when only local anesthetic is infused as part of an opioid-free analgesic regimen in an overall accelerated recovery protocol.

The use of peripheral regional analgesia has shown beneficial effects for postoperative analgesia in several studies. A preincisional paravertebral block provided good postoperative pain control and reduced the prevalence of chronic pain after breast surgery [39]. A meta-analysis found that epidural analgesia and peripheral nerve block for total knee arthroplasty provided comparable pain relief and rehabilitation, although peripheral nerve blocks had a smaller side-effect profile [40]. However, a study comparing single-injection versus continuous femoral nerve block with continuous infusions in the context of an established clinical pathway demonstrated improved analgesia and decreased opioid requirements for the first two postoperative days, but there was no difference in hospital length of stay or long-term functional recovery [41].

Complications

Epidural analgesia has been associated with several complications, including respiratory depression, epidural abscess, meningitis, epidural hematoma, and direct spinal cord injury. Respiratory depression related to neuraxial opioids has been reported by multiple authors and in the ASA closed claims database [42]. This complication is directly related to the dose of neuraxial opioid and the concurrent use of other opioids or centrally acting sedatives. Epidural abscesses and fatal meningitis have been reported in association with epidural analgesia. Meticulous attention to sterile technique during placement and subsequent management, as well as limiting the duration of catheter use, may help to reduce this risk. Epidural hematoma is a severe complication of epidural analgesia. The risk of this

complication is elevated in patients with pre-existing coagulation abnormalities and in those receiving medical anticoagulants. Use of the American Society of Regional Anesthesia guidelines may help to reduce this risk [43]. Detection of epidural hematoma requires vigilance and attention to details such as neurologic examination during the postoperative period while the epidural is in place and if abnormalities occur after catheter removal. Prompt detection does not guarantee a good outcome, but improves the patient's chances. Direct spinal cord injury may occur during epidural catheter placement [44]. There is controversy regarding the utility of avoiding placement of epidural catheters while patients are anesthetized as a means of avoiding this complication.

Regional analgesia offers many benefits, although it is not without risk. Complications can be difficult, challenging, and potentially catastrophic. Some blocks have a long history, and their potential risks and benefits have been clearly defined, as have methods for avoiding complications. Other new blocks or approaches may not have an extensive list of reported complications. This may reflect increased safety or simply lack of sufficient time, experience, or reporting of complications for newer techniques.

Some complications are relatively universal to all regional analgesic techniques. Local anesthetic toxicity may produce a number of untoward events. Intramuscular injections of local anesthetic are associated with myotoxicity and myonecrosis. In most cases this is minor; however, frequent or prolonged injection may produce permanent muscular injury [45]. Injection of local anesthetic into cerebrospinal fluid can lead to neurotoxicity or transient neurologic symptoms related to the local anesthetic or any preservatives used in preparing the drug for storage. Intravascular local anesthetic injection may produce a significant range of side effects including tinnitus, visual changes, sedation, seizure, and severe cardiotoxicity leading to arrhythmia and cardiac arrest. In most cases, careful frequent aspiration during injection, using a test dose containing local anesthetic and epinephrine, and allowing sufficient time to elapse after injection of the test dose, can help detect either intravascular or subarachnoid injection. In addition, visual confirmation of local anesthetic spread without evidence of vascular uptake during ultrasound-guided blocks may also prevent intravascular injection. However, these precautions do not always reveal improper needle placement. If large amounts of local anesthetic are administered intravenously, the consequences can be severe. Recent work has demonstrated that the use of Intralipid may be helpful in some settings during resuscitation from local anesthetic overdose [46]. Additional information regarding the role of Intralipid may be found at www.lipidrescue.org.

Brachial plexus blocks have been associated with a wide variety of complications. The cervical paravertebral block originally described by Kappis and Pippa with improvements made by Boezaart has theoretical benefits over the traditional interscalene block [47,48]. At present, there have been no reports of direct intravascular injection or brachial plexus injury using the cervical paravertebral approach. However, the cervical paravertebral approach to the brachial plexus has been associated with Horner's syndrome, dyspnea, superficial skin infection, posterior neck pain, subclavian artery puncture, spinal or epidural anesthesia, and spinal cord injury. The risk of these latter complications may be increased with the use of small, sharp needles, which are more likely to bend and move off course or pierce the dura or other neural structures. Interscalene blocks have been associated with intravascular injections, phrenic nerve injury, spinal or epidural anesthesia, intraneural injection, and direct spinal cord injury. It has been recommended that needles longer than 25–50 mm should not be used for interscalene blocks as this is typically a very superficial block. Performance of interscalene blocks under general anesthesia is relatively contraindicated and the needle should always have a slight caudad direction to decrease the risk of entering and passing through the C6–7 neural foramen [49]. Supraclavicular blocks have primarily been implicated in the development of ipsilateral pneumothorax, and a variety of approaches to reduce the potential risk of this complication have been described. A retrospective analysis of 2020 subclavian supraclavicular blocks in a single center over 11 years reported no incidence of pneumothorax or other major complication [50]. Contemporary approaches to supraclavicular brachial plexus block using ultrasound guidance may further increase the safety and utility of the supraclavicular approach, with the ability to visualize the major vessels, the brachial plexus, the first rib, and the dome of the lung. Infraclavicular blocks have been associated with vascular puncture and hematoma as well as pneumothorax. In rare cases, proximal spread of local anesthetic may produce ipsilateral hemidiaphragmatic dysfunction with resultant respiratory embarrassment [51]. Axillary blocks have been associated with hematoma formation, infection during continuous nerve block, and direct nerve injury. Reported rates of complications associated with this approach to the brachial plexus range from 1% to as high as 19% [52,53]. Thoracic paravertebral blocks have been associated with some unique complications or side effects such as the simultaneous appearance of Harlequin and Horner's syndromes [54]. They have also been associated with hypotension, vascular puncture, pleural puncture, pneumothorax, spinal and epidural anesthesia, and postdural puncture headache [55–57]. Lumbar paravertebral blocks have been associated with a variety of unique complications related to the deep location of the structures to be blocked and the close proximity of the retroperitoneal and peritoneal spaces. In a report of two cases, the lumbar plexus was approached at the L3 level using a loss-of-resistance technique [58]. Within 1 day, both patients developed intense low back pain, and it was discovered that the block needle had penetrated the renal capsule and had produced a renal subcapsular hematoma. There have been a number of case reports and case series of patients experiencing bleeding complications related to the use of enoxaparin either before or after performance of a lumbar paravertebral block [59,60]. It is worth noting that in these cases patients reported low back pain and had anemia without frank evidence of neurologic dysfunction. Lumbar paravertebral blocks have also been associated with the development of spinal and epidural anesthesia.

Lower extremity blocks commonly used for postoperative analgesia include femoral, obturator, sciatic, and popliteal. Femoral nerve blocks have been associated with very few complications beyond hematoma formation and occasional persistent paresthesias, and have a relative paucity of reported complications [27]. Using continuous femoral catheters, colonization of the catheters is extremely common, while frank infection is rare [61]. Sciatic nerve block is performed using a variety of approaches including the approach of Labat, parasacral, anterior, lateral, subgluteal, and supine lithotomy. The anterior approach has been associated with the highest rate of failure and complications. A probable direct neural injury occurred after a high-pressure injection and was manifested as a prolonged sciatic nerve block and subsequent neuropraxia of the common peroneal nerve with persistent pain radiating along the sciatic nerve. Other reported complications include the development of hematoma following continuous catheter removal in patients receiving enoxaparin [62]. Popliteal nerve blocks have not been associated with a significant number of reported complications. For example, peripheral neuropathy was seen in 3 of 952 popliteal nerve blocks, although long-term outcomes were not specifically identified [63].

Avoiding complications is most often the direct result of particular attention to detail regarding the indications for the block, patient selection, paying careful attention to issues regarding anticoagulation and antisepsis, using good block technique, choosing the best drug combination, and monitoring during and after the procedure. Although patient factors play a role, it is frequently the regional anesthesiologist who plays the biggest role in avoiding or producing significant complications.

Multimodal analgesia

Multimodal analgesia is the practice of using two or more analgesics for the treatment of pain. It is thought that using more than one analgesic will result in an additive or a synergistic effect. Further, it is thought that by combining different analgesics with different pharmacologic properties, there will be a reduction in the amount of each analgesic required, which will possibly reduce drug-specific adverse effects. Opioids, NSAIDs, local anesthetics, ketamine, and α_2-agonists have all been used to provide multimodal analgesia. Multimodal analgesia has been shown to reduce overall pain scores following a variety of surgical procedures, including orthopedic, gynecologic, and abdominal surgeries.

Several meta-analyses have been conducted to evaluate the effectiveness of multimodal analgesia for postoperative pain.

A critical appraisal of acute postsurgical pain management practice was undertaken in 2006 and many of these studies were critically reviewed [64]. The evidence suggested that multimodal analgesia techniques involving multiple dosing or infusions of nonspecific NSAIDS or COX-2 inhibitors produced an opioid-sparing effect and improved pain control after surgical procedures. However, the opioid dose reduction did not translate into a decrease in opioid-related adverse events or side effects. Paracetamol or single-dose NSAID regimens do not appear to produce an opioid-sparing effect or improved pain control after surgical procedures. NSAIDs, when used in combination with intravenous morphine PCA, reduce total opioid requirement in the postoperative period.

Gabapentin has been studied as a component of multimodal pain regimens, with promising results including reduced pain at rest and with movement and reduced opioid requirements [65]. Gabapentin reduced acute pain and prevented some chronic pain after surgical procedures when used with local anesthetics for perioperative pain control [66,67].

Pre-emptive analgesia

The search for an effective means of providing consistent and reliable pre-emptive analgesia has been the "holy grail" of perioperative analgesia. The theory that an intervention or medication(s) given prior to a surgical insult would be able to alter the cascade of events occurring after injury and result in diminished postoperative pain and a reduced risk of developing chronic pain has been investigated from numerous vantage points. In many cases, interventions have been successful in decreasing postoperative pain or the duration of severe postoperative pain, but a real reduction in the incidence of chronic pain following surgery has been difficult to achieve in most cases.

Gabapentin has been studied for its utility as a pre-emptive analgesic for a variety of surgical procedures including spine surgery, orthopedic procedures, and major abdominal procedures. It had significant opioid-sparing effects and decreased pain scores during the postoperative period if given prior to surgical procedures. The efficacious gabapentin dose ranged from 300 to 1200 mg given orally 1–2 hours before surgery [68–72]. However, the optimal dosing regimen has yet to be determined. Gabapentin studies vary with regard to the amount of medication and the number of doses used for pre-emptive analgesia. However, gabapentin has consistently proven its function as a pre-emptive analgesic.

Pregabalin is most commonly used for the treatment of neuropathic pain. It has not been extensively studied as a pre-emptive analgesic. However, studies investigating the efficacy of pregabalin as a pre-emptive analgesic for dental pain, and for laparoscopic hysterectomy and other gynecological procedures, have suggested that pregabalin may reduce overall postsurgical pain scores and reduce the amount of opioid analgesics required postoperatively [73].

NSAIDs have been used for pre-emptive analgesia with good success. Celecoxib given during the perioperative period has been shown to reduce recovery time, total opioid use, and postoperative pain [74]. Traditional NSAIDs used during the pre- and perioperative period have also been shown to decrease the postoperative opioid requirements and the opioid-related side effects.

The use of intravenous and epidural ketamine as a preemptive analgesic has been studied. It has been suggested that subanesthetic doses of intravenous ketamine ($0.25\,\mathrm{mg\,kg^{-1}}$ bolus followed by $0.5\,\mathrm{mg\,kg^{-1}\,h^{-1}}$ intraoperative infusion) reduce postoperative pain and opioid requirements [75,76].

Dexmedetomine and clonidine are intravenous α_2-agonists that have been used as pre-emptive analgesics with good results. Preoperative intravenous dexmedetomidine significantly reduced the opioid requirement for postoperative pain control [77]. Studies investigating the role of epidural clonidine as a pre-emptive analgesic have demonstrated its ability to lower the total opioid requirement in the immediate postoperative period, with reduced sedation and pain scores [78,79]. Intravenous, transdermal, and oral administration of clonidine have also been studied.

Preincisional utilization of epidural analgesia has been widely studied for its efficacy in reducing postoperative pain and total postoperative opioid requirement. Studies have shown that epidural local anesthetic, opioid, or a combination of both, when administered prior to surgical incision, results in significantly better postoperative pain control when compared to those patients receiving no medications in the epidural space. Surgical procedures in which pre-emptive epidural analgesia has been used with success include abdominal surgery, thoracic surgery, lumbar laminectomy and fusion, gynecologic surgery, and orthopedic surgery. Patients who received pre-emptive epidural analgesia had lower overall postsurgical pain scores, prolonged time to first rescue medication, and reduced total postoperative opioid requirement. The time interval between epidural administration of analgesia and incision ranged from immediately before incision to 25 minutes before incision [80–83].

Epidural morphine and intravenous ketamine administered individually provided good pre-emptive analgesia, but the combination of epidural morphine and intravenous ketamine given preoperatively produced the most effective reduction of postoperative pain scores and cumulative postoperative morphine consumption in patients undergoing gastrectomy [84]. The dose of epidural morphine was $0.06\,\mathrm{mg\,kg^{-1}}$ 40 minutes before incision followed by a maintenance intraoperative infusion of $0.02\,\mathrm{mg\,kg^{-1}\,h^{-1}}$ until skin closure. Intravenous ketamine was given as a bolus of $1\,\mathrm{mg\,kg^{-1}}$ 10 minutes before incision followed by a maintenance intraoperative infusion of $0.5\,\mathrm{mg\,kg^{-1}\,h^{-1}}$ until skin closure. Naloxone was administered intravenously immediately after surgery to prevent lasting effects of the morphine. Epidural ketamine alone, given before surgical incision, did not result in a reduction in postoperative meperidine consumption [85].

Chronic postoperative pain

Chronic pain following surgical procedures is common and has been described after a wide variety of surgical procedures [27,86]. This includes, but is not limited to, pain following mastectomy, thoracotomy, nephrectomy, hernia repair, spine surgery, and amputation. In some cases, postsurgical pain may have a detrimental effect on overall quality of life, and it can be disabling. Attempts to prevent this have met with limited success, but ongoing efforts to prevent this potentially devastating complication have continued along numerous fronts. These efforts have been successful in a very limited number of situations thus far.

Chronic pain following breast surgery is common and occurs more often after breast-conserving surgery than radical surgery. A variety of perioperative factors have been considered as potential causes of persistent pain following breast surgery. The most important seem to be intensity of acute postoperative pain and the type of operation. Regional lymph node involvement and radiotherapy have also been identified as important factors. Paravertebral blocks may be used as a sole anesthetic, but are more commonly used before or after induction of general anesthesia to provide postoperative analgesia. The success of thoracic paravertebral blocks for breast surgery pain appears to be an exception to the generally poor experience with pre-emptive analgesia for many other types of surgical procedures. In one study, preincisional paravertebral blocks provided good postoperative pain control and reduced the prevalence of chronic pain after breast surgery [39]. The investigation followed 60 patients for 1 year following breast cancer surgery, with 30 in the paravertebral block group and 30 in the control group. One month after surgery, the intensity of motion-related pain was lower in the paravertebral group. Six months after surgery, the prevalence of any pain symptoms was lower in the paravertebral group. Twelve months after surgery, the prevalence of pain symptoms, intensity of motion-related pain, and intensity of pain at rest was lower in the paravertebral group. This was independent of whether or not an axillary dissection had been performed. It was emphasized that the importance of surgical sparing of the intercostobrachial nerves during axillary dissection was still vital. In a much shorter observation period, the use of EMLA (lidocaine and prilocaine) cream on the breast and axilla, initiated before surgery and continued for 4 days postoperatively, was reported to reduce the incidence of chronic pain in the area of surgery 3 months after surgery [87]. Additional studies with more participants will be required to determine if this indeed has solved the problem related to breast surgery.

Chronic pain following both open and laparoscopic hernia repair is extremely common and often has devastating effects on patients' ability to work or engage in normal activities of daily living. Several techniques have been evaluated in attempts to reduce the incidence of this devastating complication of what is an otherwise relatively minor surgery, including preoperative NSAIDs, anticonvulsants, paravertebral blocks, spinal anesthesia, epidural anesthesia, local infiltration, and postoperative local anesthetic infusions. Despite all of these approaches, no consistently effective means of producing effective pre-emptive analgesia or preventing or eliminating chronic pain following hernia repair has thus far been identified.

The incidence of phantom limb pain following both traumatic and elective amputation is extremely common, approaching 80% in some surveys. In those experiencing phantom limb pain, more than a quarter have pain at least 20 days per month. The high incidence has led to a variety of attempts to limit or eliminate the pain. In planned amputation, psychological counseling may be useful in decreasing psychologic distress. Various surgical techniques for handling the severed nerve and vasculature have been proposed, although none has been proven to reduce postamputation pain. Postoperative compression wrapping or hard casting to reduce stump edema may facilitate rehabilitation, but it is not certain that this reduces pain. Epidural infusions of morphine and bupivacaine, alone or in combination, have been demonstrated to prevent phantom limb pain in patients with pre-existing limb pain. In addition, clonidine has been an effective analgesic when applied epidurally. A perioperative epidural infusion of diamorphine, bupivacaine, and clonidine in patients with pre-existing limb pain was evaluated for preventing postoperative phantom limb pain in a prospective controlled study of 24 patients undergoing lower limb amputation [88]. An epidural infusion containing bupivacaine 75 mg, clonidine 150 mg and diamorphine 5 mg in 60 mL normal saline was given at $1–4\,mL\,h^{-1}$ 24–48 hours preoperatively and maintained for at least 3 days postoperatively ($n = 13$). The control group ($n = 11$) received on-demand opioid analgesia. Pain was assessed by visual analog scale at 7 days, 6 months, and 1 year. At 1-year follow-up, one epidural patient and eight controls had phantom pain, and two patients in the epidural group versus eight controls had phantom limb sensation. There was no significant difference between groups in the incidence of stump pain. In one study of patients amputated for nonmalignant disease, a threefold reduction in the incidence of phantom pain 1 year after amputation was found after 72 hours of preoperative treatment with an epidural infusion of morphine and bupivacaine [89]. A more recent investigation, however, failed to replicate these results [90,91]. A small case series using 0.25% bupivacaine infusion through nerve sheath catheters for analgesia following upper extremity amputation in six patients reported complete analgesia in all patients by postoperative day 2, low opioid consumption, and phantom limb pain in three patients during follow-up evaluation. It was concluded that continuous local anesthetic perfusion of amputated nerves via a catheter placed under direct vision provided excellent postoperative analgesia [92]. A similar trial found that 72-hour postoperative perineural infusions of bupivacaine provided effective pain relief, but did not prevent residual or phantom limb pain in patients undergoing lower extremity amputation secondary to ischemic changes produced by peripheral vascular disease [93]. The preoperative application of opioids, local anesthetics, α-agonists and excitatory amino-acid receptor antagonists to prevent central nervous system consequences of amputation is being tested in animal models and humans.

Ambulatory analgesia

Analgesia following outpatient surgery is typically achieved with oral drugs. In some cases, minor surgical procedures may have little or no pain associated with them and may not require any analgesics. However, in most cases, oral analgesics ranging from NSAIDs to strong opioids may be prescribed. In some situations NSAIDs and/or an anticonvulsant such as gabapentin may be given preoperatively as part of a multimodal analgesic regimen intended to produce pre-emptive analgesia. The most commonly employed oral analgesics are combinations such as codeine/paracetamol, hydrocodone/paracetamol, and oxycodone/paracetamol taken in doses of 1–2 tablets every 4–6 hours. Less commonly, small doses of extended-release oxycodone or hydromorphone are prescribed.

In recent years, there has been increased use of various wound infusion devices to provide analgesia. These typically consist of a multiorifice catheter inserted into the surgical wound, which is then infused with dilute local anesthetic via either an elastomeric or an electric infusion pump. These pumps have well-established efficacy and have been used in a variety of settings ranging from abdominal surgery to orthopedic procedures [94,95]. They have the advantage of simple continuous use and may reduce or eliminate the need for opioids, with a resultant decrease in undesirable side effects. Infusion devices are capable of infusing one or two catheters, and may have adjustable rates and the ability to deliver on-demand bolus doses. Although there is a theoretical risk of local-anesthetic toxicity either from accumulation or from inadvertant large doses, this is extremely uncommon under normal circumstances. In most cases, infusion catheters may be removed by the patient or a family member after appropriate education and with ready access to medical advice or care if needed. These catheters have a small risk of catheter-related infection. Recently several case series of shoulder arthroscopy patients who developed severe chondrolysis after receiving large doses of intra-articular local anesthetics have been published, raising concerns about the safety of using these devices in the shoulder surgery patient [96,97].

The use of regional anesthesia/analgesia to provide acute postoperative analgesia in the outpatient setting is extremely common and effective. This is especially useful for patients undergoing extremity procedures, often orthopedic or podiatric, that are amenable to regional anesthesia as a primary anesthetic technique. The patient is often able to skip first-stage recovery and go directly to second-stage recovery, resulting in faster discharge from the surgical center. In some cases, blocks are performed in conjunction with a general anesthetic for the sole purpose of providing postoperative analgesia. These blocks may be done either as single-shot techniques using short- or long-acting local anesthetics, or as continuous techniques with perineural catheters to deliver continuous or intermittent bolus doses of local anesthetic. The consequent ability to markedly reduce or eliminate the use of opioid analgesics often helps to reduce undesirable side effects, improve analgesia, and facilitate rapid discharge from the outpatient surgery facility [98]. The use of neuraxial techniques is not favored, as the duration of action must be limited to facilitate rapid discharge. In addition, the potentially devastating side effects such as respiratory depression and death occurring after administration of neuraxial opioids in an unmonitored outpatient setting make these techniques impractical for outpatient use.

There is a wide variety of nonpharmacologic techniques that may be employed to provide analgesia. These range from simple comfort measures or distraction to transcutaneous electrical nerve stimulation (TENS), massage, and others with proven efficacy and physiologic benefit. The use of cold to reduce swelling and decrease pain is a well-established technique. Modern passive and active devices, such as Cryo Cuff and Game Ready, which have fitted cooling sleeves and a means of circulating ice water to maintain cool temperatures in conjunction with compression for orthopedic procedures involving the knee and shoulder, are common. These devices maintain specific temperatures to reduce the risk of cold-related injury. TENS has demonstrated efficacy in providing improved analgesia and reducing the need for opioids after a variety of surgical procedures. Although not commonly used, it is an effective modality in some patients and may be a useful alternative when opioids are poorly tolerated [99,100].

Inadequate analgesia and drug- or anesthesia-related side effects are common causes of unexpected admission or readmission following planned outpatient surgical procedures [101,102]. Although NSAIDs or opioid/paracetamol combinations are often sufficient to provide adequate analgesia, this does not always occur, and alternative approaches should be available.

Inpatient analgesia for special populations

Opioid-tolerant patients

There are numerous instances when patients with opioid tolerance present for planned or emergent surgery. Opioid tolerance may result from chronic use of opioids for non-cancer or cancer pain, prolonged hospitalization, or illicit use. Regardless of the etiology, opioid-tolerant patients pose a special challenge with respect to management of postoperative pain. Chronic opioid use produces numerous systemic changes that affect pain perception. These include hormonal changes, reduced thresholds to develop a pain response, and neurotransmitter and information processing changes at the spinal cord [103,104]. Opioid-tolerant patients typically require postoperative opioid doses in excess and sometimes far in excess of what is normally encountered. Chronic opioid users require a certain amount of postoperative opioid just to meet their daily preoperative consumption. In many cases, this amount alone is more than is commonly used to provide adequate postoperative analgesia to opioid-naive patients. Once the daily requirement is met, significant increases in total daily dose are required to provide adequate analgesia. This may be as much as 2–4 times the patient's preoperative requirement [105]. This amount often causes concern among prescribers unfamiliar with these patients, and in many cases patients never receive adequate analgesia. While markedly increased doses of opioids are commonly needed, this does always occur. In some cases, the surgical procedure relieves pain and the opioid requirements may be reduced. With postoperative PCA use, it is often useful to replace the normal daily opioid intake with a basal infusion rate and then allow the patient to use the demand button to obtain adequate analgesia. If able to tolerate oral intake, patients should be re-started on their preoperative opioid analgesic as a baseline, with additional oral or intravenous opioids to provide postoperative analgesia.

Opioid-tolerant patients are often excellent candidates for alternative analgesic approaches or multimodal approaches that minimize their need for opioids [106]. Use of local anesthetics for wound infiltration, peripheral nerve block, or epidural analgesia provides analgesia with a drug to which patients are not tolerant and is often sufficient as long as their daily opioid requirement is maintained to prevent withdrawal. Epidural opioids may be beneficial, but increased amounts may be required with this delivery approach, just as they would be with oral or intravenous drug. A multimodal approach with both pharmacologic (NSAIDs, anticonvulsants, or α-agonists) and nonpharmacologic approaches (heat, ice, TENS, elevation, massage, distraction, biofeedback, and others) may be helpful.

Opioid-tolerant patients should ideally be identified preoperatively, so that appropriate planning can occur, either during the preoperative visit or rarely as a preoperative consultation. In either situation, patients should be advised of the clinical analgesic issues, presented with analgesic alternatives, understand the challenges, and have their questions answered. They should also be advised to take their morning dose of opioid preoperatively.

Children
Postoperative analgesia for the pediatric patient entails consideration of numerous special factors. Initial considerations include age, general health, drug choice, avoidance of toxicity, block or catheter placement, infusion management, coanalgesics, and pain evaluation. The parents' and/or nurses' assessment of the child's pain are important, because many children may not be able to communicate effectively regarding their pain. The pain practitioner must utilize age-appropriate assessment tools in order to obtain the most accurate assessments. The extent of the surgical procedure will also help to determine the analgesic regimen. Minor surgical procedures often only require paracetamol or NSAIDs for adequate postoperative pain control.

Morphine is commonly used for pediatric postoperative pain management. The usual morphine infusion is 0.02–0.03 mg kg^{-1} h^{-1}. Boluses can be given at 0.05 mg kg^{-1} every 2–3 hours. While morphine is an excellent choice for postoperative analgesia, it increases the risks of apnea, postoperative nausea and vomiting, constipation, and pruritus. Premature infants and neonates should be given morphine and other opioids with extreme caution to avoid apnea. Careful monitoring and titration are required. Intravenous PCA has been used with success in children above the age of 5 years. Intravenous PCA can be administered with a continuous rate and a demand dosing regimen or only demand dosing. Providing a continuous infusion can prevent gaps in analgesic delivery [107,108].

Regional anesthesia is increasingly popular in pediatric surgery. The many benefits of regional techniques, such as reduction in the amount of systemic analgesics required in the postoperative period, better postoperative pain scores, and less analgesic-specific adverse reactions, are not unique to children. Regional techniques can be utilized for a variety of surgical procedures including middle ear surgery, ophthalmologic procedures, urologic procedures, circumcisions, abdominal surgeries, orthopedic procedures, thoracic surgery, and cardiac surgery. Local wound infiltration either before incision or prior to closure can reduce systemic analgesic requirements. Lidocaine and bupivacaine are commonly used local anesthetics for this purpose. The maximum recommended dose is 7 mg kg^{-1} for lidocaine and 2.5 mg kg^{-1} for bupivacaine. Epinephrine 10 µg kg^{-1} can be added to prolong the local anesthetic effects. Nerve blocks and continuous peripheral nerve catheters are often used for pediatric orthopedic procedures. Local wound infiltration, ilioinguinal nerve block, and caudal analgesia are effective in the early postoperative period following subumbilical surgery. A caudal block is a commonly utilized regional technique for many subumbilical procedures. Local anesthetic with the addition of S-ketamine, clonidine, morphine, midazolam, neostigmine, and buprenorphine can create a long-lasting caudal block. Epidural analgesia with local anesthetic, with or without the addition of opioid or clonidine, is an effective therapy for major abdominal surgery [109]. Studies have suggested that ropivacaine and levobupivacaine are the local anesthetics of choice for regional anesthesia in the pediatric population owing to the reduced cardiac and CNS toxicity as well as less motor blockade. This is particularly true in infants and neonates. Bupivacaine is commonly used for continuous epidural infusions at $0.2\,mg\,kg^{-1}\,h^{-1}$ for infants and neonates and $0.4\,mg\,kg^{-1}\,h^{-1}$ for older children [110].

Kidney failure

Patients with severe renal insufficiency and renal failure can receive postoperative analgesia using all currently available techniques, and there are no specific contraindications. However, choice of drugs, dosing intervals, total doses, metabolism, and elimination are all major considerations. Many opioids (e.g., morphine, hydromorphone, codeine, oxycodone, meperidine) have active metabolites that are eliminated primarily via the kidney. These drugs should be limited or avoided if possible in favor of drugs with inactive metabolites or those primarily eliminated via the liver such as fentanyl. Peripheral nerve or plexus blocks or neuraxial analgesia may be appropriate options, but concerns about coagulation status may prevent the use of these techniques. These coagulation abnormalities are typically thought to be related to platelet dysfunction in the face of a normal platelet count, and in some cases to the use of heparin during dialysis. If epidural analgesia is selected, renally impaired patients may warrant increased observation to detect any bleeding complications. Local anesthetics in appropriate doses pose little additional risk in these patients and can be used in a variety of ways to improve postoperative analgesia.

Liver failure

Patients with hepatic failure have a variety of problems that complicate the provision of acute postoperative pain care. These include abnormal metabolism of commonly used analgesics with the potential for significant accumulation of active compound and the need for dose reduction [111]. In addition, decreased production of coagulation factors with accompanying bleeding disorders may prevent the use of neuraxial analgesia or peripheral nerve blocks. Hepatic insufficiency may be present for a variety of reasons and in some cases may occur in the immediate perioperative period due to hepatic resection, trauma, or other surgical procedures producing decreased hepatic blood flow or injury. In most cases, the necessary clinical action is to reduce the amount of drug given, because of likely accumulation. There are no specific guidelines to guide exact drug dosing as they relate to liver function. Codeine should be avoided altogether because it requires conversion to morphine in the liver, and that conversion may be impaired with moderate to severe disease. Dextropropoxyphene has been associated with liver toxicity in patients with liver disease. Meperidine may precipitate seizures at low doses in patients with hepatic encephalopathy. Constipation in association with opioids should be avoided as it my increase ammonia absorption and precipitate encephalopathy. Nonopioid analgesics are also affected. The plasma half-life of paracetamol is increased significantly in severe liver failure. The elimination half-life of aspirin and ibuprofen are not affected to a significant degree by hepatic disease, but naproxen has a

greatly increased elimination half-life and the dose may need to be reduced by 50%. Tramadol requires liver metabolism for bioactivation to the active metabolite, and therefore this drug should be avoided. Antiepileptics such as gabapentin or pregabalin may be part of a multimodal analgesic regimen in the patient with hepatic disease, but at present there are no data regarding their use to improve postoperative pain control. In general, gabapentin does not undergo any hepatic metabolism and is renally excreted. There should therefore be no specific contraindication to this compound. Pregabalin also undergoes minimal metabolism, and approximately 90% of the administered dose is recovered as unchanged pregabalin in the urine.

Heart failure

Postoperative analgesia in patients with congestive heart failure may be challenging for many reasons. The challenges relate to drugs being used for congestive heart failure, such as vasodilators to diminish blood pressure or anticoagulants to maintain cardiac stent patency. In addition, altered drug metabolism or elimination due to diminished hepatic or renal blood flow may produce undesirable side effects from commonly employed analgesic drugs and doses. In general, analgesics should be started in small doses and increased based on actual need. Ideally, drugs that have inactive metabolites are preferred over those with active metabolites that may accumulate.

Summary

Optimal postoperative analgesia is the product of a good understanding of the available options, consideration of the multidimensional character of pain, consideration of special patient characteristics or risks, and careful selection and expert use of individual drugs, techniques, or combinations thereof. Major approaches to treating postoperative pain include systemic analgesics, regional anesthesia, and multimodal analgesia, all of which may need adjustment in specific patient populations.

Among systemic analgesics, opioids are the most efficacious drugs for treating acute pain. Postoperatively, opioids are commonly administered using intravenous patient-controlled analgesia (PCA), and then switched to oral dosing when postoperative oral intake has resumed. It is important to be able to rapidly and accurately convert the dose of one opioid to another and from one route of administration to another. Morphine and hydromorphone are the most commonly used opioids in PCA. Pain control and patient satisfaction are improved with PCA compared with nurse-administered parenteral opioids. An inherent safety feature of PCA is that patients who are oversedated will not self-administer more medication. This safety feature is absent in patients receiving basal opioid infusions or when the PCA device is activated by another person. Opioid side effects (commonly pruritus, nausea, vomiting, constipation, urinary retention, and respiratory depression) occur regardless of route of administration. Nonsteroidal anti-inflammatory drugs (NSAIDs) are effective as a sole analgesic for mild to moderate postoperative pain. However, they have limited efficacy, and are used in combination with opioids for moderate–severe pain, where they decrease postoperative opioid requirements and opioid-related side effects. Ketamine has been used in conjunction with PCA, but its effectiveness in improving postoperative analgesia and reducing opioid requirements and opioid side effects is controversial.

Postoperative pain treatment with regional, neuraxial, and local anesthesia is common. There is growing use of peripheral nerve block analgesia for outpatient surgery, which may enable converting an inpatient procedure to an outpatient procedure. Brachial plexus blocks, as single-shot injections with long-acting local anesthetics or continuous catheters for prolonged analgesia, are routinely used. Lumbar plexus and peripheral nerve blocks are used for lower-extremity surgery. Epidural analgesia, including both continuous infusions and/ or patient-controlled administration, provides effective postoperative pain relief for many types of surgical procedures. Combinations of local anesthetics (typically bupivacaine,

levobupivacaine, or ropivacaine) and opioids (typically morphine, hydromorphone, or fentanyl) are most frequently used. Intrathecal opioids also produce prolonged, high-quality analgesia. Local anesthetics infused through catheters placed in or near surgical wounds, joints, various nerves, and nerve plexuses, using elastometric pumps or disposable electronic infusion devices, have become commonplace. The use of regional anesthesia/analgesia for acute postoperative analgesia in outpatients is common and effective. Therapy for chronic postoperative pain presents more challenges.

Although postoperative analgesia is far from perfect, and many patients still experience significant postoperative pain, there is unquestionable ability to provide high-quality postoperative pain control. It requires the will and the financial resources to apply multidisciplinary multimodal analgesic techniques to the broad spectrum of patients and disease processes encountered in the perioperative period. Ongoing research and new discoveries will no doubt change current practice and provide better tools to provide excellent acute postoperative pain control and reduce the risk of developing chronic life-limiting pain following major injury or surgery.

References

1. Ahles TA, Blanchard EB, Ruckdeschel JC. The multidimensional nature of cancer-related pain. *Pain* 1983; **17**: 277–88.

2. Ballantyne JC, Carr DB, Chalmers TC, *et al.* Postoperative patient-controlled analgesia: meta-analyses of initial randomized control trials. *J Clin Anesth* 1993; **5**: 182–93.

3. Walder B, Schafer M, Henzi I, Tramer MR. Efficacy and safety of patient-controlled opioid analgesia for acute postoperative pain: a quantitative systematic review. *Acta Anaesthesiol Scand* 2001; **45**: 795–804.

4. Sveticic G, Farzanegan F, Zmoos P, *et al.* Is the combination of morphine with ketamine better than morphine alone for postoperative intravenous patient-controlled analgesia? *Anesth Analg* 2008; **106**: 287–293.

5. Murdoch CJ, Crooks BA, Miller CD. Effect of the addition of ketamine to morphine in patient-controlled analgesia. *Anaesthesia* 2002; **57**: 484–8.

6. Joint Commission. Patient controlled analgesia by proxy. Sentinel Event Alert 33, December 20, 2004. www. jointcommission.org/SentinelEvents/ SentinelEventAlert/sea_33.htm (accessed May 31, 2010).

7. Institute for Safe Medication Practices. Safety issues with patient-controlled analgesia [Parts 1 & 2]. *Nurse Advise-ERR* 2005; **3** (1 & 2). www.ismp.org/ newsletters/nursing/backissues.asp (accessed May 31, 2010).

8. Rathmell JP, Wu C, Sinatra RS, *et al.* Acute post-surgical pain management: a critical appraisal of current practice. *Reg Anesth Pain Med* 2006; **31**: 1–42.

9. Webb AR, Leong S, Myles PS, Burn SJ. The addition of a Tramadol infusion to morphine patient-controlled analgesia after abdominal surery: a double-blinded, placebo-controlled randomized trial. *Anesth Analg* 2002; **95**: 1713–18.

10. Hadi MA, Kamaruljan HS, Saedah A, Abdullah NM. A comparative study of intravenous patient-controlled analgesia morphine and tramadol in patients undergoing major operation. *Med J Malaysia* 2006; **61**: 570–6.

11. Ng KF, Yuen TS, Ng VM. A comparison of postoperative cognitive function and pain relief with fentanyl or tramadol patient-controlled analgesia. *J Clin Anesth* 2006; **18**: 205–10.

12. Chin KR, Sundram H, Marcotte P. Bleeding risk with ketorolac after lumbar microdiscectomy. *Spinal Disord Tech* 2007; **20**: 123–6.

13. Gupta A, Daggett C, Ludwick J, Wells W, Lewis A. Ketorolac after congenital heart surgery: does it increase the risk of significant bleeding complications? *Paediatr Anaesth* 2005; **15**: 139–42.

14. Lumawig JM, Yamazaki A, Watanabe K. Dose-dependent inhibition of diclofenac sodium on posterior lumbar interbody fusion rates. *Spine J* 2009; **9**: 343–9.

15. Sucato DJ, Lovejoy JF, Agrawal S, *et al.* Postoperative ketorolac does not predispose to pseudoarthrosis following posterior spinal fusion and instrumentation for adolescent idiopathic scoliosis. *Spine* 2008; **33**: 1119–24.

16. Zakine J, Samarcq D, Lorne E, *et al.* Postoperative ketamine administration decreases morphine consumption in major abdominal surgery: a prospective, randomized, double-blind, controlled study. *Anesth Analg* 2008; **106**: 1856–61.

17. Bell RF, Dahl JB, Moore RA, Kalso E. Perioperative ketamine for acute postoperative pain. *Cochrane Database Syst Rev* 2006; (1): CD004603.

18. Lavand'homme PM, Roelants F, Waterloos H, Collet V, DeKock MF. An evaluation of the postoperative antihyperalgesic and analgesic effects of intrathecal clonidine administered

during elective cesarean delivery. *Anesth Analg* 2008; **107**: 948–55.

19. YaDeau JT, LaSala VR, Paroli L, *et al.* Clonidine and analgesic duration after popliteal fossa nerve blockade: Randomized, double blind, placebo-controlled study. *Anesth Analg* 2008; **106**: 1916–20.

20. Gómez-Vázquez ME, Hernández-Salazar E, Hernández-Jiménez A, *et al.* Clinical analgesic efficacy and side effects of dexmedetomidine in the early postoperative period after arthroscopic knee surgery. *J Clin Anesth* 2007; **19**: 576–82.

21. McCartney CJ, Duggan E, Apatu E. Should we add clonidine to local anesthetic for peripheral nerve blockade? A qualitative systematic review of the literature. *Reg Anesth Pain Med* 2007; **32**: 330–8.

22. Ilfeld BM, Mariano ER, Williams BA, Woodard JN, Macario A. Hospitalization costs of total knee arthroplasty with a continuous femoral nerve block provided only in the hospital versus on an ambulatory basis. *Reg Anesth Pain Med* 2007; **32**: 46–54.

23. Ilfeld BM, Vandenborne K, Duncan PW, *et al.* Ambulatory continuous interscalene nerve blocks decrease the time to discharge readiness after total shoulder arthroplasty: a randomized, triple masked, placebo-controlled study. *Anesthesiology* 2006; **105**: 999–1007.

24. Ilfeld BM, Wright TW, Enneking FK, Vandenborne K. Total elbow arthroplasty as an outpatient procedure using a continuous infraclavicular nerve block at home: a prospective case report. *Reg Anesth Pain Med* 2006; **31**: 172–6.

25. Behera BK, Puri GD, Ghai B. Patient-controlled epidural analgesia with fentanyl and bupivacaine provides better analgesia than intravenous morphine patient-controlled analgesia for early thoracotomy pain. *J Postgrad Med* 2008; **54**: 86–90.

26. Viscusi ER, Martin G, Hartrick CT, *et al.* Forty-eight hours of postoperative pain relief after total hip arthroplasty with a novel, extended-release epidural morphine formulation. *Anesthesiology* 2005; **102**: 1014–22.

27. Horlocker TT, Burton AW, Connis RT, *et al.* Practice guidelines for the prevention, detection and management of respiratory depression associated with neuraxial opioid administration. American Society of Anesthesiologists Task Force on Neuraxial Opioids. *Anesthesiology* 2009; **110**: 218–30.

28. Wang JK. Pain relief by intrathecal injection of serotonin or morphine. *Ann Anesthesiol Fr* 1978; **19**: 371–2.

29. Rathmell JP, Lair TR, Nauman B. The role of intrathecal drugs in the treatment of acute pain. *Anesth Analg* 2005; **101**: S30–S43.

30. Forastiere E, Sofra M, Giannerelli D, Fabrizi L, Simone G. Effectiveness of continuous wound infusion of 0.5% ropivacaine by the On-Q pain relief system for postoperative pain management after open nephrectomy. *Br J Anaesth* 2008; **101**: 841–7.

31. Sherwinter DA, Ghaznavi AM, Spinner D, *et al.* Continuous infusion of intraperitoneal bupivacaine after laparoscopic surgery: a randomized controlled trial. *Obes Surg* 2008; **18**: 1581–6.

32. Eider JB, Hoh DJ, Wang MY. Postoperative continuous paravertebral anesthetic infusion for pain control in lumbar spinal fusion surgery. *Spine* 2008; **33**: 210–18.

33. Wheatley GH, Rosenbaum DH, Paul MC, *et al.* Improved pain management outcomes with continuous infusion of a local anesthetic after thoracotomy. *J Thorac Cardiovasc Surg* 2005; **130**: 464–8.

34. Cheng GS, Choy LP, Ilfeld BM. Regional anesthesia at home. *Curr Opin Anaesthesiol* 2008; **21**: 488–93.

35. Fredrickson MJ, Ball CM, Dalgleish AJ. Successful continuous interscalene analgesia for ambulatory shoulder surgery in a private practice setting. *Reg Anesth Pain Med* 2008: **33**: 122–8.

36. Ballantyne JC, Carr DB, deFerranti S, *et al.* The comparative effects of postoperative analgesic therapies on pulmonary outcome: Cumulative meta-analyses of randomized, controlled trials. *Anesth Analg* 1998; **86**: 598–612.

37. Block BM, Liu SS, Rowlingson AJ, *et al.* Efficacy of postoperative epidural analgesia: a meta-analysis. *JAMA* 2003; **18**: 2455–63.

38. Werawatganon T, Charuluxanun S. Patient controlled intravenous opioid analgesia versus continuous epidural analgesia for pain after intra-abdominal surgery (Review). *Cochrane Database Syst Rev* 2005; **25**: CD004088.

39. Kairaluoma PM, Bachmann MS, Rosenberg PH, Pere PJ. Preincisional paravertebral block reduces the prevalance of chronic pain after breast surgery. *Anesth Analg* 2006; **103**: 703–8.

40. Fowler SJ, Symons J, Sabato S, Myles PS. Epidural analgesia compared with peripheral nerve blockade after major knee surgery: a systematic review and meta-analysis of randomized trials. *Br J Anaesth* 2008; **100**: 154–64.

41. Salinas FV, Liu SS, Mulroy MF. The effect of single-injection femoral nerve block versus continuous femoral nerve block after total knee arthroplasty on hospital length of stay and long-term functional recovery within an established clinical pathway. *Anesth Analg* 2006; **102**: 1234–9.

42. Cashman JN, Dolin SJ. Respiratory and haemodynamic effects of acute postoperative pain management: evidence from published data. *Br J Anaesth* 2004; **93**: 212–23.

43. Horlocker TT, Wedel DJ, Benzon H, *et al.* Regional anesthesia in the anticoagulated patient: Defining the risks (the second ASRA Consensus Conference on Neuraxial Anesthesia and Anticoagulation). *Reg Anesth Pain Med* 2003; **28**: 172–97.

44. Kao MC, Tsai SK, Tsou MY, *et al.* Paraplegia after inadvertent intracord catheterization. *Anesth Analg* 2004; **99**: 580–3.

45. Hogan Q, Dotson R, Erickson S, Kettler R, Hogan K. Local anesthetic myotoxocity: a case and review. *Anesthesiology* 1994: **80**: 942–7.

46. Weinberg G. Lipid rescue resuscitation from local anesthetic cardiac toxicity. *Toxicol Rev* 2006; **25**: 139–45.

47. Kappis M. Conduction anesthesia of abdomen, breast, arm, and neck with paraverterbral injection [in German]. *Munchener Medizinische Wochenschrift* 1912; **59**: 794–6.

48. Boezaart AP, Korn R, Rosenquist RW. Paravertebral approach to the brachial plexus: an anatomic improvement in

technique. *Reg Anesth Pain Med* 2003;
28: 241–4.

49. Benumof JL. Permanent loss of cervical spinal cord function associated with interscalene block performed under general anesthesia. *Anesthesiology* 2000; **93**: 1541–4.

50. Franco CD, Gloss FJ, Voronov G, Tyler SF, Stojiljkovic LS. Supraclavicular block in the obese population: an analysis of 2020 blocks. *Anesth Analg* 2006; **102**: 1252–4.

51. Gentili ME, Deleuze A, Estebe JP, *et al.* Severe respiratory failure after infraclavicular block with 0.75% ropivacaine: a case report. *J Clin Anesth* 2002; **14**: 459–61.

52. Winchell SW, Wolfe R. The incidence of neuropathy following upper extremity nerve blocks. *Reg Anesth Pain Med* 1985; **10**: 12–15.

53. Urban MK, Urquhart B. Evaluation of brachial plexus anesthesia for upper extremity surgery. *Reg Anesth Pain Med* 1994; **19**: 175–82.

54. Burlacu CL, Buggy DJ. Coexisting Harlequin and Horner syndromes after high thoracic paravertebral anaesthesia. *Br J Anaesth* 2005; **95**: 822–4.

55. Lonnqvist PA, MacKenzie J, Soni AK, Conacher ID. Paravertebral blockade. Failure rate and complications. *Anaesthesia* 1995; **50**: 813–15.

56. Lin HM, Chelly JE. Post-dural headache associated with thoracic paravertebral blocks. *J Clin Anesth* 2006; **18**: 376–8.

57. Lekhak B, Bartley C, Conacher ID, Nouraei SM. Total spinal anesthesia in association with insertion of a paravertebral catheter. *Br J Anaesth* 2001; **86**: 280–2.

58. Aida S, Takahashi H, Shimoji K. Renal subscapsular hematoma after lumbar plexus block. *Anesthesiology* 1996; **84**: 452–5.

59. Klein SM, D'Ercole F, Greengrass RA, Warner DS. Enoxaparin associated with psoas hematoma and lumbar plexopathy after lumbar plexus block. *Anesthesiology* 1997; **87**: 1576–9.

60. Weller RS, Gerancher JC, Crews JC, Wade KL. Extensive retroperitoneal hematoma without neurologic deficit in two patients who underwent lumbar plexus block and were later anticoagulated. *Anesthesiology* 2003; **98**: 581–5.

61. Cuvillon P, Ripart J, Lalourcey L, *et al.* The continuous femoral nerve block catheter for postoperative analgesia: bacterial colonization, infectious rate and adverse effects. *Anesth Analg* 2001; **93**: 1045–9.

62. Bickler P, Brandes J, Lee M, *et al.* Bleeding complications from femoral and sciatic nerve catheters in patients receiving low molecular weight heparin. *Anesth Analg* 2006; **103**: 1036–7.

63. Auroy Y, Benhamou D, Bargues L, *et al.* Major complications of regional anesthesia in France: the SOS regional anesthesia hotline service. *Anesthesiology* 2002; **97**: 1274–80.

64. Rathmell JP, Wu CL, Sinatra RS, *et al.* Acute postsurgical pain management: a critical appraisal of current practice. *Reg Anesth Pain Med* 2006; **31**: S1–42.

65. Hurley RW, Cohen SP, Williams KA, Rowlingson AJ, Wu CL. The analgesic effects of perioperative gabapentin on postoperative pain: a meta-analysis. *Reg Anesth Pain Med* 2006; **31**: 237–47.

66. Fassoulaki A, Melemeni A, Stamatakis E, Petropoulos G, Sarantopoulos C. A combination of gabapentin and local anesthetics attenuates acute and late pain after abdominal hysterectomy. *Eur J Anaesthesiol* 2007; **24**: 521–8.

67. Fassoulaki A, Triga A, Melemeni A, Sarantopoulos C. Multimodal analgesia with gabapentin and local anesthetics prevents acute and chronic pain after breast surgery for cancer. *Anesth Analg* 2005; **101**: 1427–32.

68. Pandey CK, Prive S, Singh S, *et al.* Preemptive use of gabapentin significantly decreases postoperative pain and rescue analgesia requirements in laparoscopic cholecystectomy. *Can J Anesth* 2004; **51**: 358–63.

69. Mathiesen O, Meiniche S, Dahl JB. Gabapentinand postoperative pain: A qualitative and quantitative systematic review, withfocus on procedure. *BMC Anesthesiol* 2007; **7**: 6.

70. Turan A, Memis D, Karamanlioǒlu B, *et al.* The analgesic effects of gabapentin in monitored anesthesia care for ear-nose-throat surgery. *Anesth Analg* 2004; **99**: 375–8.

71. Menigaux C, Adams F, Guignard B, Sessler DI, Chauvin M. Preoperative gabapentin decreases anxiety and improves early functional recovery from knee surgery. *Anesth Analg* 2005; **100**: 1394–9.

72. Ho K-Y, Gan TJ, Habib AS. Gabapentin and postoperative pain – a systematic review of randomized controlled trials. *Pain* 2006; **126**: 91–101.

73. Agarwal A, Gautam S, Gupta D, *et al.* Evaluation of a single preoperative dose of pregabalin for attenuation of postoperative pain after laparoscopic cholecystectomy. *Br J Anaesth* 2008; **101**: 700–4.

74. Derry S, Barden J, McQuay HJ, Moore RA. Single dose oral celecoxib for acute postoperative pain in adults. *Cochrane Database Syst Rev* 2008; (4): CD004233.

75. De Kock M, Lavand'homme P, Waterloos H. 'Balanced analgesia' in the perioperative period: is there a place for ketamine? *Pain* 2001; **92**: 373–80.

76. Lavand'homme P, De Kock M, Waterloos H. Intraoperative epidural analgesia combined with ketamine provides effective preventive analgesia in patients undergoing major digestive surgery. *Anesthesiology* 2005; **103**: 813–20.

77. Unlugenc H, Gundez M, Guler T, Yagmur O, Isik G. The effect of pre-anaesthetic administration of intravenous dexmedetomidine on postoperative pain in patients receiving patient-controlled morphine. *Eur J Anaesthesiol* 2005; **22**: 386–91.

78. Persec J, Persec Z, Bukuvić D, *et al.* Effects of clonidine preemptive analgesia on acute postoperative pain in abdominal surgery. *Coll Antropol* 2007; **31**: 1071–5.

79. Samsó E, Vallés J, Pol O, Gallart L, Puig MM. Comparative assessment of the anaesthetic and analgesic effects of intramuscular and epidural clonidine in humans. *Can J Anaesth* 1996; **43**: 1195–202.

80. Bong CL, Samuel M, Ng JM, Ip-Yam C. Effects of preemptive epidural analgesia on post-thoracotomy pain. *J of Cardiothoracic Vasc Anesth* 2005; **19**: 786–93.

81. Sekar C, Rajasekaran S, Kannan R, *et al.* Preemptive analgesia for postoperative

pain relief in lumbosacral spine surgeries: a randomized controlled trial. *The Spine J* 2004; **4**: 261–4.

82. Beilin B, Bessler H, Mayburd E, *et al.* Effects of preemptive analgesia on pain and cytokine production in the postoperative period. *Anesthesiology* 2003; **98**: 151–5.

83. Katz J, Cohen L, Schmid R, Chan VWS, Wowket A. Postoperative morphine use and hyperalgesia are reduced by preoperative but not intraoperative epidural analgesia: implications for preemptive analgesia and the prevention of central sensitization. *Anesthesiology* 2003; **98**: 1449–60.

84. Aida S, Yamakura T, Baba H, *et al.* Preemptive analgesia by intravenous low-dose ketamine and epidural morphine in gastrectomy: a randomized double-blind study. *Anesthesiology* 2000; **92**: 1624–30.

85. Kucuk N, Kizilkaya M, Tokdemir M. Preoperative epidural ketamine does not have a postoperative opioid sparing effect. *Anesth Analg* 1998; **87**: 103–6.

86. Kehlet H, Jensen TS, Woolf CJ. Persistent postsurgical pain: risk factors and prevention. *Lancet* 2006; **367**: 1618–25.

87. Fassoulaki A, Sarantopoulos C, Melemeni A, Hogan Q. EMLA reduces acute and chronic pain after breast surgery for cancer. *Reg Anesth Pain Med* 2000; **25**: 350–5.

88. Jahangiri M, Jayatunga AP, Bradley JW, Dark CH. Prevention of phantom pain after major lower limb amputation by epidural infusion of diamorphine, clonidine and bupivacaine. *Ann R Coll Surg Engl* 1995; **77**: 71.

89. Bach S, Noreng MF, Tjellden NU. Phantom limb pain in amputees during the first 12 months following limb amputation, after preoperative lumbar epidural blockade. *Pain* 1988; **33**: 297–301.

90. Ktaz J. Phantom limb pain. *Lancet* 1997; **350**: 1338–9.

91. Nikolajsen L, Ilkjaer S, Christensen JH, Kroner K, Jensen TS. Randomised trial of epidural bupivacaine and morphine in prevention of stump and phantom pain in lower-limb amputation. *Lancet* 1997; **350**: 1353–7.

92. Enneking FK, Scarborough MT, Radson EA. Local anesthetic infusion through nerve sheath catheters for analgesia following upper extremity amputation. Clinical report. *Reg Anesth* 1997; **22**: 351–6.

93. Pinzur MS, Garla PG, Pluth T, Vrbos L. Continuous postoperative infusion of a regional anesthetic after an amputation of the lower extremity. A randomized clinical trial. *J Bone Joint Surg Am* 1997; **79**: 1752–3.

94. Polglase AL, McMurrick PJ, Simpson PJ, *et al.* Continuous wound infusion of local anesthetic for the control of pain after elective abdominal colorectal surgery. *Dis Colon Rectum* 2007; **50**: 2158–67.

95. Alford JW, Fadale PD. Evaluation of postoperative bupivacaine infusion for pain management after anterior cruciate ligament reconstruction. *Arthroscopy* 2003; **19**: 855–61.

96. Bailie DS, Ellenbecker T. Severe chondrolysis after shoulder arthroscopy: a case series. *J Shoulder Elbow Surg* 2009; **18**: 742–7.

97. Hansen BP, Beck CL, Beck EP, Townsley RW. Postarthroscopic glenohumeral chondrolysis. *Am J Sports Med* 2007; **35**: 1619–20.

98. Ilfeld BM, Enneking FK. Continuous peripheral nerve blocks at home: a review. *Anesth Analg* 2005; **100**: 1822–33.

99. Erdogan M, Erdogan A, Erbil N, Karakaya HK, Demircan A. Prospective, randomized, placebo-controlled study of the effect of TENS on postthoracotomy pain and pulmonary function. *World J Surg* 2005; **29**: 1563–70.

100. Bjordal JM, Johnson MI, Ljunggreen AE. Transcutaneous electrical nerve stimulation (TENS) can reduce postoperative analgesic consumption. A meta-analysis with assessment of optimal treatment parameters for postoperative pain. *Eur J Pain* 2003; **7**: 181–88.

101. Mandal A, Imran D, McKinnel T, Rao GS. Unplanned admissions following ambulatory plastic surgery – a retrospective study. *Ann R Coll Surg Engl* 2005; **87**: 466–8.

102. Greenburg AG, Greenburg JP, Tewel A, *et al.* Hospital admission following ambulatory surgery. *Am J Surg* 1996; **172**: 21–3.

103. Lim G, Wang S, Zeng Q, *et al.* Expression of spinal NMDA receptor and PKCgamma after chronic morphine is regulated by spinal glucocorticoid receptor. *J Neurosci* 2005; **25**: 11145–54.

104. Lim G, Wang S, Zeng Q, Sung B, Mao J. Evidence for a long-term influence on morphine tolerance after previous morphine exposure: role of neuronal glucocorticoid receptors. *Pain* 2005; **114**: 81–92.

105. Carroll IR, Angst MS, Clark JD. Management of perioperative pain in patients chronically consuming opioids. *Reg Anesth Pain Med* 2004; **29**: 576–91.

106. Gordon D, Inturrisi CE, Greensmith JE, *et al.* Perioperative pain management in the opioid-tolerant individual. *J Pain* 2008; **9**: 383–7.

107. Feldman D, Reich N, Foster MMT. Pediatric anesthesia and postoperative analgesia. *Ped Clinics N Amer* 1998; **45**: 1525–37.

108. Duedahl TH, Hansen EH. A qualitative systematic review of morphine treatment in children with postoperative pain. *Pediatric Anesthesia* 2007; **17**: 756–74.

109. Howard R, Carter B, Curry J, *et al.* Postoperative pain. *Ped Anesth* 2008; **18**: 36–63.

110. Bosenberg A. Pediatric regional anesthesia update. *Ped Anesth* 2004; **14**: 398–402.

111. Rhee C, Broadbent AM. Palliation and liver failure: palliative medications dosage guidelines. *J Palliat Med* 2007; **10**: 677–85.

Clinical applications: evidence-based anesthesia practice

Control of blood pressure and vascular tone

Arthur Wallace

Introduction

A stable hemodynamic system results from an inherently stable cardiovascular system combined with a control system based on the autonomic nervous system. As suppressing autonomic response is a fundamental component of anesthesia, when the autonomic nervous system is inhibited, the autonomic control of blood pressure and heart rate is either reduced or eliminated altogether. Another result of anesthesia inhibiting the autonomic nervous system is a less stable hemodynamic system in response to vasodilation, changes in blood volume, changes in patient position, changes in temperature, hypoxia, or pain. In essence, the anesthesiologist must become the "autonomic nervous system" for the patient under general anesthesia.

The pharmacologic control of blood pressure and vascular tone can be addressed using a number of approaches. The choice of an inotrope or vasoactive compound should be based on an understanding of the cardiovascular system, the cause of the hemodynamic perturbation being treated, and the pharmacology of the drug. The appropriate management of hemodynamic perturbations must be based on a guess at the etiology of the hemodynamic perturbation, the pathophysiology of the patient, the pharmacology of the drugs, and how these factors interact. The response to a drug is a complex combination of the direct pharmacologic actions, the hemodynamic response, and the autonomic response. There are a set of basic anatomic and physiologic functions that must be understood in order to master hemodynamics and to allow the diagnosis and optimal treatment of hemodynamic problems.

This chapter provides an overview of hemodynamics, autonomic control, and cardiac physiology, including ventricular function and ventricular energetics, before discussing the physiologic and pharmacologic factors that go into the choice of inotropes, vasocontrictors, vasodilators, and their use to control blood pressure and vascular tone.

The effects of anesthesia on cardiovascular stability

The cardiovascular system, because of the Frank–Starling mechanism, is inherently stable. The distribution of blood between the pulmonary and systemic circulations is maintained without any outside inputs [1]. The preload dependence of cardiac output, which is defined by the Frank–Starling mechanism, makes the relative distribution of pulmonary and systemic blood volumes inherently stable, and it is controlled by ventricular mechanics. Unfortunately, hemodynamic perturbations, whether from changes in blood volume, positional changes of the patient, or vasodilation of vascular beds as metabolic requirements change, are not handled well solely by the Frank–Starling mechanism of the heart. As vascular beds vasodilate in response to changes in metabolic load, or venous beds dilate, or blood volume changes in response to hemorrhage, cardiac output and blood pressure change without the control of the autonomic nervous system. The autonomic nervous system controls vascular tone, which affects both systemic vascular resistance (SVR) and venous capacity [2], the relative distribution of blood flow to organs, and the inotropic and chronotropic state of the heart. The combination of an inherently stable cardiovascular system combined with a control system based on the autonomic nervous system, makes a very stable hemodynamic system. Patients are able to change their position in gravitational fields (e.g., standing up), exercise, and have acute changes in blood volume with relatively minor changes in blood pressure and cardiac output, because of the combination of the inherently stable cardiovascular system and regulation by the autonomic nervous system [1,3,4].

Anesthesia and many medications administered to patients inhibit the autonomic nervous system and reduce hemodynamic stability. The entire point of anesthesia is to reduce the body's response to surgical stimuli, and suppressing autonomic response is a fundamental component of anesthesia. Anesthetics inhibit the heart rate and blood pressure response to pain [5]. When patients undergo general anesthesia, the systemic vasculature vasodilates, decreasing SVR, venous capacity vessels dilate, reducing central venous pressure and venous return, filling pressures drop, blood pressure drops, and breathing frequently stops. Vasodilation in response to anesthesia is sufficient to drop the core temperature by vasodilating the skin, causing a redistribution and mixing of peripheral and

Anesthetic Pharmacology, 2nd edition, ed. Alex S. Evers, Mervyn Maze, Evan D. Kharasch. Published by Cambridge University Press. © Cambridge University Press 2011.

central blood volumes [6]. General anesthesia inhibits the autonomic nervous system, reducing or eliminating the autonomic control of blood pressure and heart rate [7]. Heart rates, in response to synthetic opioid (fentanyl, sufentanil, remifentanil, etc.) stimulation of vagal reflexes, may become profoundly bradycardic [8]. Sufentanil can increase vagal effects to the point of asystole [9]. The carotid baroreceptor reflexes are inhibited by anesthesia [10]. Unfortunately one result of anesthesia inhibiting the autonomic nervous system is a less stable hemodynamic system in response to vasodilation, changes in blood volume, changes in patient position, changes in temperature, hypoxia, or pain. The anesthesiologist takes over the functions of the autonomic nervous system for the patient under general anesthesia, and is responsible for maintaining blood pressure, cardiac output, blood volume, temperature, bladder function, respiration, and other autonomic functions.

The autonomic nervous system

The autonomic nervous system is divided into sympathetic and parasympathetic systems (see Chapter 22, Fig. 22.1). Parasympathetic efferents (outputs) arise from the dorsal motor nucleus of X and form into the vagus nerve [11]. The most common vagal effect on hemodynamics is slowing of the heart in response to vagal stimulation. One of the more common hemodynamic perturbations caused by the parasympathetic nervous system is fainting from vasovagal effects. This reflex can be quite profound during ophthalmic surgery, with the occulocardiac reflex causing brief asystole. The most common autonomic effects of the sympathetic nervous system in anesthetic care are either vasodilation in response to inhibition of sympathetic tone with induction of general anesthesia, or tachycardia and hypertension with sympathetic stimulation in response to pain. The hypertensive and tachycardiac response of the sympathetic nervous system to surgical stimulation is used to monitor depth of anesthesia. Autonomic control of the cardiovascular system relies on multiple pressure sensors and output control systems. Sympathetic afferents arise from the carotid sinus baroreceptors and form into the carotid sinus nerve, then form the glossopharyngeal nerve and synapse in the nucleus tractus solitarius (NTS) in the medulla oblongata [12]. There are also afferent sympathetic nerves (inputs) from the aortic arch, right atrium, left atrium, and pulmonary artery and venous baroreceptors [13–16]. Projections then go from the NTS to the dorsal motor nucleus of X [17] and the intermediolateral column [18]. Sympathetic efferents from the intermediolateral column synapse in the sympathetic chain ganglion prior to sending efferents to the blood vessels to control SVR and venous capacity. Sympathetic efferents also project to the heart to control inotropic state.

Figure 65.1 shows a system diagram for autonomic control of hemodynamics. The NTS compares the pressure measured by the baroreceptors to a set point, and sends signals to the dorsal motor nucleus of X, for parasympathetic outputs [17], and to the intermediolateral column [18], which controls sympathetic outputs. The parasympathetic and sympathetic outputs combine to control the cardiovascular system. Intermediolateral column nuclei are predominantly in the thoracic cord (T1–T12), with cardioaccelerator fibers from T1–T5. The output of the cardiovascular system (blood pressure) is then detected by the baroreceptors and fed back to the NTS [12]. Closed-loop control, based on measurement of blood pressure by the baroreceptors and regulation by the sympathetic and parasympathetic nervous systems, maintains blood pressure, given changes in blood volume, metabolic demand, and vasodilation. Figure 65.1 shows the complete input and output system. There are multiple interactions between the control systems, with carotid reflexes inhibiting many cardiopulmonary reflexes. Figure 65.2 shows an example of the response curves for the interaction of left and right carotid baroreceptors. The use of anesthetics, including local anesthetics placed in the thoracic epidural space, can profoundly inhibit this system.

Hemodynamics

Hemodynamic instability is common after the induction of anesthesia and can be used to demonstrate the key elements in correcting hemodynamic problems. The first step is to identify the etiology of the problem. Is the etiology vascular volume, SVR, chronotropy (heart rate), inotropy (ventricular systolic function), lusiotropy (ventricular diastolic function), or some extrinsic problem such as tamponade (a lusiotropic problem), or tension pneumothorax (a problem with venous return)? The diagnosis can usually be obtained by a combination of brief history and statistical likelihood among common potential causes. A young patient who has just had the induction of anesthesia most likely has a decrease in SVR and venodilation lowering preload. The most common therapy would be an infusion of volume. A previously healthy patient with trauma most likely has a low blood volume. An elderly patient with pre-existing coronary artery disease who has just had the induction of anesthesia may have a low preoperative blood volume and vasodilation. The therapy would be volume and possibly a vasoconstrictor. If the hypotension persists despite first attempts at therapy, other etiologies such as ventricular dysfunction and/or myocardial ischemia need to be addressed. If the first approach at therapy does not work, additional information should be obtained. Therapy should be guided to correct the problem. Vasodilation, blood volume, or cardiac problems should be investigated separately.

Vasodilation causes two problems, which should be viewed separately. Arteriolar vasodilation lowers SVR and afterload. Venous dilation dilates systemic veins, increasing their unstressed vascular volume, decreasing central venous pressure, and decreasing preload, which lowers cardiac output. Both changes in SVR caused by arteriolar dilation and changes in unstressed vascular volume caused by venous dilation must be addressed when "vasodilation" occurs. SVR and blood volume must be increased to compensate for "vasodilation."

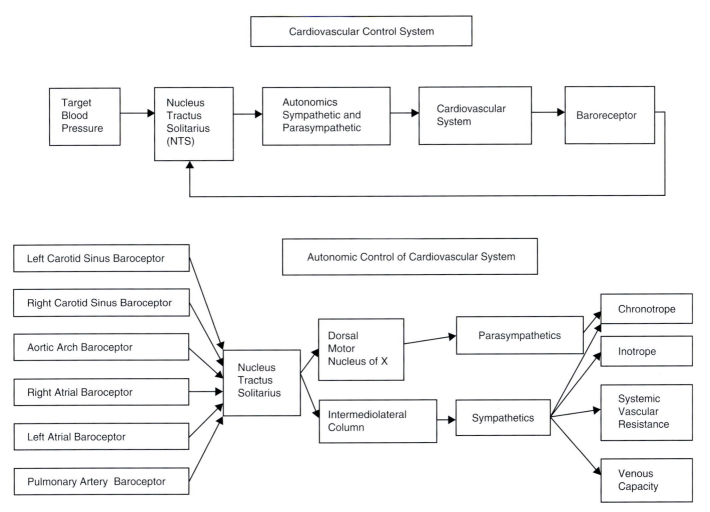

Figure 65.1. Autonomic control of hemodynamics. The top panel shows the basics of the closed-loop control system. Blood pressure measured by the baroreceptors is fed back to the nucleus tractus solitarius (NTS) to achieve closed-loop control and increased stability. The lower panel shows the complete control system with multiple inputs to the NTS as well as the two output systems (sympathetic and parasympathetic) and the multiple output variables in the cardiovascular system.

The next important point to note is that drugs have three basic effects. They have the direct effect noted in the package insert on the autonomic nervous or vascular systems. They may also have direct effects on blood vessels and the heart. Finally, the hemodynamic changes may cause reflex effects, making the net response even more complex. The combined effect is complex because it is rare that each component can be isolated. For example, inhaled anesthetics inhibit autonomic tone [5,20], have direct vasodilatory effects [21], inhibit ventricular function [22], dilate coronary arteries [23,24], and may cause sympathetic stimulation through irritant receptors (desflurane) [25,26], all of which may lead to reflex compensation in response to decreases in blood pressure. The net result of this combination of autonomic, vasodilatory, and cardiac effects is both dose- and time-dependent, and complex to predict in magnitude. A patient with low blood volume may not tolerate the vasodilation following induction of anesthesia. Figure 65.3 illustrates a fundamentally important concept. Patients with an intact autonomic nervous system can maintain normal blood pressure if blood volume is decreased by 10% [3,4]. At a certain point, further decreases in blood volume result in a decrease in blood pressure. Patients with an inhibited autonomic nervous system (such as those under general anesthesia) decrease their blood pressure with all decreases in blood volume. If a patient is already on the decreasing slope of this relationship, then induction of general anesthesia (with a shift from the solid to the dashed line) may result in dramatic and possibly lethal decreases in blood pressure.

The vascular system

The most common hemodynamic problems are the result of vascular problems, either blood volume, venous capacity, or SVR. It is very difficult, if not impossible, to have sufficient cardiac function to compensate for a vasculature that is not functioning properly. Profound vasodilation from anaphylaxis

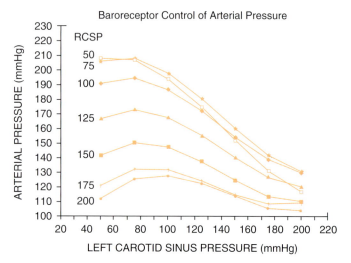

Figure 65.2. Interaction of left and right carotid sinus baroreceptor systems, demonstrating inhibition of one carotid sinus baroreceptor reflex by high pressure in the contralateral system. Denervation or low contralateral pressure allows full reflex control by the ipsilateral reflex. Reproduced with permission from Greene *et al.* [19].

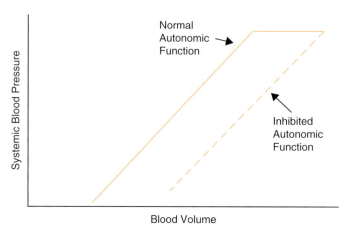

Figure 65.3. Effect of hemorrhage on blood pressure with and without inhibition of autonomic function. A 10% hemorrhage has little effect on blood pressure if autonomic function is intact. With inhibited autonomic function, reduction in blood volume reduces blood pressure.

or septic shock can progress to cardiac failure. Rapidly correcting the vascular problem is essential to prevent the progression to cardiac failure. Profound volume depletion will rapidly lead to hypotension, which will result in poor coronary perfusion, myocardial ischemia, myocardial infarction, ventricular stunning, arrhythmias, and ultimately cardiac failure. The most common hemodyamic problems are the result of vascular problems, either blood volume or resistance. An example will make the point clearer. Suppose SVR, which is normally 900–1200 dynes·sec/cm^5 (90–120 MPa·s/m^3), is reduced during shock to 400 dynes·sec/cm^5. What would the cardiac output need to be to have a reasonable blood pressure?

$$SVR = \frac{(MAP - CVP)}{CO} \times 80 \qquad (65.1)$$

where SVR is systemic vascular resistance, MAP is mean arterial pressure, CVP is central venous pressure, and CO is cardiac output. The 80 converts the units to dynes·sec/cm^5. Rearranging, the cardiac output would be given by

$$CO = \frac{(MAP - CVP)}{SVR} \times 80 \qquad (65.2)$$

Substituting in SVR = 400 dynes·sec/cm^5 and some typical values (MAP = 60 mmHg, CVP = 10 mmHg) gives a cardiac output of 10 liters per minute! Unless the heart is able to produce a cardiac output of 10 L min^{-1}, the blood pressure will be quite low. The effect of SVR or afterload on cardiac output requirements is a fundamentally important point. For the heart to work efficiently, the SVR must be reasonable and the blood volume adequate. The first steps in solving hemodynamic problems is to assess blood volume for adequacy and SVR for reasonableness.

Ventricular function

The next important point in control of blood pressure and vascular tone is ventricular function. Decisions on hemodynamic management must consider the effects of the drug not only on blood pressure and cardiac output but also on ventricular function, ventricular energetics, oxygen consumption, and efficiency. A brief review of ventricular mechanics and energetics is essential to understand these effects. There are many different models that have been used to explain ventricular mechanics. The most successful has been the Sagawa model of pressure–volume analysis [27–29]. Pressure–volume analysis plots simultaneously measured pressure and volume data on a single graph. Sagawa and colleagues applied the techniques of pressure–volume analysis used in thermodynamics of engines to the heart [27]. A simple linear relationship was identified between end-systolic pressure and volume. The end-systolic pressure–volume relationship is an afterload-independent measure of systolic ventricular function [27] that completely describes the systolic properties of the ventricle [29], while the end-diastolic pressure–volume relationship completely describes the passive diastolic properties of the ventricle. Together the end-systolic and end-diastolic pressure–volume relationships provide a complete description of the mechanical properties of the ventricle. The ventricle operates between the end-systolic and end-diastolic pressure–volume relationships.

Ventricular function and energetics

Pressure–volume analysis also describes myocardial energetics, oxygen consumption, and efficiency [30]. The area of the pressure–volume relationship describes the work performed by the ventricle [31]. The stroke work performed by the ventricle is the integral of pressure with respect to volume integrated from the end-diastolic volume to the end-systolic volume [32,33].

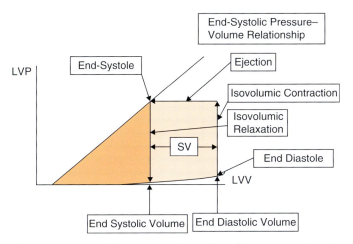

Figure 65.4. Ventricular pressure–volume relationship: gray area is stroke work; black area is potential energy. LVP, left ventricular pressure; LVV, left ventricular volume; SV, stroke volume.

The pressure–volume plot of an ejecting beat is shown in Fig. 65.4, and the definition of stroke work is given by:

$$\text{Stroke work} = \int_{EDV}^{ESV} P(v)\mathrm{d}v \qquad (65.3)$$

where ESV is end-systolic volume and EDV is end-diastolic volume, $P(v)$ is the pressure at a given volume and $\mathrm{d}v$ is the change in volume. The gray area in Fig. 65.4 represents the stroke work for a single ejecting beat. End-diastolic volume is the lower right corner of the gray area. Tracing around the plot in a counterclockwise direction starting at end-diastole, there is initial isovolumic contraction. When left ventricular pressure exceeds aortic pressure, the aortic valve opens and left ventricular ejection begins. When the pressure in the left ventricle drops below aortic pressure, end-systole occurs, followed by isovolumic relaxation. Once left ventricular pressure drops below left atrial pressure, the mitral valve opens and ventricular filling begins. Stroke volume is the difference between end-diastolic volume and end-systolic volume. The integral of pressure with respect to volume between end-diastole and end-systole represents the work of ejection (stroke work: the gray area in Fig. 65.4).

Another concept is that of potential energy (Fig. 65.5). Consider an isovolumic nonejecting beat. If the ventricle is forced to contract without ejecting, it still consumes energy on each beat. In a nonejecting beat, there is only potential energy of the pressurized ventricle on each beat. No external work is performed because there is no ventricular ejection. The potential energy of the ventricle is given by the area of the black triangle (Fig. 65.5). In a nonejecting beat no external work is done but energy is consumed (Fig. 65.5A). All energy in a nonejecting beat is potential energy of the pressurized ventricle and is given by the area to the left of the isovolumic relaxation line (Fig. 65.5A). In an ejecting beat, there is both potential energy of the pressurized blood at end-systole (black triangle) and the external work of the ejected blood (gray square) (Fig. 65.5B).

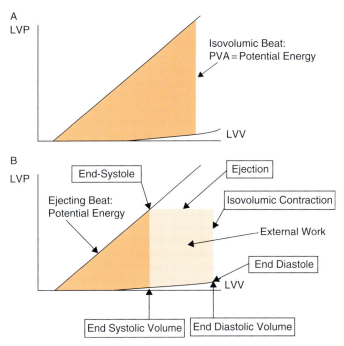

Figure 65.5. Ventricular pressure–volume relationship. (A) The pressure–volume relationship of an isovolumic contraction: no external work is done; the black area represents the potential energy of an isovolumic contraction with energy stored in the pressurized blood in the ventricle. (B) The pressure–volume relationship of an ejecting beat: the black area is the potential energy of the pressurized blood at the end of systole; the gray area is the external work from the ejection; the sum of the gray and black areas is the total energy of the contraction and is proportional to the total oxygen consumed to pump blood. LVP, left ventricular pressure; LVV, left ventricular volume; SV, stroke volume.

Ventricular function, energetics, and oxygen consumption

There is a very close relationship between ventricular energetics described by the pressure–volume analysis and oxygen consumption [34]. Total oxygen consumption per beat can be described by the area between the end-systolic pressure–volume relationship and the end-diastolic pressure–volume relationship for each beat [35]. The total area in Fig. 65.6A, which is the sum of the potential energy and the external work, gives the total energy for each beat, and the total energy is proportional to oxygen consumption for each beat. The relationship between the pressure–volume area and oxygen consumption per beat can be used to analyze ventricular performance. Prior to doing that, let us derive one more term. The efficiency of ventricular function can be calculated by the ratio of external work divided by total energy consumed per beat [33]. Total work is equal to the total energy consumed per beat and is proportional to the total oxygen consumed per beat. The total energy consumed per beat is equal to the sum of the external work and the potential energy per beat. The efficiency can therefore be derived from the oxygen consumed to pump blood divided by the total oxygen consumed per beat [33]:

$$TotalWork = PotentialEnergy + ExternalWork$$

$$Efficiency = \frac{ExternalWork}{TotalWork}$$

$$Efficiency = \frac{ExternalWork}{ExternalWork + PotentialEnergy}$$

$$Efficiency = \frac{OxygenConsumedtoPump}{TotalOxygenConsumedperBeat} \quad (65.4)$$

Pressure–volume analysis allows the rapid evaluation of a complex physiologic system. For example, what are the effects of changing afterload on ventricular energetics? In the standard pressure–volume plot, with external work and potential energy, total oxygen consumption is the sum of the black and gray areas (Fig. 65.6A). The efficiency is the gray area divided by the sum of the black and gray areas. Let us examine the effect of an increase in afterload, such as could be accomplished clinically by administering a vasoconstrictor such as phenylephrine (Fig. 65.6B). Total energy consumption (sum of gray and black areas) is increased, but stroke volume is decreased and cardiac output decreased. The efficiency, as calculated by the ratio of oxygen consumed to pump blood divided by total oxygen consumed, would decrease. Thus administering a vasoconstrictor raised afterload, lowered stroke volume, lowered cardiac output, increased total oxygen consumption, and lowered ventricular efficiency. Conversely, afterload reduction (nitroprusside) would increase both stroke volume and cardiac output, decrease total oxygen consumption, and improve efficiency (Fig. 65.6C).

Understanding ventricular energetics and ventricular function is important in solving hemodynamic problems. The ventricle works as part of the vascular system. It is a profound mistake to attempt to solve hemodynamic problems by focusing exclusively on the heart. The heart, while important, is too often viewed as the cause and solution of all hemodynamic problems. Most hemodynamic problems are not primarily cardiac in nature. Most hemodynamic problems are fundamentally vascular problems: SVR, venous capacity, or blood volume. Moreover, vascular problems are extremely common causes of death. For example, hypovolemia is a vascular problem. Inotropic support alone will not solve the problem of hypovolemia. The profound vasodilation of anaphylaxis or septic shock is primarily a vascular problem. Tamponade is a vascular problem in that the heart cannot fill because of decreased diastolic compliance. Vascular problems frequently lead to low blood pressure, which lowers coronary blood flow, which leads to myocardial ischemia, arrhythmias, and finally death. The primary problem is vascular and the primary solution should be to correct the vasculature.

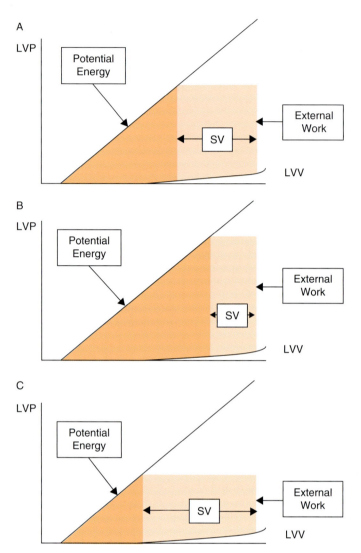

Figure 65.6. Ventricular pressure–volume relationship with pharmacologic changes in afterload. (A) Baseline pressure–volume relationship: black area is potential energy; gray area is external work; total of gray and black area is total energy consumed and is proportional to total oxygen consumed; efficiency is gray area divided by sum of gray and black areas. (B) Effect of increased afterload by vasoconstriction with phenylephrine: notice the increase in total energy and total oxygen consumption with a reduction in stroke volume and cardiac output; total energy (black area + gray area) is increased; total oxygen consumption is increased; efficiency is reduced (gray area/(black area + gray area)). (C) Effect of reduction in afterload by vasodilation with nitroprusside: notice the decrease in total energy and total oxygen consumption with an increase in stroke volume and cardiac output; efficiency is increased (gray area/(black area + gray area)); cardiac output is increased while reducing oxygen consumption and improving efficiency. LVP, left ventricular pressure; LVV, left ventricular volume; SV, stroke volume.

Impedance and optimal hemodynamics

Optimal vascular function is essential to optimal ventricular performance [32]. The heart fundamentally is a pump that transfers blood from the venous system to the arterial system. In all physical systems, including the cardiovascular system, maximal energy transfer of a system is achieved when the output impedance of the source equals the input impedance of the load [32]. Impedance is the opposition of a system to a driving function. In the cardiovascular system, vascular resistance is the simplest form of impedance. Impedance matching is the practice of attempting to make the output impedance Z_S of a source equal to the input impedance Z_L of the load, in order to maximize the power transfer. Impedance matching provides maximal energy transfer between source and load in all physical systems including electrical, mechanical, and hemodynamic.

In the cardiovascular system, impedance matching between the venous system and the heart in diastole, and between the arterial system and the heart in systole, is essential to achieve optimal energy transfer [32,36,37]. If the afterload is too high, cardiac output is depressed. If the afterload is too low, blood pressure will be too low to maintain coronary perfusion, resulting in myocardial ischemia. Afterload describes the impedance of the ventricle in systole and that of the arterial system. Preload is the relationship between the impedance of the venous system and that of the ventricle in diastole. Both preload and afterload must be optimized to match the venous and arterial systems to the ventricle for optimal performance.

Pressure–volume analysis and impedance matching to the vasculature

Figure 65.7A shows a schematic of the cardiovascular system. The impedance of the heart can be described by the pressure–volume relationship [32,33]. The end-diastolic pressure–volume relationship describes the input impedance to the heart. The end-systolic pressure–volume relationship describes the output impedance of the heart. The end-diastolic and end-systolic pressure–volume relationships describe the diastolic and systolic elastances of the ventricle. The slope of the ventricular diastolic pressure–volume relationship is about 0.1 mmHg mL^{-1} [10,38,39]. The elastance of the venous system is about 0.1 mmHg mL^{-1} [2,15,40]. The normal venous system has a very similar elastance to the ventricular diastolic elastance, providing impedance matching between the venous system and the ventricle in diastole [40]. The slope of the systolic pressure–volume relationship normally is about 2.0 mmHg mL^{-1}, which is very similar to the arterial elastance of 2.0 mmHg mL^{-1}, once again matching the output systolic impedance of the heart to the input impedance of the arterial system [10,38–40]. The heart in essence changes its elastance from that of the venous system (0.1 mmHg mL^{-1}) to that of the arterial system (2.0 mmHg mL^{-1}) on each beat (Fig. 65.7B) [32,36,41]. The contraction of the heart can be described as a change in ventricular elastance between the elastance of the venous system and the elastance of the arterial system. If the elastance of the venous system and the diastolic elastance of the heart are equal, there will be maximal transfer of energy from the venous system to the heart (i.e., optimal filling). If the elastance of the ventricle at end-systole equals that of the

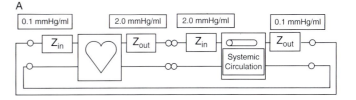

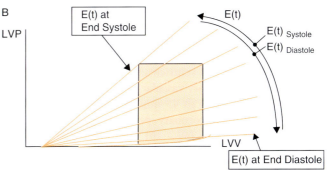

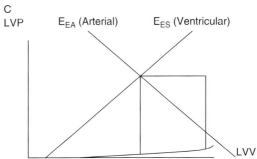

Figure 65.7. Optimization of cardiac function by impedance matching of vasculature to ventricle. (A) Schematic diagram of cardiovascular system with input (Z_{in}) and output (Z_{out}) impedance of heart as well as input (Z_{in}) and output (Z_{out}) impedance of vasculature: optimal energy transfer and cardiac function occurs when $Z_{out} = Z_{in}$; output impedance of venous system should equal the diastolic input impedance of heart; output impedance of heart during systole should equal input impedance of arterial vasculature. (B) Ventricular pressure–volume relationship with variation in elastance: ventricular elastance (pressure–volume) changes with the cardiac cycle, varying from end-diastole to end-systole and then back to end-diastole with each contraction. (C) Relationship between ventricular end-systolic elastance (E_{ES}) and arterial elastance (E_{EA}): when $E_{EA} = E_{ES}$, ventricular systolic output impedance equals arterial input impedance and there is optimal energy transfer and optimal cardiac output.

arterial system, there will be optimal energy transfer (i.e., optimal ejection).

Hemodynamic problems and impedance

Solutions of hemodynamic problems should be thought of as optimizing energy transfer from the venous system to the heart and from the heart to the arterial system, by matching the impedance of the venous system to diastolic impedance of the heart and matching the impedance of the arterial system to the systolic impedance of the heart [40]. Figure 65.7C shows the maximization of cardiac function by matching the arterial elastance E_{EA} to the end-systolic pressure–volume relationship E_{ES}. Maximum cardiac function with minimal energy consumption and maximum efficiency can only be achieved when the venous impedance matches the diastolic elastance

Summary

Factors involved in the control of blood pressure and vascular tone include vascular mechanics, autonomic function, hemodynamics, ventricular function, heart rate, and the vasculature. Anesthesia dramatically influences autonomic, vascular, and ventricular function.

Solving hemodynamic problems requires identification of the root cause. It may appear counterintuitive, but the heart does not cause most hemodynamic problems and should not be the primary focus of an evaluation. Rather, most hemodyamic issues are frequently the result of vascular problems, most commonly blood volume followed by systemic vascular resistance (SVR). Initial steps are to determine whether the etiology of the problem is vascular volume (hypotension and tachycardia are the result of volume depletion until proven otherwise), SVR, chronotropy (heart rate), inotropy (ventricular systolic function), lusiotropy (ventricular diastolic function), or some extrinsic problem such as tamponade (a lusiotropic problem), or tension pneumothorax (a problem with venous return). Vasodilation, blood volume, or cardiac problems should be investigated separately.

Solutions of hemodynamic problems should be thought of as optimizing energy transfer from the venous system to the heart, and from the heart to the arterial system, by matching the impedance of the venous system to diastolic impedance of the heart, and optimizing the impedance of the arterial system to the systolic impedance of the heart. Cardiogenic causes of low cardiac output such as diastolic dysfunction, systolic dysfunction, and myocardial ischemia need to be rapidly identified and corrected. External causes such as tamponade or tension pneumothorax should be viewed as essentially diastolic dysfunction, and must be rapidly corrected. The effect of SVR (afterload) on cardiac output is a fundamentally important concept. For the heart to work efficiently, the SVR must be reasonable and the blood volume adequate. Pulmonary hypertension raises right ventricular afterload and can lead to right ventricular failure and hemodynamic collapse.

A primary role of the anesthesiologist is to correct hemodynamic problems through appropriate pharmacologic and nonpharmacologic control of blood pressure and vascular tone. The choice of an inotrope or vasoactive drug should be based on an understanding of the cardiovascular system, the cause of the hemodynamic perturbation being treated, and the pharmacology of the drug.

References

1. Greene AS, Shoukas AA. Changes in canine cardiac function and venous return curves by the carotid baroreflex. *Am J Physiol* 1986; **251**: H288–96.

2. Shoukas AA, Sagawa K. Control of total systemic vascular capacity by the carotid sinus baroreceptor reflex. *Circ Res* 1973; **33**: 22–33.

3. Katoh N, Sheriff DD, Siu CO, Sagawa K. Relative importance of four pressoregulatory mechanisms after 10% bleeding in rabbits. *Am J Physiol* 1989; **256**: H291–6.

4. Hosomi H, Sagawa K. Sinovagal interaction in arterial pressure restoration after 10% hemorrhage. *Am J Physiol* 1979; **237**: R203–9.

5. Daniel M, Weiskopf RB, Noorani M, Eger EI. Fentanyl augments the blockade of the sympathetic response to incision (MAC-BAR) produced by desflurane and isoflurane: desflurane and isoflurane MAC-BAR without and with fentanyl. *Anesthesiology* 1998; **88**: 43–9.

6. Matsukawa T, Sessler DI, Sessler AM, et al. Heat flow and distribution during induction of general anesthesia. *Anesthesiology* 1995; **82**: 662–73.

7. Latson TW, McCarroll SM, Mirhej MA, et al. Effects of three anesthetic induction techniques on heart rate variability. *J Clin Anesth* 1992; **4**: 265–76.

8. Gravlee GP, Ramsey FM, Roy RC, et al. Rapid administration of a narcotic and neuromuscular blocker: a hemodynamic comparison of fentanyl, sufentanil, pancuronium, and vecuronium. *Anesth Analg* 1988; **67**: 39–47.

9. Starr NJ, Sethna DH, Estafanous FG. Bradycardia and asystole following the rapid administration of sufentanil with vecuronium. *Anesthesiology* 1986; **64**: 521–3.

10. Wallace A, Lam HW, Mangano DT. Linearity, load dependence, hysteresis, and clinical associations of systolic and diastolic indices of left ventricular function in man. Multicenter Study of Perioperative Ischemia (McSPI) Research Group. *J Card Surg* 1995; **10**: 460–7.

11. Contreras RJ, Gomez MM, Norgren R. Central origins of cranial nerve parasympathetic neurons in the rat. *J Comp Neurol* 1980; **190**: 373–94.

12. Lipski J, McAllen RM, Spyer KM. The sinus nerve and baroreceptor input to the medulla of the cat. *J Physiol* 1975; **251**: 61–78.

13. Ciriello J, Calaresu FR. Projections from buffer nerves to the nucleus of the solitary tract: an anatomical and electrophysiological study in the cat. *J Auton Nerv Syst* 1981; **3**: 299–310.

14. Brunner MJ, Greene AS, Kallman CH, Shoukas AA. Interaction of canine carotid sinus and aortic arch baroreflexes in the control of total peripheral resistance. *Circ Res* 1984; **55**: 740–50.

15. Shoukas AA, Brunner MJ, Greene AS, MacAnespie CL. Aortic arch reflex control of total systemic vascular capacity. *Am J Physiol* 1987; **253**: H598–603.

16. Hirooka Y, Sakai K, Kishi T, Takeshita A. Adenovirus-mediated gene transfer into the NTS in conscious rats. A new approach to examining the central control of cardiovascular regulation. *Ann N Y Acad Sci* 2001; **940**: 197–205.

17. Ter Horst GJ, Postema F. Forebrain parasympathetic control of heart activity: retrograde transneuronal viral labeling in rats. *Am J Physiol* 1997; **273**: H2926–30.

18. Mtui EP, Anwar M, Gomez R, Reis DJ, Ruggiero DA. Projections from the nucleus tractus solitarii to the spinal cord. *J Comp Neurol* 1993; **337**: 231–52.

19. Greene AS, Brunner MJ, Shoukas AA. Interaction of right and left carotid sinus baroreflexes in the dog. *Am J Physiol* 1986; **250**: H96–107.

20. Antognini JF, Berg K. Cardiovascular responses to noxious stimuli during isoflurane anesthesia are minimally affected by anesthetic action in the brain. *Anesth Analg* 1995; **81**: 843–8.

21. Hickey RF, Sybert PE, Verrier ED, Cason BA. Effects of halothane, enflurane, and isoflurane on coronary blood flow autoregulation and coronary vascular reserve in the canine heart. *Anesthesiology* 1988; **68**: 21–30.

22. Sahlman L, Henriksson BA, Martner J, Ricksten SE. Effects of halothane, enflurane, and isoflurane on coronary vascular tone, myocardial performance, and oxygen consumption during controlled changes in aortic and left atrial pressure. Studies on isolated working rat hearts in vitro. *Anesthesiology* 1988; **69**: 1–10.

23. Cutfield GR, Francis CM, Foex P, Jones LA, Ryder WA. Isoflurane and large coronary artery haemodynamics. A study in dogs. *Br J Anaesth* 1988; **60**: 784–90.

24. Cason BA, Verrier ED, London MJ, Mangano DT, Hickey RF. Effects of isoflurane and halothane on coronary vascular resistance and collateral myocardial blood flow: their capacity to induce coronary steal. *Anesthesiology* 1987; **67**: 665–75.

25. Bunting HE, Kelly MC, Milligan KR. Effect of nebulized lignocaine on airway irritation and haemodynamic changes during induction of anaesthesia with desflurane. *Br J Anaesth* 1995; **75**: 631–3.

26. Schutz N, Petak F, Barazzone-Argiroffo C, Fontao F, Habre W. Effects of volatile anaesthetic agents on enhanced airway tone in sensitized guinea pigs. *Br J Anaesth* 2004; **92**: 254–60.

27. Sagawa K, Suga H, Shoukas AA, Bakalar KM. End-systolic pressure/volume ratio: a new index of ventricular contractility. *Am J Cardiol* 1977; **40**: 748–53.

28. Sagawa K. The end-systolic pressure–volume relation of the ventricle: definition, modifications and clinical use. *Circulation* 1981; **63**: 1223–7.

29. Sagawa K, Maughan L, Suga H, Sunagawa K. *Cardiac Contraction and the Pressure–Volume Relationship.* New York, NY: Oxford University Press, 1988.

30. Suga H, Hisano R, Hirata S, *et al.* Heart rate-independent energetics and systolic pressure–volume area in dog heart. *Am J Physiol* 1983; **244**: H206–14.

31. Denslow S. Relationship between PVA and myocardial oxygen consumption can be derived from thermodynamics. *Am J Physiol* 1996; **270**: H730–40.

32. Sunagawa K, Maughan WL, Sagawa K. Optimal arterial resistance for the maximal stroke work studied in isolated canine left ventricle. *Circ Res* 1985; **56**: 586–95.

33. Burkhoff D, Sagawa K. Ventricular efficiency predicted by an analytical model. *Am J Physiol* 1986; **250**: R1021–7.

34. Khalafbeigui F, Suga H, Sagawa K. Left ventricular systolic pressure–volume area correlates with oxygen consumption. *Am J Physiol* 1979; **237**: H566–9.

35. Suga H. Total mechanical energy of a ventricle model and cardiac oxygen consumption. *Am J Physiol* 1979; **236**: H498–505.

36. Sunagawa K, Sagawa K, Maughan WL. Ventricular interaction with the loading system. *Ann Biomed Eng* 1984; **12**: 163–89.

37. Maughan WL, Sunagawa K, Burkhoff D, Sagawa K. Effect of arterial impedance changes on the end-systolic pressure–volume relation. *Circ Res* 1984; **54**: 595–602.

38. Wallace A, Lam HW, Nose PS, Bellows W, Mangano DT. Changes in systolic and diastolic ventricular function with cold cardioplegic arrest in man. The Multicenter Study of Perioperative Ischemia (McSPI) Research Group. *J Card Surg* 1994; **9**: 497–502.

39. Wallace AW, Ratcliffe MB, Nose PS, *et al.* Effect of induction and reperfusion with warm substrate-enriched cardioplegia on ventricular function [In Process Citation]. *Ann Thorac Surg* 2000; **70**: 1301–7.

40. Rose WC, Shoukas AA. Two-port analysis of systemic venous and arterial impedances. *Am J Physiol* 1993; **265**: H1577–87.

41. Sunagawa K, Sagawa K. Models of ventricular contraction based on time-varying elastance. *Crit Rev Biomed Eng* 1982; **7**: 193–228.

42. Suga H, Yasumura Y, Nozawa T, *et al.* Ventricular systolic pressure–volume area (PVA) and contractile state (Emax) determine myocardial oxygen demand. *Adv Exp Med Biol* 1988; **222**: 421–30.

43. Ferro G, Spinelli L, Duilio C, *et al.* Diastolic perfusion time at ischemic threshold in patients with stress-induced ischemia. *Circulation* 1991; **84**: 49–56.

44. Sasse SA, Chen PA, Mahutte CK. Relationship of changes in cardiac output to changes in heart rate in medical ICU patients. *Intensive Care Med* 1996; **22**: 409–14.

45. Biddle TL, Benotti JR, Creager MA, *et al.* Comparison of intravenous milrinone and dobutamine for congestive heart failure secondary to either ischemic or dilated cardiomyopathy. *Am J Cardiol* 1987; **59**: 1345–50.

46. Aranda JM, Schofield RS, Pauly DF, *et al.* Comparison of dobutamine versus milrinone therapy in hospitalized patients awaiting cardiac transplantation: a prospective, randomized trial. *Am Heart J* 2003; **145**: 324–9.

47. Burger AJ, Elkayam U, Neibaur MT, *et al.* Comparison of the occurrence of ventricular arrhythmias in patients with acutely decompensated congestive heart failure receiving dobutamine versus nesiritide therapy. *Am J Cardiol* 2001; **88**: 35–9.

48. McCance AJ, Forfar JC. Myocardial ischaemia and ventricular arrhythmias precipitated by physiological concentrations of adrenaline in patients with coronary heart disease. *Br Heart J* 1991; **66**: 316–19.

49. Reid JL, Whyte KF, Struthers AD. Epinephrine-induced hypokalemia: the role of beta adrenoceptors. *Am J Cardiol* 1986; **57**: 23F–27F.

50. Kreisman SH, Ah Mew N, Arsenault M, *et al.* Epinephrine infusion during moderate intensity exercise increases glucose production and uptake. *Am J Physiol Endocrinol Metab* 2000; **278**: E949–57.

51. O'Connor CM, Gattis WA, Uretsky BF, *et al.* Continuous intravenous dobutamine is associated with an increased risk of death in patients with advanced heart failure: insights from the Flolan International Randomized Survival Trial (FIRST). *Am Heart J* 1999; **138**: 78–86.

52. Silver MA, Horton DP, Ghali JK, Elkayam U. Effect of nesiritide versus dobutamine on short-term outcomes in the treatment of patients with acutely decompensated heart failure. *J Am Coll Cardiol* 2002; **39**: 798–803.

53. Nanas JN, Tsagalou EP, Kanakakis J, *et al.* Long-term intermittent dobutamine infusion, combined with oral amiodarone for end-stage heart failure: a randomized double-blind study. *Chest* 2004; **125**: 1198–204.

54. Stanek B, Sturm B, Frey B, *et al.* Bridging to heart transplantation: prostaglandin E1 versus prostacyclin versus dobutamine. *J Heart Lung Transplant* 1999; **18**: 358–66.

55. Elis A, Bental T, Kimchi O, Ravid M, Lishner M. Intermittent dobutamine treatment in patients with chronic refractory congestive heart failure: a randomized, double-blind, placebo-controlled study. *Clin Pharmacol Ther* 1998; **63**: 682–5.

56. Gruner Svealv B, Tang MS, Waagstein F, Andersson B. Pronounced improvement in systolic and diastolic ventricular long axis function after treatment with metoprolol. *Eur J Heart Fail* 2007; **9**: 678–83.

57. Hjalmarson A, Fagerberg B. MERIT-HF mortality and morbidity data. *Basic Res Cardiol* 2000; **95**: I98–103.

58. Maggioni AP, Sinagra G, Opasich C, *et al.* Treatment of chronic heart failure with beta adrenergic blockade beyond controlled clinical trials: the BRING-UP experience. *Heart* 2003; **89**: 299–305.

59. Janosi A, Ghali JK, Herlitz J, *et al.* Metoprolol CR/XL in postmyocardial infarction patients with chronic heart failure: experiences from MERIT-HF. *Am Heart J* 2003; **146**: 721–8.

60. Randomised trial of intravenous atenolol among 16 027 cases of suspected acute myocardial infarction. ISIS-1. First International Study of Infarct Survival Collaborative Group. *Lancet* 1986; **2**: 57–66.

61. Metoprolol in acute myocardial infarction. Patients and methods. The MIAMI Trial Research Group. *Am J Cardiol* 1985; **56**: 3G–9G.

62. Herlitz J, Waldenstrom J, Hjalmarson A. Infarct size limitation after early intervention with metoprolol in the MIAMI Trial. *Cardiology* 1988; **75**: 117–22.

63. Wallace A, Layug B, Tateo I, *et al.* Prophylactic atenolol reduces postoperative myocardial ischemia. *McSPI Research Group Anesthesiology* 1998; **88**: 7–17.

64. Mangano DT, Layug EL, Wallace A, Tateo I. Effect of atenolol on mortality and cardiovascular morbidity after noncardiac surgery. Multicenter Study of Perioperative Ischemia Research Group. *N Engl J Med* 1996; **335**: 1713–20.

65. Poldermans D, Boersma E, Bax JJ, *et al.* Bisoprolol reduces cardiac death and myocardial infarction in high-risk patients as long as 2 years after successful major vascular surgery. *Eur Heart J* 2001; **22**: 1353–8.

66. Poldermans D, Boersma E, Bax JJ, *et al.* The effect of bisoprolol on perioperative mortality and myocardial infarction in high-risk patients undergoing vascular surgery. Dutch Echocardiographic Cardiac Risk Evaluation Applying Stress Echocardiography Study Group. *N Engl J Med* 1999; **341**: 1789–94.

67. Wallace AW, Galindez D, Salahieh A, *et al.* Effect of clonidine on cardiovascular morbidity and mortality after noncardiac surgery. *Anesthesiology* 2004; **101**: 284–93.

68. Parker JD, Bart BA, Webb DJ, *et al.* Safety of intravenous nitroglycerin after administration of sildenafil citrate to men with coronary artery disease: a double-blind, placebo-controlled, randomized, crossover trial. *Crit Care Med* 2007; **35**: 1863–8.

69. Levin RL, Degrange MA, Bruno GF, Del Mazo CD, Taborda DJ, Griotti JJ, Boullon FJ. Methylene blue reduces mortality and morbidity in vasoplegic patients after cardiac surgery. *Ann Thorac Surg* 2004; **77**: 496–9.

Clinical applications: evidence-based anesthesia practice

Cardiac protection and pharmacologic management of myocardial ischemia

Eric Jacobsohn, Waiel Almoustadi, and Chinniampalayam Rajamohan

Introduction

The acute coronary syndrome (ACS) – which includes ST-elevation myocardial infarction (STEMI), non-ST-elevation myocardial infarction (NSTEMI), and unstable angina (UA) – arises following rupture of a coronary artery plaque and subsequent local activation of coagulation and thrombus formation. There are key differences in the management of STEMI and NSTEMI/UA. This chapter reviews diagnostic criteria and risk stratification utilized in the determination of an appropriate interventional approach. Percutaneous coronary intervention (PCI) may be required, and a number of pharmacologic therapies have a role in the management of ACS, including anticoagulants, thrombolytic drugs, analgesics, platelet glycoprotein (GP) IIb/IIIa antagonists, and antiplatelet therapy. Possible adjunctive therapies include nitrates, β-blockers, calcium channel blockers (CCBs), angiotensin-converting enzyme (ACE) inhibitors, aldosterone antagonists, statins, antiarrhythmic drugs, insulin (for diabetic patients), magnesium sulfate, and inotropic therapy. In considering perioperative cardioprotective strategies, the roles of β-blockers, statins, and antiplatelet therapy as well as thoracic sympathectomy are discussed in detail. Cardioplegia is used for cardiopulmonary bypass (CPB) techniques for cardiac surgery and the various techniques which have been investigated or are currently in use are discussed.

Definition and diagnosis of acute coronary syndromes

The acute coronary syndrome encompasses NSTEMI, STEMI, and UA [1]. The pathological definition of a myocardial infarction is myocardial cell death caused by prolonged ischemia. In the clinical setting a myocardial infarction is diagnosed if one of the five criteria listed in Table 66.1 is met.

The genesis of ACS involves rupture or fissuring of a coronary artery plaque that exposes the underlying subendothelial matrix, leading to the local activation of coagulation and thrombus formation. There is significant overlap between the pathophysiology of STEMI and NSTEMI. STEMI usually

Table 66.1. Criteria for diagnosing myocardial infarction

1. Rise and/or fall of cardiac biomarkers (preferably troponin) with at least one value > 99th percentile of the upper reference limit (URL) *plus* evidence of myocardial ischemia as recognized by one of the following:

    a. symptoms of ischemia

    b. ECG changes indicative of ischemia (ST-T wave changes, new LBBB)

    c. pathological Q waves

    d. imaging evidence of new loss of myocardium or new regional wall motion abnormalities

2. Sudden cardiac death with evidence of ischemia, including symptoms of ischemia, ECG changes (new ST elevation or LBBB) or definite new thrombus by coronary angiogram or autopsy, and death occurring before a blood sample for biomarker could be drawn or biomarker was drawn before appearance in the blood

3. Post-PCI myocardial infarction, defined as cardiac biomarkers > 3 × 99th percentile of the URL

4. Post-CABG myocardial infarction, evidenced by biomarkers > 5 × 99th percentile of the URL, *plus* one of the following:

    a. a new pathological Q wave

    b. a new LBBB

    c. angiographic evidence of new or native graft occlusion

    d. new imaging evidence of loss of viable myocardium

5. Postmortem pathological findings of acute myocardial infarction

Any one of the five criteria constitutes a diagnosis of myocardial infarction.

results from complete occlusion of a coronary artery in the absence of significant collaterals, and results in ST elevation at the J point in two contiguous ECG leads (defined as 2 mm elevation in men and 1.5 mm in women in V_2–V_3, or > 1 mm

Anesthetic Pharmacology, 2nd edition, ed. Alex S. Evers, Mervyn Maze, Evan D. Kharasch. Published by Cambridge University Press. © Cambridge University Press 2011.

Table 66.2. Characteristics of cardiac markers for diagnosing myocardial infarction

Serum cardiac marker	Test first becomes positive (hours)	Peak level (hours)	Sensitivity (%)	Specificity (%)	Positive predictive value (%)	Negative predictive value (%)
CK single assay	3–8	12–24	35	80	20	90
CK serial assays			95	68	30	99
CK-MB single assay	4–6	12–24	35	85	25	90
CK-MB serial assays			95	95	73	99
Troponin I/T measured 4 hours after onset of chest pain	4–10	8–28	35	96	56	91
Troponin I/T measured 10 hours after onset of chest pain			89	95	72	98

in any other lead) or new onset of left bundle branch block (LBBB) in the setting of ischemic symptoms. NSTEMI results from partial or incomplete occlusion of a coronary artery, an occlusion with significant collaterals, or ischemia with sufficient severity and duration to result in myocardial necrosis. The initial ECG does not show ST-segment elevation. There is the typical increase in cardiac biomarkers. UA presents with prolonged rest symptoms (> 20 minutes, new onset of exertional angina, or an acceleration of symptoms in a patient with known coronary artery disease, CAD), in the absence of elevated cardiac biomarkers.

Defining the clinical phenotype of ACS involves evaluation of acute chest pain beginning with a clinical history that focuses on the characteristics of pain, time of onset, duration of symptoms, and exploring symptoms of masquerading pathologies. The pain may be referred to the arms, jaw, neck, shoulder, back, or abdomen, but may be absent or atypical in some, especially diabetic or female patients. The physical examination should include the vital signs and a detailed cardiac and peripheral vasculature examination. The physical examination in patients with ACS is often normal. Ominous physical findings include a new mitral regurgitant murmur, a murmur suggestive of a ventricular septal defect (VSD), pulmonary rales, a third heart sound, or new jugular venous distension. Although the diagnosis of ACS is usually straightforward, the astute clinician should always consider the possible differential diagnosis, including potential lethal conditions that could masquerade as an ACS. These conditions include aortic dissection (which may have typical ECG changes of ACS if a coronary artery is involved), pulmonary embolism, and pneumothorax. Other potential causes of chest pain include pneumonia, myocarditis, pericarditis, gastrointestinal pathology, anxiety, and others.

Troponin is the preferred biomarker for the diagnosis (Table 66.2) [2]. Troponin T and I have similar sensitivity and specificity, but unlike troponin I levels, troponin T levels may be elevated in patients with renal or muscle disease. Patients with

a normal CK-MB level but elevated troponin are considered to have sustained minor myocardial damage, whereas patients with elevated CK-MB and troponin have had a larger ACS. Myoglobin is very sensitive, can be detected as early as 2 hours, but falls rapidly. It has a low cardiac specificity but is useful for ruling out a myocardial infarction in the early hours of chest pain.

Pharmacologic and interventional management of ACS

It is crucial to differentiate between STEMI and NSTEMI/UA, as they have different priorities and management principles (Fig. 66.1). In STEMI there is usually a complete occlusion of a coronary artery, and expeditious reperfusion is required. In NSTEMI/UA the obstruction is often incomplete, and the management is directed at preventing further coagulation and platelet aggregation by using anticoagulant, antiplatelet, and other adjuvant anti-ischemic therapies. A delayed, non-emergent interventional approach is often taken, except in high-risk NSTEMI, where early intervention may be indicated. Risk stratification is therefore an important tool to help guide therapy and to prognosticate. There are many ACS risk scores. The commonly used Thrombolysis in Myocardial Infarction (TIMI) risk scores for STEMI and NSTEMI/UA are summarized in Table 66.3 [3,4].

Management of STEMI
Immediate therapy
The patient should immediately be given 325 mg of soluble aspirin (acetylsalicylic acid) [5,6]. Recent evidence suggests that adding at least 300 mg of clopidogrel to aspirin may further improve the outcome [7,8] without increasing the bleeding risk, especially in those patients who subsequently

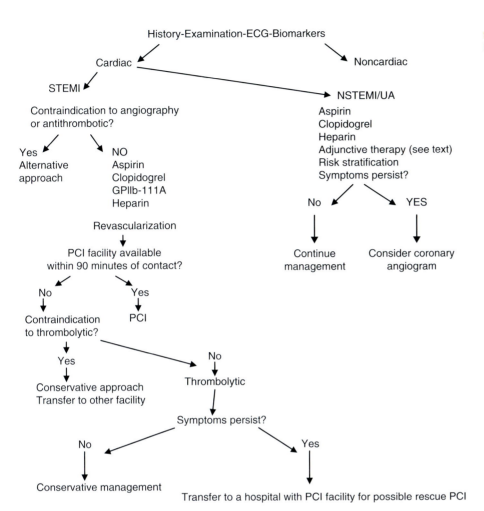

Figure 66.1. Clinical approach to management of NSTEMI/UA and STEMI.

need thrombolytic therapy. Sublingual nitroglycerin may be considered for symptom relief, and also to rule out the possibility of coronary vasospasm. Morphine is the analgesic of choice for patients whose symptoms are not relieved by nitrates or where pain recurs despite anti-ischemic therapy.

Reperfusion

Reperfusion is achieved by either PCI or thrombolysis. Earlier reperfusion is associated with less myocardial necrosis and a better prognosis than thrombolysis. There is minimal benefit to pharmacologic reperfusion after 12 hours, while recent data indicate that the benefit of primary PCI in reducing the infarct size may extend beyond 12–24 hours [9]. In PCI-capable health networks, medical-contact-to-balloon time should be less than 90 minutes. If this is not feasible, immediate fibrinolytic therapy should be considered.

(1) **Primary PCI** – This is defined as urgent balloon angioplasty (with or without stenting). It results in vessel patency in about 90% of patients.

(2) **Fibrinolytic therapy** – In centers where immediate PCI is not available, fibrinolytic therapy should be considered. The various drugs include the first-generation drug streptokinase, the second-generation drug tissue plasminogen

activator (tPA), and the third-generation drugs reteplase and tenecteplase (TNK). Although streptokinase is less effective at reperfusion, it has a lower incidence of intracerebral bleeding, and this may make it the preferred choice in elderly patients. Fibrinolysis results in approximately a 50–60% vessel patency rate, preserves left ventricular (LV) function, and improves survival [10]. There are limitations to fibrinolytic therapy, including contraindications (recent stroke, intracranial neoplasm, active internal bleeding, suspected aortic dissection and others), failure to reperfuse, reocclusion of the culprit vessel with reinfarction, and late presentation (> 12 hours), where this therapy has no proven benefits.

(3) **Rescue PCI** – This is a PCI after a failed thrombolytic therapy. In this group of patients, rescue PCI has been shown to reduce morbidity and mortality by up to 50% [11].

(4) **Facilitated PCI** – This is a planned PCI after initial drugs are given to try and improve the subsequent PCI success rate. Drugs include reduced-dose fibrinolytics, GPIIb/IIIa inhibitors, or a combination of these. Despite the theoretical advantages of facilitated PCI, a clinical trial was terminated prematurely because of higher in-hospital mortality rate in the facilitated PCI group [12]. Facilitated PCI should be

Table 66.3. TIMI risk scores for STEMI and NSTEMI/UA

TIMI score for STEMI

Score calculation	Points	Score	Risk of death by 30 days (%)
History of DM, HTN, or angina	1	0	0.8
Anterior STEMI or LBBB	1	1	1.6
Time to treatment > 4 h	1	2	2.2
Weight < 67 kg	1	3	4.4
HR > 100 min^{-1}	2	4	7.3
Killip class 2–4	2	5	12.4
Age > 65–74	2	6	16.1
Age > 75	3	7	23.4
SBP < 100 mmHg	3	8	26.8
		> 8	35.9

TIMI score for NSTEMI/UA

Score calculation	Points	Score	Death, myocardial infarction, or urgent revascularization by 14 days
Age > 65	1	0–1	5%
> 3 risk factors for ACS	1	2	8%
Known CAD (> 50% stenosis)	1	3	13%
Aspirin use in past 7 days	1	4	20%
> 2 episodes of angina in 24 h	1	5	26%
ST elevation > 0.5 mm	1	6–7	41%
(+) Cardiac enzymes	1		

STEMI score: low risk = 1–3; intermediate risk = 4; high risk >4
NSTEMI score: low risk = 1–2; intermediate risk = 3–4; high risk >4

considered only in high-risk patients where PCI is not available within 90 minutes and the bleeding risk is low.

(5) **Emergency CABG** (coronary artery bypass graft) – This is the treatment of choice for patients in whom the primary rescue PCI was intended, but critical left main or severe three-vessel disease, not amenable to angioplasty, is discovered.

Anticoagulant therapy

Anticoagulation maintains the vessel patency after reperfusion, with additional benefits being prevention of deep vein thrombosis (DVT)/pulmonary embolism (PE) and ventricular thrombus [13]. Patients who have undergone reperfusion with fibrinolytic therapy should receive anticoagulant therapy for a minimum of 48 hours.

Heparin remains the most commonly used anticoagulant for ACS. The commonest and most economical heparin is unfractionated heparin (UFH). However, a major drawback with UFH is the significant variability that necessitates close monitoring of aPTT, heparin resistance, and the risk of heparin-induced thrombocytopenia (HIT). These drawbacks, together with the requirement for continuous intravenous administration, make it less than ideal after ACS. However, UFH remains the drug of choice if there is a significant risk of bleeding and if urgent surgical intervention is likely. Unlike UFH, the low-molecular-weight heparin (LMWH) preparations do not routinely require continuous monitoring and have a predictable dose–response. Enoxaparin has been extensively compared to UFH following fibrinolytic therapy, and has been shown in some studies to be associated with reduced mortality, reinfarction, and readmission rates, with no increase in bleeding [14,15]. Because increased intracranial hemorrhage may occur with LMWH in patients over 75 years of age, dose reduction is required in this age group [16]. The same considerations are required in other patients with or at risk of renal dysfunction.

Fondaparinux is a synthetic pentasaccharide that is a selective, indirect inhibitor of factor Xa. Its 100% bioavailability after subcutaneous injection, half-life of 15–18 hours, and predictable anticoagulant effect facilitates once-daily administration without routine monitoring. There is no or a very low incidence of HIT. In patients with STEMI, fondaparinux had no difference in the incidence of major bleeding when compared to UFH or LMWH, and an improved mortality [17]. However, in the primary PCI patients, there was no benefit and significant increase in the angiography catheter thrombosis rate. The use of fondaparinux during STEMI appears attractive and will continue to evolve.

Direct thrombin inhibitors (DTIs) are primarily indicated for patients with HIT or at risk for HIT. Clinical trial evidence has demonstrated that a DTI such as bivalirudin is safe and effective in the setting of ACS, regardless of HIT status [18]. In recent studies DTIs used in STEMI have shown reduced reinfarction but not mortality, and there has been a suggestion that they may replace GPIIb/IIIa inhibitors in high-risk patients with STEMI [18].

Platelet glycoprotein IIb/IIIa antagonists

These compounds inhibit the binding of fibrinogen to the GPIIb/IIIa receptors on the platelet surface, inhibiting cross-bridging of platelets and preventing platelet activation and aggregation. The three intravenous drugs include the long-acting monoclonal antibody abciximab, and the small molecular inhibitors eptifibatide and tirofiban. These drugs are indicated in patients who have PCI as the primary therapy for STEMI. The drugs are generally administered at the time of PCI, although early administration of tirofiban and eptifibatide in the emergency department prior to the PCI may increase PCI patency rates. The addition of these drugs to thrombolytic therapy provides no benefit but increases the risk of bleeding [19]. The need for these drugs is declining as the use of loading doses of clopidogrel and newer anticoagulants becomes more established.

Management of NSTEMI and unstable angina

The treatment paradigm in NSTEMI/UA is directed towards inhibition of platelet aggregation, anticoagulation, and antianginal therapy [20]. Fibrinolytic drugs have no beneficial effect in NSTEMI/UA and may increase the risk of myocardial infarction. Risk stratification of NSTEMI/UA helps in identifying patients who may require earlier invasive therapy (Table 66.3). Other reasons for early angiography and interventional therapy include persistent symptoms despite full medical management, hemodynamic instability, depressed LV function, and prior CABG/PCI within the last 6 months.

Antiplatelet therapy

As with STEMI, 325 mg of soluble aspirin should immediately be administered to all patients with NSTEMI/UA. Aspirin should be continued indefinitely [6]. The addition of clopidogrel to aspirin is recommended for all patients with NSTEMI/UA (conservative and interventionally managed patients) as it improves prognosis [21]. A loading dose

of 300 mg is followed by a maintenance dose of 75 mg daily for at least 1 year, especially in patients who have had a PCI [22]. Indefinite therapy may be required in the case of drug-eluting stents [23].

Anticoagulation

(1) **Unfractionated heparin** – In an early study of UA, the combination of UFH and aspirin reduced the incidence of ischemic events compared to aspirin alone [24]. UFH is administered using a weight-adjusted algorithm, and the aPTT is maintained between 45 and 75 seconds. Most of the trials that evaluated the use of UFH in NSTEMI/UA have continued therapy for between 2 and 5 days. At present, the optimal duration of therapy remains undefined. As in STEMI, UFH remains the drug of choice if there is a significant possibility that CABG surgery may be required.

(2) **Low-molecular-weight heparin** – The advantages of LMWH have been discussed in management of STEMI, and also apply to patients with NSTEMI/UA [20]. Although some controversy still exists about the role of these drugs versus UFH in NSTEMI, many studies suggest that LMWH is more effective than UFH in the management of patients with NSTEMI/UA. The outcomes suggest less recurrent ischemia and improved mortality, including those patients who have a higher risk score and who ultimately require early interventional therapy [25].

(3) **Factor Xa inhibitors** – In a recent trial comparing fondaparinux to enoxaparin in patients with NSTEMI/UA who were treated conservatively, fondaparinux was associated with a significantly lower mortality at 30 and 180 days [26]. Its pharmacokinetics makes it a very attractive drug in ACS; its role in NSTEMI/UA continues to evolve.

(4) **Direct thrombin inhibitors** – Bivalirudin is a synthetic analog of hirudin that binds reversibly to thrombin and inhibits clot-bound thrombin. In a recent large meta-analysis of 25 457 patients, bivalirudin had a comparable risk of death, myocardial infarction, revascularization, and composite ischemic endpoints to the heparin plus a GPIIb/IIIa antagonist [27]. However, the risk of major bleeding was lower with bivalirudin.

Platelet glycoprotein IIb/IIIa antagonists

The role of this class of drugs may be much diminished in the new era of routine clopidogrel loading. The recent ACC/AHA guidelines suggest that either clopidogrel or GPIIb/IIIa inhibitor can be used in low-risk patients; combination therapy is favorable in high-risk patients, including diabetics and troponin-positive patients [20]. However, there is no single approach to these complex patients, and therapy will depend on the assessment of each patient's risk for ischemic complications versus the risk of bleeding.

Adjunctive therapies for treating STEMI and NSTEMI/UA

Nitrates

In STEMI, nitrates may be useful to determine whether any ST elevation is due to spasm while arrangements for reperfusion therapy are being initiated. Although there was some suggestion of a mortality benefit in the pre-reperfusion era, studies in the modern era of ACS management have shown no outcome benefit. Nitrates are an important component of anti-ischemic therapy in the patient with NSTEMI/UA. Sublingual nitroglycerin should first be administered, and patients who are unresponsive to this should be converted to intravenous therapy.

β-Blockers

β-Blockers have a favorable myocardial oxygen supply–demand profile and have an antiarrhythmic effect. In the pre-reperfusion era of STEMI, they were shown to reduce mortality. Although still beneficial, the effect has been less obvious in the post-reperfusion era. More recently the COMMIT study has even suggested that acute β-blocker therapy in STEMI may increase mortality in patients with or at risk for cardiogenic shock [28]. As a result of this, the 2007 ACC/AHA guidelines suggest avoiding β-blockers in the first 24 hours, and that they be introduced judiciously thereafter [20]. In the case of NSTEMI/UA, a cardioselective β-blocker should be started as early as possible unless there is an absolute contraindication.

Calcium channel blockers

Although CCBs have a favorable myocardial oxygen supply–demand profile, they have an extremely limited role in ACS. The only indications for CCBs in ACS are in cocaine-induced ACS, variant angina, supraventricular tachycardia, refractory angina after full β-blockade/nitrate therapy, and as an alternative to β-blockade where absolute contraindications to β-blockade exist (such as true asthma, decompensated or acute heart failure, shock, hypotension, heart block, and allergy). The nondihydropyridine CCBs (verapamil or diltiazem) are the preferred drugs, as they reduce heart rate and contractility.

ACE inhibitors and ARBs

An ACE inhibitor should be started on all patients after STEMI unless there is a contraindication. Patients with LV dysfunction, heart failure, and diabetes have been shown to benefit the most from this therapy with respect to reducing morbidity and mortality [29]. However, even patients with normal cardiac function benefit from ACE inhibition [30]. Although the data for ACE inhibition after NSTEMI/UA are less compelling, current recommendations include this therapy for these patients who have LV dysfunction, but it should be considered for all patients considering the potential beneficial effect in CAD. Angiotensin receptor blockers (ARBs) are indicated in patients intolerant of an ACE inhibitor.

Aldosterone antagonists

This class of drugs should be considered in all post-ACS patients who have significantly reduced LV function. Reduced hospitalization and death have been shown in two studies, but there is a serious risk of hyperkalemia, especially when combined with ACE inhibitors or ARBs are used in patients with renal insufficiency [31].

Lipid-lowering drugs

Statins are a cornerstone of primary and secondary prevention after ACS. In all patients with ACS, early aggressive lipid-lowering therapy should be started. Several studies (performed mostly after NSTEMI/UA) have shown improved morbidity and mortality including reinfarction, unstable angina, unplanned revascularization, stroke, and death [32]. Early aggressive statin therapy likely has a beneficial effect due to their lipid-independent effects ("pleiotropic effects"), which include anti-inflammatory and antithrombotic effects, enhancement of fibrinolysis, reduction of ischemic–reperfusion injury, decreased platelet reactivity, and restoration of endothelial function.

Antiarrhythmogenic drugs/AICD

A large meta-analysis showed that ventricular arrhythmias contributed to an increase in 30-day and 6-month mortality after NSTEMI [33]. These should be treated with appropriate antiarrhythmic medications. Another study that examined early automatic implantable cardioverter-defibrillator (AICD) implantation after STEMI failed to show reduction in all-cause mortality at 6 months [34]. The current recommendations are for these patients to generally wait 6 months after revascularization before AICD evaluation [35].

Diabetes control

Diabetic patients who are treated with aggressive insulin therapy have been shown to have a lower mortality at 1 year compared with standard therapy [36]. The 2007 ACC/AHA guidelines emphasize vigorous lifestyle modification as well as pharmacotheraputic measures to achieve a near-normal HbA1c level (< 7%) [20].

Magnesium sulfate

There was an increased interest in use of magnesium sulfate in patients with ACS after a trial that showed a 24% reduction in mortality [37]. However, a recent Cochrane review concluded that magnesium did not reduce mortality, that it possibly reduced the incidence of tachyarrhythmias, but that hypotension, bradycardia, and flushing were increased [38]. Currently magnesium is mostly used for hypomagnesaemia and in the treatment of torsades de pointes.

Hemodynamic support

Inotropic drugs such as β-stimulants, phosphodiesterase 3 inhibitors, and calcium sensitizers improve cardiac contractility, but they all increase myocardial oxygen consumption. Intra-aortic balloon pump (IABP) counterpulsation increases coronary perfusion pressure and reduces LV afterload. In ACS, inotrope use should be minimized. However, patients with cardiogenic shock will require IABP with or without inotropic therapy.

Perioperative β-blocker therapy

The potential cardioprotective effects of β-blockade were initially demonstrated over many years of clinical and laboratory research. The mechanism of cardioprotection is manifold, and includes a reduction in heart rate, an increase in diastolic coronary perfusion (as a result of increased diastolic time), and reduced myocardial contractility. β-Blockers likely have little influence on the primary variables influencing plaque stability (inflammation, lipid accumulation, and others), but they may reduce shear stress on the plaque as a result of their hemodynamic and sympatholyic effects. They also have anti-arrhythmic effects, especially when the myocardium is ischemic. In this respect they have been shown to reduce circulating free fatty acids by inhibiting lipolysis; this may reduce ventricular fibrillation.

In the late 1980s, a series of small studies suggested that β-blocker therapy used in certain high-catecholamine states in the perioperative period improved surrogate endpoints such as ST-T segment changes, ischemia, hypertension, and arrhythmias. The first randomized study to investigate morbidity and mortality endpoints was published in 1996. In a group of vascular and nonvascular surgical patients, the investigators showed that there was an improved morbidity and mortality with either oral or intravenous atenolol started soon before surgery [39]. However, the study had significant methodological flaws. It was soon followed by a trial from the Netherlands where high-risk vascular surgery patients were treated with a perioperative protocol using bisoprolol [40]. Unlike the previous study, the β-blockade was started many days in advance of surgery and the dose titrated to ensure a slow heart rate. In this study there was a very striking reduction in perioperative cardiac mortality, and the trial was stopped early. Like the previous trial, it too has been widely debated, criticized for some methodological flaws, and the results have not been duplicated since. However, these two studies led to a dramatic change in practice. They were hailed by organized medicine as breakthroughs in perioperative safety and outcome. Hospitals were soon required to measure β-blocker compliance rates.

However, some investigators called for more inclusive and larger trials before advocating routine β-blocker use in patients at risk for CAD [41]. Several questions remained unanswered, including what entailed adequate β-blockade. Was adequate β-blockade a heart rate of 50–60 beats per minute, a

suppression of the heart's response to stress, a reduction of cardiac output at rest and in response to stress, a protection of the myocyte from the toxic effects of catecholamines, possible anti-inflammatory or their other "pleiotropic" effects, or a combination of the above factors [42]? In addition, some systematic reviews of β-blocker therapy questioned their efficacy [43]. These uncertainties were reflected in the 2007 ACC/AHA guidelines, which suggested that β-blockers reduced perioperative ischemia but only *may* reduce the risk of myocardial infarction and death [44]. At the same time as β-blockers were being questioned in the treatment of ACS, the publication of the large COMMIT study from China showed that early β-blockade in STEMI reduced the risk of reinfarction and ventricular fibrillation, but increased the risk of cardiogenic shock, especially when administered early [28]. The conclusions of COMMIT (and the subsequent ACC/AHA guidelines) were that β-blockers should not be started routinely, but only when the hemodynamics were stable [45].

Despite the state of the evidence, clinical practice evolved to such an extent that doing a large perioperative β-blocker study in the USA seemed fraught with concerns of how ethical consent could be obtained – i.e., could β-blockers be withheld from these patients [46]? This sentiment was not universally held. The Perioperative Ischemia Evaluation (POISE) study would provide valuable new information [47]. This randomized controlled trial involved patients in 190 hospitals in 23 countries outside the USA. It randomized 8351 patients with or at risk of atherosclerotic disease who were undergoing noncardiac surgery to receive either extended-release metoprolol or placebo; the design was similar to the initial β-blocker study [39] in that treatment was started 2–4 hours before surgery and continued for 30 days. The primary endpoint was a composite of cardiovascular death, nonfatal myocardial infarction, and nonfatal cardiac arrest (Fig. 66.2). Fewer patients in the metoprolol group than in the placebo group reached the primary endpoint (5.8% vs. 6.9%, hazard ratio 0.84, 95% CI 0.70–0.99, $p = 0.0399$). Similarly, fewer patients in the metoprolol group than in the placebo group had a myocardial infarction (4.2% vs. 5.7%, hazard ratio 0.73, 95% CI 0.60–0.89, $p = 0.0017$). There was also a reduction in atrial fibrillation and the need for revascularization in the metoprolol group. There was no increase in the incidence of heart failure in the metoprolol group. However, there were *more* overall deaths in the metoprolol group (3.1% vs. 2.3%, hazard ratio 1.33, 95% CI 1.03–1.74, $p = 0.0317$). More patients in the metoprolol group than in the placebo group had a stroke (1.0% vs. 0.5%, hazard ratio 2.17, 95% CI 1.26–3.74, $p = 0.0053$). In the metoprolol group, there was an increase in patients dying from sepsis and an increased incidence of bradycardia and hypotension. Therefore, the statistically significant reductions in the important primary outcomes of cardiac death, nonfatal myocardial infarction, and cardiac arrest were more than offset by an increase in overall death and stroke. As most strokes were ischemic, it is likely that the

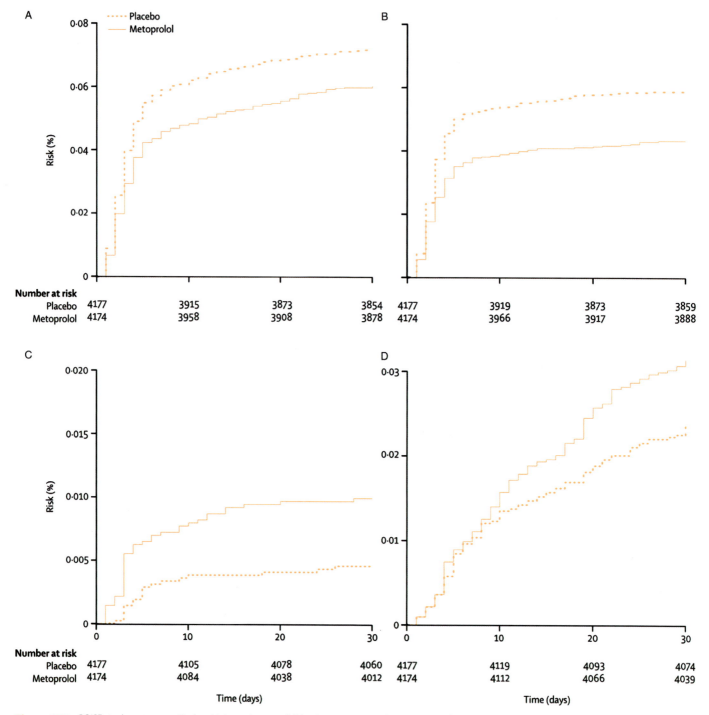

Figure 66.2. POISE study outcomes: Kaplan–Meier estimates of (A) primary outcome (a composite of cardiovascular death, nonfatal myocardial infarction, and nonfatal cardiac arrest), (B) myocardial infarction, (C) stroke, (D) death. Reproduced with permission from POISE Study Group [47].

increase in stroke rate is related to the hypotensive effect of β-blockade.

Although some authors suggested that the dose of metoprolol was too high [48], it is the accepted dose for non-heart failure. The type of β-blockers used in POISE may however have had an effect. In a recent study examining the benefits of long-term β-blockers as secondary prevention after myocardial infarction, there was a higher mortality with metoprolol than with atenolol or acebutolol [49]. How this applies to the perioperative period and the POISE study results is unclear. It is also known that there are certain genotypes that may be resistant to β-blocker therapy [50], but genetic factors were not examined in the POISE study. There is debate about whether high heart rates were controlled tightly enough in POISE.

However, previous to POISE it was controversial whether or not this was critically important [51]. In a meta-analysis by Beattie *et al.*, perioperative β-blockade was not associated with fewer myocardial infarctions but did result in a significant reduction when it was aggressive (arbitrarily defined rate $< 100\,min^{-1}$) [52]. On the other hand, a meta-analysis of mostly the same studies by Biccard *et al.* showed no such association [53]. The POISE investigators did several meta-analyses of the β-blocker trials and presented these within their manuscript. In their meta-analysis of eight trials, β-blockers did not show a significant effect on death, but when one trial that had a very large reduction in mortality (and that was stopped early) was excluded, β-blockers resulted in an increased risk of death. β-Blocker therapy reduced the risk of myocardial infarction and increased the risk of nonfatal stroke.

Where does this leave perioperative physicians and β-blockers therapy? The patient who is taking chronic β-blockers is unaffected; acute withdrawal of these drugs can lead to serious morbidity and mortality [54]. Similarly, current evidence does not propose that patients with CAD should not receive chronic β-blockade. However, if the CAD is only recognized at the preoperative visit, it is probably inappropriate to start therapy at that time. Ideally, in patients with CAD who need β-blockers for their CAD, therapy should be started well in advance of surgery so that the appropriate dosage can be determined and the patient's hemodynamic status be shown to be stable on the new therapy.

Perioperative statin therapy

One of the other strategies for perioperative cardiac protection is the use of statin (3-hydroxy-3-methylglutaryl coenzyme A reductase inhibitors) therapy. As previously discussed, their pleiotropic properties exert beneficial effects over and above the effect on lipids [55]. Statins have proved to be very safe, and death attributable to statin therapy is in the range of 1/1 000 000 patient years of use. Other reported severe side effects, including rhabdomyolysis and acute liver failure, are also exceedingly rare; the incidence of these events in the perioperative-use setting is unknown. There is an emerging consensus that perioperative statin withdrawal can cause rebound effects leading to cardiac morbidity [56,57]. The mechanism is shown in Fig. 66.3 [58].

There is emerging evidence that statins significantly reduce cardiovascular morbidity and mortality after noncardiac surgery [59–61]. However, most of these are retrospective studies. Since withdrawal of statins leading to ischemia or infarction has a mechanistically sound explanation, they should not be stopped before surgery. Statins should be restarted immediately in the postoperative period. In the intubated patient they should be given via the nasogastric tube. For patients who are strictly nil per mouth or per tube (a requirement that applies to very few patients), there is currently no other approved route of administration. In those patients at risk for CAD and who

meet the criteria for statins, therapy should be started well in advance of surgery. In patients who are at risk for CAD and who present for imminent surgery, the decision to start statins should be individualized. The benefit-versus-risk assessment in this population would suggest that it would likely be safe, but this cannot be definitively stated until larger prospective trials are completed.

Perioperative antiplatelet therapy

The management of aspirin and clopidogrel in the perioperative period will depend on whether they are prescribed for primary or secondary prevention, and also on the risk of bleeding versus the risk of discontinuing therapy. Many patients take aspirin for primary prevention of ACS and ischemic stroke. In a recent meta-analysis of six trials involving over 50 000 patients, aspirin nonadherence or withdrawal was associated with a threefold increased risk of major adverse events, and an 89-fold increase in risk for patients with coronary stents [62]. The authors concluded that aspirin should only be discontinued when bleeding risk clearly outweighs the benefit. The mechanism of the increased risk of ACS or acute stroke is not well defined, and may either represent a withdrawal of the protective effect in a susceptible plaque/vessel or a rebound hypercoagulable state [63].

The evidence for aspirin as a cardioprotective drug in the perioperative period is not well defined [64]. In patients having carotid endarterectomy, aspirin reduces stroke and myocardial infarction [65]. There have been no randomized controlled trials to quantify the bleeding risk due aspirin. In a meta-analysis by Burger *et al.*, up to 10.2% of acute cardiovascular syndromes may have been due to aspirin withdrawal [66]. The median time to acute stroke was 14 days, 8 days for ACS, and 25 days for peripheral arterial withdrawal syndromes. Aspirin was found to possibly increase the rate of bleeding complications by a factor of 1.5, but it did not lead to an increased severity of bleeding (with possible exceptions in neurological and prostatic operations with a high risk for bleeding). It was concluded that low-dose aspirin should only be stopped if the bleeding risks/sequelae exceed the cardiovascular risks of withdrawal. Whether aspirin should be started in patients at risk for CAD who are not taking aspirin has not been studied. Current primary prevention evidence suggests that this would be a safe intervention, but again the bleeding risk will need to be assessed.

Clopidogrel inhibits the binding of adenosine diphosphate (ADP) to its platelet receptor and the subsequent ADP-mediated activation of the GPIIb/IIIa complex. The platelet aggregation is irreversibly affected. If administered for primary prevention in place of aspirin, clopidogrel should ideally be discontinued 7–10 days prior to elective surgery. However, serious thrombotic risks are associated with clopidogrel withdrawal when it is used as secondary prevention, especially in patients with coronary stents [67]. The duration of required

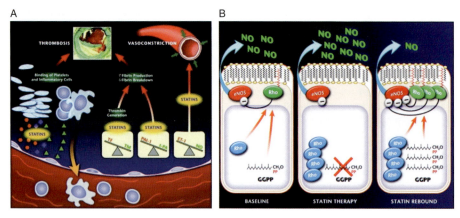

Figure 66.3. Perioperative statin therapy. (A) Statin therapy decreases endothelial adhesion molecules and tissue factor (TF), whereas thrombomodulin (TM) expression is increased. Tissue plasminogen activator (tPA)/plasminogen activator inhibitor 1 (PAI-1) ratio is normalized, while nitric oxide (NO) bioavailability is restored. All these effects lead to restoration of the physiologic properties of the endothelium. ET-1, endothelin. (B) Withdrawal from chronic statins modulates NO bioavailability. At baseline, Rho (small guanosine triphosphatase family) is active, associated to geranylgeranylpyrophosphate (GGPP). After initiation of statin treatment, formation of GGPP is interrupted, and Rho is inactive in its cytosolic form, which results in endothelial NO synthetase (eNOS) upregulation. After discontinuation of chronic statin therapy, GGPP becomes available, and Rho is transferred to the membrane, causing downregulation of eNOS production below baseline levels. Reproduced with permission from Le Manach et al. [55].

dual antiplatelet therapy varies depending on the type of stent, and catastrophic results have occurred when stopping clopidogrel even more than 12 months after drug-eluting stent implantation. Some now suggest that patients with drug-eluting stents be maintained on aspirin and clopidogrel indefinitely. Therefore, the perioperative decision regarding potentially stopping clopidogrel is very difficult and must involve the surgeon, internist, neurologist (where appropriate), anesthesiologist, and primary care physician.

Thoracic sympathectomy

Thoracic sympathectomy may benefit cardiac function by improving myocardial oxygen supply–demand balance. Thoracic epidural anesthesia (TEA) with local anesthetics has been shown to decrease determinants of myocardial oxygen demand, improve LV function, improve anginal symptoms, and in animal models to decrease infarct size. In patients with multivessel ischemic heart disease, TEA partly normalizes the myocardial blood flow in response to sympathetic stimulation [68]. TEA improves diastolic function in patients undergoing cardiac surgery [69]. Thoracic sympathectomy has been shown to have favorable effects on the myocardial β-receptor function at the time of cardiac surgery [70]. There have been many studies examining the effect of TEA on surrogate outcomes after cardiac and noncardiac surgery, many of which have shown beneficial effects. A meta-analysis by Liu et al. assessed the effects of neuraxial techniques on outcome after CABG: there was no effect on mortality or myocardial infarction, shorter time to extubation, decreased pulmonary complications, decreased arrhythmias, and better pain control [71]. Djaiani et al. showed that regional techniques resulted in better analgesia, shorter postoperative ventilation, reduced

supraventricular arrhythmias, and less perioperative myocardial infarction after cardiac surgery [72]. A recent randomized controlled trial compared TEA to morphine patient-controlled analgesia (PCA) after cardiac surgery and showed that it did not offer any major advantages with respect to length of stay, quality of recovery, and morbidity [73]. Thus, the TEA studies have been inconsistent and are disappointing, with relatively small numbers of patients [74]. The question whether thoracic symapathectomy using regional anesthetic techniques influences outcome after cardiac surgery is yet to be answered. Similarly, in major noncardiac surgery, the effect of epidural anesthesia on major outcomes has yielded conflicting results [75,76]. In a recent population-based cohort study in over 250 000 patients, epidural anesthesia or analgesia was associated with a very small reduction in 30-day mortality (1.7% vs. 2.0%, relative risk 0.89, 95% CI 0.81–0.98, $p = 0.02$), corresponding to a number needed to treat (NNT) of 477 patients [77]. The authors concluded that the data must be used with caution and do not provide compelling evidence for epidurals as a means of improving postoperative survival.

Cardioplegia

Cardioplegia rapidly arrests the heart for a still operative field, conserves cellular adenosine triphosphate (ATP) stores, induces cardiac hypothermia to further reduce energy consumption, and provides other drugs that may further protect from ischemia–reperfusion injury [78]. In 1978, the concept of cold, hyperkalemic blood cardioplegia was described. Common commercial cardioplegia preparations, such as the modified St. Thomas preparations, deliver between 15 and 20 mEq L^{-1} potassium to induce a depolarized cardiac arrest. It is rapid and reversible. However, this hyperkalemic arrest leads to a several pathophysiologic processes, including Ca^{2+}-activated dysrhythmogenic currents, abnormal regulation of intracellular second messengers, activation of cytosolic and membrane-bound enzyme systems, impaired myocardial contraction and the potential for Ca^{2+}-induced reperfusion injury. The disadvantages of hyperkalemic arrest are mostly related to Ca^{2+} overload, the potential for endothelial damage at high potassium concentrations, temperature sensitivity requiring greater concentrations for normothermic arrest, the potential for systemic hyperkalemia, and sustained metabolic activity. Hypocalcemia-induced depolarizing arrest with a solution containing zero calcium, combined with low sodium and procaine, has been tried as an alternative to hyperkalemic arrest. However, zero-calcium and low-sodium solutions appear to affect the cell membrane, leading to loosening of gap junctions and the intercalated disc, which can have adverse effects during the reperfusion phase; this technique of cardioplegia is now rarely used. Because of the problems inherent in depolarized arrest, polarized or hyperpolarized arrest is a theoretical alternative. Here membrane potential (E_m) is kept close to, or more negative than, the resting membrane potential. This more physiologic state has several theoretic advantages. The transmembrane ion gradients remain balanced at or close to E_m, which prevents the ionic imbalance seen during hyperkalemic arrest. Few pumps or channels are activated, metabolic demand remains low, and myocyte energy stores are maintained. Adenosine and K_{ATP} channel activators are examples employing this strategy.

The cardioplegia solutions are delivered either by antegrade administration into aortic root or coronary arteries, or retrograde through coronary sinus cannulation, or by a combination. Reduced postoperative morbidity has been demonstrated with combined antegrade and retrograde blood cardioplegia versus antegrade crystalloid cardioplegia alone [79]. In another trial, no difference between cold antegrade blood and cold retrograde blood cardioplegia could be demonstrated [80]. A recent survey of practice in the United Kingdom found that all these techniques were being employed, and that the data favoring one technique over the other were fraught with methodological challenges [81].

Standard techniques of intermittent cold cardioplegia may have some deleterious effects on myocardial enzyme systems and delay in the recovery of postoperative myocardial metabolism and function. In the early 1990s, it became clear that the heart could be maintained at a temperature of 37 °C throughout the crossclamp period, and that the postclamp myocardial metabolic dysfunction could be reduced. A trial of warm versus cold cardioplegia in 2000 CABG patients showed a lower incidence of postoperative low cardiac output syndrome in the warm group, but no differences in mortality or myocardial infarction [82]. Controversy still exists regarding the optimal temperature, although many centers have reduced the use of cold cardioplegia (9 °C) in favor of tepid cardioplegia [83]. Complement activation occurs during CPB, and anticomplement therapies have been studied as adjuncts to cardioplegia [84]. Antileukotriene and anti-TNF strategies have been employed with variable results [85]. Nitric oxide has been extensively studied for its adjunctive role in cardioplegia. Although reperfusion injury is reduced by some nitric oxide donors [86], other studies have shown that this may be harmful by producing peroxynitrite [87]. Insulin-enhanced cardioplegia has also been extensively studied, with limited or no improvement in functional cardiac recovery [88,89]. Cyclosporine A has been investigated as a cardioplegia additive for its nonspecific mitochondrial permeability transition pore inhibition [90,91]. β-Blockers have been used in combination with cardioplegia solutions and have shown promising surrogate endpoints [92–93]. Pretreatment with the purine nucleoside autocoid adenosine has been shown to reduce the severity of acute post-reperfusion myocardial infarction [95]. Although sodium/hydrogen exchange inhibition should reduce myocardial reperfusion, the cardioprotective effect of the sodium/hydrogen exchanger inhibitor cariporide failed to show an overall benefit [96]. Adenosine has been successfully used in cardioplegia, and has shown promise as an alternative or adjunct to high-potassium cardioplegia [97,98].

Summary

Acute coronary syndromes (ACS) consist of unstable angina (UA), ST-elevation myocardial infarction (STEMI), and non-ST-elevation myocardial infarction (NSTEMI). The treatment of STEMI is expeditious reperfusion therapy with percutaneous coronary intervention (PCI). If PCI is not available or unlikely to be expeditious, thrombolysis may be indicated. Adjuvant medical therapy consists of antiplatelet, anticoagulant, anti-ischemic, and anti-heart-failure medications. The initial treatment of NSTEMI is aggressive medical therapy, with PCI reserved for patients with high TIMI risk scores. There is no role for thrombolysis in NSTEMI/UA.

The landmark Perioperative Ischemia Evaluation (POISE) trial showed that acute β-blocker therapy in patients at risk for coronary artery disease having major surgery was not associated with improved overall outcome. If chronic β-blocker treatment is indicated in a patient presenting for surgery it should be started well in advance of surgery. Patients on chronic β-blockers should not have therapy interrupted at the time of surgery, as serious withdrawal effects can occur. Patients taking statins may have improved perioperative cardiovascular outcomes, although there are no conclusive data yet on starting perioperative statin therapy for this indication. Chronic statin therapy should be continued, as acute withdrawal can have deleterious effects. Acute aspirin withdrawal can lead to myocardial infarction. Patients on aspirin for primary or secondary prevention should only have therapy stopped if the consequences of even a small amount of bleeding outweigh the cardioprotective effect. In the case of clopidogrel, there is an increased risk of bleeding but a very serious risk of interrupting therapy. Management for each patient should be individualized and the decision made with the help of the appropriate perioperative consultants.

Epidural anesthesia with local anesthetics causes a thoracic sympathectomy which may favorably affect myocardial oxygen supply–demand ratio. However, there are no conclusive clinical data supporting this anesthetic technique solely to improve major perioperative cardiac outcomes. Cardioplegia arrests the heart, providing a still operative field, conserving energy, and protecting the myocardium. The optimal administration route of cardioplegia preparations, temperature, and adjunctive therapy all remain subject to debate. Polarized or hyperpolarized arrest has been proposed as a theoretical alternative to overcome the problems associated with depolarized arrest.

References

1. Alpert JS, Thygesen K, Jaffe A, White HD. The universal definition of myocardial infarction: a consensus document: ischaemic heart disease. *Heart* 2008; **94**: 1335–41.

2. Achar SA, Kundu S, Norcross WA. Diagnosis of acute coronary syndrome. *Am Fam Physician* 2005; **72**: 119–26.

3. Morrow DA, Antman EM, Charlesworth A, *et al.* TIMI risk score for ST-elevation myocardial infarction: a convenient, bedside, clinical score for risk assessment at presentation: an intravenous nPA for treatment of infarcting myocardium early II trial substudy. *Circulation* 2000; **102**: 2031–7.

4. Antman EM, Cohen M, Bernink PJ, *et al.* The TIMI risk score for unstable angina/non-ST elevation MI: a method for prognostication and therapeutic decision making. *JAMA* 2000; **284**: 835–42.

5. Antman EM, Hand M, Armstrong PW, *et al.* 2007 focused update of the ACC/AHA 2004 Guidelines for the Management of Patients With ST-Elevation Myocardial Infarction: a report of the American College of Cardiology/American Heart Association Task Force on Practice Guidelines. *Circulation* 2008; **117**: 296–329.

6. Randomised trial of intravenous streptokinase, oral aspirin, both, or neither among 17,187 cases of suspected acute myocardial infarction: ISIS-2. ISIS-2 (Second International Study of Infarct Survival) Collaborative Group. *Lancet* 1988; **2**: 349–60.

7. Chen ZM, Jiang LX, Chen YP, *et al.* Addition of clopidogrel to aspirin in 45,852 patients with acute myocardial infarction: randomised placebo-controlled trial. *Lancet* 2005; **366**: 1607–21.

8. Sabatine MS, McCabe CH, Gibson CM, Cannon CP. Design and rationale of Clopidogrel as Adjunctive Reperfusion Therapy-Thrombolysis in Myocardial Infarction (CLARITY-TIMI) 28 trial. *Am Heart J* 2005; **149**: 227–33.

9. Parodi G, Ndrepepa G, Kastrati A, *et al.* Ability of mechanical reperfusion to salvage myocardium in patients with acute myocardial infarction presenting beyond 12 hours after onset of symptoms. *Am Heart J* 2006; **152**: 1133–9.

10. Long-term effects of intravenous thrombolysis in acute myocardial infarction: final report of the GISSI study. Gruppo Italiano per lo Studio della Streptochi-nasi nell'Infarto Miocardico (GISSI). *Lancet* 1987; **2**: 871–4.

11. Gershlick AH, Stephens-Lloyd A, Hughes S, *et al.* Rescue angioplasty after failed thrombolytic therapy for acute myocardial infarction. *N Engl J Med* 2005; **353**: 2758–68.

12. Assessment of the Safety and Efficacy of a New Treatment Strategy with Percutaneous Coronary Intervention (ASSENT-4 PCI) investigators. Primary versus tenecteplase-facilitated percutaneous coronary intervention in patients with ST-segment elevation acute myocardial infarction (ASSENT-4 PCI): randomised trial. *Lancet* 2006; **367**: 569–78.

13. McCann CJ, Menown IB. New anticoagulant strategies in ST elevation myocardial infarction: trials and clinical implications. *Vasc Health Risk Manag* 2008; **4**: 305–13.

14. Assessment of the Safety and Efficacy of a New Thrombolytic Regimen (ASSENT)-3 Investigators. Efficacy and safety of tenecteplase in combination with enoxaparin, abciximab, or unfractionated heparin: the ASSENT-3 randomised trial in acute myocardial infarction. *Lancet* 2001; **358**: 605–13.

15. Antman EM, Louwerenburg HW, Baars HF, *et al.* Enoxaparin as adjunctive antithrombin therapy for ST-elevation myocardial infarction: results of the ENTIRE-Thrombolysis in Myocardial Infarction (TIMI) 23 Trial. *Circulation* 2002; **105**: 1642–9.

16. Wallentin L, Goldstein P, Armstrong PW, *et al.* Efficacy and safety of tenecteplase in combination with the low-molecular-weight heparin enoxaparin or unfractionated heparin in the prehospital setting: the Assessment of the Safety and Efficacy of a New Thrombolytic Regimen (ASSENT)-3 PLUS randomized trial in acute myocardial infarction. *Circulation* 2003; **108**: 135–42.

17. Yusuf S, Mehta SR, Chrolavicius S, *et al.* Effects of fondaparinux on mortality and reinfarction in patients with acute ST-segment elevation myocardial infarction: the OASIS-6 randomized trial. *JAMA* 2006; **295**: 1519–30.

18. De Luca G, Marino P. Advances in antithrombotic therapy as adjunct to reperfusion therapies for ST-segment elevation myocardial infarction. *Thromb Haemost* 2008; **100**: 184–95.

19. Faxon DP. Use of antiplatelet agents and anticoagulants for cardiovascular disease: current standards and best practices. *Rev Cardiovasc Med* 2005; **6**: S3–14.

20. Anderson JL, Adams CD, Antman EM, *et al.* ACC/AHA 2007 guidelines for the management of patients with unstable angina/non-ST-elevation myocardial infarction: a report of the American College of Cardiology/American Heart Association Task Force on Practice Guidelines. *J Am Coll Cardiol* 2007; **50**: e1–157.

21. Fox KA, Mehta SR, Peters R, *et al.* Benefits and risks of the combination of clopidogrel and aspirin in patients undergoing surgical revascularization for non-ST-elevation acute coronary syndrome: the Clopidogrel in Unstable angina to prevent Recurrent ischemic Events (CURE) Trial. *Circulation* 2004; **110**: 1202–8.

22. Beinart SC, Kolm P, Veledar E, *et al.* Long-term cost effectiveness of early and sustained dual oral antiplatelet therapy with clopidogrel given for up to one year after percutaneous coronary intervention results: from the Clopidogrel for the Reduction of Events During Observation (CREDO) trial. *J Am Coll Cardiol* 2005; **46**: 761–9.

23. Casterella PJ, Tcheng JE. Review of the 2005 American College of Cardiology, American Heart Association, and Society for Cardiovascular Interventions guidelines for adjunctive pharmacologic therapy during percutaneous coronary interventions: practical implications, new clinical data, and recommended guideline revisions. *Am Heart J* 2008; **155**: 781–90.

24. Oler A, Whooley MA, Oler J, Grady D. Adding heparin to aspirin reduces the incidence of myocardial infarction and death in patients with unstable angina. A meta-analysis. *JAMA* 1996; **276**: 811–15.

25. Galli M. The treatment of acute coronary syndromes of the "non-ST elevation" type with enoxaparin: the TIMI 11B study. Thrombolysis in Myocardial Infarct. *Ital Heart J Suppl* 2000; **1**: 575–6.

26. Fifth Organization to Assess Strategies in Acute Ischemic Syndromes Investigators, Yusuf S, Mehta SR, *et al.* Comparison of fondaparinux and enoxaparin in acute coronary syndromes. *N Engl J Med* 2006; **354**: 1464–76.

27. Singh S, Molnar J, Arora R. Efficacy and safety of bivalirudin versus heparins in reduction of cardiac outcomes in acute coronary syndrome and percutaneous coronary interventions. *Cardiovasc Pharmacol Ther* 2007; **12**: 283–91.

28. Chen ZM, Pan HC, Chen YP, *et al.* Early intravenous then oral metoprolol in 45,852 patients with acute myocardial infarction: randomised placebo-controlled trial. *Lancet* 2005; **366**: 1622–32.

29. Pedrazzini G, Santoro E, Latini R, *et al.* Causes of death in patients with acute myocardial infarction treated with angiotensin-converting enzyme inhibitors: findings from the Gruppo Italiano per lo Studio della Sopravvivenza nell'Infarto (GISSI)-3 trial. *Am Heart J* 2008; **155**: 388–94.

30. Yusuf S, Sleight P, Pogue J, *et al.* Effects of an angiotensin-converting-enzyme inhibitor, ramipril, on cardiovascular events in high-risk patients. The Heart Outcomes Prevention Evaluation Study Investigators. *N Engl J Med* 2000; **342**: 145–53.

31. Pitt B, Bakris G, Ruilope LM, *et al.* Serum potassium and clinical outcomes in the Eplerenone Post-Acute Myocardial Infarction Heart Failure Efficacy and Survival Study (EPHESUS). *Circulation* 2008; **118**: 1643–50.

32. Cannon CP, Braunwald E, McCabe CH, *et al.* Intensive versus moderate lipid lowering with statins after acute coronary syndromes. *N Engl J Med* 2004; **350**: 1495–1504.

33. Al-Khatib SM, Granger CB, Huang Y, *et al.* Sustained ventricular arrhythmias among patients with acute coronary syndromes with no ST-segment elevation: incidence, predictors, and outcomes. *Circulation* 2002; **106**: 309–12.

34. Hohnloser SH, Kuck KH, Dorian P, *et al.* Prophylactic use of an implantable cardioverter-defibrillator after acute myocardial infarction. *N Engl J Med* 2004; **351**: 2481–8.

35. Hallstrom AP, Wyse DG, McAnulty J, for the CAST and AVID Investigators. Clinical criteria for predicting benefit of ICD/PM in post myocardial infarction patients: an AVID and CAST analysis. *J Interv Card Electrophysiol* 2008; **23**: 159–66.

36. Malmberg K, Norhammar A, Wedel H, Ryden L. Glycometabolic state at admission: important risk marker of mortality in conventionally treated patients with diabetes mellitus and acute myocardial infarction: long-term results from the Diabetes and Insulin-Glucose Infusion in Acute Myocardial Infarction (DIGAMI) study. *Circulation* 1999 May; **99**: 2626–32.

37. Woods KL, Fletcher S. Long-term outcome after intravenous magnesium sulphate in suspected acute myocardial infarction: the second Leicester Intravenous Magnesium Intervention Trial (LIMIT-2). *Lancet* 1994; **343**: 816–19.

38. Li J, Zhang Q, Zhang M, Egger M. *Cochrane Database Syst Rev* 2007; (2): CD002755.

39. Mangano DT, Layug EL, Wallace A, Tateo I. Effect of atenolol on mortality and cardiovascular morbidity after noncardiac surgery. Multicenter Study of Perioperative Ischemia Research Group. *N Engl J Med* 1996; **335**: 1713–20.

40. Poldermans D, Boersma E, Bax JJ, *et al.* The effect of bisoprolol on perioperative mortality and myocardial infarction in high-risk patients undergoing vascular surgery. Dutch Echocardiographic Cardiac Risk Evaluation Applying Stress Echocardiography Study Group. *N Engl J Med* 1999; **341**: 1789–94.

41. Leslie K, Devereaux PJ. A large trial is vital to prove perioperative beta-blockade effectiveness and safety before widespread use. *Anesthesiology* 2004; **101**: 803.

42. Yeager MP, Fillinger MP, Hettleman BD, Hartman GS. Perioperative beta-blockade and late cardiac outcomes: a complementary hypothesis. *J Cardiothorac Vasc Anesth* 2005; **19**: 237–41.

43. Devereaux PJ, Beattie WS, Choi PT, *et al.* How strong is the evidence for the use of perioperative beta blockers in non-cardiac surgery? Systematic review and meta-analysis of randomised controlled trials. *BMJ* 2005; **331**: 313–21.

44. Fleisher LA, Beckman JA, Brown KA, *et al.* ACC/AHA 2007 Guidelines on Perioperative Cardiovascular Evaluation and Care for Noncardiac Surgery: executive summary: a report of the American College of Cardiology/ American Heart Association Task Force on Practice Guidelines. *Circulation* 2007; **116**: 1971–96.

45. Antman EM, Hand M, Armstrong PW, *et al.* 2007 Focused update of the ACC/ AHA 2004 Guidelines for the Management of Patients With ST-Elevation Myocardial Infarction: a report of the American College of Cardiology/American Heart Association Task Force on

Practice Guidelines. *Circulation* 2008; **117**: 296–329.

46. London MJ. Quo vadis, perioperative beta blockade? Are you "POISE'd" on the brink? *Anesth Analg* 2008; **106**: 1025–30.

47. POISE Study Group. Effects of extended-release metoprolol succinate in patients undergoing non-cardiac surgery (POISE trial): a randomised controlled trial. *Lancet* 2008; **371**: 1839–47.

48. Fleisher LA, Poldermans D. Perioperative beta blockade: where do we go from here? *Lancet* 2008; **371**: 1813–14.

49. Rinfret S, Abrahamowicz M, Tu J, et al. A population-based analysis of the class effect of beta-blockers after myocardial infarction. *Am Heart J* 2007; **153**: 224–30.

50. Zaugg M, Bestmann L, Wacker J, et al. Adrenergic receptor genotype but not perioperative bisoprolol therapy may determine cardiovascular outcome in at-risk patients undergoing surgery with spinal block: the Swiss Beta Blocker in Spinal Anesthesia (BBSA) study: a double-blinded, placebo-controlled, multicenter trial with 1-year follow-up. *Anesthesiology* 2007; **107**: 33–44.

51. Sear JW, Giles JW, Howard-Alpe G, Foex P. Perioperative beta-blockade, 2008: what does POISE tell us, and was our earlier caution justified? *Br J Anaesth* 2008; **101**: 135–8.

52. Beattie WS, Wijeysundera DN, Karkouti K, McCluskey S, Tait G. Does tight heart rate control improve beta-blocker efficacy? An updated analysis of the noncardiac surgical randomized trials. *Anesth Analg* 2008; **106**: 1039–48.

53. Biccard BM, Sear JW, Foex P. Meta-analysis of the effect of heart rate achieved by perioperative beta-adrenergic blockade on cardiovascular outcomes. *Br J Anaesth* 2008; **100**: 23–8.

54. Shammash JB, Trost JC, Gold JM, et al. Perioperative beta-blocker withdrawal and mortality in vascular surgical patients. *Am Heart J* 2001; **141**: 148–53.

55. Le Manach Y, Coriat P, Collard CD, Riedel B. Statin therapy within the perioperative period. *Anesthesiology* 2008; **108**: 1141–6.

56. Le Manach Y, Godet G, Coriat P, et al. The impact of postoperative discontinuation or continuation of chronic statin therapy on cardiac outcome after major vascular surgery. *Anesth Analg* 2007; **104**: 1326–33.

57. Pan W, Pintar T, Anton J, et al. Statins are associated with a reduced incidence of perioperative mortality after coronary artery bypass graft surgery. *Circulation* 2004; **110**: II45–9.

58. Spencer FA, Allegrone J, Goldberg RJ, et al. Association of statin therapy with outcomes of acute coronary syndromes: the GRACE study. *Ann Intern Med* 2004; **140**: 857–66.

59. Poldermans D, Bax JJ, Kertai MD, et al. Statins are associated with a reduced incidence of perioperative mortality in patients undergoing major noncardiac vascular surgery. *Circulation* 2003; **107**: 1848–51.

60. Lindenauer PK, Pekow P, Wang K, Gutierrez B, Benjamin EM. Lipid-lowering therapy and in-hospital mortality following major noncardiac surgery. *JAMA* 2004; **291**: 2092–9.

61. Hindler K, Shaw AD, Samuels J, et al. Improved postoperative outcomes associated with preoperative statin therapy. *Anesthesiology* 2006; **105**: 1260–72.

62. Biondi-Zoccai GG, Lotrionte M, Agostoni P, et al. A systematic review and meta-analysis on the hazards of discontinuing or not adhering to aspirin among 50,279 patients at risk for coronary artery disease. *Eur Heart J* 2006; **27**: 2667–74.

63. Vial JH, McLeod LJ, Roberts MS. Rebound elevation in urinary thromboxane B2 and 6-keto-PGF1 alpha excretion after aspirin withdrawal. *Adv Prostaglandin Thromboxane Leukot Res* 1991; **21A**: 157–60.

64. Poldermans D, Hoeks SE, Feringa HH. Pre-operative risk assessment and risk reduction before surgery. *J Am Coll Cardiol* 2008; **51**: 1913–24.

65. Lindblad B, Persson NH, Takolander R, Bergqvist D. Does low-dose acetylsalicylic acid prevent stroke after carotid surgery? A double-blind, placebo-controlled randomized trial. *Stroke* 1993; **24**: 1125–8.

66. Burger W, Chemnitius JM, Kneissl GD, Rucker G. Low-dose aspirin for secondary cardiovascular prevention: cardiovascular risks after its perioperative withdrawal versus bleeding risks with its continuation. Review and meta-analysis. *J Intern Med* 2005; **257**: 399–414.

67. Smith SC, Feldman TE, Hirshfeld JW, et al. ACC/AHA/SCAI 2005 Guideline Update for Percutaneous Coronary Intervention-Summary Article: a Report of the American College of Cardiology/American Heart Association Task Force on Practice Guidelines (ACC/AHA/SCAI Writing Committee to Update the 2001 Guidelines for Percutaneous Coronary Intervention). *J Am Coll Cardiol* 2006; **47**: 216–35.

68. Nygård E, Kofoed KF, Freiberg J, et al. Effects of high thoracic epidural analgesia on myocardial blood flow in patients with ischemic heart disease. *Circulation* 2005; **111**: 2165–70.

69. Schmidt C, Hinder F, Van Aken H, et al. The effect of high thoracic epidural anesthesia on systolic and diastolic left ventricular function in patients with coronary artery disease. *Anesth Analg* 2005; **100**: 1561–9.

70. Lee TW, Grocott HP, Schwinn D, Jacobsohn E, Winnipeg High-Spinal Anesthesia Group. 2High spinal anesthesia for cardiac surgery: effects on beta-adrenergic receptor function, stress response, and hemodynamics. *Anesthesiology* 2003; **98**: 499–510.

71. Liu SS, Block BM, Wu CL. Effects of perioperative central neuraxial analgesia on outcome after coronary artery bypass surgery: a meta-analysis. *Anesthesiology* 2004; **101**: 153–61.

72. Djaiani G, Fedorko L, Beattie WS. Regional anesthesia in cardiac surgery: a friend or a foe? *Semin Cardiothorac Vasc Anesth* 2005; **9**: 87–104.

73. Hansdottir V, Philip J, Olsen MF, et al. Thoracic epidural versus intravenous patient-controlled analgesia after cardiac surgery: a randomized controlled trial on length of hospital stay and patient-perceived quality of recovery. *Anesthesiology* 2006; **104**: 142–51.

74. Hemmerling TM, Carli F, Noiseux N. Thoracic epidural anaesthesia for

cardiac surgery: are we missing the point? *Br J Anaesth* 2008; **100**: 3–5.

75. Rodgers A, Walker N, Schug S, *et al.* Reduction of postoperative mortality and morbidity with epidural or spinal anaesthesia: results from overview of randomised trials. *BMJ* 2000; **321**: 1493.

76. Park WY, Thompson JS, Lee KK. Effect of epidural anesthesia and analgesia on perioperative outcome: a randomized, controlled Veterans Affairs cooperative study. *Ann Surg* 2001; **234**: 560–9.

77. Wijeysundera DN, Beattie WS, Austin PC, Hux JE, Laupacis A. Epidural anaesthesia and survival after intermediate-to-high risk non-cardiac surgery: a population-based cohort study. *Lancet* 2008; **372**: 562–9.

78. Nicolini F, Beghi C, Muscari C, *et al.* Myocardial protection in adult cardiac surgery: current options and future challenges. *Review Eur J Cardiothorac Surg* 2003; **24**: 986–93.

79. Flack JE, Cook JR, May SJ, *et al.* Does cardioplegia type affect outcome and survival in patients with advanced left ventricular dysfunction? Results from the CABG Patch Trial. *Circulation* 2000; **102**: 84–9.

80. Dagenais F, Pelletier LC, Carrier M. Antegrade/retrograde cardioplegia for valve replacement: a prospective study. *Ann Thorac Surg* 1999; **68**: 1681–5.

81. Jacob S, Kallikourdis A, Sellke F, Dunning J. Is blood cardioplegia superior to crystalloid cardioplegia? *Interact Cardiovasc Thorac Surg* 2008; **7**: 491–8.

82. Naylor CD, Lichtenstein SV, Fremes SE, Warm Investigators. Randomized trial of normothermic versus hypothermic coronary bypass surgery. *Lancet* 1994; **343**: 559–63.

83. Hayashida N, Weisel RD, Shirai T, *et al.* Tepid antegrade and retrograde cardioplegia. *Ann Thorac Surg* 1995; **59**: 723–9.

84. Fung M, Loubser PG, Undar A, *et al.* Inhibition of complement, neutrophil, and platelet activation by an anti-factor D monoclonal antibody in simulated cardiopulmonary bypass circuits. *J Thorac Cardiovasc Surg* 2001; **122**: 113–22.

85. Vermeiren GLJ, Claeys MJ, Van Bockstaele D, *et al.* Reperfusion injury after focal myocardial ischemia: polymorphonuclear leukocyte activation and its clinical implications. *Resuscitation* 2002; **45**: 35–61.

86. Carrier M, Pellerin M, Perrault LP, *et al.* Cardioplegic arrest with L-arginine improves myocardial protection: results of a prospective randomised clinical trial. *Ann Thorac Surg* 2002; **73**: 837–42.

87. Nakamura M, Thourani VH, Ronson RS, *et al.* Glutathione reverses endothelial damage from peroxynitrite, the byproduct of nitric oxide degradation, in crystalloid cardioplegia. *Circulation* 2000; **102**: 332–8.

88. Hynninen M, Borger MA, Rao V, *et al.* The effect of insulin cardioplegia on atrial fibrillation after high-risk coronary bypass surgery: a double-blinded, randomized, controlled trial. *Anesth Analg* 2001; **92**: 810–16.

89. Rao V, Christakis GT, Weisel RD, *et al.* . The Insulin Cardioplegia Trial: myocardial protection for urgent coronary artery bypass grafting. *J Thorac Cardiovasc Surg* 2002; **123**: 928–35.

90. Nakagawa T, Shimizu S, Watanabe T, *et al.* Cyclophilin D-dependent mitochondrial permeability transition regulates some necrotic but not apoptotic cell death. *Nature* 2005; **434**: 652–8.

91. Oka N, Wang L, Mi W, Caldarone CA. Inhibition of mitochondrial remodeling by cyclosporine A preserves myocardial performance in a neonatal rabbit model of cardioplegic arrest. *J Thorac Cardiovasc Surg* 2008; **135**: 585–93.

92. Bessho R, Chambers DJ. Myocardial protection with oxygenated esmolol cardioplegia during prolonged normothermic ischemia in the rat. *J Thorac Cardiovasc Surg* 2002; **124**: 340–51.

93. Scorsin M, Mebazaa A, Al Attar N, *et al.* Efficacy of esmolol as a myocardial protective agent during continuous retrograde blood. *J Thorac Cardiovasc Surg* 2003; **125**: 1022–9.

94. Fannelop T, Dahle GO, Matre K, *et al.* Esmolol before 80 min of cardiac arrest with oxygenated cold blood cardioplegia alleviates systolic dysfunction. An experimental study in pigs. *Eur J Cardiothorac Surg* 2008; **33**: 9–17.

95. Mangano DT, Miao Y, Tudor IC, *et al.* Post-reperfusion myocardial infarction: long-term survival improvement using adenosine regulation with acadesine. *J Am Coll Cardiol* 2006; **48**: 206–14.

96. Theroux P, Chaitman BR, Danchin N, *et al.* Inhibition of the sodium-hydrogen exchanger with cariporide to prevent myocardial infarction in high-risk ischemic situations: main results of the GUARDIAN trial. *Circulation* 2000; **102**: 3032–8.

97. Corvera JS, Kin H, Dobson GP, *et al.* Polarized arrest with warm or cold adenosine/lidocaine blood cardioplegia is equivalent to hypothermic potassium blood cardioplegia. *J Thorac Cardiovasc Surg* 2005; **129**: 599–606.

98. Jakobsen Ø, Muller S, Aarsaether E, Steensrud T, Sørlie DG. Adenosine instead of supranormal potassium in cardioplegic solution improves cardioprotection. *Eur J Cardiothorac Surg* 2007; **32**: 493–500.

Management of patients with chronic alcohol or drug use

Howard B. Gutstein

Introduction

The high prevalence of drug and polydrug abuse necessitates that practicing anesthesiologists are familiar with the physiology and pharmacology of a wide variety of addictive drugs and emerging drugs of abuse (or drug combinations), which can impact anesthetic management profoundly. This chapter explores how alcoholics and drug users are affected by anesthesia. Specifically, alcohol, opoids, benzodiazepines/barbiturates, cocaine, amphetamines, and psychedelic drugs and their complications are examined, to enable anesthesiologists to anticipate possible patient problems and to manage outcomes.

Drug abuse is one of the most overwhelming problems facing society today. Addiction has been defined as the compulsive, uncontrolled use of drugs regardless of the physical or social consequences, as well as a strong tendency to relapse when abstinent. The cost to society, in terms of economics, social disruption, as well as health, is enormous. Abused drugs affect multiple organ systems and have many important implications for anesthetic care. Abuse of multiple drugs at once (polydrug abuse) is common, complicating medical management. Psychiatric disorders are also more common among drug abusers, possibly because these individuals are trying to "self-medicate" their underlying disorders [1]. Direct and indirect (trauma, infection, nutritional disorders) effects of addiction increase disease burden and lead to disproportionately frequent interactions with anesthesiologists. Thus it is essential for the practicing anesthesiologist to be familiar with the pharmacology of the wide variety of addictive drugs. Whether the anesthesiologist knows it or not, these patients make up a substantial portion of his or her practice. This chapter starts by presenting a brief synopsis of current theories of addiction. Addictive drugs are then considered by broad category, starting with depressant drugs, moving to psychostimulants, and concluding with hallucinogenic drugs and inhalants.

Theories of addiction

Drug addiction is formally defined as a chronic relapsing disorder characterized by (1) compulsion to seek and take the drug, (2) loss of control in limiting drug intake, and (3) emergence of a negative emotional state (e.g., dysphoria, anxiety, irritability) when access to the drug is prevented (also defined as dependence) [2]. Addictive behavior has been characterized by the "4 Cs": **compulsive** drug use, loss of **control** over drug-taking behavior, **craving**, and **continued use** despite harm. Clearly, the occasional but limited use of a drug with the potential for abuse or dependence is distinct both behaviorally and physiologically from uncontrolled drug use and the emergence of a chronic drug-dependent state.

The rewarding effects of drugs and motivation to continue taking drugs are mediated by a brain circuit called the mesolimbic dopamine system [3]. Increases in dopamine release in this circuit have been found to underlie the rewarding effects of all addictive drugs, including nicotine. Historically, theories of addiction have focused on the rewarding effects of drugs, postulating that a compulsive pattern of drug taking evolves, characterized by intoxication and the development of tolerance to this intoxication, with a resulting escalation in drug intake [4].

More recently, greater attention has been devoted to the contribution of aversive symptoms of withdrawal and the biology of the abstinent state [5]. For example, the brain reward system is progressively downregulated as drug use escalates, requiring more and more drug to achieve a positive emotional state [6]. Increased drug use also enhances the negative affective consequences of abstinence, resulting in profound dysphoria, physical discomfort, and somatic withdrawal signs. Intense preoccupation with obtaining drugs (i.e., craving) also develops. Craving often precedes somatic signs of withdrawal and is associated not only with obtaining the drug and its positive reinforcing effects, but also with avoiding the negative reinforcing or aversive effects of withdrawal.

Anesthetic Pharmacology, 2nd edition, ed. Alex S. Evers, Mervyn Maze, Evan D. Kharasch. Published by Cambridge University Press. © Cambridge University Press 2011.

These general mechanisms are common to all stimulant and depressant addictive drugs. However, these drugs vary widely in the disruptiveness of behavior they induce in addicts, both to obtain drugs and while under the influence.

Drug dependence has multiple meanings in the minds of both patients and clinicians. Particularly confusing has been the use of the term *physical dependence*, referring to physiological adaptations that occur with repeated drug exposure. Upon discontinuation of drug use, these adaptations result in withdrawal symptoms that can be mild (such as mild fatigue with cocaine) or severe (such as a flu-like state with opioids or hyperthermia and seizures with alcohol). These changes are distinct from adaptations in brain reward systems that result in addiction [5]. Thus, an individual can become physically dependent upon a drug without being addicted and, conversely, can be addicted without suffering from physical dependence. Unfortunately, the emphasis on distinguishing physical dependence from addiction has diminished attention on the role that motivational aspects of opioid withdrawal play in the genesis of the addicted state. Clearly, the negative emotional effects of drug withdrawal (sometimes incorrectly, in the author's opinion, described as "psychological dependence") are a key element of addiction [6] and may eventually provide a key to understanding mechanisms underlying drug addiction.

An area of great controversy in anesthesiology has been the risk of addiction in chronic pain patients. The scientific literature on this topic is actually quite limited. However, based on the available data, it appears that only a minority of patients undergoing chronic pain treatment with opioids are at high risk of developing addiction, and this risk is similar to the risk of addiction in the general population [7,8]. However, a recent meta-analysis suggested that chronic pain patients with a prior history of substance abuse had a 20-fold increase in the risk of addiction or aberrant drug-related behaviors during opioid therapy [9]. Thus, careful screening and patient selection is imperative prior to instituting chronic opioid therapy. A related concern of addicts undergoing surgery is that opioid analgesics will cause them to relapse. Two small studies of methadone-maintained individuals did not show evidence of relapse perioperatively or when cancer pain was treated with opioids [10,11]. In fact, it has been suggested that untreated or undertreated pain could play a significant role in sustaining drug use in addicts [12].

Depressant drugs

Alcohol

Alcohol has been commonly abused throughout human history. It has been estimated that 5% of the population of the United States meets standard definitions of alcoholism [13]. Alcohol can initially cause behavioral disinhibiton, but ultimately central nervous system (CNS)-depressant effects dominate, leading to ataxia, sedation, and in extreme cases coma.

Alcohol is a very "dirty" drug, affecting multiple target proteins. The majority of these are ion channels, such as γ-aminobutyric acid type A (GABA$_A$) receptors, the nicotinic acetylcholine receptor, N-methyl-D-aspartate (NMDA) and kainate types of glutamate receptors, BK potassium channels, as well as N and P/Q type calcium channels. Alcohol also activates several isoforms of adenylate cyclase [14]. This wide diversity of targets correlates with the wide diversity of pathological effects alcohol has upon multiple organ systems, all of which have important implications for anesthetic management. Alcoholics have up to a threefold increase in postoperative morbidity, and prolonged hospitalization [15]. This increase may not be as severe in alcoholics who are not actively drinking.

Alcohol is rapidly absorbed from the stomach and distributed into the total body water. Peak blood levels occur 30 minutes after ingestion. Alcohol is metabolized by sequential oxidation in the liver to acetate. This metabolic pathway saturates at relatively low blood alcohol levels, resulting in zero-order elimination kinetics, or elimination of a constant amount of alcohol per unit time. This amount is approximately one-half to one mixed drink per hour for an adult [13]. Alcohol also induces the activity of the cytochrome P450 (CYP) enzyme CYP2E1, which increases the metabolism of drugs such as paracetamol (acetaminophen), chlorzoxazone, and volatile anesthetics [16]. CYP2E1 can also metabolize ethanol, but normally accounts for less than 2% of alcohol metabolism. It is important to note that *decreased* metabolism of CYP2E1 substrates can be observed during acute binge drinking, due to competition by large amounts of ethanol for the CYP enzymes. CYP2E1 induction can increase the damage caused by other toxins, such as carbon tetrachloride, which can be abused as an inhalant.

Medicines used to treat alcoholism can also present unique management challenges to anesthesiologists. Disulfiram inhibits aldehyde dehydrogenase activity. If the patient consumes ethanol, this leads to acetaldehyde poisoning, making the patient sick [17]. Binge drinking while taking disulfiram can be life-threatening, presenting with hypotension, nausea, vomiting, and confusion. Disulfiram also inhibits several CYP enzymes, which can diminish the metabolism of phenytoin, barbiturates, and theophylline. The opiod receptor antagonists naltrexone and nalmefene are also used to treat alcoholism, and could complicate postoperative analgesic management [18]. Acamprosate, a GABA analog, is also used for the treatment of alcoholism [19]. Little is known about the implications of acamprosate for anesthetic management.

Chronic alcohol abuse leads to toxic effects on many organ systems [20]. Alcohol is a direct neurotoxin, as its effectiveness for neurolytic blocks demonstrates. Neurotoxicity may underlie a number of the CNS effects of alcohol, including cerebellar and cortical degeneration, peripheral neuropathy, and autonomic dysfunction. Nutritional deficiencies in thiamine and B vitamins cause Wernicke–Korsakoff syndrome, and may underlie neuropathies (e.g., beriberi due to thiamine deficiency) [21]. Prophylactic correction of potential nutritional deficits should be part of the routine care of alcoholic patients. The incidence of stroke is also increased in alcoholics. This could be due to either the cardiovascular toxicity of alcohol (hypertension, arrhythmia, thrombus), hepatic toxicity (coagulopathy), or trauma associated with inebriation or gait instability. Careful assessment for neurologic signs of stroke or cranial hemorrhage should be performed in any alcoholic presenting with altered mental status.

The cardiovascular toxicity of alcohol can cause a dilated cardiomyopathy and arrhythmias [22]. The most common arrhythmias are atrial fibrillation and supraventricular tachycardias. Fibrillation can predispose to thrombus formation and either stroke or pulmonary embolus. Ventricular tachycardia can be observed in alcohol-dependent individuals. Conventional therapies are used to treat these arrhythmias, although they may be more resistant to treatment than arrhythmias of idiopathic origin. It is estimated that 5–10% of hypertension is due to alcoholism, which is commensurate with the overall incidence of alcoholism in the population. The reasons why hypertension develops are thought to be either a direct pressor effect of alcohol or that hypertension is a sign of withdrawal, and alcoholics may usually be in mild withdrawal at physician appointments.

Alcohol has significant effects on the gastrointestinal system. The liver is possibly the most severely affected organ. Fatty liver is common in alcoholics, and can occasionally cause fat embolus and death. The amount of alcohol consumed and the duration of drinking behavior are the most important predisposing factors for alcoholic hepatitis, not the pattern of drinking (e.g., binge vs. continuous) or the specific beverage. It is extremely important to test for hepatitis preoperatively, as the perioperative mortality of patients with alcoholic hepatitis has been reported to be as high as 50% [23]. End-stage liver disease with cirrhosis and esophageal varices is also common, and also associated with high operative mortality [24]. Patients can be coagulopathic due to deficiencies in vitamin-K-dependent clotting factors, encephalopathic due to accumulation of ammonia, can develop hepatorenal syndrome leading to concomitant renal failure, and can be hypoglycemic due to diminished glycogen stores in the liver. Severe binge drinkers can also become hypoglycemic during alcohol withdrawal.

Acute and chronic pancreatitis is also common in alcoholics. The main presenting symptom of acute pancreatitis is severe abdominal pain. Acute hemorrhagic pancreatitis can also cause shock. In addition to causing chronic pain, chronic pancreatitis destroys both exocrine and endocrine functions of the pancreas, causing malabsorption and hyperglycemia. Malabsorption can aggravate nutritional deficiencies and require pancreatic enzyme replacement, while hyperglycemia can require insulin. Gastritis and esophageal varices can cause significant gastrointestinal bleeding. Increased gastric secretions and ileus due to inflammation and/or opioid use can increase the risk of gastric aspiration upon induction.

Hematologic abnormalities associated with alcoholism include anemia, leukopenia, mild thrombocytopenia, and coagulopathy. Of these, coagulopathy is the most clinically significant, and can be caused both by cirrhotic liver disease [25] and potentially by direct effects of alcohol on the blood [26]. Coagulopathy can usually be corrected emergently by administration of fresh frozen plasma. Vitamin K can also be given. In refractory cases, the use of activated recombinant factor VII may help provide hemostasis [27].

Anesthetic management of the alcoholic varies depending on the state of intoxication. The acutely intoxicated patient is already partially anesthetized! Anesthetic and analgesic requirements will be decreased, patients should be considered as "full stomachs," and, as mentioned above, close scrutiny for signs of chronic alcoholic disease should be undertaken.

Despite the prevalence of chronic ethanol use, and the high incidence of ethanol intoxication in trauma patients presenting for surgery, there are relatively few investigations of acute and chronic ethanol effects on anesthetic requirements in humans. It is commonly believed that MAC and sedative-hypnotic requirements are greater in patients with chronic ethanol use who are not acutely intoxicated, but data are inconsistent. One study demonstrated no differences in thiopental dose requirements for anesthetic induction, pharmacokinetics, or pharmacodynamics between healthy controls and abstinent chronic alcoholics [28]. In contrast, propofol dose requirements for anesthetic induction were mildly (20–30%) increased in chronic alcoholics, but there was no difference in propofol blood concentrations at which induction endpoints occurred, suggesting a pharmacokinetic rather than a pharmacodynamic mechanism [29]. Also, the EEG response to midazolam at the same degree of brain receptor occupancy was reduced in chronic alcoholics, suggesting reduced sensitivity to benzodiazepines [30]. Cardiomyopathy or arrhythmia may slow induction times and require invasive or echocardiographic hemodynamic monitoring in the perioperative period. Regional anesthetic techniques can be considered if feasible for the procedure, as long as the patient is cooperative and not coagulopathic.

Drug doses should be chosen considering the pharmacokinetic and pharmacodynamic variables outlined above. Neuromuscular blockade should be monitored if used, and the use of drugs that do not undergo hepatic metabolism should be considered. Rapid sequence induction should be considered, and suspicion of varices is a relative contraindication to nasogastric tube placement. Intraoperative management may be complicated by arrhythmias, hypotension, or hypertension. These events can be managed conventionally, although hypertension under anesthesia should also include alcohol withdrawal in the differential diagnosis.

Alcohol withdrawal is unique among abused drugs in that it is potentially life-threatening. Thus, prophylactic treatment of withdrawal should be considered part of the anesthetic plan to avoid unpleasant surprises later. Like all withdrawal syndromes, alcohol withdrawal has signs and symptoms opposite to the acute effects of alcohol. Patients may be tremulous, irritable, anxious, and nauseated. Tachycardia, hypertension, and sweating may be present. Seizures and hallucinations can occur 6–48 hours after the last drink. Withdrawal symptoms are usually not life-threatening unless other complications, such as infection, trauma, malnutrition, or electrolyte disturbance also occur. Approximately 5% of patients will develop the potentially fatal syndrome of delirium tremens 2–3 days after the last drink. This syndrome consists of severe agitation, confusion, dilated pupils, fever and sweating, nausea, diarrhea, and tachycardia [31]. Mortality is about 10%, generally due to arrhythmias or hypotension. Prophylactic treatment of withdrawal includes benzodiazepine administration and maintenance of hydration and electrolyte balance. Clonidine can also be a useful adjunct, and use of a clonidine patch perioperatively should be considered. Severe cases may require phenothiazines such as haloperidol for delirium and agitation, as well as aggressive intravenous hydration and electrolyte normalization. Postoperative analgesic management should take the patient's metabolic derangements into consideration, as well as reducing opioid doses, because of potential interactions between clonidine, benzodiazepines, and opioid analgesics.

Alcohol rapidly crosses the placenta. Fetal levels equilibrate with maternal blood in less than 1 hour. Chronic alcohol abuse by the mother can cause the fetal alcohol syndrome, currently a leading cause of mental retardation. Craniofacial abnormalities are also common in this syndrome, and there have been case reports of upper airway obstruction and difficult intubation. Drugs are eliminated in the newborn at half to two-thirds of adult rates, so the effects of alcohol may persist in the fetus even when the mother does not appear intoxicated. Ethanol intoxication in the newborn can require immediate resuscitation in the delivery suite, possibly including airway management. Intoxication is characterized by a depressed, floppy infant, hypotension, hypoglycemia, and acidosis. Titration of benzodiazepines and appropriate fluid resuscitation are the mainstays of prophylaxis and treatment.

Opioids

Opioid addiction has undergone a recent resurgence with the advent of long-acting opioids for chronic pain (such as controlled-release oxycodone [OxyContin]). Opioids remain the most commonly used drugs for perioperative pain management, so tolerance to their analgesic effects poses a significant problem. Unlike alcohol, the withdrawal syndrome is not life-threatening. Opioids act via μ-opioid receptors, so their adverse physiological effects are somewhat more targeted. Expected complications of sedation, respiratory depression, nausea, and itching are mediated by opioid receptors in the CNS [32]. However, drug administration and associated lifestyle choices can also induce pathology. For example, intravenous heroin administration causes cellulitis, abscesses, and in severe cases sepsis. Tetanus occurs rarely, but is often fatal

because of the advanced stage at presentation. Transverse myelitis with paraplegia and sensory loss has been observed. The etiology of this rare complication is unclear, but it is felt to be due to either an allergic reaction to the opioid or a contaminant, or hypotension caused by high opioid doses. Stroke has also been reported due to septic embolization.

Pneumonia is common in addicts, due to aspiration or poor nutrition. In Asia, heavy opium smokers can develop abnormalities in pulmonary function known as "opium lung." A ground-glass appearance of the lower lobes on chest radiographs is pathognomonic. Pulmonary hypertension can occur after septic lung infarction or septic pulmonary embolism. Injections of contaminants, such as cotton fibers or talc, can also cause embolization as well as pulmonary edema and anaphylactic reactions. Pulmonary edema can also arise from congestive heart failure secondary to valve damage caused by subacute bacterial endocarditis. Opioids cause delayed gastric emptying, which can increase the risk of aspiration [32]. Opioids do not directly damage the liver, but viral hepatitis from needle sharing is common in intravenous opioid abusers, and can cause substantial perioperative mortality and morbidity [23]. If liver function is impaired, opioid metabolism can also be prolonged. Chronic opioid abuse can also cause adrenocortical insufficiency due to suppression of adrenocorticotropic hormone (ACTH) secretion, but this is relatively uncommon.

Anesthetic management of opioid abusers is fairly straightforward. The acutely intoxicated patient will have decreased analgesic requirements. Aspiration precautions should be taken with acutely intoxicated patients, and possibly with chronic abusers. After induction, gastric decompression should be considered. Withdrawal is not life-threatening, and can easily be managed using long-acting opioids perioperatively. Hypotension is common, and could be a sign of either overmedication or withdrawal.

Conversely, perioperative management of opioid-dependent patients is far from straightforward. Profound tolerance makes determining adequate analgesic doses of opioids difficult and unpredictable. The potential for withdrawal symptoms to develop as well as for opioid-induced hyperalgesia to occur (see below) further complicates matters. However, the vast majority of patients can be successfully managed in a structured, straightforward manner. First, reassure the patient that pain will be adequately controlled. If the patient is maintained on long-acting opioids such as methadone or buprenorphine, make sure that the patient takes the usual dose before surgery. During long cases, or when patients will be nil-by-mouth after surgery, intravenous supplementation with equivalent opioid doses [33,34] is necessary to avoid withdrawal. The management of patients chronically taking buprenorphine can be complicated by the high affinity of this partial agonist for the opioid receptor [32]. It is possible that buprenorphine could compete with short-acting opioid agonists, increasing the doses of short-acting opioids required for acute analgesia. Conversely, if buprenorphine is withdrawn, overdose could theoretically occur [35]. In hospitalized patients, buprenorphine can be discontinued or changed to methadone to simplify management. It is important to remember that buprenorphine can precipitate withdrawal in patients using other opioids, so it is best to restart buprenorphine when the patient is already in mild withdrawal.

All patients should be provided with adequate opioid doses to effectively treat their pain, regardless of whether or not they are addicts. However, because of the variables mentioned above, proper doses for dependent patients will have to be determined on a case-by-case basis. Since tolerance to life-threatening side effects such as respiratory depression may not develop at the same rate as analgesic tolerance, caution should be used and naloxone should be readily available. To minimize the potential risks of large opioid doses, regional anesthesia, including local infiltration/instillation, and nonopioid adjuvant therapies should be aggressively utilized. Useful adjuvants include the NMDA antagonists dextromethorphan and ketamine (0.25–0.5 mg kg^{-1}), nonsteroidal anti-inflammatory drugs such as paracetamol (1000 mg preoperatively and/or postoperatively), ketorolac (30–60 mg), the α_2-receptor agonists clonidine and dexmedetomidine, and the anticonvulsant gabapentin (1200 mg) [34,36].

Recently, there has been a resurgence of interest in the concept that chronic opioid use could induce a hyperalgesic state. Opioid-induced hyperalgesia was first reported over 100 years ago [37]. Numerous animal studies have shown that opioid administration may increase the sensitivity to pain and potentially aggravate pre-existing pain [38]. Evidence for abnormal or paradoxical pain responses in opioid-treated patients includes case reports and observations of patients in clinical settings [39,40].

A review of opioid-induced hyperalgesia summarized findings from 139 studies [38]. Although most of these studies were performed in animals or volunteers tested with experimental pain procedures, the authors concluded that opioid-induced hyperalgesia occurred in humans in three clinical situations: (1) former opioid addicts maintained on methadone, (2) patients receiving high doses of opioids for surgical procedures, and (3) patients with a history of high-dose opioid treatment or a prior history of addiction who may require high therapeutic doses of opioids in a time of acute need (e.g., after surgery or trauma) [38]. Self-reports of pain score in patients undergoing detoxification from high-dose opioids showed that 21 out of 23 patients reported a significant decrease in pain after detoxification, suggesting that pain sensitization may be associated with chronic opioid use [41].

Increases in postoperative pain as well as increased postoperative opioid consumption have been observed in two controlled studies in which high doses of opioids were used during surgery [42], but other studies have failed to observe similar effects [43]. Taken together, these findings suggest that chronic or high-dose opioid treatment might be an important contributing factor to the perception of pain in the clinical setting.

Thus, opioid addicts could be more sensitive to pain in addition to being tolerant to opioid analgesic effects. This presents quite a conundrum for the clinician. Regional blockade for intra- and postoperative pain management could be very useful if the patient is cooperative and does not have infection at the injection site or pre-existing neurologic signs. Adjuvants such as nonsteroidal anti-inflammatory drugs, α_2-agonists, and local anesthetic infiltration should also be used whenever possible [44,45]. Even when patients are profoundly tolerant, improved analgesia may be obtained by using a different opioid, or "opioid rotation." This strategy is effective because cross-tolerance between different opioids is not complete. The reasons for this are not known. However, it is known that different opioid ligands bind to their receptors differently. It has been postulated that conformational differences lead to different interactions with downstream signaling molecules, which may bypass some of the changes that have induced tolerance. The new opioid can be started at roughly half the dose-equivalent of the old one, as the patient should be less tolerant to the new opioid. Methadone has proven particularly useful in opioid rotation, because there is the least cross-tolerance with other opioids. The mechanism is not entirely clear, but may relate to methadone NMDA receptor antagonist properties. Opioid dose equivalents, as well as a comprehensive review of chronic pain treatment with opioids, are provided by Ballantyne and Mao [33]. NMDA antagonists have been proposed as adjuvants to minimize and/or reverse tolerance development [46]. This strategy has been limited by the psychotomimetic effects of many of these drugs. Dextromethorphan is a NMDA antagonist without these side effects, but unfortunately has not proven as clinically efficacious as once hoped.

Newborns of opioid-addicted mothers have a high incidence of prematurity and neonatal distress, which may require resuscitation [47]. It is not clear whether these complications are due to drug effects or maternal lifestyle. Respiratory depression is actually not that common in these infants, as tolerance develops in utero. However, it is very important that withdrawal is aggressively treated in the neonate. Symptoms in the neonate are irritability, tremors, poor feeding, gooseflesh, and constant crying. Left untreated, many of these infants will convulse. Circulatory collapse can also occur. Once maintenance opioid requirements are established, doses can be tapered by 10–20% per day. Profound opioid tolerance in toddlers born to heroin-addicted mothers has also been observed, requiring careful consideration of pain management options.

Cannabinoids

Marijuana is the only commonly abused cannabinoid, but has been tried by roughly half of high-school graduates [48]. Delta-9-tetrahydrocannabinol (THC) is the active compound and acts through CB$_1$ (CNS) and CB$_2$ (peripheral) receptors. An endogenous ligand for these receptors, anandamide, has been identified in the brain [49]. THC is effective clinically as an antiemetic and for reducing intraocular pressure in glaucoma patients. Animal studies have shown that marijuana induces similar changes in brain reward systems as other addictive substances. Marijuana induces a euphoric feeling, also causing people to "mellow out." Increased appetite and giddiness also occur. High doses of marijuana can cause anxiety and psychosis, but these effects are very transient, unlike those from other abused drugs (e.g., cocaine and amphetamines: see below). Tolerance to marijuana's effects can develop rapidly, but also dissipate rapidly. Withdrawal signs can occur, but only in heavy users who suddenly stop. The withdrawal syndrome is relatively mild, consisting of irritability, nausea, and insomnia.

The anesthetic implications of marijuana use are minor compared with other abused drugs. Smoking can lead to pulmonary pathology similar to tobacco, but takes that frequency of use to occur. Hypotension can occur during anesthesia, possibly due to reductions in anesthetic requirements. There is no evidence that marijuana withdrawal has hemodynamic consequences during anesthesia. Postoperatively, conventional analgesics can be used. Marijuana may help reduce postoperative nausea and vomiting, and irritability can be managed with mild sedatives.

Benzodiazepines and barbiturates

Benzodiazepines are commonly used sedatives that act at specific benzodiazepine receptors that modulate the GABA$_A$ receptor [50]. Barbiturates, which act directly upon the GABA$_A$ receptor, have been largely supplanted by benzodiazepines in clinical practice, but are still available and have a high abuse potential. These drugs are commonly abused by individuals addicted to other drugs to reduce withdrawal symptoms. Polydrug abuse can complicate the clinical presentation of addicts, and should always be suspected regardless of the history obtained.

Benzodiazepines and barbiturates cause relatively little direct end-organ damage. Barbiturates induce numerous hepatic enzymes, and can increase the metabolism of many drugs. It is also important to note whether patients are taking anticoagulants, as barbiturates can increase warfarin metabolism. As the barbiturate is weaned, metabolism of warfarin may decrease, and patients become coagulopathic if the warfarin dose is not reduced. Overdose can lead to delirium, stupor, respiratory depression, hypoxia, and ultimately cardiovascular collapse. Flumazenil can acutely antagonize the effects of benzodiazepines but not barbiturates. Physostigmine may reverse delirium in barbiturate overdose. Barbiturate injection can cause phlebitis and venous sclerosis because of high pH.

These patients are appropriate candidates for regional or general anesthesia. Acute benzodiazepine or barbiturate intoxication greatly reduces the doses of induction and maintenance drugs needed. In this situation, normal anesthetic doses can cause profound hypotension. In the chronic abuser, tolerance develops and higher induction doses of benzodiazepine or barbiturates may therefore be needed. In addition, hepatically metabolized drugs may need to be administered more frequently. Use of

long-acting benzodiazepines should be considered to mitigate withdrawal symptoms. However, it is important to note that these drugs can potentiate opioid-induced respiratory depression. Withdrawal symptoms, consisting of sweating, cramps, vomiting, convulsions, and insomnia, can be avoided by establishing an appropriate baseline dose of benzodiazepines and reducing this dose by 10–20% per day [21].

Stimulants

Cocaine

Cocaine has become one of the most commonly abused drugs in the world. In the United States, it is estimated that 10% of the population has tried cocaine at least once, and 1% use cocaine chronically [48]. One-fifth of the chronic users are cocaine addicts. Cocaine has been used for over 100 years as a local anesthetic and vasoconstrictor. The pioneering physicians who introduced cocaine also discovered the euphoria, excitement, and feelings of increased mental and physical capacity induced by the drug, and consequently its addictive potential.

The CNS-stimulating effect of cocaine is caused by inhibiting presynaptic catecholamine reuptake. Accumulation of extracellular dopamine in the mesolimbic dopamine system may lead to the feelings of euphoria, alertness, and heightened sensation [51]. Overdoses can cause hallucinations and paranoid reactions. Cocaine is abused by inhalation, smoking, or intravenous injection. Injected cocaine is commonly combined with heroin ("speedball"). Smoking "crack" cocaine ("freebasing") rapidly produces high drug concentrations in the brain due to rapid absorption over the large surface area of the lung and direct delivery to the brain without dilution by the systemic circulation. Preparing cocaine as the free base for smoking removes contaminants, also increasing drug delivery. Thus, smoking crack cocaine is the most likely route to produce addiction. Contradicting street lore, cocaine can be effectively absorbed from the gastrointestinal tract, much to the surprise of many addicts who swallowed cocaine packets to avoid detection and arrest and subsequently overdosed. Cocaine is metabolized by plasma and liver esterases, and has a serum half-life of about 50 minutes. However, addicts report craving cocaine far sooner, perhaps reflecting the rapid decrease in plasma cocaine concentrations [48]. The withdrawal syndrome consists of craving, dysphoria, depression, fatigue, and bradycardia, and can be treated symptomatically with benzodiazepines.

Overdoses present with severe agitation, seizures, vertigo, and delirium. These signs can be managed with benzodiazepines. Severe overdoses can lead to coma. Severe hypertension can cause intracranial bleeding or stroke. Fever, tachycardia, dysrhythmias, and cardiac ischemia are also common. A neuroleptic-malignant syndrome has been reported with cocaine intoxication, and rarely with amphetamine and LSD overdose [52]. Cocaine-induced ischemia may be due to vasospasm [53], and thus treatment with with β-blockers may worsen the problem. Calcium channel blockers avoid cardiac depression and increase coronary blood flow in this situation. Smooth-muscle spasm can also cause wheezing and pulmonary edema.

Acutely intoxicated patients have increased anesthetic requirements, and may be combative. Sympathetic stimulation during induction should be avoided, and patients closely monitored for fever, arrhythmias, and cardiac ischemia. Chronic users may have decreased anesthetic requirements; however, the risks of arrhythmia and ischemia remain [54]. Sympathetic tone is decreased, and indirect-acting sympathomimetics such as ephedrine will be less effective. Regional techniques and conventional opioid medication can be used in these patients. Opioid doses may need to be increased in patients who are also abusing heroin. Cocaine withdrawal is uncomfortable but not dangerous, and can be treated symptomatically with benzodiazepines.

In pregnancy, cocaine may increase the risk of premature labor, placental abruption, and uterine rupture. Maternal vasoconstriction can also decrease placental blood flow, leading to fetal distress [55]. A wide variety of congenital abnormalities have been associated with maternal cocaine abuse. Infants may need to be resuscitated accordingly, and withdrawal signs treated with appropriate doses of benzodiazepines.

Amphetamines

Amphetamines are also CNS stimulants, but unlike cocaine they stimulate presynaptic catecholamine release, rather than block reuptake [56]. Two main patterns of abuse, binge ("sprees") and chronic high-dose intake, are seen. Amphetamine causes a rush of power, energy, and euphoria much like that of cocaine. However, addicts deteriorate clinically and socially much faster than cocaine abusers. Animal studies have demonstrated neurotoxic effects of amphetamines on dopaminergic and serotonergic neurons, which could represent a possible reason for the more rapid deterioration [57]. Tolerance develops rapidly to the rush and the sympathomimetic effects of amphetamines, leading to rapid dose escalation. Cross-tolerance between the different amphetamine drugs is profound. The withdrawal syndrome is similar to that caused by cocaine.

Acutely intoxicated amphetamine addicts can present with hyperactivity, confusion, delirium, hallucinations, aggressive behavior, paranoia, schizophrenia-like symptoms, or seizures [58]. Fever, tachycardia, hypertension, and arrhythmias are common, and should be treated aggressively. Moderate amphetamine doses can cause significant hyperthermia requiring aggressive cooling intraoperatively. Chronic amphetamine use also causes a chronic vasculitis, which can lead to aneurysm formation, stroke, renal and splenic infarcts, and in rare cases blindness [59]. Weight loss, malnutrition, dehydration, and poor dentition may also be present [21].

Regional anesthesia may be difficult in these patients because of the behavioral abnormalities. Sedatives as well as

antipsychotic drugs may be needed to manage these signs. Hypertension, tachycardia, and arrhythmias need to be aggressively treated. Renal damage may decrease drug clearance, and should be screened for. Requirements for induction and maintenance anesthetic drugs are increased. However, marked increases in peripheral vascular resistance caused by amphetamines combined with dehydration may lead to profound hypotension during anesthetic induction. Hypotension is best managed with direct-acting sympathetic drugs, as the effects of indirect-acting sympathomimetics will be increased in an unpredictable fashion. Also, amphetamines may potentiate opioid analgesia.

Chronic amphetamine addicts have decreased anesthetic requirements, and indirect-acting sympathomimetics will have a decreased effect. Arrhythmias are less likely, but hypotension during induction is more common due to decreased sympathetic vascular responses and dehydration. Postoperatively, opioid effectiveness could be potentiated by amphetamines. Benzodiazepines used to treat agitation or the withdrawal syndrome may also potentiate opioid-induced respiratory depression.

Effects on the fetus are similar to those of cocaine, and are aggravated by inadequate prenatal care received by most addicts [60]. Management considerations for the newborn are similar to those described for cocaine.

Psychedelics ("party drugs")

These drugs are abused for their euphoric and hallucinogenic effects. Abused psychedelics can be classified into four groups: indoleamines, or compounds related to lysergic acid diethyeamide (LSD), phenylethylamines such as methylenedioxymethamphetamine (MDMA; "ecstasy"), NMDA antagonists such as phencyclidine (PCP), and belladonna alkaloids such as scopolamine.

Indoleamines include LSD, psilocybin ("magic mushrooms"), and N,N-dimethyltryptamine (DMT). These drugs act primarily through the 5-HT$_2$ subtype of serotonin receptors, although they have high affinity toward multiple serotonin receptor subtypes [48]. The half-life of LSD is 3 hours, but psychedelic effects can persist for 12 hours. Tolerance to the hallucinogenic effects occurs, as well as cross-tolerance between drugs of this class. No withdrawal syndrome has been noted, although episodes of hallucinations and dysphoria ("flashbacks") can occur long after drug use has been discontinued. LSD can cause mild hypertension, tachycardia, and hyperthermia, as well as wheezing and salivation. LSD also has significant analgesic effects.

Phenylethylamines, such as MDMA ("ecstasy"), mescaline, and methylenedioxyamphetamine (MDA), are structurally closely related to amphetamines and share many of their stimulant effects. However, these drugs are taken mainly for their psychedelic actions, which are also mediated by 5-HT$_2$ receptor activation. Like amphetamines, these drugs also cause degeneration of serotonergic neurons in rats. Physiological effects and anesthetic considerations are similar to those described above for amphetamines and cocaine.

NMDA receptor antagonists such as PCP and ketamine ("special K") have marked hallucinogenic effects. In low doses, PCP also induces euphoria and giddiness. These drugs are taken orally, and PCP can also be smoked, sometimes in conjunction with marijuana. PCP undergoes hepatic metabolism and renal excretion, and has a half-life of 3 days. Prolonged psychosis can be seen after only one dose of PCP, perhaps because of its high lipid solubility. PCP overdose can induce a dissociated state much like ketamine, although with extremely violent behavior. Sweating, fever, rigidity, and other signs of sympathetic activation are also seen. Hyperreflexia and convulsions can occur, and severe cases can present with coma that lasts for up to 10 days [61]. Animal studies have shown that these drugs are reinforcing and induce tolerance and dependence. Dependence has been reported in humans, but is unusual as most people use these drugs intermittently. The cardiovascular effects of PCP are similar to the well-known sympathetic stimulating effect of ketamine, causing hypertension and tachycardia. Fever and increased salivation can also be seen.

The belladonna alkaloids include the clinically used anticholinergics atropine and scopolamine. These drugs are not commonly abused presently. However, plants such as jimson-weed (North America) and trumpet lily (Australia) contain belladonna alkaloids, and have been abused [62]. Signs are characterized by the classic mnemonic "dry as a bone, red as a beet, and mad as a hatter." Confusion and a schizophrenia-like syndrome can be observed at higher doses, and may respond to treatment with physostigmine, a centrally acting cholinergic agonist. In addition to characteristic cardiovascular effects, a generalized myocardial conduction delay can develop that requires pacing [21]. Dehydration, urinary retention, and constipation are also seen. Higher doses may induce seizures and respiratory depression.

Injuries are common in patients abusing hallucinogens, because of their altered sense of reality. Uncooperative and unpredictable behavior may argue against the use of regional anesthesia. Sedatives may be needed to help control behavior. Neuroleptics can actually increase agitation and confusion in patients on LSD, but may be useful in other settings. LSD has also been found to have mild inhibitory effects on cholinesterase and monoamine oxidase (MAO). There have been no reports of prolonged succinylcholine action or toxicity of ester local anesthetics, but this is something of which to be aware. However, if physostigmine has been given to patients abusing belladonna alkaloids, the effect of succinylcholine could be markedly prolonged. Augmented effects of sympathomimetics as a consequence of MAO inhibition could be observed. Neuroleptic-malignant syndrome has been reported with LSD intoxication, but not with other psychedelic substances. Hemodynamic instability and arrhythmias may be seen intraoperatively. Emergence can be particularly stormy in these patients, often accompanied by significant hemodynamic changes, arrhythmias, and "postoperative panic." Postoperative opioid doses may need to be reduced because of analgesic effects of the hallucinogen as well as synergistic interactions with benzodiazepines needed for sedation.

The effects of these drugs on the fetus have not been extensively studied. It is known that PCP abuse can increase the incidence of preterm labor and fetal distress [60]. Treatment of direct drug effects in the infant is supportive.

Inhalants

Inhalants are a diverse group of compounds that are volatile at room temperature. These drugs include glue, cleaning fluid, organic solvents, and Freon ("frost freaking") [63]. The drug is placed in a bag and the fumes inhaled, resulting in euphoria, visual and auditory hallucinations, as well as destructive behavior. Extremely high doses can cause stupor and convulsions. These drugs are readily available, easy to use, and relatively inexpensive. Unfortunately, for these reasons inhalants are commonly abused by children [48]. Tolerance is seen to the effects of organic solvents, but there is no evidence for the development of dependence. Inhalant abuse can cause severe liver damage as well as renal failure, both of which can profoundly impact anesthetic management. Patients may have a solvent odor on their breath. Arrhythmias may occur, which should respond to conventional therapies. Regional anesthesia may be a preferred option in cooperative patients. Conventional methods of postoperative pain management can be used, and irritability can be treated symptomatically.

Summary

Addictive behavior is characterized by compulsive drug use, loss of control over drug-taking behavior, craving, and continued use despite harm. However, an individual can become physically dependent upon a drug without being addicted and, conversely, can be addicted without suffering from physical dependence, as drug tolerance and dependence are not the same as addiction. The pervasiveness of drug abuse and addiction mandates that anesthesiologists are aware of typical and emerging drug abuse patterns, be they regional or national trends. Both single and polydrug abuse, of both licit and illicit substances, are common. Vigilance about the possibility of patient drug abuse and addiction will ensure that perioperative problems can be anticipated and managed to achieve the best possible outcomes.

The most commonly abused depressant drug is ethanol. Active alcoholics have nearly a threefold increase in postoperative morbidity and prolonged hospitalization. Acute intoxication decreases anesthetic requirements, and chronic use is considered to increase anesthetic requirements, although this has been disputed. Increased gastric secretions and ileus can increase the risk of aspiration, and rapid sequence induction should be considered. Suspicion of esophageal varices is a relative contraindication to nasogastric tube placement.

Hypertension under anesthesia should include alcohol withdrawal in the differential diagnosis, and withdrawal should be managed with benzodiazepines. Coagulopathy due to liver dysfunction can be corrected with fresh frozen plasma or vitamin K. Naltrexone and nalmefene, opioid antagonists used occasionally to treat alcoholism, can complicate perioperative opioid use. Fetal alcohol syndrome is a leading cause of mental retardation and craniofacial abnormalities, including possible upper airway obstruction and difficult intubation.

Opioid addiction and tolerance have undergone a recent resurgence with the advent of long-acting opioids for chronic pain (such as OxyContin and methadone). Chronic pain patients with a prior history of substance abuse have a 20-fold increase in the risk of addiction or aberrant drug-related behaviors during opioid therapy. Perioperatively, acute opioid intoxication decreases analgesic requirements. Chronic opioid use or abuse makes analgesic management difficult, because of tolerance. Use of adjuvants, regional techniques, and opioid rotation are recommended. Patients who are maintained on long-acting opioids such as methadone or buprenorphine should continue to receive their usual regimen before and after surgery. Opioid withdrawal syndrome is not life-threatening and can be managed using long-acting opioids perioperatively.

Chronic benzodiazepine use can cause tolerance to, and require higher doses of, benzodiazepine or barbiturates, while acute benzodiazepine intoxication greatly reduces the required doses of induction and maintenance anesthetics. Long-acting benzodiazepines are used to pevent withdrawal symptoms.

Cocaine and amphetamines are central nervous system and sympathetic stimulants with significant anesthetic implications. Patients acutely intoxicated with cocaine have increased anesthetic requirements and may be combative. Sympathetic stimulation during induction should be avoided, and patients closely monitored for fever, arrhythmias, and cardiac ischemia. Chronic users may have decreased anesthetic requirements, but the risks of arrhythmia and ischemia remain. In pregnancy, cocaine may increase the risk of premature labor, placental abruption, and uterine rupture. Maternal vasoconstriction can also decrease placental blood flow, leading to fetal distress. Infants may need to be resuscitated accordingly, and withdrawal signs treated with appropriate doses of benzodiazepines.

Chronic amphetamine addicts have decreased anesthetic requirements, and indirect-acting sympathomimetics will have a decreased effect. Arrhythmias are less likely, but hypotension during induction is more common due to decreased sympathetic vascular responses and dehydration. Opioid effects can be potentiated by amphetamines. Tolerance develops rapidly to the rush and the sympathomimetic effects of amphetamines, leading to rapid dose escalation. Cross-tolerance between the different amphetamine drugs is profound. The withdrawal syndrome is similar to that caused by cocaine. Hypotension in acute amphetamine intoxication is best managed with direct-acting sympathetic drugs, as the effects of indirect-acting sympathomimetics will be increased in an unpredictable fashion. Also, amphetamines may potentiate opioid analgesia. Amphetamine effects on the fetus are similar to those of cocaine, and are aggravated by inadequate prenatal care received by most addicts. Management considerations for the newborn are similar to those described for cocaine.

References

1. Khantzian EJ. The self medication hypothesis of addictive disorders: focus on heroin and cocaine dependence. *Am J Psychiatry* 1985; **142**: 1259–64.

2. Koob GF, LeMoal M. Drug abuse: hedonic homeostatic dysregulation. *Science* 1997; **278**: 52–8.

3. Self DW. Regulation of drug-taking and -seeking behaviors by neuroadaptations in the mesolimbic dopamine system. *Neuropharmacology* 2004; **47**: 242–55.

4. Nestler EJ, Aghajanian GK. Molecular and cellular basis of addiction. *Science* 1997; **278**: 58–63.

5. Koob GF, Le Moal M. Plasticity of reward neurocircuitry and the 'dark side' of drug addiction. *Nat Neurosci* 2005; **8**: 1442–4.

6. Koob GF, Le Moal M. Addiction and the brain antireward system. *Annu Rev Psychol* 2008; **59**: 29–53.

7. Katz NP, Adams EH, Chilcoat H, *et al.* Challenges in the development of prescription opioid abuse-deterrent formulations. *Clin J Pain* 2007; **23**: 648–60.

8. Weaver M, Schnoll S. Abuse liability in opioid therapy for pain treatment in patients with an addiction history. *Clin J Pain* 2002; **18**: S61–9.

9. Fishbain DA, Cole B, Lewis J, Rosomoff HL, Rosomoff RS. What percentage of chronic nonmalignant pain patients exposed to chronic opioid analgesic therapy develop abuse/addiction and/or aberrant drug-related behaviors? A structured evidence-based review. *Pain Med* 2008; **9**: 444–59.

10. Kantor TG, Cantor R, Tom E. A study of hospitalized surgical patients on methadone maintenance. *Drug Alcohol Depend* 1980; **6**: 163–73.

11. Manfredi PL, Gonzales GR, Cheville AL, Kornick C, Payne R. Methadone analgesia in cancer pain patients on chronic methadone maintenance therapy. *J Pain Symptom Manage* 2001; **21**: 169–74.

12. Karasz A, Zallman L, Berg K, *et al.* The experience of chronic severe pain in patients undergoing methadone maintenance treatment. *J Pain Symptom Manage* 2004; **28**: 517–25.

13. Fleming M, Mihic SJ, Harris RA. Ethanol. In: Brunton L, Lazo J, Parker K, eds., *Goodman and Gilman's The Pharmacological Basis of Therapeutics*, 11th edn. New York, NY: McGraw-Hill, 2006: 591–606.

14. Diamond I, Gordon AS. Cellular and molecular neuroscience of alcoholism. *Physiol Rev* 1997; **77**: 1–20.

15. Tonnesen H, Kehlet H. Preoperative alcoholism and postoperative morbidity. *Br J Surg* 1999; **86**: 869–74.

16. Kharasch ED, Thummel KE. Identification of cytochrome P450 2E1

as the predominant enzyme catalyzing human liver microsomal defluorination of sevoflurane, isoflurane, and methoxyflurane. *Anesthesiology* 1993; **79**: 795–807.

17. Johansson B. A review of the pharmacokinetics and pharmacodynamics of disulfiram and its metabolites. *Acta Psychiatr Scand Suppl* 1992; **369**: 15–26.

18. Johnson BA, Ait-Daoud N. Neuropharmacological treatments for alcoholism: scientific basis and clinical findings. *Psychopharmacology* 2000; **149**: 327–44.

19. Mason BJ. Acamprosate. *Recent Dev Alcohol* 2003; **16**: 203–15.

20. Lieber CS. Medical disorders of alcoholism. *New Eng J Med* 1995; **333**: 1058–65.

21. Caldwell T. Anesthesia for patients with behavioral and environmental disorders. In: Katz J, Benumof J, Kadis L, eds., *Anesthesia and Uncommon Diseases*, 2nd edn. Philadelphia, PA: WB Saunders, 1981.

22. Piano MR, Schwertz DW. Alcoholic heart disease: a review. *Heart Lung* 1994; **23**: 3–17.

23. Friedman LS. The risk of surgery in patients with liver disease. *Hepatology* 1999; **29**: 1617–23.

24. Ziser A, Plevak DJ, Wiesner RH, *et al.* Morbidity and mortality in cirrhotic patients undergoing anesthesia and surgery. *Anesthesiology* 1999; **90**: 42–53.

25. Lisman T, Leebeek FW. Hemostatic alterations in liver disease: a review on pathophysiology, clinical consequences, and treatment. *Digestive Surgery* 2007; **24**: 250–8.

26. Engstrom M, Schott U, Reinstrup P. Ethanol impairs coagulation and fibrinolysis in whole blood: a study performed with rotational thromboelastometry. *Blood Coagul & Fibrinolysis* 2006: **17**: 661–5.

27. Agarwal N, Spahr JE, Rodgers GM. Successful management of intra-abdominal hemorrhage in the presence of severe alcoholic liver disease with activated recombinant factor VII (rFVIIa; NovoSeven): a case report and review of the literature on approved and off-label use of rFVIIa. *Blood Coagul & Fibrinolysis* 2007; **18**: 205–7.

28. Swerdlow BN, Holley FO, Maitre PO, Stanski DR. Chronic alcohol intake does not change thiopental anesthetic requirement, pharmacokinetics, or pharmacodynamics. *Anesthesiology* 1990; **72**: 455–61.

29. Fassoulaki A, Farinotti R, Servin F, Desmonts JM. Chronic alcoholism increases the induction dose of propofol in humans. *Anesth Anal* 1993; **77**: 553–6.

30. Lingford-Hughes AR, Wilson SJ, *et al.* GABA-benzodiazepine receptor function in alcohol dependence: a combined 11C-flumazenil PET and pharmacodynamic study. *Psychopharmacology* 2005; **180**: 595–606.

31. Isbell H, Fraser HF, Wikler A, Belleville RE, Eisenman AJ. An experimental study of the etiology of rum fits and delirium tremens. *Q J Stud Alcohol* 1955; **16**: 1–33.

32. Gutstein H, Akil H. Opioid Analgesics. In: Brunton L, Lazo J, Parker K, eds., *Goodman & Gilman's The Pharmacological Basis of Therapeutics*, 11 edn. New York, NY: McGraw-Hill, 2006: 547–90.

33. Ballantyne JC, Mao J. Opioid therapy for chronic pain. *N Engl J Med* 2003; **349**: 1943–53.

34. Carroll IR, Angst MS, Clark JD. Management of perioperative pain in patients chronically consuming opioids. *Reg Anesth Pain Med* 2004; **29**: 576–91.

35. Alford DP, Compton P, Samet JH. Acute pain management for patients receiving maintenance methadone or buprenorphine therapy. *Ann Intern Med* 2006; **144**: 127–34.

36. Brill S, Ginosar Y, Davidson EM. Perioperative management of chronic pain patients with opioid dependency. *Curr Opin Anaesthesiol* 2006; **19**: 325–31.

37. Rossbach M. Ueber die Gewohnung an Gifte. *Pflugers Archiv fur die Gesamte Physiologie des Menschen und der Tiere* 1880; **21**: 213–25.

38. Angst MS, Clark JD. Opioid-induced hyperalgesia: a qualitative systematic review. *Anesthesiology* 2006; **104**: 570–87.

39. Chang G, Chen L, Mao J. Opioid tolerance and hyperalgesia. *Med Clin North Am* 2007; **91**: 199–211.

40. Arner S, Rawal N, Gustafsson LL. Clinical experience of long-term treatment with epidural and intrathecal opioids: a nationwide survey. *Acta Anaesthesiol Scand* 1988; **32**: 253–9.

41. Baron MJ, McDonald PW. Significant pain reduction in chronic pain patients after detoxification from high-dose opioids. *J Opioid Manag* 2006; **2**: 277–82.

42. Guignard B, Bossard AE, Coste C, *et al.* Acute opioid tolerance: intraoperative remifentanil increases postoperative pain and morphine requirement. *Anesthesiology* 2000; **93**: 409–17.

43. Cortinez LI, Brandes V, Munoz HR, Guerrero ME, Mur M. No clinical evidence of acute opioid tolerance after remifentanil-based anaesthesia. *Br J Anaesth* 2001; **87**: 866–9.

44. Mitra S, Sinatra RS. Perioperative management of acute pain in the opioid-dependent patient. *Anesthesiology* 2004; **101**: 212–27.

45. Peng PWH, Tumber PS, Gourlay D. Review article: Perioperative pain management of patients on methadone therapy. *Can J Anesth* 2005; **52**: 513–23.

46. Trujillo K, Akil H. Excitatory amino acids and drugs of abuse: A role for N-methyl-D-aspartate receptors in drug tolerance, sensitization and physical dependence. *Drug Alcohol Depend* 1994; **38**: 139–54.

47. Ludlow J, Christmas T, Paech MJ, Orr B. Drug abuse and dependency during pregnancy: anaesthetic issues. *Anaesth Intensive Care* 2007; **35**: 881–93.

48. O'Brien CP. Drug addiction and drug abuse. In: Brunton L, Lazo J, Parker K, eds., *Goodman and Gilman's The Pharmacological Basis of Therapeutics*, 11th edn. New York, NY: McGraw-Hill, 2006: 607–27.

49. Maldonado R, Rodriguez de Fonseca F. Cannabinoid addiction: behavioral models and neural correlates. *J Neurosci* 2002; **22**: 3326–31.

50. Reves J, Glass P, Lubarsky D, McEvoy M. Intravenous Nonopioid Anesthetics. In: Miller R, ed., *Miller's Anesthesia*. Philadelphia, PA: Elsevier, 2006: 317–78.

51. Nestler EJ. Molecular mechanisms of opiate and cocaine addiction. *Curr Opin Neurobiol* 1997; **7**: 713–19.

convey protection. Anaphylaxis is defined as any severe, systemic allergic reaction of rapid onset which may cause death or other adverse outcomes that is caused by classical IgE/antigen-mediated reactions. **Anaphylactoid** is a term used to precisely describe reactions that produce a similar clinical picture as anaphylaxis but are not IgE-mediated [14–16]. However, both IgE- and IgG-mediated reactions are commonly referred to as anaphylactic reactions. Currently, anaphylaxis is best considered as a life-threatening, acute, unpredictable ADR [6,7]. Although anaphylaxis accounts for only a small proportion of reported ADRs, it is associated with substantial morbidity and mortality, and increased healthcare costs [4,9].

Clinical manifestations of anaphylaxis

Acute cardiovascular and pulmonary dysfunction are the *sine qua non* of anaphylaxis. Cardiovascular manifestations include arrhythmias, hypotension, and cardiac arrest. Patients may also manifest vasodilatory shock (low systemic vascular resistance) and acute pulmonary vasoconstriction with right heart failure. Allergy practice guidelines suggest that in adults the diagnosis of anaphylaxis is a systolic blood pressure < 90 mmHg or >30% decrease from baseline after exposure to known allergens. Respiratory manifestations include acute bronchospasm and upper airway edema (angioedema) [15–17].

Diagnosing anaphylaxis is problematic in the perioperative period, however, because there are multiple potential contributors to cardiovascular and/or pulmonary dysfunction [18–20]. Wheezing and increased airway pressures can occur after endotracheal intubation or airway manipulation in patients with asthma, reactive airway disease, or smoking, due to pre-existing airway inflammation [21–23]. Bronchospasm commonly occurs following intubation, with reported frequencies as high as 30% in patients with reactive airway disease (asthma) [21,24,25]. Angioedema can also occur following angiotensin-converting enzyme (ACE) inhibitor administration [26,27]. Although flushing, rashes, and other cutaneous manifestations can occur, they may be missed during surgery as patients are often covered.

The situation is further complicated by the fact that many anesthetic drugs directly produce vasodilation, hypotension, and alterations in sympathoadrenergic responses [28,29]. Diagnosing anaphylaxis requires a high index of suspicion when acute cardiopulmonary dysfunction occurs following drug or blood product administration [15,16].

Drugs implicated

The drugs most often reported to cause perioperative anaphylaxis include antibiotics, blood products, neuromuscular blocking drugs (NMBDs), polypeptides (aprotinin, latex, and protamine), and volume expanders [20,22,30]. A precise incidence of perioperative anaphylaxis is unknown, because most reporting is retrospective. In surgical patients, the incidence of anaphylaxis is reported to range between 1/3500 and 1/20 000, with a mortality rate of 4% and an additional 2% surviving

with severe brain damage [15,16]. A report from 2004 suggests an incidence of 1/10 000 to 1/20 000 [31]. In cardiac surgery, Levy reported eight reactions in 1743 patients over a 12-month period for a rate of 0.46%; causative drugs were protamine ($n = 4$), vancomycin ($n = 2$), blood, and metocurine [32]. Ford and colleagues reported 23 patients who developed anaphylaxis during cardiac surgery in Australia, of whom 86% were documented to have an immunologic basis for their reaction [33]. These 23 patients were from a database of 1346 patients investigated for reactions during anesthesia over a 20-year period. Antibiotics ($n = 7$), colloid volume expanders ($n = 6$), and muscle relaxants ($n = 4$) were most often implicated, but blood products ($n = 2$), protamine ($n = 3$), and morphine ($n = 1$) were also implicated. Mertes *et al.* reported 789 patients evaluated for perioperative anaphylaxis in France [20]. Allergic reactions were confirmed in 518 cases (66%) by immunologic testing. NMBDs ($n = 306$, 58.2%), latex ($n = 88$, 16.7%), and antibiotics ($n = 79$, 15.1%) were the drugs most commonly reported. Among the NMBDs, rocuronium ($n = 132$, 43.1%) and succinylcholine ($n = 69$, 22.6%) were the drugs most often implicated. From Norway, 83 intraoperative reactions were evaluated by case history, tryptase measurements, specific immunoassays, and skin tests [34]. IgE-mediated anaphylaxis was established in 71% of cases, with NMBDs the most frequent allergen (93.2%) followed by latex (3.6%). The authors estimated the incidence of reactions to NMBDs at 1/5200 general anesthetics (95% CI 1/3000 to 1/14 000).

Common perioperative drug allergies

Antibiotics

Reports on the incidence of antibiotic allergy vary. The incidence of anaphylaxis with penicillins is reported as 0.004–0.015%, but this commonly used reference is from 1968 [35]. Anaphylaxis to cephalosporins is uncommon, at 0.0001–0.1% [36]. Vancomycin is a potent mast-cell degranulating drug that releases histamine to produce hypotension and flushing following intravenous administration [37,38]. The risks of cephalosporin reactions in patients with penicillin allergy are complex and have been recently reviewed [30]. Gruchalla and Pirmohamed suggest that most patients with a history of penicillin allergy will tolerate cephalosporins, but that indiscriminate administration cannot be recommended, especially for patients who have had serious acute reactions to any β-lactam antibiotic [4]. If a patient has a penicillin-allergy history that is consistent with anaphylaxis and penicillin skin testing is unavailable, then cephalosporins should be used cautiously, with graded dose escalation. A patient who has experienced an allergic reaction to a specific cephalosporin should not receive that cephalosporin again. Unfortunately patient histories are often unreliable in this circumstance.

Blood products

Blood products contain proteins and cellular antigens that can cause various immune-mediated reactions, including allergic, anaphylactic, and acute hemolytic transfusion reactions as well as transfusion-related acute lung injury (TRALI) [39–42]. In one study, the incidence of allergic transfusion reactions was 17% (273/1613) over a 9-year period, including anaphylaxis in 21 patients (7.7% of allergic reactions, or 1.3% of all transfusion reactions). Other reports estimate allergic transfusion reactions occur in 1/4124 blood components transfused, or 1/2338 transfusion episodes [43]. TRALI is the most serious event and has a high mortality when it occurs. TRALI is estimated to occur in 1/4000 to 1/557 000 transfused red blood cell units and 1/432 to 1/88 000 transfused platelet units [44].

TRALI is a life-threatening acute hypersensitivity response that presents with acute respiratory failure, bilateral pulmonary edema, hypoxemia, and hypotension [45]. The onset commonly occurs within 1–2 hours of transfusion [39,45,46]. The mortality rate from TRALI ranges from 5% to 25%. FDA data suggest that it is the third most common cause of transfusion-associated mortality, accounting for 9% of reported deaths [45]. TRALI is an immune-mediated event produced by antibodies in the donor plasma directed against antigens (including HLA-specific antigens or leukoagglutinins) on recipient neutrophils [45]. Hemolytic transfusion reactions are also routinely antibody-mediated and can potentially present with shock or a hypotensive event. [39]. Acute hemolytic transfusion reactions occur in 1/33 000 to 1/500 000 units transfused, with a fatality rate of 2–6% [47–50].

Drug additives/preservatives

Allergic and other adverse reactions to intravenously administered medications may be caused by additives, including sulfites and parabens [51,52]. Drug additives are used as preservatives in many parenteral solutions, and may be responsible for producing allergic reactions. Sulfiting agents are widely used as preservatives and antioxidants in intravenous and other solutions. Sulfiting agents include sulfur dioxide, sodium or potassium sulfite, bisulfite, and metabisulfite [52]. The FDA allows the addition of sulfites to foods and drugs. Allergic reactions to sulfites can develop from exposure to oral or parenteral sulfites. Exposure to oral sulfites typically occurs from ingestion of foods and beverages that contain sulfites, such as beer, wine, and salads at salad bars. In allergic patients who ingest sulfites, pH changes occur, generating sulfur dioxide and producing bronchospasm, coughing, or asthma [52]. Of greater concern in the perioperative setting are potential allergic reactions. The problem we face as clinicians is a lack of data on the incidence and risk of hypersensitivity reactions to intravenous sulfites.

Parabens are preservatives included in multidose vials of local anesthetics that can produce hypersensitivity reactions. They are aliphatic esters of parahydroxybenzoic acid and include methylethyl, propyl, and butyl parabens. Sodium benzoate, structurally related to the parabens, may produce allergic reactions through cross-reactivity. Interestingly, some drugs administered in the perioperative setting may contain a greater concentration of preservatives than of the active drug. In a solution of pancuronium where there is a 1% concentration of methylparaben, this implies there are 10 mg of methylparaben and only 1 mg of pancuronium per milliliter.

Heparin

The formation of IgG antibodies that bind heparin/PF4 complexes on the platelet surface to form immune complexes is common after heparin administration. Platelet activation by the Fc domain of the IgG in the immune complexes cause aggregation and further activation, releasing microparticles that produce a procoagulant effect. This syndrome is heparin-induced thrombocytopenia (HIT). Reports suggest that 7–50% of heparin-treated patients generate heparin/PF4 antibodies [53]. Cardiac surgical and orthopedic surgical patients are most often affected in the perioperative setting. This is likely due to the tremendous platelet activation that occurs in this patient population. Allergic and anaphylactic reactions to heparin can occur but, given the antigenicity of heparin, they are surprisingly infrequent [54–61]. IgG may be an important mechanism for anaphylaxis in these patients, and may explain the combined occurrence of HIT and hypersensitivity [55].

Severe allergic reactions following intravenous heparin administration in the United States and Germany were reported in early 2008 and caused major concerns about the safety of heparin. Although the reactions were initially thought to involve a component in unfractionated heparin, the causal agent was identified as a contaminant called oversulfated chondroitin sulfate (OSCS). This molecule directly activates the kinin–kallikrein pathway in human plasma, leading to the generation of bradykinin, a potent vasoactive mediator. In addition, OSCS induces generation of C3a and C5a, potent anaphylatoxins derived from complement proteins [62].

Neuromuscular blocking drugs

Neuromuscular blocking drugs (NMBDs) have been reported as a major cause of perioperative anaphylaxis. Most drugs are relatively low-molecular-weight compounds that are not antigenic by themselves. However, in the circulation they may bind to bigger proteins including albumin, α_2-macroglobulin, or other host proteins to become antigens [63]. Because NMBDs are charged biquarternary molecules they can function as complete antigens, an important characteristic that is unusual among drugs [64]. Although reported cases of anaphylaxis to NMBDs are relatively rare, their potential antigenicity has led to concern that they may produce significant immune-mediated adverse drug reactions. Although underreporting of anaphylaxis to NMBDs has been suggested, the severity of anaphylaxis and the potential adverse outcomes that occur following this syndrome make this unlikely [65]. Rocuronium is the drug often thought to have a potential risk for anaphylaxis; however, adverse drug events reported to the FDA have not demonstrated a difference in the risk of anaphylaxis with rocuronium versus vecuronium [66]. Rocuronium is a steroid-derived drug that can produce a direct positive weal and flare responses following skin testing [67–69]. In volunteers, 50% and 40% of the subjects had a positive skin reaction to prick testing with undiluted rocuronium and vecuronium, respectively [69]. Because skin testing is used to identify the causative agent following anaphylaxis, false-positive skin tests for NMBDs may lead to inflated estimates of the incidence of NMBD-induced anaphylaxis.

Polypeptides
Aprotinin
Aprotinin is a bovine-derived protease inhibitor administered to reduce bleeding in cardiac surgery. The risk of anaphylaxis is reported as 2.7% in re-exposed patients from several studies [70–73]. The risk of anaphylaxis is increased in patients with prior aprotinin exposure, and a history of prior exposure should be determined before aprotinin administration. The risk of a fatal reaction appears to be greater on re-exposure within 12 months, and therefore test doses and loading doses should only be performed when the conditions for rapid cannulation are present with re-exposure. Aprotinin is currently removed from marketing in the USA and Europe because of other concerns.

Latex
Latex is a common environmental antigen that has been widely implicated as an important cause of perioperative anaphylaxis. Healthcare workers, other workers with occupational exposure to latex, children with spina bifida and urogenital abnormalities, and individuals with certain food allergies have been recognized as individuals at increased risk for anaphylaxis to latex [14,74,75]. Brown *et al.* reported a 24% incidence of irritant or contact dermatitis and a 12.5% incidence of latex-specific IgE positivity in anesthesiologists [76]. Of this group, 10% were clinically asymptomatic although IgE-positive; the authors suggested that such individuals are in the early stages of sensitization and may prevent progression to symptomatic disease by avoiding latex exposure. A history of atopy was also a significant risk factor for latex sensitization. Patients with a history of allergy to certain fruits including avocado, banana, chestnut, kiwi, mango, passion fruit, strawberry, and stone fruits may also be at greater risk for allergy to latex [77–79]. Multiple attempts are being made to reduce the latex exposure of both healthcare workers and patients. In the latex-allergic patient, strict avoidance of latex from gloves and other sources needs to be considered, following the recommendations of Holzman [80,81]. Because latex is such a ubiquitous environmental antigen, this represents a daunting task.

Latex anaphylaxis appears to have reached a plateau, perhaps due to decreased presence of latex in surgical products and labeling warnings about the presence of latex in medical products enforced by the FDA [15,16]. Latex allergy should be considered in patients who develop intraoperative anaphylaxis after surgical intervention without another identifiable cause [82]. Latex (rubber) hypersensitivity continues to present a significant medical problem.

Protamine
Diabetic patients receiving protamine-containing insulin, as neutral protamine Hagedorn (NPH) or protamine insulin, have a 10- to 30-fold increased risk for anaphylactic reactions to protamine when it is used for heparin reversal [30]. The incidence of anaphylaxis to protamine is 0.6–2% in this patient population [83,84]. Because protamine is often administered concomitantly with blood products, protamine is frequently implicated as the causative agent in adverse reactions, especially in cardiac surgical patients. Platelet and other allogeneic blood transfusions can produce a series of adverse reactions via multiple mechanisms, and blood products have a greater potential for allergic reactions than protamine. Although antigen avoidance is one of the most important considerations in preventing anaphylaxis, this is not always possible, especially with certain drugs where alternatives are not available. Protamine is an important example of where alternatives are under investigation, but are not currently available.

Management of the allergic patient

Patients with an allergic history have been suggested to have an increased risk for anaphylaxis. The risk of anaphylaxis appears to be greater in patients receiving an intravenous anesthetic and in patients with a history of allergy or atopy. A study from Australia evaluated 1000 patients by questionnaire to determine the incidence of previous anesthesia, allergy, and atopy [85]. The patients who had reactions showed a higher incidence of allergy, atopy, asthma, and previous adverse reactions than the general population. The incidence was higher in females than in males. In a group of 85 patients with life-threatening reactions, 46% noted a history of allergy or atopy. Although the incidence of allergy and atopy was higher in anesthetized patients who had drug reactions, the incidence is not sufficiently great to make pretreatment of patients with a history of allergy or atopy a reasonable prophylactic maneuver.

In a North American study, Moscicki *et al.* reported 27 patients referred for evaluation of anaphylaxis after induction of general anesthesia in which thiobarbiturates, muscle relaxants, or antibiotics were administered intravenously [86]. Skin testing by prick and intracutaneous methods was performed with dilutions of the thiobarbiturates and muscle relaxants; β-lactam reagents were used in patients who had also received these drugs. No skin-test reactivity was noted in 16 normal subjects. Skin tests were positive in 13 patients (thiobarbiturates in five, muscle relaxants in six, and antibiotics in two). Two patients were dermatographic and yielded indeterminate skin-test results. Eleven of the 27 patients subsequently had general anesthesia and all patients received a premedication regimen of prednisone and diphenhydramine. Of three patients with negative skin tests, one experienced an arrhythmia, but no other signs attributable to anaphylaxis were noted. One patient with dermatographism had general anesthesia without a reaction. Positive skin tests implicated an agent that was avoided in seven patients; one of these patients experienced delayed urticaria/angioedema after the completion of general anesthesia. Thus, no patients developed anaphylaxis during subsequent general anesthesia for which agents producing positive skin tests were avoided, and a premedication regimen was used. In this patient population, the incidence of atopy in the 27 was 44.4%; the reported incidence of atopy in the US population was 5–22%.

Antihistamines, test doses, pretreatment, and anaphylaxis

Test doses are often administered before giving the full therapeutic dose to test for a reaction. Test doses are used empirically in clinical practice, but they may cause anaphylaxis. When a test dose is given, monitoring for acute cardiopulmonary dysfunction is important [20]. However, nonreactive test doses can be followed by anaphylaxis when the full dose is administered, as previously reviewed with aprotinin [71,72]. Although antihistamines are widely used in pretreatment, patients receiving both antihistamines and corticosteroids can still have anaphylaxis [72,84]. Most studies regarding pretreatment protocols are derived from radiocontrast media reactions that are not immunologically mediated [87].

Therapy

Airway maintenance with 100% oxygen, intravascular volume expansion, and epinephrine are important to treat the hypotension and hypoxemia associated with vasodilation, increased capillary permeability, and bronchospasm in anaphylaxis [88]. A representative protocol for management of perioperative anaphylaxis is presented in Box 68.1. Published guidelines including the advanced cardiopulmonary life-support recommendations from the American Heart Association for treating anaphylaxis often include intramuscular epinephrine, an issue not relevant in most perioperative management [89]. Absorption and subsequent achievement of maximum plasma concentration after subcutaneous administration is slower and may be significantly delayed with shock. They recommend intravenous epinephrine if anaphylaxis appears to be severe with immediate life-threatening manifestations [89].

Vasopressin or other V_1 agonists are important therapeutic considerations to treat the associated vasodilatory shock that can occur with anaphylaxis [90]. Vasodilatory shock is caused by activation of vasodilator mechanisms and the inability of sympathetic α-adrenergic mechanisms to compensate [90]. This may be further complicated by excessive nitric oxide formation that contributes to the profound vascular collapse, as well as activation of potassium channels (K_{ATP} and K_{Ca}) in

vascular smooth muscle that occurs despite catecholamine therapy [90]. Vasopressin and its analogs are uniquely effective because they have different vasoconstrictive mechanisms than α_1-adrenergic drugs, including blocking K_{ATP} channels in vascular smooth muscle and interfering with other signaling pathways [90,91]. Vasopressin's efficacy is documented in both case reports and experimental models of anaphylactic shock [92–94]. Although methylene blue has been reported for treating anaphylactic shock, this selective nitric oxide synthetase inhibitor has not been shown to be consistently effective [91,95].

Evaluation of patients following anaphylaxis

Following an anaphylactic reaction, a blood sample should be obtained for serum and sent for tryptase determination. Plasma levels of tryptase, a mast-cell mediator, are increased in IgE-mediated reactions, and correlate with histamine release [96]. A blood sample should be measured within 2 hours of the reaction and repeated at 24 hours to demonstrate a return to normal values [96]. Mast-cell tryptase can also be released by drugs like vancomycin, and may be negative in the case of patients who have IgG antibodies causing reactions [38]. Histamine measurements are not diagnostic for anaphylaxis; rather tryptase has replaced histamine as the mediator to measure. However, patients with mastocytosis and abnormal proliferation of mast cells may also have elevated tryptase levels [97]. In-vitro testing is not widely available for drugs administered perioperatively. Skin testing is the method most often reported to evaluate patients following anaphylaxis in the perioperative setting [98]. Skin testing includes prick and intradermal administration of suspected antigens [98,99]. Anesthesiologists should consider consulting an allergist to help them evaluate patients following reactions.

FDA reporting mechanisms: MedWatch

To improve the detection of previously unknown serious adverse drug reactions and knowledge about regulatory actions taken in response to reporting of these events, the FDA introduced the MedWatch program in 1993 (www.fda.gov/safety/medwatch). The FDA has responsibility for assuring the safety and efficacy of all regulated medical products marketed in the USA, including drugs, biologics, medical and radiation-emitting devices, and special nutritional products (e.g., medical foods, dietary supplements, and infant formulas).

The purpose of the MedWatch program is to enhance the effectiveness of postmarketing surveillance of medical products as they are used in clinical practice, and to rapidly identify significant health hazards associated with these products. The program has four goals: (1) to increase awareness of drug- and device-induced disease, (2) to clarify what should and should not be reported to the agency, (3) to make it easier to report by operating a single system for health professionals to report adverse events and product problems to the agency, and (4) to provide regular feedback to the healthcare community about safety issues involving medical products. The program is intended to encourage healthcare professionals to report

Box 68.1. Potential treatment plan for anaphylaxis: therapeutic protocol and pharmacologic intervention

Reproduced with permission from AnaphylaxisWeb.com
Therapy is divided into initial and secondary treatment. Therapy must be individualized, and the following is provided as a potential guide when these life-threatening events occur.

Initial therapy

Stop administration of the antigen
Drug or blood infusions should be immediately stopped. From a practical perspective, this may not always be possible. Limiting antigen administration may prevent further recruitment of activated mast cells and basophils.

Maintain the airway with 100% oxygen
Profound ventilation–perfusion abnormalities producing hypoxemia can occur with anaphylactic reactions. Always administer 100% oxygen along with airway support as needed. Patients may not initially be intubated but may require endotracheal intubation if severe cardiopulmonary collapse occurs. Arterial blood gases should be drawn and followed during resuscitation. Patients not intubated who develop laryngeal edema may require tracheostomy.

Discontinue all sedatives, hypnotics, or anesthetic drugs
These drugs interfere with the body's compensatory response to shock and cardiovascular dysfunction. Inhalational anesthetic drugs are not the bronchodilators of choice in treating bronchospasm following anaphylaxis, especially during hypotension.

Administer intravascular volume
Hypovolemia rapidly ensues during anaphylactic shock, with up to 40% loss of intravascular fluid into the interstitial space, as demonstrated by hemoconcentration. Therefore, volume expansion is extremely important in conjunction with epinephrine in correcting the acute hypotension. Initially, in an adult, 25–50 mL kg^{-1} of lactated Ringer's solution, normal saline, or colloid solutions should be administered, keeping in mind that additional volume may be necessary with persistent hypotension. Refractory hypotension following volume and epinephrine administration requires additional hemodynamic monitoring including transesophageal echocardiography to acutely determine the underlying mechanism of ventricular dysfunction, and it can be an extremely useful tool in patients who develop acute cardiovascular collapse. Fulminant noncardiogenic pulmonary edema with loss of intravascular volume can occur following anaphylaxis. This condition requires intravascular volume repletion with careful hemodynamic monitoring until the capillary defect improves. Colloid volume expansion has not been proven to be more effective than crystalloid volume expansion for treating anaphylactic shock.

Administer epinephrine for shock
Epinephrine is the drug of choice when resuscitating patients during anaphylactic shock. α_1-Adrenergic effects produce vasoconstriction of both vascular capacitance and arterial resistance vessels to reverse hypotension; β_2-receptor stimulation bronchodilates and inhibits mediator release by increasing cyclic AMP in mast cells and basophils. The route of epinephrine administration and the dose depends upon the patient's condition. Rapid and timely intervention with common sense must be used when treating anaphylaxis. Furthermore, during anesthesia patients may have altered sympathoadrenergic responses to acute anaphylactic shock, while patients during spinal or epidural anesthesia may be partially "sympathectomized," requiring even larger doses of catecholamines. This is also a consideration regarding patients who are receiving β-adrenergic blocking agents.

In hypotensive patients, 5–10 μg intravenous boluses of epinephrine (0.05–0.1 mL of 1:10 000 epinephrine) should be titrated for restoring blood pressure. Additional volume and incremental doses of epinephrine should be administered until hypotension is corrected. Although an epinephrine infusion represents an ideal method of administering epinephrine, it is usually impossible to infuse the drug through peripheral intravenous access during acute volume resuscitation. With cardiovascular collapse, full intravenous cardiopulmonary resuscitative doses of epinephrine, 0.25–0.5 mg (5–10 μg kg^{-1}), should be administered and repeated until hemodynamic stability occurs. Higher doses may be required in the patient who is "sympathectomized" following spinal or epidural anesthesia. Patients with laryngeal edema without hypotension should receive subcutaneous epinephrine. Epinephrine should not be administered intravenously to patients with normal blood pressures. If intravenous access is not available, then epinephrine can be administered down the endotracheal tube. The cardiovascular system is the major target organ in anaphylaxis, and shock must be aggressively treated.

Secondary treatment

Administer antihistamines
Since H_1 receptors mediate many of the adverse effects of histamine, the intravenous administration of 0.5–1 mg kg^{-1} of an H_1 antagonist such as diphenhydramine may be useful in treating acute anaphylaxis. Antihistamines do not inhibit anaphylactic reactions or inhibit histamine release but compete with histamine at receptor sites. H_1 antagonists are indicated in all forms of anaphylaxis. The H_1 antagonists presently available for parenteral administration may have antidopaminergic effects and should be given slowly to prevent precipitous hypotension in potentially hypovolemic patients. The indication for administering an H_2 antagonist once anaphylaxis has occurred remains unclear.

Consider administering catecholamine infusions
Catecholamine infusions are life-saving therapeutic modalities when treating anaphylaxis with persistent hypotension. The catecholamines used clinically to treat different forms of shock including anaphylaxis include dopamine, dobutamine, epinephrine, norepinephrine, and isoproterenol. The

Box 68.1. *(cont.)*

currently available catecholamines have different effects on α, β_1, and β_2-adrenoceptors and variable effects on heart rate, rhythm, systemic vascular resistance, and pulmonary vascular resistance. Patients during anaphylactic shock are vasodilated with low systemic vascular resistance, necessitating therapy with catecholamines that have α-adrenergic effects. Epinephrine stimulates α, β_1, and β_2 receptors and is often the mainstay therapy for anaphylaxis and for patients who have had cardiac surgery. Dopamine, a precursor of norepinephrine, undergoes biosynthetic transformation to norepinephrine when administered in high doses, and by virtue of its ability to stimulate renal dopaminergic receptors, dopamine also increases renal perfusion. Patients with heart failure or in shock can have neurotransmitter depletion and be less responsive to indirect-acting catecholamines, such as dopamine. Norepinephrine at doses as high as 1 μg kg^{-1} min^{-1} has been administered to cardiac surgical patients to maintain systemic arterial blood pressure without evidence of renal dysfunction. Dobutamine, a synthetic catecholamine, stimulates primarily β_1 receptors. Isoproterenol, a β_1-, β_2-selective drug, produces tachyarrhythmias as well as systemic vasodilation and is used primarily in right ventricular failure for pulmonary hypertension and/or in status asthmaticus. Catecholamine administration also stimulates β_1-adrenoceptors, resulting in an increase in heart rate. The first-line catecholamines that should be used to treat anaphylactic shock include epinephrine and norepinephrine.

Epinephrine infusions may be useful in patients with persistent hypotension or bronchospasm after initial resuscitation. Epinephrine infusions should be started at 4–8 μg min^{-1} (0.05–0.1 μg kg^{-1} min^{-1}) and titrated to correct hypotension. Norepinephrine infusions may be required in patients with refractory hypotension due to decreased systemic vascular resistance. It may be started at 4–8 μg min^{-1} (0.05–0.1 μg kg^{-1} min^{-1}) and adjusted to correct hypotension. Isoproterenol infusions can be used in patients with refractory bronchospasm, pulmonary hypertension, or right ventricular dysfunction. The usual starting dose is 0.5–1 μg min^{-1}. Isoproterenol has profound β_2-adrenergic effects that can produce systemic vasodilation; therefore, it must be used cautiously in hypotensive or hypovolemic patients.

Consider phosphodiesterase inhibitors
Aminophylline, a phosphodiesterase inhibitor, is a weak bronchodilator that also increases right and left ventricular contractility and decreases pulmonary vascular resistance. Aminophylline may be useful in patients with persistent bronchospasm and hemodynamic stability; however, the newer cAMP-specific phosphodiesterase inhibitors (e.g., milrinone) have increasing importance in treating right ventricular failure and pulmonary hypertension. An intravenous loading dose of 5–6 mg kg^{-1} of aminophylline given over 20 minutes should be followed by an infusion of 0.5–0.9 mg kg^{-1} h^{-1}.

Administer corticosteroids
Indications for corticosteroid administration during anaphylaxis are not well defined. Experimental evidence suggests that they will decrease arachidonic acid metabolites by inducing synthesis of nuclear regulatory proteins to inhibit phospholipid membrane breakdown. In addition, they may alter the activation and migration of other inflammatory cells (i.e., polymorphonuclear leukocytes) following an acute reaction. Corticosteroids may require 12–24 hours to work, and despite their unproven efficacy in treating acute reactions they are often administered as adjuncts to therapy when refractory bronchospasm or refractory shock occurs following resuscitative therapy. Recommended doses of corticosteroids are 0.25–1 g of hydrocortisone in IgE-mediated reactions. Alternatively, 1–2 g of methylprenisolone (30–35 mg kg^{-1}) may be useful in reactions thought to be complement-mediated, such as catastrophic pulmonary vasoconstriction following protamine transfusion reactions. Administering corticosteroids after an anaphylactic reaction may also be important in attenuating the late-phase reactions reported to occur 12–24 hours after anaphylaxis.

Consider sodium bicarbonate
Acidosis rapidly develops in patients with persistent hypotension. This diminishes the effect of epinephrine on the heart and systemic vasculature. Therefore, with refractory hypotension or acidemia, sodium bicarbonate 0.5–1 mEq kg^{-1} should be given and repeated every 5 minutes or as dictated by arterial blood gases.

Evaluate the airway
Because profound laryngeal edema may be a sequela of anaphylactic reactions, the airway should be evaluated before extubation of the trachea. Persistent facial edema suggests airway edema. The tracheas of these patients should remain intubated until the edema subsides. Assessment for a significant air leak after endotracheal tube cuff deflation ("leak test") may be useful in assessing airway patency prior to extubation of the trachea. If there is any question of airway edema, then direct laryngoscopy should be performed before extubation of the trachea.

Additional considerations
Bronchospasm refractory to therapy should be treated with inhaled β_2-adrenergic drugs (albuterol or terbutaline) administered by metered-dose inhaler, or through an endotracheal tube in the critically ill patient. For refractory bronchospasm and/or status asthmaticus, urgent cardiopulmonary support may have a role.

serious adverse events suspected to be caused by products regulated by the FDA. Serious events are those that lead to death, hospitalization, significant or permanent disability, or congenital anomaly, or that require medical or surgical intervention to prevent one of these events. Physicians may report adverse drug reactions by telephone, fax, or mail, or through the MedWatch website (www.fda.gov/safety/medwatch/howtoreport).

Summary

Allergic and anaphylactic reactions are important problems for the perioperative management of patients. These reactions are immune-mediated adverse responses and occur because of prior sensitization to an offending antigen. The pathophysiology of acute allergic reactions involves mast-cell- and basophil-mediated release of inflammatory mediators when an antigen interacts with membrane-bound IgE. The most life-threatening form of an adverse reaction is anaphylaxis. Common intraoperative manifestations of anaphylaxis include hypotension, cardiac arrest, acute bronchospasm and upper airway edema. Diagnosing anaphylaxis in the perioperative period is problematic, however, because of the presence of multiple potential contributors to cardiovascular and/or pulmonary dysfunction. Furthermore, cutaneous manifestations may be missed during surgery, as patients are usually covered.

Patients often receive a broad spectrum of drugs and other substances, all of which may produce allergic reactions. Perioperative anaphylaxis may be due to antibiotics, blood products, neuromuscular blocking drugs (NMBDs), polypeptides (aprotinin, latex, and protamine), drug additives/preservatives, and volume expanders. The risk of anaphylaxis appears to be greater in patients receiving an intravenous anesthetic and in patients with a history of allergy or atopy. Although the incidence of allergy and atopy is higher in anesthetized patients who have drug reactions, the incidence is not sufficiently great to make pretreatment of patients with a history of allergy or atopy a routine prophylactic maneuver.

Patients with anaphylaxis should have airway maintenance with 100% oxygen and should be treated with intravascular volume expansion and intravenous epinephrine. When cardiovascular collapse unresponsive to epinephrine occurs, intravenous vasopressin should be administered. In cases of suspected allergic or anaphylactic reactions, serum tryptase levels should be sent within 2 hours of the event and 24 hours later (to demonstrate return to normal). Tryptase levels have replaced histamine levels in the diagnosis of anaphylaxis.

Allergic and anaphylactic reactions represent a continuing challenge, and developing diagnostic testing to prevent reactions, as well as rapid diagnosis and treatment, is important in preventing adverse clinical outcomes. The FDA's MedWatch program is intended to encourage healthcare professionals to report serious adverse events suspected to be caused by drugs, medical devices, special nutritional products, and other products regulated by the FDA, to ensure that the detection of previously unknown serious adverse drug reactions can be improved.

References

1. Levy JH. Anaphylactic reactions during anesthesia. *Anesth Analg* 1992; **74**: 167.

2. Bigby M, Jick S, Jick H, Arndt K. Drug-induced cutaneous reactions: a report from the Boston Collaborative Drug Surveillance Program on 15,438 consecutive inpatients, 1975 to 1982. *JAMA* 1986; **256**: 3358–63.

3. Gruchalla RS. 10. Drug allergy. *J Allergy Clin Immunol* 2003; **111**: S548–59.

4. Gruchalla RS, Pirmohamed M. Clinical practice: antibiotic allergy. *N Engl J Med* 2006; **354**: 601–9.

5. Fiszenson-Albala F, Auzerie V, Mahe E, *et al.* A 6-month prospective survey of cutaneous drug reactions in a hospital setting. *Br J Dermatol* 2003; **149**: 1018–22.

6. Kay AB. Allergy and allergic diseases. First of two parts. *N Engl J Med* 2001; **344**: 30–7.

7. Kay AB. Allergy and allergic diseases. Second of two parts. *N Engl J Med* 2001; **344**: 109–13.

8. Bani D, Nistri S, Mannaioni PF, Masini E. Cardiac anaphylaxis: pathophysiology and therapeutic perspectives. *Curr Allergy Asthma Rep* 2006; **6**: 14–19.

9. Pumphrey RS. Lessons for management of anaphylaxis from a study of fatal reactions. *Clin Exp Allergy* 2000; **30**: 1144–50.

10. Romano A, Mayorga C, Torres MJ, *et al.* Immediate allergic reactions to cephalosporins: cross-reactivity and selective responses. *J Allergy Clin Immunol* 2000; **106**: 1177–83.

11. Torres MJ, Gonzalez FJ, Mayorga C, *et al.* IgG and IgE antibodies in subjects allergic to penicillins recognize different parts of the penicillin molecule. *Int Arch Allergy Immunol* 1997; **113**: 342–4.

12. Cohen SG, Zelaya-Quesada M. Portier, Richet, and the discovery of anaphylaxis: a centennial. *J Allergy Clin Immunol* 2002; **110**: 331–6.

13. Portier MM. De l'action anaphylactique de certains venins. *C R Soc Biol* 1902; **54**: 170–2.

14. Lieberman P, Kemp SF, Oppenheimer J, *et al.* The diagnosis and management of anaphylaxis: an updated practice parameter. *J Allergy Clin Immunol* 2005; **115**: S483–523.

15. Sampson HA, Munoz-Furlong A, Bock SA, *et al.* Symposium on the definition and management of anaphylaxis: summary report. *J Allergy Clin Immunol* 2005; **115**: 584–91.

16. Sampson HA, Munoz-Furlong A, Campbell RL, *et al.* Second symposium on the definition and management of anaphylaxis: summary report: second National Institute of Allergy and Infectious Disease/Food Allergy and Anaphylaxis Network symposium. *Ann Emerg Med* 2006; **47**: 373–80.

17. Smith PL, Kagey Sobotka A, Bleecker ER, *et al.* Physiologic manifestations of human anaphylaxis. *J Clin Invest* 1980; **66**: 1072–80.

18. Levy JH. *Anaphylactic Reactions in Anesthesia and Intensive Care*, 2nd edn. Stoneham: Butterworth-Heinemann Publishers, 1992.

19. Weiss ME, Adkinson NF, Hirshman CA. Evaluation of allergic drug reactions in the perioperative period. *Anesthesiology* 1989; **71**: 483–6.

20. Mertes PM, Laxenaire MC, Alla F. Anaphylactic and anaphylactoid reactions occurring during anesthesia in France in 1999–2000. *Anesthesiology* 2003; **99**: 536–45.

21. Pizov R, Brown RH, Weiss YS, *et al.* Wheezing during induction of general anesthesia in patients with and without asthma. A randomized, blinded trial. *Anesthesiology* 1995; **82**: 1111–16.

22. Tirumalasetty J, Grammer LC. Asthma, surgery, and general anesthesia: a review. *J Asthma* 2006; **43**: 251–4.

23. Busse WW, Lemanske RF. Asthma. *N Engl J Med* 2001; **344**: 350–62.

24. Warner DO, Warner MA, Barnes RD, *et al.* Perioperative respiratory complications in patients with asthma. *Anesthesiology* 1996; **85**: 460–7.

25. Olsson GL. Bronchospasm during anaesthesia. A computer-aided incidence study of 136,929 patients. *Acta Anaesthesiol Scand* 1987; **31**: 244–52.

26. Kaplan AP. Clinical practice. Chronic urticaria and angioedema. *N Engl J Med* 2002; **346**: 175–9.

27. Levy JH, O'Donnell PS. The therapeutic potential of a kallikrein inhibitor for treating hereditary angioedema. *Expert Opin Investig Drugs* 2006; **15**: 1077–90.

28. Reich DL, Hossain S, Krol M, *et al.* Predictors of hypotension after induction of general anesthesia. *Anesth Analg* 2005; **101**: 622–8.

29. Marone G, Bova M, Detoraki A, *et al.* The human heart as a shock organ in anaphylaxis. *Novartis Found Symp* 2004; **257**: 133–49.

30. Levy JH, Adkinson NF. Anaphylaxis during cardiac surgery: implications for clinicians. *Anesth Analg* 2008; **106**: 392–403.

31. Mertes PM, Laxenaire MC. Allergy and anaphylaxis in anaesthesia. *Minerva Anestesiol* 2004; **70**: 285–91.

32. Levy JH. Anaphylactic/anaphylactoid reactions during cardiac surgery. *J Clin Anesth* 1989; **1**: 426–30.

33. Ford SA, Kam PC, Baldo BA, Fisher MM. Anaphylactic or anaphylactoid reactions in patients undergoing cardiac surgery. *J Cardiothorac Vasc Anesth* 2001; **15**: 684–8.

34. Harboe T, Guttormsen AB, Irgens A, Dybendal T, Florvaag E. Anaphylaxis during anesthesia in Norway: a 6-year single-center follow-up study. *Anesthesiology* 2005; **102**: 897–903.

35. Idsoe O, Guthe T, Willcox RR, de Weck AL. Nature and extent of penicillin side-reactions, with particular reference to fatalities from anaphylactic shock. *Bull World Health Organ* 1968; **38**: 159–88.

36. Kelkar PS, Li JT. Cephalosporin allergy. *N Engl J Med* 2001; **345**: 804–9.

37. Levy JH, Kettlekamp N, Goertz P, Hermens J, Hirshman CA. Histamine release by vancomycin: a mechanism for hypotension in man. *Anesthesiology* 1987; **67**: 122–5.

38. Veien M, Szlam F, Holden JT, *et al.* Mechanisms of nonimmunological histamine and tryptase release from human cutaneous mast cells. *Anesthesiology* 2000; **92**: 1074–81.

39. Despotis GJ, Zhang L, Lublin DM. Transfusion risks and transfusion-related pro-inflammatory responses. *Hematol Oncol Clin North Am* 2007; **21**: 147–61.

40. Gilstad CW. Anaphylactic transfusion reactions. *Curr Opin Hematol* 2003; **10**: 419–23.

41. Sandler SG, Zantek ND. Review: IgA anaphylactic transfusion reactions. Part II. Clinical diagnosis and bedside management. *Immunohematol* 2004; **20**: 234–8.

42. Vassallo RR. Review: IgA anaphylactic transfusion reactions. Part I. Laboratory diagnosis, incidence, and supply of IgA-deficient products. *Immunohematol* 2004; **20**: 226–33.

43. Domen RE, Hoeltge GA. Allergic transfusion reactions: an evaluation of 273 consecutive reactions. *Arch Pathol Lab Med* 2003; **127**: 316–20.

44. Kleinman S, Caulfield T, Chan P, *et al.* Toward an understanding of transfusion-related acute lung injury: statement of a consensus panel. *Transfusion* 2004; **44**: 1774–89.

45. Silliman CC, Ambruso DR, Boshkov LK. Transfusion-related acute lung injury. *Blood* 2005; **105**: 2266–73.

46. Sheppard CA, Logdberg LE, Zimring JC, Hillyer CD. Transfusion-related acute lung injury. *Hematol Oncol Clin North Am* 2007; **21**: 163–76.

47. Goodnough LT, Shander A, Brecher ME. Transfusion medicine: looking to the future. *Lancet* 2003; **361**: 161–9.

48. Goodnough LT, Brecher ME, Kanter MH, AuBuchon JP. Transfusion medicine. First of two parts: blood transfusion. *N Engl J Med* 1999; **340**: 438–47.

49. Sazama K. Reports of 355 transfusion-associated deaths: 1976 through 1985. *Transfusion* 1990; **30**: 583–90.

50. Stainsby D, Russell J, Cohen H, Lilleyman J. Reducing adverse events in blood transfusion. *Br J Haematol* 2005; **131**: 8–12.

51. Spergel JM, Fiedler J. Food allergy and additives: triggers in asthma. *Immunol Allergy Clin North Am* 2005; **25**: 149–67.

52. Madan V, Walker SL, Beck MH. Sodium metabisulfite allergy is common but is it relevant? *Contact Dermatitis* 2007; **57**: 173–6.

53. Levy JH, Tanaka KA, Hursting MJ. Reducing thrombotic complications in the perioperative setting: an update on heparin-induced thrombocytopenia. *Anesth Analg* 2007; **105**: 570–82.

54. Berkun Y, Haviv YS, Schwartz LB, Shalit M. Heparin-induced recurrent anaphylaxis. *Clin Exp Allergy* 2004; **34**: 1916–18.

55. Hewitt RL, Akers DL, Leissinger CA, Gill JI, Aster RH. Concurrence of anaphylaxis and acute heparin-induced thrombocytopenia in a patient with heparin-induced antibodies. *J Vasc Surg* 1998; **28**: 561–5.

56. Bottio T, Pittarello G, Bonato R, Fagiolo U, Gerosa G. Life-threatening anaphylactic shock caused by porcine heparin intravenous infusion during mitral valve repair. *J Thorac Cardiovasc Surg* 2003; **126**: 1194–5.

57. Juhl D, Eichler P, Lubenow N, *et al.* Incidence and clinical significance of anti-PF4/heparin antibodies of the IgG, IgM, and IgA class in 755 consecutive patient samples referred for diagnostic testing for heparin-induced thrombocytopenia. *Eur J Haematol* 2006; **76**: 420–6.

58. al-Eryani AY, al-Momen AK, Fayed DF, Allam AK. Successful heparin desensitization after heparin-induced anaphylactic shock. *Thromb Res* 1995; **79**: 523–6.

59. Bernstein IL. Anaphylaxis to heparin sodium; report of a case, with immunologic studies. *J Am Med Assoc* 1956; **161**: 1379–81.

60. Chernoff AI. Anaphylactic reaction following injection of heparin. *N Engl J Med* 1950; **242**: 315–19.

61. Tejedor Alonso MA, Lopez Revuelta K, Garcia Bueno MJ, *et al.* Thrombocytopenia and anaphylaxis secondary to heparin in a hemodialysis patient. *Clin Nephrol* 2005; **63**: 236–40.

62. Kishimoto TK, Viswanathan K, Ganguly T, *et al.* Contaminated heparin associated with adverse clinical events and activation of the contact system. *N Engl J Med* 2008; **358**: 2457–67.

63. Baldo BA, Pham NH, Zhao Z. Chemistry of drug allergenicity. *Curr Opin Allergy Clin Immunol* 2001; **1**: 327–35.

64. Baldo BA, Fisher MM. Substituted ammonium ions as allergenic determinants in drug allergy. *Nature* 1983; **306**: 262–4.

65. Levy JH. Anaphylactic reactions to neuromuscular blocking drugs: are we making the correct diagnosis? *Anesth Analg* 2004; **98**: 881–2.

66. Bhananker SM, O'Donnell JT, Salemi JR, Bishop MJ. The risk of anaphylactic reactions to rocuronium in the United States is comparable to that of vecuronium: an analysis of food and drug administration reporting of adverse events. *Anesth Analg* 2005; **101**: 819–22.

67. Levy JH, Adelson D, Walker B. Wheal and flare responses to muscle relaxants in humans. *Agents Actions* 1991; **34**: 302–8.

68. Levy JH, Gottge M, Szlam F, Zaffer R, McCall C. Weal and flare responses to intradermal rocuronium and cisatracurium in humans. *Br J Anaesth* 2000; **85**: 844–9.

69. Dhonneur G, Combes X, Chassard D, Merle JC. Skin sensitivity to rocuronium and vecuronium: a randomized controlled prick-testing study in healthy volunteers. *Anesth Analg* 2004; **98**: 986–9.

70. Beierlein W, Scheule AM, Dietrich W, Ziemer G. Forty years of clinical aprotinin use: a review of 124 hypersensitivity reactions. *Ann Thorac Surg* 2005; **79**: 741–8.

71. Dietrich W, Spath P, Ebell A, Richter JA. Prevalence of anaphylactic reactions to aprotinin: analysis of two hundred forty-eight reexposures to aprotinin in heart operations. *J Thorac Cardiovasc Surg* 1997; **113**: 194–201.

72. Dietrich W, Spath P, Zuhlsdorf M, *et al.* Anaphylactic reactions to aprotinin reexposure in cardiac surgery: relation to antiaprotinin immunoglobulin G and E antibodies. *Anesthesiology* 2001; **95**: 64–71.

73. Jaquiss RD, Huddleston CB, Spray TL. Use of aprotinin in pediatric lung transplantation. *J Heart Lung Transplant* 1995; **14**: 302–7.

74. Pumphrey RS. Allergy to Hevea latex. *Clin Exp Immunol* 1994; **98**: 358–60.

75. Peixinho C, Tavares-Ratado P, Tomas MR, Taborda-Barata L, Tomaz CT. Latex allergy: new insights to explain different sensitization profiles in different risk groups. *Br J Dermatol* 2008; **159**: 132–6.

76. Brown RH, Schauble JF, Hamilton RG. Prevalence of latex allergy among anesthesiologists: identification of sensitized but asymptomatic individuals. *Anesthesiology* 1998; **89**: 292–9.

77. Blanco C, Carrillo T, Castillo R, Quiralte J, Cuevas M. Latex allergy: clinical features and cross-reactivity with fruits. *Ann Allergy* 1994; **73**: 309–14.

78. Isola S, Ricciardi L, Saitta S, *et al.* Latex allergy and fruit cross-reaction in subjects who are nonatopic. *Allergy Asthma Proc* 2003; **24**: 193–7.

79. Garcia Ortiz JC, Moyano JC, Alvarez M, Bellido J. Latex allergy in fruit-allergic patients. *Allergy* 1998; **53**: 532–6.

80. Holzman RS. Latex allergy: an emerging operating room problem. *Anesth Analg* 1993; **76**: 635–41.

81. Holzman RS. Clinical management of latex-allergic children. *Anesth Analg* 1997; **85**: 529–33.

82. Poley GE, Slater JE. Latex allergy. *J Allergy Clin Immunol* 2000; **105**: 1054–62.

83. Levy JH, Schwieger IM, Zaidan JR, Faraj BA, Weintraub WS. Evaluation of patients at risk for protamine reactions. *J Thorac Cardiovasc Surg* 1989; **98**: 200–4.

84. Levy JH, Zaidan JR, Faraj B. Prospective evaluation of risk of protamine reactions in patients with NPH insulin-dependent diabetes. *Anesth Analg* 1986; **65**: 739–42.

85. Laforest M, More D, Fisher M. Predisposing factors in anaphylactoid reactions to anaesthetic drugs in an Australian population: the role of allergy, atopy and previous anaesthesia. *Anaesth Intensive Care* 1980; **8**: 454–9.

86. Moscicki RA, Sockin SM, Corsello BF, Ostro MG, Bloch KJ. Anaphylaxis during induction of general anesthesia: subsequent evaluation and management. *J Allergy Clin Immunol* 1990; **86**: 325–32.

87. Marshall GD, Lieberman PL. Comparison of three pretreatment protocols to prevent anaphylactoid reactions to radiocontrast media. *Ann Allergy* 1991; **67**: 70–4.

88. Pumphrey RS, Roberts IS. Postmortem findings after fatal anaphylactic reactions. *J Clin Pathol* 2000; **53**: 273–6.

89. 2005 American Heart Association guidelines for cardiopulmonary resuscitation and emergency cardiovascular care. Part 10.6: Anaphylaxis. *Circulation 2005*; **112** (24 suppl): IV-143–5.

90. Landry DW, Oliver JA. The pathogenesis of vasodilatory shock. *N Engl J Med* 2001; **345**: 588–95.

91. Cauwels A, Janssen B, Buys E, Sips P, Brouckaert P. Anaphylactic shock depends on PI3K and eNOS-derived NO. *J Clin Invest* 2006; **116**: 2244–51.

92. Tsuda A, Tanaka KA, Huraux C, *et al.* The in vitro reversal of histamine-induced vasodilation in the human internal mammary artery. *Anesth Analg* 2001; **93**: 1453–9.

93. Krismer AC, Dunser MW, Lindner KH, *et al.* Vasopressin during

cardiopulmonary resuscitation and different shock states: a review of the literature. *Am J Cardiovasc Drugs* 2006; **6**: 51–68.

94. Kill C, Wranze E, Wulf H. Successful treatment of severe anaphylactic shock with vasopressin. Two case reports. *Int Arch Allergy Immunol* 2004; **134**: 260–1.

95. Evora PR. Should methylene blue be the drug of choice to treat vasoplegias caused by cardiopulmonary bypass and anaphylactic shock? *J Thorac Cardiovasc Surg* 2000; **119**: 632–4.

96. The diagnosis and management of anaphylaxis. Joint Task Force on Practice Parameters, American Academy of Allergy, Asthma and Immunology, American College of Allergy, Asthma and Immunology, and the Joint Council of Allergy, Asthma and Immunology. *J Allergy Clin Immunol* 1998; **101**: S465–528.

97. Schwartz LB. Diagnostic value of tryptase in anaphylaxis and mastocytosis. *Immunol Allergy Clin North Am* 2006; **26**: 451–63.

98. Fisher MM, Bowey CJ. Intradermal compared with prick testing in the diagnosis of anaesthetic allergy. *Br J Anaesth* 1997; **79**: 59–63.

99. Fisher M. Skin testing and the anaesthetist. *Br J Anaesth* 2001; **86**: 734–5.

Clinical applications: evidence-based anesthesia practice

Pediatric pharmacology

Greg B. Hammer and Brian J. Anderson

Introduction

The provision of perioperative care for neonates, infants, and children demands appreciation of developmental changes regarding the pharmacology of anesthetic drugs. Despite this, these patients remain therapeutic orphans, and the paucity of well-conducted pharmacokinetic and pharmacodynamic studies results in extrapolation of dosing from adult or nonhuman data. Young children are not simply small adults; they have unique physiology that changes remarkably with age, especially in the first year of life. For example, neonates and infants have a high percentage of body water, and therefore drugs that are distributed in water have a high volume of distribution in these patients. Other developmental processes impact drug absorption, distribution, clearance, and potency. Drug toxicity may be enhanced in this population; for example, cardiac output is highly dependent on heart rate in infants, and anesthetic drugs that cause a reduction in heart rate may disproportionately depress blood pressure and blood flow to tissues.

The pediatric population is commonly divided into three age groups. Neonates are aged less than 4 weeks after birth; this group is commonly subdivided into those born prematurely (before 37 weeks gestational age) and term neonates ($\geq$ 37 weeks gestation). Infants include those between 4 weeks and 1 year of age, while children are aged greater than 1 year. These divisions are useful because each group is typified by characteristic pharmacokinetic and pharmacodynamic differences.

This chapter will target issues related to neonates, infants, and children that affect the pharmacokinetics and pharmacodynamics of drugs used in the perioperative period in this unique and vulnerable population.

The rationale for providing anesthesia and analgesia to neonates

Those who are used to bearing an accustomed pain, even if they be weak and old, bear it more easily than the young and strong who are unaccustomed [1].

Contrary to popular modern belief, the ancient Greeks recognized that neonates, infants, and children tolerated pain poorly compared to adults. The understanding, assessment, and management of acute pain in pediatrics has lagged behind that of pain in adults until very recent times. Even in the late twentieth century pediatric patients received less analgesia postoperatively than adults; there was an established view that neonates were neither capable of perceiving pain nor able to remember painful stimuli. Anesthetic techniques in pediatrics reflected this view and ignored the possibility that pain during surgery caused adverse physiological effects that could compromise recovery and subsequent development. The primary indication for anesthesia was the prevention of movement during surgery. This was achieved with little more than controlled ventilation and neuromuscular blocking drugs [2]. Debate about the nature of consciousness in neonates and fear of adverse effects attributable to anesthetic drugs contributed to this practice. These latter fears have returned with the suggestion that some drugs commonly used in anesthesia may cause neuronal apoptosis in neonates [3].

Improvements in pediatric anesthesia and analgesia have resulted from a greater understanding of the developmental physiology of pain, along with reliable and valid techniques for measuring pain and a growing number of pharmacokinetic/pharmacodynamic studies in pediatrics [4]. It was assumed, for example, that the incomplete myelination of peripheral nerves was associated with impaired sensation in neonates. However, Anand and colleagues demonstrated simple and complex behavioral responses to painful stimuli, including reflex withdrawal, facial grimacing, and crying [5]. The behavioral response to a standard noxious stimulus in the neonate may be unpredictable, but the stress response associated with noxious stimuli is impressive and consistent [6]. Infants undergoing surgery without adequate anesthesia suffer a significant hormonal and metabolic response, which adversely affects postoperative recovery [7].

Developmental pharmacokinetics

Important developmental changes in the determinants of pharmacokinetics occur during infancy. These include drug

Anesthetic Pharmacology, 2nd edition, ed. Alex S. Evers, Mervyn Maze, Evan D. Kharasch. Published by Cambridge University Press. © Cambridge University Press 2011.

Table 69.1. Pharmacokinetic changes in infancy

Absorption

Uptake of inhalation drugs is rapid

Age-dependent changes in structure and function of the gastrointestinal tract affect oral absorption

    Skin thickness, perfusion, hydration in infancy increases percutaneous absorption

    Rectal absorption is erratic and variable with unpredictable effect on first-pass metabolism

Distribution

    Prediction is by weight out of infancy

    Changes in body composition affect drug distribution volumes

Water

    "Wet" at birth – extracellular fluid 50% volume

    Adult is "dry" – extracellular fluid 25% of weight within 3 months

Fat

    "Skinny" at birth – fat 10% of weight

    Adult fat – 20% of weight within 3 months

Clearance

    "Size" is predicted by $W^{3/4}$ out of infancy

    Maturation to adult rates in first year of life

Kidney

    30% of size-predicted value at birth

Liver

    20–50% of size-predicted value at birth

Plasma esterases

    100% at birth

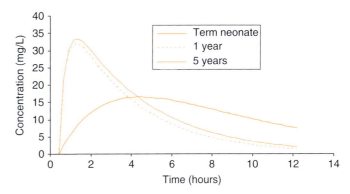

Figure 69.1. Simulated mean predicted time–concentration profiles for a term neonate, a 1-year-old infant, and a 5-year-old child given paracetamol elixir. Reproduced with permission from Anderson *et al.* [8].

absorption, distribution, binding, entry into the brain across the blood–brain barrier (BBB), and metabolism. These changes are summarized in Table 69.1.

Absorption

The majority of drugs used in anesthesia are administered either by the intravenous route or by inhalation. Drugs are given by extravascular routes (oral, nasal, rectal, intramuscular, transdermal, pulmonary) when no intravenous access is available in the preoperative or postoperative period. Chemical, physical, mechanical, and biological barriers must be overcome in order for drugs given by these routes to reach the systemic circulation.

The principal site of absorption for drugs given orally is the small intestine. The rate at which a drug leaves the stomach is the determinant of speed of drug absorption. There may also

be a lag time before the drug gets to the small intestine, where it is rapidly absorbed. The rate at which most drugs are absorbed when given by the oral route is slower in neonates and young infants than in older children because gastric emptying is delayed (Fig. 69. 1). The time (T_{max}) at which maximum concentration (C_{max}) is achieved is prolonged. Gastric emptying and intestinal motor motility mature through infancy, and normal adult rates may not be reached until 6–8 months [9]. Gastric pH is elevated (> 4) in neonates, increasing the bioavailability of acid-labile compounds (e.g., penicillin G) and decreasing the bioavailability of weak acids (e.g., phenobarbital) when given orally [10,11]. The infant gut is more permeable to large molecules (e.g., proteins, high-molecular-weight drugs) than that of older children.

Absorption of drugs administered via the rectal route is erratic and variable. Drugs given rectally may have reduced first-pass hepatic extraction because the venous drainage is directly into the inferior and middle hemorrhoidal veins, which are not part of the splanchnic circulation. The bioavailability of nasal, buccal, and sublingual routes is also less certain in infants and young children than in adults because of poor patient cooperation. Nasal midazolam, for example, has a bitter taste; as with the fentanyl oralet, buccal and sublingual routes are associated with more swallowed drug than in older, more cooperative patients.

The larger relative skin surface area, increased cutaneous perfusion, and thinner stratum corneum in neonates increases absorption of topically applied drugs (corticosteroids, local anesthetic creams, antiseptics). Neonates manifest a tendency to form methemoglobin because they have reduced levels of methemoglobin reductase and fetal hemoglobin is more readily oxidized than adult hemoglobin. This, combined with increased absorption through the neonatal epidermis, has resulted in reluctance to use lidocaine/prilocaine cream (EMLA) in this age group. EMLA, however, has been shown to be safe in neonates when applied as a one-time dose, and

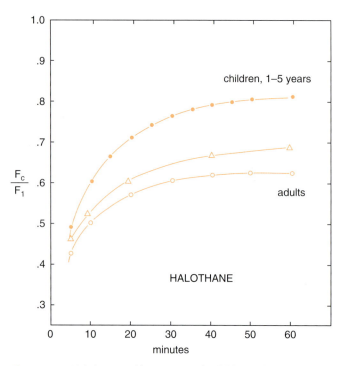

Figure 69.2. Halothane equilibration curves for children and adults, expressed as the ratio of exhaled (F_E) to inspired (F_I) gas. Reproduced with permission from Salanitre and Rackow [15].)

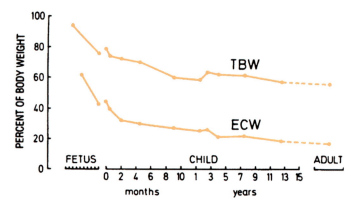

Figure 69.3. Body water compartment changes during growth. ECW, extracellular water; TBW, total body water. Reproduced with permission from Friis-Hansen [19].

has been shown to be efficacious for pain related to circumcision [12,13].

One might expect decreased absorption of drugs administered by intramuscular injection in neonates, because of their reduced muscle bulk, skeletal muscle blood flow, and muscular contractions. This is not necessarily the case, however, because neonates also have a high density of skeletal muscle capillaries [14].

Pulmonary absorption is generally more rapid in infants and children than in adults (Fig. 69.2) [15]. Developmental changes in lung physiology, architecture, and mechanics play a role. Other factors causing a more rapid "wash-in" of inhalational anesthetics include the greater fraction of cardiac output distributed to the vessel-rich tissue group (e.g., the lungs) and the lower tissue/blood solubility of inhaled anesthetics in neonates and infants [16]. Because solubility determines the volume of distribution, it has considerable effect on the uptake of inhalation drugs in children. An inhalation drug with a greater volume of distribution will take longer to reach a steady-state concentration when delivered at a constant rate. The solubilities ($\lambda_{\text{blood/gas}}$) in blood of halothane, isoflurane, enflurane, and methoxyflurane are 18% less in neonates than in adults, which is attributable to altered serum albumin, globulin, cholesterol, and triglyceride concentrations. The solubilities of these same drugs in the vessel-rich tissue group in neonates are approximately one-half of those in adults [17]. The latter may be due to the greater water content and decreased protein and lipid concentration in neonatal tissues.

Accordingly, a given F_E/F_I ratio (i.e., equilibration) is achieved more rapidly in infants than in adults (Fig. 69.2). This may increase the toxicity of inhaled anesthetics in neonates (e.g., bradycardia, cardiac depression due to halothane). Age has little effect on the solubility of the less soluble drugs, nitrous oxide and sevoflurane [18].

Induction of anesthesia will be slowed, on the other hand, by right-to-left shunting of blood in neonates. This may be caused by cyanotic congenital cardiac disease (e.g., pulmonary atresia, hypoplastic left heart syndrome) or intrapulmonary conditions (e.g., atelectasis, congenital vascular malformations).

Distribution

Total body water constitutes 85% of body weight in the preterm neonate and 75% in term neonates. This decreases to approximately 60% at 5 months and remains relatively constant thereafter [19]. The reduction in percentage of body water is primarily related to the decrease in extracellular fluid (ECF). ECF constitutes 45% of body weight at birth and 26% at 1 year (Fig. 69.3). There is a further reduction in ECF during childhood until the adult value of 18% is reached. Polar drugs such as aminoglycosides and nondepolarizing neuromuscular blocking drugs (NMBDs) distribute rapidly into the ECF but enter cells more slowly. The initial dose of such drugs is usually higher in the neonate and infant compared to older children and adults because of the greater ECF volume in the former. For example, equivalent intubation conditions are provided by succinylcholine 3–4 mg kg^{-1} in infants, 2 mg kg^{-1} in children, and 1 mg kg in^{-1} in adolescents and adults.

The percentage of body weight contributed by fat is 3% in a 1.5 kg premature neonate and 12% in a term neonate; this proportion doubles by 4–5 months of age. "Baby fat" is lost when infants start walking and protein mass increases (20% in a term neonate, 50% in an adult). Relative body proportions change dramatically over the first few years of life and significantly affect volumes of distribution of drugs. For example, thiopental has a short-lived effect after an induction dose owing to its rapid redistribution into muscle and fat. The redistribution half-life of thiopental is increased in neonates because of their low body-fat and muscle mass.

Protein and tissue binding

Acidic drugs (e.g., barbiturates) tend to bind mainly to albumin, while basic drugs (e.g., diazepam, amide local anesthetic drugs) bind to globulins, lipoproteins, and glycoproteins. Plasma protein binding of many drugs is decreased in the newborn infant relative to adults, but the clinical impact of this decrease is minor for most drugs compared to the effect of reduced clearance in this age group [20]. Reduced protein binding in neonates is important for drugs with more than 95% protein binding, a high extraction ratio, and a narrow therapeutic index (e.g., lidocaine).

α_1-acid glycoprotein (AAG) concentrations are reduced in neonates, increase during early infancy, and are similar to those in adults by 6 months [21]. Because AAG is an acute-phase reactant, serum concentrations increase after surgical stress. Mean preoperative AAG concentrations of 0.38 (SD 0.16) g L^{-1} increased to 0.76 (SD 0.18) g L^{-1} in infants by day 4 after surgery and stayed at that concentration through to day 7 [22]. This change causes an increase in total plasma concentrations for low- to intermediate-extraction drugs such as bupivacaine. The unbound drug concentration, however, does not change, because clearance of the unbound drug is affected only by the intrinsic metabolizing capacity of the liver. Any increase in unbound concentration observed during long-term drug administration is attributable to reduced clearance rather than AAG concentration [20].

Binding to albumin is reduced in neonates compared with infants, children, and adults. Plasma albumin concentrations are lowest in premature infants, and other fetal proteins such as α-fetoprotein (synthesized by the embryonic yolk sac, fetal gastrointestinal tract, and liver, having 40% homology with albumin) have reduced affinity for drugs. In addition, increased concentrations of free fatty acids and unconjugated bilirubin compete with acidic drugs for albumin binding sites. Neonates also have a tendency to manifest a metabolic acidosis that alters ionization and binding properties of plasma proteins. Serum albumin concentrations approximate adult values by 5 months of age, and binding capacity approaches adult values by 1 year of age [23].

Low concentrations of binding proteins, including AAG and albumin, may be especially relevant when a highly bound drug is injected rapidly and in a large dose. Decreased binding of thiopental to plasma albumin may contribute to the observation that the induction dose of thiopental is lower in neonates than in older age groups (13% of the drug is unbound in newborns, compared to 7% in adults).

Most drugs cross physiologic membranes as a result of passive diffusion along concentration gradients. This process is influenced by factors such as molecular size, ionization, tissue binding, and lipophilicity. P-glycoprotein, a member of the ATP-binding cassette family of transporters, is capable of producing a biologic barrier to membrane passage. This glycoprotein is an efflux transporter capable of extruding selected toxins and xenobiotics from cells at diverse site that include the BBB, hepatocytes, renal tubular cells, and erythrocytes. The level of expression of P-glycoprotein appears to be low in neonatal rats, and this may explain increased brain/plasma phenobarbital ratios in neonates [24,25]. However, pore density and blood flow distribution differences may also explain this observation.

Maturational changes in tissue binding also affect drug distribution. Tissue binding increases the volume of distribution. Myocardial digoxin concentrations in infants are six times higher than those in adults despite similar serum concentrations [26]. Erythrocyte/plasma concentration ratios of digoxin in infants are one-third smaller during digitalization than during maintenance digoxin therapy [27]. These findings are consistent with a greater apparent volume of distribution of digoxin in infants and may partly explain the unusually large therapeutic doses needed in infants.

The blood–brain barrier (BBB)

The BBB is a lipid membrane interface between the endothelial cells of the brain blood vessels and the ECF of the brain. Brain uptake of drugs is dependent on lipid solubility and blood flow, i.e., uptake is enhanced by high lipid solubility and cerebral blood flow. It was postulated that BBB permeability to water-soluble drugs such as morphine changes with maturation. This concept originated from a study of neonates less than 4 days of age who developed ventilatory depression following intramuscular injection of morphine 0.05 mg kg^{-1}, a dose associated with minimal ventilatory depression in adults [28]. In this study, ventilatory depression in neonates following intramuscular administration of the more lipid-soluble meperidine 0.5 mg kg^{-1} was similar to that expected in adults, suggesting that lipid-soluble drugs cross the immature and mature BBB comparably. Fentanyl, a lipid-soluble drug, has similar respiratory-depressant effects in infants and adults when plasma concentrations are comparable [29]. However, the increased neonatal respiratory depression observed after morphine could be due to pharmacokinetic rather than BBB age-related changes. For example, the volume of distribution of morphine is reduced in term neonates, and initial plasma concentrations of morphine may be higher in neonates than in adults [30]. Respiratory depression is the same in children from 2 to 570 days of age at the same morphine plasma concentration [31].

Drug metabolism

The majority of drug metabolism (clearance) occurs in the liver, where lipid-soluble compounds are converted to more water-soluble compounds. The latter are generally excreted in the bile or urine. Water-soluble drugs may be excreted unchanged in the kidneys by glomerular filtration and/or renal tubular secretion. Many of these processes are immature in the neonate and mature within the first year of life, during which time most enzyme systems appear to evolve and approximate adult rates when scaled using allometric models (see below). Selected processes appear to mature later during childhood; isoniazid acetylation (*N*-acetyltransferase) given to children with tuberculosis has activity at 4 years of age equivalent to that observed in adults [32].

Hepatic elimination

Drugs are metabolized in the liver by phase I and phase II reactions. Phase I metabolic processes involve oxidative, reductive, or hydrolytic reactions that are commonly catalyzed by the mixed function oxidase system. Phase II pathways involve conjugation. The different pathways develop at different rates, and maturity of some components may take several months.

The cytochrome P450 (CYP) is the major enzyme system for oxidation of drugs (Table 69.2). There are distinct patterns associated with isoform-specific developmental expression of CYPs. Some CYPs appear to be switched on at birth, while others have a later onset of expression [34]. CYP2E1 activity increases after birth, CYP2D6 becomes detectable soon thereafter, the CYP3A4 and CYP2C family appear during the first week (Fig. 69.4), and CYP1A2 is the last to appear. The immaturity of the CYP systems in neonates may have important effects on the risk of drug toxicity in these patients.

Neonates are dependent on the immature CYP3A4 for levobupivacaine clearance and CYP1A2 for ropivacaine clearance, dictating reduced epidural infusion rates in this age group [36]. Toxicity associated with prolonged bupivacaine infusion in neonates can be avoided by reducing infusion rates according to the reduced clearance in neonates and young infants.

The toxic metabolite of paracetamol (acetaminophen), *N*-acetyl-p-benzoquinone imine (NAPQI) is formed by CYP2E1, 1A2, and 3A4. This metabolite binds to intracellular hepatic macromolecules to produce cell necrosis and damage. CYP2E1 activity surges after birth, but data suggest that infants less than 90 days old have decreased clearance of CYP2E1 substrates compared with older infants, children, and adults. CYP3A4 appears during the first week, whereas CYP1A2 is the last to appear. The lower activity of CYP in neonates may contribute to the low occurrence of paracetamol-induced hepatotoxicity seen in neonates [37].

Fentanyl is metabolized by oxidative *N*-dealkylation (CYP3A4) into norfentanyl, which is then hydroxylated. All metabolites of fentanyl are inactive. A small amount of fentanyl is eliminated by the kidney. Fentanyl clearance is 70–80% of adult values in term neonates and reaches adult values (approximately 50 L h^{-1} [70 kg]$^{-1}$) within the first 2 weeks of life [20]. Termination of effect in neonates is rapid after low-dose administration because the volume of distribution is large in neonates (~ 5.9 L kg^{-1} in term neonates) compared to adults (1.6 L kg^{-1}). High-dose therapy results in prolonged effect in neonates due to reduced clearance. Fentanyl clearance

Table 69.2. Examples of some drugs metabolized using the cytochrome P450 system

Cytochrome P450	Substrate
CYP1A2	Ondansetron, paracetamol, caffeine, ropivacaine
CYP2A6	Methoxyflurane
CYP3A4	Fentanyl, levobupivacaine
CYP2C9	Ibuprofen, warfarin
CYP2C19	Omeprazole, phenytoin, diazepam
CYP2D6	Codeine, metoprolol, tramadol, amitriptyline
CYP2E1	Alcohol, enflurane, halothane, paracetamol

From Sweeney and Bromilow [33].

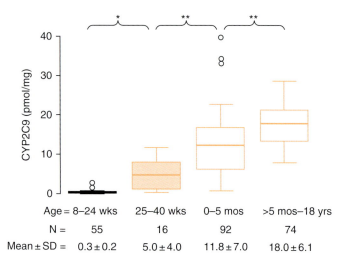

Figure 69.4. Developmental expression of human hepatic CYP2C9 enzyme. Reproduced with permission from Koukouritaki *et al.* [35].

is reduced when intra-abdominal pressure is increased (e.g., omphalocele) due to decreased hepatic blood flow and decreased hepatic extraction.

Knowledge of maturation of phase II enzymes remains incomplete. Some phase II pathways are mature at birth (sulfate conjugation), while others are not (acetylation, glycination, glucuronidation). Morphine is largely metabolized to morphine-3-glucuronide and morphine-6-glucuronide [38]. In-vitro studies using liver microsomes from fetuses aged 15–27 weeks indicated that morphine glucuronidation was approximately 10–20% of that seen with adult microsomes [39]. Morphine glucuronidation has been demonstrated in premature infants as young as 24 weeks. Clearance maturation is related to postmenstrual age and increases

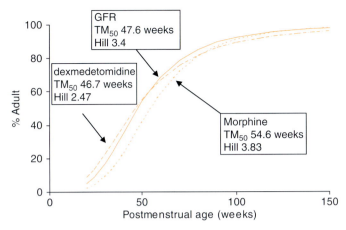

Figure 69.5. Maturation of morphine [40] and dexmedetomidine [41] (phase II conjugation), and glomerular filtration rate [42], over the first year of life. Rates are scaled to a 70 kg person, and the relationship between age and rate is described using the Hill equation. Maturation of the many CYP enzyme systems is believed to be more rapid.

to reach 87% of adult rates by 1 year (Fig. 69.5) [30]. The neonate can use sulfate conjugation as an alternative route for substrates such as morphine or paracetamol before glucuronidation (or maturity of CYP activity) develops. The sulfate pathway is the dominant metabolic route for paracetamol in infancy [43].

Renal elimination

Drugs and their metabolites are excreted by the kidneys by two processes, glomerular filtration and tubular secretion. The glomerular filtration rate (GFR) is approximately 30% that of adults at birth in term neonates and is 90% at 1 year (Fig. 69.5) [42]. Proximal tubular secretion reaches adult rates by 7 months age [44]. Aminoglycosides are almost exclusively cleared by renal elimination, and maintenance dosing is predicted by postmenstrual age because this predicts the time course of development of renal function [45]. Penicillin is actively secreted by the para-amino hippurate pathway, which is immature in neonates, resulting in an increased elimination half-life for penicillin and related compounds [46]. Slightly acidic urine at birth (pH 6–6.5) decreases the elimination of weak acids.

The immaturity of renal clearance pathways for caffeine results in prolonged effect of the prodrug theophylline, used to treat or prevent postoperative apnea in preterm neonates. N-methylation of theophylline to produce caffeine in the newborn is well developed at birth, whereas oxidative demethylation by CYP1A2, responsible for caffeine metabolism, is deficient. Theophylline is effective for the management of postoperative apnea in the premature neonate partly because the metabolite, caffeine, is cleared slowly by the immature kidney.

Extrahepatic elimination

Some drugs are metabolized at extrahepatic sites. Remifentanil and, to a lesser extent, atracurium are rapidly broken down by nonspecific esterases in tissue and erythrocytes. Remifentanil clearance is approximately 150 L h^{-1} (70 kg)$^{-1}$ in all age groups. Expressed per kilogram of body weight, clearance is greater in

term neonates (4.5 L h^{-1} kg^{-1}) than in infants (3.7 L h^{-1} kg^{-1}) or adults (2.1 L h^{-1} kg^{-1}). The rate constant representing hydrolysis by plasma esterases of propacetamol to paracetamol is size-related, but not age-related [47]. The ester group of local anesthetics are metabolized by plasma pseudocholinesterase, which is present in reduced concentrations in neonates [48]. The in-vitro plasma half-life of 2-chloroprocaine in umbilical cord blood is twice that in maternal blood, but there are no in-vivo studies examining the effects of age.

Developmental pharmacodynamics

There are few data describing age-related pharmacodynamic changes despite recognition that the number, affinity, and type of receptors and the availability of natural ligands change with age. Some examples of altered pharmacodynamics in infants are shown in Table 69.3. Opioid receptors are not fully developed in the newborn rat and mature into adulthood, but increased human neonatal sensitivity to morphine is attributable to pharmacokinetic rather than pharmacodynamic differences [49]. Neonates have an increased sensitivity to the effects of NMBDs [50]. The reason for this is unknown, but it is consistent with the observation that there is a threefold reduction in the release of acetylcholine from the infant rat phrenic nerve [51].

γ-Aminobutyric acid (GABA) is the neurotransmitter at most inhibitory synapses in the human central nervous system. The GABA$_A$ receptor complex is the site of action for benzodiazepines, barbiturates, and numerous anesthetic drugs [52]. At birth the cerebellum only contains one-third the number of GABA$_A$ receptors found in an adult; these receptors also have reduced binding affinity for benzodiazepines in neonates [53]. Major changes in receptor binding and subunit expression occur during postnatal development [54]. The GABA$_A$ receptor complex, identified by positron emission tomography, becomes more prevalent from birth to 2 years and the values then decrease to 50% of peak values by 17 years [54]. These changes are consistent with age-related MAC changes of inhalational anesthetics and possibly contribute to higher midazolam doses required in young children for sedation (Fig. 69.6) [56]. The amount of drug going to the brain (and subsequent anesthetic effect) may also be affected by changes in regional blood flow. Mean cerebral blood flow increases during infancy and early childhood to reach a peak of about 70 mL min^{-1} (100 g)$^{-1}$ at about 3–8 years of age. Cerebral blood flow subsequently decreases with age from early childhood.

There are numerous additional examples of increased or decreased drug effect unrelated to pharmacokinetics in neonates, infants, and children. Bronchodilators have reduced effect in infants because of immaturity of bronchial smooth muscle at this age. The effect of anesthetic gases

Table 69.3. Pharmacodymanic changes in infancy

Neuromuscular blocking drugs – increased sensitivity in neonates

    Reduced acetylcholine from presynaptic junction

MAC increased in infancy

    GABA$_A$ receptor numbers increased

    Regional blood flow changes with age

Bronchodilators ineffective under 1 year

    Immaturity of bronchial smooth muscle

Calcium is an effective inotrope in neonates

    Cardiac calcium stores in the endoplasmic reticulum are reduced

Neural blockade from amide local anesthetic drugs shorter duration and require a larger weight-scaled dose

    Myelination, spacing of nodes of Ranvier

    Length of nerve exposed

    Size-related factors

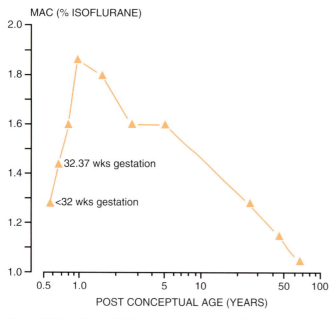

Figure 69.6. Isoflurane MAC changes with age. Reproduced with permission from LeDez et al. [55].

on bronchodilation in neonates and infants has not been studied. Cardiac calcium stores in the endoplasmic reticulum are reduced in the neonatal heart because of immaturity. Exogenous calcium has greater impact on contractility in this age group than in older children or adults. There are some data

to suggest greater sensitivity to warfarin in children, but the mechanism has not been determined [57]. Cyclosporine induces greater immunosuppression in infants than in older children and adults; this is possibly related to the T-lymphocyte response in infants [58]. Amide local anesthetic drugs induce shorter block duration and require a larger weight-scaled dose to achieve similar dermatome levels when given by subarachnoid block to infants. This may be due, in part, to myelination, spacing of nodes of Ranvier, the length of nerve exposed, and size-related factors.

Developmental pharmacogenomics, polymorphism, and receptors

Pharmacogenomics is the development and discovery of new drugs based on genome information. This may influence either pharmacokinetics or pharmacodynamics. Pharmacogenetics is the genetically determined variability in metabolism of drugs. There is large interindividual pharmacokinetic variability associated with polymorphisms of the genes encoding for metabolic enzymes. Genetic variability influencing plasma cholinesterase activity and succinylcholine metabolism is a well-known example.

Polymorphism of CYP2D6 is inherited as an autosomal recessive trait. Homozygous individuals are deficient in the metabolism of a variety of important groups of drugs – β-adrenoceptor blocking drugs, antidepressants, neuroleptic drugs, and opioids. Poor metabolizers have reduced morphine production from codeine [59]. Tramadol is also metabolized by hepatic O-demethylation (CYP2D6) to O-desmethyl tramadol (M1); the M1 metabolite has a μ-opioid affinity approximately 200 times greater than tramadol. CYP2D6 isoenzyme activity is important for the analgesic effect attributable to tramadol. The nature of the CYP2D6 polymorphism can be related to an activity score, and differences can be observed as early as 45 weeks postconceptual age. Clearance is reduced in the premature neonate, where the CYP2D6 polymorphism has little impact (Fig. 69.7). Maturation of the CYP2D6 pathway is rapid after 40 weeks' gestation when compared to glucuronide conjugation.

Candidate genes involved in pain perception, processing, and management, including opioid receptors, transporters, and other targets of pharmacotherapy, are under investigation. For example, the single nucleotide polymorphism A118G of the μ-opioid receptor gene has been associated with decreased potency of morphine and morphine-6-glucuronide as well as decreased analgesic effects and higher alfentanil dose demands in carriers of the mutated G118 allele. These genetic differences may explain why some patients need higher opioid doses, and the adverse effects profile may be modified by these mutations.

Pharmacokinetic modeling of age and size

Empiric size models for young children have led to the idea that there is an enhanced capacity of children to metabolize drugs due to proportionally larger livers and kidneys than their adult counterparts. This erroneous notion arises because clearance, expressed per kilogram of body weight, is larger in children than adults (Fig. 69.8). It has been suggested that a standard individual of 70 kg weight be used as a reference size for pharmacokinetic measures and that nonlinear scaling be used to compare individuals to this size standard [62]. Growth and development are two major aspects of children not readily apparent in adults. These aspects can be investigated using readily observable demographic factors such as weight and age.

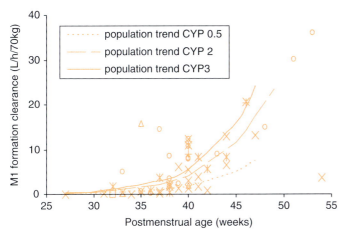

Figure 69.7. Tramadol M1 metabolite formation clearance (CYP2D6) increases with postmenstrual age. The rate of increase varies with genotype expression. Adapted with permission from Allegaert K *et al.*

There is a nonlinear relationship between weight and drug elimination. The log of basal metabolic rate (BMR) plotted against the log of body weight produces a straight line with a slope of ¾ in homeotherms, poikilotherms, and unicellular organisms [63]. This factor for size can be expressed using allometry as:

$$Fsize = \left(W/70\right)^{PWR} \tag{69.1}$$

Weight (W) is expressed as a fraction of a standard adult weight (70 kg). A great many physiological, structural, and time-related variables scale predictably within and between species with weight (W) exponents (PWR) of 0.75, 1, and 0.25, respectively. These exponents have applicability to pharmacokinetic parameters such as clearance (CL), volume (V), and half-time. Clearance, a metabolic process, scales with an exponent of ¾, volumes of distribution with an exponent of 1, and half-life with an exponent of ¼.

By choosing weight as the primary covariate and by using this empirical exponent of ¾ for clearance, secondary covariates can be investigated within a given dataset describing time–concentration profiles in a population. Babies must grow from an immature form to reach a size that allows reproduction. This maturation factor cannot be explained by allometry. The addition of a model describing maturation is required. The sigmoid hyperbolic model (familiar to anesthetists for describing the oxygen dissociation curve) has been found useful for describing this maturation factor (MF) [64]:

$$MF = \frac{PMA^{Hill}}{TM_{50}^{Hill} + PMA^{Hill}} \tag{69.2}$$

The TM_{50} describes the maturation half-time, while the Hill coefficient relates to the slope of this maturation profile. Maturation of clearance begins before birth, suggesting that postmenstrual age (PMA) would be a better predictor of drug elimination than postnatal age (PNA).

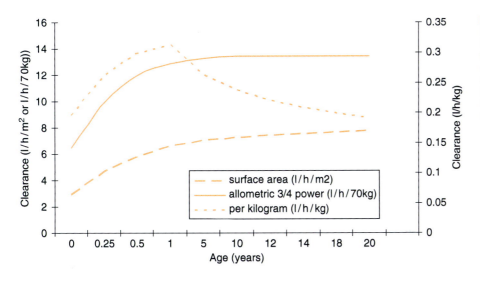

Figure 69.8. Age-related clearance changes for a hypothetical drug. All three models show an increase in clearance over the first year of life due to maturation of metabolic pathways. Clearance expressed using the per-kilogram model then decreases with age after 1 year to reach adult levels in adolescence. This course is not evident with the allometric ¾ power and surface-area models. Reproduced with permission from Anderson *et al.* [61].

Lastly, a factor for organ function (*OF*) accounts for pathological variation once size and maturation are accounted for. Drug clearance, for example, may be altered in renal failure. Metabolic processes are slower when temperature is reduced. Pharmacokinetic parameters (*P*) can be described in an individual as the product of these influences [65]:

$$P = Pstd \cdot Fsize \cdot MF \cdot OF \qquad (69.3)$$

where *Pstd* is the typical parameter for an adult weighing 70 kg. Examples of clearance maturation, scaled to a 70 kg person, for morphine and dexmedetomidine are shown alongside glomerular filtration rate in Fig. 69.5.

Summary

The pharmacology of drugs used in the perioperative period is significantly different in neonates, infants, and children versus adults. The growth in body weight and length and changes in physiology that occur during infancy and childhood impact drug absorption, distribution, and metabolism. Concomitant changes affect protein binding and receptor physiology and alter the efficacy of drugs during this time. The first year of life is the most critical period during which the majority of these maturational changes take place. An understanding of the basic elements of pediatric pharmacology will guide the practitioner in safe and efficacious treatment in this population.

Orally administered drugs are often absorbed more slowly by neonates and young infants than by older children, due to delayed gastric emptying. Furthermore, neonatal gastric pH is higher, affecting the bioavailability of orally administered acid-labile compounds and weak acids. Absorption of drugs administered via rectal, nasal, buccal, and sublingual routes is variable, while absorption of topically applied medications is increased. Inhalational anesthetics are generally absorbed more rapidly in infants and children than in adults; however, induction of anesthesia is slower in the presence of neonatal right-to-left shunting of blood, which may result from cyanotic congenital cardiac disease or intrapulmonary conditions.

Extracellular fluid constitutes a much greater proportion of body weight in neonates than in older children and adults, hence the requirement in neonates for higher initial doses of polar drugs which distribute rapidly into the extracellular fluid with relatively slower entry to the cells. Drugs which redistribute to muscle and fat are also affected by the changes in relative proportions of these body constituents during development and maturation.

Newborn infants display reduced levels of plasma protein binding of many drugs relative to adults. This generally has little clinical impact compared to the effect of reduced clearance in this age range. It is, however, an important factor in neonates for drugs with greater than 95% protein binding, a high extraction ratio, and a narrow therapeutic index. Tissue binding also undergoes maturational changes which affect drug distribution.

Many of the processes involved in metabolism and clearance of drugs mature during the first year of life. Developmental expression of the components of the cytochrome P450 (CYP) enzyme system varies in an isoform-dependent manner, and immaturity of CYPs can affect the risk of drug toxicity in neonates. Reduced infusion rates can circumvent the increased risk of toxicity that arises from reduced clearance for some drugs (e.g., bupivacaine). Conversely, immature metabolism may reduce the formation of some toxic metabolites, possibly contributing to the low occurrence of paracetamol-induced hepatotoxicity in neonates. In the kidneys, the glomerular filtration rate is greatly reduced in neonates, but reaches 90% that of adult rates by 1 year of age; proximal tubular secretion rates equal those of an adult by the age of 7 months. Changes in extrahepatic metabolism by enzymes in tissue, erythrocytes, and plasma also affect the pharmacokinetics of some drugs. Polymorphisms in genes encoding metabolic enzymes are associated with interindividual variability in drug pharmacokinetics. Receptor quantity, affinity, and type, as well as availability of natural ligands, also undergo developmental changes, affecting the pharmacodynamics of certain drugs such as benzodiazepines.

References

1. Chadwick J, Mann WN. *The Medical Works of Hippocrates: a New Translation from the Original Greek Made Especially for English Readers.* Oxford: Blackwell Scientific Publications, 1950: 153.

2. Betts EK, Downes JJ. Anesthetic considerations in newborn surgery. *Seminars in Anesthesiology* 1984; **3**: 59–74.

3. Davidson A, Soriano S. Does anaesthesia harm the developing brain: evidence or speculation? *Paediatr Anaesth* 2004; **14**: 199–200.

4. Walker SM. Pain in children: recent advances and ongoing challenges. *Br J Anaesth* 2008; **101**: 101–10.

5. Anand KJ, Sippell WG, Aynsley-Green A. Randomised trial of fentanyl anaesthesia in preterm babies undergoing surgery: effects on the stress response. *Lancet* 1987; **1**: 62–6.

6. Wolf AR. Pacifiers, passive behaviour and pain. *Lancet* 1992; **339**: 275–6.

7. Anand KJ, Hansen DD, Hickey PR. Hormonal-metabolic stress responses in neonates undergoing cardiac surgery. *Anesthesiology* 1990; **73**: 661–70.

8. Anderson BJ, van Lingen RA, Hansen TG, Lin YC, Holford NH. Acetaminophen developmental pharmacokinetics in premature neonates and infants: a pooled population analysis. *Anesthesiology* 2002; **96**: 1336–45.

9. Carlos MA, Babyn PS, Marcon MA, Moore AM. Changes in gastric emptying in early postnatal life. *J Pediatr* 1997; **130**: 931–7.

10. Agunod M, Yamaguchi N, Lopez R, Luhby AL, Glass GB. Correlative study of hydrochloric acid, pepsin, and intrinsic factor secretion in newborns and infants. *Am J Dig Dis* 1969; **14**: 400–14.

11. Huang NN, High RH. Comparison of serum levels following the administration of oral and parenteral preparations of penicillin to infants and children of various age groups. *J Pediatr* 1953; **42**: 657–8.

12. Taddio A, Shennan AT, Stevens B, Leeder JS, Koren G. Safety of lidocaine-prilocaine cream in the treatment of preterm neonates. *J Pediatr* 1995; **127**: 1002–5.

13. Taddio A, Stevens B, Craig K, *et al.* Efficacy and safety of lidocaine-prilocaine cream for pain during circumcision. *N Engl J Med* 1997; **336**: 1197–201.

14. Carry MR, Ringel SP, Starcevich JM. Distribution of capillaries in normal and diseased human skeletal muscle. *Muscle Nerve* 1986; **9**: 445–54.

15. Salanitre E, Rackow H. The pulmonary exchange of nitrous oxide and halothane in infants and children. *Anesthesiology* 1969; **30**: 388–94.

16. Lerman J. Pharmacology of inhalational anaesthetics in infants and children. *Paediatr Anaesth* 1992; **2**: 191–203.

17. Lerman J, Schmitt Bantel BI, *et al.* Effect of age on the solubility of volatile anesthetics in human tissues. *Anesthesiology* 1986; **65**: 307–11.

18. Malviya S, Lerman J. The blood/gas solubilities of sevoflurane, isoflurane, halothane, and serum constituent concentrations in neonates and adults. *Anesthesiology* 1990; **72**: 793–6.

19. Friis-Hansen B. Body water compartments in children: changes during growth and related changes in body composition. *Pediatrics* 1961; **28**: 169–81.

20. Anderson BJ, McKee AD, Holford NH. Size, myths and the clinical pharmacokinetics of analgesia in paediatric patients. *Clin Pharmacokinet* 1997; **33**: 313–27.

21. Luz G, Innerhofer P, Bachmann B, *et al.* Bupivacaine plasma concentrations during continuous epidural anesthesia in infants and children. *Anesth Analg* 1996; **82**: 231–4.

22. Booker PD, Taylor C, Saba G. Perioperative changes in alpha 1-acid glycoprotein concentrations in infants undergoing major surgery. *Br J Anaesth* 1996; **76**: 365–8.

23. Kearns GL, Reed MD. Clinical pharmacokinetics in infants and children: a reappraisal. *Clin Pharmacokinet* 1989; **17**: 29–67.

24. Tsai CE, Daood MJ, Lane RH, *et al.* P-glycoprotein expression in mouse brain increases with maturation. *Biol Neonate* 2002; **81**: 58–64.

25. Painter MJ, Pippenger C, Wasterlain C, *et al.* Phenobarbital and phenytoin in neonatal seizures: metabolism and tissue distribution. *Neurology* 1981; **31**: 1107–12.

26. Park MK, Ludden T, Arom KV, Rogers J, Oswalt JD. Myocardial vs serum digoxin concentrations in infants and adults. *Am J Dis Child* 1982; **136**: 418–20.

27. Gorodischer R, Jusko WJ, Yaffe SJ. Tissue and erythrocyte distribution of digoxin in infants. *Clin Pharmacol Ther* 1976; **19**: 256–63.

28. Way WL, Costley EC, Way EL. Respiratory sensitivity of the newborn infant to meperidine and morphine. *Clin Pharmacol Ther* 1965; **6**: 454–61.

29. Hertzka RE, Gauntlett IS, Fisher DM, Spellman MJ. Fentanyl-induced ventilatory depression: effects of age. *Anesthesiology* 1989; **70**: 213–18.

30. Bouwmeester NJ, Anderson BJ, Tibboel D, Holford NH. Developmental pharmacokinetics of morphine and its metabolites in neonates, infants and young children. *Br J Anaesth* 2004; **92**: 208–17.

31. Lynn AM, Nespeca MK, Opheim KE, Slattery JT. Respiratory effects of intravenous morphine infusions in neonates, infants, and children after cardiac surgery. *Anesth Analg* 1993; **77**: 695–701.

32. Pariente-Khayat A, Rey E, Gendrel D, *et al.* Isoniazid acetylation metabolic ratio during maturation in children. *Clin Pharmacol Ther* 1997; **62**: 377–83.

33. Sweeney BP, Bromilow J. Liver enzyme induction and inhibition: implications for anaesthesia. *Anaesthesia* 2006; **61**: 159–77.

34. Hines RN, McCarver DG. The ontogeny of human drug-metabolizing enzymes: phase I oxidative enzymes. *J Pharmacol Exp Ther* 2002; **300**: 355–60.

35. Koukouritaki SB, Manro JR, Marsh SA, *et al.* Developmental expression of human hepatic CYP2C9 and CYP2C19. *J Pharmacol Exp Ther* 2004; **308**: 965–74.

36. Berde C. Convulsions associated with pediatric regional anesthesia. *Anesth Analg* 1992; **75**: 164–6.

37. Palmer GM, Atkins M, Anderson BJ, *et al.* I.V. acetaminophen pharmacokinetics in neonates after multiple doses. *Br J Anaesth* 2008; **101**: 523–30.

38. de Wildt SN, Kearns GL, Leeder JS, van den Anker JN. Glucuronidation in humans. Pharmacogenetic and developmental aspects. *Clin Pharmacokinet* 1999; **36**: 439–52.

39. Pacifici GM, Sawe J, Kager L, Rane A. Morphine glucuronidation in human fetal and adult liver. *Eur J Clin Pharmacol* 1982; **22**: 553–8.

40. Anand KJ, Anderson BJ, Holford NH, *et al.* Morphine pharmacokinetics and pharmacodynamics in preterm and term neonates: secondary results from the NEOPAIN trial. *Br J Anaesth* 2008; **101**: 680–9.

41. Potts AL, Warman GR, Anderson BJ. Dexmedetomidine disposition in children: a population analysis. *Paediatr Anaesth* 2008; **18**: 722–30.

42. Rhodin MM, Anderson BJ, Peters AM, *et al.* Human renal function maturation: a quantitative description using weight and postmenstrual age. *Pediatr Nephrol* 2009; **24**: 67–76.

43. Alam SN, Roberts RJ, Fischer LJ. Age-related differences in salicylamide and acetaminophen conjugation in man. *J Pediatr* 1977; **90**: 130–5.

44. Arant BS. Developmental patterns of renal functional maturation compared in the human neonate. *J Pediatr* 1978; **92**: 705–12.

45. Langhendries JP, Battisti O, Bertrand JM, *et al.* Adaptation in neonatology of the once-daily concept of aminoglycoside administration: evaluation of a dosing chart for amikacin in an intensive care unit. *Biol Neonate* 1998; **74**: 351–62.

46. Besunder JB, Reed MD, Blumer JL. Principles of drug biodisposition in the

neonate. A critical evaluation of the pharmacokinetic-pharmacodynamic interface (Part I). *Clin Pharmacokinet* 1988; **14**: 189–216.

47. Anderson BJ, Pons G, Autret Leca E, Allegaert K, Boccard E. Pediatric intravenous paracetamol (propacetamol) pharmacokinetics: a population analysis. *Paediatr Anaesth* 2005; **15**: 282–92.

48. Zsigmond EK, Downs JR. Plasma cholinesterase activity in newborns and infants. *Can Anaesth Soc J* 1971; **18**: 278–85.

49. Freye E. Development of sensory information processing: the ontogenesis of opioid binding sites in nociceptive afferents and their significance in the clinical setting. *Acta Anaesthesiol Scand Suppl* 1996; **109**: 98–101.

50. Fisher DM, O'Keeffe C, Stanski DR, *et al.* Pharmacokinetics and pharmacodynamics of D-tubocurarine in infants, children, and adults. *Anesthesiology* 1982; **57**: 203–8.

51. Meakin G, Morton RH, Wareham AC. Age-dependent variation in response to tubocurarine in the isolated rat diaphragm. *Br J Anaesth* 1992; **68**: 161–3.

52. Franks NP, Lieb WR. Molecular and cellular mechanisms of general anaesthesia. *Nature* 1994; **367**: 607–14.

53. Brooks-Kayal AR, Pritchett DB. Developmental changes in human gamma-aminobutyric acid$_A$ receptor subunit composition. *Ann Neurol* 1993; **34**: 687–93.

54. Chugani DC, Muzik O, Juhasz C, *et al.* Postnatal maturation of human GABA$_A$ receptors measured with positron emission tomography. *Ann Neurol* 2001; **49**: 618–26.

55. LeDez KM, Lerman J. The minimum alveolar concentration (MAC) of isoflurane in preterm neonates. *Anesthesiology* 1987; **67**: 301–7.

56. Marshall J, Rodarte A, Blumer J, *et al.* Pediatric pharmacodynamics of midazolam oral syrup. Pediatric Pharmacology Research Unit Network. *J Clin Pharmacol* 2000; **40**: 578–89.

57. Takahashi H, Ishikawa S, Nomoto S, *et al.* Developmental changes in pharmacokinetics and pharmacodynamics of warfarin enantiomers in Japanese children. *Clin Pharmacol Ther* 2000; **68**: 541–55.

58. Marshall JD, Kearns GL. Developmental pharmacodynamics of cyclosporine. *Clin Pharmacol Ther* 1999; **66**: 66–75.

59. Williams DG, Hatch DJ, Howard RF. Codeine phosphate in paediatric medicine. *Br J Anaesth* 2001; **86**: 413–21.

60. Allegaert K, van den Anker JN, de Hoon JN, *et al.* Covariates of tramadol disposition in the first months of life. *Br J Anaesth* 2008; **100**: 525–32.

61. Anderson BJ, Meakin GH. Scaling for size: some implications for paediatric anaesthesia dosing. *Paediatr Anaesth* 2002; **12**: 205–19.

62. Holford NHG. A size standard for pharmacokinetics. *Clin Pharmacokinet* 1996; **30**: 329–32.

63. West GB, Brown JH, Enquist BJ. A general model for the origin of allometric scaling laws in biology. *Science* 1997; **276**: 122–6.

64. Anderson BJ, Holford NH. Mechanism-based concepts of size and maturity in pharmacokinetics. *Annu Rev Pharmacol Toxicol* 2008; **48**: 303–32.

65. Tod M, Jullien V, Pons G. Facilitation of drug evaluation in children by population methods and modelling. *Clin Pharmacokinet* 2008; **47**: 231–43.

Clinical applications: evidence-based anesthesia practice

Geriatric pharmacology

Jeffrey H. Silverstein

Introduction

Experience anesthetizing increasingly large numbers of elderly patients provides the impetus to focus on pharmacogeriatrics in anesthesiology [1,2]. Although elderly patients (65 years and older) are underrepresented in the pharmacology literature relative to other distinct population groups, anesthesiologists have accumulated significant evidence that allows adjustment of drug selection and dosing to achieve quality anesthesia, rapid emergence, and minimal side effects for the elderly. In the absence of specific information, it is generally prudent to "start low and go slow" when administering drugs to aged patients, as the elderly normally require less. However, understanding the mechanisms can help the practitioner adjust to individual patients. This chapter presents general pharmacology associated with aging as a foundation for a discussion of the most commonly used anesthetic drugs and the knowledge available to guide expert practice in caring for the elderly.

Aging has been described as a progressive loss of those physiologic processes necessary to maintain homeostasis (homeostenosis), death being the ultimate failure of these mechanisms. Aging might also be characterized as the composite of all changes that occur in an organism with the passage of time. A balance in favor of longevity over senescence (the progressive loss of physiological functions with aging) defines successful aging [3]. While it may be intellectually useful to define aging as a discrete phenomenon, it is becoming increasingly clear that there are important interactions between age-related changes and specifically identifiable disease processes [4]. Chronological age is a modifier of almost all disease processes. Clinicians use chronological age as a starting point, then evaluate disease, to understand whether the patient is aging successfully or not.

General geriatric pharmacokinetics and pharmacodynamics

Anesthesiologists use drugs with such immediate effects that drug interactions are observed and managed in real time, requiring both knowledge and facileness. From a practical perspective, the phenomena of adverse drug reactions and interactions are substantially magnified in patients of advanced age. The multiple drugs that are consumed by the elderly may also influence anesthetic drugs, but this extremely deep and varied body of knowledge is beyond the scope of this chapter.

Absorption

Passive gastric absorption is not markedly altered in the elderly. Drugs that inhibit intestinal motility have a greater effect than age. The importance of age in transdermal absorption is not completely resolved. Due to erratic absorption and a tendency to develop sterile infiltrates, intramuscular and subcutaneous injection are generally not recommended for elderly patients [5].

Body composition

Total body water is considered decreased by 10–15% in the elderly [6]. These data are old, however, and there is insufficient current information on measured total and extracellular water volumes, particularly with changing weight patterns and obesity-related alterations in total body and extracellular water [7]. Elderly patients may be dehydrated due to decreased thirst [6].

Most drugs used by anesthesiologists are described by multicompartment kinetic models. A decrease in total body water, in combination with changes in the distribution of cardiac output, results in a decreased central-compartment volume in elderly patients [8]. Initial plasma concentrations following rapid intravenous administration may be increased because of the decreased size of the central compartment, yet the steady-state distribution volume may be larger due to increased body fat. Body fat increases and muscle mass decreases in the elderly, by 20–40%, so lipophilic drugs will have a large volume of distribution [6]. Even in the healthy and exercising elderly, muscle loss is noted. There is no general rule for estimating muscle mass in the elderly; physical examination remains the best method. Overmedication based on a failure to adjust for weight is a concern [9].

Changes in serum proteins include a small decrease in plasma albumin and a slight increase in α_1-acid glycoprotein (AAG) (which binds amine drugs) concentrations. While these

---

Anesthetic Pharmacology, 2nd edition, ed. Alex S. Evers, Mervyn Maze, Evan D. Kharasch. Published by Cambridge University Press. © Cambridge University Press 2011.

alterations can affect circulating free drug concentrations and therefore pharmacodynamics and elimination, in practice they do not appear to have an important impact on geriatric pharmacology [10]. Plasma protein levels have not been identified as a major concern in geriatric anesthetic pharmacology.

Metabolism: hepatic function

Hepatic blood flow declines by 20–53% in elderly subjects, while liver mass is reduced by 11–36%, the endoplasmic reticulum is diminished, the hepatic extracellular space is increased, and bile flow is decreased [1]. Phase I drug metabolism is catalyzed mainly by microsomal cytochrome P450 (CYP) enzymes and may be decreased in the elderly, even though CYP enzyme activity is relatively preserved. Phase II reactions comprise conjugations with endogenous compounds such as glucuronic acid, and appear to be unaltered in old age [1]. Hepatically eliminated drugs are frequently divided into those that are flow-limited versus those that are capacity (metabolism)-limited. In general, age reduces the clearance of flow-limited drugs by about 30–40%, similar to the decrease in hepatic blood flow, but there is no alteration for capacity-limited drugs.

Renal function

Glomerular filtration rate (GFR) is reported to decrease by 1 mL per year. In a large study, about 30% of participants had no change in GFR with aging, while others showed much greater decrements [11]. The principal formula used to estimate creatinine clearance, the Cockcroft–Gault equation, was derived from a retrospective cohort that included primarily elderly patients with renal dysfunction, and it is particularly inaccurate for elderly women. Overall, it appears that there is a small decrease in GFR with aging, but in the absence of disease it probably decreases less than previously thought. Aging per se appears not to diminish renal drug excretion significantly.

Cardiopulmonary function

In the absence of disease, cardiac output is generally maintained in the elderly. However, many patients have coexisting diseases and circulation times appear increased. Thus initial drug effect may be delayed. For this reason, to prevent relative overdose, and (as noted below) to mitigate the adverse cardiovascular impact of some induction drugs, slower bolus injection in the elderly is prudent.

Clinical pharmacology for geriatric anesthesia patients

This section reviews the impact of senescence on specific anesthetic drugs, with the goal of providing clinical guidance. In evaluating an elderly patient, interactions between polypharmacy and comorbidities are factored into assessing how altered pharmacodynamic sensitivity, and even modest changes in pharmacokinetics, will modify the anesthetic plan.

For more information on specific drugs, the reader is referred to more in-depth reviews.

Opioids

There is more information regarding the pharmacogeriatrics of opioids than most other drugs in anesthesiology. Opiates have been used since ancient times, yet μ-, δ-, and κ-opioid receptors were not identified until the early 1970s. Differences in activity and efficacy of the various opioids appear related to relative stimulation of the various opioid receptors as well as genetic differences in opioid receptor sensitivity. Work primarily in rodents indicates that brain opioid receptor density decreases with aging, but there is more variability noted in receptor affinity [12]. Opioid elimination occurs mainly by hepatic metabolism, with renal excretion of metabolites and of some parent drugs. Important factors that influence opioid metabolism are genetics, sex, age, and environmental factors including concurrent medications, diet, and disease. Metabolites of some opioids (codeine, morphine, meperidine) are pharmacologically active, accounting for both persistent analgesia and many side effects. Metabolite pharmacokinetics can be a major factor in opioid choices for the elderly.

The primary risk of opioids is respiratory depression, the incidence of which is markedly increased with age [13]. Interestingly, morphine was more problematic than meperidine, and there was almost no respiratory depression in patients receiving fentanyl (Fig. 70.1).

Fentanyl

Fentanyl is a highly selective μ-receptor agonist with few other significant effects, metabolized by CYP3A4 to inactive and nontoxic metabolites [14]. Early studies suggested that the terminal elimination half-life ($t_{1/2\beta}$) was prolonged in the elderly. As no change was found in volume of distribution

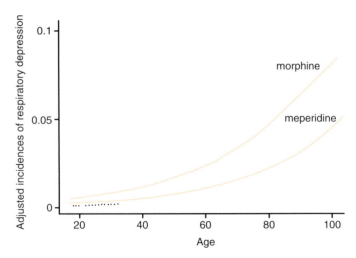

Figure 70.1. Adjusted incidences of respiratory depression by type of opioid and age. The graph illustrates how the incidence of respiratory depression increases with age for morphine and meperidine. The fentanyl group was not included in the adjusted analysis because of the small number of patients who had respiratory depression in this group. Reproduced with permission from Cepeda *et al.* [13].

(V_d) in the elderly, investigators concluded that clearance was therefore decreased, suggesting that fentanyl would last longer in the elderly [15]. Subsequent studies found minimal influence of aging on fentanyl pharmacokinetics, with the exception of a transient concentration increase following the start of drug infusion that was attributed to decreased rapid intercompartmental clearance [16].

Aging has a greater effect on fentanyl pharmacodynamics than pharmacokinetics. The EC_{50} for suppression of the electroencephalogram, used as a measure of fentanyl potency, was decreased approximately 50% from ages 20 to 85 [17]. Available evidence suggests that elderly patients are significantly more sensitive to fentanyl and therefore should receive reduced doses, but the offset of drug effect should be similar to younger patients.

Fentanyl is also available in a number of unique dosage forms including oral transmucosal, transdermal, and iontophoretic transdermal delivery systems. Oral transmucosal fentanyl citrate is a lozenge, marketed for control of breakthrough cancer pain. No change with aging was found in the pharmacokinetics of oral transmucosal fentanyl citrate, including absorption characteristics from the buccal mucosa; however, only healthy older patients were studied [18].

The fentanyl patch adheres to skin and releases drug from a reservoir through a copolymer membrane at a nearly constant amount per unit time. Fentanyl plasma concentrations depend on the rates of release and penetration through the skin layers. The mean half-time (time for plasma concentrations to double after patch application) was 4.2 hours in younger patients (25–38 years), compared with 11.1 hours in elderly patients (64–82 years) [19]. Mean maximum plasma concentrations were slightly but not statistically significantly higher in the younger patients (1.9 vs. 1.5 ng mL^{-1}) [19]. In contrast, a study using a 20 cm^2 fentanyl 24-hour transdermal patch in healthy elderly and young subjects found higher serum concentrations and, of note, had to remove the patch early from all the elderly patients [20]. As general evidence suggests that fentanyl clearance is not significantly altered by aging, it appears that alterations in the elderly integumentary system favor increased absorption of fentanyl over a longer period of time. Indeed, the time course of fentanyl absorption through the skin is delayed in the elderly, but subcutaneous fat acts as secondary reservoir, leading to prolonged release even after removal of the patch [21].

A novel parenteral delivery system for fentanyl is the iontophoretic transdermal system (ITS) [22]. This is a small patient-controlled analgesia (PCA) device incorporated into a credit-card size patch that is applied to a hairless skin area. An imperceptible current of 170 milliamperes actively delivers a fentanyl hydrochloride 40 μg dose into the vasculature over a 10-minute interval. The unit is programmed to lock out further doses after either 80 doses or 24 hours, whichever is reached first. A recent review of this device indicated that good analgesia was achieved and that age was not a major factor in the side-effect profile. A lower incidence of nausea, fever, and headache was observed in patients over 65 years of age [23].

Morphine

Morphine is metabolized by glucuronidation to morphine-3-glucuronide, which is essentially inactive, and to morphine-6-glucuronide (M6G). Although M6G passes the blood–brain barrier extremely slowly, it is an effective analgesic. M6G is currently under clinical investigation as a primary analgesic for moderate postoperative pain [24]. M6G is associated with a reduction in the severity of opioid side effects, such as reduced postoperative nausea and vomiting and reduced respiratory depression [25]. M6G is eliminated by the kidney. In general, the elderly have significantly decreased GFR, although there is tremendous variability in this process. In patients with elevated creatinine concentrations, there was accumulation of both morphine glucuronides [26].

Probably a more important and perhaps less well understood aspect of morphine pharmacology is that the peak effect occurs approximately 90 minutes after a bolus dose. This has been confirmed using numerous endpoints and is suggested to result from morphine interaction with the efflux transporter P-glycoprotein, which transports morphine out of the central nervous system (CNS) [27]. When onset time was not considered and morphine was administered in 2–3 mg doses every 5 minutes, elderly patients required similar quantities of morphine to younger patients [28]. The failure to wait for peak effect was considered to be responsible for this finding [27].

Meperidine

Meperidine is a relatively weak μ-agonist with only approximately 10% effectiveness of morphine. The half-life of meperidine is approximately 3 hours. It is metabolized in the liver to normeperidine, which has a half-life of 15–30 hours and causes agitation and seizures at high concentrations. Meperidine has a complex pharmacology that includes local anesthetic activity [29], negative inotropic effects [30], and intrinsic anticholinergic properties which can result in increased heart rate. Meperidine is associated with severe serotonergic reactions when combined with monoamine oxidase (MAO) A inhibitors. Renal excretion is reduced in elderly patients, particularly for normeperidine [31]. The result is that normeperidine will likely accumulate with repeated doses in elderly patients. Meperidine has been associated with development of postoperative delirium in elderly patients [32]. Aside from the treatment of postoperative shivering with single small doses, meperidine is not a good drug for use with the elderly.

Remifentanil

Remifentanil is an ultra-short-acting synthetic opioid. While most opioids are metabolized in the liver, remifentanil is an ester which undergoes rapid hydrolysis by nonspecific tissue and plasma esterases. Thus remifentanil accumulation does not occur, and its context-sensitive half-life remains at 4 minutes after a 4-hour infusion. Remifentanil has been extremely well evaluated in special populations, including the elderly.

Pharmacokinetic and pharmacodynamic models for remifentanil in the elderly have been well developed, and computer simulation used to model experimental data and the complex age-related changes on remifentanil pharmacology [33,34]. In an investigation of 62 individuals in three age groups, young (20–40 years), middle-aged (40–65 years), and elderly (> 65 years), the general findings were that the volume of the central compartment (V_1) decreased linearly by approximately 25% and clearance (CL_1) decreased 33%, respectively, from age 20 to 85 (Fig. 70.2A,B). The elderly were significantly more sensitive, using EEG suppression as an endpoint, with both the remifentanil EC_{50} and plasma/effect-site equilibration-rate constant (k_{e0}) decreased by approximately 50% over the age range studied (Fig. 70.2C,D). The slower $t_{1/2}k_{e0}$ in elderly subjects results in less rapid equilibration, but this is somewhat balanced by the higher blood concentrations found in elderly subjects because of the smaller central compartment. The onset and offset are slower in elderly individuals, although the blood concentrations are similar to younger patients. The peak drug effect is expected in about 90 seconds after a bolus injection in a young individual as opposed to 2–3 minutes in an elderly patient. Nomograms for calculating the bolus and infusion dose of remifentanil are presented as a function of age and lean body mass (Fig. 70.2E,F). Elderly subjects need about half of the bolus dose as younger subjects for the same drug effect. As with fentanyl and alfentanil, this is because of increased pharmacodynamic sensitivity in the elderly rather than pharmacokinetics. Elderly subjects require an infusion rate about one-third that of younger subjects, because of the combined impact of increased sensitivity and decreased clearance. The simulation also suggests that elderly patients can be expected to recover from remifentanil about as fast as younger subjects, provided the dose has been appropriately reduced.

Other opioids

There are no specific studies examining the pharmacokinetics and pharmacodynamics of methadone or hydropmorphone in elderly subjects. However, as the increased brain sensitivity to opioid drug effect appears to be a class effect for opioids, it seems prudent to reduce the doses of these drugs by about 50% in elderly patients. The balance of available information for both alfentanil and sufentanil suggests that the elderly are significantly more sensitive to both opioids but that there are only modest pharmacokinetic differences between young and old patients [35–38]. However, this statement is not made without controversy. A series of articles suggested that there is no difference in alfentanil sensitivity in the elderly but rather a major difference in protein binding, yet prolonged infusions of alfentanil required approximately a 50% reduction in dose. There was no influence of age on sufentanil requirements for mechanically ventilated patients in the intensive care unit [39]. The central-compartment volume of sufentanil was significantly decreased in elderly patients [36]. This would predict an increase in the effects of sufentanil in the first few minutes after a bolus dose, but not subsequently.

Opioid antagonists are employed with some frequency in the elderly. Naloxone has an elimination half-life of 1–1.5 hours. There are no reports of altered pharmacokinetics or pharmacodynamics for naloxone or naltrexone. The longer-acting opioid antagonist nalmefene was found to have a higher initial concentration, attributed to a smaller central compartment, but no differences were observed for elimination half-life [40].

Clinical summary

Opioid doses in the elderly should be reduced about 50%, primarily because they are more sensitive. Pharmacokinetic changes are important only when long-term infusions are contemplated. Meperidine should probably not be used in the elderly except in small doses for shivering. The dose of naloxone is not significantly altered in aging.

Sedative-hypnotics

Sedative-hypnotics are drugs whose primary effect is CNS depression. Most are thought to work primarily through the γ-aminobutyric acid A ($GABA_A$) receptors in the CNS, although some have specific action upon excitatory amino acid receptors as well. $GABA_A$ receptor systems have been well characterized, but there is not much information on alterations associated with aging.

Propofol

Aging effects on propofol pharmacology have been well characterized. Propofol pharmacodynamics are significantly altered with aging [41]. EC50 values for loss of consciousness were 2.35, 1.8, and 1.25 $\mu g\ mL^{-1}$ in healthy volunteers who were 25, 50, and 75 years old, respectively, i.e., nearly a 50% decrease (Fig. 70.3) Age-related changes were found for both induction doses and infusions. Using a fixed dose of propofol, patients older than 70 years reached significantly deeper EEG stages than younger patients, needed a longer time to reach the deepest EEG stage, and needed more time until a lighter EEG stage was regained [42]. A particularly important finding in this study was that the baseline EEG characteristics of elderly patients were changed, so the total power, mainly in deep EEG stages, was significantly smaller due to a distinctly smaller absolute power of the delta frequency band. Older patients needed less propofol for steady-state maintenance of a defined stage of hypnosis than younger patients. Propofol doses used to achieve a specific EEG endpoint were found to decrease significantly with age, from 5.9 ± 1.7 mg $kg^{-1}\ h^{-1}$ for 31- to 50-year-old patients to 3.5 ± 1.4 mg $kg^{-1}\ h^{-1}$ for those older than 70 [43].

Evaluation of propofol pharmacokinetics in the elderly suggests that both clearance and volume of the central compartment decrease with age. Elimination clearance decreases linearly after age 60 [44]. When the pharmacokinetic and pharmacodynamic changes are considered together, current

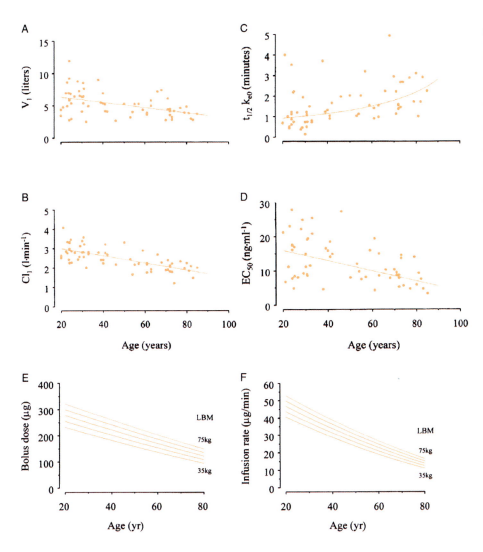

Figure 70.2. (A, B) Individual Bayesian estimates of V_1 and CL_1 for remifentanil as a function of age (dots). The linear relationship between age, V_1, and CL_1 (lines) is estimated by linear regression. (C, D) Individual Bayesian estimates of k_{e0} and EC_{50} (dots) for remifentanil. The relationship between age, k_{e0}, and EC_{50} (lines) is estimated by NONMEM for the complex pharmacodynamic model. The relation between k_{e0} and age has been transformed to show the increase in equilibration half-life ($t_{1/2}$ k_{e0}) [34]. (E, F) Nomogram for calculating the intravenous bolus dose (upper) and intravenous infusion rate (lower) required to cause 50% of the maximum electroencephalographic effect as a function of age and lean body mass (LBM) [33].

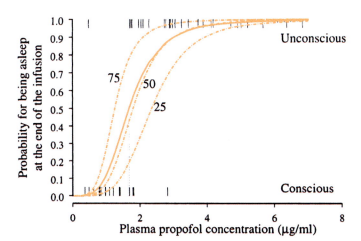

Figure 70.3. Influence of age on propofol pharmacodynamics. The solid line represents a logistic regression fit through all the data with the age-independent model. The dotted lines are the logistic regression fits predicted by the age-adjusted regression model for 25-, 50-, and 75-year-old participants. Reproduced with permission from Schnider *et al.* [41].

literature suggests a 20% reduction in the induction dose of propofol, if given as a bolus (1.5–1.8 mg kg^{-1}) [45]. Doses as low as 0.8–1.2 mg kg^{-1} in the elderly may be appropriate [46,47]. Because initial effect-site concentrations are not affected by elimination, but elimination declines in the elderly, propofol pharmacokinetics in the elderly become progressively more significant after about 1 hour (Fig. 70.4A) [44]. Propofol infusion rates to achieve a persistent level of moderate sedation are lower in the elderly (Fig. 70.4B). Recent data indicate that propofol clearance is considerably more altered by age in females than in males [48]. Based on these data, a pharmacokinetic model for target-controlled infusion systems was proposed that employs both sex and age as major covariates. Of particular note is that outliers both above and below the norms were found in both young and old patients, indicating that alterations in clearance are not only a phenomenon of the elderly.

Age has no effect on the rate of Bispectral Index reduction with increasing propofol concentration, whereas with increasing age systolic blood pressure decreases to a greater degree but more slowly [46]. This greater hemodynamic effect of

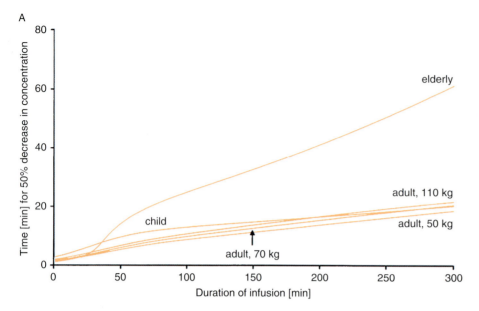

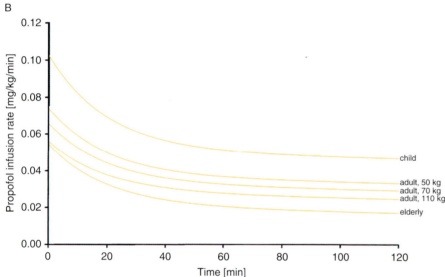

Figure 70.4. Influence of age on propofol pharmacokinetics and dose requirements. (A) Propofol infusion rates required to maintain a concentration of 1 μg mL^{-1} in a child (20 kg body weight, 5 years of age), a lean adult (50 kg, 30 years), an adult of average weight (70 kg, 70 years), an obese adult (110 kg, 30 years), and an elderly individual (65 kg, 80 years). (B) Time required for a 50% decrease in concentration after continuous infusion of variable length (context-sensitive half-time). Simulations were performed for a child, a lean adult, an adult of average weight, an obese adult, and an elderly individual (as in A), based on the final model parameters. Reproduced with permission from Schüttler and Ihmsen [44].

propofol in the elderly can be minimized by infusing a bolus over a longer period of time.

Thiopental

Although both are GABAergic agonists, and propofol and thiopental produce similar effects, they affect different regions of the brain [49]. There are no age-related changes in thiopental brain responsiveness or pharmacodynamics [50]. Nevertheless, thiopental doses do need to be decreased in the elderly because of a reduction in the central volume of distribution [51]. The optimal dose in an 80-year-old patient was suggested to be 2.1 mg kg^{-1}, or 80% of the dose needed for a young adult [45]. Awakening after a bolus dose of thiopental may be delayed in older relative to young patients, mainly because of a decreased central volume of distribution [50]. Except in disease states, however, thiopental clearance is not reduced in

the elderly, and awakening should therefore only be prolonged in the elderly after a bolus and not after a constant infusion. As with propofol, slower administration of a bolus induction dose will generally result in less acute hemodynamic alterations.

Midazolam

There is no decrease in the affinity or density of CNS benzodiazepine receptors with age in rats [52]. However, benzodiazepine binding in both young and old rats was enhanced by chronic, but not acute, stress, and recovery following cessation of stress was delayed in older animals [53]. To the extent that age does alter benzodiazepine binding, it is a modifier of chronic stress.

In humans, midazolam has been found to have significantly different kinetics in elderly patients [54]. Clearance is reduced in the elderly by as much as 30% from that of a young

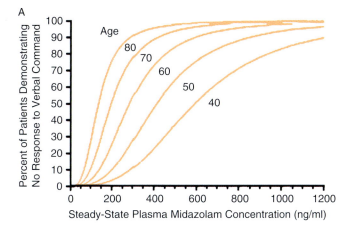

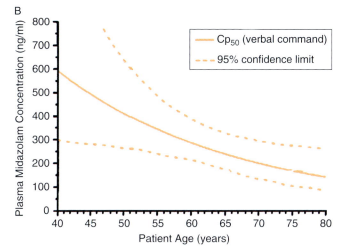

Figure 70.5. Influence of age on midazolam pharmacodynamics. (A) Simulated quantal concentration–response curves generated by a parameterized pharmacodynamic model for midazolam. (B) Midazolam Cp50 (EC50) for response to verbal command as a function of age. Confidence limits are included to indicate the effect of the net uncertainty in the mean model parameters estimates on the Cp50 calculation. The increasing width of the confidence limits on the calculated Cp50 values associated with patient age less than approximately 55 years is presumed to be due to the relatively small number of subjects studied. Reproduced with permission from Jacobs *et al.* [56].

adult due to a loss of functional hepatic tissue and a decrease in hepatic perfusion. Midazolam undergoes significant metabolism, primarily to hydroxymidazolam, which is pharmacologically active, renally excreted, and may accumulate in patients with diminished renal function. A particularly poignant example of how long a benzodiazepine can last was provided in a recent case report of a patient misdiagnosed as suffering from anoxic encephalopathy when the primary problem was drug-induced delirium and coma [55]. Elderly patients are significantly more sensitive to midazolam than younger patients, primarily because of a pharmacodynamic difference (Fig. 70.5) [56]. A 75% reduction in dose from the 20-year-old to the 90-year-old has been recommended [45].

Paradoxical reactions to midazolam occur in which patients become agitated rather than sedated. Flumazenil may reverse

these episodes [57]. There is a general sense that midazolam sedation is associated with the production of confusion, but a recent double-blind placebo-controlled study of 65 patients undergoing upper gastrointestinal endoscopy suggested that midazolam was a good sedative for this procedure in the elderly [58].

Etomidate

Etomidate is a carboxylated imidazole derivative with anesthetic and amnestic, but not analgesic properties, which is frequently considered an ideal drug in the elderly because it is associated with less hemodynamic instability than propofol or thiopental. A smaller initial volume of distribution and reduced clearance in the elderly was reported, as well as a significant increase in pharmacodynamic sensitivity, which together mean that the elderly may only require 0.2 mg kg^{-1} (compared with 0.3–0.4 mg kg^{-1} for young adults) [59].

Clinical summary

The dose of induction drugs should be significantly decreased in the elderly, and the induction dose should be infused more slowly to minimize hemodynamic consequences. Propofol appears to have both pharmacokinetic and pharmacodynamic differences between the young and old, while the primary alterations for thiopental are pharmacokinetic. Elderly patients can be very sensitive to midazolam and may have paradoxical reactions.

Neuromuscular blocking drugs

The neuromuscular blocking drugs inhibit transmission at the neuromuscular junction, resulting in paralysis of the affected skeletal muscles. While there are drugs that act presynaptically via the inhibition of acetylcholine synthesis or release (botulinum toxin and tetrodotoxin), all the drugs of interest to anesthesiologists exert their effect postsynaptically. A number of factors associated with senescence may influence the pharmacology of neuromuscular blocking drugs in the elderly. On average, there is a 25–35% decrease in muscle mass. Beyond the average muscle loss, some elderly patients have significant muscle loss and weakness, resulting in a state defined as frail [60]. Aging is associated with structural changes at the neuromuscular junction [61]. One of the intriguing alterations is the presence of extrajunctional acetylcholine receptors in elderly muscle, although these have no known impact on neuromuscular function [62].

Interestingly, the alterations described above do not significantly alter the pharmacodynamics of neuromuscular blocking drugs. Studies of the relationship between the depth of neuromuscular blockade and plasma drug concentration show little if any difference with age. The ED95 for neuromuscular blockade is essentially the same for young and old patients for all currently used neuromuscular blockers [63].

In contrast, the pharmacokinetics of muscle relaxants are significantly altered with age. The onset of neuromuscular

Table 70.1. Neuromuscular blocking drugs: time to onset of maximal block in young adult and elderly patients

Neuromuscular blocking drug	Dose (mg kg^{-1})	Onset (minutes)		Difference (seconds)
		Young adult patients	*Elderly patients*	
Succinylcholine	1	1.2 [0.1]	1.6 [0.1]	24
Mivacurium	0.15	2.1 (0.8)	2.0 (0.5)	−3
Vecuronium	0.1	3.7 [0.2]	4.9 [0.5]	73
	0.1	2.6 (0.7) *	3.5 (1.1)	57
Rocuronium	0.6	4.1 (1.5)	4.5 (2.4)	24
	1	1.0 (0.2) *	1.3 (0.4)	17
Cisatracurium	0.1	3.0 *	4.0	60
	0.1	2.5 (0.6) *	3.4 (1.0)	54
Pipecuronium	0.07	4.5 (1.5) *	6.9 (2.6)	144
Doxacurium	0.025	7.7 (1.0) *	11.2 (1.1)	210

Data are mean (SD) or [SEM]
*Statistically significant difference when compared to elderly patients
Modified with permission from Lien and Suzuki [64].

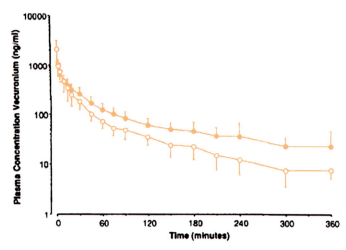

Figure 70.6. Plasma concentration versus time course in elderly (●) and in younger (O) patients after a single intravenous dose (0.1 mg kg^{-1}) of vecuronium. Values are mean ± SD; $n = 8$ in each group. Reproduced with permission from Lien *et al.* [66].

block is dependent on a number of factors, including muscle mass and cardiac output, that may be altered in elderly patients. Experimentally, investigators report that onset of maximal block is delayed to various degrees in the elderly (Table 70.1) The majority of neuromuscular blockers are metabolized or eliminated by hepatic and/or renal mechanisms which are, as noted above, altered in the elderly, and there are age-related alterations in neuromuscular blocker elimination kinetics. For long-acting relaxants (e.g., pancuronium), elimination is primarily renal and the prolonged clearance is consistent with reported decreases in renal function with age [65]. The intermediate-acting relaxants either rely to a greater degree on hepatic metabolism (vecuronium and rocuronium) or via Hofmann elimination (atracurium). Hepatically metabolized drugs (vecuronium and rocuronium) manifest prolonged recovery (Fig. 70.6). For example, spontaneous recovery from vecuronium was longer (50% recovery time 97 ± 29 vs. 40 ± 14 min), the elimination half-life was prolonged (125 ± 55 vs. 78 ± 21 min), and plasma clearance was reduced (2.6 ± 0.6 vs. 5.6 ± 3.2 mL kg^{-1} min^{-1}) in elderly compared with younger patients. Although not completely universal, this type of result has been reported for most neuromuscular blocking drugs (Table 70.1) There are minor differences between elderly and young patients in the pharmacokinetics of atracurium and cisatracurium. Onset time is similarly prolonged, but the recovery profile after a single bolus dose is not significantly changed in elderly patients [67].

Anticholinesterase drugs

The anticholinesterase drugs are used primarily to counteract the effects of neuromuscular blocking drugs. The clearance of anticholinesterases may be prolonged in the elderly, but this is actually beneficial, given their clinical application. The dose of edrophonium in the elderly does not have to be adjusted to obtain the same degree of recovery as younger adults [68–70]. The geropharmacology of neostigmine is less clear. Several studies indicate no significant difference in the dose of neostigmine necessary to reverse a doxacurium-induced block [71], but there is a report that more neostigmine was needed to reverse vecuronium in an elderly population [72]. The duration of action of neostigmine and pyridostigmine is prolonged in the aged patient [73]. Geriatric patients appear more susceptible to cardiac arrhythmias associated with the reversal of neuromuscular blockade [74,75].

Clinical summary

The doses of neuromuscular blockers are not altered in the elderly, but the clinician must wait slightly longer for the full effect. The dose of anticholinesterase reversal drugs is not altered by aging.

Volatile anesthetics

Despite 150 years of use and extensive research, a comprehensive description of the mechanism of action of volatile anesthetics remains elusive. It has been suggested that development of anesthetics with faster kinetics, better molecular stability, and less flammability may have resulted in drugs with less molecular specificity [76]. Excellent reviews on target molecules for volatile anesthetics are available [77,78].

The principal physiologic mechanisms involved in the uptake and distribution of volatile anesthetics are minute ventilation and cardiac output. These, along with the blood/gas partition coefficient of the drug, determine the rate of equilibration between the alveolar partial pressure and the inspired anesthetic partial pressure. Senescence is associated with major changes in both cardiovascular and pulmonary function; however, in healthy elderly patients, baseline cardiac output is maintained. Minute ventilation is typically controlled during anesthesia. So while it has been known since early in anesthetic practice that age decreases the dose (concentration) of volatile anesthetics, this is thought to be exclusively pharmacodynamic. Furthermore, there are essentially no publications suggesting significant pharmacokinetic alterations in volatile anesthetics for elderly patients.

The minimum alveolar concentration (MAC) is the alveolar concentration of inhaled anesthetic that prevents movement in half of subjects in response to a surgical incision, and is the inhalational equivalent of a median effective dose (ED50). If the stimulus or response is changed, the MAC will be appropriately altered, with more intense stimuli requiring more anesthetic while less intense stimuli/responses (e.g. response to verbal command, as in MAC-awake) have much lower levels of MAC. Age is a major modifier of anesthetic action. Two retrospective analyses found a MAC reduction of approximately 6% per decade of life (after 1 year of age) [79], which was also seen for MAC-awake [80]. This was consistent across halothane, enflurane, isoflurane, sevoflurane, desflurane, and nitrous oxide. MAC as a fraction of MAC at age 40 for halothane, isoflurane, sevoflurane, and desflurane, was calculated to be $1.32 \times 10^{-0.00303 \cdot age}$ (Fig. 70.7). This formula suggests that, on average, volatile anesthetic MAC decreases 6.7% per decade. MAC for nitrous oxide decreases about 7.7% per year [73]. MAC-awake decreased with age proportionate to MAC. For desflurane, isoflurane, and sevoflurane, MAC-awake/MAC is 0.343 ± 0.017, or about one-third of normal MAC [80]. A more complicated single nomogram is available to determine MAC alterations in aging for multiple drugs [81]. Age is now factored into the MAC equivalents displayed by some sophisticated gas monitors.

There are few studies of the impact of volatile anesthetics on physiologic functions of the elderly. The clinical impression is that in appropriate doses, the impact of volatile anesthetics is qualitatively similar in elderly and younger patients. This perception is supported by a study of 30 patients aged 70 and older, which used the formation of the lidocaine metabolite monoethylglycinexylidide (MEGX), cytosolic liver enzyme α-glutathione-S-transferase (α-GST), and gastric mucosal tonometry as sensitive markers of hepatic function and splanchnic perfusion [82]. Overall hepatocyte function was well preserved in these elderly patients during desflurane and sevoflurane anesthesia, as determined by the MEGX formation test. There was a mild disturbance of hepatocellular integrity, indicated by a transient increase of α-GST levels, and brief changes of gastric tonometry variables, which were interpreted as a reduction in splanchnic perfusion. There was no difference between the two anesthetics.

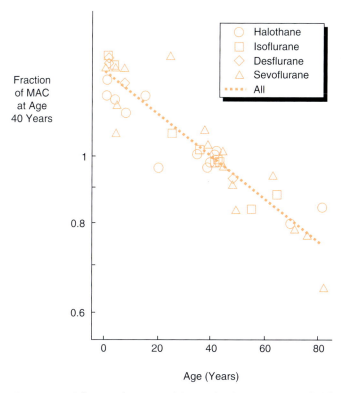

Figure 70.7. Influence of age on minimum alveolar concentration (MAC). MAC values are expressed as a fraction of the value at age 40. Least squares regression provided an estimate of MAC as a function of age: MAC as a fraction of MAC at age 40 = $1.32 \times 10^{-0.00303 \cdot age}$ ($r^2 = 0.85$). MAC decreased by 6.7% per decade. Reproduced with permission from Eger [80].

Clinical summary

MAC is significantly reduced for all volatile anesthetics. Monk *et al.* reported that cumulative deep hypnotic time and intraoperative hypotension were significant independent predictors of increased mortality [83]. This highly disputed result has become part of an evolving exploration of cognitive problems following surgery and anesthesia and concerns about the toxicity of anesthetics, both volatile and intravenous. At the moment, there is no compelling evidence to avoid volatile anesthetics in elderly patients.

Summary

An understanding of the mechanisms of aging, and of the general pharmacology associated with aging, can help to guide expert practice in caring for the elderly. Changes of particular concern to the anesthesiologist include alterations in absorption, body composition, metabolism, and hepatic, renal, and cardiovascular function. Intramuscular and subcutaneous injection are generally not recommended for elderly patients, given erratic absorption and a tendency to develop sterile infiltrates. In the absence of disease, cardiac output is generally maintained in the elderly. However, many patients have coexisting diseases, and circulation times appear increased, so that initial drug effect may be delayed. It is therefore prudent to employ slower bolus injection in the elderly. Increases in body fat and decreases in muscle mass also mean that lipophilic drugs will have a large volume of distribution. Furthermore, a decrease in total body water, in combination with changes in the distribution of cardiac output, results in a decreased central-compartment volume. For hepatically eliminated drugs, age tends to reduce the clearance of those that are flow-limited, but there is no alteration for capacity-limited drugs. Aging per se appears not to diminish renal drug excretion significantly. Changes in serum proteins do not appear to have an important impact on geriatric anesthetic pharmacology.

Major changes in pharmacology are best appreciated by drug class. Opioid doses in the elderly should be reduced about 50%. Pharmacokinetic changes are important only when long-term infusions are contemplated. Meperidine should probably not be used in the elderly except in small doses for shivering. The dose of naloxone is not significantly altered in aging. The primary risk of opioids is respiratory depression, and the incidence of this is markedly increased with age.

The dose of sedative-hypnotic induction drugs should be significantly decreased in the elderly, and the induction dose should be infused more slowly to minimize hemodynamic consequences. Propofol appears to have both pharmacokinetic and pharmacodynamic differences between the young and old, while the primary alterations for thiopental are pharmacokinetic. Elderly patients can be very sensitive to midazolam and may have paradoxical reactions.

Doses of neuromuscular blockers do not need to be altered in the elderly, but the clinician must wait slightly longer for the full effect. Aging does not alter the dose of anticholinesterase reversal drugs, although geriatric patients appear more susceptible to cardiac arrhythmias associated with the reversal of neuromuscular blockade.

Volatile-anesthetic MAC is significantly reduced with aging for all anesthetics. The existence and occurrence of cognitive problems following surgery and anesthesia and concerns about the toxicity of anesthetics, both volatile and intravenous, is currently unresolved, as is any differential sensitivity of elderly patients. At the moment, there is no compelling evidence to avoid volatile anesthetics in elderly patients

Ever-increasing numbers of elderly patients mean that geriatrics should be at the forefront of future anesthesia research efforts.

References

1. McLean AJ, Le Couteur DG. Aging biology and geriatric clinical pharmacology. *Pharmacol Rev* 2004; **56**: 163–84.

2. Silverstein JH. The practice of geriatric anesthesia. In: Silverstein JH, Rooke GA, Reeves JG, McLeskey CH, eds., *Geriatric Anesthesiology*, 2nd edn. New York, NY: Springer, 2008: 3–14.

3. Rowe JW, Kahn RL. Successful aging. *Gerontologist* 1997; **37**: 433–40.

4. Lakatta EG, Levy D. Arterial and cardiac aging: major shareholders in cardiovascular disease enterprises: Part II: the aging heart in health: links to heart disease. *Circulation* 2003; **107**: 346–54.

5. Turnheim K. Pharmacokinetic dosage guidelines for elderly subjects. *Expert Opin Drug Metab Toxicol* 2005; **1**: 33–48.

6. Beaufrere B, Morio B. Fat and protein redistribution with aging: metabolic considerations. *Eur J Clin Nutr* 2000; **54**: S48–53.

7. Chumlea WC, Schubert CM, Sun SS, *et al.* A review of body water status and the effects of age and body fatness in children and adults. *J Nutr Health Aging* 2007; **11**: 111–18.

8. Shafer SL. *Pharmacokinetics and pharmacodynamics of the elderly, Geriatric Anesthesiology*. McLeskey CH, ed. Baltimore, MD: Williams & Wilkins, 1997: 123–42.

9. Campion EW, Avorn J, Reder VA, Olins NJ. Overmedication of the low-weight elderly. *Arch Intern Med* 1987; **147**: 945–7.

10. Benet LZ, Hoener BA. Changes in plasma protein binding have little clinical relevance. *Clin Pharmacol Ther* 2002; **71**: 115–21.

11. Lindeman RD. Renal physiology and pathophysiology of aging. *Contrib Nephrol* 1993; **105**: 1–12.

12. Ueno E, Liu DD, Ho IK, Hoskins B. Opiate receptor characteristics in brains from young, mature and aged mice. *Neurobiol Aging* 1988; **9**: 279–83.

13. Cepeda MS, Farrar JT, Baumgarten M, *et al.* Side effects of opioids during short-term administration: effect of age, gender, and race. *Clin Pharmacol Ther* 2003; **74**: 102–12.

14. Feierman DE, Lasker JM. Metabolism of fentanyl, a synthetic opioid analgesic, by human liver microsomes. Role of CYP3A4. *Drug Metab Dispos* 1996; **24**: 932–9.

15. Bentley JB, Borel JD, Nenad RE, Gillespie TJ. Age and fentanyl pharmacokinetics. *Anesth Analg* 1982; **61**: 968–71.

16. Singleton MA, Rosen JI, Fisher DM. Pharmacokinetics of fentanyl in the elderly. *Br J Anaesth* 1988; **60**: 619–22.

17. Scott JC, Ponganis KV, Stanski DR. EEG quantitation of narcotic effect: the comparative pharmacodynamics of fentanyl and alfentanil. *Anesthesiology* 1985; **62**: 234–41.

18. Kharasch ED, Hoffer C, Whittington D. Influence of age on the pharmacokinetics and pharmacodynamics of oral transmucosal fentanyl citrate. *Anesthesiology* 2004; **101**: 738–43.

19. Thompson JP, Bower S, Liddle AM, Rowbotham DJ. Perioperative pharmacokinetics of transdermal fentanyl in elderly and young adult patients. *Br J Anaesth* 1998; **81**: 152–4.

20. Holdsworth MT, Forman WB, Killilea TA, *et al.* Transdermal fentanyl disposition in elderly subjects. *Gerontology* 1994; **40**: 32–7.

21. Davis MP, Srivastava M. Demographics, assessment and management of pain in the elderly. *Drugs Aging* 2003; **20**: 23–57.

22. Herndon CM. Iontophoretic drug delivery system: focus on fentanyl. *Pharmacotherapy* 2007; **27**: 745–54.

23. Viscusi ER, Siccardi M, Damaraju CV, Hewitt DJ, Kershaw P. The safety and efficacy of fentanyl iontophoretic transdermal system compared with morphine intravenous patient-controlled analgesia for postoperative pain management: an analysis of pooled data from three randomized, active-controlled clinical studies. *Anesthesia and Analgesia* 2007; **105**: 1428–36.

24. Joshi GP. Morphine-6-glucuronide, an active morphine metabolite for the potential treatment of post-operative pain. *Curr Opin Investig Drugs* 2008; **9**: 786–99.

25. Dahan A, van DE, Smith T, Yassen A. Morphine-6-glucuronide (M6G) for postoperative pain relief. *Eur J Pain* 2008; **12**: 403–11.

26. Wolff T, Samuelsson H, Hedner T. Concentrations of morphine and morphine metabolites in CSF and plasma during continuous subcutaneous morphine administration in cancer pain patients. *Pain* 1996; **68**: 209–16.

27. Shafer SL, Flood P. *The Pharmacology of Opioids, Geriatric Anesthesiology*, 2nd edn. Silverstein JH, Rooke GA, Reves JG, McLeskey CH, eds., New York, NY: Springer, 2008: 209–28.

28. Aubrun F, Salvi N, Coriat P, Riou B. Sex- and age-related differences in morphine requirements for postoperative pain relief. *Anesthesiology* 2005; **103**: 156–60.

29. Wagner LE, Eaton M, Sabnis SS, Gingrich KJ. Meperidine and lidocaine block of recombinant voltage-dependent Na+ channels: evidence that meperidine is a local anesthetic. *Anesthesiology* 1999; **91**: 1481–90.

30. Upton RN, Huang YF, Mather LE, Doolette DJ. The relationship between the myocardial kinetics of meperidine and its effect on myocardial contractility: model-independent analysis and optimal

31. Odar-Cederlof I, Boreus LO, Bondesson U, Holmberg L, Heyner L. Comparison of renal excretion of pethidine (meperidine) and its metabolites in old and young patients. *Eur J Clin Pharmacol* 1985; **28**: 171–5.

32. Marcantonio ER, Juarez G, Goldman L, *et al.* The relationship of postoperative delirium with psychoactive medications. *J Am Med Assoc* 1994; **272**: 1518–22.

33. Minto CF, Schnider TW, Shafer SL. Pharmacokinetics and pharmacodynamics of remifentanil. II. Model application. *Anesthesiology* 1997; **86**: 24–33.

34. Minto CF, Schnider TW, Egan TD, *et al.* Influence of age and gender on the pharmacokinetics and pharmacodynamics of remifentanil. I. Model development. *Anesthesiology* 1997; **86**: 10–23.

35. Scott JC, Stanski DR. Decreased fentanyl and alfentanil dose requirements with age. A simultaneous pharmacokinetic and pharmacodynamic evaluation. *J Pharmacol Exp Ther* 1987; **240**: 159–66.

36. Matteo RS, Schwartz AE, Ornstein E, Young WL, Chang WJ. Pharmacokinetics of sufentanil in the elderly surgical patient. *Can J Anaesthesiol* 1990; **37**: 852–6.

37. Helmers JH, van LL, Zuurmond WW. Sufentanil pharmacokinetics in young adult and elderly surgical patients. *Eur J Anaesthesiol* 1994; **11**: 181–5.

38. Helmers H, Van Peer A, Woestenborghs R, Noorduin H, Heykants J. Alfentanil kinetics in the elderly. *Clin Pharmacol Ther* 1984; **36**: 239–43.

39. Hofbauer R, Tesinsky P, Hammerschmidt V, *et al.* No reduction in the sufentanil requirement of elderly patients undergoing ventilatory support in the medical intensive care unit. *Eur J Anaesthesiol* 1999; **16**: 702–7.

40. Frye RF, Matzke GR, Jallad NS, Wilhelm JA, Bikhazi GB. The effect of age on the pharmacokinetics of the opioid antagonist nalmefene. *Br J Clin Pharmacol* 1996; **42**: 301–6.

41. Schnider TW, Minto CF, Shafer SL, *et al.* The influence of age on propofol pharmacodynamics. *Anesthesiology* 1999; **90**: 1502–16.

42. Schultz A, Grouven U, Zander I, *et al.* Age-related effects in the EEG during propofol anaesthesia. *Acta Anaesthesiol Scand* 2004; **48**: 27–34.

43. Kreuer S, Schreiber JU, Bruhn J, Wilhelm W. Impact of patient age on propofol consumption during propofol-remifentanil anaesthesia. *Eur J Anaesthesiol* 2005; **22**: 123–8.

44. Schüttler J, Ihmsen H. Population pharmacokinetics of propofol: a multicenter study. *Anesthesiology* 2000; **92**: 727–38.

45. Shafer SL. The pharmacology of anesthetic drugs in elderly patients. *Anesthesiol Clin North Am* 2000; **18**: 1–29.

46. Kazama T, Ikeda K, Morita K, *et al.* Comparison of the effect-site k(e0)s of propofol for blood pressure and EEG bispectral index in elderly and younger patients. *Anesthesiology* 1999; **90**: 1517–27.

47. McEvoy MD, Reves JG. *Intravenous Hypnotic Anesthetics, Geriatric Anesthesiology*, 2nd edn. Silverstein JH, Rooke GA, Reves JG, McLeskey CH, eds., New York, NY: Springer, 2008: 229–45.

48. White M, Kenny GN, Schraag S. Use of target controlled infusion to derive age and gender covariates for propofol clearance. *Clin Pharmacokinet* 2008; **47**: 119–27.

49. Veselis RA, Feshchenko VA, Reinsel RA, *et al.* Thiopental and propofol affect different regions of the brain at similar pharmacologic effects. *Anesth Analg* 2004; **99**: 399–408.

50. Stanski DR, Maitre PO. Population pharmacokinetics and pharmacodynamics of thiopental: the effect of age revisited. *Anesthesiology* 1990; **72**: 412–22.

51. Avram MJ, Krejcie TC, Henthorn TK. The relationship of age to the pharmacokinetics of early drug distribution: the concurrent disposition of thiopental and indocyanine green. *Anesthesiology* 1990; **72**: 403–11.

52. Barnhill JG, Greenblatt DJ, Miller LG, *et al.* Kinetic and dynamic components

of increased benzodiazepine sensitivity in aging animals. *J Pharmacol Exp Ther* 1990; **253**: 1153–61.

53. Barnhill JG, Miller LG, Greenblatt DJ, *et al.* Benzodiazepine receptor binding response to acute and chronic stress is increased in aging animals. *Pharmacology* 1991; **42**: 181–7.

54. Seppala M, Alihanka J, Himberg JJ, *et al.* Midazolam and flunitrazepam: pharmacokinetics and effects on night time respiration and body movements in the elderly. *Int J Clin Pharmacol Ther Toxicol* 1993; **31**: 170–6.

55. Dunn WF, Adams SC, Adams RW. Iatrogenic delirium and coma: a "near miss". *Chest* 2008; **133**: 1217–20.

56. Jacobs JR, Reves JG, Marty J, *et al.* Aging increases pharmacodynamic sensitivity to the hypnotic effects of midazolam. *Anesth Analg* 1995; **80**: 143–8.

57. Weinbroum AA, Szold O, Ogorek D, Flaishon R. The midazolam-induced paradox phenomenon is reversible by flumazenil. Epidemiology, patient characteristics and review of the literature. *Eur J Anaesthesiol* 2001; **18**: 789–97.

58. Christe C, Janssens JP, Armenian B, Herrmann F, Vogt N. Midazolam sedation for upper gastrointestinal endoscopy in older persons: a randomized, double-blind, placebo-controlled study. *J Am Geriatr Soc* 2000; **48**: 1398–403.

59. Arden JR, Holley FO, Stanski DR. Increased sensitivity to etomidate in the elderly: initial distribution versus altered brain response. *Anesthesiology* 1986; **65**: 19–27.

60. Fried LP, Tangen CM, Walston J, *et al.* Frailty in older adults: evidence for a phenotype. *J Gerontol A Biol Sci Med Sci* 2001; **56**: M146–56.

61. Frolkis VV, Martynenko OA, Zamostyan VP. Aging of the neuromuscular apparatus. *Gerontology* 1976; **22**: 244–79.

62. Oda K. Age changes of motor innervation and acetylcholine receptor distribution on human skeletal muscle fibres. *J Neurol Sci* 1984; **66**: 327–38.

63. Slavov V, Khalil M, Merle JC, *et al.* Comparison of duration of neuromuscular blocking effect of atracurium and vecuronium in young and elderly patients. *Br J Anaesth* 1995; **74**: 709–11.

64. Lien CA, Suzuki T. Relaxants and their reversal agents. In: Silverstein JH, Rooke GA, Reeves JG, McLeskey CH, eds., *Geriatric Anesthesiology*, 2nd edn. New York, NY: Springer, 2008.

65. Duvaldestin P, Saada J, Berger JL, D'Hollander A, Desmonts JM. Pharmacokinetics, pharmacodynamics, and dose-response relationships of pancuronium in control and elderly subjects. *Anesthesiology* 1982; **56**: 36–40.

66. Lien CA, Matteo RS, Ornstein E, Schwartz AE, Diaz J. Distribution, elimination, and action of vecuronium in the elderly. *Anesth Analg* 1991; **73**: 39–42.

67. Ornstein E, Lien CA, Matteo RS, *et al.* Pharmacodynamics and pharmacokinetics of cisatracurium in geriatric surgical patients. *Anesthesiology* 1996; **84**: 520–5.

68. Matteo RS, Young WL, Ornstein E, *et al.* Pharmacokinetics and pharmacodynamics of edrophonium in elderly surgical patients. *Anesth Analg* 1990; **71**: 334–9.

69. McCarthy GJ, Mirakhur RK, Maddineni VR, McCoy EP. Dose-responses for edrophonium during antagonism of vecuronium block in young and older adult patients. *Anaesthesia* 1995; **50**: 503–6.

70. Kitajima T, Ishii K, Ogata H. Edrophonium as an antagonist of vecuronium-induced neuromuscular block in the elderly. *Anaesthesia* 1995; **50**: 359–61.

71. Koscielniak-Nielsen ZJ, Law-Min JC, Donati F, *et al.* Dose-response relations of doxacurium and its reversal with neostigmine in young adults and healthy elderly patients. *Anesth Analg* 1992; **74**: 845–50.

72. McCarthy GJ, Cooper R, Stanley JC, Mirakhur RK. Dose-response relationships for neostigmine antagonism of vecuronium-induced neuromuscular block in adults and the elderly. *Br J Anaesth* 1992; **69**: 281–3.

73. Young WL, Matteo RS, Ornstein E. Duration of action of neostigmine and pyridostigmine in the elderly. *Anesth Analg* 1988; **67**: 775–8.

74. Qaseem A, Snow V, Fitterman N, *et al.* Risk assessment for and strategies to reduce perioperative pulmonary complications for patients undergoing noncardiothoracic surgery: a guideline from the American College of Physicians. *Ann Intern Med* 2006; **144**: 575–80.

75. Muravchick S, Owens WD, Felts JA. Glycopyrrolate and cardiac dysrhythmias in geriatric patients after reversal of neuromuscular blockade. *Can Anaesth Soc J* 1979; **26**: 22–5.

76. Kelz MB, Yang J, Eckenhoff RG. *Mechanisms of General Anesthetic Action, Anesthesiology*. Longnecker DE, Brown DL, Newman MF, Zapol WM, eds., New York, NY: McGraw Hill Medical, 2008: 718–38.

77. Grasshoff C, Rudolph U, Antkowiak B. Molecular and systemic mechanisms of general anaesthesia: the "multi-site and multiple mechanisms" concept. *Curr Opin Anaesthesiol* 2005; **18**: 386–91.

78. Campagna JA, Miller KW, Forman SA. Mechanisms of actions of inhaled anesthetics. *N Engl J Med* 2003; **348**: 2110–24.

79. Mapleson WW. Effect of age on MAC in humans: a meta-analysis. *Br J Anaesth* 1996; **76**: 179–85.

80. Eger EI. Age, minimum alveolar anesthetic concentration, and minimum alveolar anesthetic concentration-awake. *Anesth Analg* 2001; **93**: 947–53.

81. Lerou JG. Nomogram to estimate age-related MAC. *Br J Anaesth* 2004; **93**: 288–91.

82. Suttner SW, Surder C, Lang K, *et al.* Does age affect liver function and the hepatic acute phase response after major abdominal surgery? *Intensive Care Med* 2001; **27**: 1762–9.

83. Monk TG, Saini V, Weldon BC, Sigl JC. Anesthetic management and one-year mortality after noncardiac surgery. *Anesth Analg* 2005; **100**: 4–10.

Emerging concepts of anesthetic neuroprotection and neurotoxicity

Brian P. Head and Piyush Patel

Introduction

General anesthetics cause a profound suppression of neuronal activity, and they reduce the brain's metabolic rate substantially. Although the means by which these effects are attained are not clear, the available data indicate that anesthetics interact with and modulate specific protein targets. Chief amongst these targets are the γ-aminobutyric acid A (GABA$_A$) receptors, two-pore potassium channels, and the N-methyl-D-aspartate (NMDA) subtype of glutamate receptors. Anesthetics have effects that can positively modulate GABA$_A$ receptors and two-pore potassium channels and can also antagonize the NMDA receptor. These molecular targets also play a critical role in two fundamentally different pathophysiologic processes, namely **neuronal injury** in the developing brain and **neuroprotection** in the setting of cerebral ischemia. The mechanisms by which general anesthetics can have diametrically opposite effects on neuronal viability are the focus of the present chapter. The pathophysiology of cerebral ischemia and the neuroprotective efficacy of anesthetics is presented first, followed by a discussion of anesthetic neurotoxicity during brain development and in old age.

Cerebral ischemia and anesthetic neuroprotection

Cerebral ischemia is broadly classified into two categories: global ischemia and focal ischemia. **Global ischemia** is characterized by a complete cessation of cerebral blood flow (e.g., cardiac arrest). In this situation, neuronal depolarization occurs within 5 minutes. Selectively vulnerable neurons within the hippocampus and cerebral cortex are the first to die. The window of opportunity for the restoration of flow is very small because death of neurons is rapid. **Focal ischemia** is characterized by a region of dense ischemia (the so-called *core*) that is surrounded by a larger variable zone that is less ischemic (the *penumbra*). Within the core, flow reduction is severe enough to result in relatively rapid neuronal death. Flow reduction in the penumbra is sufficient to render the electroencephalogram (EEG) isoelectric but not severe enough to kill neurons rapidly. If, however, the flow is not restored, death and infarction will also occur in the penumbra, albeit at a much slower rate. Because of this slow rate of neuronal death, the window of opportunity for therapeutic intervention that is designed to salvage neurons is considerably longer in the setting of focal ischemia.

A variety of experimental models of cerebral ischemia have been employed in the study of anesthetic neuroprotection. These include global and forebrain ischemia (bilateral carotid artery occlusion, with or without vertebral artery ligation, and systemic hypotension), focal ischemia (temporary or permanent middle cerebral artery occlusion), and hemispheric ischemia (unilateral carotid artery occlusion in combination with systemic hypoxia).

Pathophysiology of cerebral ischemia

Energy failure is the central event in the pathophysiology of ischemia. Maintenance of normal ionic gradients across the cell membrane is an adenosine triphosphate (ATP)-requiring active process. When ATP levels reach critically low levels, ionic homeostasis is no longer maintained; this leads to rapid influx of sodium, efflux of POTASSIUM, and depolarization of the membrane (Fig. 71.1). Simultaneously, depolarization of presynaptic terminals leads to a massive release of the excitatory neurotransmitter glutamate. Glutamate activates NMDA and AMPA glutamate receptors, the result being membrane depolarization and influx of calcium and sodium. Calcium entry also occurs via voltage-gated calcium channels (VGCCs). In addition, calcium is released from the endoplasmic reticulum. The net result is an increase in intracellular calcium to levels that are toxic to the cell. Excessive glutamate-mediated injury is referred to as **excitotoxicity**.

Calcium is a ubiquitous second messenger in cells, and it is a required cofactor for the activation of a number of enzyme systems. The rapid, uncontrolled increase in cytosolic calcium levels initiates the activation of a number of cellular enzymes (proteases, lipases, endonucleases) that contribute to injury. Free radicals that are generated in response to mitochondrial injury exacerbate neuronal damage.

Anesthetic Pharmacology, 2nd edition, ed. Alex S. Evers, Mervyn Maze, Evan D. Kharasch. Published by Cambridge University Press. © Cambridge University Press 2011.

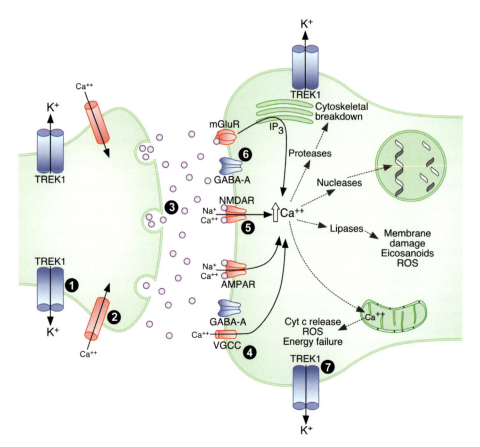

Figure 71.1. Excitotoxic injury during cerebral ischemia. Ischemia results in the depolarization of presynaptic terminals and the subsequent uncontrolled release of glutamate, which activates NMDA receptors (NMDAR), metabotropic glutamate receptors (mGluR), and AMPA receptors (AMPAR). This results in the influx of calcium into the neuron. Calcium also enters via the voltage-gated calcium channels (VGCC) and from the endoplasmic reticulum. The massive increase in neuronal calcium leads to the unregulated activation of a variety of enzymes, which subsequently leads to mitochondrial injury, release of reactive oxygen species (ROS), DNA strand breakage, and neuronal death. Anesthetics modulate this pathophysiologic cascade at multiple points, as indicated by the numerals 1–7. TREK1 is a two-pore K^+ channel.

In neurons in which ATP production is severely compromised, death is rapid. This type of death is referred to as **necrosis**. Neuronal death is, however, a dynamic process in which neurons continue to die for several weeks after the initial ischemia. The delayed neuronal death occurs by **apoptosis**. Apoptosis is a cellular program in which the coordinated activation of a variety of proteases, called caspases, leads to the breakdown of key cellular constituents. Pathologically, the neuron undergoing apoptosis (or programmed cell death, PCD) manifests chromatin condensation, cell shrinkage, membrane blebbing, and apoptotic bodies. The neuron is fragmented in the later stages of the process and is then resorbed. A fundamental difference between apoptosis and necrosis is that the former does not provoke inflammation whereas inflammation is a hallmark of the latter.

Influence of anesthetics on the ischemic brain
Barbiturates

The approach to the problem of cerebral ischemia was initially focused on reducing the brain's requirement for energy. The rationale was that by reducing ATP requirements, the brain would be able to tolerate ischemia for a longer time. Such a supply–demand concept had already been proven to be relevant in the case of cardiac ischemia. Therefore, the drugs investigated first were those that could render the EEG isoelectric (such drugs would be capable of reducing ATP requirements by 50%).

Barbiturates can produce isoelectricity of the EEG and they have been studied extensively. In the setting of global ischemia, barbiturates in EEG burst suppression doses do not reduce ischemia injury [1]. This is not particularly surprising, because the EEG is rendered isoelectric rapidly after the occurrence of global ischemia. In this situation, barbiturates would not be expected to provide much benefit. Barbiturates have been found to be efficacious in the treatment of focal ischemia. A number of investigators have shown that barbiturates can reduce the extent of cerebral injury produced by occlusion of the middle cerebral artery [2]. In humans, thiopental loading has been demonstrated to reduce neurologic deficits after cardiopulmonary bypass. The protective efficacy ascribed to the barbiturates has been questioned on the basis that reduction in injury produced by barbiturate anesthesia might have been a function of anesthesia-induced hypothermia rather than barbiturates per se [3]. Although other studies, in which brain temperature was rigidly controlled, have confirmed the protective efficacy of barbiturates [2], it should be noted that the magnitude of the protective efficacy is modest. In addition, doses that produce burst suppression of the EEG may not be necessary to achieve protection; a dose of barbiturate that is approximately a third of the dose required to achieve EEG suppression can yield a reduction in injury that is of similar magnitude to that achieved with much larger dose [4].

Volatile anesthetics

There is general agreement that volatile anesthetics reduce ischemic cerebral injury. Isoflurane neuroprotection has been demonstrated in a variety of experimental models of ischemia, including hemispheric [5], focal [6], and near-complete ischemia [7]. Similarly, the available data suggest that both sevoflurane [8,9] and desflurane [10,11] can reduce ischemic cerebral injury. There does not appear to be a substantial difference among the volatile drugs with regard to neuroprotective efficacy.

In most of the studies cited above, injury was evaluated a few days after the ischemic insult. Postischemic neuronal injury is a dynamic process in which neurons continue to die for a long time after the initial ischemic insult [12]. Therefore, therapeutic strategies that are neuroprotective after short recovery periods may not produce long-lasting neuroprotection because of the continual loss of neurons in the postischemic period. Volatile anesthetics do produce neuroprotection after short recovery periods. However, isoflurane's neuroprotective efficacy was not sustained when the recovery period was extended to 2 weeks [13]. There is a gradual expansion of the infarction such that neuroprotection is no longer apparent after a longer recovery period. This infarct expansion has been attributed to ongoing apoptosis; indeed, the simultaneous administration of isoflurane and inhibitors of apoptosis produced sustained protection [14,15]. More recent work has shown that, under some circumstances, sustained neuroprotection with volatile drugs can be achieved. In a model of hemispheric ischemia combined with hypotension, sevoflurane produced neuroprotection that was apparent even 4 weeks after ischemia [16]. Similarly, in a model of reversible focal ischemia, sustained neuroprotection with isoflurane was observed [17]. In models of neonatal hypoxia–ischemia, volatile drugs significantly reduce cerebral injury; this reduction is accompanied by an improvement in neurologic function that is apparent as late as 10 weeks after ischemia [18].

How can these discrepant results be reconciled? A closer examination of the models that were employed in these studies indicates that the durability of anesthetic neuroprotection is dependent upon the severity of ischemia and the age of animals. In studies in which adult models are utilized, durable protection is achieved provided that the ischemic insult is either mild [16] or moderate in severity [17]. In models in which the injury is severe, durable protection is not achieved [13,14]. By contrast, sustained neuroprotection can be achieved in neonatal animals even when the injury is severe [18]. Although the impact of age on protection is not clearly defined, the greater plasticity of the neonatal brain may allow protective programs, endogenous to neurons, to limit brain

damage. A logical extension of this premise is that anesthetic protection might be limited in the aged brain. The lack of protective efficacy of isoflurane in brain slices from aged animals is consistent with this premise [19].

Propofol

A number of investigators have shown that propofol can reduce ischemic cerebral injury. In a model of focal ischemia, propofol significantly reduced the extent of cerebral infarction [20]. In fact, the ability of propofol to reduce injury is similar to that achieved with pentobarbital [21]. Propofol neuroprotection, like that of isoflurane, is not sustained beyond a period of 1 week [22]. By contrast, sustained neuroprotection with propofol can be achieved provided that the severity of injury is very mild [16]. In this regard, the neuroprotective efficacy of propofol is similar to that of volatile drugs.

Etomidate

Etomidate is an anesthetic drug whose administration does not result in significant hemodynamic perturbation. Its use as a drug to protect the brain against ischemic injury has been advocated, given its ability to significantly reduce cerebral metabolism. Experimental studies have shown, surprisingly, that etomidate actually increased the volume of brain infarction [23]. This injury-enhancing effect of etomidate has been attributed to its ability to reduce nitric oxide levels in ischemic brain tissue (either by inhibiting nitric oxide synthase or by directly scavenging nitric oxide). In patients undergoing temporary intracranial artery clipping, etomidate administration is associated with a greater reduction in tissue PO_2 than desflurane administration [24]. Based on these investigations, the use of etomidate as a means to reduce ischemic cerebral injury cannot be recommended.

Lidocaine

Lidocaine, by virtue of its ability to block sodium channels and delay the onset of neuronal depolarization during ischemia [25], has been evaluated in several models of focal ischemia. Gelb and colleagues were amongst the first to show that lidocaine can reduce injury [26]. More recent data have confirmed this original observation. In a model of focal ischemia, clinically used concentrations of lidocaine reduced the extent of cerebral infarction and improved neurologic outcome [27]. Importantly, this neuroprotection was sustained for several weeks. In spite of these supportive data, the use of lidocaine for purposes of cerebral protection in the operating room setting has not gained wide acceptance.

Ketamine

Glutamate excitotoxicity, mediated in part by excessive activation of NMDA receptors, plays a major role in the pathophysiology of ischemic cerebral injury. Ketamine is a potent NMDA receptor antagonist, and its ability to reduce ischemic injury has been extensively evaluated. Ketamine reduces neuronal damage in in-vitro models of hypoxia and glucose-oxygen deprivation [28,29]. In vivo, ketamine has been shown to reduce the extent of ischemic infarction after focal ischemia [30,31] and selective neuronal necrosis after global ischemia [32,33]. The neuroprotective efficacy of (S+) ketamine may be greater than that of the more commonly used racemic mixture. To date, whether the neuroprotective effect of ketamine is sustained after long-term recovery has not been evaluated.

Xenon

The noble gas xenon is currently undergoing trials as an anesthetic adjunct in patients. Xenon exerts its anesthetic effects by noncompetitive antagonism of the NMDA subtype of glutamate receptors [34]. Of importance to the present discussion are the data that indicate that xenon has neuroprotective efficacy. In in-vitro models of NMDA toxicity and oxygen-glucose deprivation, xenon significantly attenuated the extent of injury [35]. In rodents subjected to focal ischemia, xenon reduced the extent of cerebral infarction [36]. Of considerable interest are the studies of neonatal hypoxic-ischemic encephalopathy; in this model, xenon not only improved neurologic outcome but also led to histologic protection [37]. In combination with either hypothermia [38] or the α_2-agonist dexmedetomidine [39], xenon afforded protection that was greater than either intervention alone. Like volatile anesthetics, xenon can also precondition the brain against ischemic injury [40]. Collectively, these data demonstrate the neuroprotective efficacy of xenon in a variety of models of cerebral ischemia. Whether xenon protection is sustained in other models of ischemia after long recovery periods has yet to be determined. Nonetheless, there is a significant potential that xenon might provide a means by which intraoperative ischemic cerebral injury can be reduced.

Mechanisms of anesthetic neuroprotection
Excitotoxicity

Anesthetics are pleiotropic drugs and they impact the pathophysiology of cerebral ischemia at multiple levels. Volatile anesthetics reduce ischemia-induced glutamate release [41], antagonize postsynaptic glutamate receptors [42], and enhance GABA$_A$-mediated hyperpolarization [43]. In addition, they increase the levels of antiapoptotic proteins such as Bcl-2 that reduce mitochondrial permeability transition, cytochrome c release, and subsequent activation of cascades that lead to apoptosis [16]. More recent data have also indicated that anesthetics can "precondition" the brain. Exposure of the brain to anesthetics, either immediately or up to 1–4 days prior to the induction of ischemia, attenuates injury [44]. Such preconditioning has been demonstrated for isoflurane [45] and sevoflurane. The means by which preconditioning is effected include the activation of sarcolemmal and mitochondrial K$_{ATP}$ channels, activation of adenosine receptors [46], and the activation of signaling cascades, such as ERK1/2, Akt, PKC, and p38 signaling pathways [47,48], that have prosurvival effects.

Of interest, however, is the observation that isoflurane-mediated preconditioning may be gender-specific, with male subjects being preconditioned [49]. The potential molecular targets of anesthetic neuroprotection are shown in Fig. 71.1.

Neurogenesis

The concept that neuronal proliferation and growth is restricted to the development of the central nervous system (CNS), and that the adult brain is incapable of regeneration, was first advanced by Ramon y Cajal. A wide body of evidence now indicates that new neurons are generated (neurogenesis) not only in the neonatal but also in the adult brain. There are two primary regions of the brain in which neurogenesis is active: the dentate gyrus (DG) of the hippocampus and the subventricular zone (SVZ). In the former, neurogenesis occurs in the subgranular zone; radial glia-like cells give rise to neuroblasts, which then migrate to the molecular layer of the DG and differentiate into neurons [50]. Approximately 6000 neuroblasts are added to the DG per day and, at any given time about 6% of the total number of neurons in the DG are newborn [51]. Neuroblasts generated in the SVZ migrate along an astrocyte scaffold into the olfactory bulb and differentiate into neurons. The newborn neurons are integrated into neuronal networks, receive synaptic input, and make appropriate connections with target neurons.

A number of factors influence the rate of neurogenesis. Neurogenesis declines with age, and this is probably a function of the change in the microenvironment of the progenitor cells in the DG and SVZ. Environmental enrichment, exercise, trophic factors (fibroblast growth factor [FGF], epidermal growth factor [EGF], brain-derived neurotrophic factor [BDNF]), and neurotransmitters influence neurogenesis [52]. With respect to the latter, NMDA receptor activation negatively regulates proliferation [53], while blockade of NMDA receptors accelerates proliferation. GABA$_A$ activity not only acts as a negative feedback regulator of proliferation but also modulates the differentiation of neuronal precursor cells [54].

Neurogenesis is dramatically increased with a variety of forms of brain injury, including ischemia, trauma, hypoglycemia, and epilepsy. Both focal and global cerebral ischemia accelerate neurogenesis in the DG [55]. The proliferation peaks between 7 and 10 days post-injury and returns to basal levels in a few weeks. While a majority of the newborn cells undergo death, the surviving neuroblasts differentiate into neurons and are integrated into the network of the DG [56]. Within the SVZ, neurogenesis is also accelerated after ischemia. Of considerable interest are the observations that indicate that migration of the neuroblasts, which in normal circumstances is to the olfactory bulb, is redirected to the areas of injury. For example, in a focal ischemia model, neuroblasts from the SVZ migrate to the striatum, a region of the brain that is injured in this model [57]. Moreover, the new neurons differentiate into striatal cells and are integrated into the synaptic network in the striatum [58]. However, only a small fraction of neuroblasts (less than 1%) survive. The extent to which neurogenesis contributes to replacement of injured neurons and to functional recovery after stroke remains to be clarified. Although NMDA receptor antagonism increases proliferation in the normal brain, it reduces neuronal injury and neurogenesis in the postischemic brain [59]. Similarly, AMPA receptor blockade attenuates postischemic neurogenesis [60]. It is probable that the extent of neurogenesis in the setting of ischemia is dependent, not only upon the modulation of glutamatergic signaling, but also on the impact of this modulation on the extent of injury, possible neuroprotection, and the impact of glutamate on the elaboration of other factors such as nitric oxide and trophic factors.

Given the potent effects of anesthetics on NMDA and $GABA_A$ receptor signaling, it is possible that anesthetics might also modulate neurogenesis. Isoflurane significantly reduces the rate of neuronal progenitor cell proliferation in vitro [61]. In the developing brain, isoflurane reduces neurogenesis transiently, and the rate of proliferation returns to basal levels 4 weeks after exposure [62]. By contrast, in a recent investigation, propofol, dexmedetomidine, isoflurane, and ketamine anesthesia had no impact on neurogenesis in the hippocampus in both the young and old rodent brain [63]. This surprising result may be a function of evaluation of neurogenesis after too short an interval (2 hours) post anesthesia. Sevoflurane anesthesia during forebrain ischemia has been shown to increase hippocampal neurogenesis 1–2 weeks after ischemia [64]. A limitation of such studies is that it is difficult to separate the effects of anesthesia per se on neurogenesis from the protective effect of anesthetics on hippocampal injury. With significant neuroprotection, the reduction in injury might reduce the stimulus to neurogenesis, as has been reported for AMPA receptor antagonism during global ischemia [60]. With lack of protection with severe ischemic injury, neurogenesis might be reduced significantly because of the injury to the pool of neuronal progenitor cells. By this logic, with moderate injury and moderate anesthetic-mediated neuroprotection, neurogenesis would be increased [64].

Anesthetic neurotoxicity in the developing brain

A fundamental premise of general anesthesia is that anesthetics produce a reversible state of unconsciousness and unresponsiveness. Implicit in this premise is that the brain and spinal cord are neurophysiologically the same before and after anesthesia. Recent experimental data have questioned the complete reversibility of anesthesia. In certain circumstances, anesthetic exposure in neonatal animals leads to neuronal death. Given the large number of neonates and infants that undergo surgery and anesthesia, the implications of these data for anesthesia in humans are readily apparent. Although the relevance of these findings to humans is a subject of heated debate, the

unequivocal demonstration of neuronal death in animals exposed to clinically relevant concentrations of anesthetics has provoked significant concern amongst anesthesia care providers and patients.

Anesthetic neurotoxicity

The adverse impact from halothane exposure on the developing brain was reported two decades ago [65] when it was demonstrated that long-term exposure to halothane, beginning in utero and continuing for several days in the postnatal period, led to impaired synaptogenesis, reduced dendritic branching, suppressed axonal growth, and reduced myelination in rodents. Yet these studies did not achieve notoriety because the manifestation of CNS toxicity required prolonged exposure to halothane, a situation not encountered in clinical practice.

Interest in anesthetic neurotoxicity was renewed by the demonstration that drugs which antagonize NMDA receptors and agonize $GABA_A$ receptors produce widespread neurodegeneration in the developing brain [66]. These data led to a re-evaluation of anesthetic neurotoxicity, because commonly used anesthetic drugs have these effects on NMDA and $GABA_A$ receptors [67]. In a seminal investigation, it was demonstrated that exposure to isoflurane (0.75–1.5%) resulted in substantial neurodegeneration in a number of structures of the brain, including the hippocampus and neocortex [68]. In addition, electrophysiologic function in the hippocampus was significantly reduced by anesthetics. Impaired cognitive function has been demonstrated as late as 8 months after isoflurane exposure at postnatal day 5 [69]. Similar impairment of cognitive function at 8–10 weeks of age has also been shown in rodents given a combination of thiopental or propofol and ketamine at postnatal day 10 [70]. These effects cannot be attributed to a disturbance in physiologic function (e.g., hypotension, hypoxia, or hypercarbia) because blood gas tensions have been reported to be normal [71]. Moreover, anesthetic neurotoxicity has also been demonstrated in vitro in hippocampal slice preparations wherein blood flow is moot. In slices from 7-day-old pups, a 6-hour exposure to isoflurane significantly increased neuronal death [72]. In primate cortical neurons, ketamine induced neurotoxicity [73], and this toxicity also occurred in neonatal monkeys in vivo [74]. Anesthesia-induced injury has now also been demonstrated in the spinal cord; exposure to a combination of isoflurane and nitrous oxide resulted in significant increase in neuronal apoptosis in the ventral horn of the spinal cord [75].

By contrast, anesthesia-induced toxicity was not observed in three mammalian species, mice, rabbits, and piglets [76]. In fetal sheep exposed to isoflurane, midazolam, and thiopental, neuronal injury was not apparent [77]. An important limitation of these two studies is that the extent of injury was evaluated 48 hours [76] and 6 days [77] after exposure. This time period may well be too long to observe neuronal apoptosis, given that apoptotic neurons are rapidly removed from the brain (within 24 hours).

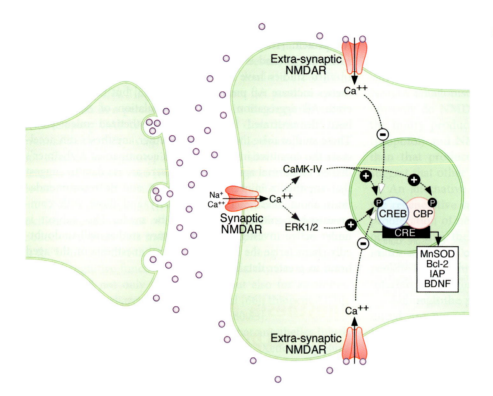

Figure 71.3. The "yin–yang" NMDA receptor (NMDAR) signaling. Neuronal activity increases synaptic NMDAR activation, the result of which is downstream activation of the kinases CaM kinase IV and ERK1/2. These in turn cause phosphorylation of the transcription factor CREB and a CREB binding protein (CBP) and the transcription of genes that enhance survival. By contrast, excessive glutamate release during ischemia leads to diffusion of glutamate from the cleft and activation of extrasynaptic NMDAR. Signaling via extrasynaptic NMDAR inhibits CREB phosphorylation, thereby reducing the levels of prosurvival genes. Inhibition of synaptic NMDAR during synaptogenesis reduces neuronal survival by decreasing CREB activation. Inhibition of extrasynaptic NMDAR during ischemia limits the deleterious signaling initiated by this receptor, and thereby enhances neuronal survival.

During ischemia, excessive release of glutamate leads to the diffusion of glutamate away from the synaptic cleft and the activation of *extrasynaptic* NMDA receptors (Fig. 71.3). The consequence of extrasynaptic NMDA receptor signaling is a reduction in the activation of CREB, thereby curtailing an important survival pathway. A logical extension of these observations is that physiologic blockade of NMDA receptors would reduce survival and increase neuronal death. At the same time, NMDA receptor blockade during ischemia would be expected to reduce extrasynaptic NMDA receptor signaling and enhance survival.

Such a mechanism may be operative in the "yin–yang" effects of anesthetics (Fig. 71.4). During development, synaptic activity is important in neuronal survival. Blockade of synaptic NMDA receptors by anesthetics during this period would be expected to damage neurons. At the same time, during cerebral ischemia, anesthetic NMDA receptor blockade would be of benefit in reducing excitotoxicity and in reducing extrasynaptic NMDA receptor activation. Although there is a paucity of experimental support for this proposition, the demonstration of the adverse and beneficial effects of NMDA receptor blockade (depending upon the context) makes this plausible.

Summary

Anesthetics cause a profound suppression of brain activity, and this effect is mediated primarily by the modulation of GABA$_A$ and NMDA receptors and the two-pore potassium channels. Neuronal activity is critical to neuronal survival,

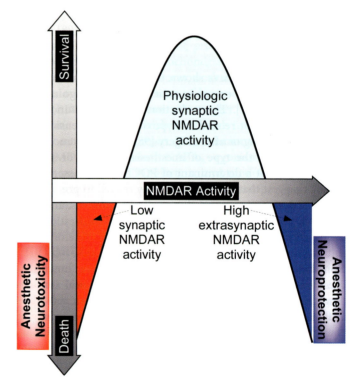

Figure 71.4. The yin–yang effect of anesthetics. During synaptogenesis, glutamatergic signaling is essential to neuronal development and survival. Anesthetic blockade of synaptic NMDA receptors (NMDAR) results in a reduction of synaptic NMDAR activation, reduced glutamatergic signaling, and neuronal apoptosis. By contrast, in the setting of cerebral ischemia, excessive glutamate release leads to extrasynaptic NMDAR activation. Administration of anesthetics during ischemia results in the blockade of extrasynaptic NMDAR, thereby reducing excitotoxicity and neuronal death. Adapted from Hardingham and Bading [107].

particularly during synaptic formation in brain development. Suppression of neuronal activity during synaptogenesis in neonatal subjects can cause neuronal death. By contrast, in pathologic conditions, particularly cerebral ischemia, anesthetics can reduce excitotoxicity and can protect the brain against ischemic injury. These effects are also mediated by the GABA$_A$ and NMDA receptors. Therefore, whether anesthetics injure or protect the brain depends upon the context in which anesthetics are evaluated. In addition, anesthetics can also potentially increase the formation of Aβ protein in the brain. This

accumulation of Aβ protein can adversely impact cognitive function in aged subjects. Collectively, the available information indicates that anesthetics are not completely benign and that they do not produce a completely reversible state of unconsciousness. However, the benefits of general anesthesia for suppression of pain during surgery greatly outweigh the potential adverse effects. An understanding of the mechanisms of anesthetic neurotoxicity at the extremes of age is important for the development of therapeutic approaches to mitigate this toxicity.

References

1. Todd MM, Chadwick HS, Shapiro HM, et al. The neurologic effects of thiopental therapy following experimental cardiac arrest in cats. Anesthesiology 1982; 57: 76–86.

2. Warner DS, Zhou J, Ramani R, Todd MM. Reversible focal ischemia in the rat: effects of halothane, isoflurane, and methohexital anesthesia. J Cereb Blood Flow Metab 1991; 11: 794–802.

3. Drummond JC. Do barbiturates really protect the brain? Anesthesiology 1993; 78: 611–13.

4. Warner DS, Takaoka S, Wu B, et al. Electroencephalographic burst suppression is not required to elicit maximal neuroprotection from pentobarbital in a rat model of focal cerebral ischemia. Anesthesiology 1996; 84: 1475–84.

5. Baughman VL, Hoffman WE, Thomas C, Miletich DJ, Albrecht RF. Comparison of methohexital and isoflurane on neurologic outcome and histopathology following incomplete ischemia in rats. Anesthesiology 1990; 72: 85–94.

6. Soonthon-Brant V, Patel PM, Drummond JC, et al. Fentanyl does not increase brain injury after focal cerebral ischemia in rats. Anesth Analg 1999; 88: 49–55.

7. Nellgard B, Mackensen GB, Pineda J, et al. Anesthetic effects on cerebral metabolic rate predict histologic outcome from near-complete forebrain ischemia in the rat. Anesthesiology 2000; 93: 431–6.

8. Warner DS, McFarlane C, Todd MM, Ludwig P, McAllister AM. Sevoflurane and halothane reduce focal ischemic brain damage in the rat. Anesthesiology 1993; 79: 985–92.

9. Werner C, Mollenberg O, Kochs E, Schulte JE. Sevoflurane improves neurological outcome after incomplete cerebral ischaemia in rats. Br J Anaesth 1995; 75: 756–60.

10. Engelhard K, Werner C, Reeker W, et al. Desflurane and isoflurane improve neurological outcome after incomplete cerebral ischaemia in rats. Br J Anaesth 1999; 83: 415–21.

11. Haelewyn B, Yvon A, Hanouz JL, et al. Desflurane affords greater protection than halothane against focal cerebral ischaemia in the rat. Br J Anaesth 2003; 91: 390–6.

12. Du C, Hu R, Csernansky C, Hsu C, Choi D. Very delayed infarction after mild focal cerebral ischemia: a role for apoptosis? J Cereb Blood Flow Metab 1996; 16: 195–201.

13. Kawaguchi M, Kimbro JR, Drummond JC, et al. Isoflurane delays but does not prevent cerebral infarction in rats subjected to focal ischemia. Anesthesiology 2000; 92: 1335–42.

14. Inoue S, Davis DP, Drummond JC, Cole DJ, Patel PM. The combination of isoflurane and caspase 8 inhibition results in sustained neuroprotection in rats subject to focal cerebral ischemia. Anesth Analg 2006; 102: 1548–55.

15. Inoue S, Drummond JC, Davis DP, Cole DJ, Patel PM. Combination of isoflurane and caspase inhibition reduces cerebral injury in rats subjected to focal cerebral ischemia. Anesthesiology 2004; 101: 75–81.

16. Engelhard K, Werner C, Eberspacher E, et al. Sevoflurane and propofol influence the expression of apoptosis-regulating proteins after cerebral ischaemia and reperfusion in rats. Eur J Anaesthesiol 2004; 21: 530–7.

17. Sakai H, Sheng H, Yates RB, et al. Isoflurane provides long-term protection against focal cerebral ischemia in the rat. Anesthesiology 2007; 106: 92–9.

18. McAuliffe JJ, Joseph B, Vorhees CV. Isoflurane-delayed preconditioning reduces immediate mortality and improves striatal function in adult mice after neonatal hypoxia-ischemia. Anesth Analg 2007; 104: 1066–77.

19. Zhan X, Fahlman CS, Bickler PE. Isoflurane neuroprotection in rat hippocampal slices decreases with aging: changes in intracellular Ca^{2+} regulation and N-methyl-D-aspartate receptor-mediated Ca2+ influx. Anesthesiology 2006; 104: 995–1003.

20. Gelb AW, Bayona NA, Wilson JX, Cechetto DF. Propofol anesthesia compared to awake reduces infarct size in rats. Anesthesiology 2002; 96: 1183–90.

21. Pittman JE, Sheng H, Pearlstein RD, et al. Comparison of the effects of propofol and pentobarbital on neurologic outcome and cerebral infarction size after temporary focal ischemia in the rat. Anesthesiology 1997; 87: 1139–44.

22. Bayona NA, Gelb AW, Jiang Z, et al. Propofol neuroprotection in cerebral ischemia and its effects on low-molecular-weight antioxidants and skilled motor tasks. Anesthesiology 2004; 100: 1151–9.

23. Drummond JC, McKay LD, Cole DJ, Patel PM. The role of nitric oxide synthase inhibition in the adverse effects of etomidate in the setting of focal cerebral ischemia in rats. Anesth Analg 2005; 100: 841–6.

24. Hoffman WE, Charbel FT, Edelman G, Misra M, Ausman JI. Comparison of

the effect of etomidate and desflurane on brain tissue gases and pH during prolonged middle cerebral artery occlusion. *Anesthesiology* 1998; **88**: 1188–94.

25. Seyfried FJ, Adachi N, Arai T. Suppression of energy requirement by lidocaine in the ischemic mouse brain. *J Neurosurg Anesthesiol* 2005; **17**: 75–81.

26. Shokunbi MT, Gelb AW, Wu XM, Miller DJ. Continuous lidocaine infusion and focal feline cerebral ischemia. *Stroke* 1990; **21**: 107–11.

27. Lei B, Popp S, Capuano-Waters C, Cottrell JE, Kass IS. Lidocaine attenuates apoptosis in the ischemic penumbra and reduces infarct size after transient focal cerebral ischemia in rats. *Neuroscience* 2004; **125**: 691–701.

28. Mathews KS, Toner CC, McLaughlin DP, Stamford JA. Comparison of ketamine stereoisomers on tissue metabolic activity in an in vitro model of global cerebral ischaemia. *Neurochem Int* 2001; **38**: 367–72.

29. Zhan RZ, Qi S, Wu C, et al. Intravenous anesthetics differentially reduce neurotransmission damage caused by oxygen-glucose deprivation in rat hippocampal slices in correlation with N-methyl-D-aspartate receptor inhibition. *Crit Care Med* 2001; **29**: 808–13.

30. Chang ML, Yang J, Kem S, et al. Nicotinamide and ketamine reduce infarct volume and DNA fragmentation in rats after brain ischemia and reperfusion. *Neurosci Lett* 2002; **322**: 137–40.

31. Lin SZ, Chiou AL, Wang Y. Ketamine antagonizes nitric oxide release from cerebral cortex after middle cerebral artery ligation in rats. *Stroke* 1996; **27**: 747–52.

32. Zhang C, Shen W, Zhang G. N-methyl-D-aspartate receptor and L-type voltage-gated Ca(2+) channel antagonists suppress the release of cytochrome c and the expression of procaspase-3 in rat hippocampus after global brain ischemia. *Neurosci Lett* 2002; **328**: 265–8.

33. Reeker W, Werner C, Mollenberg O, Mielke L, Kochs E. High-dose S(+)-ketamine improves neurological

outcome following incomplete cerebral ischemia in rats. *Can J Anaesth* 2000; **47**: 572–8.

34. Franks NP, Dickinson R, de Sousa SL, Hall AC, Lieb WR. How does xenon produce anaesthesia? *Nature* 1998; **396**: 324.

35. Wilhelm S, Ma D, Maze M, Franks NP. Effects of xenon on in vitro and in vivo models of neuronal injury. *Anesthesiology* 2002; **96**: 1485–91.

36. Homi HM, Yokoo N, Ma D, et al. The neuroprotective effect of xenon administration during transient middle cerebral artery occlusion in mice. *Anesthesiology* 2003; **99**: 876–81.

37. Dingley J, Tooley J, Porter H, Thoresen M. Xenon provides short-term neuroprotection in neonatal rats when administered after hypoxia-ischemia. *Stroke* 2006; **37**: 501–6.

38. Ma D, Hossain M, Chow A, et al. Xenon and hypothermia combine to provide neuroprotection from neonatal asphyxia. *Ann Neurol* 2005; **58**: 182–93.

39. Rajakumaraswamy N, Ma D, Hossain M, et al. Neuroprotective interaction produced by xenon and dexmedetomidine on in vitro and in vivo neuronal injury models. *Neurosci Lett* 2006; **409**: 128–33.

40. Ma D, Hossain M, Pettet GK, et al. Xenon preconditioning reduces brain damage from neonatal asphyxia in rats. *J Cereb Blood Flow Metab* 2006; **26**: 199–208.

41. Patel PM, Drummond JC, Goskowicz R, Sano T, Cole DJ. The volatile anesthetic isoflurane reduces ischemia induced release of glutamate in rats. *J Cereb Blood Flow Metab* 1993; **13**: S685.

42. Harada H, Drummond JC, Cole DJ, Kelly PJ, Patel PM. Isoflurane reduces NMDA toxicity in vivo in the rat cerebral cortex. *Anesth Analg* 1999; **89**: 1442–7.

43. Bickler PE, Warner DS, Stratmann G, Schuyler JA. gamma-Aminobutyric acid-A receptors contribute to isoflurane neuroprotection in organotypic hippocampal cultures. *Anesth Analg* 2003; **97**: 564–71.

44. Payne RS, Akca O, Roewer N, Schurr A, Kehl F. Sevoflurane-induced preconditioning protects against cerebral ischemic neuronal damage in

rats. *Brain Res* 2005; **1034**: 147–52.

45. Xiong L, Zheng Y, Wu M, et al. Preconditioning with isoflurane produces dose-dependent neuroprotection via activation of adenosine triphosphate-regulated potassium channels after focal cerebral ischemia in rats. *Anesth Analg* 2003; **96**: 233–7.

46. Zheng S, Zuo Z. Isoflurane preconditioning reduces purkinje cell death in an in vitro model of rat cerebellar ischemia. *Neuroscience* 2003; **118**: 99–106.

47. Bickler PE, Fahlman CS. The inhaled anesthetic, isoflurane, enhances Ca2+-dependent survival signaling in cortical neurons and modulates MAP kinases, apoptosis proteins and transcription factors during hypoxia. *Anesth Analg* 2006; **103**: 419–29.

48. Bickler PE, Zhan X, Fahlman CS. Isoflurane preconditions hippocampal neurons against oxygen-glucose deprivation: role of intracellular Ca2+ and mitogen-activated protein kinase signaling. *Anesthesiology* 2005; **103**: 532–9.

49. Kitano H, Young JM, Cheng J, et al. Gender-specific response to isoflurane preconditioning in focal cerebral ischemia. *J Cereb Blood Flow Metab* 2007; **27**: 1377–86.

50. Cameron HA, Woolley CS, McEwen BS, Gould E. Differentiation of newly born neurons and glia in the dentate gyrus of the adult rat. *Neuroscience* 1993; **56**: 337–44.

51. Cameron HA, McKay RD. Adult neurogenesis produces a large pool of new granule cells in the dentate gyrus. *J Comp Neurol* 2001; **435**: 406–17.

52. Lichtenwalner RJ, Parent JM. Adult neurogenesis and the ischemic forebrain. *J Cereb Blood Flow Metab* 2006; **26**: 1–20.

53. Cameron HA, McEwen BS, Gould E. Regulation of adult neurogenesis by excitatory input and NMDA receptor activation in the dentate gyrus. *J Neurosci* 1995; **15**: 4687–92.

54. Yuan TF. GABA effects on neurogenesis: an arsenal of regulation. *Sci Signal* 2008; **1**: jc1.

55. Choi YS, Lee MY, Sung KW, *et al.* Regional differences in enhanced neurogenesis in the dentate gyrus of adult rats after transient forebrain ischemia. *Mol Cells* 2003; **16**: 232–8.

56. Tanaka R, Yamashiro K, Mochizuki H, *et al.* Neurogenesis after transient global ischemia in the adult hippocampus visualized by improved retroviral vector. *Stroke* 2004; **35**: 1454–9.

57. Parent JM, Vexler ZS, Gong C, Derugin N, Ferriero DM. Rat forebrain neurogenesis and striatal neuron replacement after focal stroke. *Ann Neurol* 2002; **52**: 802–13.

58. Arvidsson A, Collin T, Kirik D, Kokaia Z, Lindvall O. Neuronal replacement from endogenous precursors in the adult brain after stroke. *Nat Med* 2002; **8**: 963–70.

59. Bernabeu R, Sharp FR. NMDA and AMPA/kainate glutamate receptors modulate dentate neurogenesis and CA3 synapsin-I in normal and ischemic hippocampus. *J Cereb Blood Flow Metab* 2000; **20**: 1669–80.

60. Arvidsson A, Kokaia Z, Lindvall O. N-methyl-D-aspartate receptor-mediated increase of neurogenesis in adult rat dentate gyrus following stroke. *Eur J Neurosci* 2001; **14**: 10–18.

61. Sall J, Bickler P, Stratmann G, McKleroy W. Isoflurane is toxic to isolated neural progenitor cells from rat hippocampus (abstract). *J Neurgsurg Anesth* 2006; **18**: 288.

62. Head BP, Patel HH, Niesman IR, *et al.* Inhibition of p75 neurotrophin receptor attenuates isoflurane-mediated neuronal apoptosis in the neonatal central nervous system. *Anesthesiology* 2009; **110**: 813–25.

63. Tung A, Herrera S, Fornal CA, Jacobs BL. The effect of prolonged anesthesia with isoflurane, propofol, dexmedetomidine, or ketamine on neural cell proliferation in the adult rat. *Anesth Analg* 2008; **106**: 1772–7.

64. Engelhard K, Winkelheide U, Werner C, *et al.* Sevoflurane affects neurogenesis after forebrain ischemia in rats. *Anesth Analg* 2007; **104**: 898–903.

65. Levin ED, Uemura E, Bowman RE. Neurobehavioral toxicology of halothane in rats. *Neurotoxicol Teratol* 1991; **13**: 461–70.

66. Olney JW, Ishimaru MJ, Bittigau P, Ikonomidou C. Ethanol-induced apoptotic neurodegeneration in the developing brain. *Apoptosis* 2000; **5**: 515–21.

67. Franks NP, Lieb WR. Molecular and cellular mechanisms of general anaesthesia. *Nature* 1994; **367**: 607–14.

68. Jevtovic-Todorovic V, Hartman RE, Izumi Y, *et al.* Early exposure to common anesthetic agents causes widespread neurodegeneration in the developing rat brain and persistent learning deficits. *J Neurosci* 2003; **23**: 876–82.

69. Stratmann G, Bell J, Alvi RS, *et al.* Neonatal isoflurane anesthesia causes a permanent neurocognitive deficit in rats. *J Neurgsurg Anesth* 2006; **18**: 288.

70. Fredriksson A, Ponten E, Gordh T, Eriksson P. Neonatal exposure to a combination of N-methyl-D-aspartate and gamma-aminobutyric acid type A receptor anesthetic agents potentiates apoptotic neurodegeneration and persistent behavioral deficits. *Anesthesiology* 2007; **107**: 427–36.

71. Yon JH, Daniel-Johnson J, Carter LB, Jevtovic-Todorovic V. Anesthesia induces neuronal cell death in the developing rat brain via the intrinsic and extrinsic apoptotic pathways. *Neuroscience* 2005; **135**: 815–27.

72. Wise-Faberowski L, Zhang H, Ing R, Pearlstein RD, Warner DS. Isoflurane-induced neuronal degeneration: an evaluation in organotypic hippocampal slice cultures. *Anesth Analg* 2005; **101**: 651–7.

73. Wang C, Sadovova N, Hotchkiss C, *et al.* Blockade of N-methyl-D-aspartate receptors by ketamine produces loss of postnatal day 3 monkey frontal cortical neurons in culture. *Toxicol Sci* 2006; **91**: 192–201.

74. Slikker W, Zou X, Hotchkiss CE, *et al.* Ketamine-induced neuronal cell death in the perinatal rhesus monkey. *Toxicol Sci* 2007; **98**: 145–58.

75. Sanders RD, Xu J, Shu Y, *et al.* General anesthetics induce apoptotic neurodegeneration in the neonatal rat spinal cord. *Anesth Analg* 2008; **106**: 1708–11.

76. Loepke A, McCann JC, Miles L. General anesthesia does not cause widespread neuronal cell death in the neonatal brain – a study in three mammalian species. *Anesthesiology* 2004; A: 1504.

77. McClaine RJ, Uemura K, de la Fuente SG, *et al.* General anesthesia improves fetal cerebral oxygenation without evidence of subsequent neuronal injury. *J Cereb Blood Flow Metab* 2005; **25**: 1060–9.

78. Vutskits L, Gascon E, Tassonyi E, Kiss JZ. Effect of ketamine on dendritic arbor development and survival of immature GABAergic neurons in vitro. *Toxicol Sci* 2006; **91**: 540–9.

79. Vutskits L, Gascon E, Tassonyi E, Kiss JZ. Clinically relevant concentrations of propofol but not midazolam alter in vitro dendritic development of isolated gamma-aminobutyric acid-positive interneurons. *Anesthesiology* 2005; **102**: 970–6.

80. Spahr-Schopfer I, Vutskits L, Toni N, *et al.* Differential neurotoxic effects of propofol on dissociated cortical cells and organotypic hippocampal cultures. *Anesthesiology* 2000; **92**: 1408–17.

81. Webb SJ, Monk CS, Nelson CA. Mechanisms of postnatal neurobiological development: implications for human development. *Dev Neuropsychol* 2001; **19**: 147–71.

82. Young C, Jevtovic-Todorovic V, Qin YQ, *et al.* Potential of ketamine and midazolam, individually or in combination, to induce apoptotic neurodegeneration in the infant mouse brain. *Br J Pharmacol* 2005; **146**: 189–97.

83. Honegger P, Matthieu JM. Selective toxicity of the general anesthetic propofol for GABAergic neurons in rat brain cell cultures. *J Neurosci Res* 1996; **45**: 631–6.

84. Ma D, Williamson P, Januszewski A, *et al.* Xenon mitigates isoflurane-induced neuronal apoptosis in the developing rodent brain. *Anesthesiology* 2007; **106**: 746–53.

85. Olney JW. New insights and new issues in developmental neurotoxicology. *Neurotoxicology* 2002; **23**: 659–68.

86. Ikonomidou C, Bosch F, Miksa M, *et al.* Blockade of NMDA receptors and apoptotic neurodegeneration in the developing brain. *Science* 1999; **283**: 70–4.

87. Ben-Ari Y. Excitatory actions of gaba during development: the nature of the nurture. *Nat Rev Neurosci* 2002; **3**: 728–39.

88. Olney JW, Young C, Wozniak DF, Ikonomidou C, Jevtovic-Todorovic V. Anesthesia-induced developmental neuroapoptosis. Does it happen in humans? *Anesthesiology* 2004; **101**: 273–5.

89. Olney JW, Wozniak DF, Farber NB, *et al.* The enigma of fetal alcohol neurotoxicity. *Ann Med* 2002; **34**: 109–19.

90. Lu LX, Yon JH, Carter LB, Jevtovic-Todorovic V. General anesthesia activates BDNF-dependent neuroapoptosis in the developing rat brain. *Apoptosis* 2006; **11**: 1603–15.

91. Anand KJ, Soriano SG. Anesthetic agents and the immature brain: are these toxic or therapeutic? *Anesthesiology* 2004; **101**: 527–30.

92. Anand KJ. Anesthetic neurotoxicity in newborns: should we change clinical practice? *Anesthesiology* 2007; **107**: 2–4.

93. Bhutta AT, Venkatesan AK, Rovnaghi CR, Anand KJ. Anaesthetic neurotoxicity in rodents: is the ketamine controversy real? *Acta Paediatr* 2007 Nov; **96**: 1554–6.

94. Todd MM. Anesthetic neurotoxicity: the collision between laboratory neuroscience and clinical medicine. *Anesthesiology* 2004; **101**: 272–3.

95. Mellon RD, Simone AF, Rappaport BA. Use of anesthetic agents in neonates and young children. *Anesth Analg* 2007; **104**: 509–20.

96. Abildstrom H, Rasmussen LS, Rentowl P, *et al.* Cognitive dysfunction 1–2 years after non-cardiac surgery in the elderly. ISPOCD group. International Study of Post-operative Cognitive Dysfunction. *Acta Anaesthesiol Scand* 2000; **44**: 1246–51.

97. Johnson T, Monk T, Rasmussen LS, *et al.* Postoperative cognitive dysfunction in middle-aged patients. *Anesthesiology* 2002; **96**: 1351–7.

98. Moller JT, Cluitmans P, Rasmussen LS, *et al.* Long-term postoperative cognitive dysfunction in the elderly ISPOCD1 study. ISPOCD investigators. International Study of Post-operative Cognitive Dysfunction. *Lancet* 1998; **351**: 857–61.

99. Rasmussen LS, Johnson T, Kuipers HM, *et al.* Does anaesthesia cause postoperative cognitive dysfunction? A randomised study of regional versus general anaesthesia in 438 elderly patients. *Acta Anaesthesiol Scand* 2003; **47**: 260–6.

100. Culley DJ, Baxter MG, Crosby CA, Yukhananov R, Crosby G. Impaired acquisition of spatial memory 2 weeks after isoflurane and isoflurane-nitrous oxide anesthesia in aged rats. *Anesth Analg* 2004; **99**: 1393–7.

101. Culley DJ, Baxter MG, Yukhananov R, Crosby G. Long-term impairment of acquisition of a spatial memory task following isoflurane-nitrous oxide anesthesia in rats. *Anesthesiology* 2004; **100**: 309–14.

102. Bianchi SL, Tran T, Liu C, *et al.* Brain and behavior changes in 12-month-old Tg2576 and nontransgenic mice exposed to anesthetics. *Neurobiol Aging* 2008; **29**: 1002–10.

103. Uemura K, Kuzuya A, Shimohama S. Protein trafficking and Alzheimer's disease. *Curr Alzheimer Res* 2004; **1**: 1–10.

104. Xie Z, Dong Y, Maeda U, *et al.* The common inhalation anesthetic isoflurane induces apoptosis and increases amyloid beta protein levels. *Anesthesiology* 2006; **104**: 988–94.

105. Xie Z, Dong Y, Maeda U, *et al.* The inhalation anesthetic isoflurane induces a vicious cycle of apoptosis and amyloid beta-protein accumulation. *J Neurosci* 2007; **27**: 1247–54.

106. Eckenhoff RG, Johansson JS, Wei H, *et al.* Inhaled anesthetic enhancement of amyloid-beta oligomerization and cytotoxicity. *Anesthesiology* 2004; **101**: 703–9.

107. Hardingham GE, Bading H. The yin and yang of NMDA receptor signalling. *Trends Neurosci* 2003; **26**: 81–9.

108. Pokorska A, Vanhoutte P, Arnold FJ, *et al.* Synaptic activity induces signalling to CREB without increasing global levels of cAMP in hippocampal neurons. *J Neurochem* 2003; **84**: 447–52.

Index

Page numbers in *italic* refer to figures/tables
Greek letters are spelled out (e.g., alpha)

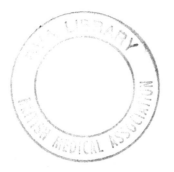